D0851062

AMERICA'S
TOP DOCTORS®
A CASTLE CONNOLLY GUIDE

11th Edition

The Best in American Medicine

America's trusted source for identifying Top Doctors

For more information, please contact:

Castle Connolly Medical Ltd., 42 West 24th St, New York, New York 10010
212-367-8400x10
E-mail: info@castleconnolly.com
Web site: http://www.castleconnolly.com.

Library of Congress Control Number: 2010940313

| ISBN | 0-9845670-8-9; | 978-0-9845670-8-9 | (paperback) |
| ISBN | 0-9845670-9-7; | 978-0-9845670-9-6 | (hardcover) |

Printed in the United States of America

Table of Contents

Table of Contents

Table of Contents

Table of Contents

Table of Contents

Table of Contents

Table of Contents

Table of Contents

Table of Contents

Table of Contents

Table of Contents

Table of Contents

Table of Contents

Table of Contents

Appendices

Indices

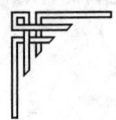

The Best in American Medicine
www.CastleConnolly.com

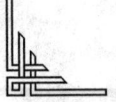
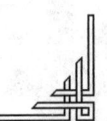

About The Publishers

John K. Castle, the Chairman of Castle Connolly Medical Ltd., has spent much of the last three decades involved with healthcare institutions and issues. Mr. Castle served as Chairman of the Board of New York Medical College for eleven years, an institution where he served on the Board of Trustees for twenty-two years.

Mr. Castle has been extensively involved in other healthcare and voluntary activities as well. He served for five years as a commissioner and officer of the Joint Commission formerly known as (JCAHO), the body which accredits most public and private hospitals throughout the United States. Mr. Castle has also served as a trustee of five different hospitals in the metropolitan New York region, including NewYork Presbyterian Hospital, where he continues to serve.

Mr. Castle has also served as the Chairman of the Columbia Presbyterian Science Advisory Council and as a Director of the Whitehead Institute for Biomedical Research. He is a Fellow of New York Academy of Medicine and has served as a Trustee of the Academy. He was Chairman of the United Hospital Fund of New York's Capital Campaign and continues as Director Emeritus of the United Hospital Fund. He is a Life Member of the MIT Corporation, the governing body of the Massachusetts Institute of Technology.

Mr. Castle received his bachelor's degree from the Massachusetts Institute of Technology, his MBA as a Baker Scholar with High Distinction from Harvard, and two Honorary Doctorate degrees.

Mr. Castle's goal, as is the goal of Dr. John Connolly and all the Castle Connolly team, is to publish *America's Top Doctors*®, *America's Top Doctors*® *for Cancer, Top Doctors: New York Metro Area*, and other materials as well as build websites to help the public identify the very best in healthcare resources.

John J. Connolly, Ed.D., - the nation's foremost expert on identifying top physicians, is the President & CEO of Castle Connolly Medical Ltd. publisher of *America's Top Doctors®* and other consumer guides to help people find the best healthcare. He is also Vice-Chairman of Castle Connolly Graduate Medical Ltd., which publishes review manuals to assist resident physicians and fellows in preparing for their board exams.

Dr. Connolly served as President of New York Medical College, the nation's second largest private medical college, for more than ten years. He is a Fellow of the New York Academy of Medicine, a Fellow of the New York Academy of Sciences, a Director of the Northeast Business Group on Health, a member of the President's Council of the United Hospital Fund, and a member of the Board of Advisors of the Whitehead Institute for Biomedical Research.

Dr. Connolly has served as trustee of two hospitals and as Chairman of the Board of one. He is extensively involved in healthcare and community activities and has served on a number of voluntary and corporate boards including the Board of the American Lyme Disease Foundation, of which he is a founder and past chairman, and the Culinary Institute of America for over 20 years where he is now Chairman Emeritus. He also served as a director and Chairman of the Professional Examination Service and is presently on the board of the American Swiss Foundation. His current corporate board service includes: Baker and Taylor; Morton's of Chicago; Dearborn Risk Management and Perkins & Marie Callender's. He holds a Bachelor of Science degree from Worcester State College, a Master's degree from the University of Connecticut, and a Doctor of Education degree in College and University Administration from Teacher's College, Columbia University. He also has been awarded honorary doctorates by Mercy College (LHD) and Worcester State University.

Dr. Connolly has appeared on or been interviewed by over 100 television and radio stations nationwide including "Good Morning America" (ABC-TV), "The Today Show" (NBC-TV), "20/20" (ABC-TV), "48 Hours" (CBS-TV), Fox Cable News, "Morning News" (CNN) and "Weekend Today in New York" (WNBC-TV). *The New York Times, The Chicago Tribune, The Daily News* (New York), *The Boston Herald* and other newspapers, as well as many national and regional magazines, have featured Castle Connolly Guides and/or Dr. Connolly in stories. He is the author and/or editor of seven books.

Medical Advisory Board

Castle Connolly Medical Ltd. is pleased to have associated with a distinguished group of medical leaders who offer invaluable advice and wisdom in our efforts to assist consumers in making good healthcare choices. We thank each member of the Medical Advisory Board for their valuable contributions.

Jeremiah A. Barondess, M.D.
President Emeritus
New York Acadmey of Medicine
Professor of Clinical Medicine
Emeritus,
Weill-Cornell Medical College

Roger Bulger, M.D.
National Institutes of Health (ret.)

Menard M. Gertler, M.D., D.Sc.
Clinical Prof. of Medicine
Cornell University
Medical School

Leo Hennikoff, M.D.
President and CEO (Ret.)
Rush Presbyterian-St. Luke's
Medical Center

Yutaka Kikkawa, M.D.
Professor and Chairman (Emeritus)
Department of Pathology, University
of California,
Irvine
College of Medicine

David Paige, M.D.
Professor
Bloomberg School of Public Health,
Johns Hopkins University

Ronald Pion, M.D.
Chairman and CEO
Medical Telecommunications
Associates

Richard L. Reece, M.D.
Editor
Physician Practice Options

Leon G. Smith, M.D.
Professor of Medicine & Preventive
Medicine
New Jersey Medical School

Helen Smits, M.D.
Former Deputy Director
Health Care Financing
Administration (HCFA)

Ralph Snyderman, M.D.
Former President and CEO
Duke University Health System

Foreword

The challenge of finding the best healthcare is a formidable one for most Americans and for others who seek medical care in the United States. While this country offers the best medical care in the world, many people are overwhelmed by its complexity and bureaucracy.

While most of us are fortunate and never need to venture beyond our local communities to find medical specialists able to meet our healthcare needs, the needs of many patients cannot be met in their local areas. For them, the search for the top specialists can be as important as life itself!

This great nation is fortunate in possessing some of the world's leading medical centers and specialty hospitals where cutting edge research is conducted and innovative new therapies are practiced daily. These health centers employ and train many of the world's most skilled physicians. The organization which I formerly headed, the Association of Academic Health Centers, serves as a forum of exchange for these centers of medical excellence and, therefore, I know them well. However, I also know well the difficulty and challenges that patients and their families face in identifying and locating the tremendous wealth of medical talent and dedication that lies within the walls of these outstanding facilities.

Castle Connolly Medical Ltd. has dedicated extensive time and resources to identify-ing the best healthcare this nation has to offer. They have done this not to serve physicians or hospitals, but to serve healthcare consumers. Their efforts will be vital and important resources to Americans and others who seek the best medical care available in this country—wherever it is being practiced.

Roger Bulger, M.D.
Former President, Association of Academic Health Centers (AAHC)
Washington DC

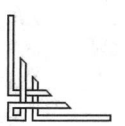
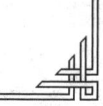

The Best in American Medicine
www.CastleConnolly.com

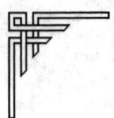

The Best in American Medicine
www.CastleConnolly.com

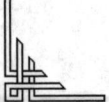
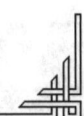

Introduction

There are times in life when the nature of a disease or medical condition that afflicts you or a loved one warrants identifying the top doctor—the very best specialist anywhere in the nation—to diagnose or treat that particular medical problem. At times like these, you need Castle Connolly's *America's Top Doctors®*, the national guide designed to assist you under just these circumstances.

While the overall quality of medical care throughout the United States is generally of very high quality and in many places is superb, there are still those rare, complex or extremely difficult problems that demand resources beyond the ordinary or that require talents that are exceptional.

This guide identifies those top medical specialists throughout the country who possess the skill and experience to address these problems. Top specialists who provide excellent care tend to be located predominantly, although not exclusively, at major medical centers, specialty hospitals and leading teaching hospitals. These exceptional physicians are acknowledged as such by their peers and are recognized for their expertise by the medical profession.

The top specialists we have identified are not the only excellent physicians who are caring for patients in this nation. Since there are more than 720,000 doctors in the United States, we cannot identify every top specialist. Therefore, we have included narrative to assist those using this guide who may not find the specialist they need within its listings. Clearly, there are many primary care physicians and other well-trained specialists in communities and hospitals throughout the United States.

Most physicians in this guide are board certified not only in a specialty, but also in a subspecialty or in multiple subspecialties. Board or subspecialty certification alone, however, does not distinguish them from excellent specialists at hospitals in your community, many of whom are also board certified in both a specialty and a subspecialty.

However, the majority of physicians included in this guide have trained at the top medical centers under medical pioneers who possess state-of-the-art knowledge in a specific disease or problem and have often devised new techniques and therapeutic approaches, many of which are life-saving procedures or cures. These doctors most often practice their science and art at leading hospitals and, more specifically, in programs at hospitals that are recognized for their excellence in a given field. Many others have been trained at leading centers in other nations since the U.S. is not alone in pioneering new medical knowledge, although its position as the leader in "high-tech" medicine is generally acknowledged.

Introduction

Another major characteristic distinguishing the majority of physicians in this guide from those at local hospitals is their continued focus and training. Rather than practicing at a community hospital (or even at a leading regional hospital) and developing a general, broad-based practice, these physicians continued their training in a particular disease, syndrome or subspecialty to such a degree that they developed extensive knowledge and unique skills in treating that particular problem.

Often that focused, advanced training is accompanied by active involvement in clinical research. This is an additional reason why the physicians listed in this guide are located at only a few hundred of the more than six thousand hospitals in the United States. It is difficult, although not impossible, to conduct important clinical research in isolation or without an environment supportive of research. It takes time, money, residents, research associates, technicians, equipment and more to produce significant clinical research. Certainly there have been individuals who have made important and lasting contributions to research with little or none of this support, but those instances are rare. Today, for the most part, major advances in medicine occur in the labs and on the floors of major medical centers and specialty hospitals, in medical schools and in clinical labs created and financed for that purpose by commercial enterprises.

How Physicians Were Selected For Inclusion In This Guide

Castle Connolly's Top Doctors™ selection process begins with surveys of physicians and healthcare professionals. Each year, Castle Connolly surveys thousands of physicians and other healthcare professionals and asks them to identify excellent doctors in every specialty in their region and throughout the nation. When we began the research for the first edition of America's Top Doctors® 20 years ago, we surveyed over 230,000 of the nation's leading medical specialists, department chairs, residency program directors, vice presidents of medical affairs and presidents of the nation's leading medical centers and specialty hospitals. In addition to mail and online surveys, the Castle Connolly physician-led research team makes thousands of phone calls each year, talking with leading specialists, chairs of clinical departments and vice presidents of medical affairs, seeking to identify top specialists for every disease and procedure.

The Castle Connolly physician-led research team carefully reviews the credentials of every physician being considered for inclusion in Castle Connolly Guides, magazine features and website. The review includes, among other factors, scrutiny of medical education, training, hospital appointments, administrative posts, professional achievements, and malpractice and disciplinary history. Information on outcomes, procedure volume and malpractice is becoming increasingly available, but the public disclosure varies from state to state. Castle Connolly uses its best efforts to gather the information that is available and use it effectively. Ultimately, however, it is the professional judgment of the Castle Connolly editors, the Chief Medical and Research Officer and the research staff, which determines Castle Connolly Top Doctor™ selection.

Physicians may also be removed from the Castle Connolly lists if, in the judgment of the selection team, that is warranted. Some of the reasons physicians are removed include retirement, change in practice (taking a full time administrative post, for example), unavailability to patients, malpractice or disciplinary issues, negative physician or patient feedback, professional demeanor or a change in the "mix" of specialists Castle Connolly will present for a given community. Being removed from a Castle Connolly list does not necessarily indicate something negative about the physician.

Castle Connolly does not claim to identify every excellent physician in the nation or a region; it is impossible to identify them all. Those identified by Castle Connolly are clearly among the very best in the nation. That is why our guides, websites and other distribution channels for this critical information describe a process whereby consumers can identify excellent physicians using their own efforts. Furthermore, there are many excellent physicians on the regional level, especially in primary care, that are not included in this guide. Included in this guide are the nation's top referral specialists and those skilled at treating a specific condition or disease; they are found primarily at teaching hospitals, major medical centers and leading specialty hospitals.

How do we accomplish this enormous task? Over the years, the Castle Connolly physician-led research team developed its extensive database of physicians across the nation through periodic mail, telephone and email surveys. This cumulative database is systematically maintained and continuously updated. Surveyed physicians nominate top doctors in both their own and related specialties – especially those to whom they would refer their own patients. Each year this database is supplemented by further mail surveys and telephone interviews with leaders in the various medical specialties and leading physicians at major medical centers.

To augment our large mail, telephone and online polling process, additional surveys are conducted among the following carefully selected groups: directors of graduate medical programs, directors of clinical services at member hospitals of the Council of Teaching Hospitals (COTH), board members of medical specialty academies, associations and societies and deans and chairs of departments at medical schools

Building on years of prior research, thousands of top doctors included in earlier editions of our guides are invited to offer their nominations for Castle Connolly *America's Top Doctors®*. Beginning in 2011, and moving forward, the nomination process invited every licensed MD and DO across the country to participate. This involved contacting over 50,000 physicians and healthcare executives, a nationwide distribution of nomination notifications via various media channels and partnering with US News and World Report as a means of expanding our process to physicians across the country.

Over 55,000 physicians have been nominated through this process this year. Extensive biographical forms were sent to those physicians most frequently nominated for completion. After careful review of their professional backgrounds, the Castle Connolly research staff conducted further research to check disciplinary, certification and license histories.

We do not intentionally include physicians simply because they have important titles. While a position as a chief of service or a department head at a teaching hospital is an important post, such positions are achieved through a combination of many talents including administrative skills, seniority and factors that are not as important for inclusion in this guide as is skill in clinical care. The same is true of leaders of county medical societies, professional associations or even specialty groups. While these are significant positions and acknowledge a leadership among peers, these titles are not essential to clinical skill recognition.

The same perspective applies to research expertise. Many physicians listed in the Guide are engaged in clinical research and make significant contributions to their fields, with some devoting a substantial portion of their time to research. However, we avoided including those physicians who solely conduct research and who do not provide patient care.

The result of this extensive research effort is a list of outstanding, highly skilled physicians who are recognized as among the best in their specialties and in the nation; a list which consumers/patients can use to find the very best specialists to meet their particular needs.

Lastly, this book differs from the regional Castle Connolly Guides in two important ways. First, Castle Connolly *America's Top Doctors® 11th Edition* is national, not regional, in scope. Second, the regional Guides are based on the generally accurate premise that healthcare is local and most people find their healthcare where they live and work. However, Castle Connolly *America's Top Doctors® 11th Edition* is designed to meet the needs of those people who cannot find the right specialists locally but who can and will travel anywhere in the country to be cared for by a top specialist at an outstanding hospital. This guide will assist readers in that important search and, for that reason, does not include primary care physicians.

Using This Guide To Find Top Specialists

This guide is organized and planned to be as user-friendly as possible. Still, as with anything as complex as medical specialties, subspecialties and the myriad of diseases and problems that specialists treat, there needs to be a system to organize the physicians' names, the diseases and problems they manage and their special expertise.

To organize the specialists in this guide, we have followed the American Board of Medical Specialties (ABMS) format. The ABMS is the authoritative body for the recognition of medical specialties. Without the ABMS as the official controlling body there would be hundreds of unregulated medical specialties.

The ABMS recognizes twenty-five specialties and more than ninety subspecialties. The listing of ABMS specialties and subspecialties can be found in Appendix A. In addition to ABMS recognized specialties, there are at least one hundred other groups calling themselves "medical specialists" that are not recognized by the ABMS. Some of these groups are working toward recognition and have exams and other standards for membership. Others are organizations of physicians interested in a particular problem or area of medicine that exist to exchange information but have no intention of seeking ABMS recognition. Some groups calling themselves "boards" really have little authority or meaningful standards. Thus, while a physician may state he/she is, for example, a specialist in cosmetic surgery, there is no ABMS recognized specialty by that name. Therefore, you have no idea whether this physician has any special training and expertise or is simply trying to recruit paying patients to a lucrative aspect of surgical practice.

You can get information on a doctor's credentials from the doctor, from the doctor's hospital (Medical Affairs Office) or from your health plan if a doctor is in the network. You can also get this information from numerous Web sites, including www.castleconnolly.com. You can check on a physician's board certification by calling the ABMS at (866) 275-2267 or by logging on to its Web site at www.abms.org.

If you seek a particular type of specialist or subspecialist, turn to the section of this guide covering that medical specialty or subspecialty. There you will be able to further restrict your search to a specific geographic region or, if you prefer, to search throughout the nation.

Using This Guide To Find Top Specialists

To make your search easier, we have organized the specialties and subspecialties into the following regions: New England, Mid Atlantic, Midwest, Southeast, Southwest, Great Plains and Mountains, and West Coast and Pacific. To find an outstanding cardiologist in St. Louis, for example, look under Cardiovascular Disease and then under the Midwest region. (See Pages 38-39 for geographical regions and states.)

A second way to use this guide is to look at the Special Expertise Index, which lists the areas of special expertise of included physicians. This list of special expertise indicates more than 2,000 medical topics including diseases, therapeutic approaches and techniques. You can look up the particular disease, problem or technique you are interested in and locate a physician in that manner. We assume that many people using this guide will know what their particular problem is and will begin their exploration with this index. However, we encourage you to read the entire text since it will help you to better understand how to find the right physician for yourself or a family member, especially if one is not found in this guide.

Choosing An Appropriate Specialist

It may seem that choosing the correct specialist to treat a particular medical problem is simply a matter of finding a top doctor in a specific medical specialty. For treatment of a problem with your vision, you would choose an ophthalmologist. A skin or hair problem would require treatment by a dermatologist and a broken bone would need the care of an orthopaedic surgeon.

Sometimes, however, the type of specialist needed may not be obvious. For example, back surgery may be performed by either an orthopaedic surgeon or a neurosurgeon. Different aspects of sports medicine, as another example, are practiced by orthopaedic surgeons who treat sports-related injuries in both adults and children, pediatricians who treat only children or internists and family practitioners whose focus is on prevention of injuries.

In some cases, several specialists with expertise in different areas of medical practice all become involved in treating the same patient's health problem. For example, a person with diabetes might need care from an endocrinologist, a cardiologist and an ophthalmologist. In other situations, doctors trained in different specialties may use varied approaches or differing therapies to manage a disease or condition. Such is the case, for example, with prostate cancer: a patient could be treated by a urologist, a medical oncologist, or a radiation oncologist. The urologist might provide the patient with a surgical treatment option, while the medical oncologist would treat the patient with chemotherapy and the radiotherapist would use radiation therapy and/or radioactive seed implantation. All approaches could be successful, or one might be preferable to another, depending on the patient and his condition. Therefore, a wise patient will thoroughly explore all options before making a choice.

Finding the right specialist is also important in terms of the quality of your care. For example, many orthopaedic surgeons will operate on hands, but it is clearly preferable to have someone trained and certified specifically in hand surgery (a subspecialty of both orthopaedic surgery and plastic surgery) to perform that delicate surgery. Similarly, a dermatologist may indicate that his/her practice includes cosmetic surgery; however, there is no approved ABMS dermatology subspecialty or fellowship training in cosmetic surgery. While many dermatologists do pursue additional training in cosmetic surgery, it should be understood that dermatologic practice is limited to cutaneous procedures ranging from the removal of skin tumors to laser resurfacing. On the other hand, some board certified otolaryngologists have additional training that enables them to perform cosmetic surgery procedures on the head and neck.

Choosing the right type of specialist is as important as selecting the right doctor. For example, the diagnosis of melanoma, a very serious, potentially life threatening form of skin cancer, is missed in many cases. Therefore, if you have a skin lesion that might possibly be melanoma, you should be certain that the pathologist reading your slides is board certified in the subspecialty of dermatopathology.

These examples illustrate this important principle: always seek the best healthcare. Look for the best-trained doctors, not those who simply can do the job. That doesn't mean that you need to consult a doctor listed in this guide every time you have a health problem. It does mean you should be certain that the physicians who care for you, whether in your community or at a world-class medical center, are trained appropriately and are qualified to provide the care you require. Remember, when it comes to healthcare no one wants second best!

Given this complexity, how do you find the right specialist to provide your care? The first and most important person to look to for guidance is your primary care physician. He/she will assess your medical condition, determine the appropriate type of specialist to recommend and perhaps refer you to a specific doctor or doctors. You should always ask your primary care physician why a particular specialist is being recommended, since that specialist may be a colleague in your doctor's medical group or may be the only (or the most conveniently located) specialist of the type in your health plan. Ask how well your primary care physician knows the specialist, whether they have a long-standing professional relationship and if other patients referred to the specialist had successful outcomes. Be sure to ask for several recommendations, if possible, to provide you with some choice among specialists.

If you do not have a primary care doctor, try to learn as much as you can about your medical problem and the type of specialist best suited to treat it. However, keep in mind that many diseases or conditions present with symptoms that often are indistinguishable from those of other diseases or conditions, making them difficult to diagnose precisely even for physicians armed with the results of diagnostic tests.

Using This Guide To Find Top Specialists

Judging The Qualifications Of A Physician

The specialists listed in Castle Connolly *America's Top Doctors*® are clearly among the best in the nation and have been identified through a rigorous research process and thorough screening by the Castle Connolly research team. Through our extensive surveys and research we have done much of the work in finding a top referral specialist for you. But how do you judge the qualifications of a physician who may not be listed in this Guide? If you are trying to find a specialist on your own, how should you go about it? How can you tell when a physician has the appropriate training in a specialty and how do you distinguish what is meaningful and what is not from among all those plaques and certificates on a doctor's wall?

The following pages will outline that process for you. In fact, what is written here reflects much of the logic that underlies the selection of physicians for this book.

The following material will help you not only in finding a top specialist in this Guide, but it also should be helpful to you in choosing among the many specialists, primary care doctors and other physicians that you will need to consult throughout your life.

The reality is that few of us see only one doctor in our lifetime. Each of us may be cared for by a primary care physician, an ophthalmologist, an orthopaedic surgeon, a dermatologist, a surgeon or a number of other specialists. The choices can be many and they can be among the most important choices that we make in our lives.

Education

Your review of your prospective doctor's education and training should begin with medical school. While you may feel that the institution at which someone earned a bachelor's degree could be an indication of the quality of the doctor, most people in the medical field do not believe it plays a major role. A degree from a highly selective undergraduate college or university will help an aspiring doctor gain admission to a medical school, but once there, all students are peers. However, the information on undergraduate colleges, if important to you, is available in *The Official ABMS Directory of Board Certified Medical Specialists*® and other medical directories.

American medical schools are highly standardized, at least in terms of basic quality. A group known as the Liaison Committee for Medical Education (LCME) accredits all U.S. medical schools that grant medical degrees (MDs) and osteopathic degrees (DOs). Most also are accredited by the appropriate state agency, if one exists, and by regional accrediting agencies that accredit colleges and universities of all kinds.

Furthermore, U.S. medical schools have universally high standards for admission, including success on the undergraduate level and on the Medical College Admissions Tests (MCATs). Although frequently criticized for being slow to change and for training too many specialists, the system of medical education in the United States has insured high quality in medical practice. One recent positive change is a strong effort in most medical schools to diversify the composition of the student body. While these schools have been less successful in enrolling racial minorities, the number of women in U.S. medical schools has increased to the point that women now make up about 50 percent of most classes. In certain specialties preferred by women medical graduates (pediatrics, for example) it is possible that in coming years the majority of specialists will be female.

Most doctors practicing in the United States are graduates of U.S. medical schools, but there are two other groups of doctors who make up a relatively small portion of the total physician population. They are (1) foreign nationals who graduated from foreign schools and (2) U.S. nationals who graduated from foreign schools. (Canadian medical schools are not considered foreign).

Foreign Medical Graduates

Foreign medical schools vary greatly in quality. Even some of the oldest and finest European schools have become virtually "open door," with huge numbers of unscreened students making teaching and learning difficult. Others are excellent and provided the model for our system of medical education.

The fact that someone graduated from a foreign school does not mean that he/she is a poor doctor. Foreign schools, like U.S. schools, produce good doctors and poor doctors. Foreign medical graduates must pass the same exam taken by U.S. graduates for licensure, but the failure rate for foreign graduates is significantly higher. In the first year of using the new United States Medical Licensing Exam (USMLE), 93 percent of U.S. medical school graduates passed Step II, the clinical exam, as compared with 39 percent of the foreign graduates. It is clear that the quality of foreign schools, if not individual doctors, is not the same as U.S. medical schools, at least as measured by our standards. Nonetheless, many communities and patients have been well served by foreign medical graduates practicing in this country—often in areas where it has been difficult to attract graduates of American schools. In fact, almost one-third of physicians practicing in the U.S. are foreign trained.

In addition, many foreign medical schools and their teaching hospitals are world renowned for their leadership in medical care, research and teaching and many of the technologies and techniques we utilize in the U.S. today have been developed and perfected in foreign countries.

Residency

Most doctors practicing today have at least three years of postgraduate training (following the MD or DO) in an approved residency program. This not only is an important step in the process of becoming a competent doctor, but it is also a requirement for board (specialty) certification. Most people assume that a prospective doctor needs to complete a three-year residency program to obtain a medical license. That is not an accurate assumption! New York State, for example, requires only one postgraduate year. However, since all approved residencies last at least three years and some, such as those in neurosurgery, general surgery, orthopaedic surgery and urology, may extend for five or more years, it is important to know the details of a doctor's training. Licensure alone is not enough of a basis upon which to make a decision.

Without undertaking extensive and detailed research on every residency program, the best assessment you can make of a doctor's residency program is to see if it took place in a large medical center whose name you recognize. The more prestigious institutions tend to attract the best medical students, sometimes regardless of the quality of the individual residency program. If in doubt about a doctor's training, ask the doctor if the residency he/she completed was in the specialty of the practice; if not, ask why not.

It is also important to be certain that a doctor completed a residency that has been approved by the appropriate governing board of the specialty, such as the American Board of Surgery, the American Board of Radiology, or the American Osteopathic Board of Pediatrics. These board groups are listed in Appendix A. If you are really concerned about a doctor's training, you should call the hospital that offered the residency and ask if the residency program was approved by the appropriate specialty group. If still in doubt, consult the publication *Directory of Graduate Medical Education Programs*, often called the "green book," found in medical school or hospital libraries, which lists all approved residencies.

Board Certification

With an MD or DO degree and a license, an individual may practice in any medical specialty with or without additional training. For example, doctors with a license but no special training may call themselves cardiologists, pediatricians or gynecologists. This is why board certification is such an important factor. The American Board of Medical Specialties (ABMS) recognizes 25 specialties and more than 90 subspecialties. Visit www.abms.org or call 866-275-2267 for more information. Eighteen boards certify in 106 specialties under the aegis of the American Osteopathic Association (AOA). Visit www.osteopathic.org or call 800-621-1773 for more information. Doctors who have qualified for such specialization are called board certified; they have completed an approved residency and passed the board's exam. (See Appendix A for the approved ABMS and AOA lists). While many doctors who are not board certified do call themselves "specialists," board certification is the best standard by which to measure competence and training. Throughout this Guide a description of each specialty and subspecialty is provided as an introduction to the listing of physicians in that specialty.

You can be confident that doctors who are board certified have, at a minimum, the proper training in their specialty and have demonstrated their proficiency through supervision and testing. While there are many non-board certified doctors who are highly competent, it is more difficult to assess the level of their training. While board certification alone does not guarantee competence, it is a standard that reflects successful completion of an appropriate training program. If it is impossible to find a doctor in your area who is board certified in a particular subspecialty, for example, geriatric medicine or sports medicine, at least be certain the physician is board certified in a related specialty such as internal medicine or orthopaedic surgery.

Board certified doctors are referred to as Diplomates of the Board. Some of the colleges of medical specialties (e.g., the American College of Radiology, the American College of Surgeons) have multiple levels of recognition. The first is basic membership and the second, more prestigious and difficult to obtain, is status as a Fellow. Fellowship status in the colleges is meaningful and is based on experience, professional achievement and recognition by one's peers, including extensive experience in patient care. It should be viewed as a significant professional qualification.

Board Eligibility

Many doctors who have been more recently trained are waiting to take the boards. They are sometimes described as "board eligible," a common term that the ABMS advocates abandoning because of its ambiguity. Board eligible means that the doctor has completed an approved residency and is qualified to sit for the related board's exam.

Each member board of the ABMS has its own policy regarding the use and recognition of the board eligible term. Therefore, the description "board eligible" should not be viewed as a genuine qualification, especially if a doctor has been out of medical school long enough to have taken the certification exam. To the boards, a doctor is either board certified or not. Furthermore, most of the specialty boards permit unlimited attempts to pass the exam and, in some cases, doctors who have failed the exam twice or even ten times continue to call themselves board eligible. In osteopathic medicine, the board eligible status is recognized only for the first six years after completion of a residency.

In addition to the approved lists of specialties and subspecialties of the ABMS and AOA, there are a wide variety of other doctors and groups of doctors who call themselves specialists. At present there are at least 100 such groups called "self-designated medical specialties." They range from doctors who are working to create a recognized body of knowledge and subspecialty training to less formal groups interested in a particular approach to the practice of medicine. These groups may or may not have standards for membership. There is no way to determine the true extent of their members' training and neither the ABMS or the AOA recognizes them. While you should be cautious of doctors who claim they are specialists in these areas, many do have advanced training and the groups at least offer a listing of people interested in a particular approach to medical care. Rely on board certification to assure yourself of basic competence, and use membership in one of these groups to indicate strong interest and possible additional training in a particular aspect of medicine. A list of these self-designated medical specialties may be found in Appendix B.

Recertification

A relatively new focus of the specialty boards is the area of recertification. Until recently, board certification lasted for an unlimited time. Now, almost all the boards have put time limits on the certification period. For example, in Internal Medicine and Anesthesiology, the time limit is ten years; in Family Practice, six, and under some circumstances, seven years. These more stringent standards reflect an increasing emphasis on recertification by both the medical boards and state agencies responsible for licensing doctors.

Since the policies of the boards vary widely, it is a good procedure to ask a doctor if certification was awarded and when. If the date was seven to ten years ago, ask if he/she has been recertified. Unfortunately, many boards permit "grandfathering," whereby already certified doctors do not have to be recertified, and recertification requirements apply only to newly certified doctors. Appendix A contains a list of the names and addresses of the boards and the certification period for each board specialty. Even if recertification is not required, it is good professional practice for doctors to undertake the process. It assures you, the patient, that they are attempting to stay current.

Many states have a continuing medical education requirement for doctors. These states typically require a minimum number of continuing medical education (CME) credits for a doctor to maintain a medical license. Seven states require 150 CME credits over a three-year period. Osteopathic doctors are required to take 120 hours of CME credits within three years to maintain certification.

Fellowships

The purpose of a fellowship is to provide advanced training in the clinical techniques and research of a particular specialty. Fellowships usually, but not always, are designed to lead to board certification in a subspecialty such as cardiology, which is a subspecialty of internal medicine. Many physicians listed in this Guide have had fellowship training. In the U.S. there are a variety of fellowship programs available to doctors, which fall into two broad categories: approved and unapproved. Approved fellowships are those that are approved by the appropriate medical specialty board (e.g., the American Board of Radiology) and lead to subspecialty certificates. Fellowship programs that are unapproved are often in the same areas of training as those that are approved, but they do not lead to subspecialty certificates. Unfortunately, all too often, an unapproved fellowship exists only to provide relatively inexpensive labor for the research and/or patient care activities of a clinical department in a medical school or hospital. In such cases, the learning that takes place is secondary and may be a good deal less than in an approved fellowship. On the other hand, any fellowship is better than none at all and some unapproved fellowships have that status for a valid reason that should not reflect negatively on the program. For example, the fellowship may have been recently created, with approval being sought. To check that a fellowship is an approved one, call the hospital where the training took place or call the medical board for that specialty.

Some physicians may have completed more than one fellowship and may be boarded in two or more subspecialties. Also, some physicians may pursue fellowship training and subspecialty certification, but then choose to practice in their primary field of certification. For example, a doctor who is board certified in internal medicine also may have obtained board certification in cardiology, but may choose to practice primarily internal medicine rather than cardiology. For the most part, the physicians in this Guide practice in their subspecialties.

Professional Reputation

There are doctors who meet every professional standard on paper, but who are simply not good doctors. In all probability the medical community has ascertained that and, while the individual may still practice medicine, his/her reputation will reflect that collective assessment. There are also doctors who are outstanding leaders in their fields because of research or professional activities but who are not particularly strong, or perhaps even active, in patient care. It is important to distinguish that kind of professional reputation from a reputation as a competent, caring doctor in delivering patient care, or in the case of this Guide, as an outstanding practitioner in a given specialty.

Using This Guide To Find Top Specialists

Hospital Appointment

Most doctors are on the medical staff of one or more hospitals and are known as "attendings;" some are not. If a doctor does not have admitting privileges or is not on the attending staff of a hospital, you may wish to consider choosing a different doctor. It can be very difficult to ascertain whether or not the lack of hospital appointment is for a good reason. For example, it is understandable that some doctors who are raising families or heading toward retirement choose not to meet the demands (meetings, committees, etc.) of being an attending. However, if you need care in a hospital, the lack of such an appointment means that another doctor will have to oversee that care. In some specialties, such as dermatology and psychiatry, doctors may conduct their entire practice in the office and a hospital appointment is not as essential, or as good a criterion for assessment, as in other specialties.

While mistakes are made, most hospitals are quite careful about admissions to their medical staffs. The best hospitals are highly selective, so a degree of screening (or "credentialing") has been done for you. In other words, the best doctors practice at the best hospitals. Since caring for a patient in a hospital is often a team effort involving a number of specialists, the reputation of the hospital to which the doctor admits patients carries special weight. Hospital medical staffs review their colleagues' credentials and authorize performance of specific procedures. In addition, they typically review and reappoint their medical staff every two or three years. In effect, this is an additional screening to protect patients. It is especially true of hospitals that have what are known as closed staffs, where it is impossible to obtain admitting privileges unless there is a vacancy that the administration and medical staff deem necessary to fill. If you are having a surgical procedure and are concerned about the doctor's skill or experience, it may be worthwhile to call the Medical Affairs office at the doctor's hospital to see if he/she is authorized to perform that procedure in that hospital.

The reasons for a hospital's selectivity are easy to understand: no hospital wishes to expose itself to liability and every hospital wants to have the best reputation possible in order to attract patients. Obviously, the quality of the medical staff is immensely important in creating that reputation.

Physicians listed in this guide are primarily on the staffs of major medical centers, usually teaching hospitals, and leading specialty hospitals, e.g. children's, cancer, heart, psychiatric, etc. There are many excellent physicians on the staffs of community hospitals that call themselves "medical centers," but they are not physicians who typically attract complex cases and referrals from outside their area.

To learn about a hospital visit its website. It is also useful to review a hospital's accreditation status under the Joint Commission on the Accreditation of Healthcare Organizations at www.JCAHO.com. A new website created by the federal government, www.hospitalcompare.com, offers some measures of comparative hospital quality and may be of interest as well.

A last and very important reason why a hospital appointment is an essential requirement in your choice of doctor is that some states permit doctors to practice without malpractice insurance. If you are injured as a result of a doctor's poor care, you could be without recourse. However, few hospitals permit doctors to practice in them unless they carry malpractice insurance. This not only protects the hospital, but the patient as well.

Medical School Faculty Appointment

Many doctors have appointments on the faculties of medical schools. There is a range of categories from "straight" appointments, meaning full-time appointment as professor, associate professor, assistant professor or instructor, to clinical ranks that may reflect lesser degrees of involvement in teaching or research. If someone carries what is known as a straight academic rank (i.e. "professor of surgery," without clinical in the title), this usually means that the individual is engaged full-time in medical school research, teaching activities and patient care. The title "clinical professor of surgery" usually indicates a less direct involvement in medical school activities such as teaching and research.

Doctors who are full-time academicians may be in the forefront of new techniques and research, but they are not necessarily better doctors. Nonetheless, you would be assured that they have the support of other faculty, residents and medical students.

When you are seeking a subspecialist, a doctor's relationship to a medical school becomes more meaningful since medical school faculties tend to be made up of subspecialists. You are less likely to find large numbers of general or primary care practitioners engaged full-time on a medical school faculty. The newest approaches and techniques in medicine, for the most part, are explored and developed by medical school faculties in their laboratories and clinical practice settings. This is where they practice their subspecialties, as well as teach and conduct research. Such leading specialists are not necessarily better doctors than community doctors; rather, they are trained to provide a different kind of medical care. Obviously the type of medical care users of this guide are seeking is that different kind of care available primarily from top subspecialists at leading hospitals and medical centers.

Medical Society Membership

Most medical society memberships sound very prestigious and some are; however, there are many societies that are not selective and which virtually any doctor can join. In addition, membership in many of the more prestigious societies is based on research and publication or on leadership in the field and may have little to do with direct patient care. While it is clearly an honor to be invited to join these groups, membership may be less than helpful in discerning whether a doctor can deliver the excellent clinical care you require.

Experience

Experience is difficult to assess. Obviously, in most cases, an older doctor has more experience; on the other hand, a younger doctor has been more recently immersed in the challenge of medical school, residency, or even a fellowship, and may be the most up-to-date. If a doctor is board certified, you may assume that assures at least a minimal amount of experience, but since it could be as little as a year, check the date of graduation from medical school or completion of residency to know precisely how long a doctor has been in practice.

There is a good deal of evidence that there is a positive relationship between quantity of experience and quality of care. It may be that, the more a doctor performs a procedure, the better he/she becomes at it. That is why it is important to ask a doctor about his or her experience with the procedure that you need. Does the doctor see and treat similar cases every day, every week or only rarely? Of course, with some rare diseases, rarely is the only possible answer, but it is relative frequency that is critical. Major metropolitan areas, especially New York and San Francisco, became leaders in the treatment of AIDS because of the number of patients seen in those metropolitan areas. Doctors in the suburbs of New York City (especially in New York's Westchester, Nassau and Suffolk counties) and in Fairfield County, Connecticut became leaders in the research and treatment of Lyme disease because that region is the epicenter of the disease.

In some states, data is available on volume or numbers of certain procedures performed at hospitals. Likewise, The Leapfrog Group (www.leapfroggroup.org) compares hospitals' performance on the national standards of safety, quality and efficiency - areas of healthcare that are most relevant to consumers and this information is later used to improve hospital quality, save healthcare spending and assist hospital employees with purchasing strategies. The federal government has posted outcome data for hospitals, but for a limited number of procedures, on a website www.hospitalcompare.hhs.gov/hospital-search.aspx or http://bit.ly/jdvCzW. There is a good deal of controversy, however, on the validity and usefulness of such data. Opponents cite the fact that some of the data is produced from Medicare patient records only and, thus, is based solely on an elderly population that does not represent the total activity of a hospital or doctor. Proponents of the use of such volume data agree that it is not perfect, but suggest it can be one useful criterion in selecting the best places to receive care for these specific problems

The one type of experience you should specifically want to know about is that dealing with any special procedure, particularly a surgical one, that has recently been developed and introduced into practice. For example, in the 1980's many doctors using laparoscopic cholecystectomy, a then new surgical technique for removing gallbladders, experienced a high percentage of problems because they were not properly trained. This prompted the American Board of Surgery to announce new standards for the training of surgeons using this technique. Do not hesitate to ask about your doctor's training in a procedure and how frequently and with what degree of success he/she has performed it. Practice may not lead to perfection, but it does improve skills and enhance the probability of success.

In some cases, relatively young doctors have recently completed residency or fellowship training under recognized leaders who have developed new approaches or techniques for dealing with a particular problem. They may have learned the new techniques from their mentors and may be far ahead of the field (and ahead of more senior and distinguished colleagues) in using those approaches. So age and experience must be considered and weighed along with other factors when choosing a physician.

Second Opinions

Second opinions are a valuable medical tool, too infrequently used in many instances and overused in others. Clearly, you do not want to seek another doctor's opinion on every ailment or problem that you face, but a second opinion should be pursued in the following situations:

• before major surgery

• if the diagnosis is serious or life threatening

• if a rare disease is diagnosed

• if a diagnosis is uncertain

• if the number of tests or procedures recommended might be excessive

• if a test result has serious implications (e.g., a positive Pap smear)

• if the treatment suggested is risky or expensive

• if you are uncomfortable with the diagnosis and/or treatment

• if a course of treatment is not successful

• if you question your doctor's competence

• if your insurance company requires it

Most doctors will be supportive if you request a second opinion and many will recommend it. In many cases, insurance companies will pay for second opinions, but check ahead of time to make sure your insurance plan does cover them. In an HMO you may have to be more assertive because one way HMOs control costs is by limiting second opinions. Often, the opinion of a second doctor will confirm the opinion of the first, but the reassurance may be worth the time and extra cost. On the other hand, if the second opinion differs from the first, you have two alternatives: seek the opinion of a third doctor, or educate yourself as much as possible by talking to both doctors, reading up on the problem, and trusting your instincts about which diagnosis is correct.

Office And Practice Arrangements

Although clearly not as important as training or reputation, a specialist's office and practice arrangements often are of significance to patients. Practice arrangements include office hours, office location, billing procedures and accessibility among the many factors that result in how well the office is run.

Some specialists only will see new patients who are referred to them by another doctor. Therefore, you may need to have your treating physician contact the specialist's office to arrange for your initial visit. Your health plan may also require that your primary care doctor provide a referral.

If English is not your first language, it may be advisable to determine whether someone in the specialist's office speaks your primary language or if a translator can be present during appointments. This will ease communication and assure that all questions, responses and instructions are understood.

Accessibility of the specialist's office may be a concern if you are wheelchair-bound, are elderly or cannot climb stairs or negotiate narrow corridors. Convenient parking may also be important to you.

Other arrangements that may need to be made in advance of your first visit or discussed with the specialist's office staff concern payment. You may wish to ask the following:

- Does the specialist accept your health insurance coverage?

- Is the specialist within your plan's network and will you need to pay a
  co-payment? Or, is the specialist out-of-network and will you have to pay for
  your care out-of-pocket, meet a deductible or submit a form for reimbursement?

- Are credit cards an acceptable mode of payment?

- Does the specialist accept Medicare, Medicaid or no-fault insurance? Does the
  specialist treat workers' compensation cases?

- If you are a non-resident of the United States, will you need to arrange for the transfer or exchange of currency to pay the specialist's fee?

When you are choosing a top specialist, these issues may be of lesser or greater importance, depending on the problem and type of care warranted. If you are traveling a great distance to have a specific procedure performed by a top specialist at a major medical center, continuing long-term monitoring or follow-up care by that physician may not be required or may not be feasible and such things as office practice arrangements are of less importance. On the other hand, if you have a chronic problem that needs to be monitored with follow-up care provided by the same top specialist, then such issues as accessibility of the doctor's office, appointment hours, waiting times and courtesy and professionalism of the staff become more significant.

Personal Chemistry

One element of the doctor-patient relationship that we stress in our guides is chemistry between doctor and patient, a part of which is often referred to as a doctor's "bedside manner." While this factor is of major import in a long-term relationship such as one you would have with your primary care physician, it is of less importance when you see a specialist only once or twice. However, since many people using this book may have chronic conditions that require ongoing care, it is important to give the matter some consideration.

It is vital that there is a sense of mutual trust and respect between patient and doctor; a judgment that individuals must make for themselves. Among the many talented doctors listed in this guide, there are very likely some to whom you would relate well and others with whom you may not feel as comfortable.

Patients prefer doctors who listen, demonstrate concern, are responsive to patient needs and spend sufficient time with them. The qualities of physicians in this regard, even the excellent ones in this guide, vary immensely.

You, the patient, are the only one who can assess these qualities because individuals react differently to various personalities. It is important for you to carefully judge your feelings towards a physician, especially if you are embarking on a long-term relationship. You should feel you can be open, trusting and responsive to your physician and that your relationship will be a positive one. Otherwise, find another doctor, since not doing so could adversely affect your care.

Once you have used this guide to identify the top specialist(s) best suited to treat your condition, there is much you can do to maximize the value of your first visit.

The Best in American Medicine
www.CastleConnolly.com

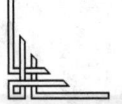
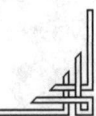

Maximizing Your First Appointment With A Top Doctor

After your research is done and you've secured an appointment for an initial consultation with a top doctor known for his/her expertise in the diagnosis or treatment of your particular medical condition, what should you do?

Whether your visit to the specialist's office is a car ride or a plane trip away, there undoubtedly will be arrangements to make before your appointment. You may have to take time off from work, arrange for childcare while you are away and make travel plans and hotel reservations, but there are a number of other important steps to take to assure that you and the specialist make the best use of the time you spend together.

Have you done everything you can to prepare yourself and the specialist for the consultation? The following checklist will help you maximize the value of your visit to the specialist and will go a long way toward focusing you on the task at hand—getting the best advice or treatment for your health problem from one of the top doctors in the medical specialty related to your condition.

Gathering The Facts

- Does the specialist have all the information needed to make a diagnosis of or treatment plan for your condition?

- Have your medical records, test results and X-rays been sent ahead of time to allow for their review by the specialist in advance of your first appointment?

- Have you written out your medical history, including that of your siblings, parents and grandparents, emphasizing the particular problem for which you are visiting this specialist?

- Are you prepared with a written list of questions?

- Do you understand the answers?

A specialist becoming newly involved in your care needs to learn as much as possible about the state of your health in a very limited time. Since top doctors are extremely busy people with many demands on their time, you should make certain that all relevant records and case summaries are obtained and sent to the specialist well in advance of your appointment.

Obtaining Your Records

All healthcare providers, including hospitals, doctors and their staffs, are under legal obligation to maintain the privacy of your medical records. In order to obtain release of those records, you must make a request in writing. If you need to obtain records from a number of providers, you should write one clear and concise letter authorizing release of your records and including your name, address, telephone number, date of birth, identification number and any other identifying information such as a hospital chart number. You then can make photocopies of this letter, but be sure to sign and date each copy as if it were an original. You also may want to specifically name those test results (e.g., pathology slides) or X-ray films (not just written reports or summaries) that must be included in addition to making a general request for your records. It's also a good idea to indicate the date of your appointment so the office staff can respond in a timely manner.

Although state laws require the timely release of medical records, hospital medical records departments and doctors' offices often take several weeks to pull and review patient charts and get them in the mail either to you or to another doctor. In addition to written authorization, you may be asked to pay the costs involved in copying your records, test results and X-ray films because many doctors' offices will not release the originals. Consider placing a call in advance to determine the procedure for releasing your records, how long you can expect it to take and the costs involved so that you can save time by including payment with your release authorization letter. Be sure to allow sufficient time in advance of your consultation appointment for your request to be processed. Since you often must wait several weeks for an appointment with a specialist, allow at least that amount of time to obtain your records.

Even after making your written requests, you should follow up each letter with a telephone call to be sure that your records actually are sent. You should not assume that your request for records will be promptly fulfilled by an often overburdened, although well-intentioned, office staff.

Remember, the more information the specialist has about your condition, the fewer repeat or additional tests or procedures you will need to undergo, the lower the costs of your consultation and, most important, the more expeditiously the specialist will be able to render an opinion.

The Facts And Only The Facts

Be thorough and organized in documenting your personal and familial medical histories, the medications you take and in relaying information about your condition. Even seemingly minor bits of information may provide subtle clues to the nature of your medical problem and the optimal way in which to treat it. It's also advisable to bring a list with you of names, addresses and telephone numbers of all physicians who have cared for you, especially those you have seen regarding your current medical problem.

Even though thoroughness is essential to presenting a clear picture of your medical condition, bear in mind that the specialist needs to get to your core health concerns as quickly as possible. Therefore, if you have a complex medical history, you may want to ask your current doctors to provide treatment summaries in addition to copies of your medical records. Hospital records should include your admission history and physical exam, dictated consultation and operation notes and discharge summaries for all hospitalizations. You may also be able to get a cumulative lab and X-ray summary for your hospital stays.

Unlike X-rays, which can be copied at reasonable cost, original pathology slides must be transported by mail or hand-carried. Your specialist may wish to have the pathologist with whom he/she works speak directly with the pathologist who initially interpreted your slides as part of the process of evaluating your case.

Being Prepared

You are likely to be a bit nervous when you meet with the specialist you have chosen. Anxiety about your health and concern about your future care may cause you to forget information you should provide or miss hearing or understanding important information that the specialist communicates. Therefore, you may want to write down all relevant information so that you do not leave out anything of importance when you meet with the specialist or complete forms in the office. You also may want to write out your questions in advance so you don't forget anything.

To avoid leaving out important details of your condition or past treatment, prepare a concise, chronological summary before your consultation takes place. You may wish to type it and provide a copy to the specialist for inclusion in your chart. Highlight major medical results or significant events in the course of an illness or treatment if these will enlighten the doctor about your condition. Your personal perspective on the state of your health is vital to a full understanding of your medical problem.

It is possible that the specialist will use language that you do not understand or may speak quickly assuming certain knowledge on your part about your condition or its treatment. Don't hesitate to ask for clarification as often or repeatedly as you may need to in order to fully comprehend what you are being told. If you are concerned that you may forget what the doctor tells you, ask the doctor's permission to take notes or ask if you might bring along a tape recorder so you can later replay what was said, especially any instructions you are given. You may prefer to bring along a relative or close friend to serve as a "second set of ears," but, again, seek the doctor's permission to do so in advance of your appointment.

Following this process will assure that you and the specialist you are consulting get the most from your appointment. After all, you both have the same goal: restoring you to optimal health and well being.

What To Do If You Can't Get An Appointment

At times it may be difficult, perhaps even impossible, to secure an appointment with the specific specialist you have identified. There are a number of reasons why this may occur. For example, the specialist may not be taking any new patients or may have such a busy schedule that it takes several weeks or months to get an appointment. He/she may only see patients during very limited hours because of teaching, research or other responsibilities or currently may have other limitations related to the acceptance of new patients.

However, bear in mind that the doctors in this guide are the leaders in their specialties and therefore they work with and train the very best and brightest in their specialties. So, if you are unable to consult with a particular doctor, consider making an appointment with one of his/her outstanding colleagues. You can do this by asking a member of the doctor's office staff to refer you to an associate who is a member of the practice group or to another excellent physician who is specially trained to address your particular medical issue.

You can be comfortable knowing that you will receive high quality care from another specialist who practices in the same top setting.

Utilizing Special Resources

The following information on special resources has been included to meet the needs of healthcare consumers who have extraordinarily difficult or unique health problems, and have been unable to identify the resources to address their problems. These patients and their doctors may need to search for very new, cutting-edge, perhaps even experimental and not yet approved therapies. In such cases the search may lead to clinical trials; tests of new drugs and new medical devices or innovative therapeutic approaches. Fortunately, these situations are rare, but when they do occur, they are critical.

In addition to the outstanding private and public hospitals recognized in this guide, the U.S. government maintains its own unique, expert source of patient care and clinical research at the National Institutes of Health (NIH). In fact, the NIH operates its own hospital at which the care provided is usually related to clinical studies its researchers are undertaking.

In addition to those at the NIH, clinical trials also are conducted at leading medical centers and other organizations throughout the country. These facilities may be testing a new drug therapy, a new use for an existing medication or a medical device to deal with a problem that is not being resolved through the use of more traditional approaches.

This section will guide you in utilizing these special resources.

The Clinical Trial As A Treatment Option

For some patients the best medical treatment may only be available through clinical trials (also called treatment studies), which are designed to develop improved ways to use current medical treatments or to find new medical treatments by studying their effects on humans. Treatments are studied to determine if they are safe, effective and better treatments than conventional or standard therapies. Only if they meet all three of these criteria are they made available to the general public.

Many people are frightened by the term "clinical trial" because it conveys the notion of being a "guinea pig" in an experiment. Contrary to popular belief, however, most new treatments are extensively studied by scientists in the laboratory before they are ever tested by physicians in clinical settings. Among the factors that keep patients from participating in clinical trials are: lack of awareness about clinical trials as a treatment option; fear of side effects or adverse reactions to treatment; refusal of insurance companies to pay for experimental treatments; failure of a physician to inform the patient about clinical trials; difficulty finding suitable clinical trials; unavailability of clinical trials for certain medical problems; distance of the patient from major medical centers conducting clinical trials; disruption of personal and family life; and the decision to stop medical treatment altogether.

Despite these and other obstacles, many people do seek out clinical trials. One of the most pressing reasons to participate is the opportunity to obtain treatment that might not be available otherwise. New medical treatments can offer participants hope for a cure, an extended lifespan, or an improvement in how they feel. Some participants also take comfort in knowing that others may benefit from their contribution to medical knowledge.

Deciding if a clinical trial is the right treatment option for you is no simple matter. Certainly, you will want to talk about it with your doctor(s) and other professionals involved in your care, as well as with family members and friends. But in order to fully benefit from what others have to say — based on either their professional knowledge or personal experience — you need to understand exactly what a clinical trial is and what your role as a volunteer will be.

Understanding Clinical Trials

Clinical trials are conducted for just about every medical condition, including life-threatening diseases such as AIDS or cancer; chronic illnesses such as diabetes and asthma; psychiatric disorders such as depression or anxiety; behavioral problems such as smoking and substance abuse; and even common ailments such as hair loss and acne. Chances are, there is at least one trial (and probably more) that may be appropriate for you.

With more than 100 different types of cancer, it is understandable that a large number of clinical trials are cancer-related. Extensive information about clinical trials for cancer can be found on www.cancer.gov, the Web site of the National Cancer Institute (NCI). NCI is part of the NIH. CenterWatch, an online clinical trials listing service, identifies over 14,000 clinical trials that are actively recruiting patients. Veritas Medicine, another useful online organization, allows individuals to perform personalized searches of its clinical trials database. See Appendix D for "Selected Resources" for more information on clinical trials.

Most clinical trials study new medical treatments, combinations of treatments, or improvements in conventional treatments using drugs, surgery and other medical procedures, medical devices, radiation or other therapies. Newer types of clinical trials, called screening or prevention trials, study how to prevent the incidence or recurrence of disease through the use of medicines, vitamins, minerals or other supplements; and how to screen for disease, especially in its early stages. Another type of trial studies how to improve the quality of life for patients, including both their physical and emotional well-being.

Clinical trials are sponsored both by the federal government (through the National Institutes of Health, the National Cancer Institute and many others) and by private industry through pharmaceutical and biotechnology companies, and through healthcare institutions (hospitals or health maintenance organizations) and community-based physician-investigators. The National Cancer Institute sponsors clinical trials at more than 1000 sites in the United States. Trials are carried out in major medical research centers such as teaching hospitals as well as in community hospitals, specialized medical clinics (for example, those for the treatment of AIDS or Alzheimer's disease) and in doctors' offices.

Though clinical trials often involve hospitalized patients, a fair number of trials are conducted on an outpatient basis. Many trials are part of a cooperative network which may include as few as one or two sites or hundreds of locations, although one center generally assumes responsibility for overall coordination of the research. More than 45 research-oriented institutions, recognized for their scientific excellence, have been designated by the NCI as comprehensive or clinical cancer centers. See Appendix D "Selected Resources" to find out how to locate these centers.

Clinical research is based on a protocol (established rules or procedures) describing who will be studied, how and when medications, procedures and/or treatments will be administered and how long the study will last. Trials that are conducted simultaneously at different sites use the same protocol to ensure that all patients are treated identically and all data are collected uniformly so that study findings can be compared.

Clinical trials generally are conducted in four phases. The first phase begins testing of the treatment on a small group of human subjects after rigorous and successful animal testing has been concluded. Phases Two and Three involve a broader test group and are designed to further evaluate the treatment's safety and more accurately determine appropriate dosage, application methods and side effects. The fourth phase, conducted after the treatment has been approved by the FDA for widespread use, monitors its long-term efficacy and is used to determine if any restrictions should be placed on the population of patients to whom the treatment is administered, or if any adverse effects result from interactions with other medications.

Some clinical trials test one treatment on one group of subjects, while others compare two or more groups of subjects. In such comparison studies participants are divided into two groups: the control group that receives the standard treatment and the experimental or treatment group which receives the new treatment. For example, the control group may undergo a surgical procedure while the experimental or treatment group undergoes a surgical procedure plus radiation to determine which treatment modality is more effective. To ensure that patient characteristics do not unduly influence the study findings, patients may be randomly assigned to either the control or the experimental group, meaning that each patient's assignment is based purely on chance. In cases in which a standard treatment does not exist for a particular disease, the experimental group of patients receives the new treatment and the control group receives no treatment at all, or receives a placebo, an inactive medicine or procedure that has no treatment value and is sometimes called a "dummy" pill or a "sugar" pill. It is important to keep in mind that patients are never put into a control group without any treatment if there is a known treatment that could help them. Also, whether a patient is receiving an investigational drug or a placebo, he/she receives the same level and quality of medical care as those receiving the investigational treatment.

Questions to ask your doctor and the trial's research team if you are considering participating in a clinical trial:

- Who is sponsoring the trial?

- How many patients will be involved?

- Will the trial be testing a single treatment or a combination of treatments?

- Will there be one treatment group or more than one treatment group?

- If more than one treatment group, how are patients assigned to each group?

- Has this treatment been studied in previous clinical trials? What were the findings?

Protecting the Rights of Participants

The safety of those who participate in clinical trials is a serious matter and is the number one priority of medical investigators. All clinical research, regardless of type of sponsorship, is guided by the same ethical and legal codes that govern the medical profession and the practice of medicine. Most clinical research is federally funded or federally regulated (at least in part) with built-in safeguards for patients. According to federal government regulations (and some state laws), every clinical trial in the United States must be approved and monitored by an Institutional Review Board (IRB), which is an independent committee of physicians, statisticians, community advocates and others (representing at least five distinct disciplines) to ensure that the protocol is being followed.

Government regulations require researchers to fully inform participants about all aspects of a clinical trial before they agree to participate through a process called informed consent. To be sure that you understand your role in a clinical trial, you should jot down any questions beforehand so as not to forget them. You should also consider bringing along a friend or family member for support and additional input, and perhaps even tape recording the conversation (after asking permission to do so) to make sure you do not forget or misunderstand anything. Each participant in a clinical trial must be given a written consent form, which should be available in English and other languages. The consent form explains the following:

- Why the research is being done.

- What the researchers hope to accomplish.

- What types of treatment interventions (and other tests or procedures) will be performed.

- How long the study will continue.

- What the expected benefits and the possible risks are.

- What other treatments are available.

- What costs will be covered by the study, by the patient or by third-party payers such as Medicare, Medicaid or private insurance.

Patients also are informed that they may leave the trial, or exclude themselves from any part of it, at any time. Informed consent means exactly what the term implies: you agree to join a clinical trial only after you completely understand exactly what your participation will involve for the duration of the study. By law, each patient must be provided with a copy of the signed consent form, which also must include the name and telephone number of a contact person for questions or additional information. Informed consent is a continuous process, so do not hesitate to ask questions before, during or after the trial.

The investigators must protect the privacy of each participant in a clinical trial by ensuring that all medical records are kept confidential except for inspection by the sponsoring agency, the Food and Drug Administration and other agencies involved in regulating the drug or treatment, and all data are collected anonymously by assigning a numeric code or initials to each individual.

During the course of the trial, participants are regularly seen by members of the research team to monitor their health and well-being. Participants also should be responsible for their own health by following the treatment plan (such as taking the proper dosage of medications on time), keeping all scheduled visits and informing members of the healthcare team about any symptoms that occur. If during the course of the trial, the treatment proves to be ineffective or harmful, the patient is free to leave the study and still obtain conventional care. Conversely, as soon as there is evidence that one treatment modality is better than another, all patients in the trial are given the benefit of the new information.

Questions to ask the sponsors about your rights as a participant in a clinical trial:

- Who is responsible for approving and monitoring this research? Is there an IRB?

- Who informs me about the trial process? Do I sign a consent form? Will I receive a copy?

- May I leave the trial at any time? Have previous patients dropped out? Why?

- Whom do I contact if I am experiencing any difficulty with this trial?

Enrolling In Clinical Trials

Each clinical trial has its own guidelines, called eligibility criteria, for determining who can participate. Treatment studies recruit participants who have a disease or other medical condition, while screening and prevention studies generally recruit healthy volunteers. Inclusion criteria (those that allow you to participate in a study) and exclusion criteria (those that keep you from participating in a study) ensure that the study will answer the research questions posed in the research protocol while maintaining the safety of participants. The disease being studied is a primary factor in selecting suitable patients, but other factors such as the patient's gender, age, treatment history and other diagnosed medical conditions may also be important. Unfortunately, eligibility also may depend upon ability to pay. Many health plans do not cover all of the costs associated with clinical trials because they define these trials as experimental procedures. However, trials sometimes pay volunteers for their time and/or reimburse them for travel, childcare, meals and lodging.

To prevent people who qualify from being excluded from clinical trials for financial reasons, agencies such as the National Cancer Institute are working with health plans to find solutions and a growing number of states require insurance companies to pay for all routine patient care costs in cancer trials. To encourage more senior citizens to participate in cancer trials, Medicare plans to revise its payment policy to cover those trials.

When choosing a clinical trial you should determine the factors that are most important to you. For instance, patients generally prefer to participate in trials near their homes so that they can maintain their usual day-to-day activities, be surrounded by family and friends and avoid travel and lodging costs. If travel or temporary relocation becomes necessary, try to find a trial site that is near to some family member or friend or one that is in a locale similar to your own city or town. Many organizations, such as the National Cancer Institute, will work with patients and their families to identify support networks for them wherever they participate.

Questions to ask the trial's sponsor about eligibility criteria:

- What are the inclusion and exclusion criteria for the clinical trial(s) I am considering?

- How can I improve my chances of being accepted?
  Can I change my health plan to one that will cover the trial's costs?
  Can I relocate to another city or state?

- If I am not eligible for one trial, what other trials are being conducted for my condition?

- Will I be paid for my time or reimbursed for my out-of-pocket expenses?

Participating In A Clinical Trial

Clinical trials are conducted by a research team led by a principal investigator (usually a physician) and are comprised of physicians, nurses and other health professionals such as social workers, psychologists and nutritionists. As a participant you may be required to commit a fair amount of time to a clinical trial, often more than with standard treatment. Initially, you will probably be given a physical examination and asked for your medical history. During the trial, you will have regular or periodic visits to the trial site which may include diagnostic and laboratory tests. You also may be asked to follow fixed schedules for medications and other interventions and to keep detailed records of your symptoms and health condition. Generally, clinical trials last from six to twenty-six weeks, though some (called maintenance trials) can last up to a year to determine if a treatment will prevent the relapse of a medical condition.

Participants in clinical trials should remain under the care of their regular physician(s) since clinical trials tend to provide short-term treatment for a specific medical condition and do not generally provide comprehensive primary care. In fact, some trials require that a patient's regular physician sign a consent form before the patient is enrolled. In addition, your regular physician can collaborate with the research team to make sure there are no adverse reactions between your other medications or treatments and the investigational treatment.

Questions to ask the research team or your physician about your role in a clinical trial:

- Who are the members of the health team?
  Who will be in charge of my care?

- How long will the trial last?

- How does treatment in the trial compare with or differ from the standard treatment?

- Will I be hospitalized? How often? For how long a period of time?

- What will occur during each visit?
  What treatments or procedures will I be given?

- Will I still be able to see my regular physician(s)?
  Will my doctor and the research team collaborate?

- Can I be put in touch with other patients who have participated in this trial?

Weighing The Benefits And Risks Of A Clinical Trial

If you are considering participation in a clinical trial, you need to consider the medical, emotional and financial ramifications of participation. Of course, the obvious benefit of a clinical trial is the chance that a new treatment may improve your health and prognosis. You will have access to drugs and other medical interventions before they are widely available to the public and you will obtain expert and specialized medical care at leading healthcare facilities. Many patients receive an added psychological benefit by taking an active role in their treatment.

It is important to bear in mind that some medical interventions used in clinical trials may carry potential risks depending upon the type of treatment and the patient's condition. While many side effects or adverse reactions are temporary (such as hair loss and nausea caused by some anti-cancer drugs), other more serious reactions can be permanent and even life-threatening (for example, heart, liver or kidney damage).

Deciding whether or not to participate in a clinical trial is often a matter of determining if the trial's potential benefits outweigh its possible risks. This is a highly personal decision that may be difficult to make in situations involving experimental treatment in which limited medical information may be available.

Questions to ask the research team about the benefits and risks of a clinical trial:

- What other treatment option(s) do I have at this time?
  Is there any chance that a more promising treatment may be available soon?

- What are the short and long-term benefits and risks as compared with standard treatment?

- Will I experience any known side effects or adverse reactions?
  Will these be temporary, long-term or permanent?
  Relatively minor or perhaps life-threatening?

- If I am harmed in any way by the new treatment, what other treatments will I be entitled to?
  Who will pay for subsequent treatment?

Getting Information On Clinical Trials

The more information you have about a clinical trial, the easier it will be to make a decision about whether or not it is right for you, and the more confident you will be that you made an appropriate decision. In addition to the "Selected Resources" appendix in this guide, the staff at your local public library, community hospital, or major medical center can assist you in locating the information you need from books, consumer organizations and on the Internet.

Learning About The National Institutes Of Health(NIH)

The National Institutes of Health (NIH) comprise one of the world's leading medical research centers and the Federal government's principal agency for biomedical research. An agency of the United States Department of Health, United States Public Health Service, NIH encompasses 25 separate institutions and centers with its main campus located in Bethesda, Maryland. Research is also conducted at several field units across the country and abroad.

Patient Care At The NIH

The Warren Grant Magnuson Clinical Center, NIH's principal medical research center and hospital located in Bethesda, Maryland, provides medical care only to patients participating in clinical research programs. Two categories of patients participate in the Clinical Center studies: children and adults who wish to improve their own health, such as those with newly diagnosed medical problems, ongoing medical problems or family history of disease; and healthy volunteers wishing to advance knowledge about the causes, progress and treatment of disease. The patient's case must fit into an ongoing NIH research project for which the patient has the precise kind or stage of illness under investigation. General diagnostic and treatment services common to community hospitals are not available.

The Magnuson Clinical Center is the world's largest biomedical research hospital and ambulatory care facility, housing 1,600 laboratories conducting basic and clinical research. There are 1,200 tenured physicians, dentists and researchers on staff along with 660 nurses and 570 allied healthcare professionals (dieticians, imaging technologists, medical technologists, medical records and clerical staff, pharmacists and therapists).

The Center's hospital is specially designed for medical research and accommodates 540 carefully selected patients who are participating in clinical research programs. Its 350-bed facility has 24 inpatient care units to which 7,000 patients are admitted annually. The Center also has an Ambulatory Care Research Facility (ACRF) that serves 68,000 outpatient visits each year. A new facility, called the Mark O. Hatfield Clinical Research Center, which began accepting patients in early 2005, has 242 beds for inpatient care and 90 day-hospital stations for outpatient care. The Mark O. Hatfield Center carries out the latest biomedical research that results in new forms of disease diagnosis, prevention and treatment, which is then incorporated into improved methods of patient care.

This is a fine example of Translational Medicine where excellent research discoveries are translated into new and improved methods of clinical treatment. In other words, the laboratory discoveries are brought to the bedside.

The Clinical Center also maintains a Children's Inn for pediatric outpatients and their families. This family-centered residence operates 24 hours a day, 7 days a week, 365 days a year.

In an effort to bring clinical research to the community, NIH supports approximately 80 General Clinical Research Centers (GCRCs) around the country, located within hospitals of major academic medical centers.

It is important to note that, as part of the federal government, the Warren Grant Magnuson Clinical Center provides treatment in clinical trials at no cost to its patients. In some cases, patients receive a stipend to help cover the costs of traveling to Bethesda for treatment and follow-up care. Travel costs for the initial screening visit, however, are not covered.

Areas Of Clinical Study At The NIH

At the Magnuson Clinical Center alone, NIH physician-scientists conduct nearly 1,000 studies each year. Among the areas of study are cancer and related diseases.

Not all of these clinical areas are under investigation at any given time, however. The Patient Recruitment and Public Liaison Office (PRPL) at the NIH Clinical Center assists patients, their families and their physicians in obtaining information about participation in NIH clinical trials. Trained nurses are available to answer questions about the research programs and admission procedures.

Cancer Care At The Warren Grant Magnuson Clinical Center

The National Cancer Institute (NCI) is the largest of the biomedical research institutes and centers at NIH. There, clinical studies are designed to evaluate new and promising ways to prevent, detect, diagnose and treat cancer. The Warren Grant Magnuson Clinical Center provides a separate outpatient division for cancer patients and also has several designated inpatient units.

If you are interested in entering a cancer study at the Magnuson Clinical Center (or at the General Clinical Research Centers), you should first discuss treatment options with a physician. As a general rule, patients interested in participating in clinical studies must be referred by a physician. However, in some instances, self-referral may be permitted.

Patients with medical problems other than cancer or healthy volunteers who wish to participate in a clinical study should contact the particular NIH institute responsible for the clinical area involved.

Cancer Care At The NCI Clinical Centers And Comprehensive Cancer Centers

You may also obtain clinical oncology services (education, screening, diagnosis or treatment) or participate in clinical trials at one of the 22 Cancer Centers or 39 Comprehensive Cancer Centers designated by the NCI for their scientific excellence and extensive resources devoted to cancer and cancer-related problems. Centers are located in 32 states, with the majority of sites in California, New York and Pennsylvania. You can find out about clinical trials at the NCI-designated centers by contacting NCI's Clinical Studies Support Center (CSSC) or by calling each center directly. Information about other cancer-related services at these centers also may be obtained from the center itself. For more information, you can visit the National Cancer Institute's website at www.cancer.gov.

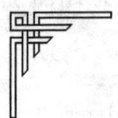

The Best in American Medicine
www.CastleConnolly.com

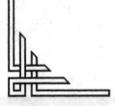
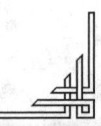

How To Use This Guide

Locating A Specialist

This guide is organized to make finding the right specialists for you or your loved ones as simple as possible. Physicians' biographies are presented by specialty and are organized by geographic region within each specialty or subspecialty. Thus, you may search for a particular type of specialist or subspecialist in one or more regions or throughout the nation.

A second way to locate the right specialist is to use the **"Specialty & Special Expertise Index"** beginning on page 1281. This index is organized according to diseases, conditions, procedures or techniques as well as the doctor's specialty. For example, you can locate a top specialist for diabetes or for Mohs' surgery by looking for those terms in the **"Specialty & Special Expertise Index."**

If you already know a specialist's name, you can find his/her listing by using the **"Alphabetical Listing of Doctors"** beginning on page 1453.

SAMPLE PHYSICIAN LISTING

Smith, John MD [Ped] - **Spec Exp:** Asthma Allergy; **Hospital:** Children's Hosp (page 120);

Name [Specialty]   Special Expertise(s)   Admitting Hospital & Hospital Information Page

Address: 300 Ridge Road Boston, MA 12345; **Phone:** (617) 555-2343; **Board Cert:** Ped 75;

Office Address   Office Phone   Board Certification(s)

Med School: Harvard Med Sch 70; **Resid:** Ped, Children's Hosp 73;

Medical School   Residency(ies)

Fellow: AM, Children's Hosp 74; **Fac Appt:** Assoc Prof Ped, The Med Sch

Fellowship(s)   Faculty Appointment

Geographic Regions And States

To assist you in using Castle Connolly *America's Top Doctors*® in the most efficient and effective manner, the Guide is divided into seven geographic regions. This will help you to locate a specialist in your local or neighboring region. For example, if you live in Mississippi in the Southeast region and you are willing and able to travel to Louisiana in the Southwest region to consult with a specialist in neurology, you can review just those two regions, under the section headed "NEUROLOGY." However, if you prefer to review the information on neurologists throughout the country, you can search the entire neurology section. Or, you can consult the "SPECIAL EXPERTISE INDEX" in the back of this Guide and choose a neurologist who has specific expertise to meet your particular needs.

The geographic regions are as follows:

> New England
>
> Mid Atlantic
>
> Southeast
>
> Midwest
>
> Great Plains and Mountains
>
> Southwest
>
> West Coast and Pacific

The states that are included in each region are listed on the following page and a map of the regions is also provided. Please note that not all regions are represented in all specialties. For example, in "Geriatric Psychiatry" there are no listings in the Southwest region.

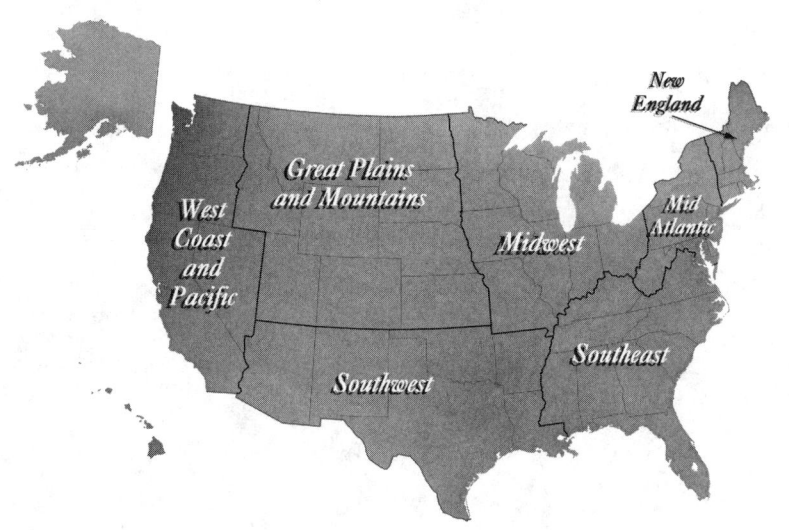

West Coast and Pacific:
Alaska
California
Hawaii
Nevada
Oregon
Washington

Great Plains and Mountains:
Colorado
Idaho
Kansas
Montana
Nebraska
North Dakota
South Dakota
Utah
Wyoming

Southwest:
Arizona
Arkansas
Louisiana
New Mexico
Oklahoma
Texas

Midwest:
Illinois
Indiana
Iowa
Michigan
Minnesota
Missouri
Ohio
Wisconsin

New England:
Connecticut
Maine
Massachusetts
New Hampshire
Rhode Island
Vermont

Mid Atlantic:
Delaware
Maryland
New Jersey
New York
Pennsylvania
Washington, DC
West Virginia

Southeast:
Alabama
Florida
Georgia
Kentucky
Mississippi
North Carolina
South Carolina
Tennessee
Virginia

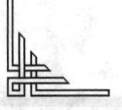
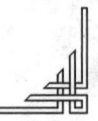

The Best in American Medicine
www.CastleConnolly.com

Medical Specialties

In the pages that follow, each list of doctors in a medical specialty or subspecialty is preceded by a brief description of that specialty (or subspecialty) and the training required for board certification.

Critical Care Medicine has been excluded because in emergency situations there is neither time nor opportunity for choice. A number of other specialities not relevant to most patients (e.g., Forensic Psychiatry) have not been included as well.

The following descriptions of medical specialties and subspecialties were provided by the American Board of Medical Specialties (ABMS), an organization comprised of the 24 medical specialty boards that provide certification in 25 medical specialties. A complete listing of all specialists certified by the ABMS can be found in *The Official ABMS Directory of Board Certified Medical Specialists*, and is published by *Marquis Who's Who*. It is available (either in a multi-volume directory or on CD-ROM) in most public libraries, hospital libraries, university libraries and medical libraries. The ABMS also operates a toll-free phone line at 1-866-275-2267 and a website at www.abms.org to verify the certification status of individual doctors.

The following important policy statement, approved by the ABMS Assembly on March 19, 1987, remains valid.

The Purpose Of Certification

The intent of the certification process, as defined by the member boards of the American Board of Medical Specialties, is to provide assurance to the public that a certified medical specialist has successfully completed an approved educational program and an evaluation, including an examination process designed to assess the knowledge, experience and skills requisite to the provision of high quality patient care in that specialty.

Medical Specialties

Medical Specialty and Subspecialty Descriptions and Abbreviations

The following medical specialties and subspecialties are indicated in the doctors' listings by their abbreviations. Specialties are indicated in bold, subspecialties in italics, and the four primary care specialties in bold capitals. To review the official American Board of Medical Specialties (ABMS) organization of specialties, refer to Appendix A.

Addiction Psychiatry   *AdP*

Deals with habitual psychological and physiological dependence on a substance or practice which is beyond voluntary control.

Adolescent Medicine   *AM*

Involves the primary care treatment of adolescents and young adults.

Allergy & Immunology   **A&I**

Diagnosis and treatment of allergies, asthma, and skin problems such as hives and contact dermatitis.

Anesthesiology   **Anes**

Provides pain relief in maintenance or restoration of a stable condition during and following an operation. Anesthesiologists also diagnose and treat acute and long standing pain problems.

Cardiac Electrophysiology (Clinical)   *CE*

Involves complicated technical procedures to evaluate heart rhythms and determine appropriate treatment for them.

Cardiovascular Disease   *Cv*

Involves the diagnosis and treatment of disorders of the heart, lungs, and blood vessels.

Child & Adolescent Psychiatry   *ChAP*

Deals with the diagnosis and treatment of mental diseases in children and adolescents.

Child Neurology   *ChiN*

Diagnosis and medical treatment of disorders of the brain, spinal cord, and nervous system in children.

Clinical Genetics   **CG**

Deals with identifying the genetic causes of inherited diseases and ailments and preventing, when possible, their occurrence.

Colon and Rectal Surgery   **CRS**

Surgical treatment of diseases of the intestinal tract, colon and rectum, anal canal, and perianal area.

Critical Care Medicine   *CCM*

Involves diagnosing and taking immediate action to prevent death or further injury of a patient. Examples of critical injuries include shock, heart attack, drug overdose, and massive bleeding.

Dermatology   **D**

Diagnosis and treatment of benign and malignant disorders of the skin, mouth, external genitalia, hair and nails, as well as a number of sexually transmitted diseases.

Diagnostic Radiology   *DR*

Involves the study of all modalities of radiant energy in medical diagnoses and therapeutic procedures utilizing radiologic guidance.

Endocrinology, Diabetes & Metabolism   *EDM*

Involves the study and treatment of patients suffering from hormonal and chemical disorders.

FAMILY MEDICINE   **FP**

Deals with and oversees the total healthcare of individual patients and their family members. Family practitioners are more common in rural areas and may perform procedures more commonly performed by specialists (e.g., minor surgery).

Forensic Psychiatry   *FPsy*

Concerns the evaluation of certain diagnostic groups of patients that include those with sexual disorders, antisocial personality disorders, paranoid disorders, and addictive disorders.

Gastroenterology   *Ge*

The study, diagnosis and treatment of diseases of the digestive organs including the stomach, bowels, liver, and gallbladder.

Geriatric Medicine   *Ger*

Deals with diseases of the elderly and the problems associated with aging.

Geriatric Psychiatry   *GerPsy*

Involves the diagnosis, prevention, and treatment of mental illness in the elderly.

Gynecologic Oncology   *GO*

Deals with cancers of the female genital tract and reproductive systems.

Hand Surgery   *HS*

Involves the treatment of injury to the hand through surgical techniques.

Hematology   *Hem*

Involves the diagnosis and treatment of diseases and disorders of the blood, bone marrow, spleen, and lymph glands.

Infectious Disease   *Inf*

The study and treatment of diseases caused by a bacterium, virus, fungus, or animal parasite.

INTERNAL MEDICINE   **IM**

Diagnosis and nonsurgical treatment of diseases, especially those of adults. Internists may act as primary care specialists, highly trained family doctors, or they may subspecialize in specialties such as cardiology or nephrology.

Maternal & Fetal Medicine   *MF*

Involves the care of women with high-risk pregnancies and their unborn fetuses.

Medical Specialties

Medical Oncology *Onc*
Refers to the study and treatment of tumors and other cancers.

Neonatal-Perinatal Medicine *NP*
Involves the diagnosis and treatments of infants prior to, during, and one month beyond birth.

Nephrology *Nep*
Concerned with disorders of the kidneys, high blood pressure, fluid and mineral balance, dialysis of body wastes when the kidneys do not function, and consultation with surgeons about kidney transplantation.

Neurological Surgery **NS**
Involves surgery of the brain, spinal cord, and nervous system.

Neurology **N**
Diagnosis and medical treatment of disorders of the brain, spinal cord, and nervous system.

Neuroradiology *NRad*
Involves the utilization of imaging procedures during diagnosis as they relate to the brain, spine and spinal cord, head, neck, and organs of special sense in adults and children.

Nuclear Medicine **NuM**
Evaluation of the functions of all the organs in the body and treatment of thyroid disease, benign and malignant tumors, and radiation exposure through the use of radioactive substances.

Nuclear Radiology *NR*
Involves the use of radioactive substances to diagnose and treat certain functions and diseases of the body.

OBSTETRICS & GYNECOLOGY **ObG**
Deals with the medical aspects of and intervention in pregnancy and labor and the overall health of the female reproductive system.

Occupational Medicine *OM*
Concentrates on the effect of the work environment on the health of employees.

Ophthalmology **Oph**
Diagnosis and treatment of diseases of and injuries to the eye.

Orthopaedic Surgery **OrS**
Involves operations to correct injuries which interfere with the form and function of the extremities, spine, and associated structures.

Otolaryngology **Oto**
Explores and treats diseases in the interrelated areas of the ears, nose and throat.

Otology/Neurotology *ON*
Concentrates on the management, prevention, cure and care of patients with diseases of the ear and temporal bone, including disorders of hearing and balance.

Pain Medicine   *PM*

Involves providing a high level of care for patients experiencing problems with acute or chronic pain in both hospital and ambulatory settings.

Pediatric Cardiology   *PCd*

Involves the diagnosis and treatment of heart disease in children.

Pediatric Critical Care Medicine   *PCCM*

Involves the care of children who are victims of life threatening disorders such as severe accidents, shock, and diabetes acidosis.

Pediatric Dermatology   *PD*

Diagnosis and treatment of benign and malignant disorders of the skin, mouth, external genitalia, hair and nails in children.

Pediatric Endocrinology   *PEn*

Involves the study and treatment of children with hormonal and chemical disorders.

Pediatric Gastroenterology   *PGe*

The study, diagnosis, and treatment of diseases of the digestive tract in children.

Pediatric Hematology-Oncology   *PHO*

The study and treatment of cancers of the blood and blood-forming parts of the body in children.

Pediatric Infectious Disease   *PInf*

The study and treatment of diseases caused by a virus, bacterium, fungus, or animal parasite in children.

Pediatric Nephrology   *PNep*

Deals with the diagnosis and treatment of disorders of the kidneys in children.

Pediatric Otolaryngology   *POto*

Involves the diagnosis and treatment of disorders of the ear, nose, and throat which affect children.

Pediatric Pulmonology   *PPul*

Involves the diagnosis and treatment of diseases of the chest, lungs, and chest tissue in children.

Pediatric Radiology   *PR*

Involves diagnostic imaging as it pertains to the newborn, infant, child, and adolescent.

Pediatric Rheumatology   *PRhu*

Involves the treatment of diseases of the joints and connective tissues in children.

Pediatric Surgery   *PS*

Treatment of disease, injury, or deformity in children through surgical techniques.

PEDIATRICS   **Ped**

Diagnosis and treatment of diseases of childhood and monitoring of the growth, development, and well-being of preadolescents.

Medical Specialties

Physical Medicine & Rehabilitation   **PMR**

The use of physical therapy and physical agents such as water, heat, light electricity, and mechanical manipulations in the diagnosis, treatment, and prevention of disease and body disorders.

Plastic Surgery   **PlS**

Involves reconstructive and cosmetic surgery of the face and other body parts.

Preventive Medicine   **PrM**

A specialty focusing on the prevention of illness and on the health of groups rather than individuals.

Psychiatry   **Psyc**

Examination, treatment, and prevention of mental illness through the use of psychoanalysis and/or drugs.

Public Health & General Preventive Medicine   *PHGPM*

Involves the investigation of the causes of epidemic disease and the prevention of a wide variety of acute and chronic illness.

Pulmonary Disease   *Pul*

Involves the diagnosis and treatment of diseases of the chest, lungs, and airways.

Radiation Oncology   *RadRo*

Involves the use of radiant energy and isotopes in the study and treatment of disease, especially malignant cancer.

Reproductive Endocrinology   *RE*

Deals with the endocrine system (including the pituitary, thyroid, parathyroid, adrenal glands, placenta, ovaries, and testes) and how its failure relates to infertility.

Rheumatology   *Rhu*

Involves the treatment of diseases of the joints, muscles, bones and associated structures.

Sleep Medicine   *Sleep Med*

Involves the investigation and treatment of patients with sleep disorders.

Spinal Cord Injury Medicine   *SpCdInj*

Involves the prevention, diagnosis, treatment and management of traumatic spinal cord injuries.

Sports Medicine   *SM*

Refers to the practice of an orthopaedist or other physician who specializes in injuries to the bone or other soft tissues (muscles, tendons, ligaments) caused by participation in athletic activity.

Surgery   **S**

Treatment of disease, injury, and deformity by surgical procedures.

Surgery of the Hand   *SHd*

Involves providing appropriate care for all structures in the upper extremity directly affecting the hand and wrist function.

Surgical Critical Care — SCC

Involves specialized care in the management of the critically ill patient, particularly the trauma victim and postoperative patient in the emergency department, intensive care unit, trauma unit, burn unit, and other similar settings.

Thoracic Surgery (includes open heart surgery) — TS

Involves surgery on the heart, lungs, and chest area.

Urology — U

Diagnosis and treatment of diseases of the genitals in men and disorders of the urinary tract and bladder in both men and women.

Vascular & Interventional Radiology — VIR

Involves diagnosing and treating diseases by percutaneous methods guided by various radiologic imaging modalities.

Vascular Surgery — VascS

Involves the operative treatment of disorders of the blood vessels excluding those to the heart, lungs, or brain.

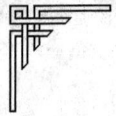

The Best in American Medicine
www.CastleConnolly.com

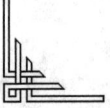
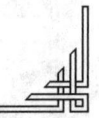

The Training Of A Specialist

Excerpted from "Which Medical Specialist For You?" American Board of Medical Specialties, Evanston, IL, Revised 2000

Everyone knows that a "medical doctor" is a physician who has had years of training to understand the diagnosis, treatment and prevention of disease. The basic training for a physician specialist includes four years of premedical education in a college or university, four years of medical school, and after receiving the M.D. degree, at least three years of specialty training under supervision (called a "residency"). Training in subspecialties can take an additional one to three years.

Some specialists are primary care doctors such as family physicians, general internists and general pediatricians. Other specialists concentrate on certain body systems, specific age groups, or complex scientific techniques developed to diagnose or treat certain types of disorders. Specialties in medicine developed because of the rapidly expanding body of knowledge about health and illness and the constantly evolving new treatment techniques for disease.

A subspecialist is a physician who has completed training in a general medical specialty and then takes additional training in a more specific area of that specialty called a subspecialty. This training increases the depth of knowledge and expertise of the specialist in that particular field. For example, cardiology is a subspecialty of internal medicine, pediatric surgery is a subspecialty of surgery and pediatrics, and child and adolescent psychiatry is a subspecialty of psychiatry. The training of a subspecialist within a specialty requires an additional one or more years of full-time education.

The training, or residency, of a specialist begins after the doctor has received the M.D. degree from a medical school. Resident physicians dedicate themselves for three to seven years to full-time experience in hospital and/or ambulatory care settings, caring for patients under the supervision of experienced specialists. Educational conferences and research experience are often part of that training. In years past, the first year of post-medical school training was called an internship, but is now called residency.

Licensure

The legal privilege to practice medicine is governed by state law and is not designed to recognize the knowledge and skills of a trained specialist. A physician is licensed to practice general medicine and surgery by a state board of medical examiners after passing a state or national licensure examination. Each state or territory has its own procedures to license physicians and sets the general standards for all physicians in that state or territory.

Who Credentials A Specialist And Subspecialist?

Specialty boards certify physicians as having met certain published standards. There are 24 specialty boards that are recognized by the American Board of Medical Specialties (ABMS) and the American Medical Association (AMA). All of the specialties and subspecialties recognized by the ABMS and the AMA are listed in the brief descriptions that follow. Remember, a subspecialist first must be trained and certified as a specialist.

In order to be certified as a medical specialist by one of these recognized boards a physician must complete certain requirements. Generally, these include:

1 Completion of a course of study leading to the M.D. or D.O. (Doctor of Osteopathy) degree from a recognized school of medicine.

2 Completion of three to seven years of full-time training in an accredited residency program designed to train specialists in the field.

3 Many specialty boards require assessments and documentation of individual performance from the residency training director, or from the chief of service in the hospital where the specialist has practiced.

4 All of the ABMS Member Boards require that a person seeking certification have an unrestricted license to practice medicine in order to take the certification examination.

5 Finally, each candidate for certification must pass a written examination given by the specialty board. Fifteen of the 24 specialty boards also require an oral examination conducted by senior specialists in that field. Candidates who have passed the exams and other requirements are then given the status of "Diplomate" and are certified as specialists. A similar process is followed for specialists who want to become subspecialists.

All of the ABMS Member Boards now, or will soon, issue only time-limited certificates which are valid for six to ten years. In order to retain certification, diplomates must become "recertified," and must periodically go through an additional process involving continuing education in the specialty, review of credentials and further examination. Boards that may not yet require recertification have provided voluntary recertification with similar requirements.

How To Determine If A Physician Is A Certified Specialist

Certified specialists are listed in *The Official ABMS Directory of Board Certified Medical Specialists* published by *Marquis Who's Who*. The ABMS Directory can be found in most public libraries, hospital libraries, university libraries and medical libraries, and is also available on CD-ROM. Alternatively, you could ask for that information from your county medical society, the American Board of Medical Specialties, or one of the specialty boards.

The ABMS operates a toll free number (1-866-275-2267) to verify the certification status of individual physicians. Additionally, information about the ABMS organization and links to an electronic directory of certified specialists can be accessed through the ABMS Web site at www.abms.org.

Almost all board certified specialists also are members of their medical specialty societies. These societies are dedicated to furthering standards, practice and professional and public education within individual medical specialties. Some, such as the American College of Surgeons and the American College of Obstetricians and Gynecologists, require board certification for full membership. A physician who has attained full membership is called a "Fellow" of the society and is entitled to use this designation in all formal communications such as certificates, publications, business cards, stationery and signage. Thus, "John Doe, M.D., F.A.C.S." (Fellow of the American College of Surgeons) is a board certified surgeon. Similarly, F.A.A.D. (Fellow of the American Academy of Dermatology) following the M.D. or D.O. in a physician's title would likely indicate board certification in that specialty.

The Partnership For Excellence Program

Among the more than 6,000 acute care and specialty hospitals in the United States, many have extraordinary capabilities for superior patient care. These hospitals, renowned for their use of state-of-the-art equipment and up-to-the-minute technology, also attract outstanding physicians and other healthcare professionals. Many of their physicians are among those in the listings in this Guide.

To assist you in your search for top specialists and to supplement the information contained in the physician listings that follow, we invited a select group of these fine institutions to profile their services, special programs and centers of excellence in the *Partnership for Excellence* program. This special section contains pages sponsored by the included hospitals. This paid sponsorship program is totally separate from the physician selection process, which is based upon nominations by physicians and a completely independent review by our physician led research team.

The *Partnership for Excellence* program provides an overview of the programs and services offered by the included hospitals with information related to their accreditation and sponsorship. Most also provide their physician referral numbers, should you wish to ask the hospitals for recommendations of doctors not listed in Castle Connolly *America's Top Doctors*® 11th Edition.

In addition to the *Partnership for Excellence* program, profiled hospitals were also invited to highlight their special programs or services that focus on a particular disease or medical condition. These can be found in the "Centers of Excellence" sections that are interspersed throughout this book following the medical specialties and/or subspecialties to which they relate. Sponsored pages in the centers of excellence sections reflect the depth of commitment of these hospitals, which provide the staff, resources and financial support necessary to develop these special programs.

By visiting our website **www.CastleConnolly.com**, you may also link to the websites of these outstanding hospitals for even more detailed information on their cancer programs. We believe you will find this informaton helpful in your search for the best healthcare—from both physicians and hospitals—through out the United States!

Participating Hospitals

- **Continuum Health Partners**
- **Cleveland Clinic Foundation**
- **Dana-Farber/Brigham and Women's Cancer Center**
- **Fox Chase Cancer Center**
- **H Lee Moffitt Cancer Center & Research Institute**
- **Hospital for Special Surgery**
- **The Johns Hopkins Hospital**
- **Maimonides Medical Center**
- **Mount Sinai Medical Center**
- **New York Eye & Ear Infirmary**
- **New York-Presbyterian Hospital**
- **NYU Langone Medical Center**
- **NYU Rusk Institute of Rehabilitation**
- **Penn Medicine**
- **St. Francis Hospital -The Heart Center**
- **UHealth - University of Miami Health System**
- **UHealth - Bascom Palmer Eye Institute**
- **UHealth - University of Miami Hospital**
- **UHealth - University of Miami Hospitals & Clinics/Sylvester Comprehensive Cancer Center**
- **University Hospitals Case Medical Center**
- **USC University Hospital**
- **Vanderbilt University Medical Center**

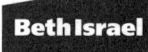

| Beth Israel | Roosevelt Hospital | St. Luke's Hospital | NY Eye & Ear Infirmary |

Sponsorship: Voluntary Not-for-profit   **Beds:** 2,208 certified beds
Accreditation: Joint Commission of Accreditation of Healthcare Organizations (JCAHO), Accreditation Council for Graduate Medical Education, Medical Society of New York, in conjunction with the Accreditation Council for Continuing Medical Education

A STRONG PARTNERSHIP WITH A PROUD HERITAGE

Continuum Health Partners is a partnership of five venerable health care providers: Beth Israel Medical Center-Manhattan, Beth Israel Medical Center-Brooklyn, St. Luke's Hospital, Roosevelt Hospital, and The New York Eye and Ear Infirmary. Each of the five partner institutions was established more than a century ago by individuals committed to improving health and health care in their communities. Today, the system represents over 4,000 physicians and dentists and is superbly equipped to respond to the health care needs of the populations we serve. Our providers also see patients in group and private practice settings and in ambulatory centers in New York City and Westchester County.

LOCATIONS

Continuum Health Partners has campuses in Manhattan and Brooklyn. Beth Israel Medical Center has two divisions: the Milton and Caroll Petrie Division on First Avenue at 16th Street, and the Brooklyn Division on Kings Highway at East 32nd Street. Beth Israel's Phillips Ambulatory Care Center, a state-of-art outpatient center, is located at 10 Union Square East at 14th Street. St. Luke's Hospital is on Amsterdam Avenue at 114th Street, and Roosevelt Hospital is on Tenth Avenue at 59th Street. The New York Eye and Ear Infirmary is located on Second Avenue and 14th Street.

ACADEMIC AFFILIATIONS

Beth Israel Medical Center is the University Hospital and Manhattan Campus for the Albert Einstein College of Medicine. St. Luke's-Roosevelt Hospital Center is an Academic Affiliate of Columbia University College of Physicians and Surgeons. The New York Eye and Ear Infirmary is the primary teaching center of the New York Medical College and affiliated teaching hospitals in the areas of ophthalmology and otolaryngology.

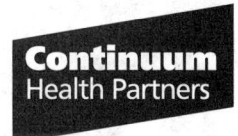

For a referral to a great doctor in your neighborhood, call (800) 420-4004. Our Physician Referral Service can help you find a primary care physician or specialist affiliated with Beth Israel, St. Luke's, Roosevelt or The New York Eye and Ear Infirmary. Visit our Website at www.chpnyc.org

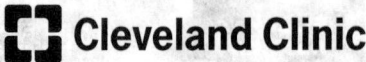 **Cleveland Clinic**

Every life deserves world class care.

Cleveland Clinic
9500 Euclid Avenue
Cleveland, OH 44195

clevelandclinic.org/topdocs

Offering Same-Day Appointments
Call 800.274.2009.

Cleveland Clinic is one of the largest and busiest health centers in America. Founded in 1921, it integrates clinical and hospital care with research and education in a private, non-profit group practice. Cleveland Clinic is ranked among the top four hospitals in America in *U.S. News & World Report's* annual survey, and has been ranked No. 1 in America for heart care 17 years in a row.

At Cleveland Clinic and Cleveland Clinic Florida, 2,700 full-time salaried physicians representing 120 medical specialties and subspecialties provide for more than 3.5 million outpatient visits and approximately 50,000 hospital admissions a year, for patients from throughout the United States and more than 80 countries. A major inpatient and outpatient surgery center, it performs more than 71,000 cases a year.

The main campus of Cleveland Clinic occupies 50 buildings on 180 acres east of downtown Cleveland, Ohio. Cleveland Clinic also includes a system of eight full-service Community Hospitals, and 18 family health and surgery centers in surrounding communities.

Cleveland Clinic has a growing international presence. It serves patients at Cleveland Clinic Canada, in Toronto. It manages Sheikh Kahlifah Medical City, in Abu Dhabi, and is in the process of constructing Cleveland Clinic Abu Dhabi — a comprehensive clinic and hospital in Dubai.

Cleveland Clinic was founded by four physicians who had served in World War One and hoped to replicate the organizational efficiency of military medicine. They established Cleveland Clinic as a not-for-profit group practice with a mission of patient care, research and education. Cleveland Clinic has grown through the years by adhering to that model.

Cleveland Clinic's integrated structure enables it to control costs, measure and improve quality, and provide access to high-quality healthcare services across a broad regional system.

Treatment Guides
Cleveland Clinic has developed comprehensive treatment guides for many diseases and conditions. To download our free treatment guides, visit clevelandclinic.org/treatmentguides.

Online Medical Second Opinion
Cleveland Clinic's My**Consult** Online Medical Second Opinion program securely connects patients to our physician specialists for more than 1,000 life-changing or life-threatening diagnoses all by the click of a mouse. To learn more, log onto eclevelandclinic.org/myconsult or call 800.223.2273, ext. 43223.

Special Assistance for Out-of-State Patients
Cleveland Clinic Global Patient Services offers a complimentary Medical Concierge service for patients who travel from outside of Ohio. Call 800.223.2273, ext. 55580 or email medicalconcierge@ccf.org.

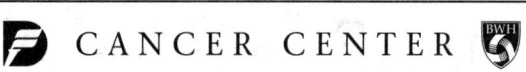

DANA-FARBER/BRIGHAM AND WOMEN'S

CANCER CENTER

Focused on cancer. Focused on life.

75 Francis Street
Boston, MA 02115

450 Brookline Avenue
Boston, MA 02215

1-877-DFCI-BWH (877-332-4294)

www.dfbwcc.org

Accreditations: NCI-designated Comprehensive Cancer Center; Joint Commission on Accreditation of Healthcare Organizations (JCAHO); National Comprehensive Cancer Network (NCCN); American Nurses Credentialing Center (ANCC) Magnet Recognition

General Overview:
Dana-Farber/Brigham and Women's Cancer Center brings together one of the world's top cancer centers with one of the world's leading teaching hospitals. Our 13 sub-specialized treatment centers are each devoted to a major type of adult cancer. Together, these centers are dedicated to providing the most advanced care for every form of cancer. Dana-Farber/Brigham and Women's Cancer Center is the highest ranked cancer center in New England and was named among the top five cancer centers in the nation by *U.S. News and World Report.*

Academic and Clinical Affiliations:
Dana-Farber Cancer Institute and Brigham and Women's Hospital are major teaching hospitals of Harvard Medical School. Dana-Farber/Brigham and Women's Cancer Center is a member of the National Comprehensive Cancer Network (NCCN) and Dana-Farber/Harvard Cancer Center, an NCI-designated Comprehensive Cancer Center. We also are among the nation's leading recipients of research funding from the National Cancer Institute.

Medical Staff:
Our treatment centers offer advanced chemotherapy, extensive clinical trials, innovative radiation oncology, and surgical expertise in all solid tumors – including the latest approaches in minimally invasive and image-guided surgery.

Our patients benefit from being cared for by a team of specialists who sees their kind of cancer every day. This approach enables us to offer every patient specialized treatment options and a personalized approach to cancer care.

Pioneering, Comprehensive Medical Care:
Dana-Farber/Brigham and Women's Cancer Center offers patients access to more than 700 clinical trials, many of them developed here. Our physicians, scientists, and researchers have made groundbreaking discoveries in targeted therapies and combined approaches to treatment, including major findings in breast, lung, and gastrointestinal cancers. These discoveries have changed the way many cancers are treated. Today, we are currently leading one of the world's most comprehensive cancer genetics studies. We also offer a wide variety of support services, integrative therapies, and survivorship programs for patients and their families and lead many efforts to prevent the development of cancers in high-risk patients.

Access is One Call Away: 1-877-DFCI-BWH (877-332-4294)
Schedule an appointment with any specialist in our 13 treatment centers with just one phone call.

FOX CHASE
CANCER CENTER

333 Cottman Avenue
Philadelphia, PA 19111-2497
Phone: 1-888-FOX CHASE • Fax: 215-728-2702
www.foxchase.org

Sponsorship	Independent Nonprofit
Beds	100 licensed beds
Accreditation	The Joint Commission; American Hospital Association; American College of Surgeons Commission on Cancer with commendation; College of American Pathology; American College of Radiology; American Nurses Credentialing Center's Magnet designation

Overview

Fox Chase Cancer Center is one of the leading cancer research and treatment centers in the United States. Founded in 1904 in Philadelphia as one of the nation's first cancer hospitals, Fox Chase was also among the first institutions to be designated a National Cancer Institute Comprehensive Cancer Center in 1974. Fox Chase researchers have won the highest awards in their fields, including two Nobel Prizes. Fox Chase physicians are also routinely recognized in national rankings, and the Center's nursing program has received Magnet status for nursing excellence three consecutive times, having been the first hospital in Pennsylvania and the nation's first cancer hospital to earn this distinction from the American Nurses Credentialing Center. Today, Fox Chase conducts a broad array of nationally competitive basic, translational, and clinical research, with special programs in cancer prevention, detection, survivorship, and community outreach.

- Fox Chase's 100-bed hospital is one of the few in the country devoted entirely to adult cancer care.
- Fox Chase sees more than 7,900 new patients a year. Annual hospital admissions exceed 4,800, and outpatient visits to physicians total about 82,000 a year.
- Fox Chase's board-certified specialists are recognized nationally and internationally in medical, radiation and surgical oncology, diagnostic imaging, diagnostic pathology, pain management, oncology nursing and oncology social work.
- The staff provides a coordinated approach to meet the treatment needs of each patient. Special multidisciplinary centers provide consultations and treatment recommendations for specific types of cancer.
- The nursing staff of specially trained oncology nurses maintains excellent nurse-to-patient ratios.
- Fox Chase investigators have received numerous awards and honors, including Nobel Prizes in medicine and chemistry, a Kyoto Prize, a Lasker Clinical Research Award, memberships in the National Academy of Sciences and General Motors Cancer Research Foundation Prizes.
- Fox Chase maintains the first known cancer affiliate network in the United States. Established in 1986, Fox Chase Cancer Center Partners is a select group of 21 community hospitals in Pennsylvania and New Jersey with Fox Chase-affiliated cancer programs.
- Fox Chase is a founding member of the National Comprehensive Cancer Network, an alliance of the nation's leading academic cancer centers that is dedicated to improving the quality and effectiveness of cancer care.

For more about Fox Chase physicians and services, visit our website, www.foxchase.org, or call 1-888-FOX CHASE.

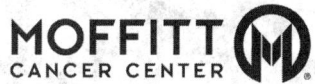

MOFFITT CANCER CENTER

H. Lee Moffitt Cancer Center & Research Institute
12902 Magnolia Drive | Tampa, Florida 33612
Telephone: 813-745-4673 | www.MOFFITT.org

Sponsorship:	Free-standing cancer center, not-for-profit corporation
Beds:	206
Accreditations:	JCAHO, the American College of Surgeons Commission on Cancer, the American College of Radiology and the National Accreditation Program for Breast Centers (among others).

One of the fastest growing cancer centers in the United States, Moffitt Cancer Center & Research Institute is Florida's only National Cancer Institute (NCI) Comprehensive Cancer Center. As a private, not-for-profit corporation with more than 2 million square feet dedicated to research and patient care the Center includes a 206 bed-hospital, a 36-bed blood and marrow transplant unit, an outpatient clinic with a complete digital imaging center, a state-of-the-art radiation therapy department, infusion center, 14 operating rooms, two research buildings, and off site locations including a screening center for high risk patients and a 50,000 square foot outpatient center that enables further growth and service to cancer patients. Moffitt has also created a network of strategic partners composed of 17 affiliate hospitals within the state of Florida and beyond, along with practice affiliations represented by more than 400 oncologists.

Moffitt partners or collaborates with academic centers including: University of South Florida, University of Florida, FAMU, Burnham Institute, Florida Atlantic University, Florida State University, Florida Institute for Human and Machine Cognition, Scripps Florida, Translational Genomics Research Institute/Arizona, University of Central Florida.

Moffitt supports a staff of more than 300 physicians, known as the Moffitt Medical Group. Most are fellowship trained and among the best in their respective fields. The Center's clinical services are organized into disease-oriented interdisciplinary programs with a full complement of services.

Moffitt is at the forefront of personalized medicine with its commitment to Total Cancer Care™ - a system of care enabling researchers and treatment teams to identify and meet all of the needs of patients and their families. Total Cancer Care encompasses all aspects of the disease including prevention, genetic predisposition, the impact of lifestyle and the uses of integrative medicine during treatment.

The foundation of this approach is the Total Cancer Care™ research protocol, a longitudinal study that enrolls patients from Moffitt and from numerous cancer treatment sites within Florida and from other states. The partnership among patients, doctors and researchers is designed to advance cancer care by maintaining a repository of human tissue specimens and clinical data. This data will further the discovery of biomarkers that can be used to identify those at high risk, facilitate early detection, improve prognoses, allow drug targeting and toxicity predictions, and match individuals to the best treatment and to the right clinical trials.

Referral Information: To make an appointment please call the New Patient Appointment Center at 813-745-3980 or go on-line to www.MOFFITT.org

HOSPITAL FOR SPECIAL SURGERY

535 East 70th Street • New York, NY 10021
Physician Referral: 800.854.0071 • www.HSS.edu

Specialists in Mobility

Sponsorship: Private, Non-Profit
Beds: 205
Accreditation: The Joint Commission
Web Site: HSS.edu

FIRST IN ITS FIELD

Founded in 1863, Hospital for Special Surgery is a leading specialty hospital for orthopedics, rheumatology, and rehabilitation.

FIRST IN JOINT REPLACEMENTS

HSS performs more knee replacements and more hip surgeries than any other hospital in the nation. HSS pioneered designs and surgical techniques for the modern artificial knee replacement in the 1970's and has been leading total knee replacement ever since.

PIONEERING MINIMALLY INVASIVE SURGERY

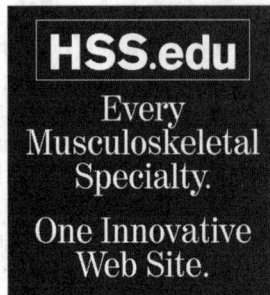

HSS.edu
Every Musculoskeletal Specialty.

One Innovative Web Site.

HSS surgeons pioneered the techniques, special instruments, and smaller implants that made minimally invasive total hip and knee replacements possible. HSS also pioneered minimally invasive spine surgery techniques that reduce the need for spinal fusion. With 35 state-of-the-art musculoskeletal operating rooms, HSS is a world leader in orthopedic surgery, performing over 25,000 procedures per year. HSS anesthesiologists, world leaders in regional anesthesia, developed special pain blocks required for minimally invasive surgery. HSS surgeons are innovators in hand, elbow, shoulder, and spine surgery techniques and are leading experts in arthroscopy and hip preservation.

GLOBAL LEADERS IN RHEUMATOLOGY

HSS rheumatologists are international authorities and pioneering researchers in all rheumatological and autoimmune conditions and treatments, including lupus, rheumatoid arthritis, juvenile rheumatoid arthritis, osteoarthritis, scleroderma, gout, uveitis, and Antiphospholipid Syndrome. Cutting edge research and treatment centers include the Mary Kirkland Center for Lupus Research, the Mary Kirkland Center for Lupus Care, the Barbara Volcker Center for Women and Rheumatic Diseases, the Scleroderma and Vasculitis Center, and the Gosden Robinson Inflammatory Arthritis Center.

WORLD'S MOST EXPERIENCED MUSCULOSKELETAL RADIOLOGISTS

HSS is the world's largest academic center dedicated to musculoskeletal imaging. Our experts developed novel MRI techniques that detect early failure of joint arthroplasty and implants. HSS innovations in ultrasound and MRI also allow earlier diagnosis of autoimmune conditions and arthritis.

Ranked #1 in the Nation for Orthopedics in
U.S.News & World Report
"America's Best Hospitals" 2011-12 issue.
Among the top ranked in
Orthopedics & Rheumatology
for 21 consecutive years

Designated a Magnet Hospital for
Nursing Excellence since 2002

#1 Hospital in NYC
in a study on patient satisfaction
by *Consumer Reports*

A National Institutes of Health
Core Center for Musculoskeletal
Repair and Regeneration

Official Hospital of the NY Mets, NY Giants,
NY Knicks, NY Liberty, NY Red Bulls,
Nets Basketball, The PGA of America,
St. John's Athletics, and
CUNY Athletic Conference.
HSS doctors and physical
therapists also work closely with
the Association of Tennis Professionals,
US Rowing, USA Swimming and other
professional and college teams

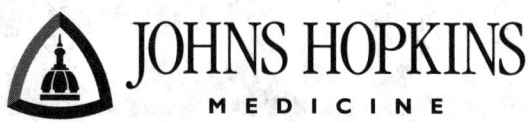

JOHNS HOPKINS

MEDICINE

Baltimore, Maryland
www.hopkinsmedicine.org

Johns Hopkins Medicine unites physicians and scientists of the Johns Hopkins University School of Medicine with the organizations, health professionals and facilities of the Johns Hopkins Health System, including the world-renowned Johns Hopkins Hospital. All share a single mission: to improve the health of the community and the world by setting the standard of excellence in medical education, research and clinical care.

We heal. Ranked as America's top hospital year after year by *U.S. News & World Report*, The Johns Hopkins Hospital and its related facilities serve as beacons of hope for thousands of patients in our community, in our nation and throughout the world.

We discover. Research is the foundation of clinical care. Johns Hopkins physicians and researchers consistently receive more research grants from the National Institutes of Health than faculty at any other institution. Johns Hopkins has been home to four Nobel laureates, 11 Lasker awardees, 17 National Academy of Sciences members and 33 members of the Institute of Medicine.

We teach. The Johns Hopkins University School of Medicine educates and trains medical students, graduate students and postdoctoral fellows from around the world.

Our Centers of Excellence include
- Asthma & Allergy Center
- Brady Urological Institute
- Children's Center
- Sidney Kimmel Comprehensive Cancer Center
- Comprehensive Transplant Center
- Heart and Vascular Institute
- Institute for Basic Biomedical Sciences
- Solomon H. Snyder Department of Neuroscience
- McKusick-Nathans Institute of Genetic Medicine
- Wilmer Eye Institute

To find a physician or make an appointment at Johns Hopkins, call 410-735-7575 in Baltimore.

For calls outside Baltimore, call 410-735-4872.

For calls outside the United States, call +01-410-955-8032.

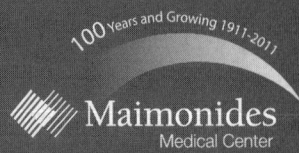
Sponsorship:	Voluntary, Not-for-Profit
Beds:	705 acute, 70 psychiatric
Accreditation:	The Joint Commission
	American College of Surgeons
	American Council of Graduate Medical Education (ACGME)

Maimonides Medical Center is among the largest independent teaching hospitals in the US and trains more than 450 fellows and residents each year. Widely recognized for major achievements in medical technology and patient safety, Maimonides is a conductor of clinical trials for new treatments and therapies, and cited for clinical excellence by numerous health care evaluation services.

CENTERS OF EXCELLENCE

Cancer Center
Maimonides Cancer Center offers a fully integrated approach that includes prevention, screening, diagnostics, treatment, palliative care and clinical research. Staffed by leading physicians, nurses and social workers, the Center provides compassionate, patient-centered, state-of-the-art care.

Cardiac Institute
Maimonides is in the top 2% of hospitals in the nation for heart attack outcomes. Its renowned Cardiac Institute includes Catheterization Labs, state-of-the-art ORs, an electrophysiology lab, two ICUs, a Chest Pain Observation Unit, Advanced Cardiac Care Unit, Congestive Heart Failure Program, and Atrial Fibrillation Center.

Jaffe Stroke Center
The Jaffe Stroke Center at Maimonides received the *Gold Plus Quality Award* from the American Stroke Association. Currently the site of clinical trials for new stroke medications, medical devices and protocols, the Stroke Center offers interventional neuroradiology techniques and telemedicine.

Infants & Children's Hospital
The Maimonides Infants & Children's Hospital of Brooklyn, one of only five accredited children's hospitals in NYC, includes comprehensive inpatient services and more than 30 pediatric subspecialties. The Children's Hospital also has a Child Life Program, Pediatric ICU, Neonatal ICU and Pediatric ER.

Vascular Institute
The Vascular Institute at Maimonides provides comprehensive diagnostic, clinical and vascular surgical services for patients with circulatory complications. The Vascular Institute is one of only five centers in New York certified to train vascular surgeons.

Stella & Joseph Payson Birthing Center
Maimonides delivers more babies than any other hospital in New York State. With excellent outcomes, the Payson Birthing Center includes a Perinatal Testing Center, offers the services of doulas, and includes midwifery in a home-like setting – while utilizing the most advanced technology.

Geriatrics Program
Maimonides serves one of the oldest populations in New York City, with one in four patients over the age of 75. The Geriatrics Program is fully equipped to meet the special needs of seniors and encompasses inpatient and outpatient services.

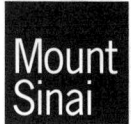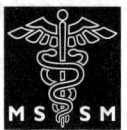

THE MOUNT SINAI MEDICAL CENTER
One Gustave L. Levy Place
Fifth Avenue and 100th Street
New York, NY 10029-6574
Physician Referral: 1-800-MD-SINAI (637-4624)
www.mountsinai.org

Sponsorship: Voluntary Not-for-Profit
Beds: 1,171
Accreditation: The Joint Commission;
Commission for Accreditation of Rehabilitation Facilities;
Magnet Award for Nursing Excellence

For nearly 160 years, The Mount Sinai Medical Center has been a leader in patient care and translational research. Generations of patients have benefitted as our teams of physicians and scientists have always worked together to translate laboratory research into newer and better treatments.

Located between the Upper East Side and East and Central Harlem—New York City's most and least affluent communities—Mount Sinai provides a broad range of services that meet the needs of every patient. The Medical Center consists of The Mount Sinai Hospital and Mount Sinai School of Medicine, both of which continue to be ranked among the nation's best by *U.S. News & World Report.*

In 2011, Mount Sinai was again named among America's Best Hospitals, earning a spot on *U.S. News & World Report* "Honor Roll," and ranking 16 out of 5,000 hospitals nationwide. We also ranked highly in 12 specialties: geriatric care; digestive disorders; cardiology and heart surgery; rehabilitation; diabetes and endocrinology; ear, nose and throat; psychiatry; neurology and neurosurgery; kidney disorders; gynecology; urology; and cancer. In addition, our School of Medicine was ranked 18th by the *Best Graduate Schools* edition.

Under the direction of Valentin Fuster, MD, PhD, **Mount Sinai Heart** incorporates world-class resources, innovative thinking and interdisciplinary programs in support of its mission to prevent and treat cardiovascular disease. Ours was the first hospital in the country to perform successfully two unique procedures for atrial fibrillation: a non-surgical procedure to tie off the left atrial appendage, and a visually guided laser balloon catheter to ablate the condition. In a statewide study, our Cardiac Catheterization Laboratory was deemed both the busiest and, with the lowest 30-day risk-adjusted mortality rate, the safest. Building on the expertise of our internationally renowned physicians David H. Adams, MD; Michael L. Marin, MD; Jagat Narula, MD; Samin K. Sharma, MD; Eric A. Rose, MD; Vivek Y. Reddy, MD; and many other prominent cardiac surgeons, interventionalists, and cardiologists, we provide patients with the most advanced approach to care.

The Tisch Cancer Institute coordinates a full-service diagnostic and treatment program for cancer patients. Current clinical programs include those in cancer of the liver, breast, prostate, and head and neck, as well as hematological malignancies, such as myeloproliferative disorders. In 2011, we opened the Dubin Breast Center, which provides state-of-the-art detection and treatment, and addresses every aspect of breast health, in one centralized location.

Recognized as a national leader in organ transplantation, **The Recanati/Miller Transplantation Institute** is one of the few places in the country that provides multi-organ transplantation. Our surgeons were the first in New York State to perform many combined transplant procedures, including liver and kidney transplantation, pediatric liver transplantation, and living adult- and pediatric-donor liver transplantation.

Geriatrics and Palliative Medicine specialists at Mount Sinai promote healthy aging and provide a balanced and integrated approach to improving the quality of life for New York's elderly. Ranked first in the country for geriatrics by *U.S. News & World Report* in 2011, we remain a national pioneer in geriatric medicine.

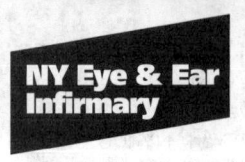

Continuum Health Partners, Inc.

THE NEW YORK EYE AND EAR INFIRMARY

310 East 14th Street
New York, New York 10003
Tel. 212.979.4000   Fax. 212.228.0664
www.nyee.edu

BEDS:	69; Operating Rooms: 17; Surgical Cases: 27,000+ a year
Sponsorship:	Voluntary Not-for-Profit
Accreditation:	The Joint Commission
	College of American Pathologists

GENERAL OVERVIEW

The New York Eye and Ear Infirmary is one of the world's leading facilities for the diagnosis and treatment of diseases of the eyes, ears, nose, throat and related conditions. Founded in 1820, it is the first and most historic specialty hospital in the nation, as well as one of the busiest.

ACADEMIC AND CLINICAL AFFILIATIONS

A voluntary, not-for-profit institution, the Infirmary is a member of Continuum Health Partners, Inc. and an affiliated teaching hospital of New York Medical College. There are highly regarded residency programs in ophthalmology and otolaryngology, plus some two dozen post-graduate fellowship positions.

THE MEDICAL STAFF

The Medical Staff includes more than 600 board-certified attending physicians and surgeons throughout the metropolitan area. Many are renowned for their breakthrough research introducing widely practiced techniques.

SPECIALTIES

Ophthalmology: Within this area are subspecialties of cataract, glaucoma, retina, cornea and external disease, ocular plastic surgery, pediatric ophthalmology and strabismus, neuro-ophthalmology. ocular tumor and uveitis. Laser, photography, fluorescein angiography and electrophysiological testing are among the most advanced services available anywhere.

Otolaryngology: The department is in the forefront of treatment modalities using highly sophisticated endoscopic and laser equipment. Subspecialties include rhinology, laryngology, head & neck surgery, otology/neurotology, facial plastic surgery, pediatric otolaryngology, audiology, speech therapy and hearing aid dispensing.

Plastic & Reconstructive Surgery: Microsurgical capabilities and premium patient accommodations provide an optimum environment for facial plasty, liposuction, breast surgery and repair of defects from disease or trauma.

RELATED SERVICES

New York Eye Trauma Center: An advanced program for emergency treatment of eye injuries, it also is the Eye Injury Registry of New York State and leading collector of data which will help develop preventative strategies.

Ambulatory Surgery: A comprehensive Ambulatory Surgery Center is designed to expedite admission testing, pre-op preparation and post-op recovery in an efficient and comfortable setting.

Pediatric Specialty Care: Services of eye and ear, nose and throat specialists are coordinated with other professional and support staff especially sensitive to the youngest patients.

RESEARCH AND EDUCATION

The New York Eye and Ear Infirmary is a national and international leader in research in its specialties, achieving many "firsts" in successful surgical procedures and medical treatments. Laboratories include Cell Culture, Ocular Imaging, and Microsurgical Education. Over a hundred studies and clinical trials are currently being conducted.

Physician Referral: Call 1.800.449.HOPE (4673)

⌐ NewYork-Presbyterian
⌐ The University Hospital of Columbia and Cornell

Affiliated with Columbia University College of Physicians and Surgeons and Weill Cornell Medical College

NewYork-Presbyterian Hospital	NewYork-Presbyterian Hospital
Columbia University Medical Center	Weill Cornell Medical Center
622 West 168th Street	525 East 68th Street
New York, NY 10032	New York, NY 10065

1-877-NYP-WELL (1-877-697-9355)   www.nyp.org

Sponsorship:	Voluntary Not-for-Profit
Beds:	2,409
Accreditation:	Joint Commission on Accreditation of Healthcare Organizations (JCAHO), Commission on Accreditation of Rehabilitation Facilities (CARF) and College of American Pathologists (CAP)

For 11 consecutive years, NewYork-Presbyterian Hospital has been listed on the prestigious "Honor Roll" of the *U.S. News & World Report* "Best Hospitals" survey and is ranked #1 in the New York metro area. NewYork-Presbyterian has the most physicians listed in *New York Magazine's* "Best Doctors" issue and is recognized for having more top doctors than any other hospital in the nation.

Overview

NewYork-Presbyterian Hospital is one of the foremost academic medical centers in the world and one of the most comprehensive healthcare institutions in the nation, with more than 6,100 physicians, some 117,00 discharges, and nearly 1.5 million outpatient visits annually. The Hospital enjoys a unique affiliation with two of the nation's leading Ivy League medical schools—the Joan and Sanford I. Weill Medical College of Cornell University and the Columbia University College of Physicians and Surgeons.

NewYork-Presbyterian Hospital Features Renowned CENTERS OF EXCELLENCE Including:

Morgan Stanley Children's Hospital and the Komansky Center for Children's Health— One of the largest, most comprehensive children's hospitals in the world, providing highly sophisticated pediatric medical, surgical, and intensive care services in a family-friendly, compassionate environment.

NewYork-Presbyterian Cancer Centers—Through a multidisciplinary team approach, we deliver seamless care and offer the latest therapeutic options and clinical trials for all cancer types.

NewYork-Presbyterian Digestive Disease Services—Our collaborative team manages and treats patients with digestive cancers and nonmalignant digestive diseases, such as inflammatory bowel disease and, pancreatic and biliary disorders, with compassionate care.

NewYork-Presbyterian Heart—Advances in cardiac care—from clinical cardiology, to interventional procedures, to surgical solutions—offer outstanding outcomes to adult and pediatric heart patients.

NewYork-Presbyterian Neuroscience Centers—Expert teams provide the most sophisticated diagnostic and treatment services for Alzheimer's disease, multiple sclerosis, Parkinson's disease, aneurysms, epilepsy, brain tumors, strokes, and other neurological disorders.

NewYork-Presbyterian Psychiatry—NewYork-Presbyterian Hospital's behavioral health and psychiatric services for adults, children, and adolescents offer a full continuum of programs at all levels of care.

NewYork-Presbyterian Transplant Institute—Our experts are internationally known for performing adult and pediatric heart, liver, kidney, pancreas, lung, bone marrow/stem cell, and intestinal and ex vivo transplantation.

NewYork-Presbyterian Vascular Care Center—We provide comprehensive, multidisciplinary preventive, diagnostic, and treatment services for aortic aneurysm, carotid artery disease, blood clots, and peripheral vascular diseases.

William Randolph Hearst Burn Center — NewYork-Presbyterian Hospital is home to the largest and busiest burn center in the nation, caring for more than 900 inpatients and 4,000 outpatients annually.

In addition, we offer extraordinary expertise, comprehensive programs, and specialized resources in the fields of AIDS, gene therapy, reproductive medicine and infertility, trauma care, and women's health.

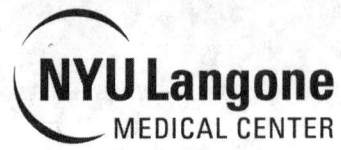

NYU LANGONE MEDICAL CENTER

NYU Langone Medical Center is one of the nation's premier centers of excellence in health care, biomedical research, and medical education. For over 170 years, Medical Center physicians and researchers have made countless contributions to the practice and science of health care.

NYU Langone is comprised of Tisch Hospital, Rusk Institute of Rehabilitation Medicine, Hospital for Joint Diseases, and NYU School of Medicine.

In a culture where treating the whole person and not simply the disease is the norm, NYU Langone Medical Center is renowned for clinical excellence across a wide array of specialties, including cardiology, cardiac and vascular surgery, cancer, musculoskeletal (including orthopaedics and rehabilitation), neurosurgery and children's services.

As an academic medical center, NYU Langone's clinical services are continually informed and enhanced by hundreds of basic and clinical research projects, as well as by major initiatives in translational research that promise to speed the transfer of laboratory discoveries to the patient's bedside.

We have brought together some of our most outstanding basic and translational scientists with clinicians to create six centers of excellence focused on addiction, brain aging, cancers of the skin, multiple sclerosis, musculoskeletal disease, and urologic disease. By applying the expertise and resources of multiple disciplines to specific health problems, our centers of excellence have a transformative effect on the quality of both our research and our patient care.

Additional Areas of Expertise:

Adult Cardiovascular Services
Behavioral Health
Cardiac Surgery
Child and Adolescent Psychiatry
Colon and Rectal Surgery
Dermatology
Gastroenterology
Hematology/Oncology
Infectious Diseases
Internal Medicine
Maternal and Fetal Medicine
Minimally Invasive Surgery
Neonatal-Perinatal Medicine
Obstetrics and Gynecology

Orthopaedic Services
Otolaryngology
Pediatric Subspecialties
Program for IVF Reproductive
Psychiatry
Pulmonology
Radiology
Radiation Oncology
Reconstructive Plastic Surgery
Rheumatology
Thoracic Surgery
Urology
Vascular Surgery

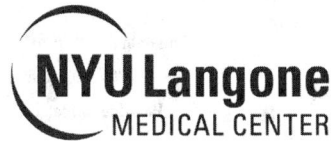

RUSK INSTITUTE OF REHABILITATION MEDICINE
400 East 34th Street *(between 1st Avenue and FDR Drive)*
New York, NY 10016
HJD: 301 East 17th Street *(at 2nd Avenue)*
New York, NY 10003
www.RUSKINSTITUTE.org • 212-263-8830

RUSK INSTITUTE OF REHABILITATION MEDICINE

The Rusk Institute of Rehabilitation Medicine at NYU Langone Medical Center (Rusk) is ranked among the nation's top 10 "Best Hospitals" for the 22nd consecutive year in U.S. News & World Report, as well as #1 rehabilitation program in New York. Rusk is internationally renowned for the treatment of adults and children with disabilities, providing the full continuum of inpatient and outpatient rehabilitation care across all specialties: physical, occupational, speech/swallowing and vocational therapy, psychology, music and recreational therapy, nutrition, nursing, and social work.

Rusk's CARF-Accredited Brain Injury Rehabilitation Program is tailored for patients who have medical, physical, cognitive, and behavioral changes as a result of a brain injury or neurological illness.

The Amputee Program provides specialized limb deficiency rehabilitation to patients who have undergone amputations.

The Joan and Joel Smilow Cardiac and Pulmonary Rehabilitation & Prevention Center offers a model of transitional care for patients with cardiac and lung conditions.

Orthopaedic/Musculoskeletal Rehabilitation is offered for patients with back, neck, hip, elbow and shoulder disorders, arthritis-related joint pain, conditions affecting the bones, tendon, ligaments and muscles, and for pre- and post-surgical patients.

The Spinal Cord Injury program offers a comprehensive, patient-centered array of specialized and innovative clinical and educational programs to optimize quality of life.

Sports Injury Rehabilitation addresses the needs of patients with sports-related conditions, including post-operative rehabilitation for patients who require orthopaedic surgery.

Rusk's CARF-Accredited Stroke Program offers an interdisciplinary team with specialized training in the medical, nursing or therapeutic care and treatment of stroke patients.

Vestibular Rehabilitation addresses the evaluation and treatment of patients suffering from dizziness and imbalance.

The Women's Health Program addresses issues that uniquely affect women, including pelvic floor muscle dysfunction/pain, urinary incontinence, cancer rehabilitation and lymphedema, and prenatal and postpartum musculoskeletal conditions.

Chest Physical Therapy cares for individuals with lung congestion, secretion retention or areas of lung collapse.

The Outpatient Rehabilitation Psychology Service provides care to patients with neurological and medical conditions on an outpatient basis.

Speech-Language Pathology & Swallowing is dedicated to patients with communication disorders due to neurological problems as well as diagnosis and management of swallowing and feeding disorders.

Vocational Services provides disabled individuals with the competencies needed to return to school or work and to lead a productive life.

Penn Medicine

OVERVIEW

For more than two centuries, Penn physicians and scientists have been committed to the highest standards of patient care, education and research. That commitment has been recognized throughout the greater Philadelphia region and across the nation.

Penn Medicine received over $400 million in research grant funding from the National Institutes of Health in 2010, with several departments ranking first nationally. *U.S.News & World Report* also consistently ranks Penn Medicine, the Perelman School of Medicine and the School of Nursing among the nation's best.

What Sets Penn Apart?

Penn's physicians and scientists are united in the health system's mission to expand the frontiers of medicine through new discoveries in the detection, treatment and prevention of human disease. Because they develop and test new treatments through clinical trials, their patients gain access to the very latest advances and future generations will benefit from the work they do today.

Penn continues to lead the way in discovering new treatment methods for diseases once considered incurable, including groundbreaking research in cancer, cardiac, neurosciences, orthopaedics, genetics and imaging.

Over the past 30 years, Penn physicians and scientists have participated in many important discoveries, including:

- The first general vaccine against pneumonia.
- The introduction of total intravenous feeding.
- The development of cognitive therapy.
- The development of magnetic resonance imaging and other imaging technologies.
- The discovery of the Philadelphia chromosome, which revolutionized cancer research by making the connection between genetic abnormalities and cancer.
- The development of a cure for atrial fibrillation.
- Pioneering new procedures in robotic-assisted surgery.
- Developing immunotherapies that use the body's own immune system to fight cancer and reduce treatment side-effects.
- Pioneering groundbreaking studies using genetically modified T cells to treat patients with B cell Chronic Lymphocytic Leukemia (CLL) and other B cell malignancies.

Locations

Patients are seen at:

- Hospital of the University of Pennsylvania
- Penn Presbyterian Medical Center
- Pennsylvania Hospital
- Penn Medicine Bucks County
- Penn Medicine Cherry Hill
- Penn Medicine Radnor
- Penn Medicine Rittenhouse
- PennCare, a primary care physician network, provides services in the local communities in Bucks, Chester, Delaware, Montgomery and Philadelphia counties in Pennsylvania and in Southern New Jersey.
- Hospice and home care services are provided by Penn Home Care and Hospice Services.

On the Web

Visit PennMedicine.org for the latest patient education with explanation of surgical procedures and follow-up care, screening tools, drug interactions and descriptions as well as an encyclopedia of health information.

To learn more about Penn physicians or services, call 800.789.PENN or visit PennMedicine.org

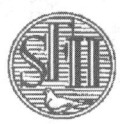

St. Francis Hospital The Heart Center®
100 Port Washington Blvd.
Roslyn, New York 11576
www.stfrancisheartcenter.com
(516) 562-6000   1-888-HEARTNY

St. Francis Hospital, The Heart Center® is New York State's only specialty designated cardiac center, offering one of the leading cardiac care programs in the nation. Founded in 1922 by the Franciscan Missionaries of Mary, the Hospital is recognized as an innovator in the delivery of specialized cardiovascular services in an environment where excellence and compassion are emphasized. St. Francis also offers a superb program in non-cardiac surgery, including some of the most advanced technology and minimally invasive techniques available for vascular, prostate, ear-nose-throat (ENT), abdominal, oncologic, and orthopedic surgery.

Cardiac Diagnostics and Treatment
St. Francis Hospital performs one of the highest volumes of cardiac surgical, interventional and arrhythmia procedures in the nation and has been consistently recognized for its outstanding quality of care. In 2011-12, St. Francis Hospital was ranked one of America's best hospitals by *U.S. News & World Report*.

Cardiac surgery: In 2010, 1,630 open-heart surgeries were performed at St. Francis Hospital. The Hospital's seven cardiothoracic surgeons have the combined experience of over 20,000 open-heart procedures in the last 10 years alone and are experts in all types of heart surgery, from conventional, open-heart bypass to off-pump coronary artery bypass (OPCAB) to the newest, minimally invasive valve procedures, including surgical techniques designed to treat certain cardiac arrhythmias or irregular heart rhythms.

Cardiac catheterization: In 2010, St. Francis interventional cardiologists performed 8,593 cardiac catheterizations and 3,425 percutaneous coronary interventions (angioplasty and insertion of stents). The Hospital is also recognized as one of the East Coast's highest volume centers for catheter-based techniques to close atrial septal defects (ASDs) and patent foramen ovale (PFO).

Arrhythmia and Pacemaker Center: St. Francis has a leading national program for pacemaker implantation and the diagnosis and treatment of cardiac rhythm abnormalities. The Center has unparalleled expertise in radiofrequency cardiac ablation, including treatment of atrial fibrillation.

Research and Technology: At the St. Francis Cardiac Research Institute, a team of world-renowned researchers is working with the latest non-invasive imaging technology, including advanced techniques and world-class expertise in cardiac CT angiography, cardiac magnetic resonance imaging, cardiac PET/CT and three-dimensional echocardiography. This multimodality approach to investigating the heart's function and disease processes is aimed at improving methods of diagnosing heart disease.

Prevention and Education
St. Francis Hospital's satellite campus, The DeMatteis Center for Cardiac Research and Education, in Greenvale, New York, is one of the few freestanding campuses in the U.S. dedicated to the prevention of heart disease. It is the site of community health lectures, as well as the largest medically staffed cardiac fitness and rehabilitation program on Long Island.

Physician referral: **1-888-HEARTNY**
Sponsorship: Voluntary not-for-profit
Beds: 364
Accreditation: Awarded accreditation from the Joint Commission.

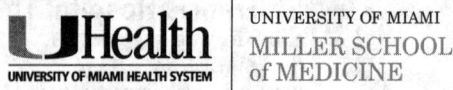

UHealth

UNIVERSITY OF MIAMI
MILLER SCHOOL
of MEDICINE

305-243-4000 • 1-877-243-4340
www.uhealthsystem.com

UHEALTH

For almost 60 years, the University of Miami has been a vital part of South Florida's health care landscape. Now, known by the name UHealth – University of Miami Health System, we continue our leading role as South Florida's source for breakthrough medicine and the region's unequivocal health care leader. Backed by up-to-the-minute research, award-winning community service, and top-ranked physicians practicing in more than 100 medical specialties and subspecialties, UHealth provides health care for the 21st Century.

LEONARD M. MILLER SCHOOL OF MEDICINE

The University of Miami's Leonard M. Miller School of Medicine serves as the "engine" driving UHealth. Driven by the vision of University President Donna Shalala, (the former U.S. Secretary of Health and Human Services,) and Dean Pascal J. Goldschmidt, the Miller School of Medicine has attracted international leaders from dozens of fields. Moreover, this renowned team is transforming thousands of lives by helping our patients – and the beneficiaries of our research – live longer and live healthier.

TOP DOCTORS

UHealth's 1,500 doctors are among the nation's most respected. More than 400 of them are listed as "best doctors" in regional and national rankings.* Providing care to one of the most diverse patient populations in the world and delivering services in five counties stretching from the Palm Beaches to the Florida Keys, UHealth physicians keep Florida healthy.

*Based on listings provided by Best Doctors®, Castle Connolly Medical Ltd., and Florida Super Doctors.

INNOVATIVE RESEARCH

Currently, UHealth physicians and scientists are involved in more than 1,500 ongoing studies, many of which lead to clinical trials that directly change the standard for care. They work every day to uncover new information, build better understanding, and develop new cures. It's what sets us apart, and it's why patients from all over the world choose UHealth.

UHealth's physicians and health care professionals provide care at more than 30 facilities, including:

- University of Miami Hospital
- Sylvester Comprehensive Cancer Center
- Bascom Palmer Eye Institute
- Diabetes Research Institute
- The Miami Project to Cure Paralysis
- Mailman Center for Child Development
- John P. Hussman Institute for Human Genetics
- Interdisciplinary Stem Cell Institute

In affiliation with:

- Jackson Memorial Hospital
- Holtz Children's Hospital
- Miami VA Medical Center

UHealth: Top-ranked doctors and hospitals providing the finest health care at more than 30 convenient South Florida locations, including our hospitals: University of Miami Hospital, Bascom Palmer Eye Institute, and Sylvester Comprehensive Cancer Center. UHealth is powered by the research and education of the University of Miami Miller School of Medicine.

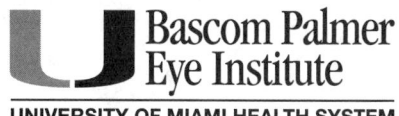

UNIVERSITY OF MIAMI HEALTH SYSTEM

INTERNATIONALLY ACCLAIMED

Bascom Palmer Eye Institute is committed to the protection and preservation of the treasured gift of sight. The Institute's full-time faculty of internationally-respected physicians and scientists are skilled in every ophthalmic subspecialty. Bascom Palmer Eye Institute, which serves as the Department of Ophthalmology for the University of Miami Miller School of Medicine in Miami, Florida, is recognized as one of the world's finest and most progressive centers for ophthalmic care, research and education.

BASCOM PALMER EYE INSTITUTE RANKED #1 IN USA

Bascom Palmer Eye Institute continues to be ranked as one of the nation's best ophthalmic hospitals by board-certified ophthalmologists from across the United States. In 2011, Bascom Palmer was named the #1 eye hospital in the United States by *U.S. News & World Report* for the eighth year in a row. Bascom Palmer is also recognized as having the Best Overall Program, Best Clinical (Patient) Care and Best Residency Education Program by *Ophthalmology Times*, which annually ranks the top ophthalmology programs in the United States.

BASCOM PALMER RESEARCHERS ADVANCE OPHTHALMIC CARE AND TREATMENT

Consistent with its mission to resolve diseases and disorders of the eye, the physicians and scientists of Bascom Palmer Eye Institute develop new theories, therapeutic techniques and surgical instruments. Many of the institute's innovations have advanced the course of ophthalmic practices worldwide, including:

- Discovering a new treatment for wet macular degeneration and introducing the use of bevacizumab (Avastin) as a remarkable breakthrough therapy.
- Alerting ophthalmologists around the world of fungal infections affecting contact lens users, significantly reducing the number of new infections.
- Performing the first successful vitreous surgery – and inventing miniature surgical instrumentation required for this procedure.
- Unraveling the mystery of normal tension glaucoma.
- Establishing predictive tests and new treatments for complicated retinal detachments.

To schedule an appointment please call (800) 329-7000 or visit www.bascompalmer.org

Miami	**Palm Beach Gardens**	**Naples**	**Plantation**
900 NW 17th Street	7101 Fairway Drive,	311 9th Street North	1000 South Pine Island Road
Miami, FL 33136	Palm Beach Gardens, FL 33418	Naples, FL 34102	Plantation, FL 33324
(305) 326-6000	(561) 515-1500	(239) 659-3937	(954) 465-2700

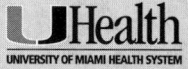
UNIVERSITY OF MIAMI HEALTH SYSTEM

UNIVERSITY OF MIAMI
MILLER SCHOOL
of MEDICINE

UHealth: Top-ranked doctors and hospitals providing the finest health care at more than 30 convenient South Florida locations, including our hospitals: University of Miami Hospital, Bascom Palmer Eye Institute, and Sylvester Comprehensive Cancer Center. UHealth is powered by the research and education of the University of Miami Miller School of Medicine.

www.uhealthsystem.com

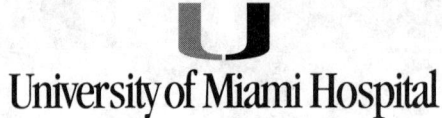
A HOSPITAL FOR THE 21ST CENTURY

University of Miami Hospital is the only university-owned, multi-specialty, acute care hospital in South Florida and part of UHealth – University of Miami Health System. Here, physicians on the faculty of the Miller School of Medicine and private practice physicians, plan and provide care, investigate new treatments still in the clinical research phase, and utilize the most advanced technologies available.

BREAKTHROUGH MEDICINE HAPPENS HERE

UHealth physicians participate in hundreds of ongoing studies, many of which culminate in clinical trials underway at University of Miami Hospital. These studies give our patients access to up-to-the-minute breakthroughs straight from the laboratory. Currently, our physicians are investigating new approaches to prevention, diagnosis, and treatment in a number of areas, including: cardiology, sports medicine, orthopaedics, neurology, urology, gynecology, and otolaryngology.

TOP TECHNOLOGY

To provide better diagnoses, deliver more effective treatments, and promote faster recoveries, University of Miami Hospital has invested in the latest technology. At our new cardiac catheterization and electrophysiology labs, we use the Stereoaxis Magnetic Navigation System and the Siemens Artis Zeego Robot to accurately and safely guide catheters through the most delicate vessels. Surgeons representing multiple specialties at University of Miami Hospital use the da Vinci Surgical System® to increase the speed and precision of their procedures. And our 128-slice CT scanner produces the highest-resolution 3D images available.

PRIORITIZING THE PATIENT EXPERIENCE

In addition to all-private rooms and a team of nurses trained to deliver high quality, compassionate care, University of Miami Hospital offers 24-hour access to personal patient representatives; physical, occupational, and speech therapists; and an on-site pharmacy. We even have a specially outfitted ambulance for transferring patients from other facilities.

> **To make an appointment, please call 305-689-5000.**

University of Miami Hospital Services

- Ambulatory Care
- Bariatric Center of Excellence
- Behavioral Health
- Breast Care Center
- Cardiac Rehabilitation
- Cardiac Services
- Critical Care (46 beds)
- Dermatology
- Emergency Room
- Endocrinology
- Gastrointestinal Center
- Gynecology/Women's Services
- Hepatology
- Hyperbaric Medicine
- Infertility Center
- International Medicine
- Laser & Laparoscopic Surgery
- Minimally Invasive Robotic Surgery
- Nephrology
- Neurology & Neurosurgery
- Oral & Maxillofacial Surgery
- Orthopaedics – Joint Center
- Otolaryngology (ENT)
- Outpatient Rehabilitation
- Pain Management Center
- Physical & Occupational Therapy
- Plastic & Reconstructive Surgery
- Podiatry
- Progressive Care Unit
- Pulmonary Medicine
- Radiation Oncology
- Sports Medicine Program
- Urology
- Vascular Surgery
- VITAS Hospice & Palliative Care
- Wound Healing Center

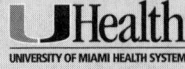

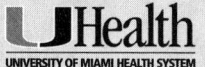

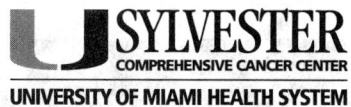

UNIVERSITY OF MIAMI HEALTH SYSTEM

DRIVEN TO BEAT CANCER

Sylvester Comprehensive Cancer Center serves as the cancer treatment and research hub of UHealth – University of Miami Health System. For nearly 20 years, Sylvester has grown with unstoppable momentum and singular focus – to develop and implement cancer breakthroughs and save lives.

Gaining the attention and respect of physicians and scientists from around the world, Sylvester has emerged as a magnet for today's leading cancer experts, attracting among the most innovative cancer professionals across a full spectrum of disciplines. Drawn to its entrepreneurial spirit, its unique international flair, and its awe-inspiring knowledge base, the team at Sylvester represents the future of university-based cancer care and research. It represents the real-world possibility to find the cure.

MORE CANCER SPECIALISTS. MORE SPECIALIZED CARE.

Patients who receive care from specialized hospitals often have better outcomes. At Sylvester we recognize the value of specialization, so we maintain a singular focus on cancer…only cancer. With more cancer experts than any other South Florida facility – more than 250 physicians and scientists, all faculty of the Miller School of Medicine – we have earned a reputation for delivering the most advanced treatment options available. This recognition has contributed to intense demand for care at Sylvester and more than a quarter million patient visits annually.

PHASE I CLINICAL TRIALS PROGRAM

Sylvester created South Florida's only academic phase I testing center dedicated to drug development for cancer patients. This novel program provides the necessary foundation to speed promising therapies from the laboratory to patients in need of care.

Phase I trials are the first studies in humans and an important step to transition novel treatments from the laboratories to the patients' bedside. The Phase I Clinical Trials Program assists physicians and scientists to establish important collaborative relationships that often translate into more treatment choices for patients.

Sylvester has assembled 15 multidisciplinary teams with focused expertise in specific types of cancers, including:

- Bone & Soft Tissue Cancers
- Breast Cancer
- Colorectal Cancer
- Eye Cancer
- Gynecologic Cancer
- Head & Neck Cancer
- Leukemia, Lymphoma & Myeloma
- Lung Cancer
- Melanoma & Related Skin Cancers
- Neurological Cancer
- Pancreatic, Liver & Related Cancers
- Pediatric Cancer
- Prostate, Bladder & Kidney Cancers
- Stomach & Esophageal Cancers
- Thyroid & Other Endocrine Cancers

As a leader in cancer research and treatment, Sylvester Comprehensive Cancer Center, with outpatient locations in Deerfield Beach and Kendall, is part of UHealth – University of Miami Health System, which includes more than 1,200 physicians, 30 outpatient locations, University of Miami Hospital, and the nation's top-ranked eye hospital, Bascom Palmer Eye Institute.

1475 N.W. 12th Avenue
Miami, Florida 33136
800-545-2292
www.sylvester.org

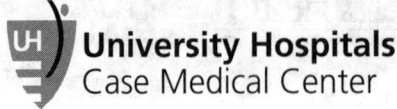

University Hospitals
Case Medical Center

11100 Euclid Avenue
Cleveland, OH 44106
1-866-UH4-CARE (1-866-844-2273)
UHhospitals.org

Sponsorship: Voluntary Not-for-Profit
Beds: 1,032
Accreditation: Full Joint Commission – ANNS Magnet Status

Overview

Founded in 1866, University Hospitals Case Medical Center, our physicians, nurses, and staff work with a devotion to the UH mission – To Heal. To Teach. To Discover. Ranked among the top hospitals in 11 medical specialties by U.S.News & World Report, UH Case Medical Center is located in Northeast Ohio near the shores of Lake Erie and in the heart of Cleveland's University Circle. University Hospitals Case Medical Center is a 1,032-bed hospital specializing in adult and pediatric medical and surgical specialties.

Shaping the Future of Health Care

As the primary affiliate of Case Western Reserve University School of Medicine, UH Case Medical Center is recognized as one of the nation's great centers of academic medicine and the only in Northeast Ohio named by Thomson Reuters as one of the top 15 major teaching hospitals in the country. UH Case Medical Center clinical researchers and physicians are at the forefront of medical research, education and innovation.

University Hospitals Seidman Cancer Center is one of only 12 freestanding cancer hospitals designated by the National Cancer Institute as a Comprehensive Cancer Center through our affiliation with Case Western Reserve University School of Medicine and offers more than 300 clinical trials. University Hospitals Rainbow Babies & Children's Hospital is the region's largest group of medical professionals providing care to children and is recognized by U.S.News & World Report as one of America's Best Children's Hospitals. It boasts a Neonatal Intensive Care Unit ranked among the best in the world. University Hospitals MacDonald Women's Hospital is the only hospital in Ohio solely dedicated to women's health specializing in high-risk pregnancy, infertility, gyn-oncology and breast health.

To schedule an appointment with any University Hospitals physician, call
1-866-UH4-CARE (1-866-844-2273) or visit UHhospitals.org.

Keck Medical Center of USC

1500 San Pablo Street
Los Angeles, CA 90033
1 800.USC.CARE
KeckMedicalCenterofUSC.org

THE NEW NAME IN WORLD-CLASS MEDICINE

The University of Southern California's (USC) renowned doctors and nationally ranked hospitals have a new name: Keck Medical Center of USC. Our new name is a symbol of USC's commitment to change lives through the spark of scientific discovery and the healing power of compassion. This innovative team includes the newly renamed Keck Hospital of USC (formerly USC University Hospital), USC Norris Cancer Hospital, and 500 faculty physicians of the Keck School of Medicine of USC. The Keck Medical Center of USC brings hope back to health care, connecting patients with some of the brightest medical minds in the country.

OUR HOSPITALS

Keck Hospital of USC is conveniently located just off the San Bernardino and Golden State freeways near downtown Los Angeles. Among the hospital's advanced services are heart, lung, and vascular care; weight loss and digestive disorders; urology; gynecology; transplantation; orthopedics; and neurology and neurosurgery.

USC Norris Cancer Hospital is one of only a few facilities in Southern California built exclusively for cancer patient care and research. The hospital is part of the nationally recognized USC Norris Comprehensive Cancer Center—one of the original eight comprehensive cancer centers designated by the National Cancer Institute.

HONORS AND RECOGNITION

- *U.S. News & World Report* again named USC University Hospital as one of "America's Best Hospitals" in 2011-12.

- Many USC doctors are cited in "Best Doctors," and extensive polls of medical specialists in the U.S.

- USC hospitals are accredited by The Joint Commission.

SPECIALTIES & RESEARCH

The Keck Medical Center of USC is known throughout the region for expertise and excellence in:

+ Alzheimer's/dementia
+ Bariatric surgery
+ Brain tumor care
+ Breast cancer
+ Cardiovascular medicine and surgery
+ Cardiac arrhythmia
+ Epilepsy surgery
+ Esophageal, digestive, and colorectal diseases
+ Gynecology
+ Hip and knee replacement surgery
+ Liver, pancreatic, and hepatic diseases
+ Lung cancer
+ Neurosurgery
+ Ophthalmology
+ Organ transplantation
+ Orthopedics
+ Plastic and reconstructive surgery
+ Prostate cancer
+ Sports medicine
+ Stroke care
+ Valvular and aortic diseases
+ Women's health

VANDERBILT ▼ UNIVERSITY
MEDICAL CENTER

1211 Medical Center Drive | Nashville, TN 37232 | (615) 322-5000 | VanderbiltHealth.com

Overview

Vanderbilt University Medical Center (VUMC) has built a strong reputation throughout the U.S. as a leader in patient care, research and education over its 136-year history. VUMC specializes in applying new discoveries and innovations into patient care and medical education while offering every patient compassionate, personalized care.

In 2010, VUMC had more than 1.5 million outpatient visits and nearly 52,000 admissions. Our Emergency Department, Level 1 Trauma Center, Burn Center and Lifeflight air ambulance service provide trauma care for a three-state region.

Elite National Rankings

VUMC is consistently ranked among the nation's best by *U.S. News & World Report*'s Best Hospitals listing. In 2011, VUMC was ranked in the top 1% of America's highest performing health care providers on the Best Hospitals Honor Roll. In addition, its Monroe Carell Jr. Children's Hospital at Vanderbilt is listed among the nation's best children's hospitals, ranking in 10 of 10 specialties.

Specialty Programs

Monroe Carell Jr. Children's Hospital at Vanderbilt
Vanderbilt-Ingram Cancer Center
Heart and Vascular Institute
Neurosciences
Orthopaedics
Women's Health

Discovery, Innovation and Collaboration

VUMC thrives on a culture of collaboration that produces world-leading discovery and innovation. Learn more.

Recently our institution has produced:
- One of the nation's most advanced electronic medical records
- Leading programs in personalizing care for heart disease, cancer and other conditions based on each patient's DNA
- A program developing new drugs for schizophrenia, Parkinson's disease and more

My Health at Vanderbilt

VUMC patients can manage their care through our secure, convenient electronic medical record system, My Health at Vanderbilt. This free service is just one of the ways we're making healthcare more efficient and personal.

Physician
Listings

The Best in American Medicine
www.CastleConnolly.com

Adolescent Medicine
a subspecialty of Pediatrics

An internist or pediatrician who specializes in adolescent medicine is a multidiciplinary healthcare specialist trained in the unique physical, psychological and social characteristics of adolescents, their healthcare problems and needs.

Training Required: Three years in internal medicine OR three years in pediatrics *plus* additional training and examination for certification in adolescent medicine

ADOLESCENT MEDICINE

New England

Emans, Sarah Jean H MD [AM] - **Spec Exp:** Pediatric Gynecology; Adolescent Gynecology; **Hospital:** Children's Hospital - Boston; **Address:** Childrens Hosp, Dept Adolescent Med, 300 Longwood Ave, Boston, MA 02115-5724; **Phone:** 617-355-7170; **Board Cert:** Pediatrics 1993; Adolescent Medicine 2009; **Med School:** Harvard Med Sch 1970; **Resid:** Pediatrics, Chldns Hosp 1973; **Fellow:** Adolescent Medicine, Chldns Hosp 1975; **Fac Appt:** Prof Ped, Harvard Med Sch

Mid Atlantic

Diaz, Angela MD [AM] - **Spec Exp:** Adolescent Gynecology; Abuse/Neglect; **Hospital:** Mount Sinai Med Ctr (page 63); **Address:** 320 E 94th St Fl 2, New York, NY 10128-5604; **Phone:** 212-423-2900; **Board Cert:** Pediatrics 1987; **Med School:** Columbia P&S 1981; **Resid:** Pediatrics, Mt Sinai Med Ctr 1984; **Fellow:** Adolescent Medicine, Mt Sinai Med Ctr 1985; **Fac Appt:** Prof Ped, Mount Sinai Sch Med

Ginsburg, Kenneth R MD [AM] - **Spec Exp:** Behavioral Disorders; Adolescent Behavior-High Risk; **Hospital:** Chldns Hosp of Philadelphia; **Address:** 3550 Market St Fl 4, Philadelphia, PA 19104; **Phone:** 215-590-3537; **Board Cert:** Adolescent Medicine 2009; **Med School:** Albert Einstein Coll Med 1987; **Resid:** Pediatrics, Chldns Hosp 1990; **Fac Appt:** Assoc Prof Ped, Univ Pennsylvania

Murray, Pamela J MD [AM] - **Spec Exp:** Adolescent Gynecology; Menstrual Disorders; **Hospital:** Ruby Memorial - WVU Hosp; **Address:** Physician's Office Center, 1 Stadium Drive, Morgantown, WV 26505; **Phone:** 304-598-4835; **Board Cert:** Pediatrics 1983; Adolescent Medicine 2009; **Med School:** Med Coll PA 1978; **Resid:** Pediatrics, Chldns Hosp 1981; **Fellow:** Public Health, Univ New South Wales 1987; **Fac Appt:** Prof Ped, W VA Univ

Slap, Gail MD [AM] - **Spec Exp:** Chronic Illness; Developmental Disorders; **Hospital:** Chldns Hosp of Philadelphia; **Address:** Childrens Hosp Philadelphia, Main Bldg, 34th St & Civic Center Blvd, Philadelphia, PA 19104; **Phone:** 215-590-5868; **Board Cert:** Internal Medicine 1980; Adolescent Medicine 1994; **Med School:** Univ Pennsylvania 1977; **Resid:** Internal Medicine, Hosp Univ Penn 1980; **Fellow:** Adolescent Medicine, Chldns Hosp 1982; **Fac Appt:** Prof Ped, Univ Pennsylvania

Midwest

Bravender, Terrill D MD [AM] - **Spec Exp:** Eating Disorders; Nutrition; **Hospital:** Nationwide Chldn's Hosp; **Address:** 495 E Main St, Columbus, OH 43215; **Phone:** 614-722-2450; **Board Cert:** Pediatrics 2004; Adolescent Medicine 2007; **Med School:** Univ Mich Med Sch 1992; **Resid:** Pediatrics, Duke Med Ctr 1996; **Fellow:** Adolescent Medicine, Chldns Hosp 1998; **Fac Appt:** Asst Prof Med, Ohio State Univ

Kokotailo, Patricia K MD [AM] - **Spec Exp:** Adolescent Gynecology; Substance Abuse; **Hospital:** Univ WI Hosp & Clins; **Address:** UW Health, Univ Station Clinic, 2880 University Ave, Ste 9010, Madison, WI 53705; **Phone:** 608-263-6421; **Board Cert:** Pediatrics 1987; Adolescent Medicine 2009; **Med School:** Northwestern Univ 1982; **Resid:** Pediatrics, Johns Hopkins Hosp 1985; **Fellow:** Adolescent Medicine, Johns Hopkins Hosp 1989; **Fac Appt:** Prof Ped, Univ Wisc

Singh, Nimi MD [AM] - **Spec Exp:** Anxiety & Depression; Eating Disorders; Nutrition; Autism; **Address:** 2535 University Ave SE, Minneapolis, MN 55414; **Phone:** 612-672-2350; **Board Cert:** Pediatrics 2009; Adolescent Medicine 2005; **Med School:** Mount Sinai Sch Med 1989; **Resid:** Pediatrics, Rainbow Babies & Chldn's Hosp 1992; **Fellow:** Adolescent Medicine, Univ Wash Med Ctr 1997; **Fac Appt:** Asst Prof Ped, Univ Minn

Great Plains and Mountains

Bermudez, Ovidio B MD [AM] - **Spec Exp:** Eating Disorders; Obesity; **Address:** Eating Recovery Center, 8140 E Fifth Ave, Lawry, CO 80230; **Phone:** 877-825-8584; **Board Cert:** Pediatrics 2005; Adolescent Medicine 2009; **Med School:** Dominican Republic 1985; **Resid:** Pediatrics, Med Coll Penn Hosp 1988; **Fellow:** Adolescent Medicine, Univ Alabama 1990; **Fac Appt:** Clin Prof Ped, Univ Okla Coll Med

Kaplan, David W MD [AM] - **Spec Exp:** Anxiety Disorders; Adolescent Gynecology; Depression; **Hospital:** Chldn's Hosp - Aurora (CO); **Address:** Chldns Hosp, 13123 E 16th Ave, Aurora, CO 80045; **Phone:** 720-777-6131; **Board Cert:** Pediatrics 1975; Public Health & Genl Preventive Med 1980; Adolescent Medicine 2009; **Med School:** Case West Res Univ 1970; **Resid:** Pediatrics, Univ Colorado Med Ctr 1972; Pediatrics, Chldns Hosp Med Ctr 1975; **Fellow:** Public Health & Genl Preventive Med, Harvard Sch Pub Hlth 1976; **Fac Appt:** Prof Ped, Univ Colorado

Sigel, Eric J MD [AM] - **Spec Exp:** Eating Disorders; **Hospital:** Chldn's Hosp - Aurora (CO); **Address:** Children's Hosp, Adolescent Med Clinic, 13123 E 16th Ave, Aurora, CO 80045; **Phone:** 720-777-6131; **Board Cert:** Pediatrics 2007; Adolescent Medicine 2005; **Med School:** Case West Res Univ 1989; **Resid:** Pediatrics, Rainbow Babies & Chldns Hosp 1992; **Fellow:** Adolescent Medicine, Chldns Hosp 1993; **Fac Appt:** Assoc Prof Ped, Univ Colorado

Southwest

Hergenroeder, Albert C MD [AM] - **Spec Exp:** Pediatric & Adolescent Sports Medicine; Eating Disorders; Adolescent Gynecology; **Hospital:** Texas Chldns Hosp; **Address:** Texas Chldns Hosp, Adol Med, 6701 Fannin St, Clinical Care Ctr, 1710.00 Fl 11, Houston, TX 77030; **Phone:** 832-822-4887; **Board Cert:** Pediatrics 1993; Sports Medicine 2004; Adolescent Medicine 2009; **Med School:** Univ Pittsburgh 1980; **Resid:** Pediatrics, Duke Univ Med Ctr 1983; **Fellow:** Adolescent Medicine, Univ Wash Affil Hosp 1985; **Fac Appt:** Prof Ped, Baylor Coll Med

West Coast and Pacific

Anderson, Martin M MD [AM] - **Hospital:** UCLA Ronald Reagan Med Ctr; **Address:** UCLA Med Ctr, Dept Pediatrics, 10833 Le Conte Ave, 12-358MDCC, Los Angeles, CA 90095; **Phone:** 310-825-9346; **Board Cert:** Pediatrics 1986; Adolescent Medicine 2009; **Med School:** UC Davis 1980; **Resid:** Pediatrics, Mott Chldns Hosp 1983; **Fellow:** Adolescent Medicine, UCSF Med Ctr 1986; UCLA Med Ctr 1998; **Fac Appt:** Prof Ped, UCLA

Irwin Jr, Charles E MD [AM] - **Spec Exp:** Eating Disorders; Adolescent Gynecology; **Hospital:** UCSF Med Ctr; **Address:** UCSF Chldns Hosp, 400 Parnassus Ave Fl 2, Box 0314, San Francisco, CA 94143; **Phone:** 415-353-2002; **Board Cert:** Pediatrics 1993; Adolescent Medicine 2002; **Med School:** UCSF 1971; **Resid:** Pediatrics, UCSF Med Ctr 1974; **Fellow:** Adolescent Medicine, UCSF Med Ctr 1977; **Fac Appt:** Prof Ped, UCSF

Adolescent Medicine

MacKenzie, Richard G MD [AM] - **Spec Exp:** Eating Disorders; Menstrual Disorders; **Hospital:** Chldns Hosp - Los Angeles; **Address:** 5000 Sunset Blvd, Fl 4, Los Angeles, CA 90027-5861; **Phone:** 323-361-2153; **Med School:** McGill Univ 1966; **Resid:** Internal Medicine, Royal Victoria Hosp-Montreal 1969; **Fellow:** Adolescent Medicine, Chidrens Hosp 1970; **Fac Appt:** Assoc Prof Ped, USC Sch Med

Staggers, Barbara C MD [AM] - **Spec Exp:** Adolescent Behavior-High Risk; **Hospital:** Chldns Hosp - Oakland; **Address:** 5400 Telegraph Ave, Oakland, CA 94618; **Phone:** 510-428-3387; **Board Cert:** Adolescent Medicine 2011; **Med School:** UCSF 1980; **Resid:** Pediatrics, Chldns Hosp 1983; **Fellow:** Adolescent Medicine, UCSF Med Ctr 1985

Allergy & Immunology

An allergist-immunologist is trained in evaluation, physical and laboratory diagnosis and management of disorders involving the immune system. Selected examples of such conditions include asthma, anaphylaxis, rhinitis, eczema and adverse reactions to drugs, foods and insect stings as well as immune deficiency diseases (both acquired and congenital), defects in host defense and problems related to autoimmune disease, organ transplantation or malignancies of the immune system. As our understanding of the immune system develops, the scope of this specialty is widening.

Training programs are available at some medical centers to provide individuals with expertise in both allergy/immunology and adult rheumatology, or in both allergy/immunology and pediatric pulmonology. Such individuals are candidates for dual certification.

Training Required: Two years in allergy/immunology OR prior certification in internal medicine or pediatrics *plus* additional training and examination

ALLERGY & IMMUNOLOGY

New England

Castells, Maria C MD/PhD [A&I] - **Spec Exp:** Drug Allergy; Food Allergy; Anaphylaxis; Mast Cell Diseases; **Hospital:** Brigham and Women's Hosp (page 57); **Address:** Brigham & Women's Hosp, Allergy Div, 850 Boylston St, Ste 540, Chestnut Hill, MA 02467; **Phone:** 617-732-9850; **Board Cert:** Internal Medicine 2004; Allergy & Immunology 2005; **Med School:** Spain 1979; **Resid:** Internal Medicine, Kansas Univ Med Ctr 1988; Allergy & Immunology, Medical Coll Virginia 1990; **Fac Appt:** Assoc Prof Med, Harvard Med Sch

MacLean, James A MD [A&I] - **Spec Exp:** Asthma; Allergy; Urticaria; **Hospital:** Mass Genl Hosp, N Shore Med Ctr - Salem Hosp; **Address:** Mass General Allergy Assocs, 55 Fruit St, Cox 201, Boston, MA 02114-2621; **Phone:** 617-726-3850; **Board Cert:** Internal Medicine 1988; Allergy & Immunology 2001; **Med School:** McGill Univ 1985; **Resid:** Internal Medicine, Royal Victoria Hosp 1989; **Fellow:** Allergy & Immunology, Mass Genl Hosp 1991; Immunopathology, Mass Genl Hosp 1994; **Fac Appt:** Asst Prof A&I, Harvard Med Sch

Umetsu, Dale T MD/PhD [A&I] - **Spec Exp:** Asthma; Immune Deficiency; Eczema; Food Allergy; **Hospital:** Children's Hospital - Boston; **Address:** Div Immunology, Children's Hosp, 1 Blackfan Cir, Karp Labs, rm 10127, Boston, MA 02115; **Phone:** 617-919-2439; **Board Cert:** Pediatrics 1984; Allergy & Immunology 1985; **Med School:** NYU Sch Med 1979; **Resid:** Pediatrics, Chldns Hosp 1982; **Fellow:** Allergy & Immunology, Chldns Hosp 1984; **Fac Appt:** Prof Ped, Harvard Med Sch

Wong, Johnson T MD [A&I] - **Spec Exp:** Asthma; Rhinosinusitis; Urticaria; Immune Deficiency; **Hospital:** Mass Genl Hosp, Newton - Wellesley Hosp; **Address:** 8 Hawthorne Pl, Ste 104, Boston, MA 02114; **Phone:** 617-742-5730; **Board Cert:** Internal Medicine 1983; Allergy & Immunology 1985; **Med School:** UCSF 1980; **Resid:** Internal Medicine, UCLA-Wadsworth VA Hosp 1983; **Fellow:** Allergy & Immunology, Mass Genl Hosp 1986; **Fac Appt:** Asst Prof Med, Harvard Med Sch

Mid Atlantic

Buchbinder, Ellen MD [A&I] - **Spec Exp:** Asthma & Allergy; Rhinitis; Hives; Food & Drug Allergy; **Hospital:** Mount Sinai Med Ctr (page 63); **Address:** 111B E 88th St, New York, NY 10128; **Phone:** 212-410-3246; **Board Cert:** Internal Medicine 1981; Allergy & Immunology 1983; **Med School:** Tulane Univ 1978; **Resid:** Internal Medicine, New England Deaconess Hosp 1981; **Fellow:** Allergy & Immunology, Mass Genl Hosp 1983; **Fac Appt:** Asst Clin Prof Med, Mount Sinai Sch Med

Chandler, Michael MD [A&I] - **Spec Exp:** Asthma; Sinus Disorders; Airway Disorders; **Hospital:** Mount Sinai Med Ctr (page 63); **Address:** 115 E 61st St Fl 12, New York, NY 10065; **Phone:** 212-486-6715; **Board Cert:** Internal Medicine 1984; Allergy & Immunology 1987; **Med School:** Wayne State Univ 1981; **Resid:** Internal Medicine, Northwestern Meml Hosp 1984; **Fellow:** Allergy & Immunology, Northwestern Meml Hosp 1986; **Fac Appt:** Asst Clin Prof Med, Mount Sinai Sch Med

Cunningham-Rundles, Charlotte MD/PhD [A&I] - **Spec Exp:** Immunotherapy; Immunodeficiency Disorders; **Hospital:** Mount Sinai Med Ctr (page 63); **Address:** 5 E 98th St, New York, NY 10029; **Phone:** 212-659-9268; **Board Cert:** Internal Medicine 1972; **Med School:** Columbia P&S 1969; **Resid:** Internal Medicine, Bellevue Hosp Ctr 1972; **Fellow:** Allergy & Immunology, NYU Med Ctr 1974; **Fac Appt:** Prof Med, Mount Sinai Sch Med

Ein, Daniel MD [A&I] - **Spec Exp:** Asthma & Allergy; Sinus Disorders; Chemical Exposure; Immune Deficiency; **Hospital:** G Washington Univ Hosp; **Address:** GWU Med Faculty Assocs, 2150 Pennsylvania Ave NW Fl Ground, Washington, DC 20037; **Phone:** 202-741-2770; **Board Cert:** Internal Medicine 1980; Allergy & Immunology 1989; **Med School:** Albert Einstein Coll Med 1964; **Resid:** Internal Medicine, Mass Genl Hosp 1969; **Fellow:** Immunology, Natl Cancer Inst 1968; **Fac Appt:** Clin Prof Med, Geo Wash Univ

Fishman, Henry J MD [A&I] - **Spec Exp:** Asthma & Allergy; Chemical Exposure; **Hospital:** G Washington Univ Hosp; **Address:** 2141 K St NW, Ste 206, Washington, DC 20037; **Phone:** 202-833-3500; **Board Cert:** Internal Medicine 1982; Allergy & Immunology 1985; **Med School:** Univ Rochester 1979; **Resid:** Internal Medicine, Geo Wash Med Ctr 1982; **Fellow:** Allergy & Immunology, Georgetown Univ Hosp 1984; **Fac Appt:** Asst Clin Prof Med, Georgetown Univ

Kaliner, Michael A MD [A&I] - **Spec Exp:** Asthma & Allergy; Sinusitis; Rhinitis; **Hospital:** W MD Hosp Ctr; **Address:** Institute for Asthma and Allergy, 5454 Wisconsin Ave, Ste 700, Chevy Chase, MD 20815; **Phone:** 301-986-9262; **Board Cert:** Internal Medicine 1974; Allergy & Immunology 1993; **Med School:** Univ MD Sch Med 1967; **Resid:** Internal Medicine, UCSF Med Ctr 1970; **Fellow:** Allergy & Immunology, Harvard Univ 1973; **Fac Appt:** Clin Prof Med, Geo Wash Univ

Mazza, David S MD [A&I] - **Spec Exp:** Asthma; Sinus Disorders; Eczema; **Hospital:** St. Luke's - Roosevelt Hosp Ctr - Roosevelt Div (page 55); **Address:** 7 Lexington Ave, Ste P3, New York, NY 10010-5517; **Phone:** 212-677-7170; **Board Cert:** Pediatrics 1983; Allergy & Immunology 2008; **Med School:** Univ VT Coll Med 1977; **Resid:** Pediatrics, NYU-Bellevue Hosp 1980; **Fellow:** Pediatric Allergy & Immunology, Bellevue Hosp 1982; **Fac Appt:** Assoc Prof Ped, Columbia P&S

Metcalfe, Dean D MD [A&I] - **Spec Exp:** Mast Cell Diseases; Food Allergy; Anaphylaxis; **Hospital:** Natl Inst of Hlth - Clin Ctr; **Address:** Natl Inst Allergy & Infectious Disease, Allergic Disease Lab, 10 Center Drive Bldg 10 - rm 11C207, Bethesda, MD 20892-1881; **Phone:** 301-496-2165; **Board Cert:** Internal Medicine 1975; Allergy & Immunology 1977; Rheumatology 1980; **Med School:** Univ Tenn Coll Med 1972; **Resid:** Internal Medicine, Univ Mich Hosps 1974; Allergy & Immunology, Natl Inst Allergy & Infectious Dis-NIH 1977; **Fellow:** Rheumatology, Peter Bent Brigham Hosp 1979

Phillips, S Michael MD [A&I] - **Spec Exp:** Allergy; Autoimmune Disease; Immunodeficiency Disorders; **Hospital:** Penn Presby Med Ctr - UPHS (page 68); **Address:** 51 N 39th St Mutch Bldg Fl 5, Allergy & Immunology Section, Philadelphia, PA 19104; **Phone:** 215-662-2775; **Board Cert:** Internal Medicine 1974; Allergy & Immunology 1979; **Med School:** Univ Wisc 1966; **Resid:** Internal Medicine, Hosp Univ Penn 1968; **Fellow:** Immunology, Hosp Univ Penn 1969; Immunology, Peter Bent Brigham Hosp 1972; **Fac Appt:** Prof Med, Univ Pennsylvania

Shepherd, Gillian M MD [A&I] - **Spec Exp:** Food & Drug Allergy; Rhinosinusitis & Asthma; Urticaria; Insect Allergies; **Hospital:** NY-Presby/Weill Cornell Med Ctr, NY (page 65); **Address:** 235 E 67th St, Ste 203, New York, NY 10065; **Phone:** 212-288-9300; **Board Cert:** Internal Medicine 1979; Allergy & Immunology 1981; **Med School:** NY Med Coll 1976; **Resid:** Internal Medicine, Lenox Hill Hosp 1979; **Fellow:** Allergy & Immunology, New York Hosp-Cornell 1981; **Fac Appt:** Assoc Clin Prof Med, Cornell Univ-Weill Med Coll

Slankard, Marjorie MD [A&I] - **Spec Exp:** Sinus Disorders; Asthma; Food Allergy; Hereditary Angioedema; **Hospital:** NY-Presby/Columbia Univ Med Ctr, NY (page 65), Valley Hosp; **Address:** 16 E 60th St, Ste 321, New York, NY 10022-1002; **Phone:** 212-326-8410; **Board Cert:** Internal Medicine 1974; Allergy & Immunology 1977; **Med School:** Univ MO-Columbia Sch Med 1971; **Resid:** Internal Medicine, New York Hosp 1974; Internal Medicine, Rockefeller Univ Hosp 1974; **Fellow:** Immunology, New York Hosp-Cornell 1976; Immunology, Mount Sinai Med Ctr 1980; **Fac Appt:** Clin Prof Med, Columbia P&S

Allergy & Immunology

Southeast

Benenati, Susan V MD [A&I] - **Spec Exp:** Asthma; Latex Allergy; Sinus Disorders; Nasal Allergy; **Hospital:** Baptist Hosp of Miami, South Miami Hosp; **Address:** 6705 Red Rd, Ste 318, Coral Gables, FL 33143; **Phone:** 305-665-1623; **Board Cert:** Internal Medicine 1988; Allergy & Immunology 1999; **Med School:** Univ S Fla Coll Med 1984; **Resid:** Internal Medicine, Indiana Univ Med Ctr 1988; **Fellow:** Allergy & Immunology, Johns Hopkins Hosp 1990

Bonner, James R MD [A&I] - **Spec Exp:** Asthma; Urticaria; Food Allergy; Infectious Disease; **Hospital:** Univ of Ala Hosp at Birmingham, Birmingham, Alabama VA Med Ctr; **Address:** Alabama Allergy & Asthma Center, 10 Old Montgomery Highway, Ste 100, Birmingham, AL 35209; **Phone:** 205-871-9661; **Board Cert:** Internal Medicine 1974; Infectious Disease 1976; Allergy & Immunology 1979; **Med School:** Univ Mich Med Sch 1971; **Resid:** Internal Medicine, Univ Ala Med Ctr 1974; **Fellow:** Allergy & Immunology, Univ Ala Med Ctr 1977; **Fac Appt:** Prof Med, Univ Alabama

DeShazo, Richard D MD [A&I] - **Spec Exp:** Immunodeficiency Disorders; Allergy; Rheumatology; Pediatric Allergy & Immunology; **Hospital:** Univ Mississippi Med Ctr, G.V. (Sonny) Montgomery VA Med Ctr - Jackson; **Address:** Univ Mississippi Med Ctr, Dept Med, 2500 N State St, Jackson, MS 39216; **Phone:** 601-984-5600; **Board Cert:** Internal Medicine 1974; Allergy & Immunology 1977; Rheumatology 1982; Geriatric Medicine 2005; **Med School:** Univ Alabama 1971; **Resid:** Internal Medicine, Walter Reed Genl Hosp 1974; **Fellow:** Microbiology, Walter Reed Army Inst Rsch 1975; Clinical Immunology, Walter Reed Genl Hosp 1977; **Fac Appt:** Prof Med, Univ Miss

Friedman, Stuart A MD [A&I] - **Spec Exp:** Asthma; Sinus Disorders; Allergy; **Hospital:** Boca Raton Regl Hosp, Delray Med Ctr; **Address:** 5162 Linton Blvd, Ste 201, Delray Beach, FL 33484-6567; **Phone:** 561-495-2580; **Board Cert:** Internal Medicine 1980; Allergy & Immunology 1983; **Med School:** Spain 1976; **Resid:** Internal Medicine, Winthrop Univ Hosp 1980; **Fellow:** Immunology, Univ Cincinnati 1982

Ledford, Dennis K MD [A&I] - **Spec Exp:** Asthma; **Hospital:** University Comm Hosp, Tampa Genl Hosp; **Address:** Univ S Florida Coll Med, Dept Allergy & Immunology, 13801 Bruce B Downs Blvd, Ste 502, Tampa, FL 33613-4745; **Phone:** 813-971-9743; **Board Cert:** Internal Medicine 1980; Rheumatology 1984; Allergy & Immunology 1985; Clinical & Laboratory Immunology 1986; **Med School:** Univ Tenn Coll Med 1976; **Resid:** Internal Medicine, City of Memphis Hosp 1980; **Fellow:** Rheumatology, NYU Hosp-Bellevue 1982; Allergy & Immunology, Univ S Florida Coll Med 1985; **Fac Appt:** Assoc Prof A&I, Univ S Fla Coll Med

Lieberman, Phillip L MD [A&I] - **Spec Exp:** Asthma; Rhinitis; Anaphylaxis; **Hospital:** Baptist Memorial Hospital-Memphis, Methodist Univ Hosp - Memphis; **Address:** 7205 Wolf River Blvd, Ste 200, Germantown, TN 38138; **Phone:** 901-757-6100; **Board Cert:** Internal Medicine 1970; Allergy & Immunology 2003; **Med School:** Univ Tenn Coll Med 1965; **Resid:** Internal Medicine, Memphis City Hosps 1969; **Fellow:** Allergy & Immunology, Northwestern Univ Affil Hosp 1971; **Fac Appt:** Clin Prof A&I, Univ Tenn Coll Med

Lockey, Richard F MD [A&I] - **Spec Exp:** Asthma & Allergy; Rhinitis; Immune Deficiency; Hereditary Angioedema; **Hospital:** University Comm Hosp, Tampa Genl Hosp; **Address:** 13801 Bruce B Downs Blvd, Ste 502, Tampa, FL 33613; **Phone:** 813-971-9743; **Board Cert:** Internal Medicine 1970; Allergy & Immunology 1974; **Med School:** Temple Univ 1965; **Resid:** Internal Medicine, Univ Mich Hosp 1968; **Fellow:** Allergy & Immunology, Univ Mich Hosp 1970; **Fac Appt:** Prof Med, Univ S Fla Coll Med

Pacin, Michael P MD [A&I] - **Spec Exp:** Insect Allergies; Asthma; Rhinitis; **Hospital:** Baptist Hosp of Miami, South Miami Hosp; **Address:** Florida Ctr Asthma & Allergy, 9035 Sunset Drive, Ste 202, Miami, FL 33173; **Phone:** 305-279-3366; **Board Cert:** Internal Medicine 1974; Allergy & Immunology 1979; **Med School:** Washington Univ, St Louis 1969; **Resid:** Internal Medicine, Jewish Hosp 1971; Internal Medicine, Jackson Meml Hosp 1972; **Fellow:** Allergy & Immunology, Long Beach VA Hosp 1974

Sullivan, Timothy J MD [A&I] - **Spec Exp:** Drug Allergy; Anaphylaxis; Asthma; Urticaria; **Hospital:** Northside Hosp, St. Joseph's Hosp - Atlanta; **Address:** 5555 Peachtree Dunwoody Rd, Ste 125, Atlanta, GA 30342; **Phone:** 404-255-2918; **Board Cert:** Allergy & Immunology 1979; **Med School:** Univ Miami Sch Med 1966; **Resid:** Internal Medicine, Barnes Hosp 1971; **Fellow:** Allergy & Immunology, Barnes Hosp 1973; **Fac Appt:** Assoc Clin Prof Ped, Med Coll GA

Sundy, John S MD/PhD [A&I] - **Spec Exp:** Asthma; Allergic Rhinitis; Immunotherapy; Gout; **Hospital:** Duke Univ Hosp, Durham Regional Hosp; **Address:** Duke Univ Medical Center, Box 3278, Durham, NC 27710; **Phone:** 919-668-2169; **Board Cert:** Internal Medicine 2006; Allergy & Immunology 2009; Rheumatology 2008; **Med School:** Hahnemann Univ 1991; **Resid:** Internal Medicine, Duke Univ Med Ctr 1993; **Fellow:** Rheumatology, Duke Univ Med Ctr 1996; Allergy & Immunology, Duke Univ Med Ctr 1998; **Fac Appt:** Assoc Prof Med, Duke Univ

Midwest

Baker Jr, James Russell MD [A&I] - **Spec Exp:** Immune Deficiency-Thyroid; **Hospital:** Univ of Michigan Hosp; **Address:** UM Allergy Specialty Clin, 24 Frank Lloyd Wright Drive, Ste H-2100, PO Box 442, Ann Arbor, MI 48106; **Phone:** 734-647-2777; **Board Cert:** Internal Medicine 1981; Allergy & Immunology 1983; Clinical & Laboratory Immunology 1986; **Med School:** Loyola Univ-Stritch Sch Med 1978; **Resid:** Internal Medicine, Walter Reed Army Med Ctr 1981; **Fellow:** Allergy & Immunology, Walter Reed Army Med Ctr/NIAID 1984; **Fac Appt:** Prof A&I, Univ Mich Med Sch

Ballas, Zuhair K MD [A&I] - **Hospital:** Univ Iowa Hosp & Clinics; **Address:** UIHC Dept of Internal Med, 200 Hawkins Drive, Iowa City, IA 52242; **Phone:** 319-356-8133; **Board Cert:** Internal Medicine 1977; Allergy & Immunology 1981; Diagnostic Lab Immunology 1988; **Med School:** Amer Univ Beirut 1974; **Resid:** Internal Medicine, Rutgets Med Sch Affil Hosp 1975; Internal Medicine, Jefferson Univ Hosp 1976; **Fellow:** Allergy & Immunology, Johns Hopkins Univ Hosp 1978; Allergy & Immunology, Fred Hutchinson Cancer Rsch Ctr 1980; **Fac Appt:** Prof A&I, Univ Iowa Coll Med

Bernstein, David Isaac MD [A&I] - **Spec Exp:** Occupational Asthma; Asthma; Rhinosinusitis; **Hospital:** Univ Hosp - Cincinnati; **Address:** 8444 Winton Rd, Cincinnati, OH 45231; **Phone:** 513-931-0775; **Board Cert:** Internal Medicine 1980; Allergy & Immunology 1983; Diagnostic Lab Immunology 1988; **Med School:** Univ Cincinnati 1977; **Resid:** Internal Medicine, Cleveland Clinic 1980; **Fellow:** Allergy & Immunology, Northwestern Univ 1982; **Fac Appt:** Clin Prof Med, Univ Cincinnati

Bernstein, Jonathan A MD [A&I] - **Spec Exp:** Asthma; Occupational Asthma; Drug Allergy; Eczema; **Hospital:** Univ Hosp - Cincinnati; **Address:** 8444 Winton Rd, Cincinnati, OH 45267-0563; **Phone:** 513-931-0775; **Board Cert:** Internal Medicine 1988; Allergy & Immunology 2001; **Med School:** Univ Cincinnati 1985; **Resid:** Internal Medicine, Cleveland Clinic 1988; **Fellow:** Allergy & Immunology, Northwestern Univ 1990; **Fac Appt:** Assoc Prof Med, Univ Cincinnati

Busse, William MD [A&I] - **Spec Exp:** Asthma; Autoimmune Disease; Rhinitis; **Hospital:** Univ WI Hosp & Clins; **Address:** 451 Junction Rd, Madison, WI 53717; **Phone:** 608-263-6180; **Board Cert:** Internal Medicine 1972; Allergy & Immunology 1974; **Med School:** Univ Wisc 1966; **Resid:** Internal Medicine, Cincinnati Genl Hosp 1968; Internal Medicine, Cincinnati Genl Hosp 1971; **Fellow:** Allergy & Immunology, Univ Wisconsin 1973; **Fac Appt:** Prof Med, Univ Wisc

Allergy & Immunology

Grammer, Leslie C MD [A&I] - **Spec Exp:** Asthma; Sinusitis; Drug Allergy; **Hospital:** Northwestern Meml Hosp, Rehab Inst of Chicago; **Address:** Northwestern Med Faculty Fdn, Amb Care Ctr, 675 N St Clair Fl 18 - Ste 18-250, Chicago, IL 60611-5975; **Phone:** 312-695-8624; **Board Cert:** Internal Medicine 1979; Allergy & Immunology 1981; Diagnostic Lab Immunology 1986; Occupational Medicine 1989; **Med School:** Northwestern Univ 1976; **Resid:** Internal Medicine, Northwestern Meml Hosp 1979; **Fellow:** Allergy & Immunology, Northwestern Meml Hosp 1981; **Fac Appt:** Prof Med, Northwestern Univ

Greenberger, Paul A MD [A&I] - **Spec Exp:** Asthma; Anaphylaxis; Drug Allergy; Hypersensitivity Pneumonitis; **Hospital:** Northwestern Meml Hosp, Jesse Brown VA Med Ctr; **Address:** Northwestern Med Faculty Fdn, Ambulatory Care Ctr, 675 N St Clair Fl 18 - Ste 18-250, Chicago, IL 60611; **Phone:** 312-695-8624; **Board Cert:** Internal Medicine 1976; Allergy & Immunology 1979; Diagnostic Lab Immunology 1986; **Med School:** Indiana Univ 1973; **Resid:** Internal Medicine, Jewish Hosp 1976; **Fellow:** Allergy & Immunology, Northwestern Meml Hosp 1978; **Fac Appt:** Prof Med, Northwestern Univ

Korenblat, Phillip E MD [A&I] - **Spec Exp:** Allergy; Asthma; Anaphylaxis; **Hospital:** Barnes-Jewish West County Hosp, Missouri Baptist Med Ctr; **Address:** 1040 N Mason Rd, Ste 115, St Louis, MO 63141-6361; **Phone:** 314-542-0606; **Board Cert:** Internal Medicine 1971; Allergy & Immunology 1974; **Med School:** Univ Ark 1960; **Resid:** Internal Medicine, Jewish Hosp 1965; **Fellow:** Allergy & Immunology, Scripps Clin Rsch Fdn 1966; **Fac Appt:** Clin Prof Med, Washington Univ, St Louis

Routes, John M MD [A&I] - **Spec Exp:** Immunodeficiency Disorders; Asthma; Allergy; **Hospital:** Chldns Hosp - Wisconsin; **Address:** Children's Hosp Wisconsin, 9000 W Wisconsin Ave, Ste 440, Milwaukee, WI 53226; **Phone:** 414-266-6840; **Board Cert:** Internal Medicine 1984; Allergy & Immunology 1987; **Med School:** Indiana Univ 1981; **Resid:** Internal Medicine, Univ Utah Affil Hosps 1984; **Fellow:** Allergy & Immunology, Natl Jewish Hosp 1989; Infectious Disease, Natl Jewish Hosp 1990; **Fac Appt:** Prof Ped, Med Coll Wisc

Sanders, Georgiana MD [A&I] - **Spec Exp:** Asthma; Food Allergy & Eczema; Rhinitis; **Hospital:** Univ of Michigan Hosp, St. Joseph Mercy Hosp - Ann Arbor; **Address:** Domino's Farms Allergy Specialy Clin, 24 Frank Lloyd Wright Dr, Ste H-2100, PO Box 442, Ann Arbor, MI 48105; **Phone:** 734-936-5634; **Board Cert:** Pediatrics 1982; Allergy & Immunology 1985; **Med School:** Univ Cincinnati 1975; **Resid:** Pediatrics, Chldns Hosp Mich 1978; Pediatrics, Boston City Hosp 1979; **Fellow:** Allergy & Immunology, Univ of Michigan Hosp 1984; **Fac Appt:** Asst Clin Prof Med, Univ Mich Med Sch

Wood, John A MD [A&I] - **Spec Exp:** Asthma; **Hospital:** St. Luke's Hosp - Chesterfield, MO; **Address:** 224 S Woodsmill Rd, Ste 500S, Chesterfield, MO 63017; **Phone:** 314-878-6260; **Board Cert:** Internal Medicine 1972; Pulmonary Disease 1978; Allergy & Immunology 1979; **Med School:** Univ Okla Coll Med 1968; **Resid:** Internal Medicine, Univ Hosp 1970; Internal Medicine, Barnes Hosp-Wash Univ Sch Med 1971; **Fellow:** Pulmonary Disease, Wash Univ Sch Med 1977; Allergy & Immunology, Wash Univ Sch Med 1977; **Fac Appt:** Asst Prof Med, Washington Univ, St Louis

Southwest

Freeman, Theodore M MD [A&I] - **Spec Exp:** Insect Allergies; Asthma; Rhinitis; **Hospital:** Methodist Hosp-San Antonio; **Address:** 5282 Medical Ctr Drive, Ste 500, Westgate Med Ctr Plaza, San Antonio, TX 78229; **Phone:** 210-614-7594; **Board Cert:** Internal Medicine 1983; Allergy & Immunology 1987; Clinical & Laboratory Immunology 1988; **Med School:** Univ S Fla Coll Med 1980; **Resid:** Internal Medicine, Keesler Med Ctr 1983; **Fellow:** Allergy & Immunology, Wilford Hall Med Ctr 1986; Diagnostic Lab Immunology, Mass Genl Hosp 1987; **Fac Appt:** Assoc Prof Med, Uniformed Srvs Univ, Bethesda

Gruchalla, Rebecca S MD/PhD [A&I] - **Spec Exp:** Asthma & Allergy; Drug Allergy; Immun-odeficiency Disorders; **Hospital:** UT Southwestern Med Ctr at Dallas, Chldns Med Ctr of Dallas; **Address:** Div Allergy & Immunology, 5323 Harry Hines Blvd, Dallas, TX 75390-8872; **Phone:** 214-645-2800; **Board Cert:** Internal Medicine 1988; Allergy & Immunology 2001; **Med School:** Univ Tex SW, Dallas 1985; **Resid:** Internal Medicine, Hosp Univ Penn 1988; **Fellow:** Allergy & Immunology, Univ Tex SW Med Ctr 1990; **Fac Appt:** Prof Med, Univ Tex SW, Dallas

Lewis, John C MD [A&I] - **Spec Exp:** Asthma; Rhinosinusitis; Mast Cell Diseases; Eosinophil Disorders; **Hospital:** Mayo Clinic - Scottsdale; **Address:** Mayo Clinic, Div Allergy & Immunology, 13400 E Shea Blvd, Scottsdale, AZ 85259-5404; **Phone:** 480-301-8227; **Board Cert:** Internal Medicine 1985; Allergy & Immunology 2001; **Med School:** Loyola Univ-Stritch Sch Med 1982; **Resid:** Internal Medicine, Wilford Hall USAF Med Ctr 1985; **Fellow:** Allergy & Immunology, Mayo Clinic 1990; **Fac Appt:** Asst Prof Med, Mayo Med Sch

Schubert, Mark S MD/PhD [A&I] - **Spec Exp:** Asthma & Allergy; Sinus Disorders; **Hospital:** Banner Good Samaritan Regl Med Ctr - Phoenix, St. Joseph's Hosp & Med Ctr - Phoenix; **Address:** Asthma Allergy Clinic, 300 W Clarendon Rd, Ste 120, Phoenix, AZ 85013-2517; **Phone:** 602-277-3337; **Board Cert:** Internal Medicine 1987; Allergy & Immunology 2009; **Med School:** Univ Ariz Coll Med 1983; **Resid:** Neurological Surgery, Barrow Neurological Inst 1985; Internal Medicine, Good Samaritan Med Ctr 1987; **Fellow:** Allergy Immunology & Rheumatology, Stanford Univ Med Ctr 1989; **Fac Appt:** Assoc Clin Prof Med, Univ Ariz Coll Med

West Coast and Pacific

Altman, Leonard C MD [A&I] - **Spec Exp:** Urticaria; Asthma; Sinusitis; Allergy; **Hospital:** Univ Wash Med Ctr, Seattle Chldns Hosp; **Address:** 4540 Sand Point Way NE, Ste 200, Seattle, WA 98105-3941; **Phone:** 206-527-1200; **Board Cert:** Internal Medicine 1975; Allergy & Immunology 1979; **Med School:** Harvard Med Sch 1969; **Resid:** Internal Medicine, Univ Wash Affil Hosps 1971; Internal Medicine, Univ Wash Affil Hosps 1975; **Fellow:** Allergy & Immunology, Natl Inst Hlth 1974; **Fac Appt:** Clin Prof Med, Univ Wash

Henderson Jr, William R MD [A&I] - **Spec Exp:** Asthma; Allergic Rhinitis; **Hospital:** Univ Wash Med Ctr; **Address:** 1959 NE Pacific St, Box 356166, Seattle, WA 98195-6166; **Phone:** 206-598-4615; **Board Cert:** Internal Medicine 1976; Allergy & Immunology 1979; **Med School:** UCSF 1973; **Resid:** Internal Medicine, Stanford Med Ctr 1975; Internal Medicine, Natl Inst Hlth 1976; **Fellow:** Allergy & Immunology, Natl Inst Hlth 1978; **Fac Appt:** Prof Med, Univ Wash

Meltzer, Eli O MD [A&I] - **Spec Exp:** Asthma & Allergy; Sinus Disorders; Rhinitis; **Hospital:** Rady Children's Hosp - San Diego, Sharp Meml Hosp; **Address:** Allergy & Asthma Medical & Research Ctr, 5776 Ruffin Rd, San Diego, CA 92123; **Phone:** 858-292-1144; **Board Cert:** Pediatrics 1969; Allergy & Immunology 1972; Pediatric Allergy & Immunology 1969; **Med School:** Jefferson Med Coll 1964; **Resid:** Pediatrics, St Christophers Hosp Chldn 1967; **Fellow:** Pediatric Allergy & Immunology, National Jewish Hosp 1969; **Fac Appt:** Clin Prof Ped, UCSD

Montanaro, Anthony MD [A&I] - **Spec Exp:** Asthma; Allergy; Immunodeficiency Disorders; **Hospital:** OR Hlth & Sci Univ; **Address:** OHSU Div Allergy & Clin Immunology, 3181 SW Sam Jackson Park Rd, MC OP-34, Portland, OR 97239-2098; **Phone:** 503-494-4300; **Board Cert:** Internal Medicine 1981; Allergy & Immunology 1993; Rheumatology 1984; **Med School:** Univ Wash 1978; **Resid:** Internal Medicine, Mercy Med Ctr 1981; **Fellow:** Allergy Immunology & Rheumatology, Oregon Hlth Sci Univ 1983; **Fac Appt:** Prof Med, Oregon Hlth & Sci Univ

Allergy & Immunology

Ostrom, Nancy K MD [A&I] - **Spec Exp:** Asthma & Allergy; **Hospital:** Rady Children's Hosp - San Diego; **Address:** Allergy/Asthma Med Group & Research Ctr, 5776 Ruffin Rd, San Diego, CA 92123; **Phone:** 858-292-1144; **Board Cert:** Pediatrics 1984; Allergy & Immunology 1987; **Med School:** Mayo Med Sch 1980; **Resid:** Pediatrics, Mayo Clinic 1983; **Fellow:** Allergy & Immunology, Mayo Clinic 1985; **Fac Appt:** Assoc Clin Prof Ped, UCSD

Tamaroff, Marc A MD [A&I] - **Spec Exp:** Sinus Disorders; Asthma; Rhinitis; Immune Deficiency; **Hospital:** Long Beach Meml Med Ctr, Lakewood Reg Med Ctr; **Address:** 3816 Woodruff Ave, Ste 209, Long Beach, CA 90808-2145; **Phone:** 562-496-4749; **Board Cert:** Internal Medicine 1979; Allergy & Immunology 1983; **Med School:** Univ Ariz Coll Med 1974; **Resid:** Internal Medicine, St Mary Med Ctr 1977; **Fellow:** Allergy & Immunology, UCLA Med Ctr 1979; **Fac Appt:** Assoc Clin Prof Med, UCLA

Wasserman, Stephen I MD [A&I] - **Spec Exp:** Asthma; Rhinitis; Sinus Disorders; Urticaria; **Hospital:** UCSD Med Ctr, VA San Diego Hlthcre Sys; **Address:** UCSD, MC 0637, Stein Bldg-rm 244, 9500 Gilman Drive, La Jolla, CA 92093-0637; **Phone:** 858-822-4261; **Board Cert:** Internal Medicine 1973; Allergy & Immunology 1975; **Med School:** UCLA 1968; **Resid:** Internal Medicine, Peter Bent Brigham Hosp 1970; **Fellow:** Allergy & Immunology, R Breck-PB Brigham Hosps 1974; **Fac Appt:** Prof Med, UCSD

Cardiovascular Disease
a subspecialty of Internal Medicine

Cardiovascular Disease: An internist specializing in diseases of the heart, lungs and blood vessels and manages complex cardiac conditions such as heart attacks and life-threatening, abnormal heartbeat rhythms.

Cardiac Electrophysiology: A field of special interest within the subspecialty of cardiovascular disease which involves intricate technical procedures to evaluate heart rhythms and determine appropriate treatment for them.

Interventional Cardiology: An area of medicine within the subspecialty of cardiology which uses specialized imaging and other diagnostic techniques to evaluate blood flow and pressure in the coronary arteries and chambers of the heart, and uses technical procedures and medications to treat abnormalities that impair the function of the heart.

Training Required: Three years in internal medicine *plus* additional training and examination for certification in cardiovascular disease, clinical electrophysiology or interventional cardiology

CARDIOVASCULAR DISEASE

New England

Balady, Gary MD [Cv] - **Spec Exp:** Preventive Cardiology; **Hospital:** Boston Med Ctr; **Address:** Boston Med Ctr, Dept Cardiology, 732 Harrison Ave, Preston Family Bldg Fl 3, Boston, MA 02118; **Phone:** 617-638-7490; **Board Cert:** Internal Medicine 1982; Cardiovascular Disease 1985; **Med School:** UMDNJ-Rutgers Med Sch 1979; **Resid:** Internal Medicine, Boston Univ Med Ctr 1982; **Fellow:** Cardiovascular Disease, Boston Univ Med Ctr 1985; **Fac Appt:** Prof Med, Boston Univ

Cabin, Henry S MD [Cv] - **Spec Exp:** Interventional Cardiology; Cardiac Catheterization; **Hospital:** Yale-New Haven Hosp, Yale Med Group; **Address:** 11 Harrison Ave, Branford, CT 06405; **Phone:** 203-483-8300; **Board Cert:** Internal Medicine 1978; Cardiovascular Disease 1983; **Med School:** Yale Univ 1975; **Resid:** Internal Medicine, Yale-New Haven Hosp 1978; **Fellow:** Internal Medicine, Natl Heart Lung and Blood Inst 1981; Cardiovascular Disease, Yale-New Haven Hosp 1982; **Fac Appt:** Prof Med, Yale Univ

Catherwood, Edward MD [Cv] - **Hospital:** Dartmouth - Hitchcock Med Ctr; **Address:** Dartmouth-Hitchcock Medical Ctr, Div Cardiology, 1 Medical Center Drive, Lebanon, NH 03756; **Phone:** 603-650-7607; **Board Cert:** Internal Medicine 1978; Cardiovascular Disease 1981; Critical Care Medicine 2009; **Med School:** Jefferson Med Coll 1975; **Resid:** Internal Medicine, Hahnemann Univ Hosp 1978; **Fellow:** Cardiovascular Disease, Hahnemann Univ Hosp 1980; **Fac Appt:** Asst Prof Med, Dartmouth Med Sch

DeNofrio, David MD [Cv] - **Spec Exp:** Transplant Medicine-Heart; Heart Failure; **Hospital:** Tufts Med Ctr; **Address:** Tufts Med Ctr, Cardiovascular Div, 800 Washington St, Box 5931, Boston, MA 02111; **Phone:** 617-636-8068; **Board Cert:** Internal Medicine 2001; Cardiovascular Disease 2005; **Med School:** Tufts Univ 1988; **Resid:** Internal Medicine, Barnes Hosp 1991; **Fellow:** Cardiovascular Disease, Duke Univ Med Ctr 1995

Hutter Jr, Adolph M MD [Cv] - **Hospital:** Mass Genl Hosp; **Address:** 55 Fruit St, Yawkey Ctr, rm 5B, Boston, MA 02114-3139; **Phone:** 617-726-2884; **Board Cert:** Internal Medicine 1969; Cardiovascular Disease 1971; **Med School:** Univ Wisc 1963; **Resid:** Internal Medicine, Strong Meml Hosp 1968; **Fellow:** Cardiovascular Disease, Mass Genl Hosp 1970; **Fac Appt:** Prof Med, Harvard Med Sch

Johnson, Paula A MD [Cv] - **Spec Exp:** Heart Disease in Women; Women's Health; **Hospital:** Brigham and Women's Hosp (page 57); **Address:** Brigham & Womens Hosp, 75 Francis St, PB5-534, Boston, MA 02115; **Phone:** 857-307-4000; **Board Cert:** Internal Medicine 1988; Cardiovascular Disease 2001; **Med School:** Harvard Med Sch 1985; **Resid:** Internal Medicine, Brigham & Womens Hosp 1988; **Fellow:** Cardiovascular Disease, Brigham & Womens Hosp 1991; **Fac Appt:** Assoc Prof Med, Harvard Med Sch

Kirshenbaum, James M MD [Cv] - **Spec Exp:** Cardiac Catheterization; Coronary Artery Disease; Congestive Heart Failure; **Hospital:** Brigham and Women's Hosp (page 57); **Address:** Brigham & Womens Hosp, Div Cardiology, 75 Francis St-SH5, Boston, MA 02115; **Phone:** 857-307-1967; **Board Cert:** Internal Medicine 1982; Cardiovascular Disease 1985; **Med School:** Harvard Med Sch 1979; **Resid:** Internal Medicine, Peter Bent Brigham Hosp 1982; **Fellow:** Cardiovascular Disease, Brigham & Womens Hosp 1985; **Fac Appt:** Assoc Prof Med, Harvard Med Sch

Konstam, Marvin A MD [Cv] - **Spec Exp:** Transplant Medicine-Heart; Heart Failure; Coronary Angioplasty/Stents; **Hospital:** Tufts Med Ctr; **Address:** Tufts Med Ctr, Div Cardiology, 800 Washington St, Box 108, Boston, MA 02111; **Phone:** 617-636-6293; **Board Cert:** Internal Medicine 1979; Cardiovascular Disease 1981; Diagnostic Radiology 1980; **Med School:** Columbia P&S 1975; **Resid:** Diagnostic Radiology, Mass Genl Hosp 1978; Internal Medicine, Mass Genl Hosp 1979; **Fellow:** Cardiovascular Disease, Brigham & Women's Hosp 1981; **Fac Appt:** Prof Med, Tufts Univ

Kuvin, Jeffrey T MD [Cv] - **Spec Exp:** Preventive Cardiology; Congenital Heart Disease; Echocardiography; **Hospital:** Tufts Med Ctr; **Address:** 750 Washington St, Box 315, Boston, MA 02111; **Phone:** 617-636-5846; **Board Cert:** Internal Medicine 2005; Cardiovascular Disease 2009; **Med School:** Emory Univ 1992; **Resid:** Internal Medicine, New England Med Ctr Hosps 1996; **Fellow:** Cardiovascular Disease, New England Med Ctr Hosps 1999; **Fac Appt:** Assoc Prof Med, Tufts Univ

Liang, Bruce T MD [Cv] - **Spec Exp:** Ischemic Heart Disease; Congestive Heart Failure; **Hospital:** Univ of Conn Hlth Ctr, John Dempsey Hosp; **Address:** Univ Connecticut Health Ctr, Cardiopulmonary & Hypertension Service, 263 Farmington Ave, Farmington, CT 06030-2202; **Phone:** 860-679-3343; **Board Cert:** Internal Medicine 1985; Cardiovascular Disease 1987; **Med School:** Harvard Med Sch 1982; **Resid:** Internal Medicine, Hosp Univ Penn 1985; **Fellow:** Cardiovascular Disease, Brigham & Womens Hosp 1987; **Fac Appt:** Prof Med, Univ Conn

Loscalzo, Joseph MD/PhD [Cv] - **Spec Exp:** Coronary Artery Disease; Peripheral Vascular Disease; **Hospital:** Brigham and Women's Hosp (page 57); **Address:** Brigham & Women's Hosp, Div Cardiology, 75 Francis St, Boston, MA 02115; **Phone:** 617-732-6340; **Board Cert:** Internal Medicine 1981; Cardiovascular Disease 1983; **Med School:** Univ Pennsylvania 1978; **Resid:** Internal Medicine, Peter Bent Brigham Hosp 1981; **Fellow:** Cardiovascular Disease, Brigham & Women's Hosp 1983; **Fac Appt:** Prof Med, Harvard Med Sch

Manning, Warren MD [Cv] - **Spec Exp:** Heart Valve Disease; Echocardiography; **Hospital:** Beth Israel Deaconess Med Ctr - Boston; **Address:** BIDMC, Dept Non-Invasive Cardiology, 330 Brookline Ave, Boston, MA 02215-5400; **Phone:** 617-667-2192; **Board Cert:** Internal Medicine 1986; Cardiovascular Disease 1989; **Med School:** Harvard Med Sch 1983; **Resid:** Internal Medicine, Beth Israel Hosp 1986; **Fellow:** Cardiovascular Disease, Beth Israel Hosp 1989; **Fac Appt:** Prof Med, Harvard Med Sch

O'Gara, Patrick T MD [Cv] - **Spec Exp:** Heart Valve Disease; Coronary Artery Disease; Aortic Diseases & Dissection; **Hospital:** Brigham and Women's Hosp (page 57); **Address:** Brigham & Womens Hosp, Cardiovascular Div, 75 Francis St, Boston, MA 02115; **Phone:** 857-307-1990; **Board Cert:** Internal Medicine 1981; Cardiovascular Disease 1983; **Med School:** Northwestern Univ 1978; **Resid:** Internal Medicine, Mass Genl Hosp 1981; **Fellow:** Cardiovascular Disease, Mass Genl Hosp 1983; **Fac Appt:** Assoc Prof Med, Harvard Med Sch

Palacios, Igor F MD [Cv] - **Spec Exp:** Interventional Cardiology; **Hospital:** Mass Genl Hosp; **Address:** Mass Genl Hosp, Cardiac Unit, 55 Fruit St, GRB 800, Boston, MA 02114; **Phone:** 617-726-8424; **Board Cert:** Internal Medicine 1979; Cardiovascular Disease 1981; Interventional Cardiology 2009; **Med School:** Venezuela 1969; **Resid:** Cardiovascular Disease, Hosp Univ de Caracas 1973; **Fellow:** Cardiovascular Disease, Mass Genl Hosp-Harvard 1980; **Fac Appt:** Assoc Prof Med, Harvard Med Sch

Pfeffer, Marc Alan MD [Cv] - **Hospital:** Brigham and Women's Hosp (page 57); **Address:** Brigham & Women's Hosp, 75 Francis St, Boston, MA 02115; **Phone:** 617-732-5681; **Board Cert:** Internal Medicine 1979; Cardiovascular Disease 1981; **Med School:** Univ Okla Coll Med 1976; **Resid:** Internal Medicine, Peter Bent Brigham Hosp 1979; **Fellow:** Cardiovascular Disease, Peter Bent Brigham Hosp 1980; **Fac Appt:** Prof Med, Harvard Med Sch

Cardiovascular Disease

Phillips, Robert A MD/PhD [Cv] - **Spec Exp:** Hypertension; Coronary Artery Disease; Heart Valve Disease; **Hospital:** UMass Memorial Med Ctr; **Address:** U Mass Memorial, 55 Lake Ave North, S3-836, Worcester, MA 01655; **Phone:** 508-334-3452; **Board Cert:** Internal Medicine 1983; Cardiovascular Disease 1985; **Med School:** Mount Sinai Sch Med 1980; **Resid:** Internal Medicine, Columbia Presby Med Ctr 1983; **Fellow:** Cardiovascular Disease, Mt Sinai Med Ctr 1985; Hypertension, Mt Sinai Med Ctr 1986; **Fac Appt:** Prof Med, Univ Mass Sch Med

Ridker, Paul M MD [Cv] - **Spec Exp:** Coronary Artery Disease; Preventive Cardiology; Cholesterol/Lipid Disorders; **Hospital:** Brigham and Women's Hosp (page 57); **Address:** Brigham & Women's Hosp, Div Preventive Medicine, 640 Center St, Jamaica Plains, MA 02130; **Phone:** 617-278-0869; **Board Cert:** Internal Medicine 1989; **Med School:** Harvard Med Sch 1986; **Resid:** Internal Medicine, Brigham & Women's Hosp 1989; **Fellow:** Cardiovascular Disease, Brigham & Women's Hosp 1991; **Fac Appt:** Assoc Prof Med, Harvard Med Sch

Roberts, Barbara H MD [Cv] - **Spec Exp:** Heart Disease in Women; Preventive Cardiology; **Hospital:** Miriam Hosp; **Address:** The Miriam Hosp - Women's Cardiac Ctr, 164 Summit Ave, Fain Med Bldg, Providence, RI 02906; **Phone:** 401-793-5750; **Board Cert:** Internal Medicine 1975; Cardiovascular Disease 1975; **Med School:** Case West Res Univ 1968; **Resid:** Internal Medicine, Yale-New Haven Hosp 1971; **Fellow:** Cardiovascular Disease, PB Brigham Hosp-Harvard 1975; **Fac Appt:** Assoc Clin Prof Med, Brown Univ

Stevenson, Lynne W MD [Cv] - **Spec Exp:** Heart Failure; Transplant Medicine-Heart; **Hospital:** Brigham and Women's Hosp (page 57); **Address:** Brigham & Women's Hospital, 75 Francis St, Boston, MA 02115; **Phone:** 857-307-4000; **Board Cert:** Internal Medicine 1982; Cardiovascular Disease 1985; **Med School:** Stanford Univ 1979; **Resid:** Internal Medicine, UCLA Med Ctr 1982; **Fellow:** Cardiovascular Disease, UCLA Med Ctr 1984; **Fac Appt:** Prof Med, Harvard Med Sch

Zusman, Randall M MD [Cv] - **Spec Exp:** Hypertension; Cholesterol/Lipid Disorders; Atrial Fibrillation; Coronary Artery Disease; **Hospital:** Mass Genl Hosp; **Address:** Massachusettes Hospital, Yawkey Ctr, 55 Fruit St, Ste 5928, Boston, MA 02114; **Phone:** 617-726-7790; **Board Cert:** Internal Medicine 1976; Cardiovascular Disease 1983; **Med School:** Yale Univ 1973; **Resid:** Internal Medicine, Mass General Hosp 1978; Internal Medicine, Natl Heart, Lung, & Blood Inst (NHBLI) 1977; **Fellow:** Cardiovascular Disease, Mass General Hosp 1979; **Fac Appt:** Assoc Prof Med, Harvard Med Sch

Mid Atlantic

Andersen, Holly S MD [Cv] - **Spec Exp:** Preventive Cardiology; Women's Health; Mitral Valve Prolapse; **Hospital:** NY-Presby/Weill Cornell Med Ctr, NY (page 65); **Address:** 125 E 72nd St, New York, NY 10021; **Phone:** 212-628-6100; **Board Cert:** Internal Medicine 2002; Cardiovascular Disease 2005; **Med School:** Univ Rochester 1989; **Resid:** Internal Medicine, Ny Presby-Cornell Med Ctr 1992; **Fellow:** Cardiovascular Disease, NY Presby-Cornell Med Ctr 1995; **Fac Appt:** Assoc Clin Prof Med, Cornell Univ-Weill Med Coll

Blumenthal, David S MD [Cv] - **Spec Exp:** Heart Valve Disease; Preventive Cardiology; Coronary Artery Disease; **Hospital:** NY-Presby/Weill Cornell Med Ctr, NY (page 65); **Address:** 407 E 70th St, Fl 1, New York, NY 10021-5302; **Phone:** 212-861-3222; **Board Cert:** Internal Medicine 1978; Cardiovascular Disease 1981; **Med School:** Cornell Univ-Weill Med Coll 1975; **Resid:** Internal Medicine, NY Hosp 1978; Internal Medicine, NY Hosp 1981; **Fellow:** Cardiovascular Disease, Johns Hopkins Hosp 1980; **Fac Appt:** Clin Prof Med, Cornell Univ-Weill Med Coll

Blumenthal, Roger S MD [Cv] - **Spec Exp:** Preventive Cardiology; Hypertension; Cardiovascular Disease/Young Adult; **Hospital:** Johns Hopkins Hosp (page 61); **Address:** Johns Hopkins Hospital, Div Cardiology, 600 N Wolfe St Blalock Bldg - rm 524C, Baltimore, MD 21287; **Phone:** 410-955-7376; **Board Cert:** Internal Medicine 1988; Cardiovascular Disease 2003; **Med School:** Cornell Univ-Weill Med Coll 1985; **Resid:** Internal Medicine, Johns Hopkins Hosp 1988; **Fellow:** Cardiovascular Disease, Johns Hopkins Hosp 1992; **Fac Appt:** Assoc Prof Med, Johns Hopkins Univ

Borer, Jeffrey S MD [Cv] - **Spec Exp:** Heart Valve Disease; Heart Failure; Nuclear Cardiology; **Hospital:** SUNY Downstate Med Ctr, NY-Presby/Weill Cornell Med Ctr, NY (page 65); **Address:** SUNY Downstate Med Ctr, Div Cardiology, 445 Lenox Rd, Brooklyn, NY 11226; **Phone:** 212-289-7777; **Board Cert:** Internal Medicine 1973; Cardiovascular Disease 1975; **Med School:** Cornell Univ-Weill Med Coll 1969; **Resid:** Internal Medicine, Mass Genl Hosp 1971; **Fellow:** Cardiovascular Disease, Natl Heart, Lung & Blood Inst 1974; Cardiovascular Disease, Guy's Hosp 1975; **Fac Appt:** Prof Med, SUNY Downstate

Bove, Alfred A MD/PhD [Cv] - **Spec Exp:** Diving Medicine; Heart Failure; Sports Medicine; **Hospital:** Temple Univ Hosp; **Address:** Temple Univ Hosp, Div Cardiology, 3401 N Broad St, Parkinson Pavillon Fl 9, Philadelphia, PA 19140; **Phone:** 215-707-5757; **Board Cert:** Internal Medicine 1971; Cardiovascular Disease 1983; Undersea & Hyperbaric Medicine 2010; **Med School:** Temple Univ 1966; **Resid:** Internal Medicine, Temple Univ Hosp 1970; **Fellow:** Physiology, Temple Univ Hosp 1970; Physiology, Mayo Clinic 1971; **Fac Appt:** Prof Emeritus Med, Temple Univ

Brozena, Susan C MD [Cv] - **Spec Exp:** Transplant Medicine-Heart; Congestive Heart Failure; Heart Disease in Women; **Hospital:** Hosp Univ Penn - UPHS (page 68); **Address:** Perelman Ctr for Advanced Medicine, 3400 Civic Ctr Blvd, East Pavilion Fl 2, Philadelphia, PA 19104; **Phone:** 215-615-0800; **Board Cert:** Internal Medicine 1984; Cardiovascular Disease 1987; Advanced Heart Failure & Transplant Cardiology 2010; **Med School:** Temple Univ 1981; **Resid:** Internal Medicine, Temple Univ Hosp 1984; **Fellow:** Cardiovascular Disease, Temple Univ Hosp 1986; **Fac Appt:** Assoc Prof Med, Univ Pennsylvania

Cohen, Howard A MD [Cv] - **Spec Exp:** Interventional Cardiology; Carotid Artery Stent Placement; **Hospital:** Lenox Hill Hosp; **Address:** Lenox Hill Hospital, Interventional Cardiology, 130 E 77th St Fl 9, New York, NY 10075; **Phone:** 212-434-2606; **Board Cert:** Internal Medicine 1976; Cardiovascular Disease 1977; **Med School:** NYU Sch Med 1970; **Resid:** Internal Medicine, Bellevue Hosp Ctr 1974; **Fellow:** Cardiovascular Disease, Johns Hopkins Hosp 1976

Coppola, John T MD [Cv] - **Spec Exp:** Cardiac Catheterization; Angioplasty; **Hospital:** NYU Langone Med Ctr (page 66), Bellevue Hosp Ctr; **Address:** 275 7th Ave Fl 3, New York, NY 10001; **Phone:** 646-660-9999; **Board Cert:** Internal Medicine 1981; Cardiovascular Disease 1983; Interventional Cardiology 2009; **Med School:** NY Med Coll 1978; **Resid:** Internal Medicine, St Vincent Catholic Med Ctr 1981; **Fellow:** Cardiovascular Disease, St Vincent Catholic Med Ctr 1983

Devereux, Richard B MD [Cv] - **Spec Exp:** Marfan's Syndrome; **Hospital:** NY-Presby/Weill Cornell Med Ctr, NY (page 65); **Address:** 525 E 68th St, rm K-415, New York, NY 10065; **Phone:** 212-746-4655; **Board Cert:** Internal Medicine 1974; Cardiovascular Disease 1977; **Med School:** Univ Pennsylvania 1971; **Resid:** Internal Medicine, New York Hosp 1974; **Fellow:** Cardiovascular Disease, Hosp Univ Penn 1976; **Fac Appt:** Prof Med, Cornell Univ-Weill Med Coll

Edmundowicz, Daniel MD [Cv] - **Spec Exp:** Preventive Cardiology; Cholesterol/Lipid Disorders; **Hospital:** UPMC Passavant-McCandless, UPMC Presby, Pittsburgh; **Address:** Cardiovascular Inst at Univ Center, 120 Lytton Ave, Ste 302, Pittsburgh, PA 15213; **Phone:** 412-802-3014; **Board Cert:** Internal Medicine 2005; Cardiovascular Disease 2008; **Med School:** Hahnemann Univ 1990; **Resid:** Internal Medicine, Temple Univ Hosp 1993; **Fellow:** Cardiovascular Disease, Univ Pittsburgh Med Ctr 1996; **Fac Appt:** Assoc Prof Med, Univ Pittsburgh

Cardiovascular Disease

Eisen, Howard J MD [Cv] - **Spec Exp:** Transplant Medicine-Heart; Congestive Heart Failure; **Hospital:** Hahnemann Univ Hosp; **Address:** Drexel Univ Coll Med, Div Cardiology, 230 N Broad St, Ste 740, Philadelphia, PA 19102; **Phone:** 215-762-3829; **Board Cert:** Internal Medicine 1984; Cardiovascular Disease 1987; Advanced Heart Failure & Transplant Cardiology 2010; **Med School:** Univ Pennsylvania 1981; **Resid:** Internal Medicine, Hosp Univ Penn 1984; **Fellow:** Cardiovascular Disease, Barnes Jewish Hosp 1987; **Fac Appt:** Prof Med, Drexel Univ Coll Med

Follansbee, William P MD [Cv] - **Spec Exp:** Nuclear Cardiology; **Hospital:** UPMC Presby, Pittsburgh; **Address:** A429PUH UPMC Cardiovascular Inst, 200 Lothrop St, Ste 5B, Pittsburgh, PA 15213; **Phone:** 412-647-3437; **Board Cert:** Internal Medicine 1977; Cardiovascular Disease 1981; **Med School:** Univ Pennsylvania 1974; **Resid:** Internal Medicine, Hosp Univ Penn 1979; **Fellow:** Cardiovascular Disease, Hosp Univ Penn 1978; **Fac Appt:** Prof Med, Univ Pittsburgh

Friedman, Sanford MD [Cv] - **Spec Exp:** Preventive Cardiology; **Hospital:** Mount Sinai Med Ctr (page 63); **Address:** 941 Park Ave, New York, NY 10028; **Phone:** 212-988-3772; **Board Cert:** Internal Medicine 1980; Cardiovascular Disease 1977; **Med School:** Tufts Univ 1971; **Resid:** Internal Medicine, Mt Sinai Med Ctr 1974; **Fellow:** Cardiovascular Disease, Mt Sinai Med Ctr 1976; **Fac Appt:** Assoc Clin Prof Med, Mount Sinai Sch Med

Fuster, Valentin MD/PhD [Cv] - **Spec Exp:** Coronary Artery Disease; Heart Valve Disease; Congenital Heart Disease; Preventive Cardiology; **Hospital:** Mount Sinai Med Ctr (page 63); **Address:** One Gustave Levy Pl, Box 1030, New York, NY 10029-6500; **Phone:** 212-241-7911; **Board Cert:** Internal Medicine 1976; Cardiovascular Disease 1977; **Med School:** Spain 1967; **Resid:** Internal Medicine, Mayo Clin 1972; Cardiovascular Disease, Mayo Clin 1974; **Fellow:** Cardiovascular Disease, Univ Edinburgh 1971; **Fac Appt:** Prof Med, Mount Sinai Sch Med

Gardin, Julius M MD [Cv] - **Spec Exp:** Echocardiography; Geriatric Cardiology; Preventive Cardiology; Cholesterol/Lipid Disorders; **Hospital:** Hackensack Univ Med Ctr; **Address:** Hackensack Univ Med Ctr, Dept Medicine, 30 Prospect Ave, 1 Main, rm 1647, Hackensack, NJ 07601; **Phone:** 201-996-3500; **Board Cert:** Internal Medicine 1975; Cardiovascular Disease 1977; **Med School:** Univ Mich Med Sch 1972; **Resid:** Internal Medicine, Univ Mich Hosp 1975; **Fellow:** Cardiovascular Disease, Georgetown Univ Hosp 1977; **Fac Appt:** Prof Med, UMDNJ-Univ Med Dent NJ

Gliklich, Jerry MD [Cv] - **Spec Exp:** Heart Valve Disease; Arrhythmias; **Hospital:** NY-Presby/Columbia Univ Med Ctr, NY (page 65); **Address:** 173 Fort Washington Ave, New York, NY 10032; **Phone:** 212-305-5588; **Board Cert:** Internal Medicine 1978; Cardiovascular Disease 1981; **Med School:** Columbia P&S 1975; **Resid:** Internal Medicine, NY Hosp 1978; **Fellow:** Cardiovascular Disease, Columbia-Presby Med Ctr 1981; **Fac Appt:** Clin Prof Med, Columbia P&S

Goldberg, Nieca MD [Cv] - **Spec Exp:** Heart Disease in Women; Preventive Cardiology; Echocardiography; Women's Health; **Hospital:** NYU Langone Med Ctr (page 66), Lenox Hill Hosp; **Address:** 207 E 84th St, New York, NY 10028; **Phone:** 212-289-2045; **Board Cert:** Internal Medicine 1987; Cardiovascular Disease 2005; **Med School:** SUNY Downstate 1984; **Resid:** Internal Medicine, St Lukes Roosevelt Hosp Ctr 1987; **Fellow:** Cardiovascular Disease, SUNY Hlth Sci Ctr 1990; **Fac Appt:** Assoc Clin Prof Med, NYU Sch Med

Gottdiener, John S MD [Cv] - **Spec Exp:** Echocardiography; **Hospital:** Univ of MD Med Ctr; **Address:** 22 S Greene St, rm S3B08, Baltimore, MD 21201; **Phone:** 410-328-6190; **Board Cert:** Internal Medicine 1975; Cardiovascular Disease 1979; **Med School:** Georgetown Univ 1970; **Resid:** Internal Medicine, Univ NC Hosp 1972; **Fellow:** Cardiovascular Disease, Georgetown Univ Hosp 1976; **Fac Appt:** Prof Med, Univ MD Sch Med

Gottlieb, Stephen Scott MD [Cv] - **Spec Exp:** Heart Failure; Transplant Medicine-Heart; **Hospital:** Univ of MD Med Ctr; **Address:** Univ Maryland Med Ctr, Cardiology, 419 W Redwood St, Ste 520, Baltimore, MD 21201; **Phone:** 410-328-8788; **Board Cert:** Internal Medicine 1984; Cardiovascular Disease 1987; **Med School:** Brown Univ 1981; **Resid:** Internal Medicine, Univ Chicago Hosps 1984; **Fellow:** Cardiovascular Disease, Mt Sinai Hosp 1985; **Fac Appt:** Prof Med, Univ MD Sch Med

Greenberg, Mark A MD [Cv] - **Spec Exp:** Interventional Cardiology; Cardiac Catheterization; Heart Valve Disease; **Hospital:** Montefiore Med Ctr - Div. Moses; **Address:** 111 E 210th St, Division of Cardiology, Bronx, NY 10467; **Phone:** 718-920-4212; **Board Cert:** Internal Medicine 1976; Cardiovascular Disease 1979; **Med School:** Univ IL Coll Med 1973; **Resid:** Internal Medicine, Montefiore Hosp Med Ctr 1976; **Fellow:** Cardiovascular Disease, Montefiore Hosp Med Ctr 1978; **Fac Appt:** Clin Prof Med, Albert Einstein Coll Med

Halperin, Jonathan L MD [Cv] - **Spec Exp:** Peripheral Vascular Disease; Atrial Fibrillation; **Hospital:** Mount Sinai Med Ctr (page 63); **Address:** 1190 5th Ave, New York, NY 10029; **Phone:** 212-241-7243; **Board Cert:** Internal Medicine 1980; Cardiovascular Disease 1981; **Med School:** Boston Univ 1975; **Resid:** Internal Medicine, Mass Genl Hosp 1977; **Fellow:** Vascular Medicine, Boston Univ Med Ctr 1978; Cardiovascular Disease, Boston Univ Med Ctr 1980; **Fac Appt:** Prof Med, Mount Sinai Sch Med

Herling, Irving M MD [Cv] - **Spec Exp:** Cholesterol/Lipid Disorders; Preventive Cardiology; Heart Valve Disease; **Hospital:** Hosp Univ Penn - UPHS (page 68); **Address:** Perelman Center for Advanced Medicine, 3400 Civic Center Blvd, East Pavilion Fl 2, Philadelphia, PA 19104-4206; **Phone:** 215-615-0800; **Board Cert:** Internal Medicine 1977; Cardiovascular Disease 1979; **Med School:** Univ Pennsylvania 1974; **Resid:** Internal Medicine, Hosp Univ Penn 1977; **Fellow:** Cardiovascular Disease, Hosp Univ Penn 1979; **Fac Appt:** Assoc Prof Med, Univ Pennsylvania

Horn, Evelyn M MD [Cv] - **Spec Exp:** Pulmonary Hypertension; Heart Failure; Ventricular Assist Device (LVAD); Heart Disease-Complex; **Hospital:** NY-Presby/Weill Cornell Med Ctr, NY (page 65); **Address:** Perkins Heart Failure Ctr-Weill Cornell, 520 E 70th St, Starr 4, New York, NY 10021; **Phone:** 212-746-2381; **Board Cert:** Internal Medicine 1983; Cardiovascular Disease 1985; **Med School:** Mount Sinai Sch Med 1980; **Resid:** Internal Medicine, Mt Sinai Hosp 1983; **Fellow:** Cardiovascular Disease, Cedars-Sinai Med Ctr 1985; **Fac Appt:** Clin Prof Med, Cornell Univ-Weill Med Coll

Inra, Lawrence A MD [Cv] - **Spec Exp:** Coronary Artery Disease; Heart Valve Disease; Cholesterol/Lipid Disorders; Hypertension; **Hospital:** NY-Presby/Weill Cornell Med Ctr, NY (page 65), Hosp For Special Surgery (page 60); **Address:** 407 E 70th St, New York, NY 10021; **Phone:** 212-249-1011; **Board Cert:** Internal Medicine 1979; Cardiovascular Disease 1981; **Med School:** Johns Hopkins Univ 1976; **Resid:** Internal Medicine, NY Hosp 1979; **Fellow:** Cardiovascular Disease, Mt Sinai Hosp 1981; **Fac Appt:** Assoc Clin Prof Med, Cornell Univ-Weill Med Coll

Jessup, Mariell L MD [Cv] - **Spec Exp:** Congestive Heart Failure; Transplant Medicine-Heart; **Hospital:** Hosp Univ Penn - UPHS (page 68), Penn Presby Med Ctr - UPHS (page 68); **Address:** Perelman Center for Advanced Medicine, 3400 Civic Center Blvd, Philadelphia, PA 19104; **Phone:** 215-615-0808; **Board Cert:** Internal Medicine 1979; Cardiovascular Disease 1981; Advanced Heart Failure & Transplant Cardiology 2010; **Med School:** Hahnemann Univ 1976; **Resid:** Internal Medicine, Hahnemann Hosp 1979; **Fellow:** Cardiovascular Disease, Hosp Univ Penn 1982; **Fac Appt:** Prof Med, Univ Pennsylvania

Cardiovascular Disease

Katz, Stuart D MD [Cv] - **Spec Exp:** Heart Failure; Transplant Medicine-Heart; **Hospital:** NYU Langone Med Ctr (page 66); **Address:** NYU Cardiology Assocs, 530 First Ava, Ste 9U, New York, NY 10016; **Phone:** 212-263-7751; **Board Cert:** Internal Medicine 1986; Cardiovascular Disease 1989; Advanced Heart Failure & Transplant Cardiology 2010; **Med School:** SUNY Downstate 1983; **Resid:** Internal Medicine, Francis Scott Key Med Ctr 1986; **Fellow:** Cardiovascular Disease, Montefiore Med Ctr 1989; **Fac Appt:** Prof Med, NYU Sch Med

Kostis, John B MD [Cv] - **Spec Exp:** Hypertension; Coronary Artery Disease; Cholesterol/Lipid Disorders; **Hospital:** Robert Wood Johnson Univ Hosp - New Brunswick; **Address:** UMDNJ-Robert Wood Johnson Med School, 1 Robert Wood Johnson Pl, Box 19, New Brunswick, NJ 08903-0019; **Phone:** 732-235-7685; **Board Cert:** Internal Medicine 1973; Cardiovascular Disease 1973; **Med School:** Greece 1960; **Resid:** Internal Medicine, Evanglismos Hosp 1964; Internal Medicine, Cumberland Med Ctr 1967; **Fellow:** Cardiovascular Disease, Philadelphia Genl Hosp 1969; **Fac Appt:** Prof Med, UMDNJ-RW Johnson Med Sch

Landzberg, Joel S MD [Cv] - **Spec Exp:** Preventive Cardiology; Coronary Artery Disease; Heart Failure; Heart Valve Disease; **Hospital:** Hackensack Univ Med Ctr, Valley Hosp; **Address:** 333 Old Hook Rd, Ste 200, Westwood, NJ 07675-3200; **Phone:** 201-664-0201; **Board Cert:** Internal Medicine 1986; Cardiovascular Disease 1989; Interventional Cardiology 2002; **Med School:** Columbia P&S 1983; **Resid:** Internal Medicine, Vanderbilt Univ Hosp 1986; **Fellow:** Cardiology Research, Moffit Hosp 1987; Cardiovascular Disease, Brigham & Womens Hosp 1991; **Fac Appt:** Assoc Clin Prof Med, UMDNJ-NJ Med Sch, Newark

Mather, Paul J MD [Cv] - **Spec Exp:** Heart Failure; Transplant Medicine-Heart; **Hospital:** Thomas Jefferson Univ Hosp; **Address:** Jefferson Heart Inst, 925 Chestnut St, Mezzanine Fl, Philadelphia, PA 19107; **Phone:** 215-955-5050; **Board Cert:** Internal Medicine 2002; Cardiovascular Disease 2005; **Med School:** Temple Univ 1988; **Resid:** Internal Medicine, Temple Univ 1991; **Fellow:** Cardiovascular Disease, Temple Univ 1994; **Fac Appt:** Assoc Prof Med, Temple Univ

Meller, Jose MD [Cv] - **Spec Exp:** Cardiac Catheterization; Hypertension; Angioplasty; **Hospital:** Mount Sinai Med Ctr (page 63); **Address:** 941 Park Ave, New York, NY 10028; **Phone:** 212-988-3772; **Board Cert:** Internal Medicine 1973; Cardiovascular Disease 1975; **Med School:** Chile 1969; **Resid:** Internal Medicine, Elmhurst Hosp 1971; Internal Medicine, Mt Sinai Med Ctr 1972; **Fellow:** Cardiovascular Disease, Mt Sinai Med Ctr 1974; **Fac Appt:** Prof Med, Mount Sinai Sch Med

Naccarelli, Gerald V MD [Cv] - **Spec Exp:** Pacemakers; Arrhythmias; **Hospital:** Penn State Milton S Hershey Med Ctr; **Address:** Heart & Vascular Institute, 500 University Drive, rm H1511, PO Box 850, MC HO47, Hershey, PA 17033; **Phone:** 717-531-3907; **Board Cert:** Internal Medicine 1979; Cardiovascular Disease 1981; **Med School:** Penn State Coll Med 1976; **Resid:** Internal Medicine, NC Bapt Hosp 1978; Internal Medicine, Hershey Med Ctr 1979; **Fellow:** Cardiovascular Disease, Indiana Univ Med Ctr 1982; **Fac Appt:** Prof Med

Parrillo, Joseph E MD [Cv] - **Spec Exp:** Septic Shock; Heart Failure; **Hospital:** Cooper Univ Hosp; **Address:** Cooper Medical Ctr, Div Cardiology, 1 Cooper Plaza, Dorrance Bldg, Ste D384, Camden, NJ 08103; **Phone:** 856-968-8349; **Board Cert:** Internal Medicine 1975; Allergy & Immunology 1977; Cardiovascular Disease 1981; Critical Care Medicine 2005; **Med School:** Cornell Univ-Weill Med Coll 1972; **Resid:** Internal Medicine, Mass General Hosp 1975; Allergy & Immunology, Natl Inst Hlth 1978; **Fellow:** Cardiovascular Disease, Mass General Hosp 1980; **Fac Appt:** Prof Med, UMDNJ-RW Johnson Med Sch

Poon, Michael MD [Cv] - **Spec Exp:** Coronary Artery Disease; Pulmonary Hypertension; Cardiac CT Angiography; Cardiac Imaging; **Hospital:** Stony Brook Univ Med Ctr, Mount Sinai Med Ctr (page 63); **Address:** Stony Brook Health Science Ctr, Level 4, rm 120, Stony Brook, NY 11794; **Phone:** 631-444-5400; **Board Cert:** Cardiovascular Disease 2007; **Med School:** Mount Sinai Sch Med 1987; **Resid:** Internal Medicine, Mount Sinai Med Ctr 1991; **Fellow:** Cardiovascular Disease, Mount Sinai Med Ctr 1993; **Fac Appt:** Prof Med, SUNY Stony Brook

Reis, Steven E MD [Cv] - **Spec Exp:** Heart Disease in Women; Congestive Heart Failure; Metabolic Syndrome; Preventive Cardiology; **Hospital:** UPMC Presby, Pittsburgh, Magee-Womens Hosp - UPMC; **Address:** UPMC Cardiovascular Inst at Univ Ctr, 120 Lytton Ave, Ste 100B, Pittsburgh, PA 15213; **Phone:** 412-802-3000; **Board Cert:** Internal Medicine 2000; Cardiovascular Disease 2000; **Med School:** Harvard Med Sch 1987; **Resid:** Internal Medicine, Brigham & Womens Hosp 1990; **Fellow:** Cardiovascular Disease, Johns Hopkins Hosp 1994; **Fac Appt:** Assoc Prof Med, Univ Pittsburgh

Russell, Stuart D MD [Cv] - **Spec Exp:** Heart Failure; **Hospital:** Johns Hopkins Hosp (page 61); **Address:** Johns Hopkins Hosp, Carnegie 568, 600 N Wolfe St, Baltimore, MD 21287; **Phone:** 410-955-5708; **Board Cert:** Internal Medicine 2006; Cardiovascular Disease 2007; Advanced Heart Failure & Transplant Cardiology 2010; **Med School:** Univ Wash 1991; **Resid:** Internal Medicine, Johns Hopkins Hosp 1994; **Fellow:** Cardiovascular Disease, Duke Univ Med Ctr 1997; **Fac Appt:** Assoc Prof Med, Johns Hopkins Univ

Saunders, Elijah MD [Cv] - **Spec Exp:** Hypertension-Complex; Coronary Disease in Black Populations; **Hospital:** Univ of MD Med Ctr; **Address:** Univ MD Med Sch, Div Hypertension, 419 W Redwood St, Ste 620, Baltimore, MD 21201; **Phone:** 410-328-4366; **Med School:** Univ MD Sch Med 1960; **Resid:** Internal Medicine, Univ Maryland Med Ctr; **Fellow:** Cardiovascular Disease, Univ Maryland Med Ctr; **Fac Appt:** Prof Med, Univ MD Sch Med

Schulman, Steven P MD [Cv] - **Hospital:** Johns Hopkins Hosp (page 61); **Address:** Johns Hopkins Outpatient Ctr, 601 N Caroline St, Baltimore, MD 21287; **Phone:** 410-955-7378; **Board Cert:** Internal Medicine 1986; Cardiovascular Disease 1989; **Med School:** Johns Hopkins Univ 1981; **Resid:** Internal Medicine, Johns Hopkins Hosp 1984; **Fellow:** Cardiovascular Disease, Johns Hopkins Hosp 1988; **Fac Appt:** Assoc Prof Med, Johns Hopkins Univ

Schwartz, Allan MD [Cv] - **Hospital:** NY-Presby/Columbia Univ Med Ctr, NY (page 65); **Address:** 173 Fort Washington Ave, Ste 4-600C, New York, NY 10032; **Phone:** 212-305-5367; **Board Cert:** Internal Medicine 1977; Cardiovascular Disease 1979; **Med School:** Columbia P&S 1974; **Resid:** Internal Medicine, Columbia-Presby Med Ctr 1976; **Fellow:** Cardiovascular Disease, Mass Genl Hosp 1978; **Fac Appt:** Clin Prof Med, Columbia P&S

Schwartz, William J MD [Cv] - **Spec Exp:** Coronary Artery Disease; Cardiac Catheterization; Congestive Heart Failure; **Hospital:** Mount Sinai Med Ctr (page 63), Lenox Hill Hosp; **Address:** Mt Sinai Multispecialty Physicians, 150 E 77th St, Ste 1E, New York, NY 10075; **Phone:** 212-439-6000; **Board Cert:** Internal Medicine 1978; Cardiovascular Disease 1981; **Med School:** Albert Einstein Coll Med 1975; **Resid:** Internal Medicine, Bronx Municipal Hosp 1978; **Fellow:** Cardiovascular Disease, Bronx Municipal Hosp 1979

Shlofmitz, Richard A MD [Cv] - **Spec Exp:** Interventional Cardiology; Cardiac Catheterization; **Hospital:** St. Francis Hosp - The Heart Ctr (page 69); **Address:** 100 Port Washington Blvd, Ste 105, Roslyn, NY 11576; **Phone:** 516-390-9640; **Board Cert:** Internal Medicine 1984; Cardiovascular Disease 1987; **Med School:** NYU Sch Med 1980; **Resid:** Internal Medicine, North Shore Univ Hosp 1984; **Fellow:** Cardiovascular Disease, Columbia Presby Med Ctr 1987

Cardiovascular Disease

Silvestry, Frank E MD [Cv] - **Spec Exp:** Heart Valve Disease; Ischemic Heart Disease; Non-Invasive Cardiology; **Hospital:** Hosp Univ Penn - UPHS (page 68); **Address:** 250 King of Prussia Rd, Radnor, PA 19087; **Phone:** 610-902-2273; **Board Cert:** Cardiovascular Disease 2008; **Med School:** Univ Pennsylvania 1990; **Resid:** Internal Medicine, Hosp Univ Penn 1994; **Fellow:** Cardiology Research, Hosp Univ Penn 1997; **Fac Appt:** Assoc Prof Med, Univ Pennsylvania

Steingart, Richard MD [Cv] - **Spec Exp:** Heart Failure; Nuclear Cardiology; Heart Disease in Cancer Patients; Cardiac Effects of Cancer/Cancer Therapy; **Hospital:** Meml Sloan-Kettering Cancer Ctr; **Address:** 1275 York Ave, New York, NY 10065; **Phone:** 800-525-2225; **Board Cert:** Internal Medicine 1977; Cardiovascular Disease 1979; **Med School:** Mount Sinai Sch Med 1974; **Resid:** Internal Medicine, Yale-New Haven Hosp 1977; **Fellow:** Cardiovascular Disease, Mt Sinai Med Ctr 1979; **Fac Appt:** Prof Med, Cornell Univ-Weill Med Coll

Tenenbaum, Joseph MD [Cv] - **Spec Exp:** Heart Valve Disease; Coronary Artery Disease; Atrial Fibrillation; **Hospital:** NY-Presby/Columbia Univ Med Ctr, NY (page 65); **Address:** 173 Ft Washington Ave Fl 4, Irving Pavilion, New York, NY 10032; **Phone:** 212-305-5288; **Board Cert:** Internal Medicine 1977; Cardiovascular Disease 1979; **Med School:** Harvard Med Sch 1974; **Resid:** Internal Medicine, Columbia-Presby Med Ctr 1977; **Fellow:** Cardiovascular Disease, Mt Sinai Hosp 1979; **Fac Appt:** Prof Med, Columbia P&S

Waxman, Harvey L MD [Cv] - **Spec Exp:** Arrhythmias; Cardiac Catheterization; Heart Valve Disease; **Hospital:** Penn Presby Med Ctr - UPHS (page 68); **Address:** Penn Presby Med Ctr, Philadelphia Heart Inst, 39th & Market Sts, 4PHI, Philadelphia, PA 19104; **Phone:** 215-662-9000; **Board Cert:** Internal Medicine 1977; Cardiovascular Disease 1979; Cardiac Electrophysiology 2002; **Med School:** Mount Sinai Sch Med 1974; **Resid:** Internal Medicine, Bellevue Hosp 1977; **Fellow:** Cardiovascular Disease, Jackson Meml Hosp 1979; Cardiac Electrophysiology, Hosp Univ Penn 1980; **Fac Appt:** Clin Prof Med, Univ Pennsylvania

Weitz, Howard H MD [Cv] - **Spec Exp:** Preventive Cardiology; **Hospital:** Thomas Jefferson Univ Hosp; **Address:** Jefferson Heart Institute, 925 Chestnut St, Mezzanine Level, Philadelphia, PA 19107; **Phone:** 215-955-4194; **Board Cert:** Internal Medicine 1981; Cardiovascular Disease 1985; **Med School:** Thomas Jefferson Univ 1978; **Resid:** Internal Medicine, Thos Jefferson Univ Hosp 1982; **Fellow:** Cardiovascular Disease, Thos Jefferson Univ Hosp 1984; **Fac Appt:** Prof Med, Thomas Jefferson Univ

Southeast

Bashore, Thomas M MD [Cv] - **Spec Exp:** Heart Valve Disease; Pulmonary Hypertension; Congenital Heart Disease-Adult; **Hospital:** Duke Univ Hosp; **Address:** Duke Univ Med Ctr, PO Box 3012, Durham, NC 27710-0001; **Phone:** 919-684-2407; **Board Cert:** Internal Medicine 1975; Cardiovascular Disease 1977; **Med School:** Ohio State Univ 1972; **Resid:** Internal Medicine, NC Meml Hosp 1975; **Fellow:** Cardiovascular Disease, Duke Univ Med Ctr 1977; **Fac Appt:** Prof Med, Duke Univ

Bass, Theodore A MD [Cv] - **Spec Exp:** Interventional Cardiology; Coronary Artery Disease; **Hospital:** Shands Jacksonville; **Address:** Shands Jacksonville Cardiovascular Ctr, 655 W 8th St ACC Bldg Fl 5, Jacksonville, FL 32209; **Phone:** 904-244-2655; **Board Cert:** Internal Medicine 1979; Cardiovascular Disease 1981; Interventional Cardiology 2001; **Med School:** Brown Univ 1976; **Resid:** Internal Medicine, Mayo Clinic 1979; **Fellow:** Cardiovascular Disease, University Hosp 1981; **Fac Appt:** Prof Med, Univ Fla Coll Med

Borzak, Steven L MD [Cv] - **Spec Exp:** Coronary Artery Disease; Arrhythmias; Heart Failure; Cholesterol/Lipid Disorders; **Hospital:** JFK Med Ctr - Atlantis, Bethesda Memorial Hosp; **Address:** Florida Cardiology Group, 110 JFK Drive, Ste 110, Atlantis, FL 33462-1146; **Phone:** 561-641-9541; **Board Cert:** Internal Medicine 1987; Cardiovascular Disease 2001; **Med School:** Univ IL Coll Med 1984; **Resid:** Internal Medicine, Michael Reese Hosp 1988; **Fellow:** Cardiovascular Disease, Brigham & Womens Hosp 1991; **Fac Appt:** Prof Med, Nova SE Univ, Coll Osteo Med

Bourge, Robert C MD [Cv] - **Spec Exp:** Heart Failure; Transplant Medicine-Heart; Pulmonary Hypertension; Nuclear Cardiology; **Hospital:** Univ of Ala Hosp at Birmingham; **Address:** UAB Cardiology, THT 321-K, 1530 3rd Ave S, Birmingham, AL 35294-0001; **Phone:** 205-934-3624; **Board Cert:** Internal Medicine 1982; Cardiovascular Disease 1985; Nuclear Medicine 1987; **Med School:** Louisiana State U, New Orleans 1979; **Resid:** Internal Medicine, Univ Alabama Hosps 1982; Nuclear Medicine, Univ Alabama Hosps 1985; **Fellow:** Cardiovascular Disease, Univ Alabama Hosps 1984; **Fac Appt:** Prof Med, Univ Alabama

Byrd III, Benjamin F MD [Cv] - **Spec Exp:** Congenital Heart Disease; Echocardiography; Heart Valve Disease; **Hospital:** Vanderbilt Univ Med Ctr (page 76); **Address:** Vanderbilt Heart & Vascular Inst, 1215 21st Ave, MCE S Tower, Ste 5209, Nashville, TN 37232; **Phone:** 615-322-2318; **Board Cert:** Internal Medicine 1981; Cardiovascular Disease 1983; **Med School:** Vanderbilt Univ 1977; **Resid:** Psychiatry, Harvard/Mass Mental Hlth 1979; Internal Medicine, Vanderbilt Univ Hosp 1981; **Fellow:** Cardiovascular Disease, Vanderbilt Univ Hosp 1983; Cardiovascular Disease, UCSF 1984; **Fac Appt:** Prof Med, Vanderbilt Univ

Califf, Robert M MD [Cv] - **Spec Exp:** Coronary Artery Disease; Cholesterol/Lipid Disorders; Heart Failure; **Hospital:** Duke Univ Hosp; **Address:** Duke Univ Med Ctr 3701, 200 Trent Drive, 1117 Davison Bldg, Durham, NC 27710; **Phone:** 919-668-8820; **Board Cert:** Internal Medicine 1984; Cardiovascular Disease 1985; **Med School:** Duke Univ 1978; **Resid:** Internal Medicine, UCSF Med Ctr 1980; **Fellow:** Cardiovascular Disease, Duke Univ Med Ctr 1983; **Fac Appt:** Prof Med, Duke Univ

Chizner, Michael A MD [Cv] - **Spec Exp:** Preventive Cardiology; Coronary Artery Disease; Cardiac Catheterization; Coronary Angioplasty/Stents; **Hospital:** Broward General Med Ctr, Imperial Point Med Ctr; **Address:** 1625 SE 3rd Ave, Ste 300, Fort Lauderdale, FL 33316; **Phone:** 954-355-5001; **Board Cert:** Internal Medicine 1977; Cardiovascular Disease 1979; **Med School:** Cornell Univ-Weill Med Coll 1974; **Resid:** Internal Medicine, New York Hosp 1977; **Fellow:** Cardiovascular Disease, Georgetown Affil Hosps 1979; **Fac Appt:** Clin Prof Med, Univ Miami Sch Med

Clements Jr, Stephen D MD [Cv] - **Spec Exp:** Cardiac Catheterization; Echocardiography; Heart Valve Disease; **Hospital:** Emory Univ Hosp; **Address:** Emory Clinic, 1365 Clifton Rd NE A Bldg - Ste 2200, Atlanta, GA 30322; **Phone:** 404-778-3468; **Board Cert:** Internal Medicine 1971; Cardiovascular Disease 1975; **Med School:** Med Coll GA 1966; **Resid:** Internal Medicine, Grady Meml Hosp 1970; **Fellow:** Cardiovascular Disease, Emory Univ Hosp 1971; **Fac Appt:** Prof Med, Emory Univ

Corrigan, Victor E MD [Cv] - **Spec Exp:** Cardiac Catheterization; Interventional Cardiology; Transplant Medicine-Heart; **Hospital:** Piedmont Hosp, St. Joseph's Hosp - Atlanta; **Address:** Piedmont Heart Inst, 275 Collier Rd, Ste 300, Atlanta, GA 30309; **Phone:** 404-605-2800; **Board Cert:** Internal Medicine 1986; Cardiovascular Disease 1989; Interventional Cardiology 2009; **Med School:** Med Coll GA 1983; **Resid:** Internal Medicine, Emory Univ Hosp 1986; **Fellow:** Cardiovascular Disease, Emory Univ Hosp 1988

Cardiovascular Disease

Gandy Jr, Winston H MD [Cv] - **Spec Exp:** Echocardiography; Cardoiovascular Imaging; Preventive Cardiology; **Hospital:** Piedmont Hosp; **Address:** Piedmont Heart Institute-Perimeter, 1140 Hammond Drive K Bldg - Ste 300, Atlanta, GA 30328; **Phone:** 404-851-5400; **Board Cert:** Internal Medicine 1989; Cardiovascular Disease 2002; Echocardiography 2008; **Med School:** Howard Univ 1986; **Resid:** Internal Medicine, Emory Univ Affil Hosps 1989; **Fellow:** Cardiovascular Disease, Univ Alabama 1992

Hare, Joshua M MD [Cv] - **Spec Exp:** Heart Failure; Stem Cell Therapy in Heart Failure; **Hospital:** Univ of Miami Hosp (page 72); **Address:** University of Miami, PO Box 016960, Building BRB, R-125, Miami, FL 33101; **Phone:** 305-243-4813; **Board Cert:** Cardiovascular Disease 2006; **Med School:** Johns Hopkins Univ 1988; **Resid:** Internal Medicine, Johns Hopkins Hosp 1991; **Fellow:** Cardiovascular Disease, Brigham & Women's Hosp 1993

Harrison, J Kevin MD [Cv] - **Spec Exp:** Interventional Cardiology; Heart Valve Disease; **Hospital:** Duke Univ Hosp; **Address:** Duke Univ Med Ctr, Box 3331, Durham, NC 27710; **Phone:** 919-681-3763; **Board Cert:** Internal Medicine 1988; Cardiovascular Disease 2001; Interventional Cardiology 2003; **Med School:** NYU Sch Med 1984; **Resid:** Internal Medicine, Johns Hopkins Hosp 1987; **Fellow:** Cardiovascular Disease, Duke Univ Med Ctr 1990; **Fac Appt:** Prof Med, Duke Univ

Iskandrian, Ami E MD [Cv] - **Spec Exp:** Nuclear Cardiology; Coronary Artery Disease; Heart Valve Disease; **Hospital:** Univ of Ala Hosp at Birmingham; **Address:** UAB Cardiology, 318 LHRB, 1900 University Blvd, Birmingham, AL 35294-0006; **Phone:** 205-934-0545; **Board Cert:** Internal Medicine 1974; Cardiovascular Disease 1975; Nuclear Cardiology 1999; **Med School:** Iraq 1965; **Resid:** Internal Medicine, Univ Baghdad Affil Hosp 1971; Internal Medicine, Hahnemann Univ Hosp 1973; **Fellow:** Cardiovascular Disease, Hahnemann Univ Hosp 1975; **Fac Appt:** Prof Med, Univ Alabama

Linton, MacRae F MD [Cv] - **Spec Exp:** Cholesterol/Lipid Disorders; Preventive Cardiology; Metabolic Syndrome; **Hospital:** Vanderbilt Univ Med Ctr (page 76); **Address:** Vanderbilt Heart & Vascular Inst, 1215 21st Ave, MCE S Tower, Ste 5209, Nashville, TN 37232-8802; **Phone:** 615-322-2318; **Board Cert:** Internal Medicine 1988; **Med School:** Univ Tenn Coll Med 1985; **Resid:** Internal Medicine, Vanderbilt Univ Med Ctr 1988; **Fellow:** Endocrinology, UCSF Med Ctr 1991; **Fac Appt:** Prof Med, Vanderbilt Univ

Miller, D Douglas MD [Cv] - **Spec Exp:** Heart Disease in Women; Nuclear Cardiology; **Hospital:** Med Coll of GA Hosp and Clin (MCG Health Inc); **Address:** Medical College of Georgia, 1120 15th St BBR Bldg - rm 6518, Augusta, GA 30912; **Phone:** 706-721-4997; **Med School:** McGill Univ 1978; **Resid:** Internal Medicine, Montreal Genl Hosp 1981; Cardiovascular Disease, Montreal Heart Inst 1982; **Fellow:** Cardiovascular Disease, Emory Univ Med Ctr 1984; Nuclear Cardiology, Mass Genl Hosp-Harvard 1986; **Fac Appt:** Prof Med, Med Coll GA

Myerburg, Robert J MD [Cv] - **Spec Exp:** Arrhythmias; Pacemakers; Heart Attack; **Hospital:** Jackson Meml Hosp (page 70); **Address:** Univ Miami School Med, Div Cardiology, PO Box 016960 (D-39), Miami, FL 33101-6960; **Phone:** 305-585-5523; **Board Cert:** Internal Medicine 1968; Cardiovascular Disease 1970; **Med School:** Univ MD Sch Med 1961; **Resid:** Internal Medicine, Charity Hosp 1966; **Fellow:** Cardiovascular Disease, Grady Meml Hosp 1968; Cardiac Electrophysiology, Columbia P&S 1970; **Fac Appt:** Prof Med, Univ Miami Sch Med

Nocero Jr, Michael A MD [Cv] - **Spec Exp:** Nuclear Cardiology; **Hospital:** Florida Hosp - Orlando; **Address:** 1745 N Mills Ave, Orlando, FL 32803; **Phone:** 407-841-7151; **Board Cert:** Internal Medicine 1972; Cardiovascular Disease 1976; **Med School:** NYU Sch Med 1966; **Resid:** Internal Medicine, Bellevue Hosp Ctr NYU 1971; **Fellow:** Cardiovascular Disease, Bellevue Hosp Ctr NYU 1973

O'Connell Jr, John B MD [Cv] - **Spec Exp:** Congestive Heart Failure; Transplant Medicine-Heart; **Hospital:** St. Joseph's Hosp - Atlanta; **Address:** St Joseph Heart & Vascular Institute, 5665 Peachtree Dunwoody Rd, Atlanta, GA 30342; **Phone:** 678-843-5801; **Board Cert:** Internal Medicine 1978; Cardiovascular Disease 1981; **Med School:** Loyola Univ-Stritch Sch Med 1974; **Resid:** Internal Medicine, McGaw Hosp 1978; **Fellow:** Cardiovascular Disease, Loyola Univ 1980

O'Connor, Christopher M MD [Cv] - **Spec Exp:** Heart Failure; **Hospital:** Duke Univ Hosp; **Address:** Duke Univ Med Ctr, Box 3356, Durham, NC 27710; **Phone:** 919-681-6195; **Board Cert:** Internal Medicine 1988; Cardiovascular Disease 1989; **Med School:** Univ MD Sch Med 1983; **Resid:** Internal Medicine, Duke Univ Med Ctr 1986; **Fellow:** Cardiovascular Disease, Duke Univ Med Ctr 1989; **Fac Appt:** Prof Med, Duke Univ

O'Neill, William Walter MD [Cv] - **Spec Exp:** Interventional Cardiology; Heart Valve Disease; **Hospital:** Univ of Miami Hosp & Clins/Sylvester Comp Canc Ctr (page 73); **Address:** Univ Miami Dept Medicine, 1600 NW 10 Ave, R-MSB 1122A, Miami, FL 33136; **Phone:** 305-243-9483; **Board Cert:** Internal Medicine 1980; Cardiovascular Disease 1983; **Med School:** Wayne State Univ 1977; **Resid:** Internal Medicine, Wayne State Univ Affil Hosps 1980; **Fellow:** Cardiovascular Disease, Univ Mich Med Ctr 1982; **Fac Appt:** Prof Med, Univ Miami Sch Med

Oparil, Suzanne MD [Cv] - **Spec Exp:** Hypertension; Heart Disease in Women; **Hospital:** Univ of Ala Hosp at Birmingham; **Address:** UAB Cardiology, 1530 3rd Ave S, ZRB 1034, Birmingham, AL 35294; **Phone:** 205-801-7563; **Board Cert:** Internal Medicine 1970; **Med School:** Columbia P&S 1965; **Resid:** Internal Medicine, Columbia Presby Med Ctr 1967; Internal Medicine, Mass Genl Hosp 1968; **Fellow:** Cardiovascular Disease, Mass Genl Hosp 1971; **Fac Appt:** Prof Med, Univ Alabama

Pepine, Carl J MD [Cv] - **Spec Exp:** Coronary Artery Disease; Hypertension; Heart Disease in Women; **Hospital:** Shands at Univ of FL; **Address:** Univ Florida, Div Cardiovascular Med, 7120 NW 11th Pl, Gainesville, FL 32605; **Phone:** 352-265-0820; **Board Cert:** Internal Medicine 1971; Cardiovascular Disease 1973; **Med School:** UMDNJ-NJ Med Sch, Newark 1966; **Resid:** Internal Medicine, Jefferson Univ Hosp 1968; Internal Medicine, Naval Hosp-Thomas Jefferson Univ 1969; **Fellow:** Cardiovascular Disease, Naval Hosp-Thomas Jeff Univ 1971; **Fac Appt:** Prof Med, Univ Fla Coll Med

Phillips III, Harry R MD [Cv] - **Spec Exp:** Cardiac Catheterization; **Hospital:** Duke Univ Hosp; **Address:** Duke Univ Med Ctr, Box 3126, Durham, NC 27710; **Phone:** 919-681-4804; **Board Cert:** Internal Medicine 1978; Cardiovascular Disease 1979; Interventional Cardiology 2001; **Med School:** Duke Univ 1975; **Resid:** Internal Medicine, Mass Genl Hosp 1977; **Fellow:** Cardiovascular Disease, Mass Genl Hosp 1979

Powers, Eric R MD [Cv] - **Spec Exp:** Heart Valve Disease; Interventional Cardiology; Coronary Artery Disease; **Hospital:** MUSC Med Ctr; **Address:** MUSC Heart & Vascular Ctr, 25 Courtenay Drive, ART 7052, MSC 592, Charleston, SC 29425-5920; **Phone:** 843-792-1952; **Board Cert:** Internal Medicine 1977; Cardiovascular Disease 1979; Interventional Cardiology 2000; **Med School:** Harvard Med Sch 1974; **Resid:** Internal Medicine, Mass Genl Hosp 1976; **Fellow:** Cardiovascular Disease, Mass Genl Hosp 1979; **Fac Appt:** Prof Med, Med Univ SC

Rogers, Joseph Gordon MD [Cv] - **Spec Exp:** Congestive Heart Failure; Transplant Medicine-Heart; **Hospital:** Duke Univ Hosp; **Address:** DUMC, Box 3034, Durham, NC 27710; **Phone:** 919-681-3398; **Board Cert:** Cardiovascular Disease 2005; **Med School:** Univ Nebr Coll Med 1988; **Resid:** Internal Medicine, Univ Nebraska Med Ctr 1991; **Fellow:** Cardiovascular Disease, Wash Univ Med Ctr 1995; **Fac Appt:** Assoc Prof Med, Duke Univ

Cardiovascular Disease

Smith Jr, Sidney C MD [Cv] - **Spec Exp:** Cholesterol/Lipid Disorders; Coronary Artery Disease; Invasive Cardiology; **Hospital:** NC Memorial Hosp - UNC; **Address:** 300 Meadowmont Village Cir, Ste 313, Chapel Hill, NC 27517; **Phone:** 919-966-7244; **Board Cert:** Internal Medicine 1972; Cardiovascular Disease 1973; **Med School:** Yale Univ 1967; **Resid:** Internal Medicine, Peter Bent Brigham Hosp 1969; **Fellow:** Cardiovascular Disease, Peter Bent Brigham Hosp 1971; Research, Harvard Med Sch 1971; **Fac Appt:** Prof Med, Univ NC Sch Med

Vetrovec, George MD [Cv] - **Spec Exp:** Interventional Cardiology; **Hospital:** Med Coll of VA Hosp; **Address:** 1200 E Broad St, rm 607, Box 980036, West Hospital, Richmond, VA 23298; **Phone:** 804-828-8885; **Board Cert:** Internal Medicine 1974; Cardiovascular Disease 1977; Interventional Cardiology 2010; **Med School:** Univ VA Sch Med 1970; **Resid:** Internal Medicine, Med Coll Virginia Hosp 1974; **Fellow:** Cardiovascular Disease, Med Coll Virginia Hosp 1976; **Fac Appt:** Prof Med, Med Coll VA

Vignola, Paul MD [Cv] - **Spec Exp:** Interventional Cardiology; **Hospital:** Aventura Hosp & Med Ctr; **Address:** Aventura Hosp, Cardiac Cath Lab, 21097 NE 27th Ct, Ste 480, Aventura, FL 33180; **Phone:** 786-428-1059; **Board Cert:** Internal Medicine 1974; Cardiovascular Disease 1977; Interventional Cardiology 2009; **Med School:** Yale Univ 1971; **Resid:** Internal Medicine, Yale-New Haven Hosp 1974; **Fellow:** Cardiovascular Disease, Harvard/Mass Genl Hosp 1976; **Fac Appt:** Assoc Clin Prof Med, Univ Miami Sch Med

Wells, Gretchen L MD/PhD [Cv] - **Spec Exp:** Heart Valve Disease; Congenital Heart Disease-Adult; Heart Disease in Pregnancy; Cardiac Effects of Chemotherapy; **Hospital:** Wake Forest Univ Baptist Med Ctr; **Address:** Wake Forest Baptist Med Ctr, Dept Cardiology, Medical Center Blvd, Winston-Salem, NC 27157-1045; **Phone:** 336-716-6674; **Board Cert:** Cardiovascular Disease 2000; **Med School:** Univ Alabama 1994; **Resid:** Internal Medicine, NC Baptist Hosp 1997; **Fellow:** Cardiovascular Disease, Wake Forest Univ 2000; **Fac Appt:** Assoc Prof Med, Wake Forest Univ

Midwest

Armstrong, William F MD [Cv] - **Spec Exp:** Echocardiography; Non-Invasive Cardiology; **Hospital:** Univ of Michigan Hosp; **Address:** 1500 E Med Ctr Drive, rm L3119, Ann Arbor, MI 48109; **Phone:** 734-647-7321; **Board Cert:** Internal Medicine 1979; Cardiovascular Disease 1981; **Med School:** Med Coll VA 1976; **Resid:** Internal Medicine, Med Coll Va Hosp 1979; **Fellow:** Cardiovascular Disease, Indiana Univ Hosp 1982; **Fac Appt:** Prof Med, Univ Mich Med Sch

Bonow, Robert O MD [Cv] - **Spec Exp:** Heart Valve Disease; Coronary Artery Disease; Nuclear Cardiology; **Hospital:** Northwestern Meml Hosp; **Address:** Bluhm Cardiovascular Inst, 675 N St Clair St, Galter 19-100, Chicago, IL 60611; **Phone:** 312-695-4965; **Board Cert:** Internal Medicine 1976; Cardiovascular Disease 1981; **Med School:** Univ Pennsylvania 1973; **Resid:** Internal Medicine, Hosp Univ Penn 1976; **Fellow:** Cardiovascular Disease, Natl Inst Health-NHLBI 1979; **Fac Appt:** Prof Med, Northwestern Univ

Braverman, Alan C MD [Cv] - **Spec Exp:** Marfan's Syndrome; Aortic Diseases & Dissection; Aneurysm; Heart Valve Disease; **Hospital:** Barnes-Jewish Hosp; **Address:** Wash Univ Med Sch, Div Cardiovascular Disease, 660 S Euclid Ave, Box 8086, St Louis, MO 63110; **Phone:** 314-362-1291; **Board Cert:** Internal Medicine 1988; Cardiovascular Disease 2001; **Med School:** Univ MO-Kansas City 1985; **Resid:** Internal Medicine, Brigham & Womens Hosp 1988; Internal Medicine, Brigham & Womens Hosp 1991; **Fellow:** Cardiovascular Disease, Brigham & Womens Hosp 1990; **Fac Appt:** Prof Med, Washington Univ, St Louis

Burket, Mark W MD [Cv] - **Spec Exp:** Peripheral Vascular Disease; Coronary Artery Disease; Percutaneous Vascular Interventions; **Hospital:** Univ of Toledo Med Ctr; **Address:** 3000 Arlington Ave, Ste 1192, Toledo, OH 43614; **Phone:** 419-383-3697; **Board Cert:** Internal Medicine 1982; Cardiovascular Disease 1985; **Med School:** Ohio State Univ 1979; **Resid:** Internal Medicine, Ohio State Univ 1982; **Fellow:** Cardiovascular Disease, Med Coll Ohio 1985; **Fac Appt:** Prof Med, Med Univ Ohio at Toledo

Cerqueira, Manuel MD [Cv] - **Spec Exp:** Cardiac Imaging; Nuclear Cardiology; Coronary Artery Disease; **Hospital:** Cleveland Clin (page 56); **Address:** Cleveland Clinic, 9500 Euclid Ave, MC JB3, Cleveland, OH 44195; **Phone:** 216-444-2665; **Board Cert:** Internal Medicine 1981; Nuclear Medicine 1984; Cardiovascular Disease 1989; **Med School:** NYU Sch Med 1976; **Resid:** Internal Medicine, Bellevue Hosp Ctr 1980; Cardiovascular Disease, Yale-New Haven Hosp 1982; **Fellow:** Nuclear Medicine, Yale-New Haven Hosp 1983; **Fac Appt:** Prof Med, Cleveland Cl Coll Med/Case West Res

Chaitman, Bernard R MD [Cv] - **Spec Exp:** Nuclear Cardiology; Echocardiography; **Hospital:** St. Louis Univ Hosp; **Address:** Univ Club Tower, 1034 S Brentwood Blvd, Ste 1550, St Louis, MO 63117; **Phone:** 314-725-4668; **Board Cert:** Internal Medicine 1973; Cardiovascular Disease 1975; Echocardiography 2001; Cardiovascular Computed Tomography 2009; **Med School:** McGill Univ 1969; **Resid:** Internal Medicine, Royal Victoria Hosp 1972; **Fellow:** Cardiovascular Disease, Univ Oregon Hosps 1974; Cardiovascular Disease, Univ of Montreal 1975; **Fac Appt:** Prof Med, St Louis Univ

Connolly, Heidi M MD [Cv] - **Spec Exp:** Congenital Heart Disease; Heart Disease in Pregnancy; **Hospital:** Mayo Med Ctr & Clin - Rochester; **Address:** Mayo Clin, 200 First St SW, Rochester, MN 55905; **Phone:** 507-284-1226; **Board Cert:** Internal Medicine 1989; Cardiovascular Disease 2001; **Med School:** Ireland 1986; **Resid:** Internal Medicine, Mayo Clinic 1989; **Fellow:** Cardiovascular Disease, Mayo Clinic 1991; **Fac Appt:** Assoc Prof Med, Mayo Med Sch

Cooper, Christopher J MD [Cv] - **Spec Exp:** Interventional Cardiology; **Hospital:** Univ of Toledo Med Ctr; **Address:** University of Toledo, 3000 Arlington Ave, Ste 1192, Toledo, OH 43614; **Phone:** 419-383-3697; **Board Cert:** Internal Medicine 2004; Cardiovascular Disease 2005; Interventional Cardiology 2009; **Med School:** Univ Cincinnati 1988; **Resid:** Internal Medicine, Brigham & Womens Hosp 1991; **Fellow:** Cardiovascular Disease, Brigham & Women's Hosp-Harvard Med Sch 1994; **Fac Appt:** Prof Med, Univ Toledo, Med Univ OH

Davidson, Michael MD [Cv] - **Spec Exp:** Preventive Cardiology; Cholesterol/Lipid Disorders; **Hospital:** Univ of Chicago Med Ctr; **Address:** 150 E Huron St, Avenue Hotel Bldg, Ste 900, Chicago, IL 60611; **Phone:** 773-834-4150; **Board Cert:** Internal Medicine 1984; Cardiovascular Disease 1987; **Med School:** Ohio State Univ 1981; **Resid:** Internal Medicine, Rush Presby-St Lukes Med Ctr 1984; **Fellow:** Cardiovascular Disease, Rush Presby-St Lukes Med Ctr 1986; **Fac Appt:** Clin Prof Med, Univ Chicago-Pritzker Sch Med

Eagle, Kim A MD [Cv] - **Spec Exp:** Aortic Diseases & Dissection; Acute Coronary Syndromes; Heart Attack; Peripheral Vascular Disease; **Hospital:** Univ of Michigan Hosp; **Address:** Dominos Farms, 24 Frank Lloyd Wright Drive, Ann Arbor, MI 48106-0363; **Phone:** 734-998-7400; **Board Cert:** Internal Medicine 1982; Cardiovascular Disease 1987; **Med School:** Tufts Univ 1979; **Resid:** Internal Medicine, Yale New Haven Hosp 1983; **Fellow:** Cardiovascular Disease, Mass Genl Hosp-Harvard 1986; **Fac Appt:** Asst Prof Med, Univ Mich Med Sch

Cardiovascular Disease

Geltman, Edward M MD [Cv] - **Spec Exp:** Congestive Heart Failure; Transplant Medicine-Heart; Non-Invasive Cardiology; **Hospital:** Barnes-Jewish Hosp, Barnes-Jewish West County Hosp; **Address:** Washington Univ Sch of Med, Cardiovascular Division, 660 S Euclid Ave, Box 8086, St Louis, MO 63110; **Phone:** 314-362-1291; **Board Cert:** Internal Medicine 1974; Cardiovascular Disease 1979; Advanced Heart Failure & Transplant Cardiology 2010; **Med School:** NYU Sch Med 1971; **Resid:** Internal Medicine, Bellevue Hosp 1974; **Fellow:** Cardiovascular Disease, Barnes Jewish Hosp 1978; **Fac Appt:** Prof Med, Washington Univ, St Louis

Gibbons, Raymond J MD [Cv] - **Spec Exp:** Nuclear Cardiology; Heart Attack; **Hospital:** Mayo Med Ctr & Clin - Rochester; **Address:** Mayo Clinic, Div Cardiovascular Disease, 200 First St SW, Rochester, MN 55905; **Phone:** 507-284-2541; **Board Cert:** Internal Medicine 1979; Cardiovascular Disease 1981; **Med School:** Harvard Med Sch 1976; **Resid:** Internal Medicine, Mass Genl Hosp 1978; **Fellow:** Cardiovascular Disease, Duke Univ Med Ctr 1981; **Fac Appt:** Prof Med, Mayo Med Sch

Grubb, Blair P MD [Cv] - **Spec Exp:** Autonomic Disorders; **Hospital:** Univ of Toledo Med Ctr, St. Vincent's Mercy Med Ctr - Toledo; **Address:** 3000 Arlington Rd, Ste 1192, Toledo, OH 43614-2598; **Phone:** 419-383-3697; **Board Cert:** Internal Medicine 1985; Cardiovascular Disease 1987; **Med School:** Dominican Republic 1980; **Resid:** Internal Medicine, Grtr Baltimore Med Ctr 1985; **Fellow:** Cardiovascular Disease, MS Hershey Med Ctr/Penn State 1987; Cardiac Electrophysiology, MS Hershey Med Ctr/Penn State 1988; **Fac Appt:** Prof Med, Univ SD Sch Med

Hauptman, Paul J MD [Cv] - **Spec Exp:** Heart Failure; **Hospital:** St. Louis Univ Hosp; **Address:** SLUCare Cardiology, Univ Club Tower, 1034 S Brentwood Blvd, Ste 1120, Saint Louis, MO 63117; **Phone:** 314-977-4663; **Board Cert:** Cardiovascular Disease 2003; **Med School:** Cornell Univ 1987; **Resid:** Internal Medicine, Brigham & Womens Hosp 1990; **Fellow:** Cardiovascular Disease, Mt Sinai Hosp 1992; Cardiovascular Disease, Brigham & Womens Hosp 1993; **Fac Appt:** Prof Med, St Louis Univ

Hayes, Sharonne N MD [Cv] - **Spec Exp:** Heart Disease in Women; Preventive Cardiology; Cholesterol/Lipid Disorders; Echocardiography; **Hospital:** Mayo Med Ctr & Clin - Rochester; **Address:** Mayo Clin Women's Heart Clin, 200 First St SW, Rochester, MN 55905; **Phone:** 507-284-3683; **Board Cert:** Internal Medicine 1986; Cardiovascular Disease 1989; **Med School:** Northwestern Univ 1983; **Resid:** Internal Medicine, Mayo Clin 1986; **Fellow:** Cardiovascular Research, Mayo Clin 1987; Cardiovascular Disease, Mayo Clin 1990; **Fac Appt:** Assoc Prof Med, Mayo Med Sch

Heroux, Alain MD [Cv] - **Spec Exp:** Transplant Medicine-Heart; Heart Failure; **Hospital:** Loyola Univ Med Ctr; **Address:** 2160 S 1st Ave Bldg 111 - rm 1110, Maywood, IL 60153; **Phone:** 708-327-2738; **Med School:** Canada 1981; **Resid:** Internal Medicine, Laval Univ Med Ctr 1985; Cardiovascular Disease, Royal Victory Hosp 1987; **Fellow:** Univ Virginia Med Coll 1989; **Fac Appt:** Asst Prof Med, Rush Med Coll

Jaffe, Allan S MD [Cv] - **Spec Exp:** Ischemic Heart Disease; Heart Disease & Depression; **Hospital:** Mayo Med Ctr & Clin - Rochester; **Address:** Mayo Clinic-Gonda 5-468, Div Cardiovascular Disease, 200 First St SW, Rochester, MN 55905; **Phone:** 507-284-2511; **Board Cert:** Internal Medicine 1976; Cardiovascular Disease 1979; **Med School:** Univ MD Sch Med 1973; **Resid:** Internal Medicine, Barnes Hosp 1975; Internal Medicine, Wash Univ 1976; **Fellow:** Cardiovascular Disease, Barnes Hosp 1978; **Fac Appt:** Prof Med, Mayo Med Sch

Johnson, Maryl R MD [Cv] - **Spec Exp:** Congestive Heart Failure; Transplant Medicine-Heart; **Hospital:** Univ WI Hosp & Clins, Meriter Hosp; **Address:** Univ Wisconsin Hosp/Clins-Cardio, 600 Highland Ave, rm E5-582, MC 5710, Madison, WI 53792-0001; **Phone:** 608-263-0080; **Board Cert:** Internal Medicine 1981; Cardiovascular Disease 1983; **Med School:** Univ Iowa Coll Med 1977; **Resid:** Internal Medicine, Univ Iowa Hosp 1981; **Fellow:** Cardiovascular Disease, Univ Iowa Hosp 1982; **Fac Appt:** Prof Med, Univ Wisc

Kereiakes, Dean J MD [Cv] - **Spec Exp:** Coronary Angioplasty/Stents; Congestive Heart Failure; Interventional Cardiology; **Hospital:** Christ Hosp, The - Cincinnati; **Address:** 2123 Auburn Ave, Ste 136, Cincinnati, OH 45219; **Phone:** 513-721-8881; **Board Cert:** Internal Medicine 1981; Cardiovascular Disease 1985; **Med School:** Univ Cincinnati 1978; **Resid:** Internal Medicine, UCSF Med Ctr 1982; Internal Medicine, Mass Genl Hosp 1981; **Fellow:** Cardiovascular Disease, UCSF 1984; Coronary Angioplasty, Sequoia Hosp 1984; **Fac Appt:** Clin Prof Med, Ohio State Univ

Klein, Lloyd W MD [Cv] - **Spec Exp:** Coronary Artery Disease; Angiography-Coronary; Interventional Cardiology; Coronary Syndrome-Acute; **Hospital:** Gottlieb Meml Hosp, Adv Illinois Masonic Med Ctr; **Address:** Clinical Cardiology Assocs, 675 W North Ave, POB Bldg Fl 4 - Ste 406, Melrose Park, IL 60160; **Phone:** 708-681-7862; **Board Cert:** Internal Medicine 1980; Cardiovascular Disease 1983; Interventional Cardiology 2009; **Med School:** Univ Cincinnati 1977; **Resid:** Internal Medicine, Einstein-Bronx Muni Hosp 1980; **Fellow:** Cardiovascular Disease, Mt Sinai Hosp 1982; **Fac Appt:** Prof Med, Rush Med Coll

Labovitz, Arthur J MD [Cv] - **Spec Exp:** Echocardiography; Heart Failure; **Hospital:** St. Louis Univ Hosp; **Address:** 3365 Vista Ave, St Louis, MO 63141; **Phone:** 314-977-6190; **Board Cert:** Internal Medicine 1981; Cardiovascular Disease 1983; **Med School:** Hahnemann Univ 1978; **Resid:** Internal Medicine, Hahnemann Med Ctr 1981; **Fellow:** Cardiovascular Disease, St Louis Univ Hosp 1983; **Fac Appt:** Prof Med, Washington Univ, St Louis

Liebson, Philip R MD [Cv] - **Spec Exp:** Hypertension; Cholesterol/Lipid Disorders; Preventive Cardiology; **Hospital:** Rush Univ Med Ctr; **Address:** University Cardiologists, 1724 W Harrison St, Ste 1159, Chicago, IL 60612; **Phone:** 312-942-5020; **Board Cert:** Internal Medicine 1977; Cardiovascular Disease 1974; **Med School:** SUNY Downstate 1960; **Resid:** Infectious Disease, New York VA Hosp 1964; **Fellow:** Cardiovascular Disease, Cornell Univ Med Ctr 1967; **Fac Appt:** Prof Med, Rush Med Coll

Mehlman, David J MD [Cv] - **Spec Exp:** Echocardiography; Heart Valve Disease; Coronary Artery Disease; **Hospital:** Northwestern Meml Hosp; **Address:** Northwestern Cardiovascular Inst, 675 N St Clair St, Galter Bldg Fl 19 - Ste 100, Chicago, IL 60611; **Phone:** 312-695-4965; **Board Cert:** Internal Medicine 1976; Cardiovascular Disease 1979; **Med School:** Johns Hopkins Univ 1973; **Resid:** Internal Medicine, Johns Hopkins Hosp 1976; **Fellow:** Cardiovascular Disease, Univ Chicago Hosps 1978; **Fac Appt:** Assoc Prof Med, Northwestern Univ

Moran, John F MD [Cv] - **Spec Exp:** Coronary Artery Disease; Congestive Heart Failure; Cholesterol/Lipid Disorders; **Hospital:** Loyola Univ Med Ctr; **Address:** 2160 S 1st Ave, Bldg 110 - Ste 6210, Maywood, IL 60153; **Phone:** 708-327-2784; **Board Cert:** Internal Medicine 1971; Cardiovascular Disease 1973; **Med School:** Loyola Univ-Stritch Sch Med 1964; **Resid:** Internal Medicine, Univ Illinois Med Ctr 1967; **Fellow:** Cardiovascular Disease, Univ Chicago Hosps 1969; **Fac Appt:** Prof Med, Loyola Univ-Stritch Sch Med

Nishimura, Rick A MD [Cv] - **Spec Exp:** Echocardiography; Pericardial Disease; **Hospital:** Mayo Med Ctr & Clin - Rochester, St. Mary's Hosp - Rochester MN (Mayo); **Address:** Mayo Clinic-Gonda 5-368, 200 First St SW, Rochester, MN 55905; **Phone:** 507-284-8342; **Board Cert:** Internal Medicine 1981; Cardiovascular Disease 1983; **Med School:** Rush Med Coll 1978; **Resid:** Internal Medicine, Mayo Clin 1980; **Fellow:** Cardiovascular Disease, Mayo Clin 1983; **Fac Appt:** Prof Med, Mayo Med Sch

Cardiovascular Disease

Nissen, Steven E MD [Cv] - **Spec Exp:** Cholesterol/Lipid Disorders; Intravascular Ultrasound; Cardiac Intensive Care; **Hospital:** Cleveland Clin (page 56); **Address:** 9500 Euclid Ave, MC J2-3, Cleveland, OH 44195; **Phone:** 216-445-6852; **Board Cert:** Internal Medicine 1981; Cardiovascular Disease 1983; **Med School:** Univ Mich Med Sch 1978; **Resid:** Internal Medicine, UC Davis Med Ctr 1981; **Fellow:** Cardiovascular Disease, Univ Kentucky-Chandler Med Ctr 1983; **Fac Appt:** Prof Med, Cleveland Cl Coll Med/Case West Res

Rahko, Peter S MD [Cv] - **Spec Exp:** Congestive Heart Failure; Heart Valve Disease; Echocardiography; Echocardiography - Transesophageal; **Hospital:** Univ WI Hosp & Clins, Meriter Hosp; **Address:** 600 Highland Ave, rm G7-343 CSC, MC 3248, Madison, WI 53792-3248; **Phone:** 608-263-1530; **Board Cert:** Internal Medicine 1982; Cardiovascular Disease 1985; **Med School:** Univ Minn 1979; **Resid:** Internal Medicine, Indiana Univ Med Ctr 1982; **Fellow:** Cardiovascular Disease, Univ Pittsburgh 1985; **Fac Appt:** Prof Med, Univ Wisc

Reiss, Craig MD [Cv] - **Spec Exp:** Ischemic Heart Disease; Heart Valve Disease; Preventive Cardiology; Coronary Artery Disease; **Hospital:** Barnes-Jewish Hosp, Barnes-Jewish West County Hosp; **Address:** Wash Univ Med Sch, Div Cardiovascular Disease, 660 S Euclid Ave, Box 8086, St Louis, MO 63110; **Phone:** 314-362-1291; **Board Cert:** Internal Medicine 1986; Cardiovascular Disease 1989; **Med School:** Univ MO-Kansas City 1983; **Resid:** Internal Medicine, Brigham & Women's Hosp 1989; **Fellow:** Cardiovascular Disease, Brigham & Women's Hosp 1988; **Fac Appt:** Assoc Prof Med, Washington Univ, St Louis

Rich, Stuart MD [Cv] - **Spec Exp:** Pulmonary Hypertension; Heart Failure; **Hospital:** Univ of Chicago Med Ctr; **Address:** 5841 S Maryland Ave, MC 5403, Chicago, IL 60637; **Phone:** 773-702-6049; **Board Cert:** Internal Medicine 1978; Cardiovascular Disease 1981; **Med School:** Loyola Univ-Stritch Sch Med 1974; **Resid:** Internal Medicine, Barnes-Jewish Hosp 1978; **Fellow:** Cardiovascular Disease, Univ Chicago Hosp 1980; **Fac Appt:** Prof Med, Rush Med Coll

Rosenbush, Stuart W MD [Cv] - **Spec Exp:** Cardiac Catheterization; Coronary Angioplasty/Stents; Coronary Artery Disease; Heart Failure; **Hospital:** Rush Univ Med Ctr, Skokie/North Shore Univ Htlh Syst; **Address:** Univ Cardiologists, 1725 W Harrison St, Ste 1159, Chicago, IL 60612-3835; **Phone:** 312-942-5020; **Board Cert:** Internal Medicine 1979; Cardiovascular Disease 1981; Interventional Cardiology 2000; **Med School:** Univ IL Coll Med 1976; **Resid:** Internal Medicine, Michael Reese Hosp 1979; **Fellow:** Cardiovascular Disease, Rush Presby-St Lukes Med Ctr 1981; **Fac Appt:** Asst Prof Med, Rush Med Coll

Safian, Robert D MD [Cv] - **Spec Exp:** Interventional Cardiology; **Hospital:** Beaumont Hosp-Royal Oak; **Address:** Beaumont Heart Ctr, 3601 W 13 Mile Rd Fl 3, Royal Oak, MI 48073; **Phone:** 248-898-4163; **Board Cert:** Internal Medicine 1983; Cardiovascular Disease 1987; Interventional Cardiology 2010; **Med School:** Univ Fla Coll Med 1979; **Resid:** Pathology, Univ Miami Med Ctr 1981; Internal Medicine, UCSD Med Ctr 1983; **Fellow:** Cardiovascular Disease, Beth Israel Hosp-Harvard 1987

Sanborn, Timothy MD [Cv] - **Spec Exp:** Interventional Cardiology; Gene Therapy-Cardiac Angiogenesis; Heart Valve Disease; Carotid Artery Stent Placement; **Hospital:** Evanston/North Shore Univ Hlth Sys; **Address:** 2650 Ridge Ave, Walgreen Bldg Fl 3, Evanston, IL 60201; **Phone:** 847-570-2250; **Board Cert:** Internal Medicine 1980; Cardiovascular Disease 2003; Interventional Cardiology 2009; **Med School:** Northwestern Univ 1977; **Resid:** Internal Medicine, Boston City Hosp 1980; **Fellow:** Cardiovascular Disease, Boston Univ Med Ctr 1983; **Fac Appt:** Prof Med, Northwestern Univ

Shapiro, Jerrold MD [Cv] - **Spec Exp:** Echocardiography; Preventive Cardiology; **Hospital:** Swedish Covenant Hosp; **Address:** 4801 W Peterson Ave, Ste 610, Chicago, IL 60646; **Phone:** 773-283-5900; **Board Cert:** Internal Medicine 1976; Cardiovascular Disease 1977; **Med School:** Univ IL Coll Med 1968; **Resid:** Internal Medicine, Ill Masonic Med Ctr 1972; **Fellow:** Cardiovascular Disease, Northwestern Meml Hosp 1974

Shea, Richard J MD [Cv] - **Spec Exp:** Heart Valve Disease; Echocardiography; Nuclear Cardiology; Echocardiography-Transesophageal; **Hospital:** Franciscan St. Francis Hlth-Indianapolis, Comm Hosp S - Indianapolis; **Address:** Indiana Heart Physicians, 5330 East Stop 11 Road, Indianapolis, IN 46237; **Phone:** 317-893-1664; **Board Cert:** Cardiovascular Disease 2009; **Med School:** Georgetown Univ 1989; **Resid:** Internal Medicine, Fitzsimons Army Med Ctr 1992; **Fellow:** Cardiovascular Disease, Washington Hosp Ctr 1995

Simon, Daniel I MD [Cv] - **Spec Exp:** Interventional Cardiology; **Hospital:** Univ Hosps Case Med Ctr (page 74); **Address:** UH Case Medical Center, 11100 Euclid Ave, Cleveland, OH 44106-5038; **Phone:** 216-844-3800; **Board Cert:** Cardiovascular Disease 2003; Interventional Cardiology 2010; **Med School:** Harvard Med Sch 1987; **Resid:** Internal Medicine, Brigham & Womens Hosp 1989; Interventional Cardiology, Beth Isreal 1995; **Fellow:** Cardiovascular Disease, Brigham & Womens Hosp 1992; **Fac Appt:** Prof Med, Case West Res Univ

Sorrentino, Matthew MD [Cv] - **Spec Exp:** Preventive Cardiology; Hypertension; **Hospital:** Univ of Chicago Med Ctr; **Address:** 5841 S Maryland Ave, MC 6080, Chicago, IL 60637; **Phone:** 773-702-9461; **Board Cert:** Internal Medicine 1987; Cardiovascular Disease 2001; **Med School:** Univ Chicago-Pritzker Sch Med 1984; **Resid:** Internal Medicine, Univ Chicago Hosps 1989; **Fellow:** Cardiovascular Disease, Univ Chicago Hosps 1991; **Fac Appt:** Assoc Prof Med, Univ Chicago-Pritzker Sch Med

Stein, James H MD [Cv] - **Spec Exp:** Preventive Cardiology; Echocardiography; Cholesterol/Lipid Disorders; **Hospital:** Univ WI Hosp & Clins; **Address:** UW Heart & Vascular Clin G3/4, 600 Highland Ave, Madison, WI 53792; **Phone:** 608-263-1530; **Board Cert:** Internal Medicine 2003; Cardiovascular Disease 2007; **Med School:** Yale Univ 1990; **Resid:** Internal Medicine, Univ Chicago Hosps 1993; **Fellow:** Cardiovascular Disease, Rush-Presby St Lukes Med Ctr 1996; **Fac Appt:** Prof Med, Univ Wisc

Stewart, William J MD [Cv] - **Spec Exp:** Heart Valve Disease; Echocardiography; **Hospital:** Cleveland Clin (page 56); **Address:** Div Cardiovascular Medicine, 9500 Euclid Ave, Desk J1-5, Cleveland, OH 44195; **Phone:** 216-444-5923; **Board Cert:** Internal Medicine 1980; Cardiovascular Disease 1983; **Med School:** Univ Cincinnati 1977; **Resid:** Internal Medicine, Univ Mich Hosp 1980; **Fellow:** Cardiovascular Disease, Boston Univ Med Ctr 1982; Cardiovascular Disease, Mass Genl Hosp 1984; **Fac Appt:** Assoc Prof Med, Cleveland Cl Coll Med/Case West Res

Volgman, Annabelle S MD [Cv] - **Spec Exp:** Heart Disease in Women; Arrhythmias; Atrial Fibrillation; Preventive Cardiology; **Hospital:** Rush Univ Med Ctr, Rush Oak Park Hosp; **Address:** Rush Heart Ctr for Women, 1725 W Harrison St, Professional Bldg, Ste 1159, Chicago, IL 60612; **Phone:** 312-942-5020; **Board Cert:** Cardiovascular Disease 2006; **Med School:** Columbia P&S 1984; **Resid:** Internal Medicine, Univ Chicago Hosps 1987; **Fellow:** Cardiovascular Disease, Northwestern Meml Hosp 1989; Cardiac Electrophysiology, Northwestern Meml Hosp 1990; **Fac Appt:** Assoc Prof Med, Rush Med Coll

Cardiovascular Disease

von der Lohe, Elisabeth MD [Cv] - **Spec Exp:** Heart Disease in Women; Interventional Cardiology; Pulmonary Hypertension; **Hospital:** IU Health University Hosp, IU Health Methodist Hosp; **Address:** Krannert Institute of Cardiology, 1801 N Senate Blvd, Ste E400, Indianapolis, IN 46202; **Phone:** 317-962-0500; **Board Cert:** Internal Medicine 2000; Cardiovascular Disease 2001; Interventional Cardiology 2003; **Med School:** Germany 1978; **Resid:** Internal Medicine, Marien Hosp 1981; **Fellow:** Cardiovascular Disease, Klinikum Aachen 1986; **Fac Appt:** Clin Prof Med, Indiana Univ

Wagoner, Lynne E MD [Cv] - **Spec Exp:** Congestive Heart Failure; Heart Disease in Women; Transplant Medicine-Heart; Pulmonary Hypertension; **Hospital:** Mercy Hosp - Fairfield, Christ Hosp, The - Cincinnati; **Address:** 2123 Auburn Ave, Ste 624, Cincinnati, OH 45219; **Phone:** 513-751-4222; **Board Cert:** Internal Medicine 1989; Cardiovascular Disease 2003; **Med School:** E Carolina Univ 1986; **Resid:** Internal Medicine, Pitt Co Meml Hosp 1989; **Fellow:** Cardiovascular Disease, Univ Utah Affil Hosp 1994

Walsh, Mary N MD [Cv] - **Spec Exp:** Heart Disease in Women; Nuclear Cardiology; Congestive Heart Failure; Transplant Medicine-Heart; **Hospital:** St. Vincent Indianapolis Hosp; **Address:** The Care Group at St Vincent, 8333 Naab Rd, Ste 400, Indianapolis, IN 46260; **Phone:** 317-338-6666; **Board Cert:** Internal Medicine 1986; Cardiovascular Disease 2001; Advanced Heart Failure & Transplant Cardiology 2010; **Med School:** Univ Minn 1983; **Resid:** Internal Medicine, Univ Tex SW Med Ctr 1986; **Fellow:** Cardiovascular Disease, Wash Univ 1989; **Fac Appt:** Asst Clin Prof Med, Indiana Univ

Weaver, W Douglas MD [Cv] - **Spec Exp:** Heart Attack; Angioplasty; Cholesterol/Lipid Disorders; **Hospital:** Henry Ford Hosp, Henry Ford- W Bloomfield Hosp; **Address:** Henry Ford Hosp, 2799 W Grand Blvd, Cardiology K-14, Detroit, MI 48202-2689; **Phone:** 313-916-4420; **Board Cert:** Internal Medicine 1974; Cardiovascular Disease 1977; **Med School:** Tufts Univ 1971; **Resid:** Internal Medicine, Univ Wash Hosps 1974; **Fellow:** Cardiovascular Disease, Univ Wash Hosps 1976

Webb, Gary D MD [Cv] - **Spec Exp:** Congenital Heart Disease-Adult; **Hospital:** Cincinnati Chldns Hosp Med Ctr; **Address:** The Heart Inst, Cincinatti Chldn's Hosp, 3333 Burnett Ave, MC 2003, Cincinatti, OH 45229; **Phone:** 513-803-7329; **Med School:** McGill Univ 1967; **Resid:** Internal Medicine, Royal Victoria Hosp 1972; **Fellow:** Cardiovascular Disease, Toronto Genl Hosp 1974

Wilkoff, Bruce L MD [Cv] - **Spec Exp:** Defibrillator Cable Extraction; **Hospital:** Cleveland Clin (page 56); **Address:** Cleveland Clinic, 9500 Euclid Ave, Desk J2-2, Cleveland, OH 44195; **Phone:** 216-444-6697; **Board Cert:** Internal Medicine 1982; Cardiovascular Disease 1985; **Med School:** Ohio State Univ 1979; **Resid:** Internal Medicine, Univ Hosps 1982; **Fellow:** Cardiovascular Disease, Univ Hosps 1984; Cerebrovascular Disease, Ohio State Univ 1986

Williams Sr, Kim A MD [Cv] - **Spec Exp:** Nuclear Cardiology; Coronary Artery Disease; **Hospital:** Harper Univ Hosp; **Address:** Wayne St Univ Sch Med, Harper Univ Hosp, 3990 John R St, 4 Hudson, Detroit, MI 48201; **Phone:** 313-745-2620; **Board Cert:** Internal Medicine 1982; Cardiovascular Disease 1985; Nuclear Medicine 1986; **Med School:** Univ Chicago-Pritzker Sch Med 1979; **Resid:** Internal Medicine, Emory Univ 1982; **Fellow:** Cardiovascular Disease, Univ Chicago 1984; Nuclear Medicine, Univ Chicago 1986; **Fac Appt:** Prof Med, Wayne State Univ

Young, James B MD [Cv] - **Spec Exp:** Transplant Medicine-Heart; Heart Failure; Ventricular Assist Device (LVAD); Amyloid Heart Disease; **Hospital:** Cleveland Clin (page 56); **Address:** 9500 Euclid Ave Desk NA-21, Cleveland, OH 44195; **Phone:** 216-444-2270; **Board Cert:** Internal Medicine 1977; Cardiovascular Disease 1979; **Med School:** Baylor Coll Med 1974; **Resid:** Internal Medicine, Baylor Affil Hosp 1977; Internal Medicine, Methodist Hosp 1980; **Fellow:** Cardiovascular Disease, Baylor Affl Hosp 1979; **Fac Appt:** Prof Med, Cleveland Cl Coll Med/Case West Res

Great Plains and Mountains

Anderson, Jeffrey L MD [Cv] - **Spec Exp:** Arrhythmias; Cholesterol/Lipid Disorders; Cardiac MRI; **Hospital:** LDS Hosp, Salt Lake Regional Med Ctr; **Address:** Intermountain Med Ctr, 5121 S Cottonwood St, Murray, UT 84107-5701; **Phone:** 801-507-4757; **Board Cert:** Internal Medicine 1975; Cardiovascular Disease 1979; Cardiac Electrophysiology 2002; **Med School:** Harvard Med Sch 1972; **Resid:** Internal Medicine, Mass Genl Hosp 1974; **Fellow:** Research, Natl Inst Hlth 1976; Cardiovascular Disease, Stanford Univ Med Ctr 1978; **Fac Appt:** Prof Med, Univ Utah

Benjamin, Ivor J MD [Cv] - **Spec Exp:** Arrhythmias; **Hospital:** Univ Utah Hlth Care; **Address:** Div Cardiology, 30 N 1900 E, rm 4A100, Salt Lake City, UT 84132; **Phone:** 801-581-7715; **Board Cert:** Internal Medicine 1985; Cardiovascular Disease 1989; **Med School:** Johns Hopkins Univ 1982; **Resid:** Internal Medicine, Yale-New Haven Hosp 1985; **Fellow:** Cardiology Research, Yale-New Haven Hosp 1988; Echocardiography, Michael Reese Hosp 1989; **Fac Appt:** Prof Med, Univ Utah

Lindenfeld, JoAnn MD [Cv] - **Spec Exp:** Congestive Heart Failure; Transplant Medicine-Heart; Heart Disease in Women; **Hospital:** Univ of CO Hosp - Anschutz Inpatient Pav; **Address:** 12605 E 16th Ave, B120, Aurora, CO 80045; **Phone:** 720-848-5300; **Board Cert:** Internal Medicine 1976; Cardiovascular Disease 1979; Advanced Heart Failure & Transplant Cardiology 2010; **Med School:** Univ Mich Med Sch 1973; **Resid:** Internal Medicine, UCSD Med Ctr 1977; **Fellow:** Cardiovascular Disease, Univ Tex 1979; **Fac Appt:** Prof Med, Univ Colorado

Southwest

Abi-samra, Freddy M MD [Cv] - **Spec Exp:** Arrhythmias; Atrial Fibrillation; **Hospital:** Ochsner Med Ctr-New Orleans; **Address:** Oschner Med Ctr, Cardiovascular, 1514 Jefferson Hwy Fl 3rd, Clinic Tower, New Orleans, LA 70121; **Phone:** 504-842-4145; **Board Cert:** Internal Medicine 1984; Cardiovascular Disease 1985; **Med School:** Lebanon 1979; **Resid:** Internal Medicine, Amer Univ Med Ctr 1981; Cardiovascular Disease, Metro Genl Hosp 1984; **Fellow:** Hypertension, Cleveland Clin Fdn 1982; Cardiac Electrophysiology, Cleveland Clin Fdn 1986

Ballantyne, Christie M MD [Cv] - **Spec Exp:** Preventive Cardiology; Cholesterol/Lipid Disorders; **Hospital:** Methodist Hosp - Houston; **Address:** Methodist Hospital, DeBakey Heart & Vascular Ctr, 6565 Fannin St, Houston, TX 77030; **Phone:** 713-798-5034; **Board Cert:** Internal Medicine 1985; Cardiovascular Disease 1987; **Med School:** Baylor Coll Med 1982; **Resid:** Internal Medicine, Univ Tex SW Med Ctr 1985; **Fellow:** Cardiovascular Disease, Baylor Coll Med 1988; **Fac Appt:** Prof Med, Baylor Coll Med

Carabello, Blase A MD [Cv] - **Spec Exp:** Heart Valve Disease; **Hospital:** DeBakey VA Med Ctr-Houston; **Address:** Houston VA Medical Ctr, 2002 Holcombe Blvd, MS 111MCL, Houston, TX 77030; **Phone:** 713-794-7070; **Board Cert:** Internal Medicine 1977; Cardiovascular Disease 1979; **Med School:** Temple Univ 1973; **Resid:** Internal Medicine, Mass Genl Hosp 1976; **Fellow:** Cardiovascular Disease, Peter Bent Brigham Hosp 1978; **Fac Appt:** Prof Med, Baylor Coll Med

Freeman, Gregory L MD [Cv] - **Spec Exp:** Interventional Cardiology; Angioplasty; **Hospital:** Univ Hlth Syst-San Antonio; **Address:** Cardiology Clinical Associates, 4411 Medical Drive, Ste 300, San Antonio, TX 78229; **Phone:** 210-614-5400; **Board Cert:** Internal Medicine 1979; Cardiovascular Disease 1983; **Med School:** Loyola Univ-Stritch Sch Med 1976; **Resid:** Internal Medicine, Cook County Hosp 1979; **Fellow:** Cardiovascular Disease, Loyola Univ Med Ctr 1981; Research, UCSD Sch Med 1983; **Fac Appt:** Prof Med, Univ Tex, San Antonio

Cardiovascular Disease

Gould, K Lance MD [Cv] - **Spec Exp:** Preventive Cardiology; PET Imaging; Cholesterol/Lipid Disorders; **Hospital:** Meml Hermann Hosp - Texas Med Ctr; **Address:** Univ Texas - PET Imaging Ctr, 6431 Fannin St, rm 4.256 MSB, Houston, TX 77030-1501; **Phone:** 713-500-6611; **Med School:** Case West Res Univ 1964; **Resid:** Internal Medicine, Univ Wash Med Ctr 1967; Cardiovascular Disease, Univ Wash Med Ctr 1964; **Fellow:** Cardiovascular Disease, Univ Wash Med Ctr 1971; **Fac Appt:** Prof Med, Univ Tex, Houston

Krajcer, Zvonimir MD [Cv] - **Spec Exp:** Peripheral Vascular Disease; Carotid Artery Disease; Aneurysm-Abdominal & Thoracic Aortic; **Hospital:** St. Luke's Episcopal Hosp-Houston; **Address:** 6624 Fannin St, Ste 2780, Houston, TX 77030; **Phone:** 713-791-4158; **Board Cert:** Internal Medicine 1975; Cardiovascular Disease 1977; **Med School:** Slovenia 1970; **Resid:** Internal Medicine, Northwestern Medical Ctr 1974; **Fellow:** Cardiovascular Disease, St Luke's Episcopal Hosp 1977; **Fac Appt:** Clin Prof Med, Baylor Coll Med

Massin, Edward K MD [Cv] - **Spec Exp:** Congestive Heart Failure; Transplant Medicine-Heart; Coronary Artery Disease; **Hospital:** St. Luke's Episcopal Hosp-Houston; **Address:** Cardiology Consultants Houston, 6624 Fannin St, Ste 2310, Houston, TX 77030-2335; **Phone:** 713-796-2668; **Board Cert:** Internal Medicine 1973; Cardiovascular Disease 1973; **Med School:** Washington Univ, St Louis 1965; **Resid:** Internal Medicine, Barnes Hosp 1967; **Fellow:** Cardiovascular Disease, Univ CO Med Ctr 1971; **Fac Appt:** Clin Prof Med, Baylor Coll Med

McPherson, David D MD [Cv] - **Spec Exp:** Echocardiography; Congenital Heart Disease-Adult; Heart Valve Disease; **Hospital:** Univ Hlth Syst-San Antonio; **Address:** 6431 Fannin St, MSB 1252, Houston, TX 77030; **Phone:** 713-500-6553; **Board Cert:** Internal Medicine 2005; Cardiovascular Disease 2007; **Med School:** Univ Alberta 1978; **Resid:** Internal Medicine, Dalhousie Univ 1981; **Fellow:** Cardiovascular Disease, Dalhousie Univ 1983; Cardiovascular Disease, Iowa Univ Med 1984; **Fac Appt:** Prof Med, Northwestern Univ

Nagueh, Sherif F MD [Cv] - **Spec Exp:** Echocardiography; Heart Failure; **Hospital:** Methodist Hosp - Houston; **Address:** Methodist DeBakey Heart & Vascular Ctr, 6550 Fannin St, Ste 1901, Smith Tower, Houston, TX 77030; **Phone:** 713-441-1100; **Board Cert:** Internal Medicine 2003; Cardiovascular Disease 2007; **Med School:** Egypt 1986; **Resid:** Internal Medicine, Baylor Coll Med 1993; **Fellow:** Cardiovascular Disease, Baylor Coll Med 1996; **Fac Appt:** Prof Med, Cornell Univ-Weill Med Coll

Quinones, Miguel A MD [Cv] - **Spec Exp:** Echocardiography; Heart Valve Disease; **Hospital:** Methodist Hosp - Houston; **Address:** Methodist DeBakey Cardiology Assocs, 6550 Fannin St, rm 1901, Smith Tower, Houston, TX 77030; **Phone:** 713-441-1100; **Board Cert:** Internal Medicine 1972; Cardiovascular Disease 1974; **Med School:** Puerto Rico 1968; **Resid:** Internal Medicine, Harlem Hosp 1971; **Fellow:** Cardiovascular Disease, Baylor Coll Med 1974; **Fac Appt:** Prof Med, Univ Tex, Houston

Ramee, Stephen R MD [Cv] - **Spec Exp:** Interventional Cardiology; Angioplasty; Carotid Artery Stent Placement; Renovascular Disease; **Hospital:** Ochsner Med Ctr-New Orleans; **Address:** Ochsner Medical Ctr-Cardiology, 1514 Jefferson Hwy, New Orleans, LA 70121; **Phone:** 504-842-3724; **Board Cert:** Internal Medicine 1983; Cardiovascular Disease 1985; **Med School:** Geo Wash Univ 1980; **Resid:** Internal Medicine, Letterman Army Med Ctr 1983; **Fellow:** Cardiovascular Disease, Letterman Army Med Ctr 1985

Smart, Frank W MD [Cv] - **Spec Exp:** Congestive Heart Failure; Transplant Medicine-Heart; Ventricular Assist Device (LVAD); Pulmonary Hypertension; **Hospital:** Ochsner Baptist Med Ctr, Touro Infirmary; **Address:** LSU Cardiology, 1542 Tulane Ave, Box T4M2, New Orleans, LA 70112; **Phone:** 504-412-1366; **Board Cert:** Internal Medicine 1988; Cardiovascular Disease 2001; Advanced Heart Failure & Transplant Cardiology 2010; **Med School:** Louisiana State U, New Orleans 1985; **Resid:** Internal Medicine, Ochsner Fdn Hosp 1988; **Fellow:** Cardiovascular Disease, Baylor Coll Med 1991; **Fac Appt:** Prof Med, Louisiana State U, New Orleans

Stainback III, Raymond F MD [Cv] - **Spec Exp:** Stroke; Coronary Artery Disease; Heart Valve Disease; Echocardiography-Transesophageal; **Hospital:** St. Luke's Episcopal Hosp-Houston; **Address:** Hall-Garcia Cardiology Assoc, 6624 Fannin St Ste 2480, Houston, TX 77030-2309; **Phone:** 713-529-5530; **Board Cert:** Cardiovascular Disease 2007; Echocardiography 2008; **Med School:** Baylor Coll Med 1987; **Resid:** Internal Medicine, Vanderbilt Univ Med Ctr 1990; **Fellow:** Cardiovascular Disease, Vanderbilt Univ Med Ctr 1993; Echocardiography, UCSF Med Ctr 1995; **Fac Appt:** Asst Clin Prof Med, Baylor Coll Med

Thames, Marc D MD [Cv] - **Spec Exp:** Coronary Artery Disease; Congestive Heart Failure; **Hospital:** Scottsdale Hlthcare - Shea; **Address:** Cardiovascular Consultants, 3805 E Bell Rd, Ste 3100, Phoenix, AZ 85032-3356; **Phone:** 602-867-8644; **Board Cert:** Internal Medicine 1974; Cardiovascular Disease 1979; **Med School:** Med Coll VA 1970; **Resid:** Internal Medicine, Peter Bent Brigham Hosp 1974; **Fellow:** Cardiology Research, Peter Bent Brigham Hosp 1975; Cardiovascular Disease, Mayo Clinic 1977

Wilansky, Susan MD [Cv] - **Spec Exp:** Heart Disease in Women; Heart Disease in Pregnancy; Echocardiography; Heart Valve Disease; **Hospital:** Mayo Clinic - Scottsdale; **Address:** Mayo Clinic, Div Cardiology, 13400 E Shea Blvd, Scottsdale, AZ 85259; **Phone:** 480-301-8200; **Board Cert:** Cardiovascular Disease 1989; **Med School:** McMaster Univ 1979; **Resid:** Internal Medicine, Univ Toronto Hosp 1983; **Fellow:** Cardiovascular Disease, Univ Toronto 1985; Echocardiography, Univ Toronto 1986; **Fac Appt:** Assoc Prof Med, Mayo Med Sch

Zoghbi, William A MD [Cv] - **Spec Exp:** Echocardiography; **Hospital:** Methodist Hosp - Houston; **Address:** 6550 Fannin St, Ste 1901, Smith Tower, Houston, TX 77030; **Phone:** 713-441-1100; **Board Cert:** Internal Medicine 1982; Cardiovascular Disease 1985; **Med School:** Meharry Med Coll 1979; **Resid:** Internal Medicine, Baylor Coll Affil Hosps 1982; **Fellow:** Cardiovascular Disease, Baylor Coll Med 1985

West Coast and Pacific

Bairey, Cathleen Noel MD [Cv] - **Spec Exp:** Preventive Cardiology; Heart Disease in Women; **Hospital:** Cedars-Sinai Med Ctr; **Address:** Cedars-Sinai Women's Heart Ctr, 444 S San Vicente Blvd, Ste 600, Los Angeles, CA 90048; **Phone:** 310-423-9680; **Board Cert:** Internal Medicine 1984; Cardiovascular Disease 1987; **Med School:** Harvard Med Sch 1981; **Resid:** Internal Medicine, UCSF Med Ctr 1984; **Fellow:** Cardiovascular Disease, Cedars-Sinai Med Ctr 1986; **Fac Appt:** Assoc Clin Prof Med, UCLA

Blanchard, Daniel G MD [Cv] - **Spec Exp:** Echocardiography; Hypertension; **Hospital:** UCSD Med Ctr; **Address:** Perlman Medical Office, 9350 Campus Point Dr, Ste 1D, Box 0986, La Jolla, CA 92037; **Phone:** 858-657-8530; **Board Cert:** Internal Medicine 1988; Cardiovascular Disease 2002; **Med School:** UCSD 1985; **Resid:** Internal Medicine, UCSD Med Ctr 1988; **Fellow:** Cardiovascular Disease, USCD Med Ctr 1991; **Fac Appt:** Prof Med, UCSD

Cardiovascular Disease

Brindis, Ralph G MD [Cv] - **Spec Exp:** Acute Coronary Syndromes; Interventional Cardiology; **Hospital:** Kaiser Permanente Oakland Med Ctr, Alta Bates Summit Med Ctr-Oakland; **Address:** Hospital Bldg Fl 2, 280 W MacArthur Blvd, Oakland, CA 94611; **Phone:** 510-752-6474; **Board Cert:** Internal Medicine 1980; Cardiovascular Disease 1983; **Med School:** Emory Univ 1977; **Resid:** Internal Medicine, Herbert C Moffitt Hosp 1980; Internal Medicine, Fort Miley VA Hosp 1981; **Fellow:** Cardiovascular Disease, Herbert C Moffitt Hosp 1983; **Fac Appt:** Prof Med, UCSF

Budoff, Matthew J MD [Cv] - **Spec Exp:** Cholesterol/Lipid Disorders; Preventive Cardiology; Cardiac Imaging; **Hospital:** LAC - Harbor - UCLA Med Ctr, Little Co of Mary-Torrance Hosp; **Address:** 1124 W Carson St, Torrance, CA 90502; **Phone:** 310-222-5101; **Board Cert:** Internal Medicine 2003; Cardiovascular Disease 2007; **Med School:** Geo Wash Univ 1990; **Resid:** Internal Medicine, UCLA/Harbor Med Ctr 1993; **Fellow:** Cardiovascular Disease, UCLA/Harbor Med Ctr 1997; **Fac Appt:** Assoc Prof Med, UCLA

Dichek, David A MD [Cv] - **Spec Exp:** Gene Therapy; Coronary Artery Disease; **Hospital:** Univ Wash Med Ctr; **Address:** Univ Washington, Dept Cardiology, 1959 NE Pacific St, Box 356171, Seattle, WA 98195; **Phone:** 206-598-4300; **Board Cert:** Internal Medicine 1987; Cardiovascular Disease 2004; **Med School:** UCLA 1984; **Resid:** Internal Medicine, Mass Genl Hosp 1987; **Fellow:** Cardiovascular Disease, NIH/Johns Hopkins Hosp 1992; **Fac Appt:** Prof Med, Univ Wash

Elkayam, Uri MD [Cv] - **Spec Exp:** Congestive Heart Failure; Heart Disease in Pregnancy; Heart Valve Disease; Cardiomyopathy; **Hospital:** LAC & USC Med Ctr; **Address:** USC Cardiovascular Medicine, 2020 Zonal Ave, rm 331, Los Angeles, CA 90033; **Phone:** 323-226-7541; **Board Cert:** Internal Medicine 1989; Cardiovascular Disease 2009; **Med School:** Israel 1973; **Resid:** Internal Medicine, Tel Aviv Sowaski Med Ctr 1976; **Fellow:** Cardiovascular Disease, Albert Einstein Hosp 1978; Cardiovascular Disease, Cedars Sinai Med Ctr 1979; **Fac Appt:** Prof Med, USC Sch Med

Fishbein, Daniel P MD [Cv] - **Spec Exp:** Congestive Heart Failure; Transplant Medicine-Heart; **Hospital:** Univ Wash Med Ctr; **Address:** Univ Wash, Div Cardiology, 1959 NE Pacific St, Box 356171, Seattle, WA 98195; **Phone:** 206-598-4300; **Board Cert:** Internal Medicine 1983; Cardiovascular Disease 1987; **Med School:** Albert Einstein Coll Med 1980; **Resid:** Internal Medicine, Univ Wash Med Ctr 1983; **Fellow:** Cardiovascular Disease, Univ Wash Med Ctr 1987; Interventional Cardiology, Univ Wash Med Ctr 1989; **Fac Appt:** Assoc Prof Med, Univ Wash

Fonarow, Gregg C MD [Cv] - **Spec Exp:** Cardiomyopathy; Congestive Heart Failure; Transplant Medicine-Heart; Preventive Cardiology; **Hospital:** UCLA Ronald Reagan Med Ctr; **Address:** UCLA Cardiomyopathy Ctr, 200 UCLA Medical Plaza, Ste 224, Los Angeles, CA 90095; **Phone:** 310-825-8816; **Board Cert:** Cardiovascular Disease 2003; **Med School:** UCLA 1987; **Resid:** Internal Medicine, UCLA Med Ctr 1990; **Fellow:** Cardiovascular Disease, UCLA Med Ctr 1993; **Fac Appt:** Prof Med, UCLA

French, William J MD [Cv] - **Spec Exp:** Heart Failure; Interventional Cardiology; Coronary Artery Disease; Cholesterol/Lipid Disorders; **Hospital:** LAC - Harbor - UCLA Med Ctr; **Address:** Harbor-UCLA Med Ctr, 1000 W Carson St, Torrance, CA 90509-2004; **Phone:** 310-222-2415; **Board Cert:** Internal Medicine 1973; Cardiovascular Disease 1979; Interventional Cardiology 2002; **Med School:** Univ VT Coll Med 1968; **Resid:** Internal Medicine, Harlem Hosp-Columbia 1971; Nephrology, Grad Hosp Univ Penn 1972; **Fellow:** Critical Care Medicine, Hollywood Pres Hosp-USC 1975; Cardiovascular Disease, Harbor-UCLA Med Ctr 1977; **Fac Appt:** Prof Med, UCLA

Hunt, Sharon Ann MD [Cv] - **Spec Exp:** Transplant Medicine-Heart; **Hospital:** Stanford Univ Hosp & Clinics; **Address:** Stanford Univ Div Cardiovascular Med, 300 Pasteur Drive, CVRB 265, Stanford, CA 94305; **Phone:** 650-498-6605; **Board Cert:** Internal Medicine 1977; Cardiovascular Disease 1979; Advanced Heart Failure & Transplant Cardiology 2010; **Med School:** Stanford Univ 1972; **Resid:** Internal Medicine, Stanford Univ Hosp 1974; **Fellow:** Cardiovascular Disease, Stanford Univ 1976; **Fac Appt:** Prof Med, Stanford Univ

Johnson, Allen D MD [Cv] - **Spec Exp:** Congenital Heart Disease-Adult; Congestive Heart Failure; **Hospital:** Scripps Green Hosp; **Address:** Scripps Clinic-Torrey Pines, 10666 N Torrey Pines Rd, SW 206, La Jolla, CA 92037; **Phone:** 858-554-8836; **Board Cert:** Internal Medicine 1973; Cardiovascular Disease 1973; **Med School:** Johns Hopkins Univ 1965; **Resid:** Internal Medicine, Johns Hopkins Hosp 1970; **Fellow:** Cardiovascular Disease, UCSD Med Ctr 1972; **Fac Appt:** Clin Prof Med, Univ SD Sch Med

Judelson, Debra R MD [Cv] - **Spec Exp:** Hypertension; Cholesterol/Lipid Disorders; Heart Disease in Women; **Hospital:** Cedars-Sinai Med Ctr, Brotman Med Ctr; **Address:** Women's Heart Institute, Cardiovascular Med Group Southern CA, 414 N Camden Drive, Ste 1100, Beverly Hills, CA 90210-4532; **Phone:** 310-278-3400 x155; **Board Cert:** Internal Medicine 1979; Cardiovascular Disease 1981; **Med School:** Harvard Med Sch 1976; **Resid:** Internal Medicine, Kaiser Foundation Hosp 1979; **Fellow:** Cardiovascular Disease, Kaiser Foundation Hosp 1981

Kaul, Sanjiv MD [Cv] - **Spec Exp:** Cardiac Imaging; Echocardiography; Coronary Artery Disease; Preventive Cardiology; **Hospital:** OR Hlth & Sci Univ; **Address:** OHSU Cardiovascular Med, 3181 SW Sam Jackson Park Rd, MC UHN62, Portland, OR 97239; **Phone:** 503-494-8750; **Board Cert:** Internal Medicine 1980; Cardiovascular Disease 1983; **Med School:** India 1975; **Resid:** Internal Medicine, Univ Vermont Med Ctr 1980; Cardiovascular Disease, Wadsworth VA Hosp-UCLA 1982; **Fellow:** Cardiovascular Disease, Mass Genl Hosp 1984; **Fac Appt:** Prof Med, Oregon Hlth & Sci Univ

Kobashigawa, Jon A MD [Cv] - **Spec Exp:** Transplant Medicine-Heart; Congestive Heart Failure; Heart Valve Disease; **Hospital:** Cedars-Sinai Med Ctr, UCLA Ronald Reagan Med Ctr; **Address:** California Heart Ctr, 8336 Wilshire Blvd, Ste 302, Beverly Hills, CA 90211; **Phone:** 310-794-1200; **Board Cert:** Internal Medicine 1983; Cardiovascular Disease 1987; **Med School:** Mount Sinai Sch Med 1980; **Resid:** Internal Medicine, UCLA Med Ctr 1983; **Fellow:** Cardiovascular Disease, UCLA Med Ctr 1986; **Fac Appt:** Clin Prof Med, UCLA

Lewis, Sandra J MD [Cv] - **Spec Exp:** Heart Disease in Women; Preventive Cardiology; Congestive Heart Failure; **Hospital:** Legacy Good Samaritan Med Ctr, Legacy Emanuel Hospitals; **Address:** Northwest Cardiovascular Inst, 2222 NW Lovejoy St, Ste 606, Portland, OR 97210; **Phone:** 503-229-7554; **Board Cert:** Internal Medicine 1980; Cardiovascular Disease 1985; **Med School:** Stanford Univ 1977; **Resid:** Internal Medicine, Stanford Univ Med Ctr 1980; **Fellow:** Cardiovascular Disease, Stanford Univ Med Ctr 1983; **Fac Appt:** Assoc Clin Prof Med, Oregon Hlth & Sci Univ

Redberg, Rita F MD [Cv] - **Spec Exp:** Echocardiography; Heart Disease in Women; Preventive Cardiology; **Hospital:** UCSF Med Ctr; **Address:** UCSF Cardiology, 535 Mission Bay Blvd S, San Francisco, CA 94158; **Phone:** 415-353-2873; **Board Cert:** Internal Medicine 1985; Cardiovascular Disease 1989; **Med School:** Univ Pennsylvania 1982; **Resid:** Internal Medicine, Columbia-Presby Med Ctr 1985; **Fellow:** Cardiovascular Disease, Columbia-Presby Med Ctr 1988; **Fac Appt:** Prof Med, UCSF

Cardiovascular Disease

Schnittger, Ingela MD [Cv] - **Spec Exp:** Echocardiography; Echocardiography-Transesophageal; **Hospital:** Stanford Univ Hosp & Clinics; **Address:** 300 Pasteur Drive, rm H2157, Stanford, CA 94305-5233; **Phone:** 650-723-5196; **Board Cert:** Internal Medicine 1980; Cardiovascular Disease 1983; **Med School:** Sweden 1975; **Resid:** Internal Medicine, Stanford Univ Hosp 1980; **Fellow:** Cardiovascular Disease, Stanford Univ 1983; **Fac Appt:** Prof Med, Stanford Univ

Shah, Prediman K MD [Cv] - **Spec Exp:** Coronary Artery Disease; Cholesterol/Lipid Disorders; Preventive Cardiology; Heart Valve Disease; **Hospital:** Cedars-Sinai Med Ctr; **Address:** Cedars-Sinai Med Ctr, 8700 Beverly Blvd, Ste 5531, Los Angeles, CA 90048; **Phone:** 310-423-3884; **Board Cert:** Internal Medicine 1975; Cardiovascular Disease 1977; **Med School:** India 1969; **Resid:** Internal Medicine, All India Inst Med Scis 1971; Internal Medicine, Montefiore Hosp 1974; **Fellow:** Cardiovascular Disease, Montefiore Hosp 1976; Research, Cedars Sinai Med Ctr 1977; **Fac Appt:** Prof Med, UCLA

Skolnick, Alan E MD [Cv] - **Spec Exp:** Nuclear Cardiology; **Hospital:** Providence Alaska Med Ctr; **Address:** Alaska Heart Institute, 3841 Piper St, Ste T-100, Anchorage, AK 99508; **Phone:** 907-561-3211; **Board Cert:** Internal Medicine 2002; Cardiovascular Disease 2005; Nuclear Cardiology 1998; **Med School:** Albert Einstein Coll Med 1989; **Resid:** Internal Medicine, Beth Israel Hosp 1992; **Fellow:** Cardiovascular Disease, Boston Univ Med Ctr 1994

Tobis, Jonathan Marvin MD [Cv] - **Spec Exp:** Interventional Cardiology; **Hospital:** UCLA Ronald Reagan Med Ctr; **Address:** 200 UCLA Medical Plaza, Ste 365C, Los Angeles, CA 90095; **Phone:** 310-825-8811; **Board Cert:** Internal Medicine 1976; Cardiovascular Disease 1979; Interventional Cardiology 2009; **Med School:** Albert Einstein Coll Med 1973; **Resid:** Internal Medicine, Lincoln Hosp 1975; Internal Medicine, Univ CA Irvine Med Ctr 1976; **Fellow:** Cardiovascular Disease, Univ CA Irvine Med Ctr 1978; **Fac Appt:** Prof Med, UCLA-David Geffen Sch Med

CARDIAC ELECTROPHYSIOLOGY

New England

Batsford, William P MD [CE] - **Spec Exp:** Arrhythmias; **Hospital:** Yale-New Haven Hosp, Yale Med Group; **Address:** Yale Univ School Medicine, Section Cardiovascular Medicine, 333 Cedar St, 3 FMP, Box 208017, New Haven, CT 06520-8017; **Phone:** 203-785-4126; **Board Cert:** Internal Medicine 1972; Cardiovascular Disease 1977; **Med School:** Albany Med Coll 1969; **Resid:** Internal Medicine, Hosp Univ Penn 1972; **Fac Appt:** Prof Med, Yale Univ

Buxton, Alfred E MD [CE] - **Spec Exp:** Arrhythmias; **Hospital:** Beth Israel Deaconess Med Ctr - Boston; **Address:** 185 Pilgrim Rd, Baker Bldg Fl 4, Boston, MA 02115; **Phone:** 617-667-8800; **Board Cert:** Internal Medicine 1977; Cardiovascular Disease 1981; Cardiac Electrophysiology 2002; **Med School:** Univ Pennsylvania 1973; **Resid:** Internal Medicine, Hosp Univ Penn 1977; **Fellow:** Cardiovascular Disease, Hosp Univ Penn 1980; Cardiac Electrophysiology, Hosp Univ Penn 1981

Estes, N.A. Mark MD [CE] - **Spec Exp:** Arrhythmias; **Hospital:** Tufts Med Ctr; **Address:** Tufts Medical Ctr, Div Cardiology, 860 Washington St, Box 197, Boston, MA 02111; **Phone:** 617-636-6156; **Board Cert:** Internal Medicine 1980; Cardiovascular Disease 1983; Cardiac Electrophysiology 2002; **Med School:** Univ Cincinnati 1977; **Resid:** Internal Medicine, New England Deaconess Hosp 1980; **Fellow:** Cardiovascular Disease, New England Med Ctr 1980; Cardiac Electrophysiology, Mass General Hosp 1983

Josephson, Mark Eric MD [CE] - **Spec Exp:** Arrhythmias; **Hospital:** Beth Israel Deaconess Med Ctr - Boston; **Address:** 185 Pilgrim Rd Baker Bldg Fl 4, Boston, MA 02215; **Phone:** 617-667-8800; **Board Cert:** Internal Medicine 1973; Cardiovascular Disease 1975; Cardiac Electrophysiology 2002; **Med School:** Columbia P&S 1969; **Resid:** Internal Medicine, Mt Sinai Med Ctr 1971; **Fellow:** Cardiovascular Disease, Hosp Univ Penn 1975; **Fac Appt:** Prof Med, Harvard Med Sch

Link, Mark S MD [CE] - **Spec Exp:** Arrhythmias; Ventricular Tachycardia Ablation; Heart Disease in Athletes; Sudden Death Prevention; **Hospital:** Tufts Med Ctr; **Address:** Tufts Med Ctr, 800 Washington St, Box 197, Boston, MA 02111; **Phone:** 617-636-5902; **Board Cert:** Internal Medicine 1989; Cardiovascular Disease 2007; Cardiac Electrophysiology 2008; **Med School:** Tufts Univ 1986; **Resid:** Internal Medicine, NY Presby Hosp/Columbia 1989; **Fellow:** Cardiovascular Disease, New England Med Ctr 1996; Cardiac Electrophysiology, New England Med Ctr 1997; **Fac Appt:** Prof Med, Tufts Univ

Ruskin, Jeremy N MD [CE] - **Spec Exp:** Arrhythmias; **Hospital:** Mass Genl Hosp; **Address:** Cardiac Arrhythmia Service, Mass General Hosp, 55 Fruit St, Boston, MA 02114; **Phone:** 617-726-8514; **Board Cert:** Internal Medicine 1974; Cardiovascular Disease 1975; Cardiac Electrophysiology 2003; **Med School:** Harvard Med Sch 1971; **Resid:** Internal Medicine, Beth Israel Hosp 1974; Cardiovascular Disease, Mass Genl Hosp 1977; **Fac Appt:** Assoc Prof Med, Harvard Med Sch

Stevenson, William G MD [CE] - **Spec Exp:** Arrhythmias; **Hospital:** Brigham and Women's Hosp (page 57); **Address:** Brigham & Womens Hosp, Cardiovascular Div, 75 Francis St, Boston, MA 02115; **Phone:** 857-307-1948; **Board Cert:** Internal Medicine 1982; Cardiovascular Disease 1985; Cardiac Electrophysiology 2005; **Med School:** Tulane Univ 1979; **Resid:** Internal Medicine, UCLA Med Ctr 1982; **Fellow:** Cardiovascular Disease, UCLA Med Ctr 1984; Cardiac Electrophysiology, UCLA Med Ctr 1985; **Fac Appt:** Prof Med, Harvard Med Sch

Mid Atlantic

Berger, Ronald D MD/PhD [CE] - **Spec Exp:** Catheter Ablation; **Hospital:** Johns Hopkins Hosp (page 61); **Address:** Johns Hopkins Medicine Outpatient Ctr, 600 N Wolfe St Carnegie Bldg - Ste 592, C Medicine, Baltimore, MD 21287; **Phone:** 410-502-0550; **Board Cert:** Cardiovascular Disease 2004; Cardiac Electrophysiology 2006; **Med School:** Harvard Med Sch 1987; **Resid:** Internal Medicine, Brigham & Women's Hosp 1990; **Fellow:** Cardiovascular Disease, Johns Hopkins Hosp 1993; **Fac Appt:** Prof Med, Johns Hopkins Univ

Callans, David J MD [CE] - **Spec Exp:** Arrhythmias; Pacemakers; **Hospital:** Hosp Univ Penn - UPHS (page 68); **Address:** Hosp Univ Penn, 3400 Spruce St Founders Bldg Fl 9, Philadelphia, PA 19104; **Phone:** 215-662-6052; **Board Cert:** Internal Medicine 1989; Cardiovascular Disease 2005; Cardiac Electrophysiology 2005; **Med School:** Johns Hopkins Univ 1986; **Resid:** Internal Medicine, Hosp Univ Penn 1989; Cardiovascular Disease, Hosp Univ Penn 1999; **Fac Appt:** Prof Med, Univ Pennsylvania

Chinitz, Larry MD [CE] - **Spec Exp:** Arrhythmias; Pacemakers; Defibrillators; Atrial Fibrillation; **Hospital:** NYU Langone Med Ctr (page 66); **Address:** 403 E 34th St, Heart Rhythm Center, 4th Fl, New York, NY 10016-6402; **Phone:** 212-263-7149; **Board Cert:** Internal Medicine 1982; Cardiovascular Disease 1985; **Med School:** NYU Sch Med 1979; **Resid:** Internal Medicine, Bellevue Hosp Ctr 1983; **Fellow:** Cardiovascular Disease, NYU Med Ctr/Bellevue Hosp Ctr 1986; Cardiac Electrophysiology, Montefiore Hosp 1985; **Fac Appt:** Assoc Prof Med, NYU Sch Med

Cardiac Electrophysiology

Cohen, Martin B MD [CE] - **Spec Exp:** Interventional Cardiology; Pacemakers; Defibrillators; Coronary Angioplasty/Stents; **Hospital:** Westchester Med Ctr, White Plains Hosp Ctr; **Address:** 19 Bradhurst Ave, Ste 700, Cardiology Assocs, Hawthorne, NY 10532-2140; **Phone:** 914-593-7800; **Board Cert:** Internal Medicine 1983; Cardiovascular Disease 1985; Cardiac Electrophysiology 2006; Interventional Cardiology 2004; **Med School:** SUNY Downstate 1980; **Resid:** Internal Medicine, Univ Hosp 1983; **Fellow:** Cardiovascular Disease, Univ Hosp 1985; Interventional Cardiology, Westchester Co Med Ctr 1986; **Fac Appt:** Assoc Clin Prof Med, NY Med Coll

Curtis, Anne B MD [CE] - **Spec Exp:** Pacemakers; Arrhythmias; Defibrillators; **Hospital:** Erie County Med Ctr; **Address:** Erie Co Med Ctr, Dept Medicine, 462 Grider St, Buffalo, NY 14215; **Phone:** 716-898-4328; **Board Cert:** Internal Medicine 1982; Cardiovascular Disease 1985; Cardiac Electrophysiology 2002; **Med School:** Columbia P&S 1979; **Resid:** Internal Medicine, Columbia- Presby Hosp 1982; **Fellow:** Cardiovascular Disease, Duke Univ Med Ctr 1985; Cardiac Electrophysiology, Duke Univ Med Ctr 1986; **Fac Appt:** Prof Med, Univ S Fla Coll Med

Epstein, Andrew E MD [CE] - **Spec Exp:** Arrhythmias; Defibrillators; Catheter Ablation; Genetic Arrhythmias; **Hospital:** Hosp Univ Penn - UPHS (page 68), VA Med Ctr - Philadelphia; **Address:** Electrophysiology Section, Hosp Univ Penn, 3400 Spruce St, 9 Founders, Philadelphia, PA 19104; **Phone:** 215-662-6052; **Board Cert:** Internal Medicine 1980; Cardiovascular Disease 1983; Cardiac Electrophysiology 2006; **Med School:** Univ Rochester 1977; **Resid:** Internal Medicine, Barnes Hosp 1980; **Fellow:** Cardiovascular Disease, Univ Ala Hosp 1982; **Fac Appt:** Prof Med, Univ Pennsylvania

Gomes, J Anthony MD [CE] - **Spec Exp:** Arrhythmias; Heart Attack; Atrial Fibrillation; Pacemakers; **Hospital:** Mount Sinai Med Ctr (page 63); **Address:** Mount Sinai Medical Ctr, One Gustave L Levy Pl, Box 1030, New York, NY 10029-6500; **Phone:** 212-241-7272; **Board Cert:** Internal Medicine 1974; Cardiovascular Disease 1975; **Med School:** India 1970; **Resid:** Internal Medicine, Mt Sinai Med Ctr 1973; **Fellow:** Cardiovascular Disease, Mt Sinai Med Ctr 1975; Cardiac Electrophysiology, USPHS Cardio-Pulmonary Lab 1976; **Fac Appt:** Prof Med, Mount Sinai Sch Med

Halperin, Henry R MD [CE] - **Spec Exp:** Catheter Ablation; Pacemakers; **Hospital:** Johns Hopkins Hosp (page 61); **Address:** 600 N Wolfe St, Blalock 524A, Cardiology Division, Baltimore, MD 21287; **Phone:** 410-955-2412; **Board Cert:** Internal Medicine 1981; Cardiovascular Disease 1983; Cardiac Electrophysiology 2009; **Med School:** Louisiana State U, Shrevport 1977; **Resid:** Internal Medicine, LSU Charity Hosp; **Fellow:** Cardiovascular Disease, Johns Hopkins Hosp; **Fac Appt:** Prof Med, Johns Hopkins Univ

Lerman, Bruce MD [CE] - **Spec Exp:** Catheter Ablation; Defibrillators; Arrhythmias; **Hospital:** NY-Presby/Weill Cornell Med Ctr, NY (page 65); **Address:** NY Weill Cornell Med Ctr, 520 E 70th St, Starr 4, New York, NY 10021-9800; **Phone:** 212-746-2169; **Board Cert:** Internal Medicine 1980; Cardiovascular Disease 1985; Cardiac Electrophysiology 2002; **Med School:** Loyola Univ-Stritch Sch Med 1977; **Resid:** Internal Medicine, Northwestern Univ Hosp 1980; Internal Medicine, Univ Michigan Med Ctr 1981; **Fellow:** Cardiovascular Disease, Hosp Univ Penn 1982; Cardiovascular Disease, Johns Hopkins Hosp 1983; **Fac Appt:** Prof Med, Cornell Univ-Weill Med Coll

Levine, Joseph H MD [CE] - **Spec Exp:** Arrhythmias; Sudden Death Prevention; Atrial Fibrillation; Pacemakers; **Hospital:** St. Francis Hosp - The Heart Ctr (page 69); **Address:** 100 Port Washington Blvd, Roslyn, NY 11576; **Phone:** 516-622-1011; **Board Cert:** Internal Medicine 1983; Cardiovascular Disease 1987; Cardiac Electrophysiology 2003; **Med School:** Univ Rochester 1980; **Resid:** Internal Medicine, Yale-New Haven Hosp 1983; **Fellow:** Cardiovascular Disease, Johns Hopkins Hosp 1986; Cardiac Electrophysiology, Hosp Univ Penn 1986

Marchlinski, Francis E MD [CE] - **Spec Exp:** Pacemakers; Arrhythmias; **Hospital:** Hosp Univ Penn - UPHS (page 68); **Address:** Hosp University Penn, Div Cardiology, 3400 Spruce St Founders Bldg Fl 9, Philadelphia, PA 19104-4206; **Phone:** 215-662-6052; **Board Cert:** Internal Medicine 1979; Cardiovascular Disease 1981; Cardiac Electrophysiology 2002; **Med School:** Univ Pennsylvania 1976; **Resid:** Internal Medicine, Hosp Univ Penn 1979; **Fellow:** Cardiovascular Disease, Hosp Univ Penn 1982; **Fac Appt:** Prof Med, Univ Pennsylvania

Mehta, Davendra MD/PhD [CE] - **Spec Exp:** Arrhythmias; Congenital Heart Disease-Adult; Atrial Fibrillation; Heart Failure; **Hospital:** Mount Sinai Med Ctr (page 63), James J. Peters VA Med Ctr-Bronx; **Address:** One Gustave L Levy Pl, Box 1030, New York, NY 10029-6501; **Phone:** 212-241-7272; **Board Cert:** Cardiovascular Disease 2009; Cardiac Electrophysiology 2009; **Med School:** India 1979; **Resid:** Internal Medicine, Leicester Royal Infirmary 1983; **Fellow:** Cardiovascular Disease, Groby Road Hosp 1986; Electrocardiography, St George's Hosp 1989; **Fac Appt:** Prof Med, Mount Sinai Sch Med

Tomaselli, Gordon F MD [CE] - **Spec Exp:** Arrhythmias; Sudden Death Prevention; **Hospital:** Johns Hopkins Hosp (page 61); **Address:** Johns Hopkins Medicine Outpatient Center, 601 N Caroline St, Baltimore, MD 21287; **Phone:** 410-502-0550; **Board Cert:** Internal Medicine 1985; Cardiac Electrophysiology 2005; Cardiovascular Disease 1989; **Med School:** Albert Einstein Coll Med 1982; **Resid:** Internal Medicine, UCSF Med Ctr 1985; **Fellow:** Cardiovascular Disease, Johns Hopkins Hosp 1986; **Fac Appt:** Prof Med, Johns Hopkins Univ

Southeast

DeLurgio, David B MD [CE] - **Spec Exp:** Arrhythmias; Atrial Fibrillation; Sudden Death Prevention; Heart Failure; **Hospital:** Emory Univ Hosp Midtown, Emory Univ Hosp; **Address:** Emory Univ Hosp Midtown, 550 Peachtree St NE Fl 6, Atlanta, GA 30308; **Phone:** 404-686-2504; **Board Cert:** Cardiovascular Disease 2007; Cardiac Electrophysiology 2008; **Med School:** UCLA 1990; **Resid:** Internal Medicine, Emory Univ Med Ctr 1993; **Fellow:** Cardiovascular Disease, UCLA Med Ctr 1995; **Fac Appt:** Assoc Prof Med, Emory Univ

DiMarco, John P MD/PhD [CE] - **Spec Exp:** Arrhythmias; Pacemakers; Defibrillators; **Hospital:** Univ of Virginia Health Sys; **Address:** Univ Virginia Hlth Scis Ctr, PO Box 800158, Charlottesville, VA 22908-0158; **Phone:** 434-924-2031; **Board Cert:** Internal Medicine 1978; Cardiovascular Disease 1981; Cardiac Electrophysiology 2005; **Med School:** Case West Res Univ 1975; **Resid:** Internal Medicine, Mass Genl Hosp 1977; Critical Care Medicine, Case West Res Univ 1978; **Fellow:** Cardiovascular Disease, Mass Genl Hosp 1980; Cardiac Electrophysiology, Mass Genl Hosp 1981; **Fac Appt:** Prof Med, Univ VA Sch Med

Ellenbogen, Kenneth A MD [CE] - **Spec Exp:** Arrhythmias; Pacemakers; Defibrillators; **Hospital:** Med Coll of VA Hosp, Henrico Doctors Hosp; **Address:** Dept Electrophysiology, PO Box 980053, Richmond, VA 23298; **Phone:** 804-828-7565; **Board Cert:** Internal Medicine 1983; Cardiovascular Disease 1985; Cardiac Electrophysiology 2005; **Med School:** Johns Hopkins Univ 1980; **Resid:** Internal Medicine, Johns Hopkins Hosp 1983; **Fellow:** Cardiovascular Disease, Duke Univ Med Ctr 1986; **Fac Appt:** Prof Med, Med Coll VA

Interian Jr, Alberto MD [CE] - **Spec Exp:** Arrhythmias; **Hospital:** Mercy Hosp, Jackson Meml Hosp (page 70); **Address:** Mercy Arrhythmia & Syncope Ctr, 3641 S Miami Ave, Ste 221, Bayside Pavillion Bldg, Miami, FL 33133; **Phone:** 305-285-2685; **Board Cert:** Internal Medicine 1985; Cardiovascular Disease 1987; Cardiac Electrophysiology 2000; **Med School:** Univ Miami Sch Med 1982; **Resid:** Internal Medicine, Univ Miami Hosps 1985; **Fellow:** Cardiovascular Disease, Univ Miami Hosps 1988; **Fac Appt:** Prof Med, Univ Miami Sch Med

Cardiac Electrophysiology

Kay, G Neal MD [CE] - **Spec Exp:** Arrhythmias; Atrial Fibrillation; Pacemakers; **Hospital:** Univ of Ala Hosp at Birmingham; **Address:** UAB, Div Cardiovascular Disease, 1530 3rd Ave S, FOT 930, Birmingham, AL 35294; **Phone:** 205-934-1335; **Board Cert:** Internal Medicine 1983; Cardiovascular Disease 1989; Cardiac Electrophysiology 2006; **Med School:** Univ Mich Med Sch 1979; **Resid:** Internal Medicine, Univ Alabama Hosp 1983; **Fellow:** Cardiovascular Disease, Duke Univ Med Ctr 1986; **Fac Appt:** Prof Med, Univ Alabama

Onufer, John R MD [CE] - **Spec Exp:** Atrial Fibrillation; Catheter Ablation; Pacemakers; Defibrillators; **Hospital:** Henrico Doctors Hosp; **Address:** Virginia Cardiovascular Specialists, 7611 Forest Ave, Ste 100, Richmond, VA 23229; **Phone:** 804-288-4827; **Board Cert:** Internal Medicine 1987; Cardiovascular Disease 2001; Cardiac Electrophysiology 2002; **Med School:** Washington Univ, St Louis 1984; **Resid:** Internal Medicine, Barnes Jewish Hosp 1987; **Fellow:** Cardiovascular Disease, Washington Univ 1990; Cardiac Electrophysiology, Washington Univ 1991

Sorrentino, Robert A MD [CE] - **Spec Exp:** Arrhythmias; Defibrillators; Pacemakers; Heart Failure; **Hospital:** Med Coll of GA Hosp and Clin (MCG Health Inc); **Address:** Medical College of Georgia, 1120 15th St BBR Bldg - rm 6518, Augusta, GA 30912-0004; **Phone:** 706-721-4997; **Board Cert:** Internal Medicine 1988; Cardiovascular Disease 2002; Cardiac Electrophysiology 2008; **Med School:** Albany Med Coll 1985; **Resid:** Internal Medicine, Duke Univ Med Ctr 1988; **Fellow:** Cardiovascular Disease, Duke Univ Med Ctr 1991; **Fac Appt:** Prof Med, Med Coll GA

Midwest

Anderson, Mark E MD/PhD [CE] - **Spec Exp:** Arrhythmias; **Hospital:** Univ Iowa Hosp & Clinics; **Address:** 200 Hawkins Drive, rm SE308 GH, Iowa City, IA 52242-1081; **Phone:** 319-356-2745; **Board Cert:** Internal Medicine 2005; Cardiovascular Disease 2005; **Med School:** Univ Minn 1989; **Resid:** Internal Medicine, Stanford Univ Med Ctr 1991; **Fellow:** Cardiovascular Disease, Stanford Univ Sch Med 1994; Cardiac Electrophysiology, Stanford Univ Sch Med 1996; **Fac Appt:** Prof Med, Univ Iowa Coll Med

Donahue, J Kevin MD [CE] - **Spec Exp:** Arrhythmias; Catheter Ablation; Defibrillators; Ventricular Tachycardia Ablation; **Hospital:** MetroHealth Med Ctr; **Address:** MetroHealth Hosp, 2500 MetroHealth Drive, R-653, Dept Heart & Vascular, Cleveland, OH 44109; **Phone:** 216-778-2328; **Board Cert:** Cardiovascular Disease 2009; Cardiac Electrophysiology 2001; **Med School:** Washington Univ, St Louis 1992; **Resid:** Internal Medicine, Hosp Univ Penn 1996; **Fellow:** Cardiac Electrophysiology, Johns Hopkins Hosp 1997; **Fac Appt:** Assoc Prof Med, Case West Res Univ

Faddis, Mitchell N MD/PhD [CE] - **Spec Exp:** Arrhythmias; **Hospital:** Barnes-Jewish Hosp; **Address:** Barnes Jewish Hosp, Dept Cardiology, Ctr for Avanced Medicine Fl 8, 1 Barnes Hosp Pl, St Louis, MO 63110; **Phone:** 314-362-1291; **Board Cert:** Internal Medicine 2006; Cardiovascular Disease 2009; Cardiac Electrophysiology 2000; **Med School:** Washington Univ, St Louis 1993; **Resid:** Internal Medicine, Barnes Jewish Hosp 1995; **Fellow:** Cardiovascular Disease, Barnes Jewish Hosp 1996; **Fac Appt:** Assoc Prof Med, Washington Univ, St Louis

Hammill, Stephen C MD [CE] - **Spec Exp:** Pacemakers; Arrhythmias; **Hospital:** Mayo Med Ctr & Clin - Rochester; **Address:** Mayo Clinic, 200 First St SW, Rochester, MN 55905; **Phone:** 507-284-2129; **Board Cert:** Internal Medicine 1978; Cardiovascular Disease 1981; Cardiac Electrophysiology 2005; **Med School:** Univ Colorado 1974; **Resid:** Internal Medicine, Univ Colo Hlth Sci Ctr 1977; **Fellow:** Cardiovascular Disease, Duke Univ Med Ctr 1981; **Fac Appt:** Prof Med, Mayo Med Sch

Hayes, David L MD [CE] - **Spec Exp:** Pacemakers; **Hospital:** Mayo Med Ctr & Clin - Rochester; **Address:** Mayo Clinic, 200 1st St SW, Rochester, MN 55905; **Phone:** 507-284-2511; **Board Cert:** Internal Medicine 1980; Cardiovascular Disease 1981; **Med School:** Univ MO-Kansas City 1977; **Resid:** Internal Medicine, Mayo Clin 1980; **Fellow:** Cardiovascular Disease, Mayo Clin 1982; **Fac Appt:** Prof Med, Mayo Med Sch

Lindsay, Bruce MD [CE] - **Spec Exp:** Arrhythmias; **Hospital:** Cleveland Clin (page 56); **Address:** Cleveland Clinic, Desk J2-2, 9500 Euclid Ave, Cleveland, OH 44195; **Phone:** 216-444-4293; **Board Cert:** Internal Medicine 1980; Cardiovascular Disease 1987; Cardiac Electrophysiology 2002; **Med School:** Jefferson Med Coll 1976; **Resid:** Internal Medicine, Univ Michigan Medical Ctr 1980; **Fellow:** Cardiovascular Disease, Barnes-Jewish Hosp 1985; **Fac Appt:** Assoc Prof Med

Love, Charles J MD [CE] - **Spec Exp:** Defibrillator Cable Extraction; Pacemakers; **Hospital:** Ohio St Univ Med Ctr; **Address:** Heart & Lung Inst Fl 2, 473 W 12 Ave, Columbus, OH 43210; **Phone:** 614-293-4947; **Board Cert:** Internal Medicine 1986; Cardiovascular Disease 1989; Cardiac Electrophysiology 2004; **Med School:** Univ Pittsburgh 1983; **Resid:** Internal Medicine, Ohio State Univ Hosp 1986; **Fellow:** Cardiac Electrophysiology, Ohio State Univ Hosp 1988; **Fac Appt:** Prof Med, Ohio State Univ

Miller, John M MD [CE] - **Spec Exp:** Arrhythmias; Catheter Ablation; Atrial Fibrillation; **Hospital:** IU Health Methodist Hosp, IU Health University Hosp; **Address:** Krannert Inst Cardiology, 1800 N Senate Blvd, MPC 2, Ste 4000, Indianapolis, IN 46202; **Phone:** 317-962-0101; **Board Cert:** Internal Medicine 1982; Cardiovascular Disease 1985; Cardiac Electrophysiology 2003; **Med School:** Penn State Coll Med 1979; **Resid:** Internal Medicine, NC Meml Hosp 1982; **Fellow:** Cardiovascular Disease, Hosp Univ Penn 1985; **Fac Appt:** Prof Med, Indiana Univ

Morady, Fred MD [CE] - **Spec Exp:** Arrhythmias; WPW Syndrome; **Hospital:** Univ of Michigan Hosp; **Address:** Specialty Electrophysiology, 1500 E Med Ctr Drive, SPC 3rd FL 5856, Ann Arbor, MI 48109; **Phone:** 734-647-7321; **Board Cert:** Internal Medicine 1978; Cardiovascular Disease 1981; Cardiac Electrophysiology 2005; **Med School:** UCSF 1975; **Resid:** Internal Medicine, UCSF Med Ctr 1978; **Fellow:** Cardiovascular Disease, UCSF Med Ctr 1980; **Fac Appt:** Prof Med, Univ Mich Med Sch

Prystowsky, Eric N MD [CE] - **Spec Exp:** Arrhythmias; Catheter Ablation; Atrial Fibrillation; **Hospital:** St. Vincent Indianapolis Hosp; **Address:** The Care Group, 8333 Naab Rd, Ste 400, Indianapolis, IN 46260; **Phone:** 317-338-6666; **Board Cert:** Internal Medicine 1976; Cardiovascular Disease 1979; Cardiac Electrophysiology 2005; **Med School:** Mount Sinai Sch Med 1973; **Resid:** Internal Medicine, Mt Sinai Hosp 1976; **Fellow:** Cardiovascular Disease, Duke Univ Med Ctr 1979

Schuger, Claudio D MD [CE] - **Spec Exp:** Arrhythmias; Defibrillators; **Hospital:** Henry Ford Hosp; **Address:** Henry Ford Hosp, Div Cardiology, 2799 W Grand Blvd, Ste 322, Detroit, MI 48202; **Phone:** 313-916-2417; **Board Cert:** Cardiac Electrophysiology 2008; Cardiovascular Disease 2007; **Med School:** Argentina 1977; **Resid:** Internal Medicine, Hacarmel Hosp 1982; **Fellow:** Cardiovascular Disease, Bikur Cholim Hosp 1985; Cardiac Electrophysiology, Harper Hosp 1990; **Fac Appt:** Prof Med, Wayne State Univ

Tchou, Patrick J MD [CE] - **Spec Exp:** Arrhythmias; **Hospital:** Cleveland Clin (page 56); **Address:** Dept Cardiology, 9500 Euclid Ave, Ste J2-2, Cleveland, OH 44195; **Phone:** 216-444-6792; **Board Cert:** Internal Medicine 1982; Cardiovascular Disease 1985; Cardiac Electrophysiology 2002; **Med School:** Case West Res Univ 1979; **Resid:** Internal Medicine, Metro Genl Hosp 1982; **Fellow:** Cardiovascular Disease, Metro Genl Hosp 1984; Cardiac Electrophysiology, Mt Sinai Med Ctr 1985; **Fac Appt:** Prof Med, Ohio State Univ

Cardiac Electrophysiology

Waldo, Albert MD [CE] - **Spec Exp:** Arrhythmias; Syncope; Long QT Interval Syndrome; Atrial Fibrillation; **Hospital:** Univ Hosps Case Med Ctr (page 74); **Address:** Univ Hosps Case Med Ctr, Div Cardiovascular Medicine, 11100 Euclid Ave, MS LKS-5038, Cleveland, OH 44106-1736; **Phone:** 216-844-7690; **Board Cert:** Internal Medicine 1971; Cardiovascular Disease 1975; **Med School:** SUNY Downstate 1962; **Resid:** Internal Medicine, Baltimore City Hosp 1965; Internal Medicine, Kings Co Hosp 1966; **Fellow:** Cardiovascular Disease, Columbia Presby Med Ctr 1968; Cardiac Electrophysiology, Columbia Presby Med Ctr 1969; **Fac Appt:** Prof Med, Case West Res Univ

Wilber, David J MD [CE] - **Spec Exp:** Atrial Fibrillation; Catheter Ablation; Sudden Death Prevention; **Hospital:** Loyola Univ Med Ctr; **Address:** Loyola Univ Med Ctr, Cardiovascular Inst, 2160 S First Ave Bldg 110 - rm 6232, Maywood, IL 60153; **Phone:** 708-216-2642; **Board Cert:** Internal Medicine 1980; Cardiovascular Disease 1985; Cardiac Electrophysiology 2002; **Med School:** Northwestern Univ 1977; **Resid:** Internal Medicine, Northwestern Meml Hosp 1980; **Fellow:** Cardiovascular Disease, Univ Mich Med Sch 1984; Cardiac Electrophysiology, Mass Genl Hosp 1986; **Fac Appt:** Prof Med, Loyola Univ-Stritch Sch Med

Great Plains and Mountains

Lewkowiez, Laurent MD [CE] - **Spec Exp:** Arrhythmias; Ventricular Tachycardia Ablation; Atrial Fibrillation; **Address:** Franklin Medical Offices, 2045 Franklin St, Denver, CO 80205; **Phone:** 303-338-4545; **Board Cert:** Cardiovascular Disease 2010; Cardiac Electrophysiology 2003; **Med School:** Univ SC Sch Med 1992; **Resid:** Internal Medicine, Univ Colorado Affil Hosp 1996; **Fellow:** Nuclear Cardiology, Univ Colorado 1998; Cardiac Electrophysiology, Univ Colorado 2001; **Fac Appt:** Asst Prof Med, Univ Colorado

Southwest

Snyder, David W MD [CE] - **Hospital:** E Jefferson Genl Hosp; **Address:** East Jefferson Cardiology Consultants, 4200 Houma Blvd Fl 2nd, Metairie, LA 70002; **Phone:** 504-454-4102; **Board Cert:** Cardiac Electrophysiology 2002; Cardiovascular Disease 1981; Internal Medicine 1978; **Med School:** Duke Univ 1975; **Resid:** Internal Medicine, Barnes-Jewish Hosp 1978; **Fellow:** Cardiovascular Disease, Barnes-Jewish Hosp 1978

West Coast and Pacific

Cannom, David S MD [CE] - **Spec Exp:** Arrhythmias; **Hospital:** Good Samaritan Hosp - LA; **Address:** 1245 Wilshire Blvd, Ste 703, Los Angeles, CA 90017; **Phone:** 213-977-0419; **Board Cert:** Internal Medicine 1980; Cardiovascular Disease 1975; **Med School:** Univ Minn 1967; **Resid:** Internal Medicine, Yale-New Haven Hosp 1969; **Fellow:** Cardiovascular Disease, Stanford Univ 1973; **Fac Appt:** Clin Prof Med, UCLA

Feld, Gregory K MD [CE] - **Hospital:** UCSD Med Ctr; **Address:** 4168 Front St, MC 8649, San Diego, CA 92103-8649; **Phone:** 619-543-5428; **Board Cert:** Internal Medicine 1980; Cardiovascular Disease 1983; Cardiac Electrophysiology 2002; **Med School:** Dartmouth Med Sch 1977; **Resid:** Internal Medicine, Wadsworth VA Hosp 1981; **Fellow:** Cardiothoracic Research, Wadsworth VA Hosp 1984; **Fac Appt:** Prof Med, UCSD

Gang, Eli S MD [CE] - **Spec Exp:** Arrhythmias; **Hospital:** Cedars-Sinai Med Ctr, Brotman Med Ctr; **Address:** 414 N Camden Drive, Ste 1100, Beverly Hills, CA 90210; **Phone:** 310-278-3400; **Board Cert:** Internal Medicine 1978; Cardiovascular Disease 1981; **Med School:** Columbia P&S 1975; **Resid:** Internal Medicine, Roosevelt Hosp 1978; **Fellow:** Cardiovascular Disease, Columbia Presby Hosp 1979; **Fac Appt:** Clin Prof Med, UCLA

Higgins, Steven MD [CE] - **Spec Exp:** Arrhythmias; Defibrillators; **Hospital:** Scripps Meml Hosp - La Jolla, Tri-City Med Ctr - Oceanside; **Address:** 9850 Genesee Ave, Ste 940, La Jolla, CA 92037; **Phone:** 858-658-0088; **Board Cert:** Cardiovascular Disease 1985; Cardiac Electrophysiology 1992; **Med School:** Univ Rochester 1979; **Resid:** Internal Medicine, Univ CO Med Ctr 1982; **Fellow:** Cardiovascular Disease, Univ CO Med Ctr 1985

Swerdlow, Charles D MD [CE] - **Spec Exp:** Defibrillators; Arrhythmias; Pacemakers; WPW Syndrome; **Hospital:** Cedars-Sinai Med Ctr, UCLA Ronald Reagan Med Ctr; **Address:** 414 N Camden Drive, Ste 700, Beverly Hills, CA 90210; **Phone:** 310-278-3400; **Board Cert:** Internal Medicine 1979; Cardiovascular Disease 1981; Cardiac Electrophysiology 2004; **Med School:** Harvard Med Sch 1976; **Resid:** Internal Medicine, LAC-Harbor Genl Hosp 1979; **Fellow:** Cardiovascular Disease, Stanford Univ Med Ctr 1981; **Fac Appt:** Clin Prof Med, UCLA

Wang, Paul J MD [CE] - **Spec Exp:** Arrhythmias; Atrial Fibrillation; Defibrillators; **Hospital:** Stanford Univ Hosp & Clinics; **Address:** Stanford Univ Cardiovascular Med, 300 Pasteur Drive, Stanford, CA 94305; **Phone:** 650-723-7111; **Board Cert:** Internal Medicine 1986; Cardiovascular Disease 1989; Cardiac Electrophysiology 2002; **Med School:** Columbia P&S 1983; **Resid:** Internal Medicine, NY Presby-Columbia Med Ctr 1986; **Fellow:** Cardiovascular Disease, Brigham & Women's Hosp 1989; **Fac Appt:** Prof Med, Stanford Univ

INTERVENTIONAL CARDIOLOGY

New England

Diver, Daniel J MD [IC] - **Spec Exp:** Angioplasty; Coronary Artery Disease; **Hospital:** St. Francis Hosp & Med Ctr; **Address:** St Francis Hosp - Div Cardiology, 114 Woodland St, Hartford, CT 06105; **Phone:** 860-714-4019; **Board Cert:** Internal Medicine 1984; Cardiovascular Disease 1989; **Med School:** Johns Hopkins Univ 1981; **Resid:** Internal Medicine, Johns Hopkins Hosp 1984; **Fellow:** Cardiovascular Disease, Beth Israel Hosp/Harvard 1987; **Fac Appt:** Prof Med, Univ Conn

Gibson, C Michael MD [IC] - **Spec Exp:** Acute Coronary Syndromes; Clinical Trials; **Hospital:** Beth Israel Deaconess Med Ctr - Boston; **Address:** Beth Israel Deaconess Med Ctr, 185 Pilgrim Rd, Room Deaconess 319, Boston, MA 02215; **Phone:** 617-667-8800; **Board Cert:** Internal Medicine 1989; Cardiovascular Disease 2002; Interventional Cardiology 2002; **Med School:** Univ Chicago-Pritzker Sch Med 1986; **Resid:** Internal Medicine, Brigham & Womens Hosp 1989; Internal Medicine, Brigham & Womens Hosp 1993; **Fellow:** Cardiovascular Disease, Beth Israel Deaconess Med Ctr 1992; **Fac Appt:** Assoc Prof Med, Harvard Med Sch

Jacobs, Alice K MD [IC] - **Spec Exp:** Interventional Cardiology; Cardiac Catheterization; Heart Disease in Women; **Hospital:** Boston Med Ctr; **Address:** Boston Univ Med Ctr, Dept Cardiology, 88 E Newton St, rm C822, Boston, MA 02118; **Phone:** 617-638-8707; **Board Cert:** Internal Medicine 1978; Endocrinology 1979; Cardiovascular Disease 1985; **Med School:** St Louis Univ 1975; **Resid:** Internal Medicine, St Louis Univ Hosp 1977; **Fellow:** Endocrinology, UCSD Med Ctr 1980; Cardiovascular Disease, Boston Univ Med Ctr 1982; **Fac Appt:** Prof Med, Boston Univ

Laham, Roger MD [IC] - **Spec Exp:** Angioplasty; **Hospital:** Beth Israel Deaconess Med Ctr - Boston; **Address:** Beth Israel Deaconess Med Ctr, 185 Pilgrim Rd, Baker 4, Boston, MA 02215; **Phone:** 617-667-8800; **Board Cert:** Internal Medicine 2004; Cardiovascular Disease 2005; Interventional Cardiology 2010; **Med School:** Amer Univ Beirut 1989; **Resid:** Internal Medicine, Duke Univ Med Ctr 1992; **Fellow:** Cardiovascular Disease, Harvard Med Sch 1995; **Fac Appt:** Assoc Prof Med, Harvard Med Sch

Interventional Cardiology

Rosenfield, Kenneth MD [IC] - **Spec Exp:** Angioplasty & Stent Placement; **Hospital:** Mass Genl Hosp, Anna Jaques Hosp; **Address:** Mass Genl Hosp, 55 Fruit St, Ste GRB800, Boston, MA 02114; **Phone:** 617-724-1935; **Board Cert:** Internal Medicine 1985; Cardiovascular Disease 1989; Interventional Cardiology 2002; **Med School:** Univ Mass Sch Med 1982; **Resid:** Internal Medicine, Kaiser Fdn Hosp 1985; **Fellow:** Cardiovascular Disease, New Eng Med Ctr 1988; Interventional Cardiology, St Elizabeth's Med Ctr 1989

Williams, David O MD [IC] - **Spec Exp:** Cardiac Catheterization; **Hospital:** Brigham and Women's Hosp (page 57); **Address:** Brigham & Women's Hosp, Cardiovascular Div, 1620 Tremont St Fl 3, Boston, MA 02115; **Phone:** 617-732-5089; **Board Cert:** Internal Medicine 1972; Cardiovascular Disease 1975; Interventional Cardiology 1999; **Med School:** Hahnemann Univ 1969; **Resid:** Internal Medicine, Hahnemann Univ Hosp 1972; **Fellow:** Cardiovascular Disease, UC Davis Med Ctr 1974; **Fac Appt:** Prof Med, Brown Univ

Zelman, Richard MD [IC] - **Spec Exp:** Angioplasty & Stent Placement; **Hospital:** Cape Cod Hosp; **Address:** 40 Quinlan Way, Ste 104, Hyannis, MA 02601; **Phone:** 508-862-7645; **Board Cert:** Internal Medicine 1986; Cardiovascular Disease 1989; Interventional Cardiology 2009; **Med School:** Univ Tex, San Antonio 1983; **Resid:** Internal Medicine, Brigham & Womens Hosp 1986; **Fellow:** Cardiovascular Disease, Brigham & Womens Hosp 1989

Mid Atlantic

Chang, Gene MD [IC] - **Spec Exp:** Cardiac Catheterization; Angioplasty & Stent Placement; Atrial Septal Defect; **Hospital:** Penn Presby Med Ctr - UPHS (page 68); **Address:** Penn Presby Med Ctr, Philadelphia Heart Inst, 39th & Market Sts, 4PHI, Philadelphia, PA 19104; **Phone:** 215-662-9000; **Board Cert:** Cardiovascular Disease 2008; Interventional Cardiology 2009; **Med School:** Tufts Univ 1991; **Resid:** Internal Medicine, New England Deaconess Hosp 1994; **Fellow:** Cardiovascular Disease, Hosp U Penn 1998; Interventional Cardiology, Hosp U Penn 1999; **Fac Appt:** Asst Clin Prof Med, Univ Pennsylvania

Farah, Tony G MD [IC] - **Spec Exp:** Cardiac Catheterization; **Hospital:** Allegheny General Hosp; **Address:** Cardiology Assocs, 490 E North Ave, Ste 307, Pittsburgh, PA 15212; **Phone:** 412-359-5822; **Board Cert:** Internal Medicine 1987; Cardiovascular Disease 1989; Interventional Cardiology 2009; **Med School:** Lebanon 1984; **Resid:** Internal Medicine, Allegheny Genl Hosp 1987; **Fellow:** Cardiovascular Disease, Allegheny Genl Hosp 1990; **Fac Appt:** Asst Prof Med, Med Coll PA

Gray, William A MD [IC] - **Spec Exp:** Percutaneous Valve Repair; Peripheral Vascular Disease; Patent Foramen Ovale; **Hospital:** NY-Presby/Columbia Univ Med Ctr, NY (page 65); **Address:** Ctr for Interventional Vascular Therapy, 173 Fort Washington Ave Fl 4, New York, NY 10032; **Phone:** 212-305-7060; **Board Cert:** Internal Medicine 1987; Cardiovascular Disease 2002; Interventional Cardiology 2011; **Med School:** Temple Univ 1984; **Resid:** Internal Medicine, Rhode Island Hosp 1988; **Fellow:** Cardiovascular Disease, Brown Univ 1992; **Fac Appt:** Assoc Clin Prof Med, Columbia P&S

Herrmann, Howard C MD [IC] - **Spec Exp:** Cardiac Catheterization; Angioplasty & Stent Placement; Heart Valve Disease; Atrial Septal Defect; **Hospital:** Hosp Univ Penn - UPHS (page 68), Penn Presby Med Ctr - UPHS (page 68); **Address:** Hosp Univ Penn, Div Cardiovascular Med, 3400 Spruce St, 9038 Gates Pavillion, Philadelphia, PA 19104-4283; **Phone:** 215-662-2180; **Board Cert:** Internal Medicine 1984; Cardiovascular Disease 1987; Interventional Cardiology 2009; **Med School:** Harvard Med Sch 1981; **Resid:** Internal Medicine, Mass General Hosp 1984; **Fellow:** Cardiovascular Disease, Mass General Hosp 1987; **Fac Appt:** Prof Med, Univ Pennsylvania

Lee, Joon S MD [IC] - **Spec Exp:** Cardiac Catheterization; **Hospital:** UPMC Presby, Pittsburgh; **Address:** UPMC Presbyterian, Div Cardiology, 200 Lothrop St, Ste A333, Pittsburgh, PA 15213; **Phone:** 412-647-1385; **Board Cert:** Internal Medicine 2005; Cardiovascular Disease 2005; Interventional Cardiology 2009; **Med School:** Duke Univ 1988; **Resid:** Internal Medicine, Mass General Hosp 1991; **Fellow:** Cardiovascular Disease, Mass General Hosp 1996; **Fac Appt:** Asst Prof Med, Univ Pittsburgh

Leon, Martin MD [IC] - **Hospital:** NY-Presby/Columbia Univ Med Ctr, NY (page 65); **Address:** 173 Ft Washington Ave Fl 4, New York, NY 10032; **Phone:** 212-305-7060; **Board Cert:** Internal Medicine 1979; Cardiovascular Disease 1983; **Med School:** Yale Univ 1975; **Resid:** Internal Medicine, Yale-New Haven Hosp 1978; **Fellow:** Cardiovascular Disease, Yale-New Haven Hosp 1980

Moses, Jeffrey W MD [IC] - **Spec Exp:** Angiography-Coronary; Angioplasty & Stent Placement; Heart Valve Disease; **Hospital:** NY-Presby/Columbia Univ Med Ctr, NY (page 65); **Address:** 161173 Fort Washington Fl 4, New York, NY 10032; **Phone:** 212-305-7060; **Board Cert:** Internal Medicine 1977; Cardiovascular Disease 1981; Interventional Cardiology 2009; **Med School:** Univ Pennsylvania 1974; **Resid:** Internal Medicine, Penn Presby Med Ctr 1977; **Fellow:** Cardiovascular Disease, Penn Presby Med Ctr 1980

Parikh, Manish A MD [IC] - **Spec Exp:** Coronary Angioplasty/Stents; **Hospital:** Lenox Hill Hosp; **Address:** 16 E 60th St, Ste 322, New York, NY 10022; **Phone:** 212-326-8532; **Board Cert:** Cardiovascular Disease 2010; Interventional Cardiology 2010; **Med School:** UMDNJ-NJ Med Sch, Newark 1990; **Resid:** Internal Medicine, New York Hosp 1993; **Fellow:** Cardiovascular Disease, New York Hosp 1997; **Fac Appt:** Asst Prof Med, Cornell Univ-Weill Med Coll

Petrossian, George A MD [IC] - **Spec Exp:** Carotid Artery Stent Placement; Peripheral Vascular Disease; Coronary Angioplasty/Stents; Renovascular Disease; **Hospital:** St. Francis Hosp - The Heart Ctr (page 69), South Nassau Comm Hosp; **Address:** New York Cardiology Group, 1405 Old Northern Blvd Fl 1st, Roslyn, NY 11576-1353; **Phone:** 516-484-6777; **Board Cert:** Internal Medicine 1986; Cardiovascular Disease 1989; Interventional Cardiology 2010; **Med School:** Mount Sinai Sch Med 1983; **Resid:** Internal Medicine, Columbia-Presby Med Ctr 1987; **Fellow:** Cardiovascular Disease, Columbia -Presby Med Ctr 1989; Interventional Cardiology, Mass Genl Hosp 1990

Pichard, Augusto MD [IC] - **Spec Exp:** Angioplasty & Stent Placement; Cardiac Catheterization; **Hospital:** Washington Hosp Ctr; **Address:** 110 Irving St NW, Ste 4B1 NW, Washington, DC 20010; **Phone:** 202-877-5975; **Board Cert:** Internal Medicine 1975; Cardiovascular Disease 1977; Interventional Cardiology 1999; **Med School:** Chile 1969; **Resid:** Internal Medicine, Univ Chile 1970; Internal Medicine, Catholic Univ 1971; **Fellow:** Cardiovascular Disease, Cleveland Clinic 1973; **Fac Appt:** Clin Prof Med, Geo Wash Univ

Reiner, Jonathan S MD [IC] - **Spec Exp:** Angioplasty & Stent Placement; **Hospital:** G Washington Univ Hosp; **Address:** GWU Med Faculty Assocs, 2150 Pennsylvania Ave NW, rm 4-417, Washington, DC 20037; **Phone:** 202-741-3333; **Board Cert:** Internal Medicine 1989; Cardiovascular Disease 2004; Interventional Cardiology 1999; **Med School:** Georgetown Univ 1986; **Resid:** Internal Medicine, North Shore Univ Hosp 1989; **Fellow:** Cardiovascular Disease, George Wash Univ Sch Med 1993; **Fac Appt:** Asst Prof Med, Geo Wash Univ

Resar, Jon R MD [IC] - **Spec Exp:** Percutaneous Coronary Intervention; Percutaneous Valve Repair; Percutaneous ASD/PFO closure; **Hospital:** Johns Hopkins Hosp (page 61); **Address:** Johns Hopkins Hosp, Dept Cardiology, 600 N Wolfe St, Carnegie 568, Baltimore, MD 21287; **Phone:** 410-614-1132; **Board Cert:** Internal Medicine 1988; Cardiovascular Disease 2000; Interventional Cardiology 2009; **Med School:** Med Coll Wisc 1985; **Resid:** Internal Medicine, Johns Hopkins Hosp 1988; **Fellow:** Cardiovascular Disease, Johns Hopkins Hosp 1990; Interventional Cardiology, Johns Hopkins Hosp; **Fac Appt:** Assoc Prof Med, Johns Hopkins Univ

Interventional Cardiology

Roubin, Gary MD/PhD [IC] - **Spec Exp:** Coronary Angioplasty/Stents; Carotid Artery Stent Placement; Peripheral Vascular Disease; **Hospital:** Lenox Hill Hosp; **Address:** 130 E 77th St Fl 9th, New York, NY 10075; **Phone:** 212-434-6836; **Med School:** Australia 1975; **Resid:** Internal Medicine, Royal Prince Albert Hosp 1979; Cardiovascular Disease, Hallstrom Inst of Cardiology 1981; **Fellow:** Cardiology Research, Natl Heart Fdn 1983; Interventional Cardiology, Emory Univ 1985; **Fac Appt:** Clin Prof Med, NYU Sch Med

Sacchi, Terrence J MD [IC] - **Spec Exp:** Arrhythmias; Cardiac Catheterization; Coronary Angioplasty/Stents; Percutaneous Coronary Intervention; **Hospital:** New York Methodist Hosp; **Address:** NY Methodist Hospital, Buckley 2, 506 6th St, Brooklyn, NY 11215; **Phone:** 718-780-7830; **Board Cert:** Internal Medicine 1979; Cardiovascular Disease 1981; Interventional Cardiology 2009; **Med School:** Albany Med Coll 1976; **Resid:** Internal Medicine, St Vincents Hosp 1979; **Fellow:** Cardiovascular Disease, Georgetown Univ Hosp 1981; Interventional Cardiology, Mercy Hosp 1987; **Fac Appt:** Assoc Clin Prof Med, SUNY Downstate

Shani, Jacob MD [IC] - **Spec Exp:** Cardiac Catheterization; Angioplasty & Stent Placement; Percutaneous Valve Repair; **Hospital:** Maimonides Med Ctr (page 62); **Address:** Maimonides Med Ctr, Cardiac Cath Lab, 4802 10th Ave, Brooklyn, NY 11219-2844; **Phone:** 718-283-7480; **Board Cert:** Internal Medicine 1981; Cardiovascular Disease 1983; Interventional Cardiology 2009; **Med School:** Israel 1977; **Resid:** Internal Medicine, Maimonides Med Ctr 1981; **Fellow:** Cardiovascular Disease, Beth Israel Hosp 1983; **Fac Appt:** Prof Med, SUNY Downstate

Shorofsky, Stephen R MD/PhD [IC] - **Spec Exp:** Arrhythmias; **Hospital:** Univ of MD Med Ctr; **Address:** 22 Greene St, Ste N3W77, Baltimore, MD 21201; **Phone:** 410-328-6056; **Board Cert:** Internal Medicine 1988; Cardiovascular Disease 2001; Cardiac Electrophysiology 2004; **Med School:** Univ Chicago-Pritzker Sch Med 1985; **Resid:** Internal Medicine, Univ Chicago Hosps 1988; **Fellow:** Cardiovascular Disease, Univ Chicago Hosps 1991; **Fac Appt:** Assoc Prof Med, Univ MD Sch Med

Stone, Gregg W MD [IC] - **Spec Exp:** Angioplasty & Stent Placement; Coronary Artery Disease; **Hospital:** NY-Presby/Columbia Univ Med Ctr, NY (page 65); **Address:** 111 E 59th St Fl 11, New York, NY 10022; **Phone:** 646-434-4131; **Board Cert:** Internal Medicine 1985; Cardiovascular Disease 1987; **Med School:** Johns Hopkins Univ 1982; **Resid:** Internal Medicine, NY Hosp-Cornell Medical Ctr 1985; **Fellow:** Cardiovascular Disease, Cedars-Sinai Medical Ctr 1988; Coronary Angioplasty, Mid-America Heart Inst 1989

Southeast

Applegate, Robert J MD [IC] - **Spec Exp:** Cardiac Catheterization; Angioplasty; **Hospital:** Wake Forest Univ Baptist Med Ctr; **Address:** Wake Forest, Div Cardiology, Medical Center Blvd, Winston-Salem, NC 27157-1045; **Phone:** 336-716-6674; **Board Cert:** Internal Medicine 1983; Cardiovascular Disease 1987; Interventional Cardiology 2009; **Med School:** Univ VA Sch Med 1980; **Resid:** Internal Medicine, Oregon Hlth Sci Univ Hosp 1983; **Fellow:** Pharmacology, Univ Texas Hlth Sci Ctr 1984; Cardiovascular Disease, Univ Texas Hlth Sci Ctr 1986; **Fac Appt:** Prof Med, Wake Forest Univ

Bittl, John A MD [IC] - **Spec Exp:** Cardiac Catheterization; Invasive Cardiology; **Hospital:** Munroe Regional Med Ctr; **Address:** Ocala Heart Inst, 1500 SW 1st Ave, Ocala, FL 34471; **Phone:** 352-351-7206; **Board Cert:** Internal Medicine 1982; Cardiovascular Disease 1985; Interventional Cardiology 2001; **Med School:** Johns Hopkins Univ 1979; **Resid:** Internal Medicine, UCLA Med Ctr 1982; **Fellow:** Cardiovascular Disease, Brigham-Womens Hosp 1984

Douglas Jr, John S MD [IC] - **Spec Exp:** Angioplasty & Stent Placement; Cardiac Catheterization; Coronary Artery Disease; **Hospital:** Emory Univ Hosp; **Address:** Emory Univ Hosp-Div Cardiology, 1364 Clifton Rd, rm F606, Atlanta, GA 30322; **Phone:** 404-727-7040; **Board Cert:** Internal Medicine 1972; Cardiovascular Disease 1975; Interventional Cardiology 2009; **Med School:** Washington Univ, St Louis 1967; **Resid:** Internal Medicine, NC Memorial Hosp 1969; Internal Medicine, Grady Memorial Hosp 1972; **Fellow:** Cardiovascular Disease, Emory Affil Hosps 1974; **Fac Appt:** Prof Med, Emory Univ

Heldman, Alan W MD [IC] - **Spec Exp:** Cardiomyopathy-Hypertrophic; Coronary Restenosis; Stem Cell Therapy in Heart Failure; **Hospital:** Univ of Miami Hosp (page 72); **Address:** Univ Miami Dept Cardiology, 1295 NW 14th St Fl 2 - Ste A, Miami, FL 33136; **Phone:** 305-243-5554; **Board Cert:** Interventional Cardiology 1999; **Med School:** Univ Alabama 1988; **Resid:** Internal Medicine, Johns Hopkins Hosp 1991; **Fellow:** Cardiovascular Disease, Johns Hopkins Hosp 1994; Interventional Cardiology, Johns Hopkins Hosp 1995; **Fac Appt:** Prof Med, Univ Miami Sch Med

Kandzari, David E MD [IC] - **Spec Exp:** Angioplasty & Stent Placement; Peripheral Arterial Disease; Clinical Trials; **Hospital:** Piedmont Hosp; **Address:** Piedmont Heart Institute, 275 Collier Rd NW, Ste 300, Atlanta, GA 30309; **Phone:** 404-605-2800; **Board Cert:** Cardiovascular Disease 2003; Interventional Cardiology 2005; **Med School:** Duke Univ 1995; **Resid:** Internal Medicine, Johns Hopkins Hosp 1998; **Fellow:** Cardiovascular Disease, Duke Univ 2002; Interventional Cardiology, Duke Univ 2004

Khawaja, Shazib N MD [IC] - **Spec Exp:** Peripheral Vascular Disease; Vascular Medicine; Echocardiography; Nuclear Cardiology; **Hospital:** Tanner Med Ctr; **Address:** 705 Dixie St, Ste 401, Carrollton, GA 30117; **Phone:** 770-836-9326; **Board Cert:** Cardiovascular Disease 2001; Interventional Cardiology 2003; Vascular Medicine 2007; **Med School:** Univ S Ala Coll Med 1995; **Resid:** Internal Medicine, Albany Med Ctr 1998; **Fellow:** Cardiovascular Disease, Dartmouth Hitchcock Med Ctr 2000; Interventional Cardiology, Univ Minnesota Med Ctr 2002; **Fac Appt:** Asst Clin Prof Med, Emory Univ

Knopf, William D MD [IC] - **Spec Exp:** Coronary Angioplasty/Stents; Angioplasty; Carotid Artery Stent Placement; Angiogenesis; **Hospital:** Piedmont Hosp; **Address:** Piedmont Heart Inst, 275 Collier Rd, Ste 300, Atlanta, GA 30309; **Phone:** 404-605-2800; **Board Cert:** Internal Medicine 1982; Cardiovascular Disease 1985; Interventional Cardiology 2009; **Med School:** Emory Univ 1979; **Resid:** Internal Medicine, Parkland Hosp 1982; **Fellow:** Cardiovascular Disease, Emory Univ Hosp 1985; **Fac Appt:** Assoc Clin Prof Med, Med Coll GA

Margolis, James MD [IC] - **Spec Exp:** Cardiac Catheterization; Angioplasty & Stent Placement; **Hospital:** Jackson Meml Hosp (page 70); **Address:** Jackson Med Group Specialty Physicians, 9380 SW 150th St, Ste 290B, Miami Beach, FL 33176; **Phone:** 305-256-5018; **Board Cert:** Internal Medicine 1973; Cardiovascular Disease 1975; **Med School:** Univ IL Coll Med 1968; **Resid:** Internal Medicine, Barnes Hosp 1972; **Fellow:** Cardiovascular Disease, Duke Med Ctr 1974; **Fac Appt:** Clin Prof Med, Univ Miami Sch Med

Matar, Fadi MD [IC] - **Spec Exp:** Angioplasty; **Hospital:** Tampa Genl Hosp, St. Joseph's Hosp - Tampa; **Address:** 509 S Armenia Ave, Ste 200, Tampa, FL 33609; **Phone:** 813-353-1515; **Board Cert:** Cardiovascular Disease 2007; Interventional Cardiology 2009; **Med School:** Amer Univ Beirut 1987; **Resid:** Internal Medicine, Maryland Genl Hosp 1990; **Fellow:** Cardiovascular Disease, Wash Hosp Ctr 1994; **Fac Appt:** Asst Prof Med, Univ S Fla Coll Med

Interventional Cardiology

Morris, Douglas C MD [IC] - **Spec Exp:** Angioplasty; Cardiac Catheterization; Heart Valve Disease; **Hospital:** Emory Univ Hosp, Emory Univ Hosp Midtown; **Address:** Emory Clinic - Cardiology, 1365 Clifton Rd NE, A Bldg Fl 2, Atlanta, GA 30322; **Phone:** 404-778-5299; **Board Cert:** Internal Medicine 1973; Cardiovascular Disease 1975; **Med School:** Baylor Coll Med 1968; **Resid:** Internal Medicine, Vanderbilt Univ Med Ctr 1970; Internal Medicine, Vanderbilt Univ Med Ctr 1973; **Fellow:** Cardiovascular Disease, Emory Univ Hosps 1975; **Fac Appt:** Prof Med, Emory Univ

Reddy, Bhagat K MD [IC] - **Spec Exp:** Angioplasty & Stent Placement; Carotid Artery Stent Placement; Peripheral Vascular Disease; Intravascular Ultrasound; **Hospital:** Piedmont Hosp; **Address:** Piedmont Heart Inst, 275 Collier Rd NW, Ste 300, Atlanta, GA 30309; **Phone:** 404-605-2800; **Board Cert:** Cardiovascular Disease 2002; Interventional Cardiology 2003; Vascular Medicine 2004; **Med School:** India 1995; **Resid:** Internal Medicine, Robert Packer Hosp 1999; **Fellow:** Cardiovascular Disease, Med Coll Ohio 2002; Interventional Cardiology, Vanderbilt Univ 2003

Midwest

Bach, Richard G MD [IC] - **Spec Exp:** Cardiac Catheterization; Acute Coronary Syndromes; Cardiomyopathy-Hypertrophic; **Hospital:** Barnes-Jewish Hosp; **Address:** Washington Univ Sch Med, Cardiovascular Div, 660 S Euclid Ave, Campus Box 8086, St Louis, MO 63110; **Phone:** 314-362-1963; **Board Cert:** Internal Medicine 1987; Cardiovascular Disease 2001; Interventional Cardiology 2000; **Med School:** NYU Sch Med 1984; **Resid:** Internal Medicine, Bellvue Hosp/NYU Med Ctr 1987; **Fellow:** Cardiovascular Disease, Bellvue Hosp/NYU Med Ctr 1990; Interventional Cardiology, NYU Med Ctr 1991; **Fac Appt:** Assoc Prof Med, Washington Univ, St Louis

Dieter, Robert S MD [IC] - **Spec Exp:** Vascular Medicine; Peripheral Vascular Disease; Angioplasty & Stent Placement; Renal Artery Stenosis; **Hospital:** Loyola Univ Med Ctr; **Address:** Loyola Univ MC, Dept Cardiology, EMS Bldg, 2150 S First Ave, Maywood, IL 60153; **Phone:** 708-216-4466; **Board Cert:** Internal Medicine 2000; Cardiovascular Disease 2002; Interventional Cardiology 2003; **Med School:** Univ IL Coll Med 1996; **Resid:** Internal Medicine, UIC Med Ctr 1999; Cardiovascular Disease, Univ Wisconsin 2002; **Fellow:** Interventional Cardiology, Univ Wisconsin; Vascular Medicine, Georgetown Univ; **Fac Appt:** Asst Prof Med, Loyola Univ-Stritch Sch Med

Ellis, Stephen G MD [IC] - **Spec Exp:** Angioplasty & Stent Placement; Angiogenesis; **Hospital:** Cleveland Clin (page 56); **Address:** Cleveland Clinic, Div Cardiovasc Med, 9500 Euclid Ave, Desk J2-3, Cleveland, OH 44195; **Phone:** 216-445-6712; **Board Cert:** Internal Medicine 1981; Cardiovascular Disease 1985; Interventional Cardiology 2009; **Med School:** UCLA 1978; **Resid:** Internal Medicine, Cedars-Sinai Med Ctr 1981; **Fellow:** Cardiovascular Disease, Stanford Univ Med Ctr 1985; Interventional Cardiology, Emory Univ Hosp 1986; **Fac Appt:** Prof Med, Cleveland Cl Coll Med/Case West Res

Feldman, Ted E MD [IC] - **Spec Exp:** Angioplasty; **Hospital:** Evanston/North Shore Univ Hlth Sys; **Address:** ENH Med Group, Cardiology, 2650 Ridge Ave Walgreen Bldg Fl 3, Evanston, IL 60201; **Phone:** 847-570-2250; **Board Cert:** Internal Medicine 1981; Cardiovascular Disease 1985; Interventional Cardiology 2009; **Med School:** Indiana Univ 1978; **Resid:** Internal Medicine, Rush-Presby-St Lukes Hosp 1982; **Fellow:** Cardiovascular Disease, Univ Chicago 1985; **Fac Appt:** Prof Med, Northwestern Univ

Henry, Timothy D MD [IC] - **Spec Exp:** Acute Coronary Syndromes; Angiogenesis; **Hospital:** Abbott - Northwestern Hosp; **Address:** Minneapolis Heart Inst, 920 E 28th St, Ste 100, Minneapolis, MN 55407; **Phone:** 612-863-3900; **Board Cert:** Internal Medicine 1985; Cardiovascular Disease 1989; Interventional Cardiology 2000; **Med School:** UCSF 1982; **Resid:** Internal Medicine, Univ Colorado Hosp 1985; **Fellow:** Cardiovascular Disease, Univ Minnesota 1990; Interventional Cardiology, Univ Minnesota 1991; **Fac Appt:** Prof Med, Univ Minn

Holmes Jr, David R MD [IC] - **Spec Exp:** Heart Attack; Acute Coronary Syndromes; Angioplasty & Restenosis; **Hospital:** Mayo Med Ctr & Clin - Rochester; **Address:** Mayo Clinic, Div Cardiovasc Dis, 200 First St SW, Rochester, MN 55905; **Phone:** 507-255-2504; **Board Cert:** Internal Medicine 1974; Cardiovascular Disease 1977; Interventional Cardiology 1999; **Med School:** Med Coll Wisc 1971; **Resid:** Internal Medicine, Mayo Clinic 1974; **Fellow:** Cardiovascular Disease, Mayo Clinic 1977; **Fac Appt:** Prof Med, Mayo Med Sch

Lasala, John M MD/PhD [IC] - **Spec Exp:** Coronary Artery Disease; Coronary Angioplasty/Stents; Cardiac Catheterization; Aortic Diseases & Dissection; **Hospital:** Barnes-Jewish Hosp; **Address:** Washington Univ School of Medicine, 660 Euclid Ave, Box 8086, St Louis, MO 63110; **Phone:** 314-747-4535; **Board Cert:** Internal Medicine 1986; Cardiovascular Disease 1989; Interventional Cardiology 2009; **Med School:** Univ Conn 1983; **Resid:** Internal Medicine, Barnes Jewish Hosp 1986; **Fellow:** Cardiovascular Disease, Yale-New Haven Hosp 1989; Interventional Cardiology, Yale-New Haven Hosp 1990; **Fac Appt:** Assoc Prof Med, Washington Univ, St Louis

Losordo, Douglas W MD [IC] - **Spec Exp:** Stem Cell Therapy in Heart Failure; Angiogenesis; Angioplasty & Stent Placement; Heart Attack; **Hospital:** Northwestern Meml Hosp; **Address:** 675 N St Clair St, Galter Bldg Fl 11 - Ste 240, Chicago, IL 60611; **Phone:** 312-695-0072; **Board Cert:** Internal Medicine 1986; Cardiovascular Disease 1989; Interventional Cardiology 2002; **Med School:** Univ VT Coll Med 1983; **Resid:** Internal Medicine, St Elizabeth's Med Ctr 1986; **Fellow:** Cardiovascular Disease, St Elizabeth's Med Ctr 1989; **Fac Appt:** Prof Med, Northwestern Univ-Feinberg Sch Med

Schreiber, Theodore L MD [IC] - **Spec Exp:** Coronary Angioplasty/Stents; Carotid Artery Disease; Aortic Diseases & Dissection; **Hospital:** Harper Univ Hosp; **Address:** Harper Univ Hosp, 3990 John R St, Webber Bldg - Ste 9370, Detroit, MI 48201; **Phone:** 313-745-7025; **Board Cert:** Internal Medicine 1981; Cardiovascular Disease 1983; Interventional Cardiology 2000; **Med School:** Cornell Univ-Weill Med Coll 1978; **Resid:** Internal Medicine, NY Hosp-Cornell Med Ctr 1981; **Fellow:** Cardiovascular Disease, NY Hosp-Cornell Med Ctr 1983; **Fac Appt:** Assoc Prof Med, Wayne State Univ

Whitlow, Patrick MD [IC] - **Spec Exp:** Cardiac Catheterization; **Hospital:** Cleveland Clin (page 56); **Address:** Cleveland Clinic, Dept Cardiology, 9500 Euclid Ave, Desk J2-3, Cleveland, OH 44195; **Phone:** 216-444-1746; **Board Cert:** Internal Medicine 1979; Cardiovascular Disease 1981; Interventional Cardiology 1999; **Med School:** Duke Univ 1976; **Resid:** Internal Medicine, Parkland Meml Hosp 1979; **Fellow:** Cardiovascular Disease, Univ Alabama Hosp 1979

Southwest

Bailey, Steven R MD [IC] - **Spec Exp:** Coronary Artery Disease; Coronary Angioplasty/Stents; Congenital Heart Disease; Heart Valve Disease; **Hospital:** Univ Hlth Syst-San Antonio, Christus Santa Rosa Med Ctr Hosp; **Address:** 8300 Floyd Curl Drive Fl 3, San Antonio, TX 78229-3900; **Phone:** 210-567-4601; **Board Cert:** Internal Medicine 1981; Cardiovascular Disease 1983; Interventional Cardiology 2009; **Med School:** Oregon Hlth & Sci Univ 1978; **Resid:** Internal Medicine, Fitzsimmons AMC 1981; **Fellow:** Cardiovascular Disease, Fitzsimmons AMC 1983; **Fac Appt:** Prof Med, Univ Tex, San Antonio

Kleiman, Neal Stephen MD [IC] - **Spec Exp:** Angioplasty; **Hospital:** Methodist Hosp - Houston; **Address:** 6550 Fannin St, Ste 1901, Smith Tower, Houston, TX 77030; **Phone:** 713-441-1100; **Board Cert:** Internal Medicine 1984; Cardiovascular Disease 1987; Interventional Cardiology 2009; **Med School:** Columbia P&S 1981; **Resid:** Internal Medicine, Baylor Coll Med 1984; **Fellow:** Interventional Cardiology, Baylor Coll Med 1987; **Fac Appt:** Assoc Prof Med, Baylor Coll Med

Interventional Cardiology

Perin, Emerson C MD/PhD [IC] - **Spec Exp:** Stem Cell Therapy in Heart Failure; Angiogenesis; **Hospital:** St. Luke's Episcopal Hosp-Houston; **Address:** Southwest Cardiology Consultants, 6624 Fannin St, Ste 2220, St Lukes Medical Tower Fl 22, Houston, TX 77030-2334; **Phone:** 713-791-9400; **Board Cert:** Internal Medicine 1988; Cardiovascular Disease 2010; **Med School:** Brazil 1983; **Resid:** Internal Medicine, Jackson Meml Hosp 1988; **Fellow:** Cardiovascular Disease, St Luke's Episcopal Hosp 1991; **Fac Appt:** Asst Prof Med, Baylor Coll Med

Smalling, Richard Warren MD/PhD [IC] - **Spec Exp:** Coronary Artery Disease; Peripheral Vascular Disease; Heart Valve Disease; Congenital Heart Disease; **Hospital:** Meml Hermann Hosp - Texas Med Ctr; **Address:** 6431 Fannin St, MSB 1.246, Houston, TX 77030-1501; **Phone:** 713-500-6559; **Board Cert:** Internal Medicine 1978; Cardiovascular Disease 1981; Interventional Cardiology 2009; **Med School:** Univ Tex, Houston 1975; **Resid:** Internal Medicine, UCSD Med Ctr 1978; **Fellow:** Cardiovascular Disease, UCSD Med Ctr 1980; **Fac Appt:** Prof Med, Univ Tex, Houston

West Coast and Pacific

Mahmud, Ehtisham MD [IC] - **Spec Exp:** Cardiac Catheterization; Carotid Artery Stent Placement; Stem Cell Therapy in Heart Failure; Gene Therapy; **Hospital:** UCSD Med Ctr; **Address:** 9434 Medical Center Drive, MC 7784, La Jolla, CA 92037; **Phone:** 619-543-5990; **Board Cert:** Cardiovascular Disease 2010; Interventional Cardiology 2001; **Med School:** Univ Alberta 1989; **Resid:** Internal Medicine, UC San Diego 1995; **Fellow:** Cardiovascular Disease, UC San Diego 1999; Interventional Cardiology, Emory Univ 2000; **Fac Appt:** Asst Prof Med, UCSD

Teirstein, Paul S MD [IC] - **Spec Exp:** Coronary Angioplasty/Stents; Heart Valve Disease; **Hospital:** Scripps Green Hosp; **Address:** Scripps Clinic, 10666 N Torrey Pines Rd, Mail Drop S1056, La Jolla, CA 92037; **Phone:** 858-554-9905; **Board Cert:** Internal Medicine 1983; Cardiovascular Disease 1987; Interventional Cardiology 2009; **Med School:** Mount Sinai Sch Med 1980; **Resid:** Internal Medicine, Brigham & Womens Hosp 1983; **Fellow:** Cardiovascular Disease, Stanford Univ 1986; Interventional Cardiology, Mid-Amer Heart Inst 1987

Yeung, Alan C MD [IC] - **Spec Exp:** Mitral Valve Disease; Coronary Artery Disease; **Hospital:** Stanford Univ Hosp & Clinics; **Address:** Stanford Univ Med Ctr, Div Interventional Cardiology, 300 Pasteur Drive, rm H2103, MC 5218, Stanford, CA 94305-5218; **Phone:** 650-723-0180; **Board Cert:** Internal Medicine 1987; Cardiovascular Disease 1989; Interventional Cardiology 2010; **Med School:** Harvard Med Sch 1984; **Resid:** Internal Medicine, Mass Gen Hosp 1987; **Fellow:** Cardiovascular Disease, Brigham & Womens Hosp 1990; **Fac Appt:** Prof Med, Stanford Univ

Cleveland Clinic

Every life deserves world class care.

Cleveland Clinic
Heart & Vascular Institute
9500 Euclid Avenue
Cleveland, OH 44195

Cardiovascular Disease

Cleveland Clinic's Sydell and Arnold Miller Family Heart & Vascular Institute is one of the largest and most experienced cardiovascular specialty groups in the world, providing patients with expert medical management and a full range of therapies. Our areas of expertise combine research, education and clinical practice to provide innovative and scientifically based treatments for cardiovascular disease. *U.S.News & World Report* has ranked Cleveland Clinic best in the nation for heart care every year since 1995.

Patients come to the Heart & Vascular Institute from every state in the country and from around the world. In 2010, our staff recorded more than 370,000 patient visits, completed more than 13,000 procedures, performed more than 4,000 open cardiac surgeries and more than 1,300 thoracic surgeries.

Clinical Trials and Research

Our Heart & Vascular Institute is a recognized leader in multicenter and international trials. An outstanding clinical infrastructure and strong commitment to basic science places Cleveland Clinic on the cutting edge of treatment and research in cardiovascular disease. Currently, Cleveland Clinic is conducting more than 200 trials and clinical research projects. Our researchers are investigating new alternative treatment options for patients with severe aortic valve stenosis and are researching non-invasive repair of the mitral and tricuspid valves.

History of Innovations

Cleveland Clinic doctors and researchers have helped define the modern era of cardiovascular care, having pioneered coronary angiography and saphenous vein bypass surgery. Today, our staff continues this proud tradition of innovation and discovery to shape the future of cardiovascular care.

clevelandclinic.org/
hearttopdocs

Offering Same-Day Appointments
Call 800.274.2009.

Treatment Guides

Cleveland Clinic has developed comprehensive treatment guides for many diseases and conditions. To download our free treatment guides, visit clevelandclinic.org/treatmentguides.

Online Medical Second Opinion

Cleveland Clinic's My**Consult** Online Medical Second Opinion program securely connects patients to our physician specialists for more than 1,000 life-changing or life-threatening diagnoses all by the click of a mouse. To learn more, log onto eclevelandclinic.org/myconsult or call 800.223.2273, ext. 43223.

Special Assistance for Out-of-State Patients

Cleveland Clinic Global Patient Services offers a complimentary Medical Concierge service for patients who travel from outside of Ohio. Call 800.223.2273, ext. 55580 or email medicalconcierge@ccf.org.

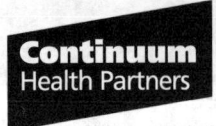

Beth Israel Medical Center
Roosevelt Hospital
St. Luke's Hospital
New York Eye & Ear

Cardiac Services

(800) 420-4004

Continuum Health Partners offers outstanding cardiac programs at its member hospitals—Beth Israel Medical Center, Roosevelt Hospital and St. Luke's Hospital—with a constant dedication to clinical excellence.

The Continuum hospitals offer the full array of clinical expertise needed to diagnose and treat the many conditions that can affect the heart, including coronary artery disease, heart valve insufficiencies, congenital and non-congenital structural abnormalities, hypertension, heart failure, heart rhythm abnormalities and hypertrophic cardiomyopathy.

We are strong believers in prevention and early detection, and our experts provide complete cardiac diagnostic testing, utilizing state-of-the-art echocardiography, nuclear and non-nuclear stress testing, angiography, PET scanning and more. We also offer programs for coronary artery disease prevention, smoking cessation, treatment centers for obesity and diabetes, and complementary techniques for relaxation and stress reduction, such as massage therapy and therapeutic touch.

Our state-of-the-art cardiac catheterization labs are available around the clock for emergency cardiac cases—when every minute counts—offering life-saving angioplasty to patients arriving in our emergency departments with acute heart attack conditions.

Our cardiac surgery outcomes have been recognized by the New York State Department of Health as having some of the lowest mortality rates in New York City, and our programs have maintained a consistent level of performance since their inception.

Some of the unique features in the cardiac programs at the Continuum hospitals include a nationally recognized arrhythmia service, CT angiography for non-invasive cardiac angiograms, minimally invasive radial artery harvesting for bypass surgery, medical and surgical management of hypertrophic cardiomyopathy, nationally and internationally recognized experts in heart failure, hypertension, and a commitment to research to find the cures of tomorrow.

Continuum Health Partners, Inc.

Beth Israel   **Roosevelt Hospital**   **St. Luke's Hospital**   **NY Eye & Ear Infirmary**

www.chpnyc.org

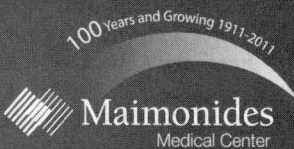
Having pioneered numerous heart care innovations through the years, the Cardiac Institute offers diagnostic studies and therapeutic treatments, procedures and surgeries. It has been ranked by the Centers for Medicare and Medicaid Services among the few hospitals achieving excellent ratings in both heart attack and heart failure patient outcomes.

Cardiology
Among the most published and respected in the field, the Maimonides cardiology team continuously sets higher standards for patient care. Edgar Lichstein, MD, Chair of Medicine, has been chief investigator of NIH-sponsored cardiac drug trials, and our Congestive Heart Failure (CHF) Program is among the most effective in the nation.

Interventional Cardiology
Led by Cardiac Institute Chair Jacob Shani, MD, numerous therapeutic devices have been developed and implemented here. Our Electrophysiology Lab has a superb record of achievement in diagnosing and treating arrhythmias. A close collaboration with the Department of Emergency Medicine ensures that chest pain patients are evaluated immediately and that interventional procedures are used to stop heart attacks in progress whenever necessary.

Cardiothoracic Surgery
The Maimonides Cardiothoracic Surgery program has an illustrious history, setting a national standard for advances in cardiothoracic. Under the direction of Greg Ribakove, MD, minimally invasive and robotic heart surgeries are offered in state-of-the-art facilities. In collaboration with Electrophysiology, Cardiothoracic Surgery has established an Atrial Fibrillation Center of Excellence. Maimonides provides one of the most prestigious cardiothoracic residency programs in the US.

Historic Moments
- In 1967, the first successful human heart transplant in the nation was performed at Maimonides.
- The intra-aortic balloon pump was developed here in 1970.
- Surgical techniques that protect the spine during cardiothoracic surgery were perfected here in 1982.
- Revolutionary cardiac catheterization devices were invented here in 1992 and 1997.
- Maimonides was the first hospital in the US to implement fully automatic external cardiac defibrillators in 2001.

The Centers for Medicare and Medicaid Services, an agency of the federal government, recently published the latest data on 30-day mortality rates for hospitals across the country. Maimonides Medical Center achieved better-than-expected results in all three categories measured – heart attack, heart failure and pneumonia – a distinction only 20 hospitals in the U.S. achieved. In fact, Maimonides was 9th lowest for heart failure, 8th lowest for heart attack, and the single lowest for patients being treated for pneumonia.

Maimonides Medical Center
Passionate about medicine.
Compassionate about people.

www.maimonidesmed.org/cardiac

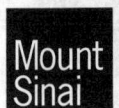 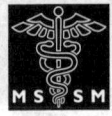

**MOUNT SINAI
SCHOOL OF
MEDICINE**

THE MOUNT SINAI MEDICAL CENTER
MOUNT SINAI HEART—CARDIOVASCULAR HEALTH

One Gustave L. Levy Place
Fifth Avenue and 100th Street
New York, NY 10029-6574
Physician Referral: 1-800-MD-SINAI (637-4624)
www.mountsinai.org/heart

At **MOUNT SINAI HEART**, we take both a personal and a global view of cardiovascular health. Our integrated system of care brings together the world's most accomplished physicians, research scientists, and educators who deliver creative programs and an unwavering commitment to the prevention and treatment of cardiovascular disease. With access to the latest discoveries and a diversity of the most experienced minds, our doctors ensure that patients receive the best individualized care. The rapid translation of innovative research into prevention, diagnosis, and therapy means that patients receive multidisciplinary treatment of unprecedented quality. Our programs treat patients from the earliest stages of life (our pediatric cardiologists can detect cardiac disease in the unborn fetus) well into the advanced elderly years (through specialized geriatric cardiology).

We specialize in consultative cardiology, cardiac catheterization, heart and lung transplantation, cardiovascular surgery, heart failure, pulmonary hypertension, lipid management, and hypertension, as well as:

Noninvasive diagnostic imaging – State-of-the-art echocardiography, nuclear cardiology, PET, CT, and MRI technology;

Coronary artery disease – We are ranked as New York State's safest and highest volume center for coronary angioplasty and other catheter-based procedures;

Cardiac rhythm disturbances – Expert management of all aspects of heart rhythm disorders is provided under the auspices of pioneers in the field, including for atrial fibrillation (AFib), the most common abnormal heart rhythm, and ventricular tachycardias, the most common cause of sudden cardiac death, as well as implantable devices, such as pacemakers and defibrillators;

Valvular heart disease – Medical and surgical options, including a leading valve-repair program and long-term follow-up care;

Aortic diseases – Pioneering techniques for stent-graft repair of thoracic and abdominal aortic aneurysms and for surgical correction of the most complex aortic pathology;

Congenital heart disease – Expertise in pediatric cardiology and in minimally invasive approaches to the correction of congenital heart defects in children and adults;

Cardiac failure and transplantation – A multidisciplinary team approach to comprehensive, compassionate care for patients with the most advanced forms of heart failure and cardiomyopathy;

Comprehensive cardiac disease prevention and rehabilitation – A unique synergism provides unparalleled patient care and breakthroughs in cardiovascular disease prevention and treatment, while promoting cardiovascular health globally through six projects around the world;

LEADING SURGEONS, INNOVATIVE TREATMENTS
Under the direction of internationally renowned cardiologist Valentin Fuster, MD, PhD, Mount Sinai Heart is recognized worldwide for expert evaluation, management, and prevention of cardiovascular disease through integrated patient care, education, and research. Mount Sinai Heart encompasses the Zena and Michael A. Wiener Cardiovascular Institute and the Marie-Josée and Henry R. Kravis Center for Cardiovascular Health at Mount Sinai, both preeminent resources for the study and treatment of heart and blood vessel diseases.

Vascular medicine and surgery – Noninvasive diagnostic procedures and an interdisciplinary approach to disease management, including medical, surgical, catheter-based, and gene therapy techniques for arterial obstruction, limb salvage, venous, and lymphatic diseases. A pioneer in large-artery stenting, Mount Sinai fostered the development of stenting of abdominal aortic aneurysms.

Mount Sinai's Cardiac Catheterization Laboratory – Studies the heart with the most precise technologies available, including diagnostic angiography, angioplasty, and biopsy. In a statewide study, our Cath Lab was found to be the safest, with the lowest 30-day risk-adjusted mortality rate for percutaneous coronary intervention (angioplasty), as well as the busiest.

NewYork-Presbyterian
The University Hospital of Columbia and Cornell

Affiliated with Columbia University College of Physicians and Surgeons and Weill Cornell Medical College

NewYork-Presbyterian Hospital
Columbia University Medical Center
622 West 168th Street
New York, NY 10032

NewYork-Presbyterian Hospital
Weill Cornell Medical Center
525 East 68th Street
New York, NY 10065

1-877-NYP-WELL (1-877-697-9355)   www.nyp.org/heart

NewYork-Presbyterian Heart

NewYork-Presbyterian Hospital has leading clinical programs for patients with coronary artery disease and a wide range of other heart disorders, with particular expertise in the management of:

- Aortic aneurysms: ruptures, acute dissections, and trauma, with rapid diagnosis and effective medical and surgical interventions

- Heart failure: featuring a robust mechanical circulatory support program. Patients come from all over the world for placement of ventricular assist devices to be used long-term or as a bridge to transplant. NewYork-Presbyterian Hospital/Columbia University Medical Center is one of the world's leading institutions for heart transplantation and is one of the few centers offering patients a total artificial heart

- Cardiac rhythm abnormalities: with experienced electrophysiologists who diagnose and treat atrial fibrillation and other arrhythmias using pacemakers, implantable cardioverter defibrillators, ablation, and novel approaches to restore normal heart rhythm

- Valve disorders: using minimally invasive surgical approaches whenever possible. NewYork-Presbyterian Hospital investigators led the PARTNER Trial, which in 2011 demonstrated that transcatheter aortic valve implantation (TAVI) was as effective as conventional open-heart surgery for reducing mortality among high-risk patients with aortic stenosis

- Heart disorders in the elderly: NewYork-Presbyterian Hospital surgeons have earned a reputation for performing heart surgery on the very elderly (over age 80), achieving excellent outcomes

- Patients who require surgery may receive treatment using a robotic approach, delivered using the Siemens Artis zeego® medical imaging system. This system provides surgeons with exceptional visualization of blood vessels.

A Reputation for Excellence

At NewYork-Presbyterian Hospital, the optimal care of patients with heart disease is achieved by combining an experienced team of clinicians with the latest advances in technology. Basic science and clinical research efforts are aimed at developing more effective ways to prevent, diagnose, and treat cardiac disorders. NewYork-Presbyterian Hospital features renowned cardiac care programs in the following areas:

- Cardiac diagnostics
- Electrophysiology
- Clinical cardiology
- Interventional cardiology
- Cardiac assist devices
- Cardiothoracic surgery, including transplantation
- Mitral Valve Repair

NewYork-Presbyterian Hospital is designated by the Society of Chest Pain Centers as an Accredited Chest Pain Center, dedicated to reducing heart-related deaths by improving the response time for the diagnosis and treatment of chest pain.

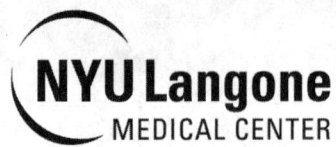

CARDIAC SURGERY

NYU Langone Medical Center is one of the largest cardiac surgery centers in the tri-state area, and a nationally recognized leader in advanced treatment and technology for adult, pediatric and congenital heart disease. World renowned surgeons at the Medical Center pioneered minimally invasive heart surgery and valve repair or replacement, and have since performed over 5,000 minimally invasive procedures. They also perform state-of-the-art surgical procedures for structural and valvular heart disease, coronary artery disease, congenital heart disease, and aortic aneurysm disease, while specializing in cardiac surgery for high-risk and elderly patients

Center for Structural and Valvular Heart Disease
Mitral Valve Repair. NYU Langone's heart surgeons introduced mitral valve repair to the U.S. more than 30 years ago, and have since performed over 3,800 mitral valve repairs, the most in the country.
High Risk Cardiac Surgery. Our cardiac surgery team specializes in the surgical care of high-risk patients, including re-operative surgery in the elderly, coronary bypass surgery, heart valve repair or replacement, surgical repair of the failing heart, and ventricular assist device implantation.
Minimally Invasive Cardiac Surgery. NYU Langone is in the vanguard of minimally invasive cardiac surgery, the benefits of which include reduced pain, lower risk of bleeding and infection, and a quicker recovery.

Center for Aortic Diseases
The Medical Center is committed to a multidisciplinary approach in the treatment of complex aortic disease, and the long-term management of patients with residual aortic dissection and connective tissue disorders. A wide range of treatment and therapeutic options is offered, including open surgery and stent graft therapy for patients with aortic aneurysms, aortic dissections and inherited diseases of the aorta, like Marfan's syndrome.

Center for Pediatric and Adult Congenital Heart Disease
The Division of Pediatric and Adult Congenital Cardiac Surgery treats patients of all ages with inherited and acquired cardiac defects. Our surgeons are experts in reconstructive procedures for complex cardiovascular disorders. The Division maintains a highly experienced team of specialists in pediatric and adult cardiology, neonatal and pediatric cardiac intensive care, pediatric cardiac anesthesiology, nursing, and extracorporeal perfusion.

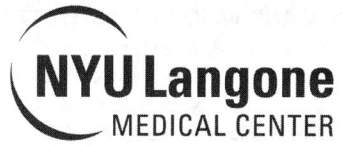

CARDIAC AND VASCULAR INSTITUTE

The Cardiac and Vascular Institute (CVI) at NYU Langone Medical Center continues to lead in developing new techniques for repairing heart valves, curing heart rhythm disorders, treating aortic diseases and congestive heart failure. CVI is consistently ranked among the leading heart and heart surgery centers in U.S. News & World Report's annual 'Best Hospitals' rankings.

Cardiac Catheterization
CVI offers superior catheter-based diagnosis and evaluation of cardiac health. Our laboratory provides a full range of procedures to evaluate, diagnose, and recommend treatment options.

Cardiac Rehabilitation and Prevention
The Joan and Joel Smilow Cardiac and Pulmonary Rehabilitation and Prevention Center focuses on individualized patient care in a state-of-the-art facility.

Cardiac Surgery
CVI is a nationally recognized leader in advanced treatments for adult and congenital heart disease. Our team has performed over 5,000 minimally invasive surgical procedures since pioneering the technique in 1996, and offers over 30 years of experience in mitral valve repair, valve replacement and aortic aneurysm repair, specializing in high-risk and elderly patients.

Cardiology
The Leon H. Charney Division of Cardiology is a leader in cardiovascular biomedical research, patient care and education. We are advancing the field of cardiovascular medicine and continually contribute to NYU Langone's comprehensive cardiovascular center of excellence.

Heart Failure
We offer the most advanced echocardiograms, pacemaker or defibrillator implantations, open heart surgeries (including promising new procedures to reshape the hearts of patients with chronic heart failure), and left ventricular assist devices (LVADs).

Nuclear Cardiology/Stress
The Nuclear Cardiology/Stress Laboratory performs a range of tests that assist cardiologists in the diagnosis and assessment of many forms of heart disease.

Vascular Surgery
We offer minimally invasive diagnostic and treatment approaches and have treated thousands of patients with conditions ranging from arterial aneurysms to deep vein thrombosis, as well as carotid stenosis and limb salvage. We offer minimally invasive vein surgery, endovascular aortic surgery, thoracic aneurysm correction and abdominal aneurysm interventions.

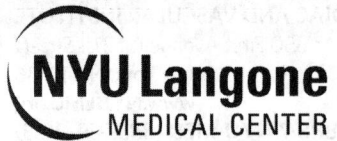

ADULT CARDIOVASCULAR SERVICES

The Cardiac and Vascular Institute (CVI) at NYU Langone Medical Center continues to lead in developing new techniques for repairing heart valves, curing heart rhythm disorders, and treating aortic diseases and congestive heart failure. CVI is consistently ranked among the leading heart and heart surgery centers in U.S. News & World Report's annual 'Best Hospitals.'

Cardiac Catheterization
The Cardiac Catheterization Laboratory offers superior catheter-based diagnosis and evaluation of cardiac health. It provides a full range of procedures to evaluate heart muscle, valves, and coronary arteries and recommends appropriate treatment as needed.

Cardiac Rehabilitation and Prevention
The Joan and Joel Smilow Cardiac Rehabilitation and Prevention Center focuses on individualized patient care in a state-of-the-art facility.

Cardiac Surgery
The Division of Cardiac Surgery is a nationally recognized leader with a multidisciplinary approach in performing more than 5,000 minimally invasive heart surgery procedures since pioneering the technique in 1996. Moreover it offers over 30 years experience in mitral valve repairs as well as heart valve replacements and aortic aneurysm repairs.

Cardiology
The Leon H. Charney Division of Cardiology is a leader in cardiovascular biomedical research, patient care and education. Clinicians and researchers are advancing the field of cardiovascular medicine and contributing to the reputation of NYU Langone Medical Center as a comprehensive cardiovascular center of excellence.

Heart Failure
The cardiologists and surgeons at the Heart Failure Center offer advanced echocardiograms, pacemaker/defibrillator implantations, open heart surgeries and ventricular assist devices.

Nuclear Cardiology/Stress
The Nuclear Cardiology/Stress Laboratory performs a range of tests that assist cardiologists in the diagnosis and assessment of many forms of heart disease.

Vascular Surgery
The Division of Vascular and Endovascular Surgery has treated thousands of patients for arterial aneurysms, deep vein thrombosis, carotid stenosis and limb salvage, emphasizing minimally invasive diagnostic and treatment approaches.

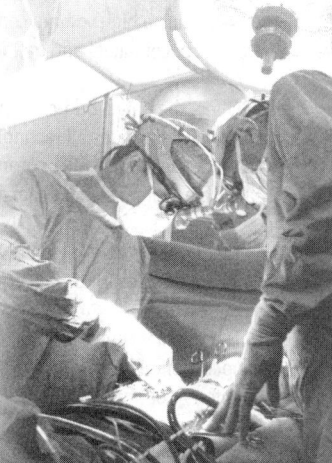

![Penn Medicine logo]

Penn Medicine

Philadelphia, PA 19104
800.789.PENN
PennMedicine.org

PENN HEART AND VASCULAR

Penn Heart and Vascular combines the renowned expertise of its clinicians, researchers and educators to bring hope to and provide a better quality of life for patients whose options are limited by conventional medicine. Penn Medicine is leading heart and vascular care beyond those limits, delivering advanced patient care every day.

World-Class Heart and Vascular Care

Penn Heart and Vascular is recognized as one of the nation's leading cardiovascular programs offering patients a wide range of diagnostic, medical, interventional and surgical treatment options that are not available anywhere else in the region, including but not limited to:

- Consultations and 2nd opinions
- Preventive approaches to treat cardiovascular risk factors
- Complex lipid disease management
- Heart failure management
- Familial cardiomyopathy diagnosis and evaluation
- Pulmonary hypertension management
- Cardiac interventions
- Implantable cardiac defibrillators and pacemakers
- Ablation therapy for heart rhythm disorders
- Transcatheter Aortic Valve Replacement (TAVR)
- Minimally invasive valve repair and replacement
- Endovascular stent graft repair for thoracic aortic aneurysms
- Congenital heart repair
- Mechanical assist devices
- Heart transplantation

State-of-the-Art Technology and Research

- Among the few surgical institutions in the nation with a fully incorporated research facility, Penn ensures the future progress of cardiovascular research.

- Pioneering the most advanced techniques and devices, such as ablation therapy for ventricular tachycardia and atrial
- Offering a full-range of surgical options including transcatheter, minimally invasive robotic, off-pump, port access and bloodless techniques, Penn offers patients every option.
- Conducting numerous clinical studies, such as mechanical assist devices and percutaneous approaches to treating valve disease, Penn brings the latest treatments to patients first.
- Serving as the lead national site for several trials, including endovascular stent graft repair for thoracic aortic aneurysms, Penn cardiac and vascular surgeons collaborate to improve patient care.
- Implanting the first temporary total artificial heart in the region, Penn continues to bring a new generation of ventricular assist devices to the treatment of late-stage heart failure.

A National and Regional Referral Center

- Penn Heart and Vascular is among the nation's top 3 adult heart transplant centers, performing more adult heart transplants than all other Philadelphia area hospitals combined.
- Penn offers the most advanced mechanical assist device options for patients with end-stage heart failure and for those patients awaiting heart transplantation.
- The Hospital of the University of Pennsylvania has the largest EP program on the east coast and one of the two largest single-hospital programs in the country.
- The Hospital of the University of Pennsylvania (HUP) was the first in the region to use implantable devices for patients at risk for recurrent sustained VT or fibrillation and to improve cardiac function in patients with heart failure.

- Penn has the largest valve program in the region with a nationally recognized team of physician who perform more minimally invasive valve repairs and replacements with better patient outcomes.
- Penn is one of the largest valve centers in the U.S. for advanced port access surgery for mitral valve repair or replacement.
- Penn is participating in landmark clinical trials, including trials to develop the latest mechanical-assist devices and pioneer transcatheter-based approaches to heart valve replacement.

Recognized Expertise

- Penn Heart and Vascular at the Hospital of the University of Pennsylvania is ranked 10th in the nation, and best in the Philadelphia region, for cardiology and heart surgery by *U.S.News & World Report*
- The Hospital of the University of Pennsylvania and Penn Presbyterian Medical Center are recognized *Blue Distinction Centers for Cardiac Care* by Independence Blue Cross.
- *Best Doctors in America*® lists more doctors from Penn Medicine than any other academic medical center or health system in the Philadelphia region.

St. Francis Hospital The Heart Center®

100 Port Washington Blvd.
Roslyn, New York 11576
www.stfrancisheartcenter.com
(516) 562-6000 1-888-HEARTNY

A Leader in Cardiac Care

St. Francis Hospital, The Heart Center® is New York State's only specialty designated cardiac center and is one of the busiest heart centers in the nation. Located in Roslyn, New York, on Long Island's North Shore, St. Francis Hospital has been ranked among the best hospitals in the United States for the fifth consecutive year by *U.S. News & World Report* in heart and heart surgery and geriatrics, and neurology and neurosurgery.

St. Francis Hospital:

• Has a highly experienced team of physicians and surgeons with one of the highest volumes in the nation for cardiac surgery, interventional and arrhythmia procedures.

• Offers innovative approaches to cardiac surgery, including minimally invasive procedures and off-pump coronary artery bypass surgery, designed to minimize trauma and reduce surgical complications

• Performs one of the region's highest volumes of catheter-based techniques to close atrial septal defects (ASDs) and patent foramen ovale (PFO)

• Operates a nationally recognized Arrhythmia and Pacemaker Center staffed with electrophysiologists with over a decade of experience in radiofrequency ablation, a permanent cure for certain arrhythmias, including atrial fibrillation

• Maintains a high volume center for the implantation of cardiac pacemakers and defibrillators

• Offers the only world-class program in cardiac imaging that fully integrates all technologies, including advanced methods in cardiac MRI, coronary CT angiography, PET/CT and three-dimensional echocardiography

• Has received the Magnet Award for excellence in nursing services for the second time

• Is a premier center for clinical trials and studies of the application of image-guided methods of diagnosis and treatment of heart disease

St. Francis Hospital has near-perfect patient satisfaction ratings, with over 99 percent of patients saying they would recommend the Hospital to family and friends.

"Our large cardiac caseload and our growing research program put us in an excellent position to introduce new techniques that can benefit thousands of people in need each year."

–Alan D. Guerci, M.D.
President and Chief Executive Officer
St. Francis Hospital, The Heart Center®

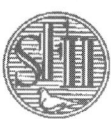

St. Francis Hospital The Heart Center®
100 Port Washington Blvd.
Roslyn, New York 11576
www.stfrancisheartcenter.com
(516) 562-6000   1-888-HEARTNY

Noninvasive Cardiac Imaging

Using the latest in noninvasive cardiac imaging technology, St. Francis Hospital's physicians can evaluate blood flow, heart muscle strength, anatomy, and coronary artery blockages, allowing them to more effectively guide a patient's course of treatment.

Among the most recent advances in St. Francis Hospital's range of services are:

Coronary CT Angiography

St. Francis Hospital was the first hospital on Long Island to offer Multidetector Computed Tomography (MDCT) for noninvasive coronary artery imaging. Now, with installation of more advanced technology, St. Francis can minimize radiation exposure for every patient.

Cardiac MRI

The only center on Long Island with a dedicated Cardiac MRI program and world-class expertise in cardiac MRI, St. Francis Hospital uses MRI to evaluate heart anatomy, function, blood flow, scarring and inflammation using advanced techniques on two state-of-the-art scanners. Cardiac MRI allows physicians to evaluate effects of heart attack and coronary artery blockages and noncoronary causes of heart failure to determine whether or not patients will benefit from heart surgery or other therapies. World-renowned cardiac MRI authority Nathaniel Reichek, M.D., leads St. Francis Hospital's clinical and research applications with cardiac MRI.

Three-Dimensional Echocardiography

St. Francis Hospital is an internationally recognized leader in three-dimensional echocardiography for quantifying the effects of heart disease and is the leading center in the New York metropolitan area in this field. By creating three-dimensional reconstructions of the heart and blood flow within it, this technology provides diagnostic information that far surpasses that available with conventional echocardiography in many patients.

Nuclear Imaging

Conventional nuclear imaging involves the injection of nuclear isotopes and imaging by a gamma camera that circles the patient's body, improving the accuracy of stress testing. St. Francis Hospital offers the latest advances in nuclear cardiology, such as positron emission tomography of the heart with CT attenuation correction (PET/CT). The nuclear cardiology laboratory at St. Francis Hospital is also a leader in developing new types of computer analysis to improve the value of all forms of cardiac nuclear imaging, and was among the first facilities in the U.S. to receive accreditation from The Intersocietal Commission for the Accreditation of Nuclear Medicine Laboratories.

Noninvasive Imaging at St. Francis Hospital

Noninvasive imaging services at St. Francis Hospital include:

• Multidetector computed tomographic coronary angiography
• Cardiac MRI
• SPECT/CT nuclear Imaging
• Cardiac PET/CT imaging
• Transesophageal echocardiography
• Three-dimensional echocardiography
• Stress testing with nuclear, echocardiographic or MRI imaging.

St. Francis Hospital's leading-edge noninvasive imaging technology is also being applied in its research programs on cardiovascular disease. Drawing on its depth of experience with various imaging modalities, the Hospital has launched a multi-disciplinary effort at its St. Francis Cardiac Research Institute to improve methods for the diagnosis and treatment of cardiac disease. Past research efforts at the Hospital include The St. Francis Heart Study–a pioneering effort and the largest study of CT calcium scoring to be conducted at any single center—which supported the use of CT calcium scoring for atherosclerotic plaque detection as a tool in cardiac risk evaluation.

Vanderbilt Heart and Vascular Institute

Medical Center East | 1215 21st Ave. S. | Nashville, TN 37232 | (615) 322-2318 | VanderbiltHeart.com

Overview

Vanderbilt Heart is the top provider of cardiology and heart surgery in Middle Tennessee and southern Kentucky. We are the only program in either state ranked in the nation's top 50 by *U.S. News & World Report*.

We treat patients with many kinds of cardiovascular disease, including very complex cases. We offer a wide range of services at our main Vanderbilt campus in Nashville as well as 23 locations in Tennessee and Kentucky.

Treatment Programs

Vanderbilt Heart offers the latest in heart treatments and programs. These include programs for acquired and inherited heart disease in adults; arrhythmia; atrial fibrillation; cardiac surgery; congestive heart failure; general cardiology; heart transplant; interventional cardiology and radiology; heart disease prevention; valve repair and replacement; vascular surgery; and heart disease in women.

Our Team

Our team of cardiologists, surgeons, nurses and staff is highly skilled and specialized in many areas of heart care. We value a culture of collaboration that ensures each patient receives personalized, compassionate care from a team of experts.

DISCOVERY AND INNOVATION

Our PREDICT program is the first of its kind in a U.S. academic medical center. PREDICT uses genetic tests to find which blood-thinning and cholesterol-lowering drugs will be most effective for each patient. The information goes into our advanced electronic medical record, which allows our doctors to choose the right dose of the right drug, the first time.

We are the only center in Tennessee to study a new way to replace the aortic valve without open-heart surgery. This minimally invasive technique allows for a smaller incision, requires less time to perform and can reduce recovery time. Learn more.

When heart attack patients are on their way to Vanderbilt, we use a proven therapy that cools the body. This prevents brain damage, which can make for a better recovery.

Vanderbilt University Medical Center was the first hospital in the region to offer a novel approach to cardiac surgery that's raising our standard of care. Our Hybrid Operating Room/Catheterization Lab houses equipment and monitoring devices for open-heart surgeries such as coronary bypass as well as less invasive procedures such as angioplasty and stenting. If a patient needs two kinds of heart procedures, they can be done at the same time. This can cut down on complications and costs.

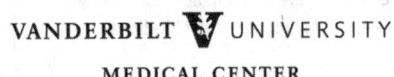

VANDERBILT UNIVERSITY
MEDICAL CENTER

Child Neurology
a subspecialty of Neurology

A neurologist specializes in the diagnosis and treatment of all types of disease or impaired function of the brain, spinal cord, peripheral nerves, muscles and autonomic nervous system, as well as the blood vessels that relate to these structures. A child neurologist has special skills in the diagnosis and management of neurologic disorders of the neonatal period, infancy, early childhood and adolescence.

Training Required: Four years

CHILD NEUROLOGY

New England

Bourgeois, Blaise MD [ChiN] - **Spec Exp:** Epilepsy/Seizure Disorders; **Hospital:** Children's Hospital - Boston; **Address:** Chldn's Hosp-Boston, Fegan 9, 300 Longwood Ave, Boston, MA 02115; **Phone:** 617-355-2413; **Board Cert:** Pediatrics 1981; Child Neurology 1990; Clinical Neurophysiology 1992; **Med School:** Switzerland 1971; **Resid:** Neurology, Washington Univ/Barnes Jewish Hosp 1979; Child Neurology, Washington Univ/Barnes Jewish Hosp 1981; **Fellow:** Neurological Pharmacology, Washington Univ/Barnes Jewish Hosp 1982; **Fac Appt:** Prof N, Harvard Med Sch

Darras, Basil T MD [ChiN] - **Spec Exp:** Neuromuscular Disorders; Cerebral Palsy; **Hospital:** Children's Hospital - Boston; **Address:** 300 Longwood Ave, Childrens Hosp, Neurology, Fegan 11, Boston, MA 02115; **Phone:** 617-355-8235; **Board Cert:** Clinical Genetics 1987; Pediatrics 1988; Child Neurology 1992; Neuromuscular Medicine 2008; **Med School:** Greece 1977; **Resid:** Pediatrics, Nassau County Med Ctr 1982; Child Neurology, Tufts-New England Med Ctr 1985; **Fellow:** Clinical Genetics, Yale Univ Sch Med 1988; **Fac Appt:** Prof N, Harvard Med Sch

Griesemer, David A MD [ChiN] - **Spec Exp:** Epilepsy/Seizure Disorders; Brain Injury; **Hospital:** Tufts Med Ctr, Floating Hosp for Children at Tufts Med Ce; **Address:** Tufts Med Ctr, 800 Washington St, Box 330, Boston, MA 02111; **Phone:** 617-636-8100; **Board Cert:** Child Neurology 1992; **Med School:** Johns Hopkins Univ 1976; **Resid:** Pediatrics, Johns Hopkins Hosp 1978; **Fellow:** Child Neurology, Univ Michigan Hosp 1985; **Fac Appt:** Prof N, Tufts Univ

Holmes, Gregory L MD [ChiN] - **Spec Exp:** Epilepsy/Seizure Disorders; **Hospital:** Dartmouth - Hitchcock Med Ctr; **Address:** Dartmouth-Hitchcock Med Ctr, Dept Neurology, 1 Medical Center Drive, Lebanon, NH 03756; **Phone:** 603-650-4211; **Board Cert:** Pediatrics 1979; Neurology 1980; **Med School:** Univ VA Sch Med 1974; **Resid:** Pediatrics, Yale-New Haven Hosp 1976; **Fellow:** Pediatric Neurology, Univ Virginia 1979; **Fac Appt:** Prof N, Dartmouth Med Sch

Mandelbaum, David E MD/PhD [ChiN] - **Spec Exp:** Epilepsy/Seizure Disorders; Neonatal Neurology; Autism; **Hospital:** Rhode Island Hosp, Women & Infants Hosp of RI; **Address:** Dept of Neurology, 593 Eddy St George Bldg, Providence, RI 02903; **Phone:** 401-444-5685; **Board Cert:** Child Neurology 1987; Pediatrics 1987; Clinical Neurophysiology 2003; Neurodevelopmental Disabilities 2001; **Med School:** Columbia P&S 1980; **Resid:** Pediatrics, Yale-New Haven Hosp 1982; Neurology, Neuro Inst-Columbia 1983; **Fellow:** Child Neurology, Neuro Inst-Columbia 1985; **Fac Appt:** Prof Ped, Brown Univ

Pomeroy, Scott L MD/PhD [ChiN] - **Spec Exp:** Neuro-Oncology; Brain Tumors; **Hospital:** Children's Hospital - Boston, Dana-Farber Cancer Inst (page 57); **Address:** Chldns Hosp, Dept Neurology-Fegan 11, 300 Longwood Ave, Boston, MA 02115; **Phone:** 617-355-6386; **Board Cert:** Child Neurology 1988; **Med School:** Univ Cincinnati 1982; **Resid:** Pediatrics, Chldns Hosp 1984; Neurology, Barnes Hosp/Washington Univ 1985; **Fellow:** Pediatric Neurology, St Louis Chldns Hosp 1987; Neurological Biology, Washington Univ 1990; **Fac Appt:** Prof N, Harvard Med Sch

Sahin, Mustafa MD/PhD [ChiN] - **Spec Exp:** Tuberous Sclerosis; Cerebrovascular Malformations; Sturge-Weber Syndrome; Cortical Malformations; **Hospital:** Children's Hospital - Boston; **Address:** Childrens Hosp Boston, 300 Longwood Ave, Fegan 11, Boston, MA 02115; **Phone:** 617-355-8994; **Board Cert:** Child Neurology 2001; **Med School:** Yale Univ 1995; **Resid:** Pediatrics, Chldns Hosp 1997; Child Neurology, Chldns Hosp 2000; **Fac Appt:** Asst Prof N, Harvard Med Sch

Shaywitz, Bennett A MD [ChiN] - **Spec Exp:** Learning Disorders; Dyslexia; Headache; **Hospital:** Yale-New Haven Hosp, Yale Med Group; **Address:** Yale Univ Sch Med, Dept Peds, 333 Cedar St, Box 208064, New Haven, CT 06520-8064; **Phone:** 203-785-4641; **Board Cert:** Pediatrics 1968; Child Neurology 1973; **Med School:** Washington Univ, St Louis 1963; **Resid:** Pediatrics, Bronx Muni Hosp Ctr 1967; **Fellow:** Child Neurology, Albert Einstein Coll Med 1970; **Fac Appt:** Prof Ped, Yale Univ

Volpe, Joseph J MD [ChiN] - **Spec Exp:** Neonatal Neurology; Cerebral Palsy; **Hospital:** Children's Hospital - Boston, Mass Genl Hosp; **Address:** 300 Longwood Ave, Fegan 11, Boston, MA 02115-5724; **Phone:** 617-355-8994; **Board Cert:** Pediatrics 1970; Child Neurology 1974; **Med School:** Harvard Med Sch 1964; **Resid:** Pediatrics, Mass Genl Hosp 1966; Neurology, Mass Genl Hosp 1971; **Fellow:** Research, Natl Inst Child Hlth Human Dev 1968; **Fac Appt:** Prof N, Harvard Med Sch

Mid Atlantic

Allen, Jeffrey MD [ChiN] - **Spec Exp:** Neuro-Oncology; Brain Tumors; **Hospital:** NYU Langone Med Ctr (page 66); **Address:** Hassenfeld Childrens Ctr, 160 E 32nd St Fl 2nd - Ste L3, New York, NY 10016; **Phone:** 212-263-9907; **Board Cert:** Child Neurology 1977; **Med School:** Harvard Med Sch 1969; **Resid:** Pediatrics, Montreal Chldns Hosp 1973; Pediatric Neurology, Montreal Neur Inst/McGill 1976; **Fac Appt:** Prof Ped, NYU Sch Med

Bergman, Ira MD/PhD [ChiN] - **Spec Exp:** Complex Diagnosis; Neuro-Oncology; **Hospital:** Chldns Hosp of Pittsburgh - UPMC; **Address:** Chldns Hosp Pittsburgh, 4401 Penn Ave, Pittsburgh, PA 15224; **Phone:** 412-692-5520; **Board Cert:** Pediatrics 1981; Child Neurology 1980; **Med School:** Univ Chicago-Pritzker Sch Med 1974; **Resid:** Pediatrics, Mass Genl Hosp 1976; **Fellow:** Neurology, Mass Genl Hosp 1979; **Fac Appt:** Assoc Prof Ped, Univ Pittsburgh

Comi, Anne M MD [ChiN] - **Spec Exp:** Sturge-Weber Syndrome; **Hospital:** Kennedy Krieger Inst, Johns Hopkins Hosp (page 61); **Address:** Kennedy-Krieger Institute, 707 N Broadway, Baltimore, MD 21205; **Phone:** 443-923-9150; **Board Cert:** Child Neurology 2000; **Med School:** SUNY Buffalo 1993; **Resid:** Pediatrics, Childrens Hosp Buffalo 1996; Pediatric Neurology, Johns Hopkins Hospital 1999; **Fac Appt:** Assoc Prof N, Johns Hopkins Univ

Crawford, Thomas O MD [ChiN] - **Spec Exp:** Neuromuscular Disorders; Muscular Dystrophy; Ataxia Telangiectasia; **Hospital:** Johns Hopkins Hosp (page 61); **Address:** Pediatric Neurology, 200 N Wolfe St, Ste 2158, Baltimore, MD 21287; **Phone:** 410-955-4259; **Board Cert:** Pediatrics 1986; Child Neurology 1990; **Med School:** USC Sch Med 1980; **Resid:** Pediatrics, LAC-USC Med Ctr 1984; Child Neurology, Chldns Hosp 1987; **Fellow:** Neuromuscular Medicine, Johns Hopkins Hosp 1988; **Fac Appt:** Assoc Prof N, Johns Hopkins Univ

De Vivo, Darryl C MD [ChiN] - **Spec Exp:** Metabolic Disorders; Neuromuscular Disorders; Spinal Muscular Atrophy (SMA); **Hospital:** NY-Presby/Columbia Univ Med Ctr, NY (page 65); **Address:** Neurological Institute, 710 W 168th St, rm 201, New York, NY 10032; **Phone:** 212-305-5244; **Board Cert:** Child Neurology 1972; **Med School:** Univ VA Sch Med 1964; **Resid:** Pediatrics, Mass Genl Hosp 1966; Neurology, Mass Genl Hosp 1967; **Fellow:** Neurology, Natl Inst Hlth 1969; Child Neurology, Children's Hosp 1970; **Fac Appt:** Prof N, Columbia P&S

Duffner, Patricia K MD [ChiN] - **Spec Exp:** Brain Tumors; Krabbe Disease; Cancer Survivors-Late Effects of Therapy; **Hospital:** Women's & Chldn's Hosp of Buffalo, The; **Address:** Women & Childrens Hosp, Dept Neurology, 219 Bryant St, Buffalo, NY 14222-2006; **Phone:** 716-878-7819; **Board Cert:** Pediatrics 1977; Child Neurology 1979; **Med School:** SUNY Buffalo 1972; **Resid:** Pediatrics, Buffalo Chldns Hosp 1975; **Fellow:** Child Neurology, SUNY Buffalo 1978; **Fac Appt:** Prof N, SUNY Buffalo

Child Neurology

Eviatar, Lydia MD [ChiN] - **Spec Exp:** Balance Disorders; Tourette's Syndrome; Headache; Cerebral Palsy; **Hospital:** Steven & Alexandra Cohen Chldn's Med Ctr of NY; **Address:** 410 Lakeville Rd, Ste 105, New Hyde Park, NY 11042-1433; **Phone:** 516-465-5255; **Board Cert:** Pediatrics 1969; Child Neurology 1977; **Med School:** Israel 1961; **Resid:** Pediatrics, Tel Hashomer Hosp 1966; Neurology, Montefiore Med Ctr 1977; **Fellow:** Developmental-Behavioral Pediatrics, UCLA Med Ctr 1967; Pediatric Neurology, UCLA Med Ctr 1969; **Fac Appt:** Prof N, Albert Einstein Coll Med

Finkel, Richard S MD [ChiN] - **Spec Exp:** Neuromuscular Disorders; **Hospital:** Chldns Hosp of Philadelphia; **Address:** Children's Hosp of Philadelphia, Neurology Division, 34th St & Civic Ctr Blvd, Philadelphia, PA 19104; **Phone:** 215-590-2763; **Board Cert:** Pediatrics 1984; Child Neurology 1986; Neuromuscular Medicine 2008; **Med School:** Washington Univ, St Louis 1978; **Resid:** Pediatrics, Chldn's Hosp 1980; **Fellow:** Neurology, Chldn's Hosp/ Brigham & Women's Hosp 1983; **Fac Appt:** Clin Prof Ped, Univ Pennsylvania

Ichord, Rebecca N MD [ChiN] - **Spec Exp:** Stroke in Children; Brain Injury; **Hospital:** Chldns Hosp of Philadelphia; **Address:** Children's Hosp of Philadelphia, Wood Ctr Fl 6, 34th & Civic Ctr Blvd, Philadelphia, PA 19104-4318; **Phone:** 215-590-4142; **Board Cert:** Pediatrics 1984; Child Neurology 1992; **Med School:** Geo Wash Univ 1979; **Resid:** Pediatrics, Children's Natl Med Ctr 1983; **Fellow:** Developmental-Behavioral Pediatrics, Johns Hopkins Hosp 1985; Child Neurology, Johns Hopkins Hosp 1991; **Fac Appt:** Assoc Prof N, Univ Pennsylvania

Kosofsky, Barry MD/PhD [ChiN] - **Spec Exp:** Developmental Disorders; Autism; Stroke; **Hospital:** NY-Presby/Weill Cornell Med Ctr, NY (page 65); **Address:** NY-Cornell Med Ctr, Dept Pediatrics, 525 E 68th St, Box 91, New York, NY 10065; **Phone:** 212-746-3278; **Board Cert:** Child Neurology 1993; **Med School:** Johns Hopkins Univ 1985; **Resid:** Pediatrics, Chldns Hosp 1987; Child Neurology, Mass Genl Hosp 1990; **Fellow:** Neurological Biology, Mass Genl Hosp 1992; **Fac Appt:** Prof Ped, Cornell Univ-Weill Med Coll

Legido, Agustin MD/PhD [ChiN] - **Spec Exp:** Mitochondrial Disorders; Neonatal Neurology; Epilepsy; **Hospital:** St. Christopher's Hosp for Chldn; **Address:** St Christopher's Hospital, Dept Neurology, 3601 A St, Philadelphia, PA 19134; **Phone:** 215-427-5452; **Board Cert:** Pediatrics 2011; Child Neurology 1991; **Med School:** Spain 1980; **Resid:** Pediatrics, St Christopher's Chldns Hosp 1989; Neurology, Hosp Univ Penn 1990; **Fellow:** Child Neurology, Chldns Hosp 1988; **Fac Appt:** Prof Ped, Drexel Univ Coll Med

Maytal, Joseph MD [ChiN] - **Spec Exp:** Epilepsy/Seizure Disorders; Migraine; **Hospital:** Steven & Alexandra Cohen Chldn's Med Ctr of NY; **Address:** Dept Pediatric Neurology, 410 Lakeville Rd, Ste 105, New Hyde Park, NY 11042; **Phone:** 516-465-5255; **Board Cert:** Pediatrics 1986; Child Neurology 1988; **Med School:** Israel 1979; **Resid:** Pediatrics, Brookdale Hosp 1983; Child Neurology, Montefiore Med Ctr 1986; **Fellow:** Neurological Physiology, Albert Einstein Med Coll 1987; **Fac Appt:** Clin Prof N, Albert Einstein Coll Med

Mink, Jonathan W MD/PhD [ChiN] - **Spec Exp:** Movement Disorders; Tourette's Syndrome; Dystonia; **Hospital:** Univ of Rochester Strong Meml Hosp; **Address:** Univ Rochester, Child Neurology, 601 Elmwood Ave, Box 631, Rochester, NY 14642; **Phone:** 585-275-2808; **Board Cert:** Child Neurology 2007; **Med School:** Washington Univ, St Louis 1989; **Resid:** Pediatrics, St Louis Chldns Hosp 1991; Neurology, Barnes Hosp 1992; **Fellow:** Child Neurology, St Louis Chldns Hosp 1994; **Fac Appt:** Prof N, Univ Rochester

Nass, Ruth MD [ChiN] - **Spec Exp:** Autism; ADD/ADHD; Learning Disorders; Migraine; **Hospital:** NYU Langone Med Ctr (page 66); **Address:** 577 First Ave, New York, NY 10016; **Phone:** 212-263-7753; **Board Cert:** Pediatrics 1980; Child Neurology 1981; **Med School:** Albert Einstein Coll Med 1975; **Resid:** Pediatrics, NY Hosp 1977; Child Neurology, Columbia-Presby 1980; **Fellow:** Neurology, NY Hosp 1982; **Fac Appt:** Prof N, NYU Sch Med

Packer, Roger J MD [ChiN] - **Spec Exp:** Brain Tumors; Neurofibromatosis; **Hospital:** Chldns Natl Med Ctr; **Address:** Chldns Natl Med Ctr, Dept Neurology, 111 Michigan Ave NW, Washington, DC 20010-2978; **Phone:** 202-476-6230; **Board Cert:** Child Neurology 1982; Pediatrics 1982; **Med School:** Northwestern Univ 1976; **Resid:** Pediatrics, Chldns Med Ctr 1978; Neurology, Chldns Hosp-Univ Penn 1981; **Fac Appt:** Prof N, Geo Wash Univ

Phillips, Peter C MD [ChiN] - **Spec Exp:** Brain Tumors; Neuro-Oncology; **Hospital:** Chldns Hosp of Philadelphia; **Address:** Chldns Hosp Philadelphia, 34th St & Civic Center Blvd, CTRB Bldg - Ste 4027, Philadelphia, PA 19104; **Phone:** 215-590-5188; **Board Cert:** Pediatrics 1985; Child Neurology 1986; **Med School:** Univ Conn 1978; **Resid:** Pediatrics, Chldns Hosp 1980; Pediatric Neurology, Neuro Inst 1983; **Fellow:** Neuro-Oncology, Meml Sloan Kettering Cancer Ctr 1986; **Fac Appt:** Prof N, Univ Pennsylvania

Riviello Jr, James J MD [ChiN] - **Spec Exp:** Epilepsy/Seizure Disorders; Epilepsy in Tuberous Sclerosis; Electrical Status Epilepticus Of Sleep; **Hospital:** NYU Langone Med Ctr (page 66); **Address:** NYU Epilepsy and Neurology Center, 223 E 34th St, New York, NY 10016; **Phone:** 646-558-0871; **Board Cert:** Pediatrics 1984; Child Neurology 1985; Clinical Neurophysiology 2006; **Med School:** Tufts Univ 1978; **Resid:** Pediatrics, St Christopher Hosp Chldn 1980; Neurology, Temple Univ Hosp 1983; **Fellow:** Pediatric Neurology, St Christopher Hosp Chldn 1983; **Fac Appt:** Prof N, NYU Sch Med

Santos, Cesar C MD [ChiN] - **Spec Exp:** Epilepsy; Sleep Disorders; Stroke in Children; Clinical Trials; **Hospital:** Georgetown Univ Hosp; **Address:** Georgetown Univ Hosp, Peds-Child Neuro, 3800 Reservoir Rd NW Fl 2, Pasquerilla Healthcare Ctr, Washington, DC 20007; **Phone:** 202-444-8785; **Board Cert:** Pediatrics 2004; Child Neurology 2004; Clinical Neurophysiology 2005; **Med School:** Philippines 1982; **Resid:** Pediatrics, St Lukes Roosevelt Hosp 1988; **Fellow:** Neurology, Duke Univ Med Ctr 1991; Neurological Physiology, Duke Univ 1992; **Fac Appt:** Prof N, Wake Forest Univ

Shinnar, Shlomo MD/PhD [ChiN] - **Spec Exp:** Epilepsy/Seizure Disorders; Headache; **Hospital:** Montefiore Med Ctr - Div. Moses; **Address:** Montefiore Med Ctr, Children's Hospital, 111 E 210th St Fl 4, Bronx, NY 10467-2401; **Phone:** 718-920-4378; **Board Cert:** Neurology 1984; Pediatrics 1984; Clinical Neurophysiology 2005; **Med School:** Albert Einstein Coll Med 1978; **Resid:** Pediatrics, Johns Hopkins Hosp 1980; Neurology, Johns Hopkins Hosp 1983; **Fac Appt:** Prof N, Albert Einstein Coll Med

Southeast

Dure, Leon S MD [ChiN] - **Spec Exp:** Huntington's Disease; Tourette's Syndrome; Movement Disorders; **Hospital:** Children's Hospital - Birmingham, Univ of Ala Hosp at Birmingham; **Address:** UAB Pediatric Neurology, 1600 7th Ave S, CHB 314, Birmingham, AL 35233-0011; **Phone:** 205-996-7850; **Board Cert:** Child Neurology 1991; **Med School:** Baylor Coll Med 1984; **Resid:** Pediatrics, Columbia Presby Hosp 1986; Child Neurology, Texas Chldns Hosp 1989; **Fellow:** Child Neurology, Univ Michigan Affil Hosp 1990; **Fac Appt:** Prof N, Univ Alabama

Goldstein, Edward M MD [ChiN] - **Spec Exp:** Neuromuscular Disorders; Headache; Cerebral Palsy; Botox Therapy; **Hospital:** Chldns Hlthcare Atlanta @ Scottish Rite; **Address:** 5505 Peachtree Dunwoody Rd, Ste 500, Atlanta, GA 30342; **Phone:** 404-256-3535; **Board Cert:** Child Neurology 1994; **Med School:** Johns Hopkins Univ 1985; **Resid:** Pediatrics, Johns Hopkins Hosp 1987; Neurology, Johns Hopkins Hosp 1990; **Fellow:** Neuromuscular Disease, Emory Univ 1993; **Fac Appt:** Assoc Clin Prof N, Mercer Univ Sch Med

Child Neurology

Greenwood, Robert S MD [ChiN] - **Spec Exp:** Neurofibromatosis; Epilepsy; **Hospital:** NC Memorial Hosp - UNC; **Address:** 101 Manning Drive, CB Box #7025, Chapel Hill, NC 27599; **Phone:** 919-966-2528; **Board Cert:** Pediatrics 1974; Child Neurology 1979; **Med School:** Univ Tex Med Br, Galveston 1968; **Resid:** Pediatrics, Chldns Hosp 1971; Child Neurology, Chldns Hosp 1975; **Fellow:** Child Neurology, Chldns Hosp 1977; **Fac Appt:** Prof N, Univ NC Sch Med

Lavenstein, Bennett L MD [ChiN] - **Spec Exp:** Movement Disorders; Neuromuscular Disorders; **Hospital:** Chldns Natl Med Ctr, Inova Fairfax Hosp for Chldn; **Address:** 8501 Arlington Blvd, Ste 200, Fairfax, VA 22031; **Phone:** 571-226-8368; **Board Cert:** Pediatrics 1977; Child Neurology 1979; **Med School:** Univ MD Sch Med 1974; **Resid:** Pediatrics, Univ of MD Hlth System 1977; Neurology, Georgetown Univ Hosp 1979; **Fellow:** Neuromuscular Medicine, Natl Inst Hlth; **Fac Appt:** Assoc Clin Prof N, Univ VA Sch Med

Tennison, Michael MD [ChiN] - **Spec Exp:** Epilepsy; Headache; Neurophysiology; Neurogenetics; **Hospital:** NC Memorial Hosp - UNC; **Address:** UNC Chapel Hill- Pediatric Neurology, Campus Box 7025, Chapel Hill, NC 27599-7025; **Phone:** 919-966-2528; **Board Cert:** Pediatrics 1979; Child Neurology 1983; **Med School:** Harvard Med Sch 1975; **Resid:** Pediatrics, UCLA Affil Hosp 1978; Pediatric Neurology, Univ NC Hosp 1981; **Fellow:** Clinical Neurophysiology, Univ NC Hosp; **Fac Appt:** Prof N, Univ NC Sch Med

Weig, Spencer G MD [ChiN] - **Spec Exp:** Epilepsy; Neuromuscular Disorders; Neurophysiology; **Hospital:** NC Memorial Hosp - UNC; **Address:** UNC Chapel Hill- Pediatric Neurology, Campus Box 7025, Chapel Hill, NC 27599-7025; **Phone:** 919-966-2528; **Board Cert:** Pediatrics 1983; Child Neurology 1987; **Med School:** Mount Sinai Sch Med 1973; **Resid:** Pediatrics, Duke Univ Med Ctr 1975; Child Neurology, NC Meml Hosp 1986; **Fellow:** Electroencephalography, Univ Mass Med Ctr 1987; **Fac Appt:** Prof N, Univ NC Sch Med

Wheless, James W MD [ChiN] - **Spec Exp:** Epilepsy/Seizure Disorders; **Hospital:** Le Bonheur Chldns Med Ctr, St. Jude Children's Research Hosp; **Address:** 50 N Dunlap St, Ste L-80400, Memphis, TN 38103; **Phone:** 901-287-5060; **Board Cert:** Pediatrics 1987; Child Neurology 1989; Clinical Neurophysiology 2007; **Med School:** Univ Okla Coll Med 1982; **Resid:** Pediatrics, Univ Oklahoma Med Ctr 1985; **Fellow:** Pediatric Neurology, Chldns Meml Hosp 1988; Epilepsy, Med Coll Georgia Affil Hosp 1989; **Fac Appt:** Prof N, Univ Tenn Coll Med

Midwest

Brunstrom, Janice MD [ChiN] - **Spec Exp:** Cerebral Palsy; **Hospital:** St. Louis Chldns Hosp; **Address:** Washington Univ Sch Med, Dept Ped Neuro, 660 S Euclid Ave, Box 8111, St Louis, MO 63110; **Phone:** 314-454-6120; **Board Cert:** Pediatrics 2003; Child Neurology 2005; **Med School:** Med Coll VA 1987; **Resid:** Neurology, St Louis Chldns Hosp 1989; Neurology, Barnes Jewish Hosp 1990; **Fellow:** Child Neurology, St Louis Chldns Hosp 1995; **Fac Appt:** Asst Prof N, Washington Univ, St Louis

Cohen, Bruce H MD [ChiN] - **Spec Exp:** Brain Tumors; Mitochondrial Disorders; Neurometabolic Disorders; **Hospital:** Akron Children's Hosp; **Address:** 215 W Bowery St, rm 400, Akron, OH 44308; **Phone:** 330-543-6048; **Board Cert:** Pediatrics 2004; Child Neurology 1990; **Med School:** Albert Einstein Coll Med 1982; **Resid:** Pediatrics, Chldns Hosp 1984; Child Neurology, Neurologic Inst-Columbia 1987; **Fellow:** Pediatric Neuro-Oncology, Chldns Hosp 1989; **Fac Appt:** Prof Ped, NE Ohio Univ

Edgar, Terence MD [ChiN] - **Spec Exp:** Neuromuscular Disorders; Cerebral Palsy; Epilepsy; **Hospital:** St. Vincent Hosp - Green Bay; **Address:** Prevea Health, 1821 S Webster Fl 3, Green Bay, WI 54301; **Phone:** 920-272-1270; **Board Cert:** Pediatrics 2010; Child Neurology 2006; **Med School:** South Africa 1984; **Resid:** Pediatrics, Univ Wisconsin Hosp & Clin 1995; Child Neurology, Univ Wisconsin Hosp & Clin 1996; **Fellow:** Neuromuscular Disease, Univ Wisconsin Hosp & Clin 1996; Epilepsy, Mayo Clinic 2010

Epstein, Leon G MD [ChiN] - **Spec Exp:** Migraine; **Hospital:** Children's Mem Hosp -Chicago; **Address:** Chldns Meml Hosp, Div Neurology, 2300 Childrens Plaza, Box 51, Chicago, IL 60614; **Phone:** 773-880-4352; **Board Cert:** Child Neurology 1979; **Med School:** Wayne State Univ 1973; **Resid:** Neurology, St Josephs Mercy Hosp 1974; Neurology, Univ Arizona Med Ctr 1976; **Fellow:** Neurology, Columbia Presby Med Ctr 1978; **Fac Appt:** Prof Ped, Northwestern Univ

Hershey, Andrew D MD/PhD [ChiN] - **Spec Exp:** Headache; Migraine; **Hospital:** Cincinnati Chldns Hosp Med Ctr; **Address:** Children's Hospital, Dept Neurology, 3333 Burnet Ave, Cincinnati, OH 45229; **Phone:** 513-636-4222; **Board Cert:** Child Neurology 2008; **Med School:** Univ Wash 1992; **Resid:** Pediatrics, St Louis Children's Hosp 1995; Neurology, St Louis Children's Hosp 1997; **Fac Appt:** Prof Ped, Univ Cincinnati

Keating, Gesina F MD [ChiN] - **Spec Exp:** Brain Tumors; Spinal Tumors; Cancer Survivors-Late Effects of Therapy; Chiari's Deformity; **Hospital:** Mayo Med Ctr & Clin - Rochester; **Address:** 200 First St SW, Mayo Clinic, Rochester, MN 55905; **Phone:** 507-284-2511; **Board Cert:** Child Neurology 2008; **Med School:** Mayo Med Sch 1991; **Resid:** Pediatric Neurology, Mayo Clinic 1996; Pediatrics, Vanderbilt Univ Med Ctr 1999; **Fellow:** Pediatric Neuro-Oncology, Beth Israel Med Ctr 2000

Kotagal, Suresh MD [ChiN] - **Spec Exp:** Sleep Disorders/Apnea; **Hospital:** Mayo Med Ctr & Clin - Rochester, St. Mary's Hosp - Rochester MN (Mayo); **Address:** Mayo Clinic, 200 First St SW, Rochester, MN 55905-0002; **Phone:** 507-266-0774; **Board Cert:** Pediatrics 1979; Child Neurology 1982; **Med School:** India 1974; **Resid:** Child Neurology, Chldns Hosp Mich 1976; Pediatrics, St Louis Univ 1979; **Fellow:** Sleep Medicine, Stanford Univ 1982; **Fac Appt:** Prof N, Mayo Med Sch

Kovnar, Edward H MD [ChiN] - **Spec Exp:** Epilepsy/Seizure Disorders; Neurophysiology; Developmental Disorders; **Hospital:** Chldns Hosp - Wisconsin; **Address:** Advanced Healthcare, SC, 3003 W Good Hope Rd, Milwaukee, WI 53209-0996; **Phone:** 414-352-8828; **Board Cert:** Pediatrics 1984; Child Neurology 1984; Clinical Neurophysiology 2004; Neurodevelopmental Disabilities 2005; **Med School:** Washington Univ, St Louis 1977; **Resid:** Pediatrics, Chldns Hosp 1979; Neurology, Barnes Hosp 1980; **Fellow:** Pediatric Neurology, Chldns Hosp 1982; Clinical Neurophysiology, Chldns Hosp 1991

Noetzel, Michael MD [ChiN] - **Spec Exp:** Cerebral Palsy; Brain Injury; Movement Disorders; **Hospital:** St. Louis Chldns Hosp; **Address:** 660 S Euclid Ave, Box 8111, St Louis, MO 63110; **Phone:** 314-454-6120; **Board Cert:** Child Neurology 1984; Pediatrics 1984; **Med School:** Univ VA Sch Med 1977; **Resid:** Pediatrics, St Louis Chldns Hosp 1979; Neurology, Barnes Hosp 1980; **Fellow:** Child Neurology, St Louis Chldns Hosp 1982; **Fac Appt:** Prof Ped, Washington Univ, St Louis

Patterson, Marc C MD [ChiN] - **Spec Exp:** Neurogenetics; Developmental Delay; Metabolic Disorders; **Hospital:** Mayo Med Ctr & Clin - Rochester; **Address:** Mayo Clinic, Dept Neurology, 200 First St SW, Rochester, MN 55905; **Phone:** 507-266-0774; **Board Cert:** Child Neurology 2004; Neurodevelopmental Disabilities 2001; **Med School:** Australia 1981; **Resid:** Neurology, Univ Queenland 1988; Child Neurology, Mayo Clinic 1990; **Fellow:** Metabolic Neurology, Natl Inst Health 1992; Pediatrics, Mayo Cilnic 1993; **Fac Appt:** Prof N, Mayo Med Sch

Child Neurology

Scher, Mark S MD [ChiN] - **Spec Exp:** Epilepsy; Neonatal Neurology; **Hospital:** UH Rainbow Babies & Chldns Hosp (page 74), Univ Hosps Case Med Ctr (page 74); **Address:** UH Rainbow Babies & Children's Hospital, Pediatric Neurology, 11100 Euclid Ave, MS 6090, Cleveland, OH 44106; **Phone:** 216-844-3691; **Board Cert:** Pediatrics 1986; Child Neurology 1983; **Med School:** SUNY Downstate 1976; **Resid:** Pediatrics, NY Presby Hosp 1978; **Fellow:** Pediatric Neurology, Univ MN Med Ctr 1980; Epilepsy, Stanford Univ Med Ctr 1983; **Fac Appt:** Prof N, Case West Res Univ

Tonsgard, James MD [ChiN] - **Spec Exp:** Epilepsy/Seizure Disorders; Tuberous Sclerosis; **Hospital:** Univ of Chicago Med Ctr; **Address:** Univ Chicago Med Ctr, 5841 S Maryland Ave, MC 3055, Chicago, IL 60637-1463; **Phone:** 773-702-6487; **Board Cert:** Pediatrics 1981; **Med School:** Yale Univ 1975; **Resid:** Pediatrics, Yale-New Haven Hosp 1977; Neurology, Univ Chicago Hosp 1980; **Fellow:** Child Neurology, Univ Chicago Hosp 1981; **Fac Appt:** Assoc Prof Ped, Univ Chicago-Pritzker Sch Med

Tuxhorn, Ingrid E MD [ChiN] - **Spec Exp:** Epilepsy; Gravet Syndrome; **Hospital:** UH Rainbow Babies & Chldns Hosp (page 74), Univ Hosps Case Med Ctr (page 74); **Address:** UH Rainbow Babies & Children's Hospital, Pediatric Epileptology, 11100 Euclid Ave, MS 6009, Cleveland, OH 44106; **Phone:** 216-286-6644; **Board Cert:** Pediatrics 1985; **Med School:** Africa 1975; **Resid:** Pediatrics, Baystate Med Ctr 1982; Pediatrics, Yale-New Haven Hosp 1983; **Fellow:** Pediatric Neurology, U Mass Meml Med Ctr 1990; Neurological Physiology, Cleveland Clinic 1992; **Fac Appt:** Prof N, Case West Res Univ

Wiznitzer, Max MD [ChiN] - **Hospital:** UH Rainbow Babies & Chldns Hosp (page 74); **Address:** Rainbow Babies & Chldns Hosp, 11100 Euclid Ave, MS RBC6090, Cleveland, OH 44106; **Phone:** 216-844-3691; **Board Cert:** Pediatrics 1982; Child Neurology 1986; Neurodevelopmental Disabilities 2004; **Med School:** Northwestern Univ 1977; **Resid:** Pediatrics, Chldns Hosp Med Ctr 1980; **Fellow:** Developmental-Behavioral Pediatrics, Cincinnati Med Ctr 1981; Pediatric Neurology, Chldns Hosp 1984; **Fac Appt:** Assoc Prof Ped, Case West Res Univ

Wyllie, Elaine MD [ChiN] - **Spec Exp:** Epilepsy/Seizure Disorders; **Hospital:** Cleveland Clin (page 56); **Address:** Div Ped Neurology, 9500 Euclid Ave, Desk S51, Cleveland, OH 44195; **Phone:** 216-444-5559; **Board Cert:** Pediatrics 1982; Child Neurology 1986; **Med School:** Indiana Univ 1978; **Resid:** Pediatrics, Indiana Univ Med Ctr 1980; Pediatrics, Case West Med Ctr 1981; **Fellow:** Child Neurology, Cleveland Clinic 1984; Clinical Neurophysiology, Cleveland Clinic 1985; **Fac Appt:** Prof Ped, Cleveland Cl Coll Med/Case West Res

Yamada, Kelvin MD [ChiN] - **Spec Exp:** Epilepsy; **Hospital:** St. Louis Chldns Hosp; **Address:** St Louis Chldns Hosp-Neurology Div, 660 S Euclid Ave, Campus Box 8111, Saint Louis, MO 63110; **Phone:** 314-454-6120; **Board Cert:** Pediatrics 2004; Child Neurology 1990; Clinical Neurophysiology 2004; Sleep Medicine 2007; **Med School:** Baylor Coll Med 1983; **Resid:** Pediatrics, Baylor Coll Affil Hosp 1985; Neurology, Barnes-Jewish Hosp 1986; **Fellow:** Child Neurology, St Louis Chldn's Hosp 1990; **Fac Appt:** Prof Ped, Washington Univ, St Louis

Great Plains and Mountains

Bale Jr, James F MD [ChiN] - **Spec Exp:** Infections-Neurologic; Infections-Congenital; **Hospital:** Primary Children's Med Ctr, Univ Utah Hlth Care; **Address:** Primary Chldns Med Ctr, 100 N Mario Capecchi Drive, Salt Lake City, UT 84113; **Phone:** 801-587-7575; **Board Cert:** Pediatrics 2002; Child Neurology 1982; **Med School:** Univ Mich Med Sch 1975; **Resid:** Pediatrics, Univ Utah Hosps 1977; Neurology, Univ Utah Hosps 1980; **Fellow:** Infectious Disease, Univ Utah 1981; Neurovirology, UCSF-VA Med Ctr 1982; **Fac Appt:** Prof N, Univ Utah

Southwest

Iannaccone, Susan T MD [ChiN] - **Spec Exp:** Neuromuscular Disorders; **Hospital:** Chldns Med Ctr of Dallas, UT Southwestern Med Ctr at Dallas; **Address:** 1935 Med District Drive, F5.06, Dallas, TX 75207; **Phone:** 214-456-2768; **Board Cert:** Pediatrics 1975; Child Neurology 1976; **Med School:** SUNY Hlth Sci Ctr 1969; **Resid:** Pediatrics, St Louis Chldns Hosp 1972; Neurology, Strong Meml Hosp 1975; **Fellow:** Neurology, Strong Meml Hosp 1975

Sharp, Gregory B MD [ChiN] - **Spec Exp:** Epilepsy; **Hospital:** UAMS Med Ctr, Arkansas Chldns Hosp; **Address:** 1 Children's Way, Little Rock, AR 72202; **Phone:** 501-364-1100; **Board Cert:** Pediatrics 2011; Child Neurology 1993; **Med School:** Univ Ark 1984; **Resid:** Pediatrics, Univ Ark Chldns Hosp 1987; **Fellow:** Pediatric Neurology, Mayo Clinic 1990; **Fac Appt:** Prof Ped, Univ Ark

West Coast and Pacific

Ashwal, Stephen MD [ChiN] - **Spec Exp:** Metabolic Disorders; **Hospital:** Loma Linda Univ Med Ctr; **Address:** Pediatric Neurosciences Ctr, 2195 Club Ctr Drive, Ste A, San Bernadino, CA 92408; **Phone:** 909-835-1810; **Board Cert:** Pediatrics 1975; Child Neurology 1978; **Med School:** NYU Sch Med 1970; **Resid:** Pediatrics, Bellevue Hosp 1973; **Fellow:** Child Neurology, Univ Minn Med Ctr 1976; **Fac Appt:** Prof Ped, Loma Linda Univ

Ferriero, Donna MD [ChiN] - **Spec Exp:** Neuroendocrinology; **Hospital:** UCSF Med Ctr; **Address:** UCSF Med Ctr, 350 Parnassus Ave, Ste 609, San Francisco, CA 94117; **Phone:** 415-353-7596; **Board Cert:** Pediatrics 1986; Child Neurology 1987; **Med School:** UCSF 1979; **Resid:** Pediatrics, Mass Genl Hosp 1982; Child Neurology, UCSF Med Ctr 1985; **Fellow:** Neurological Endocrinology, UCSF Med Ctr 1987; **Fac Appt:** Prof N, UCSF

Fisher, Paul G MD [ChiN] - **Spec Exp:** Neuro-Oncology; Brain Tumors; **Hospital:** Lucile Packard Chldn's Hosp; **Address:** Stanford Cancer Ctr-Dept Neurology, 750 Welch Rd, Ste 317, MC 5, Palo Alto, CA 94304; **Phone:** 650-721-5889; **Board Cert:** Pediatrics 2003; Child Neurology 2008; **Med School:** UCSF 1989; **Resid:** Pediatrics, Johns Hopkins Univ Hosp 1991; Neurology, Johns Hopkins Univ Hosp 1994; **Fellow:** Neuro-Oncology, Children's Hosp 1994; **Fac Appt:** Assoc Prof Ped, Stanford Univ

Gospe Jr, Sidney M MD/PhD [ChiN] - **Spec Exp:** Epilepsy; Neuromuscular Disorders; Neurotoxicology; **Hospital:** Seattle Chldns Hosp; **Address:** Chldns Hosp/Regl Med Ctr, Dept Neurology, 4800 Sand Point Way NE, MS B5552, Seattle, WA 98195; **Phone:** 206-987-2078; **Board Cert:** Pediatrics 2005; Child Neurology 2010; **Med School:** Duke Univ 1981; **Resid:** Pediatrics, Baylor Coll Med 1983; **Fellow:** Child Neurology, Baylor Coll Med 1986; **Fac Appt:** Prof N, Univ Wash

Haas, Richard H MD [ChiN] - **Spec Exp:** Mitochondrial Disorders; Neurometabolic Disorders; **Hospital:** UCSD Med Ctr, Rady Children's Hosp - San Diego; **Address:** UCSD Sch Med, Div Ped Neuro, 9500 Gilman Drive, MC 0935, La Jolla, CA 92093-0935; **Phone:** 858-822-6700; **Board Cert:** Child Neurology 1983; Pediatrics 1985; **Med School:** England, UK 1972; **Resid:** Pediatrics, Univ London 1979; Child Neurology, Univ Colo Hlth Sci Ctr 1981; **Fellow:** Biochemical Mental Retardation, Univ Colo Hlth Sci Ctr 1981; **Fac Appt:** Prof Ped, UCSD

Lott, Ira T MD [ChiN] - **Spec Exp:** Down Syndrome; **Hospital:** Chldns Hosp Orange Co, UC Irvine Med Ctr; **Address:** 455 S Main St, Attn: PSF Neurology, Orange, CA 92868; **Phone:** 714-532-7601; **Board Cert:** Pediatrics 1975; Child Neurology 1977; **Med School:** Ohio State Univ 1967; **Resid:** Pediatrics, Mass Genl Hosp 1969; **Fellow:** Research, Natl Inst Hlth 1971; Neurology, Harvard-Mass Genl Hosp 1974; **Fac Appt:** Prof N, UC Irvine

Child Neurology

Mitchell, Wendy G MD [ChiN] - **Spec Exp:** Epilepsy/Seizure Disorders; Opsoclonus-Ataxia in Children; Neurodegenerative Disorders; **Hospital:** Chldns Hosp - Los Angeles; **Address:** Chldns Hosp Los Angeles, Dept Neuro, 4650 Sunset Blvd, MS 82, Los Angeles, CA 90027-6062; **Phone:** 323-361-2498; **Board Cert:** Pediatrics 1978; Child Neurology 1983; **Med School:** UCSF 1973; **Resid:** Pediatrics, Moffit Hosp-UCSF 1975; Child Neurology, Univ North Carolina 1981; **Fellow:** Behavioral Pediatrics, Mt Zion Hosp 1976; Univ North Carolina 1978; **Fac Appt:** Prof N, USC Sch Med

Pinter, Joseph David MD [ChiN] - **Spec Exp:** Down Syndrome; Tourette's Syndrome; Epilepsy; **Hospital:** Doernbecher Chldns Hosp/OHSU; **Address:** OHSU, Dept Child Neurology, 707 SW Gaines Rd, MC CDRCP, Portland, OR 97239; **Phone:** 503-494-5856; **Board Cert:** Child Neurology 2008; **Med School:** UCLA 1990; **Resid:** Pediatrics, Univ Washington/Cedars Sinai Med Ctr 1993; Child Neurology, Chldn's Hosp 1996; **Fellow:** Neurological Science, UCSF Med Ctr 1999; **Fac Appt:** Assoc Prof N, Oregon Hlth & Sci Univ

Roddy, Sarah M MD [ChiN] - **Spec Exp:** Tourette's Syndrome; **Hospital:** Loma Linda Chldns Hosp; **Address:** Pediatric Neuroscience Ctr, 2195 Club Ctr Drive, Ste A, San Bernadino, CA 92408; **Phone:** 909-835-1810; **Board Cert:** Child Neurology 1987; Pediatrics 1987; **Med School:** Loma Linda Univ 1980; **Resid:** Pediatrics, Loma Linda Univ Med Ctr 1983; **Fellow:** Pediatric Neurology, Loma Linda Univ Med Ctr 1986; **Fac Appt:** Assoc Prof N, Loma Linda Univ

Rosser, Tena L MD [ChiN] - **Spec Exp:** Neurocutaneous Disorders; Neurofibromatosis; Tuberous Sclerosis; **Hospital:** Chldns Hosp - Los Angeles; **Address:** Chldns Hosp Los Angeles, Dept Neurology, 4650 Sunset Blvd, MS 82, Los Angeles, CA 90027; **Phone:** 323-361-2471; **Board Cert:** Pediatrics 2007; Child Neurology 2003; **Med School:** Univ NC Sch Med 1996; **Resid:** Pediatrics, Chldn's Natl Med Ctr 1999; **Fellow:** Child Neurology, Chldn's Natl Med Ctr 2003; **Fac Appt:** Asst Prof N, USC-Keck School of Medicine

Sankar, Raman MD/PhD [ChiN] - **Spec Exp:** Epilepsy/Seizure Disorders; Headache; Migraine; **Hospital:** Mattel Chldns Hosp at UCLA, UCLA Ronald Reagan Med Ctr; **Address:** UCLA Sch Med-Div Ped Neurology, 22-474 MDCC, Box 951752, Los Angeles, CA 90095-1752; **Phone:** 310-825-6196; **Board Cert:** Child Neurology 2005; **Med School:** Tulane Univ 1986; **Resid:** Pediatrics, Chldns Hosp 1988; Neurology, UCLA Med Ctr 1989; **Fellow:** Child Neurology, UCLA Med Ctr 1991; **Fac Appt:** Prof Ped, UCLA

Trauner, Doris A MD [ChiN] - **Spec Exp:** Autism; Speech Disorders; **Hospital:** Rady Children's Hosp - San Diego; **Address:** UCSD Med Ctr, Div Ped Neurology, 9500 Gilman Drive, Dept 0935, La Jolla, CA 92093-0935; **Phone:** 858-966-5819; **Board Cert:** Pediatrics 1978; Child Neurology 1979; Neurodevelopmental Disabilities 2001; **Med School:** Med Coll VA 1972; **Resid:** Pediatrics, UCSD Med Ctr 1974; Neurology, UCSD Med Ctr 1975; **Fellow:** Child Neurology, Univ Chicago 1977; **Fac Appt:** Prof Ped, UCSD

Clinical Genetics

A specialist trained in diagnostic and therapeutic procedures for patients with genetically-linked diseases. This specialist uses modern cytogenetic, radiologic and biochemical testing to assist in specialized genetic counseling, implements needed therapeutic interventions and provides prevention through prenatal diagnosis.

A clinical geneticist demonstrates competence in providing comprehensive diagnostic, management and counseling services for genetic disorders.

A medical geneticist plans and coordinates large scale screening programs for inborn errors of metabolism, hemoglobinopathies, chromosome abnormalities and neural tube defects.

Training Required: Two or four years

CLINICAL GENETICS

New England

Bale, Allen E MD [CG] - **Spec Exp:** Cancer Genetics; **Hospital:** Yale-New Haven Hosp, Yale Med Group; **Address:** 333 Cedar St, SHM Bldg - rm I321, New Haven, CT 06519; **Phone:** 203-785-5745; **Board Cert:** Internal Medicine 1983; Clinical Genetics 1987; Clinical Molecular Genetics 2006; **Med School:** Univ Mass Sch Med 1979; **Resid:** Internal Medicine, Western Penn Hosp 1983; **Fellow:** Medical Genetics, Natl Inst of Health 1987; **Fac Appt:** Assoc Prof CG, Yale Univ

Bianchi, Diana MD [CG] - **Spec Exp:** Prenatal Genetic Diagnosis; Fetal Abnormalities; Twin to Twin Transfusion Syndrome (TTTS); **Hospital:** Tufts Med Ctr; **Address:** Tufts Med Ctr/Floating Hosp for Children, Div of Genetics, 800 Washington St, Box 394, Boston, MA 02111; **Phone:** 617-636-1468; **Board Cert:** Pediatrics 1985; Clinical Genetics 1987; Neonatal-Perinatal Medicine 1987; **Med School:** Stanford Univ 1980; **Resid:** Pediatrics, Chldns Hosp 1983; **Fellow:** Neonatology, Chldns Hosp 1986; Clinical Genetics, Harvard Med Sch 1987; **Fac Appt:** Prof Ped, Tufts Univ

Holmes, Lewis B MD [CG] - **Spec Exp:** Birth Defects; Inherited Disorders; Prenatal Diagnosis; **Hospital:** Mass Genl Hosp, Brigham and Women's Hosp (page 57); **Address:** Mass Genl Hosp, Dept Pediatrics, 175 Cambridge St Fl 5 - rm 504, Boston, MA 02114; **Phone:** 617-726-1742; **Board Cert:** Pediatrics 1968; Clinical Genetics 1982; **Med School:** Duke Univ 1963; **Resid:** Pediatrics, Mass Genl Hosp 1965; **Fellow:** Pediatric Endocrinology, Mass Genl Hosp 1966; **Fac Appt:** Prof Ped, Harvard Med Sch

Mahoney, Maurice J MD [CG] - **Spec Exp:** Fetal Therapy; Prenatal Diagnosis; **Hospital:** Yale-New Haven Hosp, Yale Med Group; **Address:** Yale Genetics Consultation Serv, 333 Cedar St, rm WWW330, New Haven, CT 06520-8005; **Phone:** 203-785-2661; **Board Cert:** Pediatrics 1967; Clinical Genetics 1982; Clinical Biochemical Genetics 1982; **Med School:** Univ Pittsburgh 1962; **Resid:** Pediatrics, Johns Hopkins Hosp 1965; Pediatrics, Childrens Hosp 1966; **Fellow:** Clinical Genetics, Yale Univ Sch Med 1970; **Fac Appt:** Prof CG, Yale Univ

Pauker, Susan Perlmutter MD [CG] - **Spec Exp:** Prenatal Diagnosis; Marfan's Syndrome; **Hospital:** Beth Israel Deaconess Med Ctr - Boston, Brigham and Women's Hosp (page 57); **Address:** 133 Brookline Ave, Boston, MA 02215-3904; **Phone:** 617-421-3320; **Board Cert:** Pediatrics 1976; Clinical Genetics 1987; **Med School:** Tufts Univ 1971; **Resid:** Pediatrics, Mass Genl Hosp 1973; **Fellow:** Clinical Genetics, Mass Genl Hosp 1975; **Fac Appt:** Assoc Clin Prof Ped, Harvard Med Sch

Seashore, Margretta MD [CG] - **Spec Exp:** Inherited Metabolic Disorders; **Hospital:** Yale-New Haven Hosp, Yale Med Group; **Address:** Yale Univ Sch Med, Dept Genetics, 333 Cedar St, rm 305, Box 208005, New Haven, CT 06520-8005; **Phone:** 203-785-2660; **Board Cert:** Pediatrics 1970; Clinical Biochemical Genetics 1982; Clinical Genetics 1982; **Med School:** Yale Univ 1965; **Resid:** Pediatrics, Yale-New Haven Hosp 1968; **Fellow:** Clinical Genetics, Yale-New Haven Hosp 1970; **Fac Appt:** Prof CG, Yale Univ

Mid Atlantic

Anyane-Yeboa, Kwame MD [CG] - **Spec Exp:** Dysmorphology; Prenatal Diagnosis; **Hospital:** Morgan Stanley Children's Hosp of NY-Presby, NY (page 65), St. Luke's - Roosevelt Hosp Ctr - Roosevelt Div (page 55); **Address:** Morgan Stanley Children's Hospital of NY, 3959 Broadway, rm 601A, New York, NY 10032; **Phone:** 212-305-6731; **Board Cert:** Pediatrics 1979; Clinical Genetics 1982; **Med School:** Ghana 1972; **Resid:** Pediatrics, Harlem Hosp 1977; **Fellow:** Clinical Genetics, Babies Hosp-Columbia Presby 1980; **Fac Appt:** Assoc Prof Ped, Columbia P&S

Bialer, Martin G MD/PhD [CG] - **Spec Exp:** Marfan's Syndrome; Neurofibromatosis; Metabolic Genetic Disorders; Cancer Genetics; **Hospital:** Steven & Alexandra Cohen Chldn's Med Ctr of NY, NS-LIJ Hlth Sys; **Address:** 1554 Northern Blvd, Ste 204, Manhasset, NY 11030; **Phone:** 516-365-3996; **Board Cert:** Pediatrics 1987; Clinical Biochemical Genetics 1990; Clinical Genetics 1990; **Med School:** Med Univ SC 1983; **Resid:** Pediatrics, N Shore Univ Hosp 1986; **Fellow:** Clinical Genetics, Univ VA Hlth Sci Ctr 1989; **Fac Appt:** Clin Prof Ped, NYU Sch Med

Davis, Jessica G MD [CG] - **Spec Exp:** Marfan's Syndrome; Mental Retardation; Neurofibromatosis; Ehlers-Danlos Syndrome; **Hospital:** NY-Presby/Weill Cornell Med Ctr, NY (page 65), Hosp For Special Surgery (page 60); **Address:** 505 E 70th St, Box 128, New York, NY 10065; **Phone:** 646-962-2205; **Board Cert:** Clinical Genetics 1984; **Med School:** Columbia P&S 1959; **Resid:** Pediatrics, St Luke's Hosp 1962; Clinical Genetics, Albert Einstein Coll Med 1965; **Fellow:** Cytogenetics, Albert Einstein Coll Med 1966; Pediatrics, Albert Einstein Col Med 1968; **Fac Appt:** Assoc Clin Prof Ped, Cornell Univ-Weill Med Coll

Desnick, Robert J MD/PhD [CG] - **Spec Exp:** Inherited Metabolic Disorders; Fabry's Disease; Gaucher Disease; Porphyria; **Hospital:** Mount Sinai Med Ctr (page 63), Beth Israel Med Ctr - Petrie Division (page 55); **Address:** Mt Sinai Sch Med, Box 1498, Fifth Ave @ 100th St, New York, NY 10029; **Phone:** 212-241-6947; **Board Cert:** Clinical Genetics 1982; Clinical Molecular Genetics 2009; Clinical Biochemical Genetics 1982; **Med School:** Univ Minn 1971; **Resid:** Pediatrics, Univ Minn Hosps 1973; **Fac Appt:** Prof CG, Mount Sinai Sch Med

Desposito, Franklin MD [CG] - **Spec Exp:** Birth Defects; Genetic Disorders; **Hospital:** Univ Hosp-UMDNJ—Newark, Saint Barnabas Med Ctr; **Address:** 90 Bergen St, Ste 5400, Newark, NJ 07103; **Phone:** 973-972-3300; **Board Cert:** Pediatrics 1986; Clinical Genetics 1982; Clinical Cytogenetics 1990; Clinical Molecular Genetics 2010; **Med School:** Ros Franklin Univ/Chicago Med Sch 1957; **Resid:** Pediatrics, Long Island Jewish Hosp 1961; **Fellow:** Hematology, Univ Wisc Sch Med 1963; **Fac Appt:** Prof Ped, UMDNJ-NJ Med Sch, Newark

Driscoll, Deborah A MD [CG] - **Spec Exp:** Prenatal Genetic Diagnosis; Fetal Abnormalities; Adolescent Gynecology; **Hospital:** Hosp Univ Penn - UPHS (page 68); **Address:** Chldns Hosp of Philadelphia, Clin Genetics Ctr, 3400 Spruce St, Philadelphia, PA 19104; **Phone:** 215-662-3232; **Board Cert:** Obstetrics & Gynecology 2008; Clinical Genetics 1990; **Med School:** NYU Sch Med 1983; **Resid:** Obstetrics & Gynecology, Hosp Univ Penn 1987; **Fellow:** Clinical Genetics, Hosp Univ Penn 1989; **Fac Appt:** Prof ObG, Univ Pennsylvania

Gilbert, Fred MD [CG] - **Spec Exp:** Cancer Genetics; Prenatal Diagnosis; **Hospital:** NY-Presby/Weill Cornell Med Ctr, NY (page 65), Brooklyn Hosp Ctr-Downtown; **Address:** 1300 York Ave, Box 128, New York, NY 10065; **Phone:** 646-962-2205; **Board Cert:** Clinical Genetics 1982; Clinical Cytogenetics 1982; Clinical Molecular Genetics 2006; **Med School:** Albert Einstein Coll Med 1966; **Resid:** Internal Medicine, Barnes Hosp 1968; Internal Medicine, Natl Inst Hlth 1971; **Fellow:** Clinical Genetics, Yale-New Haven Hosp 1974; **Fac Appt:** Assoc Prof Ped, Cornell Univ-Weill Med Coll

Clinical Genetics

Gross, Susan MD [CG] - **Spec Exp:** Prenatal Diagnosis; Prenatal Ultrasound; Reproductive Genetics; **Hospital:** Montefiore Med Ctr - Div. Moses, Jacobi Med Ctr; **Address:** Jacobi Med Ctr, Dept of OB/GYN, 1400 Pelham Pkwy S, Ste BS26, Bronx, NY 10461; **Phone:** 718-918-6310; **Board Cert:** Obstetrics & Gynecology 2010; Clinical Genetics 2010; **Med School:** Univ Toronto 1985; **Resid:** Obstetrics & Gynecology, Univ Toronto Hosp 1991; **Fellow:** Maternal & Fetal Medicine, Univ Toronto 1992; Clinical Genetics, Univ Tenn 1994; **Fac Appt:** Prof ObG, Albert Einstein Coll Med

Kronn, David F MD [CG] - **Spec Exp:** Bone Disorders-Metabolic; Bone Disorders-Inherited; **Hospital:** Westchester Med Ctr, Children's & Women's Phys.of Westchester; **Address:** Regional Med Genetics Ctr, Children/Women's Physicians of Westchester, 503 Grasslands Rd, Ste 200, Valhalla, NY 10595; **Phone:** 914-304-5300; **Board Cert:** Clinical Genetics 2007; Pediatrics 2002; Clinical Biochemical Genetics 1999; **Med School:** Ireland 1989; **Resid:** Pediatrics, NYU Med Ctr 1996; **Fellow:** Clinical Genetics, NYU Med Ctr 1996; **Fac Appt:** CG, NY Med Coll

Marion, Robert W MD [CG] - **Spec Exp:** Spina Bifida; Williams Syndrome; Marfan's Syndrome; Down Syndrome; **Hospital:** Montefiore Med Ctr - Div. Moses, Blythedale Children's Hosp; **Address:** 3415 Bainbridge Ave, Bronx, NY 10467; **Phone:** 718-741-2323; **Board Cert:** Pediatrics 1985; Clinical Genetics 1987; **Med School:** Albert Einstein Coll Med 1979; **Resid:** Pediatrics, Montefiore Med Ctr 1982; **Fellow:** Clinical Genetics, Montefiore Med Ctr 1984; **Fac Appt:** Prof Ped, Albert Einstein Coll Med

Ostrer, Harry MD [CG] - **Spec Exp:** Genetic Disorders; Hereditary Cancer; **Hospital:** NYU Langone Med Ctr (page 66); **Address:** NYU Medical Ctr, 550 1st Ave, rm MSB136, New York, NY 10016; **Phone:** 212-263-5746; **Board Cert:** Clinical Genetics 1984; Pediatrics 1985; Clinical Cytogenetics 1990; Clinical Molecular Genetics 2010; **Med School:** Columbia P&S 1976; **Resid:** Pediatrics, Johns Hopkins Hosp 1978; Clinical Genetics, Natl Inst Health 1981; **Fellow:** Molecular Genetics, Johns Hopkins Hosp 1983; **Fac Appt:** Prof Ped, NYU Sch Med

Pyeritz, Reed E MD/PhD [CG] - **Spec Exp:** Marfan's Syndrome; Hereditary Hemorrhagic Telangiectasia; Inherited Disorders; **Hospital:** Hosp Univ Penn - UPHS (page 68), Chldns Hosp of Philadelphia; **Address:** Univ Penn, Div Medical Genetics, 3400 Spruce St, Penn Tower 1115, Philadelphia, PA 19104; **Phone:** 215-662-4740; **Board Cert:** Internal Medicine 1978; Clinical Genetics 2004; **Med School:** Harvard Med Sch 1975; **Resid:** Internal Medicine, Peter Bent Brigham Hosp 1977; Clinical Genetics, Johns Hopkins Hosp 1978; **Fac Appt:** Prof Med, Univ Pennsylvania

Rosenbaum, Kenneth MD [CG] - **Spec Exp:** Birth Defects; **Hospital:** Chldns Natl Med Ctr, Shady Grove Adven Hosp; **Address:** Chldns Natl Med Ctr, Dept Med Genetics, 111 Michigan Ave NW, rm 1950, Washington, DC 20010; **Phone:** 202-476-6287; **Board Cert:** Pediatrics 1976; Clinical Genetics 1982; Clinical Cytogenetics 1982; **Med School:** Univ Louisville Sch Med 1971; **Resid:** Pediatrics, Childrens Natl Med Ctr 1974; **Fellow:** Clinical Genetics, Johns Hopkins Hosp 1977; **Fac Appt:** Assoc Prof Ped, Geo Wash Univ

Shapiro, Lawrence R MD [CG] - **Spec Exp:** Dysmorphology; Prenatal Diagnosis; Hereditary Cancer; Developmental Disorders; **Hospital:** Westchester Med Ctr, Nyack Hosp; **Address:** Children/Women's Physicians Westchester, 503 Grasslands Ave, Ste 200, Valhalla, NY 10595; **Phone:** 914-304-5300; **Board Cert:** Pediatrics 1967; Clinical Genetics 1982; Clinical Cytogenetics 1982; **Med School:** NYU Sch Med 1962; **Resid:** Pediatrics, Chldns Hosp 1964; Pediatrics, Bellevue Hosp 1965; **Fellow:** Clinical Genetics, Mount Sinai Med Ctr 1968; **Fac Appt:** Prof Ped, NY Med Coll

Zackai, Elaine MD [CG] - **Spec Exp:** Craniosynostosis; Cytogenetic Disorders; **Hospital:** Chldns Hosp of Philadelphia; **Address:** Chldns Hosp Philadelphia, Dept Clinical Genetics, 34th St & Civic Center Blvd, rm 8C05, Philadelphia, PA 19104; **Phone:** 215-590-2920; **Board Cert:** Pediatrics 1977; Clinical Genetics 1982; Clinical Cytogenetics 1982; **Med School:** NYU Sch Med 1968; **Resid:** Pediatrics, Chldns Hosp 1970; **Fellow:** Clinical Genetics, Chldns Hosp 1971; Clinical Genetics, Yale Univ Med Sch 1972; **Fac Appt:** Prof Ped, Univ Pennsylvania

Southeast

Driscoll, Daniel J MD/PhD [CG] - **Spec Exp:** Prader-Willi Syndrome; Obesity-Pediatric; Angelman Syndrome; **Hospital:** Shands at Univ of FL; **Address:** Pediatric Genetics & Metabolism, Univ FL Hlth Sicence Ctr, PO Box 100296, Gainesville, FL 32610-0296; **Phone:** 352-294-5050; **Board Cert:** Pediatrics 1987; Clinical Genetics 1990; Clinical Cytogenetics 1990; **Med School:** Albany Med Coll 1983; **Resid:** Pediatrics, Johns Hopkins Hosp 1986; **Fellow:** Clinical Genetics, Johns Hopkins Hosp 1989; **Fac Appt:** Prof Ped, Univ Fla Coll Med

Fernhoff, Paul M MD [CG] - **Spec Exp:** Birth Defects; Metabolic Genetic Disorders; **Hospital:** Chldns Hlthcare Atlanta @ Scottish Rite, Emory Univ Hosp; **Address:** Emory Childrens Ctr-Medical Genetics, 2165 N Decatur Rd NE, Decatur, GA 30033-5307; **Phone:** 404-778-8500; **Board Cert:** Pediatrics 1976; Clinical Genetics 1982; **Med School:** Jefferson Med Coll 1971; **Resid:** Pediatrics, Children's Hosp 1974; **Fellow:** Clinical Genetics, Emory Univ Hosp 1979; **Fac Appt:** Assoc Prof Ped, Emory Univ

Korf, Bruce R MD/PhD [CG] - **Spec Exp:** Inherited Disorders; Neuro-Genetics; Neurofibromatosis; **Hospital:** Univ of Ala Hosp at Birmingham; **Address:** UAB Dept Genetics, 720 20th St S, KAUL 230, Birmingham, AL 35294-0024; **Phone:** 205-934-4983; **Board Cert:** Clinical Genetics 1984; Child Neurology 1986; Pediatrics 1988; Clinical Molecular Genetics 2010; **Med School:** Cornell Univ-Weill Med Coll 1980; **Resid:** Pediatrics, Chldns Hosp 1982; Child Neurology, Chldns Hosp 1985; **Fellow:** Clinical Genetics, Chldns Hosp 1985; **Fac Appt:** Prof CG, Univ Alabama

Saul, Robert MD [CG] - **Spec Exp:** Birth Defects; Neurofibromatosis; **Hospital:** Self Regional Healthcare; **Address:** Greenwood Genetic Ctr, 106 Gregor Mendel Cir, Research Bldg, Greenwood, SC 29646; **Phone:** 864-941-8119; **Board Cert:** Pediatrics 1981; Clinical Genetics 1982; **Med School:** Univ Colorado 1976; **Resid:** Pediatrics, Duke Med Ctr 1979; **Fellow:** Clinical Genetics, Greenwood Genetics Ctr 1981; **Fac Appt:** Clin Prof Ped, Univ SC Sch Med

Stevenson, Roger E MD [CG] - **Spec Exp:** Birth Defects; Mental Retardation; **Hospital:** Self Regional Healthcare; **Address:** Greenwood Genetic Ctr, 1113 Gregor Mendel Cir, Research Bldg, Greenwood, SC 29646; **Phone:** 864-941-8146; **Board Cert:** Pediatrics 1971; Clinical Genetics 1982; Clinical Cytogenetics 1984; **Med School:** Wake Forest Univ 1966; **Resid:** Pediatrics, Johns Hopkins Hosp 1969; **Fellow:** Clinical Genetics, Johns Hopkins Hosp 1972

Sutphen, Rebecca MD [CG] - **Spec Exp:** Genetic Disorders; Hereditary Cancer; Cancer Risk Assessment; **Hospital:** H Lee Moffitt Cancer Ctr & Research Inst (page 59); **Address:** 3650 Spectrum Blvd, Ste 100, Tampa, FL 33612; **Phone:** 813-396-9234; **Board Cert:** Clinical Molecular Genetics 2010; Clinical Cytogenetics 2009; Clinical Genetics 2010; **Med School:** Temple Univ 1990; **Resid:** Pediatrics, All Children's Hosp 1993; **Fellow:** Clinical Genetics, Univ S Fla Coll Med 1995; **Fac Appt:** Prof CG, Univ S Fla Coll Med

Ward, Jewell C MD/PhD [CG] - **Spec Exp:** Inborn Errors of Metabolism; Metabolic Genetic Disorders; Phenylketonuria (PKU); Reproductive Genetics; **Hospital:** Le Bonheur Chldns Med Ctr; **Address:** 777 Washington Ave, Ste P-110, Memphis, TN 38105; **Phone:** 901-866-8818; **Board Cert:** Clinical Genetics 1982; Clinical Biochemical Genetics 1982; **Med School:** Indiana Univ 1971; **Resid:** Pediatrics, Ohio's Chldns Hosp 1974; **Fellow:** Medical Genetics, Indiana Univ Affil Hosp 1975; Medical Genetics, Johns Hopkins Univ Hosp 1979; **Fac Appt:** Prof Ped, Univ Tenn Coll Med

Clinical Genetics

Midwest

Bartholomew, Dennis W MD [CG] - **Spec Exp:** Genetic Disorders; **Hospital:** Nationwide Chldn's Hosp; **Address:** Nationwide Chldn's Hosp: Timken Hall, 700 Children's Drive Fl Second, Columbus, OH 43205; **Phone:** 614-722-3537; **Board Cert:** Pediatrics 1986; Clinical Biochemical Genetics 1990; Clinical Genetics 1987; **Med School:** Northwestern Univ 1980; **Resid:** Pediatrics, David Grant Med Ctr 1983; **Fellow:** Genetics, Johns Hopkins Hosp 1987; **Fac Appt:** Clin Prof Ped, Ohio State Univ

Burton, Barbara MD [CG] - **Spec Exp:** Marfan's Syndrome; Phenylketonuria (PKU); Lysosomal Diseases; Inborn Errors of Metabolism; **Hospital:** Children's Mem Hosp -Chicago, Northwestern Meml Hosp; **Address:** Chldns Meml Hosp, Dept Genetics, 2300 Children's Plaza, Box 59, Chicago, IL 60614-3363; **Phone:** 773-880-4462; **Board Cert:** Pediatrics 1978; Clinical Genetics 1982; Clinical Biochemical Genetics 1982; **Med School:** Northwestern Univ 1973; **Resid:** Pediatrics, Chldns Meml Hosp 1975; **Fellow:** Clinical Genetics, Chldns Meml Hosp 1977; **Fac Appt:** Prof Ped, Northwestern Univ

Charrow, Joel MD [CG] - **Spec Exp:** Biochemical Genetics; Lysosomal Diseases; Neurofibromatosis; **Hospital:** Children's Mem Hosp -Chicago; **Address:** Chldns Meml Hosp-Div Genetics, 2300 Chldn's Plaza, Box 16, Chicago, IL 60614-3318; **Phone:** 773-880-4462; **Board Cert:** Pediatrics 1980; Clinical Genetics 1982; Clinical Biochemical Genetics 1987; **Med School:** Mount Sinai Sch Med 1976; **Resid:** Pediatrics, Chldns Meml Hosp 1979; **Fellow:** Clinical Genetics, Chldns Meml Hosp-Northwestern Univ 1981; **Fac Appt:** Prof Ped, Northwestern Univ

Elias, Sherman MD [CG] - **Spec Exp:** Prenatal Diagnosis; Reproductive Genetics; **Hospital:** Northwestern Meml Hosp; **Address:** 250 E Superior, Ste 03-2306, Chicago, IL 60611-2914; **Phone:** 312-472-3636; **Board Cert:** Obstetrics & Gynecology 2010; Clinical Genetics 2004; **Med School:** Univ KY Coll Med 1972; **Resid:** Obstetrics & Gynecology, Univ Louisville Hosp 1976; **Fellow:** Clinical Genetics, Yale Univ 1975; Clinical Genetics, Northwestern Univ 1978; **Fac Appt:** Prof ObG, Northwestern Univ

Pergament, Eugene MD/PhD [CG] - **Spec Exp:** Prenatal Genetic Diagnosis; Down Syndrome; Genetic Preimplantation Diagnosis; **Hospital:** Northwestern Meml Hosp; **Address:** 680 N Lake Shore Drive, Ste 1230, Chicago, IL 60611; **Phone:** 312-981-4360; **Board Cert:** Clinical Genetics 1982; Clinical Cytogenetics 1984; **Med School:** Univ Chicago-Pritzker Sch Med 1970; **Resid:** Pediatrics, Univ Chicago 1972; **Fac Appt:** Prof ObG, Northwestern Univ

Rubinstein, Wendy S MD/PhD [CG] - **Spec Exp:** Breast Cancer; Colon Cancer; Pancreatic Cancer; **Hospital:** Evanston/North Shore Univ Hlth Sys; **Address:** Ctr for Medical Genetics, 1000 Central St, Ste 620, Evanston, IL 60201; **Phone:** 847-570-1029; **Board Cert:** Internal Medicine 2003; Clinical Genetics 2010; Clinical Molecular Genetics 2010; **Med School:** Mount Sinai Sch Med 1989; **Resid:** Internal Medicine, Strong Meml Hosp 1992; **Fellow:** Clinical Genetics, Univ Pittsburgh Hosp 1996; Clinical Molecular Genetics, Univ Pittsburgh Hosp 1996; **Fac Appt:** Assoc Clin Prof Med, Univ Chicago-Pritzker Sch Med

Saal, Howard M MD [CG] - **Spec Exp:** Craniofacial Disorders; Cleft Palate/Lip; Neurofibromatosis; **Hospital:** Cincinnati Chldns Hosp Med Ctr; **Address:** Chldns Hosp Med Ctr, Div Human Genetics, 3333 Burnet Ave Bldg E5 - rm 5430, MC 4006, Cincinnati, OH 45229-3039; **Phone:** 513-636-4760; **Board Cert:** Clinical Genetics 1984; Clinical Cytogenetics 1984; Pediatrics 1985; **Med School:** Wayne State Univ 1979; **Resid:** Pediatrics, Univ Conn Hlth Ctr 1982; **Fellow:** Medical Genetics, Univ Washington 1984; **Fac Appt:** Prof Ped, Univ Cincinnati

Shulman, Lee P MD [CG] - **Spec Exp:** Prenatal Diagnosis; Breast Cancer Genetics; Ovarian Cancer Genetics; **Hospital:** Northwestern Meml Hosp, Rush Univ Med Ctr; **Address:** Northwestern Univ Dept Ob/Gyn, Division Clinical Genetics, 250 E Superior St, Ste 05-2168, Chicago, IL 60611; **Phone:** 312-472-4683; **Board Cert:** Obstetrics & Gynecology 1999; Clinical Genetics 1990; **Med School:** Cornell Univ 1983; **Resid:** Obstetrics & Gynecology, N Shore Univ Hosp 1987; **Fellow:** Reproductive Genetics, Univ Tenn Med Ctr 1989; **Fac Appt:** Prof ObG, Northwestern Univ

Weaver, David D MD [CG] - **Spec Exp:** Bone Disorders-Inherited; Genetic Disorders; Inherited Disorders; Weaver Syndrome; **Hospital:** Riley Hosp for Children, IU Health North Hosp; **Address:** 975 W Walnut St, IB 130, Indianapolis, IN 46202-5251; **Phone:** 317-274-1057; **Board Cert:** Pediatrics 1978; Clinical Genetics 1982; **Med School:** Oregon Hlth & Sci Univ 1966; **Resid:** Pediatrics, Oregon HSU Affil Hosp 1972; **Fellow:** Clinical Genetics, Univ Washington 1974; Metabolic Diseases, Oregon Health Scis Univ 1976; **Fac Appt:** Prof Emeritus CG, Indiana Univ

Whelan, Alison MD [CG] - **Spec Exp:** Gynecologic Cancer Risk; Colon & Rectal Cancer Risk; Hereditary Cancer; **Hospital:** Barnes-Jewish Hosp, St. Louis Chldns Hosp; **Address:** Washington Univ Sch Med, 660 S Euclid Ave, Campus Box 8116, St Louis, MO 63110; **Phone:** 314-454-6093; **Board Cert:** Internal Medicine 1989; Clinical Genetics 2010; **Med School:** Washington Univ, St Louis 1986; **Resid:** Internal Medicine, Barnes Hosp 1989; Pediatrics, Wash Univ Sch Med 1994; **Fellow:** Research, Wash Univ Sch Med 1991; Clinical Genetics, Wash Univ Sch Med 1994; **Fac Appt:** Prof Med, Washington Univ, St Louis

Great Plains and Mountains

Carey, John C MD [CG] - **Spec Exp:** Neurofibromatosis; Birth Defects; Hearing Loss; **Hospital:** Primary Children's Med Ctr, Univ Utah Hlth Care; **Address:** Div Med Genetics, 50 N Med Drive Bldg SOM - rm 2C412, Salt Lake City, UT 84113; **Phone:** 801-581-8943; **Board Cert:** Pediatrics 1979; Clinical Genetics 1982; **Med School:** Georgetown Univ 1972; **Resid:** Pediatrics, UCSF Med Ctr 1975; **Fellow:** Clinical Genetics, UCSF Med Ctr 1979; **Fac Appt:** Prof Ped, Univ Utah

Hoyme, H Eugene MD [CG] - **Spec Exp:** Fetal Alcohol Syndrome; Cytogenetic Disorders; Dysmorphology; **Hospital:** Sanford USD Med Ctr; **Address:** PO Box 5039, 1305 W 18th St, Sioux Falls, SD 57117-5039; **Phone:** 605-333-6447; **Board Cert:** Pediatrics 1980; Clinical Genetics 1984; Clinical Cytogenetics 1987; **Med School:** Univ Chicago-Pritzker Sch Med 1976; **Resid:** Pediatrics, UCSD Med Ctr 1979; **Fellow:** Dysmorphology, UCSD Med Ctr 1981; **Fac Appt:** Prof Ped, Univ SD Sch Med

Opitz, John MD [CG] - **Spec Exp:** Skeletal Dysplasia; Sexual Differentiation Disorders; Mental Retardation; **Hospital:** Univ Utah Hlth Care; **Address:** Univ Utah, Div Med Genetics, 50 N Medical Drive, rm SOM 2C412, Salt Lake City, UT 84132; **Phone:** 801-581-8943; **Board Cert:** Pediatrics 1964; Clinical Genetics 1982; **Med School:** Univ Iowa Coll Med 1959; **Resid:** Pediatrics, SUI Hosp 1961; Pediatrics, Univ Wisc Hosps 1962; **Fellow:** Clinical Genetics, Univ Wisc Hosps 1964; **Fac Appt:** Prof Ped, Univ Utah

Southwest

Beaudet, Arthur L MD [CG] - **Spec Exp:** Genetic Biochemical Disorders; **Hospital:** Texas Chldns Hosp; **Address:** Clinical Care Center, 6701 Fannin St, Fl 16, MC CC 1560, Houston, TX 77030; **Phone:** 832-822-4280; **Board Cert:** Pediatrics 1973; Clinical Genetics 1982; Clinical Biochemical Genetics 1982; Clinical Molecular Genetics 2010; **Med School:** Yale Univ 1967; **Resid:** Pediatrics, Johns Hopkins Hosp 1969; **Fellow:** Biochemical Genetics, Natl Inst Hlth 1971; **Fac Appt:** Prof CG, Baylor Coll Med

Clinical Genetics

Craigen, William J MD/PhD [CG] - **Spec Exp:** Biochemical Genetics; Mitochondrial Disorders; **Hospital:** Texas Chldns Hosp, Ben Taub Genl Hosp; **Address:** Texas Children's Genetic Clinic, 6701 Fannin St, Fl 16, MC CC 1560, Houston, TX 77030; **Phone:** 832-822-4280; **Board Cert:** Clinical Genetics 2010; Clinical Biochemical Genetics 2010; **Med School:** Baylor Coll Med 1988; **Resid:** Pediatrics, Baylor Coll Med 1990; Pediatrics, Baylor Coll Med 1992; **Fellow:** Clinical Genetics, Baylor Coll Med 1990; **Fac Appt:** Assoc Prof CG, Baylor Coll Med

Cunniff, Christopher M MD [CG] - **Spec Exp:** Genetic Disorders; Developmental Disorders; Sexual Differentiation Disorders; Fetal Alcohol Syndrome; **Hospital:** Univ Med Ctr - Tucson; **Address:** Univ Ariz Dept Pediatric Genetics, 1501 N Campbell Ave, PO Box 245073, Tucson, AZ 85724; **Phone:** 520-626-5175; **Board Cert:** Pediatrics 2010; Clinical Genetics 1990; **Med School:** Univ Alabama 1984; **Resid:** Pediatrics, MC Hosp Vermont 1987; **Fellow:** Clinical Genetics, UCSD 1989; **Fac Appt:** Prof Ped, Univ Ariz Coll Med

Mulvihill, John J MD [CG] - **Spec Exp:** Genetic Disorders; Neurofibromatosis; Fertility in Cancer Survivors; **Hospital:** Chldns Hosp OU Med Ctr; **Address:** Chldn's Hosp-OU Med Ctr, Dept Ped Genetics, Dept Pediatric Genetics, 1200 N Phillips Ave, Ste 12100, Oklahoma City, OK 73104; **Phone:** 405-271-8685; **Board Cert:** Pediatrics 1975; Clinical Genetics 1982; **Med School:** Univ Wash 1969; **Resid:** Pediatrics, Johns Hopkins Hosp 1974; **Fellow:** Research, NCI-Natl Inst Hlth 1972; **Fac Appt:** Prof CG, Univ Okla Coll Med

Northrup, Hope MD [CG] - **Spec Exp:** Biochemical Genetics; Neuro-Genetics; Dysmorphology; **Hospital:** Meml Hermann Hosp - Texas Med Ctr, LBJ General Hosp; **Address:** Univ TX Med Sch, Dept Peds-Div Med Genetics, rm MSB-3.144, Box 20708, 6431 Fannin St, Houston, TX 77030; **Phone:** 713-500-5760; **Board Cert:** Pediatrics 1988; Clinical Genetics 1990; Clinical Biochemical Genetics 1990; **Med School:** Med Univ SC 1983; **Resid:** Pediatrics, Chldns Med Ctr-Univ Tex SW 1986; **Fellow:** Medical Genetics, Inst Molec Gene-Baylor Coll Med 1989; **Fac Appt:** Prof Ped, Univ Tex, Houston

Plon, Sharon E MD/PhD [CG] - **Spec Exp:** Hereditary Cancer; Cancer Risk Assessment; Breast Cancer Risk Assessment; Ovarian Cancer Genetics; **Hospital:** Texas Chldns Hosp, St. Luke's Episcopal Hosp-Houston; **Address:** Texas Chldn's Hosp, 1102 Bates St, MC FC1200, Houston, TX 77030; **Phone:** 832-824-4539; **Board Cert:** Clinical Genetics 2006; **Med School:** Harvard Med Sch 1987; **Resid:** Internal Medicine, Univ Washington Affil Hosp 1988; **Fellow:** Molecular Genetics, National Cancer Inst 1990; Medical Genetics, Fred Hutchinson Cancer Research Ctr 1993; **Fac Appt:** Prof CG, Baylor Coll Med

West Coast and Pacific

Boles, Richard G MD [CG] - **Spec Exp:** Mitochondrial Disorders; Vomiting-Cyclic; **Hospital:** Chldns Hosp - Los Angeles; **Address:** 4650 Sunset Blvd, MS 90, Los Angeles, CA 90027; **Phone:** 323-361-2178; **Board Cert:** Clinical Genetics 2010; Clinical Biochemical Genetics 2010; Pediatrics 2009; **Med School:** UCLA 1987; **Resid:** Pediatrics, Harbor-UCLA Med Ctr 1990; **Fellow:** Genetics and Metabolism, Yale Univ 1993; **Fac Appt:** Assoc Prof Ped, USC Sch Med

Cassidy, Suzanne MD [CG] - **Spec Exp:** Prader-Willi Syndrome; Connective Tissue Disorders; Neurocutaneous Disorders; **Hospital:** UCSF Med Ctr; **Address:** 533 Parnassus Ave, rm U-100A, Box 0706, San Francisco, CA 94143; **Phone:** 415-476-2757; **Board Cert:** Pediatrics 1982; Clinical Genetics 1983; **Med School:** Vanderbilt Univ 1976; **Resid:** Pediatrics, Univ Wash Affil Prgms 1979; **Fellow:** Clinical Genetics, Univ Wash 1981; **Fac Appt:** Prof Ped, UC Irvine

Cederbaum, Stephen D MD [CG] - **Spec Exp:** Inborn Errors of Metabolism; Genetic Disorders; **Hospital:** UCLA Ronald Reagan Med Ctr; **Address:** 635 Charles E Young Drive S, rm 347, Los Angeles, CA 90095-7332; **Phone:** 310-825-0402; **Board Cert:** Clinical Genetics 1982; Clinical Biochemical Genetics 1982; **Med School:** NYU Sch Med 1964; **Resid:** Internal Medicine, Barnes-Jewish Hosp 1966; **Fellow:** Clinical Genetics, Univ Wash 1970; **Fac Appt:** Prof Emeritus CG, UCLA

Curry, Cynthia J MD [CG] - **Hospital:** Chldns Hosp Central CA, Comm Regl Med Ctr - Fresno; **Address:** UCSF Fresno, 155 N Fresno St, Fresno, CA 93701; **Phone:** 559-227-4472; **Board Cert:** Pediatrics 1973; Clinical Genetics 1982; **Med School:** Yale Univ 1967; **Resid:** Pediatrics, Univ Wash Orth Chldns Hosp 1969; Pediatrics, Univ Minn Hosp 1970; **Fellow:** Dysmorphology, UCSF Med Ctr 1976; **Fac Appt:** Prof CG, UCSF

Falk, Rena MD [CG] - **Spec Exp:** Prenatal Diagnosis; Mental Retardation; Prenatal Genetic Diagnosis; **Hospital:** Cedars-Sinai Med Ctr; **Address:** 8700 Beverly Blvd, PACT 400, Los Angeles, CA 90048; **Phone:** 310-423-9914; **Board Cert:** Pediatrics 1976; Clinical Genetics 1982; Clinical Cytogenetics 1984; **Med School:** UCLA 1971; **Resid:** Pediatrics, Cedars-Sinai Med Ctr 1973; **Fellow:** Clinical Genetics, UCLA Med Schl 1975; UCLA 1977; **Fac Appt:** Prof Ped, UCLA

Graham Jr, John M MD [CG] - **Spec Exp:** Dysmorphology; Craniofacial Disorders; Mental Retardation; **Hospital:** Cedars-Sinai Med Ctr; **Address:** 8700 Beverly Blvd, PACT-Suite 400, Los Angeles, CA 90048; **Phone:** 310-423-9909; **Board Cert:** Pediatrics 1982; Clinical Genetics 1982; **Med School:** Med Univ SC 1975; **Resid:** Pediatrics, Boston Chldns Hosp-Harvard 1977; **Fellow:** Developmental-Behavioral Pediatrics, Boston Chldns Hosp 1978; Dysmorphology, Univ Wash 1980; **Fac Appt:** Prof Ped, UCLA

Grody, Wayne W MD/PhD [CG] - **Spec Exp:** Genetic Disorders; Hereditary Cancer; **Address:** UCLA School Medicine, Div, Med Genetic & Molecular Pathology, 10833 Le Conte Ave, Los Angeles, CA 90095-1732; **Phone:** 310-825-5648; **Board Cert:** Clinical Genetics 1990; Anatomic & Clinical Pathology 1987; Clinical Biochemical Genetics 1990; Molecular Genetic Pathology 2001; **Med School:** Baylor Coll Med 1977; **Resid:** Pathology, UCLA Med Ctr 1986; **Fellow:** Clinical Genetics, UCLA Med Ctr 1987; **Fac Appt:** Prof CG, UCLA

Hudgins, Louanne MD [CG] - **Spec Exp:** Congenital Anomalies-Limb; Prenatal Diagnosis; **Hospital:** Stanford Univ Hosp & Clinics; **Address:** Stanford Univ Med Ctr, Div Medical Genetics, 300 Pasteur Drive, rm H315, Stanford, CA 94305; **Phone:** 650-723-6858; **Board Cert:** Pediatrics 2004; Clinical Genetics 2010; **Med School:** Univ Kansas 1984; **Resid:** Pediatrics, Univ Conn Hlth Ctr 1987; **Fellow:** Clinical Genetics, Univ Conn 1990; **Fac Appt:** Prof Ped, Stanford Univ

Jonas, Adam J MD [CG] - **Spec Exp:** Biochemical Genetics; Inherited Disorders; **Hospital:** LAC - Harbor - UCLA Med Ctr; **Address:** Harbor-UCLA Med Ctr, Div Med Genetics, 1000 W Carson St, Box 17, Torrance, CA 90509-2910; **Phone:** 310-222-2301; **Board Cert:** Pediatrics 1982; Clinical Biochemical Genetics 1987; Clinical Genetics 1990; **Med School:** UCSD 1976; **Resid:** Pediatrics, Chldns Ortho Hosp 1978; Pediatrics, Univ Hosp 1979; **Fellow:** Genetics and Metabolism, UCSD Sch Med 1982; **Fac Appt:** Prof Ped, UCLA

Jones, Marilyn MD [CG] - **Spec Exp:** Dysmorphology; Craniofacial Disorders; **Hospital:** Rady Children's Hosp - San Diego, UCSD Med Ctr; **Address:** 3020 Chldns Way, MC 5031, San Diego, CA 92123-2746; **Phone:** 858-966-5840; **Board Cert:** Pediatrics 1979; Clinical Genetics 2006; **Med School:** Columbia P&S 1974; **Resid:** Internal Medicine, UCSD Med Ctr 1977; Pediatrics, UCSD Med Ctr 1978; **Fellow:** Dysmorphology, UCSD Med Ctr 1979

Clinical Genetics

Morris, Colleen A MD [CG] - **Spec Exp:** Williams Syndrome; Inherited Disorders; Fetal Alcohol Syndrome; **Hospital:** Univ Med Ctr - Las Vegas; **Address:** Univ Nevada Sch Medicine, Dept Pediatrics/Genetics, 2040 W Charleston Blvd, Ste 401, Las Vegas, NV 89102; **Phone:** 702-671-2200; **Board Cert:** Pediatrics 1986; Clinical Genetics 1987; **Med School:** Loyola Univ-Stritch Sch Med 1981; **Resid:** Pediatrics, Phoenix Hosp 1984; **Fellow:** Clinical Genetics, Univ Utah Sch Med 1986; **Fac Appt:** Prof Ped, Univ Nevada

Nussbaum, Robert MD [CG] - **Spec Exp:** Genetic Disorders; **Hospital:** UCSF Med Ctr; **Address:** Inst Human Genetics, 513 Parnassus Ave, rm HSE901E, San Francisco, CA 94143-0794; **Phone:** 415-476-3200; **Board Cert:** Internal Medicine 1978; Clinical Genetics 1982; Clinical Molecular Genetics 2004; **Med School:** Harvard Med Sch 1975; **Resid:** Internal Medicine, Barnes Hosp 1978; **Fellow:** Clinical Genetics, Baylor Univ 1983

Randolph, Linda MD [CG] - **Spec Exp:** Dysmorphology; Skeletal Dysplasia; Prenatal Genetic Diagnosis; Neurofibromatosis; **Hospital:** Chldns Hosp - Los Angeles, Van Nuys Comm Hosp; **Address:** 4650 Sunset Blvd, MS 90, Los Angeles, CA 90027; **Phone:** 323-361-2178; **Board Cert:** Pediatrics 1987; Clinical Genetics 1987; Clinical Cytogenetics 1990; **Med School:** Geo Wash Univ 1982; **Resid:** Pediatrics, Chldns Natl Med Ctr 1985; **Fellow:** Clinical Molecular Genetics, Harbor-UCLA Med Ctr/Cedar-Sinai Med Ctr 1989; **Fac Appt:** Asst Prof Ped, USC-Keck School of Medicine

Rimoin, David L MD/PhD [CG] - **Spec Exp:** Skeletal Dysplasia; Marfan's Syndrome; Birth Defects; **Hospital:** Cedars-Sinai Med Ctr; **Address:** 8700 Beverly Blvd, PACT 400, Los Angeles, CA 90048; **Phone:** 310-423-9914; **Board Cert:** Internal Medicine 1968; Clinical Genetics 1984; **Med School:** McGill Univ 1961; **Resid:** Internal Medicine, Royal Victoria Hosp 1963; Internal Medicine, Johns Hopkins Hosp 1964; **Fellow:** Clinical Genetics, Johns Hopkins Hosp 1967; **Fac Appt:** Prof Ped, UCLA

Seaver, Laurie H MD [CG] - **Spec Exp:** Birth Defects; Fetal Alcohol Syndrome; Dysmorphology; Prenatal Diagnosis; **Hospital:** Kapiolani Med Ctr for Women & Chldn, Queen's Med Ctr - Honolulu; **Address:** Hawaii Community Genetics, 1441 Kapiolani Blvd, Ste 1800, Honolulu, HI 96814; **Phone:** 808-973-3403; **Board Cert:** Pediatrics 2005; Clinical Genetics 2010; **Med School:** Univ Ariz Coll Med 1987; **Resid:** Pediatrics, Univ Ariz 1990; **Fellow:** Clinical Genetics, Univ Ariz Coll Med 1993; **Fac Appt:** Assoc Prof Ped, Univ Hawaii JA Burns Sch Med

Weitzel, Jeffrey N MD [CG] - **Spec Exp:** Breast Cancer; Ovarian Cancer; Hereditary Cancer; **Hospital:** City of Hope Natl Med Ctr; **Address:** City of Hope Cancer Ctr, 1500 E Duarte Rd, Duarte, CA 91010; **Phone:** 626-256-8662; **Board Cert:** Internal Medicine 1986; Medical Oncology 1989; Clinical Genetics 2009; **Med School:** Univ Minn 1983; **Resid:** Internal Medicine, Univ Minn Hosps 1986; Hematology, Hammersmith Hosp 1987; **Fellow:** Hematology & Oncology, Tufts-New England Med Ctr 1992; Clinical Genetics, Tufts-New England Med Ctr 1996; **Fac Appt:** Assoc Clin Prof Med, USC Sch Med

Wilcox Jr, William R MD/PhD [CG] - **Spec Exp:** Inborn Errors of Metabolism; Skeletal Dysplasia; Fabry's Disease; Rare Genetic Disorders; **Hospital:** Cedars-Sinai Med Ctr; **Address:** Cedars Sinai Med Ctr, Dept Med Genetics, 8700 Beverly Blvd, PACT 400, Los Angeles, CA 90048; **Phone:** 310-423-9914; **Board Cert:** Clinical Genetics 2010; Clinical Biochemical Genetics 2010; Clinical Molecular Genetics 2010; **Med School:** UCLA 1988; **Resid:** Pediatrics, UCLA Med Ctr 1991; **Fellow:** Clinical Genetics, Cedars-Sinai Med Ctr 1994; **Fac Appt:** Prof Ped, UCLA

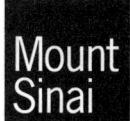 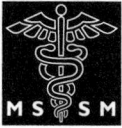

MOUNT SINAI
SCHOOL OF
MEDICINE

**THE MOUNT SINAI MEDICAL CENTER
GENETICS AND GENOMIC SCIENCES**
One Gustave L. Levy Place
Fifth Avenue and 100th Street
New York, NY 10029-6574
Physician Referral: 212-241-6947
www.mountsinaimedicalgenetics.org

THE DEPARTMENT OF GENETICS AND GENOMIC SCIENCES at The Mount Sinai Medical Center is one of the largest medical genetics centers in the nation, providing expert diagnostic, therapeutic, and counseling services for patients and families with or at risk for genetics disorders or birth defects. The department performs sophisticated diagnostic tests in its state-of-the-art molecular, biochemical, and cytogenetics laboratories, which are New York State and Clinical Laboratory Improvement Amendments (CLIA) licensed, and certified by the College of American Pathologists (CAP).

The department has more than 50 internationally recognized faculty members, including physicians, counselors, and laboratory geneticists who are certified by the American Board of Medical Genetics or the American Board of Genetic Counseling.

Programs and services offered by the department include:

- Clinical Genetic Disorders Program
- Program for Inherited Metabolic Diseases
- Reproductive Genetic Counseling Program
- Cancer Genetic Counseling Program
- Mount Sinai Center for Jewish Genetic Diseases
- International Center for Fabry Disease
- Mount Sinai Comprehensive Gaucher Disease Treatment Center
- Porphyria Comprehensive Diagnostic and Treatment Center
- Congenital Anomalies and Craniofacial Program
- Cardiovascular Genetics Program
- Niemann Pick Disease Center

Advances In Diagnosis And Disease Treatment – In the past several years, Mount Sinai researchers have identified genes responsible for various genetic diseases and developed new treatments for inherited disorders. The following are some examples and results of this important work:

- We have identified genes involved in over a dozen diseases, most recently a debilitating juvenile arthritis, several dystonias, and an inherited form of obesity. The identification of these genes leads to precise diagnosis, understanding disease pathogenesis, and new treatments for these diseases. We have also recently identified a gene linked to prostate cancer.

GROUNDBREAKING RESEARCH AND NEW FORMS OF TREATMENT
There are more than 10,000 known genetic disorders, and current research is identifying the genetic susceptibilities and causative genes for many of these diseases. The faculty of the Department of Genetics and Genomic Sciences at Mount Sinai is performing research to develop new and improved methods for the diagnosis, prevention, and treatment of rare and common diseases. The Human Genome Project, and advances in gene analysis technology and stem cell biology, have accelerated this research.

- Our researchers helped identify eight genes involved in causing Noonan syndrome, a common genetic disorder that causes congenital heart defects. Affected families can now receive early diagnosis and prevention.

- Research pioneered by the Department of Genetics and Genomic Sciences resulted in the development of a safe, effective, FDA-approved treatment for Fabry disease, an inherited metabolic disorder that can cause kidney failure, heart disease, stroke, and premature death.

- Departmental faculty have developed a treatment for Niemann-Pick Type B disease, a hereditary disorder that results in death in childhood or early adulthood.

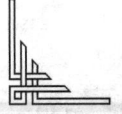

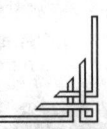

The Best in American Medicine
www.CastleConnolly.com

Colon & Rectal Surgery

A colon and rectal surgeon is trained to diagnose and treat various diseases of the intestinal tract, colon, rectum, anal canal and perianal area by medical and surgical means. This specialist also deals with other organs and tissues (such as the liver and gallbladder) involved with primary
intestinal disease.

Colon and rectal surgeons have the expertise to diagnose and often manage anorectal conditions such as hemorrhoids, fissures (painful tears in the anal lining), abscesses and fistulae (infections located around the anus and rectum) in the office setting. They also treat problems of the intestine and colon and perform endoscopic procedures to evaluate and treat problems such as cancer, polyps (precancerous growths) and inflammatory conditions.

Training Required: Six years (including general surgery)

COLON & RECTAL SURGERY

New England

Bleday, Ronald MD [CRS] - **Spec Exp:** Colon & Rectal Cancer; **Hospital:** Brigham and Women's Hosp (page 57), Dana-Farber Cancer Inst (page 57); **Address:** Brigham & Women's Hosp, Dept Surgery, 75 Francis St, ASB II, Boston, MA 02115; **Phone:** 617-732-8460; **Board Cert:** Surgery 2009; Colon & Rectal Surgery 2003; **Med School:** McGill Univ 1982; **Resid:** Surgery, Rhode Island Hosp 1989; Surgical Oncology, Brigham & Womens Hosp 1986; **Fellow:** Endoscopy, Mass Genl Hosp 1990; Colon & Rectal Surgery, Univ Minn 1991; **Fac Appt:** Assoc Prof S, Harvard Med Sch

Hackford, Alan W MD [CRS] - **Hospital:** Caritas St Elizabeth's Med Ctr-Boston; **Address:** St Elizabeth's Med Ctr, Dept Surgery, 736 Cambridge St, Boston, MA 02135; **Phone:** 617-789-2442; **Board Cert:** Colon & Rectal Surgery 1985; Surgery 2002; **Med School:** Univ Conn 1977; **Resid:** Surgery, New England Med Ctr 1982; **Fellow:** Colon & Rectal Surgery, Lahey Clinic 1984; **Fac Appt:** Prof S, Tufts Univ

Harnsberger, Jeffrey R MD [CRS] - **Spec Exp:** Colon & Rectal Cancer; Inflammatory Bowel Disease; **Hospital:** Dartmouth - Hitchcock Med Ctr, Elliot Hosp; **Address:** Dartmouth-Hitchcock Manchester, 100 Hitchcock Way, Manchester, NH 03104; **Phone:** 603-695-2840; **Board Cert:** Surgery 2001; Colon & Rectal Surgery 2005; **Med School:** Med Coll OH 1987; **Resid:** Surgery, Dartmouth-Hitchkock Med Ctr 1992; **Fellow:** Colon & Rectal Surgery, St Louis Univ Med Ctr 1993; **Fac Appt:** Asst Prof S, Dartmouth Med Sch

Hyman, Neil H MD [CRS] - **Spec Exp:** Inflammatory Bowel Disease; Colon & Rectal Cancer; **Hospital:** Fletcher Allen Health Care- Med Ctr Campus; **Address:** FAHC 111 Colchester Ave, Burlington, VT 05401; **Phone:** 802-847-3339; **Board Cert:** Surgery 2008; Colon & Rectal Surgery 2003; **Med School:** Univ VT Coll Med 1984; **Resid:** Surgery, Mt Sinai Med Ctr 1989; **Fellow:** Colon & Rectal Surgery, Cleveland Clinic 1990; **Fac Appt:** Prof S, Univ VT Coll Med

Longo, Walter E MD [CRS] - **Spec Exp:** Colon & Rectal Cancer; Gastrointestinal Surgery; Inflammatory Bowel Disease; **Hospital:** Yale-New Haven Hosp, Yale Med Group; **Address:** Dept Surgery/Gastroenterology, 330 Cedar St, rm LH118, Box 208062, New Haven, CT 06520-8062; **Phone:** 203-785-2616; **Board Cert:** Surgery 2001; Colon & Rectal Surgery 2006; **Med School:** NY Med Coll 1984; **Resid:** Surgery, Yale-New Haven Hosp 1990; **Fellow:** Research, Yale-New Haven Hosp 1988; Colon & Rectal Surgery, Cleveland Clinic 1991; **Fac Appt:** Prof S, Yale Univ

Nagle, Deborah A MD [CRS] - **Spec Exp:** Colon & Rectal Cancer; Anal Cancer; Laparoscopic Surgery; **Hospital:** Beth Israel Deaconess Med Ctr - Boston; **Address:** Beth Israel Deaconess Med Ctr, 330 Brookline Ave Stoneman Bldg - rm 932, Boston, MA 02215; **Phone:** 617-667-4159; **Board Cert:** Colon & Rectal Surgery 2006; Surgery 2004; **Med School:** Univ Pennsylvania 1988; **Resid:** Surgery, Graduate Hosp 1993; Colon & Rectal Surgery, Thos Jefferson Univ Hosp 1994; **Fac Appt:** Prof CRS, Univ Pennsylvania

Orkin, Bruce A MD [CRS] - **Spec Exp:** Colon & Rectal Cancer; Laparoscopic Surgery; **Hospital:** Tufts Med Ctr; **Address:** Tufts Med Ctr, Div Colon & Rectal Surg, 860 Washington St, Box 6190, Boston, MA 02111; **Phone:** 617-636-6190; **Board Cert:** Colon & Rectal Surgery 2001; Surgery 2008; **Med School:** Univ Minn 1981; **Resid:** Surgery, Mayo Clinic 1986; **Fellow:** Surgical Research, Mayo Clinic 1988; Colon & Rectal Surgery, Cleveland Clinic 1989; **Fac Appt:** Prof S, Tufts Univ

Read, Thomas E MD [CRS] - **Spec Exp:** Colon & Rectal Cancer; Inflammatory Bowel Disease; Laparoscopic Surgery; Diverticulitis; **Hospital:** Lahey Clin; **Address:** Department of Colon and Rectal Surgery, Lahey Clinic Medical Center, 41 Mall Road, Burlington, MA 01805; **Phone:** 781-744-8971; **Board Cert:** Surgery 2005; Colon & Rectal Surgery 2008; **Med School:** UCSF 1988; **Resid:** Surgery, UCSF Med Ctr 1995; **Fellow:** Colon & Rectal Surgery, Lahey Clinic 1996; **Fac Appt:** Prof S, Tufts Univ

Roberts, Patricia L MD [CRS] - **Spec Exp:** Diverticulitis; Colon & Rectal Cancer; Inflammatory Bowel Disease; Crohn's Disease; **Hospital:** Lahey Clin; **Address:** 41 Mall Rd, Burlington, MA 01805; **Phone:** 781-744-8243; **Board Cert:** Colon & Rectal Surgery 2003; **Med School:** Boston Univ 1981; **Resid:** Surgery, Boston City Hosp 1986; **Fellow:** Colon & Rectal Surgery, Lahey Clinic 1988; **Fac Appt:** Prof S, Tufts Univ

Schoetz Jr, David J MD [CRS] - **Spec Exp:** Inflammatory Bowel Disease/Crohn's; Colon & Rectal Cancer; Incontinence-Fecal; Anorectal Disorders; **Hospital:** Lahey Clin; **Address:** Lahey Clin Med Ctr, Dept Colon & Rectal Surg, 41 Mall Rd, Burlington, MA 01805-0001; **Phone:** 781-744-8889; **Board Cert:** Surgery 2001; Colon & Rectal Surgery 1983; **Med School:** Med Coll Wisc 1974; **Resid:** Surgery, Boston Univ Med Ctr 1981; Surgery, Boston Univ Med Ctr 1978; **Fellow:** Colon & Rectal Surgery, Lahey Clin 1982; **Fac Appt:** Prof S, Tufts Univ

Shah, Nishit S MD [CRS] - **Spec Exp:** Anorectal Disorders; Colon & Rectal Cancer; Inflammatory Bowel Disease; **Hospital:** Rhode Island Hosp; **Address:** University Surgical Associates Inc., 2 Dudley St, Ste 370, Providence, RI 02905; **Phone:** 401-553-8322; **Board Cert:** Surgery 2001; Colon & Rectal Surgery 2004; **Med School:** England, UK 1989; **Resid:** Surgery, Univ Pittsburgh Med Ctr 1995; **Fellow:** Colon & Rectal Surgery, Cleveland Clinic 1996

Shellito, Paul C MD [CRS] - **Spec Exp:** Colon & Rectal Cancer; Ulcerative Colitis; Anorectal Disorders; **Hospital:** Mass Genl Hosp; **Address:** 15 Parkman St, Ste Wang 460, Mass General, Boston, MA 02114-3117; **Phone:** 617-724-0365; **Board Cert:** Surgery 2002; Colon & Rectal Surgery 1994; **Med School:** Harvard Med Sch 1977; **Resid:** Surgery, Mass Genl Hosp 1983; Surgery, Auckland Univ Med Sch 1981; **Fellow:** Colon & Rectal Surgery, Univ Minn 1985; **Fac Appt:** Asst Prof S, Harvard Med Sch

Mid Atlantic

Efron, Jonathan E MD [CRS] - **Spec Exp:** Colon & Rectal Cancer; Incontinence-Fecal; Inflammatory Bowel Disease; Anorectal Disorders; **Hospital:** Johns Hopkins Hosp (page 61), Johns Hopkins Bayview Med Ctr (page 61); **Address:** Johns Hopkins Hosp, 600 N Wolfe St, Baltimore, MD 21287; **Phone:** 410-933-1233; **Board Cert:** Surgery 2008; Colon & Rectal Surgery 2009; **Med School:** Univ MD Sch Med 1993; **Resid:** Surgery, LIJ Medical Ctr 1999; **Fellow:** Colon & Rectal Surgery, Cleveland Clinic 2000; Research, Cleveland Clinic 2001; **Fac Appt:** Assoc Prof S, Johns Hopkins Univ

Eisenstat, Theodore E MD [CRS] - **Spec Exp:** Colon Cancer; Inflammatory Bowel Disease; Anorectal Disorders; Hemorrhoids; **Hospital:** Robert Wood Johnson Univ Hosp - New Brunswick, JFK Med Ctr - Edison; **Address:** 3900 Park Ave, Ste 101, Edison, NJ 08820-3032; **Phone:** 732-494-6640; **Board Cert:** Surgery 1974; Colon & Rectal Surgery 1994; **Med School:** NY Med Coll 1968; **Resid:** Surgery, Thomas Jefferson Univ Hosp 1971; Surgery, Pennsylvania Hosp 1973; **Fellow:** Colon & Rectal Surgery, Muhlenberg Med Ctr 1978; **Fac Appt:** Clin Prof S, UMDNJ-RW Johnson Med Sch

Colon & Rectal Surgery

Fry, Robert D MD [CRS] - **Spec Exp:** Colon & Rectal Cancer; Inflammatory Bowel Disease/Crohn's; Anal Cancer; Hemorrhoids; **Hospital:** Pennsylvania Hosp-UPHS (page 68), Hosp Univ Penn - UPHS (page 68); **Address:** Pennsylvania Hospital, Div Colon & Rectal Surgery, 700 Spruce St, Ste 305, Philadelphia, PA 19106-4023; **Phone:** 215-662-2078; **Board Cert:** Surgery 2006; Colon & Rectal Surgery 1998; **Med School:** Washington Univ, St Louis 1972; **Resid:** Surgery, Barnes Jewish Hosp 1977; **Fellow:** Colon & Rectal Surgery, Cleveland Clinic 1978; **Fac Appt:** Prof S, Univ Pennsylvania

Gearhart, Susan L MD [CRS] - **Spec Exp:** Colon & Rectal Cancer-Hereditary; Incontinence-Fecal; Inflammatory Bowel Disease/Crohn's; **Hospital:** Johns Hopkins Hosp (page 61); **Address:** Johns Hopkins Hosp, Dept of Surgery, 600 N Wolfe St, Blalock 658, Baltimore, MD 21287; **Phone:** 410-955-7323; **Board Cert:** Surgery 2002; Colon & Rectal Surgery 2003; **Med School:** Loyola Univ-Stritch Sch Med 1993; **Resid:** Surgery, John Hopkins Hospital 2000; **Fellow:** Colon & Rectal Surgery, Cleveland Clin 2002; **Fac Appt:** Asst Prof S, Johns Hopkins Univ

Geisler, Daniel P MD [CRS] - **Spec Exp:** Colon & Rectal Cancer & Surgery; Minimally Invasive Surgery; Rectal Cancer/Sphincter Preservation; Anal Cancer; **Hospital:** Allegheny General Hosp; **Address:** Allegheny Cancer Center, 320 East North Ave, Ste 261, Pittsburgh, PA 15212; **Phone:** 412-359-3901; **Board Cert:** Surgery 2003; Colon & Rectal Surgery 2005; **Med School:** St Louis Univ 1996; **Resid:** Surgery, Univ Oklahoma Hlth Sci Ctr 2001; **Fellow:** Colon & Rectal Surgery, Lankenau Hosp 2002; Minimally Invasive Surgery, Saint Vincent Hlth Ctr 2003; **Fac Appt:** Assoc Prof S, Cleveland Cl Coll Med/Case West Res

Goldstein, Scott D MD [CRS] - **Spec Exp:** Colon & Rectal Cancer; Inflammatory Bowel Disease; Laparoscopic Surgery; **Hospital:** Thomas Jefferson Univ Hosp; **Address:** 1100 Walnut St Fl 5 - Ste 500, Philadelphia, PA 19107; **Phone:** 215-955-5869; **Board Cert:** Surgery 1984; Colon & Rectal Surgery 1985; **Med School:** SUNY Buffalo 1978; **Resid:** Surgery, Lenox Hill Hosp 1983; Colon & Rectal Surgery, UMDNJ Med Ctr 1984; **Fac Appt:** Assoc Prof S, Thomas Jefferson Univ

Gorfine, Stephen R MD [CRS] - **Spec Exp:** Anal Disorders & Reconstruction; Hemorrhoids; Rectal Cancer; Anal Cancer; **Hospital:** Mount Sinai Med Ctr (page 63), Lenox Hill Hosp; **Address:** 25 E 69th St, New York, NY 10021-4925; **Phone:** 212-517-8600; **Board Cert:** Internal Medicine 1981; Surgery 2007; Colon & Rectal Surgery 1988; **Med School:** Univ Mass Sch Med 1978; **Resid:** Internal Medicine, Mt Sinai Hosp 1981; Surgery, Mt Sinai Hosp 1985; **Fellow:** Colon & Rectal Surgery, Ferguson Hosp 1987; **Fac Appt:** Clin Prof S, Mount Sinai Sch Med

Guillem, Jose MD [CRS] - **Spec Exp:** Colon & Rectal Cancer; Rectal Cancer/Sphincter Preservation; Colon & Rectal Cancer-Hereditary; Peritoneal Mucinous Carcinomatosis; **Hospital:** Meml Sloan-Kettering Cancer Ctr; **Address:** 1275 York Avenue, New York, NY 10065; **Phone:** 212-639-8278; **Board Cert:** Colon & Rectal Surgery 2005; Surgery 2004; **Med School:** Yale Univ 1983; **Resid:** Surgery, Columbia-Presby Med Ctr 1990; **Fellow:** Colon & Rectal Surgery, Lahey Clinic 1991; **Fac Appt:** Prof CRS, Cornell Univ-Weill Med Coll

Medich, David MD [CRS] - **Spec Exp:** Colon & Rectal Cancer; Ulcerative Colitis; Inflammatory Bowel Disease/Crohn's; **Hospital:** UPMC Passavant-McCandless; **Address:** UPMC Cancer Ctr at UPMC Pasavant, Ground FL, South Pavilion, 9100 Babcock Blvd, Pittsburgh, PA 15237; **Phone:** 877-684-7189; **Board Cert:** Surgery 2004; Colon & Rectal Surgery 2006; **Med School:** Ohio State Univ 1987; **Resid:** Surgery, Univ Pittsburgh 1990; **Fellow:** Research, Univ Pittsburgh 1993; Colon & Rectal Surgery, Cleveland Clinic 1994; **Fac Appt:** Assoc Prof CRS, Drexel Univ Coll Med

Milsom, Jeffrey W MD [CRS] - **Spec Exp:** Inflammatory Bowel Disease; Laparoscopic Surgery; Colon & Rectal Cancer; Crohn's Disease; **Hospital:** NY-Presby/Weill Cornell Med Ctr, NY (page 65); **Address:** NY Cornell Med Ctr, Div Colorectal Surgery, 1315 York Ave Fl 2, New York, NY 10065-5304; **Phone:** 212-746-6030; **Board Cert:** Colon & Rectal Surgery 1986; **Med School:** Univ Pittsburgh 1979; **Resid:** Surgery, Roosevelt Hosp 1981; Surgery, Univ Virginia Med Ctr 1984; **Fellow:** Colon & Rectal Surgery, Ferguson Hosp 1985; **Fac Appt:** Prof S, Cornell Univ-Weill Med Coll

Pello, Mark J MD [CRS] - **Spec Exp:** Colon & Rectal Cancer; Inflammatory Bowel Disease; Laparoscopic Surgery; **Hospital:** Cooper Univ Hosp; **Address:** 3 Cooper Plaza, Ste 411, Camden, NJ 08103; **Phone:** 856-342-2270; **Board Cert:** Surgery 1997; Colon & Rectal Surgery 1980; **Med School:** Jefferson Med Coll 1975; **Resid:** Surgery, Cooper Med Ctr 1979; Colon & Rectal Surgery, Wm Beaumont Hosp 1980; **Fac Appt:** Assoc Prof S, UMDNJ-RW Johnson Med Sch

Procaccino Jr, John A MD [CRS] - **Spec Exp:** Inflammatory Bowel Disease/Crohn's; Colon & Rectal Cancer; Anorectal Disorders; Colon & Rectal Cancer-Familial Polyposis; **Hospital:** N Shore Univ Hosp, Long Island Jewish Med Ctr; **Address:** Chief, Division of Colon & Rectal Surg, 900 Northern Blvd, Ste 100, Great Neck, NY 11021; **Phone:** 516-730-2100; **Board Cert:** Colon & Rectal Surgery 2003; Surgery 2009; **Med School:** NYU Sch Med 1984; **Resid:** Surgery, N Shore Univ Hosp 1989; **Fellow:** Colon & Rectal Surgery, Cleveland Clinic 1990; **Fac Appt:** Asst Clin Prof S, Cornell Univ-Weill Med Coll

Rombeau, John L MD [CRS] - **Spec Exp:** Colon & Rectal Cancer; Inflammatory Bowel Disease/Crohn's; Ulcerative Colitis; Rectal Cancer/Sphincter Preservation; **Hospital:** Temple Univ Hosp; **Address:** Dept Surg, 3401 N Broad St, Parkinson Pavilion Fl 4, Philadelphia, PA 19104-5103; **Phone:** 215-707-3133; **Board Cert:** Colon & Rectal Surgery 1977; **Med School:** Loma Linda Univ 1967; **Resid:** Surgery, Good Samaritan Hosp 1971; Surgery, LAC-USC Med Ctr 1975; **Fellow:** Colon & Rectal Surgery, Cleveland Clinic 1976; Nutrition & Metabolism, Brigham & Women's Hosp 1984; **Fac Appt:** Prof S, Temple Univ

Stein, David E MD [CRS] - **Spec Exp:** Colon & Rectal Cancer & Surgery; Laparoscopic Surgery; Inflammatory Bowel Disease; Anorectal Disorders; **Hospital:** Hahnemann Univ Hosp, St. Francis Hosp; **Address:** 245 N 15th St, Ste 413, Philadelphia, PA 19102; **Phone:** 215-762-1545; **Board Cert:** Surgery 2004; Colon & Rectal Surgery 2004; **Med School:** SUNY Downstate 1997; **Resid:** Surgery, T Jefferson Univ Hosp 2002; **Fellow:** Colon & Rectal Surgery, Cleveland Clinic 2003; **Fac Appt:** Asst Prof S, Drexel Univ Coll Med

Steinhagen, Randolph MD [CRS] - **Spec Exp:** Colostomy Avoidance; Colon & Rectal Cancer; Inflammatory Bowel Disease/Crohn's; Ulcerative Colitis; **Hospital:** Mount Sinai Med Ctr (page 63), St. John's Riverside Hosp-Andrus Pavil; **Address:** Div Colon & Rectal Surgery, 5 E 98th St Fl 14, Box 1259, New York, NY 10029-6501; **Phone:** 212-241-3547; **Board Cert:** Surgery 2002; Colon & Rectal Surgery 1985; **Med School:** Wayne State Univ 1977; **Resid:** Surgery, Mount Sinai Hosp 1982; **Fellow:** Colon & Rectal Surgery, Cleveland Clinic 1983; **Fac Appt:** Prof S, Mount Sinai Sch Med

Whelan, Richard L MD [CRS] - **Spec Exp:** Laparoscopic Surgery; Colon & Rectal Cancer; **Hospital:** St. Luke's - Roosevelt Hosp Ctr - Roosevelt Div (page 55); **Address:** 425 W 59th St, Ste 7B, New York, NY 10019; **Phone:** 212-523-8172; **Board Cert:** Surgery 1997; Colon & Rectal Surgery 1989; **Med School:** Columbia P&S 1982; **Resid:** Surgery, Columbia Presby Hosp 1987; **Fellow:** Colon & Rectal Surgery, Univ Minn Med Ctr 1988; **Fac Appt:** Assoc Clin Prof S, Columbia P&S

Colon & Rectal Surgery

Southeast

Beck, Sandra J MD [CRS] - **Hospital:** Univ of Kentucky Albert B. Chandler Hosp; **Address:** U Kentucky Chandler Hosp, Dept Surgery, 800 Rose St, Lexington, KY 40536; **Phone:** 859-323-6346 x232; **Board Cert:** Surgery 2002; Colon & Rectal Surgery 2003; **Med School:** Wright State Univ 1995; **Resid:** Surgery, Allegheny Gen Hosp 2001; **Fellow:** Colon & Rectal Surgery, Cleveland Clinic 2002; **Fac Appt:** Asst Prof S, Univ KY Coll Med

Galandiuk, Susan MD [CRS] - **Spec Exp:** Colon & Rectal Cancer; Inflammatory Bowel Disease/Crohn's; **Hospital:** Univ of Louisville Hosp, Norton Hosp; **Address:** 401 E Chestnut St, Ste 710, Louisville, KY 40202; **Phone:** 502-583-8303; **Board Cert:** Surgery 2008; Colon & Rectal Surgery 2002; **Med School:** Germany 1982; **Resid:** Surgery, Cleveland Clinic Fdtn 1988; **Fellow:** Research, Univ Louisville Hosp 1989; Colon & Rectal Surgery, Mayo Clin 1990; **Fac Appt:** Prof CRS, Univ Louisville Sch Med

Golub, Richard W MD [CRS] - **Spec Exp:** Colon & Rectal Cancer; Laparoscopic Surgery; Hemorrhoids; **Hospital:** Sarasota Meml Hosp, Doctors Hosp - Sarasota; **Address:** Surgical Specialists, 3333 Cattlemen Rd, Ste 206, Sarasota, FL 34232; **Phone:** 941-341-0042; **Board Cert:** Surgery 2000; Colon & Rectal Surgery 2003; **Med School:** Albert Einstein Coll Med 1984; **Resid:** Surgery, Univ Hosp 1990; **Fellow:** Colon & Rectal Surgery, Grant Medical Center 1991

Hartmann, Rene F MD [CRS] - **Spec Exp:** Laparoscopic Surgery; Rectovaginal Fistula; Colon Cancer; Inflammatory Bowel Disease; **Hospital:** Mercy Hosp, Baptist Hosp of Miami; **Address:** Laparoscopic Ctr of S Florida, 9195 Sunset Drive, Ste 230, Miami, FL 33173; **Phone:** 305-271-0300; **Board Cert:** Colon & Rectal Surgery 1994; **Med School:** Venezuela 1971; **Resid:** Surgery, Jackson Meml Hosp 1976; Surgery, Orange Meml Hosp 1977; **Fellow:** Colon & Rectal Surgery, Grant Hosp 1978; **Fac Appt:** Assoc Clin Prof S, Univ Miami Sch Med

Mantyh, Christopher R MD [CRS] - **Spec Exp:** Colon & Rectal Cancer & Surgery; Rectal Cancer/Sphincter Preservation; Incontinence-Fecal; Colon & Rectal Cancer-Familial Polyposis; **Hospital:** Duke Univ Hosp; **Address:** DUMC, Box 3117, Durham, NC 27710; **Phone:** 919-681-3977; **Board Cert:** Surgery 2010; Colon & Rectal Surgery 2000; **Med School:** Univ Wisc 1991; **Resid:** Surgery, Duke Univ Med Ctr 1998; **Fellow:** Colon & Rectal Surgery, Cleveland Clinic 1999; **Fac Appt:** Assoc Prof CRS, Univ Wisc

Marcet, Jorge E MD [CRS] - **Spec Exp:** Colon & Rectal Cancer; Crohn's Disease; Anal Disorders & Reconstruction; **Hospital:** Tampa Genl Hosp; **Address:** USF Dept Surgery, 1 Tample General Circle, Ste F-145, Tampa, FL 33606; **Phone:** 813-844-4545; **Board Cert:** Surgery 2001; Colon & Rectal Surgery 2003; **Med School:** Cornell Univ-Weill Med Coll 1985; **Resid:** Surgery, St Luke's-Roosevelt Med Ctr 1990; **Fellow:** Colon & Rectal Surgery, Columbia Presby Hosp 1990; Colon & Rectal Surgery, St Luke's-Roosevelt Hosp 1991; **Fac Appt:** Assoc Prof S, Univ S Fla Coll Med

Nogueras, Juan J MD [CRS] - **Spec Exp:** Colon & Rectal Cancer; Inflammatory Bowel Disease/Crohn's; Incontinence-Fecal; Laparoscopic Surgery; **Hospital:** Cleveland Clin - Weston; **Address:** Cleveland Clinic, Dept Colorectal Surgery, 2950 Cleveland Clinic Blvd, Weston, FL 33331; **Phone:** 954-659-5251; **Board Cert:** Surgery 2007; Colon & Rectal Surgery 2003; **Med School:** Jefferson Med Coll 1982; **Resid:** Surgery, Columbia Presby Med Ctr 1987; **Fellow:** Colon & Rectal Surgery, Univ Minn 1991

Vernava III, Anthony M MD [CRS] - **Spec Exp:** Colon & Rectal Cancer; Colon & Rectal Cancer-Familial Polyposis; Inflammatory Bowel Disease; Crohn's Disease; **Hospital:** Physicians Regl Hlthcare Med Ctr-Pine Ridge; **Address:** Physicians Regl Med Grp, 6101 Pine Ridge Rd, Naples, FL 34119; **Phone:** 239-348-4531; **Board Cert:** Surgery 2007; Colon & Rectal Surgery 1989; **Med School:** St Louis Univ 1982; **Resid:** Surgery, St Louis Univ Med Ctr 1988; Colon & Rectal Surgery, Univ Minnesota Med Ctr 1989; **Fellow:** Colon & Rectal Surgery, St Marks Hosp 1990; Colon & Rectal Surgery, Natl Cancer Ctr 1989

Wexner, Steven D MD [CRS] - **Spec Exp:** Colon & Rectal Cancer; Inflammatory Bowel Disease/Crohn's; Laparoscopic Surgery; Incontinence-Fecal; **Hospital:** Cleveland Clin - Weston; **Address:** 2950 Cleveland Clinic Blvd, Weston, FL 33331-3609; **Phone:** 954-659-5278; **Board Cert:** Surgery 2005; Colon & Rectal Surgery 2006; **Med School:** Cornell Univ-Weill Med Coll 1982; **Resid:** Surgery, Roosevelt Hosp 1987; **Fellow:** Colon & Rectal Surgery, Univ Minn 1988; **Fac Appt:** Prof S, Cleveland Cl Coll Med/Case West Res

Wise, Paul E MD [CRS] - **Spec Exp:** Colon & Rectal Cancer & Surgery; Minimally Invasive Surgery; Colon & Rectal Cancer-Hereditary; Crohn's Disease; **Hospital:** Vanderbilt Univ Med Ctr (page 76); **Address:** Vanderbilt Univ Med Ctr, Dept of General Surgery, D-5248 Medical Center N, Nashville, TN 37232; **Phone:** 615-343-4612; **Board Cert:** Surgery 2004; Colon & Rectal Surgery 2005; **Med School:** Johns Hopkins Univ 1996; **Resid:** Surgery, Vanderbilt Univ Med Ctr 2003; **Fellow:** Colon & Rectal Surgery, Barnes-Jewish Hosp 2004; **Fac Appt:** Asst Prof S, Vanderbilt Univ

Midwest

Abcarian, Herand MD [CRS] - **Spec Exp:** Rectal Cancer/Sphincter Preservation; Inflammatory Bowel Disease; Anorectal Disorders; Incontinence-Fecal; **Hospital:** Univ of IL Med Ctr at Chicago, Gottlieb Meml Hosp; **Address:** University of Illinois, Dept of Colorectal Surgery, 1801 W Taylor St, Ste 3F, Chicago, IL 60612; **Phone:** 312-413-2708; **Board Cert:** Surgery 1972; Colon & Rectal Surgery 1972; **Med School:** Iran 1965; **Resid:** Surgery, Cook County Hosp 1971; Colon & Rectal Surgery, Cook County Hosp 1972; **Fac Appt:** Prof S, Univ IL Coll Med

Birnbaum, Elisa H MD [CRS] - **Spec Exp:** Colon & Rectal Cancer; Inflammatory Bowel Disease/Crohn's; Pelvic Organ Prolapse; Rectovaginal Fistula; **Hospital:** Barnes-Jewish Hosp; **Address:** Washington Univ Sch Med, Div Colorectal Surgery, 660 S Euclid, Box 8109, St Louis, MO 63110; **Phone:** 314-454-7177; **Board Cert:** Surgery 2009; Colon & Rectal Surgery 2003; **Med School:** Univ IL Coll Med 1985; **Resid:** Surgery, LIJ Med Ctr 1990; **Fellow:** Colon & Rectal Surgery, Barnes Jewish Hosp 1991; **Fac Appt:** Prof S, Washington Univ, St Louis

Church, James MD [CRS] - **Spec Exp:** Colon & Rectal Cancer-Familial Polyposis; Anorectal Disorders; Incontinence-Fecal; Inflammatory Bowel Disease; **Hospital:** Cleveland Clin (page 56); **Address:** Cleveland Clinic, 9500 Euclid Ave, MC A-30, Cleveland, OH 44195; **Phone:** 216-444-7000; **Med School:** New Zealand 1974; **Resid:** Surgery, Aukland Hosps 1980; **Fellow:** Research, Aukland Hosps 1983; Colon & Rectal Surgery, Cleveland Clinic 1984; **Fac Appt:** Prof CRS, Cleveland Cl Coll Med/Case West Res

Delaney, Conor P MD/PhD [CRS] - **Spec Exp:** Laparoscopic Surgery; Colon & Rectal Cancer; Inflammatory Bowel Disease/Crohn's; Rectal Cancer/Sphincter Preservation; **Hospital:** Univ Hosps Case Med Ctr (page 74); **Address:** 11100 Euclid Ave, Cleveland, OH 44106-5047; **Phone:** 216-844-8087; **Board Cert:** Surgery 1998; Colon & Rectal Surgery 1998; **Med School:** Ireland 1989; **Resid:** Surgery, Univ Hosp 1993; Surgery, Univ Hosp 1999; **Fellow:** Research, Univ of Pittsburgh 1995; Colon & Rectal Surgery, Cleveland Clinic 2000; **Fac Appt:** Prof S, Cleveland Cl Coll Med/Case West Res

Colon & Rectal Surgery

Dietz, David W MD [CRS] - **Spec Exp:** Colon & Rectal Cancer; Anal Cancer; Anorectal Disorders; Pelvic Floor Disorders; **Hospital:** Cleveland Clin (page 56); **Address:** Cleveland Clinic, Colorectal Surgery, 9500 Euclid Ave, Desk A30, Cleveland, OH 44195; **Phone:** 216-445-6597; **Board Cert:** Surgery 2001; Colon & Rectal Surgery 2002; **Med School:** Jefferson Med Coll 1993; **Resid:** Surgery, Cleveland Clinic 1999; Colon & Rectal Surgery, Cleveland Clinic 2001

Fleshman Jr, James W MD [CRS] - **Spec Exp:** Colon & Rectal Cancer; Laparoscopic Surgery; Inflammatory Bowel Disease; **Hospital:** Barnes-Jewish Hosp, Barnes-Jewish West County Hosp; **Address:** Wash Univ Sch Med, Div Colorectal Surgery, 660 S Euclid Ave, Box 8109, St Louis, MO 63110; **Phone:** 314-454-7177; **Board Cert:** Colon & Rectal Surgery 1988; Surgery 2002; **Med School:** Washington Univ, St Louis 1980; **Resid:** Surgery, Jewish Hospital 1986; **Fellow:** Colon & Rectal Surgery, Univ Toronto 1987; **Fac Appt:** Prof S, Washington Univ, St Louis

Foley, Eugene F MD [CRS] - **Spec Exp:** Colon & Rectal Cancer; Ulcerative Colitis; **Hospital:** Univ WI Hosp & Clins; **Address:** Univ WI Hosp & Clins, 600 Highland Ave, Madison, WI 53792-7375; **Phone:** 608-263-2521; **Board Cert:** Surgery 2003; Colon & Rectal Surgery 2005; **Med School:** Harvard Med Sch 1985; **Resid:** Surgery, New England Deaconess Hosp 1991; **Fellow:** Colon & Rectal Surgery, Lahey Clinic 1993; **Fac Appt:** Prof S, Univ Wisc

Kodner, Ira J MD [CRS] - **Spec Exp:** Colon & Rectal Cancer; Inflammatory Bowel Disease/Crohn's; Laparoscopic Surgery; **Hospital:** Barnes-Jewish Hosp; **Address:** Wash Univ Sch Med, Div Colorectal Surgery, 660 S Euclid Ave, Box 8109, St Louis, MO 63110; **Phone:** 314-454-7177; **Board Cert:** Surgery 1975; Colon & Rectal Surgery 1975; **Med School:** Washington Univ, St Louis 1967; **Resid:** Surgery, Barnes-Jewish Hosp 1974; **Fellow:** Colon & Rectal Surgery, Cleveland Clinic 1975; Medical Ethics, Univ Chicago Hosps & Hlth Sys 2004; **Fac Appt:** Prof S, Washington Univ, St Louis

Lavery, Ian C MD [CRS] - **Spec Exp:** Colon & Rectal Cancer; Inflammatory Bowel Disease; Pediatric Gastrointestinal Surgery; **Hospital:** Cleveland Clin (page 56); **Address:** 9500 Euclid Ave, Desk A30, Cleveland, OH 44195; **Phone:** 216-444-6930; **Board Cert:** Colon & Rectal Surgery 1998; **Med School:** Australia 1967; **Resid:** Surgery, Princess Alexandra Hosp 1974; Colon & Rectal Surgery, Cleveland Clinic 1977; **Fac Appt:** Prof S, Case West Res Univ

Lederman, Eric D MD [CRS] - **Spec Exp:** Colon & Rectal Cancer; Anorectal Disorders; Crohn's Disease; Diverticulitis; **Hospital:** Missouri Baptist Med Ctr; **Address:** Suburban Surgical Assocs, 555 N New Ballas Rd, Ste 265, St Louis, MO 63141-6886; **Phone:** 314-991-4644; **Board Cert:** Surgery 2010; Colon & Rectal Surgery 2008; **Med School:** Washington Univ, St Louis ; **Resid:** Surgery, Albany Med Ctr 1999; **Fellow:** Colon & Rectal Surgery, St Louis Univ Hosp 2001

Lowry, Ann C MD [CRS] - **Spec Exp:** Anal Sphincter Repair; Rectovaginal Fistula; Inflammatory Bowel Disease; **Hospital:** Abbott - Northwestern Hosp, Fairview Southdale Hosp; **Address:** 1055 W Gate Drive, Ste 190, St Paul, MN 55114; **Phone:** 651-312-1700; **Board Cert:** Colon & Rectal Surgery 1988; **Med School:** Tufts Univ 1977; **Resid:** Surgery, New Eng Med Ctr Hosps 1982; **Fellow:** Colon & Rectal Surgery, Univ Minn Affil Hosps 1987; **Fac Appt:** Clin Prof S, Univ Minn

Ludwig, Kirk A MD [CRS] - **Spec Exp:** Colon & Rectal Cancer & Surgery; Pelvic Organ Prolapse; Rectal Cancer/Sphincter Preservation; Incontinence-Fecal; **Hospital:** Froedtert and Med Ctr of WI; **Address:** 9200 W Wisconsin Ave, Dept Surgery, Milwaukee, WI 53226; **Phone:** 414-805-5783; **Board Cert:** Surgery 2005; Colon & Rectal Surgery 2007; **Med School:** Univ Cincinnati 1988; **Resid:** Surgery, Med Coll Wisc 1994; **Fellow:** Colon & Rectal Surgery, Cleveland Clinic 1996; **Fac Appt:** Assoc Prof S, Med Coll Wisc

Madoff, Robert D MD [CRS] - **Spec Exp:** Colon & Rectal Cancer; Inflammatory Bowel Disease; Incontinence/Pelvic Floor Disorders; **Address:** 420 Delaware St SE, MC MMC88, Minneapolis, MN 55455; **Phone:** 612-624-9708; **Board Cert:** Colon & Rectal Surgery 2002; **Med School:** Columbia P&S 1979; **Resid:** Surgery, Univ Minn Hosps 1987; **Fellow:** Colon & Rectal Surgery, Univ Minn Hosps 1988; **Fac Appt:** Prof S, Univ Minn

Mutch, Matthew G MD [CRS] - **Spec Exp:** Colon & Rectal Cancer; Inflammatory Bowel Disease; Incontinence/Pelvic Floor Disorders; Rectovaginal Fistula; **Hospital:** Barnes-Jewish Hosp; **Address:** Washington U Med Sch, Dept Surgery, 660 S Euclid Ave, Ste 14102, Box 8109, St Louis, MO 63110-1010; **Phone:** 314-454-7177; **Board Cert:** Surgery 2002; Colon & Rectal Surgery 2003; **Med School:** Washington Univ, St Louis 1994; **Resid:** Surgery, Barnes Jewish Hosp 2001; **Fellow:** Research, Barnes Jewish Hosp 1998; Colon & Rectal Surgery, Lahey Clinic 2002; **Fac Appt:** Assoc Prof S, Washington Univ, St Louis

Nelson, Heidi MD [CRS] - **Spec Exp:** Colon & Rectal Cancer; Gastrointestinal Cancer; **Hospital:** Mayo Med Ctr & Clin - Rochester, Rochester Methodist Hosp; **Address:** Mayo Clinic, Gonda 9 South, 200 First St SW, Rochester, MN 55905; **Phone:** 507-284-3329; **Board Cert:** Surgery 2007; Colon & Rectal Surgery 1989; **Med School:** Univ Wash 1981; **Resid:** Surgery, Oregon Hlth Sci Univ Hosp 1987; Colon & Rectal Surgery, Oregon Hlth Sci Univ Hosp 1985; **Fellow:** Colon & Rectal Surgery, Mayo Clin 1988; **Fac Appt:** Prof S, Mayo Med Sch

Pemberton, John H MD [CRS] - **Spec Exp:** Inflammatory Bowel Disease/Crohn's; Colon & Rectal Cancer; **Hospital:** St. Mary's Hosp - Rochester MN (Mayo), Rochester Methodist Hosp; **Address:** Mayo Clinic, Div Colon & Rectal Surg, 200 First St SW, Gonda 9-S, Rochester, MN 55905; **Phone:** 507-284-2359; **Board Cert:** Surgery 2001; Colon & Rectal Surgery 1985; **Med School:** Tulane Univ 1976; **Resid:** Surgery, Mayo Clinic 1983; **Fellow:** Colon & Rectal Surgery, Mayo Clinic 1984; **Fac Appt:** Prof S, Mayo Med Sch

Rafferty, Janice F MD [CRS] - **Spec Exp:** Colon & Rectal Cancer; Ulcerative Colitis; Crohn's Disease; Anal Disorders & Reconstruction; **Hospital:** Univ Hosp - Cincinnati, Christ Hosp, The - Cincinnati; **Address:** Univ Cincinnati, Colon & Rectal Surgery, 2123 Auburn Ave, Ste 524, Cincinnati, OH 45219; **Phone:** 513-929-0104; **Board Cert:** Surgery 2004; Colon & Rectal Surgery 2008; **Med School:** Ohio State Univ 1988; **Resid:** Surgery, Univ CincinnatiHosp 1995; Colon & Rectal Surgery, Barnes Jewish Hosp 1996; **Fac Appt:** Assoc Prof S, Univ Cincinnati

Remzi, Feza H MD [CRS] - **Spec Exp:** Colon & Rectal Cancer & Surgery; Inflammatory Bowel Disease; Laparoscopic Surgery; **Hospital:** Cleveland Clin (page 56); **Address:** Cleveland Clinic, 9500 Euclid Ave, Dept A30, Cleveland, OH 44195; **Phone:** 216-445-5020; **Board Cert:** Surgery 2006; Colon & Rectal Surgery 2007; **Med School:** Turkey 1989; **Resid:** Colon & Rectal Surgery, Cleveland Clinic 1996; Colon & Rectal Surgery, Cleveland Clinic 1997

Rothenberger, David A MD [CRS] - **Spec Exp:** Colon & Rectal Cancer; **Hospital:** Univ Minn Med Ctr, Fairview - Riverside Campus; **Address:** Univ Minnesota Med Ctr, Dept Surg, 420 Delaware St SE MMC 88, Minneapolis, MN 55455; **Phone:** 612-624-9708; **Board Cert:** Colon & Rectal Surgery 2006; **Med School:** Tufts Univ 1973; **Resid:** Surgery, St Paul-Ramsey Med Ctr 1978; **Fellow:** Colon & Rectal Surgery, Univ Minnesota Hosps 1979; **Fac Appt:** Prof S, Univ Minn

Saclarides, Theodore J MD [CRS] - **Spec Exp:** Rectal Cancer/Sphincter Preservation; Laparoscopic Surgery; Inflammatory Bowel Disease; **Hospital:** Rush Univ Med Ctr, Skokie/North Shore Univ Hlth Syst; **Address:** University Surgeons, 1725 W Harrison St, Ste 810, Chicago, IL 60612-3832; **Phone:** 312-942-6500; **Board Cert:** Surgery 2007; Colon & Rectal Surgery 1989; **Med School:** Univ Miami Sch Med 1982; **Resid:** Surgery, Rush Univ Med Ctr 1987; **Fellow:** Colon & Rectal Surgery, Mayo Clinic 1988; **Fac Appt:** Prof S, Rush Med Coll

Colon & Rectal Surgery

Stryker, Steven J MD [CRS] - **Spec Exp:** Colon & Rectal Cancer; Inflammatory Bowel Disease; Laparoscopic Surgery; **Hospital:** Northwestern Meml Hosp; **Address:** 676 N Saint Clair St, Ste 1525A, Chicago, IL 60611-2862; **Phone:** 312-943-5427; **Board Cert:** Surgery 2004; Colon & Rectal Surgery 1986; **Med School:** Northwestern Univ 1978; **Resid:** Surgery, Northwestern Meml Hosp 1983; **Fellow:** Colon & Rectal Surgery, Mayo Clinic 1985; **Fac Appt:** Clin Prof S, Northwestern Univ

Trudel, Judith L MD [CRS] - **Spec Exp:** Colon & Rectal Cancer; Anorectal Disorders; **Hospital:** St. John's Hosp-Maplewood MN, St. Joseph's Hosp; **Address:** Colon & Rectal Surgery Assoc, 1055 Westgate Drive, Ste 190, St Paul, MN 55114; **Phone:** 651-312-1620; **Board Cert:** Surgery 2007; Colon & Rectal Surgery 2006; **Med School:** Canada 1979; **Resid:** Surgery, Montreal Genl Hosp 1984; **Fellow:** Colon & Rectal Surgery, Cleveland Clinic 1986; **Fac Appt:** Assoc Prof S, Univ Minn

Wolff, Bruce G MD [CRS] - **Spec Exp:** Inflammatory Bowel Disease; Crohn's Disease; Colon & Rectal Cancer; **Hospital:** Mayo Med Ctr & Clin - Rochester; **Address:** Mayo Clinic, Gonda 9 South, 200 First St SW, Rochester, MN 55905; **Phone:** 507-284-3329; **Board Cert:** Surgery 2000; Colon & Rectal Surgery 2001; **Med School:** Duke Univ 1973; **Resid:** Surgery, NY Hosp-Cornell Med Ctr 1981; **Fellow:** Colon & Rectal Surgery, Mayo Clinic 1982; **Fac Appt:** Prof S, Mayo Med Sch

Great Plains and Mountains

Blatchford, Garnet J MD [CRS] - **Spec Exp:** Colon Cancer; Anal Disorders & Reconstruction; **Hospital:** Alegent Hlth - Immanuel Med Ctr; **Address:** Colon & Rectal Surgery Inc, 9850 Nicholas St, Ste 100, Omaha, NE 68114; **Phone:** 402-343-1122; **Board Cert:** Colon & Rectal Surgery 2009; **Med School:** Univ Nebr Coll Med 1983; **Resid:** Surgery, Univ Nebraska Med Ctr 1988; Colon & Rectal Surgery, Creighton Univ 1990; **Fac Appt:** Assoc Prof S, Creighton Univ

Schatz, Lisa Shawn MD [CRS] - **Hospital:** Rose Med Ctr; **Address:** Rocky Mountain Surgical Associates, 4545 E 9th Ave, Ste 460, Denver, CO 80220; **Phone:** 303-388-2922; **Board Cert:** Surgery 2001; Colon & Rectal Surgery 2002; **Med School:** Case West Res Univ 1995; **Resid:** Surgery, Univ Hosps of Cleveland 2000; Colon & Rectal Surgery, Ochsner Clinic 2001; **Fac Appt:** Assoc Clin Prof CRS, Univ Colorado

Thorson, Alan G MD [CRS] - **Spec Exp:** Colon & Rectal Cancer; Rectal Cancer/Sphincter Preservation; Incontinence-Fecal; Laparoscopic Surgery; **Hospital:** Nebraska Meth Hosp, Bergan Mercy Med Ctr-Alegant Hlth; **Address:** 9850 Nicholas St, Ste 100, Omaha, NE 68114-2191; **Phone:** 402-343-1122; **Board Cert:** Colon & Rectal Surgery 1999; **Med School:** Univ Nebr Coll Med 1979; **Resid:** Surgery, Univ Nebraska Affil Hosp 1984; Colon & Rectal Surgery, Univ Minn Affil Hosp 1985; **Fac Appt:** Clin Prof S, Creighton Univ

Williams, Shauna Tseu MD [CRS] - **Hospital:** St. Luke's Boise Med Ctr, St. Alphonsus Regl Med Ctr; **Address:** 1072 N Liberty St, Ste 201, Boise, ID 83704; **Phone:** 208-377-2273; **Board Cert:** Surgery 2009; Colon & Rectal Surgery 2010; **Med School:** Univ Hawaii JA Burns Sch Med 1984; **Resid:** Surgery, Univ Oregon Hlth Sci Ctr 1990; **Fellow:** Colon & Rectal Surgery, Mayo Clinic 1991

Southwest

Adkins, Terrance P MD [CRS] - **Spec Exp:** Colon & Rectal Cancer; Inflammatory Bowel Disease; **Hospital:** Tucson Med Ctr; **Address:** Southwestern Surgery Assoc, 1951 N Wilmot Rd Bldg 2, Tucson, AZ 85712; **Phone:** 520-795-5845; **Board Cert:** Surgery 2001; Colon & Rectal Surgery 2004; **Med School:** Univ Tex SW, Dallas 1985; **Resid:** Surgery, Univ Utah Med Ctr 1991; **Fellow:** Colon & Rectal Surgery, Univ Texas Med Ctr 1992; **Fac Appt:** Asst Clin Prof S, Univ Ariz Coll Med

Bailey, H Randolph MD [CRS] - **Spec Exp:** Rectal Cancer/Sphincter Preservation; Inflammatory Bowel Disease; Incontinence-Fecal; Endometriosis-Intestine; **Hospital:** Methodist Hosp - Houston, St. Luke's Episcopal Hosp-Houston; **Address:** Colon & Rectal Clinic, Smith Twr, 6550 Fannin St, Ste 2307, Houston, TX 77030-2717; **Phone:** 713-790-9250; **Board Cert:** Surgery 1974; Colon & Rectal Surgery 2004; **Med School:** Univ Tex SW, Dallas 1968; **Resid:** Surgery, Hermann Hosp-Univ Tex Med Sch 1973; **Fellow:** Colon & Rectal Surgery, Ferguson-Droste Hosp 1974; **Fac Appt:** Clin Prof S, Univ Tex, Houston

Beck, David E MD [CRS] - **Spec Exp:** Colon & Rectal Cancer; Minimally Invasive Surgery; Inflammatory Bowel Disease; **Hospital:** Ochsner Med Ctr-New Orleans; Ochsner Med Ctr-Baton Rouge; **Address:** 1514 Jefferson Hwy, Fl 4th, 1514 Jefferson Hwy, 4th Fl, rm 04 East, New Orleans, LA 70121-2429; **Phone:** 504-842-4060; **Board Cert:** Colon & Rectal Surgery 1987; **Med School:** Univ Miami Sch Med 1979; **Resid:** Surgery, Wilford Hall USAF Med Ctr 1984; **Fellow:** Colon & Rectal Surgery, Cleveland Clinic Fdn 1986; **Fac Appt:** Assoc Clin Prof S, Louisiana State U, New Orleans

Haas, Eric M MD [CRS] - **Spec Exp:** Laparoscopic Surgery; Colon & Rectal Cancer; Inflammatory Bowel Disease/Crohn's; Incontinence-Fecal; **Hospital:** Methodist Hosp - Houston, St. Luke's Episcopal Hosp-Houston; **Address:** Colorectal Surgical Assocs, 7900 Fannin St, Ste 2700, Houston, TX 77054; **Phone:** 713-790-0600; **Board Cert:** Surgery 2003; Colon & Rectal Surgery 2004; **Med School:** Univ Tex, Houston 1997; **Resid:** Surgery, St Joseph Hosp 2002; **Fellow:** Colon & Rectal Surgery, Texas affil Hosps 2003

Heppell, Jacques P MD [CRS] - **Spec Exp:** Colon & Rectal Cancer; Inflammatory Bowel Disease; Anorectal Disorders; **Hospital:** Mayo Clinic - Phoenix; **Address:** Mayo Clinic, GENS/CB/Distribution 13, 5777 E Mayo Blvd, Phoenix, AZ 85054; **Phone:** 480-342-2697; **Board Cert:** Surgery 2004; Colon & Rectal Surgery 1995; **Med School:** Univ Montreal 1974; **Resid:** Surgery, Univ Montreal Med Ctr 1979; **Fellow:** Colon & Rectal Surgery, Mayo Clinic 1983; **Fac Appt:** Prof S, Mayo Med Sch

Hicks, Terry C MD [CRS] - **Spec Exp:** Colon & Rectal Cancer; **Hospital:** Ochsner Med Ctr-New Orleans; **Address:** Ochsner Clinic, Div Colorectal Surgery, 1514 Jefferson Hwy, New Orleans, LA 70121; **Phone:** 504-842-5884; **Board Cert:** Colon & Rectal Surgery 2002; **Med School:** Univ Tex, San Antonio 1977; **Resid:** Surgery, Univ Louisville Med Ctr 1982; Colon & Rectal Surgery, Ochsner Clinic 1983; **Fac Appt:** Assoc Prof S, Louisiana State U, New Orleans

Huber Jr, Philip J MD [CRS] - **Spec Exp:** Colon & Rectal Cancer; Inflammatory Bowel Disease; **Hospital:** Med City Dallas Hosp, TX Hlth Presby Hosp Dallas; **Address:** 7777 Forest Lane, Ste C-204, Dallas, TX 75230; **Phone:** 972-566-6115; **Board Cert:** Colon & Rectal Surgery 1993; **Med School:** Columbia P&S 1972; **Resid:** Surgery, Parkland Hosp 1977; Colon & Rectal Surgery, Presby Hosp 1978

West Coast and Pacific

Beart Jr, Robert W MD [CRS] - **Spec Exp:** Colon & Rectal Cancer; Rectal Cancer/Sphincter Preservation; **Hospital:** Glendale Mem Hosp & Hlth Ctr; **Address:** Colorectal Surgery Inst, 222 W Eulalia St, Ste 100A, Glendale, CA 91204; **Phone:** 818-244-8161; **Board Cert:** Colon & Rectal Surgery 1995; **Med School:** Harvard Med Sch 1971; **Resid:** Surgery, Univ Colo Med Ctr 1976; Colon & Rectal Surgery, Mayo Clinic 1978; **Fellow:** Transplant Surgery, Univ Colo Med Ctr 1975; **Fac Appt:** Prof Emeritus S, USC Sch Med

Colon & Rectal Surgery

Chiu, Yanek S MD [CRS] - **Hospital:** CA Pacific Med Ctr-Pacific Campus; **Address:** 3838 California St, Ste 616, San Francisco, CA 94118; **Phone:** 415-668-0411; **Board Cert:** Colon & Rectal Surgery 1997; **Med School:** Boston Univ 1971; **Resid:** Surgery, Boston Med Ctr 1976; **Fellow:** Colon & Rectal Surgery, Mayo Clinic 1978; **Fac Appt:** Assoc Clin Prof CRS, UCSF

Coutsoftides, Theodore MD [CRS] - **Spec Exp:** Laparoscopic Surgery; Inflammatory Bowel Disease; Anal Sphincter Repair; **Hospital:** St. Joseph's Hosp - Orange; **Address:** 1310 W Stewart Drive, Ste 605, Orange, CA 92868-3857; **Phone:** 714-532-2544; **Board Cert:** Colon & Rectal Surgery 1977; **Med School:** Israel 1970; **Resid:** Surgery, Cleveland Clinic 1973; Surgery, Royal Victoria Hosp 1976; **Fellow:** Colon & Rectal Surgery, Cleveland Clinic 1977; **Fac Appt:** Assoc Prof S, UC Irvine

Lee, Patrick Y H MD [CRS] - **Hospital:** Providence Portland Med Ctr, Legacy Good Samaritan Med Ctr; **Address:** Surgical Specialty Group, Colon & Rectal Clinic, 9155 SW Barnes Rd, Ste 839, Portland, OR 97225; **Phone:** 503-222-1615; **Board Cert:** Surgery 2004; Colon & Rectal Surgery 2007; **Med School:** Northwestern Univ-Feinberg Sch Med 1988; **Resid:** Surgery, Oregon Hlth Sci Ctr 1994; **Fellow:** Colon & Rectal Surgery, Cleveland Clinic 1995

Ramamoorthy, Sonia L MD [CRS] - **Spec Exp:** Colon & Rectal Cancer; Diverticulitis; Incontinence/Pelvic Floor Disorders; Inflammatory Bowel Disease; **Hospital:** UCSD Med Ctr; **Address:** UCSD, Dept Surgery, 3855 Hlth Sci Drive, MC 0987, La Jolla, CA 92093; **Phone:** 858-822-6277; **Board Cert:** Surgery 2002; Colon & Rectal Surgery 2005; **Med School:** Boston Univ 1996; **Resid:** Surgery, UCSD Med Ctr 2001; **Fellow:** Colon & Rectal Surgery, Barnes-Jewish Hosp 2002; Research, UCSD Med Ctr 2006; **Fac Appt:** Asst Prof S, UCSD

Senagore, Anthony MD [CRS] - **Spec Exp:** Laparoscopic Surgery; Colon & Rectal Cancer; Anorectal Disorders; Inflammatory Bowel Disease/Crohn's; **Hospital:** USC Norris Cancer Hosp (page 75); **Address:** USC North Cancer Hosp, 1441 Eastlake Ave, Ste 7418, Los Angeles, CA 90033; **Phone:** 323-865-3690; **Board Cert:** Surgery 2006; Colon & Rectal Surgery 2009; Surgical Critical Care 2006; **Med School:** Mich State Univ 1981; **Resid:** Surgery, Butterworth Hosp 1987; Colon & Rectal Surgery, Ferguson Hosp 1989; **Fac Appt:** Prof S

Sokol, Thomas P MD [CRS] - **Spec Exp:** Colon & Rectal Cancer & Surgery; Incontinence-Fecal; Constipation; Gastrointestinal Motility Disorders; **Hospital:** Cedars-Sinai Med Ctr; **Address:** 8737 Beverly Blvd, Ste 402, Los Angeles, CA 90048-1828; **Phone:** 310-854-3580; **Board Cert:** Colon & Rectal Surgery 2008; **Med School:** Ros Franklin Univ/Chicago Med Sch 1980; **Resid:** Surgery, Habor UCLA Med Ctr 1985; **Fellow:** Colon & Rectal Surgery, Carle Fdn Hosp/Univ Ill 1986; **Fac Appt:** Assoc Clin Prof S, UCLA

Stamos, Michael J MD [CRS] - **Spec Exp:** Rectal Cancer/Sphincter Preservation; Laparoscopic Surgery; Inflammatory Bowel Disease; Colon & Rectal Cancer; **Hospital:** UC Irvine Med Ctr; **Address:** UC Irvine Med Ctr, Div Colon & Rectal Surg, 333 City Blvd W, Ste 700, Orange, CA 92868-2993; **Phone:** 714-456-6262; **Board Cert:** Surgery 2010; Colon & Rectal Surgery 2003; **Med School:** Case West Res Univ 1985; **Resid:** Surgery, Jackson Meml Hosp 1990; Colon & Rectal Surgery, Ochsner Clinic 1991; **Fac Appt:** Prof S, UC Irvine

Varma, Madhulika G MD [CRS] - **Spec Exp:** Colon & Rectal Cancer & Surgery; Inflammatory Bowel Disease; Pelvic Floor Disorders; Laparoscopic Surgery; **Hospital:** UCSF - Mt Zion Med Ctr; **Address:** Center for Colorectal Surgery, 2330 Post St, Ste 260, San Francisco, CA 94115-1799; **Phone:** 415-885-3606; **Board Cert:** Colon & Rectal Surgery 2010; Surgery 2007; **Med School:** Brown Univ 1991; **Resid:** Surgery, UCSF Med Ctr 1998; **Fellow:** Colon & Rectal Surgery, Univ Minnesota Med Ctr 2000; Research, UCSF Med Ctr 2001; **Fac Appt:** Asst Prof S, UCSF

Welton, Mark L MD [CRS] - **Spec Exp:** Ulcerative Colitis; Crohn's Disease; Colon & Rectal Cancer; Anal Cancer; **Hospital:** Stanford Univ Hosp & Clinics; **Address:** The Cancer Ctr, 875 Blake Wilbur Drive, Stanford, CA 94305; **Phone:** 650-723-5461; **Board Cert:** Surgery 2000; Colon & Rectal Surgery 2005; **Med School:** UCLA 1984; **Resid:** Surgery, UCLA Med Ctr 1992; **Fellow:** Colon & Rectal Surgery, Barnes Jewish Hosp 1993; **Fac Appt:** Assoc Prof S, Stanford Univ

Wong, Ronald J MD [CRS] - **Spec Exp:** Laparoscopic Surgery; **Hospital:** Queen's Med Ctr - Honolulu; **Address:** Queen's Physicians' Office Bldg 1, 1380 Lusitana St, Ste 614, Honolulu, HI 96813; **Phone:** 808-524-1856; **Board Cert:** Surgery 2008; **Med School:** Univ Hawaii JA Burns Sch Med 1981; **Resid:** Surgery, Univ Hawaii 1985; Surgery, Catholic Med Ctr 1987; **Fellow:** Colon & Rectal Surgery, Suburban Hosp 1989; Research, Cornell Univ Med Ctr 1988; **Fac Appt:** Clin Prof S, Univ Hawaii JA Burns Sch Med

Worsey, Michael J MD [CRS] - **Spec Exp:** Colon & Rectal Cancer; Inflammatory Bowel Disease; **Hospital:** Scripps Meml Hosp - La Jolla; **Address:** Advanced Surgical Assocs, 9834 Genesee Ave, Ste 201, La Jolla, CA 92037; **Phone:** 858-558-2272; **Board Cert:** Surgery 2008; Colon & Rectal Surgery 2009; **Med School:** England, UK 1985; **Resid:** Surgery, Bristol Royal Infirm/Royal Gwent Hosp 1989; Surgery, Univ Pittsburgh Med Ctr 1997; **Fellow:** Colon & Rectal Surgery, Cleveland Clin 1998

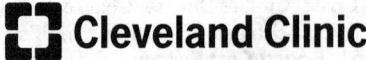

Cleveland Clinic

Every life deserves world class care.

Cleveland Clinic
Digestive Disease Institute
9500 Euclid Avenue
Cleveland, OH 44195

Colorectal Surgery

Cleveland Clinic's Digestive Disease Institute (DDI) is one of the largest digestive programs in the country and is ranked No. 2 in the nation by *U.S.News & World Report*. DDI is the first to fully integrate its departments of Colorectal Surgery, Gastroenterology & Hepatology, General Surgery and Nutrition. Combining these disciplines in one location facilitates unprecedented patient care, multidisciplinary education and collaborative research. In 2010, DDI physicians performed over 27,000 surgical cases and 38,000 endoscopic cases. Transplant surgeons completed over 170 digestive disease-related organ transplants, including liver, pancreas and intestinal transplantation, achieving outstanding outcomes.

Highlights of the Department of Colorectal Surgery:

- The first ileoanal pouch for ulcerative colitis was performed at Cleveland Clinic in the 1980s.

- Our colorectal surgeons performed the world's first colon resection entirely through a single incision in the belly button in 2008.

- We performed the world's first single-incision procto-colectomy and ileoanal pouch anastomosis (removing the entire large intestine and rectum) in 2009, leaving only a coin-sized scar in the patient's abdomen.

- We have an international reputation for excellence in inflammatory bowel disease, performing the most Crohn's disease operations, especially the bowel-conserving strictureplasty. We also perform the world's highest volume of J-Pouch surgeries and are the nation's largest referral center for repairing failed pelvic pouches.

- Our team performs more colon and rectal cancer surgeries than any other hospital in Ohio and one of the highest volumes in the nation.

- Led by a team of female physicians, our pelvic floor center treats the entire spectrum of bowel disorders, including fecal incontinence and chronic constipation.

clevelandclinic.org/colontopdocs

Offering Same-Day Appointments
Call 800.274.2009.

Treatment Guides

Cleveland Clinic has developed comprehensive treatment guides for many diseases and conditions. To download our free treatment guides, visit clevelandclinic.org/treatmentguides.

Online Medical Second Opinion

Cleveland Clinic's My**Consult** Online Medical Second Opinion program securely connects patients to our physician specialists for more than 1,000 life-changing or life-threatening diagnoses all by the click of a mouse. To learn more, log onto eclevelandclinic.org/myconsult or call 800.223.2273, ext. 43223.

Special Assistance for Out-of-State Patients

Cleveland Clinic Global Patient Services offers a complimentary Medical Concierge service for patients who travel from outside of Ohio. Call 800.223.2273, ext. 55580 or email medicalconcierge@ccf.org.

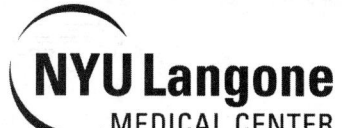

550 First Avenue (*at 31st Street*)
New York, NY 10016
www.NYULMC.org
Physician Referral: **888-7-NYU-MED** (*888-769-8633*)

COLON AND RECTAL SURGERY

About the Division of Colon and Rectal Surgery
Colorectal surgeons at NYU Langone Medical Center perform more than 5,000 outpatient and inpatient procedures each year using laser, laparoscopic, endoscopic and other minimally invasive techniques. Candidates for surgery receive same-day care that includes imaging, radiation and nutritional support. We specialize in the following areas:

Adrenalectomies
Our surgeons are skilled at performing adrenalectomies, the surgical removal of one or both of the adrenal glands. This procedure is usually advised for patients with tumors of the adrenal glands, which may be malignant or benign. Adrenalectomy, once performed by conventional (open) surgery, is now routinely done laparoscopically through four very small incisions, which allows patients to usually be discharged within 36 hours.

Colorectal Cancer
We offer the most advanced screening options available for the diagnosis of colon cancer, the second leading cause of cancer death in the U.S. Additionally, we continue to investigate colorectal cancer screenings in special populations such as women, veterans, immigrants, minorities and patients with HIV, and offer the use of virtual colonoscopy for the detection of colorectal polyps and cancer.

Laparoscopic Techniques
Surgeons at NYU Langone use tiny incisions to remove a segment of the colon, which dramatically speeds recovery and reduces the need for pain medication. Laparoscopic techniques are used to treat pancreatic tumors, splenic related conditions, hiatus hernias, small bowel tumors and adrenalectomies.

Liver Lesions
Our surgeons treat liver lesions with painless radiofrequency ablation. Minimally invasive resections and open liver surgery are also routinely performed.

Robotic Surgery
NYU Langone was the first hospital in New York City to use the minimally invasive da Vinci Si HD robotic surgical system, which allows a 40 percent higher definition view of the surgical field.

Virtual Colonoscopy
The Medical Center offers the latest developments in colon cancer detection, including virtual colonoscopy. This noninvasive procedure makes use of sophisticated imaging techniques to generate a 3-D reconstruction of the inner surface of the colon, which can then be evaluated for abnormalities by specially trained radiologists.

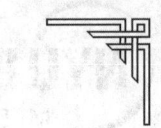

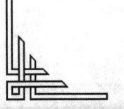
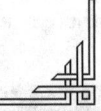

The Best in American Medicine
www.CastleConnolly.com

Dermatology

A dermatologist is trained to diagnose and treat pediatric and adult patients with benign and malignant disorders of the skin, mouth, external genitalia, hair and nails, as well as a number of sexually transmitted diseases. The dermatologist may have additional training and experience in the diagnosis and treatment of skin cancers, melanomas, moles and other tumors of the skin, the management of contact dermatitis and other allergic and nonallergic skin disorders, and in the recognition of the skin manifestations of systemic (including internal malignancy) and infectious diseases. Dermatologists may have special training in dermatopathology and in the surgical techniques used in dermatology. They also have expertise in the management of cosmetic disorders of the skin such as hair loss and scars, and the skin changes associated with aging.

Training Required: Four years.

Certification in the following subspecialties requires additional training and examination.

Dermatopathology: A dermatopathologist has the expertise to diagnose and monitor diseases of the skin including infectious, immunologic, degenerative and neoplastic diseases. This entails the examination and interpretation of specially prepared tissue sections, cellular scrapings and smears of skin lesions by means of routine and special (electron and fluorescent) microscopes.

Pediatric Dermatology: A dermatologist trained to diagnose and treat pediatric patients with dermatologic diseases.

DERMATOLOGY

New England

Anderson, Richard Rox MD [D] - **Spec Exp:** Birthmarks/Hemangiomas; **Hospital:** Mass Genl Hosp; **Address:** Dermatology Laser Center, 50 Staniford St, Ste 250, Boston, MA 02114; **Phone:** 617-724-6960; **Board Cert:** Dermatology 2009; **Med School:** Harvard Med Sch 1984; **Resid:** Dermatology, Mass Genl Hosp 1991; **Fellow:** Dermatologic Research, Mass Genl Hosp 1988; **Fac Appt:** Assoc Prof D, Harvard Med Sch

Arndt, Kenneth MD [D] - **Spec Exp:** Skin Laser Surgery; Cosmetic Dermatology; **Hospital:** Beth Israel Deaconess Med Ctr - Boston, New England Bapt Hosp; **Address:** Skincare Phys, 1244 Boylston St, Ste 302, Chestnut Hill, MA 02467; **Phone:** 617-731-1600; **Board Cert:** Dermatology 1966; **Med School:** Yale Univ 1961; **Resid:** Dermatology, Mass Genl Hosp 1965; **Fellow:** Dermatology, Harvard Med Sch 1965; **Fac Appt:** Clin Prof D, Harvard Med Sch

Bolognia, Jean L MD [D] - **Spec Exp:** Melanoma; Skin Cancer; **Hospital:** Yale-New Haven Hosp, Yale Med Group; **Address:** 2 Church St S, Ste 305, New Haven, CT 06519; **Phone:** 203-789-1249; **Board Cert:** Dermatology 2005; **Med School:** Yale Univ 1980; **Resid:** Internal Medicine, Yale-New Haven Hosp 1982; Dermatology, Yale-New Haven Hosp 1985; **Fellow:** Dermatology, Yale-New Haven Hosp 1987; **Fac Appt:** Prof D, Yale Univ

Del Giudice, Stephen M MD [D] - **Spec Exp:** Skin Cancer; Phototherapy; Psoriasis; Acne; **Hospital:** Concord Hospital; **Address:** Dartmouth Hitchcock Concord Dermatology, 253 Pleasant St, Concord, NH 03301; **Phone:** 603-226-6119; **Board Cert:** Dermatology 1987; **Med School:** Tufts Univ 1981; **Resid:** Dermatology, Yale-New Haven Hosp 1987

Dover, Jeffrey MD [D] - **Spec Exp:** Cosmetic Dermatology; Skin Laser Surgery; **Hospital:** Beth Israel Deaconess Med Ctr - Boston, New England Bapt Hosp; **Address:** 1244 Boylston St, Ste 302, Chesnut Hill, MA 02467; **Phone:** 617-731-1600; **Board Cert:** Dermatology 1985; **Med School:** Univ Ottawa 1981; **Resid:** Dermatology, Univ Toronto 1984; Dermatology, St Johns Hosp 1985; **Fellow:** Dermatology, Mass Genl Hosp-Harvard 1987; **Fac Appt:** Assoc Prof D, Yale Univ

Dufresne, Raymond G MD [D] - **Spec Exp:** Mohs' Surgery; **Hospital:** Rhode Island Hosp; **Address:** University Dermatology, 593 Eddy St, APC 10, Providence, RI 02903; **Phone:** 401-444-7024; **Board Cert:** Internal Medicine 1983; Dermatology 1986; **Med School:** Vanderbilt Univ 1980; **Resid:** Internal Medicine, Vanderbilt Univ Med Ctr 1983; Dermatology, Vanderbilt Univ Med Ctr 1986; **Fellow:** Mohs Surgery, Cleveland Clinic 1987; **Fac Appt:** Prof D, Brown Univ

Edelson, Richard L MD [D] - **Spec Exp:** Cutaneous Lymphoma; Immune Deficiency-Skin Disorders; **Hospital:** Yale-New Haven Hosp, Yale Med Group; **Address:** 2 Church St S, Ste 305, New Haven, CT 06519; **Phone:** 203-789-1249; **Board Cert:** Dermatology 1977; **Med School:** Yale Univ 1970; **Resid:** Dermatology, Mass Genl Hosp 1972; Dermatology, Natl Inst Hlth 1975; **Fac Appt:** Prof D, Yale Univ

Falanga, Vincent MD [D] - **Spec Exp:** Wound Healing/Care; Collagen Vascular Diseases; Scleroderma; **Hospital:** Roger Williams Med Ctr; **Address:** Roger Williams Med Ctr, Dept Dermatology, 50 Maude St Elmhurst Bldg, Providence, RI 02908; **Phone:** 401-456-2521; **Board Cert:** Internal Medicine 1980; Dermatology 1982; **Med School:** Harvard Med Sch 1977; **Resid:** Internal Medicine, Univ Miami Med Ctr 1980; **Fellow:** Dermatology, Hosp Univ Penn 1982; **Fac Appt:** Prof D, Boston Univ

Fewkes, Jessica L MD [D] - **Spec Exp:** Mohs' Surgery; Skin Cancer-Head & Neck; Melanoma-Head & Neck; Cosmetic Dermatology; **Hospital:** Mass Eye & Ear Infirmary, Mass Genl Hosp; **Address:** Facial & Cosmetic Surgery Center, Mass Eye & Ear Infirmary, 243 Charles St, 9th Fl, Boston, MA 02114; **Phone:** 617-573-3789; **Board Cert:** Dermatology 1982; **Med School:** UCSF 1978; **Resid:** Dermatology, Mass Genl Hosp 1982; **Fellow:** Chemosurgery, Duke Univ Med Ctr 1983; **Fac Appt:** Asst Prof D, Harvard Med Sch

Gellis, Stephen MD [D] - **Spec Exp:** Pediatric Dermatology; Melanoma; Pigmented Lesions; **Hospital:** Children's Hospital - Boston; **Address:** Chldn's Hosp-Boston, 300 Longwood Ave, Fegan-6, Boston, MA 02115-5737; **Phone:** 617-355-6117; **Board Cert:** Pediatrics 1978; Dermatology 1979; Pediatric Dermatology 2006; **Med School:** Harvard Med Sch 1973; **Resid:** Pediatrics, Chldn's Hosp 1976; Dermatology, Mass Genl Hosp 1978; **Fac Appt:** Asst Prof D, Harvard Med Sch

Gilchrest, Barbara MD [D] - **Spec Exp:** Photoaging; Melanoma; Skin Cancer; **Hospital:** Boston Med Ctr; **Address:** Boston Med Ctr- Dermatolgy Dept, 609 Albany St, Ste 8B, Doctor's Off Bldg, Boston, MA 02118; **Phone:** 617-638-7420; **Board Cert:** Internal Medicine 1975; Dermatology 1978; **Med School:** Harvard Med Sch 1971; **Resid:** Internal Medicine, Boston City Hosp 1973; Dermatology, Harvard Med Sch 1976; **Fellow:** Photo Biology, Harvard Med Sch 1975; **Fac Appt:** Prof D, Boston Univ

Gottlieb, Alice B MD/PhD [D] - **Spec Exp:** Psoriasis; Psoriatic Arthritis; Atopic Dermatitis; Clinical Trials; **Hospital:** Tufts Med Ctr; **Address:** 800 Washington St, Box 114, Boston, MA 02111; **Phone:** 617-636-0156; **Board Cert:** Internal Medicine 1982; Dermatology 2001; Rheumatology 1984; **Med School:** Cornell Univ-Weill Med Coll 1980; **Resid:** Internal Medicine, New York Hosp 1982; Dermatology, New York Hosp 1993; **Fellow:** Rheumatology, Hosp Special Surgery 1984; **Fac Appt:** Prof D, Tufts Univ

Kane, Kay S MD [D] - **Spec Exp:** Pediatric Dermatology; **Hospital:** Children's Hospital - Boston; **Address:** 1244 Boylston St, Route 9, Chestnut Hill, MA 02467; **Phone:** 617-731-1600; **Board Cert:** Dermatology 2005; **Med School:** Harvard Med Sch 1993; **Resid:** Dermatology, Mass General Hosp 1997; **Fac Appt:** Asst Prof D, Harvard Med Sch

Kupper, Thomas S MD [D] - **Spec Exp:** Melanoma; Cutaneous Lymphoma; Skin Cancer; **Hospital:** Brigham and Women's Hosp (page 57), Dana-Farber Cancer Inst (page 57); **Address:** Brigham & Women's Hosp, Dept Dermatology, 77 Avenue Louis Pasteur, Ste 671, Boston, MA 02115; **Phone:** 617-525-5550; **Board Cert:** Dermatology 1989; **Med School:** Yale Univ 1981; **Resid:** Surgery, Yale-New Haven Hosp 1983; Dermatology, Yale-New Haven Hosp 1989; **Fac Appt:** Prof D, Harvard Med Sch

Leffell, David J MD [D] - **Spec Exp:** Mohs' Surgery; Melanoma; Skin Cancer; Skin Laser Surgery; **Hospital:** Yale-New Haven Hosp, Yale Med Group; **Address:** 40 Temple St, Ste 5a, New Haven, CT 06520; **Phone:** 203-785-3466; **Board Cert:** Internal Medicine 1984; Dermatology 2009; **Med School:** McGill Univ 1981; **Resid:** Internal Medicine, New York Hosp 1984; Dermatology, Yale-New Haven Hosp 1986; **Fellow:** Dermatology, Yale Sch Med 1987; Dermatologic Surgery, Univ Michigan Med Ctr 1988; **Fac Appt:** Prof D, Yale Univ

Maloney, Mary E MD [D] - **Spec Exp:** Mohs' Surgery; Skin Cancer; Dermatologic Surgery; **Hospital:** UMass Memorial Med Ctr; **Address:** UMass Meml Med Ctr-Hahnemann Campus, 281 Lincoln St, Worcester, MA 01605; **Phone:** 508-334-5962; **Board Cert:** Dermatology 1982; **Med School:** Univ VT Coll Med 1977; **Resid:** Internal Medicine, Hartford Hospital 1979; Dermatology, Dartmouth-Hitchcock Med Ctr 1982; **Fellow:** Dermatologic Surgery, UCSF Med Ctr 1983; **Fac Appt:** Prof D, Univ Mass Sch Med

Dermatology

McDonald, Charles J MD [D] - **Spec Exp:** Cutaneous Lymphoma; Autoimmune Disease; Melanoma; Psoriasis; **Hospital:** Rhode Island Hosp, Miriam Hosp; **Address:** Rhode Island Hosp, Dept Dermatology, 593 Eddy St, APC-10, Providence, RI 02903-4923; **Phone:** 401-444-7959; **Board Cert:** Dermatology 1966; **Med School:** Howard Univ 1960; **Resid:** Internal Medicine, Hosp St Raphael 1963; Dermatology, Yale New Haven Hosp 1965; **Fellow:** Clinical Oncology, Yale New Haven Hosp 1966; **Fac Appt:** Prof D, Brown Univ

Mihm Jr, Martin C MD [D] - **Spec Exp:** Melanoma; Vascular Birthmarks; Dermatopathology; **Hospital:** Brigham and Women's Hosp (page 57); **Address:** Skin Care & Dermatopathology Assocs, 1 Broadway Fl 14, Cambridge, MA 02142; **Phone:** 617-401-2231; **Board Cert:** Dermatology 1969; Dermatopathology 1974; Anatomic Pathology 1974; **Med School:** Univ Pittsburgh 1961; **Resid:** Internal Medicine, Mt Sinai Hosp 1964; Dermatology, Mass Genl Hosp 1967; **Fellow:** Anatomic Pathology, Mass Genl Hosp 1972; **Fac Appt:** Clin Prof Path, Harvard Med Sch

Neel, Victor A MD/PhD [D] - **Spec Exp:** Mohs' Surgery; Skin Cancer; Cosmetic Dermatology; **Hospital:** Mass Genl Hosp; **Address:** 50 Staniford St, Ste 270, Boston, MA 02114; **Phone:** 617-726-1869; **Board Cert:** Dermatology 2009; **Med School:** Cornell Univ-Weill Med Coll 1995; **Resid:** Pediatrics, Rhode Island Hosp 1997; Dermatology, Rhode Island Hosp 2000; **Fellow:** Mohs Surgery, UCLA Med Ctr 2001

Olbricht, Suzanne M MD [D] - **Spec Exp:** Skin Cancer; Mohs' Surgery; Muir-Torre Syndrome; **Hospital:** Lahey Clin; **Address:** Lahey Clinic, 41 Mall Rd, Burlington, MA 01805; **Phone:** 781-744-8348; **Board Cert:** Internal Medicine 1979; Dermatology 1983; **Med School:** Baylor Coll Med 1976; **Resid:** Internal Medicine, Mass General Hosp 1979; Dermatology, Mass General Hosp 1983; **Fellow:** Mohs Surgery, Mass General Hosp 1991; **Fac Appt:** Assoc Prof D, Harvard Med Sch

Sober, Arthur Joel MD [D] - **Spec Exp:** Melanoma; Skin Cancer; Merkel Cell Carcinoma; Mohs' Surgery; **Hospital:** Mass Genl Hosp; **Address:** 50 Staniford St, Ste 200, Boston, MA 02114; **Phone:** 617-726-2914; **Board Cert:** Internal Medicine 1974; Dermatology 1975; **Med School:** Geo Wash Univ 1968; **Resid:** Internal Medicine, Beth Israel Hosp 1970; Dermatology, Mass General Hosp 1974; **Fellow:** Immunology, Peter Bent Brigham Hosp 1976; **Fac Appt:** Prof D, Harvard Med Sch

Stern, Robert S MD [D] - **Spec Exp:** Psoriasis; Phototherapy; Drug Allergy; Skin Cancer; **Hospital:** Beth Israel Deaconess Med Ctr - Boston; **Address:** Beth Israel Deaconess Med Ctr, Dept Dermatology, 330 Brookline Ave, Boston, MA 02215-5400; **Phone:** 617-667-3689; **Board Cert:** Dermatology 1977; **Med School:** Yale Univ 1970; **Resid:** Dermatology, Mass Genl Hosp 1976; **Fellow:** Epidemiology, NIH 1973; **Fac Appt:** Prof D, Harvard Med Sch

Tsao, Hensin MD/PhD [D] - **Spec Exp:** Melanoma; Melanoma Genetics; Skin Cancer; **Hospital:** Mass Genl Hosp; **Address:** Mass Genl Hosp, Dept Dermatology, 55 Fruit St, Edwards Bldg, rm 211, Boston, MA 02114-2543; **Phone:** 617-726-2914; **Board Cert:** Dermatology 2006; **Med School:** Columbia P&S 1993; **Resid:** Dermatology, Brigham & Women's Hosp 1996; **Fellow:** Dermatology, Mass Genl Hosp 1997; **Fac Appt:** Assoc Prof D, Harvard Med Sch

Mid Atlantic

Alster, Tina MD [D] - **Spec Exp:** Skin Laser Surgery; Scar Revision; Birthmarks/Hemangiomas; **Hospital:** Georgetown Univ Hosp; **Address:** 1430 K St NW, Ste 200, Washington Inst of Derm Laser Surgery, Washington, DC 20005; **Phone:** 202-628-8855; **Board Cert:** Dermatology 1990; **Med School:** Duke Univ 1986; **Resid:** Dermatology, Yale Univ 1989; **Fellow:** Dermatologic Laser Surgery, Boston Univ Hosp 1990; **Fac Appt:** Clin Prof D, Georgetown Univ

Anhalt, Grant J MD [D] - **Spec Exp:** Blistering Diseases; Pemphigus; Autoimmune Disease; **Hospital:** Johns Hopkins Hosp (page 61); **Address:** Hopkins at Green Spring Station, 10751 Falls Rd, Ste 304, Lutherville, MD 21093; **Phone:** 410-321-5900; **Board Cert:** Dermatology 2009; Clinical & Laboratory Dematologic Immunology 1987; **Med School:** Canada 1975; **Resid:** Internal Medicine, Hlth Scis Ctr 1977; Dermatology, Univ Mich Med Ctr 1980; **Fellow:** Immunology, Univ Mich Med Ctr 1981; **Fac Appt:** Prof D, Johns Hopkins Univ

Avram, Marc R MD [D] - **Spec Exp:** Hair Restoration/Transplant; Skin Laser Surgery; Cosmetic Dermatology; Botox Therapy; **Hospital:** NY-Presby/Weill Cornell Med Ctr, NY (page 65), Univ Hosp of Bklyn at Long Island Coll Hosp; **Address:** 905 5th Ave, New York, NY 10021-2650; **Phone:** 212-734-4007; **Board Cert:** Dermatology 2005; Hair Restoration Surgery 1997; **Med School:** SUNY Downstate 1989; **Resid:** Dermatology, Mass Genl Hosp 1994; **Fac Appt:** Assoc Prof D, Cornell Univ-Weill Med Coll

Belsito, Donald V MD [D] - **Spec Exp:** Contact Dermatitis; Cutaneous Lymphoma; Occupational Skin Diseases; Atopic Dermatitis; **Hospital:** NY-Presby/Columbia Univ Med Ctr, NY (page 65); **Address:** Columbia Dermatology Associates, 16 E 60th St, New York, NY 10022; **Phone:** 212-305-5293; **Board Cert:** Internal Medicine 1979; Dermatology 1983; Clinical & Laboratory Dematologic Immunology 1985; **Med School:** Cornell Univ-Weill Med Coll 1976; **Resid:** Internal Medicine, Case West Res Univ Hosps 1979; Dermatology, NYU Med Ctr 1982; **Fac Appt:** Clin Prof D, Columbia P&S

Bernstein, Robert M MD [D] - **Spec Exp:** Hair Restoration/Transplant; Hair Loss in Women; **Hospital:** NY-Presby/Columbia Univ Med Ctr, NY (page 65); **Address:** 110 E 55th St Fl 11, New York, NY 10022; **Phone:** 212-826-2400; **Board Cert:** Dermatology 1982; Hair Restoration Surgery 1998; **Med School:** UMDNJ-NJ Med Sch, Newark 1978; **Resid:** Dermatology, Montefiore Med Ctr 1982; **Fac Appt:** Clin Prof D, Columbia P&S

Bickers, David MD [D] - **Spec Exp:** Skin Cancer; Photodynamic Therapy; Psoriasis; Phototherapy; **Hospital:** NY-Presby/Columbia Univ Med Ctr, NY (page 65); **Address:** 16 E 60th St, Ste 300, New York, NY 10022-1002; **Phone:** 212-326-8465; **Board Cert:** Dermatology 1974; **Med School:** Univ VA Sch Med 1967; **Resid:** Dermatology, NYU Med Ctr 1973; **Fellow:** Pharmacology, Rockefeller Univ Hosp 1974; **Fac Appt:** Prof D, Columbia P&S

Brandt, Fredric S MD [D] - **Spec Exp:** Botox Therapy; Cosmetic Dermatology; **Address:** Laser & Skin Surgery Ctr, 323 E 34th St Fl 6, New York, NY 10016; **Phone:** 212-889-7096; **Board Cert:** Internal Medicine 1978; Dermatology 1981; **Med School:** Hahnemann Univ 1975; **Resid:** Internal Medicine, VA Hosp 1981; Dermatology, Univ Miami Hosps 1983

Braun III, Martin MD [D] - **Spec Exp:** Mohs' Surgery; Skin Cancer; **Hospital:** G Washington Univ Hosp, Washington Hosp Ctr; **Address:** 2112 F St NW, Ste 701, Washington, DC 20037; **Phone:** 202-293-7618; **Board Cert:** Dermatology 1977; Dermatopathology 1982; **Med School:** Univ MD Sch Med 1970; **Resid:** Dermatology, Univ Mich Med Ctr 1976; **Fellow:** Mohs Surgery, Precept w/ Dr Frederic Mohs 1975; **Fac Appt:** Clin Prof D, Geo Wash Univ

Brodland, David MD [D] - **Spec Exp:** Mohs' Surgery; Skin Cancer; Reconstructive Surgery-Skin; **Hospital:** UPMC Shadyside, Jefferson Reg Med Ctr - Pittsburgh; **Address:** South Hills Med Bldg, 575 Coal Valley Rd, Ste 360, Clairton, PA 15025; **Phone:** 412-466-9400; **Board Cert:** Dermatology 1989; **Med School:** Southern IL Univ 1985; **Resid:** Dermatology, Mayo Grad Sch Med 1989; **Fellow:** Mohs Surgery, John A Zitelli MD 1990; **Fac Appt:** Asst Clin Prof D, Univ Pittsburgh

Dermatology

Cohen, Bernard A MD [D] - **Spec Exp:** Pediatric Dermatology; Skin Laser Surgery; Hemangiomas; Vascular Malformations; **Hospital:** Johns Hopkins Hosp (page 61); **Address:** Johns Hopkins Div Ped Dermatology, Rubenstein Child Health Bldg, 200 N Wolfe St Fl 1, Baltimore, MD 21287; **Phone:** 410-955-2049; **Board Cert:** Pediatrics 1982; Dermatology 1984; Pediatric Dermatology 2004; **Med School:** Johns Hopkins Univ 1977; **Resid:** Pediatrics, Johns Hopkins Hosp 1980; Dermatology, Johns Hopkins Hosp 1984; **Fac Appt:** Prof D, Johns Hopkins Univ

Cotsarelis, George MD [D] - **Spec Exp:** Hair Loss; Scalp Disorders; **Hospital:** Hosp Univ Penn - UPHS (page 68); **Address:** Perelman Ctr for Advanced Medicine, Ste 1-330S, 3400 Civic Ctr Blvd, Philadelphia, PA 19104; **Phone:** 215-662-2737; **Board Cert:** Dermatology 2001; **Med School:** Univ Pennsylvania 1987; **Resid:** Dermatology, Hosp Univ Penn 1992; **Fellow:** Dermatology, Hosp Univ Penn; **Fac Appt:** Prof D, Univ Pennsylvania

DeLeo, Vincent A MD [D] - **Spec Exp:** Photosensitive Skin Diseases; Contact Dermatitis; Facial Rejuvenation; Eczema; **Hospital:** St. Luke's - Roosevelt Hosp Ctr - Roosevelt Div (page 55), Beth Israel Med Ctr - Petrie Division (page 55); **Address:** 1090 Amsterdam Ave Fl 11, New York, NY 10025; **Phone:** 212-523-5898; **Board Cert:** Dermatology 1976; **Med School:** Louisiana State U, New Orleans 1969; **Resid:** Dermatology, Columbia-Presby Med Ctr 1976; **Fac Appt:** Clin Prof D, Columbia P&S

Dzubow, Leonard M MD [D] - **Spec Exp:** Mohs' Surgery; Skin Cancer; **Address:** 101 Chesley Drive, Media, PA 19063; **Phone:** 484-621-0082; **Board Cert:** Internal Medicine 1978; Dermatology 2009; **Med School:** Univ Pennsylvania 1975; **Resid:** Internal Medicine, Hosp Univ Penn 1978; Dermatology, NYU-Skin Cancer Unit 1980; **Fellow:** Mohs Surgery, NYU-Skin Cancer Unit 1981

Franks Jr, Andrew G MD [D] - **Spec Exp:** Lupus/SLE; Raynaud's Disease; Scleroderma; Dermatomyositis; **Hospital:** NYU Langone Med Ctr (page 66); **Address:** NYU Dermatologic Assocs, Faculty Practice Tower, 530 First Ave Fl 7 - Ste 7R, New York, NY 10016; **Phone:** 212-263-5889; **Board Cert:** Internal Medicine 1975; Dermatology 1977; Rheumatology 1978; **Med School:** NY Med Coll 1971; **Resid:** Internal Medicine, Beth Israel Med Ctr 1974; Dermatology, Columbia-Presby Med Ctr 1975; **Fellow:** Rheumatology, Columbia-Presby Med Ctr 1977; **Fac Appt:** Prof D, NYU Sch Med

Geronemus, Roy MD [D] - **Spec Exp:** Skin Laser Surgery; Cosmetic Dermatology; Mohs' Surgery; Skin Cancer; **Hospital:** NYU Langone Med Ctr (page 66), New York Eye & Ear Infirm (page 64); **Address:** 317 E 34 St, Ste 11N, New York, NY 10016-4974; **Phone:** 212-686-7306; **Board Cert:** Dermatology 1983; **Med School:** Univ Miami Sch Med 1979; **Resid:** Dermatology, NYU-Skin Cancer Unit 1983; **Fellow:** Mohs Surgery, NYU-Skin Cancer Unit 1984; **Fac Appt:** Clin Prof D, NYU Sch Med

Gordon, Marsha MD [D] - **Spec Exp:** Cosmetic Dermatology; Botox Therapy; Facial Rejuvenation; **Hospital:** Mount Sinai Med Ctr (page 63); **Address:** 5 E 98th St Fl 5, New York, NY 10029-6574; **Phone:** 212-241-9728; **Board Cert:** Dermatology 1988; **Med School:** Univ Pennsylvania 1984; **Resid:** Dermatology, Mt Sinai Hosp 1988; **Fac Appt:** Clin Prof D, Mount Sinai Sch Med

Grossman, Melanie MD [D] - **Spec Exp:** Skin Laser Surgery; Tattoo Removal; Facial Rejuvenation; Cosmetic Dermatology; **Hospital:** NY-Presby/Columbia Univ Med Ctr, NY (page 65); **Address:** 161 Madison Ave, Ste 4NW, New York, NY 10016-5405; **Phone:** 212-725-8600; **Board Cert:** Dermatology 2010; **Med School:** NYU Sch Med 1988; **Resid:** Internal Medicine, Yale-New Haven Hosp 1989; Dermatology, Columbia-Presby Med Ctr 1992; **Fellow:** Laser Surgery, Mass Genl Hosp 1995; **Fac Appt:** Asst Clin Prof D, Columbia P&S

Halpern, Allan C MD [D] - **Spec Exp:** Skin Cancer; Melanoma; Melanoma Early Detection/Prevention; **Hospital:** Meml Sloan-Kettering Cancer Ctr; **Address:** 160 E 53rd St Fl 2, Dermatology, New York, NY 10022; **Phone:** 212-610-0766; **Board Cert:** Internal Medicine 1984; Dermatology 1988; **Med School:** Albert Einstein Coll Med 1981; **Resid:** Internal Medicine, Montefiore Hosp 1985; Dermatology, Hosp Univ Penn 1989; **Fellow:** Epidemiology, Hosp Univ Penn 1989; **Fac Appt:** Assoc Prof Med, Cornell Univ-Weill Med Coll

James, William D MD [D] - **Spec Exp:** Contact Dermatitis; Acne; Rosacea; **Hospital:** Hosp Univ Penn - UPHS (page 68); **Address:** Univ Penn Dept Dermatology, 3400 Spruce St, 2 Maloney, Philadelphia, PA 19104; **Phone:** 215-662-4282; **Board Cert:** Dermatology 1981; Diagnostic Lab Immunology 1985; **Med School:** Indiana Univ 1977; **Resid:** Dermatology, Letterman Army Med Ctr 1981; **Fac Appt:** Prof D, Univ Pennsylvania

Kalb, Robert E MD [D] - **Spec Exp:** Psoriasis; Phototherapy; **Hospital:** Buffalo General Hosp; **Address:** Buffalo Medical Group, 325 Essjay Rd, Ste 210, Williamsville, NY 14221; **Phone:** 716-630-1102; **Board Cert:** Dermatology 1986; **Med School:** SUNY Downstate 1982; **Resid:** Dermatology, Columbia Presby Med Ctr 1986; **Fac Appt:** Clin Prof D, SUNY Buffalo

Kress, Douglas W MD [D] - **Spec Exp:** Pediatric Dermatology; **Hospital:** Chldns Hosp of Pittsburgh - UPMC; **Address:** Children's Dermatology Ctr, 11279 Perry Hwy, Ste 108, Wexford, PA 15090; **Phone:** 724-933-9190; **Board Cert:** Dermatology 2006; Pediatric Dermatology 2004; **Med School:** Jefferson Med Coll 1992; **Resid:** Dermatology, Univ Pittsburgh Med Ctr 1996; **Fellow:** Pediatric Dermatology, Children's Hosp 2003; **Fac Appt:** Assoc Clin Prof D, Univ Pittsburgh

Kriegel, David MD [D] - **Spec Exp:** Mohs' Surgery; Botox Therapy; Skin Laser Surgery; Cosmetic Dermatology; **Hospital:** Mount Sinai Med Ctr (page 63); **Address:** 250 W 57th St, Ste 825, New York, NY 10107-0809; **Phone:** 212-489-6669; **Board Cert:** Dermatology 2003; **Med School:** Boston Univ 1987; **Resid:** Dermatology, New England Med Ctr 1991; **Fellow:** Mohs Surgery, Stony Brook Univ Hosp 1993; **Fac Appt:** Assoc Prof D, Mount Sinai Sch Med

Lebwohl, Mark MD [D] - **Spec Exp:** Skin Cancer; Psoriasis; Cutaneous Lymphoma; Pseudoxanthoma Elasticum; **Hospital:** Mount Sinai Med Ctr (page 63); **Address:** 5 E 98th St, Fl 5, New York, NY 10029-6501; **Phone:** 212-241-9728; **Board Cert:** Internal Medicine 1981; Dermatology 1983; **Med School:** Harvard Med Sch 1978; **Resid:** Internal Medicine, Mt Sinai Hosp 1981; Dermatology, Mt Sinai Hosp 1983; **Fellow:** Dermatology, Mt Sinai Hosp 1983; **Fac Appt:** Prof D, Mount Sinai Sch Med

Lessin, Stuart R MD [D] - **Spec Exp:** Cutaneous Lymphoma; Skin Cancer; Melanoma Risk Assessment; Mycosis Fungoides; **Hospital:** Bryn Mawr Hosp; **Address:** Bryn Mawr Skin & Cancer Ctr, 919 Conestoga Rd, Rosemont, PA 19010; **Phone:** 610-525-5028; **Board Cert:** Dermatology 1986; **Med School:** Temple Univ 1982; **Resid:** Dermatology, Hosp Univ Penn 1986; **Fellow:** Molecular Biology, Wistar Inst 1987; **Fac Appt:** Prof D, Temple Univ

Lowitt, Mark H MD [D] - **Spec Exp:** Skin Cancer; Melanoma; Acne; Eczema; **Hospital:** Greater Baltimore Med Ctr; **Address:** 6565 N Charles St, Ste 315, Baltimore, MD 21204; **Phone:** 410-321-1195; **Board Cert:** Dermatology 2003; **Med School:** Tulane Univ 1987; **Resid:** Internal Medicine, New England Deaconess Hosp 1990; **Fellow:** Dermatology, Univ Maryland 1993; **Fac Appt:** Assoc Clin Prof D, Univ MD Sch Med

Miller, Stanley J MD [D] - **Spec Exp:** Skin Cancer; Mohs' Surgery; Melanoma; **Hospital:** Johns Hopkins Hosp (page 61), Univ of MD Med Ctr; **Address:** Charles Towson Bldg, 1104 Kenilworth Drive, Ste 201, Towson, MD 21204; **Phone:** 443-279-0340; **Board Cert:** Dermatology 1989; **Med School:** Univ VT Coll Med 1984; **Resid:** Dermatology, UCSD Med Ctr 1989; **Fellow:** Dermatologic Surgery, Univ Penn 1991; **Fac Appt:** Assoc Prof D, Johns Hopkins Univ

Dermatology

Nigra, Thomas P MD [D] - **Spec Exp:** Hair Loss; Psoriasis; Skin Cancer; Vitiligo; **Hospital:** Washington Hosp Ctr, Natl Rehab Hosp; **Address:** Dermatology Assocs, 110 Irving St NW, Ste 2B28, Washington, DC 20010; **Phone:** 202-877-6227; **Board Cert:** Dermatology 1973; **Med School:** Univ Pennsylvania 1967; **Resid:** Dermatology, Mass Genl Hosp 1973; Dermatology, Natl Inst of Health 1971; **Fac Appt:** Clin Prof D, Geo Wash Univ

Orlow, Seth J MD/PhD [D] - **Spec Exp:** Pediatric Dermatology; Birthmarks/Hemangiomas; Psoriasis/Eczema; **Hospital:** NYU Langone Med Ctr (page 66); **Address:** 530 1st Ave, Ste 7R, New York, NY 10016-6402; **Phone:** 212-263-5889; **Board Cert:** Dermatology 2009; Pediatric Dermatology 2004; **Med School:** Albert Einstein Coll Med 1986; **Resid:** Pediatrics, Mt Sinai Hosp 1987; Dermatology, Yale-New Haven Hosp 1989; **Fellow:** Pediatric Dermatology, Yale-New Haven Hosp 1990; **Fac Appt:** Prof D, NYU Sch Med

Prioleau, Philip G MD [D] - **Spec Exp:** Melanoma; Skin Cancer; Mohs' Surgery; **Hospital:** NY-Presby/Weill Cornell Med Ctr, NY (page 65); **Address:** 1035 Fifth Ave, Ste C, New York, NY 10028; **Phone:** 212-794-3548; **Board Cert:** Surgery 1973; Anatomic Pathology 1979; Dermatopathology 1980; Dermatology 1983; **Med School:** Med Univ SC 1967; **Resid:** Surgery, Univ Va Hosp 1972; Plastic Surgery, Duke Univ Hosp 1975; **Fellow:** Pathology, Barnes Jewish Hosp 1980; Dermatopathology, NYU Med Ctr 1981; **Fac Appt:** Assoc Prof D, Cornell Univ-Weill Med Coll

Ramsay, David L MD [D] - **Spec Exp:** Cutaneous Lymphoma; Skin Cancer; **Hospital:** NYU Langone Med Ctr (page 66); **Address:** 530 1st Ave, Ste 7G, New York, NY 10016-6402; **Phone:** 212-683-6283; **Board Cert:** Dermatology 1974; **Med School:** Indiana Univ 1969; **Resid:** Dermatology, NYU Med Ctr 1973; **Fellow:** Dermatology, Univ Ill Hosp 1973; **Fac Appt:** Clin Prof D, NYU Sch Med

Rigel, Darrell S MD [D] - **Spec Exp:** Melanoma; Skin Cancer; Cosmetic Dermatology; **Hospital:** NYU Langone Med Ctr (page 66), Mount Sinai Med Ctr (page 63); **Address:** 35 E 35th Street, Ste 208, New York, NY 10016-3823; **Phone:** 212-684-5964; **Board Cert:** Dermatology 1983; **Med School:** Geo Wash Univ 1978; **Resid:** Dermatology, NYU Med Ctr 1982; **Fellow:** Dermatologic Surgery, NYU Med Ctr 1983; **Fac Appt:** Clin Prof D, NYU Sch Med

Rook, Alain H MD [D] - **Spec Exp:** Cutaneous Lymphoma; Immune Deficiency-Skin Disorders; Mycosis Fungoides; **Hospital:** Hosp Univ Penn - UPHS (page 68); **Address:** Hosp Univ Penn, Dept Dermatology, Perelman Center Fl 1 - Ste 330-S, 3400 Civic Center Blvd, Philadelphia, PA 19104-4283; **Phone:** 215-662-2737; **Board Cert:** Internal Medicine 1979; Nephrology 1980; Dermatology 2001; **Med School:** Univ Mich Med Sch 1975; **Resid:** Internal Medicine, McGill Univ Med Ctr 1977; Dermatology, Hosp Univ Penn 1989; **Fellow:** Nephrology, McGill Univ Med Ctr 1979; Immunology, NIH 1986; **Fac Appt:** Prof D, Univ Pennsylvania

Sarnoff, Deborah S MD [D] - **Spec Exp:** Mohs' Surgery; Skin Cancer; Dermatologic Surgery; Skin Laser Surgery; **Hospital:** NYU Langone Med Ctr (page 66); **Address:** 31 Northern Blvd, Greenvale, NY 11548; **Phone:** 516-484-9000; **Board Cert:** Dermatology 1984; **Med School:** Geo Wash Univ 1980; **Resid:** Dermatology, NYU Med Ctr 1984; **Fellow:** Dermatologic Surgery, NYU Med Ctr 1986; **Fac Appt:** Clin Prof D, NYU Sch Med

Schultz, Neal MD [D] - **Spec Exp:** Cosmetic Dermatology; Melanoma Early Detection/Prevention; Skin Laser Surgery; Tattoo Removal; **Hospital:** Mount Sinai Med Ctr (page 63), Lenox Hill Hosp; **Address:** 1130 Park Ave, New York, NY 10128; **Phone:** 212-369-9600; **Board Cert:** Dermatology 1978; **Med School:** Columbia P&S 1973; **Resid:** Internal Medicine, Mt Sinai Hosp 1975; Dermatology, Mt Sinai Hosp 1978; **Fac Appt:** Asst Clin Prof D, Mount Sinai Sch Med

Shupack, Jerome L MD [D] - **Spec Exp:** Rare Skin Disorders; Psoriasis; Eczema; Blistering Diseases; **Hospital:** NYU Langone Med Ctr (page 66); **Address:** 530 1st Ave, HCC 7F, New York, NY 10016-6402; **Phone:** 212-263-7344; **Board Cert:** Dermatology 1970; **Med School:** Columbia P&S 1963; **Resid:** Internal Medicine, Mt Sinai Hosp 1965; Dermatology, NYU Med Ctr 1970; **Fac Appt:** Prof D, NYU Sch Med

Soter, Nicholas A MD [D] - **Spec Exp:** Urticaria; Psoriasis; Vasculitis; **Hospital:** NYU Langone Med Ctr (page 66); **Address:** Dermatologic Assocs-Langone, 530 1st Ave, Ste 7-R, New York, NY 10016-6402; **Phone:** 212-263-5889; **Board Cert:** Dermatology 1970; Diagnostic Lab Immunology 1985; **Med School:** Univ Tex SW, Dallas 1965; **Resid:** Dermatology, Baylor Med Ctr 1968; Dermatology, Mass Genl Hosp 1969; **Fac Appt:** Prof D, NYU Sch Med

Stanley, John R MD [D] - **Spec Exp:** Blistering Diseases; Pemphigus; **Hospital:** Hosp Univ Penn - UPHS (page 68); **Address:** Univ of Pennsylvania, Dept Dermatology, Perelman Ctr for Advanced Medicine Fl 1, 3400 Civic Ctr Blvd, Ste 330-South, Philadelphia, PA 19104; **Phone:** 215-662-2737; **Board Cert:** Dermatology 1978; Clinical & Laboratory Dematologic Immunology 1985; **Med School:** Harvard Med Sch 1974; **Resid:** Dermatology, NYU Med Ctr 1978; **Fac Appt:** Prof D, Univ Pennsylvania

Werth, Victoria P MD [D] - **Spec Exp:** Autoimmune Disease; Lupus/SLE; Connective Tissue Disorders; Blistering Diseases; **Hospital:** Hosp Univ Penn - UPHS (page 68); **Address:** Perelman Ctr of Advanced Medicine Fl 1, 3400 Civic Ctr Blvd, Ste 330-South, Philadelphia, PA 19104; **Phone:** 215-662-2737; **Board Cert:** Internal Medicine 1983; Dermatology 1986; Diagnostic Lab Immunology 1989; **Med School:** Johns Hopkins Univ 1980; **Resid:** Internal Medicine, Northwestern Meml Hosp 1983; Dermatology, NYU Med Ctr 1986; **Fellow:** Immunological Dermatology, NYU Sch Med 1988; **Fac Appt:** Prof D, Univ Pennsylvania

Yan, Albert C MD [D] - **Spec Exp:** Pediatric Dermatology; Hemangiomas; Genetic Disorders-Skin; Atopic Dermatitis; **Hospital:** Chldns Hosp of Philadelphia, Hosp Univ Penn - UPHS (page 68); **Address:** Chldn's Hosp of Philadelphia, Dept Dermatology, 3550 Market St, Ste 2044, Philadelphia, PA 19104; **Phone:** 215-590-2169; **Board Cert:** Dermatology 2008; Pediatrics 2004; Pediatric Dermatology 2004; **Med School:** Univ Pennsylvania 1993; **Resid:** Pediatrics, Chldn's Hosp 1996; Dermatology, Hosp Univ Penn 1999; **Fac Appt:** Assoc Prof Ped, Univ Pennsylvania

Zitelli, John MD [D] - **Spec Exp:** Mohs' Surgery; Skin Cancer; Melanoma; **Hospital:** UPMC Shadyside, Jefferson Reg Med Ctr - Pittsburgh; **Address:** South Hills Med Bldg, 575 Coal Valley Rd, Ste 360, Clairton, PA 15025; **Phone:** 412-466-9400; **Board Cert:** Dermatology 2009; **Med School:** Univ Pittsburgh 1976; **Resid:** Dermatology, Univ Hlth Ctr Hosp 1979; **Fellow:** Mohs Surgery, Univ Wisconsin 1980; **Fac Appt:** Assoc Clin Prof D, Univ Pittsburgh

Southeast

Amonette, Rex A MD [D] - **Spec Exp:** Skin Cancer; Mohs' Surgery; **Address:** Memphis Dermatology Clin, 1455 Union Ave, Memphis, TN 38104-6727; **Phone:** 901-726-6655; **Board Cert:** Dermatology 1974; **Med School:** Univ Ark 1966; **Resid:** Dermatology, Univ Tenn Med Ctr 1971; **Fellow:** Mohs Surgery, NYU Med Ctr 1972; **Fac Appt:** Clin Prof D, Univ Tenn Coll Med

Brody, Harold J MD [D] - **Spec Exp:** Cosmetic Dermatology; Dermatologic Surgery; Facial Rejuvenation; Skin Laser Surgery-Resurfacing; **Hospital:** Emory Univ Hosp Midtown; **Address:** 1218 W Paces Ferry Rd NW, Ste 200, Atlanta, GA 30327; **Phone:** 404-525-7409; **Board Cert:** Dermatology 1978; **Med School:** Med Univ SC 1974; **Resid:** Dermatology, Emory Affil Hosps 1978; **Fac Appt:** Clin Prof D, Emory Univ

Dermatology

Burton III, Claude S MD [D] - **Spec Exp:** Leg Ulcers; Wound Healing/Care; Hemangiomas; Skin Laser Surgery; **Hospital:** Duke Univ Hosp; **Address:** Duke Univ Med Ctr, Box 3511, Durham, NC 27710; **Phone:** 919-681-5442; **Board Cert:** Internal Medicine 1982; Dermatology 1984; **Med School:** Duke Univ 1979; **Resid:** Internal Medicine, Duke Univ Med Ctr 1982; Dermatology, Duke Univ Med Ctr 1984; **Fac Appt:** Prof D, Duke Univ

Callen, Jeffrey P MD [D] - **Spec Exp:** Lupus/SLE; Dermatomyositis; Vasculitis; Psoriasis; **Hospital:** Univ of Louisville Hosp, Kosair Chldn's Hosp; **Address:** 310 E Broadway, Ste 200, Louisville, KY 40202; **Phone:** 502-583-1749; **Board Cert:** Internal Medicine 1975; Dermatology 2009; **Med School:** Univ Mich Med Sch 1972; **Resid:** Internal Medicine, Univ Mich Med Ctr 1975; Dermatology, Univ Mich Med Ctr 1977; **Fac Appt:** Prof Med, Univ Louisville Sch Med

Camisa, Charles MD [D] - **Spec Exp:** Psoriasis; Oral Dermatology; Lichen Planus; Cutaneous T-cell Lymphoma; **Address:** Riverchase Dermatology, 1015 Crosspointe Drive, Naples, FL 34110; **Phone:** 239-596-9075; **Board Cert:** Dermatology 1981; Clinical & Laboratory Dematologic Immunology 1987; **Med School:** Mount Sinai Sch Med 1977; **Resid:** Dermatology, NYU Med Ctr 1981; **Fac Appt:** Assoc Prof D, Univ S Fla Coll Med

Cohen, Bernard H MD [D] - **Spec Exp:** Hair Restoration/Transplant; Hair Loss; **Hospital:** Jackson Meml Hosp (page 70); **Address:** 4425 Ponce de Leon Blvd, Ste 230, Coral Gables, FL 33146; **Phone:** 305-476-9544; **Board Cert:** Dermatology 1972; Hair Restoration Surgery ; **Med School:** Columbia P&S 1967; **Resid:** Dermatology, NYU Med Ctr 1971; **Fac Appt:** Clin Prof D, Univ Miami Sch Med

Cook, Jonathan L MD [D] - **Spec Exp:** Skin Cancer; Mohs' Surgery; Reconstructive Surgery-Skin; Skin Laser Surgery; **Hospital:** Duke Univ Hosp; **Address:** Duke Univ Med Ctr, 5324 McFarland Drive, Ste 400, Durham, NC 27707; **Phone:** 919-684-6805; **Board Cert:** Dermatology 2005; **Med School:** Med Univ SC 1992; **Resid:** Dermatology, Emory Univ Hosp 1996; **Fellow:** Dermatologic Surgery, Hosp Univ Penn 1997; **Fac Appt:** Prof D, Duke Univ

Eichler, Craig J MD [D] - **Spec Exp:** Skin Cancer; Dermatologic Surgery; **Hospital:** Physicians Regl Hlthcare Med Ctr-Pine Ridge; **Address:** 6101 Pine Ridge Rd, Naples, FL 34119; **Phone:** 239-348-4335; **Board Cert:** Dermatology 2003; **Med School:** Univ Fla Coll Med 1989; **Resid:** Dermatology, Univ Texas Med Branch 1993

Elmets, Craig A MD [D] - **Spec Exp:** Psoriasis/Eczema; Phototherapy; Skin Cancer; Photodynamic Therapy; **Hospital:** Univ of Ala Hosp at Birmingham, Birmingham, Alabama VA Med Ctr; **Address:** Univ of Alabama-Birmingham-Derm Dept, 1530 3rd Ave S EFH Bldg - rm 414, Birmingham, AL 35294; **Phone:** 205-996-7546; **Board Cert:** Internal Medicine 1978; Dermatology 2009; Clinical & Laboratory Dematologic Immunology 1989; **Med School:** Univ Iowa Coll Med 1975; **Resid:** Internal Medicine, Kansas Med Ctr 1978; Dermatology, Univ Iowa Hosps 1980; **Fellow:** Immunological Dermatology, Univ Texas Hlth Sci Ctr 1982; **Fac Appt:** Prof D, Univ Alabama

Fenske, Neil A MD [D] - **Spec Exp:** Skin Cancer; Melanoma; Psoriasis; **Hospital:** H Lee Moffitt Cancer Ctr & Research Inst (page 59), Tampa Genl Hosp; **Address:** 12901 Bruce B Downs Blvd, MDC-79, Tampa, FL 33612; **Phone:** 813-974-4744; **Board Cert:** Dermatology 1977; Dermatopathology 1984; **Med School:** St Louis Univ 1973; **Resid:** Dermatology, Wisc Hlth Sci Ctr 1977; **Fac Appt:** Prof Med, Univ S Fla Coll Med

Flowers, Franklin P MD [D] - **Spec Exp:** Mohs' Surgery; Dermatopathology; **Hospital:** Shands at Univ of FL; **Address:** Shands Healthcare, PO Box 100383, Gainesville, FL 32610-0383; **Phone:** 352-265-8001; **Board Cert:** Dermatology 1976; Dermatopathology 1981; **Med School:** Univ Fla Coll Med 1971; **Resid:** Dermatology, Ohio State Univ 1975; **Fellow:** Mohs Surgery, Univ Alabama 1993; **Fac Appt:** Prof Med, Univ Fla Coll Med

Garrett, Algin MD [D] - **Spec Exp:** Skin Cancer; Mohs' Surgery; **Hospital:** Med Coll of VA Hosp; **Address:** Stonypoint Medical Park, 9000 Stonypoint Pkwy Fl 2, Richmond, VA 23235; **Phone:** 804-560-8991; **Board Cert:** Dermatology 1983; **Med School:** Penn State Coll Med 1978; **Resid:** Internal Medicine, VA Med Ctr 1980; Dermatology, Med Col VA 1983; **Fellow:** Mohs Surgery, Cleveland Clin Fdn 1988; **Fac Appt:** Prof D, Va Commonwealth Univ Sch Med

Green, Howard A MD [D] - **Spec Exp:** Mohs' Surgery; Skin Cancer; **Hospital:** St. Mary's Med Ctr - W Palm Bch; **Address:** 120 Butler St, Ste A, West Palm Beach, FL 33407-6106; **Phone:** 561-659-1510; **Board Cert:** Internal Medicine 1988; Dermatology 2004; **Med School:** Boston Univ 1985; **Resid:** Internal Medicine, Jefferson Univ Hosp 1988; Dermatology, Harvard Affil Hosps 1992; **Fellow:** Mohs Surgery, Boston Univ Med Ctr 1993

Grichnik, James M MD/PhD [D] - **Spec Exp:** Melanoma; Skin Cancer; **Hospital:** Univ of Miami Hosp & Clins/Sylvester Comp Canc Ctr (page 73); **Address:** 1501 NW 10th Ave BRB Bldg - rm 912, Miami, FL 33136; **Phone:** 305-243-6045; **Board Cert:** Dermatology 2003; **Med School:** Harvard Med Sch 1990; **Resid:** Dermatology, Duke Univ Med Ctr 1994; **Fac Appt:** Prof D, Univ Miami Sch Med

Johr, Robert MD [D] - **Spec Exp:** Pigmented Lesions; Melanoma; Pediatric Dermatology; **Hospital:** Boca Raton Regl Hosp, Univ of Miami Hosp & Clins/Sylvester Comp Canc Ctr (page 73); **Address:** 1050 NW 15th St, Ste 201A, Boca Raton, FL 33486-1341; **Phone:** 561-368-4545; **Board Cert:** Dermatology 1981; **Med School:** Mexico 1975; **Resid:** Dermatology, Roswell Park Cancer Ctr 1977; Dermatology, Metro Med Ctr 1979; **Fac Appt:** Clin Prof D, Univ Miami Sch Med

Jorizzo, Joseph L MD [D] - **Spec Exp:** Rheumatologic Dermatology; Immune Deficiency-Skin Disorders; Complex Diagnosis; **Hospital:** Wake Forest Univ Baptist Med Ctr; **Address:** Wake Forest Univ Sch Med, Dept Derm, 4618 Country Club Rd, Winston-Salem, NC 27104; **Phone:** 336-716-3926; **Board Cert:** Dermatology 1979; **Med School:** Boston Univ 1975; **Resid:** Dermatology, Univ N Carolina Hosps 1979; **Fellow:** Dermatology, Dermatology Inst 1980; **Fac Appt:** Prof D, Wake Forest Univ

Kirsner, Robert S MD/PhD [D] - **Spec Exp:** Wound Healing/Care; Leg Ulcers; **Hospital:** Univ of Miami Hosp (page 72), Jackson Meml Hosp (page 70); **Address:** Univ Miami, Dept Dermatology, 1295 NW 14th St South Bldg - Ste M, Miami, FL 33125; **Phone:** 305-243-6704; **Board Cert:** Dermatology 2005; **Med School:** Univ Miami Sch Med 1988; **Resid:** Internal Medicine, Univ Miami-Jackson Meml Hosp 1990; Dermatology, Univ Miami-Jackson Meml Hosp 1995; **Fellow:** Wound Healing, Univ Miami-Jackson Meml Hosp 1992; **Fac Appt:** Prof D, Univ Miami Sch Med

Leshin, Barry MD [D] - **Spec Exp:** Skin Cancer; Mohs' Surgery; **Address:** 1450 Professional Prak Drive, Ste 150, Winston-Salem, NC 27103; **Phone:** 336-724-2434; **Board Cert:** Dermatology 2009; **Med School:** Univ Tex, Houston 1981; **Resid:** Dermatology, Univ Iowa Hosp 1985; **Fellow:** Dermatologic Surgery, Univ Iowa Hosp 1986; **Fac Appt:** Clin Prof PlS, Wake Forest Univ

McMichael, Amy J MD [D] - **Spec Exp:** Hair Loss; Ethnic Skin Disorders; Pigmented Lesions; Skin Cancer; **Hospital:** Wake Forest Univ Baptist Med Ctr; **Address:** Wake Forest Univ Baptist Med Ctr, 4618 Country Club Rd, Winston-Salem, NC 27104; **Phone:** 336-716-3926; **Board Cert:** Dermatology 2004; **Med School:** Univ Pennsylvania 1990; **Resid:** Dermatology, Univ Mich Hosps 1994

Nouri, Keyvan MD [D] - **Spec Exp:** Mohs' Surgery; Skin Cancer; **Hospital:** Univ of Miami Hosp & Clins/Sylvester Comp Canc Ctr (page 73); **Address:** 1475 NW 12th Ave, Miami, FL 33163; **Phone:** 305-243-4183; **Board Cert:** Dermatology 1997; **Med School:** Boston Univ 1993; **Resid:** Dermatology, Univ Miami 1997; **Fellow:** Dermatologic Surgery, NYU Med Ctr 1999; **Fac Appt:** Prof D, Univ Miami Sch Med

Dermatology

Olsen, Elise A MD [D] - **Spec Exp:** Cutaneous Lymphoma; Hair Loss; Hirsutism; **Hospital:** Duke Univ Hosp; **Address:** Trent and Erwin Road, Box 3294, Durham, NC 27710; **Phone:** 919-684-3432; **Board Cert:** Dermatology 1983; **Med School:** Baylor Coll Med 1978; **Resid:** Internal Medicine, Univ NC Meml Hosp 1980; Dermatology, Duke Univ Med Ctr 1983; **Fac Appt:** Prof D, Duke Univ

Resnik, Sorrel MD [D] - **Spec Exp:** Hair Restoration/Transplant; Skin Laser Surgery; Cosmetic Dermatology; **Hospital:** Baptist Hosp of Miami; **Address:** Miami Dermatology & Laser Inst, 7800 SW 87th Ave, Ste B-200, Miami, FL 33173-3570; **Phone:** 305-279-6060; **Board Cert:** Dermatology 1966; **Resid:** Dermatology, Univ Penn 1965; **Fac Appt:** Clin Prof D, Univ Miami Sch Med

Russell, Mark A MD [D] - **Spec Exp:** Skin Cancer; Mohs' Surgery; Melanoma; **Hospital:** Univ of Virginia Health Sys; **Address:** Univ Virginia Hlth, Dept Dermatology, 1221 Lee St, Box 800718, Charlottesville, VA 22908; **Phone:** 434-924-5115; **Board Cert:** Dermatology 2005; Dermatopathology 2001; **Med School:** Ohio State Univ 1993; **Resid:** Dermatology, Vanderbilt Univ Med Ctr 1997; **Fellow:** Mohs Surgery, Vanderbilt Univ Med Ctr 1999; Dermatopathology, Univ Virginia Hlth System 2000; **Fac Appt:** Assoc Prof Med, Univ VA Sch Med

Sherertz, Elizabeth F MD [D] - **Spec Exp:** Eczema; Contact Dermatitis; Occupational Skin Diseases; **Address:** 1400 West Gate Ctr Drive, Ste 200, Winston-Salem, NC 27103; **Phone:** 336-774-8636; **Board Cert:** Dermatology 1982; **Med School:** Univ VA Sch Med 1978; **Resid:** Dermatology, Duke Univ Med Ctr 1982; **Fac Appt:** Clin Prof D, Wake Forest Univ

Sobel, Stuart A MD [D] - **Spec Exp:** Skin Cancer; Cosmetic Dermatology; **Hospital:** Meml Regl Hosp, Joe DiMaggio Chldns Hosp; **Address:** 4340 Sheridan St, Ste 101, Hollywood, FL 33021-3511; **Phone:** 954-983-5533; **Board Cert:** Dermatology 2009; **Med School:** Tufts Univ 1972; **Resid:** Dermatology, Mt Sinai Hosp 1976

Sokoloff, Daniel O MD [D] - **Spec Exp:** Skin Cancer; Cosmetic Dermatology; **Hospital:** Good Sam Med Ctr - W Palm Beach, St. Mary's Med Ctr - W Palm Bch; **Address:** Palm Beach Dermatology, 4475 Medical Center Way, Ste 2, West Palm Beach, FL 33407; **Phone:** 561-863-1000; **Board Cert:** Dermatology 1982; **Med School:** Geo Wash Univ 1977; **Resid:** Dermatology, Baylor Med Ctr 1982

Thiers, Bruce H MD [D] - **Spec Exp:** Cutaneous Lymphoma; Skin Cancer; Psoriasis; **Hospital:** MUSC Med Ctr; **Address:** MUSC Dept Dermatology, 135 Rutledge Ave Fl 11, MS 578, Charleston, SC 29425; **Phone:** 843-792-9784; **Board Cert:** Dermatology 1978; **Med School:** SUNY Buffalo 1974; **Resid:** Dermatology, SUNY Buffalo Med Ctr 1978; **Fac Appt:** Prof D, Med Univ SC

Midwest

Arpey, Christopher J MD [D] - **Spec Exp:** Mohs' Surgery; Skin Cancer; Skin Laser Surgery; Wound Healing/Care; **Hospital:** Mayo Med Ctr & Clin - Rochester; **Address:** Mayo Clinic - Dept Dermatology, 200 First St SW, Rochester, MN 55905; **Phone:** 507-284-2536; **Board Cert:** Dermatology 2001; Internal Medicine 1989; **Med School:** Univ Rochester 1986; **Resid:** Internal Medicine, Univ Iowa Hosps & Clinics 1989; Dermatology, Univ Hosps 1992; **Fellow:** Mohs Surgery, Univ Iowa Hosps & Clinics 1994; **Fac Appt:** Prof D, Mayo Med Sch

Bailin, Philip L MD [D] - **Spec Exp:** Mohs' Surgery; Skin Laser Surgery; Skin Cancer; **Hospital:** Cleveland Clin (page 56); **Address:** 9500 Euclid Ave A Bldg Fl 6, MC A-61, Cleveland, OH 44195-5032; **Phone:** 216-444-2115; **Board Cert:** Dermatology 1975; **Med School:** Northwestern Univ 1968; **Resid:** Dermatology, Cleveland Clin Fdn 1974; **Fellow:** Dermatopathology, Armed Forces Inst Pathology 1975; Mohs Surgery, Univ Wisc Hosp & Clin

Barbosa, Victoria H MD [D] - **Spec Exp:** Ethnic Skin Disorders; Hair Loss; Pigmented Lesions; Acne; **Hospital:** Rush Univ Med Ctr; **Address:** Rush Univ Med Ctr, 30 N Michigan Ave, Ste 1429, Chicago, IL 60602; **Phone:** 312-407-0000; **Board Cert:** Dermatology 2007; **Med School:** Yale Univ 1994; **Resid:** Dermatology, Yale-New Haven Hosp 1998; **Fac Appt:** Asst Prof D, Rush Med Coll

Bayliss, Susan J MD [D] - **Spec Exp:** Pediatric Dermatology; Eczema; Vascular Malformations; Hemangiomas/Birthmarks; **Hospital:** St. Louis Chldns Hosp; **Address:** St Louis Children's Hosp, 1 Children's Pl, rm 3N48, St Louis, MO 63110; **Phone:** 314-454-6187; **Board Cert:** Dermatology 1980; Pediatric Dermatology 2006; **Med School:** Univ Tex Med Br, Galveston 1977; **Resid:** Pediatrics, St Louis Children's Hosp 1980; **Fac Appt:** Prof Med, Washington Univ, St Louis

Cornelius, Lynn A MD [D] - **Spec Exp:** Melanoma; **Hospital:** Barnes-Jewish Hosp; **Address:** Washington Univ Dept Dermatology, 4921 Parkview Place, Campus Box 8123, St Louis, MO 63110; **Phone:** 314-362-2643; **Board Cert:** Dermatology 1989; **Med School:** Univ MO-Columbia Sch Med 1984; **Resid:** Dermatology, Barnes Jewish Hosp-Wash Univ 1989; **Fellow:** Immunological Dermatology, Emory Univ Med Ctr 1992; **Fac Appt:** Assoc Prof D, Washington Univ, St Louis

Crutchfield III, Charles Edward MD [D] - **Spec Exp:** Skin Cancer; Psoriasis; Eczema; Cosmetic Dermatology; **Hospital:** Regions Hosp - St Paul; **Address:** Crutchfield Dermatology, 1185 Town Center Drive, Ste 101, Eagan, MN 55123; **Phone:** 651-209-3600; **Board Cert:** Dermatology 2008; **Med School:** Mayo Med Sch 1994; **Resid:** Dermatology, Univ Minnesota Affil Hosp 1998; **Fac Appt:** Assoc Clin Prof D, Univ Minn

Fivenson, David P MD [D] - **Spec Exp:** Blistering Diseases; Wound Healing/Care; Lupus/SLE; Behcet's Syndrome; **Hospital:** St. Joseph Mercy Hosp - Ann Arbor; **Address:** 3001 Miller Rd, Ann Arbor, MI 48103; **Phone:** 734-222-9630; **Board Cert:** Dermatology 1989; Clinical & Laboratory Dematologic Immunology 1991; **Med School:** Univ Mich Med Sch 1984; **Resid:** Dermatology, Univ Cincinnati Med Ctr 1989; **Fellow:** Immunological Dermatology, UCSD Med Ctr 1986; **Fac Appt:** Assoc Clin Prof Med, Mich State Univ

Fosko, Scott W MD [D] - **Spec Exp:** Mohs' Surgery; Skin Cancer; Dermatologic Surgery; **Hospital:** St. Louis Univ Hosp; **Address:** 1755 S Grand Blvd, Ste 210, St Louis, MO 63104; **Phone:** 314-256-3420; **Board Cert:** Internal Medicine 1989; Dermatology 2001; **Med School:** Univ MD Sch Med 1986; **Resid:** Internal Medicine, Univ Va Med Ctr 1989; Dermatology, Yale-New Haven Hosp 1992; **Fellow:** Mohs Surgery, Hosp UPenn 1993; **Fac Appt:** Prof D, St Louis Univ

Garden, Jerome M MD [D] - **Spec Exp:** Skin Laser Surgery; Facial Rejuvenation; Vascular Birthmarks; **Hospital:** Northwestern Meml Hosp, Children's Mem Hosp -Chicago; **Address:** 150 E Huron St, Ste 1200, Chicago, IL 60611-2946; **Phone:** 312-280-0890; **Board Cert:** Dermatology 1984; **Med School:** Northwestern Univ 1980; **Resid:** Internal Medicine, Northwestern Univ Affil Hosp 1981; Dermatology, Northwestern Univ Affil Hosp 1984; **Fac Appt:** Prof D, Northwestern Univ

Hanke, C William MD [D] - **Spec Exp:** Mohs' Surgery; Skin Laser Surgery; Cosmetic Dermatology; Photodynamic Therapy; **Hospital:** St. Vincent Carmel Hosp; **Address:** Laser & Skin Surgery Ctr of Indiana, 13400 N Meridian St, Ste 290, Carmel, IN 46032-1486; **Phone:** 317-660-4900; **Board Cert:** Dermatology 2009; Dermatopathology 1982; **Med School:** Univ Iowa Coll Med 1971; **Resid:** Dermatology, Cleveland Clinic 1978; Dermatopathology, Indiana Univ 1982; **Fellow:** Cutaneous Oncology, Cleveland Clinic 1979; **Fac Appt:** Clin Prof D, Indiana Univ

Hruza, George J MD [D] - **Spec Exp:** Skin Laser Surgery; Mohs' Surgery; Cosmetic Surgery; **Hospital:** St. Luke's Hosp - Chesterfield, MO, St. Louis Univ Hosp; **Address:** Laser & Derm Surg Ctr, 1001 Chesterfield Pkwy E, Ste 101, St Louis, MO 63017; **Phone:** 314-878-3839; **Board Cert:** Dermatology 1986; **Med School:** NYU Sch Med 1982; **Resid:** Dermatology, NYU Med Ctr-Skin Cancer Unit 1986; **Fellow:** Laser Surgery, Mass Genl Hosp-Harvard 1987; Mohs Surgery, Univ Wisc Affil Hosp 1988; **Fac Appt:** Clin Prof D, St Louis Univ

Dermatology

Johnson, Timothy M MD [D] - **Spec Exp:** Melanoma; Mohs' Surgery; **Hospital:** Univ of Michigan Hosp; **Address:** Univ Michigan Dermatology, 1910 Taubman Ctr, 1500 E Medical Center Drive, Ann Arbor, MI 48109-5314; **Phone:** 734-936-4190; **Board Cert:** Dermatology 1988; **Med School:** Univ Tex, Houston 1984; **Resid:** Dermatology, Univ Texas Med Ctr 1988; **Fellow:** Cutaneous Oncology, Univ Mich Med Ctr 1989; Mohs Surgery, Univ Oregon Hlth Sci Ctr 1990; **Fac Appt:** Prof D, Univ Mich Med Sch

Krunic, Aleksandar L MD [D] - **Spec Exp:** Mohs' Surgery; Skin Cancer; Melanoma; Dermatologic Surgery; **Hospital:** Univ of IL Med Ctr at Chicago; **Address:** 1801 W Taylor St, Ste 3E, Chicago, IL 60612; **Phone:** 312-996-8666; **Board Cert:** Dermatology 2003; **Med School:** Yugoslavia 1988; **Resid:** Dermatology, Univ Chicago Hosp 2003; **Fellow:** Mohs Surgery, Duke Univ Med Ctr 1997; Mohs Surgery, Univ Texas SW Med Ctr 2004; **Fac Appt:** Assoc Clin Prof D, Univ IL Coll Med

Lim, Henry W MD [D] - **Spec Exp:** Phototherapy; Vitiligo; Cutaneous Lymphoma; Skin Cancer; **Hospital:** Henry Ford Hosp; **Address:** Henry Ford Hosp, Dept Derm, 3031 W Grand Blvd, Ste 800, Detroit, MI 48202-3141; **Phone:** 313-916-4060; **Board Cert:** Dermatology 2005; Clinical & Laboratory Dematologic Immunology 1985; **Med School:** SUNY Downstate 1975; **Resid:** Dermatology, NYU Med Ctr 1979; **Fellow:** Immunological Dermatology, NYU Med Ctr 1980; **Fac Appt:** Prof Path, Wayne State Univ

Liu, Vincent MD [D] - **Hospital:** Univ Iowa Hosp & Clinics; **Address:** UI Hosp-Dept of Dermatology, 200 Hawkins Dr 30000-PFP, Iowa City, IA 52242; **Phone:** 319-356-7546; **Board Cert:** Dermatology 2009; Dermatopathology 2001; **Med School:** Univ Pennsylvania 1996; **Resid:** Dermatology, Mass Genl Hosp 2000; **Fellow:** Dermatopathology, Mass Genl Hosp 2001; **Fac Appt:** Assoc Clin Prof D, Univ Iowa Coll Med

Lowe, Lori MD [D] - **Spec Exp:** Dermatopathology; Skin Cancer; **Hospital:** Univ of Michigan Hosp; **Address:** Univ Michigan Dept Pathology, 1301 Catherine Rd, M3261-Med Sci 1, Ann Arbor, MI 48109-5602; **Phone:** 734-764-4460; **Board Cert:** Dermatology 1990; Dermatopathology 1991; **Med School:** Univ Tex, Houston 1985; **Resid:** Dermatology, Univ Tex Hlth Sci Ctr 1990; **Fellow:** Dermatopathology, Univ Colo Hlth Sci Ctr 1991; **Fac Appt:** Prof D, Univ Mich Med Sch

Lucky, Anne W MD [D] - **Spec Exp:** Pediatric Dermatology; Acne; **Hospital:** Cincinnati Chldns Hosp Med Ctr; **Address:** Derm Assocs Cincinnati, 7691 Five Mile Rd, Ste 312, Cincinnati, OH 45230; **Phone:** 513-232-3332; **Board Cert:** Pediatrics 1975; Pediatric Endocrinology 1978; Dermatology 1981; Pediatric Dermatology 2004; **Med School:** Yale Univ 1970; **Resid:** Pediatrics, Boston Chldns Hosp 1973; Dermatology, Yale-New Haven Hosp 1981; **Fellow:** Pediatric Endocrinology, Natl Inst Hlth 1976; **Fac Appt:** Prof D, Univ Cincinnati

Mutasim, Diya F MD [D] - **Spec Exp:** Immune Deficiency-Skin Disorders; Dermatopathology; **Hospital:** Univ Hosp - Cincinnati; **Address:** 222 Piedmont Ave, Ste 5300, Cincinnati, OH 45219; **Phone:** 513-475-7630; **Board Cert:** Dermatology 1990; Dermatology 1990; Dermatopathology 1993; **Med School:** Lebanon 1979; **Resid:** Dermatology, Johns Hopkins Hosp 1989; **Fellow:** Dermatopathology, Johns Hopkins Hosp 1990; **Fac Appt:** Prof D, Univ Cincinnati

Neuburg, Marcelle MD [D] - **Spec Exp:** Mohs' Surgery; Skin Cancer; Pigmented Lesions; **Hospital:** Froedtert and Med Ctr of WI; **Address:** Dept Dermatology, 9200 W Wisconsin Ave, Milwaukee, WI 53226; **Phone:** 414-805-5300; **Board Cert:** Internal Medicine 1985; Dermatology 1988; **Med School:** Oregon Hlth & Sci Univ 1982; **Resid:** Internal Medicine, Georgetown Univ Hosp 1985; Dermatology, Boston Univ Sch Med Ctr 1988; **Fellow:** Mohs Surgery, Tufts New England Med Ctr 1990; **Fac Appt:** Prof D, Med Coll Wisc

Otley, Clark C MD [D] - **Spec Exp:** Mohs' Surgery; Skin Cancer; Skin Cancer in Transplant Patients; Dermatologic Surgery; **Hospital:** Mayo Med Ctr & Clin - Rochester; **Address:** Mayo Clinic, 200 First St SW, Rochester, MN 55905; **Phone:** 507-284-3579; **Board Cert:** Dermatology 2004; **Med School:** Duke Univ 1991; **Resid:** Dermatology, Mass Genl Hosp 1995; **Fellow:** Dermatologic Surgery, Mayo Clinic 1996; **Fac Appt:** Assoc Prof D, Mayo Med Sch

Paller, Amy S MD [D] - **Spec Exp:** Genetic Disorders-Skin; Immune Deficiency-Skin Disorders; Atopic Dermatitis; Pediatric Dermatology; **Hospital:** Children's Mem Hosp -Chicago; **Address:** 2300 Children's Plaza, Box 107, Chicago, IL 60614; **Phone:** 773-327-3446; **Board Cert:** Pediatrics 1982; Dermatology 2007; Pediatric Dermatology 2004; **Med School:** Stanford Univ 1978; **Resid:** Pediatrics, Chldns Meml Hosp 1981; Dermatology, Northwestern Meml Hosp 1983; **Fellow:** Research, Univ NC Hosp 1984; **Fac Appt:** Prof D, Northwestern Univ

Rhodes, Arthur R MD [D] - **Spec Exp:** Melanoma; Melanoma Risk Assessment; Melanoma Early Detection/Prevention; Pediatric Dermatology; **Hospital:** Rush Univ Med Ctr; **Address:** Rush Univ Dermatology Patient Svcs, 1725 W Harrison St, Ste 264, Chicago, IL 60612; **Phone:** 312-942-2195; **Board Cert:** Internal Medicine 1972; Dermatology 2009; **Med School:** Columbia P&S 1969; **Resid:** Internal Medicine, Beth Israel Hosp 1972; Dermatology, Mass Genl Hosp 1978; **Fac Appt:** Prof D, Rush Med Coll

Shea, Christopher R MD [D] - **Spec Exp:** Melanoma; Cutaneous Lymphoma; Pigmented Lesions; **Hospital:** Univ of IL Med Ctr at Chicago; **Address:** Univ Chicago Med Ctr, 5758 S Maryland Ave, MC 9815, Chicago, IL 60637; **Phone:** 773-702-6559; **Board Cert:** Anatomic Pathology 1998; Dermatology 2009; Dermatopathology 1991; **Med School:** Georgetown Univ 1983; **Resid:** Dermatology, Mass Genl Hosp 1986; Anatomic Pathology, Georgetown Univ Hosp 1981; **Fellow:** Dermatology, Mass Genl Hosp 1989; Dermatopathology, NY Presby Hosp/Weill Cornell 1991; **Fac Appt:** Prof Med, Univ IL Coll Med

Treadwell, Patricia A MD [D] - **Spec Exp:** Pediatric Dermatology; Vascular Birthmarks; **Hospital:** Riley Hosp for Children; **Address:** 1001 W 10th St, Bryce Bldg - rm B2101, Indianapolis, IN 46202; **Phone:** 317-944-2801; **Board Cert:** Pediatrics 1982; Dermatology 1983; **Med School:** Cornell Univ-Weill Med Coll 1977; **Resid:** Pediatrics, Riley Hosp 1980; Dermatology, Indiana Univ Med Ctr 1983; **Fac Appt:** Prof D, Indiana Univ

Voorhees, John MD [D] - **Spec Exp:** Psoriasis; Photoaging; **Hospital:** Univ of Michigan Hosp; **Address:** Univ Michigan, Dept Dermatology, 1500 E Med Ctr Drive, rm 1910 Taubman Ctr, Ann Arbor, MI 48109-5314; **Phone:** 734-936-4054; **Board Cert:** Dermatology 1970; **Med School:** Univ Mich Med Sch 1963; **Resid:** Dermatology, Univ Mich Hosp 1969; **Fac Appt:** Prof D, Univ Mich Med Sch

Wheeland, Ronald G MD [D] - **Spec Exp:** Skin Laser Surgery; Mohs' Surgery; Cosmetic Dermatology; Cutaneous Lymphoma; **Hospital:** Univ of Missouri Hosp; **Address:** One Hospital Drive, One University Missouri Hospital Drive, Columbia, MO 65212; **Phone:** 573-882-4800 x2; **Board Cert:** Dermatology 2009; Dermatopathology 1978; **Med School:** Univ Ariz Coll Med 1973; **Resid:** Dermatology, Univ Ok Hlth Sci Ctr 1977; **Fellow:** Dermatopathology, Univ Ok Hlth Sci Ctr 1978; Mohs Surgery, Cleveland Clin Fnd 1984; **Fac Appt:** Prof D, Univ MO-Columbia Sch Med

Witman, Patricia Mary MD [D] - **Spec Exp:** Pediatric Dermatology; **Hospital:** Nationwide Chldn's Hosp; **Address:** 555 S 18th St, Nationwide Chldn's Hosp, Columbus, OH 43205; **Phone:** 614-722-4579; **Board Cert:** Dermatology 2007; Pediatric Dermatology 2006; **Med School:** Med Coll Wisc 1994; **Resid:** Dermatology, Froedtert Meml Hosp 1998; **Fellow:** Pediatric Dermatology, UCSF Med Ctr 2002; **Fac Appt:** Asst Prof D, Ohio State Univ

Dermatology

Wood, Gary S MD [D] - **Spec Exp:** Cutaneous Lymphoma; Melanoma; Skin Cancer; **Hospital:** Univ WI Hosp & Clins, Wm S Middleton Mem Vet Hosp-Madison; **Address:** Univ Wisconsin Health, Dept Dermatology, 1 S Park St Fl 7, Madison, WI 53715-1375; **Phone:** 608-287-2620; **Board Cert:** Anatomic Pathology 1983; Dermatology 1986; Dermatopathology 1987; **Med School:** Univ IL Coll Med 1979; **Resid:** Anatomic Pathology, Stanford Univ Med Ctr 1983; Dermatology, Stanford Univ Med Ctr 1985; **Fellow:** Immunopathology, Stanford Univ Med Ctr 1981; **Fac Appt:** Prof D, Univ Wisc

Zelickson, Brian D MD [D] - **Spec Exp:** Skin Laser Surgery; **Hospital:** Abbott - Northwestern Hosp, Fairview Southdale Hosp; **Address:** 825 Nicollet Mall, Med Arts Bldg - Ste 1002, Minneapolis, MN 55402; **Phone:** 612-338-0711; **Board Cert:** Dermatology 2009; **Med School:** Mayo Med Sch 1986; **Resid:** Dermatology, Mayo Clinic 1990; **Fac Appt:** Asst Prof D, Univ Minn

Great Plains and Mountains

Bowen, Glen M MD [D] - **Spec Exp:** Melanoma; Cutaneous Lymphoma; Clinical Trials; Mohs' Surgery; **Hospital:** Univ Utah Hlth Care, Cottonwood Hosp & Med Ctr; **Address:** Huntsman Cancer Inst, 50 N Medical Drive, rm 4A330, Salt Lake City, UT 84132; **Phone:** 801-585-0197; **Board Cert:** Dermatology 2005; **Med School:** Univ Utah 1990; **Resid:** Dermatology, Univ Michigan Med Ctr 1993; **Fellow:** Immunological Dermatology, Univ Michigan Med Ctr 1995; Mohs Surgery, Univ Utah 2001; **Fac Appt:** Assoc Prof D, Univ Utah

Krueger, Gerald MD [D] - **Spec Exp:** Psoriasis; **Hospital:** Univ Utah Hlth Care; **Address:** Univ Utah Hlth Sci Ctr, Dept Derm, 30 N 1900 E, rm 4A330 SOM, Salt Lake City, UT 84132; **Phone:** 801-581-6465; **Board Cert:** Dermatology 1973; **Med School:** Loma Linda Univ 1966; **Resid:** Dermatology, Univ Colorado Med Ctr 1972; **Fac Appt:** Prof D, Univ Utah

Sontheimer, Richard D MD [D] - **Spec Exp:** Immune Deficiency-Skin Disorders; Lupus/SLE; Dermatomyositis; **Hospital:** Univ Utah Hlth Care; **Address:** Univ Hlth Care, Dept Dermatology, 30 N 1900 E, rm 4A330, Salt Lake City, UT 84132; **Phone:** 801-581-6465; **Board Cert:** Internal Medicine 1976; Dermatology 1979; Clinical & Laboratory Dematologic Immunology 1985; **Med School:** Univ Tex SW, Dallas 1972; **Resid:** Internal Medicine, Univ Utah Affil Hosps 1976; Dermatology, Parkland Meml Hosp 1979; **Fellow:** Research, Southwestern Med Sch 1978; **Fac Appt:** Prof D, Univ Utah

Southwest

Butler, David F MD [D] - **Spec Exp:** Skin Cancer; **Hospital:** Scott & White Mem Hosp; **Address:** Scott White Meml Hosp, Dept Dermatology, 409 W Adams St, Temple, TX 76501; **Phone:** 254-742-3724; **Board Cert:** Dermatology 1985; **Med School:** Univ Tex Med Br, Galveston 1980; **Resid:** Dermatology, Walter Reed Army Med Ctr 1985; **Fac Appt:** Assoc Prof D, Texas Tech Univ

Carney, John M MD [D] - **Spec Exp:** Mohs' Surgery; Skin Cancer; **Hospital:** UAMS Med Ctr; **Address:** Southwest Med Arts Bldg, 11321 Interstate 30, Ste 201, Little Rock, AR 72209; **Phone:** 501-455-4700; **Board Cert:** Dermatology 1984; **Med School:** Northwestern Univ 1979; **Resid:** Dermatology, Univ Hosps 1984; **Fellow:** Physiology, Harvard Med Sch 1985; Dermatologic Surgery, Univ Tenn Med Ctr 1986

Cather, Jennifer Clay MD [D] - **Spec Exp:** Cutaneous Lymphoma; Cutaneous T-cell Lymphoma; Psoriasis; **Hospital:** Baylor Univ Medical Ctr-Dallas; **Address:** Modern Dermatology, 9101 N Central Expy Ste 150, Dallas, TX 75231; **Phone:** 214-265-1818; **Board Cert:** Dermatology 1999; **Med School:** Univ Tex SW, Dallas 1994; **Resid:** Dermatology, UT Derm Hosp 2000; **Fellow:** Research, MD Anderson Canc Ctr 1997

Cockerell, Clay J MD [D] - **Spec Exp:** Dermatopathology; **Hospital:** UT Southwestern Med Ctr at Dallas; **Address:** Cockerell & Assocs, 2330 Butler St, Ste 115, Dallas, TX 75235; **Phone:** 214-530-5200; **Board Cert:** Dermatology 2008; Dermatopathology 1986; **Med School:** Baylor Coll Med 1981; **Resid:** Dermatology, NYU Langone Med Ctr 1985; **Fellow:** Dermatopathology, NYU Langone Med Ctr 1986; **Fac Appt:** Prof DP, Univ Tex SW, Dallas

Curiel, Clara N MD [D] - **Spec Exp:** Skin Cancer; Cutaneous Lymphoma; **Hospital:** Univ Med Ctr - Tucson; **Address:** 3838 N Campbell Ave, Tucson, AZ 85719; **Phone:** 520-694-2873; **Board Cert:** Dermatology 2008; **Med School:** Venezuela 1992; **Resid:** Dermatology, Boston Univ Med Ctr 2000; **Fellow:** Dermatology, Boston Univ Med Ctr 2001; **Fac Appt:** Asst Prof D, Univ Ariz Coll Med

Duvic, Madeleine MD [D] - **Spec Exp:** Cutaneous Lymphoma; Skin Cancer; Alopecia Areata; **Hospital:** UT MD Anderson Cancer Ctr, St. Luke's Episcopal Hosp-Houston; **Address:** UT MD Anderson Cancer Center, Dept of Dermatology, 1515 Holcombe Blvd, Unit 1452, Houston, TX 77030; **Phone:** 713-745-4615; **Board Cert:** Dermatology 1981; Internal Medicine 1982; **Med School:** Duke Univ 1977; **Resid:** Dermatology, Duke Univ Med Ctr 1980; Internal Medicine, Duke Univ Med Ctr 1982; **Fellow:** Geriatric Medicine, Duke Univ Med Ctr 1984; **Fac Appt:** Prof D, Univ Tex, Houston

Hansen, Ronald C MD [D] - **Spec Exp:** Pediatric Dermatology; **Hospital:** Phoenix Children's Hosp; **Address:** Phoenix Childrens Hosp, Dermatology Clinic F, 1919 E Thomas Rd, Phoenix, AZ 85006; **Phone:** 602-546-0895; **Board Cert:** Pediatrics 1974; Dermatology 1980; **Med School:** Univ Iowa Coll Med 1968; **Resid:** Pediatrics, Childrens Hosp 1970; Pediatrics, Stanford Univ Med Ctr 1972; **Fellow:** Dermatology, Univ Arizona 1980; **Fac Appt:** Prof D, Univ Ariz Coll Med

Levy, Moise L MD [D] - **Spec Exp:** Pediatric Dermatology; Vascular Birthmarks; Genetic Disorders-Skin; Blistering Diseases; **Hospital:** Seton Med Ctr; **Address:** 1301 Barbara Jordan Blvd, Pediatrics Bldg - Ste 200, Austin, TX 78723; **Phone:** 512-628-1920; **Board Cert:** Pediatrics 1985; Dermatology 1986; Pediatric Dermatology 2004; **Med School:** Univ Tex, Houston 1979; **Resid:** Pediatrics, Univ Tex Affil Hosp 1983; Dermatology, Baylor Coll Med 1986; **Fac Appt:** Prof D, Baylor Coll Med

Lim Quan, Katherine K MD [D] - **Spec Exp:** Mohs' Surgery; Skin Cancer; **Hospital:** Chandler Regional Med Ctr; **Address:** 1100 S Dobson Rd, Ste 223, Shea, Chandler, AZ 85286; **Phone:** 480-214-0388; **Board Cert:** Dermatology 2006; **Med School:** Northwestern Univ 1992; **Resid:** Dermatology, Mayo Clinic 1996; **Fellow:** Mohs Surgery, Mayo Clinic 1997

Menter, M Allan MD [D] - **Spec Exp:** Psoriasis; Cosmetic Dermatology; Eczema; **Hospital:** Baylor Univ Medical Ctr-Dallas, UT Southwestern Med Ctr at Dallas; **Address:** 3900 Junius St, Ste 145, Dallas, TX 75246; **Phone:** 972-386-7546 x400; **Board Cert:** Dermatology 1978; **Med School:** South Africa 1966; **Resid:** Dermatology, Pretoria Genl Hosp 1971; Dermatology, Guys Hosp 1972; **Fellow:** Dermatology, St Johns Hosp 1973; Dermatology, Univ Texas SW 1979; **Fac Appt:** Clin Prof D, Univ Tex SW, Dallas

Orengo, Ida F MD [D] - **Spec Exp:** Melanoma; Mohs' Surgery; **Hospital:** St. Luke's Episcopal Hosp-Houston, DeBakey VA Med Ctr-Houston; **Address:** Baylor College of Medicine, 6620 Main St, Ste 1425, Houston, TX 77030; **Phone:** 713-798-6925; **Board Cert:** Dermatology 2009; **Med School:** Harvard Med Sch 1988; **Resid:** Dermatology, Baylor Coll Med 1991; **Fac Appt:** Assoc Prof D, Baylor Coll Med

Perone, Jennifer Beth MD [D] - **Spec Exp:** Mohs' Surgery; **Hospital:** UT Southwestern Med Ctr at Dallas; **Address:** North TX Prof Building, 2817 S Mayhill Rd, Ste 115, Denton, TX 76208; **Phone:** 940-591-0900; **Board Cert:** Dermatology 2003; **Med School:** NYU Sch Med 1999; **Resid:** Dermatology, Duke Univ Med Ctr 2003; **Fellow:** Mohs Surgery, UT Southwestern Med Ctr-Dalla 2006

Dermatology

Taylor, R Stan MD [D] - **Spec Exp:** Mohs' Surgery; Melanoma; Skin Cancer; **Hospital:** UT Southwestern Med Ctr at Dallas, Parkland Hlth & Hosp Sys; **Address:** Univ Tex SW Med Sch, Dept Derm, 5323 Harry Hines Blvd, MC 9192, Dallas, TX 75390-7208; **Phone:** 214-645-8950; **Board Cert:** Dermatology 1989; **Med School:** Univ Tex Med Br, Galveston 1985; **Resid:** Dermatology, Univ Mich Med Ctr 1989; **Fellow:** Immunological Dermatology, Univ Mich 1990; Mohs Surgery, Oregon Hlth Sci Univ 1991; **Fac Appt:** Prof D, Univ Tex SW, Dallas

West Coast and Pacific

Bennett, Richard G MD [D] - **Spec Exp:** Mohs' Surgery; Skin Cancer; Hidradenitis Suppurativa; Dermatofibrosarcoma Protruberans; **Hospital:** Keck Med Ctr of USC (page 75), UCLA Ronald Reagan Med Ctr; **Address:** 1301 20th St, Ste 570, Santa Monica, CA 90404-2080; **Phone:** 310-315-0171; **Board Cert:** Dermatology 1975; **Med School:** Case West Res Univ 1970; **Resid:** Dermatology, Hosp Univ Penn 1974; **Fellow:** Mohs Surgery, NYU Med Ctr 1977; **Fac Appt:** Clin Prof D, UCLA

Berg, Daniel MD [D] - **Spec Exp:** Skin Cancer; Mohs' Surgery; Skin Laser Surgery; Cosmetic Dermatology; **Hospital:** Univ Wash Med Ctr; **Address:** 4225 Roosevelt Way NE, Box 354697, Seattle, WA 98105; **Phone:** 206-598-6647; **Board Cert:** Dermatology 2009; **Med School:** Univ Toronto 1985; **Resid:** Internal Medicine, Sunnybrook Med Ctr 1988; Dermatology, Duke Univ Med Ctr 1991; **Fellow:** Dermatologic Surgery, Univ Toronto 1992; Dermatologic Surgery, Univ British Columbia 1994; **Fac Appt:** Prof D, Univ Wash

Eichenfield, Lawrence F MD [D] - **Spec Exp:** Eczema; Acne; Vascular Birthmarks; Pediatric Dermatology; **Hospital:** Rady Children's Hosp - San Diego, UCSD Med Ctr; **Address:** Chldns Hosp, Ped & Adolescent Dermatology, 8010 Frost St, Ste 602, San Diego, CA 92123-4204; **Phone:** 858-966-6795; **Board Cert:** Dermatology 2009; Pediatric Dermatology 2004; **Med School:** Mount Sinai Sch Med 1984; **Resid:** Pediatrics, Chldns Hosp 1987; Dermatology, Hosp Univ Penn 1991; **Fac Appt:** Prof Ped, UCSD

Fitzpatrick, Richard E MD [D] - **Spec Exp:** Cosmetic Dermatology; Skin Laser Surgery-Resurfacing; Hair Restoration/Transplant; **Address:** 9339 Genesee Ave, Ste 300, La Jolla, CA 92121; **Phone:** 858-657-1002; **Board Cert:** Dermatology 2003; **Med School:** Emory Univ 1970; **Resid:** Dermatology, UCLA Med Ctr 1978; **Fac Appt:** Assoc Clin Prof D, UCSD

Frieden, Ilona J MD [D] - **Spec Exp:** Pediatric Dermatology; Vascular Birthmarks; Hemangiomas; **Hospital:** UCSF - Mt Zion Med Ctr; **Address:** UCSF, Dept Dermatology, 1701 Divisadero St, Fl 3, Box 0316, San Francisco, CA 94115; **Phone:** 415-353-7800; **Board Cert:** Dermatology 2005; Pediatrics 1983; Pediatric Dermatology 2004; **Med School:** UCSF 1977; **Resid:** Pediatrics, UCSF Med Ctr 1980; Dermatology, UCSF Med Ctr 1983; **Fac Appt:** Clin Prof D, UCSF

Friedlander, Sheila Fallon MD [D] - **Spec Exp:** Pediatric Dermatology; Infectious Disease; Vascular Malformations; Hemangiomas; **Hospital:** Rady Children's Hosp - San Diego, UCSD Med Ctr; **Address:** 8010 Frost St, Ste 602, San Diego, CA 92123; **Phone:** 858-966-6795; **Board Cert:** Pediatrics 1984; Dermatology 1990; Pediatric Dermatology 2004; **Med School:** Univ Chicago-Pritzker Sch Med 1979; **Resid:** Pediatrics, Bronx Municipal Hosp 1983; Dermatology, UCLA Med Ctr 1990; **Fellow:** Infectious Disease, Montefiore Med Ctr 1986; **Fac Appt:** Clin Prof Ped, UCSD

Glogau, Richard G MD [D] - **Spec Exp:** Cosmetic Dermatology; Skin Laser Surgery; Mohs' Surgery; Botox Therapy; **Hospital:** UCSF Med Ctr; **Address:** 350 Parnassus Ave, Ste 400, San Francisco, CA 94117; **Phone:** 415-564-1261; **Board Cert:** Dermatology 2009; Dermatopathology 1982; **Med School:** Harvard Med Sch 1973; **Resid:** Dermatology, UCSF Med Ctr 1977; **Fellow:** Chemosurgery, UCSF Med Ctr 1978; **Fac Appt:** Clin Prof D, UCSF

Greenway, Hubert T MD [D] - **Spec Exp:** Skin Cancer; Mohs' Surgery; Melanoma; **Hospital:** Scripps Green Hosp; **Address:** Scripps Clinic, Div Mohs' Surgery, 10666 N Torrey Pines Rd, MS 112A, La Jolla, CA 92037; **Phone:** 858-554-8646; **Board Cert:** Dermatology 1982; **Med School:** Med Coll GA 1974; **Resid:** Dermatology, Naval Hosp 1982; **Fellow:** Mohs Surgery, Univ Wisconsin Med Ctr 1981

Grimes, Pearl E MD [D] - **Spec Exp:** Pigmented Lesions; Ethnic Skin Disorders; Vitiligo; Cosmetic Dermatology; **Hospital:** UCLA Ronald Reagan Med Ctr; **Address:** 5670 Wilshire Blvd, Ste 650, Los Angeles, CA 90036; **Phone:** 323-467-4389; **Board Cert:** Dermatology 1979; **Med School:** Washington Univ, St Louis 1974; **Resid:** Dermatology, Howard Univ Hosp 1979; **Fac Appt:** Clin Prof D, UCLA

Hanifin, Jon M MD [D] - **Spec Exp:** Atopic Dermatitis; **Hospital:** OR Hlth & Sci Univ; **Address:** OHSU, Dept Dermatology, 3303 SW Bond Ave, MC CH16D, Portland, OR 97239; **Phone:** 503-418-3376; **Board Cert:** Dermatology 1970; **Med School:** Univ Wisc 1965; **Resid:** Dermatology, UCSF Med Ctr 1969; **Fellow:** Clinical & Laboratory Immunology, UCSF Med Ctr; **Fac Appt:** Prof D, Oregon Hlth & Sci Univ

Kilmer, Suzanne L MD [D] - **Spec Exp:** Skin Laser Surgery-Resurfacing; Facial Rejuvenation; Cosmetic Dermatology; **Hospital:** Mercy General Hosp - Sacramento; **Address:** The Laser & Skin Surgery Center, 3835 J St, Sacramento, CA 95816-5520; **Phone:** 916-456-0400; **Board Cert:** Dermatology 2009; **Med School:** UC Davis 1987; **Resid:** Dermatology, UC Davis Med Ctr 1991; **Fellow:** Laser Surgery, Mass Genl Hosp 1992; **Fac Appt:** Asst Clin Prof D, UC Davis

Kim, Youn-Hee MD [D] - **Spec Exp:** Cutaneous Lymphoma; Skin Cancer; **Hospital:** Stanford Univ Hosp & Clinics; **Address:** 875 Blake Wilbur Drive, Stanford, CA 94305; **Phone:** 650-723-6316; **Board Cert:** Dermatology 1989; **Med School:** Stanford Univ 1984; **Resid:** Dermatology, Metropolitan Hosp 1989

Koo, John Ying Ming MD [D] - **Spec Exp:** Psoriasis/Eczema; Photosensitive Skin Diseases; Phototherapy; Psychodermatology; **Hospital:** UCSF Med Ctr; **Address:** Psoriasis Day Treatment Ctr, 515 Spruce St, San Francisco, CA 94118; **Phone:** 415-476-4701; **Board Cert:** Dermatology 1988; Psychiatry 1988; **Med School:** Harvard Med Sch 1981; **Resid:** Psychiatry, UCLA Neur Psyc Inst 1985; Dermatology, UCSF Med Ctr 1988; **Fac Appt:** Prof D, UCSF

Lask, Gary P MD [D] - **Spec Exp:** Cosmetic Dermatology; Mohs' Surgery; Skin Laser Surgery-Resurfacing; Scar Revision; **Hospital:** UCLA Ronald Reagan Med Ctr; **Address:** 16260 Ventura Blvd, Ste 530, Encino, CA 91436; **Phone:** 818-788-4022; **Board Cert:** Dermatology 1983; **Med School:** Mexico 1977; **Resid:** Dermatology, ML King Jr-Drew Med Ctr 1983; **Fellow:** Mohs Surgery, ML King Jr-Drew Med Ctr 1984; **Fac Appt:** Clin Prof D, UCLA

Nghiem, Paul T MD/PhD [D] - **Spec Exp:** Merkel Cell Carcinoma; Skin Cancer; **Hospital:** Univ Wash Med Ctr; **Address:** Seattle Cancer Care Alliance, 825 Eastlake Ave E, Seattle, WA 98109; **Phone:** 206-288-1024; **Board Cert:** Dermatology 2009; **Med School:** Stanford Univ 1994; **Resid:** Dermatology, Massachusetts General Hosp 1998; **Fellow:** Research, Harvard Univ 2002; **Fac Appt:** Assoc Prof D, Univ Wash

Rubin, Mark G MD [D] - **Spec Exp:** Skin Laser Surgery; Cosmetic Dermatology; **Hospital:** UCSD Med Ctr; **Address:** 153 S Lasky Drive, Ste 1, Beverly Hills, CA 90212; **Phone:** 310-556-0119; **Board Cert:** Dermatology 1985; **Med School:** Jefferson Med Coll 1981; **Resid:** Dermatology, Henry Ford Hosp 1985; **Fac Appt:** Assoc Prof D, UCSD

Dermatology

Swanson, Neil A MD [D] - **Spec Exp:** Skin Cancer; Mohs' Surgery; Reconstructive Surgery-Skin; Cosmetic Dermatology; **Hospital:** OR Hlth & Sci Univ, VA Medical Center - Portland; **Address:** 3303 SW Bond Ave, MC CH-5D, Portland, OR 97239; **Phone:** 503-418-3376; **Board Cert:** Dermatology 1980; **Med School:** Univ Rochester 1976; **Resid:** Dermatology, Univ Michigan Med Ctr 1979; **Fellow:** Dermatology, UCSF Med Ctr 1980; **Fac Appt:** Prof D, Oregon Hlth & Sci Univ

Swetter, Susan M MD [D] - **Spec Exp:** Melanoma; Melanoma Early Detection/Prevention; Skin Cancer; **Hospital:** Stanford Univ Hosp & Clinics, VA Hlth Care Sys - Palo Alto; **Address:** Stanford Univ Med Ctr, Dept Dermatology, 875 Blake Wilbur Dr, W0069, MC 5334, Stanford, CA 94305; **Phone:** 650-723-0119; **Board Cert:** Dermatology 2001; **Med School:** Univ Pennsylvania 1990; **Resid:** Dermatology, Stanford Univ Med Ctr 1994; **Fac Appt:** Assoc Prof D, Stanford Univ

Woodley, David T MD [D] - **Spec Exp:** Autoimmune Disease; Blistering Diseases; Pemphigus; Psoriasis; **Hospital:** Keck Med Ctr of USC (page 75); **Address:** USC Dermatology, 1520 San Pablo St, Los Angeles, CA 90033; **Phone:** 323-442-6200; **Board Cert:** Dermatology 1982; Internal Medicine 1976; Clinical & Laboratory Dematologic Immunology 1993; **Med School:** Univ MO-Columbia Sch Med 1973; **Resid:** Internal Medicine, Univ Nebraska Med Ctr 1976; Dermatology, Univ NC Med Ctr 1978; **Fellow:** Dermatologic Research, Univ Paris 1980; **Fac Appt:** Prof D, USC-Keck School of Medicine

Cleveland Clinic

Every life deserves world class care.

Dermatology

Cleveland Clinic's Department of Dermatology, part of the Dermatology & Plastic Surgery Institute, offers a full array of subspecialized care for adult and pediatric patients. Our physicians diagnose and treat all disorders of the skin, hair and nails, whether primary or related to an underlying systemic illness, including industrial-related conditions.

Volume-Leading Mohs Center

The department offers a full range of procedures in the subspecialty area of dermatologic surgery. These include Mohs micrographic surgery for high-risk skin cancers (including local tissue reconstruction), laser surgery, chemical peels, soft tissue augmentation, Botox® injections, hair transplant and liposuction. We performed more than 2,000 Mohs procedures in the past year alone. Additionally, our Cutaneous Care Center provides outpatient treatment, rather than hospitalization, for patients with extensive, severe or chronic skin diseases utilizing phototherapy and excimer laser treatment. Staff dermatologists and residents are involved in research, either institutionally or through industrial support of clinical trials.

Cleveland Clinic's Department of Dermatology provides expertise in the diagnosis and management of the full spectrum of dermatologic conditions, as well as an extensive range of cosmetic evaluations and surgeries. We continue to meet our community responsibility through active participation in Skin Cancer Screening and in other activities related to National Skin Cancer Week. The Department of Dermatology also provides medical missionary assistance in developing countries. We continuously strive to improve outcomes in dermatology, not just for the patients who entrust us with their care today, but for future generations.

Cleveland Clinic
Dermatology & Plastic
Surgery Institute
9500 Euclid Avenue
Cleveland, OH 44195

clevelandclinic.org/
dermtopdocs

Offering Same-Day Appointments
Call 800.274.2009.

Treatment Guides

Cleveland Clinic has developed comprehensive treatment guides for many diseases and conditions. To download our free treatment guides, visit clevelandclinic.org/ treatmentguides.

Online Medical Second Opinion

Cleveland Clinic's My**Consult** Online Medical Second Opinion program securely connects patients to our physician specialists for more than 1,000 life-changing or life-threatening diagnoses all by the click of a mouse. To learn more, log onto eclevelandclinic.org/myconsult or call 800.223.2273, ext. 43223.

Special Assistance for Out-of-State Patients

Cleveland Clinic Global Patient Services offers a complimentary Medical Concierge service for patients who travel from outside of Ohio. Call 800.223.2273, ext. 55580 or email medicalconcierge@ccf.org.

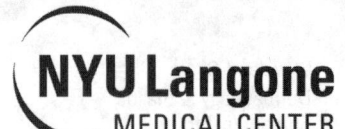

550 First Avenue *(at 31st Street)*
New York, NY 10016
www.NYULMC.org
Physician Referral: **888-7-NYU-MED** *(888-769-8633)*

DERMATOLOGY

About the Ronald O. Perelman Department of Dermatology
The Ronald O. Perelman Department of Dermatology is a national and international leader in dermatology, employing the most advanced science and medicine to diagnose and treat skin disorders. The Department provides dermatologic care for more than 100,000 patients each year, as well as conducting research into some of the most significant dermatologic problems. Services include adult and pediatric medical dermatology, dermatologic/ skin cancer surgery and cosmetic dermatology. We specialize in the following areas:

Dermatologic / Skin Cancer Surgery and Cosmetic Dermatology
NYU Langone Medical Center's dermatologists provide specialized care for the treatment of malignant and benign skin lesions and offer cutting-edge therapies for aesthetic and cosmetic concerns.

General Dermatology
Dermatologic associates offer multi-subspecialty dermatology care in private office settings for patients with disorders of the skin, hair, and nails, including inflammatory skin diseases such as psoriasis and lupus, cancers and other skin tumors, hair loss, infections and allergic skin diseases such as eczema, contact dermatitis and hives.

Pediatric and Adolescent Dermatology
The Medical Center also boasts a specialized professional practice dedicated to the treatment of diseases affecting the skin, hair, and nails of infants, children and adolescents. These disorders include acne, atopic dermatitis/eczema, hair loss, hemangiomas, moles, birthmarks, vitiligo and genetic disorders affecting the skin.

Charles C. Harris Skin and Cancer Unit / Dermatology Clinical Trials Unit
The Charles C. Harris Skin and Cancer Unit at Tisch Hospital is an outpatient dermatology teaching center combining unique patient care with superior medical education. Resident and attending physicians provide diagnosis and treatment of skin diseases that include acne, eczema and warts as well as complex medical conditions such as connective tissue disorders, pigmented lesions, skin allergies and skin cancers.

Dermatopathology
Highly trained dermatopathologists at the Medical Center examine skin tissues submitted by physicians from biopsies and surgeries to diagnose skin diseases and malignancies. One of the busiest academic skin pathology units in the country, the Dermatopathology section of the Department also provides consultative services for the review of skin pathology specimens performed elsewhere.

Endocrinology, Diabetes & Metabolism
a subspecialty of Internal Medicine

An internist who concentrates on disorders of the internal (endocrine) glands such as the thyroid and adrenal glands. This specialist also deals with disorders such as diabetes, metabolic and nutritional disorders, pituitary diseases, menstrual and sexual problems.

Training Required: Three years in internal medicine *plus* additional training and examination for certification in endocrinology, diabetes and metabolism.

ENDOCRINOLOGY, DIABETES & METABOLISM

New England

Abrahamson, Martin J MD [EDM] - **Spec Exp:** Diabetes; **Hospital:** Beth Israel Deaconess Med Ctr - Boston; **Address:** Joslin Diabetes Clinic, 1 Joslin Pl, Boston, MA 02215; **Phone:** 617-732-2501; **Board Cert:** Internal Medicine 2005; Endocrinology, Diabetes & Metabolism 2005; **Med School:** South Africa 1977; **Resid:** Internal Medicine, Groote Schuuer Hosp-Univ Cape Town 1983; **Fellow:** Endocrinology, Diabetes & Metabolism, Groote Schuuer Hosp-Univ Cape Town 1985; Research, Univ Cape Town 1987; **Fac Appt:** Assoc Prof Med, Harvard Med Sch

Axelrod, Lloyd MD [EDM] - **Spec Exp:** Diabetes; Geriatric Endocrinology; **Hospital:** Mass Genl Hosp; **Address:** 50 Stanford St Fl 3 - Ste 340, Boston, MA 02114; **Phone:** 617-726-8722; **Board Cert:** Internal Medicine 1973; Endocrinology, Diabetes & Metabolism 1973; **Med School:** Harvard Med Sch 1967; **Resid:** Internal Medicine, Peter Bent Brigham Hosp 1969; Internal Medicine, Mass Genl Hosp 1971; **Fellow:** Endocrinology, Diabetes & Metabolism, Peter Bent Brigham Hosp 1970; Endocrinology, Diabetes & Metabolism, Mass Genl Hosp 1972; **Fac Appt:** Assoc Prof Med, Harvard Med Sch

Beaser, Richard S MD [EDM] - **Spec Exp:** Diabetes; **Hospital:** Beth Israel Deaconess Med Ctr - Boston; **Address:** Joslin Clinic, 1 Joslin Pl, Boston, MA 02215; **Phone:** 617-732-2665; **Board Cert:** Internal Medicine 1980; **Med School:** Boston Univ 1977; **Resid:** Internal Medicine, Univ Mass Med Ctr 1980; **Fellow:** Diabetes, Joslin Clinic 1981; Endocrinology, Lahey Clinic 1982; **Fac Appt:** Assoc Clin Prof Med, Harvard Med Sch

Bhasin, Shalender MD [EDM] - **Spec Exp:** Reproductive Endocrinology; Sexual Dysfunction; **Hospital:** Boston Med Ctr; **Address:** Boston Med Ctr, Div Endocrinology, 670 Albany St, Boston, MA 02118; **Phone:** 617-414-2950; **Board Cert:** Internal Medicine 1981; Endocrinology, Diabetes & Metabolism 2008; **Med School:** India 1976; **Resid:** Internal Medicine, Northwestern Univ Med Ctr 1981; **Fellow:** Endocrinology, Diabetes & Metabolism, Harbor-UCLA Med Ctr 1984; **Fac Appt:** Prof Med, Boston Univ

Biller, Beverly M K MD [EDM] - **Spec Exp:** Pituitary Disorders; Cushing's Syndrome; Acromegaly; **Hospital:** Mass Genl Hosp; **Address:** Neuroendocrine Clinic Center, Zero Emerson Pl, Ste 112, Boston, MA 02114-3117; **Phone:** 617-726-3870; **Board Cert:** Internal Medicine 1986; Endocrinology 1989; **Med School:** Univ Okla Coll Med 1983; **Resid:** Internal Medicine, Beth Israel Deaconness Hosp 1986; **Fellow:** Endocrinology, Diabetes & Metabolism, Mass Genl Hosp 1989; **Fac Appt:** Assoc Prof Med, Harvard Med Sch

Braverman, Lewis E MD [EDM] - **Spec Exp:** Thyroid Disorders; **Hospital:** Boston Med Ctr, Caritas St Elizabeth's Med Ctr-Boston; **Address:** Boston Med Ctr, Dept Endocrinology, Diabetes & Nutrition, 732 Harrison Ave Fl 2, Boston, MA 02118-2309; **Phone:** 617-638-7470; **Board Cert:** Internal Medicine 1963; Nuclear Medicine 1972; **Med School:** Johns Hopkins Univ 1955; **Resid:** Internal Medicine, Boston City Hosp 1960; **Fellow:** Endocrinology, Thorndike Meml Lab-Harvard 1962; **Fac Appt:** Prof Med, Boston Univ

Comi, Richard J MD [EDM] - **Spec Exp:** Diabetes; Hypoglycemia; Thyroid Disorders; Pituitary Disorders; **Hospital:** Dartmouth - Hitchcock Med Ctr; **Address:** Dartmouth-Hitchcock Med Ctr, Dept Endocrinology, 1 Med Ctr Drive, Lebanon, NH 03756; **Phone:** 603-650-8630; **Board Cert:** Internal Medicine 1983; Endocrinology 1987; **Med School:** Harvard Med Sch 1980; **Resid:** Internal Medicine, Mass Genl Hosp 1983; **Fellow:** Endocrinology & Diabetes, Natl Inst Hlth 1986

Cushing, Gary W MD [EDM] - **Spec Exp:** Thyroid Disorders; **Hospital:** Lahey Clin; **Address:** Lahey Clin, 4 West Endocrinology, 41 Mall Rd, Burlington, MA 01805; **Phone:** 781-744-2088; **Board Cert:** Internal Medicine 1983; Endocrinology 1985; **Med School:** Univ Mass Sch Med 1980; **Resid:** Internal Medicine, St Vincent Hosp 1983; **Fellow:** Endocrinology, Beth Israel Hosp 1985; **Fac Appt:** Assoc Clin Prof Med, Tufts Univ

Daniels, Gilbert H MD [EDM] - **Spec Exp:** Thyroid Disorders; Parathyroid Disease; Adrenal Disorders; Thyroid Cancer; **Hospital:** Mass Genl Hosp; **Address:** 15 Parkman St WACC Bldg - Ste 730, Boston, MA 02114; **Phone:** 617-726-8430; **Board Cert:** Internal Medicine 1972; Endocrinology, Diabetes & Metabolism 1975; **Med School:** Harvard Med Sch 1966; **Resid:** Internal Medicine, Mass Genl Hosp 1972; **Fellow:** Biochemistry, Natl Inst Hlth 1970; Endocrinology, Diabetes & Metabolism, UCSF Med Ctr 1971; **Fac Appt:** Prof Med, Harvard Med Sch

Holick, Michael F MD/PhD [EDM] - **Spec Exp:** Bone Disorders-Metabolic; Osteoporosis; Calcium Disorders; Nutrition; **Hospital:** Boston Med Ctr; **Address:** Boston Univ Sch Med, 732 Harrison Ave Fl 2, Boston, MA 02118; **Phone:** 617-638-7470; **Board Cert:** Internal Medicine 1979; **Med School:** Univ Wisc 1976; **Resid:** Internal Medicine, Mass Genl Hosp 1979; **Fellow:** Endocrinology, Mass Genl Hosp 1980; **Fac Appt:** Prof Med, Boston Univ

Inzucchi, Silvio E MD [EDM] - **Spec Exp:** Diabetes; Pituitary Disorders; Growth Hormone Disorder-Adult; Cholesterol/Lipid Disorders; **Hospital:** Yale-New Haven Hosp, Yale Med Group; **Address:** Yale Univ Sch Med, Sect. Endocrinology, 789 Howard Ave Fl 2, New Haven, CT 06519; **Phone:** 203-737-1932; **Board Cert:** Internal Medicine 1988; Endocrinology, Diabetes & Metabolism 2006; **Med School:** Harvard Med Sch 1985; **Resid:** Internal Medicine, Yale-New Haven Hosp 1988; **Fellow:** Endocrinology, Diabetes & Metabolism, Yale-New Haven Hosp 1994; **Fac Appt:** Prof Med, Yale Univ

Kahn, Barbara B MD [EDM] - **Spec Exp:** Obesity; Nutrition; **Hospital:** Beth Israel Deaconess Med Ctr - Boston; **Address:** Beth Israel Deaconess Medical Ctr, 330 Brookline Ave, rm E/CLS747, Boston, MA 02215; **Phone:** 617-735-3324; **Board Cert:** Internal Medicine 1980; Endocrinology, Diabetes & Metabolism 1985; **Med School:** Stanford Univ 1977; **Resid:** Internal Medicine, UC Davis Med Ctr 1980; **Fellow:** Endocrinology, Diabetes & Metabolism, Natl Inst Hlth 1982; **Fac Appt:** Prof Med, Harvard Med Sch

Klibanski, Anne MD [EDM] - **Spec Exp:** Pituitary Disorders; Prolactin Disorders; Acromegaly; **Hospital:** Mass Genl Hosp; **Address:** Neuroendocrine Clin Ctr, Zero Emerson Pl Fl 1 - Ste 112, Boston, MA 02114; **Phone:** 617-726-7948; **Board Cert:** Internal Medicine 1978; Endocrinology, Diabetes & Metabolism 1981; **Med School:** NYU Sch Med 1975; **Resid:** Internal Medicine, Bellevue Hosp Ctr 1978; **Fellow:** Endocrinology, Mass Genl Hosp 1981; **Fac Appt:** Prof Med, Harvard Med Sch

Kronenberg, Henry M MD [EDM] - **Spec Exp:** Bone Disorders-Metabolic; Parathyroid Disease; **Hospital:** Mass Genl Hosp; **Address:** Endocrine Associates, 15 Parkman Street, Wang AC 730A, Boston, MA 02114; **Phone:** 617-726-8720; **Board Cert:** Internal Medicine 1973; Endocrinology, Diabetes & Metabolism 1975; **Med School:** Columbia P&S 1970; **Resid:** Internal Medicine, Mass Genl Hosp 1972; **Fellow:** Endocrinology, Mass Genl Hosp 1975; **Fac Appt:** Prof Med, Harvard Med Sch

Larsen, Philip Reed MD [EDM] - **Spec Exp:** Thyroid Disorders; **Hospital:** Brigham and Women's Hosp (page 57); **Address:** 221 Longwood Ave Fl 2, Boston, MA 02115; **Phone:** 617-732-5666; **Board Cert:** Internal Medicine 1970; **Med School:** Columbia P&S 1963; **Resid:** Internal Medicine, NY Presby-Columbia Med Ctr 1965; Internal Medicine, Cincinnati General Hosp 1967; **Fellow:** Endocrinology, NIH 1968; Endocrinology, Cincinnati General Hosp 1969; **Fac Appt:** Prof Med, Harvard Med Sch

Endocrinology, Diabetes & Metabolism

LeBoff, Meryl S MD [EDM] - **Spec Exp:** Osteoporosis; Bone Disorders-Metabolic; **Hospital:** Brigham and Women's Hosp (page 57); **Address:** 221 Longwood Ave Fl 2, Boston, MA 02115; **Phone:** 617-732-5666; **Board Cert:** Internal Medicine 1979; Endocrinology, Diabetes & Metabolism 1981; **Med School:** UMDNJ-NJ Med Sch, Newark 1975; **Resid:** Internal Medicine, USC Med Ctr 1979; **Fellow:** Endocrinology, Brigham & Womens Hosp 1982; **Fac Appt:** Assoc Prof Med, Harvard Med Sch

Lechan, Ronald M MD/PhD [EDM] - **Spec Exp:** Pituitary Disorders; Hypothalamic Dysfunction; Endocrine Cancers; Adrenal Disorders; **Hospital:** Tufts Med Ctr; **Address:** Tufts Med Ctr, 800 Washington St, Box 268, Boston, MA 02111; **Phone:** 617-636-5689; **Board Cert:** Internal Medicine 1979; Endocrinology, Diabetes & Metabolism 1981; **Med School:** Univ VT Coll Med 1976; **Resid:** Internal Medicine, Beth Israel Hosp 1978; **Fellow:** Endocrinology, Diabetes & Metabolism, Tufts-New England Med Ctr 1981; **Fac Appt:** Prof Med, Tufts Univ

Levine, Robert A MD [EDM] - **Spec Exp:** Thyroid Cancer; Thyroid Disorders; Thyroid Ultrasound; **Hospital:** St. Joseph Hosp & Trauma Ctr; **Address:** Thyroid Center of New Hampshire, 5 Coliseum Ave, Ste 209, Nashua, NH 03063; **Phone:** 603-881-7141; **Board Cert:** Internal Medicine 1984; Endocrinology, Diabetes & Metabolism 1987; **Med School:** Univ Conn 1981; **Resid:** Internal Medicine, Mt Auburn Hosp 1984; **Fellow:** Endocrinology, Yale Univ 1987

Nathan, David Matthew MD [EDM] - **Spec Exp:** Diabetes; **Hospital:** Mass Genl Hosp; **Address:** Diabetes Unit, 50 Staniford St, Box 340, Boston, MA 02114; **Phone:** 617-726-8722; **Board Cert:** Internal Medicine 1978; Endocrinology, Diabetes & Metabolism 1981; **Med School:** Mount Sinai Sch Med 1975; **Resid:** Internal Medicine, Brigham & Women's Hosp 1978; **Fellow:** Endocrinology, Diabetes & Metabolism, Mass Genl Hosp 1980; **Fac Appt:** Prof Med, Harvard Med Sch

Pearce, Elizabeth N MD [EDM] - **Spec Exp:** Thyroid Disorders; **Hospital:** Boston Med Ctr; **Address:** Boston Med Ctr, 88 E Newton St, Evans 201, Boston, MA 02118; **Phone:** 617-414-1348; **Board Cert:** Endocrinology, Diabetes & Metabolism 2002; **Med School:** Harvard Med Sch 1997; **Resid:** Internal Medicine, Beth Israel Deaconess Med Ctr 2000; **Fellow:** Endocrinology, Diabetes & Metabolism, Boston Med Ctr 2003; **Fac Appt:** Assoc Prof Med, Boston Univ

Ross, Douglas S MD [EDM] - **Spec Exp:** Thyroid Disorders; Thyroid Cancer; **Hospital:** Mass Genl Hosp; **Address:** Mass General Thyroid Assocs, Thyroid Unit ACC-730, 55 Fruit St, Boston, MA 02114; **Phone:** 617-726-3872 x2; **Board Cert:** Internal Medicine 1980; Endocrinology, Diabetes & Metabolism 1983; **Med School:** Harvard Med Sch 1977; **Resid:** Internal Medicine, Mass General Hosp 1980; **Fellow:** Endocrinology, Mass General Hosp 1983; **Fac Appt:** Assoc Prof Med, Harvard Med Sch

Seely, Ellen Wells MD [EDM] - **Spec Exp:** Pregnancy & Endocrine Disorders; Diabetes in Pregnancy; Diabetes in Women; Thyroid Disorders in Pregnancy; **Hospital:** Brigham and Women's Hosp (page 57); **Address:** Brigham & Womens Hosp, Endocrine Div, 221 Longwood Ave Fl 2, Boston, MA 02115; **Phone:** 617-732-5661; **Board Cert:** Internal Medicine 1984; Endocrinology, Diabetes & Metabolism 1987; **Med School:** Columbia P&S 1981; **Resid:** Internal Medicine, Brigham & Womens Hosp 1984; **Fellow:** Endocrinology, Diabetes & Metabolism, Brigham & Womens Hosp 1987; **Fac Appt:** Prof Med, Harvard Med Sch

Mid Atlantic

Ball, Douglas W MD [EDM] - **Spec Exp:** Thyroid Cancer; **Hospital:** Johns Hopkins Hosp (page 61); **Address:** Sidney Kimmel Cancer Ctr, 1830 E Monument St, Ste 333, Baltimore, MD 21287; **Phone:** 410-502-4926; **Board Cert:** Internal Medicine 1987; **Med School:** Geo Wash Univ 1984; **Resid:** Internal Medicine, Univ Pittsburgh 1987; **Fellow:** Endocrinology, Diabetes & Metabolism, Johns Hopkins Hosp 1991; **Fac Appt:** Assoc Prof Med, Johns Hopkins Univ

Bergman, Donald MD [EDM] - **Spec Exp:** Osteoporosis; Thyroid Disorders; Calcium Disorders; Paget's Disease of Bone; **Hospital:** Mount Sinai Med Ctr (page 63); **Address:** 1199 Park Ave, Ste 1F, New York, NY 10128; **Phone:** 212-876-7333; **Board Cert:** Internal Medicine 1975; Endocrinology, Diabetes & Metabolism 1977; **Med School:** Jefferson Med Coll 1971; **Resid:** Obstetrics & Gynecology, Mt Sinai Hosp 1972; Internal Medicine, Mt Sinai Hosp 1975; **Fellow:** Endocrinology, Diabetes & Metabolism, Mt Sinai Hosp 1977; **Fac Appt:** Clin Prof Med, Mount Sinai Sch Med

Bilezikian, John P MD [EDM] - **Spec Exp:** Osteoporosis; Bone Disorders-Metabolic; Parathyroid Disease; **Hospital:** NY-Presby/Columbia Univ Med Ctr, NY (page 65); **Address:** Columbia Metabolic Bone Disease Program, Harkness Pavilion, 180 Ft Washington Ave Fl 9 - Ste 904, New York, NY 10032; **Phone:** 212-305-2663; **Board Cert:** Internal Medicine 1975; Endocrinology, Diabetes & Metabolism 1977; **Med School:** Columbia P&S 1969; **Resid:** Internal Medicine, Columbia-Presby Hosp 1975; **Fellow:** Endocrinology, Diabetes & Metabolism, Natl Inst Health 1977; **Fac Appt:** Prof Med, Columbia P&S

Blum, Conrad B MD [EDM] - **Spec Exp:** Cholesterol/Lipid Disorders; Thyroid Disorders; Diabetes; **Hospital:** NY-Presby/Columbia Univ Med Ctr, NY (page 65); **Address:** 16 E 60th St, Ste 320, New York, NY 10022-1002; **Phone:** 212-326-8421; **Board Cert:** Internal Medicine 1976; Endocrinology, Diabetes & Metabolism 1977; **Med School:** Northwestern Univ 1971; **Resid:** Internal Medicine, Brigham Women & Chldn's Hosp 1976; **Fellow:** Endocrinology, Diabetes & Metabolism, Northwestern Univ Med Sch 1977; **Fac Appt:** Clin Prof Med, Columbia P&S

Bockman, Richard MD/PhD [EDM] - **Spec Exp:** Bone Disorders-Metabolic; Osteoporosis; Parathyroid Disease; Paget's Disease of Bone; **Hospital:** Hosp For Special Surgery (page 60), NY-Presby/Weill Cornell Med Ctr, NY (page 65); **Address:** 519 E 72nd St, Ste 206, New York, NY 10021; **Phone:** 212-606-1458; **Board Cert:** Internal Medicine 1975; **Med School:** Yale Univ 1968; **Resid:** Internal Medicine, NYU Med Ctr 1975; **Fellow:** Internal Medicine, NY-Cornell Med Ctr 1973; **Fac Appt:** Prof Med, Cornell Univ-Weill Med Coll

Brillon, David MD [EDM] - **Spec Exp:** Diabetes; Thyroid Disorders; **Hospital:** NY-Presby/Weill Cornell Med Ctr, NY (page 65); **Address:** NY Presby-Cornell, Div Endocrinology, 525 E 68th St, Box 136, New York, NY 10065; **Phone:** 212-746-6290; **Board Cert:** Internal Medicine 1983; Endocrinology, Diabetes & Metabolism 1987; **Med School:** Brown Univ 1980; **Resid:** Internal Medicine, Rochester Genl Hosp 1983; **Fellow:** Endocrinology, Rochester Genl Hosp 1986; Endocrinology, Diabetes & Metabolism, UCSD Med Ctr 1988; **Fac Appt:** Assoc Clin Prof Med, Cornell Univ-Weill Med Coll

Burman, Kenneth D MD [EDM] - **Spec Exp:** Thyroid Disorders; Thyroid Cancer; **Hospital:** Washington Hosp Ctr; **Address:** Wash Hosp Ctr, Endocrinology Section, 110 Irving St NW, rm 2A72, Washington, DC 20010; **Phone:** 202-877-6563; **Board Cert:** Internal Medicine 1973; Endocrinology, Diabetes & Metabolism 1975; **Med School:** Univ MO-Columbia Sch Med 1970; **Resid:** Internal Medicine, Barnes Hosp 1972; **Fellow:** Endocrinology, Diabetes & Metabolism, Walter Reed Hosp 1974; **Fac Appt:** Prof Med, Georgetown Univ

Calvi, Laura MD [EDM] - **Spec Exp:** Neuroendocrinology; Pituitary Disorders; **Hospital:** Univ of Rochester Strong Meml Hosp; **Address:** 601 Elmwood Ave, Box 693, Rochester, NY 14642; **Phone:** 585-273-2343; **Board Cert:** Endocrinology, Diabetes & Metabolism 2010; **Med School:** Harvard Med Sch 1995; **Resid:** Internal Medicine, Mass Genl Hosp 1998; **Fellow:** Endocrinology, Mass Genl Hosp 2000; **Fac Appt:** Assoc Prof Med, Univ Rochester

Endocrinology, Diabetes & Metabolism

Cooper, David S MD [EDM] - **Spec Exp:** Thyroid Disorders; **Hospital:** Johns Hopkins Hosp (page 61); **Address:** Div Endocrinology & Metabolism, 1830 E Monument St, Ste 333, Baltimore, MD 21287; **Phone:** 410-502-4926; **Board Cert:** Internal Medicine 1987; Endocrinology, Diabetes & Metabolism 2008; **Med School:** Tufts Univ 1973; **Resid:** Internal Medicine, Barnes Hosp 1976; **Fellow:** Endocrinology, Mass Genl Hosp 1978; **Fac Appt:** Prof Med, Johns Hopkins Univ

Davies, Terry MD [EDM] - **Spec Exp:** Thyroid Disorders in Pregnancy; Graves' Disease; Hashimoto's Disease; Thyroid Cancer; **Hospital:** Mount Sinai Med Ctr (page 63), VA NY Harbor Hlthcare Sys-Manhattan Campus; **Address:** 5 E 98th St, Box 1055, New York, NY 10029-6500; **Phone:** 212-241-7975; **Med School:** England, UK 1971; **Resid:** Internal Medicine, Univ Newcastle 1975; **Fellow:** Endocrinology, Diabetes & Metabolism, Univ Newcastle 1977; Endocrinology, Diabetes & Metabolism, Natl Inst Hlth 1979; **Fac Appt:** Prof Med, Mount Sinai Sch Med

Dobs, Adrian S MD [EDM] - **Spec Exp:** Hormonal Disorders; Hypogonadism-Male; Metabolic Disorders; Complementary Medicine; **Hospital:** Johns Hopkins Hosp (page 61); **Address:** Johns Hopkins Hosp, Div Endocrinology, 1830 E Monument St, Ste 333, Baltimore, MD 21287; **Phone:** 410-502-4926; **Board Cert:** Internal Medicine 1981; Endocrinology 1987; **Med School:** Albany Med Coll 1978; **Resid:** Internal Medicine, Montefiore Hosp 1982; **Fellow:** Endocrinology, Johns Hopkins Hosp 1984; **Fac Appt:** Prof Med, Johns Hopkins Univ

Donner, Thomas W MD [EDM] - **Spec Exp:** Diabetes; **Hospital:** Johns Hopkins Hosp (page 61); **Address:** Johns Hopkins Hosp, Div Endocrinology, 1830 E Monument St, Ste 333, Baltimore, MD 21287; **Phone:** 410-502-4926; **Board Cert:** Internal Medicine 1989; Endocrinology, Diabetes & Metabolism 2007; **Med School:** Univ VA Sch Med 1986; **Resid:** Internal Medicine, Univ Maryland 1989; **Fellow:** Endocrinology, Diabetes & Metabolism, Univ Maryland 1991; **Fac Appt:** Assoc Prof Med, Univ MD Sch Med

Felig, Philip MD [EDM] - **Spec Exp:** Diabetes; Thyroid Disorders; Osteoporosis; **Hospital:** Lenox Hill Hosp, Beth Israel Med Ctr - Petrie Division (page 55); **Address:** 1056 5th Ave, New York, NY 10028-0112; **Phone:** 212-534-5900; **Board Cert:** Internal Medicine 1968; **Med School:** Yale Univ 1961; **Resid:** Internal Medicine, Yale-New Haven Hosp 1967; **Fellow:** Endocrinology, Diabetes & Metabolism, Peter Bent Brigham Hosp 1969

Garibaldi, Luigi MD [EDM] - **Spec Exp:** Pubertal Disorders; Growth Disorders; **Hospital:** Chldns Hosp of Pittsburgh - UPMC; **Address:** Div of Endocrinology, 4401 Penn Ave, Faculty Pavilion Fl 8, Pittsburgh, PA 15224; **Phone:** 412-692-5170; **Board Cert:** Pediatrics 1986; Pediatric Endocrinology 1986; **Med School:** Italy 1973; **Resid:** Pediatrics, Gaslini Inst-Chldn's Hosp 1978; Pediatrics, Univ Michigan Affil Hosp 1985; **Fellow:** Pediatric Endocrinology, Temple Univ Hosp 1981; Pediatric Endocrinology, Univ Chicago Med Ctr 1986; **Fac Appt:** Prof Ped, Univ Pittsburgh

Greene, Loren Wissner MD [EDM] - **Spec Exp:** Thyroid Disorders; Osteoporosis; Pituitary Disorders; Diabetes; **Hospital:** NYU Langone Med Ctr (page 66), NY Downtown Hosp; **Address:** 650 First Ave Fl 7, New York, NY 10016-6402; **Phone:** 212-263-7449; **Board Cert:** Internal Medicine 1978; Endocrinology, Diabetes & Metabolism 1981; **Med School:** NYU Sch Med 1975; **Resid:** Internal Medicine, Bellevue Hosp Ctr-NYU 1978; **Fellow:** Endocrinology, Bellevue Hosp Ctr-NYU 1980; **Fac Appt:** Assoc Clin Prof Med, NYU Sch Med

Greenspan, Susan L MD [EDM] - **Spec Exp:** Osteoporosis; **Hospital:** UPMC Presby, Pittsburgh; **Address:** Univ Pittsburgh, Osteoporosis Ctr, 3471 Fifth Ave, Kaufmann Bldg - Ste 1110, Pittsburgh, PA 15213; **Phone:** 412-692-2472; **Board Cert:** Internal Medicine 1982; Endocrinology, Diabetes & Metabolism 1987; **Med School:** Harvard Med Sch 1979; **Resid:** Internal Medicine, Beth Israel Hosp 1982; **Fellow:** Endocrinology, Mass Genl Hosp 1985; Geriatric Medicine, Beth Israel Hosp 1986; **Fac Appt:** Prof Med, Univ Pittsburgh

Jacobs, Thomas MD [EDM] - **Spec Exp:** Adrenal Disorders; Pituitary Disorders; Calcium Disorders; Thyroid Disorders; **Hospital:** NY-Presby/Columbia Univ Med Ctr, NY (page 65); **Address:** 161 Fort Washington Ave, rm 210, New York, NY 10032-3713; **Phone:** 212-305-5578; **Board Cert:** Internal Medicine 1973; Endocrinology, Diabetes & Metabolism 1975; **Med School:** Johns Hopkins Univ 1968; **Resid:** Internal Medicine, Columbia Presby Hosp 1973; **Fellow:** Endocrinology, Diabetes & Metabolism, Univ Wash Med Ctr 1975; **Fac Appt:** Clin Prof Med, Columbia P&S

Kleinberg, David L MD [EDM] - **Spec Exp:** Neuroendocrinology; Pituitary Disorders; **Hospital:** NYU Langone Med Ctr (page 66); **Address:** 530 1st Ave, Ste 4C, New York, NY 10016; **Phone:** 212-263-6772; **Board Cert:** Internal Medicine 1972; Endocrinology 1975; **Med School:** Univ Miami Sch Med 1966; **Resid:** Internal Medicine, Maimonides Med Ctr 1968; Internal Medicine, Columbia-Presby Med Ctr 1971; **Fellow:** Endocrinology, Diabetes & Metabolism, Columbia-Presby Med Ctr 1970; **Fac Appt:** Prof Med, NYU Sch Med

Korytkowski, Mary T MD [EDM] - **Spec Exp:** Diabetes; Polycystic Ovarian Syndrome; Thyroid Disorders; Diabetic Vascular Disease; **Hospital:** UPMC Presby, Pittsburgh, VA Pittsburgh Hlth Care Sys-Univ Dr; **Address:** Center for Diabetes & Endocrinology, 3601 Fifth Ave, Ste 3B, Pittsburgh, PA 15213-3403; **Phone:** 412-586-9714; **Board Cert:** Internal Medicine 1985; Endocrinology 1989; **Med School:** Univ NC Sch Med 1982; **Resid:** Internal Medicine, Francis Scott Key Med Ctr 1985; **Fellow:** Endocrinology, Diabetes & Metabolism, Sinai Hosp/Johns Hopkins Hosp 1988; **Fac Appt:** Prof Med, Univ Pittsburgh

Ladenson, Paul W MD [EDM] - **Spec Exp:** Thyroid Disorders; Thyroid Cancer; **Hospital:** Johns Hopkins Hosp (page 61); **Address:** Johns Hopkins Hosp, Div Endocrinology & Metabolism, 1830 E Monument St, rm 333, Baltimore, MD 21287; **Phone:** 410-955-3663; **Board Cert:** Internal Medicine 1978; Endocrinology, Diabetes & Metabolism 1981; **Med School:** Harvard Med Sch 1975; **Resid:** Internal Medicine, Mass Genl Hosp 1978; **Fellow:** Endocrinology, Diabetes & Metabolism, Mass Genl Hosp 1980; **Fac Appt:** Prof Med, Johns Hopkins Univ

Lipson, Ace MD [EDM] - **Spec Exp:** Diabetes; **Hospital:** G Washington Univ Hosp; **Address:** 1120 19th St NW, Ste 200, Washington, DC 20036; **Phone:** 202-296-3443; **Board Cert:** Internal Medicine 1976; Endocrinology, Diabetes & Metabolism 1979; **Med School:** Washington Univ, St Louis 1973; **Resid:** Internal Medicine, George Washington Univ Med Ctr 1976; **Fellow:** Endocrinology, Johns Hopkins Hosp 1978; **Fac Appt:** Clin Prof Med, Geo Wash Univ

Mandel, Susan J MD [EDM] - **Spec Exp:** Thyroid Disorders; Endocrine Cancers; **Hospital:** Hosp Univ Penn - UPHS (page 68); **Address:** Div Endocrinology, Perelman Ctr for Advanced Medicine, 3400 Civic Ctr Blvd Fl 4 -West, Philadelphia, PA 19104; **Phone:** 215-662-2300; **Board Cert:** Internal Medicine 1989; Endocrinology 2001; **Med School:** Columbia P&S 1986; **Resid:** Internal Medicine, Columbia Presby Med Ctr 1989; **Fellow:** Endocrinology, Brigham & Womens Hosp 1992; **Fac Appt:** Prof Med, Univ Pennsylvania

McConnell, Robert John MD [EDM] - **Spec Exp:** Thyroid Disorders; Thyroid Ultrasound; **Hospital:** NY-Presby/Columbia Univ Med Ctr, NY (page 65); **Address:** 161 Fort Washington Ave, Ste 210, New York, NY 10032-3713; **Phone:** 212-305-5579; **Board Cert:** Internal Medicine 1978; Endocrinology, Diabetes & Metabolism 1981; **Med School:** Columbia P&S 1973; **Resid:** Internal Medicine, Barnes Hosp 1975; **Fellow:** Endocrinology, Diabetes & Metabolism, Columbia-Presby Hosp 1978; **Fac Appt:** Prof Med, Columbia P&S

Roberts, Michelle M MD [EDM] - **Spec Exp:** Osteoporosis; Diabetes; **Hospital:** UPMC Presby, Pittsburgh; **Address:** UPMC Presby, 3601 Fifth Ave, Ste 3B, Pittsburgh, PA 15213; **Phone:** 412-586-9714; **Board Cert:** Internal Medicine 1986; Endocrinology, Diabetes & Metabolism 1989; **Med School:** Duke Univ 1983; **Resid:** Internal Medicine, Univ Pittsburgh Med Ctr 1986; **Fellow:** Endocrinology, Diabetes & Metabolism, Univ Pittsburgh Med Ctr 1989; **Fac Appt:** Assoc Clin Prof Med, Univ Pittsburgh

Endocrinology, Diabetes & Metabolism

Rodbard, Helena W MD [EDM] - **Spec Exp:** Diabetes; Gynecomastia; **Hospital:** Shady Grove Adven Hosp, Suburban Hosp; **Address:** 3200 Tower Oaks Blvd, Ste 250, Rockville, MD 20852; **Phone:** 301-770-7373; **Board Cert:** Internal Medicine 1981; Endocrinology, Diabetes & Metabolism 1983; **Med School:** Brazil 1972; **Resid:** Internal Medicine, Washington Hosp 1981; **Fellow:** Endocrinology, Diabetes & Metabolism, Natl Inst Hlth 1979; Endocrinology, Diabetes & Metabolism, Geo Wash Univ 1982

Schutta, Mark H MD [EDM] - **Spec Exp:** Diabetes; Preventive Medicine; **Hospital:** Hosp Univ Penn - UPHS (page 68); **Address:** Penn Rodebaugh Diabetes Ctr, Perelman Ctr for Advanced Medicine, 3400 Civic Center Blvd, Ste 4-900, Philadelphia, PA 19104; **Phone:** 215-662-2300; **Board Cert:** Endocrinology, Diabetes & Metabolism 2002; **Med School:** Jefferson Med Coll 1993; **Resid:** Internal Medicine, T Jefferson Univ Hosp 1996; **Fellow:** Endocrinology, Hosp Univ Penn 1999; **Fac Appt:** Assoc Prof Med, Univ Pennsylvania

Schwartz, Stanley S MD [EDM] - **Spec Exp:** Diabetes; Metabolic Syndrome; Thyroid Disorders; **Hospital:** Lankenau Hosp, Bryn Mawr Hosp; **Address:** 233 E Lancaster Ave, Ste 305, Ardmore, PA 19003-2321; **Phone:** 610-642-6800; **Board Cert:** Internal Medicine 1976; Endocrinology, Diabetes & Metabolism 1979; **Med School:** Univ Chicago-Pritzker Sch Med 1973; **Resid:** Internal Medicine, Hosp Univ Penn 1976; **Fellow:** Endocrinology, Diabetes & Metabolism, Univ Chicago Hosps 1978; **Fac Appt:** Prof Emeritus Med, Univ Pennsylvania

Seplowitz, Alan H MD [EDM] - **Spec Exp:** Thyroid Disorders; Cholesterol/Lipid Disorders; Diabetes; **Hospital:** NY-Presby/Columbia Univ Med Ctr, NY (page 65); **Address:** 161 Fort Washington Ave, Ste 4-422, New York, NY 10032-3729; **Phone:** 212-305-5503; **Board Cert:** Internal Medicine 1975; Endocrinology 1977; **Med School:** Columbia P&S 1972; **Resid:** Internal Medicine, Columbia-Presby Med Ctr 1974; **Fellow:** Endocrinology, Diabetes & Metabolism, Columbia-Presby Med Ctr 1978; **Fac Appt:** Assoc Clin Prof Med, Columbia P&S

Shuldiner, Alan R MD [EDM] - **Spec Exp:** Diabetes; Eating Disorders/Obesity; **Hospital:** Univ of MD Med Ctr; **Address:** Univ MD Sch Med, Div Endocrinology, 660 W Redwood St, rm HH-494, Baltimore, MD 21201; **Phone:** 410-706-1623; **Board Cert:** Internal Medicine 1988; Endocrinology 1989; **Med School:** Harvard Med Sch 1984; **Resid:** Internal Medicine, Columbia-Presby Hosp 1986; **Fellow:** Endocrinology, Diabetes & Metabolism, Natl Inst Hlth 1990; **Fac Appt:** Prof Med, Univ MD Sch Med

Siris, Ethel MD [EDM] - **Spec Exp:** Osteoporosis; Paget's Disease of Bone; Bone Disorders-Metabolic; **Hospital:** NY-Presby/Columbia Univ Med Ctr, NY (page 65); **Address:** 180 Ft Washington Ave, Harkness Bldg - Ste 904, New York, NY 10032-3710; **Phone:** 212-305-9531; **Board Cert:** Internal Medicine 1974; Endocrinology, Diabetes & Metabolism 1977; **Med School:** Columbia P&S 1971; **Resid:** Internal Medicine, Columbia-Presby Med Ctr 1974; **Fellow:** Research, Natl Inst Hlth 1976; Endocrinology, Diabetes & Metabolism, Columbia-Presby Med Ctr 1977; **Fac Appt:** Prof Med, Columbia P&S

Snyder, Peter J MD [EDM] - **Spec Exp:** Pituitary Tumors; Reproductive Endocrinology-Male; **Hospital:** Hosp Univ Penn - UPHS (page 68); **Address:** Hosp Univ Pennsylvania, 3400 Civic Ctr Blvd, West Pavilion, Fl 4, Perelman Ctr, Philadelphia, PA 19104; **Phone:** 215-662-2300; **Board Cert:** Internal Medicine 1972; Endocrinology, Diabetes & Metabolism 1972; **Med School:** Harvard Med Sch 1965; **Resid:** Internal Medicine, Beth Israel Hosp 1967; Internal Medicine, Beth Israel Hosp 1970; **Fellow:** Endocrinology, Diabetes & Metabolism, Hosp Univ Penn 1971; **Fac Appt:** Prof Med, Univ Pennsylvania

Surks, Martin MD [EDM] - **Spec Exp:** Thyroid Disorders; **Hospital:** Montefiore Med Ctr - Div. Moses, N Central Bronx Hosp; **Address:** 3400 Bainbridge Ave Fl 2, Bronx, NY 10467; **Phone:** 866-633-8255; **Board Cert:** Internal Medicine 1967; Endocrinology, Diabetes & Metabolism 1977; **Med School:** NYU Sch Med 1960; **Resid:** Internal Medicine, Montefiore Hosp Med Ctr 1962; Internal Medicine, VA Hosp 1964; **Fellow:** Research, Natl Inst Arthritis-Metabolic Disease 1964; **Fac Appt:** Prof Med, Albert Einstein Coll Med

Tuttle, R Michael MD [EDM] - **Spec Exp:** Thyroid Cancer; **Hospital:** Meml Sloan-Kettering Cancer Ctr; **Address:** 1275 York Avenue, New York, NY 10065; **Phone:** 800-525-2225; **Board Cert:** Endocrinology, Diabetes & Metabolism 2004; **Med School:** Univ Louisville Sch Med 1987; **Resid:** Internal Medicine, DD Eisenhower Army Med Ctr 1990; **Fellow:** Endocrinology, Diabetes & Metabolism, Madigan Army Med Ctr 1993; **Fac Appt:** Assoc Prof Med, Cornell Univ-Weill Med Coll

Wartofsky, Leonard MD [EDM] - **Spec Exp:** Thyroid Cancer; Thyroid Disorders; **Hospital:** Washington Hosp Ctr; **Address:** 110 Irving St NW, Ste 2A62, Washington, DC 20010-2975; **Phone:** 202-877-3109; **Board Cert:** Internal Medicine 1971; Endocrinology, Diabetes & Metabolism 1972; **Med School:** Geo Wash Univ 1964; **Resid:** Internal Medicine, Barnes Jewish Hosp 1966; Internal Medicine, Montefiore Med Ctr 1967; **Fellow:** Endocrinology, Diabetes & Metabolism, Boston City Hosp 1969; **Fac Appt:** Prof Med, Georgetown Univ

Xing, Michael M MD/PhD [EDM] - **Spec Exp:** Thyroid Disorders; Thyroid Cancer; **Hospital:** Johns Hopkins Hosp (page 61); **Address:** The Johns Hopkins Hospital, Div Endocrinology & Metabolism, 1830 E Monument St, Ste 333, Baltimore, MD 21287; **Phone:** 410-502-4926; **Board Cert:** Internal Medicine 2000; Endocrinology, Diabetes & Metabolism 2003; **Med School:** China 1984; **Resid:** Internal Medicine, Greater Baltimore Med Ctr 2000; **Fellow:** Endocrinology, Johns Hopkins Hosp 2003; **Fac Appt:** Assoc Prof Med, Johns Hopkins Univ

Young, Iven MD [EDM] - **Spec Exp:** Thyroid Disorders; Osteoporosis; Pituitary Disorders; **Hospital:** NYU Langone Med Ctr (page 66); **Address:** 275 7th Ave Fl 2, New York, NY 10011; **Phone:** 212-675-9332; **Board Cert:** Internal Medicine 1966; Endocrinology, Diabetes & Metabolism 1973; **Med School:** NYU Sch Med 1959; **Resid:** Internal Medicine, VA Med Ctr 1963; **Fellow:** Endocrinology, NYU Med Ctr 1966; **Fac Appt:** Assoc Clin Prof Med, NYU Sch Med

Southeast

Ain, Kenneth B MD [EDM] - **Spec Exp:** Thyroid Cancer; Thyroid Disorders; **Hospital:** Univ of Kentucky Albert B. Chandler Hosp, Lexington VA Med Ctr-Leestown Div; **Address:** Thyroid Oncology Program, rm MN524, 800 Rose St, Lexington, KY 40536-0298; **Phone:** 859-323-3778; **Board Cert:** Internal Medicine 1984; Endocrinology, Diabetes & Metabolism 1987; **Med School:** Brown Univ 1981; **Resid:** Internal Medicine, Hahnemann Univ Hosp 1984; **Fellow:** Endocrinology, Univ Chicago 1986; Thyroid Oncology, NIDDK, Natl Inst Hlth 1990; **Fac Appt:** Prof Med, Univ KY Coll Med

Barrett, Eugene J MD [EDM] - **Spec Exp:** Diabetes; Cholesterol/Lipid Disorders; **Hospital:** Univ of Virginia Health Sys; **Address:** Univ Virginia, Dept Endocrinology, Box 800412, Charlottesville, VA 22903; **Phone:** 434-924-1825; **Board Cert:** Internal Medicine 1978; **Med School:** Univ Rochester 1975; **Resid:** Internal Medicine, Strong Meml Hosp 1977; **Fellow:** Endocrinology, Diabetes & Metabolism, New Haven Hosp 1980; **Fac Appt:** Prof Med, Univ VA Sch Med

Endocrinology, Diabetes & Metabolism

Bell, David S H MD [EDM] - **Spec Exp:** Diabetes; Thyroid Disorders; Cholesterol/Lipid Disorders; Adrenal Disorders; **Hospital:** Univ of Ala Hosp at Birmingham; **Address:** Southside Endocrinology, 1020 26th St S, rm 204, Birmingham, AL 35205; **Phone:** 205-933-2667; **Board Cert:** Internal Medicine 1987; Endocrinology, Diabetes & Metabolism 1981; **Med School:** Ireland 1970; **Resid:** Internal Medicine, Royal Victoria Hosp 1973; Endocrinology, Diabetes & Metabolism, Univ Saskatchewan Hosp 1975; **Fellow:** Endocrinology, Diabetes & Metabolism, Greater Baltimore Med Ctr 1976

Buse, John B MD/PhD [EDM] - **Spec Exp:** Diabetes; **Hospital:** NC Memorial Hosp - UNC; **Address:** Univ NC School of Medicine, CB# 7172, 8027 Burnett Womack Bldg, Chapel Hill, NC 27514; **Phone:** 919-843-3289; **Board Cert:** Internal Medicine 1989; Endocrinology, Diabetes & Metabolism 2000; **Med School:** Duke Univ 1986; **Resid:** Internal Medicine, Univ Chicago Hosps 1988; **Fellow:** Endocrinology, Diabetes & Metabolism, Univ Chicago Hosps 1991; **Fac Appt:** Prof Med, Univ NC Sch Med

Clore, John MD [EDM] - **Spec Exp:** Diabetes; Hypoglycemia; **Hospital:** Med Coll of VA Hosp; **Address:** PO Box 980155, Richmond, VA 23298; **Phone:** 804-828-2161; **Board Cert:** Internal Medicine 1985; Endocrinology, Diabetes & Metabolism 1989; **Med School:** Med Coll VA 1982; **Resid:** Internal Medicine, Med Coll Virginia 1985; **Fellow:** Endocrinology, Diabetes & Metabolism, Med Coll Virginia 1988; **Fac Appt:** Assoc Prof Med, Va Commonwealth Univ Sch Med

Dalkin, Alan C MD [EDM] - **Spec Exp:** Bone Disorders-Metabolic; Osteoporosis; **Hospital:** Univ of Virginia Health Sys; **Address:** Univ VA Hlth Sys, Div Endocrinology & Metabolism, PO Box 801406, Charlottesville, VA 22908; **Phone:** 434-243-2603; **Board Cert:** Internal Medicine 1987; Endocrinology 1989; **Med School:** Univ Mich Med Sch 1984; **Resid:** Internal Medicine, Univ Chicago Hosps 1987; **Fellow:** Endocrinology, Diabetes & Metabolism, Univ Mich Med Ctr 1990; **Fac Appt:** Assoc Prof Med, Univ VA Sch Med

Earp III, H Shelton MD [EDM] - **Spec Exp:** Cancer-Hormonal Influences; **Hospital:** NC Memorial Hosp - UNC; **Address:** UNC Lineberger Comprehensive Cancer Center, 450 West Drive, Fl 1 - rm 10-012, Chapel Hill, NC 27599; **Phone:** 919-966-3036; **Board Cert:** Internal Medicine 1976; Endocrinology, Diabetes & Metabolism 1977; **Med School:** Univ NC Sch Med 1970; **Resid:** Internal Medicine, NC Memorial Hosp 1975; **Fellow:** Endocrinology, Diabetes & Metabolism, Univ North Carolina Hosp 1977; **Fac Appt:** Prof Pharm, Univ NC Sch Med

Feinglos, Mark MD [EDM] - **Spec Exp:** Diabetes; Thyroid Disorders; **Hospital:** Duke Univ Hosp; **Address:** Duke Univ Med Ctr, Box 3921, Durham, NC 27710-0001; **Phone:** 919-684-4005; **Board Cert:** Internal Medicine 1976; Endocrinology, Diabetes & Metabolism 1977; **Med School:** McGill Univ 1973; **Resid:** Internal Medicine, Duke Univ Med Ctr 1975; **Fellow:** Endocrinology, Diabetes & Metabolism, Duke Univ Med Ctr 1977; **Fac Appt:** Prof Med, Duke Univ

Goodman, Neil F MD [EDM] - **Spec Exp:** Reproductive Endrocrinology; Polycystic Ovarian Syndrome; Hormonal Disorders; Infertility; **Hospital:** Baptist Hosp of Miami, South Miami Hosp; **Address:** 9150 SW 87th Ave, Ste 210, Miami, FL 33176-2313; **Phone:** 305-595-6855; **Board Cert:** Internal Medicine 1973; Endocrinology, Diabetes & Metabolism 1975; **Med School:** Columbia P&S 1970; **Resid:** Internal Medicine, Beth Israel Hosp 1972; **Fellow:** Endocrinology, Mass Genl Hosp 1974; **Fac Appt:** Clin Prof Med, Univ Miami Sch Med

Koch, Christian A MD [EDM] - **Spec Exp:** Endocrine Cancers; Thyroid Cancer; Growth Hormone Disorder-Adult; Pituitary Disorders; **Hospital:** Univ Mississippi Med Ctr; **Address:** 2500 N State St, Dept Endocrinlogy, Jackson, MS 39216; **Phone:** 601-984-5525; **Board Cert:** Endocrinology, Diabetes & Metabolism 2000; **Med School:** Germany 1991; **Resid:** Internal Medicine, Ohio State Univ Hosp 1997; **Fellow:** Endocrinology, Natl Inst Hlth 2001; **Fac Appt:** Prof Med, Univ Miss

Marshall, John C MD/PhD [EDM] - **Spec Exp:** Pituitary Disorders; Neuroendocrinology; Polycystic Ovarian Syndrome; **Hospital:** Univ of Virginia Health Sys; **Address:** Univ VA Hlth System, Hospital Dr, Box 800612, Charlottesville, VA 22908-0001; **Phone:** 434-924-2431; **Board Cert:** Internal Medicine 1978; Endocrinology, Diabetes & Metabolism 1981; **Med School:** England, UK 1965; **Resid:** Neurology, Natl Hosp Queen Square 1968; Cardiovascular Disease, Natl Heart Hosp 1969; **Fellow:** Endocrinology, Diabetes & Metabolism, Hammersmith Hosp 1972; Endocrinology, Diabetes & Metabolism, UCLA 1974; **Fac Appt:** Prof Med, Univ VA Sch Med

Nestler, John E MD [EDM] - **Spec Exp:** Polycystic Ovarian Syndrome; Diabetes; **Hospital:** Med Coll of VA Hosp; **Address:** Med Coll Va, Div Endocrinology, Box 980009, Richmond, VA 23298-0111; **Phone:** 804-828-2161; **Board Cert:** Internal Medicine 1982; Endocrinology 1985; **Med School:** Univ Pennsylvania 1979; **Resid:** Internal Medicine, Med Coll Virginia 1983; **Fellow:** Endocrinology, Hosp Univ Penn 1985; **Fac Appt:** Prof Med, Med Coll VA

Ober, K Patrick MD [EDM] - **Spec Exp:** Diabetes; **Hospital:** Wake Forest Univ Baptist Med Ctr; **Address:** Wake Forest Univ School of Med, Div of Endocrinology, Medical Center Blvd, Winston-Salem, NC 27157; **Phone:** 336-713-7251; **Board Cert:** Internal Medicine 1977; Endocrinology, Diabetes & Metabolism 1979; **Med School:** Univ Fla Coll Med 1974; **Resid:** Internal Medicine, N Carolina Baptist Hosp 1976; **Fellow:** Endocrinology & Metabolism, N Carolina Baptist Hosp 1978; **Fac Appt:** Prof Med, Wake Forest Univ

Ovalle, Fernando MD [EDM] - **Spec Exp:** Diabetes; Diabetes in Women; Metabolic Syndrome; **Hospital:** Univ of Ala Hosp at Birmingham; **Address:** UAB Endocrinology, 1530 3rd Ave S, FOT 702, Birmingham, AL 35294; **Phone:** 205-934-4112; **Med School:** Mexico 1989; **Resid:** Internal Medicine, Henry Ford Hosp 1995; **Fellow:** Endocrinology, Diabetes & Metabolism, Wash Univ 1997; **Fac Appt:** Assoc Prof Med, Univ Alabama

Powers, Alvin C MD [EDM] - **Spec Exp:** Diabetes; Thyroid Disorders; **Hospital:** Vanderbilt Univ Med Ctr (page 76); **Address:** Vanderbilt Diabetes Ctr, 802 Light Hall, Nashville, TN 37232-0202; **Phone:** 615-343-8332; **Board Cert:** Internal Medicine 1982; Endocrinology, Diabetes & Metabolism 1985; **Med School:** Univ Tenn Coll Med 1979; **Resid:** Internal Medicine, Duke Univ Med Ctr 1982; **Fellow:** Endocrinology, Diabetes & Metabolism, Joslin Diabetes Ctr 1983; Endocrinology, Diabetes & Metabolism, Mass Genl Hosp 1985; **Fac Appt:** Prof Med, Vanderbilt Univ

Quinn, Suzanne L MD [EDM] - **Spec Exp:** Diabetes; **Hospital:** Shands at Univ of FL, Malcolm Randall VA Med Ctr; **Address:** Shands Univ Florida, Dept Endocrinology, 2000 SW Archer Rd, Gainesville, FL 32610; **Phone:** 352-265-8230; **Board Cert:** Internal Medicine 1988; Endocrinology, Diabetes & Metabolism 2003; **Med School:** Univ Fla Coll Med 1985; **Resid:** Internal Medicine, Shands at Univ Fla 1988; **Fellow:** Endocrinology, Diabetes & Metabolism, Univ Fla 1992; **Fac Appt:** Assoc Prof Med, Univ Fla Coll Med

Skyler, Jay S MD [EDM] - **Spec Exp:** Diabetes; **Hospital:** Univ of Miami Hosp (page 72), Jackson Meml Hosp (page 70); **Address:** Diabetes Research Inst, 1450 NW 10th Ave, Ste 3054, Miami, FL 33136; **Phone:** 305-243-6146; **Board Cert:** Internal Medicine 1972; Endocrinology, Diabetes & Metabolism 1973; **Med School:** Jefferson Med Coll 1969; **Resid:** Internal Medicine, Duke Univ Med Ctr 1971; **Fellow:** Endocrinology, Diabetes & Metabolism, Duke Univ Med Ctr 1973; **Fac Appt:** Prof Med, Univ Miami Sch Med

Vance, Mary Lee MD [EDM] - **Spec Exp:** Pituitary Disorders; Adrenal Disorders; **Hospital:** Univ of Virginia Health Sys; **Address:** Univ Virginia Hlth Sys, PO Box 800601, Charlottesville, VA 22908-0601; **Phone:** 434-243-2603; **Board Cert:** Internal Medicine 1980; **Med School:** Louisiana State U, New Orleans 1977; **Resid:** Internal Medicine, Baylor Univ Med Ctr 1980; **Fellow:** Endocrinology, Univ Virginia Med Ctr 1983; **Fac Appt:** Prof Med, Univ VA Sch Med

Endocrinology, Diabetes & Metabolism

Weissman, Peter N MD [EDM] - **Spec Exp:** Diabetes; **Hospital:** Baptist Hosp of Miami; **Address:** 7867 N Kendall Drive, Ste 80, Miami, FL 33156; **Phone:** 305-595-0777; **Board Cert:** Internal Medicine 1972; Endocrinology, Diabetes & Metabolism 1972; **Med School:** NYU Sch Med 1966; **Resid:** Internal Medicine, Barnes Hosp/Wash Univ 1968; **Fellow:** Geriatric Medicine, Gerontology Rsch Ctr 1970; Endocrinology, Diabetes & Metabolism, Univ Mich Hosp 1972; **Fac Appt:** Assoc Clin Prof Med, Univ Miami Sch Med

Midwest

Bahn, Rebecca S MD [EDM] - **Spec Exp:** Graves' Disease; Graves' Disease-Eye; **Hospital:** Mayo Med Ctr & Clin - Rochester; **Address:** Mayo Clin, Div Endocrinology, 200 First St SW, Rochester, MN 55905; **Phone:** 507-284-1600; **Board Cert:** Internal Medicine 1985; Endocrinology, Diabetes & Metabolism 1987; **Med School:** Mayo Med Sch 1981; **Resid:** Internal Medicine, Mayo Clin 1984; **Fellow:** Endocrinology, Diabetes & Metabolism, Mayo Clin 1986; **Fac Appt:** Prof Med, Mayo Med Sch

Brennan, Michael D MD [EDM] - **Spec Exp:** Thyroid Disorders; Diabetes; **Hospital:** Mayo Med Ctr & Clin - Rochester; **Address:** Mayo Clin, Div Endocrinology, 200 First St SW, Rochester, MN 55905; **Phone:** 507-284-1600; **Board Cert:** Internal Medicine 1975; Endocrinology, Diabetes & Metabolism 1977; **Med School:** Ireland 1969; **Resid:** Internal Medicine, Henry Ford Hosp 1972; Internal Medicine, Mayo Clinic 1975; **Fellow:** Endocrinology, Diabetes & Metabolism, Mayo Clinic 1977; **Fac Appt:** Assoc Prof Med, Mayo Med Sch

Broadstone, Vasti Lima MD [EDM] - **Spec Exp:** Diabetes; Weight Management; **Hospital:** Floyd Meml Hosp & Hlth Svcs; **Address:** Floyd Memorial Hosp Weight Mngmt Ctr, 1850 State St, New Albany, IN 47150; **Phone:** 812-949-7151; **Board Cert:** Internal Medicine 1987; Endocrinology, Diabetes & Metabolism 2002; **Med School:** Brazil 1976; **Resid:** Internal Medicine, Wright State Univ Affil Hosps 1981; **Fellow:** Endocrinology, Diabetes & Metabolism, Univ Louisville Affil Hosps 1984

Burmeister, Lynn MD [EDM] - **Spec Exp:** Thyroid Disorders; Hashimoto's Disease; Graves' Disease; **Address:** Univ Minn Medical Ctr, Fairview, 516 Delaware St SE, Clinic 6A, Minneapolis, MN 55455; **Phone:** 612-626-1960; **Board Cert:** Internal Medicine 1988; Endocrinology 2001; **Med School:** Univ Minn 1985; **Resid:** Internal Medicine, Univ Minnesota Med Ctr 1988; **Fellow:** Endocrinology, Univ Minnesota Med Ctr 1989; **Fac Appt:** Assoc Prof Med, Univ Minn

Clutter, William E MD [EDM] - **Spec Exp:** Endocrine Cancers; Calcium Disorders; Bone Disorders-Metabolic; **Hospital:** Barnes-Jewish Hosp, Washington Univ Physicians; **Address:** Washington Univ, Div Endo, Metabolism & Lipid Rsch, 660 S Euclid Ave, Campus Box 8121, St Louis, MO 63110; **Phone:** 314-362-3500; **Board Cert:** Internal Medicine 1978; Endocrinology, Diabetes & Metabolism 1981; **Med School:** Ohio State Univ 1975; **Resid:** Internal Medicine, Barnes Jewish Hosp 1978; **Fellow:** Endocrinology, Diabetes & Metabolism, Barnes Jewish Hosp 1980; **Fac Appt:** Assoc Prof Med, Washington Univ, St Louis

Cohen, Robert M MD [EDM] - **Spec Exp:** Diabetes; Metabolic Disorders; **Hospital:** Univ Hosp - Cincinnati; **Address:** Univ Cincinnati Physicians, 222 Piedmont Ave, Ste 6000, Cincinnati, OH 45219; **Phone:** 513-475-8200; **Board Cert:** Internal Medicine 1981; Endocrinology, Diabetes & Metabolism 1983; **Med School:** Univ Rochester 1978; **Resid:** Internal Medicine, Rush-Presby-St Lukes Hosp 1981; **Fellow:** Endocrinology, Univ Chicago 1984; **Fac Appt:** Assoc Prof Med, Univ Cincinnati

Cryer, Philip E MD [EDM] - **Spec Exp:** Diabetes; Hypoglycemia; Insulinoma; **Hospital:** Barnes-Jewish Hosp, St. Louis Chldns Hosp; **Address:** Wash Univ Sch Med, Div Endo, Metab & Lipid Rsch, 660 S Euclid Ave, Box 8127, St Louis, MO 63110-1093; **Phone:** 314-362-3500; **Board Cert:** Internal Medicine 1972; Endocrinology, Diabetes & Metabolism 1972; **Med School:** Northwestern Univ 1965; **Resid:** Internal Medicine, Barnes Jewish Hosp 1972; **Fellow:** Endocrinology, Diabetes & Metabolism, Barnes Hosp-Wash Univ 1968; **Fac Appt:** Prof Med, Washington Univ, St Louis

D'Alessio, David A MD [EDM] - **Spec Exp:** Diabetes; **Hospital:** Univ Hosp - Cincinnati; **Address:** Univ Cincinnati Physicians, 222 Piedmont Ave, Ste 6000, Cincinnati, OH 45219; **Phone:** 513-475-8200; **Board Cert:** Internal Medicine 1986; Endocrinology, Diabetes & Metabolism 1989; **Med School:** Univ Wisc 1983; **Resid:** Internal Medicine, Temple Univ Med Ctr 1986; **Fellow:** Endocrinology, Univ Washington 1990; **Fac Appt:** Prof Med, Univ Cincinnati

Econs, Michael J MD [EDM] - **Spec Exp:** Osteoporosis; Paget's Disease of Bone; Bone Disorders-Metabolic; Parathyroid Disease; **Hospital:** IU Health University Hosp; **Address:** 541 N Clinical Drive, rm 459, Indianapolis, IN 46202; **Phone:** 317-274-1339; **Board Cert:** Internal Medicine 1986; Endocrinology, Diabetes & Metabolism 1989; **Med School:** UCSF 1983; **Resid:** Internal Medicine, Univ Maryland Hosp 1986; **Fellow:** Endocrinology, Duke Univ Med Ctr 1989; **Fac Appt:** Prof Med, Indiana Univ

Ehrmann, David A MD [EDM] - **Spec Exp:** Polycystic Ovarian Syndrome; Diabetes; **Hospital:** Univ of Chicago Med Ctr; **Address:** Div Endocrinology, 5758 S Maryland Ave, Module 5A Fl 5, MC 9015, Chicago, IL 60637; **Phone:** 773-702-6138; **Board Cert:** Internal Medicine 1985; Endocrinology, Diabetes & Metabolism 1987; **Med School:** Univ Mich Med Sch 1982; **Resid:** Internal Medicine, Univ Mich Med Ctr 1985; **Fellow:** Endocrinology, Diabetes & Metabolism, Univ Chicago Hosps 1987; **Fac Appt:** Assoc Prof Med, Univ Chicago-Pritzker Sch Med

Emanuele, Mary Ann MD [EDM] - **Spec Exp:** Diabetes; **Hospital:** Loyola Univ Med Ctr; **Address:** Loyola Univ Med Ctr, Dept Endocrinology, 2160 S 1st Ave Fl 54 - rm 137, Maywood, IL 60153-3304; **Phone:** 708-216-0160; **Board Cert:** Internal Medicine 1978; Endocrinology, Diabetes & Metabolism 1983; **Med School:** Loyola Univ-Stritch Sch Med 1975; **Resid:** Internal Medicine, Univ Hawaii Med Ctr 1978; **Fellow:** Endocrinology, Edward Hines Jr VA Hosp 1980; **Fac Appt:** Prof Med, Loyola Univ-Stritch Sch Med

Emanuele, Nicholas V MD [EDM] - **Hospital:** Edward Hines, Jr. VA Hosp; **Address:** Hines VA Hosp Bldg 200 Fl 4, 5000 S 5th Ave, Hines, IL 60141; **Phone:** 708-202-8387; **Board Cert:** Internal Medicine 1975; Endocrinology 1979; **Med School:** Northwestern Univ 1967; **Resid:** Internal Medicine, Hines VA Hosp 1974; **Fellow:** Endocrinology, Northwestern Univ Affil Hosp 1976

Hammer, Gary D MD [EDM] - **Spec Exp:** Adrenal Cancer; Adrenal Disorders; **Hospital:** Univ of Michigan Hosp; **Address:** Univ Michigan-Biomed Science Rsch Bldg, 109 Zina Pitcher Place, rm 1502, Ann Arbor, MI 48109-2200; **Phone:** 734-647-8906; **Board Cert:** Endocrinology, Diabetes & Metabolism 2007; **Med School:** Tufts Univ 1992; **Resid:** Internal Medicine, UCSF Med Ctr 1994; **Fellow:** Endocrinology, UCSF 1997; **Fac Appt:** Assoc Prof Med, Univ Mich Med Sch

Herman, William H MD [EDM] - **Spec Exp:** Diabetes; Diabetes in Pregnancy; **Hospital:** Univ of Michigan Hosp; **Address:** 4260 Plymouth Rd, Ann Arbor, MI 48109; **Phone:** 734-764-6831; **Board Cert:** Internal Medicine 1982; Endocrinology, Diabetes & Metabolism 1989; **Med School:** Boston Univ 1979; **Resid:** Internal Medicine, Univ Mich Med Ctr 1982; Preventive Medicine, Ctrs Dis Control 1985; **Fellow:** Endocrinology, Diabetes & Metabolism, Univ Mich Med Ctr 1988; **Fac Appt:** Prof Med, Univ Mich Med Sch

Jensen, Michael D MD [EDM] - **Spec Exp:** Eating Disorders/Obesity; Nutrition; **Hospital:** Mayo Med Ctr & Clin - Rochester; **Address:** Mayo Clin, Div Endocrinology, 200 First St SW, Rochester, MN 55905; **Phone:** 507-284-1600; **Board Cert:** Internal Medicine 1982; Endocrinology, Diabetes & Metabolism 1985; **Med School:** Univ MO-Kansas City 1979; **Resid:** Internal Medicine, Mayo Clin 1982; **Fellow:** Endocrinology, Diabetes & Metabolism, Mayo Clin 1985; **Fac Appt:** Prof Med, Mayo Med Sch

Kennedy, Laurence MD [EDM] - **Spec Exp:** Diabetes; Adrenal Disorders; Cholesterol/Lipid Disorders; **Hospital:** Cleveland Clin (page 56), Cleveland Clin - Weston; **Address:** Cleveland Clinic Main Campus, 9500 Euclid Ave, MC F20, Cleveland, OH 44195; **Phone:** 216-445-8645; **Med School:** Northern Ireland 1972; **Resid:** Internal Medicine, Queens Univ Affil Hosp 1975; **Fellow:** Endocrinology, Queens Univ Affil Hosp 1978; Endocrinology, Univ Florida 1980

Khosla, Sundeep MD [EDM] - **Spec Exp:** Osteoporosis; Bone Disorders-Metabolic; **Hospital:** Mayo Med Ctr & Clin - Rochester; **Address:** Mayo Clin, Div Endocrinology, 200 First St SW, Rochester, MN 55905; **Phone:** 507-284-1600; **Board Cert:** Internal Medicine 1985; Endocrinology 1987; **Med School:** Harvard Med Sch 1982; **Resid:** Internal Medicine, Mass Genl Hosp 1985; **Fellow:** Endocrinology, Diabetes & Metabolism, Mass Genl Hosp 1988; **Fac Appt:** Asst Prof Med, Mayo Med Sch

Kloos, Richard MD [EDM] - **Spec Exp:** Thyroid Cancer; **Hospital:** Ohio St Univ Med Ctr; **Address:** 1581 Dodd Drive, 4 Fl McCampbell Hall, Columbus, OH 43210; **Phone:** 614-292-3800; **Board Cert:** Internal Medicine 2002; Endocrinology, Diabetes & Metabolism 2005; Nuclear Medicine 2005; **Med School:** Case West Res Univ 1989; **Resid:** Internal Medicine, Metrohealth MC 1992; **Fellow:** Endocrinology, Diabetes & Metabolism, Univ Michigan 1995; Nuclear Medicine, Univ Michigan 1996; **Fac Appt:** Prof Med, Ohio State Univ

Kopp, Peter A MD [EDM] - **Spec Exp:** Thyroid Cancer; Pituitary Disorders; Parathyroid Disease; McCune-Albright Syndrome; **Hospital:** Northwestern Meml Hosp; **Address:** Northwestern Medical Faculty Foundation, 675 N St Clair St, Ste 14-100, Galter Pavillion, Chicago, IL 60611; **Phone:** 312-695-7970; **Board Cert:** Internal Medicine 2003; Endocrinology, Diabetes & Metabolism 2004; **Med School:** Switzerland 1985; **Resid:** Internal Medicine, Regl Hosp 1992; Internal Medicine, Univ Bern 1992; **Fellow:** Endocrinology, Diabetes & Metabolism, Univ Bern 1992; Endocrinology, Diabetes & Metabolism, Northwestern Univ Hosp 1997; **Fac Appt:** Assoc Prof Med, Northwestern Univ-Feinberg Sch Med

Lash, Robert W MD [EDM] - **Spec Exp:** Osteoporosis; Thyroid Disorders; Diabetes in Pregnancy; Endocrine Disorders in Pregnancy; **Hospital:** Univ of Michigan Hosp; **Address:** Taubman Health Care Center, 1500 E Med Ctr Drive, rm 3920, Ann Arbor, MI 48109-5354; **Phone:** 734-647-5871; **Board Cert:** Internal Medicine 1987; Endocrinology, Diabetes & Metabolism 1989; **Med School:** Albert Einstein Coll Med 1984; **Resid:** Internal Medicine, UCSF Med Ctr 1987; **Fellow:** Endocrinology, Natl Inst Hlth 1990; **Fac Appt:** Clin Prof Med, Univ Mich Med Sch

Licata, Angelo A MD [EDM] - **Spec Exp:** Bone Disorders-Metabolic; Osteoporosis; Calcium Disorders; **Hospital:** Cleveland Clin (page 56); **Address:** Div Endocrinology, 9500 Euclid Ave, Desk F20, Cleveland, OH 44195; **Phone:** 216-444-6248; **Board Cert:** Internal Medicine 1983; **Med School:** Univ Rochester 1973; **Resid:** Internal Medicine, Washington Univ Hosp 1974; Internal Medicine, Georgetown Univ Hosp 1978; **Fellow:** Endocrinology, Diabetes & Metabolism, Natl Inst Hlth 1976; **Fac Appt:** Asst Clin Prof Med, Case West Res Univ

Mazzone, Theodore MD [EDM] - **Spec Exp:** Cholesterol/Lipid Disorders; Diabetes; **Hospital:** Evanston/North Shore Univ Hlth Sys; **Address:** Evanston Specialty Suites, 1000 Central St, Ste 800, Chicago, IL 60201; **Phone:** 847-663-8540; **Board Cert:** Internal Medicine 1980; Endocrinology, Diabetes & Metabolism 1983; **Med School:** Northwestern Univ 1977; **Resid:** Internal Medicine, UCLA Med Ctr 1980; **Fellow:** Endocrinology, Diabetes & Metabolism, Univ Wash Med Ctr 1983; **Fac Appt:** Prof Med, Univ IL Coll Med

McGill, Janet B MD [EDM] - **Spec Exp:** Diabetes; **Hospital:** Barnes-Jewish Hosp; **Address:** 4921 Parkview Pl, CB 8127, Ste 13B, St Louis, MO 63110-1010; **Phone:** 314-747-7300; **Board Cert:** Internal Medicine 1983; Endocrinology, Diabetes & Metabolism 1987; **Med School:** Mich State Univ 1979; **Resid:** Internal Medicine, William Beaumont Hosp 1984; Endocrinology, Diabetes & Metabolism, William Beaumont Hosp 1985; **Fellow:** Diabetes, Washington Univ 1987; **Fac Appt:** Assoc Prof Med, Washington Univ, St Louis

McMahon, Marion Molly MD [EDM] - **Spec Exp:** Nutrition; Diabetes; **Hospital:** Mayo Med Ctr & Clin - Rochester; **Address:** Mayo Clin, Div Endocrinology, 200 First St SW, Rochester, MN 55905; **Phone:** 507-284-1600; **Board Cert:** Internal Medicine 1985; Endocrinology, Diabetes & Metabolism 1987; **Med School:** Univ Wisc 1981; **Resid:** Internal Medicine, Med Coll Wisc 1984; **Fellow:** Endocrinology, Diabetes & Metabolism, Mayo Clin 1987; Nutrition, New Eng Deaconess Hosp 1988

Osei, Kwame MD [EDM] - **Spec Exp:** Diabetes; Nutrition; Diabetes in Minority Populations; **Hospital:** Ohio St Univ Med Ctr; **Address:** OSU Dept Medicine, Div Endocrinology, 491 McCampbell Hall, 1581 Dodd Drive, Columbus, OH 43210; **Phone:** 614-292-3800; **Board Cert:** Internal Medicine 1982; Endocrinology, Diabetes & Metabolism 1985; **Med School:** Ghana 1976; **Resid:** Pathology, Hahnemann Hosp 1979; Internal Medicine, Episcopal Hosp 1982; **Fellow:** Endocrinology, Diabetes & Metabolism, Ohio State Univ 1984; **Fac Appt:** Prof Med, Ohio State Univ

Semenkovich, Clay F MD [EDM] - **Spec Exp:** Cholesterol/Lipid Disorders; Diabetes; Thyroid Disorders; Adrenal Disorders; **Hospital:** Barnes-Jewish Hosp; **Address:** Wash Univ Sch Med, Div Endo, Metab & Lipid Rsch, 660 S Euclid Ave, Box 8127, St Louis, MO 63110; **Phone:** 314-747-7300; **Board Cert:** Internal Medicine 1984; Endocrinology, Diabetes & Metabolism 1987; **Med School:** Washington Univ, St Louis 1981; **Resid:** Internal Medicine, Barnes-Jewish Hosp 1984; **Fellow:** Endocrinology, Diabetes & Metabolism, Wash Univ Hosp 1986; **Fac Appt:** Prof Med, Washington Univ, St Louis

Sowers, James R MD [EDM] - **Spec Exp:** Diabetes; Hypertension; Cholesterol/Lipid Disorders; **Hospital:** Univ of Missouri Hosp; **Address:** UMC, Dept Internal Med, 1 Hosp Drive, rm D109, Columbia, MO 65212; **Phone:** 573-882-2573; **Board Cert:** Internal Medicine 1974; Endocrinology, Diabetes & Metabolism 1977; **Med School:** Univ MO-Columbia Sch Med 1971; **Resid:** Internal Medicine, St Johns Mercy Med Ctr 1974; **Fellow:** Endocrinology, Wadsworth VA Hosp Ctr-UCLA 1976; **Fac Appt:** Prof Med, Univ MO-Columbia Sch Med

Watts, Nelson B MD [EDM] - **Spec Exp:** Osteoporosis; Bone Disorders-Metabolic; Paget's Disease of Bone; **Hospital:** Univ Hosp - Cincinnati; **Address:** Univ Cincinnati Physicians, 222 Piedmont Ave, Ste 6000, Cincinnati, OH 45219; **Phone:** 513-475-8200; **Board Cert:** Internal Medicine 1972; Endocrinology, Diabetes & Metabolism 2010; **Med School:** Univ NC Sch Med 1969; **Resid:** Internal Medicine, Charlotte Meml Hosp 1972; **Fellow:** Endocrinology, Diabetes & Metabolism, NC Meml Hosp 1971; **Fac Appt:** Prof Med, Univ Cincinnati

Endocrinology, Diabetes & Metabolism

Weiss, Roy E MD/PhD [EDM] - **Spec Exp:** Cushing's Syndrome; Pituitary Disorders; Thyroid Disorders; **Hospital:** Univ of Chicago Med Ctr; **Address:** Univ Chicago, Sect Endocrinology, 5758 S Maryland Ave, MC 9015, Chicago, IL 60637; **Phone:** 773-702-2373; **Board Cert:** Internal Medicine 2001; **Med School:** Israel 1985; **Resid:** Internal Medicine, Univ Chicago Hosp 1988; **Fellow:** Endocrinology, Diabetes & Metabolism, Univ Chicago Hosp 1990; **Fac Appt:** Prof Med, Univ Chicago-Pritzker Sch Med

Werner, Phillip L MD [EDM] - **Spec Exp:** Diabetes; **Hospital:** Adv Luth Genl Hosp; **Address:** 1775 Ballard Rd, Nesset Pavilion, Park Ridge, IL 60068; **Phone:** 847-318-2400; **Board Cert:** Internal Medicine 1975; Endocrinology 1977; **Med School:** Univ IL Coll Med 1972; **Resid:** Internal Medicine, Univ Illinois Affl Hosp 1975; **Fellow:** Endocrinology, Diabetes & Metabolism, Univ Wash Med Ctr 1977; **Fac Appt:** Prof Med, Ros Franklin Univ/Chicago Med Sch

Great Plains and Mountains

Eckel, Robert H MD [EDM] - **Spec Exp:** Cholesterol/Lipid Disorders; Eating Disorders/Obesity; Diabetes; **Hospital:** Univ of CO Hosp - Anschutz Inpatient Pav; **Address:** 1635 Aurora Ct, MS F732, Aurora, CO 80045; **Phone:** 720-848-2650; **Board Cert:** Internal Medicine 1976; Endocrinology, Diabetes & Metabolism 2008; **Med School:** Univ Cincinnati 1973; **Resid:** Internal Medicine, Univ Wisconsin Hosps 1976; **Fellow:** Endocrinology, Diabetes & Metabolism, Univ Washington 1979; **Fac Appt:** Prof Med, Univ Colorado

Recker, Robert Roy MD [EDM] - **Spec Exp:** Osteoporosis; Diabetes; Endocrinology; **Hospital:** Creighton Univ Med Ctr, Omaha VA Med Ctr; **Address:** Creighton Univ Osteoporosis, Div Endocrinology, 601 N 30th St, Ste 4820, Omaha, NE 68131; **Phone:** 402-280-4470; **Board Cert:** Internal Medicine 1971; **Med School:** Creighton Univ 1963; **Resid:** Internal Medicine, Creighton Affil Hosps 1969; **Fellow:** Endocrinology, Diabetes & Metabolism, Creighton Univ 1971; **Fac Appt:** Prof Med, Creighton Univ

Ridgway, E Chester MD [EDM] - **Spec Exp:** Thyroid Cancer; Thyroid Disorders; Pituitary Disorders; **Hospital:** Univ of CO Hosp - Anschutz Inpatient Pav; **Address:** UCHSC at Fitzsimons, Div Endocrinology, 1635 Aurora Court, Box 6510, MS F732, Aurora, CO 80045; **Phone:** 720-848-2650; **Board Cert:** Internal Medicine 1972; Endocrinology 1973; **Med School:** Univ Colorado 1968; **Resid:** Internal Medicine, Mass Genl Hosp 1970; **Fellow:** Endocrinology, Mass Genl Hosp 1972; **Fac Appt:** Prof Med, Univ Colorado

Southwest

Cunningham, Glenn R MD [EDM] - **Spec Exp:** Diabetes; Hypogonadism; Erectile Dysfunction; **Hospital:** St. Luke's Episcopal Hosp-Houston; **Address:** 6620 Main St, Ste 1225, Houston, TX 77030; **Phone:** 713-798-2500; **Board Cert:** Internal Medicine 1972; Endocrinology, Diabetes & Metabolism 1972; **Med School:** Univ Okla Coll Med 1966; **Resid:** Internal Medicine, Duke Univ Med Ctr 1970; Internal Medicine, VA Hosp 1971; **Fellow:** Endocrinology, Duke Univ Med Ctr 1970; **Fac Appt:** Prof Med, Baylor Coll Med

Hsueh, Willa A MD [EDM] - **Spec Exp:** Diabetes; Hypertension; **Hospital:** Methodist Hosp - Houston; **Address:** Methodist Hosp Rsch Inst, 6565 Fannin St, F8-060, Houston, TX 77030; **Phone:** 713-441-2520; **Board Cert:** Internal Medicine 1976; Endocrinology, Diabetes & Metabolism 1977; **Med School:** Ohio State Univ 1973; **Resid:** Internal Medicine, Johns Hopkins Hosp 1975; **Fellow:** Endocrinology, Diabetes & Metabolism, Johns Hopkins Hosp 1976; **Fac Appt:** Prof Med, UCLA

Lavis, Victor Ralph MD [EDM] - **Spec Exp:** Diabetes; **Hospital:** UT MD Anderson Cancer Ctr, Meml Hermann Hosp - Texas Med Ctr; **Address:** MD Anderson Cancer Ctr, 1515 Holcombe Blvd, Unit 1461, Houston, TX 77050; **Phone:** 713-792-2841; **Board Cert:** Internal Medicine 1969; Endocrinology, Diabetes & Metabolism 2008; **Med School:** Stanford Univ 1962; **Resid:** Internal Medicine, Boston Cty Hosp 1964; Internal Medicine, UCLA Med Ctr 1967; **Fellow:** Endocrinology, Diabetes & Metabolism, Univ Washington 1970; **Fac Appt:** Prof Med, Univ Tex, Houston

Reasner II, Charles A MD [EDM] - **Spec Exp:** Thyroid Disorders; **Hospital:** Univ Hlth Syst-San Antonio; **Address:** Texas Diabetes Inst, 701 S Zarzamora St, San Antonio, TX 78207; **Phone:** 210-358-7402; **Board Cert:** Internal Medicine 1983; Endocrinology 1985; **Med School:** Loma Linda Univ 1979; **Resid:** Internal Medicine, USAF Med Ctr 1983; **Fellow:** Endocrinology, Diabetes & Metabolism, Wilford Hall Med Ctr 1985; **Fac Appt:** Assoc Prof Med, Univ Tex, San Antonio

Robbins, Richard J MD [EDM] - **Spec Exp:** Thyroid Cancer; Pituitary Tumors; Pituitary Disorders; **Hospital:** Methodist Hosp - Houston; **Address:** The Methodist Hosp, 6550 Fannin St, Ste 1001, Houston, TX 77030; **Phone:** 713-441-6640; **Board Cert:** Internal Medicine 1978; Endocrinology, Diabetes & Metabolism 1983; **Med School:** Creighton Univ 1975; **Resid:** Internal Medicine, New York Hosp 1978; **Fellow:** Endocrinology, New England Med Ctr 1981; **Fac Appt:** Prof Med, Cornell Univ-Weill Med Coll

Rubenfeld, Sheldon MD [EDM] - **Spec Exp:** Thyroid Cancer; Thyroid Disorders; Diabetes; **Hospital:** St. Luke's Episcopal Hosp-Houston, Methodist Hosp - Houston; **Address:** 7515 S Main St, Ste 690, Houston, TX 77030; **Phone:** 713-795-5750; **Board Cert:** Internal Medicine 1976; Endocrinology, Diabetes & Metabolism 1979; **Med School:** Georgetown Univ 1971; **Resid:** Internal Medicine, Boston City Hosp 1972; Internal Medicine, Baylor Affil Hosps 1976; **Fellow:** Endocrinology, Baylor Affil Hosps 1978; **Fac Appt:** Clin Prof Med, Baylor Coll Med

Sherman, Steven I MD [EDM] - **Spec Exp:** Thyroid Cancer; Endocrine Cancers; **Hospital:** UT MD Anderson Cancer Ctr; **Address:** MD Anderson Cancer Ctr, 1515 Holcombe Blvd, Unit 1461, Houston, TX 77030; **Phone:** 713-792-2840; **Board Cert:** Internal Medicine 1988; Endocrinology, Diabetes & Metabolism 2007; **Med School:** Johns Hopkins Univ 1985; **Resid:** Internal Medicine, Johns Hopkins Hosp 1988; **Fellow:** Endocrinology, Diabetes & Metabolism, Johns Hopkins Hosp 1991; **Fac Appt:** Prof Med, Baylor Coll Med

Waguespack, Steven G MD [EDM] - **Spec Exp:** Thyroid Cancer; Pituitary Tumors; Hereditary Cancer; **Hospital:** UT MD Anderson Cancer Ctr; **Address:** MD Anderson Cancer Ctr, Dept Endocrine Neoplasia/Hormonal Disorders, 1515 Holcombe Blvd, Houston, TX 77030; **Phone:** 713-563-4400; **Board Cert:** Endocrinology, Diabetes & Metabolism 2002; Pediatric Endocrinology 2003; **Med School:** Univ Tex, Houston 1994; **Resid:** Internal Medicine & Pediatrics, Indiana Univ Hosps 1998; **Fellow:** Endocrinology, Diabetes & Metabolism, Indiana Univ Hosps 2001; Pediatric Endocrinology, Riley Chldns Hosp 2002; **Fac Appt:** Prof Med, Univ Tex, Houston

West Coast and Pacific

Ahmann, Andrew J MD [EDM] - **Spec Exp:** Diabetes; **Hospital:** OR Hlth & Sci Univ; **Address:** OHSU Div Endocrinology, 3181 SW Sam Jackson Park Rd, MC PPV05, Portland, OR 97239; **Phone:** 503-494-3273; **Board Cert:** Internal Medicine 1983; Endocrinology, Diabetes & Metabolism 1987; **Med School:** Univ Colorado 1980; **Resid:** Internal Medicine, Fitzsimons Army Med Ctr 1983; **Fellow:** Endocrinology, Diabetes & Metabolism, Walter Reed Army Med Ctr 1986; **Fac Appt:** Prof Med, Oregon Hlth & Sci Univ

Endocrinology, Diabetes & Metabolism

Berkson, Richard A MD [EDM] - **Spec Exp:** Diabetes; Thyroid Disorders; **Hospital:** St. Mary Med Ctr - Long Beach, Long Beach Meml Med Ctr; **Address:** 1868 Pacific Ave, Long Beach, CA 90806-6113; **Phone:** 562-595-4718; **Board Cert:** Internal Medicine 1975; Endocrinology, Diabetes & Metabolism 1977; **Med School:** SUNY Buffalo 1972; **Resid:** Internal Medicine, SUNY Buffalo Affil Hosp 1975; **Fellow:** Endocrinology, Diabetes & Metabolism, Joslin Clin 1976; Endocrinology, Diabetes & Metabolism, UCLA Med Ctr 1977; **Fac Appt:** Assoc Clin Prof Med, UCLA

Braunstein, Glenn D MD [EDM] - **Spec Exp:** Hormonal Disorders; Thyroid Cancer; Reproductive Endocrinology; Endocrine Cancers; **Hospital:** Cedars-Sinai Med Ctr; **Address:** Cedars Sinai Med Ctr, 8700 Beverly Blvd, Ste 2119, Los Angeles, CA 90048; **Phone:** 310-423-5140; **Board Cert:** Internal Medicine 1973; Endocrinology, Diabetes & Metabolism 1975; **Med School:** UCSF 1968; **Resid:** Internal Medicine, Peter Bent Bringham Hosp 1970; Endocrinology, Diabetes & Metabolism, Natl Inst Hlth-NICHHD 1972; **Fellow:** Endocrinology, Diabetes & Metabolism, LAC Harbor Genl Hosp 1973; **Fac Appt:** Prof Med, UCLA

Edelman, Steven V MD [EDM] - **Spec Exp:** Diabetes; **Hospital:** UCSD Med Ctr; **Address:** Perlman Medical Office, 9350 Campus Point Drive, La Jolla, CA 92037; **Phone:** 858-657-8440; **Board Cert:** Internal Medicine 1986; Endocrinology, Diabetes & Metabolism 2003; **Med School:** UC Davis 1982; **Resid:** Internal Medicine, UCLA-San Fernando 1985; **Fellow:** Diabetes, The Joslin Clinic 1986; Endocrinology, Diabetes & Metabolism, The Lahey Clinic 1987; **Fac Appt:** Prof Med, UCSD

Fitzgerald, Paul A MD [EDM] - **Spec Exp:** Thyroid Disorders; Diabetes; Pheochromocytoma; Pituitary Tumors; **Hospital:** UCSF Med Ctr; **Address:** 350 Parnassus Ave, Ste 710, San Francisco, CA 94117-3685; **Phone:** 415-665-1136; **Board Cert:** Internal Medicine 1975; Endocrinology, Diabetes & Metabolism 1981; **Med School:** Jefferson Med Coll 1972; **Resid:** Internal Medicine, Presby Med Ctr-Univ Colo 1975; **Fellow:** Endocrinology, Diabetes & Metabolism, UCSF Med Ctr 1978; **Fac Appt:** Clin Prof Med, UCSF

Heber, David MD [EDM] - **Spec Exp:** Nutrition & Cancer Prevention; Nutrition & Disease Prevention/Control; Nutrition & Obesity; **Hospital:** UCLA Ronald Reagan Med Ctr; **Address:** 900 Veteran Ave, Rm 12-217, UCLA Center for Human Nutrition, Los Angeles, CA 90095-1742; **Phone:** 310-206-1987; **Board Cert:** Internal Medicine 1976; Endocrinology, Diabetes & Metabolism 1977; **Med School:** Harvard Med Sch 1973; **Resid:** Internal Medicine, LAC Harbor Genl Hosp 1975; **Fellow:** Endocrinology, Diabetes & Metabolism, LAC Harbor Genl Hosp 1978; **Fac Appt:** Prof Med, UCLA

Hirsch, Irl B MD [EDM] - **Spec Exp:** Diabetes; **Hospital:** Univ Wash Med Ctr; **Address:** Univ Wash Med Ctr, Diabetes Care Ctr, 4225 Roosevelt Way NE, Ste 101, Seattle, WA 98105; **Phone:** 206-598-4882; **Board Cert:** Internal Medicine 1987; Endocrinology, Diabetes & Metabolism 1989; **Med School:** Univ MO-Columbia Sch Med 1984; **Resid:** Internal Medicine, Mt Sinai Med Ctr 1987; **Fellow:** Metabolism, Washington Univ Sch Med 1989; **Fac Appt:** Prof Med, Univ Wash

Hoffman, Andrew R MD [EDM] - **Spec Exp:** Pituitary Disorders; Pituitary Tumors; Neuroendocrinology; **Hospital:** Stanford Univ Hosp & Clinics, VA Hlth Care Sys - Palo Alto; **Address:** 300 Pasteur Drive, Div of Endocinology, Stanford, CA 94305-5103; **Phone:** 650-723-6961; **Board Cert:** Internal Medicine 1979; Endocrinology 1981; **Med School:** Stanford Univ 1976; **Resid:** Internal Medicine, Mass Genl Hosp 1978; **Fellow:** Endocrinology, Natl Inst Hlth 1980; Endocrinology, Mass Genl Hosp 1982; **Fac Appt:** Prof Med, Stanford Univ

Ipp, Eli MD [EDM] - **Spec Exp:** Diabetes; **Hospital:** LAC - Harbor - UCLA Med Ctr; **Address:** 21840 S Normandy Ave, Ste 600, Torrance, CA 90502; **Phone:** 310-222-5101; **Board Cert:** Internal Medicine 1979; Endocrinology, Diabetes & Metabolism 1981; **Med School:** South Africa 1968; **Resid:** Internal Medicine, Tel Hashomer Hosp 1974; **Fellow:** Endocrinology, Diabetes & Metabolism, Univ Tex SW Med Ctr 1978; **Fac Appt:** Prof Med, UCLA

Kamdar, Vikram V MD [EDM] - **Spec Exp:** Diabetes; Diabetic Leg/Foot; Thyroid Disorders; **Hospital:** Santa Monica - UCLA Med Ctr & Ortho Hosp, UCLA Ronald Reagan Med Ctr; **Address:** 1245 16th St, Ste 309, Santa Monica, CA 90404; **Phone:** 310-828-7172; **Board Cert:** Internal Medicine 1978; Endocrinology, Diabetes & Metabolism 1979; **Med School:** India 1971; **Resid:** Internal Medicine, Lemuel Shattuck Hosp 1972; Endocrinology, Diabetes & Metabolism, Cedars-Sinai Med Ctr 1977; **Fellow:** Endocrinology, Diabetes & Metabolism, LA Co-USC Med Ctr 1975; **Fac Appt:** Assoc Clin Prof Med, UCLA

Kandeel, Fouad MD/PhD [EDM] - **Spec Exp:** Thyroid Cancer; Endocrine Cancers; Neuroendocrinology; **Hospital:** City of Hope Natl Med Ctr; **Address:** City of Hope, Diabetes Dept, 1500 E Duarte Rd, Duarte, CA 91010; **Phone:** 626-256-4673 x62251; **Med School:** Egypt 1969; **Resid:** Internal Medicine, Birmingham & Midland Hosp for Women; Endocrinology, Diabetes & Metabolism, Queen Elizabeth Hosp; **Fac Appt:** Assoc Clin Prof Med, UCLA

Katznelson, Laurence MD [EDM] - **Spec Exp:** Neuroendocrinology; Pituitary Disorders; Acromegaly; Cushing's Syndrome; **Hospital:** Stanford Univ Hosp & Clinics, Lucile Packard Chldn's Hosp; **Address:** Stanford Comprehensive Cancer Ctr, 875 Blake Wilbur Drive, MC 5826, Stanford, CA 94305; **Phone:** 650-736-2062; **Board Cert:** Internal Medicine 1988; Endocrinology, Diabetes & Metabolism 2001; **Med School:** UCLA 1985; **Resid:** Internal Medicine, Hosp Univ Penn 1988; **Fellow:** Endocrinology, Mass Genl Hosp 1991; **Fac Appt:** Assoc Prof Med, Stanford Univ

Klonoff, David C MD [EDM] - **Spec Exp:** Diabetes; **Hospital:** Peninsula Med Ctr; **Address:** 1720 El Camino Real, Ste 130, Burlingame, CA 94010; **Phone:** 650-697-4345; **Board Cert:** Internal Medicine 1980; Endocrinology, Diabetes & Metabolism 1981; **Med School:** UCSF 1976; **Resid:** Internal Medicine, UCLA Med Ctr 1978; Internal Medicine, UCSF Hosps 1979; **Fellow:** Endocrinology, Diabetes & Metabolism, Metab Rsch Unit-UCSF Med Ctr 1981; **Fac Appt:** Clin Prof Med, UCSF

Melmed, Shlomo MD [EDM] - **Spec Exp:** Pituitary Tumors; Acromegaly; Pituitary Disorders; **Hospital:** Cedars-Sinai Med Ctr; **Address:** Cedars Sinai Med Ctr, 8700 Beverly Blvd, Ste 2015, Los Angeles, CA 90048; **Phone:** 310-423-4691; **Board Cert:** Internal Medicine 1979; Endocrinology, Diabetes & Metabolism 1983; **Med School:** South Africa 1970; **Resid:** Internal Medicine, Sheba Med Ctr 1976; **Fellow:** Endocrinology, Diabetes & Metabolism, Wadsworth VA Hosp 1980; **Fac Appt:** Prof Med, UCLA

Orwoll, Eric S MD [EDM] - **Spec Exp:** Osteoporosis; Osteoporosis in Men; **Hospital:** OR Hlth & Sci Univ; **Address:** OHSU, Bone/Mineral Unit, 3181 SW Sam Jackson Park Rd, MC PPV05, Portland, OR 97239; **Phone:** 503-494-3273; **Board Cert:** Internal Medicine 1977; Endocrinology, Diabetes & Metabolism 1979; **Med School:** Univ MD Sch Med 1974; **Resid:** Internal Medicine, Providence Med Ctr 1977; **Fellow:** Endocrinology, Diabetes & Metabolism, Univ Oregon Hlth Sci Ctr 1979; **Fac Appt:** Prof Med, Oregon Hlth & Sci Univ

Riddle, Matthew C MD [EDM] - **Spec Exp:** Diabetes; Clinical Trials; **Hospital:** OR Hlth & Sci Univ; **Address:** Oregon Hlth & Sci Univ, Div Endo, 3181 SW Sam Jackson Park Rd, MC PPV05, Portland, OR 97239-3011; **Phone:** 503-494-3273; **Board Cert:** Internal Medicine 1972; Endocrinology, Diabetes & Metabolism 1972; **Med School:** Harvard Med Sch 1964; **Resid:** Internal Medicine, Rush-Presby-St Lukes Hosp 1969; **Fellow:** Endocrinology, Diabetes & Metabolism, Rush Presby-St Lukes Hosp 1971; Endocrinology, Diabetes & Metabolism, Univ Washington Med Ctr 1973; **Fac Appt:** Prof Med, Oregon Hlth & Sci Univ

Rushakoff, Robert J MD [EDM] - **Spec Exp:** Diabetes; **Hospital:** UCSF - Mt Zion Med Ctr; **Address:** UCSF-Mt Zion Med Ctr, 1600 Divisadero St, Fl 4, Box 1616, San Francisco, CA 94143-1616; **Phone:** 415-885-3868; **Board Cert:** Internal Medicine 1985; Endocrinology, Diabetes & Metabolism 1989; **Med School:** Med Coll Wisc 1982; **Resid:** Internal Medicine, Mt Zion Hosp Med Ctr 1985; **Fellow:** Endocrinology, Mt Zion Hosp/Cell Biol 1986; Endocrinology, Cedars-Sinai Med Ctr 1987; **Fac Appt:** Prof Med, UCSF

Endocrinology, Diabetes & Metabolism

Singer, Peter A MD [EDM] - **Spec Exp:** Thyroid Disorders; Pituitary Disorders; **Hospital:** Keck Med Ctr of USC (page 75); **Address:** 1520 San Pablo St, Ste 1000, Los Angeles, CA 90033; **Phone:** 323-442-5100; **Board Cert:** Internal Medicine 1972; Endocrinology, Diabetes & Metabolism 1973; **Med School:** UCSF 1965; **Resid:** Internal Medicine, LAC-USC Med Ctr 1971; **Fellow:** Endocrinology, Diabetes & Metabolism, LAC-USC Med Ctr 1973; **Fac Appt:** Clin Prof Med, USC Sch Med

Swerdloff, Ronald S MD [EDM] - **Spec Exp:** Reproductive Endocrinology-Male; Pituitary Disorders; **Hospital:** LAC - Harbor - UCLA Med Ctr; **Address:** 1000 W Carson St, Box 446, Torrance, CA 90509-2910; **Phone:** 310-222-1867; **Board Cert:** Internal Medicine 1968; Endocrinology 1972; **Med School:** UCSF 1962; **Resid:** Internal Medicine, Univ Washington Hosp 1964; Endocrinology, Diabetes & Metabolism, NIH Gerontology Branch 1966; **Fellow:** Endocrinology, Diabetes & Metabolism, Harbor-UCLA Med Ctr 1969; **Fac Appt:** Prof Med, UCLA

Woeber, Kenneth A MD [EDM] - **Spec Exp:** Thyroid Disorders; **Hospital:** UCSF Med Ctr; **Address:** UCSF Division of Endocrinology, Campus Box 1640, San Francisco, CA 94143-1640; **Phone:** 415-885-7574; **Board Cert:** Internal Medicine 1980; Endocrinology, Diabetes & Metabolism 1973; **Med School:** South Africa 1957; **Resid:** Internal Medicine, Johannesburg Hosp 1962; **Fellow:** Endocrinology, Diabetes & Metabolism, Harvard/Boston City Hosp 1964; **Fac Appt:** Prof Med, UCSF

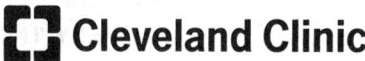

Cleveland Clinic

Every life deserves world class care.

Endocrinology, Diabetes and Metabolism

Cleveland Clinic Endocrinology & Metabolism Institute is committed to providing the highest quality healthcare for patients with endocrine, diabetes or metabolic disorders, or obesity. Our staff includes endocrinologists, endocrine surgeons, bariatric and general surgeons, psychologists, bariatricians and a cardiologist, as well as dietitians, nurse practitioners and clinical nurse specialists. We are ranked No. 5 in the nation by *U.S.News & World Report* — the highest ranking in Ohio.

We Offer Specialized Endocrine Clinics

The Endocrinology & Metabolism Institute has an array of disease-specific clinics, including:

- Thyroid/parathyroid disorders
- Pituitary disorders
- Post-pancreas transplant care
- Liver/adrenal tumor care
- Type 1 and Type 2 diabetes
- Calcium disorders
- Preventive cardiology
- Transition endocrine (pediatrics to adult)

Leading Thyroid Center

Our Thyroid Center is designed so that all specialists work together as a team to accurately and proactively diagnose and treat all forms of thyroid disorders, including thyroid cancer. We have been the leader in incorporating fine needle aspirations and ultrasounds into the realm of endocrinology.

We also offer nationally recognized pituitary care and enhanced diabetes care. Cleveland Clinic is one of the top centers in the U.S. for volume of pituitary surgeries at an institution.

Additionally, we take on all of the clinical challenges that chronic disease management continues to offer as we seek to develop healthier communities.

Cleveland Clinic
Endocrine & Metabolism Institute
9500 Euclid Avenue
Cleveland, OH 44195

clevelandclinic.org/endotopdocs

Offering Same-Day Appointments
Call 800.274.2009.

Treatment Guides

Cleveland Clinic has developed comprehensive treatment guides for many diseases and conditions. To download our free treatment guides, visit clevelandclinic.org/treatmentguides.

Online Medical Second Opinion

Cleveland Clinic's My**Consult** Online Medical Second Opinion program securely connects patients to our physician specialists for more than 1,000 life-changing or life-threatening diagnoses all by the click of a mouse. To learn more, log onto eclevelandclinic.org/myconsult or call 800.223.2273, ext. 43223.

Special Assistance for Out-of-State Patients

Cleveland Clinic Global Patient Services offers a complimentary Medical Concierge service for patients who travel from outside of Ohio. Call 800.223.2273, ext. 55580 or email medicalconcierge@ccf.org.

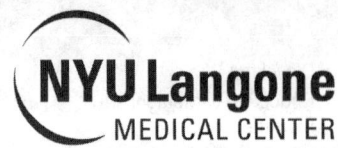

550 First Avenue (*at 31st Street*)
New York, NY 10016
www.NYULMC.org
Physician Referral: **888-7-NYU-MED** (*888-769-8633*)

WOUND CARE

About the Division of Wound Healing and Regenerative Medicine

The Division of Wound Healing and Regenerative Medicine at NYU Langone Medical Center treats chronic, non-healing wounds in a personal and caring environment that involves patients and their families at every step of the way. We are particularly dedicated to the highest standards of wound care and healing for people with diabetes, disabilities and the elderly. The Helen L. and Martin S. Kimmel Wound Healing Center specializes in treating chronic wounds, such as diabetic foot ulcers, pressure ulcers (bed sores), venous ulcers and sickle cell ulcers and is one of the only dedicated inpatient units in the world specifically for chronic wounds. We specialize in the following areas:

Clinical Care

The clinical team at the Division of Wound Healing and Regenerative Medicine—including doctors, nurses, physician assistants and social workers—brings patients the most comprehensive, innovative and compassionate care possible. Utilizing advanced, evidence-based techniques, patients have access to more than 20 types of specialists, including (but not limited to) cardiologists, vascular surgeons, plastic surgeons, orthopaedists, podiatrists and physical therapists.

Research

Researchers at the Division started a human wound cell bank, which resulted in the discovery of one of the first genes that inhibits wound healing in humans. Researchers also discovered that human skin equivalent therapy, thought to act as a skin graft, actually accelerates healing by promoting the controlled release of a series of growth factors from cells. This research has resulted in decreased amputations in persons with diabetic foot ulcers and is the only treatment approved in randomized control trials for venous ulcers.

Wound Electronic Medical Records

NYU Langone Medical Center has designed a Wound Electronic Medical Record (WEMR) system to acquire and display data and provide the decision support necessary to improve the care of patients with chronic wounds. As part of this system, photographs of wounds are taken during each clinical visit to record the progress of healing. Patients are able to view these photographs during visits, as well as a graph of the wound area, to see their improvement over time.

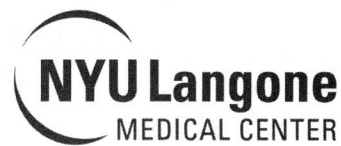

WOUND CARE

About the Division of Wound Healing and Regenerative Medicine

The Division of Wound Healing and Regenerative Medicine at NYU Langone Medical Center treats chronic, non-healing wounds in a personal and caring environment that involves patients and their families at every step of the way. We are particularly dedicated to the highest standards of wound care and healing for people with diabetes, disabilities and the elderly. The Helen L. and Martin S. Kimmel Wound Healing Center specializes in treating chronic wounds, such as diabetic foot ulcers, pressure ulcers (bed sores), venous ulcers and sickle cell ulcers and is one of the only dedicated inpatient units in the world specifically for chronic wounds. We specialize in the following areas:

Clinical Care

The clinical team at the Division of Wound Healing and Regenerative Medicine—including doctors, nurses, physician assistants and social workers—brings patients the most comprehensive, innovative and compassionate care possible. Utilizing advanced, evidence-based techniques, patients have access to more than 20 types of specialists, including (but not limited to) cardiologists, vascular surgeons, plastic surgeons, orthopaedists, podiatrists and physical therapists.

Research

Researchers at the Division started a human wound cell bank, which resulted in the discovery of one of the first genes that inhibits wound healing in humans. Researchers also discovered that human skin equivalent therapy, thought to act as a skin graft, actually accelerates healing by promoting the controlled release of a series of growth factors from cells. This research has resulted in decreased amputations in persons with diabetic foot ulcers and is the only treatment approved in randomized control trials for venous ulcers.

Wound Electronic Medical Records

NYU Langone Medical Center has designed a Wound Electronic Medical Record (WEMR) system to acquire and display data and provide the decision support necessary to improve the care of patients with chronic wounds. As part of this system, photographs of wounds are taken during each clinical visit to record the progress of healing. Patients are able to view these photographs during visits, as well as a graph of the wound area, to see their improvement over time.

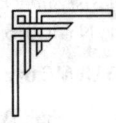

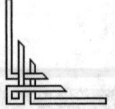

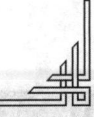

The Best in American Medicine
www.CastleConnolly.com

Gastroenterology
a subspecialty of Internal Medicine

An internist who specializes in diagnosis and treatment of diseases of the digestive organs including the stomach, bowels, liver and gallbladder. This specialist treats conditions such as abdominal pain, ulcers, diarrhea, cancer and jaundice and performs complex diagnostic and therapeutic procedures using endoscopes to see internal organs.

Training Required: Three years in internal medicine *plus* additional training and examination for certification in gastroenterology.

GASTROENTEROLOGY

New England

Aslanian, Harry R MD [Ge] - **Spec Exp:** Endoscopic Ultrasound; Esophageal Cancer; Pancreatic Cancer; Rectal Cancer; **Hospital:** Yale-New Haven Hosp; **Address:** Yale Univ School of Med, Section of Digestive Diseases, 333 Cedar St, Box 208019, New Haven, CT 06520-8019; **Phone:** 203-200-5083; **Board Cert:** Gastroenterology 2002; **Med School:** Brown Univ 1996; **Resid:** Internal Medicine, Mayo Clin 1999; **Fellow:** Gastroenterology, Yale Univ Affil Hosp 2002; Endoscopy, Yale Univ Affil Hosp 2003; **Fac Appt:** Assoc Prof Med, Yale Univ

Butterly, Lynn MD [Ge] - **Spec Exp:** Colonoscopy; Endoscopy; Colon & Rectal Cancer Detection; Colon & Rectal Cancer-Familial Polyposis; **Hospital:** Dartmouth - Hitchcock Med Ctr; **Address:** Dartmouth-Hitchcock Med Ctr, Dept Gastro, 1 Med Ctr Drive, Lebanon, NH 03756; **Phone:** 603-650-5261; **Board Cert:** Internal Medicine 1983; Gastroenterology 1985; **Med School:** Harvard Med Sch 1979; **Resid:** Internal Medicine, Mass Genl Hosp 1983; **Fellow:** Gastroenterology, Mass Genl Hosp 1985; **Fac Appt:** Asst Prof Med, Dartmouth Med Sch

Chung, Daniel C MD [Ge] - **Spec Exp:** Colonoscopy; Colon & Rectal Cancer-Familial Polyposis; Pancreatic Cancer(Familial); Pancreatic Endocrine Tumors; **Hospital:** Mass Genl Hosp; **Address:** Gastroenterology Associates, 55 Fruit St, Blake 4, Boston, MA 02114; **Phone:** 617-726-3544; **Board Cert:** Internal Medicine 2001; Gastroenterology 2003; **Med School:** Harvard Med Sch 1988; **Resid:** Internal Medicine, Mass Genl Hosp 1991; **Fellow:** Gastroenterology, Mass Genl Hosp 1995; **Fac Appt:** Assoc Prof Med, Harvard Med Sch

Chung, Raymond T MD [Ge] - **Spec Exp:** Transplant Medicine-Liver; Liver Disease; Hepatitis C; **Hospital:** Mass Genl Hosp; **Address:** Mass General Hosp, 55 Fruit St Warren Bldg Fl 10, Boston, MA 02114; **Phone:** 617-724-6006; **Board Cert:** Internal Medicine 1989; Gastroenterology 2007; **Med School:** Yale Univ 1986; **Resid:** Internal Medicine, Johns Hopkins Hosp 1989; **Fac Appt:** Assoc Prof Med, Harvard Med Sch

Dienstag, Jules L MD [Ge] - **Spec Exp:** Liver Disease; Hepatitis; Transplant Medicine-Liver; **Hospital:** Mass Genl Hosp; **Address:** Mass Genl Hosp, GI Unit, 55 Fruit St Warren Bldg Fl 10, Boston, MA 02114-2622; **Phone:** 617-726-7450; **Board Cert:** Internal Medicine 1975; **Med School:** Columbia P&S 1972; **Resid:** Internal Medicine, Univ Chicago-Billings Hosp 1974; **Fellow:** Infectious Disease, Natl Inst Hlth 1976; Virology, Mass Genl Hosp 1978; **Fac Appt:** Prof Med, Harvard Med Sch

Farraye, Francis A MD [Ge] - **Spec Exp:** Endoscopy; Inflammatory Bowel Disease; Colon & Rectal Cancer Detection; Diarrheal Diseases; **Hospital:** Boston Med Ctr; **Address:** 85 E Concord St, Ste 7711, Boston, MA 02118; **Phone:** 617-638-6525; **Board Cert:** Gastroenterology 1989; Internal Medicine 1985; **Med School:** Albert Einstein Coll Med 1982; **Resid:** Internal Medicine, Beth Israel Hosp 1985; **Fellow:** Gastroenterology, Beth Israel Hosp 1988

Fisher, Rosemarie Louise MD [Ge] - **Spec Exp:** Nutrition; Nutrition in Bowel Disorders; Inflammatory Bowel Disease/Crohn's; Endoscopy; **Hospital:** Yale-New Haven Hosp, St. Mary's Hosp - Waterbury; **Address:** 40 Temple St, Ste 1A, New Haven, CT 06510; **Phone:** 203-688-1449; **Board Cert:** Internal Medicine 1975; Gastroenterology 1977; **Med School:** Tufts Univ 1971; **Resid:** Internal Medicine, Montefiore Med Ctr 1973; **Fellow:** Gastroenterology, Yale-New Haven Hosp 1975; **Fac Appt:** Prof Med, Yale Univ

Friedman, Lawrence S MD [Ge] - **Spec Exp:** Liver Disease; **Hospital:** Newton - Wellesley Hosp, Mass Genl Hosp; **Address:** Newton-Wellesley Hosp, Dept Medicine, 2014 Washington St, Newton, MA 02462; **Phone:** 617-243-5480; **Board Cert:** Internal Medicine 1981; Gastroenterology 2005; **Med School:** Johns Hopkins Univ 1978; **Resid:** Internal Medicine, Johns Hopkins Hosp 1981; **Fellow:** Gastroenterology, Mass Genl Hosp 1984; **Fac Appt:** Prof Med, Harvard Med Sch

Gordon, Stuart R MD [Ge] - **Spec Exp:** Pancreatic & Biliary Disease; Pancreatic/Biliary Endoscopy (ERCP); Endoscopic Ultrasound; **Hospital:** Dartmouth - Hitchcock Med Ctr; **Address:** Dartmouth-Hitchcock Med Ctr, 1 Med Ctr Drive, Lebanon, NH 03756; **Phone:** 603-650-5261; **Board Cert:** Internal Medicine 2002; Gastroenterology 2005; **Med School:** Columbia P&S 1988; **Resid:** Internal Medicine, Dartmouth-Hitchcock Med Ctr 1991; **Fellow:** Gastroenterology, Dartmouth-Hitchcock Med Ctr 1994; **Fac Appt:** Assoc Prof Med, Dartmouth Med Sch

Kaplan, Lee M MD/PhD [Ge] - **Spec Exp:** Obesity; Weight Management; Liver Disease; **Hospital:** Mass Genl Hosp; **Address:** Mass Genl Hosp, Dept Gastroenterology, 55 Fruit St Bldg 4, Boston, MA 02114-2517; **Phone:** 617-724-6007; **Board Cert:** Gastroenterology 1987; Internal Medicine 1984; **Med School:** Albert Einstein Coll Med 1981; **Resid:** Internal Medicine, Mass Genl Hosp 1984; **Fellow:** Gastroenterology, Mass Genl Hosp 1987; **Fac Appt:** Assoc Prof Med, Harvard Med Sch

Levine, Joel B MD [Ge] - **Spec Exp:** Colon & Rectal Cancer Detection; Colonoscopy; Gastroesophageal Reflux Disease (GERD); **Hospital:** Univ of Conn Hlth Ctr, John Dempsey Hosp; **Address:** Univ Connecticut Hlth Ctr, Colon Cancer Prevention Prgm, 263 Farmington Ave, Farmington, CT 06030-2813; **Phone:** 860-679-4567; **Board Cert:** Internal Medicine 1973; Gastroenterology 1977; **Med School:** SUNY Downstate 1969; **Resid:** Internal Medicine, Univ Chicago Hosps 1971; Internal Medicine, Mass Genl Hosp 1974; **Fellow:** Gastroenterology, Mass Genl Hosp 1977; **Fac Appt:** Prof Med, Univ Conn

Mason, Joel B MD [Ge] - **Spec Exp:** Nutrition in Acute Illness; Nutrition in Bowel Disorders; Nutrition & Cancer Prevention; Inflammatory Bowel Disease; **Hospital:** Tufts Med Ctr; **Address:** 800 Washington St, Box 239, Boston, MA 02111-1513; **Phone:** 617-636-5623; **Board Cert:** Internal Medicine 1984; Gastroenterology 1987; **Med School:** Univ Chicago-Pritzker Sch Med 1981; **Resid:** Internal Medicine, Univ Iowa Hosps 1984; **Fellow:** Gastroenterology, Univ Chicago Hosps 1986; Nutrition, Univ Chicago Hosps 1986; **Fac Appt:** Prof Med, Tufts Univ

Nunes, David P MD [Ge] - **Spec Exp:** Liver Disease; Hepatitis; **Hospital:** Boston Med Ctr; **Address:** Boston Med Ctr, Div Gastroenterology, 830 Harrison Ave Mokley Bldg Fl 2, Ste 2100, Boston, MA 02118; **Phone:** 617-638-6525 x3; **Board Cert:** Internal Medicine 2006; Gastroenterology 2007; **Med School:** Ireland 1984; **Resid:** Gastroenterology, Federated Dublin Volunt Hosps 1987; **Fac Appt:** Assoc Prof Med, Boston Univ

Proctor, Deborah D MD [Ge] - **Spec Exp:** Inflammatory Bowel Disease; Colon Cancer Screening; Endoscopy; **Hospital:** Yale-New Haven Hosp, Yale Med Group; **Address:** 40 Temple St, Ste 1A, Temple Medical Center, 1st Fl, New Haven, CT 06519; **Phone:** 203-785-4138; **Board Cert:** Gastroenterology 2003; **Med School:** Univ Cincinnati 1982; **Resid:** Internal Medicine, Beth Israel Hosp 1990; **Fellow:** Gastroenterology, Beth Israel Hosp 1992; **Fac Appt:** Prof Med, Yale Univ

Rothstein, Richard I MD [Ge] - **Spec Exp:** Gastroesophageal Reflux Disease (GERD); Swallowing Disorders; Barrett's Esophagus; Endoscopy; **Hospital:** Dartmouth - Hitchcock Med Ctr; **Address:** Dartmouth-Hitchcock Med Ctr, Div Gastroenterology, 1 Med Ctr Drive, Lebanon, NH 03756; **Phone:** 603-650-8343; **Board Cert:** Internal Medicine 1983; Gastroenterology 1987; **Med School:** Boston Univ 1980; **Resid:** Internal Medicine, Univ Mass Med Ctr 1983; **Fellow:** Gastroenterology, Dartmouth-Hitchcock Med Ctr 1985; **Fac Appt:** Prof Med, Dartmouth Med Sch

Gastroenterology

Siegel, Corey A MD [Ge] - **Spec Exp:** Ulcerative Colitis; Crohn's Disease; Colonoscopy; Inflammatory Bowel Disease; **Hospital:** Dartmouth - Hitchcock Med Ctr; **Address:** Dartmouth-Hitchcock Med Ctr, Gastroenterology & Hepatology Div, 1 Medical Ctr Drive, Lebanon, NH 03756; **Phone:** 603-650-5261; **Board Cert:** Internal Medicine 2001; Gastroenterology 2005; **Med School:** Tufts Univ 1998; **Resid:** Internal Medicine, Dartmouth-Hitchcock Med Ctr 2002; **Fellow:** Gastroenterology, Dartmouth-Hitchcock Med Ctr 2004; Inflammatory Bowel Disease, Mass Genl Hosp 2005

Weinstock, Joel V MD [Ge] - **Spec Exp:** Endoscopy; Inflammatory Bowel Disease; **Hospital:** Tufts Med Ctr; **Address:** 800 Washington St, Box 233, Boston, MA 02111; **Phone:** 617-636-5883 x2; **Board Cert:** Internal Medicine 1976; Gastroenterology 1979; **Med School:** Wayne State Univ 1973; **Resid:** Internal Medicine, Univ Hosp Michigan 1976; **Fellow:** Gastroenterology, Univ Hosp Michigan 1978; **Fac Appt:** Prof Med, Tufts Univ

Mid Atlantic

Albert, Michael B MD [Ge] - **Spec Exp:** Inflammatory Bowel Disease; Ulcerative Colitis; Endoscopy; Colon Cancer Screening; **Hospital:** G Washington Univ Hosp; **Address:** DC Gastroenterology, 2131 K St NW, Ste 800A, Washington, DC 20037; **Phone:** 202-223-5544; **Board Cert:** Internal Medicine 1985; Gastroenterology 1987; **Med School:** Johns Hopkins Univ 1982; **Resid:** Internal Medicine, Mayo Clinic 1984; Internal Medicine, Duke Univ Med Ctr 1985; **Fellow:** Gastroenterology, G Washington Univ Med Ctr 1987; **Fac Appt:** Prof Med, Geo Wash Univ

Araya, Victor R MD [Ge] - **Spec Exp:** Transplant Medicine-Liver; Liver Disease; Clinical Trials; **Hospital:** Albert Einstein Med Ctr; **Address:** AEMC Klein Bldg - Ste 101, 5401 Old York Rd, Philadelphia, PA 19141; **Phone:** 215-456-8242; **Board Cert:** Internal Medicine 2007; Gastroenterology 2008; Transplant Hepatology 2008; **Med School:** Geo Wash Univ 1985; **Resid:** Internal Medicine, Temple Univ Hosp; **Fellow:** Gastroenterology, Univ FL Med Ctr; Transplant Hepatology, Univ FL Med Ctr

Aronchick, Craig A MD [Ge] - **Spec Exp:** Colonoscopy; Colon Cancer Screening; **Hospital:** Pennsylvania Hosp-UPHS (page 68); **Address:** 230 W Washington Square, Farm Journal Bldg, Fl 4, Philadelphia, PA 19106; **Phone:** 215-829-3561; **Board Cert:** Internal Medicine 1981; Gastroenterology 1983; **Med School:** Temple Univ 1978; **Resid:** Internal Medicine, Temple Univ Hosp 1981; **Fellow:** Gastroenterology, Hosp Univ Penn 1983

Bayless, Theodore MD [Ge] - **Spec Exp:** Inflammatory Bowel Disease/Crohn's; Ulcerative Colitis; Malabsorption Syndrome; Microscopic Colitis; **Hospital:** Johns Hopkins Hosp (page 61); **Address:** Johns Hopkins Hosp, 600 N Wolfe St, Blalock Bldg - Ste 461, Baltimore, MD 21287-0005; **Phone:** 410-933-7495; **Board Cert:** Internal Medicine 1966; **Med School:** Ros Franklin Univ/Chicago Med Sch 1957; **Resid:** Internal Medicine, Cornell-Bellevue Hosp 1958; Internal Medicine, Meml Sloan Kettering Hosp 1960; **Fellow:** Gastroenterology, Johns Hopkins Hosp 1962; **Fac Appt:** Prof Med, Johns Hopkins Univ

Borum, Marie L MD [Ge] - **Spec Exp:** Colon Cancer Screening; AIDS/HIV-Gastrointestinal Complications; Women's Health; Liver Disease; **Hospital:** G Washington Univ Hosp; **Address:** MFA Dept Medicine, 2150 Pennsylvania Ave NW Fl 3, Washington, DC 20037; **Phone:** 202-741-3333; **Board Cert:** Internal Medicine 1988; Gastroenterology 2001; **Med School:** UMDNJ-Rutgers Med Sch 1985; **Resid:** Internal Medicine, G Washington Univ Med Ctr 1988; **Fellow:** Gastroenterology, G Washington Univ Med Ctr 1991; **Fac Appt:** Prof Med, Geo Wash Univ

Brandt, Lawrence MD [Ge] - **Spec Exp:** Inflammatory Bowel Disease; Clostridium Difficile Disease; **Hospital:** Montefiore Med Ctr - Div. Moses, Montefiore Med Ctr - Div. Weiler; **Address:** 3400 Bainbridge Ave Fl 2, Bronx, NY 10467-2401; **Phone:** 866-633-8255; **Board Cert:** Internal Medicine 1972; Gastroenterology 2006; **Med School:** SUNY Downstate 1968; **Resid:** Internal Medicine, Mt Sinai Hosp 1972; **Fellow:** Gastroenterology, Mt Sinai Hosp 1972; **Fac Appt:** Prof Med, Albert Einstein Coll Med

Brown Jr, Robert S MD [Ge] - **Spec Exp:** Hepatitis; Liver Disease; Transplant Medicine-Liver; **Hospital:** NY-Presby/Columbia Univ Med Ctr, NY (page 65); **Address:** Ctr for Liver Disease & Transplantation, 622 W 168th St Fl 14 - rm 105, New York, NY 10032; **Phone:** 212-305-1305; **Board Cert:** Internal Medicine 2002; Gastroenterology 2005; Transplant Hepatology 2010; **Med School:** NYU Sch Med 1989; **Resid:** Internal Medicine, Beth Israel Deaconess Med Ctr 1992; **Fellow:** Gastroenterology, UCSF Med Ctr 1994; Hepatology, UCSF Med Ctr 1995; **Fac Appt:** Prof Med, Columbia P&S

Canto, Marcia MD [Ge] - **Spec Exp:** Endoscopy; Endoscopic Ultrasound; Pancreatic Cancer-Early Detection; **Hospital:** Johns Hopkins Hosp (page 61); **Address:** Dept of Med, Gastroenterology, 1830 E Monument St, rm 426, Baltimore, MD 21205; **Phone:** 410-614-5388; **Board Cert:** Internal Medicine 1989; Gastroenterology 2008; **Med School:** Philippines 1985; **Resid:** Internal Medicine, SUNY Hlth Sci Ctr 1991; **Fellow:** Gastroenterology, SUNY Hlth Sci Ctr 1993; **Fac Appt:** Assoc Prof Med, Johns Hopkins Univ

Carr-Locke, David L MD [Ge] - **Spec Exp:** Pancreatic/Biliary Endoscopy (ERCP); Pancreatic & Biliary Disease; Endoscopy; **Hospital:** Beth Israel Med Ctr - Petrie Division (page 55); **Address:** 1st & 16th St, New York, NY 10003; **Phone:** 212-420-4015; **Board Cert:** Internal Medicine 1974; **Med School:** England, UK 1972; **Resid:** Obstetrics & Gynecology, Orsett Hosp 1974; Internal Medicine, Leicester Hosp 1976; **Fellow:** Gastroenterology, Leicester Hosp 1978; Research, New Eng Baptist Hosp 1979; **Fac Appt:** Assoc Prof Med, Harvard Med Sch

Cohen, Jonathan MD [Ge] - **Spec Exp:** Pancreatic/Biliary Endoscopy (ERCP); Pancreatic Disease; Barrett's Esophagus; Colonoscopy; **Hospital:** NYU Langone Med Ctr (page 66); **Address:** 232 E 30th St, New York, NY 10016-8202; **Phone:** 212-889-5544; **Board Cert:** Gastroenterology 2005; **Med School:** Harvard Med Sch 1990; **Resid:** Internal Medicine, Beth Israel Hosp 1993; **Fellow:** Gastroenterology, UCLA Med Ctr 1995; Endoscopy, Wellesley Hosp 1995; **Fac Appt:** Clin Prof Med, NYU Sch Med

Cohen, Lawrence B MD [Ge] - **Spec Exp:** Gastroesophageal Reflux Disease (GERD); Esophageal Disorders; Colon & Rectal Cancer; Endoscopy; **Hospital:** Mount Sinai Med Ctr (page 63); **Address:** 311 E 79th St, Ste 2A, New York, NY 10075; **Phone:** 212-996-6633; **Board Cert:** Internal Medicine 1981; Gastroenterology 1983; **Med School:** Hahnemann Univ 1978; **Resid:** Internal Medicine, Mt Sinai Hosp 1981; **Fellow:** Gastroenterology, Mt Sinai Hosp 1983; **Fac Appt:** Assoc Clin Prof Med, Mount Sinai Sch Med

DeCross, Arthur J MD [Ge] - **Hospital:** Univ of Rochester Strong Meml Hosp; **Address:** 180 Saw Grass Drive, Rochester, NY 14620; **Phone:** 585-758-0209; **Board Cert:** Gastroenterology 2003; **Med School:** Albany Med Coll 1988; **Resid:** Internal Medicine, Strong Meml Hosp 1991; **Fellow:** Gastroenterology, Univ Virginnia Med Ctr 1994; **Fac Appt:** Assoc Prof Med, Univ Rochester

Di Marino Jr, Anthony J MD [Ge] - **Spec Exp:** Celiac Disease; Gastroesophageal Reflux Disease (GERD); Irritable Bowel Syndrome; Crohn's Disease; **Hospital:** Thomas Jefferson Univ Hosp; **Address:** Thomas Jefferson Univ, Div Gastroenterology, 132 S 10th St, Ste 480, Philadelphia, PA 19107; **Phone:** 215-955-2728; **Board Cert:** Internal Medicine 1977; Gastroenterology 1972; **Med School:** Hahnemann Univ 1968; **Resid:** Internal Medicine, Hahnemann Univ Hosp 1970; Internal Medicine, Hosp Univ Penn 1971; **Fellow:** Gastroenterology, Hosp Univ Penn 1973; **Fac Appt:** Prof Med, Thomas Jefferson Univ

Gastroenterology

Dieterich, Douglas T MD [Ge] - **Spec Exp:** Hepatitis; AIDS/HIV-Gastrointestinal Complications; Liver Disease; Endoscopy; **Hospital:** Mount Sinai Med Ctr (page 63); **Address:** 5 E 98th St Fl 11, New York, NY 10029; **Phone:** 212-241-7270; **Board Cert:** Internal Medicine 1981; Gastroenterology 1987; **Med School:** NYU Sch Med 1978; **Resid:** Internal Medicine, Bellevue Hosp Ctr-NYU 1981; **Fellow:** Gastroenterology, Bellevue Hosp Ctr-NYU 1983; **Fac Appt:** Prof Med, Mount Sinai Sch Med

Falk, Gary W MD [Ge] - **Spec Exp:** Swallowing Disorders; Esophageal Disorders; Chest Pain-Non Cardiac; Barrett's Esophagus; **Hospital:** Hosp Univ Penn - UPHS (page 68); **Address:** Hosp Univ Penn, 3400 Spruce St Ravdin Bldg Fl 3, Philadelphia, PA 19104; **Phone:** 215-662-4279; **Board Cert:** Internal Medicine 1983; Gastroenterology 1985; **Med School:** Univ Rochester 1980; **Resid:** Internal Medicine, George Washington Univ Hosp 1983; **Fellow:** Gastroenterology, Univ Michigan Med Ctr 1986; **Fac Appt:** Prof Med, Univ Pennsylvania

Fisher, Robert S MD [Ge] - **Spec Exp:** Gastrointestinal Motility Disorders; Peptic Acid Disorders; Gastrointestinal Functional Disorders; **Hospital:** Temple Univ Hosp; **Address:** 3401 N Broad St, Philadelphia, PA 19140; **Phone:** 215-707-9922; **Board Cert:** Internal Medicine 1971; Gastroenterology 1973; **Med School:** Univ Pennsylvania 1964; **Resid:** Internal Medicine, Temple Univ Med Ctr 1970; **Fellow:** Gastroenterology, Hosp Univ Penn 1972; **Fac Appt:** Prof Med, Temple Univ

Freiman, Hal MD [Ge] - **Spec Exp:** Gastroesophageal Reflux Disease (GERD); Biliary Disease; Pancreatic/Biliary Endoscopy (ERCP); Hepatitis; **Hospital:** Beth Israel Med Ctr - Petrie Division (page 55), NYU Langone Med Ctr (page 66); **Address:** 59 W 12th St, Ste 1D, New York, NY 10011-8520; **Phone:** 212-206-0074; **Board Cert:** Internal Medicine 1981; Gastroenterology 1983; **Med School:** Albany Med Coll 1978; **Resid:** Internal Medicine, St Vincent's Hosp 1981; **Fellow:** Gastroenterology, Westchester Co Med Ctr 1983; **Fac Appt:** Asst Clin Prof Med, NY Med Coll

Gerdes, Hans MD [Ge] - **Spec Exp:** Endoscopy; Endoscopic Ultrasound; Barrett's Esophagus; Gastrointestinal Cancer; **Hospital:** Meml Sloan-Kettering Cancer Ctr; **Address:** 1275 York Avenue, New York, NY 10065; **Phone:** 800-525-2225; **Board Cert:** Internal Medicine 1987; Gastroenterology 1989; **Med School:** Cornell Univ-Weill Med Coll 1983; **Resid:** Internal Medicine, New York Hosp 1986; **Fellow:** Gastroenterology, Meml Sloan Kettering Cancer Ctr 1989

Giardiello, Francis MD [Ge] - **Spec Exp:** Colon Cancer; Colon & Rectal Cancer-Familial Polyposis; Cancer Risk Assessment; **Hospital:** Johns Hopkins Hosp (page 61); **Address:** 1830 E Mounument St, rm 431, Baltimore, MD 21205; **Phone:** 410-955-7495; **Board Cert:** Internal Medicine 1983; Gastroenterology 1985; **Med School:** Tufts Univ 1980; **Resid:** Internal Medicine, Univ Michigan 1983; **Fellow:** Gastroenterology, Johns Hopkins 1985; **Fac Appt:** Prof Med, Johns Hopkins Univ

Ginsberg, Gregory G MD [Ge] - **Spec Exp:** Pancreatic/Biliary Endoscopy (ERCP); Endoscopy; Endoscopic Ultrasound; Barrett's Esophagus; **Hospital:** Hosp Univ Penn - UPHS (page 68); **Address:** Hosp U Penn, Div Gastroenterology, 3400 Civic Center Blvd, 4 S Pavillion, Philadelphia, PA 19104; **Phone:** 215-349-8222; **Board Cert:** Gastroenterology 2000; **Med School:** Jefferson Med Coll 1987; **Resid:** Internal Medicine, Georgetown Univ Med Ctr 1990; **Fellow:** Gastroenterology, Georgetown Univ Med Ctr 1992; **Fac Appt:** Clin Prof Med, Univ Pennsylvania

Goggins, Michael MD [Ge] - **Spec Exp:** Pancreatic Cancer-Early Detection; **Hospital:** Johns Hopkins Hosp (page 61); **Address:** Johns Hopkins Univ Sch Med, 1550 Orleans St, St CRB-2 Bldg - rm 342, Baltimore, MD 21231; **Phone:** 410-933-7495; **Med School:** Ireland 1988; **Resid:** Internal Medicine, St Jame's Hosp 1990; **Fellow:** Gastroenterology, St Jame's Hosp 1992; **Fac Appt:** Assoc Prof Med, Johns Hopkins Univ

Green, Peter H-R MD [Ge] - **Spec Exp:** Celiac Disease; Endoscopy; Colonoscopy; Malabsorption Syndrome; **Hospital:** NY-Presby/Columbia Univ Med Ctr, NY (page 65); **Address:** Celiac Disease Ctr, Harkness Bldg, 180 Fort Washington Ave, rm 956, New York, NY 10032-3713; **Phone:** 212-305-5590; **Med School:** Australia 1970; **Resid:** Internal Medicine, North Shore Med Ctr 1974; **Fellow:** Gastroenterology, North Shore Med Ctr 1976; Gastroenterology, Beth Israel Hosp 1977; **Fac Appt:** Clin Prof Med, Columbia P&S

Greenwald, Bruce D MD [Ge] - **Spec Exp:** Endoscopic Ultrasound; Barrett's Esophagus; Esophageal Cancer; Clinical Trials; **Hospital:** Univ of MD Med Ctr; **Address:** Univ of Maryland Hosp, Gastroenterology, 22 S Greene St Fl 3 - rm N3W62, Baltimore, MD 21201; **Phone:** 410-328-8731; **Board Cert:** Internal Medicine 2000; Gastroenterology 2000; **Med School:** Univ MD Sch Med 1987; **Resid:** Internal Medicine, Univ Virginia Hosp 1990; **Fellow:** Gastroenterology, Univ Maryland Hosp 1992; **Fac Appt:** Assoc Prof Med, Univ MD Sch Med

Haber, Gregory B MD [Ge] - **Spec Exp:** Endoscopy; Pancreatic/Biliary Endoscopy (ERCP); Endoscopic Ultrasound; Barrett's Esophagus; **Hospital:** Lenox Hill Hosp; **Address:** 100 E 77th St, New York, NY 10075; **Phone:** 212-434-6279; **Med School:** Univ Toronto 1970; **Resid:** Internal Medicine, Univ Toronto Med Ctr 1975; **Fellow:** Gastroenterology, Univ Toronto Med Ctr 1978

Haluszka, Oleh MD [Ge] - **Spec Exp:** Pancreatic/Biliary Endoscopy (ERCP); Gastrointestinal Cancer; Endoscopic Ultrasound; Endoscopy; **Hospital:** Temple Univ Hosp; **Address:** 3500 N Broad St, Philadelphia, PA 19140; **Phone:** 215-707-9577; **Board Cert:** Internal Medicine 1987; Gastroenterology 2001; **Med School:** Uniformed Srvs Univ, Bethesda 1982; **Resid:** Internal Medicine, US Naval Hosp 1987; **Fellow:** Gastroenterology, US Naval Hosp 1990; Endoscopy, Med Coll Wisconsin 1993; **Fac Appt:** Assoc Clin Prof Med, Temple Univ

Herrine, Steven K MD [Ge] - **Spec Exp:** Liver Disease; Hepatitis C; Transplant Medicine-Liver; **Hospital:** Thomas Jefferson Univ Hosp; **Address:** Jefferson University Physicians, Div Gastroenterology & Hepatology, 132 S 10th St Fl 4, Philadelphia, PA 19107; **Phone:** 215-955-8900; **Board Cert:** Internal Medicine 2003; Gastroenterology 2005; Transplant Hepatology 2006; **Med School:** Jefferson Med Coll 1990; **Resid:** Internal Medicine, Hosp U Penn 1993; **Fellow:** Gastroenterology, Thos Jefferson Univ Hosp 1995; **Fac Appt:** Prof Med, Thomas Jefferson Univ

Hoops, Timothy C MD [Ge] - **Spec Exp:** Esophageal Disorders; Endoscopy; Colonoscopy; **Hospital:** Penn Presby Med Ctr - UPHS (page 68); **Address:** Penn Presbyterian Med Ctr, 51 N 39th St, Ste 218, Philadelphia, PA 19104; **Phone:** 215-662-8900; **Board Cert:** Internal Medicine 1984; Gastroenterology 1987; **Med School:** Univ IL Coll Med 1981; **Resid:** Internal Medicine, Univ Colorado Hlth Sci Ctr 1984; **Fellow:** Gastroenterology, Univ Colorado Hlth Sci Ctr 1986; **Fac Appt:** Clin Prof Med, Univ Pennsylvania

Infantolino, Anthony MD [Ge] - **Spec Exp:** Endoscopy; Endoscopic Ultrasound; Barrett's Esophagus; Inflammatory Bowel Disease; **Hospital:** Thomas Jefferson Univ Hosp; **Address:** Jefferson University Physicians, Div Gastroenterology & Hepatology, 132 S 10th St Fl 4, Philadelphia, PA 19107; **Phone:** 215-955-8900; **Board Cert:** Internal Medicine 1988; Gastroenterology 2002; **Med School:** UMDNJ-RW Johnson Med Sch 1985; **Resid:** Internal Medicine, Thos Jefferson Univ Hosp 1988; **Fellow:** Gastroenterology, Graduate Hosp 1990; **Fac Appt:** Assoc Clin Prof Med, Thomas Jefferson Univ

Itzkowitz, Steven H MD [Ge] - **Spec Exp:** Colon & Rectal Cancer; Colon & Rectal Cancer Detection; Inflammatory Bowel Disease; Hereditary Cancer; **Hospital:** Mount Sinai Med Ctr (page 63); **Address:** 5 E 98th St, Box 1625, New York, NY 10029-6501; **Phone:** 212-241-4299; **Board Cert:** Internal Medicine 1982; Gastroenterology 1985; **Med School:** Mount Sinai Sch Med 1979; **Resid:** Internal Medicine, Bellevue Hosp/NYU Med Ctr 1982; **Fellow:** Gastroenterology, UCSF Med Ctr 1984; **Fac Appt:** Prof Med, Mount Sinai Sch Med

Gastroenterology

Jacobson, Ira MD [Ge] - **Spec Exp:** Liver & Biliary Disease; Pancreatic Disease; Colonoscopy; Hepatitis; **Hospital:** NY-Presby/Weill Cornell Med Ctr, NY (page 65); **Address:** 1305 York Ave Fl 4, New York, NY 10021-5016; **Phone:** 646-962-4040; **Board Cert:** Internal Medicine 1982; Gastroenterology 1985; Transplant Hepatology 2006; **Med School:** Columbia P&S 1979; **Resid:** Internal Medicine, UCSF Med Ctr 1982; **Fellow:** Gastroenterology, Mass Genl Hosp 1984; **Fac Appt:** Prof Med, Cornell Univ-Weill Med Coll

Kalloo, Anthony N MD [Ge] - **Spec Exp:** Endoscopy; Pancreatic Disease; **Hospital:** Johns Hopkins Hosp (page 61); **Address:** Johns Hopkins Hosp, Div Gastroenterology, 600 N Wolfe St, Blalock 465, Baltimore, MD 21231; **Phone:** 410-955-9697; **Board Cert:** Internal Medicine 1985; Gastroenterology 1987; **Med School:** Jamaica 1979; **Resid:** Internal Medicine, Howard Univ Hosp 1985; **Fellow:** Gastroenterology, VA Med Ctr/Georgetown Univ Hosp 1987; **Fac Appt:** Assoc Prof Med, Johns Hopkins Univ

Kantsevoy, Sergey V MD/PhD [Ge] - **Spec Exp:** Pancreatic Disease; Endoscopic Ultrasound; Pancreatic/Biliary Endoscopy (ERCP); **Hospital:** Mercy Med Ctr - Baltimore; **Address:** 301 St Paul Pl, Ste 718, Professional Off Bldg, Baltimore, MD 21202; **Phone:** 410-332-9356; **Board Cert:** Gastroenterology 2000; **Med School:** Russia 1983; **Resid:** Internal Medicine, Bronx-Lebanon Hosp Ctr 1995; Internal Medicine, Washington Hosp Ctr 1997; **Fellow:** Gastroenterology, Johns Hopkins Hosp 2000; **Fac Appt:** Asst Prof Med, Johns Hopkins Univ

Kastenberg, David M MD [Ge] - **Spec Exp:** Colon & Rectal Cancer Detection; Capsule Endoscopy; Celiac Disease; Nutrition & Cancer Prevention; **Hospital:** Thomas Jefferson Univ Hosp; **Address:** 132 S 10th St Main Bldg - Ste 480, Dept Gastroenterology, Phildelphia, PA 19107; **Phone:** 215-955-8900; **Board Cert:** Internal Medicine 2000; Gastroenterology 2000; **Med School:** NYU Sch Med 1987; **Resid:** Internal Medicine, Temple Univ Hosp 1990; **Fellow:** Gastroenterology, Thomas Jefferson Univ Hosp 1992; **Fac Appt:** Assoc Prof Med, Jefferson Med Coll

Katz, Philip O MD [Ge] - **Spec Exp:** Gastroesophageal Reflux Disease (GERD); Swallowing Disorders; Barrett's Esophagus; Esophageal Disorders; **Hospital:** Albert Einstein Med Ctr; **Address:** 5401 Old York Rd, Klein Bldg - Ste 202, Philadelphia, PA 19141; **Phone:** 215-456-8210; **Board Cert:** Internal Medicine 1981; Gastroenterology 1987; **Med School:** Bowman Gray 1978; **Resid:** Internal Medicine, NC Baptist Hosp 1981; **Fellow:** Gastroenterology, NC Baptist Hosp 1986; **Fac Appt:** Clin Prof Med, Thomas Jefferson Univ

Kochman, Michael L MD [Ge] - **Spec Exp:** Endoscopy; Pancreatic/Biliary Endoscopy (ERCP); Gastrointestinal Cancer; **Hospital:** Hosp Univ Penn - UPHS (page 68), Penn Presby Med Ctr - UPHS (page 68); **Address:** 3400 Spruce St Ravdin Bldg Fl 3 - Ste GI, Philadelphia, PA 19104-4206; **Phone:** 215-349-4279; **Board Cert:** Internal Medicine 1989; Gastroenterology 2003; **Med School:** Univ IL Coll Med 1986; **Resid:** Internal Medicine, Univ Illinois Med Ctr 1990; **Fellow:** Gastroenterology, Univ Michigan Med Ctr 1993; **Fac Appt:** Prof Med, Univ Pennsylvania

Korsten, Mark A MD [Ge] - **Spec Exp:** Constipation; Gastrointestinal Motility Disorders; Spinal Cord Injury & Colonic Motility; Liver Disease; **Hospital:** Mount Sinai Med Ctr (page 63), James J. Peters VA Med Ctr-Bronx; **Address:** 130 W Kingsbridge Rd, Bronx, NY 10468-3904; **Phone:** 718-584-9000 x6753; **Board Cert:** Internal Medicine 1973; Gastroenterology 1975; **Med School:** Yale Univ 1970; **Resid:** Internal Medicine, Mt Sinai Hosp 1973; **Fellow:** Gastroenterology, Mt Sinai Hosp 1975; **Fac Appt:** Prof Med, Mount Sinai Sch Med

Kotler, Donald P MD [Ge] - **Spec Exp:** Esophageal Disorders; Nutrition & AIDS; Hepatitis; **Hospital:** St. Luke's - Roosevelt Hosp Ctr - St Luke's Hosp (page 55); **Address:** 1111 Amsterdam Ave, SR 12, New York, NY 10025; **Phone:** 212-523-3670; **Board Cert:** Internal Medicine 1976; Gastroenterology 1979; **Med School:** Albert Einstein Coll Med 1973; **Resid:** Internal Medicine, Jacobi Med Ctr 1976; **Fellow:** Gastroenterology, Hosp Univ Penn 1978; **Fac Appt:** Prof Med, Columbia P&S

Kowalski, Thomas E MD [Ge] - **Spec Exp:** Pancreatic Disease; Biliary Disease; Pancreatic/Biliary Endoscopy (ERCP); Endoscopic Ultrasound; **Hospital:** Thomas Jefferson Univ Hosp; **Address:** 132 S 10th St Main Bldg, Philadelphia, PA 19107; **Phone:** 215-955-8900; **Board Cert:** Internal Medicine 2003; Gastroenterology 2003; **Med School:** SUNY Buffalo 1988; **Resid:** Internal Medicine, Johns Hopkins Hosp 1991; **Fellow:** Gastroenterology, Hosp Univ Penn 1993; Advanced Endoscopy, Hosp Univ Penn 1994; **Fac Appt:** Assoc Prof Med, Thomas Jefferson Univ

Kurtz, Robert C MD [Ge] - **Spec Exp:** Pancreatic Cancer(Familial); Gastrointestinal Cancer; Endoscopy; Nutrition & Cancer Prevention/Control; **Hospital:** Meml Sloan-Kettering Cancer Ctr; **Address:** 1275 York Avenue, New York, NY 10065; **Phone:** 212-639-7620; **Board Cert:** Internal Medicine 1971; Gastroenterology 1977; **Med School:** Jefferson Med Coll 1968; **Resid:** Internal Medicine, NY Hosp/Meml Sloan Kettering Cancer Ctr 1971; **Fellow:** Gastroenterology, Meml Sloan Kettering Cancer Ctr 1973; **Fac Appt:** Prof Med, Cornell Univ-Weill Med Coll

Lebwohl, Oscar MD [Ge] - **Spec Exp:** Endoscopy; Inflammatory Bowel Disease/Crohn's; Ulcerative Colitis; Gastrointestinal Cancer; **Hospital:** NY-Presby/Columbia Univ Med Ctr, NY (page 65); **Address:** 161 Fort Washington Ave, rm 420, New York, NY 10032-3713; **Phone:** 212-305-5363; **Board Cert:** Internal Medicine 1975; Gastroenterology 1977; **Med School:** Harvard Med Sch 1972; **Resid:** Internal Medicine, Mt Sinai Med Ctr 1975; **Fellow:** Gastroenterology, Columbia-Presby Med Ctr 1976; Hepatology, Mt Sinai Med Ctr 1977; **Fac Appt:** Clin Prof Med, Columbia P&S

Lewis, Blair MD [Ge] - **Spec Exp:** Endoscopy; Capsule Endoscopy; **Hospital:** Mount Sinai Med Ctr (page 63); **Address:** 1067 5th Ave, New York, NY 10128-0101; **Phone:** 212-369-6600; **Board Cert:** Internal Medicine 1985; Gastroenterology 1987; **Med School:** Albert Einstein Coll Med 1982; **Resid:** Internal Medicine, Montefiore Med Ctr 1985; **Fellow:** Gastroenterology, Mt Sinai Med Ctr 1987; **Fac Appt:** Clin Prof Med, Mount Sinai Sch Med

Lichtenstein, Gary R MD [Ge] - **Spec Exp:** Inflammatory Bowel Disease; Crohn's Disease; Ulcerative Colitis; **Hospital:** Hosp Univ Penn - UPHS (page 68); **Address:** Hosp U Penn, Div Gastroenterology, 3400 Civic Center Blvd, Perelman Ctr, 4 S Pavilion Fl 4 - Ste 370, Philadelphia, PA 19104-4283; **Phone:** 215-349-8222; **Board Cert:** Internal Medicine 1987; Gastroenterology 1989; **Med School:** Mount Sinai Sch Med 1984; **Resid:** Internal Medicine, Duke Univ Med Ctr 1987; **Fellow:** Gastroenterology, Hosp Univ Penn 1990; **Fac Appt:** Prof Med, Univ Pennsylvania

Lightdale, Charles J MD [Ge] - **Spec Exp:** Barrett's Esophagus; Gastrointestinal Cancer; Endoscopic Ultrasound; **Hospital:** NY-Presby/Columbia Univ Med Ctr, NY (page 65); **Address:** Columbia-Presby Med Ctr, Irving Pavilion, 161 Fort Washington Ave, rm 812, New York, NY 10032-3713; **Phone:** 212-305-3423; **Board Cert:** Internal Medicine 1972; Gastroenterology 1973; **Med School:** Columbia P&S 1966; **Resid:** Internal Medicine, Yale-New Haven Hosp 1968; Internal Medicine, NY Hosp-Cornell 1969; **Fellow:** Gastroenterology, NY Hosp-Cornell 1973; **Fac Appt:** Clin Prof Med, Columbia P&S

Lipshutz, William H MD [Ge] - **Spec Exp:** Inflammatory Bowel Disease/Crohn's; Colonoscopy; Esophageal Disorders; Gastroesophageal Reflux Disease (GERD); **Hospital:** Pennsylvania Hosp-UPHS (page 68); **Address:** 230 W Washington Sq, Farm Journal Bldg Fl 4, Philadelphia, PA 19106; **Phone:** 215-829-3561; **Board Cert:** Internal Medicine 1972; Gastroenterology 1973; **Med School:** Univ Pennsylvania 1967; **Resid:** Internal Medicine, Pennsylvania Hosp 1972; **Fellow:** Gastroenterology, Hosp Univ Penn 1971

Magun, Arthur M MD [Ge] - **Spec Exp:** Hepatitis; Ulcerative Colitis; Endoscopy; Crohn's Disease; **Hospital:** NY-Presby/Columbia Univ Med Ctr, NY (page 65); **Address:** 161 Fort Washington Ave, rm 338, New York, NY 10032-3713; **Phone:** 212-305-5287; **Board Cert:** Internal Medicine 1980; Gastroenterology 1983; **Med School:** Mount Sinai Sch Med 1977; **Resid:** Internal Medicine, Columbia-Presby Med Ctr 1980; **Fellow:** Gastroenterology, Columbia-Presby Med Ctr 1983; **Fac Appt:** Clin Prof Med, Columbia P&S

Gastroenterology

Markowitz, David D MD [Ge] - **Spec Exp:** Gastroesophageal Reflux Disease (GERD); Esophageal Disorders; Endoscopy; **Hospital:** NY-Presby/Columbia Univ Med Ctr, NY (page 65); **Address:** 161 Ft Washington Ave, Ste 853, New York, NY 10032; **Phone:** 212-305-1024; **Board Cert:** Internal Medicine 1988; Gastroenterology 2001; **Med School:** Columbia P&S 1985; **Resid:** Internal Medicine, Columbia-Presby Hosp 1988; **Fellow:** Gastroenterology, Columbia-Presby Hosp 1991; **Fac Appt:** Assoc Prof Med, Columbia P&S

Mayer, Lloyd MD [Ge] - **Spec Exp:** Inflammatory Bowel Disease/Crohn's; Ulcerative Colitis; **Hospital:** Mount Sinai Med Ctr (page 63); **Address:** 1425 Madison Ave, rm 11-20, Box 1089, New York, NY 10029; **Phone:** 212-659-9266; **Board Cert:** Internal Medicine 1979; Gastroenterology 1981; **Med School:** Mount Sinai Sch Med 1976; **Resid:** Internal Medicine, Bellevue Hosp 1979; **Fellow:** Gastroenterology, Mt Sinai Hosp 1981; **Fac Appt:** Prof Med, Mount Sinai Sch Med

Metz, David C MD [Ge] - **Spec Exp:** Peptic Acid Disorders; Neuroendocrine Tumors; Gastroesophageal Reflux Disease (GERD); Gastrointestinal Motility Disorders; **Hospital:** Hosp Univ Penn - UPHS (page 68); **Address:** Hosp Univ Penn, Div Gastroenterology, 3400 Civic Ctr Blvd, 4 S Pavilion Fl 4 - Ste 370, Philadelphia, PA 19104; **Phone:** 215-349-8222; **Board Cert:** Internal Medicine 1989; Gastroenterology 2001; **Med School:** South Africa 1982; **Resid:** Internal Medicine, Albert Einstein Med Ctr 1988; **Fellow:** Gastroenterology, Natl Inst Hlth 1991; **Fac Appt:** Prof Med, Univ Pennsylvania

Miskovitz, Paul MD [Ge] - **Spec Exp:** Endoscopy; Liver Disease; Biliary Disease; **Hospital:** NY-Presby/Weill Cornell Med Ctr, NY (page 65); **Address:** 635 Madison Ave Fl 17, New York, NY 10022; **Phone:** 212-717-4966; **Board Cert:** Internal Medicine 1978; Gastroenterology 1981; **Med School:** Cornell Univ-Weill Med Coll 1975; **Resid:** Internal Medicine, NY Hosp 1978; **Fellow:** Gastroenterology, NY Hosp 1980; **Fac Appt:** Clin Prof Med, Cornell Univ-Weill Med Coll

Munoz, Santiago J MD [Ge] - **Spec Exp:** Liver Disease; Transplant Medicine-Liver; Hepatitis; **Hospital:** Temple Univ Hosp; **Address:** Temple University Hospital, Div Gasteoenterology & Transplantation, 3401 N Broad St, Philadelphia, PA 19150; **Phone:** 215-707-9900; **Board Cert:** Internal Medicine 1985; Gastroenterology 1989; Transplant Hepatology 2006; **Med School:** Chile 1978; **Resid:** Internal Medicine, Jefferson Hosp 1985; **Fellow:** Pharmacology, Johns Hopkins Hosp 1983; Gastroenterology, Jefferson Hosp 1987; **Fac Appt:** Assoc Prof Med, Temple Univ

Navarro, Victor J MD [Ge] - **Spec Exp:** Liver Disease; Hepatitis; Transplant Medicine-Liver; **Hospital:** Thomas Jefferson Univ Hosp; **Address:** Jefferson University Physicians, Div Gastroenterology & Hepatology, 132 S 10th St Fl 4, Philadelphia, PA 19107; **Phone:** 215-955-8900; **Board Cert:** Internal Medicine 2001; Gastroenterology 2005; Transplant Hepatology 2006; **Med School:** Penn State Coll Med 1988; **Resid:** Internal Medicine, Temple Univ Hosp; **Fellow:** Gastroenterology, Yale-New Haven Hosp 1994; **Fac Appt:** Assoc Clin Prof Med, Thomas Jefferson Univ

Okolo III, Patrick I MD [Ge] - **Spec Exp:** Liver Cancer; Pancreatic Cancer; Gastrointestinal Cancer; Clinical Trials; **Hospital:** Johns Hopkins Hosp (page 61); **Address:** The John Hopkins Hospital, 600 N Wolfe St, Baltimore, MD 21287; **Phone:** 410-933-7495; **Board Cert:** Internal Medicine 2004; Gastroenterology 2008; **Med School:** Nigeria 1988; **Resid:** Internal Medicine, Indiana Univ Med Ctr 1994; **Fellow:** Gastroenterology, John Hopkins Hosp 1997; **Fac Appt:** Assoc Prof Med, Johns Hopkins Univ

Peikin, Steven MD [Ge] - **Spec Exp:** Endoscopy; **Hospital:** Cooper Univ Hosp; **Address:** Cooper Digestive Health Inst, 501 Fellowship Rd, Ste 101, Mt Laurel, NJ 08054; **Phone:** 856-642-2133; **Board Cert:** Internal Medicine 1977; Gastroenterology 1979; **Med School:** Jefferson Med Coll 1974; **Resid:** Internal Medicine, Moffit Hosps 1977; **Fellow:** Gastroenterology, Mass Genl Hosp 1980; **Fac Appt:** Prof Med

Pezzone, Michael A MD/PhD [Ge] - **Spec Exp:** Irritable Bowel Syndrome; Inflammatory Bowel Disease; Pain-Pelvic; **Hospital:** Washington Hosp, The, UPMC Presby, Pittsburgh; **Address:** 86 Wellness Way, Washington, PA 15301; **Phone:** 724-503-4637; **Board Cert:** Internal Medicine 2007; Gastroenterology 2000; **Med School:** Univ Pittsburgh 1994; **Resid:** Internal Medicine, Univ Pittsburgh Med Ctr 1997; **Fellow:** Gastroenterology, Univ Pittsburgh Med Ctr 2000; **Fac Appt:** Assoc Prof Med, Univ Pittsburgh

Pochapin, Mark B MD [Ge] - **Spec Exp:** Pancreatic Cancer; Endoscopic Ultrasound; Colon & Rectal Cancer Detection; Diarrheal Diseases; **Hospital:** NY-Presby/Weill Cornell Med Ctr, NY (page 65); **Address:** The Jay Monahan Ctr for GI Hlth, 1315 York Ave Fl Ground, New York, NY 10021; **Phone:** 212-746-4014; **Board Cert:** Gastroenterology 2004; **Med School:** Cornell Univ-Weill Med Coll 1988; **Resid:** Internal Medicine, NY Hosp-Cornell Med Ctr 1991; **Fellow:** Gastroenterology, Montefiore Med Ctr 1993; **Fac Appt:** Assoc Clin Prof Med, Cornell Univ-Weill Med Coll

Ravich, William J MD [Ge] - **Spec Exp:** Swallowing Disorders; Gastroesophageal Reflux Disease (GERD); Barrett's Esophagus; Achalasia; **Hospital:** Johns Hopkins Hosp (page 61), Greater Baltimore Med Ctr; **Address:** 10751 Falls Rd, Ste 401, Lutherville, MD 21093; **Phone:** 410-616-2840; **Board Cert:** Internal Medicine 1978; Gastroenterology 1981; **Med School:** Ros Franklin Univ/Chicago Med Sch 1975; **Resid:** Internal Medicine, Montefiore Hosp 1978; **Fellow:** Gastroenterology, Johns Hopkins Hosp 1981; **Fac Appt:** Assoc Prof Med, Johns Hopkins Univ

Reddy, K Rajender MD [Ge] - **Spec Exp:** Liver Disease; Hepatitis; Transplant Medicine-Liver; **Hospital:** Hosp Univ Penn - UPHS (page 68); **Address:** Hosp U Penn, Div Gastroenterology, 3400 Civic Center Blvd, Perelman Ctr, 4 S Pavilion Fl 4 - Ste 370, Philadelphia, PA 19104; **Phone:** 215-349-8222; **Board Cert:** Internal Medicine 1980; Gastroenterology 1983; Transplant Hepatology 2006; **Med School:** India 1972; **Resid:** Internal Medicine, NY Med Coll Hosps 1980; Gastroenterology, E Tenn State Univ 1982; **Fellow:** Hepatology, Univ Miami Hosps 1983; **Fac Appt:** Prof Med, Univ Pennsylvania

Reynolds, James C MD [Ge] - **Spec Exp:** Gastroesophageal Reflux Disease (GERD); Gastrointestinal Motility Disorders; Barrett's Esophagus; **Hospital:** Hahnemann Univ Hosp; **Address:** Drexel Gastroenterology Assocs, 219 N Broad St Fl 5, Philadelphia, PA 19107; **Phone:** 215-965-6000; **Board Cert:** Internal Medicine 1980; Gastroenterology 1985; **Med School:** Univ Fla Coll Med 1977; **Resid:** Internal Medicine, New York Hosp 1980; **Fellow:** Gastroenterology, Hosp Univ Penn 1983; **Fac Appt:** Prof Med, Drexel Univ Coll Med

Sachar, David MD [Ge] - **Spec Exp:** Inflammatory Bowel Disease-Consult; Crohn's Disease; Ulcerative Colitis; **Hospital:** Mount Sinai Med Ctr (page 63); **Address:** 5 E 98th St Fl 11, New York, NY 10029; **Phone:** 212-241-4299; **Board Cert:** Internal Medicine 1969; Gastroenterology 1972; **Med School:** Harvard Med Sch 1963; **Resid:** Internal Medicine, Beth Israel Hosp 1965; Internal Medicine, Beth Israel Hosp 1968; **Fellow:** Gastroenterology, Mount Sinai Hosp 1970; **Fac Appt:** Clin Prof Med, Mount Sinai Sch Med

Schiano, Thomas D MD [Ge] - **Spec Exp:** Liver Disease; Transplant Medicine-Liver; Transplant Medicine-Bowel; Hepatitis; **Hospital:** Mount Sinai Med Ctr (page 63); **Address:** Mount Sinai Medical Ctr, One Gustave L Levy Pl, Box 1104, New York, NY 10029; **Phone:** 212-241-8035; **Board Cert:** Internal Medicine 2000; Gastroenterology 2005; Transplant Hepatology 2006; **Med School:** Mexico 1987; **Resid:** Internal Medicine, Maimonides Med Ctr 1992; Gastroenterology, Temple Univ 1995; **Fellow:** Nutrition, Meml Sloan-Kettering Cancer Ctr 1993; Hepatology, Mt Sinai Med Ctr 1996; **Fac Appt:** Prof Med, Mount Sinai Sch Med

Gastroenterology

Shike, Moshe MD [Ge] - **Spec Exp:** Gastrointestinal Cancer; Nutrition & Cancer Prevention; Endoscopy; **Hospital:** Meml Sloan-Kettering Cancer Ctr; **Address:** 1275 York Ave, New York, NY 10065; **Phone:** 800-525-2225; **Board Cert:** Internal Medicine 1977; Gastroenterology 1981; **Med School:** Israel 1975; **Resid:** Internal Medicine, Mt Auburn Hosp 1977; **Fellow:** Gastroenterology, Toronto Genl Hosp 1981; **Fac Appt:** Prof Med, Cornell Univ-Weill Med Coll

Slivka, Adam MD/PhD [Ge] - **Spec Exp:** Pancreatic & Biliary Disease; Pancreatic Cancer; **Hospital:** UPMC Presby, Pittsburgh; **Address:** Digestive Disorders Center, 200 Lothrop St, 3rd Fl-PUH, Pittsburgh, PA 15213; **Phone:** 412-647-8666; **Board Cert:** Internal Medicine 2002; Gastroenterology 1995; **Med School:** Mount Sinai Sch Med 1988; **Resid:** Internal Medicine, Brigham & Womens Hosp 1991; **Fellow:** Gastroenterology, Brigham & Womens Hosp 1994; **Fac Appt:** Assoc Prof Med, Univ Pittsburgh

Smoot, Duane T MD [Ge] - **Spec Exp:** Colon & Rectal Cancer Detection; Gastrointestinal Cancer; Peptic Acid Disorders; **Hospital:** Howard Univ Hosp; **Address:** Howard Univ Hosp, Med, Div Gastroenterology, Ste 5100, 2041 Georgia Ave NW Tower Bldg, Washington, DC 20060; **Phone:** 202-865-6620; **Board Cert:** Internal Medicine 1987; Gastroenterology 2003; **Med School:** Howard Univ 1983; **Resid:** Internal Medicine, Univ MD Hosp 1986; **Fellow:** Gastroenterology, Univ MD Hosp 1989; **Fac Appt:** Prof Med, Howard Univ

Tobias, Hillel MD [Ge] - **Spec Exp:** Liver Disease; Hepatitis B & C; Liver & Biliary Disease; **Hospital:** NYU Langone Med Ctr (page 66); **Address:** 232 E 30th St, New York, NY 10016-8202; **Phone:** 212-889-5544; **Board Cert:** Internal Medicine 1967; Gastroenterology 1979; **Med School:** Washington Univ, St Louis 1960; **Resid:** Internal Medicine, Bellevue Hosp 1963; **Fellow:** Hepatology, Royal Free Hosp 1965; Hepatology, Mount Sinai Hosp 1967; **Fac Appt:** Prof Med, NYU Sch Med

Waye, Jerome MD [Ge] - **Spec Exp:** Endoscopy; Colon Cancer; Colonoscopy; **Hospital:** Mount Sinai Med Ctr (page 63), Lenox Hill Hosp; **Address:** 650 Park Ave, New York, NY 10065; **Phone:** 212-439-7779; **Board Cert:** Internal Medicine 1965; Gastroenterology 1970; **Med School:** Boston Univ 1958; **Resid:** Internal Medicine, Mt Sinai Hosp 1961; **Fellow:** Gastroenterology, Mt Sinai Hosp 1962; **Fac Appt:** Clin Prof Med, Mount Sinai Sch Med

Weinberg, David Seth MD [Ge] - **Spec Exp:** Colonoscopy; Cancer Risk Assessment; Cancer Prevention; Endoscopy; **Hospital:** Fox Chase Cancer Ctr (page 58); **Address:** Fox Chase Cancer Ctr, Dept Medicine, 333 Cottman Ave, Ste P3047, Philadelphia, PA 19111; **Phone:** 215-214-1424; **Board Cert:** Gastroenterology 2006; **Med School:** Cornell Univ-Weill Med Coll 1989; **Resid:** Internal Medicine, Beth Israel Hosp 1992; **Fellow:** Gastroenterology, Hosp U Penn 1995; Epidemiology, Hosp U Penn 1995; **Fac Appt:** Prof Med, Temple Univ

Southeast

Abreu, Maria T MD [Ge] - **Spec Exp:** Inflammatory Bowel Disease; Ulcerative Colitis; Crohn's Disease; **Hospital:** Univ of Miami Hosp (page 72); **Address:** Univ Miami Miller Sch Med, 1475 NW 12th Ave, Sylvester Center, Fl 1, GI Dept, Miami, FL 33136; **Phone:** 305-243-8644; **Board Cert:** Gastroenterology 2005; **Med School:** Univ Miami Sch Med 1990; **Resid:** Internal Medicine, Brigham & Women's Hosp 1992; **Fellow:** Gastroenterology, UCLA Med Ctr 1995; **Fac Appt:** Prof Med, Univ Miami Sch Med

Barkin, Jamie S MD [Ge] - **Spec Exp:** Pancreatic & Biliary Disease; Gastrointestinal Cancer; Endoscopy; **Hospital:** Mount Sinai Med Ctr - Miami, Univ of Miami Hosp & Clins/Sylvester Comp Canc Ctr (page 73); **Address:** Mount Sinai Medical Center, Gumenick Bldg, 4300 Alton Rd, Ste 2522, Miami Beach, FL 33140-2800; **Phone:** 305-674-2240; **Board Cert:** Internal Medicine 1973; Gastroenterology 1975; **Med School:** Univ Miami Sch Med 1970; **Resid:** Internal Medicine, Univ Miami Hosp 1973; **Fellow:** Gastroenterology, Univ Miami Hosp 1975; **Fac Appt:** Prof Med, Univ Miami Sch Med

Bloomer, Joseph R MD [Ge] - **Spec Exp:** Porphyria; Liver Disease; Transplant Medicine-Liver; Hepatitis B; **Hospital:** Univ of Ala Hosp at Birmingham, UAB Highlands Hosp; **Address:** UAB Liver Center, 1918 University Blvd, MCLM 284, Birmingham, AL 35294-0005; **Phone:** 205-975-5676; **Board Cert:** Internal Medicine 1972; **Med School:** Case West Res Univ 1966; **Resid:** Internal Medicine, UCSF Med Ctr 1968; **Fellow:** Hepatology, Yale Univ 1972; **Fac Appt:** Prof Med, Univ Alabama

Brazer, Scott R MD [Ge] - **Spec Exp:** Gastroesophageal Reflux Disease (GERD); Chest Pain-Non Cardiac; Colon Cancer Screening; **Hospital:** Durham Regional Hosp; **Address:** 249 E Highway 54, Ste 200, Durham, NC 27713; **Phone:** 919-806-8322; **Board Cert:** Internal Medicine 1984; Gastroenterology 1987; **Med School:** Case West Res Univ 1981; **Resid:** Internal Medicine, Duke Univ Med Ctr 1984; Internal Medicine, Duke Univ Med Ctr 1988; **Fellow:** Gastroenterology, Duke Univ 1987

Castell, Donald O MD [Ge] - **Spec Exp:** Esophageal Disorders; Gastroesophageal Reflux Disease (GERD); Gastrointestinal Motility Disorders; **Hospital:** MUSC Med Ctr; **Address:** MUSC Digestive Disease Ctr, 25 Courtenay Drive, ART-7100A, MC CMS290, Charleston, SC 29425; **Phone:** 843-876-4265; **Board Cert:** Internal Medicine 1977; Gastroenterology 1970; **Med School:** Geo Wash Univ 1960; **Resid:** Internal Medicine, US Naval Hosp 1965; **Fellow:** Gastroenterology, Tufts Univ 1969; **Fac Appt:** Prof Med, Univ SC Sch Med

DeVault, Kenneth MD [Ge] - **Spec Exp:** Gastroesophageal Reflux Disease (GERD); **Hospital:** Mayo - Jacksonville; **Address:** Mayo Clinic Davis Bldg Fl 6, 4500 San Pablo Rd S, Jacksonville, FL 32224-1865; **Phone:** 904-953-2254; **Board Cert:** Internal Medicine 1989; Gastroenterology 2003; **Med School:** Bowman Gray 1986; **Resid:** Internal Medicine, Vanderbilt Univ Med Ctr 1989; **Fellow:** Gastroenterology, Thomas Jefferson Univ Med Ctr 1992; **Fac Appt:** Prof Med, Mayo Med Sch

Drossman, Douglas A MD [Ge] - **Spec Exp:** Gastrointestinal Motility Disorders; Pain-Abdominal/Functional; Gastrointestinal Functional Disorders; **Hospital:** NC Memorial Hosp - UNC; **Address:** Univ NC, Div Digestive Diseases, 4150 Bio Informatics Bldg, Campus Box 7080, Chapel Hill, NC 27599-7080; **Phone:** 919-966-0141; **Board Cert:** Internal Medicine 1973; Gastroenterology 1979; **Med School:** Albert Einstein Coll Med 1970; **Resid:** Internal Medicine, NC Meml Hosp 1972; Internal Medicine, Bellevue Hosp Ctr-NYU 1973; **Fellow:** Psychiatry, Univ Rochester 1976; Gastroenterology, NC Meml Hosp-UNC 1978; **Fac Appt:** Prof Med, Univ NC Sch Med

Elliott, Norman L MD [Ge] - **Spec Exp:** Enteroscopy-Small Bowel; Endoscopy; **Hospital:** Emory Univ Hosp Midtown, Piedmont Hosp; **Address:** Atlanta Gastroenterology Assocs, 550 Peachtree St NE, Ste 1600, Atlanta, GA 30308; **Phone:** 404-881-1094; **Board Cert:** Internal Medicine 1982; Gastroenterology 1985; **Med School:** Yale Univ 1979; **Resid:** Internal Medicine, Emory Univ Hosp 1982; **Fellow:** Gastroenterology, Univ Alabama 1985; **Fac Appt:** Asst Clin Prof Med, Emory Univ

Gastroenterology

Estores, David S MD [Ge] - **Spec Exp:** Barrett's Esophagus; Swallowing Disorders; **Hospital:** Tampa Genl Hosp; **Address:** Ctr for Swallowing Disorders, 12901 Bruce B Downs Blvd, MDC 72, Tampa, FL 33612-4742; **Phone:** 813-974-3374; **Board Cert:** Internal Medicine 1989; Gastroenterology 2001; **Med School:** Philippines 1985; **Resid:** Internal Medicine, St Lukes Hosp 1989; **Fellow:** Gastroenterology, Univ Pittsburgh-Presby Hosp 1992

Forsmark, Christopher MD [Ge] - **Spec Exp:** Pancreatic/Biliary Endoscopy (ERCP); Celiac Disease; Pancreatic Disease; Endoscopy; **Hospital:** Shands at Univ of FL; **Address:** University of Florida, 1600 SW Archer Rd, HD 602, Box 100214, Gainesville, FL 32610; **Phone:** 352-273-9400; **Board Cert:** Internal Medicine 1986; Gastroenterology 2006; **Med School:** Johns Hopkins Univ 1983; **Resid:** Internal Medicine, UCSF Med Ctr 1987; **Fellow:** Gastroenterology, USCF Med Ctr 1990; **Fac Appt:** Prof Med, Univ Fla Coll Med

Fried, Michael W MD [Ge] - **Spec Exp:** Transplant Medicine-Liver; Liver Disease; Hepatitis; **Hospital:** NC Memorial Hosp - UNC; **Address:** UNC Gastroenterology/Hepatology, Liver Program, CB 7584, Chapel Hill, NC 27599; **Phone:** 919-966-2516; **Board Cert:** Internal Medicine 1987; Gastroenterology 1989; **Med School:** Israel 1984; **Resid:** Internal Medicine, SUNY Upstate Med Ctr 1987; **Fellow:** Gastroenterology, SUNY Upstate Med Ctr 1989; **Fac Appt:** Prof Med, Univ NC Sch Med

Hawes, Robert H MD [Ge] - **Spec Exp:** Endoscopic Ultrasound; Pancreatic/Biliary Endoscopy (ERCP); Pancreatic Disease; **Hospital:** MUSC Med Ctr; **Address:** MUSC Digestive Disease Ctr, 25 Courtenay Drive, ART-7100A, MS C290, Charleston, SC 29425; **Phone:** 843-876-4699; **Board Cert:** Internal Medicine 1985; Gastroenterology 1987; **Med School:** Indiana Univ 1980; **Resid:** Internal Medicine, Indiana Univ Hosp 1984; **Fellow:** Gastroenterology, Indiana Univ Hosp 1985; Endoscopy, Peter B Cotton/Steve Brown 1986; **Fac Appt:** Prof Med, Med Univ SC

Hoffman, Brenda J MD [Ge] - **Spec Exp:** Liver & Biliary Disease; Endoscopic Ultrasound; Gastrointestinal Cancer; Colon & Rectal Cancer-Familial Polyposis; **Hospital:** MUSC Med Ctr; **Address:** MUSC Digestive Disease Center, 25 Courteney Drive, ART7100A, MSC290, Charleston, SC 29425; **Phone:** 843-792-2301; **Board Cert:** Internal Medicine 1986; Gastroenterology 1989; **Med School:** Univ KY Coll Med 1983; **Resid:** Internal Medicine, Med Univ SC Med Ctr 1987; **Fellow:** Gastroenterology, Med Univ SC Med Ctr 1989; **Fac Appt:** Prof Med, Univ SC Sch Med

Isaacs, Kim MD/PhD [Ge] - **Spec Exp:** Inflammatory Bowel Disease; Crohn's Disease; Ulcerative Colitis; **Hospital:** NC Memorial Hosp - UNC; **Address:** Univ NC, Div Digestive Disease/Nutrition, CB# 7080, Bioinformatics Bldg, 130 Mason Farm Rd Fl 1, Chapel Hill, NC 27599-7080; **Phone:** 919-966-0140; **Board Cert:** Internal Medicine 1987; Gastroenterology 2001; **Med School:** SUNY Stony Brook 1984; **Resid:** Internal Medicine, Univ NC Hosps 1987; **Fellow:** Gastroenterology, Univ NC Hosps 1989; **Fac Appt:** Assoc Prof Med, Univ NC Sch Med

Koch, Kenneth L MD [Ge] - **Spec Exp:** Gastrointestinal Motility Disorders; Gastroparesis; Esophageal Disorders; **Hospital:** Wake Forest Univ Baptist Med Ctr; **Address:** Wake Forest Univ Baptist Med Ctr, Digestive Health Services, Medical Center Blvd, Winston-Salem, NC 27157-1015; **Phone:** 336-713-7777; **Board Cert:** Internal Medicine 1978; Gastroenterology 1983; **Med School:** Univ Iowa Coll Med 1975; **Resid:** Internal Medicine, Penn State Affil Hosps 1978; **Fellow:** Gastroenterology, Univ Florida 1980; **Fac Appt:** Prof Med, Univ NC Sch Med

Lambiase, Louis R MD [Ge] - **Spec Exp:** Pancreatic Disease; Endoscopic Ultrasound; Pain-Abdominal/Functional; Liver Disease; **Hospital:** Erlanger Med Ctr; **Address:** 979 E 3rd St, Ste C-825, Chattanooga, TN 37403; **Phone:** 423-778-4830; **Board Cert:** Internal Medicine 2002; Gastroenterology 2003; **Med School:** Univ Miami Sch Med 1987; **Resid:** Internal Medicine, Presbyterian/VA Hosps 1990; **Fellow:** Gastroenterology, Univ Fla 1993; **Fac Appt:** Prof Med, Univ Fla Coll Med

Liddle, Rodger A MD [Ge] - **Spec Exp:** Pancreatic Disease; Hormone Secreting Tumors; **Hospital:** Duke Univ Hosp, Durham VA Med Ctr; **Address:** Duke Univ Med Ctr, Box 3913, Durham, NC 27710; **Phone:** 919-681-6380; **Board Cert:** Internal Medicine 1981; Gastroenterology 1983; **Med School:** Vanderbilt Univ 1978; **Resid:** Internal Medicine, UCSF Med Ctr 1981; **Fellow:** Gastroenterology, UCSF Med Ctr 1984; **Fac Appt:** Prof Med, Duke Univ

Lind, Christopher D MD [Ge] - **Spec Exp:** Gastroesophageal Reflux Disease (GERD); Swallowing Disorders; Biliary Disease; Gastrointestinal Motility Disorders; **Hospital:** Vanderbilt Univ Med Ctr (page 76); **Address:** Vanderbilt Univ Med Ctr, Div GI, 1301 Med Ctr Drive, Ste 1660, TVC GI Clin, Nashville, TN 37232-5280; **Phone:** 615-322-0128; **Board Cert:** Internal Medicine 1984; Gastroenterology 1987; **Med School:** Vanderbilt Univ 1981; **Resid:** Internal Medicine, Univ Virginia Hosps 1985; **Fellow:** Gastroenterology, Shands/Univ Florida 1986; Gastroenterology, Univ Virginia Hosps 1988; **Fac Appt:** Prof Med, Vanderbilt Univ

Martin, Paul MD [Ge] - **Spec Exp:** Liver Disease; Hepatitis; Transplant Medicine-Liver; **Hospital:** Univ of Miami Hosp (page 72), Jackson Meml Hosp (page 70); **Address:** University of Miami, 1500 NW 12th Ave, Jackson Medical Tower E-1101, Miami, FL 33136; **Phone:** 305-243-5787; **Board Cert:** Internal Medicine 1984; Gastroenterology 1987; Transplant Hepatology 2006; **Med School:** Ireland 1978; **Resid:** Internal Medicine, St Vincent's Hosp 1982; Internal Medicine, Univ Alberta 1984; **Fellow:** Gastroenterology, Queen Univ 1986; Hepatology, Natl Inst Hlth 1989; **Fac Appt:** Prof Med, Univ Miami Sch Med

Mertz, Howard R MD [Ge] - **Spec Exp:** Endoscopic Ultrasound; Irritable Bowel Syndrome; Inflammatory Bowel Disease; **Hospital:** Saint Thomas Hosp - Nashville; **Address:** Nashville Gastrointestinal Specialists, 4230 Harding Rd, Ste 309W, Nashville, TN 37205; **Phone:** 615-383-0165; **Board Cert:** Internal Medicine 1989; Gastroenterology 2002; **Med School:** Baylor Coll Med 1986; **Resid:** Internal Medicine, Johns Hopkins Hosp 1989; **Fellow:** Gastroenterology, UCLA Med Ctr 1991; **Fac Appt:** Assoc Clin Prof Med, Vanderbilt Univ

Plevy, Scott MD [Ge] - **Spec Exp:** Inflammatory Bowel Disease; **Hospital:** NC Memorial Hosp - UNC; **Address:** 103 Mason Farm Rd, MBRB Bldg, GI Clinic, CB 7032, Rm 7200, Chapel Hill, NC 27599; **Phone:** 919-966-4318; **Board Cert:** Gastroenterology 2007; **Med School:** Columbia P&S 1988; **Resid:** Internal Medicine, Brigham-Womens Hosp 1991; **Fellow:** Gastroenterology, Univ of California 1992; Inflammatory Bowel Disease, Cedars-Sinai Med CTR 1994; **Fac Appt:** Assoc Prof Med, Univ NC Sch Med

Porayko, Michael K MD [Ge] - **Spec Exp:** Liver Disease; Transplant Medicine-Liver; Liver Cancer; Hepatitis-Chronic; **Hospital:** Vanderbilt Univ Med Ctr (page 76); **Address:** Digestive Disease Center, 1301 Medical Center Drive, Ste 1660, Nashville, TN 37232; **Phone:** 615-322-0128; **Board Cert:** Internal Medicine 1984; Gastroenterology 1987; Transplant Hepatology 2006; **Med School:** Univ IL Coll Med 1981; **Resid:** Internal Medicine, Michigan State Univ Affil Hosps 1984; **Fellow:** Gastroenterology, Lahey Clin & New England Deaconess Hosp 1987; Hepatology, Mayo Clinic 1988; **Fac Appt:** Prof Med, Vanderbilt Univ

Raiford, David S MD [Ge] - **Spec Exp:** Autoimmune Liver Disease; Steatohepatitis; Transplant Medicine-Liver; **Hospital:** Vanderbilt Univ Med Ctr (page 76); **Address:** Vanderbilt Digestive Disease Center, 1301 Medical Ctr Drive, Ste 1660, Nashville, TN 37232-5280; **Phone:** 615-322-0128; **Board Cert:** Internal Medicine 1989; Gastroenterology 2001; Transplant Hepatology 2006; **Med School:** Johns Hopkins Univ 1985; **Resid:** Internal Medicine, Johns Hopkins Hosp 1988; **Fellow:** Hepatology, Johns Hopkins Hosp 1991; **Fac Appt:** Prof Med, Vanderbilt Univ

Gastroenterology

Reuben, Adrian MD [Ge] - **Spec Exp:** Liver Disease; **Hospital:** MUSC Med Ctr; **Address:** MUSC GI & Hepatology, 25 Courtenay Drive, ART 7100A, MSC 290, Charleston, SC 29403; **Phone:** 843-792-6901; **Med School:** England, UK 1969; **Resid:** Internal Medicine, National Heart 1972; Gastroenterology, Hammersmith Hosps; **Fellow:** Hepatology, Guy's Hosp; **Fac Appt:** Prof Med, Med Univ SC

Sartor, R Balfour MD [Ge] - **Spec Exp:** Inflammatory Bowel Disease; **Hospital:** NC Memorial Hosp - UNC; **Address:** Univ NC Sch Medicine, Div Gastroenterology/Hepatology, Biomolecular Bldg-rm 7309, Box 7032, Chapel Hill, NC 27599-7032; **Phone:** 919-966-0140; **Board Cert:** Internal Medicine 1978; Gastroenterology 1981; **Med School:** Baylor Coll Med 1974; **Resid:** Internal Medicine, Baylor Affil Hosp 1977; **Fellow:** Gastroenterology, Univ NC Hosps 1981; **Fac Appt:** Prof Med, Univ NC Sch Med

Schiff, Eugene R MD [Ge] - **Spec Exp:** Hepatitis C; Liver Disease; **Hospital:** Univ of Miami Hosp (page 72), Jackson Meml Hosp (page 70); **Address:** Ctr for Liver Disease, 1500 NW 12th Ave, Jackson Medical Tower E-1101, Miami, FL 33136; **Phone:** 305-243-5787; **Board Cert:** Internal Medicine 1980; Gastroenterology 1972; **Med School:** Columbia P&S 1962; **Resid:** Internal Medicine, Cincinnati Genl Hosp 1964; Internal Medicine, Parkland Meml Hosp 1967; **Fellow:** Gastroenterology, Univ Tex SW Med Ctr 1969; **Fac Appt:** Prof Med, Univ Miami Sch Med

Scudera, Peter L MD [Ge] - **Spec Exp:** Colon & Rectal Cancer Detection; Pancreatic/Biliary Endoscopy (ERCP); Hepatitis-Chronic; **Hospital:** Inova Fair Oaks Hosp, Inova Fairfax Hosp; **Address:** 3700 Joseph Siewick Dr, Ste 308, Fairfax, VA 22033; **Phone:** 703-716-8700; **Board Cert:** Internal Medicine 1987; Gastroenterology 1989; **Med School:** Cornell Univ-Weill Med Coll 1984; **Resid:** Internal Medicine, New York Hosp 1987; **Fellow:** Gastroenterology, New York Hosp-Cornell 1989

Seidner, Douglas L MD [Ge] - **Spec Exp:** Nutrition; Malabsorption Syndrome; Nutrition in Bowel Disorders; Endoscopy; **Hospital:** Vanderbilt Univ Med Ctr (page 76); **Address:** Vanderbilt Ctr Human Nutrition, 1211 21st Ave S, 514 Med Arts Bldg, Nashville, TN 37232; **Phone:** 615-936-1288; **Board Cert:** Internal Medicine 1986; Gastroenterology 2000; **Med School:** SUNY Upstate Med Univ 1983; **Resid:** Internal Medicine, Beth Israel Deaconess Med Ctr 1986; **Fellow:** Nutrition & Metabolism, Beth Israel Deaconess Med Ctr 1987; Gastroenterology, George Washington Univ Med Ctr 1989

Shiffman, Mitchell MD [Ge] - **Spec Exp:** Transplant Medicine-Liver; Hepatitis C; Liver Disease; Liver Cancer; **Hospital:** Bon Secours Mary Immaculate Hosp; **Address:** 5855 Bremo Rd, MOB North, Ste 509, Richmond, VA 23226; **Phone:** 804-977-8920; **Board Cert:** Internal Medicine 1986; Gastroenterology 1989; **Med School:** SUNY Upstate Med Univ 1983; **Resid:** Internal Medicine, Med Coll Va Hosp 1986; **Fellow:** Gastroenterology, Med Coll Va Hosp 1988

Toskes, Phillip MD [Ge] - **Spec Exp:** Nutrition; Malabsorption Syndrome; Pancreatic Disease; **Hospital:** Shands at Univ of FL; **Address:** Univ Florida, Div Gastroenterolgy, 1600 SW Archer Rd, HD 602, Box 100214, Gainesville, FL 32610-0214; **Phone:** 352-273-9400; **Board Cert:** Internal Medicine 1970; Gastroenterology 1973; **Med School:** Univ MD Sch Med 1965; **Resid:** Internal Medicine, Univ Maryland Hosp 1968; **Fellow:** Gastroenterology, Hosp Univ Penn 1970; **Fac Appt:** Prof Med, Univ Fla Coll Med

Vaezi, Michael F MD/PhD [Ge] - **Spec Exp:** Gastroesophageal Reflux Disease (GERD); Esophageal Disorders; Achalasia; **Hospital:** Vanderbilt Univ Med Ctr (page 76); **Address:** 1301 Med Ctr Drive, Ste 1660, Nashville, TN 37232; **Phone:** 615-322-0128; **Board Cert:** Internal Medicine 2007; Gastroenterology 2009; **Med School:** Univ Alabama 1992; **Resid:** Internal Medicine, Univ AL-Birmingham Med Ctr 1995; **Fellow:** Gastroenterology, Cleveland Clin 1996; **Fac Appt:** Prof Med, Vanderbilt Univ

Wilcox, C Mel MD [Ge] - **Spec Exp:** Pancreatic & Biliary Disease; Zollinger-Ellison Syndrome; Endoscopic Therapies; Pancreatic/Biliary Endoscopy (ERCP); **Hospital:** Univ of Ala Hosp at Birmingham; **Address:** UAB-Div Gastroenterology, 1808 7th Ave South, BDB 380, Birmingham, AL 35294-0007; **Phone:** 205-975-4958; **Board Cert:** Internal Medicine 1986; Gastroenterology 2007; **Med School:** Med Coll GA 1983; **Resid:** Internal Medicine, Univ Alabama Hosps 1986; **Fellow:** Gastroenterology, UCSF 1990; **Fac Appt:** Prof Med, Univ Alabama

Yanda, Randy J MD [Ge] - **Spec Exp:** Endoscopy; Pancreatic/Biliary Endoscopy (ERCP); Colon Cancer Screening; **Hospital:** Piedmont Hosp; **Address:** Digestive Healthcare of Georgia, 95 Collier Rd NW, Ste 4055, Atlanta, GA 30309; **Phone:** 404-355-3200; **Board Cert:** Internal Medicine 1987; Gastroenterology 2001; **Med School:** Univ Iowa Coll Med 1984; **Resid:** Internal Medicine, UCSF Med Ctr 1987; **Fellow:** Gastroenterology, UCSF Med Ctr 1990

Younossi, Zobair MD [Ge] - **Spec Exp:** Liver Disease; **Hospital:** Inova Fairfax Hosp; **Address:** Ctr for Liver Diseases, Fairfax Hosp, 3300 Gallows Rd, Claude Moore Bldg, Falls Church, VA 22042; **Phone:** 703-776-3182; **Board Cert:** Gastroenterology 2005; Transplant Hepatology 2006; **Med School:** Univ Rochester 1989; **Resid:** Gastroenterology, Scripps Clin & Rsch Fdn 1993; **Fellow:** Hepatology, Scripps Clin & Rsch Fdn 1995; **Fac Appt:** Prof Med, Va Commonwealth Univ Sch Med

Midwest

Bacon, Bruce MD [Ge] - **Spec Exp:** Hepatitis C; Hepatic Iron Metabolism; Liver Disease; **Hospital:** St. Louis Univ Hosp, SSM St Mary's Hlth Ctr - St Louis; **Address:** 3660 Vista Ave, Ste 308, St Louis, MO 63110-2540; **Phone:** 314-577-6000; **Board Cert:** Internal Medicine 1978; Gastroenterology 2008; Transplant Hepatology 2006; **Med School:** Case West Res Univ 1975; **Resid:** Internal Medicine, Metro Genl Hosp 1979; **Fellow:** Gastroenterology, Metro Genl Hosp 1982; **Fac Appt:** Prof Med, St Louis Univ

Barnes, David S MD [Ge] - **Spec Exp:** Biliary Disease; Hepatitis; Liver Disease; **Hospital:** Cleveland Clin (page 56); **Address:** Cleveland Clinic, Div Gastroenterology, 9500 Euclid Ave, MC A-51, Cleveland, OH 44195; **Phone:** 216-444-1764; **Board Cert:** Internal Medicine 1984; Gastroenterology 1987; Transplant Hepatology 2006; **Med School:** Univ NC Sch Med 1981; **Resid:** Internal Medicine, U Mass Med Ctr 1984; **Fellow:** Gastroenterology, Case Western Reserve Univ 1985

Baron, Todd H MD [Ge] - **Spec Exp:** Endoscopy; Pancreatic/Biliary Endoscopy (ERCP); **Hospital:** Mayo Med Ctr & Clin - Rochester; **Address:** Mayo Clinic, 200 First St SW, Rochester, MN 55905; **Phone:** 507-284-2174; **Board Cert:** Internal Medicine 1989; Gastroenterology 2003; **Med School:** Univ Fla Coll Med 1986; **Resid:** Internal Medicine, Univ Alabama Med Ctr 1990; **Fellow:** Gastroenterology, Univ Alabama Med Ctr 1993; **Fac Appt:** Assoc Prof Med, Univ Ariz Coll Med

Brown, Kimberly A MD [Ge] - **Spec Exp:** Liver Disease; Transplant Medicine-Liver; Hepatitis C; Liver Cancer; **Hospital:** Henry Ford Hosp; **Address:** Henry Ford Hosp, Dept Gastroenterology, 2799 W Grand Blvd K-747 Bldg Fl 7, Detroit, MI 48202-2608; **Phone:** 313-916-8865; **Board Cert:** Internal Medicine 1988; Gastroenterology 2002; Transplant Hepatology 2006; **Med School:** Wayne State Univ 1985; **Resid:** Internal Medicine, Univ Michigan Med Ctr 1989; **Fellow:** Gastroenterology, Univ Michigan Med Ctr 1992

Chari, Suresh T MD [Ge] - **Spec Exp:** Pancreatic Disease; **Hospital:** Mayo Med Ctr & Clin - Rochester; **Address:** Mayo Clinic, 200 First St SW, Mayo Bldg Fl 9, Rochester, MN 55905; **Phone:** 507-284-2141; **Board Cert:** Gastroenterology 2009; **Med School:** India 1982; **Resid:** Internal Medicine, Univ Arizona Hlth Sci Ctr 1996; **Fellow:** Gastroenterology, Mayo Clinic 1999; **Fac Appt:** Prof Med, Mayo Med Sch

Gastroenterology

Chey, William D MD [Ge] - **Spec Exp:** Gastrointestinal Motility Disorders; Gastrointestinal Functional Disorders; Inflammatory Bowel Disease; Gastroesophageal Reflux Disease (GERD); **Hospital:** Univ of Michigan Hosp; **Address:** 3912 Taubman Center, SPC5362, Ann Arbor, MI 48109-5362; **Phone:** 734-936-4775; **Board Cert:** Internal Medicine 1989; Gastroenterology 2003; **Med School:** Emory Univ 1986; **Resid:** Internal Medicine, Emory Univ Med Ctr 1989; **Fellow:** Gastroenterology, Univ Mich Hosps 1993; **Fac Appt:** Prof Med, Univ Mich Med Sch

Cominelli, Fabio MD/PhD [Ge] - **Spec Exp:** Inflammatory Bowel Disease/Crohn's; Ulcerative Colitis; **Hospital:** Univ Hosps Case Med Ctr (page 74); **Address:** Univ Hosps Case Med Ctr, Div Gastroenterology, 11100 Euclid Ave, Cleveland, OH 44106-5066; **Phone:** 216-844-7344; **Med School:** Italy 1983; **Resid:** Gastroenterology, Careggi Hosp-Univ Italy 1986; **Fellow:** Gastroenterology, Harbor-UCLA Med Ctr 1989; **Fac Appt:** Prof Med, Case West Res Univ

Craig, Robert M MD [Ge] - **Spec Exp:** Inflammatory Bowel Disease/Crohn's; Liver Disease; Swallowing Disorders; Diarrheal Diseases; **Hospital:** Northwestern Meml Hosp; **Address:** 233 E Erie St, Ste 206, Chicago, IL 60611-5938; **Phone:** 312-908-9644; **Board Cert:** Internal Medicine 1972; Gastroenterology 1975; **Med School:** Northwestern Univ 1967; **Resid:** Internal Medicine, VA Rsch Hosp 1969; Internal Medicine, VA Rsch Hosp 1972; **Fellow:** Gastroenterology, Northwestern Meml Hosp 1974; **Fac Appt:** Prof Med, Northwestern Univ

Crippin, Jeffrey S MD [Ge] - **Spec Exp:** Transplant Medicine-Liver; Liver Disease; Liver Failure; Gastrointestinal Cancer; **Hospital:** Barnes-Jewish Hosp; **Address:** Barnes Jewish Hosp, Div Gastroenterology, 660 S Euclid Ave Campus Box 8124, St Louis, MO 63110; **Phone:** 314-454-8160; **Board Cert:** Internal Medicine 1987; Gastroenterology 2001; Transplant Hepatology 2006; **Med School:** Univ Kansas 1984; **Resid:** Internal Medicine, Kansas Univ Med Ctr 1988; **Fellow:** Gastroenterology, Mayo Clinic 1991; **Fac Appt:** Assoc Prof Med, Washington Univ, St Louis

Di Bisceglie, Adrian M MD [Ge] - **Spec Exp:** Hepatitis C; Hepatitis; Liver Cancer; **Hospital:** St. Louis Univ Hosp; **Address:** St Louis Univ, Div Gastroenterology, 3635 Vista Ave, St Louis, MO 63110; **Phone:** 314-577-6000; **Board Cert:** Internal Medicine 2002; Gastroenterology 2002; **Med School:** South Africa 1977; **Resid:** Internal Medicine, Baragwanath Hosp 1984; **Fellow:** Hepatology, Natl Inst Hlth 1988; **Fac Appt:** Prof Med, St Louis Univ

Early, Dayna S MD [Ge] - **Spec Exp:** Colon & Rectal Cancer Detection; Endoscopic Ultrasound; Endoscopic Therapies; **Hospital:** Barnes-Jewish Hosp, Barnes-Jewish West County Hosp; **Address:** Center for Advanced Medicine, 4921 Parkview Pl Fl 8, Saint Louis, MO 63110; **Phone:** 314-747-2066; **Board Cert:** Internal Medicine 2003; Gastroenterology 2005; **Med School:** Univ MO-Columbia Sch Med 1990; **Resid:** Internal Medicine, Vanderbilt Univ Med Ctr 1993; **Fellow:** Gastroenterology, Vanderbilt Univ Med Ctr 1995; **Fac Appt:** Prof Med, Washington Univ, St Louis

Edmundowicz, Steven A MD [Ge] - **Spec Exp:** Endoscopy; Biliary Disease; Pancreatic Disease; Pancreatic Cancer; **Hospital:** Barnes-Jewish Hosp; **Address:** Washington Univ Sch Med, Div Gastroenterology, 660 S Euclid Ave, Box 8124, St Louis, MO 63110; **Phone:** 314-747-2066; **Board Cert:** Internal Medicine 1986; Gastroenterology 1989; **Med School:** Jefferson Med Coll 1983; **Resid:** Internal Medicine, Barnes Hosp 1986; **Fellow:** Gastroenterology, Barnes Hosp/Wash Univ 1989; **Fac Appt:** Prof Med, Washington Univ, St Louis

Elliott, David MD/PhD [Ge] - **Spec Exp:** Celiac Disease; Inflammatory Bowel Disease/Crohn's; Intestinal Parasites; **Hospital:** Univ Iowa Hosp & Clinics; **Address:** Univ Iowa Hosp, Digestive Disease, 200 Hawkins Drive, rm 4501 JCP, Iowa City, IA 52242; **Phone:** 319-356-4060; **Board Cert:** Internal Medicine 2003; Gastroenterology 2003; **Med School:** Wayne State Univ 1988; **Resid:** Internal Medicine, Johns Hopkins Hosp 1991; **Fellow:** Gastroenterology, Univ Iowa Hosps 1993; **Fac Appt:** Assoc Prof Med, Univ Iowa Coll Med

Elta, Grace H MD [Ge] - **Spec Exp:** Biliary Disease; **Hospital:** Univ of Michigan Hosp; **Address:** Univ Michigan Hlth Sys, 1500 E Med Ctr Drive, 3912 Taubman Ctr, Ann Arbor, MI 48109-0362; **Phone:** 734-647-5944; **Board Cert:** Internal Medicine 1980; Gastroenterology 1983; **Med School:** Univ Mich Med Sch 1977; **Resid:** Internal Medicine, New England Med Ctr 1980; **Fellow:** Gastroenterology, New England Med Ctr 1982; **Fac Appt:** Prof Med, Univ Mich Med Sch

Gholam, Pierre M MD [Ge] - **Spec Exp:** Liver Disease; Transplant Medicine-Liver; **Hospital:** Univ Hosps Case Med Ctr (page 74); **Address:** UH Case Medical Center, 11100 Euclid Ave, WRN-5066, Cleveland, OH 44106; **Phone:** 216-844-5387; **Board Cert:** Gastroenterology 2002; Transplant Hepatology 2006; **Med School:** Lebanon 1996; **Resid:** Internal Medicine, St Lukes-Roosevelt Hosp 1999; **Fellow:** Gastroenterology, St Lukes-Roosevelt Hosp 2002; **Fac Appt:** Asst Prof Med, Case West Res Univ

Goldberg, Michael J MD [Ge] - **Spec Exp:** Colon Cancer; Inflammatory Bowel Disease; Pancreatic & Biliary Disease; Pancreatic/Biliary Endoscopy (ERCP); **Hospital:** Evanston/North Shore Univ Hlth Sys, Glenbrook Hosp-NorthShore Univ Hlth Syst; **Address:** 2650 Ridge Ave, Ste G-208, Evanston, IL 60201; **Phone:** 847-657-1900; **Board Cert:** Internal Medicine 1978; Gastroenterology 1981; **Med School:** Univ IL Coll Med 1975; **Resid:** Internal Medicine, Univ Illinois Hosp 1978; **Fellow:** Gastroenterology, Tufts-New England Med Ctr 1980; **Fac Appt:** Assoc Clin Prof Med, Northwestern Univ

Gostout, Christopher MD [Ge] - **Spec Exp:** Gastroscopy; Endoscopy; **Hospital:** Mayo Med Ctr & Clin - Rochester; **Address:** Mayo Clin, Div GI, 200 First St SW, Mayo Bldg Fl 9, Rochester, MN 55905; **Phone:** 507-284-2141; **Board Cert:** Internal Medicine 1979; Gastroenterology 1981; **Med School:** SUNY Downstate 1976; **Resid:** Internal Medicine, Mayo Clin 1979; **Fellow:** Gastroenterology, Mayo Clin 1981

Hanauer, Stephen B MD [Ge] - **Spec Exp:** Inflammatory Bowel Disease; Crohn's Disease; Ulcerative Colitis; Clinical Trials; **Hospital:** Univ of Chicago Med Ctr; **Address:** Univ Chicago Hosps, 5758 S Maryland Ave, MC 4076, Chicago, IL 60637-1426; **Phone:** 773-702-1466; **Board Cert:** Internal Medicine 1980; Gastroenterology 2010; **Med School:** Univ IL Coll Med 1977; **Resid:** Internal Medicine, Univ Chicago Hosps 1980; **Fellow:** Gastroenterology, Univ Chicago Hosps 1982; **Fac Appt:** Prof Med, Univ Chicago-Pritzker Sch Med

Jensen, Donald M MD [Ge] - **Spec Exp:** Transplant Medicine-Liver; Hepatitis C; Liver & Biliary Disease; Liver Cancer; **Hospital:** Univ of Chicago Med Ctr; **Address:** Univ of Chicago, Ctr for Liver Disease, 5841 S Maryland Ave, MC 7120, Chicago, IL 60637; **Phone:** 773-702-2300; **Board Cert:** Internal Medicine 1975; Gastroenterology 1981; **Med School:** Univ IL Coll Med 1972; **Resid:** Internal Medicine, Rush Presby St Lukes Hosp 1975; Gastroenterology, Rush Presby St Lukes Hosp 1976; **Fellow:** Gastroenterology, King's Coll Hosp 1978; **Fac Appt:** Prof Med, Univ Chicago-Pritzker Sch Med

Kahrilas, Peter J MD [Ge] - **Spec Exp:** Esophageal Disorders; Swallowing Disorders; **Hospital:** Northwestern Meml Hosp; **Address:** 675 N St Clair Fl 17 - Ste 250, Chicago, IL 60611; **Phone:** 312-695-5620; **Board Cert:** Internal Medicine 1982; Gastroenterology 1987; **Med School:** Univ Rochester 1979; **Resid:** Internal Medicine, Univ Hosp 1982; **Fellow:** Gastroenterology, Northwestern Meml Hosp 1984; Research, Med Coll Wisconsin 1986; **Fac Appt:** Prof Med, Northwestern Univ

Konicek, Frank J MD [Ge] - **Spec Exp:** Endoscopy; Inflammatory Bowel Disease/Crohn's; Pancreatic Disease; Liver Disease; **Hospital:** Swedish Covenant Hosp, Adv Illinois Masonic Med Ctr; **Address:** 3004 N Ashland Ave, Chicago, IL 60657-3012; **Phone:** 773-871-4600; **Board Cert:** Internal Medicine 1977; Gastroenterology 1975; **Med School:** Loyola Univ-Stritch Sch Med 1963; **Resid:** Internal Medicine, St Francis Hosp 1965; Internal Medicine, Hines VA Hosp 1969; **Fellow:** Gastroenterology, Hines VA Hosp 1971; **Fac Appt:** Clin Prof Med, Loyola Univ-Stritch Sch Med

Gastroenterology

Kwo, Paul Y MD [Ge] - **Spec Exp:** Hepatitis B & C; Transplant Medicine-Liver; Liver Disease; **Hospital:** IU Health University Hosp; **Address:** 975 W Walnut St, IB327, Indianapolis, IN 46202-5181; **Phone:** 317-274-3090; **Board Cert:** Gastroenterology 2005; Transplant Hepatology 2006; **Med School:** Wayne State Univ 1988; **Resid:** Internal Medicine, Univ Maryland Med Ctr 1991; **Fellow:** Gastroenterology, Mayo Clinic 1995; **Fac Appt:** Assoc Prof Med, Indiana Univ

La Russo, Nicholas F MD [Ge] - **Spec Exp:** Transplant Medicine-Liver; Liver & Biliary Disease; **Hospital:** Mayo Med Ctr & Clin - Rochester; **Address:** Mayo Clinic, Div Gastroenterology, 200 First St SW, Mayo Bldg Fl 9, Rochester, MN 55905; **Phone:** 507-284-2141; **Board Cert:** Internal Medicine 1972; Gastroenterology 1979; **Med School:** NY Med Coll 1969; **Resid:** Internal Medicine, Mayo Clinic 1972; **Fellow:** Gastroenterology, Mayo Clinic 1975; **Fac Appt:** Prof Med, Mayo Med Sch

Lashner, Bret A MD [Ge] - **Spec Exp:** Inflammatory Bowel Disease; **Hospital:** Cleveland Clin (page 56); **Address:** 9500 Euclid Ave, MC A-31, Cleveland, OH 44195; **Phone:** 216-444-6536; **Board Cert:** Internal Medicine 1983; Gastroenterology 1985; **Med School:** NYU Sch Med 1980; **Resid:** Internal Medicine, Temple Univ Hosp 1983; **Fellow:** Gastroenterology, Univ Chicago Hosps 1986; **Fac Appt:** Assoc Prof Med, Case West Res Univ

Lindor, Keith MD [Ge] - **Spec Exp:** Liver Disease; Biliary Disease; **Hospital:** Mayo Med Ctr & Clin - Rochester; **Address:** Mayo Clinic, Div Gastroenterology, 200 First St SW, Mayo Bldg Fl 9, Rochester, MN 55905; **Phone:** 507-284-2141; **Board Cert:** Internal Medicine 1982; Gastroenterology 1987; **Med School:** Mayo Med Sch 1979; **Resid:** Internal Medicine, N Carolina Baptist Hosp 1982; **Fellow:** Gastroenterology, Mayo Clin 1986; **Fac Appt:** Prof Med, Mayo Med Sch

Loftus Jr, Edward V MD [Ge] - **Spec Exp:** Inflammatory Bowel Disease; Crohn's Disease; Ulcerative Colitis; Microscopic Colitis; **Hospital:** Mayo Med Ctr & Clin - Rochester; **Address:** Mayo Clinic, Div Gastroenterology, 200 First St SW, Mayo Bldg Fl 9, Rochester, MN 55905; **Phone:** 507-284-2141; **Board Cert:** Internal Medicine 2003; Gastroenterology 2005; **Med School:** Univ Pennsylvania 1988; **Resid:** Internal Medicine, Temple Univ Hosp 1991; **Fellow:** Gastroenterology, Mayo Clinic 1995; **Fac Appt:** Prof Med, Mayo Med Sch

Lucey, Michael R MD [Ge] - **Spec Exp:** Liver Disease; Transplant Medicine-Liver; **Hospital:** Univ WI Hosp & Clins; **Address:** Univ Wisc Hosps & Clins, 1685 Highland Ave, Centennial Bldg Fl 4, Madison, WI 53705-2281; **Phone:** 608-263-7322; **Board Cert:** Internal Medicine 2001; Gastroenterology 2001; Transplant Hepatology 2006; **Med School:** Ireland 1980; **Resid:** Gastroenterology, St Bartholomews Hosp/Kings Coll Hosp 1983; Hepatology, Kings Coll Hosp 1985; **Fellow:** Gastroenterology, Univ Michigan Med Ctr 1987; **Fac Appt:** Prof Med, Univ Wisc

Meiselman, Mick S MD [Ge] - **Spec Exp:** Pancreatic & Biliary Disease; Barrett's Esophagus; Endoscopic Ultrasound; Colonoscopy; **Hospital:** Evanston/North Shore Univ Hlth Sys, Glenbrook Hosp-NorthShore Univ Hlth Syst; **Address:** 1000 Central St, Ste 800, Evanston, IL 60201; **Phone:** 847-570-2030; **Board Cert:** Internal Medicine 1982; Gastroenterology 1985; **Med School:** Northwestern Univ 1979; **Resid:** Internal Medicine, Cedars-Sinai/UCLA 1982; **Fellow:** Gastroenterology, UCSF Med Ctr 1984; **Fac Appt:** Asst Clin Prof Med, Univ Chicago-Pritzker Sch Med

Murray, Joseph A MD [Ge] - **Spec Exp:** Celiac Disease; Esophageal Disorders; **Hospital:** Mayo Med Ctr & Clin - Rochester; **Address:** Mayo Clinic, Div Gastroenterology, 200 First St SW, Mayo Bldg Fl 9, Rochester, MN 55905; **Phone:** 507-284-2141; **Board Cert:** Internal Medicine 2009; Gastroenterology 2000; **Med School:** Ireland 1983; **Resid:** Internal Medicine, St Laurences Hosp 1986; Gastroenterology, Beaumont Hosp 1988; **Fellow:** Gastroenterology, Univ Iowa Hosps & Clins 1990; **Fac Appt:** Prof Med, Mayo Med Sch

Owyang, Chung MD [Ge] - **Spec Exp:** Gastrointestinal Motility Disorders; Digestive Disorders; **Hospital:** Univ of Michigan Hosp; **Address:** Univ Mich, Div Gastroenterology, 1500 E Med Ctr Dr, Rm 3912 Taubman Ctr, Ann Arbor, MI 48109-0362; **Phone:** 734-647-5944; **Board Cert:** Internal Medicine 1976; Gastroenterology 1981; **Med School:** McGill Univ 1972; **Resid:** Internal Medicine, Montreal Genl Hosp 1975; **Fellow:** Gastroenterology, Mayo Grad Med Sch 1978; **Fac Appt:** Prof Med, Univ Mich Med Sch

Reichelderfer, Mark MD [Ge] - **Spec Exp:** Endoscopy; Inflammatory Bowel Disease; **Hospital:** Univ WI Hosp & Clins; **Address:** 1685 Highland Ave, Centennial Bldg Fl 4, Madison, WI 53705-2281; **Phone:** 608-263-4033; **Board Cert:** Internal Medicine 1977; Gastroenterology 1979; **Med School:** Columbia P&S 1974; **Resid:** Internal Medicine, Mary Imogene Bassett Hosp 1977; **Fellow:** Gastroenterology, Univ Wisc Hosps & Clin 1979; **Fac Appt:** Prof Med, Univ Wisc

Rex, Douglas K MD [Ge] - **Spec Exp:** Endoscopy; Endoscopic Ultrasound; Colon & Rectal Cancer Detection; Inflammatory Bowel Disease; **Hospital:** IU Health University Hosp; **Address:** Indiana Univ Hosp, Ste 4100, 550 N University Blvd, Indianapolis, IN 46202; **Phone:** 317-948-9763; **Board Cert:** Internal Medicine 1985; Gastroenterology 1987; **Med School:** Indiana Univ 1980; **Resid:** Internal Medicine, Indiana Univ Med Ctr 1982; Internal Medicine, Indiana Univ Hosp 1985; **Fellow:** Gastroenterology, Indiana Univ Med Ctr 1984; **Fac Appt:** Prof Med, Indiana Univ

Schulze, Konrad S MD [Ge] - **Spec Exp:** Gastroesophageal Reflux Disease (GERD); Peptic Acid Disorders; Gastroparesis; **Hospital:** Univ Iowa Hosp & Clinics; **Address:** UIHC, Dept Gastroenterology, 200 Hawkins Drive, rm 4501 JCPP, Iowa City, IA 52242; **Phone:** 319-356-4060; **Board Cert:** Internal Medicine 1987; Gastroenterology 1975; **Med School:** Germany 1968; **Resid:** Psychiatry, Boston City Hosp 1971; Internal Medicine, Montreal Genl Hosp 1974; **Fellow:** Gastroenterology, Univ Iowa 1977; **Fac Appt:** Prof Med, Univ Iowa Coll Med

Semrad, Carol E MD [Ge] - **Spec Exp:** Celiac Disease; Diarrheal Diseases; Malabsorption Syndrome; Nutrition; **Hospital:** Univ of Chicago Med Ctr; **Address:** 5841 S Maryland Ave, MC 4080.S401, Chicago, IL 60637; **Phone:** 773-702-6921; **Board Cert:** Internal Medicine 1985; Gastroenterology 1987; **Med School:** Columbia P&S 1982; **Resid:** Internal Medicine, Columbia-Presby Med Ctr 1985; **Fellow:** Gastroenterology, Columbia-Presby Med Ctr 1986; **Fac Appt:** Assoc Prof Med, Univ Chicago-Pritzker Sch Med

Shaker, Reza MD [Ge] - **Spec Exp:** Swallowing Disorders; Gastrointestinal Motility Disorders; Gastroesophageal Reflux Disease (GERD); Pancreatic/Biliary Endoscopy (ERCP); **Hospital:** Froedtert and Med Ctr of WI, Wm S Middleton Mem Vet Hosp-Madison; **Address:** Med Coll Wisconsin/Gastroenterology, 9200 W Wisconsin Ave, rm E4510, Milwaukee, WI 53226; **Phone:** 414-955-6840; **Med School:** Iran 1975; **Resid:** Internal Medicine, Kingsbrook Jewish Med Ctr 1985; **Fellow:** Gastroenterology, Med Coll Wisconsin 1988; **Fac Appt:** Prof Med, Univ Wisc

Sherman, Stuart MD [Ge] - **Spec Exp:** Pancreatic & Biliary Disease; Endoscopy; Pancreatic/Biliary Endoscopy (ERCP); **Hospital:** IU Health University Hosp; **Address:** Indiana Univ Hosp, rm 4100, 550 N University Blvd, Indianapolis, IN 46202; **Phone:** 317-944-0925; **Board Cert:** Internal Medicine 1985; Gastroenterology 1989; **Med School:** Washington Univ, St Louis 1982; **Resid:** Internal Medicine, Presby Univ Hosp 1985; **Fellow:** Gastroenterology, UCLA Med Ctr 1989; **Fac Appt:** Prof Med, Indiana Univ

Silverman, William B MD [Ge] - **Spec Exp:** Pancreatic/Biliary Endoscopy (ERCP); Liver Disease; **Hospital:** Univ Iowa Hosp & Clinics; **Address:** UIHC, Div GI/Hepatology, 200 Hawkins Drive, rm 4553 JCP, Iowa City, IA 52242; **Phone:** 319-356-4060; **Board Cert:** Internal Medicine 1988; Gastroenterology 2008; **Med School:** Belgium 1984; **Resid:** Internal Medicine, Lutheran General Hosp 1987; **Fellow:** Gastroenterology, Case Western Res Univ 1989; Gastroenterology, Indiana Univ Hosp 1990; **Fac Appt:** Prof Med, Univ Iowa Coll Med

Te, Helen MD [Ge] - **Spec Exp:** Liver Disease; Transplant Medicine-Liver; Hepatitis; **Hospital:** Univ of Chicago Med Ctr; **Address:** 5841 S Maryland Ave, MC 4076, Chicago, IL 60637; **Phone:** 773-702-2395; **Board Cert:** Internal Medicine 2006; Gastroenterology 2001; Transplant Hepatology 2006; **Med School:** Philippines 1992; **Resid:** Internal Medicine, Rush Presby Hosp 1996; **Fellow:** Gastroenterology, Univ Chicago Hosp 2000; **Fac Appt:** Assoc Prof Med, Univ Chicago-Pritzker Sch Med

Tremaine, William J MD [Ge] - **Spec Exp:** Inflammatory Bowel Disease/Crohn's; Ulcerative Colitis; Irritable Bowel Syndrome; **Hospital:** Mayo Med Ctr & Clin - Rochester, St. Mary's Hosp - Rochester MN (Mayo); **Address:** Mayo Clin, Div Gastroenterology, 200 First St SW, Mayo E-9, Rochester, MN 55905; **Phone:** 507-284-2468; **Board Cert:** Internal Medicine 1979; Gastroenterology 1981; **Med School:** Univ Miss 1976; **Resid:** Internal Medicine, Mayo Clin 1980; **Fellow:** Gastroenterology, Mayo Clin 1981; **Fac Appt:** Prof Med, Mayo Med Sch

Van Thiel, David H MD [Ge] - **Spec Exp:** Transplant Medicine-Liver; Hepatitis; Liver Disease; **Hospital:** Rush Univ Med Ctr; **Address:** Rush Univ Hepatologists, 1725 W Harrison Rd, Ste 158, Chicago, IL 60612; **Phone:** 312-942-8910; **Board Cert:** Internal Medicine 1972; Gastroenterology 1975; Transplant Hepatology 2008; **Med School:** UCLA 1967; **Resid:** Internal Medicine, NY Hosp 1969; Internal Medicine, Univ Hosp 1972; **Fellow:** Gastroenterology, Univ Hosp 1974; Research, NIH 1976; **Fac Appt:** Prof Med, Loyola Univ-Stritch Sch Med

Vargo, John J MD [Ge] - **Spec Exp:** Endoscopy; Barrett's Esophagus; Pancreatic/Biliary Endoscopy (ERCP); Pancreatic Disease; **Hospital:** Cleveland Clin (page 56); **Address:** Cleveland Clinic, 9500 Euclid Ave, MC A-31, Cleveland, OH 44195; **Phone:** 216-445-5012; **Board Cert:** Internal Medicine 1988; Gastroenterology 2001; **Med School:** Univ Rochester 1985; **Resid:** Internal Medicine, Montefiore Hosp 1988; **Fellow:** Gastroenterology, Cleveland Clinic 2000; **Fac Appt:** Assoc Prof Med, Case West Res Univ

Vege, Santhi S MD [Ge] - **Spec Exp:** Pancreatic Disease; **Hospital:** Mayo Med Ctr & Clin - Rochester; **Address:** Mayo Clinic-Div Gastroenterology, 200 First St SW, Mayo Bldg Fl 9, Rochester, MN 55905; **Phone:** 507-284-2141; **Board Cert:** Internal Medicine 2007; **Med School:** India 1975; **Resid:** Internal Medicine, Govt Genl Hosp 1978; Internal Medicine, Mayo Clin 1997; **Fellow:** Gastroenterology, Post Grad Inst 1981; Gastroenterology, Mayo Clin 1998; **Fac Appt:** Prof Med, Mayo Med Sch

Wald, Arnold MD [Ge] - **Spec Exp:** Constipation; Gastrointestinal Motility Disorders; Irritable Bowel Syndrome; Incontinence-Fecal; **Hospital:** Univ WI Hosp & Clins; **Address:** 1685 Highland Ave, Centennial Bldg Fl 4, Madison, WI 53705-2281; **Phone:** 608-263-1995; **Board Cert:** Internal Medicine 1972; Gastroenterology 1975; **Med School:** SUNY Downstate 1968; **Resid:** Internal Medicine, SUNY - Downstate Med Ctr 1971; **Fellow:** Gastroenterology, Johns Hopkins Hosp 1975; **Fac Appt:** Prof Med, Univ Wisc

Waxman, Irving MD [Ge] - **Spec Exp:** Gastrointestinal Cancer; Pancreatic Cancer; Endoscopy; Interventional Endoscopy; **Hospital:** Univ of Chicago Med Ctr; **Address:** 5758 S Maryland Ave, MS MC 9028, Chicago, IL 60637; **Phone:** 773-702-1459; **Board Cert:** Internal Medicine 1988; Gastroenterology 2003; **Med School:** Mexico 1985; **Resid:** Internal Medicine, New Eng Deaconess Hosp 1988; **Fellow:** Gastroenterology, Georgetown Univ Med Ctr 1991; Endoscopy, Univ Academic Med Ctr 1991; **Fac Appt:** Prof Med, Univ Chicago-Pritzker Sch Med

Wiesner, Russell H MD [Ge] - **Spec Exp:** Transplant Medicine-Liver; **Hospital:** Mayo Med Ctr & Clin - Rochester; **Address:** Mayo Clinic-Div Gastroenterology, 200 First St SW, Mayo Bldg Fl 9, Rochester, MN 55905; **Phone:** 507-284-2141; **Board Cert:** Internal Medicine 1978; Gastroenterology 1981; **Med School:** Med Coll Wisc 1975; **Resid:** Internal Medicine, Mayo Clin 1978

Wolfe, M Michael MD [Ge] - **Hospital:** MetroHealth Med Ctr; **Address:** MetroHealth Med Ctr, Dept Medicine, 2500 MetroHealth Drive, rm G-575, Cleveland, OH 44109; **Phone:** 216-778-8266; **Board Cert:** Internal Medicine 1979; Gastroenterology 1981; **Med School:** Ohio State Univ 1976; **Resid:** Internal Medicine, Med Coll Penn Hosp 1979; **Fellow:** Gastroenterology, Univ Florida Hosps 1982; **Fac Appt:** Prof Med, Case West Res Univ

Great Plains and Mountains

Bjorkman, David MD [Ge] - **Spec Exp:** Peptic Acid Disorders; Endoscopy; **Hospital:** Univ Utah Hlth Care; **Address:** 30 N 1900 East, Salt Lake City, UT 84132; **Phone:** 801-581-6436; **Board Cert:** Internal Medicine 1983; Gastroenterology 1985; **Med School:** Univ Utah 1980; **Resid:** Internal Medicine, Brigham & Women's Harvard 1983; **Fellow:** Gastroenterology, Brigham & Women's Harvard 1985; **Fac Appt:** Prof Med, Univ Utah

Burt, Randall W MD [Ge] - **Spec Exp:** Colon Cancer; Colon & Rectal Cancer-Familial Polyposis; **Hospital:** Univ Utah Hlth Care; **Address:** Huntsman Cancer Inst, 2000 Circle of Hope, Salt Lake City, UT 84112; **Phone:** 801-585-3281; **Board Cert:** Internal Medicine 1977; Gastroenterology 1979; **Med School:** Univ Utah 1974; **Resid:** Internal Medicine, Barnes Hosp 1977; **Fellow:** Gastroenterology, Univ Utah Med Ctr 1979; **Fac Appt:** Prof Med, Univ Utah

Everson, Gregory T MD [Ge] - **Spec Exp:** Liver Disease; Hepatitis; Transplant Medicine-Liver; **Hospital:** Univ of CO Hosp - Anschutz Inpatient Pav; **Address:** Univ Colorado-Denver, 1635 Aurora Ct, MS B-154, Aurora, CO 80045; **Phone:** 720-848-2245; **Board Cert:** Internal Medicine 1979; Gastroenterology 1983; Transplant Hepatology 2006; **Med School:** Cornell Univ-Weill Med Coll 1976; **Resid:** Internal Medicine, Creighton Univ Med Ctr 1979; **Fellow:** Gastroenterology, Univ Colorado Health Sci Ctr 1982; **Fac Appt:** Prof Med, Univ Colorado

Fang, John C MD [Ge] - **Spec Exp:** Endoscopy; Esophageal Disorders; Irritable Bowel Syndrome; Barrett's Esophagus; **Hospital:** Univ Utah Hlth Care; **Address:** 50 N Med Drive, Clinic 3, Salt Lake City, UT 84132; **Phone:** 801-581-2215; **Board Cert:** Gastroenterology 2008; **Med School:** Washington Univ, St Louis 1989; **Resid:** Internal Medicine, Temple Univ Hosp 1992; **Fellow:** Gastroenterology, Univ VA Hlth Sci Ctr 1995; **Fac Appt:** Assoc Prof Med, Univ Utah

Hunter, Ellen B MD [Ge] - **Spec Exp:** Hepatitis; **Hospital:** St. Luke's Boise Med Ctr; **Address:** 425 W Vannock St, Boise, ID 83702; **Phone:** 208-343-6458; **Board Cert:** Internal Medicine 1986; Gastroenterology 1989; **Med School:** Georgetown Univ 1983; **Resid:** Internal Medicine, Vanderbilt Univ Med Ctr 1986; **Fellow:** Gastroenterology, Mayo Clinic 1989

Sorrell, Michael MD [Ge] - **Spec Exp:** Transplant Medicine-Liver; Hepatitis; Liver Tumors; Liver Disease; **Hospital:** Nebraska Med Ctr; **Address:** 983285 Nebraska Medical Ctr, Omaha, NE 68198-3285; **Phone:** 402-559-7912; **Board Cert:** Internal Medicine 1972; **Med School:** Univ Nebr Coll Med 1959; **Resid:** Internal Medicine, Univ Nebraska Hosp 1968; Gastroenterology, Univ Nebraska Hosp 1969; **Fellow:** Hepatology, New Jersey Coll Med 1971; **Fac Appt:** Prof Med, Univ Nebr Coll Med

Young, Renee L MD [Ge] - **Spec Exp:** Inflammatory Bowel Disease; Crohn's Disease; **Hospital:** Nebraska Med Ctr; **Address:** Univ Nebraska Medical Ctr, 982000 NMC, Omaha, NE 68198-2000; **Phone:** 404-559-6209; **Board Cert:** Internal Medicine 1986; Gastroenterology 2001; **Med School:** Univ Nebr Coll Med 1983; **Resid:** Internal Medicine, Univ Nebraska Med Ctr 1986; **Fellow:** Gastroenterology, Univ Nebraska Med Ctr 1990; **Fac Appt:** Assoc Prof Med, Univ Nebr Coll Med

Gastroenterology

Southwest

Anderson, Karl MD [Ge] - **Spec Exp:** Porphyria; Liver Disease; **Hospital:** UT Med Br at Galveston; **Address:** 301 University Blvd, Galveston, TX 77555-1109; **Phone:** 409-747-6880; **Board Cert:** Internal Medicine 1972; Gastroenterology 1972; **Med School:** Johns Hopkins Univ 1965; **Resid:** Internal Medicine, Vanderbilt Univ Hosp 1967; Internal Medicine, New York Hosp-Cornell Med Ctr 1968; **Fellow:** Gastroenterology, New York Hosp-Cornell Med Ctr 1970; **Fac Appt:** Prof Med, Univ Tex Med Br, Galveston

Balart Jr, Luis A MD [Ge] - **Spec Exp:** Hepatitis C; Liver Disease; **Hospital:** Tulane Med Ctr; **Address:** Tulane Gastroenterology, 1430 Tulane Ave, SL35, New Orleans, LA 70112; **Phone:** 504-988-5800; **Board Cert:** Internal Medicine 1976; Gastroenterology 1981; **Med School:** Cuba 1973; **Resid:** Internal Medicine, Naval Regl Med Ctr 1976; **Fellow:** Gastroenterology, Ochsner Medical Fdn 1981; Hepatology, Ranchos Amigos Hosp-USC 1982; **Fac Appt:** Prof Med, Tulane Univ

Boland, C Richard MD [Ge] - **Spec Exp:** Colon & Rectal Cancer Detection; Cancer Genetics; **Hospital:** Baylor Univ Medical Ctr-Dallas; **Address:** GI Cancer Rsch Lab H-250, 3500 Gaston Ave, Dallas, TX 75246; **Phone:** 214-820-2692; **Board Cert:** Internal Medicine 1978; Gastroenterology 1981; **Med School:** Yale Univ 1973; **Resid:** Internal Medicine, USPHS Hosp 1978; **Fellow:** Gastroenterology, UCSF Med Ctr 1981; **Fac Appt:** Clin Prof Med, Univ Tex SW, Dallas

Boyer, Thomas D MD [Ge] - **Spec Exp:** Liver Disease; Hepatitis; Transplant Medicine-Liver; **Hospital:** Univ Med Ctr - Tucson; **Address:** Arizona Liver Institute, 1501 N Campbell Ave, Box 245136, Tucson, AZ 85724; **Phone:** 520-626-5952; **Board Cert:** Internal Medicine 1975; Gastroenterology 1977; Transplant Hepatology 2008; **Med School:** USC Sch Med 1969; **Resid:** Internal Medicine, LAC-USC Med Ctr 1974; **Fellow:** Hepatology, USC 1976; **Fac Appt:** Prof Med, Univ Ariz Coll Med

Bresalier, Robert MD [Ge] - **Spec Exp:** Gastrointestinal Cancer; Peptic Acid Disorders; **Hospital:** UT MD Anderson Cancer Ctr; **Address:** MD Anderson Canc Ctr, GI Med & Nutrition, 1515 Holcombe Blvd - Unit 1466, Houston, TX 77030; **Phone:** 713-745-4340; **Board Cert:** Internal Medicine 1981; Gastroenterology 1983; **Med School:** Univ Chicago-Pritzker Sch Med 1978; **Resid:** Internal Medicine, Barnes Hosp-Washington Univ 1981; **Fellow:** Gastroenterology, UCSF Med Ctr 1983; **Fac Appt:** Prof Med, Univ Tex, Houston

Bulat, Robert S MD [Ge] - **Hospital:** Tulane Med Ctr; **Address:** Tulane Univ Med Ctr, 1415 Tulane Ave, New Orleans, LA 70112; **Phone:** 504-988-3075; **Board Cert:** Internal Medicine 1995; Gastroenterology 2010; **Med School:** McMaster Univ 1990; **Resid:** Internal Medicine, Univ Toronto Med Ctr 1993; **Fellow:** Gastroenterology, McMaster Univ 1995; Gastroenterology, McMaster Univ 1997; **Fac Appt:** Prof Med, Tulane Univ

Cunningham, John T MD [Ge] - **Spec Exp:** Pancreatic Cancer; Biliary Disease; Pancreatic/Biliary Endoscopy (ERCP); **Hospital:** Univ Med Ctr - Tucson; **Address:** Univ Medical Ctr, Div Gastroenterology, 1501 N Campbell Ave, PO Box 245028, Tucson, AZ 85724-5028; **Phone:** 520-626-0195; **Board Cert:** Internal Medicine 1975; Gastroenterology 1977; **Med School:** Med Coll VA 1970; **Resid:** Internal Medicine, Med Univ S Carolina Affil Hosp 1975; **Fellow:** Gastroenterology, Med Univ S Carolina 1977; **Fac Appt:** Prof Med, Univ Ariz Coll Med

Das, Ananya MD [Ge] - **Spec Exp:** Endoscopy; Endoscopic Ultrasound; Pancreatic/Biliary Endoscopy (ERCP); Gastrointestinal Cancer; **Hospital:** Mercy Gilbert Med Ctr; **Address:** Arizona Ctr for Digestive Hlth, 2680 S Val Vista Drive, Ste 116, Gilbert, AZ 85295; **Phone:** 480-507-5678; **Board Cert:** Gastroenterology 1998; **Med School:** India 1987; **Resid:** Internal Medicine, SUNY Hlth Sci Ctr 1996; **Fellow:** Gastroenterology, Cleveland Clinic 1998; Endoscopy, Cleveland Clinic 2000; **Fac Appt:** Prof Med, Mayo Med Sch

America's Top Doctors® 11th Edition

Davis, Gary L MD [Ge] - **Spec Exp:** Liver Disease; Hepatitis; Transplant Medicine-Liver; **Hospital:** Baylor Univ Medical Ctr-Dallas; **Address:** 3410 Worth St Fl 8 - Ste 860, Transplant Services Dept, Dallas, TX 75246; **Phone:** 214-820-8500; **Board Cert:** Internal Medicine 1979; Gastroenterology 1983; **Med School:** Univ Minn 1976; **Resid:** Internal Medicine, Mayo Clinic 1979; **Fellow:** Gastroenterology, Mayo Clinic 1981; Hepatology, Natl Inst Hlth 1984; **Fac Appt:** Prof Med, Baylor Coll Med

Decker, Gustav Anton MD [Ge] - **Spec Exp:** Endoscopy; Obesity; Pancreatic Disease; Pancreatic Cancer; **Hospital:** Mayo Clinic - Scottsdale; **Address:** Mayo Clinic, Div Gastroenterology, 13400 E Shea Blvd Fl 2, Scottsdale, AZ 85259; **Phone:** 480-301-6990; **Board Cert:** Internal Medicine 1999; Gastroenterology 2003; **Med School:** South Africa 1993; **Resid:** Internal Medicine, Mayo Clinic 1999; **Fellow:** Gastroenterology, Mayo Clinic 2002; **Fac Appt:** Asst Prof Med, Mayo Med Sch

Faigel, Douglas O MD [Ge] - **Spec Exp:** Endoscopic Ultrasound; Pancreatic/Biliary Endoscopy (ERCP); Gastrointestinal Cancer; Pancreatic & Biliary Disease; **Hospital:** Mayo Clinic - Scottsdale; **Address:** Mayo Clinic, Dept Gastroenterology, 13400 E Shea Blvd Fl 2, Scottsdale, AZ 85259; **Phone:** 480-301-6990; **Board Cert:** Internal Medicine 2003; Gastroenterology 2005; **Med School:** Univ Pennsylvania 1990; **Resid:** Internal Medicine, UCSF Med Ctr 1993; **Fellow:** Gastroenterology, Hosp Univ Penn 1995

Fallon, Michael B MD [Ge] - **Spec Exp:** Liver Disease; Hepatitis C; **Hospital:** Meml Hermann Meml City Hosp; **Address:** Univ TX Professional Blg, 6411 Fannin, Ste J400, Houston, TX 77030; **Phone:** 713-704-6800; **Board Cert:** Internal Medicine 1988; Gastroenterology 2001; Transplant Hepatology 2008; **Med School:** Univ VA Sch Med 1984; **Resid:** Internal Medicine, Yale-New Haven Hosp 1988; **Fellow:** Gastroenterology, Yale-New Haven Hosp 1990; **Fac Appt:** Assoc Prof Med, Univ Alabama

Fleischer, David MD [Ge] - **Spec Exp:** Barrett's Esophagus; Esophageal Cancer; **Hospital:** Mayo Clinic - Scottsdale; **Address:** Mayo Clinic - Scottsdale, 13400 E Shea Blvd, Div Gastroenterology 2A, Scottsdale, AZ 85259; **Phone:** 480-301-8484; **Board Cert:** Internal Medicine 1975; Gastroenterology 1977; **Med School:** Vanderbilt Univ 1970; **Resid:** Internal Medicine, Metro General Hosp 1975; **Fellow:** Gastroenterology, LA Co Harbor-UCLA Med Ctr 1977; **Fac Appt:** Prof Med, Mayo Med Sch

Galati, Joseph S MD [Ge] - **Spec Exp:** Liver Disease; Transplant Medicine-Liver; Hepatitis C; Liver Cancer; **Hospital:** Methodist Hosp - Houston, St. Luke's Episcopal Hosp-Houston; **Address:** 6624 Fannin St, Ste 1990, Houston, TX 77030; **Phone:** 713-794-0700; **Board Cert:** Gastroenterology 2005; **Med School:** Grenada 1987; **Resid:** Internal Medicine, SUNY Hlth Sci Ctr-Kings Co Hosp 1991; **Fellow:** Gastroenterology, Univ Nebraska 1994; Transplant Hepatology, Univ Nebraska 1994; **Fac Appt:** Asst Prof Med, Univ Tex, Houston

Glombicki, Alan Paul MD [Ge] - **Spec Exp:** Hepatitis; Transplant Medicine-Liver; Digestive Disorders; **Hospital:** St. Luke's Episcopal Hosp-Houston, Meml Hermann Hosp - Texas Med Ctr; **Address:** 7737 SW Freeway, Ste 840, Houston, TX 77074; **Phone:** 713-777-2555; **Board Cert:** Internal Medicine 1986; Gastroenterology 1987; **Med School:** Univ IL Coll Med 1981; **Resid:** Internal Medicine, Baylor Coll Med 1984; Hepatology, Baylor Coll Med 1987; **Fellow:** Gastroenterology, Baylor Coll Med 1986; **Fac Appt:** Assoc Prof Med, Univ Tex, Houston

Leighton, Jonathan A MD [Ge] - **Spec Exp:** Capsule Endoscopy; Inflammatory Bowel Disease/Crohn's; Ulcerative Colitis; **Hospital:** Mayo Clinic - Scottsdale; **Address:** Mayo Clinic-Scottsdale, 13400 E Shea Blvd, Scottsdale, AZ 85259; **Phone:** 480-301-8000; **Board Cert:** Internal Medicine 1984; Gastroenterology 2001; **Med School:** Univ Ariz Coll Med 1981; **Resid:** Internal Medicine, UTSA Affil Hosp 1984; **Fellow:** Gastroenterology, Univ Texas Hlth Sci Ctr; **Fac Appt:** Assoc Prof Med, Mayo Med Sch

Gastroenterology

Raju, Gottumukkala S MD [Ge] - **Spec Exp:** Colon Cancer; **Hospital:** UT MD Anderson Cancer Ctr; **Address:** UT MD Anderson Cancer Center, 1515 Holcombe Blvd, Box 338, Unit 1466, Houston, TX 77030; **Phone:** 713-792-2330; **Board Cert:** Gastroenterology 2007; **Med School:** India 1986; **Resid:** Internal Medicine, Cleveland Clin 1995; **Fellow:** Gastroenterology, Univ Iowa Hosp & Clin 1997; Endoscopy, Beth Israel & Deaconess Ctr 1998; **Fac Appt:** Prof Med, Univ Tex, Houston

Schiller, Lawrence R MD [Ge] - **Spec Exp:** Diarrheal Diseases; Gastrointestinal Functional Disorders; Gastrointestinal Motility Disorders; **Hospital:** Baylor Univ Medical Ctr-Dallas; **Address:** Digestive Associates of Texas, 712 N Washington Ave, Ste 200, Dallas, TX 75246; **Phone:** 214-545-3990; **Board Cert:** Internal Medicine 1976; Gastroenterology 1981; **Med School:** Jefferson Med Coll 1972; **Resid:** Internal Medicine, Temple Univ Hosp 1976; **Fellow:** Gastroenterology, Univ Texas Hlth Sci Ctr 1980; **Fac Appt:** Clin Prof Med, Univ Tex SW, Dallas

Speeg, Kermit V MD/PhD [Ge] - **Spec Exp:** Transplant Medicine-Liver; **Hospital:** Univ Hlth Syst-San Antonio; **Address:** Dept Gastroenterology, 7703 Floyd Curl Drive, MC 7878, San Antonio, TX 78229-3900; **Phone:** 210-567-4879; **Board Cert:** Internal Medicine 1976; **Med School:** Univ Tex SW, Dallas 1972; **Resid:** Internal Medicine, Vanderbilt Univ Hosp 1974; **Fellow:** Gastroenterology, Vanderbilt Univ Hosp 1977; **Fac Appt:** Prof Med, Univ Tex, San Antonio

Stump, David L MD [Ge] - **Hospital:** Methodist Hosp-San Antonio; **Address:** Gastroenterology Clinic, 8550 Datapoint Drive, Ste LL100, San Antonio, TX 78229-3436; **Phone:** 210-615-8308; **Board Cert:** Internal Medicine 1983; Gastroenterology 1985; **Med School:** Indiana Univ 1980; **Resid:** Internal Medicine, Indiana Univ Med Ctr 1983; **Fellow:** Gastroenterology, UT San Antonio 1985

Vierling, John M MD [Ge] - **Spec Exp:** Liver Disease; Transplant Medicine-Liver; Autoimmune Liver Disease; Hepatitis B & C; **Hospital:** St. Luke's Episcopal Hosp-Houston, Baylor Clinic & Hosp-Houston; **Address:** Baylor Liver Health, 1709 Dryden, Ste 1500, Houston, TX 77030; **Phone:** 713-798-8355; **Board Cert:** Internal Medicine 1975; Gastroenterology 1979; Transplant Hepatology 2006; **Med School:** Stanford Univ 1972; **Resid:** Internal Medicine, Strong Meml Hosp 1974; Hepatology, Natl Inst Hlth 1977; **Fellow:** Gastroenterology, UCSF Med Ctr 1978; **Fac Appt:** Prof Med, Baylor Coll Med

West Coast and Pacific

Cello, John P MD [Ge] - **Spec Exp:** Endoscopy; Colonoscopy; Capsule Endoscopy; Pancreatic/Biliary Endoscopy (ERCP); **Hospital:** San Francisco Genl Hosp, UCSF Med Ctr; **Address:** San Francisco Genl Hosp-Univ California, 1001 Potrero Ave, Ste NH3D, San Francisco, CA 94110; **Phone:** 415-206-4746; **Board Cert:** Internal Medicine 1972; Gastroenterology 1977; **Med School:** Harvard Med Sch 1969; **Resid:** Internal Medicine, Peter Bent Brigham Hosp 1972; **Fellow:** Gastroenterology, UCSF Med Ctr 1977; **Fac Appt:** Prof Med, UCSF

Chang, Kenneth J MD [Ge] - **Spec Exp:** Gastrointestinal Cancer; Endoscopic Ultrasound; Interventional Endoscopy; Barrett's Esophagus; **Hospital:** UC Irvine Med Ctr; **Address:** Comprehensive Digestive Disease Ctr, 101 The City Drive South, Bldg 22C, Orange, CA 92868; **Phone:** 714-456-6187; **Board Cert:** Internal Medicine 1988; Gastroenterology 2001; **Med School:** Brown Univ 1985; **Resid:** Internal Medicine, Rhode Island Hosp 1988; **Fellow:** Gastroenterology, UC-Irvine Med Ctr 1990; **Fac Appt:** Clin Prof Med, UC Irvine

Dea, Stanley MD [Ge] - **Spec Exp:** Endoscopy; Capsule Endoscopy; Pancreatic/Biliary Endoscopy (ERCP); Endoscopic Ultrasound; **Hospital:** Olive View-UCLA Med Ctr; **Address:** Olive View-UCLA Med Ctr, 14445 Olive View Drive, rm 2B-182, Sylmar, CA 91342; **Phone:** 818-364-3205; **Board Cert:** Internal Medicine 2004; Gastroenterology 2008; **Med School:** Univ Chicago-Pritzker Sch Med 1990; **Resid:** Internal Medicine, Harbor-UCLA Med Ctr 1993; **Fellow:** Gastroenterology, UCLA Med Ctr 1995

Eisen, Glenn MD [Ge] - **Spec Exp:** Endoscopy; Liver Disease; Barrett's Esophagus; **Hospital:** Providence St Vincent Med Ctr; **Address:** Peterkort Medical Office, 9701 SW Barnes Rd, Ste 300 & 310, Portland, OR 97225; **Phone:** 503-297-8081; **Board Cert:** Internal Medicine 2002; Gastroenterology 2006; **Med School:** Albert Einstein Coll Med 1987; **Resid:** Internal Medicine, Mt Sinai Med Ctr 1991; **Fellow:** Gastroenterology, Duke Univ Med Ctr 1996; Epidemiology, Univ NC Hosp 1992; **Fac Appt:** Clin Prof Med, Oregon Hlth & Sci Univ

Ellis, Jonathan C MD [Ge] - **Hospital:** Cedars-Sinai Med Ctr; **Address:** 9090 Wilshire Blvd, Ste 101, Beverly Hills, CA 90211; **Phone:** 310-550-0400; **Board Cert:** Internal Medicine 1985; Gastroenterology 1989; **Med School:** Stanford Univ 1982; **Resid:** Internal Medicine, Cedars Sinai Med Ctr 1986; **Fellow:** Gastroenterology, UCLA 1988; **Fac Appt:** Assoc Prof Med, UCLA

Feldman, Edward Jon MD [Ge] - **Spec Exp:** Inflammatory Bowel Disease; Colonoscopy; Irritable Bowel Syndrome; Gastroesophageal Reflux Disease (GERD); **Hospital:** Cedars-Sinai Med Ctr; **Address:** 8635 W 3rd St, Ste 960W, Los Angeles, CA 90048-6101; **Phone:** 310-652-8031; **Board Cert:** Internal Medicine 1972; Gastroenterology 1977; **Med School:** Indiana Univ 1969; **Resid:** Internal Medicine, LA Co Habor Genl Hosp 1972; Internal Medicine, Hammersmith Hosp 1973; **Fellow:** Gastroenterology, UCLA Med Ctr 1976; **Fac Appt:** Clin Prof Med, UCLA

Fennerty, M Brian MD [Ge] - **Spec Exp:** Gastroesophageal Reflux Disease (GERD); **Hospital:** OR Hlth & Sci Univ; **Address:** Digestive Hlth, Ctr for Hlth & Healing, 3303 SW Bond Ave, MC CH6D, Portland, OR 97239; **Phone:** 503-494-4373; **Board Cert:** Internal Medicine 1984; Gastroenterology 2008; **Med School:** Creighton Univ 1980; **Resid:** Internal Medicine, Naval Hospital 1984; **Fellow:** Gastroenterology, Arizona Hlth Sci Ctr 1989; **Fac Appt:** Prof Med, Oregon Hlth & Sci Univ

Gerson, Lauren B MD [Ge] - **Spec Exp:** Gastroesophageal Reflux Disease (GERD); Barrett's Esophagus; Esophageal Disorders; Capsule Endoscopy; **Hospital:** Stanford Univ Hosp & Clinics; **Address:** Stanford Univ Div Gastroenterology, 450 Broadway St, Pavilion C Fl 4, MC 6341, Redwood City, CA 94063; **Phone:** 650-736-5555; **Board Cert:** Gastroenterology 2002; **Med School:** SUNY Buffalo 1990; **Resid:** Internal Medicine, California Pacific Med Ctr 1993; **Fellow:** Gastroenterology, Stanford Univ Med Ctr 1995; **Fac Appt:** Assoc Prof Med, Stanford Univ

Gish, Robert MD [Ge] - **Spec Exp:** Liver Cancer; Transplant Medicine-Liver; Hepatitis; Clinical Trials; **Hospital:** UCSD Med Ctr; **Address:** UCSD Medical Center, 200 W Arbor Drive, Ste 342, MC 8413, San Diego, CA 92103; **Phone:** 619-543-3787; **Board Cert:** Internal Medicine 1984; Gastroenterology 1987; Transplant Hepatology 2006; **Med School:** Univ Kansas 1980; **Resid:** Internal Medicine, UCSD Med Ctr 1983; **Fellow:** Gastroenterology, UCLA Med Ctr 1988; **Fac Appt:** Assoc Clin Prof Med, UCSF

Han, Steven-Huy MD [Ge] - **Spec Exp:** Transplant Medicine-Liver; Hepatitis B & C; Liver Disease; **Hospital:** UCLA Ronald Reagan Med Ctr; **Address:** UCLA Medical Ctr, 200 UCLA Medical Plaza, Ste 214, Los Angeles, CA 90095; **Phone:** 310-794-7788; **Board Cert:** Gastroenterology 2008; Transplant Hepatology 2006; **Med School:** Albany Med Coll 1990; **Resid:** Internal Medicine, Santa Clara Valley Med Ctr 1993; **Fellow:** Hepatology, USC 1996; Gastroenterology, UCLA 1998; **Fac Appt:** Assoc Prof Med, UCLA

Gastroenterology

Hillebrand, Donald J MD [Ge] - **Spec Exp:** Transplant Medicine-Liver; Liver Failure; **Hospital:** Scripps Green Hosp; **Address:** Scripps Clinic Torry Pines, 10666 N Torrey Pines Rd, N200, La Jolla, CA 92037; **Phone:** 858-554-4310; **Board Cert:** Internal Medicine 2004; Gastroenterology 2006; Transplant Hepatology 2006; **Med School:** Univ Iowa Coll Med 1990; **Resid:** Internal Medicine, Univ Iowa Hosps 1993; **Fellow:** Gastroenterology, Univ Iowa Hosps 1994

Kimmey, Michael B MD [Ge] - **Spec Exp:** Pancreatic/Biliary Endoscopy (ERCP); Endoscopy; Endoscopic Ultrasound; **Hospital:** St. Joseph Med Ctr - Tacoma, Tacoma Genl Hosp; **Address:** 1112 6th Ave, Ste 200, Tacoma, WA 98405; **Phone:** 253-272-8664; **Board Cert:** Internal Medicine 1982; Gastroenterology 1987; **Med School:** Washington Univ, St Louis 1979; **Resid:** Internal Medicine, Univ Wash Med Ctr 1982; **Fellow:** Gastroenterology, Univ Wash Med Ctr 1987; **Fac Appt:** Clin Prof Med, Univ Wash

Kozarek, Richard MD [Ge] - **Spec Exp:** Pancreatic/Biliary Endoscopy (ERCP); Inflammatory Bowel Disease; Pancreatic Disease; **Hospital:** Virginia Mason Med Ctr; **Address:** 1100 9th Ave, MS C3-GAS, PO Box 24163, Seattle, WA 98101-2756; **Phone:** 206-223-6934; **Board Cert:** Internal Medicine 1977; Gastroenterology 1979; **Med School:** Univ Wisc 1973; **Resid:** Internal Medicine, Good Samaritan Hosp 1976; **Fellow:** Gastroenterology, Univ Arizona/ VA Hosp 1978; **Fac Appt:** Clin Prof Med, Univ Wash

Lenz, Heinz Juergen MD [Ge] - **Spec Exp:** Gastrointestinal Cancer; Colon & Rectal Cancer; **Hospital:** Keck Med Ctr of USC (page 75); **Address:** 1441 East Lake Ave, NOR 3456, Los Angeles, CA 90033; **Phone:** 323-865-3105; **Board Cert:** Internal Medicine 2010; Gastroenterology 2000; **Med School:** Germany 1981; **Resid:** Internal Medicine, Univ Hamburg Affil Hosp 1987; Internal Medicine, UC San Diego Med Ctr 1989; **Fellow:** Gastroenterology, UC San Diego Med Ctr 1990; **Fac Appt:** Prof Med, USC-Keck School of Medicine

Mittal, Ravinder MD [Ge] - **Spec Exp:** Gastrointestinal Motility Disorders; Esophageal Disorders; Swallowing Disorders; **Hospital:** UCSD Med Ctr; **Address:** 9350 Campus Point Drive, MC 7788, La Jolla, CA 92037; **Phone:** 619-543-6834; **Board Cert:** Internal Medicine 1982; Gastroenterology 1985; **Med School:** India 1978; **Resid:** Internal Medicine, Lincoln Hosp 1982; **Fellow:** Gastroenterology, New Haven Hosp 1985; **Fac Appt:** Prof Med, UCSD

Ostroff, James W MD [Ge] - **Spec Exp:** Pancreatic/Biliary Endoscopy (ERCP); Colonoscopy; **Hospital:** UCSF Med Ctr, UCSF - Mt Zion Med Ctr; **Address:** 350 Parnassus Ave, Ste 410, San Francisco, CA 94117-3608; **Phone:** 415-502-2112; **Board Cert:** Internal Medicine 1980; Gastroenterology 1983; **Med School:** Cornell Univ-Weill Med Coll 1977; **Resid:** Internal Medicine, NY Hosp-Cornell Med Ctr 1980; **Fellow:** Gastroenterology, UCSF Hosps 1982; **Fac Appt:** Prof Med, UCSF

Pasricha, P Jay MD [Ge] - **Spec Exp:** Swallowing Disorders-Botox Therapy; Gastrointestinal Motility Disorders; Pancreatic Disease; Gastroparesis; **Hospital:** Stanford Univ Hosp & Clinics; **Address:** Stanford Gastroenterology/Hepatology, 300 Pasteur Drive, rm A175, Stanford, CA 94305-5309; **Phone:** 650-736-5555; **Board Cert:** Internal Medicine 1988; Gastroenterology 2006; **Med School:** India 1983; **Resid:** Internal Medicine, DC Genl Hosp 1988; **Fellow:** Pulmonary Disease, New England Med Ctr 1990; Gastroenterology, Johns Hopkins Hosp 1992; **Fac Appt:** Prof Med, Stanford Univ

Poordad, Fred F MD [Ge] - **Spec Exp:** Liver Disease; Hepatitis B & C; Transplant Medicine-Liver; **Hospital:** Cedars-Sinai Med Ctr; **Address:** Cedars Sinai Medical Ctr, Liver Diseases, West Tower, 8635 W 3rd St, Ste 590, Los Angeles, CA 90048; **Phone:** 310-423-2641; **Board Cert:** Gastroenterology 2005; Transplant Hepatology 2006; **Med School:** Canada 1990; **Resid:** Internal Medicine, St Thomas Med Ctr/Ohio State Univ Med Ctr 1993; **Fellow:** Gastroenterology, Univ S Carolina Med Ctr 1995; Hepatology, Johns Hopkins Hosp 2005; **Fac Appt:** Assoc Prof Med, UCLA-David Geffen Sch Med

Roth, Bennett E MD [Ge] - **Spec Exp:** Gastroesophageal Reflux Disease (GERD); Inflammatory Bowel Disease/Crohn's; Irritable Bowel Syndrome; Esophageal Disorders; **Hospital:** UCLA Ronald Reagan Med Ctr; **Address:** UCLA Digestive Disease Ctr, 200 UCLA Medical Plaza, Ste 365A, Los Angeles, CA 90095; **Phone:** 310-825-1597; **Board Cert:** Internal Medicine 1972; Gastroenterology 1975; **Med School:** Hahnemann Univ 1968; **Resid:** Internal Medicine, Hosp Univ Penn 1971; **Fellow:** Gastroenterology, UCLA Med Ctr 1974; **Fac Appt:** Prof Med, UCLA

Sandborn, William J MD [Ge] - **Spec Exp:** Inflammatory Bowel Disease/Crohn's; Ulcerative Colitis; Crohn's Disease; **Hospital:** UCSD Med Ctr; **Address:** Perlman Med Office, 9500 Gilman Drive, La Jolla, CA 92093-0063; **Phone:** 858-534-3320; **Board Cert:** Gastroenterology 2003; **Med School:** Loma Linda Univ 1987; **Resid:** Internal Medicine, Loma Linda Univ 1990; **Fellow:** Gastroenterology, Mayo Clin 1993; **Fac Appt:** Assoc Prof Med, Mayo Med Sch

Savides, Thomas MD [Ge] - **Spec Exp:** Gastrointestinal Cancer; Barrett's Esophagus; Colonoscopy; Endoscopic Ultrasound; **Hospital:** UCSD Med Ctr; **Address:** UCSD Med Ctr, Div Gastroenterology, 200 W Arbor Drive, MC 8788, San Diego, CA 92103-8413; **Phone:** 619-543-2347; **Board Cert:** Internal Medicine 2003; Gastroenterology 2003; **Med School:** UCSD 1987; **Resid:** Internal Medicine, UCLA Med Ctr 1990; **Fellow:** Gastroenterology, UCLA Med Ctr 1993; Gastroenterology, Indiana Univ Med Ctr 1994; **Fac Appt:** Asst Clin Prof Med, UCSD

Surawicz, Christina MD [Ge] - **Spec Exp:** Clostridium Difficile Disease; Infectious Diarrhea; **Hospital:** Harborview Med Ctr; **Address:** 325 9th Ave, Box 359866, Seattle, WA 98104-2420; **Phone:** 206-744-5021; **Board Cert:** Internal Medicine 1976; Gastroenterology 1979; **Med School:** Univ KY Coll Med 1973; **Resid:** Internal Medicine, Univ Washington Med Ctr 1976; **Fellow:** Gastroenterology, Univ Washington Med Ctr 1979; **Fac Appt:** Prof Med, Univ Wash

Targan, Stephan R MD [Ge] - **Spec Exp:** Inflammatory Bowel Disease; Crohn's Disease; **Hospital:** Cedars-Sinai Med Ctr; **Address:** Cedars-Sinai IBD Ctr, 8730 Alden Drive, Ste 3, 204 E, Los Angeles, CA 90048; **Phone:** 310-423-4100; **Board Cert:** Internal Medicine 1974; Infectious Disease 1976; Gastroenterology 1979; **Med School:** Johns Hopkins Univ 1971; **Resid:** Internal Medicine, Harbor-UCLA Med Ctr 1976; **Fellow:** Infectious Disease, Harbor-UCLA Med Ctr 1976; Gastroenterology, UCLA Med Ctr 1978; **Fac Appt:** Prof Med, UCLA

Zaman, Atif MD [Ge] - **Spec Exp:** Liver Disease; Hypertension; Hepatitis; **Hospital:** OR Hlth & Sci Univ; **Address:** OHSU, MC CH6D, 3303 SW Bond Ave, Portland, OR 97201; **Phone:** 503-494-4373; **Board Cert:** Gastroenterology 2008; **Med School:** Tufts Univ 1991; **Resid:** Internal Medicine, Baylor Coll Affil Hosp 1994; **Fellow:** Gastroenterology, Oregon Hlth Science Univ 1998; **Fac Appt:** Prof Med, Oregon Hlth & Sci Univ

Cleveland Clinic

Every life deserves world class care.

Gastroenterology

Cleveland Clinic's Digestive Disease Institute (DDI) is one of the largest digestive programs in the country and is ranked No. 2 in the nation by *U.S.News & World Report*. DDI is the first to fully integrate its departments of Colorectal Surgery, Gastroenterology & Hepatology, General Surgery, and Nutrition. Combining these disciplines in one location facilitates unprecedented patient care, multidisciplinary education and collaborative research. In 2010, DDI physicians performed over 27,000 surgical cases and 38,000 endoscopic cases. Transplant surgeons completed over 170 digestive disease-related organ transplants, including liver, pancreas and intestinal transplantation, achieving outstanding outcomes.

Highlights of our Department of Gastroenterology:

- A state-of-the-art endoscopy facility designed to improve patient satisfaction while emphasizing both safety and quality.
- Our advanced endoscopy team performs a range of endoscopic procedures annually, including endoscopic retrograde cholangiopancreatography, endoscopic ultrasound and percutaneous endoscopic gastrostomy.
- Our Center for Swallowing & Esophageal Disorders offers comprehensive treatment for swallowing and esophageal disorders.
- DDI developed the world's first Pouchitis Clinic.
- A new section of Comprehensive Gastroenterology focuses on typically underserved disorders, such as small bowel diseases, including celiac disease.
- A Chronic Abdominal Pain Clinic, provides comprehensive medical diagnostics and treatments.
- Our liver specialists have the experience and expertise to accurately diagnose and treat all forms of liver disease, including viral hepatitis, fatty liver, alcoholic liver disease, autoimmune liver diseases, genetic liver diseases and liver cancer.

clevelandclinic.org/
gastrotopdocs

Offering Same-Day Appointments
Call 800.274.2009.

Treatment Guides

Cleveland Clinic has developed comprehensive treatment guides for many diseases and conditions. To download our free treatment guides, visit clevelandclinic.org/treatmentguides.

Online Medical Second Opinion

Cleveland Clinic's My**Consult** Online Medical Second Opinion program securely connects patients to our physician specialists for more than 1,000 life-changing or life-threatening diagnoses all by the click of a mouse. To learn more, log onto eclevelandclinic.org/myconsult or call 800.223.2273, ext. 43223.

Special Assistance for Out-of-State Patients

Cleveland Clinic Global Patient Services offers a complimentary Medical Concierge service for patients who travel from outside of Ohio. Call 800.223.2273, ext. 55580 or email medicalconcierge@ccf.org.

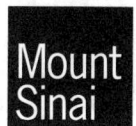
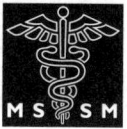

MOUNT SINAI SCHOOL OF MEDICINE

THE MOUNT SINAI MEDICAL CENTER
GASTROINTESTINAL AND SURGICAL SPECIALTIES
One Gustave L. Levy Place
Fifth Avenue and 100th Street
New York, NY 10029-6574
Physician Referral: 1-800-MD-SINAI (637-4624)
www.mountsinai.org

Mount Sinai's **DIVISIONS OF GASTROENTEROLOGY, COLON AND RECTAL SURGERY, LIVER DISEASES, PEDIATRIC GASTROENTEROLOGY, AND PEDIATRIC HEPATOLOGY** are renowned for their delivery of patient care, research, and education in diseases of the gastrointestinal (GI) tract. In 2000, the National Institutes of Health (NIH) recognized the importance of Mount Sinai as a research center with a grant for GI/Liver fellowship training. Mount Sinai is the only medical school in New York City to earn this prestigious award.

Mount Sinai's Division of Gastroenterology ranks among the top five in the country, according to the *U.S. News & World Report's* 2011–2012 "Best Hospitals" issue. Successes include breakthroughs in the medical and surgical management of the inflammatory bowel diseases (IBD): ulcerative colitis, and Crohn's disease. Mount Sinai spearheaded novel therapies for treating severe IBD and helped establish the role of colonoscopy in preventing colon cancer by removing precancerous polyps. More recent innovations include employing a tiny camera within a swallowable capsule to capture images in the stomach and intestines. Mount Sinai offers patients advanced comprehensive and interdisciplinary care; newer agents through clinical trials; services of psychologists and nutritionists; and world-class expertise in endoscopic procedures.

Division of Colon and Rectal Surgery — Continuing a long tradition of expertise in gastrointestinal disorders, Mount Sinai surgeons focus on surgical therapies for all diseases involving the colon, rectum, and anus. Highly skilled in the treatment of Crohn's disease (which was first described at Mount Sinai in 1932), ulcerative colitis, colon and rectal cancer, and diverticulitis, they specialize in the most advanced techniques of rectal surgery with an emphasis on colostomy avoidance. They also employ minimally invasive techniques and cutting-edge technologies for the treatment of hemorrhoids, fistulas, and rectal tumors.

Division of Liver Diseases — With a program that is among the largest and most successful in the world, Mount Sinai carries out a diverse portfolio of research projects. Featuring both clinical care and scientific investigations, they involve transplantation; diagnosis and treatment of viral hepatitis, including trials for revolutionary new drugs for Hepatitis B and C; treatment of scarring, or fibrosis; management of primary biliary cirrhosis, an autoimmune disease of bile ducts; treatment of liver cancer; and diagnosis and treatment of genetic liver diseases, including Wilson's disease (copper overload) and hemachromatosis (iron overload).

Division of Pediatric Gastroenterology — The division provides consultation and treatment for the full range of children's digestive and nutritional diseases. The Children's IBD Center offers comprehensive, multidisciplinary, family-centered care for pediatric patients with Crohn's disease and ulcerative colitis, and receives referrals from across the country. The division also provides care to families of infants, children, and teens who have the full range of both complex and common digestive disorders, including celiac disease, gastroesophageal reflux disease, and irritable bowel syndrome. Additionally, the division is involved in both basic science and clinical research, allowing physicians to provide state-of-the-art, evidence-based care.

Division of Pediatric Hepatology — The Transplant Program is one of the largest in the nation and was the first program in New York to perform liver transplants and, later, small bowel transplants. The division is active in clinical research in IBD, focusing on issues of genetic factors, psychosocial interactions, and drug trials in liver disease.

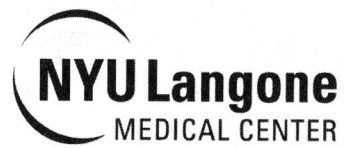

GASTROENTEROLOGY

About the Division of Gastroenterology, Department of Medicine

The Division of Gastroenterology at NYU Langone Medical Center is dedicated to the diagnosis and treatment of patients with diseases of the gastrointestinal tract. Physicians draw on their extensive knowledge and experience in the diagnosis and management of inflammatory bowel disease, peptic ulcer disease, esophageal disorders, gastrointestinal cancer, and liver, biliary and pancreatic diseases. We specialize in the following areas:

Colorectal Cancer

The Medical Center offers the most advanced screening options available for the diagnosis of colon cancer. Additionally, physicians continue to investigate colorectal cancer in special populations such as women, veterans, immigrants, minorities and patients with HIV, and offer the use of virtual colonoscopy for the detection of colorectal polyps and cancer.

Esophageal Diseases

The Esophageal Disease Center offers patients state-of-the-art diagnosis and treatment of esophageal disorders. The Center focuses on gastroesophageal reflux disease, esophageal motility disorders, Barrett's esophagus, adenocarcinoma of the esophagus and swallowing disorders. It also offers diagnostic studies on esophageal manometry, impedance testing for swallowing, pH catheter and impedance testing for reflux and BRAVO capsule pH testing, as well as such therapies as Barrett's ablation and esophageal dilations.

Gastrointestinal Cancers

NYU Cancer Institute physicians treat patients with all types of gastrointestinal cancers, including those of the esophagus, stomach, colon/rectum, small intestine, liver, pancreas, gallbladder, and biliary tract. They also treat individuals with complex recurring disease, including those originally treated elsewhere. Patients have the opportunity to participate in numerous clinical trials.

Complex Treatments and Diagnosis

Physicians in the Division of Gastroenterology are highly experienced in the use of enteroscopy and capsule endoscopy for the diagnosis of gastrointestinal bleeding of unknown origin. They have special interest in the diagnosis and treatment of patients with complex pancreatic-biliary disease through the use of ERCP and endoscopic ultrasound.

Virtual Colonoscopy

NYU Langone Medical Center is in the vanguard of advanced colon cancer detection through virtual colonoscopy. The study gives a complete evaluation of the entire surface of the colon and ensures greater accuracy and less patient discomfort.

The Best in American Medicine
www.CastleConnolly.com

Geriatric Medicine

a subspecialty of Internal Medicine or Family Practice

An internist or family physician with special knowledge of the aging process and special skills in the diagnostic, therapeutic, preventive and rehabilitative aspects of illness in the elderly. This specialist cares for geriatric patients in the patient's home, the office, long-term care settings such as nursing homes and the hospital.

Family Medicine

A family physician is concerned with the total healthcare of the individual and the family, and is trained to diagnose and treat a wide variety of ailments in patients of all ages. The family physician receives a broad range of training that includes internal medicine, pediatrics, obstetrics and gynecology, psychiatry and geriatrics. Special emphasis is placed on prevention and the primary care of entire families, utilizing consultations and community resources when appropriate.

Training Required: Three years in internal medicine or family practice *plus* additional training and examination for certification in geriatric medicine.

GERIATRIC MEDICINE

New England

Cooney Jr, Leo M MD [Ger] - **Spec Exp:** Geriatric Functional Assessment; Rheumatology; Mobility Evaluation & Treatment; **Hospital:** Yale-New Haven Hosp, Yale Med Group; **Address:** Yale-New Haven Hosp, Adler Geriatric Ctr, 20 York St, New Haven, CT 06510; **Phone:** 203-688-2204; **Board Cert:** Internal Medicine 1974; Rheumatology 1978; **Med School:** Yale Univ 1969; **Resid:** Internal Medicine, Boston City Hosp 1971; Internal Medicine, Boston City Hosp 1974; **Fellow:** Rheumatology, Boston Med Ctr 1975; **Fac Appt:** Prof Med, Yale Univ

Lipsitz, Lewis Arnold MD [Ger] - **Spec Exp:** Falls in the Elderly; Hypertension; Hypotension; Syncope; **Hospital:** Beth Israel Deaconess Med Ctr - Boston, Hebrew Senior Life; **Address:** Beth Israel Med Ctr, Gerontology, 110 Francis St, LMOB 1B, Boston, MA 02215; **Phone:** 617-632-8696; **Board Cert:** Internal Medicine 1980; Geriatric Medicine 2009; **Med School:** Univ Pennsylvania 1977; **Resid:** Internal Medicine, Beth Israel Hosp 1980; **Fellow:** Geriatric Medicine, Mass Genl Hosp 1983; **Fac Appt:** Prof Med, Harvard Med Sch

Minaker, Kenneth MD [Ger] - **Spec Exp:** Aging; Neuroendocrinology; Cardiovascular Disease; **Hospital:** Mass Genl Hosp, Brigham and Women's Hosp (page 57); **Address:** Charles River Plaza, Ste 502, 165 Cambridge St, Boston, MA 02114-2723; **Phone:** 617-726-4600; **Med School:** Univ Toronto 1972; **Resid:** Internal Medicine, Univ Toronto 1981; **Fellow:** Geriatric Medicine, Mass Gen Hosp 1983; **Fac Appt:** Assoc Prof Med, Harvard Med Sch

Oates, Daniel J MD [Ger] - **Hospital:** Boston Med Ctr; **Address:** Boston Med Ctr, Geriatrics Clinic, Yawkey Ambulatory Care Ctr Fl 3, Boston, MA 02118; **Phone:** 617-414-4639; **Board Cert:** Internal Medicine 2003; Geriatric Medicine 2005; **Med School:** Boston Univ 2000; **Resid:** Internal Medicine, Boston Med Ctr 2003; **Fellow:** Geriatric Medicine, Boston Med Ctr 2005

Tinetti, Mary E MD [Ger] - **Spec Exp:** Falls in the Elderly; Geriatric Functional Assessment; **Hospital:** Yale-New Haven Hosp, Yale Med Group; **Address:** Yale-New Haven Hosp, Adler Geriatric Ctr, 20 York St, New Haven, CT 06510; **Phone:** 203-688-6361; **Board Cert:** Internal Medicine 1981; **Med School:** Univ Mich Med Sch 1978; **Resid:** Internal Medicine, Univ Minnesota 1981; **Fellow:** Geriatric Medicine, Univ Rochester 1984; **Fac Appt:** Prof Med, Yale Univ

Mid Atlantic

Bloom, Patricia A MD [Ger] - **Spec Exp:** Complementary Medicine; Dementia; **Hospital:** Mount Sinai Med Ctr (page 63); **Address:** 1440 Madison Ave, New York, NY 10029-6542; **Phone:** 212-659-8552; **Board Cert:** Internal Medicine 1978; **Med School:** Univ Minn 1975; **Resid:** Internal Medicine, Montefiore Med Ctr 1978; **Fac Appt:** Assoc Prof Med, Mount Sinai Sch Med

Burton, John R MD [Ger] - **Hospital:** Johns Hopkins Bayview Med Ctr (page 61); **Address:** Division of Geriatric Medicine, 5505 Hopkins Bayview Cir, Baltimore, MD 21224; **Phone:** 410-550-0520; **Board Cert:** Internal Medicine 1980; Nephrology 1974; Geriatric Medicine 2005; **Med School:** McGill Univ 1965; **Resid:** Internal Medicine, Baltimore City Hosp 1971; **Fellow:** Nephrology, Mass Genl Hosp 1972; **Fac Appt:** Prof Med, Johns Hopkins Univ

Callahan, Eileen MD [Ger] - **Spec Exp:** Frail Elderly; Preventive Medicine; Dementia; **Hospital:** Mount Sinai Med Ctr (page 63); **Address:** 1440 Madison Ave, New York, NY 10029; **Phone:** 212-659-8552; **Board Cert:** Internal Medicine 2004; Geriatric Medicine 2008; Hospice & Palliative Medicine 2005; **Med School:** UMDNJ-NJ Med Sch, Newark 1991; **Resid:** Internal Medicine, St Vincents Hosp Med Ctr 1994; **Fellow:** Geriatric Medicine, Mount Sinai Hosp 1996; **Fac Appt:** Assoc Prof Med, Mount Sinai Sch Med

Finucane, Thomas E MD [Ger] - **Spec Exp:** Pain Management; Swallowing Disorders; Ethics; Palliative Care; **Hospital:** Johns Hopkins Bayview Med Ctr (page 61), Johns Hopkins Hosp (page 61); **Address:** 5505 Hopkins Bayview Cir, Level 01, Baltimore, MD 21224; **Phone:** 410-550-0925; **Board Cert:** Internal Medicine 1982; Geriatric Medicine 2008; **Med School:** Emory Univ 1978; **Resid:** Internal Medicine, George Washington Univ Hosp 1982; **Fac Appt:** Prof Med, Johns Hopkins Univ

Gambert, Steven R MD [Ger] - **Spec Exp:** Endocrinology; Osteoporosis; Aging; **Hospital:** Univ of MD Med Ctr; **Address:** Univ Maryland, Dept Med, 22 S Greene St, rm N3E09, Baltimore, MD 21201; **Phone:** 410-328-1143; **Board Cert:** Internal Medicine 1978; **Med School:** Columbia P&S 1975; **Resid:** Internal Medicine, Dartmouth Affl Hosp 1977; **Fellow:** Geriatric Medicine, Beth Israel Hosp-Harvard 1979; Endocrinology, Beth Israel Hosp-Harvard 1979; **Fac Appt:** Prof Med, Univ MD Sch Med

Lachs, Mark S MD [Ger] - **Spec Exp:** Abuse/Neglect; **Hospital:** NY-Presby/Weill Cornell Med Ctr, NY (page 65); **Address:** Irving Sherwood Wright Center on Aging, 1484 First Ave, New York, NY 10075; **Phone:** 212-746-7000; **Board Cert:** Internal Medicine 1988; Geriatric Medicine 2002; **Med School:** NYU Sch Med 1985; **Resid:** Internal Medicine, Hosp Univ Penn 1988; **Fellow:** Geriatric Medicine, Yale-New Haven Hosp 1990; **Fac Appt:** Prof Med, Cornell Univ-Weill Med Coll

Meier, Diane E MD [Ger] - **Spec Exp:** Palliative Care; **Hospital:** Mount Sinai Med Ctr (page 63); **Address:** Mt Sinai School Medicine, Box 1070, One Gustave L Levy Pl, New York, NY 10029-6501; **Phone:** 212-241-1446; **Board Cert:** Internal Medicine 1981; Geriatric Medicine 2010; Hospice & Palliative Medicine 2008; **Med School:** Northwestern Univ 1977; **Resid:** Internal Medicine, Oregon Hlth Sci Univ 1981; **Fellow:** Geriatric Medicine, VA Med Ctr 1983; **Fac Appt:** Prof Med, Mount Sinai Sch Med

Resnick, Neil M MD [Ger] - **Spec Exp:** Voiding Dysfunction; Incontinence; **Hospital:** UPMC Presby, Pittsburgh, UPMC Shadyside; **Address:** 3471 5th Ave, Kaufmann Bldg, Ste 500, Pittsburgh, PA 15213-3313; **Phone:** 412-692-2364; **Board Cert:** Internal Medicine 1980; Geriatric Medicine 2009; **Med School:** Stanford Univ 1977; **Resid:** Internal Medicine, Beth Israel Hosp 1980; **Fellow:** Geriatric Medicine, Harvard Univ 1982; Urodynamics, Harvard Univ 1984; **Fac Appt:** Prof Med, Univ Pittsburgh

Studenski, Stephanie A MD [Ger] - **Spec Exp:** Balance Disorders; Mobility Evaluation & Treatment; Falls in the Elderly; **Hospital:** UPMC Presby, Pittsburgh; **Address:** 3459 Fifth Ave Fl 4, Pittsburgh, PA 15213; **Phone:** 412-692-4200; **Board Cert:** Internal Medicine 1982; Rheumatology 1984; Geriatric Medicine 2002; **Med School:** Univ Kansas 1979; **Resid:** Internal Medicine, Duke Univ Med Ctr 1982; **Fellow:** Rheumatology, Duke Univ Med Ctr 1984; Geriatric Medicine, Duke Univ Med Ctr 1986; **Fac Appt:** Prof Med, Univ Pittsburgh

Geriatric Medicine

Southeast

Allman, Richard M MD [Ger] - **Spec Exp:** Geriatric Rehabilitation; Mobility Evaluation & Treatment; Palliative Care; **Hospital:** Univ of Ala Hosp at Birmingham; **Address:** UAB Center for Aging, 1530 3rd Ave S, CH 19-201, Birmingham, AL 35294-2041; **Phone:** 205-934-9261; **Board Cert:** Internal Medicine 1983; Geriatric Medicine 1998; **Med School:** W VA Univ 1980; **Resid:** Internal Medicine, W Va Univ Hosp 1983; **Fellow:** Internal Medicine, Johns Hopkins Univ 1985; **Fac Appt:** Prof Med, Univ Alabama

Boling, Peter A MD [Ger] - **Spec Exp:** Frail Elderly; Home Care; **Hospital:** VCU Med Ctr; **Address:** VCU Med Ctr, Div General Int Med, PO Box 980328, Richmond, VA 23298-0102; **Phone:** 804-828-9357; **Board Cert:** Internal Medicine 1984; Geriatric Medicine 2000; **Med School:** Univ Rochester 1981; **Resid:** Internal Medicine, Med Coll Va Hosp Hosp 1984; **Fac Appt:** Prof Med, Med Coll VA

Ciocon, Jerry O MD [Ger] - **Spec Exp:** Chronic Fatigue-Elderly; Pain-Musculoskeletal; Memory Disorders; Incontinence; **Hospital:** Cleveland Clin - Weston; **Address:** Cleveland Clinic, Div Geriatrics, 2950 Cleveland Clinic Blvd, Weston, FL 33331-3609; **Phone:** 954-659-5867; **Board Cert:** Internal Medicine 1985; Geriatric Medicine 2000; **Med School:** Philippines 1980; **Resid:** Internal Medicine, Mercy Hosp 1985; **Fellow:** Geriatric Medicine, LI Jewish Med Ctr 1987

Greganti, Mac A MD [Ger] - **Spec Exp:** Diagnostic Problems; Dementia; **Hospital:** NC Memorial Hosp - UNC; **Address:** Univ North Carolina Hosp, Dept Med, 125 MacNider Bldg CB#7005, Chapel Hill, NC 27599-7005; **Phone:** 919-966-3063; **Board Cert:** Internal Medicine 1987; **Med School:** Univ Miss 1972; **Resid:** Internal Medicine, Strong Meml Hosp 1975; **Fac Appt:** Prof Med, Univ NC Sch Med

Hanson, Laura C MD [Ger] - **Spec Exp:** Frailty Syndrome; Palliative Care; **Hospital:** NC Memorial Hosp - UNC; **Address:** UNC Sch Med, 5003 Old Clinic Bldg, CB 7550, Chapel Hill, NC 27599; **Phone:** 919-966-5945 x251; **Board Cert:** Internal Medicine 1989; Geriatric Medicine 2002; Hospice & Palliative Medicine 2009; **Med School:** Harvard Med Sch 1986; **Resid:** Internal Medicine, Brigham & Womens Hosp 1988; Internal Medicine, Univ North Carolina Hosp 1989; **Fellow:** Geriatric Medicine, Univ North Carolina Hosp 1991; **Fac Appt:** Assoc Prof Med, Univ NC Sch Med

Lyles, Kenneth W MD [Ger] - **Spec Exp:** Bone Disorders-Metabolic; Tumoral Calcinosis; Parathyroid Disease; Osteoporosis; **Hospital:** Duke Univ Hosp, Durham VA Med Ctr; **Address:** Duke Univ Med Center, Box 3881, Durham, NC 27710; **Phone:** 919-660-7520; **Board Cert:** Internal Medicine 1977; Endocrinology 1979; Geriatric Medicine 2000; **Med School:** Med Coll VA 1974; **Resid:** Internal Medicine, Med Coll VA 1977; **Fellow:** Endocrinology, Diabetes & Metabolism, Duke Univ Med Ctr 1979; Geriatric Medicine, Duke Univ/VA Med Ctr 1981; **Fac Appt:** Prof Med, Duke Univ

Palmer, Robert M MD [Ger] - **Spec Exp:** Geriatric Functional Assessment; Dementia; **Hospital:** Sentara Norfolk Genl Hosp; **Address:** 825 Fairfax Ave Fl 2 - rm 201, Norfolk, VA 23507; **Phone:** 757-446-7040; **Board Cert:** Internal Medicine 1975; Geriatric Medicine 2009; **Med School:** Univ Mich Med Sch 1971; **Resid:** Internal Medicine, LA County Med Ctr 1975; **Fellow:** Geriatric Medicine, UCLA Med Ctr 1986

Ritchie, Christine S MD [Ger] - **Spec Exp:** Palliative Care; **Hospital:** Univ of Ala Hosp at Birmingham; **Address:** UAB Ctr Palliative Care, Ch 19 Ave S, Ste 219, 1530 3rd Ave S, Birmingham, AL 35294-2041; **Phone:** 205-975-8197; **Board Cert:** Internal Medicine 2002; Geriatric Medicine 2006; Hospice & Palliative Medicine 2003; **Med School:** Univ NC Sch Med 1988; **Resid:** Internal Medicine, Univ Ala Sch Med 1992; **Fellow:** Geriatric Medicine, Univ Ala Sch Med 1994; **Fac Appt:** Assoc Prof Med, Univ Alabama

Midwest

Carr, David B MD [Ger] - **Spec Exp:** Polypharmacology (Excess Medications); Alzheimer's Disease; **Hospital:** Barnes-Jewish Hosp; **Address:** Wash Univ Sch Med, Div Geriatrics, 4488 Forest Park, Ste 160, St Louis, MO 63108; **Phone:** 314-286-1967; **Board Cert:** Internal Medicine 1989; Geriatric Medicine 2000; **Med School:** Univ MO-Columbia Sch Med 1985; **Resid:** Internal Medicine, Mich State Assoc Hosps 1988; **Fellow:** Geriatric Medicine, Duke Univ 1990; **Fac Appt:** Prof Med, Washington Univ, St Louis

Dale, Lowell C MD [Ger] - **Spec Exp:** Tobacco Abuse; Nutrition; **Hospital:** Mayo Med Ctr & Clin - Rochester; **Address:** Mayo Clinic, 200 First St SW, Rochester, MN 55905; **Phone:** 507-284-2439; **Board Cert:** Internal Medicine 1984; **Med School:** Univ Minn 1981; **Resid:** Internal Medicine, Mayo Clin 1984; **Fellow:** Internal Medicine, Mayo Clin 1985; **Fac Appt:** Asst Prof Med, Mayo Med Sch

Duthie Jr, Edmund H MD [Ger] - **Spec Exp:** Geriatric Functional Assessment; **Hospital:** Froedtert and Med Ctr of WI, Clement J Zablocki VA Med Ctr; **Address:** 9200 W Wisconsin Ave Fl 5, Milwaukee, WI 53226; **Phone:** 414-805-0728; **Board Cert:** Internal Medicine 1979; Geriatric Medicine 2008; **Med School:** Georgetown Univ 1976; **Resid:** Internal Medicine, Med Coll Wisc Hosps 1979; **Fellow:** Geriatric Medicine, Jewish Inst Geri Care-SUNY 1980; **Fac Appt:** Prof Med, Med Coll Wisc

Flaherty, Joseph MD [Ger] - **Spec Exp:** Drugs & Aging; **Hospital:** St. Louis Univ Hosp; **Address:** 1402 Grand Blvd, rm M238, St Louis, MO 63104; **Phone:** 314-977-8462; **Board Cert:** Internal Medicine 2003; Geriatric Medicine 2006; **Med School:** St Louis Univ 1990; **Resid:** Internal Medicine, Kansas City Univ Med Ctr 1993; **Fellow:** Geriatric Medicine, St Louis Univ 1995; **Fac Appt:** Assoc Prof Med, St Louis Univ

Gorbien, Martin J MD [Ger] - **Spec Exp:** Dementia; Alzheimer's Disease; Geriatric Functional Assessment; Palliative Care; **Hospital:** Rush Univ Med Ctr; **Address:** 1725 W Harrison St, Ste 955, Chicago, IL 60612; **Phone:** 312-942-7030; **Board Cert:** Geriatric Medicine 2008; Hospice & Palliative Medicine 2008; **Med School:** Mexico 1983; **Resid:** Internal Medicine, Mercy Hosp & Med Ctr 1987; **Fellow:** Geriatric Medicine, UCLA Med Ctr 1989; **Fac Appt:** Assoc Prof Med, Rush Med Coll

Morley, John MD [Ger] - **Spec Exp:** Endocrinology; Menopause-Male; Alzheimer's Disease; Frailty Syndrome; **Hospital:** St. Louis Univ Hosp; **Address:** St Louis Univ Hlth Sci Ctr, Div Ger Med, 3660 Vista Ave, Ste 204, St Louis, MO 63110; **Phone:** 314-977-6157; **Board Cert:** Internal Medicine 1978; Endocrinology, Diabetes & Metabolism 1981; Geriatric Medicine 2008; **Med School:** South Africa 1972; **Resid:** Internal Medicine, Johannesburg Genl Hosp 1974; Internal Medicine, Baragwanath Hosp 1976; **Fellow:** Endocrinology, Diabetes & Metabolism, Wadsworth VA Hosp-UCLA 1979; **Fac Appt:** Prof Med, St Louis Univ

Olson Jr, Jack C MD [Ger] - **Spec Exp:** Dementia; Depression; **Hospital:** Rush Univ Med Ctr; **Address:** Senior Care, Rush Univ Professional Bldg 3, 1725 W Harrison St, Ste 955, Chicago, IL 60612-3836; **Phone:** 312-942-7030; **Board Cert:** Internal Medicine 1987; **Med School:** Univ Mich Med Sch 1984; **Resid:** Internal Medicine, Univ Wisconsin Affil Hosp 1987; **Fellow:** Geriatric Medicine, Univ Wisconsin Affil Hosp 1989; **Fac Appt:** Asst Prof Med, Univ Chicago-Pritzker Sch Med

Sachs, Greg A MD [Ger] - **Spec Exp:** Memory Disorders; Alzheimer's Disease; Palliative Care; **Hospital:** IU Health University Hosp; **Address:** 1050 Wishard Blvd, Regenstrief, 4th Fl, Indianapolis, IN 46202; **Phone:** 317-630-2557; **Board Cert:** Internal Medicine 1988; Geriatric Medicine 2010; Hospice & Palliative Medicine 2010; **Med School:** Yale Univ 1985; **Resid:** Internal Medicine, Univ Chicago Hosps 1987; **Fellow:** Geriatric Medicine, Univ Chicago Hosps 1990; **Fac Appt:** Prof Med, Indiana Univ

Geriatric Medicine

Thomas, David R MD [Ger] - **Spec Exp:** Wound Healing/Care; Nutrition; Frail Elderly; **Hospital:** St. Louis Univ Hosp; **Address:** St Louis Univ Sch Med, Div Geri Med, 1402 S Grand Blvd, Ste M238, St Louis, MO 63104; **Phone:** 314-977-8462; **Board Cert:** Internal Medicine 1975; Geriatric Medicine 2009; **Med School:** Univ Miss 1971; **Resid:** Internal Medicine, Univ Miss Med Ctr 1975; **Fellow:** Geriatric Medicine, Johns Hopkins Hosp 1988; **Fac Appt:** Prof Med, St Louis Univ

Great Plains and Mountains

Kutner, Jean S MD [Ger] - **Spec Exp:** Palliative Care; Preventive Medicine; Women's Health; **Hospital:** Univ of CO Hosp - Anschutz Inpatient Pav; **Address:** 8111 E Lowry Blvd, Ste 120, Denver, CO 80230; **Phone:** 720-848-9500; **Board Cert:** Internal Medicine 2004; Geriatric Medicine 2008; Hospice & Palliative Medicine 2008; **Med School:** UCSF 1991; **Resid:** Internal Medicine, UCSF Med Ctr 1994; **Fellow:** Internal Medicine, Univ Colorado Sch Med 1996; Geriatric Medicine, Univ Colorado Sch Med 1997; **Fac Appt:** Prof Med, Univ Colorado

Schwartz, Robert S MD [Ger] - **Spec Exp:** Diabetes; Hormonal Disorders; **Hospital:** Univ of CO Hosp - Anschutz Inpatient Pav, VA Eastern CO Health Care Sys-Denver; **Address:** Univ Colorado-Seniors Clinic, 12631 E 17th Ave, MS B179, Denver, CO 80262-0001; **Phone:** 720-848-3400; **Board Cert:** Internal Medicine 1977; Endocrinology 1981; Geriatric Medicine 2000; **Med School:** Ohio State Univ 1974; **Resid:** Internal Medicine, Univ Wash Med Ctr 1977; **Fellow:** Endocrinology, Diabetes & Metabolism, Univ Wash 1980; **Fac Appt:** Prof Med, Univ Colorado

Supiano, Mark A MD [Ger] - **Spec Exp:** Hypertension; Geriatric Functional Assessment; **Hospital:** Univ Utah Hlth Care; **Address:** Univ Utah, Geriatrics Div, 30 N 1900 E, SOM AB 193, Salt Lake City, UT 84132; **Phone:** 801-587-9103; **Board Cert:** Internal Medicine 1985; Geriatric Medicine 1998; **Med School:** Univ Wisc 1982; **Resid:** Internal Medicine, Univ Mich Med Ctr 1985; **Fellow:** Geriatric Medicine, Univ Mich Med Ctr 1987; **Fac Appt:** Prof Med, Univ Utah

Southwest

Dyer, Carmel B MD [Ger] - **Spec Exp:** Elder Abuse; Dementia; Delirium; Geriatric Functional Assessment; **Hospital:** Meml Hermann Hosp - Texas Med Ctr, LBJ General Hosp; **Address:** 6431 Fannin St, rm MSB-4.200, Houston, TX 77030; **Phone:** 713-566-4646; **Board Cert:** Internal Medicine 2000; Geriatric Medicine 2000; **Med School:** Baylor Coll Med 1988; **Resid:** Internal Medicine, Baylor Affil Hosps 1991; **Fellow:** Geriatric Medicine, Baylor Affil Hosps 1993; **Fac Appt:** Prof Med, Univ Tex, Houston

Liem, Pham MD [Ger] - **Spec Exp:** Dementia; Alzheimer's Disease; Delirium; **Hospital:** UAMS Med Ctr, Cent Ark Vet Hlthcare Sys; **Address:** UAMS Thomas A Lyon Longevity Ctr, 4301 W Markham St, Slot 547-13, Little Rock, AR 72205-7101; **Phone:** 501-686-6219; **Board Cert:** Family Medicine 2006; Geriatric Medicine 2008; **Med School:** Vietnam 1973; **Resid:** Family Medicine, Univ Ark Med Sch 1980; **Fellow:** Geriatric Medicine, Univ Ark Med Sch 1982; **Fac Appt:** Prof Med, Univ Ark

Lipschitz, David A MD/PhD [Ger] - **Spec Exp:** Preventive Medicine; Nutrition; **Hospital:** St. Vincent Med Ctr; **Address:** Longevity Center-St Vincent Senior Hlth, One St Vincent Circle, Ste 210, Little Rock, AR 72205; **Phone:** 501-552-4777; **Board Cert:** Internal Medicine 1975; Hematology 1976; **Med School:** South Africa 1966; **Resid:** Internal Medicine, Johannesburg Genl Hosp 1972; **Fellow:** Hematology, Univ Washington 1974; Internal Medicine, Montefiore Hosp 1975; **Fac Appt:** Prof Med, Univ Ark

Wei, Jeanne MD/PhD [Ger] - **Spec Exp:** Cardiovascular Disease; **Hospital:** UAMS Med Ctr, John L McClellan VA Med Ctr; **Address:** UAMS Thomas A Lyon Longevity Ctr, 4301 W Markham St, Slot 547-13, Little Rock, AR 72205; **Phone:** 501-686-6219; **Board Cert:** Internal Medicine 1978; Cardiovascular Disease 1979; Geriatric Medicine 2001; **Med School:** Univ IL Coll Med 1975; **Resid:** Internal Medicine, Johns Hopkins Hosp 1977; **Fellow:** Cardiovascular Disease, Johns Hopkins Hosp 1979; Research, Natl Inst Aging 1979; **Fac Appt:** Prof Med, Univ Ark

West Coast and Pacific

Abrass, Itamar B MD [Ger] - **Spec Exp:** Geriatric Endocrinology; Endocrine Disorders; Diabetes; **Hospital:** Harborview Med Ctr, Univ Wash Med Ctr; **Address:** Harborview Medical Ctr, 325 9th Ave, Box 359860, Seattle, WA 98104; **Phone:** 206-744-4191; **Board Cert:** Internal Medicine 1974; Endocrinology, Diabetes & Metabolism 1975; **Med School:** UCSF 1966; **Resid:** Internal Medicine, Columbia-Pesby Med Ctr 1968; **Fellow:** Endocrinology, Diabetes & Metabolism, UCSD Med Ctr 1971; **Fac Appt:** Prof Med, Univ Wash

Landefeld, Charles S MD [Ger] - **Spec Exp:** Cardiovascular Disease; Incontinence; **Hospital:** UCSF Med Ctr, VA Med Ctr - San Francisco; **Address:** 3333 California St, Ste 380, San Francisco, CA 94118; **Phone:** 415-514-0715; **Board Cert:** Internal Medicine 1982; **Med School:** Yale Univ 1979; **Resid:** Internal Medicine, UCSF Med Ctr 1983; **Fellow:** Geriatric Medicine, Brigham-Womens Hosp 1985; **Fac Appt:** Prof Med, UCSF

McCormick, Wayne MD [Ger] - **Spec Exp:** Dementia; AIDS/HIV; **Hospital:** Harborview Med Ctr, Univ Wash Med Ctr; **Address:** Harborview Med Ctr, 325 9th Ave, Box 359755, Seattle, WA 98104; **Phone:** 206-744-4191; **Board Cert:** Internal Medicine 1986; Geriatric Medicine 2002; Public Health & Genl Preventive Med 1992; **Med School:** Washington Univ, St Louis 1983; **Resid:** Internal Medicine, Michael Reese Hosp 1987; **Fellow:** Geriatric Medicine, Univ Wash Med Ctr 1990; **Fac Appt:** Asst Prof Med, Univ Wash

Reuben, David B MD [Ger] - **Spec Exp:** Geriatric Functional Assessment; **Hospital:** UCLA Ronald Reagan Med Ctr, Santa Monica - UCLA Med Ctr & Ortho Hosp; **Address:** UCLA Med Ctr, 1245 16th St, Ste 309, Santa Monica, CA 90404; **Phone:** 310-319-4371; **Board Cert:** Internal Medicine 1980; Geriatric Medicine 2005; **Med School:** Emory Univ 1977; **Resid:** Internal Medicine, Rhode Island Hosp 1980; **Fellow:** Geriatric Medicine, UCLA Med Ctr 1987; **Fac Appt:** Prof Med, UCLA

Tenover, Joyce S MD/PhD [Ger] - **Spec Exp:** Menopause-Male; Prostate Disease; Polypharmacology (Excess Medications); Hormonal Disorders; **Hospital:** VA Hlth Care Sys - Palo Alto; **Address:** VA Palo Alto HCS, GRECC (182B), 3801 Miranda Ave, Palo Alto, CA 94304-1290; **Phone:** 650-493-5000 x66946; **Board Cert:** Internal Medicine 1983; Geriatric Medicine 1997; **Med School:** Geo Wash Univ 1980; **Resid:** Internal Medicine, Univ Wash Affil Hosps 1983; Internal Medicine, VA Med Ctr 1984; **Fellow:** Geriatric Medicine, VA Med Ctr 1987; **Fac Appt:** Anat

Cleveland Clinic

Every life deserves world class care.

Geriatric Medicine

Cleveland Clinic's Center for Geriatric Medicine, part of the Medicine Institute at Cleveland Clinic, specializes in diagnosing and treating frail, elderly patients with complex medical conditions and social problems.

Our Center for Geriatric Medicine consists of an inter-disciplinary team of healthcare professionals dedicated to creating comprehensive, coordinated care plans for all patients. The center offers several specialized programs to help ensure older patients receive the full scope of care necessary for optimal outcomes.

These programs include:

Geriatric Evaluation and Management Program is the cornerstone of the comprehensive care offered to senior patients and their families. It takes an in-depth look at each patient's physical and psychological health, including the person's medical history, current status, recent changes and special concerns.

Geriatric Falls Clinic provides evaluation and follow-up for the treatment and prevention of falls. The multidisciplinary assessment includes screening of vision, medical conditions, polypharmacy, nutritional status, mental alertness, physical function, balance and strength.

Aging Brain Clinic brings together a medical team that includes physicians who specialize in geriatric medicine, neurology and neurosurgery. Patients appropriate for these clinics are older adults with ventriculomegaly (hydrocephalus) and cognitive, gait and urological problems.

Geriatric Consultations

One of the special features that Cleveland Clinic offers older adults hospitalized for acute medical or surgical problems is an inpatient geriatrics assessment. These assessments can be requested by the attending physician for specific geriatric concerns, including: depression, delirium (acute confusion), dementia, falls and concerns about medications or other geriatric issues.

Cleveland Clinic
Center for Geriatric Medicine
9500 Euclid Avenue
Cleveland, OH 44195

clevelandclinic.org/
geriatrictopdocs

Offering Same-Day Appointments
Call 800.274.2009.

Treatment Guides

Cleveland Clinic has developed comprehensive treatment guides for many diseases and conditions. To download our free treatment guides, visit clevelandclinic.org/treatmentguides.

Online Medical Second Opinion

Cleveland Clinic's My**Consult** Online Medical Second Opinion program securely connects patients to our physician specialists for more than 1,000 life-changing or life-threatening diagnoses all by the click of a mouse. To learn more, log onto eclevelandclinic.org/myconsult or call 800.223.2273, ext. 43223.

Special Assistance for Out-of-State Patients

Cleveland Clinic Global Patient Services offers a complimentary Medical Concierge service for patients who travel from outside of Ohio. Call 800.223.2273, ext. 55580 or email medicalconcierge@ccf.org.

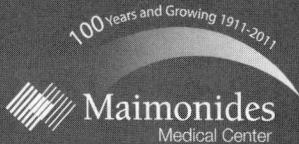

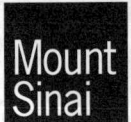 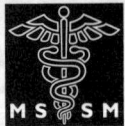

MOUNT SINAI SCHOOL OF MEDICINE

THE MOUNT SINAI MEDICAL CENTER
THE BROOKDALE DEPARTMENT OF
GERIATRICS AND PALLIATIVE MEDICINE
One Gustave L. Levy Place
Fifth Avenue and 100th Street
New York, NY 10029-6574
Physician Referral: 1-800-MD-SINAI (637-4624)
www.mountsinai.org/geriatrics
www.mountsinai.org/palliative

The Best in Clinical Care

In recognition of the care offered to older patients, The Mount Sinai Medical Center's **BROOKDALE DEPARTMENT OF GERIATRICS AND PALLIATIVE MEDICINE** is cited time and time again as the finest in the nation. In 2011, *U.S. News & World Report* ranked our geriatrics specialty #1 and our medical school program #1 in the United States.

We offer a full spectrum of patient care, including a specialized inpatient care team for the elderly to minimize complications sometimes associated with an older person's hospital stay, a primary care geriatrics practice for older adults living in the community, a hospital-based consultation service for patients throughout Mount Sinai, a number of community-linked programs and partnerships, and a palliative care team dedicated to ensuring the highest quality care and support for patients and families facing serious illnesses.

The Martha Stewart Center for Living, a modern facility designed by renowned architect C.C. Pei, provides clinical care and education for patients and serves as a training ground for physicians. Our newly opened Wiener Family Palliative Care Unit, the only one of its kind in Manhattan, provides inpatient care for patients and families facing serious and life-threatening illness.

Groundbreaking Research—Mount Sinai's researchers continue to advance the understanding, prevention, and treatment of age-related disorders. The extensive research on aging conducted by the Brookdale Department of Geriatrics and Palliative Medicine includes studies on health services, medical decision making and ethical dilemmas, palliative care, the neurobiology of aging, and clinical interventions to promote independence in old age. The department's expertise serves as a renowned educational resource for all Mount Sinai affiliates and other institutions in teaching geriatrics and palliative medicine to medical students, medical residents, geriatrics and palliative care fellows, established physicians, and health profession trainees in other disciplines.

History Of Excellence—The Mount Sinai Medical Center is a pioneer in geriatric medicine. In 1909, a Mount Sinai physician coined the term "geriatrics," and in 1914, he wrote the first textbook on medical care for older adults. Today, the Brookdale Department of Geriatrics and Palliative Medicine continues to break new ground, offering comprehensive care, disease prevention, and the promotion of healthy and productive aging. The department's enhanced expertise in assessing and managing patients with dementia greatly complements its established, interdisciplinary approach to patient care, in which medical staff and social workers address each patient's needs as a team. Our newly opened Wiener Family Palliative Care Unit, the only one of its kind in Manhattan, provides inpatient care for patients and families facing serious and life-threatening illness.

THE FIRST FREESTANDING DEPARTMENT OF GERIATRICS AT A U.S. MEDICAL SCHOOL

Mount Sinai's Brookdale Department of Geriatrics and Palliative Medicine was the first freestanding department of geriatrics established by a U.S. medical school, and it continues to be one of the very best. It offers unparalleled inpatient and outpatient care, as well as numerous treatment programs designed to meet the unique needs of older adults. Mount Sinai is also home to world-class researchers dedicated to advancing our understanding of Alzheimer's disease and other common geriatric conditions. At the department's heart are its patients. The geriatricians of The Mount Sinai Medical Center work hard to improve life and longevity for New York's elderly.

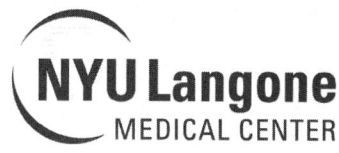

550 First Avenue *(at 31st Street)*
New York, NY 10016

www.NYULMC.org

Physician Referral: **888-7-NYU-MED** *(888-769-8633)*

GERIATRIC MEDICINE

About the Section of Geriatrics, Division of General Internal Medicine, Department of Medicine
NYU Langone Medical Center has a distinguished history as a federally designated research center and leader in the care of geriatrics. We specialize in the following areas:

Inpatient Geriatrics Services
Using a team approach, a senior geriatrician leads nurses, pharmacists, geropsychiatrists, rehabilitation experts and fellowship trainees in caring for geriatric patients with complex conditions. If screening reveals a hospitalized patient is suffering from a geriatric problem (such as cognitive impairment), special consultation is offered to the patient's health care team.

The Healthy Aging Initiative
A fundamental part of the care provided by geriatricians within NYU Langone Medical Center's faculty group practice is assessing and advising older individuals on how to avoid developing problems like cognitive or functional impairment.

The William and Sylvia Silberstein Aging and Dementia Research Center
The Silberstein Aging and Dementia Research Center is a National Institute on Aging-designated Center of Excellence in Alzheimer's treatment. The facility provides comprehensive diagnostic evaluations to determine if memory loss is "normal" or more serious; a memory enhancement program for age-related memory decline; clinical trials for mild memory loss and for Alzheimer's treatment; state-of-the-art brain imaging techniques; methods to minimize disability in Alzheimer's patients; and comprehensive counseling and support groups for patients, caregivers and family members.

The Pearl Barlow Center for Memory Evaluation and Treatment
The Pearl Barlow Center for Memory Evaluation and Treatment is the clinical care and diagnostic unit of the Silberstein Alzheimer's Institute at NYU Langone Medical Center. The Pearl Barlow Center for Memory Evaluation and Treatment is focused on patients with memory impairments caused by neurological, psychological and physical ailments, as well as memory issues resulting from medication side effects, anxiety, depression and the effects of normal aging, including Alzheimer's disease. This multidisciplinary medical approach, integrated with advanced research capabilities, is the first of its kind in New York City for the treatment of memory disorders.

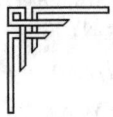

The Best in American Medicine
www.CastleConnolly.com

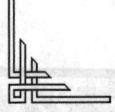
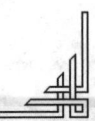

Gynecologic Oncology

a subspecialty of
Obstetrics & Gynecology

An obstetrician/gynecologist who provides consultation and comprehensive management of patients with gynecologic cancer, including those diagnostic and therapeutic procedures necessary
for the total care of the patient with gynecologic cancer and resulting complications.

Training Required: Four years *plus* two years in clinical practice before certification in obstetrics and gynecology is complete *plus* additional training and examination in gynecologic oncology.

GYNECOLOGIC ONCOLOGY

New England

Azodi, Masoud MD [GO] - **Spec Exp:** Laparoscopic Surgery; Ovarian Cancer-Early Detection; Uterine Cancer; **Hospital:** Yale-New Haven Hosp, Yale Med Group; **Address:** Smilow Cancer Hosp, 35 Park St Fl 1, New Haven, CT 06519; **Phone:** 203-200-4176; **Board Cert:** Gynecologic Oncology 2009; Obstetrics & Gynecology 2009; **Med School:** Wright State Univ 1992; **Resid:** Obstetrics & Gynecology, Aultman Hospital 1996; **Fellow:** Obstetrics & Gynecology, Yale-New Haven Hosp 1999; **Fac Appt:** Assoc Prof ObG, Yale Univ

Berkowitz, Ross S MD [GO] - **Spec Exp:** Gynecologic Cancer; **Hospital:** Brigham and Women's Hosp (page 57), Dana-Farber Cancer Inst (page 57); **Address:** Div OB/GYN Oncology, 75 Francis St, Boston, MA 02115-6110; **Phone:** 617-732-8843; **Board Cert:** Obstetrics & Gynecology 1981; Gynecologic Oncology 1982; **Med School:** Boston Univ 1973; **Resid:** Surgery, Peter Bent Brigham Hosp 1975; Obstetrics & Gynecology, Boston Hosp for Women 1978; **Fellow:** Gynecologic Oncology, Boston Hosp for Women 1980; **Fac Appt:** Prof ObG, Harvard Med Sch

Brewer, Molly A MD [GO] - **Spec Exp:** Ovarian Cancer; Gynecologic Cancer; Gynecologic Cancer-Rare; **Hospital:** Univ of Conn Hlth Ctr, John Dempsey Hosp, Hartford Hosp; **Address:** Univ Conn Hlth Ctr, Div Gyn Oncology, 263 Farmington Ave, MC2875, Farmington, CT 06032-2875; **Phone:** 860-679-2100; **Board Cert:** Obstetrics & Gynecology 2009; Gynecologic Oncology 2009; **Med School:** SUNY Upstate Med Univ 1991; **Resid:** Obstetrics & Gynecology, Oregon Hlth Scis Ctr 1995; **Fellow:** Gynecologic Oncology, MD Anderson Cancer Ctr 1997; **Fac Appt:** Prof ObG, Univ Conn

Cain, Joanna M MD [GO] - **Spec Exp:** Ovarian Cancer; Breast Cancer Risk Assessment; Uterine Cancer; Ovarian Cancer-Early Detection; **Hospital:** Women & Infants Hosp of RI, Rhode Island Hosp; **Address:** Women & Infants Hospital, 101 Dudley St, Providence, RI 02905; **Phone:** 401-274-1122 x1575; **Board Cert:** Obstetrics & Gynecology 2009; Gynecologic Oncology 2009; **Med School:** Creighton Univ 1978; **Resid:** Obstetrics & Gynecology, Univ Washington Med Ctr 1981; **Fellow:** Gynecologic Oncology, Meml Sloan Kettering Cancer Ctr 1983; **Fac Appt:** Prof ObG, Brown Univ

DeMars, Leslie R MD [GO] - **Spec Exp:** Gynecologic Cancer; Laparoscopic Surgery; **Hospital:** Dartmouth - Hitchcock Med Ctr; **Address:** Dartmouth-Hitchcock Med Ctr, Gyn-Oncology, 1 Medical Center Drive, Lebanon, NH 03756; **Phone:** 603-653-3530; **Board Cert:** Obstetrics & Gynecology 2009; Gynecologic Oncology 2009; **Med School:** Univ VT Coll Med 1987; **Resid:** Obstetrics & Gynecology, Univ NC Hosp 1991; **Fellow:** Gynecologic Oncology, Univ NC Hosp 1994; **Fac Appt:** Assoc Prof ObG, Dartmouth Med Sch

Granai, Cornelius O MD [GO] - **Spec Exp:** Gynecologic Cancer; Complementary Medicine; International Health; **Hospital:** Women & Infants Hosp of RI, Rhode Island Hosp; **Address:** Womens & Infants Hosp, 101 Dudley St, GYN Oncology Department, Providence, RI 02905; **Phone:** 401-453-7520; **Board Cert:** Obstetrics & Gynecology 2009; Gynecologic Oncology 2009; **Med School:** Univ VT Coll Med 1977; **Resid:** Obstetrics & Gynecology, Hershey Med Ctr 1981; **Fellow:** Gynecologic Oncology, Tufts Univ 1984; **Fac Appt:** Prof ObG, Brown Univ

Muto, Michael G MD [GO] - **Spec Exp:** Ovarian Cancer; Cervical Cancer; Vulvar & Vaginal Cancer; Robotic Surgery; **Hospital:** Dana-Farber Cancer Inst (page 57), Brigham and Women's Hosp (page 57); **Address:** Brigham & Womens Hosp, Div Gynecologic Oncology, 75 Francis St, Boston, MA 02115; **Phone:** 617-732-8840; **Board Cert:** Obstetrics & Gynecology 2009; Gynecologic Oncology 2008; **Med School:** Univ Mass Sch Med 1983; **Resid:** Obstetrics & Gynecology, Brigham & Women's Hosp 1987; **Fellow:** Gynecologic Oncology, Brigham & Women's Hosp 1990; **Fac Appt:** Assoc Prof ObG, Harvard Med Sch

Rutherford, Thomas J MD [GO] - **Spec Exp:** Ovarian Cancer; Uterine Cancer; Ovarian Cancer-Early Detection; Cervical Cancer; **Hospital:** Yale-New Haven Hosp, Yale Med Group; **Address:** Smilow Cancer Hosp, 35 Park St Fl 1, New Haven, CT 06519; **Phone:** 203-200-4176; **Board Cert:** Obstetrics & Gynecology 2009; Gynecologic Oncology 2009; **Med School:** Med Coll OH 1989; **Resid:** Obstetrics & Gynecology, Cooper Hosp 1993; **Fellow:** Gynecologic Oncology, Yale-New Haven Hosp 1995; **Fac Appt:** Assoc Prof ObG, Yale Univ

Santin, Alessandro MD [GO] - **Spec Exp:** Immunotherapy; Ovarian Cancer; Vulvar & Vaginal Cancer; **Hospital:** Yale-New Haven Hosp, Yale Med Group; **Address:** Yale Gynecologic Oncology, 333 Cedar St, PO Box 208063, New Haven, CT 06510; **Phone:** 203-737-2280; **Med School:** Italy 1989; **Resid:** Obstetrics & Gynecology, Univ Brescia Sch Med 1993; **Fellow:** Gynecologic Oncology, UC Irvine 1995; Gynecologic Oncology, UAMS Med Ctr 2000; **Fac Appt:** Prof ObG, Yale Univ

Schorge, John O MD [GO] - **Spec Exp:** Ovarian Cancer; Uterine Cancer; Cervical Cancer; Minimally Invasive Surgery; **Hospital:** Mass Genl Hosp; **Address:** Gillette Ctr for Gynocological Oncology, 55 Fruit St, Yawkey Ctr 9E, Boston, MA 02114; **Phone:** 617-724-6899; **Board Cert:** Obstetrics & Gynecology 2010; Gynecologic Oncology 2010; **Med School:** Vanderbilt Univ 1993; **Resid:** Obstetrics & Gynecology, Brigham & Women's Hosp 1997; **Fellow:** Gynecologic Oncology, Brigham & Women's Hosp 2000; **Fac Appt:** Assoc Prof ObG, Harvard Med Sch

Schwartz, Peter E MD [GO] - **Spec Exp:** Ovarian Cancer; Uterine Cancer; Gynecologic Surgery-Complex; Cervical Cancer; **Hospital:** Yale-New Haven Hosp, Yale Med Group; **Address:** 333 Cedar St FMB Bldg Fl 3 - Ste 328, St, New Haven, CT 06510-3289; **Phone:** 203-785-4014; **Board Cert:** Obstetrics & Gynecology 1973; Gynecologic Oncology 1979; **Med School:** Albert Einstein Coll Med 1966; **Resid:** Obstetrics & Gynecology, Yale-New Haven Hosp 1970; **Fellow:** Gynecologic Oncology, MD Anderson Cancer Ctr 1975; **Fac Appt:** Prof ObG, Yale Univ

Tarraza, Hector M MD [GO] - **Spec Exp:** Gynecologic Cancer; **Hospital:** Maine Med Ctr; **Address:** 102 Campus Drive, rm 116, Scarborough, ME 04074; **Phone:** 207-883-0069; **Board Cert:** Obstetrics & Gynecology 2009; Gynecologic Oncology 2009; **Med School:** Harvard Med Sch 1981; **Resid:** Obstetrics & Gynecology, Mass Genl Hosp 1985; **Fellow:** Gynecologic Oncology, Mass Genl Hosp 1987; **Fac Appt:** Prof ObG, Univ VT Coll Med

Mid Atlantic

Abbas, Fouad M MD [GO] - **Spec Exp:** Gynecologic Cancer; Ovarian Cancer; Cervical Cancer; **Hospital:** Sinai Hosp - Baltimore; **Address:** Sinai Hosp Baltimore, 2411 W Belvedere Ave, Ste 206, Baltimore, MD 21215; **Phone:** 410-601-9030; **Board Cert:** Obstetrics & Gynecology 2008; Gynecologic Oncology 2008; **Med School:** Univ MD Sch Med 1986; **Resid:** Obstetrics & Gynecology, John Hopkins Hosp 1990; **Fellow:** Gynecologic Oncology, John Hopkins Hosp 1992; **Fac Appt:** Asst Prof ObG, Univ MD Sch Med

Gynecologic Oncology

Abu-Rustum, Nadeem R MD [GO] - **Spec Exp:** Ovarian Cancer; Uterine Cancer; Cervical Cancer; Vulvar Disease/Cancer; **Hospital:** Meml Sloan-Kettering Cancer Ctr; **Address:** 1275 York Ave, New York, NY 10065; **Phone:** 212-639-7051; **Board Cert:** Obstetrics & Gynecology 2009; Gynecologic Oncology 2009; **Med School:** Lebanon 1990; **Resid:** Obstetrics & Gynecology, Greater Baltimore Med Ctr 1994; **Fellow:** Gynecologic Oncology, Meml Sloan-Kettering Cancer Ctr 1997; **Fac Appt:** Assoc Prof ObG, Cornell Univ-Weill Med Coll

Barakat, Richard R MD [GO] - **Spec Exp:** Laparoscopic Surgery; Ovarian Cancer; Uterine Cancer; **Hospital:** Meml Sloan-Kettering Cancer Ctr; **Address:** 1275 York Ave, rm H1305, New York, NY 10065; **Phone:** 800-525-2225; **Board Cert:** Obstetrics & Gynecology 2006; Gynecologic Oncology 2006; **Med School:** SUNY Hlth Sci Ctr 1985; **Resid:** Obstetrics & Gynecology, Bellevue Hosp 1989; **Fellow:** Gynecologic Oncology, Meml Sloan Kettering Cancer Ctr 1991; **Fac Appt:** Assoc Prof ObG, Cornell Univ-Weill Med Coll

Barnes, Willard MD [GO] - **Spec Exp:** Pelvic Tumors; Gynecologic Cancer; **Hospital:** Georgetown Univ Hosp; **Address:** Georgetown Univ Hosp, Lombardi Cancer Ctr, Dept Gyn Oncology, 3800 Reservoir Rd NW, Washington, DC 20007-2194; **Phone:** 202-444-2114; **Board Cert:** Obstetrics & Gynecology 2009; Gynecologic Oncology 2009; **Med School:** Univ Miss 1979; **Resid:** Obstetrics & Gynecology, Univ Miss Med Ctr 1983; **Fellow:** Gynecologic Oncology, Georgetown Univ Med Ctr 1985; **Fac Appt:** Assoc Prof ObG, Georgetown Univ

Barter, James MD [GO] - **Spec Exp:** Laparoscopic Surgery; Ovarian Cancer; Gynecologic Cancer; **Hospital:** Holy Cross Hospital - Silver Spring, Suburban Hosp; **Address:** 6301 Executive Blvd, Rockville, MD 20852; **Phone:** 301-770-4967; **Board Cert:** Obstetrics & Gynecology 1997; Gynecologic Oncology 1997; **Med School:** Univ VA Sch Med 1977; **Resid:** Internal Medicine, Univ Kentucky Med Ctr 1979; Obstetrics & Gynecology, Duke Univ Med Ctr 1983; **Fellow:** Gynecologic Oncology, Univ Alabama 1985; **Fac Appt:** Clin Prof ObG, Georgetown Univ

Boice, Charles R MD [GO] - **Spec Exp:** Gynecologic Cancer; Ovarian Cancer; Cervical Cancer; **Hospital:** Washington Hosp Ctr; **Address:** 10301 Georgia Ave, Ste 205, Silver Springs, MD 20902; **Phone:** 301-592-1600; **Board Cert:** Obstetrics & Gynecology 1981; Gynecologic Oncology 1982; **Med School:** Loma Linda Univ 1973; **Resid:** Obstetrics & Gynecology, Los Angeles Med Ctr 1973; Surgery, City Hope Natl Med Ctr 1978; **Fellow:** Oncology, Univ Texas-MD Anderson Cancer Ctr 1980; **Fac Appt:** Assoc Clin Prof ObG, Univ Wash

Burger, Robert MD [GO] - **Spec Exp:** Ovarian Cancer; Uterine Cancer; Cervical Cancer; Gestational Trophoblastic Disease; **Hospital:** Fox Chase Cancer Ctr (page 58); **Address:** Fox Chase Cancer Ctr, Women's Cancer Ctr, 333 Cottman Ave, Phildelphia, PA 19111; **Phone:** 215-728-2570; **Board Cert:** Obstetrics & Gynecology 2008; Gynecologic Oncology 2008; **Med School:** NYU Sch Med 1988; **Resid:** Obstetrics & Gynecology, Hosp U Penn 1992; **Fellow:** Gynecologic Oncology, UC Irvine Med Ctr 1996

Caputo, Thomas A MD [GO] - **Spec Exp:** Cervical Cancer; Ovarian Cancer; Uterine Cancer; Vulvar Disease/Cancer; **Hospital:** NY-Presby/Weill Cornell Med Ctr, NY (page 65); **Address:** NY Presby Hosp-Weill Cornell, 525 E 68th St, Ste J130, New York, NY 10021; **Phone:** 212-746-3179; **Board Cert:** Obstetrics & Gynecology 1993; Gynecologic Oncology 1977; **Med School:** UMDNJ-NJ Med Sch, Newark 1965; **Resid:** Obstetrics & Gynecology, Martland Hosp 1969; **Fellow:** Gynecologic Oncology, Emory Univ Hosp 1974; **Fac Appt:** Clin Prof ObG, Cornell Univ-Weill Med Coll

Carlson, John A MD [GO] - **Spec Exp:** Gynecologic Cancer; Ovarian Cancer; Gynecologic Surgery-Complex; **Hospital:** St. Peter's Univ Hosp; **Address:** St Peter's Univ Hosp, 254 Easton Ave Cares Bldg, New Brunswick, NJ 08901; **Phone:** 732-937-6003; **Board Cert:** Obstetrics & Gynecology 1981; Gynecologic Oncology 1982; **Med School:** Georgetown Univ 1974; **Resid:** Obstetrics & Gynecology, Hosp Univ Penn 1978; **Fellow:** Gynecologic Oncology, MD Anderson Cancer Ctr 1980; **Fac Appt:** Prof ObG, Drexel Univ Coll Med

Cornelison, Terri L MD/PhD [GO] - **Spec Exp:** Gynecologic Cancer; Ovarian Cancer; Clinical Trials; **Hospital:** Johns Hopkins Hosp (page 61); **Address:** Kelly Gynecologic Oncology Service, 600 N Wolfe St Phipps Bldg - Ste 281, Baltimore, MD 21287; **Phone:** 410-502-4245; **Board Cert:** Obstetrics & Gynecology 2007; **Med School:** Yale Univ 1985; **Resid:** Obstetrics & Gynecology, Beth Israel Hosp 1989; **Fellow:** Gynecologic Oncology, Roswell Park Cancer Inst 1992; **Fac Appt:** Asst Prof ObG, Johns Hopkins Univ

Cosin, Jonathan A MD [GO] - **Spec Exp:** Gynecologic Cancer; **Hospital:** Washington Hosp Ctr; **Address:** Washington Hosp Ctr-Dept Gyn. Onc., 110 Irving St NW, rm 5B-33, Washington, DC 20010; **Phone:** 202-877-2391; **Board Cert:** Obstetrics & Gynecology 2009; Gynecologic Oncology 2009; **Med School:** Albany Med Coll 1991; **Resid:** Obstetrics & Gynecology, Baystate Med Ctr 1995; **Fellow:** Gynecology, Meml Sloan Kettering Cancer Ctr 1993; Gynecologic Oncology, Univ Minnesota Hosp 1998; **Fac Appt:** Asst Prof ObG, Georgetown Univ

Coukos, George MD/PhD [GO] - **Spec Exp:** Ovarian Cancer; Gynecologic Cancer; Vaccine Therapy; Clinical Trials; **Hospital:** Hosp Univ Penn - UPHS (page 68); **Address:** Hosp Univ Penn, 3400 Civic Center Blvd, Jordan Ctr Fl 3W, Philadelphia, PA 19104; **Phone:** 215-662-3318; **Board Cert:** Obstetrics & Gynecology 2004; Gynecologic Oncology 2004; **Med School:** Italy 1987; **Resid:** Obstetrics & Gynecology, Hosp Univ Penn 1997; **Fellow:** Gynecologic Oncology, Hosp Univ Penn 2000; **Fac Appt:** Prof ObG, Univ Pennsylvania

Curtin, John P MD [GO] - **Spec Exp:** Uterine Cancer; Ovarian Cancer; Laparoscopic Surgery; Gestational Trophoblastic Disease; **Hospital:** NYU Langone Med Ctr (page 66); **Address:** NYU Clin Cancer Ctr, 160 E 34th St Fl 4, New York, NY 10016-6402; **Phone:** 212-731-5345; **Board Cert:** Obstetrics & Gynecology 2008; Gynecologic Oncology 2009; **Med School:** Creighton Univ 1979; **Resid:** Obstetrics & Gynecology, Univ Minn Med Ctr 1984; **Fellow:** Gynecologic Oncology, Meml Sloan-Kettering Cancer Ctr 1988; **Fac Appt:** Prof ObG, NYU Sch Med

Dottino, Peter R MD [GO] - **Spec Exp:** Laparoscopic Surgery; Gynecologic Cancer; **Hospital:** Mount Sinai Med Ctr (page 63), Hackensack Univ Med Ctr; **Address:** 800-A 5th Ave, Ste 405, New York, NY 10065; **Phone:** 212-888-8439; **Board Cert:** Obstetrics & Gynecology 2007; Gynecologic Oncology 2007; **Med School:** Georgetown Univ 1979; **Resid:** Obstetrics & Gynecology, SUNY Downstate Med Ctr 1983; **Fellow:** Gynecologic Oncology, Mt Sinai Hosp 1985

Dunton, Charles J MD [GO] - **Spec Exp:** Ovarian Cancer; Uterine Cancer; Cervical Cancer; Pap Smear Abnormalities; **Hospital:** Lankenau Hosp; **Address:** 100 E Lancaster Ave, Med Office Bldg East, Ste 661, Wynnewood, PA 19096; **Phone:** 610-649-8085; **Board Cert:** Obstetrics & Gynecology 2009; Gynecologic Oncology 2009; **Med School:** Jefferson Med Coll 1980; **Resid:** Obstetrics & Gynecology, Lankenau Hosp 1984; **Fellow:** Gynecologic Oncology, Hosp Univ Penn 1989; **Fac Appt:** Prof ObG, Jefferson Med Coll

Edwards, Robert P MD [GO] - **Spec Exp:** Ovarian Cancer; Gynecologic Cancer; Cervical Cancer; Clinical Trials; **Hospital:** Magee-Womens Hosp - UPMC; **Address:** UPP-Dept Women's Health, 300 Halket St, Ste 2130, Pittsburgh, PA 15213; **Phone:** 412-641-1153; **Board Cert:** Obstetrics & Gynecology 2009; Gynecologic Oncology 2009; **Med School:** Univ Pittsburgh 1984; **Resid:** Obstetrics & Gynecology, Magee WomensHosp-UPMC 1989; **Fellow:** Gynecologic Oncology, Univ Alabama Med Ctr 1993; **Fac Appt:** Prof ObG, Univ Pittsburgh

Fields, Abbie L MD [GO] - **Spec Exp:** Fertility Preservation in Cancer; Robotic Surgery; Cancer Genetics; Pelvic Reconstruction; **Hospital:** Washington Hosp Ctr; **Address:** Washington Hospital Center, 110 Irving St NW, rm 5B-33B, Washington, DC 20010; **Phone:** 202-877-2391; **Board Cert:** Obstetrics & Gynecology 2009; Gynecologic Oncology 2009; **Med School:** Ohio State Univ 1987; **Resid:** Obstetrics & Gynecology, Northwestern Univ 1991; **Fellow:** Gynecologic Oncology, Johns Hopkins Hosp 1993

Gynecologic Oncology

Fishman, David A MD [GO] - **Spec Exp:** Ovarian Cancer; Ovarian Cancer-Early Detection; Gynecologic Cancer; **Hospital:** Mount Sinai Med Ctr (page 63); **Address:** 5 E 98th St Fl 2, New York, NY 10029; **Phone:** 212-427-9898; **Board Cert:** Obstetrics & Gynecology 2009; Gynecologic Oncology 2009; **Med School:** Texas Tech Univ 1988; **Resid:** Obstetrics & Gynecology, Yale-New Haven Hosp 1992; **Fellow:** Gynecologic Oncology, Yale-New Haven Hosp 1994; **Fac Appt:** Prof ObG, Mount Sinai Sch Med

Follen, Michele MD/PhD [GO] - **Spec Exp:** Gynecologic Cancer; Clinical Trials; Cervical Cancer; **Hospital:** Hahnemann Univ Hosp; **Address:** 245 N 15th St NCB Bldg Fl 17 - Ste 17113, Phildelphia, PA 19102; **Phone:** 215-762-1257; **Med School:** Univ Mich Med Sch 1980; **Resid:** Obstetrics & Gynecology, Columbia-Presby Med Ctr 1983; **Fellow:** Gynecologic Oncology, MD Anderson Cancer Ctr 1986; **Fac Appt:** Prof ObG, Drexel Univ Coll Med

Giuntoli II, Robert Lawrence MD [GO] - **Spec Exp:** Gynecologic Cancer; Ovarian Cancer; Gestational Trophoblastic Disease; Immunotherapy; **Hospital:** Johns Hopkins Hosp (page 61); **Address:** Johns Hopkins Hosp, Div Gyn Onc, 600 N Wolfe St, Phipps #281, Baltimore, MD 21287-1281; **Phone:** 410-502-4245; **Board Cert:** Obstetrics & Gynecology 2005; Gynecologic Oncology 2005; **Med School:** Univ Pennsylvania 1994; **Resid:** Obstetrics & Gynecology, Duke Univ Med Ctr 1998; **Fellow:** Gynecologic Oncology, Mayo Clin 2002; **Fac Appt:** Asst Prof ObG, Johns Hopkins Univ

Herzog, Thomas J MD [GO] - **Spec Exp:** Cervical Cancer; Gynecologic Cancer; Laparoscopic Surgery; Ovarian Cancer; **Hospital:** NY-Presby/Columbia Univ Med Ctr, NY (page 65); **Address:** Herbert Irving Pavilion, 161 Fort Washington Ave, 8-837, New York, NY 10032; **Phone:** 212-305-3410; **Board Cert:** Obstetrics & Gynecology 2008; Gynecologic Oncology 2008; **Med School:** Univ Cincinnati 1986; **Resid:** Obstetrics & Gynecology, Good Samaritan Hosp 1990; **Fellow:** Gynecologic Oncology, Barnes Jewish Hosp 1993; **Fac Appt:** Prof ObG, Columbia P&S

Kelley III, Joseph L MD [GO] - **Spec Exp:** Breast Cancer; Ovarian Cancer; Cervical Cancer; Gynecologic Cancer; **Hospital:** Magee-Womens Hosp - UPMC; **Address:** Magee-Womens Hosp-UPMC, 300 Halket St, Ste 1750, Pittsburgh, PA 15213; **Phone:** 412-641-5411; **Board Cert:** Obstetrics & Gynecology 2009; Gynecologic Oncology 2008; **Med School:** St Louis Univ 1985; **Resid:** Obstetrics & Gynecology, Magee-Womens Hosp 1989; **Fellow:** Gynecologic Oncology, MD Anderson Cancer Ctr 1991; **Fac Appt:** Assoc Prof ObG, Univ Pittsburgh

King, Stephanie A MD [GO] - **Spec Exp:** Ovarian Cancer; Uterine Cancer; Cervical Cancer; Trophoblastic Tumors; **Hospital:** Fox Chase Cancer Ctr (page 58); **Address:** Fox Chase Cancer Ctr, Dept Gynecologic Oncology, 333 Cottman Ave, Philadelphia, PA 19111; **Phone:** 215-728-5628; **Board Cert:** Obstetrics & Gynecology 2009; Gynecologic Oncology 2009; **Med School:** Univ Pennsylvania 1983; **Resid:** Obstetrics & Gynecology, Hosp Univ Penn 1988; **Fac Appt:** Assoc Prof S, Drexel Univ Coll Med

Koulos, John P MD [GO] - **Spec Exp:** Uterine Cancer; Ovarian Cancer; Cervical Cancer; **Hospital:** Beth Israel Med Ctr - Petrie Division (page 55); **Address:** Beth Israel Hosp Cancer Ctr, 10 Union Square E, Ste 4C, New York, NY 10003; **Phone:** 212-844-5729; **Board Cert:** Obstetrics & Gynecology 2010; Gynecologic Oncology 2010; **Med School:** Northwestern Univ 1978; **Resid:** Obstetrics & Gynecology, Northwestern Univ Med Sch 1982; **Fellow:** Gynecologic Oncology, Meml Sloan Kettering Cancer Ctr 1984; **Fac Appt:** Assoc Prof ObG, Albert Einstein Coll Med

Lele, Shashikant B MD [GO] - **Spec Exp:** Ovarian Cancer; Reconstructive Surgery; Pelvic Surgery-Complex; **Hospital:** Roswell Park Cancer Inst, Buffalo General Hosp; **Address:** Roswell Park Cancer Inst, Dept Gynecology, Elm & Carlton Sts, Buffalo, NY 14263; **Phone:** 716-845-5776; **Board Cert:** Obstetrics & Gynecology 1976; Gynecologic Oncology 1979; **Med School:** India 1968; **Resid:** Obstetrics & Gynecology, JJ Hosp-Grant Med Ctr 1970; Obstetrics & Gynecology, Mt Sinai Hosp 1973; **Fellow:** Gynecologic Oncology, Roswell Park Cancer Inst 1976; **Fac Appt:** Clin Prof ObG, SUNY Buffalo

Lin, Jeffrey Y MD [GO] - **Spec Exp:** Gynecologic Cancer; Gynecologic Surgery; Cervical Cancer; Ovarian Cancer; **Hospital:** Sibley Mem Hosp, G Washington Univ Hosp; **Address:** Sibley Ctr for GYN Oncology, 5255 Loughboro Rd NW, Washington, DC 20016; **Phone:** 202-741-2552; **Board Cert:** Obstetrics & Gynecology 2009; Gynecologic Oncology 2009; **Med School:** Albany Med Coll 1984; **Resid:** Obstetrics & Gynecology, George Washington Med Ctr 1988; Gynecologic Oncology, Univ Rochester Affil Hosp 1991; **Fac Appt:** Prof ObG, Geo Wash Univ

Morgan, Mark A MD [GO] - **Spec Exp:** Laparoscopic Surgery; Gynecologic Surgery-Complex; Gynecologic Cancer; Uro-Gynecology; **Hospital:** Fox Chase Cancer Ctr (page 58); **Address:** Fox Chase Cancer Ctr-Department of Surgery, 333 Cottman Ave, Philadelphia, PA 19111; **Phone:** 215-214-1430; **Board Cert:** Obstetrics & Gynecology 2009; **Med School:** SUNY Downstate 1982; **Resid:** Obstetrics & Gynecology, Hosp Univ Penn 1986; **Fellow:** Gynecologic Oncology, Hosp Univ Penn 1988

Odunsi, Adekunle O MD/PhD [GO] - **Spec Exp:** Ovarian Cancer; Gynecologic Cancer; Immunotherapy; Clinical Trials; **Hospital:** Roswell Park Cancer Inst; **Address:** Roswell Park Cancer Inst, Gyn Oncology, Elm and Carlton Streets, Buffalo, NY 14263; **Phone:** 716-845-2300; **Board Cert:** Obstetrics & Gynecology 2010; Gynecologic Oncology 2010; **Med School:** Nigeria 1984; **Resid:** Obstetrics & Gynecology, Rosie Maternity & Addenbrookes Hosps 1990; Obstetrics & Gynecology, Yale-New Haven Hosp 1999; **Fellow:** Gynecologic Oncology, Roswell Park Cancer Inst 2001; **Fac Appt:** Prof ObG, SUNY Buffalo

Randall, Thomas C MD [GO] - **Spec Exp:** Gynecologic Cancer; Robotic Surgery; **Hospital:** Pennsylvania Hosp-UPHS (page 68); **Address:** Pennsylvania Hospital, Dept OB/GYN, 801 Spruce St Fl 7, Philadelphia, PA 19107; **Phone:** 215-829-2345; **Board Cert:** Obstetrics & Gynecology 2009; Gynecologic Oncology 2009; **Med School:** Johns Hopkins Univ 1987; **Resid:** Obstetrics & Gynecology, Johns Hopkins Hosp 1991; **Fellow:** Gynecologic Oncology, Hosp Univ Penn 1992; **Fac Appt:** Assoc Clin Prof ObG, Univ Pennsylvania

Rosenblum, Norman G MD/PhD [GO] - **Spec Exp:** Ovarian Cancer; Uterine Cancer; Vulvar Disease/Cancer; **Hospital:** Thomas Jefferson Univ Hosp; **Address:** 834 Chesnut St, Ste 400, Philadelphia, PA 19107-5127; **Phone:** 215-955-6200; **Board Cert:** Obstetrics & Gynecology 2010; Gynecologic Oncology 2010; **Med School:** Jefferson Med Coll 1978; **Resid:** Obstetrics & Gynecology, Hosp Univ Penn 1982; **Fellow:** Gynecologic Oncology, Hosp Univ Penn 1984; **Fac Appt:** Prof ObG, Jefferson Med Coll

Rubin, Stephen C MD [GO] - **Spec Exp:** Ovarian Cancer; Uterine Cancer; Cervical Cancer; **Hospital:** Hosp Univ Penn - UPHS (page 68); **Address:** Perelman Center, Jordan Ctr for Gynecologic Cancer, 3400 Civic Center Blvd Fl 3 W, Philadelphia, PA 19104-4283; **Phone:** 215-662-3318; **Board Cert:** Obstetrics & Gynecology 2011; Gynecologic Oncology 2011; **Med School:** Univ Pennsylvania 1976; **Resid:** Obstetrics & Gynecology, Hosp Univ Penn 1980; **Fellow:** Gynecologic Oncology, Hosp Univ Penn 1982; **Fac Appt:** Prof ObG, Univ Pennsylvania

Gynecologic Oncology

Alvarez, Ronald D MD [GO] - **Spec Exp:** Gynecologic Cancer; Ovarian Cancer; **Hospital:** Univ of Ala Hosp at Birmingham, Brookwood Med Ctr; **Address:** Univ Alabama, Div Gyn Oncology, 619 19th St S, 176F, Ste 10250, Birmingham, AL 35249; **Phone:** 205-934-4986; **Board Cert:** Obstetrics & Gynecology 2007; Gynecologic Oncology 2007; **Med School:** Louisiana State U, New Orleans 1983; **Resid:** Obstetrics & Gynecology, Univ Alabama Hosp 1987; **Fellow:** Gynecologic Oncology, Univ Alabama Hosp 1990; **Fac Appt:** Assoc Prof ObG, Univ Alabama

Berchuck, Andrew MD [GO] - **Spec Exp:** Ovarian Cancer; Uterine Cancer; **Hospital:** Duke Univ Hosp; **Address:** Duke Univ Med Center, DUMC Box 3079, Durham, NC 27710; **Phone:** 919-684-3765; **Board Cert:** Obstetrics & Gynecology 2009; Gynecologic Oncology 2009; **Med School:** Case West Res Univ 1980; **Resid:** Obstetrics & Gynecology, Case Western Reserve Univ Hosp 1984; **Fellow:** Gynecology, UT Southwestern Affil Hosp 1985; Gynecologic Oncology, Meml Sloan-Kettering Cancer Ctr 1987; **Fac Appt:** Prof ObG, Duke Univ

Bicher, Annette MD [GO] - **Spec Exp:** Ovarian Cancer; Laparoscopic Surgery; **Hospital:** Inova Fairfax Hosp; **Address:** 3289 Woodburn Rd, Ste 320, Annandale, VA 22003; **Phone:** 703-698-7100; **Board Cert:** Obstetrics & Gynecology 2009; Gynecologic Oncology 2009; **Med School:** Univ Mich Med Sch 1987; **Resid:** Obstetrics & Gynecology, George Washington Univ Med Ctr 1991; **Fellow:** Research, NCI-NIH 1992; Gynecologic Oncology, UT MD Anderson Cancer Ctr 1994

Clarke-Pearson, Daniel L MD [GO] - **Spec Exp:** Pelvic Reconstruction; Gynecologic Surgery-Complex; Gynecologic Cancer; **Hospital:** NC Memorial Hosp - UNC, Wesley Long Comm Hosp; **Address:** NC Women's Hospital, 101 Manning Drive, MS 27599, Chapel Hill, NC 27599; **Phone:** 919-966-5280; **Board Cert:** Obstetrics & Gynecology 2006; Gynecologic Oncology 2006; **Med School:** Case West Res Univ 1975; **Resid:** Obstetrics & Gynecology, Duke Univ Med Ctr 1979; **Fellow:** Gynecologic Oncology, Duke Univ Med Ctr 1981; **Fac Appt:** Prof ObG, Univ NC Sch Med

Creasman, William T MD [GO] - **Spec Exp:** Uterine Cancer; Ovarian Cancer; Cervical Cancer; Gynecologic Cancer-Rare; **Hospital:** MUSC Med Ctr; **Address:** Med Univ S Carolina-Dept ObGyn, Charleston, SC 29425; **Phone:** 843-792-4509; **Board Cert:** Obstetrics & Gynecology 1991; Gynecologic Oncology 1974; **Med School:** Baylor Coll Med 1960; **Resid:** Obstetrics & Gynecology, Rochester Med Ctr 1967; **Fellow:** Gynecologic Oncology, Anderson Hosp Tumor Inst 1969; **Fac Appt:** Prof ObG, Med Univ SC

Currie, John L MD [GO] - **Spec Exp:** Gynecologic Cancer; Pelvic Reconstruction; Gynecologic Problems of Obesity; **Hospital:** Columbus Regl Med Ctr; **Address:** John B Amos Cancer Center, 1831 5th Ave, Columbus, GA 31904; **Phone:** 706-320-8700; **Board Cert:** Obstetrics & Gynecology 1991; Gynecologic Oncology 1982; **Med School:** Univ NC Sch Med 1967; **Resid:** Gynecologic Oncology, Hosp Univ Penn 1972; **Fellow:** Gynecologic Oncology, Duke Univ Med Ctr 1980

DePriest, Paul D MD [GO] - **Spec Exp:** Ovarian Cancer-Early Detection; Cervical Cancer; Pap Smear Abnormalities; **Hospital:** Univ of Kentucky Albert B. Chandler Hosp; **Address:** Univ Kentucky Gynecologic Oncology, Whiteney Hendrickson Bldg, 800 Rose St, rm 331E1, Lexington, KY 40536; **Phone:** 859-323-5277; **Board Cert:** Obstetrics & Gynecology 2009; Gynecologic Oncology 2009; **Med School:** Univ KY Coll Med 1985; **Resid:** Obstetrics & Gynecology, Univ Kentucky Med Ctr 1989; **Fellow:** Gynecologic Oncology, Univ Kentucky Med Ctr 1991; **Fac Appt:** Prof ObG, Univ KY Coll Med

Duska, Linda R MD [GO] - **Spec Exp:** Cervical Cancer; Gynecologic Cancer; Gynecologic Surgery-Complex; Ovarian Cancer; **Hospital:** Univ of Virginia Health Sys; **Address:** Dept of Obstetrics & Gynecology, Division of Gynecologic Oncology, P. O. Box 800712, Charlottesville, VA 22908; **Phone:** 434-924-1851; **Board Cert:** Obstetrics & Gynecology 2009; Gynecologic Oncology 2009; **Med School:** NYU Sch Med 1991; **Resid:** Obstetrics & Gynecology, John Hopkins Hosp 1995; **Fellow:** Gynecologic Oncology, MA Gen Hosp 1998; **Fac Appt:** Assoc Prof ObG, Univ VA Sch Med

Finan, Michael A MD [GO] - **Spec Exp:** Ovarian Cancer; Cervical Cancer; Uterine Cancer; **Hospital:** Univ of S AL Med Ctr, Univ of S Alabama Chil and Wom Hosp; **Address:** 1660 Springhill Ave, Mobile, AL 36604; **Phone:** 251-665-8000; **Board Cert:** Obstetrics & Gynecology 2008; Gynecologic Oncology 2008; **Med School:** Louisiana State U, New Orleans 1986; **Resid:** Obstetrics & Gynecology, Univ South Fla Affil Hosps 1990; **Fellow:** Gynecologic Oncology, H Lee Moffitt Cancer Ctr 1992; **Fac Appt:** Prof ObG, Univ S Ala Coll Med

Fiorica, James V MD [GO] - **Spec Exp:** Endometriosis; Breast Cancer; Uterine Cancer; **Hospital:** Sarasota Meml Hosp; **Address:** 1888 Hillview St, Sarasota, FL 34239; **Phone:** 941-917-8383; **Board Cert:** Obstetrics & Gynecology 2009; Gynecologic Oncology 2009; **Med School:** Tufts Univ 1982; **Resid:** Obstetrics & Gynecology, Univ South Fla Affil Hosp 1986; **Fellow:** Gynecologic Oncology, Univ South Fla Affil Hosp 1989; Breast Disease, Tufts Univ 1990; **Fac Appt:** Clin Prof ObG, Univ S Fla Coll Med

Fowler Jr, Wesley C MD [GO] - **Spec Exp:** Vulvar Disease/Cancer; DES-Exposed Females; Cancer Prevention; Gynecologic Cancer; **Hospital:** NC Memorial Hosp - UNC; **Address:** UNC Chapel Hill, Div Ob/Gyn, Campus Box 7572, Chapel Hill, NC 27599-7572; **Phone:** 919-966-7822; **Board Cert:** Obstetrics & Gynecology 1991; Gynecologic Oncology 1979; **Med School:** Univ NC Sch Med 1966; **Resid:** Obstetrics & Gynecology, NC Memorial Hosp 1971; **Fellow:** Gynecologic Oncology, NC Memorial Hosp 1971; **Fac Appt:** Prof ObG, Univ NC Sch Med

Ghamande, Sharad A MD [GO] - **Spec Exp:** Ovarian Cancer; Gynecologic Surgery-Complex; Clinical Trials; **Hospital:** Med Coll of GA Hosp and Clin (MCG Health Inc), Univ HC Sys - Augusta; **Address:** MCG Health Cancer Centr, 1411 Laney Walker Blvd, Augusta, GA 30912; **Phone:** 706-721-6744; **Board Cert:** Obstetrics & Gynecology 2010; Gynecologic Oncology 2010; **Med School:** India 1990; **Resid:** Obstetrics & Gynecology, Boston Univ Hosp 1997; **Fellow:** Gynecologic Oncology, Roswell Park Cancer Inst 2000; **Fac Appt:** Assoc Prof ObG, Med Coll GA

Havrilesky, Laura J MD [GO] - **Spec Exp:** Ovarian Cancer; **Hospital:** Duke Univ Hosp; **Address:** Duke Univ Med Ctr, Gyno Oncology, Box 3079, Durham, NC 27710; **Phone:** 919-684-3765; **Board Cert:** Obstetrics & Gynecology 2005; Gynecologic Oncology 2005; **Med School:** Duke Univ 1995; **Resid:** Obstetrics & Gynecology, Duke Univ Med Ctr 1999; **Fellow:** Gynecologic Oncology, Duke Univ Med Ctr 2002; **Fac Appt:** Assoc Prof ObG, Duke Univ

Horowitz, Ira R MD [GO] - **Spec Exp:** Laparoscopic Surgery; Ovarian Cancer; Cervical Cancer; **Hospital:** Emory Univ Hosp, Emory Univ Hosp Midtown; **Address:** Emory Clinic, 1365A Clifton Rd NE, Fl 4, Atlanta, GA 30322; **Phone:** 404-778-3401; **Board Cert:** Obstetrics & Gynecology 2010; Gynecologic Oncology 2010; **Med School:** Baylor Coll Med 1980; **Resid:** Obstetrics & Gynecology, Baylor Affil Hosp 1984; **Fellow:** Gynecologic Oncology, Johns Hopkins Hosp 1987; **Fac Appt:** Prof ObG, Emory Univ

Kohler, Matthew F MD [GO] - **Spec Exp:** Gynecologic Surgery-Complex; **Hospital:** MUSC Med Ctr; **Address:** MUSC Med Ctr- Women's Hlth Ob/Gyn, 86 Jonathan Lucas St, MS 957, Charleston, SC 29425; **Phone:** 843-792-9300; **Board Cert:** Obstetrics & Gynecology 2009; Gynecologic Oncology 2009; **Med School:** Duke Univ 1987; **Resid:** Obstetrics & Gynecology, Duke Univ Med Ctr 1991; **Fellow:** Gynecologic Oncology, Duke Univ Med Ctr 1994; **Fac Appt:** Prof ObG, Med Univ SC

Gynecologic Oncology

Lancaster, Johnathan M MD/PhD [GO] - **Spec Exp:** Ovarian Cancer; Cancer Genetics; Gene Therapy; **Hospital:** H Lee Moffitt Cancer Ctr & Research Inst (page 59); **Address:** H Lee Moffitt Cancer Ctr - Gyn Oncology, 12902 Magnolia Drive, The Ctr for Women's Oncology, Tampa, FL 33612; **Phone:** 888-860-2778; **Board Cert:** Obstetrics & Gynecology 2008; Gynecologic Oncology 2008; **Med School:** Wales, UK 1997; **Resid:** Obstetrics & Gynecology, Duke Univ Med Ctr 2000; **Fellow:** Gynecologic Oncology, Duke Univ Med Ctr 2003; **Fac Appt:** Asst Prof ObG, Univ S Fla Coll Med

Lentz, Samuel S MD [GO] - **Spec Exp:** Gynecologic Cancer; Pelvic Reconstruction; Incontinence; Incontinence-Fecal; **Hospital:** Wake Forest Univ Baptist Med Ctr, Forsyth Med Ctr; **Address:** Wake Forest Univ Sch Med, Div Gyn Oncology, Medical Center Blvd, Winston-Salem, NC 27157; **Phone:** 336-716-6673; **Board Cert:** Obstetrics & Gynecology 2008; Gynecologic Oncology 2010; **Med School:** Wake Forest Univ 1978; **Resid:** Obstetrics & Gynecology, NC Baptist Hosp 1982; **Fellow:** Gynecologic Oncology, Mayo Clinic 1989; **Fac Appt:** Prof ObG, Wake Forest Univ

Lucci, Joseph A MD [GO] - **Spec Exp:** Cervical Cancer; **Hospital:** Univ of Miami Hosp & Clins/Sylvester Comp Canc Ctr (page 73), Jackson Meml Hosp (page 70); **Address:** UMHC Sylvester Comp Cancer Ctr, 1475 NW 12th Ave, Ste 3500, Miami, FL 33136; **Phone:** 305-243-2233; **Board Cert:** Obstetrics & Gynecology 2007; Gynecologic Oncology 2007; **Med School:** Univ Tex, Houston 1984; **Resid:** Obstetrics & Gynecology, St Josephs Hosp 1988; **Fellow:** Gynecologic Oncology, UC Irvine 1992; **Fac Appt:** Clin Prof ObG, Univ Miami Sch Med

Makhija, Sharmila K MD [GO] - **Spec Exp:** Ovarian Cancer; Cervical Cancer; Uterine Cancer; **Hospital:** Emory Univ Hosp; **Address:** The Emory Clinic Bldg A, 1365 Clifton Rd NE Fl 4, Atlanta, GA 30322; **Phone:** 404-778-3401; **Board Cert:** Obstetrics & Gynecology 2009; Gynecologic Oncology 2009; **Med School:** Univ Alabama 1992; **Resid:** Obstetrics & Gynecology, Univ Louisville Hosp 1996; **Fellow:** Gynecologic Oncology, Meml Sloan Kettering Cancer Ctr 1999; **Fac Appt:** Assoc Prof ObG, Emory Univ

Modesitt, Susan C MD [GO] - **Spec Exp:** Gynecologic Cancer; Ovarian Cancer; Vulvar Disease/Cancer; **Hospital:** Univ of Virginia Health Sys; **Address:** Div Gynecologic Oncology, P.O. Box 800712, Charlottesville, VA 22908-0712; **Phone:** 434-924-5197; **Board Cert:** Obstetrics & Gynecology 2005; Gynecologic Oncology 2005; **Med School:** Univ VA Sch Med 1995; **Resid:** Obstetrics & Gynecology, Univ NC Hlth Care System 1999; **Fellow:** Gynecologic Oncology, Univ TX- M.D. Anderson Cancer Ctr 2002; **Fac Appt:** Assoc Prof ObG, Univ VA Sch Med

Orr Jr, James W MD [GO] - **Spec Exp:** Gynecologic Cancer; **Hospital:** Lee Memorial Hlth Systems; **Address:** 8931 Colonial Ctr Drive, Ste 400, Fort Myers, FL 33905; **Phone:** 239-334-6626; **Board Cert:** Obstetrics & Gynecology 2008; Gynecologic Oncology 2008; **Med School:** Univ VA Sch Med 1976; **Resid:** Obstetrics & Gynecology, Univ Ala Med Ctr 1980; **Fellow:** Gynecologic Oncology, Univ Ala Med Ctr 1982; **Fac Appt:** Clin Prof ObG, Univ S Fla Coll Med

Penalver, Manuel A MD [GO] - **Spec Exp:** Gynecologic Cancer; Cervical Cancer; Pelvic Tumors; **Hospital:** Doctors' Hosp, Baptist Hosp of Miami; **Address:** South Florida Gyn Oncology, 5000 University Drive, Ste 3300, Coral Gables, FL 33146; **Phone:** 305-663-7001; **Board Cert:** Obstetrics & Gynecology 2009; Gynecologic Oncology 2009; **Med School:** Univ Miami Sch Med 1977; **Resid:** Obstetrics & Gynecology, Univ Miami/Jackson Meml Hosp 1982; **Fellow:** Gynecologic Oncology, Univ Miami/Jackson Meml Hosp 1984

Poliakoff, Steven R MD [GO] - **Spec Exp:** Ovarian Cancer; Minimally Invasive Surgery; Cancer Genetics; Robotic Surgery; **Hospital:** Mount Sinai Med Ctr - Miami, South Miami Hosp; **Address:** 6280 Sunset Dr, Ste 502, South Miami, FL 33143-4870; **Phone:** 305-596-0870; **Board Cert:** Obstetrics & Gynecology 1983; **Med School:** Univ NC Sch Med 1975; **Resid:** Obstetrics & Gynecology, Johns Hopkins Hosp 1979; **Fellow:** Gynecologic Oncology, Jackson Meml Hosp/Univ Miami 1981

Runowicz, Carolyn MD [GO] - **Spec Exp:** Ovarian Cancer; Cervical Cancer; Breast Cancer; **Hospital:** Jackson N Med Ctr; **Address:** 11200 S W 8th St SW, AHC2 Bldg Fl 6 - Ste 693, Miami, FL 33199; **Phone:** 305-348-4372; **Board Cert:** Obstetrics & Gynecology 2009; Gynecologic Oncology 2009; **Med School:** Jefferson Med Coll 1977; **Resid:** Obstetrics & Gynecology, Mount Sinai Med Ctr 1981; **Fellow:** Gynecologic Oncology, Mount Sinai Med Ctr 1983; **Fac Appt:** Prof ObG, FIU Coll Med

Soper, John T MD [GO] - **Spec Exp:** Gynecologic Cancer; Gynecologic Surgery-Complex; Gestational Trophoblastic Disease; **Hospital:** NC Memorial Hosp - UNC, Rex HlthCare; **Address:** Div Gyn-Onc, Dept OB/GYN, B110 Physicians Office Bldg, 170 Manning Drive, Chapel Hill, NC 27599-7572; **Phone:** 919-966-1195; **Board Cert:** Obstetrics & Gynecology 2009; Gynecologic Oncology 2009; **Med School:** Univ Iowa Coll Med 1978; **Resid:** Obstetrics & Gynecology, Univ Utah Med Ctr 1982; **Fellow:** Obstetrics & Gynecology, Duke Univ Med Ctr 1985; **Fac Appt:** Prof ObG, Univ NC Sch Med

Spann Jr, Cyril O MD [GO] - **Spec Exp:** Gynecologic Cancer; Ovarian Cancer; **Hospital:** Grady Hlth Sys, Emory Univ Hosp Midtown; **Address:** Dept Gynecology & Obstetrics, 69 Jesse Hill Jr Drive, Ste 400, Atlanta, GA 30303; **Phone:** 404-778-3401; **Board Cert:** Obstetrics & Gynecology 2005; Gynecologic Oncology 2005; **Med School:** Meharry Med Coll 1981; **Resid:** Obstetrics & Gynecology, Emory Univ Med Ctr 1985; **Fellow:** Gynecologic Oncology, Univ NC Meml Hosp 1989; **Fac Appt:** Prof ObG, Emory Univ

Taylor Jr, Peyton T MD [GO] - **Spec Exp:** Gynecologic Cancer; Gynecologic Surgery-Complex; **Hospital:** Univ of Virginia Health Sys; **Address:** Lee St, Cancer Cen Bldg, PO Box 800712, Charlottesville, VA 22908; **Phone:** 434-924-9933; **Board Cert:** Obstetrics & Gynecology 1994; Gynecologic Oncology 1981; **Med School:** Univ Alabama 1968; **Resid:** Obstetrics & Gynecology, Univ VA Hosp 1970; Obstetrics & Gynecology, Univ VA Hosp 1975; **Fellow:** Surgical Oncology, Natl Cancer Inst 1972; Gynecologic Oncology, Univ Va Hosp 1977; **Fac Appt:** Prof ObG, Univ VA Sch Med

Valea, Fidel A MD [GO] - **Spec Exp:** Cervical Cancer; Laparoscopic Surgery; **Hospital:** Duke Univ Hosp; **Address:** Duke Univ Med Ctr, Box 3079, Durham, NC 27710; **Phone:** 919-664-3725; **Board Cert:** Obstetrics & Gynecology 2007; Gynecologic Oncology 2007; **Med School:** SUNY Stony Brook 1985; **Resid:** Surgery, Univ NC Hosps 1987; Obstetrics & Gynecology, Univ NC Hosps 1990; **Fellow:** Gynecologic Oncology, Univ NC Hosps 1992; **Fac Appt:** Assoc Prof ObG, Duke Univ

Van Nagell Jr, John R MD [GO] - **Spec Exp:** Ovarian Cancer; Cervical Cancer; **Hospital:** Univ of Kentucky Albert B. Chandler Hosp; **Address:** 800 Rose St, Lexington, KY 40536-0001; **Phone:** 859-323-5553; **Board Cert:** Obstetrics & Gynecology 1973; Gynecologic Oncology 1976; **Med School:** Univ Pennsylvania 1967; **Resid:** Obstetrics & Gynecology, Univ Kentucky Med Ctr 1971; **Fellow:** Gynecologic Oncology, Univ Kentucky Med Ctr 1973; **Fac Appt:** Prof ObG, Univ KY Coll Med

Midwest

Cliby, William A MD [GO] - **Spec Exp:** Ovarian Cancer; **Hospital:** Mayo Med Ctr & Clin - Rochester; **Address:** Mayo Clinic, 200 First St SW, Rochester, MN 55905; **Phone:** 507-266-9323; **Board Cert:** Obstetrics & Gynecology 2010; Gynecologic Oncology 2010; **Med School:** Univ VT Coll Med 1987; **Resid:** Obstetrics & Gynecology, Duke Univ Med Ctr 1991; **Fellow:** Gynecologic Oncology, Mayo Clinic 1994; Research, Fred Hutchinson Cancer Rsch Ctr 1997; **Fac Appt:** Prof ObG, Mayo Med Sch

Copeland, Larry J MD [GO] - **Spec Exp:** Ovarian Cancer; Uterine Cancer; Gynecologic Cancer; Gynecologic Cancer-Rare; **Hospital:** Arthur G James Cancer Hosp & Research Inst, Ohio St Univ Med Ctr; **Address:** 320 W 10th Ave, Starling L Bldg, Ste 210, Columbus, OH 43210; **Phone:** 614-293-7642; **Board Cert:** Obstetrics & Gynecology 1991; Gynecologic Oncology 1981; **Med School:** Univ Western Ontario 1973; **Resid:** Obstetrics & Gynecology, McMaster Univ Affil Hosps 1977; **Fellow:** Gynecologic Oncology, MD Anderson Cancer Ctr-Univ Tex 1979; **Fac Appt:** Prof ObG, Ohio State Univ

De Geest, Koen MD [GO] - **Spec Exp:** Ovarian Cancer; Uterine Cancer; Clinical Trials; **Hospital:** Univ Iowa Hosp & Clinics; **Address:** Univ Iowa, Div Gynecological Oncology, 200 Hawkins Drive, rm 4630 JCP, Iowa City, IA 52242; **Phone:** 319-356-2015; **Board Cert:** Obstetrics & Gynecology 2008; Gynecologic Oncology 2008; **Med School:** Belgium 1977; **Resid:** Obstetrics & Gynecology, Univ Ghent 1982; **Fellow:** Gynecologic Oncology, Penn State/Hershey Med Ctr 1990; **Fac Appt:** Prof ObG, Univ Iowa Coll Med

Del Priore, Giuseppe MD [GO] - **Spec Exp:** Fertility Preservation in Cancer; **Hospital:** IU Health University Hosp; **Address:** 535 Barnhill Drive, RT 433, Indianapolis, IN 46202; **Phone:** 317-944-2130; **Board Cert:** Obstetrics & Gynecology 2010; Gynecologic Oncology 2010; **Med School:** SUNY Downstate 1987; **Resid:** Obstetrics & Gynecology, Northwestern Meml Hosp 1991; **Fellow:** Gynecologic Oncology, Univ Rochester-Strong Meml 1995; **Fac Appt:** Prof ObG, Indiana Univ

Fowler, Jeffrey M MD [GO] - **Spec Exp:** Laparoscopic Surgery; Gynecologic Cancer; Robotic Surgery; Pelvic Reconstruction; **Hospital:** Ohio St Univ Med Ctr; **Address:** Ohio State Univ, Div Gynecologic Oncology, 320 W Tenth Ave, M-210 SLH, Columbus, OH 43210; **Phone:** 614-293-3873; **Board Cert:** Obstetrics & Gynecology 2009; Gynecologic Oncology 2009; **Med School:** Northwestern Univ 1985; **Resid:** Obstetrics & Gynecology, Ohio State Univ Hosp 1989; **Fellow:** Gynecologic Oncology, Cedars-Sinai Med Ctr 1991; **Fac Appt:** Prof ObG, Ohio State Univ

Johnston, Carolyn M MD [GO] - **Spec Exp:** Gynecologic Surgery-Complex; Cervical Cancer; **Hospital:** Univ of Michigan Hosp; **Address:** Womens Hosp-Div Gyn Oncology, 1500 E Med Ctr Drive, rm L4510, Ann Arbor, MI 48109-0276; **Phone:** 734-647-8906; **Board Cert:** Obstetrics & Gynecology 2000; Gynecologic Oncology 2000; **Med School:** Yale Univ 1984; **Resid:** Obstetrics & Gynecology, Univ Chicago Hosp 1988; **Fellow:** Gynecologic Oncology, Mt Sinai Hosp 1990; **Fac Appt:** Assoc Clin Prof ObG, Univ Mich Med Sch

Lurain, John R MD [GO] - **Spec Exp:** Gestational Trophoblastic Disease; Uterine Cancer; Ovarian Cancer; Cervical Cancer; **Hospital:** Northwestern Meml Hosp; **Address:** Northwestern Medical Faculty Foundation, 250 E Superior St, Ste 04-420, Chicago, IL 60611-3056; **Phone:** 312-695-0990; **Board Cert:** Obstetrics & Gynecology 1977; Gynecologic Oncology 1981; **Med School:** Univ NC Sch Med 1972; **Resid:** Obstetrics & Gynecology, Univ Pittsburgh Magee-Womens Hosp 1975; **Fellow:** Gynecologic Oncology, Roswell Park Cancer Inst 1979; **Fac Appt:** Prof ObG, Northwestern Univ

Moore, David H MD [GO] - **Spec Exp:** Cervical Cancer; Ovarian Cancer; Laparoscopic Surgery; Robotic Surgery; **Hospital:** Franciscan St. Francis Hlth-Indianapolis, Franciscan St. Francis Hlth-Beech Grove; **Address:** Gynecologic Oncology of Indiana, 5255 E Stop 11 Rd, Ste 310, Indianapolis, IN 46237; **Phone:** 317-851-2555; **Board Cert:** Obstetrics & Gynecology 2010; Gynecologic Oncology 2009; **Med School:** Indiana Univ 1982; **Resid:** Obstetrics & Gynecology, Indiana Univ Hosp 1986; **Fellow:** Gynecologic Oncology, Univ N Carolina 1988

Mutch, David G MD [GO] - **Spec Exp:** Gynecologic Cancer; Pelvic Reconstruction; **Hospital:** Barnes-Jewish Hosp; **Address:** 4911 Barnes Jewish Hosp Plaza, CB 8064, St Louis, MO 63110; **Phone:** 314-362-3181; **Board Cert:** Obstetrics & Gynecology 2006; Gynecologic Oncology 2006; **Med School:** Washington Univ, St Louis 1980; **Resid:** Obstetrics & Gynecology, Barnes Hosp-Wash Univ 1984; **Fellow:** Gynecologic Oncology, Duke Univ Med Ctr 1987; **Fac Appt:** Prof ObG, Washington Univ, St Louis

Potkul, Ronald K MD [GO] - **Spec Exp:** Ovarian Cancer; Cervical Cancer; Robotic Surgery; Vulvar & Vaginal Cancer; **Hospital:** Loyola Univ Med Ctr; **Address:** Loyola Univ Med Ctr, 2160 S 1st Ave Bldg 112 - rm 267, Maywood, IL 60153; **Phone:** 708-327-3500; **Board Cert:** Obstetrics & Gynecology 2010; Gynecologic Oncology 2010; **Med School:** Univ Chicago-Pritzker Sch Med 1981; **Resid:** Obstetrics & Gynecology, Univ Chicago Hosps 1985; **Fellow:** Gynecologic Oncology, Georgetown Univ Hosp 1988; **Fac Appt:** Prof ObG, Loyola Univ-Stritch Sch Med

Rader, Janet S MD [GO] - **Spec Exp:** Cervical Cancer; Ovarian Cancer; Uterine Cancer; **Hospital:** Froedtert and Med Ctr of WI; **Address:** Med Coll of Wisconsin, Dept OB/GYN, 9200 W Wisconsin Ave, Milwaukee, WI 53226; **Phone:** 414-805-6606; **Board Cert:** Obstetrics & Gynecology 2009; Gynecologic Oncology 2009; **Med School:** Univ MO-Columbia Sch Med 1983; **Resid:** Obstetrics & Gynecology, Michael Reese Hosp 1987; **Fellow:** Gynecologic Oncology, Johns Hopkins Hosp 1990; **Fac Appt:** Prof ObG, Washington Univ, St Louis

Reynolds, R Kevin MD [GO] - **Hospital:** Univ of Michigan Hosp; **Address:** Women's Hosp, Div Gyn Onc, 1500 E Med Ctr Drive, rm L4510, Ann Arbor, MI 48109-0276; **Phone:** 734-764-9106; **Board Cert:** Obstetrics & Gynecology 2009; Gynecologic Oncology 2009; **Med School:** Univ New Mexico 1982; **Resid:** Obstetrics & Gynecology, Univ Vt Hosp 1986; **Fellow:** Gynecologic Oncology, Univ Mich Med Ctr 1991; **Fac Appt:** Asst Prof ObG, Univ Mich Med Sch

Rice, Laurel W MD [GO] - **Spec Exp:** Ovarian Cancer; Uterine Cancer; Cervical Cancer; **Hospital:** Univ WI Hosp & Clins; **Address:** 600 Highland Ave, Ste H4-636, Madison, WI 53792; **Phone:** 608-263-3194; **Board Cert:** Obstetrics & Gynecology 2006; Gynecologic Oncology 2006; **Med School:** Univ Colorado 1983; **Resid:** Obstetrics & Gynecology, Brigham-Womens Hosp 1987; **Fellow:** Obstetrics & Gynecology, Brigham-Womens Hosp 1989; **Fac Appt:** Assoc Prof ObG, Univ VA Sch Med

Rose, Peter G MD [GO] - **Spec Exp:** Cervical Cancer; Ovarian Cancer; Uterine Cancer; **Hospital:** Cleveland Clin (page 56), MetroHealth Med Ctr; **Address:** Cleveland Clin Fdn, 9500 Euclid Ave A-81, Cleveland, OH 44195; **Phone:** 216-444-1712; **Board Cert:** Obstetrics & Gynecology 2009; Gynecologic Oncology 2009; **Med School:** Boston Univ 1981; **Resid:** Surgery, Vanderbilt Univ Med Ctr 1983; Obstetrics & Gynecology, Ohio State Univ Med Ctr 1986; **Fellow:** Gynecologic Oncology, Roswell Park Cancer Inst 1988; **Fac Appt:** Prof ObG, Case West Res Univ

Rotmensch, Jacob MD [GO] - **Spec Exp:** Gynecologic Cancer; Ovarian Cancer; Cervical Cancer; Uterine Cancer; **Hospital:** Rush Univ Med Ctr; **Address:** Univ Gynecologic Oncology Assocs, 1725 W Harrison St, Professional Bldg, Ste 842, Chicago, IL 60612; **Phone:** 312-942-6300; **Board Cert:** Obstetrics & Gynecology 2010; **Med School:** Meharry Med Coll 1977; **Resid:** Obstetrics & Gynecology, Johns Hopkins Hosp 1981; **Fellow:** Gynecologic Oncology, Johns Hopkins Hosp 1984; **Fac Appt:** Prof ObG, Rush Med Coll

Schink, Julian C MD [GO] - **Spec Exp:** Ovarian Cancer; **Hospital:** Northwestern Meml Hosp; **Address:** Northwestern Medical Faculty Foundation, 250 E Superior St, Ste 04-420, Chicago, IL 60611; **Phone:** 312-695-0990; **Board Cert:** Obstetrics & Gynecology 2010; Gynecologic Oncology 2010; **Med School:** Univ Tex, San Antonio 1982; **Resid:** Obstetrics & Gynecology, Northwestern Univ Med Sch 1986; **Fellow:** Gynecologic Oncology, UCLA Med Ctr 1988; **Fac Appt:** Prof ObG, Northwestern Univ

Gynecologic Oncology

Smith, Donna M MD [GO] - **Spec Exp:** Cervical Cancer; Ovarian Cancer; **Hospital:** Loyola Univ Med Ctr; **Address:** Loyola Univ Medical Ctr, 2160 S 1st Ave Bldg 112 - rm 267, Maywood, IL 60153; **Phone:** 708-327-3500; **Board Cert:** Obstetrics & Gynecology 2007; Gynecologic Oncology 2007; **Med School:** Univ MO-Kansas City 1980; **Resid:** Obstetrics & Gynecology, Emory Univ Hosp 1984; **Fellow:** Gynecologic Oncology, Georgetown Univ Med Ctr 1987; **Fac Appt:** Assoc Prof ObG, Loyola Univ-Stritch Sch Med

Stehman, Frederick B MD [GO] - **Spec Exp:** Clinical Trials; Gynecologic Cancer; **Hospital:** IU Health University Hosp, Wishard Hlth Srvs; **Address:** Indiana Univ Cancer Pavilion, 535 Barnhill Drive, rm 436, Indianapolis, IN 46202; **Phone:** 317-944-2130; **Board Cert:** Obstetrics & Gynecology 2005; Gynecologic Oncology 2003; **Med School:** Univ Mich Med Sch 1972; **Resid:** Obstetrics & Gynecology, Univ Kansas Med Ctr 1975; Surgery, Univ Kansas Med Ctr 1977; **Fellow:** Gynecologic Oncology, UCLA Med Ctr 1979; **Fac Appt:** Prof Emeritus ObG, Indiana Univ

Waggoner, Steven MD [GO] - **Spec Exp:** Ovarian Cancer; Cervical Cancer; Uterine Cancer; **Hospital:** Univ Hosps Case Med Ctr (page 74); **Address:** Dept Ob/Gyn & Gyn Oncology, 11100 Euclid Ave, rm 7128, UH MacDonald Women's Hospital, Cleveland, OH 44106; **Phone:** 216-844-3954; **Board Cert:** Obstetrics & Gynecology 2008; Gynecologic Oncology 2008; **Med School:** Univ Wash 1984; **Resid:** Obstetrics & Gynecology, Univ Chicago Hosps 1988; **Fellow:** Gynecologic Oncology, Georgetown Univ 1991; **Fac Appt:** Prof ObG, Case West Res Univ

Great Plains and Mountains

Davidson, Susan MD [GO] - **Spec Exp:** Gynecologic Cancer; **Hospital:** Univ of CO Hosp - Anschutz Inpatient Pav; **Address:** Univ Colorado Hosp, Dept OB/GYN, PO Box 6510- F704, 1665 Aurora Ct, Denver, CO 80045; **Phone:** 720-848-0300; **Board Cert:** Obstetrics & Gynecology 2009; Gynecologic Oncology 2009; **Med School:** Univ Tex, San Antonio 1984; **Resid:** Obstetrics & Gynecology, Univ Texas Med Ctr 1988; **Fellow:** Gynecologic Oncology, Meml Sloan Kettering Cancer Ctr 1990; **Fac Appt:** Assoc Prof ObG, Univ Colorado

Remmenga, Steven W MD [GO] - **Spec Exp:** Ovarian Cancer; Cervical Cancer; Gynecologic Cancer; **Hospital:** Nebraska Med Ctr; **Address:** Department of Obsterics nd Gynecology, MS 0, 983255 Nebraska Med Ctr, Omaha, NE 68198-3255; **Phone:** 402-559-5068; **Board Cert:** Obstetrics & Gynecology 1998; Gynecologic Oncology 1998; **Med School:** Univ Nebr Coll Med 1981; **Resid:** Obstetrics & Gynecology, Naval Hospital 1986; **Fellow:** Gynecologic Oncology, Walter Reed Army Med Ctr 1990; **Fac Appt:** Prof ObG, Univ Nebr Coll Med

Soisson, Andrew P MD [GO] - **Spec Exp:** Cervical Cancer; HPV-Human Papilloma Virus; **Hospital:** LDS Hosp, Univ Utah Hlth Care; **Address:** Huntsman Cancer Hosp, 1950 Circle of Hope, Salt Lake City, UT 84112; **Phone:** 801-585-0100; **Board Cert:** Obstetrics & Gynecology 2006; Gynecologic Oncology 2006; **Med School:** Georgetown Univ 1981; **Resid:** Obstetrics & Gynecology, Madigan AMC 1985; **Fellow:** Gynecologic Oncology, Duke Univ Med Ctr 1990; **Fac Appt:** Assoc Prof ObG, Univ Utah

Southwest

Bodurka, Diane C MD [GO] - **Spec Exp:** Ovarian Cancer; Pelvic Surgery-Complex; **Hospital:** UT MD Anderson Cancer Ctr; **Address:** Univ Texas M.D. Anderson Cancer Center Dept of Gynecologic Oncology, 1155 Herman Pressler, Houston, TX 77030-4000; **Phone:** 713-745-3358; **Board Cert:** Gynecologic Oncology 2009; Obstetrics & Gynecology 2009; **Med School:** Georgetown Univ 1990; **Resid:** Obstetrics & Gynecology, Univ Alabama Hosp 1994; **Fellow:** Gynecologic Oncology, MD Anderson Cancer Ctr 1996; **Fac Appt:** Prof ObG, Univ Tex, Houston

Borst, Matthew MD [GO] - **Spec Exp:** Ovarian Cancer; **Hospital:** Banner Good Samaritan Regl Med Ctr - Phoenix; **Address:** Phoenix-Biltmore Cancer Ctr, 2222 E Highland Ave, Ste 400, Phoenix, AZ 85016; **Phone:** 602-253-5300; **Board Cert:** Obstetrics & Gynecology 2010; Gynecologic Oncology 2010; **Med School:** Med Coll VA 1984; **Resid:** Obstetrics & Gynecology, Cook Co Hosp 1988; **Fellow:** Gynecologic Oncology, Univ Alabama 1992

Braly, Patricia S MD [GO] - **Spec Exp:** Ovarian Cancer; Breast Cancer; **Hospital:** St. Tammany Parish Hosp, E Jefferson Genl Hosp; **Address:** Women's Cancer Care, 606 W 12th Ave, Covington, LA 70433; **Phone:** 985-892-2252; **Board Cert:** Gynecologic Oncology 1985; Obstetrics & Gynecology 1994; **Med School:** UC Irvine 1976; **Resid:** Obstetrics & Gynecology, UC Irvine Med Ctr 1980; **Fellow:** Gynecologic Oncology, UC Irvine Med Ctr 1983

Burke, Thomas W MD [GO] - **Spec Exp:** Uterine Cancer; Vulvar & Vaginal Cancer; **Hospital:** UT MD Anderson Cancer Ctr; **Address:** UT MD Anderson Cancer Ctr, 1515 Holcombe Blvd, Unit 43, Houston, TX 77030; **Phone:** 713-792-3825; **Board Cert:** Obstetrics & Gynecology 2009; Gynecologic Oncology 2009; **Med School:** Tulane Univ 1978; **Resid:** Obstetrics & Gynecology, Tripler Army Med Ctr 1982; **Fellow:** Gynecologic Oncology, Walter Reed Army Med Ctr 1986; **Fac Appt:** Prof ObG, Univ Tex, Houston

Burnett, Alexander F MD [GO] - **Spec Exp:** Laparoscopic Surgery; Fertility Preservation in Cancer; Gynecologic Cancer; **Hospital:** UAMS Med Ctr; **Address:** 4301 W Markham St, Slot 793, Little Rock, AR 72205; **Phone:** 501-686-8522; **Board Cert:** Obstetrics & Gynecology 2009; Gynecologic Oncology 2009; **Med School:** Georgetown Univ 1986; **Resid:** Obstetrics & Gynecology, Georgetown Univ Affil Hosp 1990; **Fellow:** Gynecologic Oncology, Georgetown Univ Affil Hosp 1993; **Fac Appt:** Assoc Prof ObG, Univ Ark

Chambers, Setsuko K MD [GO] - **Spec Exp:** Gynecologic Cancer; Breast Cancer; Ovarian Cancer; **Hospital:** Univ Med Ctr - Tucson; **Address:** 1515 N Campbell Ave, Arizona Cancer Center, Tucson, AZ 85724; **Phone:** 520-626-9285; **Board Cert:** Obstetrics & Gynecology 2008; Gynecologic Oncology 2008; **Med School:** Brown Univ 1980; **Resid:** Obstetrics & Gynecology, Yale-New Haven Hosp 1984; **Fellow:** Gynecologic Oncology, Yale-New Haven Hosp 1986; **Fac Appt:** Prof ObG, Univ Ariz Coll Med

Fromm, Geri-Lynn MD [GO] - **Spec Exp:** Cervical Cancer; Ovarian Cancer; Gestational Trophoblastic Disease; **Hospital:** St. Luke's Episcopal Hosp-Houston, Woman's Hosp TX; **Address:** 2223 Dorrington St, Houston, TX 77030; **Phone:** 713-665-0404; **Board Cert:** Obstetrics & Gynecology 2010; **Med School:** Northwestern Univ 1981; **Resid:** Obstetrics & Gynecology, Magee Womens Hosp 1985; **Fellow:** Gynecologic Oncology, MD Anderson Cancer Ctr 1987; **Fac Appt:** Assoc Clin Prof ObG, Baylor Coll Med

Gershenson, David M MD [GO] - **Spec Exp:** Ovarian Rare & Borderline Tumors; Uterine Cancer-Serous Carcinoma; Fertility Preservation in Cancer; Sex Cord-Stromal Tumors; **Hospital:** UT MD Anderson Cancer Ctr, St. Luke's Episcopal Hosp-Houston; **Address:** Univ Tex MD Anderson Cancer Ctr, PO Box 301439, Houston, TX 77030-1439; **Phone:** 713-745-2565; **Board Cert:** Obstetrics & Gynecology 1991; Gynecologic Oncology 1981; **Med School:** Vanderbilt Univ 1971; **Resid:** Obstetrics & Gynecology, Yale-New Haven Hosp 1975; **Fellow:** Gynecologic Oncology, MD Anderson Cancer Ctr 1979; **Fac Appt:** Prof ObG, Univ Tex, Houston

Hatch, Kenneth MD [GO] - **Spec Exp:** Cervical Cancer; Uro-Gynecology; Pelvic Organ Prolapse Repair; **Hospital:** Univ Med Ctr - Tucson, NW Med Ctr; **Address:** Arizona Cancer Center, 1515 N Campbell Ave, Tucson, AZ 85724; **Phone:** 520-626-9285; **Board Cert:** Obstetrics & Gynecology 1993; Gynecologic Oncology 1981; **Med School:** Univ Nebr Coll Med 1971; **Resid:** Obstetrics & Gynecology, Univ AL Med Ctr Birmingham 1976; **Fellow:** Gynecologic Oncology, Univ AL Med Ctr Birmingham 1978; **Fac Appt:** Prof ObG, Univ Ariz Coll Med

Gynecologic Oncology

Kline, Richard C MD [GO] - **Spec Exp:** Ovarian Cancer; Cervical Cancer; Uterine Cancer; Vulvar & Vaginal Cancer; **Hospital:** Ochsner Med Ctr-New Orleans; **Address:** Ochsner Clinic Foundation, 1514 Jefferson Hwy, New Orleans, LA 70121; **Phone:** 504-842-4165; **Board Cert:** Obstetrics & Gynecology 2009; Gynecologic Oncology 2009; **Med School:** Louisiana State U, New Orleans 1980; **Resid:** Obstetrics & Gynecology, Ochsner Fdn Hosp 1984; **Fellow:** Gynecologic Oncology, UT MD Anderson Cancer Ctr 1986

Levenback, Charles MD [GO] - **Spec Exp:** Vulvar Disease/Cancer; Cervical Cancer; Gynecologic Cancer; **Hospital:** UT MD Anderson Cancer Ctr; **Address:** 1515 Holcombe Blvd, PO Box 301439 - Unit 1362, Houston, TX 77230; **Phone:** 713-745-2563; **Board Cert:** Obstetrics & Gynecology 2009; Gynecologic Oncology 2009; **Med School:** Mount Sinai Sch Med 1983; **Resid:** Obstetrics & Gynecology, Albert Einstein Coll Med 1987; **Fellow:** Gynecologic Oncology, Meml Sloan Kettering Cancer Ctr 1989; **Fac Appt:** Prof ObG, Univ Tex, Houston

Lu, Karen Hsieh MD [GO] - **Spec Exp:** Ovarian Cancer; Ovarian Cancer-Early Detection; Uterine Cancer; Cancer Genetics; **Hospital:** UT MD Anderson Cancer Ctr; **Address:** Univ of Texas MD Anderson Cancer Ctr, 1515 Holcombe Blvd, Houston, TX 77030; **Phone:** 713-745-8902; **Board Cert:** Obstetrics & Gynecology 2003; Gynecologic Oncology 2003; **Med School:** Yale Univ 1991; **Resid:** Obstetrics & Gynecology, Brigham & Women's Hosp 1994; **Fellow:** Gynecologic Oncology, Brigham & Women's Hosp 1999; **Fac Appt:** Prof ObG, Univ Tex SW, Dallas

Magrina, Javier MD [GO] - **Spec Exp:** Gynecologic Cancer; Endometriosis; Hysterectomy Alternatives; Robotic Surgery; **Hospital:** Mayo Clinic - Scottsdale; **Address:** Mayo Clinic, 5779 E Mayo Blvd, Phoenix, AZ 85054; **Phone:** 480-342-2668; **Board Cert:** Obstetrics & Gynecology 1994; Gynecologic Oncology 1982; **Med School:** Spain 1972; **Resid:** Obstetrics & Gynecology, Mayo Clinic 1977; **Fellow:** Gynecologic Oncology, Kansas Med Ctr 1980; **Fac Appt:** Prof ObG, Mayo Med Sch

Miller, David S MD [GO] - **Spec Exp:** Gynecologic Cancer; **Hospital:** UT Southwestern Med Ctr at Dallas; **Address:** 5323 Harry Hines Blvd, Dallas, TX 75390-8585; **Phone:** 214-645-4673; **Board Cert:** Obstetrics & Gynecology 2007; Gynecologic Oncology 2007; **Med School:** Univ Okla Coll Med 1977; **Resid:** Obstetrics & Gynecology, Hosp Univ Penn 1981; **Fellow:** Reproductive Endocrinology, UCSD Med Ctr 1982; Gynecologic Oncology, Stanford Hosps & Clins 1985

Siller, Barry MD [GO] - **Spec Exp:** Cervical Cancer; **Hospital:** Meml Hermann Hosp - Texas Med Ctr; **Address:** 915 Gessner Rd, Ste 400, Medical Plaza 3, Houston, TX 77024; **Phone:** 713-242-2575; **Board Cert:** Obstetrics & Gynecology 2009; Gynecologic Oncology 2009; **Med School:** Baylor Coll Med 1988; **Resid:** Obstetrics & Gynecology, Univ Ala Med Ctr 1992; **Fellow:** Gynecologic Oncology, Univ Ala Med Ctr 1994

Sood, Anil K MD [GO] - **Spec Exp:** Gynecologic Cancer; Ovarian Cancer; **Hospital:** UT MD Anderson Cancer Ctr; **Address:** Univ Texas MD Anderson Cancer Ctr, 1515 Holcombe Blvd Ste 440, Houston, TX 77030-4000; **Phone:** 713-745-5266; **Board Cert:** Obstetrics & Gynecology 2009; Gynecologic Oncology 2009; **Med School:** Univ NC Sch Med 1991; **Resid:** Obstetrics & Gynecology, Univ FL Med Ctr 1995; **Fellow:** Gynecologic Oncology, Univ Iowa Hosps & Clin 1998

Walker, Joan L MD [GO] - **Spec Exp:** Ovarian Cancer; Cervical Cancer; Uterine Cancer; **Hospital:** OU Med Ctr; **Address:** OU Physicians, 825 NE 10th St, Ste 5200, Oklahoma City, OK 73104; **Phone:** 405-271-7770; **Board Cert:** Obstetrics & Gynecology 2009; Gynecologic Oncology 2009; **Med School:** UCLA 1982; **Resid:** Obstetrics & Gynecology, Hosp Univ Penn 1986; **Fellow:** Gynecologic Oncology, UC-Irvine 1990; **Fac Appt:** Assoc Prof ObG, Univ Okla Coll Med

West Coast and Pacific

Berek, Jonathan S MD [GO] - **Spec Exp:** Ovarian Cancer; Uterine Cancer; Cervical Cancer; Vulvar & Vaginal Cancer; **Hospital:** Stanford Univ Hosp & Clinics; **Address:** Stanford Cancer Ctr, Stanford Univ Sch Med-Clin C, 875 Blake Wilbur Drive, Stanford, CA 94305; **Phone:** 650-498-6000; **Board Cert:** Obstetrics & Gynecology 2009; Gynecologic Oncology 2009; **Med School:** Johns Hopkins Univ 1975; **Resid:** Obstetrics & Gynecology, Brigham & Womens Hosp 1979; **Fellow:** Gynecologic Oncology, UCLA Sch Med 1981; **Fac Appt:** Prof ObG, Stanford Univ

Berman, Michael L MD [GO] - **Spec Exp:** Gynecologic Cancer; Cervical Cancer; **Hospital:** UC Irvine Med Ctr, Long Beach Meml Med Ctr; **Address:** Cho Family Comprehensive Cancer Ctr, 101 The City Drive S 23 rte81 Bldg - rm 800, Orange, CA 92868-3201; **Phone:** 714-456-8000; **Board Cert:** Obstetrics & Gynecology 2005; Gynecologic Oncology 2005; **Med School:** Geo Wash Univ 1967; **Resid:** Obstetrics & Gynecology, GW Univ Hosp 1969; Obstetrics & Gynecology, LAC-Harbor Hosp 1974; **Fellow:** Gynecologic Oncology, UCLA Med Ctr 1976; **Fac Appt:** Prof ObG, UC Irvine

Bristow, Robert E MD [GO] - **Spec Exp:** Ovarian Cancer; Gynecologic Cancer; **Hospital:** UC Irvine Med Ctr; **Address:** UC Irvine Med Ctr, 101 The City Drive, Route 81 Bldg 23 - rm 800, Orange, CA 92868; **Phone:** 714-456-8000; **Board Cert:** Obstetrics & Gynecology 2009; Gynecologic Oncology 2009; **Med School:** USC Sch Med 1991; **Resid:** Obstetrics & Gynecology, Johns Hopkins Hosp 1995; **Fellow:** Gynecologic Oncology, UCLA Med Ctr 1998; **Fac Appt:** Prof ObG, UC Irvine

Carney, Michael E MD [GO] - **Spec Exp:** Gynecologic Cancer; Pelvic Surgery-Complex; Minimally Invasive Surgery; **Hospital:** Kapiolani Med Ctr for Women & Chldn; **Address:** Womens Cancer Center, 1319 Punahou St, Ste 640, Honolulu, HI 96826; **Phone:** 808-983-6090; **Board Cert:** Obstetrics & Gynecology 2009; Gynecologic Oncology 2009; **Med School:** Loyola Univ-Stritch Sch Med 1990; **Resid:** Obstetrics & Gynecology, Duke Univ Med Ctr 1994; **Fellow:** Gynecologic Oncology, Duke Univ Med Ctr 1999; **Fac Appt:** Assoc Prof ObG, Univ Hawaii JA Burns Sch Med

Chan, John K MD [GO] - **Spec Exp:** Ovarian Cancer; Pelvic Surgery-Complex; Gene Therapy; Clinical Trials; **Hospital:** UCSF Med Ctr; **Address:** UCSF Medical Center, 1600 Divisidaro St, rm A747, Box 1702, San Francisco, CA 94143-1702; **Phone:** 415-353-9600; **Board Cert:** Obstetrics & Gynecology 2006; Gynecologic Oncology 2006; **Med School:** UCLA 1995; **Resid:** Obstetrics & Gynecology, UC Irvine Med Ctr 1999; **Fellow:** Gynecologic Oncology, MD Anderson Cancer Ctr 1999; Gynecologic Oncology, UC Irvine 2003; **Fac Appt:** Assoc Prof ObG, UCSF

Di Saia, Philip J MD [GO] - **Spec Exp:** Ovarian Cancer; Gynecologic Cancer; Cervical Cancer; **Hospital:** UC Irvine Med Ctr; **Address:** 101 The City Drive Bldg 56 - rm 800, Orange, CA 92668-3201; **Phone:** 714-456-5220; **Board Cert:** Obstetrics & Gynecology 1983; Gynecologic Oncology 1974; **Med School:** Tufts Univ 1963; **Resid:** Obstetrics & Gynecology, Yale-New Haven Hosp 1967; **Fellow:** Gynecologic Oncology, MD Anderson Hosp 1971; **Fac Appt:** Prof ObG, UC Irvine

Goff, Barbara A MD [GO] - **Spec Exp:** Ovarian Cancer; Uterine Cancer; Cervical Cancer; Gynecologic Surgery-Complex; **Hospital:** Univ Wash Med Ctr; **Address:** Univ Washington, Dept Gyn/Onc, 825 Eastlake Ave E, Seattle, WA 98109; **Phone:** 206-288-2273; **Board Cert:** Obstetrics & Gynecology 2009; Gynecologic Oncology 2009; **Med School:** Univ Pennsylvania 1986; **Resid:** Obstetrics & Gynecology, Mass Genl Hosp/Brigham & Womens Hosp 1990; **Fellow:** Gynecologic Oncology, Mass Genl Hosp 1993; **Fac Appt:** Prof ObG, Univ Wash

Greer, Benjamin E MD [GO] - **Spec Exp:** Gynecologic Cancer; **Hospital:** Univ Wash Med Ctr; **Address:** Seattle Cancer Care Alliance, 825 Eastlake Ave E, MS E2102, Seattle, WA 98109; **Phone:** 206-288-2273; **Board Cert:** Obstetrics & Gynecology 2002; Gynecologic Oncology 2002; **Med School:** Univ Pennsylvania 1966; **Resid:** Obstetrics & Gynecology, Univ Colorado Med Ctr 1970; **Fac Appt:** Prof ObG, Univ Wash

Husain, Amreen MD [GO] - **Spec Exp:** Cervical Cancer; Women's Health; **Hospital:** Stanford Univ Hosp & Clinics; **Address:** Stanford Comprehensive Cancer Center, 875 Blake Wilbur Drive, Clinic C, Gynecologic Oncology Clinic, Stanford, CA 94305; **Phone:** 650-498-8080; **Board Cert:** Obstetrics & Gynecology 2009; Gynecologic Oncology 2009; **Med School:** NY Med Coll 1991; **Resid:** Obstetrics & Gynecology, Cornell Univ Med Ctr/NY Hosp 1995; **Fellow:** Gynecologic Oncology, Meml Sloan-Kettering Cancer Ctr 2000; **Fac Appt:** Assoc Prof ObG, Stanford Univ

Karlan, Beth Y MD [GO] - **Spec Exp:** Ovarian Cancer; Gynecologic Cancer; **Hospital:** Cedars-Sinai Med Ctr; **Address:** 8700 Beverly Blvd, Ste 290W, Los Angeles, CA 90048; **Phone:** 310-423-3302; **Board Cert:** Obstetrics & Gynecology 1998; Gynecologic Oncology 1998; **Med School:** Harvard Med Sch 1982; **Resid:** Obstetrics & Gynecology, Yale-New Haven Hosp 1986; **Fellow:** Gynecologic Oncology, UCLA 1989; **Fac Appt:** Prof ObG, UCLA

Muntz, Howard G MD [GO] - **Spec Exp:** Robotic Surgery; Ovarian Cancer; Gynecologic Surgery-Complex; Gestational Trophoblastic Disease; **Hospital:** Northwest Hosp - Seattle; **Address:** Women's Cancer Care of Seattle, 1560 N 115th St, Ste 101, Seattle, WA 98133; **Phone:** 206-368-6806; **Board Cert:** Obstetrics & Gynecology 2009; Gynecologic Oncology 2009; **Med School:** Harvard Med Sch 1984; **Resid:** Obstetrics & Gynecology, Brigham & Womens Hosp 1988; **Fellow:** Gynecologic Oncology, Mass General Hosp 1991; **Fac Appt:** Assoc Clin Prof ObG, Univ Wash

Pejovic, Tanja MD/PhD [GO] - **Spec Exp:** Ovarian Cancer; Gynecologic Cancer-Rare; Uterine Cancer; Cervical Cancer; **Hospital:** OR Hlth & Sci Univ; **Address:** Dept of Gyn Oncology, 3181 SW Sam Jackson Park Rd, MC KPV7, Portland, OR 97239; **Phone:** 503-418-4500; **Board Cert:** Obstetrics & Gynecology 2006; Gynecologic Oncology 2006; **Med School:** Yugoslavia 1984; **Resid:** Gynecologic Oncology, Lund Univ Affil Hosp 1995; Obstetrics & Gynecology, Yale/New Haven Hosp 2000; **Fellow:** Gynecologic Oncology, Yale/New Haven Hosp 2003; **Fac Appt:** Assoc Prof ObG, Oregon Hlth & Sci Univ

Plaxe, Steven C MD [GO] - **Spec Exp:** Ovarian Cancer; Uterine Cancer; Gestational Trophoblastic Disease; **Hospital:** UCSD Med Ctr; **Address:** Moores Cancer Center, 3855 Health Sciences Drive, MC 0987, La Jolla, CA 92093-0987; **Phone:** 858-822-6199; **Board Cert:** Obstetrics & Gynecology 2009; Gynecologic Oncology 2009; **Med School:** Mount Sinai Sch Med 1981; **Resid:** Obstetrics & Gynecology, Yale-New Haven Hosp 1985; **Fellow:** Gynecologic Oncology, Mt Sinai Med Ctr 1988; **Fac Appt:** Prof ObG, UCSD

Smith, Lloyd Herbert MD [GO] - **Spec Exp:** Ovarian Cancer; Uterine Cancer; Vulvar Disease/Cancer; Vaginal Cancer; **Hospital:** UC Davis Med Ctr, Sutter Mem Hospital-Sacramento; **Address:** UC Davis Med Ctr, Dept Ob/Gyn, 4860 Y St, Ste 2500, Sacramento, CA 95817-2307; **Phone:** 916-734-6946; **Board Cert:** Obstetrics & Gynecology 2009; Gynecologic Oncology 2009; **Med School:** UC Davis 1981; **Resid:** Obstetrics & Gynecology, UC Davis Med Ctr 1985; **Fellow:** Gynecologic Oncology, Stanford Univ Hosp 1988; **Fac Appt:** Prof ObG, UC Davis

Stern, Jeffrey L MD [GO] - **Spec Exp:** Laparoscopic Surgery; Vulvar Disease/Cancer; **Hospital:** Alta Bates Summit Med Ctr-Alta Bates Campus; **Address:** Womens Cancer Ctr Northern Calif, 2001 Dwight Way, Berkley, CA 94704; **Phone:** 510-204-5770; **Board Cert:** Obstetrics & Gynecology 1983; Gynecologic Oncology 1984; **Med School:** SUNY Upstate Med Univ 1976; **Resid:** Obstetrics & Gynecology, Johns Hopkins Hosp 1980; **Fellow:** Gynecologic Oncology, USC Med Ctr 1982

Teng, Nelson NH MD/PhD [GO] - **Spec Exp:** Ovarian Cancer; Clinical Trials; **Hospital:** Stanford Univ Hosp & Clinics; **Address:** Dept Gyn Oncology, 300 Pasteur Drive, Stanford, CA 94305-5317; **Phone:** 650-498-8080; **Board Cert:** Obstetrics & Gynecology 2003; Gynecologic Oncology 2003; **Med School:** Univ Miami Sch Med 1977; **Resid:** Obstetrics & Gynecology, UCLA Med Ctr 1981; **Fellow:** Gynecologic Oncology, Stanford Univ Sch Med 1984; **Fac Appt:** Assoc Prof ObG, Stanford Univ

Cleveland Clinic

Every life deserves world class care.

Gynecological Oncology

Cleveland Clinic Ob/Gyn & Women's Health Institute is designed to meet the unique and changing medical needs of women from adolescence to mature adulthood. Our dedicated team offers coordinated and supportive care. *U.S.News & World Report* has ranked our gynecology program No. 4 in the country. Our physicians are nationally and internally known and many serve on leadership boards for professional physician societies.

In the Section of Gynecologic Oncology, the staff employs a multidisciplinary approach to comprehensive management of gynecologic malignancies, incorporating surgery, radiation, chemotherapy and biologic therapy. We offer all types of innovative surgery, including robotics and single-port surgery. We also have a popular Gynecologic Oncology fellowship program.

Our oncologists are members of the Gynecologic Oncology Group, a non-profit organization funded by the National Cancer Institute and the only national cooperative study group devoted exclusively to the investigation of gynecologic malignancies. Extensive clinical trials of the most current treatments and techniques are available. The section also encompasses the Familial Ovarian Cancer Registry and provides complete treatment of pre-invasive lower genital tract disease.

Cleveland Clinic
Women's Health Institute
9500 Euclid Avenue
Cleveland, OH 44195

clevelandclinic.org/
gynonctopdocs

Offering Same-Day Appointments
Call 800.274.2009.

Treatment Guides

Cleveland Clinic has developed comprehensive treatment guides for many diseases and conditions. To download our free treatment guides, visit clevelandclinic.org/treatmentguides.

Online Medical Second Opinion

Cleveland Clinic's My**Consult** Online Medical Second Opinion program securely connects patients to our physician specialists for more than 1,000 life-changing or life-threatening diagnoses all by the click of a mouse. To learn more, log onto eclevelandclinic.org/myconsult or call 800.223.2273, ext. 43223.

Special Assistance for Out-of-State Patients

Cleveland Clinic Global Patient Services offers a complimentary Medical Concierge service for patients who travel from outside of Ohio. Call 800.223.2273, ext. 55580 or email medicalconcierge@ccf.org.

Hand Surgery

a subspecialty of Orthopaedics, Surgery or Plastic Surgery

A specialist trained in the investigation, preservation and restoration by medical, surgical and rehabilitative means of all structures of the upper extremity directly affecting the form and function of the hand and wrist.

For more information about the mentioned specialties or those physicians, see **Orthopaedic Surgery, Surgery** or **Plastic Surgery** section(s).

Training Required: Five years (including general surgery) in orthopaedics *plus* two years in clinical practice before final certification is achieved *plus* additional training and examination in hand surgery OR five to seven years in plastic surgery *plus* additional training and examination in hand surgery.

HAND SURGERY

New England

Akelman, Edward MD [HS] - **Spec Exp:** Carpal Tunnel Syndrome; Arthritis; Wrist/Hand Injuries; **Hospital:** Rhode Island Hosp; **Address:** 2 Dudley St, Ste 200, Rhode Island Hosp, Providence, RI 02905; **Phone:** 401-457-1510; **Board Cert:** Orthopaedic Surgery 2008; Hand Surgery 2008; **Med School:** Dartmouth Med Sch 1978; **Resid:** Surgery, Peter Bent Brigham Hosp 1980; Orthopaedic Surgery, Yale-New Haven Hosp 1984; **Fellow:** Hand Surgery, Roosevelt Hosp 1985; **Fac Appt:** Prof OrS, Brown Univ

Belsky, Mark R MD [HS] - **Spec Exp:** Arthritis; Nerve Disorders/Surgery; Elbow Surgery; **Hospital:** Newton - Wellesley Hosp; **Address:** 2000 Washington St Blue Bldg - Ste 201, Newton, MA 02462-1629; **Phone:** 617-965-4263; **Board Cert:** Orthopaedic Surgery 1982; Hand Surgery 2001; **Med School:** Tufts Univ 1974; **Resid:** Surgery, Peter Bent Brigham Hosp 1976; Orthopaedic Surgery, Tufts-New England Med Ctr 1979; **Fellow:** Hand Surgery, Roosevelt Hosp 1980; **Fac Appt:** Clin Prof OrS, Tufts Univ

Sampson, Christian E MD [HS] - **Spec Exp:** Hand Injuries; Hand & Fingers Vascular Surgery; **Hospital:** Brigham and Women's Hosp (page 57); **Address:** Brigham & Women's Hosp, Div Plastic Surg, 75 Francis St, Boston, MA 02115; **Phone:** 617-732-6297; **Board Cert:** Plastic Surgery 2004; Hand Surgery 2003; **Med School:** Boston Univ 1986; **Resid:** Surgery, Boston Univ Med Ctr 1991; Plastic Surgery, Brigham & Women's Hosp 1993; **Fellow:** Hand Surgery, Roosevelt Hosp 1994

Waters, Peter Michael MD [HS] - **Spec Exp:** Brachial Plexus Palsy; Hand-Congenital Anomaly; **Hospital:** Children's Hospital - Boston; **Address:** Chldns Hosp, Dept Ortho Surgery, 300 Longwood Ave, Hunnewell - 2, Boston, MA 02115-5724; **Phone:** 617-355-6021; **Board Cert:** Orthopaedic Surgery 2002; Hand Surgery 2004; **Med School:** Tufts Univ 1981; **Resid:** Pediatrics, Mass Genl Hosp 1983; Orthopaedic Surgery, Harvard Combined Prog 1988; **Fellow:** Hand Surgery, Brigham/Chldns Hosp 1989; **Fac Appt:** Assoc Prof OrS, Harvard Med Sch

Weiss, Arnold P MD [HS] - **Spec Exp:** Carpal Tunnel Syndrome; Wrist Surgery; Elbow Replacement; **Hospital:** Rhode Island Hosp; **Address:** Univ Orthopedics, 2 Dudley St, Ste 200, Providence, RI 02905-3248; **Phone:** 401-457-1520; **Board Cert:** Orthopaedic Surgery 2004; Hand Surgery 2004; **Med School:** Johns Hopkins Univ 1985; **Resid:** Orthopaedic Surgery, Johns Hopkins Hosp 1990; **Fellow:** Hand Surgery, Indiana Hand Ctr 1991; **Fac Appt:** Prof OrS, Brown Univ

Mid Atlantic

Athanasian, Edward MD [HS] - **Spec Exp:** Bone & Soft Tissue Tumors; Hand & Upper Extremity Tumors; Hand & Upper Extremity Surgery; **Hospital:** Hosp For Special Surgery (page 60), Meml Sloan-Kettering Cancer Ctr; **Address:** Hospital for Special Surgery, 535 E 70th St, New York, NY 10021; **Phone:** 212-606-1962; **Board Cert:** Orthopaedic Surgery 2008; Hand Surgery 2008; **Med School:** Columbia P&S 1988; **Resid:** Surgery, Beth Israel Hosp 1989; Orthopaedic Surgery, Hosp Special Surgery 1993; **Fellow:** Hand Surgery, Mayo Clinic 1994; Orthopaedic Oncology, Meml Sloan Kettering Cancer Ctr 1995; **Fac Appt:** Asst Prof OrS, Cornell Univ-Weill Med Coll

Baratz, Mark E MD [HS] - **Spec Exp:** Hand Surgery; Upper Extremity Surgery; Elbow Reconstruction; **Hospital:** Allegheny General Hosp, St. Clair Hosp; **Address:** 1307 Federal St Fl 2, Pittsburgh, PA 15212; **Phone:** 412-359-4263; **Board Cert:** Orthopaedic Surgery 2004; Hand Surgery 2004; **Med School:** Univ Pittsburgh 1984; **Resid:** Orthopaedic Surgery, Univ Hlth Ctr 1990; **Fellow:** Orthopaedic Surgery, Univ Hlth Ctr 1987; Hand Surgery, Med Coll Penn 1991; **Fac Appt:** Prof OrS, Drexel Univ Coll Med

Beredjiklian, Pedro K MD [HS] - **Spec Exp:** Hand & Wrist Surgery; Arthroscopic Surgery; Elbow Reconstruction; **Hospital:** Thomas Jefferson Univ Hosp, Riddle Meml Hosp; **Address:** Rothman Institute, 925 Chestnut Ave Fl 5, Philadelphia, PA 19107; **Phone:** 800-321-9999; **Board Cert:** Orthopaedic Sports Medicine 2011; Hand Surgery 2011; **Med School:** Columbia P&S 1992; **Resid:** Orthopaedic Surgery, Hosp U Penn 1997; **Fellow:** Hand & Microvascular Surgery, Hosp Special Surgery 1998; **Fac Appt:** Assoc Prof OrS, Thomas Jefferson Univ

Bozentka, David J MD [HS] - **Spec Exp:** Hand & Upper Extremity Surgery; Elbow Surgery; **Hospital:** Penn Presby Med Ctr - UPHS (page 68); **Address:** Penn Orthopaedic Institute, I Cupp Pavilion, 39th & Market St, Philadelphia, PA 19104; **Phone:** 215-349-5773; **Board Cert:** Orthopaedic Surgery 2006; Hand Surgery 2006; **Med School:** Jefferson Med Coll 1987; **Resid:** Orthopaedic Surgery, W Virgina Univ Hosp 1992; **Fac Appt:** Assoc Prof OrS, Univ Pennsylvania

Brushart, Thomas M MD [HS] - **Spec Exp:** Hand & Upper Extremity Surgery; Peripheral Nerve Surgery; **Hospital:** Johns Hopkins Hosp (page 61); **Address:** 601 N Caroline St, rm 5221, Baltimore, MD 21287-0882; **Phone:** 410-955-9663; **Board Cert:** Orthopaedic Surgery 1985; **Med School:** Harvard Med Sch 1978; **Resid:** Orthopaedic Surgery, Harvard Affil Hosps 1981; **Fellow:** Hand Surgery, Curtis Hand Ctr 1983; **Fac Appt:** Prof OrS, Johns Hopkins Univ

Carlson, Michelle Gerwin MD [HS] - **Spec Exp:** Sports Injuries; Hand & Upper Extremity Surgery; Pediatric Hand/Arm Surgery; Cerebral Palsy; **Hospital:** Hosp For Special Surgery (page 60), NY-Presby/Weill Cornell Med Ctr, NY (page 65); **Address:** 523 E 72nd St, Fl 4, rm 439, New York, NY 10021; **Phone:** 212-606-1546; **Board Cert:** Orthopaedic Surgery 2007; Hand Surgery 2007; **Med School:** Cornell Univ-Weill Med Coll 1987; **Resid:** Surgery, Hosp Special Surg 1992; **Fellow:** Hand Surgery, Hosp Special Surg 1993; **Fac Appt:** Assoc Prof OrS, Cornell Univ-Weill Med Coll

Culp, Randall MD [HS] - **Spec Exp:** Microsurgery; Hand & Upper Extremity Surgery; Elbow Surgery; **Hospital:** Thomas Jefferson Univ Hosp, Lankenau Hosp; **Address:** Philadelphia Hand Center, 700 S Henderson Rd, Ste 200, King of Prussia, PA 19406; **Phone:** 610-768-5959; **Board Cert:** Orthopaedic Surgery 2011; Hand Surgery 2011; **Med School:** Penn State Coll Med 1982; **Resid:** Orthopaedic Surgery, Hosp Univ Penn 1987; **Fellow:** Hand Surgery, Hosp Univ Penn 1988; **Fac Appt:** Prof OrS, Jefferson Med Coll

Egleseder Jr, W Andrew MD [HS] - **Spec Exp:** Hand & Upper Extremity Surgery; Trauma; Hand Reconstruction; **Hospital:** Univ of MD Med Ctr; **Address:** Univ Maryland Shock Trauma Ctr, 22 S Greene St, Baltimore, MD 21201; **Phone:** 410-328-6284; **Board Cert:** Orthopaedic Surgery 2010; Hand Surgery 2010; **Med School:** Univ MD Sch Med 1982; **Resid:** Orthopaedic Surgery, Univ Maryland Med Ctr 1987; **Fellow:** Hand Surgery, Univ Louisville Med Ctr 1989; **Fac Appt:** Assoc Prof OrS, Univ MD Sch Med

Glickel, Steven Z MD [HS] - **Spec Exp:** Hand & Wrist Surgery; Elbow Surgery; Peripheral Nerve Surgery; **Hospital:** St. Luke's - Roosevelt Hosp Ctr - Roosevelt Div (page 55); **Address:** 1000 10th Ave Fl 3, New York, NY 10019-1147; **Phone:** 212-523-7590; **Board Cert:** Orthopaedic Surgery 1985; Hand Surgery 2010; **Med School:** Harvard Med Sch 1976; **Resid:** Surgery, Columbia Presby Hosp 1978; Orthopaedic Surgery, Harvard Comb Ortho 1981; **Fellow:** Hand Surgery, St Luke's-Roosevelt Hosp Ctr 1983; Research, Columbia Presby Hosp 1982; **Fac Appt:** Clin Prof OrS, Columbia P&S

Hand Surgery

Goitz, Robert J MD [HS] - **Spec Exp:** Hand & Upper Extremity Surgery; **Hospital:** UPMC Mercy, Pittsburgh; **Address:** Kaufman Medical Bldg, Ste 1010, 3471 Fifth Ave, Pittsburgh, PA 15213; **Phone:** 412-605-3324; **Board Cert:** Orthopaedic Surgery 2011; Hand Surgery 2001; **Med School:** Johns Hopkins Univ 1992; **Resid:** Orthopaedic Surgery, Univ Pittsburgh Med Ctr 1997; **Fac Appt:** Assoc Prof OrS, Univ Pittsburgh

Imbriglia, Joseph E MD [HS] - **Spec Exp:** Arthritis; Carpal Tunnel Syndrome; Shoulder Surgery; Rotator Cuff Surgery; **Hospital:** UPMC Passavant-McCandless, UPMC Shadyside; **Address:** 6001 Stonewood Drive, Wexford, PA 15090-7380; **Phone:** 724-933-3850; **Board Cert:** Orthopaedic Surgery 1977; Hand Surgery 2010; **Med School:** Hahnemann Univ 1970; **Resid:** Surgery, Univ Pittsburgh Med Ctr 1972; Orthopaedic Surgery, Columbia Presby Med Ctr 1975; **Fellow:** Hand Surgery, Columbia Presby Med Ctr 1976; **Fac Appt:** Clin Prof OrS, Univ Pittsburgh

Kozin, Scott H MD [HS] - **Spec Exp:** Congenital Hand Deformities; Brachial Plexus Palsy-Pediatric; Spinal Cord Injury-Pediatric; Hand Surgery; **Hospital:** Philadelphia Shriners Hosp; **Address:** Shriners Hosp for Children, 3551 N Broad St, Philadelphia, PA 19140; **Phone:** 215-430-4074; **Board Cert:** Orthopaedic Surgery 2005; Hand Surgery 2005; **Med School:** Hahnemann Univ 1986; **Resid:** Orthopaedic Surgery, Albert Einstein Med Ctr 1991; **Fellow:** Hand Surgery, Mayo Clinic 1992; **Fac Appt:** Assoc Prof OrS, Temple Univ

Kulick, Roy G MD [HS] - **Spec Exp:** Carpal Tunnel Syndrome; Arthritis; Tendon Surgery; Hand & Upper Extremity Surgery; **Hospital:** Montefiore Med Ctr - Div. Weiler; **Address:** Montefiore Medical Center, 1200 Waters Pl Fl 11, Bronx, NY 10461; **Phone:** 718-920-2060; **Board Cert:** Orthopaedic Surgery 1980; Hand Surgery 2011; **Med School:** Cornell Univ-Weill Med Coll 1973; **Resid:** Surgery, St Lukes-Roosevelt Hosp 1975; Orthopaedic Surgery, NY Presby Hosp/Columbia Univ Med Ctr 1978; **Fellow:** Hand Surgery, Hosp for Special Surgery 1979; **Fac Appt:** Assoc Prof OrS, Albert Einstein Coll Med

Lane, Lewis B MD [HS] - **Spec Exp:** Carpal Tunnel Syndrome; Arthritis; Sports Injuries; Hand Reconstruction; **Hospital:** N Shore Univ Hosp, St. Francis Hosp - The Heart Ctr (page 69); **Address:** 600 Northern Blvd, Ste 300, Great Neck, NY 11021; **Phone:** 516-627-8717; **Board Cert:** Orthopaedic Surgery 1981; Hand Surgery 2010; **Med School:** Columbia P&S 1974; **Resid:** Surgery, NY Hosp 1975; Orthopaedic Surgery, Hosp for Special Surg 1979; **Fellow:** Research, Hosp for Special Surg 1976; Hand Surgery, St Luke's-Roosevelt Hosp Ctr 1980; **Fac Appt:** Assoc Clin Prof OrS, Albany Med Coll

Lee, W P Andrew MD [HS] - **Spec Exp:** Reconstructive Surgery; Cartilage Damage; Transplant-Hand; Pediatric Hand Surgery; **Hospital:** Johns Hopkins Hosp (page 61); **Address:** Johns Hopkins Outpatient Ctr, 601 N Carolyn St, Ste 8152F, Baltimore, MD 21287; **Phone:** 410-955-9466 x4; **Board Cert:** Hand Surgery 2005; Plastic Surgery 2005; **Med School:** Johns Hopkins Univ 1983; **Resid:** Surgery, Johns Hopkins Hosp 1989; Plastic Surgery, Mass Genl Hosp 1991; **Fellow:** Microsurgery, Johns Hopkins Hosp 1987; Hand Surgery, Indiana Hand Ctr 1993; **Fac Appt:** Prof S, Johns Hopkins Univ

Lubahn, John D MD [HS] - **Spec Exp:** Microsurgery; **Hospital:** UPMC Hamot, St. Vincent Hlth Ctr; **Address:** 300 State St, Ste 205, Erie, PA 16507; **Phone:** 814-456-6022; **Board Cert:** Orthopaedic Surgery 2000; Hand Surgery 2010; **Med School:** Case West Res Univ 1975; **Resid:** Surgery, Univ Rochester Med Ctr 1977; Orthopaedic Surgery, Univ Rochester Med Ctr 1980; **Fellow:** Hand Surgery, Univ Louisville Hosp 1981

Melone Jr, Charles P MD [HS] - **Spec Exp:** Arthritis; Wrist Surgery; Fractures; **Hospital:** Beth Israel Med Ctr - Petrie Division (page 55); **Address:** 321 E 34th St, New York, NY 10016; **Phone:** 212-340-0000; **Board Cert:** Orthopaedic Surgery 1976; Hand Surgery 2004; **Med School:** Georgetown Univ 1969; **Resid:** Surgery, Nassau Co Med Ctr 1971; Orthopaedic Surgery, Nassau Co Med Ctr 1974; **Fellow:** Hand Surgery, NYU Langone Med Ctr 1975; **Fac Appt:** Clin Prof OrS, Albert Einstein Coll Med

Osterman Jr, A Lee MD [HS] - **Spec Exp:** Upper Extremity Surgery; Wrist Surgery; Neuromuscular Disorders; **Hospital:** Thomas Jefferson Univ Hosp, Chldns Hosp of Philadelphia; **Address:** Philadelphia Hand Ctr, 700 S Henderson Rd, Ste 200, King of Prussia, PA 19406-4207; **Phone:** 610-265-3135; **Board Cert:** Orthopaedic Surgery 1980; **Med School:** Univ Pennsylvania 1973; **Resid:** Orthopaedic Surgery, Hosp Univ Penn 1978; **Fellow:** Hand Surgery, Hosp Univ Penn 1979; Microvascular Surgery, Duke Univ Med Ctr 1980; **Fac Appt:** Prof OrS, Jefferson Med Coll

Raskin, Keith B MD [HS] - **Spec Exp:** Wrist/Hand Injuries; Arthritis; Carpal Tunnel Syndrome; Elbow Surgery; **Hospital:** NYU Langone Med Ctr (page 66), NYU Hosp For Joint Diseases; **Address:** 317 E 34th St, Fl 3, New York, NY 10016; **Phone:** 212-263-4263; **Board Cert:** Orthopaedic Surgery 2002; Hand Surgery 2002; **Med School:** Geo Wash Univ 1983; **Resid:** Orthopaedic Surgery, NYU Med Ctr 1988; **Fellow:** Hand Surgery, Union Mem Hosp 1989; **Fac Appt:** Assoc Clin Prof OrS, NYU Sch Med

Rosenwasser, Melvin P MD [HS] - **Spec Exp:** Carpal Tunnel Syndrome; Sports Injuries; Elbow Surgery; Trauma; **Hospital:** NY-Presby/Columbia Univ Med Ctr, NY (page 65); **Address:** 622 W 168th St, PH 11, rm 1150, New York, NY 10032; **Phone:** 212-305-8036; **Board Cert:** Orthopaedic Surgery 1999; **Med School:** Columbia P&S 1976; **Resid:** Surgery, Roosevelt Hosp 1979; Orthopaedic Surgery, Columbia Presby Hosp 1982; **Fellow:** Hand Surgery, Columbia Presby Hosp 1983; **Fac Appt:** Prof OrS, Columbia P&S

Sotereanos, Dean G MD [HS] - **Spec Exp:** Hand & Upper Extremity Surgery; Elbow Surgery; **Hospital:** Allegheny General Hosp; **Address:** 1307 Federal St Fl 2, Pittsburgh, PA 15212; **Phone:** 412-359-4263; **Board Cert:** Orthopaedic Surgery 2003; Hand Surgery 2003; **Med School:** Hahnemann Univ 1984; **Resid:** Surgery, Univ Pittsburgh Med Ctr 1986; Orthopaedic Surgery, Univ Pittsburgh Med Ctr 1989; **Fellow:** Hand Surgery, Duke Univ Med Ctr 1990; **Fac Appt:** Assoc Prof OrS, Univ Pittsburgh

Strauch, Robert MD [HS] - **Spec Exp:** Hand Reconstruction; Hand & Elbow Nerve Disorders; Hand & Wrist Surgery; Elbow Surgery; **Hospital:** NY-Presby/Columbia Univ Med Ctr, NY (page 65); **Address:** 622 W 168th St, rm PH-11, New York, NY 10032; **Phone:** 212-305-4272; **Board Cert:** Orthopaedic Surgery 2005; Hand Surgery 2005; **Med School:** Columbia P&S 1986; **Resid:** Orthopaedic Surgery, Columbia-Presby Hosp 1991; **Fellow:** Hand Surgery, Indiana Hand Center 1992; **Fac Appt:** Prof OrS, Columbia P&S

Thoder, Joseph J MD [HS] - **Spec Exp:** Wrist/Hand Injuries; **Hospital:** Temple Univ Hosp; **Address:** Temple Univ Hosp, Dept Orthopaedics, 3501 N Broad St, Philadelphia, PA 19140; **Phone:** 215-707-2111; **Board Cert:** Orthopaedic Surgery 2011; Hand Surgery 2011; **Med School:** Temple Univ 1982; **Resid:** Orthopaedic Surgery, Temple Univ Hosp 1987; **Fellow:** Hand & Microvascular Surgery, Thos Jefferson Univ Hosp 1988; **Fac Appt:** Prof OrS, Temple Univ

Weiland, Andrew J MD [HS] - **Spec Exp:** Wrist/Hand Injuries; Hand Reconstruction; **Hospital:** Hosp For Special Surgery (page 60), NY-Presby/Weill Cornell Med Ctr, NY (page 65); **Address:** Hospital for Special Surgery, 535 E 70th St, New York, NY 10021-4872; **Phone:** 212-606-1575; **Board Cert:** Orthopaedic Surgery 1977; **Med School:** Wake Forest Univ 1968; **Resid:** Surgery, Univ Michigan Med Ctr 1970; Orthopaedic Surgery, Johns Hopkins Hosp 1975; **Fellow:** Hand Surgery, Kleinert Hosp 1975; **Fac Appt:** Prof OrS, Cornell Univ-Weill Med Coll

Hand Surgery

Wolfe, Scott W MD [HS] - **Spec Exp:** Wrist Surgery; Nerve Disorders/Surgery; Fractures; **Hospital:** Hosp For Special Surgery (page 60); **Address:** Hospital for Special Surgery, 535 E 70 St, New York, NY 10021; **Phone:** 212-606-1529; **Board Cert:** Orthopaedic Surgery 2003; Hand Surgery 2003; **Med School:** Cornell Univ-Weill Med Coll 1984; **Resid:** Surgery, St Luke's Roosevelt Hosp Ctr 1986; Orthopaedic Surgery, Hosp Special Surg 1989; **Fellow:** Hand & Microvascular Surgery, Columbia Presby Med Ctr 1990; **Fac Appt:** Prof OrS, Cornell Univ-Weill Med Coll

Southeast

Carneiro, Ronaldo D S MD [HS] - **Spec Exp:** Carpal Tunnel Syndrome; Arthritis; Dupuytren's Contracture; Hand & Wrist Surgery; **Hospital:** Physicians Regl Hlthcare Med Ctr-Pine Ridge; **Address:** 8340 Collier Blvd, Ste 303, Naples, FL 34114; **Phone:** 239-348-4040; **Board Cert:** Plastic Surgery 1990; **Med School:** Brazil 1970; **Resid:** Surgery, Union Meml Hosp 1975; Plastic Surgery, Allentown & Sacred Heart Hosp Ctr 1977; **Fellow:** Hand Surgery, Jackson Meml Hosp-Univ Miami Hosp 1977; Plastic Surgery, Univ Miami Sch Med 1978; **Fac Appt:** Assoc Clin Prof PlS, Univ S Fla Coll Med

Cendales, Linda C MD [HS] - **Spec Exp:** Transplant-Hand; Microsurgery; **Hospital:** Emory Univ Hosp, Emory Univ Hosp Midtown; **Address:** Emory Transplant Center, 1365 Clifton Road NE, Bldg B, Atlanta, GA 30322; **Phone:** 404-727-1731; **Med School:** Mexico 1992; **Resid:** Surgery, Hospital General 1996; Hand Surgery, Natl Inst Orthopaedics 1997; **Fellow:** Hand & Microvascular Surgery, Kleinert Inst, Univ Louisville 2001; Transplant Surgery, Natl Inst Hlth 2004; **Fac Appt:** Asst Prof S, Emory Univ

Friedman, David W MD [HS] - **Spec Exp:** Hand Reconstruction; Arthritis; Microsurgery; Sports Injuries; **Hospital:** Cleveland Clin - Weston; **Address:** Cleveland Clinic Florida, 2950 Cleveland Clinic Blvd, Weston, FL 33331; **Phone:** 954-659-5430; **Board Cert:** Plastic Surgery 2009; Hand Surgery 2008; **Med School:** Univ Tex SW, Dallas 1988; **Resid:** Surgery, UMDNJ Affil Hosp 1994; Plastic Surgery, NYU Med Ctr 1996; **Fellow:** Hand Surgery, NYU Med Ctr 1997

Greene, Thomas L MD [HS] - **Spec Exp:** Arthritis; Peripheral Nerve Surgery; Arthroscopic Surgery; Tendon Surgery; **Hospital:** Tampa Genl Hosp, St. Joseph's Hosp - Tampa; **Address:** 2727 W Dr Martin Luther King Jr Blvd, Ste 560, Tampa, FL 33607-6009; **Phone:** 813-873-0337; **Board Cert:** Orthopaedic Surgery 1983; Hand Surgery 2000; **Med School:** Ohio State Univ 1975; **Resid:** Surgery, Univ Michigan Med Ctr 1977; Orthopaedic Surgery, Univ Michigan Med Ctr 1980; **Fellow:** Hand Surgery, St Vincent's Hosp 1981

Grossman, John AI MD [HS] - **Spec Exp:** Brachial Plexus Palsy; Hand & Microvascular Surgery; Peripheral Nerve Surgery; Congenital Hand Deformities; **Hospital:** Miami Children's Hosp, NYU Hosp For Joint Diseases; **Address:** 8940 N Kendall Dr Ste 904E, Miami, FL 33176-2176; **Phone:** 305-666-2004; **Board Cert:** Plastic Surgery 1989; **Med School:** Univ VA Sch Med 1978; **Resid:** Surgery, Cleveland Clinic 1981; Plastic Surgery, E Virginia Affil Hosp 1985; **Fellow:** Hand Surgery, French Hand Inst 1983; **Fac Appt:** Assoc Clin Prof OrS, NYU Sch Med

Hunt III, Thomas R MD [HS] - **Spec Exp:** Hand & Wrist Surgery; Arthritis; Trauma; Hand Reconstruction; **Hospital:** Univ of Ala Hosp at Birmingham; **Address:** UAB Orthopaedic Surgery, 1313 13th St S, Ste 201, Birmingham, AL 35205-5327; **Phone:** 205-930-8339; **Board Cert:** Orthopaedic Surgery 2006; Hand Surgery 2006; **Med School:** Vanderbilt Univ 1986; **Resid:** Orthopaedic Surgery, Univ Kansas Med Ctr 1992; **Fellow:** Hand Surgery, Hosp Univ Penn 1993; **Fac Appt:** Prof S, Univ Alabama

Koman, L Andrew MD [HS] - **Spec Exp:** Pediatric Hand Surgery; Vascular Disease-Upper Extremity; Pain-Nerve Injury; **Hospital:** Wake Forest Univ Baptist Med Ctr; **Address:** Wake Forest Univ Baptist Med Ctr, Medical Ctr Blvd, Winston-Salem, NC 27157; **Phone:** 336-716-8094; **Board Cert:** Orthopaedic Surgery 1981; Hand Surgery 2010; **Med School:** Duke Univ 1974; **Resid:** Surgery, Duke Univ Med Ctr 1975; Orthopaedic Surgery, Duke Univ Med Ctr 1979; **Fellow:** Hand Surgery, Duke Univ Med Ctr 1980; **Fac Appt:** Prof OrS, Wake Forest Univ

Midwest

Bishop, Allen T MD [HS] - **Spec Exp:** Microsurgery; Brachial Plexus Palsy; **Hospital:** Mayo Med Ctr & Clin - Rochester; **Address:** Mayo Clin, Div Hand Surgery, 200 First St SW, Rochester, MN 55905; **Phone:** 507-284-0475; **Board Cert:** Orthopaedic Surgery 2000; Hand Surgery 2000; **Med School:** Mayo Med Sch 1981; **Resid:** Orthopaedic Surgery, Mayo Clin 1986; **Fellow:** Hand Surgery, St Vincent Hosp 1987; **Fac Appt:** Prof OrS, Mayo Med Sch

Carroll, Charles MD [HS] - **Spec Exp:** Carpal Tunnel Syndrome; Dupuytren's Contracture; Elbow Surgery; Shoulder Surgery; **Hospital:** Northwestern Meml Hosp; **Address:** Northwest Orthopaedic Inst, 680 N Lakeshore Drive, Ste 924, Chicago, IL 60611; **Phone:** 312-664-6848; **Board Cert:** Orthopaedic Surgery 2011; Hand Surgery 2011; **Med School:** Univ MD Sch Med 1982; **Resid:** Surgery, Johns Hopkins Hosp 1984; Orthopaedic Surgery, Johns Hopkins Hosp 1987; **Fellow:** Hand Surgery, Indiana Univ Med Ctr 1988; Shoulder Surgery, Univ Western Ontario 1988; **Fac Appt:** Assoc Clin Prof OrS, Northwestern Univ

Chung, Kevin Chi MD [HS] - **Spec Exp:** Reconstructive Surgery; Hand & Microvascular Surgery; Upper Extremity Trauma; Nail Surgery; **Hospital:** Univ of Michigan Hosp; **Address:** Univ Michigan, TC 2130-SPC 5340, 1500 E Med Ctr Drive, Ann Arbor, MI 48109; **Phone:** 734-936-5885; **Board Cert:** Hand Surgery 2007; Plastic Surgery 2007; **Med School:** Emory Univ 1987; **Resid:** Plastic Surgery, Univ Michigan Hosp & Hlth Ctr 1994; Hand Surgery, Union Meml Hosp 1995; **Fac Appt:** Assoc Prof S, Univ Mich Med Sch

Cohen, Mark S MD [HS] - **Spec Exp:** Hand Surgery; Wrist Surgery; Elbow Surgery; **Hospital:** Rush Univ Med Ctr; **Address:** Midwest Orthopedics at Rush, 1611 W Harrison St, Ste 300, Chicago, IL 60612; **Phone:** 312-432-2346; **Board Cert:** Orthopaedic Surgery 2006; Hand Surgery 2006; **Med School:** Harvard Med Sch 1986; **Resid:** Orthopaedic Surgery, UCSD Med Ctr 1992; **Fellow:** Hand Surgery, Indiana Hand Ctr 1993; **Fac Appt:** Prof OrS, Rush Med Coll

Derman, Gordon H MD [HS] - **Spec Exp:** Carpal Tunnel Syndrome; Tendon Surgery; Repetitive Motion Injuries; Nerve Disorders/Surgery; **Hospital:** Rush Univ Med Ctr, NorthShore Univ Hlth-Sys; **Address:** 1725 W Harrison St, Ste 470, Chicago, IL 60612; **Phone:** 312-432-9200; **Board Cert:** Plastic Surgery 1984; Hand Surgery 1996; **Med School:** Rush Med Coll 1975; **Resid:** Surgery, Loyola Univ Med Ctr 1981; Plastic Surgery, Univ Mich Hosp 1983; **Fellow:** Microsurgery, Rush/Presby St Luke's Med Ctr 1976; **Fac Appt:** Asst Prof S, Rush Med Coll

DeSilva, Stephen P MD [HS] - **Spec Exp:** Hand Surgery; **Hospital:** Henry Ford Hosp; **Address:** Henry Ford Hospital, 2799 West Grand Blvd Fl 12, Detroit, MI 48202; **Phone:** 248-661-7195; **Board Cert:** Orthopaedic Surgery 2002; Hand Surgery 2002; **Med School:** Johns Hopkins Univ 1983; **Resid:** Orthopaedic Surgery, Mayo Clinic 1988; **Fellow:** Hand Surgery, Union Meml Hosp 1989; **Fac Appt:** Prof OrS, Wayne State Univ

Failla, Joseph M MD [HS] - **Spec Exp:** Hand Surgery; Hand Reconstruction; **Hospital:** Providence Hosp - Southfield, Huron Valley-Sinai Hosp; **Address:** Farmbrook Med Complex, 29829 Telegraph Rd, Ste 201, Southfield, MI 48034; **Phone:** 248-352-4263; **Board Cert:** Orthopaedic Surgery 2001; Hand Surgery 2001; **Med School:** SUNY Buffalo 1982; **Resid:** Orthopaedic Surgery, SUNY-Buffalo 1987; **Fellow:** Hand Surgery, Mayo Clinic 1988

Hand Surgery

Fischer, Thomas J MD [HS] - **Spec Exp:** Microsurgery; Elbow Reconstruction; Fractures-Complex; **Hospital:** St. Vincent Indianapolis Hosp, IU Health University Hosp; **Address:** Indiana Hand to Shoulder Center, 8501 Harcourt Rd, Indianapolis, IN 46260; **Phone:** 317-875-9105; **Board Cert:** Orthopaedic Surgery 2010; Hand Surgery 2010; **Med School:** Indiana Univ 1979; **Resid:** Orthopaedic Surgery, Univ Wash Affil Hosp 1984; **Fellow:** Hand Surgery, Hand Surg Assocs 1985; Hand Surgery, Duke Univ Med Ctr 1986; **Fac Appt:** Assoc Clin Prof OrS, Indiana Univ

Gelberman, Richard H MD [HS] - **Spec Exp:** Tendon Surgery; Peripheral Nerve Surgery; **Hospital:** Barnes-Jewish Hosp; **Address:** Wash Univ Sch Med, Dept Ortho Surg, 660 S Euclid Ave, Box 8233, St Louis, MO 63110; **Phone:** 314-747-2500; **Board Cert:** Orthopaedic Surgery 2007; Hand Surgery 2007; **Med School:** Univ Tenn Coll Med 1969; **Resid:** Surgery, Univ Wisc Med Ctr 1975; **Fellow:** Hand Surgery, Duke Univ Med Ctr 1977; Pediatric Orthopaedic Surgery, Chldns Hosp-Harvard 1986; **Fac Appt:** Prof OrS, Washington Univ, St Louis

Graham, Thomas J MD [HS] - **Spec Exp:** Hand & Wrist Surgery; Elbow Surgery; Sports Injuries; Wrist/Hand Injuries; **Hospital:** Cleveland Clin (page 56); **Address:** Cleveland Clin-Dept Orthopedics, MC GCIC-10, 9500 Euclid Ave, Cleveland, OH 44195; **Phone:** 216-444-6260; **Board Cert:** Orthopaedic Surgery 2007; Hand Surgery 2007; **Med School:** Univ Cincinnati 1988; **Resid:** Orthopaedic Surgery, Univ Michigan Med Ctr 1993; **Fellow:** Hand Surgery, Indiana Hand Ctr 1994; Elbow Surgery, Mayo Clinic 1994

Harris, Gerald D MD [HS] - **Spec Exp:** Reconstructive Microvascular Surgery; **Hospital:** Northwestern Meml Hosp; **Address:** 737 N Michigan Ave, Ste 700, Chicago, IL 60611; **Phone:** 312-337-6960; **Board Cert:** Plastic Surgery 1980; Hand Surgery 2009; **Med School:** Univ IL Coll Med 1973; **Resid:** Surgery, Northwestern Meml Hosp 1977; Plastic Surgery, Northwestern Meml Hosp 1979; **Fellow:** Hand Surgery, UCSF Med Ctr 1979; **Fac Appt:** Assoc Clin Prof S, Northwestern Univ

Hastings II, Hill MD [HS] - **Spec Exp:** Wrist Surgery; Elbow Reconstruction; Fractures & Tendon Transfers; Arthritis; **Hospital:** St. Vincent Indianapolis Hosp; **Address:** Indiana Hand to Shoulder Center, 8501 Harcourt Rd, Indianapolis, IN 46260; **Phone:** 317-875-9105; **Board Cert:** Orthopaedic Surgery 1982; Hand Surgery 2010; **Med School:** USC Sch Med 1974; **Resid:** Surgery, Univ Colorado Med Ctr 1976; Orthopaedic Surgery, Mass Genl Hosp 1980; **Fellow:** Hand Surgery, St Vincent Hosp 1981; **Fac Appt:** Clin Prof OrS, Indiana Univ

Kleinman, William B MD [HS] - **Spec Exp:** Upper Extremity Surgery-Pediatric; Congenital Hand Deformities; Wrist Reconstruction; Hand Reconstruction; **Hospital:** St. Vincent Indianapolis Hosp; **Address:** Indiana Hand to Shoulder Center, 8501 Harcourt Rd, Indianapolis, IN 46260; **Phone:** 317-875-9105; **Board Cert:** Orthopaedic Surgery 1979; Hand Surgery 2000; **Med School:** Cornell Univ-Weill Med Coll 1972; **Resid:** Surgery, Univ Colorado Affil Hosp 1974; Orthopaedic Surgery, NY Orthopaedic Hosp 1977; **Fellow:** Hand Surgery, Columbia-Presby Med Ctr 1978; Microvascular Surgery, Duke Univ 1979; **Fac Appt:** Clin Prof OrS, Indiana Univ

Light, Terry R MD [HS] - **Spec Exp:** Hand-Congenital Anomaly; Hand Injuries-Pediatric; Arthritis; Thumb-Absence; **Hospital:** Loyola Univ Med Ctr, Shriners Hosp for Children-Chicago; **Address:** Loyola Univ Med Ctr, Dept Ortho Surg, 2160 S First Ave Maguire Bldg - rm 1700, Maywood, IL 60153-5590; **Phone:** 708-216-4570; **Board Cert:** Orthopaedic Surgery 1979; Hand Surgery 2010; **Med School:** Ros Franklin Univ/Chicago Med Sch 1973; **Resid:** Orthopaedic Surgery, Yale-New Haven Hosp 1977; **Fellow:** Hand Surgery, Hartford Combined Prog 1977; **Fac Appt:** Prof OrS, Loyola Univ-Stritch Sch Med

Mass, Daniel MD [HS] - **Spec Exp:** Tendon Surgery; Shoulder Reconstruction; Elbow Reconstruction; Wrist Surgery; **Hospital:** Univ of Chicago Med Ctr; **Address:** 5841 S Maryland Ave, MC 3079, Chicago, IL 60637; **Phone:** 773-834-3531; **Board Cert:** Orthopaedic Surgery 2007; Hand Surgery 2007; **Med School:** Univ Chicago-Pritzker Sch Med 1975; **Resid:** Orthopaedic Surgery, Univ Chicago Hosp 1979; **Fellow:** Hand Surgery, St Francis Hosp 1980; **Fac Appt:** Prof S, Univ Chicago-Pritzker Sch Med

Mih, Alexander D MD [HS] - **Spec Exp:** Pediatric Hand Surgery; Congenital Hand Deformities; Hand Reconstruction-Pediatric; Microsurgery; **Hospital:** IU Health University Hosp, St. Vincent Indianapolis Hosp; **Address:** Indiana Hand to Shoulder Center, 8501 Harcourt Rd, Indianapolis, IN 46260; **Phone:** 317-875-9105; **Board Cert:** Orthopaedic Surgery 2003; Hand Surgery 2003; **Med School:** Johns Hopkins Univ 1984; **Resid:** Orthopaedic Surgery, Mayo Clinic 1989; **Fellow:** Hand Surgery, Indiana Hand Ctr 1990; **Fac Appt:** Assoc Prof OrS, Indiana Univ

Nagle, Daniel J MD [HS] - **Spec Exp:** Wrist Surgery; Carpal Tunnel Syndrome; Cubital Tunnel Syndrome; **Hospital:** Northwestern Meml Hosp, Children's Mem Hosp -Chicago; **Address:** Chicago Hand Surgery, 737 N Michigan Ave, Ste 700, Chicago, IL 60611-7108; **Phone:** 312-337-6960; **Board Cert:** Orthopaedic Surgery 2007; Hand Surgery 2007; **Med School:** Belgium 1978; **Resid:** Orthopaedic Surgery, Northwestern Univ Med Sch 1983; **Fellow:** Hand Surgery, Christine Kleinert 1984; **Fac Appt:** Prof OrS, Northwestern Univ

Putnam, Matthew D MD [HS] - **Spec Exp:** Wrist Surgery; Fracture Deformities/Arm; Arthritis; Nerve Disorders/Surgery; **Hospital:** Univ Minn Med Ctr, Fairview - Riverside Campus; **Address:** 2512 S 7th St, rm 102, Minneapolis, MN 55454; **Phone:** 612-273-9400; **Board Cert:** Orthopaedic Surgery 2008; Hand Surgery 2001; **Med School:** Dartmouth Med Sch 1977; **Resid:** Surgery, Roosevelt Hosp 1979; Orthopaedic Surgery, Univ Pittsburgh 1984; **Fellow:** Hand Surgery, NYOH 1985; **Fac Appt:** Prof OrS, Univ Minn

Seitz, William H MD [HS] - **Spec Exp:** Hand & Upper Extremity Surgery; Shoulder Surgery; **Hospital:** Lutheran Med Ctr - Cleveland, Cleveland Clin (page 56); **Address:** 1730 W 25th St, Ste 2C, Cleveland, OH 44113; **Phone:** 216-363-2331; **Board Cert:** Orthopaedic Surgery 2008; Hand Surgery 2008; **Med School:** Columbia P&S 1979; **Resid:** Surgery, St Vincents Med Ctr 1981; Orthopaedic Surgery, Columbia-Presby Med Ctr 1984; **Fellow:** Hand & Microvascular Surgery, Columbia-Presby Med Ctr 1985; **Fac Appt:** Assoc Clin Prof OrS, Case West Res Univ

Steinmann, Scott P MD [HS] - **Spec Exp:** Shoulder Surgery; Elbow Surgery; Brachial Plexus Palsy; Reconstructive Microvascular Surgery; **Hospital:** Mayo Med Ctr & Clin - Rochester; **Address:** Mayo Clin, Dept Hand Surgery, 200 1st St SW, Rochester, MN 55905; **Phone:** 507-284-4577; **Board Cert:** Orthopaedic Surgery 2004; Hand Surgery 2004; **Med School:** Cornell Univ-Weill Med Coll 1988; **Resid:** Orthopaedic Surgery, Hosp Spec Surgery 1992; **Fellow:** Shoulder Surgery, Columbia-Presby Med Ctr 1995; Hand Surgery, Mayo Clin 1998; **Fac Appt:** Prof OrS, Mayo Med Sch

Stern, Peter J MD [HS] - **Spec Exp:** Hand & Wrist Surgery; Microsurgery; **Hospital:** Good Samaritan Hosp - Cincinnati, Univ Hosp - Cincinnati; **Address:** Hand Surg Specialists, 538 Oak St, Ste 200, Cincinnati, OH 45219; **Phone:** 513-961-4263; **Board Cert:** Orthopaedic Surgery 2011; Hand Surgery 2011; **Med School:** Washington Univ, St Louis 1970; **Resid:** Surgery, Beth Israel Hosp 1972; Orthopaedic Surgery, Harvard Combined Prgm 1977; **Fellow:** Hand Surgery, Univ Louisville Hosps 1979; **Fac Appt:** Prof OrS, Univ Cincinnati

Hand Surgery

Great Plains and Mountains

Idler, Richard S MD [HS] - **Spec Exp:** Upper Extremity Surgery; Microsurgery; **Hospital:** Penrose Hosp, St. Francis Med Ctr; **Address:** 3010 N Circle Drive, Ste 100, Colorado Springs, CO 80919-1174; **Phone:** 719-632-7669; **Board Cert:** Orthopaedic Surgery 1985; Hand Surgery 2010; **Med School:** Dartmouth Med Sch 1975; **Resid:** Surgery, UCLA Med Ctr 1977; Plastic Surgery, UCLA Med Ctr 1978; **Fellow:** Orthopaedic Surgery, Mass Genl Hosp-Harvard 1981; Hand Surgery, St Vincent Hosp 1982; **Fac Appt:** Asst Clin Prof OrS, Indiana Univ

Southwest

Breidenbach, Warren C MD [HS] - **Spec Exp:** Transplant-Hand; **Hospital:** Univ Med Ctr - Tucson; **Address:** UPH Clinic, 707 N Alvernon Way Fl 2, Tucson, AZ 85711; **Phone:** 520-874-2637; **Board Cert:** Plastic Surgery 1988; Hand Surgery 2003; **Med School:** Harvard Med Sch 1975; **Resid:** Plastic Surgery, McGill Univ 1982; **Fellow:** Microsurgery, Eastern Va Med Sch 1982; Hand Surgery, Univ Med Ctr 1983; **Fac Appt:** Prof PlS, Univ Ariz Coll Med

Collins, Evan D MD [HS] - **Spec Exp:** Hand & Upper Extremity Surgery; Wrist/Hand Injuries; Elbow Surgery; Sports Medicine; **Hospital:** Methodist Hosp - Houston; **Address:** Methodist Hospital, Dept Orthopaedics, 6550 Fannin St, Ste 2600, Houston, TX 77030; **Phone:** 713-441-3535; **Board Cert:** Orthopaedic Surgery 2011; Hand Surgery 2011; **Med School:** SUNY Downstate 1992; **Resid:** Surgery, Baylor College Med 1997; **Fellow:** Hand Surgery, Baylor College Med 1999

Ezaki, Marybeth MD [HS] - **Spec Exp:** Hand-Congenital Anomaly; Hand Reconstruction-Pediatric; **Hospital:** Texas Scottish Rite Hosp for Chldn; **Address:** 2222 Welborn St, Dallas, TX 75219; **Phone:** 214-559-7842; **Board Cert:** Orthopaedic Surgery 1985; **Med School:** Yale Univ 1977; **Resid:** Orthopaedic Surgery, Univ Tex SW Med Ctr 1982; **Fellow:** Hand Surgery, Weyham Pk Hosp 1982; **Fac Appt:** Assoc Prof OrS, Univ Tex SW, Dallas

Moneim, Moheb S MD [HS] - **Hospital:** Univ Hosp - New Mexico; **Address:** 1 Univ of New Mexico, Dept Orthopedics, MSC10-5600, Albuquerque, NM 87131; **Phone:** 505-272-4107; **Board Cert:** Orthopaedic Surgery 1998; Hand Surgery 2010; **Med School:** Egypt 1963; **Resid:** Orthopaedic Surgery, Duke Univ Med Ctr 1975; **Fellow:** Hand Surgery, Hosp for Spec Surgery 1976; **Fac Appt:** Prof OrS, Univ New Mexico

Rayan, Ghazi M MD [HS] - **Spec Exp:** Microsurgery; Congenital Limb Deformities; Arthritis; **Hospital:** Integris Baptist Med Ctr - OK, OU Med Ctr; **Address:** 3366 Northwest Expressway, Ste 700, Oklahoma City, OK 73112-4439; **Phone:** 405-945-4888; **Board Cert:** Orthopaedic Surgery 2000; Hand Surgery 2000; **Med School:** Egypt 1973; **Resid:** Surgery, S Baltimore Genl Hosp 1977; Orthopaedic Surgery, Union Meml Hosp 1980; **Fellow:** Hand & Microvascular Surgery, Union Meml Hosp 1980; **Fac Appt:** Clin Prof OrS, Univ Okla Coll Med

West Coast and Pacific

Abrams, Reid A MD [HS] - **Spec Exp:** Hand & Upper Extremity Surgery; Elbow Reconstruction; Fractures & Tendon Transfers; Carpal Tunnel Syndrome; **Hospital:** UCSD Med Ctr; **Address:** UCSD Med Ctr, Dept Orthopaedic Surgery, 200 W Arbor Drive, San Diego, CA 92103; **Phone:** 619-543-6312; **Board Cert:** Orthopaedic Surgery 2002; Hand Surgery 2002; **Med School:** Univ Colorado 1982; **Resid:** Orthopaedic Surgery, Univ Colo Med Ctr 1987; **Fellow:** Pediatric Orthopaedic Surgery, Chldns Hosp Hlth Ctr 1988; Hand Surgery, Brigham & Womens Hosp 1989; **Fac Appt:** Prof S, UCSD

Atkinson, Robert E MD [HS] - **Spec Exp:** Arthritis; Arthroscopic Surgery; Nerve Disorders/Surgery; **Hospital:** Queen's Med Ctr - Honolulu, Kapiolani Med Ctr @ Pali Momi; **Address:** Queen's Physicians' Office Bldg 1, 1380 Lusitana St, Ste 604, Honolulu, HI 96813; **Phone:** 808-521-8128; **Board Cert:** Orthopaedic Surgery 1985; **Med School:** Jefferson Med Coll 1977; **Resid:** Orthopaedic Surgery, Hosp Special Surgery 1982; **Fellow:** Hand Surgery, Mass Genl Hosp 1983; **Fac Appt:** Clin Prof OrS, Univ Hawaii JA Burns Sch Med

Godzik, Cathleen A MD [HS] - **Spec Exp:** Congenital Hand Deformities; Sports Injuries; Dupuytren's Contracture; Arthritis; **Hospital:** Good Samaritan Hosp - LA, California Hosp Med Ctr; **Address:** 1245 Wilshire Blvd, Ste 611, Los Angeles, CA 90017; **Phone:** 213-482-6100; **Board Cert:** Orthopaedic Surgery 2001; Hand Surgery 2001; **Med School:** NY Med Coll 1981; **Resid:** Surgery, Brown Univ Sch Med 1983; Orthopaedic Surgery, Univ Conn Sch Med 1985; **Fellow:** Hand Surgery, Joseph Boyes Hand Fell-USC 1987

Hanel, Douglas P MD [HS] - **Spec Exp:** Reconstructive Microvascular Surgery; Hand-Congenital Anomaly; Elbow Reconstruction; **Hospital:** Harborview Med Ctr, Seattle Chldns Hosp; **Address:** Harborview Medical Ctr, 325 9th Ave, Fl 6, MS 359798, Seattle, WA 98104-2420; **Phone:** 206-744-3462; **Board Cert:** Orthopaedic Surgery 2007; Hand Surgery 2007; **Med School:** St Louis Univ 1977; **Resid:** Orthopaedic Surgery, St Louis Univ Hosp 1982; **Fellow:** Hand Surgery, Univ Louisville Hosp 1983; Microsurgery, Univ Louisville Hosp 1983; **Fac Appt:** Prof OrS, Univ Wash

Hentz, Vincent R MD [HS] - **Spec Exp:** Hand & Upper Extremity Surgery; Pediatric Hand Surgery; Brachial Plexus Palsy; **Hospital:** Stanford Univ Hosp & Clinics; **Address:** Hand & Upper Extremity Surgery, 450 Broadway St, Pavilion A Fl 2, Redwood City, CA 94063; **Phone:** 650-723-5256; **Board Cert:** Plastic Surgery 1977; **Med School:** Univ Fla Coll Med 1968; **Resid:** Plastic Surgery, Stanford Univ Hosp 1974; **Fellow:** Hand Surgery, Roosevelt Hosp 1975; **Fac Appt:** Prof Emeritus S, Stanford Univ

Meals, Roy A MD [HS] - **Spec Exp:** Hand & Wrist Surgery; **Hospital:** UCLA Ronald Reagan Med Ctr; **Address:** 1030 Gayley Ave, Ste 104, Los Angeles, CA 90024; **Phone:** 310-824-1262; **Board Cert:** Orthopaedic Surgery 1980; Hand Surgery 2010; **Med School:** Vanderbilt Univ 1971; **Resid:** Surgery, Johns Hopkins Hosp 1973; Orthopaedic Surgery, Johns Hopkins Hosp 1978; **Fellow:** Hand Surgery, Mass Genl Hosp 1979; **Fac Appt:** Clin Prof S, UCLA

Slutsky, David J MD [HS] - **Spec Exp:** Preiser's Disease; Keinbocks Disease; Microsurgery; Arthroscopic Surgery; **Hospital:** LAC - Harbor - UCLA Med Ctr, Torrance Memorial Med Ctr; **Address:** The Slutsky Hand & Wrist Inst, 2808 Columbia St, Torrance, CA 90503; **Phone:** 310-618-9922; **Board Cert:** Orthopaedic Surgery 2002; Hand Surgery 2002; **Med School:** Univ Manitoba 1981; **Resid:** Orthopaedic Surgery, Univ Manitoba Med Ctr 1987; **Fellow:** Hand & Microvascular Surgery, Loma Linda Univ Med Ctr 1989; **Fac Appt:** Asst Prof OrS, UCLA

Szabo, Robert M MD [HS] - **Spec Exp:** Peripheral Nerve Surgery; Hand Injuries; Hand & Upper Extremity Tumors; **Hospital:** UC Davis Med Ctr, Mercy General Hosp - Sacramento; **Address:** UC Davis, Dept Orthopaedics, 4860 Y St, Ste 1700, Sacramento, CA 95817; **Phone:** 916-734-3678; **Board Cert:** Orthopaedic Surgery 2009; Hand Surgery 2009; **Med School:** SUNY Buffalo 1977; **Resid:** Surgery, Mt Sinai Hosp 1979; Orthopaedic Surgery, Mt Sinai Hosp 1982; **Fellow:** Hand Surgery, UCSD Med Ctr 1983; Epidemiology, UC Berkeley 1995; **Fac Appt:** Prof OrS, UC Davis

Trumble, Thomas MD [HS] - **Spec Exp:** Nerve Disorders/Surgery; Upper Extremity Trauma; **Hospital:** Overlake Hosp Med Ctr; **Address:** Bellevue Bone & Joint, 1632 116th Ave NE, Ste C, Bellevue, WA 98004; **Phone:** 425-462-9800; **Board Cert:** Orthopaedic Surgery 2009; Hand Surgery 2009; **Med School:** Yale Univ 1979; **Resid:** Orthopaedic Surgery, Yale-New Haven Hosp 1984; **Fellow:** Microvascular Surgery, Duke Univ Med Ctr 1984; Hand Surgery, Mass Genl Hosp 1985; **Fac Appt:** Prof S, Univ Wash

Cleveland Clinic

Every life deserves world class care.

Cleveland Clinic
Upper Extremity Center
9500 Euclid Avenue
Cleveland, OH 44195

clevelandclinic.org/
orthotopdocs

Offering Same-Day Appointments
Call 800.274.2009.

Hand Surgery

Cleveland Clinic's Upper Extremity Center, a center within the Department of Orthopaedic Surgery, provides a centralized, comprehensive diagnostic and treatment center for problems affecting the hand, wrist, elbow and shoulder. *U.S.News & World Report* has consistently ranked the Department of Orthopaedic Surgery among the nation's top 10 orthopaedic programs in the nation since 1992.

Surgery of the Upper Extremity

Our surgeons are experts in diagnosing and providing the operative care for a wide array of upper extremity disorders. Our center offers the newest surgical techniques, such as microsurgery and minimally invasive surgery.

Our Hand and Upper Extremity Center offers cutting-edge services and techniques. Our team focuses on the advancement of treatments and diagnostic insights by valuing education, research and the latest technologies. Our surgeons and specialists treat all disorders of the upper extremity.

Areas our specialists see and treat on a regular basis include the following:

Shoulder: fractures and dislocations, arthritis, chronic instability, replacement, rotator cuff tears, brachial plexus, injuries (occupational, sport or accidental)

Elbow: fractures and dislocations, tennis and golfer's elbow, arthritis, throwing elbow

Wrist: fractures and nonunions, dislocations, instability, carpal tunnel syndrome, tendonitis, arthritis

Hand: fractures and dislocations, trigger finger.

Treatment Guides

Cleveland Clinic has developed comprehensive treatment guides for many diseases and conditions. To download our free treatment guides, visit clevelandclinic.org/treatmentguides.

Online Medical Second Opinion

Cleveland Clinic's My**Consult** Online Medical Second Opinion program securely connects patients to our physician specialists for more than 1,000 life-changing or life-threatening diagnoses all by the click of a mouse. To learn more, log onto eclevelandclinic.org/myconsult or call 800.223.2273, ext. 43223.

Special Assistance for Out-of-State Patients

Cleveland Clinic Global Patient Services offers a complimentary Medical Concierge service for patients who travel from outside of Ohio. Call 800.223.2273, ext. 55580 or email medicalconcierge@ccf.org.

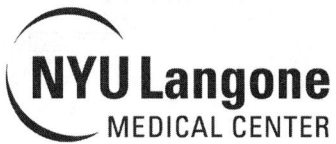

HAND SURGERY

NYU Langone Medical Center's Department of Orthopaedic Surgery provides the full continuum of care for patients with hand and wrist disorders through its specialized Division of Hand Surgery. These include fractures, congenital anomalies, soft tissue and skeletal trauma, degenerative and rheumatoid arthritis, sports-related injuries, vascular disorders, tumors and occupational disorders.

Through its Division of Hand Surgery, HJD specializes in fractures of the wrist and distal radius and reconstructive hand surgery. Hand surgery experts have particular expertise in post-traumatic injuries, arthritis and congenital, neuromuscular and neoplastic conditions. Offering one of the largest hand programs in the United States, the Division's hand specialists provide extensive care for the many problems that affect the upper extremity, including acute traumatic injuries (fractures, dislocations and tendon, nerve and vascular lacerations), post-traumatic and arthritic deformities, acquired problems (nerve compressions and tumors), congenital deformities and neuromuscular disorders such as cerebral palsy. Board-certified and fellowship-trained orthopaedists perform more than 5,000 procedures on adults and children each year.

After surgery, the outpatient Hand Therapy Unit at the Rusk Institute of Rehabilitation Medicine helps surgical patients recover full or partial use of their hands, providing comprehensive rehabilitation for a variety of ailments associated with the hand and upper body. The Unit specializes in fractures, traumatic injuries, tendonitis, sports injuries, work-related injuries, repetitive stress injuries, carpal tunnel syndrome, tendon and nerve repairs and arthritis. It is staffed by expert occupational therapists who specialize in treatment of the hand and upper extremities.

Research within the Hand Service takes place at HJD and focuses on a variety of clinical problems including wrist fractures, non-unions of the scaphoid (bone between the hand and the forearm), Kienbock's disease (the death and fracture of bone tissue due to interruption of blood supply), intercarpal subluxations (incomplete or partial dislocation) and neuropathies (disorders of the nerves) of the upper extremities.

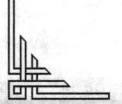
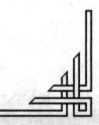

The Best in American Medicine
www.CastleConnolly.com

Hematology &
Medical Oncology

a subspecialty of Internal Medicine

Hematology: An internist with additional training who specializes in diseases of the blood, spleen and lymph glands. This specialist treats conditions such as anemia, clotting disorders, sickle cell disease, hemophilia, leukemia and lymphoma.

Medical Oncology: An internist who specializes in the diagnosis and treatment of all types of cancer and other benign and malignant tumors. This specialist decides on and administers chemotherapy for malignancy, as well as consulting with surgeons and radiotherapists on other treatments for cancer.

Training Required: Three years in internal medicine *plus* additional training and examination for certification in hematology or medical oncology.

HEMATOLOGY

New England

Anderson, Kenneth C MD [Hem] - **Spec Exp:** Multiple Myeloma; Hematologic Malignancies; **Hospital:** Dana-Farber Cancer Inst (page 57), Brigham and Women's Hosp (page 57); **Address:** 450 Brookline Ave, Ste M557, Dana-Farber Cancer Inst, Div Hematology, Boston, MA 02215; **Phone:** 617-632-2144; **Board Cert:** Internal Medicine 1980; **Med School:** Johns Hopkins Univ 1977; **Resid:** Internal Medicine, Johns Hopkins Hosp 1980; **Fellow:** Hematology & Oncology, Dana Farber Cancer Inst 1983; **Fac Appt:** Prof Med, Harvard Med Sch

Ballen, Karen K MD [Hem] - **Spec Exp:** Leukemia; Bone Marrow Transplant; **Hospital:** Mass Genl Hosp; **Address:** Mass General Hospital, Hematology/Oncology, Zero Emerson Pl, Ste 118, Boston, MA 02114; **Phone:** 617-724-1124; **Board Cert:** Internal Medicine 1989; Medical Oncology 2003; Hematology 2004; **Med School:** Dartmouth Med Sch 1986; **Resid:** Internal Medicine, Beth Israel Deaconess Med Ctr 1989; **Fellow:** Hematology & Oncology, Brigham & Women's Hosp 1992; **Fac Appt:** Assoc Prof Med, Harvard Med Sch

Comenzo, Raymond MD [Hem] - **Spec Exp:** Plasma Cell Disorders; Stem Cell Transplant; **Hospital:** Tufts Med Ctr; **Address:** 800 Washington St, Box 826, Boston, MA 02111; **Phone:** 617-636-6454; **Board Cert:** Internal Medicine 1989; Hematology 2004; Blood Banking Transfusion Medicine 1992; **Med School:** Boston Univ 1986; **Resid:** Internal Medicine, Boston City Hosp 1989; **Fellow:** Hematology & Oncology, New Engl Med Ctr 1991

Duffy, Thomas P MD [Hem] - **Spec Exp:** Mast Cell Diseases; Leukemia; Lymphoma; Mast Cell Diseases; **Hospital:** Yale-New Haven Hosp, Yale Med Group; **Address:** Yale Univ, Sect Hematology, 333 Cedar St, rm 403-WWW, Box 208021, New Haven, CT 06520-8021; **Phone:** 203-785-4744; **Board Cert:** Internal Medicine 1972; Hematology 1974; **Med School:** Johns Hopkins Univ 1962; **Resid:** Internal Medicine, Johns Hopkins Hosp 1965; **Fellow:** Hematology, Johns Hopkins Hosp 1970; **Fac Appt:** Prof Med, Yale Univ

Klingemann, Hans-Georg MD/PhD [Hem] - **Spec Exp:** Bone Marrow Transplant; Stem Cell Transplant; **Hospital:** Tufts Med Ctr; **Address:** 800 Washington St, Box 245, Boston, MA 02111; **Phone:** 617-636-6227; **Med School:** Germany 1976; **Resid:** Internal Medicine, Univ Wurzburg Med Sch 1979; **Fellow:** Hematology & Oncology, Fred Hutchinson Cancer Rsch Ctr 1986; **Fac Appt:** Prof Med, Tufts Univ

Marks, Peter W MD/PhD [Hem] - **Spec Exp:** Leukemia; Platelet Disorders; Bleeding/Coagulation Disorders; Hemophilia; **Hospital:** Yale-New Haven Hosp, Yale Med Group; **Address:** Yale Hematology, 333 Cedar St, Box 208302, New Haven, CT 06520; **Phone:** 203-200-4363; **Board Cert:** Internal Medicine 2004; Hematology 2007; Medical Oncology 2007; **Med School:** NYU Sch Med 1991; **Resid:** Internal Medicine, Brigham & Women's Hosp 1994; **Fellow:** Hematology & Oncology, Brigham & Women's Hosp 1996; **Fac Appt:** Assoc Prof Med, Yale Univ

Meehan, Kenneth MD [Hem] - **Spec Exp:** Bone Marrow Transplant; **Hospital:** Dartmouth - Hitchcock Med Ctr; **Address:** Norris Cotton Cancer Ctr, Dartmouth-Hitchcock Med Ctr, 1 Medical Center Drive, Lebanon, NH 03756; **Phone:** 603-650-4628; **Board Cert:** Internal Medicine 1989; Hematology 2004; **Med School:** Georgetown Univ 1986; **Resid:** Internal Medicine, Georgetown Univ 1989; **Fellow:** Hematology & Oncology, Dartmouth-Hitchcock Med Ctr 1992; **Fac Appt:** Assoc Prof Med, Dartmouth Med Sch

Miller, Kenneth B MD [Hem] - **Spec Exp:** Bone Marrow Transplant; Leukemia; Myelodysplastic Syndromes; **Hospital:** Tufts Med Ctr; **Address:** Tufts Med Ctr, Dept Medicine, 800 Washington St, Box 245, Boston, MA 02111; **Phone:** 617-636-2600; **Board Cert:** Internal Medicine 1976; Hematology 1980; **Med School:** NY Med Coll 1972; **Resid:** Internal Medicine, NYU Med Ctr/VA Hosp 1976; Internal Medicine, NYU Med Ctr 1976; **Fellow:** Hematology, New England Med Ctr 1979; **Fac Appt:** Prof Med, Tufts Univ

Richardson, Paul G MD [Hem] - **Spec Exp:** Multiple Myeloma; **Hospital:** Dana-Farber Cancer Inst (page 57), Brigham and Women's Hosp (page 57); **Address:** Dana Farber Cancer Inst, 44 Binney St, Boston, MA 02115; **Phone:** 617-632-2127; **Board Cert:** Hematology 1999; **Med School:** England, UK 1986; **Resid:** Internal Medicine, Baystate Med Ctr 1994; **Fellow:** Medical Oncology, Dana Farber Cancer Inst 1995; Hematology, Beth Israel Deaconess Med Ctr 1997; **Fac Appt:** Assoc Prof Med, Harvard Med Sch

Schiffman, Fred J MD [Hem] - **Spec Exp:** Hematologic Malignancies; Anemia-Cancer Related; Bleeding/Coagulation Disorders; **Hospital:** Miriam Hosp; **Address:** Comp Cancer Ctr at Miriam Hospital, 164 Summit Ave, Fain-3, Providence, RI 02906; **Phone:** 401-793-2920; **Board Cert:** Internal Medicine 1979; Hematology 1982; Medical Oncology 1987; **Med School:** NYU Sch Med 1973; **Resid:** Internal Medicine, Yale-New Haven Hosp 1975; Internal Medicine, Yale-New Haven Hosp 1979; **Fellow:** Hematology, Yale-New Haven Hosp 1981; **Fac Appt:** Prof Med, Brown Univ

Spitzer, Thomas R MD [Hem] - **Spec Exp:** Bone Marrow Transplant; Leukemia; **Hospital:** Mass Genl Hosp; **Address:** Mass Genl Hosp-Bone Marrow Tranplant Prog, 0 Emerson Pl, Ste 118, Boston, MA 02114; **Phone:** 617-724-1124; **Board Cert:** Internal Medicine 1977; Medical Oncology 1983; Hematology 1984; **Med School:** Univ Rochester 1974; **Resid:** Internal Medicine, NYew York Hosp-Cornell Med Ctr 1977; Internal Medicine, Mem Sloan Kettering Cancer Ctr 1977; **Fellow:** Hematology & Oncology, Case West Res Univ 1983; **Fac Appt:** Prof Med, Harvard Med Sch

Stone, Richard M MD [Hem] - **Spec Exp:** Leukemia; **Hospital:** Dana-Farber Cancer Inst (page 57), Brigham and Women's Hosp (page 57); **Address:** Dana Farber Cancer Inst, 44 Binney St, Mayer 1B-17, Boston, MA 02115-6084; **Phone:** 617-632-2214; **Board Cert:** Internal Medicine 1984; Medical Oncology 2008; Hematology 1988; **Med School:** Harvard Med Sch 1981; **Resid:** Internal Medicine, Brigham & Womens Hosp 1984; **Fellow:** Medical Oncology, Dana Farber Cancer Inst 1987; **Fac Appt:** Prof Med, Harvard Med Sch

Mid Atlantic

Abrams, Charles S MD [Hem] - **Spec Exp:** Bleeding/Coagulation Disorders; Thrombotic Disorders; **Hospital:** Hosp Univ Penn - UPHS (page 68); **Address:** Univ Penn, Dept Hem/Onc, Perelman Ctr for Advanced Medicine, 3400 Civic Ctr Blvd Fl 2-West, Philadelphia, PA 19104; **Phone:** 215-615-5858; **Board Cert:** Internal Medicine 1987; Medical Oncology 1989; Hematology 2005; **Med School:** Yale Univ 1984; **Resid:** Internal Medicine, Hosp Univ Penn 1987; **Fellow:** Hematology & Oncology, Hosp Univ Penn 1988; **Fac Appt:** Prof Med, Univ Pennsylvania

Allen, Steven Lee MD [Hem] - **Spec Exp:** Bleeding/Coagulation Disorders; Leukemia & Lymphoma; Multiple Myeloma; Gaucher Disease; **Hospital:** N Shore Univ Hosp; **Address:** 450 Lakeville Rd, Lake Success, NY 11042; **Phone:** 516-734-8959; **Board Cert:** Internal Medicine 1980; Hematology 1982; Medical Oncology 1983; **Med School:** Johns Hopkins Univ 1977; **Resid:** Internal Medicine, NY Hosp-Cornell 1980; **Fellow:** Hematology & Oncology, NY Hosp-Cornell 1983; **Fac Appt:** Prof Med, Albert Einstein Coll Med

Hematology

Baer, Maria R MD [Hem] - **Spec Exp:** Leukemia; Myelodysplastic Syndromes; Myeloproliferative Disorders; **Hospital:** Univ of MD Med Ctr; **Address:** Univ Maryland, Greenebaum Cancer Ctr, 22 S Greene St, rm S9D08, Baltimore, MD 21201; **Phone:** 410-328-7904; **Board Cert:** Internal Medicine 1983; Hematology 1984; **Med School:** Johns Hopkins Univ 1979; **Resid:** Internal Medicine, Vanderbilt Univ Hosp 1982; **Fellow:** Hematology, Vanderbilt Univ Hosp 1984; **Fac Appt:** Prof Med, Univ MD Sch Med

Brodsky, Robert A MD [Hem] - **Spec Exp:** Hematologic Malignancies; Autoimmune Disease; Graft vs Host Disease; **Hospital:** Johns Hopkins Hosp (page 61); **Address:** 720 Rutland Ave, Ross Bldg - rm 1025, Baltimore, MD 21205; **Phone:** 410-955-3142; **Board Cert:** Internal Medicine 2002; Hematology 2006; **Med School:** Hahnemann Univ 1989; **Resid:** Internal Medicine, Vanderbilt Univ 1991; **Fellow:** Hematology, Vanderbilt Univ Hosp 1994; Medical Oncology, Johns Hopkins Hosp 1997; **Fac Appt:** Prof Med, Johns Hopkins Univ

Cheson, Bruce D MD [Hem] - **Spec Exp:** Leukemia; Hematologic Malignancies; **Hospital:** Georgetown Univ Hosp; **Address:** GUMC - Lombardi Cancer Ctr, 3800 Reservoir Rd NW, Podium B, Washington, DC 20007; **Phone:** 202-444-7932; **Board Cert:** Internal Medicine 1974; Hematology 1976; **Med School:** Tufts Univ 1971; **Resid:** Internal Medicine, Univ Virginia Hosp 1974; **Fellow:** Hematology, New England Med Ctr Hosp 1976

Coller, Barry MD [Hem] - **Spec Exp:** Glanzmann's Thrombasthenia; Bleeding/Coagulation Disorders; **Hospital:** Rockefeller Univ, Mount Sinai Med Ctr (page 63); **Address:** Rockefeller Univ, 1230 York Ave, New York, NY 10065; **Phone:** 212-327-7490; **Board Cert:** Internal Medicine 1973; Hematology 1975; **Med School:** NYU Sch Med 1970; **Resid:** Internal Medicine, Bellevue Hosp 1972; **Fellow:** Hematology, Natl Inst Hlth Clin Ctr 1974; **Fac Appt:** Clin Prof Med, Mount Sinai Sch Med

Dang, Chi V MD/PhD [Hem] - **Spec Exp:** Anemia-Aplastic; Bone Marrow Failure Disorders; Myeloproliferative Disorders; **Hospital:** Johns Hopkins Hosp (page 61); **Address:** 1830 E Monument St, Ste 416, Baltimore, MD 21287; **Phone:** 410-614-0167; **Board Cert:** Internal Medicine 1985; Medical Oncology 1987; **Med School:** Johns Hopkins Univ 1982; **Resid:** Internal Medicine, Johns Hopkins Hosp 1985; **Fellow:** Medical Oncology, UCSF Med Ctr 1987; **Fac Appt:** Prof Med, Johns Hopkins Univ

Diuguid, David L MD [Hem] - **Spec Exp:** Bleeding/Coagulation Disorders; **Hospital:** NY-Presby/Columbia Univ Med Ctr, NY (page 65); **Address:** 161 Ft Washington Ave, Irving 10, New York, NY 10032; **Phone:** 212-305-0527; **Board Cert:** Internal Medicine 1982; Hematology 1986; Medical Oncology 1985; **Med School:** Cornell Univ-Weill Med Coll 1979; **Resid:** Internal Medicine, Boston Univ Med Ctr 1983; **Fellow:** Hematology & Oncology, New England Med Ctr 1986; **Fac Appt:** Assoc Prof Med, Columbia P&S

Filicko-OHara, Joanne E MD [Hem] - **Spec Exp:** Hematologic Malignancies; Leukemia & Lymphoma; **Hospital:** Thomas Jefferson Univ Hosp; **Address:** 925 Chestnut St, Ste 320A, Phildelphia, PA 19107; **Phone:** 215-955-8874; **Board Cert:** Hematology 2009; Medical Oncology 2000; **Med School:** Hahnemann Univ 1992; **Resid:** Internal Medicine, Thomas Jefferson Univ Hosp 1995; **Fellow:** Hematology & Oncology, Thomas Jefferson Univ Hosp 1995

Fruchtman, Steven M MD [Hem] - **Spec Exp:** Myeloproliferative Disorders; Polycythemia Rubra Vera; **Address:** 1111 Park Ave, New York, NY 10128; **Phone:** 212-427-7700; **Board Cert:** Internal Medicine 1980; Hematology 1984; **Med School:** NY Med Coll 1977; **Resid:** Internal Medicine, Univ Hosp 1981; **Fellow:** Hematology, Mount Sinai Med Ctr 1984; Hematology, Meml Sloan Kettering Cancer Ctr 1985; **Fac Appt:** Assoc Prof Med, NY Med Coll

Goldberg, Jack MD [Hem] - **Spec Exp:** Leukemia; Lymphoma; Multiple Myeloma; Bone Marrow Transplant; **Hospital:** Penn Presby Med Ctr - UPHS (page 68), Hosp Univ Penn - UPHS (page 68); **Address:** 51 N 39th St MAB Bldg Fl 1 - Ste 103A, Philadelphia, PA 19104; **Phone:** 215-662-9801; **Board Cert:** Internal Medicine 1976; Hematology 1980; Medical Oncology 1989; **Med School:** SUNY Upstate Med Univ 1973; **Resid:** Internal Medicine, Boston Univ Hosp 1975; **Fellow:** Hematology & Oncology, SUNY Syracuse Med Ctr 1977; **Fac Appt:** Clin Prof Med, Univ Pennsylvania

Isola, Luis M MD [Hem] - **Spec Exp:** Bone Marrow Transplant; Stem Cell Transplant; Myelodysplastic Syndromes; Anemia; **Hospital:** Mount Sinai Med Ctr (page 63); **Address:** Mount Sinai Med Ctr, 19 E 98th St, Ste 3D, New York, NY 10029; **Phone:** 212-241-6021; **Board Cert:** Internal Medicine 1986; Hematology 1988; **Med School:** Argentina 1979; **Resid:** Internal Medicine, Ctr for Med Education 1983; **Fellow:** Hematology, Mt Sinai Med Ctr 1985; **Fac Appt:** Assoc Prof Med, Mount Sinai Sch Med

Kempin, Sanford J MD [Hem] - **Spec Exp:** Bleeding/Coagulation Disorders; Leukemia; Lymphoma; Thrombotic Disorders; **Hospital:** Beth Israel Med Ctr - Petrie Division (page 55); **Address:** Beth Israel Comprehensive Cancer Ctr, W Side Campus, Dept Med Oncology, 325 W 15th St, New York, NY 10011; **Phone:** 212-604-6010; **Board Cert:** Internal Medicine 1976; Medical Oncology 1977; Hematology 1978; **Med School:** Belgium 1971; **Resid:** Internal Medicine, Lemuel Shattuck Hosp 1972; **Fellow:** Hematology, St Jude Chldns Hosp 1975; Medical Oncology, Meml Sloan Kettering Cancer Ctr 1976; **Fac Appt:** Asst Prof Med, NY Med Coll

Kessler, Craig M MD [Hem] - **Spec Exp:** Bleeding/Coagulation Disorders; Hemophilia; Hematologic Malignancies; **Hospital:** Georgetown Univ Hosp; **Address:** GUMC, Lombardi Cancer Ctr, 3800 Reservoir Rd NW, Washington, DC 20007; **Phone:** 202-444-8676; **Board Cert:** Internal Medicine 1976; Hematology 1980; **Med School:** Tulane Univ 1973; **Resid:** Internal Medicine, Ochsner Fdn Hosp 1976; **Fellow:** Hematology, Johns Hopkins Hosp 1978; **Fac Appt:** Prof Med, Georgetown Univ

Mangan, Kenneth F MD [Hem] - **Spec Exp:** Bone Marrow Transplant; Hematologic Malignancies; Anemia-Aplastic; Paroxysmal Nocturnal Hemoglobinuria; **Hospital:** Temple Univ Hosp, Jeanes Hosp; **Address:** Temple BMT Program, Friends Hall Physicians Bldg, 7604 Central Ave, Lower Level, Philadelphia, PA 19111-2499; **Phone:** 215-214-3129; **Board Cert:** Internal Medicine 1976; Hematology 1978; **Med School:** Geo Wash Univ 1973; **Resid:** Internal Medicine, G Washington Univ Hosps 1976; **Fellow:** Hematology, Tufts-New England Med Ctr 1977; **Fac Appt:** Prof Med, Temple Univ

Marks, Stanley M MD [Hem] - **Spec Exp:** Leukemia; Lymphoma; Multiple Myeloma; **Hospital:** UPMC Shadyside; **Address:** UPMC- Hillman Cancer Ctr, 5115 Centre Ave Fl 3, Pittsburgh, PA 15232; **Phone:** 412-235-1020; **Board Cert:** Internal Medicine 1976; Hematology 1978; **Med School:** Univ Pittsburgh 1973; **Resid:** Internal Medicine, Presby Univ Hosp 1976; **Fellow:** Hematology & Oncology, Peter Bent Brigham Hosp 1978; **Fac Appt:** Clin Prof Med, Univ Pittsburgh

Maslak, Peter G MD [Hem] - **Spec Exp:** Leukemia; Stem Cell Transplant; Myelodysplastic Syndromes; Clinical Trials; **Hospital:** Meml Sloan-Kettering Cancer Ctr; **Address:** 1275 York Avenue, New York, NY 10065; **Phone:** 800-525-2225; **Board Cert:** Internal Medicine 1987; Hematology 2000; Medical Oncology 1989; **Med School:** Mount Sinai Sch Med 1984; **Resid:** Internal Medicine, Univ Michigan Med Ctr 1987; **Fellow:** Hematology & Oncology, Meml Sloan Kettering Cancer Ctr 1990

Hematology

Mears, John Gregory MD [Hem] - **Spec Exp:** Lymphoma; Leukemia; Multiple Myeloma; Breast Cancer; **Hospital:** NY-Presby/Columbia Univ Med Ctr, NY (page 65); **Address:** 161 Ft Washington Ave, Ste 923, New York, NY 10032; **Phone:** 212-305-3506; **Board Cert:** Internal Medicine 1976; Hematology 1978; **Med School:** Columbia P&S 1973; **Resid:** Internal Medicine, Boston Univ Med Ctr 1975; **Fellow:** Hematology & Oncology, Columbia-Presby Med Ctr 1978; **Fac Appt:** Clin Prof Med, Columbia P&S

Millenson, Michael M MD [Hem] - **Spec Exp:** Leukemia & Lymphoma; Thromboembolic Disorders; Hematologic Malignancies; **Hospital:** Fox Chase Cancer Ctr (page 58); **Address:** Fox Chase Cancer Center, 333 Cottman Ave, Philadelphia, PA 19111; **Phone:** 215-728-2600; **Board Cert:** Internal Medicine 1987; Hematology 2000; Medical Oncology 2000; **Med School:** Temple Univ 1984; **Resid:** Internal Medicine, Temple Univ Hosp 1987; **Fellow:** Hematology & Oncology, Beth Israel Hosp 1991

Nimer, Stephen D MD [Hem] - **Spec Exp:** Bone Marrow Transplant; Myelodysplastic Syndromes; Leukemia; Stem Cell Transplant; **Hospital:** Meml Sloan-Kettering Cancer Ctr; **Address:** 1275 York Ave, New York, NY 10065; **Phone:** 800-525-2225; **Board Cert:** Internal Medicine 1982; Hematology 1986; Medical Oncology 1985; **Med School:** Univ Chicago-Pritzker Sch Med 1979; **Resid:** Internal Medicine, UCLA Med Ctr 1982; **Fellow:** Hematology & Oncology, UCLA Med Ctr 1986; **Fac Appt:** Prof Med, Cornell Univ-Weill Med Coll

Philipp, Claire S MD [Hem] - **Spec Exp:** Bleeding/Coagulation Disorders; **Hospital:** Robert Wood Johnson Univ Hosp - New Brunswick; **Address:** Robert Wood Johnson Med School, 125 Paterson St, CAB5231, New Brunswick, NJ 08901; **Phone:** 732-235-6531; **Board Cert:** Internal Medicine 1981; Hematology 1984; Medical Oncology 1985; **Med School:** Brown Univ 1978; **Resid:** Internal Medicine, Beth Israel Med Ctr 1981; **Fellow:** Hematology & Oncology, NYU Med Ctr 1984; **Fac Appt:** Prof Med

Porter, David L MD [Hem] - **Spec Exp:** Leukemia; Bone Marrow Transplant; Lymphoma; Gene Therapy; **Hospital:** Hosp Univ Penn - UPHS (page 68); **Address:** Perelman Ctr for Advanced Med Fl 2, 3400 Civic Center Blvd, Philadelphia, PA 19104; **Phone:** 215-615-5858; **Board Cert:** Hematology 2006; **Med School:** Brown Univ 1987; **Resid:** Internal Medicine, Univ Hosp 1990; **Fellow:** Hematology & Oncology, Brigham & Womens Hosp 1992; **Fac Appt:** Prof Med, Univ Pennsylvania

Rai, Kanti R MD [Hem] - **Spec Exp:** Leukemia; Lymphoma; Multiple Myeloma; **Hospital:** Long Island Jewish Med Ctr; **Address:** 410 Lakeville Rd, Ste 212, Long Island Jewish Med Ctr, Div of Hem-Onc, New Hyde Park, NY 10042; **Phone:** 718-470-4050; **Board Cert:** Pediatrics 1960; **Med School:** India 1955; **Resid:** Pediatrics, Lincoln Hosp 1958; Pediatrics, North Shore Univ Hosp 1959; **Fellow:** Hematology, LI Jewish Med Ctr 1960; **Fac Appt:** Prof Med, Albert Einstein Coll Med

Rao, A Koneti MD [Hem] - **Spec Exp:** Bleeding/Coagulation Disorders; Thrombotic Disorders; **Hospital:** Temple Univ Hosp; **Address:** Temple Univ Hosp, Div Hematology, Old Med Sch Bldg, 3rd Floor, 3400 N Broad St, Philadelphia, PA 19140; **Phone:** 215-707-4684; **Board Cert:** Internal Medicine 1977; Hematology 1980; **Med School:** India 1973; **Resid:** Internal Medicine, Thos Jefferson Univ Hosp 1977; **Fellow:** Hematology & Oncology, Temple Univ Hosp 1978; Hematology, Thos Jefferson Univ Hosp 1979; **Fac Appt:** Prof Med, Temple Univ

Raphael, Bruce MD [Hem] - **Spec Exp:** Lymphoma; Leukemia; Multiple Myeloma; **Hospital:** NYU Langone Med Ctr (page 66), NY Downtown Hosp; **Address:** 160 E 34th Street Ave Fl 7, NYU Clinical Cancer Ctr, New York, NY 10016-6402; **Phone:** 212-731-5185; **Board Cert:** Internal Medicine 1978; Hematology 1980; Medical Oncology 1981; **Med School:** McGill Univ 1975; **Resid:** Internal Medicine, Jewish Genl Hosp 1977; **Fellow:** Medical Oncology, Meml Sloan Kettering Cancer Ctr 1978; Hematology, NYU Med Ctr 1980; **Fac Appt:** Assoc Prof Med, NYU Sch Med

Rapoport, Aaron P MD [Hem] - **Spec Exp:** Leukemia; Lymphoma; Multiple Myeloma; **Hospital:** Univ of MD Med Ctr; **Address:** University of MD Cancer Center, 22 S Greene St, Ste N9E12, Baltimore, MD 21201; **Phone:** 410-328-1230; **Board Cert:** Internal Medicine 1989; Hematology 2002; **Med School:** Harvard Med Sch 1986; **Resid:** Internal Medicine, Strong Meml Hosp 1989; **Fellow:** Hematology, Strong Meml Hosp 1989; **Fac Appt:** Prof Med, Univ MD Sch Med

Roodman, G David MD [Hem] - **Spec Exp:** Multiple Myeloma; **Hospital:** UPMC Shadyside, VA Pittsburgh Hlth Care Sys-Univ Dr; **Address:** VA Pittsburgh Healthcare System, R&D 151-U, rm 2E113, University Drive C, Pittsburgh, PA 15240; **Phone:** 412-692-4724; **Board Cert:** Internal Medicine 1978; Hematology 1980; **Med School:** Univ KY Coll Med 1973; **Resid:** Internal Medicine, Univ Minnesota Hosp 1978; **Fellow:** Hematology, Univ Minnesota Hosp 1980; **Fac Appt:** Prof Med, Univ Pittsburgh

Rowley, Scott D MD [Hem] - **Spec Exp:** Stem Cell Transplant; Bone Marrow Transplant; Graft vs Host Disease; **Hospital:** Hackensack Univ Med Ctr; **Address:** 360 Essex St, Ste 303, Hackensack, NJ 07601; **Phone:** 201-336-8297 x8291; **Board Cert:** Internal Medicine 1981; Medical Oncology 1983; Hematology 1984; **Med School:** Univ Mass Sch Med 1978; **Resid:** Internal Medicine, Rhode Island Hosp 1981; **Fellow:** Hematology & Oncology, Rhode Island Hosp 1984; **Fac Appt:** Assoc Prof Med, UMDNJ-NJ Med Sch, Newark

Savage, David G MD [Hem] - **Spec Exp:** Stem Cell Transplant; Multiple Myeloma; Lymphoma; **Hospital:** NY-Presby/Columbia Univ Med Ctr, NY (page 65); **Address:** 177 Fort Washington Ave, Millstein Bldg Fl 6 - rm 435, New York, NY 10032; **Phone:** 212-305-9783; **Board Cert:** Internal Medicine 1977; Hematology 1982; Medical Oncology 1985; **Med School:** Columbia P&S 1974; **Resid:** Internal Medicine, Harlem Hosp/Columbia Presby Med Ctr 1977; **Fellow:** Hematology & Oncology, Harlem Hosp/Columbia Presby Med Ctr 1979; **Fac Appt:** Assoc Prof Med, Columbia P&S

Schuster, Michael W MD [Hem] - **Spec Exp:** Bone Marrow Transplant; **Hospital:** Stony Brook Univ Med Ctr; **Address:** Stony Brook University, SUNY-7099, 100 Nichols Rd, Stony Brook, NY 11794-7909; **Phone:** 631-444-3577; **Board Cert:** Internal Medicine 1984; Hematology 1986; **Med School:** Dartmouth Med Sch 1980; **Resid:** Internal Medicine, New Eng Deaconess Hosp 1983; **Fellow:** Hematology & Oncology, Beth Israel Med Ctr 1987; **Fac Appt:** Assoc Prof Med, Cornell Univ-Weill Med Coll

Schuster, Stephen J MD [Hem] - **Spec Exp:** Lymphoma; Bone Marrow Transplant; **Hospital:** Hosp Univ Penn - UPHS (page 68); **Address:** Abramson Cancer Ctr, Perelman Ctr, West Pavilion Fl 2, 3400 Civic Ctr Blvd, Philadelphia, PA 19104; **Phone:** 215-614-1846; **Board Cert:** Internal Medicine 1984; Hematology 1986; Medical Oncology 1989; **Med School:** Jefferson Med Coll 1981; **Resid:** Internal Medicine, Pennsylvania Hosp 1984; **Fellow:** Hematology & Oncology, Thos Jefferson Univ Hosp 1986; **Fac Appt:** Assoc Prof Med, Univ Pennsylvania

Slease, Robert B MD [Hem] - **Spec Exp:** Hematologic Malignancies; Hodgkin's Disease; Stem Cell Transplant; Clinical Trials; **Hospital:** Wilmington Hosp; **Address:** Cristiana Care Hlth Svs, Div Hematology, Medical Pavilion, 4701 Ogletown-Stanton Rd, Ste 4200, Newark, DE 19713; **Phone:** 302-737-7700; **Board Cert:** Internal Medicine 1975; Hematology 1978; **Med School:** Univ Kansas 1972; **Resid:** Internal Medicine, Natl Naval Med Ctr 1975; **Fellow:** Hematology, Natl Naval Med Ctr 1977; **Fac Appt:** Clin Prof Med, Jefferson Med Coll

Spivak, Jerry L MD [Hem] - **Spec Exp:** Myeloproliferative Disorders; Polycythemia Rubra Vera; Leukemia; Anemia; **Hospital:** Johns Hopkins Hosp (page 61); **Address:** 720 Rutland Ave Bldg Ross - Ste 1025, Baltimore, MD 21205; **Phone:** 410-955-3142; **Board Cert:** Internal Medicine 1971; Hematology 1974; **Med School:** Cornell Univ-Weill Med Coll 1964; **Resid:** Internal Medicine, Johns Hopkins Hosp 1966; Internal Medicine, Johns Hopkins Hosp 1972; **Fellow:** Hematology, Natl Cancer Inst 1968; Hematology, Johns Hopkins Hosp 1971; **Fac Appt:** Prof Med, Johns Hopkins Univ

Hematology

Strair, Roger MD/PhD [Hem] - **Spec Exp:** Leukemia; Lymphoma; Bone Marrow Transplant; Multiple Myeloma; **Hospital:** Robert Wood Johnson Univ Hosp - New Brunswick; **Address:** Cancer Inst of NJ, 195 Little Albany St, New Brunswick, NJ 08903; **Phone:** 732-235-6044; **Board Cert:** Internal Medicine 1984; Hematology 1986; Medical Oncology 1987; **Med School:** Albert Einstein Coll Med 1981; **Resid:** Internal Medicine, Brigham & Women's Hosp 1984; **Fellow:** Hematology & Oncology, Brigham & Women's Hosp 1988; **Fac Appt:** Assoc Prof Med, UMDNJ-RW Johnson Med Sch

Streiff, Michael B MD [Hem] - **Spec Exp:** Bleeding Coagulation Disorders; Polycythemia Rubra Vera; Clinical Trials; **Hospital:** Johns Hopkins Hosp (page 61); **Address:** Division of Hematology, 1830 E Monument St, Ste 7300, Baltimore, MD 21205; **Phone:** 410-614-0727; **Board Cert:** Internal Medicine 2002; Hematology 2004; Medical Oncology 2005; **Med School:** Johns Hopkins Univ 1988; **Resid:** Internal Medicine, Shands Hosp-Univ Fla Coll Med 1991; **Fellow:** Hematology & Oncology, Johns Hopkins Univ Hosp 1994; **Fac Appt:** Assoc Prof Med, Johns Hopkins Univ

Tallman, Martin S MD [Hem] - **Spec Exp:** Bone Marrow Transplant; Leukemia; Hairy Cell Leukemia; **Hospital:** Meml Sloan-Kettering Cancer Ctr; **Address:** 1275 York Ave, Box 380, Ste 21-100, New York, NY 10065; **Phone:** 212-639-3842; **Board Cert:** Internal Medicine 1983; Medical Oncology 1987; Hematology 1988; **Med School:** Ros Franklin Univ/Chicago Med Sch 1980; **Resid:** Internal Medicine, Evanston Hosp 1983; **Fellow:** Medical Oncology, Fred Hutchinson Cancer Ctr 1987; **Fac Appt:** Prof Med, Cornell Univ-Weill Med Coll

Wisch, Nathaniel MD [Hem] - **Spec Exp:** Lymphoma; Breast Cancer; Leukemia; Anemia-Cancer Related; **Hospital:** Lenox Hill Hosp, Mount Sinai Med Ctr (page 63); **Address:** 12 E 86th St, New York, NY 10028-0506; **Phone:** 212-861-6660; **Board Cert:** Internal Medicine 1965; Hematology 1972; Medical Oncology 1977; **Med School:** Northwestern Univ 1958; **Resid:** Internal Medicine, VA Hosp 1960; Internal Medicine, Montefiore Hosp 1961; **Fellow:** Hematology, Mount Sinai Hosp 1962; **Fac Appt:** Clin Prof Med, Mount Sinai Sch Med

Yanovich, Saul MD [Hem] - **Spec Exp:** Bone Marrow Transplant; **Hospital:** Univ of MD Med Ctr; **Address:** Greenebaum Cancer Center, 22 S Greene St, Ste N9E12, Baltimore, MD 21201; **Phone:** 410-328-1230; **Board Cert:** Internal Medicine 1980; Medical Oncology 1981; Hematology 1976; **Med School:** Colombia 1970; **Resid:** Internal Medicine, Univ Miami-Jackson Meml Hosp 1974; Hematology, Univ Miami-Jackson Meml Hosp 1976; **Fellow:** Oncology, Dana Farber Canc Ctr 1978; **Fac Appt:** Prof Med, Univ MD Sch Med

Southeast

Adams-Graves, Patricia MD [Hem] - **Spec Exp:** Sickle Cell Disease; **Hospital:** Regional Med Ctr - Memphis; **Address:** 880 Madison Ave Fl 5, Sickle Cell Center, Memphis, TN 38103; **Phone:** 901-545-8535; **Board Cert:** Internal Medicine 1989; **Med School:** Univ Louisville Sch Med 1986; **Resid:** Internal Medicine, Univ Louisville Affil Hosp 1989; **Fellow:** Hematology & Oncology, Univ Tennessee Hlth Science Ctr 1993; **Fac Appt:** Prof Med, Univ Tenn Coll Med

Bigelow, Carolyn L MD [Hem] - **Spec Exp:** Bone Marrow Transplant; Sickle Cell Disease; Leukemia; **Hospital:** Univ Mississippi Med Ctr; **Address:** Univ Mississippi Med Ctr-Div Hematology, 2500 N State St, Jackson, MS 39216; **Phone:** 601-984-5615; **Board Cert:** Internal Medicine 1982; Hematology 1988; **Med School:** Univ Miss 1979; **Resid:** Internal Medicine, Univ Mississippi Med Ctr 1982; **Fellow:** Hematology & Oncology, Univ Washington Med Ctr 1987; **Fac Appt:** Prof Med, Univ Miss

Djulbegovic, Benjamin MD/PhD [Hem] - **Spec Exp:** Multiple Myeloma; Lymphoma; Myelo-proliferative Disorders; Clinical Trials; **Hospital:** H Lee Moffitt Cancer Ctr & Research Inst (page 59), Tampa Genl Hosp; **Address:** 12901 Bruce B Downs Blvd, MDC 27, Tampa, FL 33612; **Phone:** 813-396-9178; **Board Cert:** Internal Medicine 2002; Hematology 2004; **Med School:** Bosnia 1976; **Resid:** Internal Medicine, Univ Med Ctr 1983; Internal Medicine, Univ Louisville Med Ctr 1988; **Fellow:** Univ Manchester 1985; Hematology & Oncology, Univ Louisville 1990; **Fac Appt:** Prof Med, Univ S Fla Coll Med

Files, Joe C MD [Hem] - **Spec Exp:** Bone Marrow Transplant; Stem Cell Transplant; Leukemia; **Hospital:** Univ Mississippi Med Ctr; **Address:** Univ Miss Med Ctr-Div Hematology, 2500 N State St, Jackson, MS 39216; **Phone:** 601-984-5615; **Board Cert:** Internal Medicine 1976; Hematology 1980; **Med School:** Univ Miss 1972; **Resid:** Internal Medicine, Univ Miss Med Ctr 1976; **Fellow:** Hematology, Univ Wash Sch Med 1979; **Fac Appt:** Prof Med, Univ Miss

Greer, John P MD [Hem] - **Spec Exp:** Leukemia & Lymphoma; Myelodysplastic Syndromes; Stem Cell Transplant; Clinical Trials; **Hospital:** Vanderbilt Univ Med Ctr (page 76); **Address:** 3927 The Vanderbilt Clinic, 1301 Medical Center Drive, Nashville, TN 37232; **Phone:** 615-936-8422; **Board Cert:** Pediatrics 1985; Internal Medicine 1979; Hematology 1984; Medical Oncology 1985; **Med School:** Vanderbilt Univ 1976; **Resid:** Internal Medicine, Tulane Univ Med Ctr 1979; Pediatrics, Med Coll Virginia 1981; **Fellow:** Hematology & Oncology, Vanderbilt Univ Med Ctr 1984; **Fac Appt:** Prof Med, Vanderbilt Univ

Komrokji, Rami S MD [Hem] - **Spec Exp:** Myelodysplastic Syndromes; Leukemia-Myeloid; Hodgkin's Disease; Clinical Trials; **Hospital:** H Lee Moffitt Cancer Ctr & Research Inst (page 59); **Address:** H Lee Moffitt Canc Ctr & Rsch Inst, 12902 Magnolia Drive, Tampa, FL 33612; **Phone:** 813-745-8986; **Board Cert:** Internal Medicine 2001; Hematology 2004; Medical Oncology 2004; **Med School:** Jordan 1996; **Resid:** Internal Medicine, Case Western Univ Affil Hosp 2001; **Fellow:** Hematology, Strong Meml Hosp 2004; **Fac Appt:** Assoc Prof

Laughlin, Mary J MD [Hem] - **Spec Exp:** Bone Marrow Transplant; Lymphoma; **Hospital:** Univ of Virginia Health Sys; **Address:** 1240 Lee St, Charlottesville, VA 22908; **Phone:** 434-982-6406; **Board Cert:** Internal Medicine 2003; Hematology 2004; **Med School:** SUNY Buffalo 1988; **Resid:** Internal Medicine, Duke Univ Med Ctr 1991; **Fellow:** Hematology & Oncology, Duke Univ Med Ctr 1992; Bone Marrow Transplant, Rosewell Park Cancer Inst 1994; **Fac Appt:** Assoc Prof Med, Case West Res Univ

Ortel, Thomas L MD/PhD [Hem] - **Spec Exp:** Bleeding/Coagulation Disorders; Hemophilia; Thrombotic Disorders; **Hospital:** Duke Univ Hosp; **Address:** Duke Medical Ctr, 200 Trent Dr, Clinic 2C, Durham, NC 27710; **Phone:** 919-620-3285; **Board Cert:** Internal Medicine 1988; Hematology 2002; **Med School:** Indiana Univ 1985; **Resid:** Internal Medicine, Duke Univ Med Ctr 1988; **Fellow:** Hematology & Oncology, Duke Univ Med Ctr 1989; **Fac Appt:** Prof Med, Duke Univ

Powell, Bayard L MD [Hem] - **Spec Exp:** Leukemia; Myelodysplastic Syndromes; **Hospital:** Wake Forest Univ Baptist Med Ctr; **Address:** Wake Forest Univ Baptist Med Ctr, Med Ctr Blvd-Cancer Center, Winston-Salem, NC 27157-1082; **Phone:** 336-716-7970; **Board Cert:** Internal Medicine 1983; Medical Oncology 1985; **Med School:** Univ NC Sch Med 1980; **Resid:** Internal Medicine, NC Baptist Hosp 1983; **Fellow:** Hematology & Oncology, Wake Forest Univ Sch Med 1986; **Fac Appt:** Prof Med, Wake Forest Univ

Rosenblatt, Joseph D MD [Hem] - **Spec Exp:** Lymphoma; Leukemia; Multiple Myeloma; Lymphomas-Rare; **Hospital:** Univ of Miami Hosp & Clins/Sylvester Comp Canc Ctr (page 73), Jackson Meml Hosp (page 70); **Address:** Sylvester Comprehensive Cancer Ctr, 1475 NW 12th Ave, D8-4, Ste 3300, Miami, FL 33136; **Phone:** 305-243-4909; **Board Cert:** Internal Medicine 1983; Medical Oncology 1985; **Med School:** UCLA 1980; **Resid:** Internal Medicine, UCLA Med Ctr 1983; **Fellow:** Hematology & Oncology, UCLA 1986; **Fac Appt:** Prof Med, Univ Miami Sch Med

Hematology

Schwartzberg, Lee S MD [Hem] - **Spec Exp:** Breast Cancer; Lung Cancer; Stem Cell Transplant; **Hospital:** Baptist Memorial Hospital-Memphis; **Address:** The West Clinic, 100 N Humphreys Blvd, Memphis, TN 38120; **Phone:** 901-683-0055; **Board Cert:** Internal Medicine 1983; Medical Oncology 1985; Hematology 1986; **Med School:** NY Med Coll 1980; **Resid:** Internal Medicine, North Shore Univ Hosp 1983; Internal Medicine, Meml Sloan Kettering Cancer Ctr 1985; **Fellow:** Hematology & Oncology, Meml Sloan Kettering Cancer Ctr 1984; Hematology & Oncology, Meml Sloan Kettering Cancer Ctr 1987; **Fac Appt:** Assoc Prof Med, Univ Tenn Coll Med

Sokol, Lubomir MD/PhD [Hem] - **Spec Exp:** Lymphoma; Hematologic Malignancies; **Hospital:** H Lee Moffitt Cancer Ctr & Research Inst (page 59); **Address:** H Lee Moffitt Cancer Ctr & Rsch Inst, 12902 Magnolia Drive, MS FOB3, Tampa, FL 33612; **Phone:** 813-745-8212; **Board Cert:** Internal Medicine 2000; Medical Oncology 2002; Hematology 2003; **Med School:** Czech Republic 1981; **Resid:** Radiation Oncology, Charles Univ 1984; Internal Medicine, LSU Med Ctr 1999; **Fellow:** Radiation Oncology, Charles Univ 1990; Hematology & Oncology, USF Med Ctr 2002

Solberg, Lawrence Arthur MD/PhD [Hem] - **Spec Exp:** Leukemia & Lymphoma; Myelodysplastic Syndromes; Bone Marrow Transplant; Multiple Myeloma; **Hospital:** Mayo - Jacksonville; **Address:** 4500 San Pablo Rd Mayo Bldg Fl 8, Jacksonville, FL 32224; **Phone:** 904-953-7290; **Board Cert:** Internal Medicine 1978; Hematology 1980; **Med School:** St Louis Univ 1975; **Resid:** Internal Medicine, Mayo Clinic 1978; **Fellow:** Hematology, Mayo Clinic 1980; **Fac Appt:** Prof Med, Mayo Med Sch

Telen, Marilyn J MD [Hem] - **Spec Exp:** Sickle Cell Disease; Anemias & Red Cell Disorders; Transfusion Medicine; **Hospital:** Duke Univ Hosp; **Address:** Duke Univ Med Ctr, Box 2615, Durham, NC 27710; **Phone:** 919-684-5378; **Board Cert:** Internal Medicine 1980; Hematology 1984; **Med School:** NYU Sch Med 1977; **Resid:** Internal Medicine, Erie Co Med Cr 1980; **Fellow:** Hematology, Duke Univ Med Ctr 1983; **Fac Appt:** Prof Med, Duke Univ

Williams, Michael E MD [Hem] - **Spec Exp:** Lymphoma; Multiple Myeloma; Leukemia; Mantle Cell Lymphoma; **Hospital:** Univ of Virginia Health Sys; **Address:** UVA Hlth Sys, Div Hem/Oncology, PO Box 800716, Charlottesville, VA 22908-0716; **Phone:** 434-924-9637; **Board Cert:** Internal Medicine 1982; Medical Oncology 1987; Hematology 2009; **Med School:** Univ Cincinnati 1979; **Resid:** Internal Medicine, Univ Virginia Med Ctr 1983; **Fellow:** Hematology & Oncology, Univ Virginia Med Ctr 1986; **Fac Appt:** Prof Med, Univ VA Sch Med

Zuckerman, Kenneth S MD [Hem] - **Spec Exp:** Myeloproliferative Disorders; Leukemia; Myelodysplastic Syndromes; Anemia; **Hospital:** H Lee Moffitt Cancer Ctr & Research Inst (page 59), Tampa Genl Hosp; **Address:** 12902 USF Magnolia Drive, Tampa, FL 33612-9416; **Phone:** 813-745-8090; **Board Cert:** Internal Medicine 1975; Hematology 1978; **Med School:** Ohio State Univ 1972; **Resid:** Internal Medicine, Ohio State Univ Hosps 1975; **Fellow:** Hematology, Peter Bent Brigham Hosp/Harvard Univ 1978; **Fac Appt:** Prof Med, Univ S Fla Coll Med

Midwest

Baron, Joseph M MD [Hem] - **Spec Exp:** Bleeding/Coagulation Disorders; Lymphoma; Myeloproliferative Disorders; **Hospital:** Univ of Chicago Med Ctr; **Address:** 5841 S Maryland Ave, MC 2115, Chicago, IL 60637-1463; **Phone:** 773-702-6149; **Board Cert:** Internal Medicine 1969; Hematology 1972; Medical Oncology 1975; **Med School:** Univ Chicago-Pritzker Sch Med 1962; **Resid:** Internal Medicine, Univ Chicago Hosps 1964; Internal Medicine, Univ Chicago Hosps 1968; **Fellow:** Hematology, Univ Chicago Hosps 1968; **Fac Appt:** Assoc Prof Med, Univ Chicago-Pritzker Sch Med

Blinder, Morey MD [Hem] - **Spec Exp:** Bleeding/Coagulation Disorders; Anemia; Sickle Cell Disease; **Hospital:** Barnes-Jewish Hosp; **Address:** Washington Univ School of Medicine, Hematology Division, 660 S Euclid Ave, Box 8125, St Louis, MO 63110; **Phone:** 314-362-7216; **Board Cert:** Internal Medicine 1984; Hematology 1988; Medical Oncology 1987; **Med School:** St Louis Univ 1981; **Resid:** Internal Medicine, Univ Illinois Hosp 1984; **Fellow:** Hematology & Oncology, Univ Wash Med Ctr 1986; **Fac Appt:** Assoc Prof Med, Washington Univ, St Louis

Bockenstedt, Paula MD [Hem] - **Spec Exp:** Bleeding/Coagulation Disorders; Leukemia; Von Willebrand's Disease; **Hospital:** Univ of Michigan Hosp; **Address:** Div Hematology, 1500 E Med Ctr Dr, MIB, rm C-344, Ann Arbor, MI 48109-8048; **Phone:** 734-936-6393; **Board Cert:** Internal Medicine 1981; Hematology 1984; **Med School:** Harvard Med Sch 1978; **Resid:** Internal Medicine, Brigham-Womens Hosp 1981; **Fellow:** Hematology, Brigham-Womens Hosp 1984; **Fac Appt:** Assoc Clin Prof Med, Univ Mich Med Sch

Bricker, Leslie J MD [Hem] - **Spec Exp:** Palliative Care; **Hospital:** Henry Ford Hosp; **Address:** Henry Ford Hospital, 2799 W Grand Blvd, CFP 5, 13th Fl, Detroit, MI 48202; **Phone:** 313-916-1859; **Board Cert:** Internal Medicine 1980; Hematology 1982; Medical Oncology 1983; Hospice & Palliative Medicine 2008; **Med School:** Wayne State Univ 1977; **Resid:** Internal Medicine, Sinai Hosp 1980; **Fellow:** Hematology & Oncology, Univ Mich Hosp 1983; **Fac Appt:** Assoc Prof Med, Wayne State Univ

Byrd, John C MD [Hem] - **Spec Exp:** Leukemia-Chronic Lymphocytic; **Hospital:** Arthur G James Cancer Hosp & Research Inst; **Address:** 320 W 10th Ave, B302 Starling-Loving Hall, Columbus, OH 43210; **Phone:** 614-293-3196; **Board Cert:** Hematology 2007; **Med School:** Univ Ark 1991; **Resid:** Internal Medicine, Walter Reed AMC 1994; **Fellow:** Hematology & Oncology, Walter Reed AMC 1997; **Fac Appt:** Assoc Prof Med, Ohio State Univ

Copelan, Edward A MD [Hem] - **Spec Exp:** Leukemia; Myelodysplastic Syndromes; Bone Marrow Transplant; Multiple Myeloma; **Hospital:** Cleveland Clin (page 56); **Address:** Cleveland Clinic Fdn, 9500 Euclid Ave, Cleveland, OH 44195; **Phone:** 216-445-5647; **Board Cert:** Internal Medicine 1980; Hematology 1982; Medical Oncology 1983; **Med School:** Tufts Univ 1977; **Resid:** Internal Medicine, Ohio State Univ Hosp 1980; **Fellow:** Hematology & Oncology, Ohio State Univ Hosp 1983; Bone Marrow Transplant, UCLA Med Ctr; **Fac Appt:** Prof Med, Cleveland Cl Coll Med/Case West Res

Di Persio, John F MD/PhD [Hem] - **Spec Exp:** Bone Marrow Transplant; Hematologic Malignancies; Leukemia; **Hospital:** Barnes-Jewish Hosp; **Address:** Wash Univ Sch Med, Sect Bone Marrow Transplant & Leukemia, 660 S Euclid Ave, Box 8007, St Louis, MO 63110; **Phone:** 314-454-8306; **Board Cert:** Internal Medicine 1984; Medical Oncology 1987; Hematology 1988; **Med School:** Univ Rochester 1980; **Resid:** Internal Medicine, Parkland Meml Hosp 1984; **Fellow:** Hematology & Oncology, UCLA Med Ctr 1987; **Fac Appt:** Prof Med, Washington Univ, St Louis

Erba, Harry P MD/PhD [Hem] - **Spec Exp:** Leukemia; Myelodysplastic Syndromes; Lymphoma; **Hospital:** Univ of Michigan Hosp; **Address:** Univ Michigan Medical Ctr, 1500 E Medical Center Dr, C348MIB, MC 5PC5848, Ann Arbor, MI 48109-5848; **Phone:** 734-647-8901; **Board Cert:** Internal Medicine 2004; Hematology 2004; Medical Oncology 2005; **Med School:** Stanford Univ 1988; **Resid:** Internal Medicine, Brigham & Womens Hosp 1990; **Fellow:** Hematology & Oncology, Brigham & Womens Hosp 1993; **Fac Appt:** Assoc Prof Med, Univ Mich Med Sch

Farag, Sherif S MD/PhD [Hem] - **Spec Exp:** Multiple Myeloma; Leukemia & Lymphoma; Bone Marrow Transplant; Stem Cell Transplant; **Hospital:** IU Health University Hosp; **Address:** IU Simon Cancer Center, 535 Barnhill Drive, Ste 473, Indianapolis, IN 46202; **Phone:** 317-944-0920; **Med School:** Australia 1995; **Resid:** Internal Medicine, Univ Melbourne Med Ctr; **Fellow:** Hematology & Oncology, Roswell Park Cancer Inst; **Fac Appt:** Assoc Prof Med, Indiana Univ

Hematology

Flynn, Patrick MD [Hem] - **Spec Exp:** Hematologic Malignancies; Colon & Rectal Cancer; Clinical Trials; Breast Cancer; **Hospital:** Abbott - Northwestern Hosp, Fairview Southdale Hosp; **Address:** 910 E 26th St, Minneapolis, MN 55404; **Phone:** 612-884-6300; **Board Cert:** Internal Medicine 1978; Medical Oncology 1981; Hematology 1982; **Med School:** Univ Minn 1975; **Resid:** Internal Medicine, Hennepin Co Med Ctr 1978; **Fellow:** Hematology & Oncology, Univ Minnesota Hosp 1981

Gertz, Morie MD [Hem] - **Spec Exp:** Multiple Myeloma; Amyloidosis; Waldenstrom's Macroglobulinemia; Plasma Cell Disorders; **Hospital:** Mayo Med Ctr & Clin - Rochester, Rochester Methodist Hosp; **Address:** 200 SW 1st St Fl W10, Rochester, MN 55905; **Phone:** 507-284-3725; **Board Cert:** Internal Medicine 1979; Hematology 1982; Medical Oncology 1983; **Med School:** Loyola Univ-Stritch Sch Med 1975; **Resid:** Internal Medicine, St Lukes Hosp 1979; **Fellow:** Hematology & Oncology, Mayo Clin 1982; **Fac Appt:** Prof Med, Mayo Med Sch

Godwin, John MD [Hem] - **Spec Exp:** Thrombotic Disorders; Leukemia in Elderly; Head & Neck Cancer; Lymphoma; **Hospital:** St. John's Hosp - Springfield, Memorial Med Ctr-Springfield; **Address:** SIU School Medicine, Simmons Cooper Cancer Inst, PO Box 19678, Springfield, IL 62794-9678; **Phone:** 217-545-5817; **Board Cert:** Internal Medicine 1981; Hematology 1986; **Med School:** Univ Alabama 1978; **Resid:** Internal Medicine, Baylor Coll Med 1981; Internal Medicine, Baylor Coll Med 1982; **Fellow:** Hematology, Baylor Coll Med 1983; Hematology, North Carolina Meml Hosp 1985; **Fac Appt:** Prof Med, Southern IL Univ

Gordon, Leo I MD [Hem] - **Spec Exp:** Lymphoma, Non-Hodgkin's; Hodgkin's Disease; Bone Marrow Transplant; **Hospital:** Northwestern Meml Hosp; **Address:** Div HemOnc, Northwestern Univ-Feinberg Sch Med, Robert H Lurie Comprehensive Cancer Ctr, 676 N St Clair St, Ste 850, Chicago, IL 60611-3124; **Phone:** 312-695-4546; **Board Cert:** Internal Medicine 1976; Hematology 1978; Medical Oncology 1979; **Med School:** Univ Cincinnati 1973; **Resid:** Internal Medicine, Univ Chicago Hosps 1976; **Fellow:** Hematology, Univ Minnesota Hosps 1978; Hematology & Oncology, Univ Chicago Hosps 1979; **Fac Appt:** Prof Med, Univ Chicago-Pritzker Sch Med

Gregory, Stephanie A MD [Hem] - **Spec Exp:** Lymphoma; Leukemia; Plasma Cell Disorders; Multiple Myeloma; **Hospital:** Rush Univ Med Ctr; **Address:** Rush University Medical Center, 1725 W Harrison St, Ste 834, Chicago, IL 60612; **Phone:** 312-942-5982; **Board Cert:** Internal Medicine 1972; Hematology 1972; **Med School:** Med Coll PA Hahnemann 1965; **Resid:** Internal Medicine, Rush/Presby-St Luke's Med Ctr 1969; **Fellow:** Hematology, Rush/Presby-St Luke's Med Ctr 1972; **Fac Appt:** Prof Med, Rush Med Coll

Greipp, Philip R MD [Hem] - **Spec Exp:** Multiple Myeloma; **Hospital:** Mayo Med Ctr & Clin - Rochester; **Address:** Mayo Clinic, Div Hematology, 200 First St SW Mayo Bldg Fl W-10, Rochester, MN 55905-0001; **Phone:** 507-284-3159; **Board Cert:** Internal Medicine 1974; Hematology 1994; **Med School:** Georgetown Univ 1968; **Resid:** Internal Medicine, Mayo Clin 1973; **Fellow:** Hematology, Mayo Clin 1975; **Fac Appt:** Prof Med, Mayo Med Sch

Grever, Michael R MD [Hem] - **Spec Exp:** Hematologic Malignancies; Leukemia; Drug Development; Clinical Trials; **Hospital:** Ohio St Univ Med Ctr; **Address:** 395 W 12th Ave, Rm 392, Doan Tower, Columbus, OH 43210; **Phone:** 614-293-8724; **Board Cert:** Internal Medicine 1975; Medical Oncology 1979; Hematology 1988; **Med School:** Univ Pittsburgh 1971; **Resid:** Internal Medicine, Univ of Pittsburgh 1974; **Fellow:** Hematology & Oncology, Ohio State Univ 1978; **Fac Appt:** Prof Med, Ohio State Univ

Habermann, Thomas M MD [Hem] - **Spec Exp:** Lymphoma; Hodgkin's Disease; Leukemia; **Hospital:** Mayo Med Ctr & Clin - Rochester; **Address:** Mayo Clin, 200 1st St SW, Rochester, MN 55905; **Phone:** 507-284-3159; **Board Cert:** Internal Medicine 1982; Hematology 1984; **Med School:** Creighton Univ 1979; **Resid:** Internal Medicine, Mayo Clinic 1982; **Fellow:** Hematology, Mayo Clinic 1985; **Fac Appt:** Prof Med, Mayo Med Sch

Juckett, Mark B MD [Hem] - **Spec Exp:** Bone Marrow Transplant; **Hospital:** Univ WI Hosp & Clins; **Address:** 600 Highland Ave, Ste H4/534, Madison, WI 53792; **Phone:** 608-745-5660; **Board Cert:** Internal Medicine 2001; Hematology 2004; Medical Oncology 2005; **Med School:** Univ Louisville Sch Med 1987; **Resid:** Internal Medicine, Univ Minnesota 1990; **Fellow:** Hematology & Oncology, Univ Minnesota 1992; **Fac Appt:** Assoc Prof Med, Univ Wisc

Kraut, Eric H MD [Hem] - **Spec Exp:** Hematologic Malignancies; Leukemia; Drug Development; Clinical Trials; **Hospital:** Ohio St Univ Med Ctr; **Address:** 320 W 10th Ave, A358 SL, Columbus, OH 43210; **Phone:** 614-293-2887; **Board Cert:** Internal Medicine 1975; Medical Oncology 1977; Hematology 1978; **Med School:** Temple Univ 1972; **Resid:** Internal Medicine, Univ Pittsburgh 1975; **Fellow:** Hematology & Oncology, Ohio State Univ Hosp 1977; **Fac Appt:** Prof Med, Ohio State Univ

Kuriakose, Philip MD [Hem] - **Spec Exp:** Leukemia; **Hospital:** Henry Ford Hosp; **Address:** Henry Ford Hosp, Hematology/Oncology, 2799 W Grand Blvd, K13, Detroit, MI 48202; **Phone:** 313-916-1841; **Board Cert:** Internal Medicine 1999; Medical Oncology 2002; Hematology 2002; **Med School:** India 1990; **Resid:** Internal Medicine, Christian Med Coll 1992; Internal Medicine, Henry Ford Hosp 1994; **Fellow:** Hematology & Oncology, Mayo Clinic 1995

Larson, Richard A MD [Hem] - **Spec Exp:** Leukemia & Lymphoma; Bone Marrow Transplant; Myelodysplastic Syndromes; **Hospital:** Univ of Chicago Med Ctr; **Address:** University of Chicago Medical Center, 5758 S Maryland Ave, Box 90115, Chicago, IL 60637; **Phone:** 773-702-6149; **Board Cert:** Internal Medicine 1980; Hematology 1982; Medical Oncology 1983; **Med School:** Stanford Univ 1977; **Resid:** Internal Medicine, Univ Chicago Hosps 1980; **Fellow:** Hematology & Oncology, Univ Chicago Hosps 1983; **Fac Appt:** Prof Hem & Onc, Univ Chicago-Pritzker Sch Med

Lazarus, Hillard M MD [Hem] - **Spec Exp:** Bone Marrow Transplant; Stem Cell Transplant; Leukemia; **Hospital:** Univ Hosps Case Med Ctr (page 74); **Address:** 11100 Euclid Ave, Wearn Bldg 351, Cleveland, OH 44106-5065; **Phone:** 216-844-3629; **Board Cert:** Internal Medicine 1977; Medical Oncology 1979; Hematology 1980; **Med School:** Univ Rochester 1974; **Resid:** Internal Medicine, Univ Hosps 1977; **Fellow:** Hematology & Oncology, Univ Hosps 1979; **Fac Appt:** Prof Med, Case West Res Univ

Litzow, Mark R MD [Hem] - **Spec Exp:** Bone Marrow Transplant; Leukemia; **Hospital:** Mayo Med Ctr & Clin - Rochester; **Address:** Mayo Clinic, Div Hematology, 200 First St SW, Rochester, MN 55905; **Phone:** 507-284-9448; **Board Cert:** Internal Medicine 1983; Hematology 1988; Medical Oncology 1989; **Med School:** Univ Chicago-Pritzker Sch Med 1980; **Resid:** Internal Medicine, Mayo Clinic 1984; **Fellow:** Medical Oncology, Mayo Clinic 1990; **Fac Appt:** Asst Prof Med, Mayo Med Sch

Maciejewski, Jaroslaw P MD/PhD [Hem] - **Spec Exp:** Anemia-Aplastic; Hematologic Malignancies; Stem Cell Transplant; **Hospital:** Cleveland Clin (page 56); **Address:** Cleveland Clinic, 9500 Euclid Ave, Desk R40, Cleveland, OH 44195; **Phone:** 216-445-5962; **Board Cert:** Internal Medicine 1999; Hematology 2001; **Med School:** Germany 1990; **Resid:** Internal Medicine, Univ Nevada Med Ctr 1997; **Fellow:** Hematology, Natl Inst Hlth 2000; **Fac Appt:** Prof Med, Case West Res Univ

McGlave, Philip B MD [Hem] - **Spec Exp:** Leukemia; Bone Marrow Transplant; **Address:** Univ Minn, Dept Med, Div Hem/Onc Transplanatation, 420 Delaware St SE, MMC 480, Minneapolis, MN 55455; **Phone:** 612-626-2446; **Board Cert:** Internal Medicine 1977; Hematology 1980; **Med School:** Univ IL Coll Med 1974; **Resid:** Internal Medicine, Univ Minnesota Med Ctr 1977; **Fellow:** Hematology & Oncology, Univ Minnesota Med Ctr 1980; **Fac Appt:** Prof Med, Univ Minn

Hematology

Milhem, Mohammed M MD [Hem] - **Spec Exp:** Bone Cancer; Bone Marrow Transplant; Sarcoma; Melanoma; **Hospital:** Univ Iowa Hosp & Clinics; **Address:** UIHC, 200 Hawkins Drive, C32 GH, Iowa City, IA 52242; **Phone:** 319-356-4200; **Board Cert:** Internal Medicine 2000; Hematology 2003; Medical Oncology 2003; **Med School:** Jordan 1995; **Resid:** Internal Medicine, Univ IL Med Ctr 2000; **Fellow:** Hematology & Oncology, Univ IL Med Ctr 2003; Bone Marrow Transplant, Univ IL Med Ctr 2004; **Fac Appt:** Asst Clin Prof Hem & Onc, Univ Iowa Coll Med

Mosher, Deane F MD [Hem] - **Hospital:** Univ WI Hosp & Clins; **Address:** Dept Hematology, 600 Highland Ave Fl 6, Madison, WI 53792; **Phone:** 608-263-7022; **Board Cert:** Internal Medicine 1973; Hematology 1980; **Med School:** Harvard Med Sch 1968; **Resid:** Internal Medicine, Beth Israel Hosp 1970; **Fellow:** Hematology, Harvard Med Sch 1972; **Fac Appt:** Prof Med, Univ Wisc

Nand, Sucha MD [Hem] - **Spec Exp:** Myelodysplastic Syndromes; Myeloproliferative Disorders; Leukemia; Lymphoma, Non-Hodgkin's; **Hospital:** Loyola Univ Med Ctr; **Address:** Cardinal Bernardin Cancer Ctr, 2160 S First Ave Bldg 112 - rm 345, Maywood, IL 60153-3304; **Phone:** 708-327-3217; **Board Cert:** Internal Medicine 1979; Medical Oncology 1981; Hematology 1982; **Med School:** India 1971; **Resid:** Physical Medicine & Rehabilitation, Northwestern Meml Hosp 1976; Internal Medicine, North Chicago VA Hosp 1978; **Fellow:** Hematology & Oncology, Northwestern Meml Hosp 1981; **Fac Appt:** Prof Med, Loyola Univ-Stritch Sch Med

Palascak, Joseph E MD [Hem] - **Spec Exp:** Hemophilia; Bleeding/Coagulation Disorders; Thrombotic Disorders; **Hospital:** Univ Hosp - Cincinnati; **Address:** Barrett Center, 222 Piedmont Ave Fl 2, Cincinnati, OH 45219; **Phone:** 513-475-8500; **Board Cert:** Internal Medicine 1975; Hematology 1978; **Med School:** Jefferson Med Coll 1968; **Resid:** Internal Medicine, Thomas Jefferson Univ Hosp 1971; **Fellow:** Hematology, Thomas Jefferson Univ Hosp 1972; Hematology, Thomas Jefferson Univ Hosp 1976; **Fac Appt:** Prof Med, Univ Cincinnati

Porcu, Pierluigi MD [Hem] - **Spec Exp:** Lymphoma; Lymphoma, Non-Hodgkin's; Immunotherapy; **Hospital:** Ohio St Univ Med Ctr; **Address:** 320 W 10th Ave, B320 Starling Loving Hall, Columbus, OH 43210; **Phone:** 614-293-9273; **Board Cert:** Hematology 1999; Medical Oncology 1999; **Med School:** Italy 1987; **Resid:** Internal Medicine, Indiana Univ Hosp 1996; **Fellow:** Hematology & Oncology, Indiana Univ Hosp 1999; **Fac Appt:** Asst Prof Med, Ohio State Univ

Silverstein, Roy L MD [Hem] - **Spec Exp:** Thrombotic Disorders; Bleeding/Coagulation Disorders; **Hospital:** Froedtert and Med Ctr of WI; **Address:** Froedrert & The Med Ctr of Wisconsin, 9200 W Wisconsin Ave, Ste C5038, Milwaukee, WI 53226; **Phone:** 414-805-0518; **Board Cert:** Internal Medicine 1982; Hematology 1984; Medical Oncology 1985; **Med School:** Emory Univ 1979; **Resid:** Internal Medicine, NY Hosp-Cornell Med Ctr 1982; Hematology & Oncology, NY Hosp-Cornell Med Ctr 1984; **Fac Appt:** Prof Med, Med Coll Wisc

Singhal, Seema MD [Hem] - **Spec Exp:** Multiple Myeloma; **Hospital:** Northwestern Meml Hosp; **Address:** Northwestern Div Hematology/Oncology, 676 N St Clair St, Ste 850, Chicago, IL 60611; **Phone:** 312-695-0990; **Board Cert:** Internal Medicine 2005; **Med School:** India 1989; **Resid:** Internal Medicine, King Edward Meml Hosp 1991; Hematology, King Edward Meml Hosp 1991; **Fellow:** Bone Marrow Transplant, Hadassah Univ Hosp 1992; **Fac Appt:** Prof Med, Northwestern Univ

Stiff, Patrick J MD [Hem] - **Spec Exp:** Bone Marrow Transplant; Leukemia; Lymphoma, Non-Hodgkin's; Vaccine Therapy; **Hospital:** Loyola Univ Med Ctr; **Address:** Cardinal Bernadin Cancer Ctr, 2160 S First Ave, Bldg 112, rm 255, Maywood, IL 60153; **Phone:** 708-327-3304; **Board Cert:** Internal Medicine 1978; Medical Oncology 1981; Hematology 1982; **Med School:** Loyola Univ-Stritch Sch Med 1975; **Resid:** Internal Medicine, Cleveland Clinic Fdn 1978; **Fellow:** Hematology & Oncology, Meml Sloan Kettering Cancer Ctr 1981; **Fac Appt:** Prof Med, Loyola Univ-Stritch Sch Med

Uberti, Joseph P MD/PhD [Hem] - **Spec Exp:** Bone Marrow Transplant; Stem Cell Transplant; **Hospital:** Barbara Ann Karmanos Cancer Inst; **Address:** Barbara Ann Karmanos Cancer Inst, 4100 John R St, MC HW04H0, Detroit, MI 48201; **Phone:** 313-576-8760; **Board Cert:** Internal Medicine 1986; Medical Oncology 1989; **Med School:** Wayne State Univ 1983; **Resid:** Internal Medicine, Detroit Receiving Hosp 1986; **Fellow:** Hematology & Oncology, Wayne State Univ Hosps 1988; **Fac Appt:** Prof Med, Wayne State Univ

Van Besien, Koen W MD [Hem] - **Spec Exp:** Lymphoma; Stem Cell Transplant; **Hospital:** Univ of Chicago Med Ctr; **Address:** Stem Cell Transplant Program, 5841 S Maryland Ave, Chicago, IL 60637; **Phone:** 773-702-4400; **Board Cert:** Internal Medicine 2005; Medical Oncology 2005; Hematology 2006; **Med School:** Belgium 1984; **Resid:** Internal Medicine, Univ Leuven Med Ctr 1987; **Fellow:** Hematology & Oncology, Indiana Univ Med Ctr 1990; **Fac Appt:** Prof Med, Univ Chicago-Pritzker Sch Med

Winter, Jane N MD [Hem] - **Spec Exp:** Lymphoma, Non-Hodgkin's; Hodgkin's Disease; Bone Marrow Transplant; Langerhans Cell Histiocytosis (LCH); **Hospital:** Northwestern Meml Hosp; **Address:** Northwestern Univ - Div Hem/Oncology, 675 N St Clair St, Ste 21-100, Chicago, IL 60611; **Phone:** 312-695-0990; **Board Cert:** Internal Medicine 1980; Hematology 2008; Medical Oncology 1983; **Med School:** Univ Pennsylvania 1977; **Resid:** Internal Medicine, Univ Chicago Hosps 1980; **Fellow:** Hematology & Oncology, Columbia Presby Hosp 1981; Hematology & Oncology, Northwestern Univ 1983; **Fac Appt:** Prof Med, Northwestern Univ

Great Plains and Mountains

Rodgers III, George M MD/PhD [Hem] - **Spec Exp:** Hematopathology; Anemia-Cancer Related; Bleeding/Coagulation Disorders; **Hospital:** Univ Utah Hlth Care; **Address:** Univ Utah Med Ctr - Div Hematology, 30 N 1900 E, rm 5C402, Salt Lake City, UT 84132; **Phone:** 801-585-3229; **Board Cert:** Internal Medicine 1979; Hematology 1982; Pathology 1984; **Med School:** Tulane Univ 1976; **Resid:** Internal Medicine, Baylor Affil Hosps 1979; **Fellow:** Hematology, UCSF Med Ctr 1982; **Fac Appt:** Prof Med, Univ Utah

Vose, Julie M MD [Hem] - **Spec Exp:** Lymphoma; **Hospital:** Nebraska Med Ctr; **Address:** 987630 Nebraska Med Ctr, Emile @ 42nd St, Omaha, NE 68198-7630; **Phone:** 402-559-5600; **Board Cert:** Internal Medicine 1987; Medical Oncology 2000; Hematology 2000; **Med School:** Univ Nebr Coll Med 1984; **Resid:** Internal Medicine, Univ Nebraska Med Ctr 1987; **Fellow:** Hematology & Oncology, Univ Nebraska Med Ctr 1990; **Fac Appt:** Prof Med, Univ Nebr Coll Med

Southwest

Barlogie, Bart MD/PhD [Hem] - **Spec Exp:** Bone Marrow Transplant; Plasma Cell Disorders; Multiple Myeloma; **Hospital:** UAMS Med Ctr; **Address:** UAMS-Myeloma Inst Rsch & Therapy, 4301 West Markham St, Slot 816, Little Rock, AR 72205; **Phone:** 501-526-2873; **Med School:** Germany 1969; **Resid:** Internal Medicine, Univ Muenster Med Sch; **Fellow:** Medical Oncology, MD Anderson Cancer Ctr-Tumor Inst 1976; **Fac Appt:** Prof Med, Univ Ark

Brenner, Malcolm K MD/PhD [Hem] - **Spec Exp:** Gene Therapy; Bone Marrow Transplant; **Hospital:** Methodist Hosp - Houston, Texas Chldns Hosp; **Address:** 1102 Bates Ave, Ste 1630, Houston, TX 77030; **Phone:** 832-824-4671; **Med School:** England, UK 1975; **Resid:** Internal Medicine, Cambridge Univ 1979; **Fellow:** Immunology, Clinical Rsch Ctr 1984; Hematology & Oncology, Royal Free Hosp 1986; **Fac Appt:** Prof Med, Baylor Coll Med

Hematology

Champlin, Richard E MD [Hem] - **Spec Exp:** Bone Marrow Transplant; Stem Cell Transplant; Leukemia & Lymphoma; **Hospital:** UT MD Anderson Cancer Ctr; **Address:** MD Anderson Cancer Ctr, Stem Cell Transplantation Ctr, 1515 Holcombe Blvd, Unit 0423 Blvd, Houston, TX 77030; **Phone:** 713-792-6100; **Board Cert:** Internal Medicine 1978; Hematology 1980; Medical Oncology 1981; **Med School:** Univ Chicago-Pritzker Sch Med 1975; **Resid:** Internal Medicine, LA Co Harbor/UCLA Med Ctr 1978; **Fellow:** Hematology & Oncology, LA Co Harbor/UCLA Med Ctr 1980; **Fac Appt:** Prof Med, Univ Tex, Houston

Cobos, Everardo MD [Hem] - **Spec Exp:** Bone Marrow Transplant; Bleeding/Coagulation Disorders; **Hospital:** Univ Med Ctr-Lubbock; **Address:** 602 Indiana Ave, SCRTC Dept, Lubbock, TX 779 418; **Phone:** 806-775-8600; **Board Cert:** Internal Medicine 1985; Medical Oncology 1987; Hematology 1988; **Med School:** Univ Tex, San Antonio 1981; **Resid:** Internal Medicine, Letterman Army Med Ctr 1985; **Fellow:** Hematology & Oncology, Letterman Army Med Ctr 1988; **Fac Appt:** Prof Med, Texas Tech Univ

Cooper, Barry MD [Hem] - **Spec Exp:** Leukemia; Lymphoma; Bleeding/Coagulation Disorders; **Hospital:** Baylor Univ Medical Ctr-Dallas; **Address:** 3410 Worth St, Dallas, TX 75246-2096; **Phone:** 214-370-1002; **Board Cert:** Internal Medicine 1974; Medical Oncology 1977; Hematology 1978; **Med School:** Johns Hopkins Univ 1971; **Resid:** Internal Medicine, Johns Hopkins Hosp 1973; **Fellow:** Metabolism, Natl Inst Health 1975; Hematology, Peter Bent Brigham Hosp 1977; **Fac Appt:** Clin Prof Med, Univ Tex SW, Dallas

Cortes, Jorge E MD [Hem] - **Spec Exp:** Leukemia; Myelodysplastic Syndromes; Myeloproliferative Disorders; **Hospital:** UT MD Anderson Cancer Ctr; **Address:** UT MD Anderson Cancer Center, Leukemia Center, 1515 Holcombe Blvd, Unit 357, Houston, TX 77030; **Phone:** 713-792-8760; **Med School:** Mexico 1986; **Resid:** Internal Medicine, Instituto Nacional de la Nutricion 1989; **Fellow:** Hematology, UT MD Anderson Cancer Ctr 1992; Hematology & Oncology, UT MD Anderson Cancer Ctr 1995; **Fac Appt:** Prof Med, Univ Tex, Houston

Emanuel, Peter D MD [Hem] - **Spec Exp:** Lymphoma; Leukemia; Hodgkin's Disease; Multiple Myeloma; **Hospital:** UAMS Med Ctr; **Address:** 4301 W Markham, Slot 623, Little Rock, AR 72205; **Phone:** 501-526-2272; **Board Cert:** Internal Medicine 1988; **Med School:** Univ Wisc 1985; **Resid:** Internal Medicine, Univ Alabama Hosp 1988; **Fellow:** Hematology & Oncology, Univ Alabama 1991; **Fac Appt:** Prof Med, Univ Ark

Fonseca, Rafael MD [Hem] - **Spec Exp:** Multiple Myeloma; **Hospital:** Mayo Clinic - Scottsdale; **Address:** 13400 E Shea Blvd, MCCRB 1-105, Scottsdale, AZ 85259; **Phone:** 480-301-4280; **Board Cert:** Hematology 2010; **Med School:** Mexico 1991; **Resid:** Internal Medicine, Jackson Meml Hosp 1994; **Fellow:** Hematology & Oncology, Mayo Clinic 1998; **Fac Appt:** Assoc Prof Med, Mayo Med Sch

Kantarjian, Hagop M MD [Hem] - **Spec Exp:** Leukemia; **Hospital:** UT MD Anderson Cancer Ctr; **Address:** 1400 Holcombe Blvd, Unit 428, Houston, TX 77030; **Phone:** 713-792-7026; **Board Cert:** Internal Medicine 1983; Medical Oncology 1985; **Med School:** Amer Univ Beirut 1979; **Resid:** Internal Medicine, Univ Tex MD Anderson Cancer Ctr 1983; **Fellow:** Hematology & Oncology, Univ Tex MD Anderson Cancer Ctr 1983; **Fac Appt:** Prof Med, Univ Tex, Houston

Keating, Michael MD [Hem] - **Spec Exp:** Leukemia-Chronic Lymphocytic; **Hospital:** UT MD Anderson Cancer Ctr; **Address:** MD Anderson Cancer Ctr, 1400 Holcombe Blvd, Unit 428, Houston, TX 77030-4000; **Phone:** 713-745-2376; **Med School:** Australia 1966; **Resid:** Internal Medicine, St Vincents Hosp 1973; **Fellow:** Hematology, MD Anderson Cancer Ctr 1975; **Fac Appt:** Prof Med, Univ Tex, Houston

Lin, Weei-Chin MD/PhD [Hem] - **Spec Exp:** Hematologic Malignancies; Bleeding/Coagulation Disorders; **Hospital:** Baylor Clinic & Hosp-Houston, Ben Taub Genl Hosp; **Address:** One Baylor Plaza, rm 410, Houston, TX 77030; **Phone:** 713-873-3500; **Med School:** Taiwan 1986; **Resid:** Internal Medicine, Duke Univ Med Ctr 1996; **Fellow:** Hematology & Oncology, Duke Univ Med Ctr 1999; **Fac Appt:** Assoc Prof Med, Baylor Coll Med

Lyons, Roger M MD [Hem] - **Spec Exp:** Leukemia & Lymphoma; Multiple Myeloma; Bleeding/Coagulation Disorders; Platelet Disorders; **Hospital:** Methodist Hosp-San Antonio, Methodist Spec & Transpl Hosp; **Address:** 4411 Med Drive, Ste 100, San Antonio, TX 78229-3325; **Phone:** 210-595-5300; **Board Cert:** Internal Medicine 1981; Hematology 1982; **Med School:** Canada 1967; **Resid:** Internal Medicine, Winnipeg Genl Hosp 1969; Internal Medicine, Barnes-Wohl Hosps 1972; **Fellow:** Hematology, Washington Univ Hosps 1975; **Fac Appt:** Clin Prof Med, Univ Tex, San Antonio

Maddox, Anne Marie MD [Hem] - **Spec Exp:** Hematologic Malignancies; Lung Cancer; Head & Neck Cancer; Clinical Trials; **Hospital:** UAMS Med Ctr; **Address:** Univ Arkansas Med Ctr, 4301 W Markham St, Slot 74-5, Little Rock, AR 72205; **Phone:** 501-686-8530; **Board Cert:** Internal Medicine 1979; Medical Oncology 1985; Hematology 2004; **Med School:** Dalhousie Univ 1975; **Resid:** Internal Medicine, Univ Toronto 1978; **Fellow:** Medical Oncology, TX MD Anderson Cancer Ctr 1982; **Fac Appt:** Prof, Univ Ark

Munker, Reinhold MD [Hem] - **Spec Exp:** Leukemia & Lymphoma; Bone Marrow Transplant; Hematologic Malignancies; **Hospital:** Louisiana State Univ Hosp; **Address:** LSUHSC-Shreveport, Feist-Weiller Cancer Ctr, 1501 Kings Hwy, Shreveport, LA 71130; **Phone:** 318-813-1016; **Board Cert:** Internal Medicine 2004; Hematology 2006; **Med School:** Germany 1979; **Resid:** Internal Medicine, Universit%otsklinikum Gro?hadern 1989; **Fellow:** Hematology & Oncology, Universit%otsklinikum Gro?hadern 1993; Blood Banking, Universit%otsklinikum Gro?hadern 1997; **Fac Appt:** Assoc Prof Med, Louisiana State U, Shrevport

Strauss, James F MD [Hem] - **Spec Exp:** Bleeding/Coagulation Disorders; Leukemia; Lymphoma; **Hospital:** TX Hlth Presby Hosp Dallas; **Address:** Texas Oncology at Presbyterian, 8220 Walnut Hill Ln Bldg 2 - Ste 700, Dallas, TX 75231; **Phone:** 214-739-4175; **Board Cert:** Internal Medicine 1976; Hematology 1978; Medical Oncology 1981; **Med School:** NYU Sch Med 1972; **Resid:** Internal Medicine, Baylor Univ Medical Ctr 1976; **Fellow:** Hematology, Univ Texas SW Medical Ctr 1977

Yeager, Andrew M MD [Hem] - **Spec Exp:** Bone Marrow & Stem Cell Transplant; Graft vs Host Disease; Leukemia; **Hospital:** Univ Med Ctr - Tucson; **Address:** Arizona Cancer Ctr, 1515 N Campbell Ave, Ste 2956, Tucson, AZ 85724-5024; **Phone:** 520-626-3191; **Board Cert:** Pediatrics 1979; Pediatric Hematology-Oncology 1980; **Med School:** Johns Hopkins Univ 1975; **Resid:** Pediatrics, Johns Hopkins Hosp 1978; Pediatrics, Johns Hopkins Hosp 1982; **Fellow:** Pediatric Hematology-Oncology, Johns Hopkins Hosp 1980; **Fac Appt:** Prof Med, Univ Ariz Coll Med

West Coast and Pacific

Damon, Lloyd E MD [Hem] - **Spec Exp:** Leukemia; Lymphoma; Stem Cell Transplant; **Hospital:** UCSF Med Ctr; **Address:** UCSF Comprehensive Cancer Ctr, 400 Parnassus Ave, Ste A502, Box 0324, San Francisco, CA 94143; **Phone:** 415-353-2421; **Board Cert:** Internal Medicine 1985; Medical Oncology 1987; Hematology 1988; **Med School:** Univ Mich Med Sch 1982; **Resid:** Internal Medicine, UCSF Med Ctr 1985; **Fellow:** Hematology & Oncology, UCSF Med Ctr 1988; **Fac Appt:** Prof Med, UCSF

Hematology

DeLoughery, Thomas MD [Hem] - **Spec Exp:** Thrombotic Disorders; Myeloproliferative Disorders; Bleeding/Coagulation Disorders; Platelet Disorders; **Hospital:** OR Hlth & Sci Univ; **Address:** 3303 SW Bond Ave, MC CH7M, Portland, OR 97239; **Phone:** 503-494-6594; **Board Cert:** Internal Medicine 1988; Blood Banking Transfusion Medicine 1995; Medical Oncology 2001; Hematology 2002; **Med School:** Indiana Univ 1985; **Resid:** Internal Medicine, Oregon Hlth & Science Univ 1988; **Fellow:** Hematology & Oncology, Oregon Hlth & Science Univ 1991; **Fac Appt:** Prof Med, Oregon Hlth & Sci Univ

Forman, Stephen J MD [Hem] - **Spec Exp:** Lymphoma; Leukemia; Bone Marrow Transplant; **Hospital:** City of Hope Natl Med Ctr; **Address:** City Hope Natl Med Ctr, Dept Hematology, 1500 E Duarte Rd, rm 3002, Duarte, CA 91010-3012; **Phone:** 626-256-4673 x62403; **Board Cert:** Internal Medicine 1977; **Med School:** USC Sch Med 1974; **Resid:** Internal Medicine, LAC-Harbor-UCLA Med Ctr 1976; **Fellow:** Hematology, LAC-USC Med Ctr 1978; Hematology, City of Hope Med Ctr 1979; **Fac Appt:** Clin Prof Med, USC Sch Med

Heinrich, Michael C MD [Hem] - **Spec Exp:** Hematologic Malignancies; Sarcoma; Gastrointestinal Stromal Tumors; **Hospital:** VA Medical Center - Portland, OR Hlth & Sci Univ; **Address:** 3710 SW US Veteran's Hospital Rd, MC P3RND19, Portland, OR 97239; **Phone:** 503-220-8262 x51169; **Board Cert:** Internal Medicine 1987; Hematology 2000; Medical Oncology 2001; **Med School:** Johns Hopkins Univ 1984; **Resid:** Internal Medicine, Oreg Hlth Scis Univ 1988; **Fellow:** Hematology & Oncology, Oreg Hlth Scis Univ 1991; **Fac Appt:** Prof Med, Oregon Hlth & Sci Univ

Kipps, Thomas J MD/PhD [Hem] - **Spec Exp:** Leukemia; Lymphoma, Non-Hodgkin's; **Hospital:** UCSD Med Ctr; **Address:** Moores UCSD Cancer Ctr, 3855 Health Sciences Drive, MC 0820, La Jolla, CA 92093; **Phone:** 858-822-5635; **Board Cert:** Internal Medicine 1982; Hematology 1984; **Med School:** Harvard Med Sch 1979; **Resid:** Internal Medicine, Stanford Univ Med Ctr 1981; **Fellow:** Hematology & Oncology, Stanford Univ Med Ctr 1984; **Fac Appt:** Prof Med, UCSD

Leung, Lawrence L MD [Hem] - **Spec Exp:** Bleeding/Coagulation Disorders; **Hospital:** Stanford Univ Hosp & Clinics, VA Hlth Care Sys - Palo Alto; **Address:** Stanford Cancer Center - Hematology, 875 Blake Wilbur Drive, Stanford, CA 94305; **Phone:** 650-498-6000; **Board Cert:** Internal Medicine 1978; Hematology 2009; Medical Oncology 1981; **Med School:** Columbia P&S 1975; **Resid:** Internal Medicine, New York Hosp 1978; **Fellow:** Hematology & Oncology, New York Hosp/Cornell 1981; **Fac Appt:** Prof Med, Stanford Univ

Levine, Alexandra M MD [Hem] - **Spec Exp:** Lymphoma; AIDS Related Cancers; AIDS/HIV; **Hospital:** City of Hope Natl Med Ctr; **Address:** 1500 E Duarte Rd, Needleman 213, Duarte, CA 91010; **Phone:** 626-471-7213; **Med School:** USC Sch Med 1971; **Resid:** Internal Medicine, LAC-USC Med Ctr 1974; **Fellow:** Hematology & Oncology, Grady Meml Hosp-Emory Univ 1975; Hematology, LAC-USC Med Ctr 1978; **Fac Appt:** Prof Med, USC Sch Med

Lill, Michael MD [Hem] - **Spec Exp:** Stem Cell Transplant; Lymphoma; Hematologic Malignancies; **Hospital:** Cedars-Sinai Med Ctr; **Address:** Cedars-Sinai Med Ctr-Outpt Cancer Ctr, 8700 Beverly Blvd, Ste AC 1070, Los Angeles, CA 90048; **Phone:** 310-423-1160; **Med School:** Australia 1982; **Resid:** Internal Medicine, Sir Charles Gairdner Hospital 1985; **Fellow:** Hematology, Royal Perth Hospital 1989; Hematopathology, Sir Charles Gairdner Hosp 1989; **Fac Appt:** Prof Med, UCLA

Linenberger, Michael MD [Hem] - **Spec Exp:** Bone Marrow Transplant; Leukemia & Lymphoma; Multiple Myeloma; **Hospital:** Univ Wash Med Ctr; **Address:** 825 Eastlake Ave E, MS G6-800, Seattle, WA 98109-1023; **Phone:** 206-288-1260; **Board Cert:** Internal Medicine 1985; Hematology 1988; **Med School:** Univ Kansas 1982; **Resid:** Internal Medicine, Rhode Island Hosp 1985; **Fellow:** Hematology, Univ Wash Med Ctr 1989; **Fac Appt:** Assoc Prof Med, Univ Wash

Maziarz, Richard MD [Hem] - **Spec Exp:** Leukemia; Immunotherapy; Bone Marrow Transplant; Lymphoma; **Hospital:** OR Hlth & Sci Univ; **Address:** OHSU Ctr Hematologic Malignancies, 3181 SW Sam Jackson Park Rd, Multnomah Pavilion, Ste 2502, MC L592, Portland, OR 97239; **Phone:** 503-494-5058; **Board Cert:** Internal Medicine 1982; Hematology 1988; Medical Oncology 1989; **Med School:** Harvard Med Sch 1979; **Resid:** Internal Medicine, Univ Hosp 1982; **Fellow:** Hematology & Oncology, Brigham & Womens Hosp 1988; **Fac Appt:** Prof Med, Oregon Hlth & Sci Univ

Mitchell, Beverly S MD [Hem] - **Spec Exp:** Hematologic Malignancies; Leukemia; Lymphoma; **Hospital:** Stanford Univ Hosp & Clinics; **Address:** Stanford Cancer Institute, Lorry Lokey Bldg-SIM 1, 265 Campus Drive, Ste G2167, Stanford, CA 94305; **Phone:** 650-736-7716; **Board Cert:** Internal Medicine 1973; Hematology 1978; **Med School:** Harvard Med Sch 1969; **Resid:** Internal Medicine, Univ Washington Med Ctr 1972; **Fellow:** Metabolism, Univ Zurich 1975; Hematology & Oncology, Univ Michigan 1977; **Fac Appt:** Prof Med, Stanford Univ

Nademanee, Auayporn P MD [Hem] - **Spec Exp:** Lymphoma; Hematologic Malignancies; Clinical Trials; **Hospital:** City of Hope Natl Med Ctr; **Address:** City of Hope Med Ctr-Dept Hematology, 1500 Duarte Rd, Duarte, CA 91010; **Phone:** 626-256-4673 x62691; **Board Cert:** Hematology 1982; Medical Oncology 1983; Internal Medicine 1978; **Med School:** Thailand 1973; **Resid:** Internal Medicine, Touro Infirm-Tulane Univ 1978; **Fellow:** Hematology & Oncology, Sepulveda VA Hosp 1980; Hematology & Oncology, USC Med Ctr 1981; **Fac Appt:** Prof Med, UCLA

Negrin, Robert S MD [Hem] - **Spec Exp:** Bone Marrow Transplant; **Hospital:** Stanford Univ Hosp & Clinics; **Address:** BMT Program, 300 Pasteur Drive, rm H0101, MC 5623, Stanford, CA 94305; **Phone:** 650-723-0822; **Board Cert:** Internal Medicine 1987; Hematology 2007; **Med School:** Harvard Med Sch 1984; **Resid:** Internal Medicine, Stanford Univ Hosp 1987; **Fellow:** Hematology, Stanford Univ Hosp 1990; **Fac Appt:** Prof Med, Stanford Univ

O'Donnell, Margaret R MD [Hem] - **Spec Exp:** Leukemia; Clinical Trials; **Hospital:** City of Hope Natl Med Ctr; **Address:** City of Hope National Med Ctr, 1500 E Duarte Rd, MOB-rm 3001, Duarte, CA 91010; **Phone:** 626-359-8111 x62405; **Board Cert:** Internal Medicine 1978; Hematology 1980; Medical Oncology 1979; **Med School:** Med Coll PA 1974; **Resid:** Internal Medicine, Montreal Genl Hosp 1976; Hematology, Royal Victoria Hosp-Montreal 1977; **Fellow:** Hematology & Oncology, Fred Hutchinson Cancer Ctr 1979

Saven, Alan MD [Hem] - **Spec Exp:** Leukemia; Lymphoma; **Hospital:** Scripps Green Hosp; **Address:** Scripps Green Hosp, Hematology, 10666 N Torrey Pines Rd, MS 312, La Jolla, CA 92037; **Phone:** 858-554-9489; **Board Cert:** Internal Medicine 1987; Medical Oncology 1989; **Med School:** South Africa 1982; **Resid:** Internal Medicine, Albert Einstein Med Ctr 1986; **Fellow:** Hematology & Oncology, Scripps Clinic 1987

Schiller, Gary J MD [Hem] - **Spec Exp:** Leukemia; **Hospital:** UCLA Ronald Reagan Med Ctr; **Address:** 10833 Le Conte Ave, rm 42-121 CHS, Los Angeles, CA 90095; **Phone:** 310-825-5513; **Board Cert:** Internal Medicine 1987; Medical Oncology 1989; Hematology 2000; **Med School:** USC Sch Med 1984; **Resid:** Internal Medicine, UCLA Med Ctr 1987; **Fellow:** Hematology & Oncology, UCLA Med Ctr 1990; **Fac Appt:** Prof Med, UCLA

Snyder, David S MD [Hem] - **Spec Exp:** Leukemia; Bone Marrow Transplant; Myeloproliferative Disorders; **Hospital:** City of Hope Natl Med Ctr; **Address:** 1500 E Duarte Rd, rm 1003, Duarte, CA 91010-3012; **Phone:** 626-256-4673 x62691; **Board Cert:** Internal Medicine 1980; Hematology 1984; **Med School:** Harvard Med Sch 1977; **Resid:** Internal Medicine, Beth Israel Hosp 1980; **Fellow:** Immunology, Harvard Med Sch 1982; Hematology & Oncology, New England Med Ctr 1984

MEDICAL ONCOLOGY

New England

Antin, Joseph H MD [Onc] - **Spec Exp:** Bone Marrow Transplant; Stem Cell Transplant; Leukemia; **Hospital:** Brigham and Women's Hosp (page 57), Dana-Farber Cancer Inst (page 57); **Address:** The Yawkey Center, 450 Brookline Ave, Boston, MA 02215; **Phone:** 617-632-3667; **Board Cert:** Internal Medicine 1981; Medical Oncology 1983; Hematology 1984; **Med School:** Cornell Univ-Weill Med Coll 1978; **Resid:** Internal Medicine, Peter Bent Brigham Hosp 1981; **Fellow:** Hematology & Oncology, Brigham & Womens Hosp/Dana Farber 1984; **Fac Appt:** Prof Med, Harvard Med Sch

Atkins, Michael B MD [Onc] - **Spec Exp:** Melanoma; Kidney Cancer; Immunotherapy; **Hospital:** Beth Israel Deaconess Med Ctr - Boston; **Address:** Beth Israel Deaconess Med Ctr, Cancer Clinical Trials 375 Longwood Ave, Masco Bldg Fl 4 - Ste 412, Boston, MA 02215; **Phone:** 617-632-9250; **Board Cert:** Internal Medicine 1983; Medical Oncology 1987; **Med School:** Tufts Univ 1980; **Resid:** Internal Medicine, New England Med Ctr 1983; **Fellow:** Hematology & Oncology, New England Med Ctr 1987; **Fac Appt:** Prof Med, Harvard Med Sch

Birrer, Michael J MD/PhD [Onc] - **Spec Exp:** Ovarian Cancer; Clinical Trials; Gynecologic Cancer; **Hospital:** Mass Genl Hosp; **Address:** MGH Cancer Ctr, 55 Fruit St, Yawkey 9E, Boston, MA 02114; **Phone:** 617-724-4000; **Board Cert:** Internal Medicine 1985; Medical Oncology 1987; **Med School:** Albert Einstein Coll Med 1982; **Resid:** Internal Medicine, Mass GeneralHosp 1985; **Fellow:** Medical Oncology, NIH 1987; **Fac Appt:** Prof Med, Harvard Med Sch

Bubley, Glenn J MD [Onc] - **Spec Exp:** Prostate Cancer; **Hospital:** Beth Israel Deaconess Med Ctr - Boston; **Address:** Beth Israel Deaconess Med Ctr, 330 Brookline Ave, Shapiro Bldg Fl 9, Boston, MA 02215; **Phone:** 617-735-2062; **Board Cert:** Internal Medicine 1980; Medical Oncology 1983; **Med School:** Mich State Univ 1977; **Resid:** Internal Medicine, St Francis Hosp 1980; **Fellow:** Hematology & Oncology, Beth Israel Deaconess Med Ctr 1983; **Fac Appt:** Assoc Prof Med, Harvard Med Sch

Burstein, Harold J MD [Onc] - **Spec Exp:** Breast Cancer; **Hospital:** Dana-Farber Cancer Inst (page 57), Brigham and Women's Hosp (page 57); **Address:** 450 Brookline Ave Yawkey Bldg Fl 12, Boston, MA 02215; **Phone:** 617-632-4587; **Board Cert:** Medical Oncology 2000; **Med School:** Harvard Med Sch 1994; **Resid:** Internal Medicine, Mass Genl Hosp 1997; **Fellow:** Medical Oncology, Dana Farber Cancer Inst 2000; **Fac Appt:** Assoc Prof Med, Harvard Med Sch

Canellos, George P MD [Onc] - **Spec Exp:** Lymphoma-Second Opinion; Hodgkin's Disease-Second Opinion; **Hospital:** Dana-Farber Cancer Inst (page 57), Brigham and Women's Hosp (page 57); **Address:** Dana Farber Cancer Inst, 44 Binney St, Dana 1B14, Boston, MA 02115; **Phone:** 617-632-3470; **Board Cert:** Internal Medicine 1967; Hematology 1972; Medical Oncology 1973; **Med School:** Columbia P&S 1960; **Resid:** Internal Medicine, Mass Genl Hosp 1963; Internal Medicine, Mass Genl Hosp 1966; **Fellow:** Medical Oncology, Natl Cancer Inst 1965; Hematology, Royal Post Graduate Sch of Med 1967; **Fac Appt:** Prof Med, Harvard Med Sch

Cannistra, Stephen A MD [Onc] - **Spec Exp:** Gynecologic Cancer; **Hospital:** Beth Israel Deaconess Med Ctr - Boston, Dana-Farber Cancer Inst (page 57); **Address:** Beth Israel Deaconess Med Ctr, 330 Brookline Ave, KS 158, Boston, MA 02215; **Phone:** 617-667-1909; **Board Cert:** Internal Medicine 1982; Medical Oncology 1985; **Med School:** Brown Univ 1979; **Resid:** Internal Medicine, Johns Hopkins Hosp 1982; **Fellow:** Medical Oncology, Dana-Farber Cancer Inst 1985; **Fac Appt:** Prof Med, Harvard Med Sch

Chabner, Bruce A MD [Onc] - **Spec Exp:** Breast Cancer; Colon & Rectal Cancer; **Hospital:** Mass Genl Hosp; **Address:** Mass General Hospital, 55 Fruit St, Lawrence House 214, Boston, MA 02114; **Phone:** 617-724-3200; **Board Cert:** Internal Medicine 1971; Medical Oncology 1973; **Med School:** Harvard Med Sch 1965; **Resid:** Internal Medicine, Peter Bent Brigham Hosp 1967; Internal Medicine, Yale-New Haven Hosp 1970; **Fellow:** Medical Oncology, Natl Inst Hlth 1969; **Fac Appt:** Prof Med, Harvard Med Sch

Come, Steven E MD [Onc] - **Spec Exp:** Breast Cancer; Hodgkin's Disease; **Hospital:** Beth Israel Deaconess Med Ctr - Boston, Dana-Farber Cancer Inst (page 57); **Address:** Beth Israel Deaconess Hosp, 330 Brookline Ave, Ste CC913, Boston, MA 02215-5400; **Phone:** 617-667-4599; **Board Cert:** Internal Medicine 1975; Medical Oncology 1979; **Med School:** Harvard Med Sch 1972; **Resid:** Internal Medicine, Beth Israel Hosp 1977; **Fellow:** Medical Oncology, Natl Cancer Inst 1976; **Fac Appt:** Assoc Prof Med, Harvard Med Sch

Demetri, George D MD [Onc] - **Spec Exp:** Sarcoma; Bone Tumors; **Hospital:** Dana-Farber Cancer Inst (page 57); **Address:** Dana Farber Cancer Inst, 450 Brookline Ave, MS Dana 1212, Boston, MA 02215; **Phone:** 617-632-3985; **Board Cert:** Internal Medicine 1986; Medical Oncology 1989; **Med School:** Stanford Univ 1983; **Resid:** Internal Medicine, Univ Wash Med Ctr 1986; **Fellow:** Medical Oncology, Dana Farber Cancer Inst 1989; **Fac Appt:** Assoc Prof Med, Harvard Med Sch

DeVita Jr, Vincent T MD [Onc] - **Spec Exp:** Lymphoma Consultation; Hodgkin's Disease Consultation; **Hospital:** Yale-New Haven Hosp, Yale Med Group; **Address:** Yale Cancer Ctr, 333 Cedar St, rm FMP117, New Haven, CT 06520-8028; **Phone:** 203-737-1010; **Board Cert:** Internal Medicine 1974; Hematology 1972; Medical Oncology 1973; **Med School:** Geo Wash Univ 1961; **Resid:** Internal Medicine, Geo Wash Hosp 1963; Internal Medicine, Yale-New Haven Hosp 1966; **Fellow:** Medical Oncology, Natl Cancer Inst 1965; **Fac Appt:** Prof Med, Yale Univ

Dizon, Don S MD [Onc] - **Spec Exp:** Gynecologic Cancer; Breast Cancer; **Hospital:** Women & Infants Hosp of RI; **Address:** Women & Infants Hosp, Womens Oncology Program, 101 Dudley St, Providence, RI 02905; **Phone:** 401-453-7520; **Board Cert:** Internal Medicine 2008; Medical Oncology 2002; **Med School:** Univ Rochester 1995; **Resid:** Internal Medicine, Yale-New Haven Hosp 1998; **Fellow:** Oncology, Meml Sloan Kettering Cancer Ctr 2001; **Fac Appt:** Assoc Prof Med, Brown Univ

Erban III, John K MD [Onc] - **Spec Exp:** Breast Cancer; Hematologic Malignancies; Stem Cell Transplant; **Hospital:** Tufts Med Ctr; **Address:** Tuffs Med Cancer Ctr, 800 Washington St, Mailbox 5609, Boston, MA 02111; **Phone:** 617-636-5782; **Board Cert:** Internal Medicine 1984; Medical Oncology 1989; Hematology 1999; **Med School:** Tufts Univ 1981; **Resid:** Internal Medicine, Hosp Univ Penn 1984; **Fellow:** Hematology & Oncology, New England Med Ctr 1990; **Fac Appt:** Assoc Prof Med, Tufts Univ

Ernstoff, Marc Stuart MD [Onc] - **Spec Exp:** Melanoma; Genitourinary Cancer; Skin Cancer; **Hospital:** Dartmouth - Hitchcock Med Ctr; **Address:** 1 Medical Center Drive, Lebanon, NH 03756; **Phone:** 603-650-5534; **Board Cert:** Internal Medicine 1981; Medical Oncology 1989; **Med School:** NYU Sch Med 1978; **Resid:** Internal Medicine, Albert Einstein Coll Med 1981; **Fellow:** Medical Oncology, Yale Univ Affil Hosp 1984; **Fac Appt:** Prof Med, Dartmouth Med Sch

Flaherty, Keith T MD [Onc] - **Spec Exp:** Melanoma-Advanced; Clinical Trials; **Hospital:** Mass Genl Hosp; **Address:** Massachusetts Genl Cancer Ctr, 32 Fruit St, Yawkey 9E, Boston, MA 02114; **Phone:** 617-724-4800; **Board Cert:** Internal Medicine 2000; Medical Oncology 2003; **Med School:** Johns Hopkins Univ 1997; **Resid:** Internal Medicine, Brigham & Women's Hosp 2000; **Fellow:** Hematology & Oncology, Hosp Univ Penn 2002

Medical Oncology

Foss, Francine M MD [Onc] - **Spec Exp:** Lymphoma, Cutaneous T Cell (CTCL); Stem Cell Transplant; Graft vs Host Disease; Multiple Myeloma; **Hospital:** Yale-New Haven Hosp, Yale Med Group; **Address:** Yale Cancer Ctr, 333 Cedar St, Box 208032, New Haven, CT 06520-8032; **Phone:** 203-737-5312; **Board Cert:** Internal Medicine 1985; Medical Oncology 1987; **Med School:** Univ Mass Sch Med 1982; **Resid:** Internal Medicine, Brigham & Womens Hosp 1985; **Fellow:** Medical Oncology, Natl Cancer Inst 1988; **Fac Appt:** Prof Med, Yale Univ

Freedman, Arnold S MD [Onc] - **Spec Exp:** Lymphoma; Bone Marrow Transplant; Stem Cell Transplant; **Hospital:** Brigham and Women's Hosp (page 57), Dana-Farber Cancer Inst (page 57); **Address:** Dana-Farber Cancer Inst, 44 Binney St, Ste Dana-1B, Boston, MA 02115; **Phone:** 617-632-3441; **Board Cert:** Internal Medicine 1982; Medical Oncology 1985; **Med School:** Univ Mass Sch Med 1979; **Resid:** Internal Medicine, Memorial Hosp 1982; **Fellow:** Medical Oncology, Dana Farber Cancer Inst 1985; **Fac Appt:** Assoc Prof Med, Harvard Med Sch

Fuchs, Charles S MD [Onc] - **Spec Exp:** Gastrointestinal Cancer; Esophageal Cancer; **Hospital:** Dana-Farber Cancer Inst (page 57), Brigham and Women's Hosp (page 57); **Address:** Dana Farber Cancer Inst, 450 Brookline Ave, Boston, MA 02215; **Phone:** 617-632-5840; **Board Cert:** Internal Medicine 1989; Medical Oncology 2002; **Med School:** Harvard Med Sch 1986; **Resid:** Internal Medicine, Brigham & Womens Hosp 1989; **Fellow:** Hematology & Oncology, Dana Farber Cancer Inst 1992; **Fac Appt:** Assoc Prof Med, Harvard Med Sch

Garber, Judy E MD [Onc] - **Spec Exp:** Breast Cancer; Breast Cancer Genetics; Cancer Risk Assessment; **Hospital:** Dana-Farber Cancer Inst (page 57), Brigham and Women's Hosp (page 57); **Address:** Dana Farber Cancer Inst, 44 Binney St, Mayer 2 Fl 9, Boston, MA 02115; **Phone:** 617-632-5961; **Board Cert:** Internal Medicine 1984; Medical Oncology 1987; Hematology 1988; **Med School:** Yale Univ 1981; **Resid:** Internal Medicine, Brigham & Womens Hosp 1984; **Fellow:** Hematology & Oncology, Brigham & Womens Hosp/Dana Farber Cancer Inst 1988; Cancer Epidemiology, Dana Farber Cancer Inst 1990; **Fac Appt:** Assoc Prof Med, Harvard Med Sch

Garnick, Marc B MD [Onc] - **Spec Exp:** Prostate Cancer; Urologic Cancer; **Hospital:** Beth Israel Deaconess Med Ctr - Boston; **Address:** Beth Israel Deaconess Med Ctr, SCC9, 330 Brookline Ave, Boston, MA 02215; **Phone:** 617-735-2062; **Board Cert:** Internal Medicine 1976; Medical Oncology 1979; **Med School:** Univ Pennsylvania 1972; **Resid:** Internal Medicine, Hosp Univ Penn 1974; **Fellow:** Research, Natl Inst Hlth 1976; Medical Oncology, Dana-Farber Cancer Inst 1978; **Fac Appt:** Clin Prof Med, Harvard Med Sch

Grunberg, Steven M MD [Onc] - **Spec Exp:** Lung Cancer; Head & Neck Cancer; Thyroid Cancer; Cancer Risk Assessment; **Hospital:** Fletcher Allen Health Care- Med Ctr Campus; **Address:** FAHC Division of Hematology/Oncology, 89 Beaumont Ave, Given Bldg, E214, Burlington, VT 05405; **Phone:** 802-847-8400; **Board Cert:** Internal Medicine 1978; Medical Oncology 1983; **Med School:** Cornell Univ-Weill Med Coll 1975; **Resid:** Internal Medicine, Mofitt Hosp-U Calif 1978; **Fellow:** Medical Oncology, Sidney Farber Cancer Ctr 1981; **Fac Appt:** Prof Hem & Onc, Univ VT Coll Med

Hammond, Denis B MD [Onc] - **Spec Exp:** Breast Cancer; Prostate Cancer; **Hospital:** Elliot Hosp, Catholic Med Ctr; **Address:** NH Oncology, 200 Technology Drive, Hooksett, NH 03106; **Phone:** 603-622-6484; **Board Cert:** Internal Medicine 1977; Hematology 1978; **Med School:** Tufts Univ 1973; **Resid:** Internal Medicine, SUNY Buffalo Affil Hosps 1976; **Fellow:** Hematology, Mass Genl Hosp 1977; Medical Oncology, Dartmouth Med Sch 1978

Herbst, Roy S MD/PhD [Onc] - **Spec Exp:** Lung Cancer; Head & Neck Cancer; Breast Cancer; Drug Development; **Hospital:** Yale-New Haven Hosp; **Address:** Yale Cancer Ctr, 333 Cedar St, rm WWW-221, New Haven, CT 06520; **Phone:** 203-785-6879; **Board Cert:** Medical Oncology 2007; **Med School:** Cornell Univ-Weill Med Coll 1991; **Resid:** Internal Medicine, Brigham & Women's Hosp 1994; **Fellow:** Medical Oncology, Dana Farber Cancer Inst 1996; **Fac Appt:** Assoc Prof Med, Univ Tex, Houston

Hochberg, Ephraim P MD [Onc] - **Spec Exp:** Lymphoma; Hodgkin's Disease; Lymphomatoid Granulomatosis; **Hospital:** Mass Genl Hosp; **Address:** 55 Fruit St, YAW 7B, Boston, MA 02114; **Phone:** 617-724-4000; **Board Cert:** Medical Oncology 2002; Hematology 2004; **Med School:** Case West Res Univ 1996; **Resid:** Internal Medicine, Brigham & Women's Hosp 1999; **Fellow:** Hematology & Oncology, Dana Farber Cancer Inst 2002

Hochster, Howard S MD [Onc] - **Spec Exp:** Gastrointestinal Cancer; Gynecologic Cancer; Colon & Rectal Cancer; **Hospital:** Yale-New Haven Hosp, Yale Med Group; **Address:** Smilow Cancer Center, 333 Cedar St, Box 208028, New Haven, CT 06520-8028; **Phone:** 203-785-4191; **Board Cert:** Internal Medicine 1983; Medical Oncology 1985; Hematology 1986; **Med School:** Yale Univ 1980; **Resid:** Internal Medicine, NYU Med Ctr 1983; **Fellow:** Hematology & Oncology, NYU Med Ctr 1985; Medical Oncology, Jules Bordet Inst 1986; **Fac Appt:** Prof Med, Yale Univ

Hollister Jr, Dickerman MD [Onc] - **Spec Exp:** Breast Cancer; Lung Cancer; Colon Cancer; Leukemia & Lymphoma; **Hospital:** Greenwich Hosp; **Address:** 77 Lafayette Pl, Ste 260, Greenwich, CT 06830; **Phone:** 203-863-3737; **Board Cert:** Internal Medicine 1978; Hematology 1980; Medical Oncology 1981; **Med School:** Univ VA Sch Med 1975; **Resid:** Internal Medicine, NY Hosp-Cornell Med Ctr 1978; **Fellow:** Hematology & Oncology, NY Hosp-Cornell Med Ctr 1981; **Fac Appt:** Asst Clin Prof Med, Yale Univ

Johnson, Bruce E MD [Onc] - **Spec Exp:** Lung Cancer; Thoracic Cancers; Merkel Cell Carcinoma; Mesothelioma; **Hospital:** Dana-Farber Cancer Inst (page 57), Brigham and Women's Hosp (page 57); **Address:** Dana Farber Cancer Inst, 450 Brookline Ave, Ste 1234, Boston, MA 02215; **Phone:** 617-632-4790; **Board Cert:** Internal Medicine 1982; Medical Oncology 1985; **Med School:** Univ Minn 1979; **Resid:** Internal Medicine, Univ Chicago Hosps 1982; **Fellow:** Medical Oncology, Natl Cancer Inst 1985; **Fac Appt:** Prof Med, Harvard Med Sch

Kantoff, Philip W MD [Onc] - **Spec Exp:** Genitourinary Cancer; Prostate Cancer; Testicular Cancer; **Hospital:** Dana-Farber Cancer Inst (page 57), Brigham and Women's Hosp (page 57); **Address:** Dana Farber Cancer Inst, 450 Brookline Ave, Boston, MA 02215; **Phone:** 617-632-1914; **Board Cert:** Internal Medicine 1982; Medical Oncology 1989; **Med School:** Brown Univ 1979; **Resid:** Internal Medicine, NYU/Bellevue Hosp 1982; **Fellow:** Gene Therapy Research, NIH 1986; Hematology & Oncology, NIH/Dana Farber 1986; **Fac Appt:** Prof Med, Harvard Med Sch

Kaufman, Peter A MD [Onc] - **Spec Exp:** Breast Cancer; Clinical Trials; **Hospital:** Dartmouth - Hitchcock Med Ctr; **Address:** DHMC, Dept Hem-Onc, One Medical Center Drive, Lebanon, NH 03756; **Phone:** 603-653-6181; **Board Cert:** Internal Medicine 1986; Medical Oncology 1989; **Med School:** NYU Sch Med 1983; **Resid:** Internal Medicine, Duke Univ Med Ctr 1986; **Fellow:** Hematology & Oncology, Duke Univ Med Ctr 1989; **Fac Appt:** Assoc Prof Med, Dartmouth Med Sch

Lacy, Jill MD [Onc] - **Spec Exp:** Colon & Rectal Cancer; Brain Tumors; Gastrointestinal Cancer; Pancreatic Cancer; **Hospital:** Yale-New Haven Hosp, Yale Med Group; **Address:** Yale Univ Sch Med-Div Medical Oncology, 333 Cedar St, PO Box 208032, New Haven, CT 06520-8032; **Phone:** 203-785-4191; **Board Cert:** Internal Medicine 1982; Medical Oncology 2005; **Med School:** Yale Univ 1978; **Resid:** Internal Medicine, Yale-New Haven Hosp 1981; **Fellow:** Medical Oncology, Yale-New Haven Hosp 1985; **Fac Appt:** Assoc Prof Med, Yale Univ

Medical Oncology

Legare, Robert D MD [Onc] - **Spec Exp:** Breast Cancer; Breast Cancer Risk Assessment; **Hospital:** Women & Infants Hosp of RI; **Address:** Women & Infants Hosp, 101 Dudeley St Fl 2, Providence, RI 02905; **Phone:** 401-453-7520; **Board Cert:** Internal Medicine 2005; Hematology 2006; Medical Oncology 2008; **Med School:** Tufts Univ 1990; **Resid:** Internal Medicine, Yale-New Haven Hosp 1992; **Fellow:** Hematology & Oncology, Brigham & Women's Hosp 1996; **Fac Appt:** Asst Prof Med, Brown Univ

Lynch Jr, Thomas J MD [Onc] - **Spec Exp:** Lung Cancer; Thoracic Cancers; **Hospital:** Yale-New Haven Hosp, Yale Med Group; **Address:** Smilow Cancer Hosp, 333 Cedar St, Office WWW 205, New Haven, CT 06510; **Phone:** 203-688-5864; **Board Cert:** Internal Medicine 1989; Medical Oncology 2003; **Med School:** Yale Univ 1986; **Resid:** Internal Medicine, Mass Genl Hosp 1989; **Fellow:** Medical Oncology, Dana-Farber Cancer Inst 1991; **Fac Appt:** Assoc Prof Med, Yale Univ

Mathew, Paul MD [Onc] - **Spec Exp:** Prostate Cancer; Genitourinary Cancer; **Hospital:** Tufts Med Ctr; **Address:** Tufts Med Ctr, Dept Medicine, 800 Washington St, Box 245, Boston, MA 02111; **Phone:** 617-636-8483; **Board Cert:** Internal Medicine 2000; Medical Oncology 2003; Hematology 2004; **Med School:** Nigeria 1985; **Resid:** Internal Medicine, Cook Co Hosp 1990; **Fellow:** Hematology & Oncology, Mayo Clinic 1994; **Fac Appt:** Assoc Prof Med, Boston Univ

Matulonis, Ursula A MD [Onc] - **Spec Exp:** Gynecologic Cancer; Ovarian Cancer; Breast Cancer; Fertility Preservation in Cancer; **Hospital:** Dana-Farber Cancer Inst (page 57); **Address:** Dana Farber Cancer Inst, 450 Brookline Ave, Boston, MA 02215; **Phone:** 617-632-2334; **Board Cert:** Internal Medicine 2000; Medical Oncology 2000; **Med School:** Albany Med Coll 1987; **Resid:** Internal Medicine, Univ Pittsburgh Med Ctr 1990; **Fellow:** Medical Oncology, Dana Farber Cancer Inst 1993; **Fac Appt:** Assoc Prof Med, Harvard Med Sch

Nadler, Lee M MD [Onc] - **Spec Exp:** Lymphoma; **Hospital:** Dana-Farber Cancer Inst (page 57), Brigham and Women's Hosp (page 57); **Address:** Dana Farber Cancer Inst, 450 Brookline Ave, MS Smith 339, Boston, MA 02215; **Phone:** 617-632-3331; **Board Cert:** Internal Medicine 1976; **Med School:** Harvard Med Sch 1973; **Resid:** Internal Medicine, Columbia-Presby Hosp 1975; **Fellow:** Tumor Immunology, Natl Cancer Inst 1977; Medical Oncology, Dana-Farber Cancer Inst 1978; **Fac Appt:** Prof Med, Harvard Med Sch

Ryan, David MD [Onc] - **Spec Exp:** Colon Cancer; Pancreatic Cancer; Gastrointestinal Cancer; **Hospital:** Mass Genl Hosp; **Address:** MGH Cancer Ctr, 55 Fruit St, YAW 7B, Boston, MA 02114; **Phone:** 617-724-4000; **Board Cert:** Medical Oncology 2009; **Med School:** Columbia P&S 1992; **Resid:** Internal Medicine, Columbia Presby Med Ctr 1996; **Fellow:** Hematology & Oncology, Mass Genl Hosp 1998; **Fac Appt:** Asst Prof Med, Harvard Med Sch

Schnipper, Lowell E MD [Onc] - **Spec Exp:** Breast Cancer; Lymphoma; **Hospital:** Beth Israel Deaconess Med Ctr - Boston; **Address:** Beth Israel Deaconess Med Ctr, 330 Brookline Ave, RABB 430, Boston, MA 02215; **Phone:** 617-667-1198; **Board Cert:** Internal Medicine 1973; Medical Oncology 1983; **Med School:** SUNY Downstate 1968; **Resid:** Internal Medicine, Yale-New Haven Hosp 1970; Medical Oncology, Natl Cancer Inst 1973; **Fellow:** Hematology & Oncology, Barnes Jewish Hosp 1974; **Fac Appt:** Prof Med, Harvard Med Sch

Selvaggi, Kathy J MD [Onc] - **Spec Exp:** Palliative Care; Pain-Cancer; **Hospital:** Dana-Farber Cancer Inst (page 57); **Address:** Dana Farber Cancer Inst, 450 Brookline Ave, MC SW 411, Boston, MA 02215; **Phone:** 617-632-6464; **Board Cert:** Internal Medicine 1989; Medical Oncology 2005; Hospice & Palliative Medicine 2008; **Med School:** Penn State Coll Med 1985; **Resid:** Internal Medicine, UPMC Shadyside Hosp 1989; **Fellow:** Medical Oncology, UPMC Shadyside Hosp 1992

Shulman, Lawrence N MD [Onc] - **Spec Exp:** Breast Cancer; **Hospital:** Dana-Farber Cancer Inst (page 57), Brigham and Women's Hosp (page 57); **Address:** Dana-Farber Cancer Inst, 450 Brookline Ave, MS Dana-1608, Boston, MA 02215; **Phone:** 617-632-2277; **Board Cert:** Internal Medicine 1978; Medical Oncology 1981; Hematology 1982; **Med School:** Harvard Med Sch 1975; **Resid:** Internal Medicine, Beth Israel Hosp 1977; **Fellow:** Hematology & Oncology, Beth Israel Hosp 1980; **Fac Appt:** Assoc Prof Med, Harvard Med Sch

Smith, Matthew R MD/PhD [Onc] - **Spec Exp:** Prostate Cancer; **Hospital:** Mass Genl Hosp; **Address:** Mass Genl Hosp, Hematology/Oncology, 55 Fruit St, Yawkey 7E, Boston, MA 02114; **Phone:** 617-724-5257; **Board Cert:** Medical Oncology 2007; **Med School:** Duke Univ 1992; **Resid:** Internal Medicine, Brigham & Women's Hosp 1994; **Fellow:** Medical Oncology, Dana Farber Cancer Inst 1997; **Fac Appt:** Assoc Prof Med, Harvard Med Sch

Soiffer, Robert J MD [Onc] - **Spec Exp:** Stem Cell Transplant; Bone Marrow Transplant; Leukemia; Lymphoma; **Hospital:** Dana-Farber Cancer Inst (page 57), Brigham and Women's Hosp (page 57); **Address:** Dana-Farber Cancer Inst, 450 Brookline Ave, rm D1B09, Boston, MA 02115; **Phone:** 617-632-4711; **Board Cert:** Internal Medicine 1986; Medical Oncology 1989; **Med School:** NYU Sch Med 1983; **Resid:** Internal Medicine, Brigham & Women's Hosp 1986; **Fellow:** Medical Oncology, Brigham & Women's Hosp 1989; **Fac Appt:** Prof Med, Harvard Med Sch

Strauss, Gary M MD [Onc] - **Spec Exp:** Lung Cancer; Thoracic Cancers; Melanoma; Breast Cancer; **Hospital:** Tufts Med Ctr; **Address:** Tufts Medical Ctr, Div of Hem/Onc, 800 Washington St, Box 245, Boston, MA 02111; **Phone:** 617-636-5627; **Board Cert:** Internal Medicine 1975; Medical Oncology 1979; Hematology 1980; **Med School:** Yale Univ 1972; **Resid:** Internal Medicine, Boston City Hosp 1974; Internal Medicine, Mass Genl Hosp 1977; **Fellow:** Medical Oncology, Natl Cancer Inst 1976; Hematology & Oncology, Mass General Hosp 1979; **Fac Appt:** Prof Med, Tufts Univ

Strenger, Rochelle MD [Onc] - **Spec Exp:** Breast Cancer; Hematologic Malignancies; Lymphoma; **Hospital:** Miriam Hosp; **Address:** University Medicine, Comprehensive Cancer Center, 164 Summit Ave Fain 3, Providence, RI 02906; **Phone:** 401-793-2920; **Board Cert:** Internal Medicine 1986; Medical Oncology 2009; **Med School:** Albert Einstein Coll Med 1982; **Resid:** Internal Medicine, Brigham & Women's Hosp 1985; **Fellow:** Hematology & Oncology, Brigham & Women's Hosp 1988

Sweeney, Christopher J MD [Onc] - **Spec Exp:** Genitourinary Cancer; Prostate Cancer; Testicular Cancer; **Hospital:** Dana-Farber Cancer Inst (page 57); **Address:** Dana Farber Cancer Inst, 450 Brookline Ave, Ste D-1230, Boston, MA 02215; **Phone:** 617-632-5929; **Board Cert:** Medical Oncology 2000; **Med School:** Australia 1993; **Resid:** Internal Medicine, Gundersen Lutheran Med Ctr 1997; **Fellow:** Hematology & Oncology, Indiana Univ Med Ctr 2000

Taplin, Mary-Ellen MD [Onc] - **Spec Exp:** Prostate Cancer; Genitourinary Cancer; **Hospital:** Dana-Farber Cancer Inst (page 57), Brigham and Women's Hosp (page 57); **Address:** Dana Farber Cancer Inst, 450 Brookline Ave, MS D1230, Boston, MA 02215; **Phone:** 617-632-3237; **Board Cert:** Internal Medicine 1989; Hematology 2006; Medical Oncology 2003; **Med School:** Univ Mass Sch Med 1986; **Resid:** Internal Medicine, Univ Mass Med Ctr 1990; **Fellow:** Hematology & Oncology, Beth Israel Deaconess Med Ctr 1993; **Fac Appt:** Assoc Prof Med

Treon, Steven P MD/PhD [Onc] - **Spec Exp:** Waldenstrom's Macroglobulinemia; Multiple Myeloma; **Hospital:** Dana-Farber Cancer Inst (page 57); **Address:** Dana-Farber Cancer Inst, 450 Brookline Ave, MS LG 102, Boston, MA 02115; **Phone:** 617-632-2681; **Med School:** Boston Univ 1993; **Resid:** Internal Medicine, Boston Univ Med Ctr 1995; **Fellow:** Hematology & Oncology, Mass Genl Hosp 1996; Research, Dana Farber Cancer Inst 1997; **Fac Appt:** Assoc Prof Med, Harvard Med Sch

Medical Oncology

Verschraegen, Claire F MD [Onc] - **Spec Exp:** Ovarian Cancer; Drug Discovery; Mesothelioma; **Hospital:** Fletcher Allen Health Care- Med Ctr Campus; **Address:** Univ Vermont, Hematology/Oncology, Gven E-214, UVM363, 89 Beaumont Ave, Burlington, VT 05405; **Phone:** 802-656-5487; **Board Cert:** Internal Medicine 2000; Medical Oncology 2000; **Med School:** Belgium 1982; **Resid:** Internal Medicine, Bordet 1985; Internal Medicine, Univ Texas 1991; **Fellow:** Cancer Research, Stehlin Fdn for Cancer Research 1988; Oncology, MD Anderson Cancer Ctr 1994; **Fac Appt:** Prof Med, Univ VT Coll Med

Weisberg, Tracey MD [Onc] - **Spec Exp:** Breast Cancer; **Hospital:** Maine Med Ctr; **Address:** 100 Campus Drive, Unit 108, Scarborough, ME 04074; **Phone:** 207-885-7600; **Board Cert:** Internal Medicine 1987; Medical Oncology 1989; **Med School:** SUNY Stony Brook 1983; **Resid:** Internal Medicine, Mount Sinai Hosp 1985; Internal Medicine, Hartford Hosp 1986; **Fellow:** Medical Oncology, Yale Univ Hosp 1988

Winer, Eric P MD [Onc] - **Spec Exp:** Breast Cancer; **Hospital:** Dana-Farber Cancer Inst (page 57), Brigham and Women's Hosp (page 57); **Address:** Dana Farber Cancer Inst, 450 Brookline Ave, MS Mayer 228, Boston, MA 02215; **Phone:** 617-632-3800; **Board Cert:** Internal Medicine 1987; Medical Oncology 1989; **Med School:** Yale Univ 1983; **Resid:** Internal Medicine, Yale-New Haven Hosp 1987; **Fellow:** Hematology & Oncology, Duke Univ Med Ctr 1989; **Fac Appt:** Prof Med, Harvard Med Sch

Mid Atlantic

Abraham, Jame MD [Onc] - **Spec Exp:** Breast Cancer; **Hospital:** Ruby Memorial - WVU Hosp; **Address:** WVU School of Med-Hem/Onc, PO Box 9162, Morgantown, WV 26506; **Phone:** 304-293-4229; **Board Cert:** Internal Medicine 2007; Medical Oncology 2000; **Med School:** India 1991; **Resid:** Internal Medicine, Univ Conn Sch Med 1997; **Fellow:** Medical Oncology, Natl Cancer Inst 1999

Aghajanian, Carol A MD [Onc] - **Spec Exp:** Ovarian Cancer; Gynecologic Cancer; Trophoblastic Tumors; **Hospital:** Meml Sloan-Kettering Cancer Ctr; **Address:** 1275 York Ave, Ste H905, New York, NY 10065; **Phone:** 212-639-2252; **Board Cert:** Internal Medicine 2002; Medical Oncology 2005; **Med School:** SUNY Downstate 1989; **Resid:** Internal Medicine, Mt Sinai Med Ctr 1993; **Fellow:** Medical Oncology, Meml Sloan Kettering Cancer Ctr 1995; **Fac Appt:** Assoc Prof Med, Cornell Univ-Weill Med Coll

Ahlgren, James D MD [Onc] - **Spec Exp:** Gastrointestinal Cancer; Carcinoid Tumors; **Hospital:** G Washington Univ Hosp; **Address:** Geo Wash Univ Med Ctr, Div Hem/Oncology, 2150 Pennsylvania Ave NW, Ste 1-200, Washington, DC 20037-3201; **Phone:** 202-741-2478; **Board Cert:** Internal Medicine 1980; Medical Oncology 1989; **Med School:** Georgetown Univ 1977; **Resid:** Internal Medicine, Georgetown Univ Hosp 1979; **Fellow:** Medical Oncology, Georgetown Univ Hosp 1981; **Fac Appt:** Prof Med, Geo Wash Univ

Aisner, Joseph MD [Onc] - **Spec Exp:** Lung Cancer; Solid Tumors; Thymoma; Mesothelioma; **Hospital:** Robert Wood Johnson Univ Hosp - New Brunswick; **Address:** Cancer Inst of New Jersey, 195 Little Albany St, rm 2006, New Brunswick, NJ 08903-2681; **Phone:** 732-235-6777; **Board Cert:** Internal Medicine 1973; Medical Oncology 1975; **Med School:** Wayne State Univ 1970; **Resid:** Internal Medicine, Georgetown Univ Hosp 1972; **Fellow:** Medical Oncology, Natl Cancer Inst 1975; **Fac Appt:** Prof Med, UMDNJ-RW Johnson Med Sch

Algazy, Kenneth M MD [Onc] - **Spec Exp:** Lung Cancer; Mesothelioma; Hematologic Malignancies; Head & Neck Cancer; **Hospital:** Hosp Univ Penn - UPHS (page 68), VA Med Ctr - Philadelphia; **Address:** Hosp Univ Pennsylvania, 3400 Convention Ave, The Perelman Ctr Fl 2, Philadelphia, PA 19104; **Phone:** 215-615-5810; **Board Cert:** Internal Medicine 1972; Hematology 1974; Medical Oncology 1979; **Med School:** Temple Univ 1969; **Resid:** Internal Medicine, Univ Rochester-Strong Meml Hosp 1972; **Fellow:** Hematology & Oncology, Johns Hopkins Med Ctr 1974; **Fac Appt:** Clin Prof Med, Temple Univ

Ambinder, Richard F MD/PhD [Onc] - **Spec Exp:** Lymphoma; Hodgkin's Disease; AIDS Related Cancers; **Hospital:** Johns Hopkins Hosp (page 61); **Address:** Cancer Research Bldg, 1650 Orleans St, rm CRB 389, Baltimore, MD 21231; **Phone:** 410-955-8964; **Board Cert:** Internal Medicine 1982; Medical Oncology 1985; **Med School:** Johns Hopkins Univ 1979; **Resid:** Internal Medicine, Johns Hopkins Hosp 1982; Medical Oncology, Johns Hopkins Hosp 1985; **Fac Appt:** Prof Med, Johns Hopkins Univ

Argiris, Athanassios MD [Onc] - **Spec Exp:** Lung Cancer; Head & Neck Cancer; **Hospital:** UPMC Presby, Pittsburgh, UPMC Shadyside; **Address:** UPMC Presbyterian Cancer Ctr, 5115 Centre Ave Fl 2, Pittsburgh, PA 15232; **Phone:** 412-692-4724; **Board Cert:** Medical Oncology 2000; **Med School:** Greece 1990; **Resid:** Internal Medicine, Beth Israel Med Ctr 1997; **Fellow:** Medical Oncology, Yale-New Haven Hosp 2000; **Fac Appt:** Prof Med, Univ Pittsburgh

Arlen, Philip M MD [Onc] - **Spec Exp:** Prostate Cancer-Vaccine Therapy; Vaccine Therapy-Clinical Trials Only; Clinical Trials Only; **Hospital:** Natl Inst of Hlth - Clin Ctr, Natl Naval Med Ctr; **Address:** National Cancer Inst, MSC 1750, 10 Center Drive Bldg 10 - rm 5B52, Bethesda, MD 20892-1750; **Phone:** 301-496-0629; **Board Cert:** Medical Oncology 1998; **Med School:** Med Coll GA 1991; **Resid:** Internal Medicine, Georgia Baptist Hlth Care Syst 1994; **Fellow:** Hematology & Oncology, Emory Univ Med Ctr 1994; NCI/NIH 1999

Astrow, Alan MD [Onc] - **Spec Exp:** Ovarian Cancer; Breast Cancer; Lymphoma; **Hospital:** Maimonides Med Ctr (page 62); **Address:** MMC Hematology/Oncology, 6300 8th Ave, Brooklyn, NY 11220; **Phone:** 718-765-2653; **Board Cert:** Internal Medicine 1983; Hematology 1986; Medical Oncology 1987; **Med School:** Yale Univ 1980; **Resid:** Internal Medicine, Boston City Hosp 1983; **Fellow:** Hematology & Oncology, NYU Med Ctr 1986; **Fac Appt:** Assoc Clin Prof Med, NY Med Coll

Attas, Lewis MD [Onc] - **Spec Exp:** Breast Cancer; Lymphoma; Bleeding/Coagulation Disorders; Gaucher Disease; **Hospital:** Englewood Hosp & Med Ctr, Holy Name Med Ctr; **Address:** 350 Engle St, Englewood, NJ 07631; **Phone:** 201-568-5250; **Board Cert:** Internal Medicine 1985; Medical Oncology 1987; Hematology 1988; **Med School:** Mount Sinai Sch Med 1982; **Resid:** Internal Medicine, Montefiore Hosp Med Ctr 1985; **Fellow:** Hematology & Oncology, North Shore Univ Hosp 1988; **Fac Appt:** Assoc Clin Prof Med, Mount Sinai Sch Med

Axelrod, Rita S MD [Onc] - **Spec Exp:** Head & Neck Cancer; Lung Cancer; Complementary Medicine; **Hospital:** Thomas Jefferson Univ Hosp; **Address:** Thomas Jefferson Univ Hosp, 925 Chestnut St Fl 2, Philadelphia, PA 19107; **Phone:** 215-955-8874; **Board Cert:** Internal Medicine 1976; Medical Oncology 1977; Hematology 1978; **Med School:** NYU Sch Med 1970; **Resid:** Internal Medicine, Med Coll Georgia Hosps 1973; **Fellow:** Hematology & Oncology, Hosp Univ Penn 1975; **Fac Appt:** Assoc Prof Med, Thomas Jefferson Univ

Azzoli, Christopher MD [Onc] - **Spec Exp:** Lung Cancer; Lung Cancer (advanced); **Hospital:** Meml Sloan-Kettering Cancer Ctr; **Address:** 1275 York Ave, New York, NY 10065; **Phone:** 866-675-5864; **Board Cert:** Internal Medicine 2009; Medical Oncology 2001; **Med School:** Johns Hopkins Univ 1996; **Resid:** Internal Medicine, Johns Hopkins Hosp 1999; **Fellow:** Medical Oncology, Meml Sloan Kettering Cancer Ctr 2002; **Fac Appt:** Asst Prof Med, Cornell Univ-Weill Med Coll

Medical Oncology

Bajorin, Dean F MD [Onc] - **Spec Exp:** Genitourinary Cancer; Bladder Cancer; Testicular Cancer; **Hospital:** Meml Sloan-Kettering Cancer Ctr; **Address:** 1275 York Avenue, New York, NY 10065; **Phone:** 646-497-9068; **Board Cert:** Internal Medicine 1981; Medical Oncology 1985; **Med School:** NY Med Coll 1978; **Resid:** Internal Medicine, Hartford Hosp 1981; **Fellow:** Medical Oncology, Meml Sloan Kettering Ctr 1986; **Fac Appt:** Prof Med, Cornell Univ-Weill Med Coll

Bashevkin, Michael MD [Onc] - **Spec Exp:** Solid Tumors; Bleeding/Coagulation Disorders; Hematologic Malignancies; **Hospital:** Maimonides Med Ctr (page 62); **Address:** 1660 E 14st St, Ste 501, Brooklyn, NY 11229; **Phone:** 718-382-8500 x501; **Board Cert:** Internal Medicine 1976; Hematology 1978; Medical Oncology 1979; **Med School:** SUNY Downstate 1973; **Resid:** Internal Medicine, VA Med Ctr 1976; Hematology & Oncology, Maimonides Med Ctr 1979

Belani, Chandra P MD [Onc] - **Spec Exp:** Lung Cancer; Drug Discovery; **Hospital:** Penn State Milton S Hershey Med Ctr; **Address:** Penn State Hershey Cancer Inst, 500 University Drive, MC CH72, Hershey, PA 17033; **Phone:** 717-531-1078; **Board Cert:** Internal Medicine 1986; Medical Oncology 1987; **Med School:** India 1978; **Resid:** Internal Medicine, SMS Med Hosp 1981; Internal Medicine, Good Samaritan/Univ MD Hosps 1984; **Fellow:** Hematology & Oncology, Univ Maryland Hosp 1987; **Fac Appt:** Prof Med

Biggs, David D MD [Onc] - **Spec Exp:** Breast Cancer; Kidney Cancer; Melanoma; Skin Cancer; **Hospital:** Christiana Hospital; **Address:** Hem/Med Onc Consultants, 4701 Ogletown-Stanton Rd, Ste 3400, Newark, DE 19713; **Phone:** 302-366-1200; **Board Cert:** Internal Medicine 1988; Hematology 2002; Medical Oncology 2001; **Med School:** Univ Kansas 1984; **Resid:** Internal Medicine, Med Coll Wisconsin 1989; **Fellow:** Hematology & Oncology, Hosp Univ Penn 1991; **Fac Appt:** Asst Clin Prof Med

Bosl, George MD [Onc] - **Spec Exp:** Testicular Cancer; **Hospital:** Meml Sloan-Kettering Cancer Ctr; **Address:** 1275 York Avenue, New York, NY 10065; **Phone:** 212-639-8473; **Board Cert:** Internal Medicine 1976; Medical Oncology 1979; **Med School:** Creighton Univ 1973; **Resid:** Internal Medicine, NY Hosp 1975; Internal Medicine, Meml Sloan-Kettering Cancer Ctr 1977; **Fellow:** Medical Oncology, Univ Minn Hosps 1979; **Fac Appt:** Prof Med, Cornell Univ-Weill Med Coll

Brufsky, Adam M MD/PhD [Onc] - **Spec Exp:** Breast Cancer; **Hospital:** Magee-Womens Hosp - UPMC, UPMC Presby, Pittsburgh; **Address:** Univ Pitt Cancer Inst/Magee-Women's Hosp, 300 Halket St, Ste 4628, MS 15213, Pittsburgh, PA 15213; **Phone:** 412-641-6500; **Board Cert:** Internal Medicine 2004; Medical Oncology 2005; **Med School:** Univ Conn 1990; **Resid:** Internal Medicine, Brigham & Womens Hosp 1992; **Fellow:** Medical Oncology, Dana Farber Cancer Inst 1995; Bone Marrow Transplant, Dana Farber Cancer Inst 1993; **Fac Appt:** Prof Med, Univ Pittsburgh

Carabasi, Matthew H MD [Onc] - **Spec Exp:** Bone Marrow Transplant; Stem Cell Transplant; **Hospital:** Thomas Jefferson Univ Hosp; **Address:** Dept Med Oncology, Thomas Jefferson Univ, 925 Chestnut St, Philadelphia, PA 19107; **Phone:** 215-955-8874; **Board Cert:** Internal Medicine 1983; Medical Oncology 1987; **Med School:** Jefferson Med Coll 1980; **Resid:** Internal Medicine, Hahnemann MC Hosp 1984; **Fellow:** Hematology & Oncology, Meml Sloan-Kettering Cancer Ctr 1988; Research, Meml Sloan-Kettering Cancer Ctr 1989; **Fac Appt:** Assoc Prof Med, Jefferson Med Coll

Carducci, Michael A MD [Onc] - **Spec Exp:** Urologic Cancer; Drug Discovery & Development; Vaccine Therapy; Clinical Trials; **Hospital:** Johns Hopkins Hosp (page 61); **Address:** Sidney Kimmel Cancer Ctr, 1650 Orleans St 1M59 BB Bldg, Baltimore, MD 21231; **Phone:** 410-614-3977; **Board Cert:** Internal Medicine 2001; Medical Oncology 2005; **Med School:** Wayne State Univ 1988; **Resid:** Internal Medicine, Univ Colorado Hlth Sci Ctr 1992; **Fellow:** Medical Oncology, Johns Hopkins Hosp 1995; **Fac Appt:** Prof Med, Johns Hopkins Univ

Celano, Paul MD [Onc] - **Spec Exp:** Gynecologic Cancer; Gastrointestinal Cancer; Breast Cancer; **Hospital:** Greater Baltimore Med Ctr; **Address:** GBMC Cancer Ctr, 6569 N Charles St, Ste 205, Baltimore, MD 21204; **Phone:** 443-849-3051; **Board Cert:** Internal Medicine 1984; Medical Oncology 1987; **Med School:** Mount Sinai Sch Med 1981; **Resid:** Internal Medicine, Thos Jefferson Univ Hosp 1984; **Fellow:** Medical Oncology, Thos Jefferson Univ Hosp 1985; **Fac Appt:** Asst Prof Med, Johns Hopkins Univ

Chachoua, Abraham MD [Onc] - **Spec Exp:** Lung Cancer; Thoracic Cancers; **Hospital:** NYU Langone Med Ctr (page 66); **Address:** NYU Clinical Cancer Ctr, 160 E 34th St Fl 8, New York, NY 10016; **Phone:** 212-731-5388; **Med School:** Australia 1978; **Resid:** Internal Medicine, Alfred Hosp 1982; **Fellow:** Hematology & Oncology, Alfred Hosp 1985; Hematology & Oncology, NYU Med Ctr 1988; **Fac Appt:** Assoc Prof Med, NYU Sch Med

Chanan-Khan, Asher A MD [Onc] - **Spec Exp:** Multiple Myeloma; Leukemia-Chronic Lymphocytic; **Hospital:** Roswell Park Cancer Inst; **Address:** Roswell Park Cancer Inst, Elm & Carlton Sts, Buffalo, NY 14263; **Phone:** 716-845-3221; **Board Cert:** Medical Oncology 2001; Hematology 2004; **Med School:** Pakistan 1993; **Resid:** Internal Medicine, Harlem Hosp Ctr 1997; **Fellow:** Hematology & Oncology, NYU Med Ctr 1999; **Fac Appt:** Asst Prof Med, SUNY Buffalo

Chapman, Paul B MD [Onc] - **Spec Exp:** Melanoma; Immunotherapy; Clinical Trials; Vaccine Therapy; **Hospital:** Meml Sloan-Kettering Cancer Ctr; **Address:** 1275 York Avenue, New York, NY 10065; **Phone:** 646-888-2378; **Board Cert:** Internal Medicine 1984; Medical Oncology 1987; **Med School:** Cornell Univ-Weill Med Coll 1981; **Resid:** Internal Medicine, Univ Chicago Hosps 1984; **Fellow:** Medical Oncology, Meml Sloan-Kettering Cancer Ctr 1987; **Fac Appt:** Prof Med, Cornell Univ-Weill Med Coll

Chu, Edward MD [Onc] - **Spec Exp:** Colon & Rectal Cancer; Gastrointestinal Cancer; Clinical Trials; **Hospital:** UPMC Shadyside, UPMC Presby, Pittsburgh; **Address:** Univ of Pittsburgh Cancer Institute, 5150 Centre Ave Fl 5 - rm 571, Pittsburgh, PA 15232; **Phone:** 412-648-6589; **Board Cert:** Internal Medicine 1986; Medical Oncology 1989; **Med School:** Brown Univ 1983; **Resid:** Internal Medicine, Roger Williams Hosp 1987; **Fellow:** Medical Oncology, Natl Cancer Inst 1992; **Fac Appt:** Prof Med, Univ Pittsburgh

Claxton, David F MD [Onc] - **Spec Exp:** Leukemia; Bone Marrow Transplant; Hematologic Malignancies; Anemia-Aplastic; **Hospital:** Penn State Milton S Hershey Med Ctr; **Address:** 500 University Drive, rm T4422, Hershey, PA 17033; **Phone:** 717-531-8678; **Board Cert:** Internal Medicine 1984; Medical Oncology 2004; **Med School:** McGill Univ 1978; **Resid:** Internal Medicine, Royal Victoria Hosp 1984; **Fellow:** Hematology, Royal Victoria Hosp 1986; Medical Oncology, UTMD Anderson Cancer Ctr 1989; **Fac Appt:** Prof Med

Cohen, Gary I MD [Onc] - **Spec Exp:** Hematologic Malignancies; Stem Cell Transplant; Melanoma; **Hospital:** Greater Baltimore Med Ctr; **Address:** GBMC Cancer Ctr, 6569 N Charles St, Ste 205, Baltimore, MD 21204; **Phone:** 443-849-3051; **Board Cert:** Internal Medicine 1978; Medical Oncology 1985; Hematology 1982; **Med School:** Univ MD Sch Med 1975; **Resid:** Internal Medicine, SUNY Health Sci Ctr 1978; **Fellow:** Hematology & Oncology, Dana Farber Cancer Ctr 1980

Cohen, Philip MD [Onc] - **Spec Exp:** Breast Cancer; **Hospital:** Georgetown Univ Hosp; **Address:** Georgetown Univ Hosp, Lombardi Cancer Ctr, 3800 Reservoir Rd NW, Washington, DC 20007; **Phone:** 202-444-2198; **Board Cert:** Internal Medicine 1973; Medical Oncology 1975; Hematology 1976; **Med School:** Harvard Med Sch 1970; **Resid:** Internal Medicine, Mass Genl Hosp 1972; **Fellow:** Medical Oncology, Natl Cancer Inst 1974; **Fac Appt:** Assoc Prof Med, Geo Wash Univ

Medical Oncology

Cohen, Roger B MD [Onc] - **Spec Exp:** Drug Discovery & Development; Clinical Trials; Thyroid Cancer; Lung Cancer; **Hospital:** Hosp Univ Penn - UPHS (page 68); **Address:** Hosp Univ Penn, 16 Penn Tower, 3400 Spruce St, Philadelphia, PA 19104; **Phone:** 215-662-4469; **Board Cert:** Internal Medicine 1986; Hematology 1986; Medical Oncology 2005; **Med School:** Harvard Med Sch 1980; **Resid:** Internal Medicine, Mt Sinai Hosp 1982; **Fellow:** Research, Sloan Kettering Cancer Inst 1985; Hematology, Mt Sinai Hosp 1986; **Fac Appt:** Prof Med, Univ Pennsylvania

Cohen, Seymour M MD [Onc] - **Spec Exp:** Breast Cancer; Melanoma; Lung Cancer; Lymphoma; **Hospital:** Mount Sinai Med Ctr (page 63); **Address:** 1150 5th Ave, New York, NY 10128; **Phone:** 212-249-9141; **Board Cert:** Internal Medicine 1971; Medical Oncology 1973; **Med School:** Univ Pittsburgh 1962; **Resid:** Internal Medicine, Montefiore Med Ctr 1964; Internal Medicine, Mount Sinai Med Ctr 1965; **Fellow:** Hematology, Mount Sinai Med Ctr 1966; Hematology & Oncology, LI Jewish Hosp 1969; **Fac Appt:** Assoc Clin Prof Med, Mount Sinai Sch Med

Coleman, Morton MD [Onc] - **Spec Exp:** Leukemia & Lymphoma; Hodgkin's Disease; Multiple Myeloma; Waldenstrom's Macroglobulinemia; **Hospital:** NY-Presby/Weill Cornell Med Ctr, NY (page 65); **Address:** 407 E 70th St, FL 3, New York, NY 10021-5302; **Phone:** 212-517-5900; **Board Cert:** Internal Medicine 1971; Hematology 1972; Medical Oncology 1973; **Med School:** Med Coll VA 1963; **Resid:** Internal Medicine, Grady Meml Hosp-Emory 1965; Internal Medicine, NY Hosp-Cornell 1968; **Fellow:** Hematology & Oncology, NY Hosp-Cornell 1970; **Fac Appt:** Clin Prof Med, Cornell Univ-Weill Med Coll

Cristofanilli, Massimo MD [Onc] - **Spec Exp:** Breast Cancer; Breast Cancer-Inflammatory; **Hospital:** Fox Chase Cancer Ctr (page 58); **Address:** Fox Chase Cancer Ctr, 333 Cottman Ave, rm C315, Philadelphia, PA 19111; **Phone:** 215-728-2570; **Board Cert:** Medical Oncology 2010; **Med School:** Italy 1986; **Resid:** Internal Medicine, Cabrini 1996; **Fellow:** Medical Oncology, MD Anderson Cancer Ctr 1998; **Fac Appt:** Prof Med, Univ Pennsylvania

Cullen, Kevin MD [Onc] - **Spec Exp:** Head & Neck Cancer; **Hospital:** Univ of MD Med Ctr; **Address:** Univ Md Greenbaum Cancer Ctr, 22 S Greene St, rm N9E22, Baltimore, MD 21201; **Phone:** 410-328-5506; **Board Cert:** Internal Medicine 1986; Medical Oncology 1989; **Med School:** Harvard Med Sch 1983; **Resid:** Internal Medicine, Beth Israel Hosp 1986; Internal Medicine, Hammersmith Hosp 1985; **Fellow:** Medical Oncology, Natl Cancer Inst 1988

Czuczman, Myron S MD [Onc] - **Spec Exp:** Hodgkin's Disease; Multiple Myeloma; Leukemia-Chronic Lymphocytic; Waldenstrom's Macroglobulinemia; **Hospital:** Roswell Park Cancer Inst, Buffalo General Hosp; **Address:** Roswell Park Cancer Inst, Elm & Carlton Sts, Buffalo, NY 14263; **Phone:** 716-845-7695; **Board Cert:** Internal Medicine 1988; **Med School:** Penn State Coll Med 1985; **Resid:** Internal Medicine, North Shore Univ Hosp 1988; **Fellow:** Hematology & Oncology, Meml Sloan-Kettering Cancer Ctr 1992; **Fac Appt:** Prof Med, SUNY Buffalo

Daly, Mary B MD/PhD [Onc] - **Spec Exp:** Breast Cancer; Breast Cancer Risk Assessment; Cancer Prevention; Ovarian Cancer Risk Assessment; **Hospital:** Fox Chase Cancer Ctr (page 58); **Address:** Fox Chase Cancer Ctr, 333 Cottman Ave, P1054, Philadelphia, PA 19111; **Phone:** 215-728-2791; **Board Cert:** Internal Medicine 1981; Medical Oncology 1983; **Med School:** Univ NC Sch Med 1978; **Resid:** Internal Medicine, Univ Texas Hlth Sci Ctr 1981; **Fellow:** Medical Oncology, Univ Texas Hlth Sci Ctr 1983; **Fac Appt:** Clin Prof Med, Temple Univ

Davidson, Nancy E MD [Onc] - **Spec Exp:** Breast Cancer; **Hospital:** UPMC Shadyside, Magee-Womens Hosp - UPMC; **Address:** Univ Pittsburgh Cancer Inst, 5150 Centre Ave, Ste 500, Pittsburgh, PA 15232; **Phone:** 412-623-3205; **Board Cert:** Internal Medicine 1982; Medical Oncology 1985; **Med School:** Harvard Med Sch 1979; **Resid:** Internal Medicine, Johns Hopkins Hosp 1982; **Fellow:** Medical Oncology, Natl Cancer Inst 1986; **Fac Appt:** Prof Med, Univ Pittsburgh

Dawson, Nancy MD [Onc] - **Spec Exp:** Prostate Cancer; Kidney Cancer; Bladder Cancer; **Hospital:** Georgetown Univ Hosp; **Address:** Lombardi Cancer Ctr, Georgetown Univ Hosp, 3800 Reservoir Rd NW, Washington, DC 20007; **Phone:** 202-444-9094; **Board Cert:** Internal Medicine 1982; Hematology 1984; Medical Oncology 1985; **Med School:** Georgetown Univ 1979; **Resid:** Internal Medicine, Walter Reed AMC 1982; **Fellow:** Hematology & Oncology, Walter Reed AMC 1985; **Fac Appt:** Prof Med, Georgetown Univ

Dickler, Maura MD [Onc] - **Spec Exp:** Breast Cancer; **Hospital:** Meml Sloan-Kettering Cancer Ctr; **Address:** 1275 York Ave, New York, NY 10065; **Phone:** 646-497-9064; **Board Cert:** Medical Oncology 2008; **Med School:** Univ Chicago-Pritzker Sch Med 1991; **Resid:** Internal Medicine, Univ Chicago Hosps 1994; **Fellow:** Medical Oncology, Meml Sloan Kettering Cancer Ctr 1998; **Fac Appt:** Assoc Prof Med, Cornell Univ-Weill Med Coll

DiPaola, Robert S MD [Onc] - **Spec Exp:** Genitourinary Cancer; Prostate Cancer; Urologic Cancer; **Hospital:** Robert Wood Johnson Univ Hosp - New Brunswick; **Address:** Cancer Inst of New Jersey, 195 Little Albany St, New Brunswick, NJ 08903-2681; **Phone:** 732-235-6777; **Board Cert:** Internal Medicine 2001; Medical Oncology 2005; **Med School:** Univ Utah 1988; **Resid:** Internal Medicine, Duke Univ Med Ctr 1991; **Fellow:** Hematology & Oncology, Univ Penn Hosp 1994; **Fac Appt:** Assoc Prof Med, UMDNJ-RW Johnson Med Sch

Domchek, Susan M MD [Onc] - **Spec Exp:** Breast Cancer Genetics; Breast Cancer Risk Assessment; Ovarian Cancer Genetics; **Hospital:** Hosp Univ Penn - UPHS (page 68); **Address:** 3 West Perelman Center, Abramson Cancer Ctr Univ Penn, 3400 Civic Center Blvd, Philadelphia, PA 19104; **Phone:** 215-615-3341; **Board Cert:** Medical Oncology 2001; **Med School:** Harvard Med Sch 1995; **Resid:** Internal Medicine, Mass Genl Hosp 1998; **Fellow:** Medical Oncology, Dana Farber Cancer Inst 2001; **Fac Appt:** Assoc Prof Med, Univ Pennsylvania

Donehower, Ross Carl MD [Onc] - **Spec Exp:** Pancreatic Cancer; Colon Cancer; Prostate Cancer; **Hospital:** Johns Hopkins Hosp (page 61); **Address:** Hopkins Kimmel Cancer Ctr, 1650 Orleans St, CRB-I, rm 187, Baltimore, MD 21231-1000; **Phone:** 410-955-8964; **Board Cert:** Internal Medicine 1977; Medical Oncology 1979; **Med School:** Univ Minn 1974; **Resid:** Internal Medicine, Johns Hopkins Hosp 1976; **Fellow:** Medical Oncology, Natl Inst Hlth 1980; **Fac Appt:** Prof Med, Johns Hopkins Univ

Doroshow, James H MD [Onc] - **Spec Exp:** Drug Discovery & Development; Colon Cancer; Breast Cancer; **Hospital:** Natl Inst of Hlth - Clin Ctr; **Address:** National Cancer Institute, Div Cancer Treatment & Diagnosis, 31 Center Dr, Bldg 31-rm 3A44, Bethesda, MD 20892-2440; **Phone:** 301-496-4291; **Board Cert:** Internal Medicine 1976; Medical Oncology 1977; **Med School:** Harvard Med Sch 1973; **Resid:** Internal Medicine, Mass Genl Hosp 1975; **Fellow:** Medical Oncology, Natl Cancer Inst 1978

Dutcher, Janice P MD [Onc] - **Spec Exp:** Kidney Cancer; Melanoma; Breast Cancer; Lymphoma; **Hospital:** St. Luke's - Roosevelt Hosp Ctr - Roosevelt Div (page 55); **Address:** Continuum Cancer Center of NY, 1000 Tenth Ave, Ste 11C-02, New York, NY 10019; **Phone:** 212-636-3334; **Board Cert:** Internal Medicine 1978; Medical Oncology 1983; **Med School:** UC Davis 1975; **Resid:** Internal Medicine, Rush Presbyterian Med Ctr 1978; **Fellow:** Medical Oncology, National Cancer Inst 1981; **Fac Appt:** Prof Med, NY Med Coll

Edelman, Martin J MD [Onc] - **Spec Exp:** Thoracic Cancers; Lung Cancer; Drug Discovery & Development; **Hospital:** Univ of MD Med Ctr; **Address:** Greenebaum Cancer Ctr-Univ MD, 22 S Greene St, rm N9E08, Baltimore, MD 21201; **Phone:** 410-328-2703; **Board Cert:** Internal Medicine 1986; Medical Oncology 1989; **Med School:** Albany Med Coll 1982; **Resid:** Internal Medicine, Naval Hosp 1986; **Fellow:** Hematology & Oncology, Naval Hosp 1990; **Fac Appt:** Prof Med, Univ MD Sch Med

Medical Oncology

Eisenberger, Mario MD [Onc] - **Spec Exp:** Prostate Cancer; **Hospital:** Johns Hopkins Hosp (page 61); **Address:** 1650 Orleans St, rm 1M51, Baltimore, MD 21231; **Phone:** 410-614-3511; **Board Cert:** Internal Medicine 1976; Medical Oncology 1979; **Med School:** Brazil 1972; **Resid:** Internal Medicine, Michael Reese Hosp 1975; **Fellow:** Hematology, Michael Reese Hosp 1976; Medical Oncology, Jackson Meml Hosp/Univ Miami 1979; **Fac Appt:** Prof Med, Johns Hopkins Univ

Emens, Leisha A MD/PhD [Onc] - **Spec Exp:** Breast Cancer; Immunotherapy; **Hospital:** Johns Hopkins Hosp (page 61); **Address:** 1650 Orleans St CRB1 Bldg - rm 409, Baltimore, MD 21231; **Phone:** 410-955-8964; **Board Cert:** Internal Medicine 2008; Medical Oncology 2001; Hematology 2002; **Med School:** Baylor Coll Med 1995; **Resid:** Internal Medicine, Univ TX SW Affil Hosps 1998; **Fellow:** Medical Oncology, Johns Hopkins Hosps 2001; Research, Lab of Bio Chem-NCI 1993; **Fac Appt:** Assoc Prof Med, Johns Hopkins Univ

Engstrom, Paul F MD [Onc] - **Spec Exp:** Neuroendocrine Tumors; Gastrointestinal Cancer; **Hospital:** Fox Chase Cancer Ctr (page 58); **Address:** Fox Chase Cancer Ctr, Dept Medical Oncology, 333 Cottman Ave, Philadelphia, PA 19111; **Phone:** 215-728-2986; **Board Cert:** Internal Medicine 1969; Medical Oncology 1973; **Med School:** Univ Minn 1962; **Resid:** Internal Medicine, Univ Minn Hosp 1965; **Fac Appt:** Prof Med, Temple Univ

Ettinger, David S MD [Onc] - **Spec Exp:** Lung Cancer; Sarcoma; Clinical Trials; **Hospital:** Johns Hopkins Hosp (page 61); **Address:** Bunting Blaustein Cancer Rsrch Bldg, 1650 Orleans St, rm G88, Baltimore, MD 21231-1000; **Phone:** 410-955-8847; **Board Cert:** Internal Medicine 1976; Medical Oncology 1977; **Med School:** Univ Louisville Sch Med 1967; **Resid:** Internal Medicine, Mayo Grad Schl 1971; **Fellow:** Medical Oncology, Johns Hopkins Hosp 1975; **Fac Appt:** Prof Med, Johns Hopkins Univ

Fine, Howard Alan MD [Onc] - **Spec Exp:** Brain Tumors; Neuro-Oncology; **Hospital:** Natl Inst of Hlth - Clin Ctr; **Address:** 9030 Old Georgetown Rd, Block Bldg 82, Rm 225, MSC 8202, Bethesda, MD 20892-0001; **Phone:** 301-402-6298; **Board Cert:** Internal Medicine 1987; Medical Oncology 1989; **Med School:** Mount Sinai Sch Med 1984; **Resid:** Internal Medicine, Hosp Univ Penn 1987; **Fellow:** Medical Oncology, Dana Farber Cancer Ctr 1990

Fine, Robert Lance MD [Onc] - **Spec Exp:** Pancreatic Cancer; Drug Development; Brain Tumors; Clinical Trials; **Hospital:** NY-Presby/Columbia Univ Med Ctr, NY (page 65); **Address:** 650 W 168th St Fl 20th - Ste BB20-05, New York, NY 10032; **Phone:** 212-305-1168; **Board Cert:** Internal Medicine 1983; Medical Oncology 1985; **Med School:** Univ Chicago-Pritzker Sch Med 1979; **Resid:** Internal Medicine, Stanford Univ Med Ctr 1982; **Fellow:** Medical Oncology, National Cancer Inst 1988; **Fac Appt:** Assoc Prof Med, Columbia P&S

Fisher, Richard I MD [Onc] - **Spec Exp:** Lymphoma; Hodgkin's Disease; **Hospital:** Univ of Rochester Strong Meml Hosp; **Address:** James P Wilmot Cancer Ctr, 601 Elmwood Ave, Box 704, Rochester, NY 14642; **Phone:** 585-275-5823; **Board Cert:** Internal Medicine 1973; Medical Oncology 1977; **Med School:** Harvard Med Sch 1970; **Resid:** Internal Medicine, Mass Genl Hosp 1972; **Fac Appt:** Prof Med, Univ Rochester

Flomenberg, Neal MD [Onc] - **Spec Exp:** Bone Marrow Transplant; Stem Cell Transplant; Leukemia & Lymphoma; **Hospital:** Thomas Jefferson Univ Hosp; **Address:** Thomas Jefferson Univ Hosp, 925 Chestnut St Fl 2, Philadelphia, PA 19107; **Phone:** 215-955-8874; **Board Cert:** Internal Medicine 1979; Medical Oncology 1981; Hematology 1982; **Med School:** Jefferson Med Coll 1976; **Resid:** Internal Medicine, Montefiore Med Ctr 1979; **Fellow:** Hematology & Oncology, Meml Sloan Kettering Cancer Ctr 1982; **Fac Appt:** Clin Prof Med, Thomas Jefferson Univ

Forastiere, Arlene A MD [Onc] - **Spec Exp:** Esophageal Cancer; Head & Neck Cancer; **Hospital:** Johns Hopkins Hosp (page 61); **Address:** Bunting Blaustein Cancer Research Bldg, 1650 Orleans St, rm G90, Baltimore, MD 21231; **Phone:** 410-955-8964; **Board Cert:** Internal Medicine 1978; Medical Oncology 1981; **Med School:** NY Med Coll 1975; **Resid:** Internal Medicine, Albert Einstein Med Ctr 1977; Internal Medicine, Univ Conn Health Ctr 1978; **Fellow:** Medical Oncology, Meml Sloan Kettering Cancer Ctr 1980; **Fac Appt:** Prof Med, NY Med Coll

Fox, Kevin R MD [Onc] - **Spec Exp:** Breast Cancer; **Hospital:** Hosp Univ Penn - UPHS (page 68); **Address:** 3400 Civic Ctr Blvd, 3W Perelman Ctr, Philadelphia, PA 19104; **Phone:** 215-662-7469; **Board Cert:** Internal Medicine 1985; Medical Oncology 1987; **Med School:** Johns Hopkins Univ 1981; **Resid:** Internal Medicine, Johns Hopkins Hosp 1984; **Fellow:** Hematology & Oncology, Hosp Univ Penn 1987; **Fac Appt:** Prof Med, Univ Pennsylvania

Friedberg, Jonathan MD [Onc] - **Spec Exp:** Lymphoma; Hodgkin's Disease; Clinical Trials; **Hospital:** Univ of Rochester Strong Meml Hosp; **Address:** James P Wilmot Cancer Ctr, 601 Elmwood Ave, Box 704, Rochester, NY 14642-8704; **Phone:** 585-275-4911; **Board Cert:** Medical Oncology 2000; Hematology 2000; **Med School:** Harvard Med Sch 1994; **Resid:** Internal Medicine, Mass Genl Hosp 1997; Hematology & Oncology, Dana-Farber/Partners Cancer Ctr 1999; **Fac Appt:** Prof Med, Univ Rochester

Gabrilove, Janice MD [Onc] - **Spec Exp:** Myelodysplastic Syndromes; Leukemia; Hematologic Malignancies; Myeloproliferative Disorders; **Hospital:** Mount Sinai Med Ctr (page 63); **Address:** Mount Sinai Med Ctr, One Gustave L Levy Pl, Box 1079, Dept Hem Onc, New York, NY 10029-6574; **Phone:** 212-241-9650; **Board Cert:** Internal Medicine 1980; Medical Oncology 1983; **Med School:** Mount Sinai Sch Med 1977; **Resid:** Internal Medicine, Columbia-Presby Med Ctr 1980; **Fellow:** Hematology & Oncology, Meml Sloan-Kettering Cancer Ctr 1983; **Fac Appt:** Prof Med, Mount Sinai Sch Med

Gelmann, Edward P MD [Onc] - **Spec Exp:** Prostate Cancer; Bladder Cancer; Kidney Cancer; **Hospital:** NY-Presby/Columbia Univ Med Ctr, NY (page 65); **Address:** Columbia Univ Med Ctr, Milstein Hosp Bldg 6-435, 177 Fort Washington Ave, New York, NY 10032; **Phone:** 212-305-8602; **Board Cert:** Internal Medicine 1979; Medical Oncology 1981; **Med School:** Stanford Univ 1976; **Resid:** Internal Medicine, Univ Chicago Hosps 1978; **Fellow:** Medical Oncology, National Cancer Inst 1981; **Fac Appt:** Prof Med, Columbia P&S

Geyer Jr, Charles E MD [Onc] - **Spec Exp:** Breast Cancer; **Hospital:** Allegheny General Hosp; **Address:** Allegheny Cancer Ctr, 320 E North Ave Fl ACC 3, Pittsburgh, PA 15212; **Phone:** 412-359-6147; **Board Cert:** Internal Medicine 1983; Medical Oncology 1987; **Med School:** Texas Tech Univ 1980; **Resid:** Internal Medicine, Baylor Affil Hosps 1983; **Fellow:** Medical Oncology, Baylor Affil Hosps 1985

Glick, John H MD [Onc] - **Spec Exp:** Breast Cancer; Hodgkin's Disease; Lymphoma, Non-Hodgkin's; **Hospital:** Hosp Univ Penn - UPHS (page 68); **Address:** Abramson Cancer Ctr of Univ Penn, 3400 Civic Ctr Blvd, PCAM Bldg Fl 3 - Ste 3-300S, Philadelphia, PA 19104; **Phone:** 215-662-6065; **Board Cert:** Internal Medicine 1973; Medical Oncology 1975; **Med School:** Columbia P&S 1969; **Resid:** Internal Medicine, Presbyterian Hosp 1971; **Fellow:** Medical Oncology, Natl Cancer Inst 1973; Medical Oncology, Stanford Univ 1974; **Fac Appt:** Prof Med, Univ Pennsylvania

Goldstein, Lori J MD [Onc] - **Spec Exp:** Breast Cancer; **Hospital:** Fox Chase Cancer Ctr (page 58); **Address:** Fox Chase Cancer Ctr, Dept Med Oncology, 333 Cottman Ave, Philadelphia, PA 19111; **Phone:** 215-728-2689; **Board Cert:** Internal Medicine 1985; Medical Oncology 2002; **Med School:** SUNY Upstate Med Univ 1982; **Resid:** Internal Medicine, Presby Univ Hosp 1985; **Fellow:** Medical Oncology, Natl Cancer Inst/NIH 1990; **Fac Appt:** Assoc Prof Hem & Onc, Temple Univ

Goy, Andre MD [Onc] - **Spec Exp:** Lymphoma; Hodgkin's Disease; **Hospital:** Hackensack Univ Med Ctr; **Address:** 92 2nd St, Hackensack, NJ 07601; **Phone:** 201-996-5900; **Med School:** France 1988; **Resid:** Internal Medicine, Grenoble Univ Med Ctr 1992; **Fellow:** Hematology & Oncology, Grenoble Univ Med Ctr 1993

Grana, Generosa MD [Onc] - **Spec Exp:** Breast Cancer; Cancer Genetics; Cancer Prevention; **Hospital:** Cooper Univ Hosp; **Address:** 900 Centennial Blvd, Ste M, Voorhees, NJ 08043; **Phone:** 856-325-6740; **Board Cert:** Internal Medicine 1988; Medical Oncology 2001; **Med School:** Northwestern Univ 1985; **Resid:** Internal Medicine, Temple Univ Hosp 1988; **Fellow:** Hematology & Oncology, Fox Chase Cancer Ctr 1992; **Fac Appt:** Assoc Prof Med, UMDNJ-RW Johnson Med Sch

Grossbard, Michael L MD [Onc] - **Spec Exp:** Lymphoma; Gastrointestinal Cancer; Breast Cancer; **Hospital:** St. Luke's - Roosevelt Hosp Ctr - Roosevelt Div (page 55), Beth Israel Med Ctr - Petrie Division (page 55); **Address:** 1000 10th Ave, Fl 11, Ste C02, New York, NY 10019; **Phone:** 212-523-5419; **Board Cert:** Internal Medicine 1989; Medical Oncology 2001; **Med School:** Yale Univ 1986; **Resid:** Internal Medicine, Mass Genl Hosp 1989; **Fellow:** Medical Oncology, Dana Farber Cancer Inst 1991; **Fac Appt:** Clin Prof Med, Columbia P&S

Grossman, Stuart MD [Onc] - **Spec Exp:** Brain Tumors; Neuro-Oncology; Pain-Cancer; **Hospital:** Johns Hopkins Hosp (page 61); **Address:** Cancer Research Bldg 2, rm 1M16, 1550 Orleans St, Ste 1M16, Baltimore, MD 21231; **Phone:** 410-955-8837; **Board Cert:** Internal Medicine 1976; Medical Oncology 1983; **Med School:** Univ Rochester 1973; **Resid:** Internal Medicine, Strong Meml Hosp 1976; **Fellow:** Medical Oncology, Johns Hopkins Hosp 1981; **Fac Appt:** Prof Med, Johns Hopkins Univ

Gulley, James L MD/PhD [Onc] - **Spec Exp:** Prostate Cancer-Vaccine Therapy; Vaccine Therapy-Clinical Trials Only; Clinical Trials Only; **Hospital:** Natl Inst of Hlth - Clin Ctr; **Address:** NIH Cancer Research Ctr, Bldg 10, rm 13N208, 10 Center Dr, MSC 1750, Bethesda, MD 20892; **Phone:** 301-435-2956; **Board Cert:** Internal Medicine 2009; Medical Oncology 2000; **Med School:** Loma Linda Univ 1995; **Resid:** Internal Medicine, Emory Univ Med Ctr 1998; **Fellow:** Medical Oncology, Natl Cancer Inst 2000

Haas, Naomi S Balzer MD [Onc] - **Spec Exp:** Genitourinary Cancer; Kidney Cancer; Clinical Trials; **Hospital:** Hosp Univ Penn - UPHS (page 68); **Address:** Abramson Cancer Ctr, Dept Hem/Onc, 16 Penn Tower, 3400 Spruce St, Philadelphia, PA 19104; **Phone:** 215-662-7402; **Board Cert:** Internal Medicine 1988; Medical Oncology 2005; **Med School:** NE Ohio Univ 1985; **Resid:** Internal Medicine, Abington Meml Hosp 1988; **Fellow:** Hematology & Oncology, Fox Chase Cancer Ctr 1989; **Fac Appt:** Assoc Prof Med, Univ Pennsylvania

Hageboutros, Alexandre MD [Onc] - **Spec Exp:** Gastrointestinal Cancer; Lung Cancer; Colon & Rectal Cancer; **Hospital:** Cooper Univ Hosp; **Address:** 900 Centennial Blvd, Ste M, Voorhees, NJ 08043-4689; **Phone:** 856-325-6740; **Board Cert:** Internal Medicine 2001; Hematology 2004; Medical Oncology 2005; **Med School:** Lebanon 1987; **Resid:** Internal Medicine, Cooper Hosp 1991; **Fellow:** Hematology & Oncology, Temple Univ Hosp 1992; Hematology & Oncology, Fox Chase Cancer Ctr 1994; **Fac Appt:** Assoc Prof Med, UMDNJ-NJ Med Sch, Newark

Henry, David H MD [Onc] - **Spec Exp:** AIDS Related Cancers; **Hospital:** Pennsylvania Hosp-UPHS (page 68); **Address:** 230 W Washington Square Fl 2, Philadelphia, PA 19106; **Phone:** 215-829-6088; **Board Cert:** Internal Medicine 1978; Hematology 1980; Medical Oncology 1981; **Med School:** Univ Pennsylvania 1975; **Resid:** Internal Medicine, Hosp Univ Penn 1978; **Fellow:** Hematology & Oncology, Hosp Univ Penn 1978; **Fac Appt:** Clin Prof Med, Univ Pennsylvania

Himelstein, Andrew L MD [Onc] - **Spec Exp:** Leukemia & Lymphoma; Palliative Care; **Hospital:** Christiana Hospital; **Address:** Medical Onc/Hem Consultants, 4701 Ogletown-Stanton Rd, Ste West 3400, Helen Graham Cancer Ctr, Newark, DE 19713; **Phone:** 302-366-1200; **Board Cert:** Internal Medicine 1988; Hematology 2010; Medical Oncology 2011; Hospice & Palliative Medicine 2010; **Med School:** Washington Univ, St Louis 1985; **Resid:** Internal Medicine, Mt Sinai Hosp 1988; **Fellow:** Hematology & Oncology, Colum-Presby Univ Hosp 1991; **Fac Appt:** Asst Clin Prof Med, Thomas Jefferson Univ

Hogan, Thomas F MD [Onc] - **Spec Exp:** Genitourinary Cancer; Kidney Cancer; Urologic Cancer; **Hospital:** Ruby Memorial - WVU Hosp; **Address:** MBR Cancer Ctr, Robert T Byrd Hlth Sci Ctr, 1 Medical Center Drive, Morgantown, WV 26506-8110; **Phone:** 304-293-4500; **Board Cert:** Internal Medicine 1975; Medical Oncology 1977; Anatomic Pathology 1997; **Med School:** Med Coll VA 1972; **Resid:** Internal Medicine, Thomas Jefferson Univ Hosp 1975; **Fellow:** Medical Oncology, Univ Wisconsin Affil Hosp 1977; **Fac Appt:** Prof Med, W VA Univ

Holland, James F MD [Onc] - **Spec Exp:** Breast Cancer; Colon Cancer; Lung Cancer; Pancreatic Cancer; **Hospital:** Mount Sinai Med Ctr (page 63); **Address:** Ruttenberg Cancer Ctr, 1190 5th Ave, Box 1129, New York, NY 10029; **Phone:** 212-241-6756; **Board Cert:** Internal Medicine 1955; **Med School:** Columbia P&S 1947; **Resid:** Internal Medicine, Columbia-Presby Hosp 1949; **Fellow:** Medical Oncology, Francis Delafield Hosp 1953; **Fac Appt:** Prof Med, Mount Sinai Sch Med

Horwitz, Steven MD [Onc] - **Spec Exp:** Lymphoma, Cutaneous T Cell (CTCL); **Hospital:** Meml Sloan-Kettering Cancer Ctr; **Address:** Meml Sloan-Kettering Cancer Ctr, 1275 York Ave, New York, NY 10065; **Phone:** 212-639-3045; **Board Cert:** Medical Oncology 2001; **Med School:** Case West Res Univ 1993; **Resid:** Internal Medicine, Strong Memorial Hosp 1996; **Fellow:** Medical Oncology, Stanford Univ Med Ctr 1999

Hudes, Gary R MD [Onc] - **Spec Exp:** Prostate Cancer; Genitourinary Cancer; Kidney Cancer; **Hospital:** Fox Chase Cancer Ctr (page 58); **Address:** 333 Cottman Ave, rm C307, Philadelphia, PA 19111; **Phone:** 215-728-3889; **Board Cert:** Internal Medicine 1982; Hematology 1984; Medical Oncology 1985; **Med School:** SUNY Downstate 1979; **Resid:** Internal Medicine, Graduate Hosp 1982; **Fellow:** Hematology & Oncology, Presby-Univ Penn Med Ctr 1985

Hudis, Clifford A MD [Onc] - **Spec Exp:** Breast Cancer; **Hospital:** Meml Sloan-Kettering Cancer Ctr; **Address:** 1275 York Avenue, New York, NY 10065; **Phone:** 800-525-2225; **Board Cert:** Internal Medicine 1986; Medical Oncology 2001; **Med School:** Med Coll PA Hahnemann 1983; **Resid:** Internal Medicine, Hosp Med Coll Penn 1987; **Fellow:** Medical Oncology, Meml Sloan Kettering Cancer Ctr 1991; **Fac Appt:** Prof Med, Cornell Univ-Weill Med Coll

Ilson, David H MD [Onc] - **Spec Exp:** Esophageal Cancer; Colon & Rectal Cancer; Mesothelioma; Unknown Primary Cancer; **Hospital:** Meml Sloan-Kettering Cancer Ctr; **Address:** 1275 York Avenue, New York, NY 10065; **Phone:** 212-639-8306; **Board Cert:** Internal Medicine 1989; Medical Oncology 2002; **Med School:** NYU Sch Med 1986; **Resid:** Internal Medicine, Bellevue-NYU Sch Med 1989; **Fellow:** Medical Oncology, Meml Sloan Kettering Hosp 1992; **Fac Appt:** Assoc Prof Med, Cornell Univ-Weill Med Coll

Isaacs, Claudine J MD [Onc] - **Spec Exp:** Breast Cancer; Breast Cancer Risk Assessment; **Hospital:** Georgetown Univ Hosp; **Address:** Lombardi Cancer Ctr, Podium A, 3800 Reservoir Rd NW, Washington, DC 20007; **Phone:** 202-444-3677; **Board Cert:** Internal Medicine 2002; Medical Oncology 2003; **Med School:** McGill Univ 1987; **Resid:** Internal Medicine, Montreal Genl Hosp 1990; Hematology & Oncology, McGill Univ Hosp 1992; **Fellow:** Medical Oncology, Georgetown Univ Med Ctr 1993; **Fac Appt:** Assoc Prof Med, Georgetown Univ

Medical Oncology

Jurcic, Joseph G MD [Onc] - **Spec Exp:** Leukemia; Myelodysplastic Syndromes; Clinical Trials; **Hospital:** Meml Sloan-Kettering Cancer Ctr; **Address:** 1275 York Avenue, New York, NY 10065; **Phone:** 800-525-2225; **Board Cert:** Internal Medicine 2001; Medical Oncology 2005; Hematology 2008; **Med School:** Univ Pennsylvania 1988; **Resid:** Internal Medicine, Barnes Hosp 1991; **Fellow:** Hematology & Oncology, Meml Sloan Kettering Cancer Ctr 1994; **Fac Appt:** Assoc Prof Med, Cornell Univ-Weill Med Coll

Karp, Judith MD [Onc] - **Spec Exp:** Leukemia; Clinical Trials; Myelodysplastic Syndromes; **Hospital:** Johns Hopkins Hosp (page 61); **Address:** 1650 Orleans St, CRB1 Bldg - rm 2M44, Baltimore, MD 21287; **Phone:** 410-955-8964; **Board Cert:** Internal Medicine 1976; **Med School:** Stanford Univ 1971; **Resid:** Internal Medicine, John Hopkins Hosp 1974; **Fellow:** Medical Oncology, John Hopkins Hosp 1977; **Fac Appt:** Prof Med, Johns Hopkins Univ

Kelly, William K DO [Onc] - **Spec Exp:** Prostate Cancer; Genitourinary Cancer; Urologic Cancer; Solid Tumors; **Hospital:** Thomas Jefferson Univ Hosp; **Address:** 834 Chestnut St, Ben Franklin House St, Ste 314, Philadelphia, PA 19107; **Phone:** 215-955-8874; **Board Cert:** Medical Oncology 2003; **Med School:** Philadelphia Coll Osteo Med 1986; **Resid:** Internal Medicine, Montefiore Med Ctr 1990; **Fellow:** Hematology & Oncology, Meml Sloan Kettering Cancer Ctr 1993; **Fac Appt:** Prof Med, Thomas Jefferson Univ

Kelsen, David Paul MD [Onc] - **Spec Exp:** Gastrointestinal Cancer; Neuroendocrine Tumors; Unknown Primary Cancer; Merkel Cell Carcinoma; **Hospital:** Meml Sloan-Kettering Cancer Ctr; **Address:** 1275 York Ave Howard Bldg - rm 918, New York, NY 10065; **Phone:** 212-639-8470; **Board Cert:** Internal Medicine 1976; Medical Oncology 1979; **Med School:** Hahnemann Univ 1972; **Resid:** Internal Medicine, Temple Univ Hosp 1976; **Fellow:** Medical Oncology, Meml Sloan Kettering Cancer Ctr 1978; **Fac Appt:** Prof Med, Cornell Univ-Weill Med Coll

Kemeny, Nancy MD [Onc] - **Spec Exp:** Colon Cancer; Rectal Cancer; Liver Cancer; **Hospital:** Meml Sloan-Kettering Cancer Ctr; **Address:** 1275 York Ave, rm H916, New York, NY 10065; **Phone:** 800-525-2225; **Board Cert:** Internal Medicine 1974; Medical Oncology 1981; **Med School:** UMDNJ-NJ Med Sch, Newark 1971; **Resid:** Internal Medicine, St Luke's Hosp 1974; **Fellow:** Medical Oncology, Mem Sloan Kettering Cancer Ctr 1976; **Fac Appt:** Prof Med, Cornell Univ-Weill Med Coll

Kirkwood, John M MD [Onc] - **Spec Exp:** Melanoma; Immunotherapy; **Hospital:** UPMC Shadyside, UPMC Presby, Pittsburgh; **Address:** Hillman Cancer Research Pavilion, 5115 Centre Ave, Pittsburgh, PA 15213-1862; **Phone:** 412-623-7707; **Board Cert:** Internal Medicine 1976; Medical Oncology 1981; **Med School:** Yale Univ 1973; **Resid:** Internal Medicine, Yale-New Haven Hosp 1976; **Fellow:** Medical Oncology, Dana Farber Cancer Inst 1979; **Fac Appt:** Prof Med, Univ Pittsburgh

Kressel, Bruce R MD [Onc] - **Spec Exp:** Lung Cancer; **Hospital:** G Washington Univ Hosp, Sibley Mem Hosp; **Address:** Washington Oncology-Hematology Center, 2141 K St NW, Ste 707, Washington, DC 20037; **Phone:** 202-293-5382; **Board Cert:** Internal Medicine 1976; Hematology 1978; Medical Oncology 1977; **Med School:** Tufts Univ 1973; **Resid:** Internal Medicine, George Washington Univ Med Ctr 1975; **Fellow:** Hematology & Oncology, George Washington Univ Med Ctr 1977; Oncology, George Washington Univ Med Ctr 1978; **Fac Appt:** Clin Prof Hem & Onc, Geo Wash Univ

Kris, Mark G MD [Onc] - **Spec Exp:** Lung Cancer; Mediastinal Tumors; Thymoma; Thoracic Cancers; **Hospital:** Meml Sloan-Kettering Cancer Ctr; **Address:** 1275 York Ave, New York, NY 10065; **Phone:** 212-639-7590; **Board Cert:** Internal Medicine 1980; Medical Oncology 1983; **Med School:** Cornell Univ-Weill Med Coll 1977; **Resid:** Internal Medicine, New York Hosp 1980; **Fellow:** Medical Oncology, Meml Sloan Kettering Cancer Ctr 1983; **Fac Appt:** Prof Med, Cornell Univ-Weill Med Coll

Laheru, Daniel A MD [Onc] - **Spec Exp:** Pancreatic Cancer; Gastrointestinal Cancer; Vaccine Therapy; **Hospital:** Johns Hopkins Hosp (page 61); **Address:** Bunting-Blaustein Cancer Rsch Bldg, 1650 Orleans St, rm 4M09, Baltimore, MD 21231; **Phone:** 410-955-8974; **Board Cert:** Internal Medicine 1998; Medical Oncology 2000; **Med School:** Baylor Coll Med 1995; **Resid:** Internal Medicine, Univ Utah Hosp & Clinics 1998; **Fellow:** Medical Oncology, Johns Hopkins Hosp 1998; **Fac Appt:** Assoc Prof Med, Johns Hopkins Univ

Langer, Corey J MD [Onc] - **Spec Exp:** Lung Cancer; Head & Neck Cancer; Mesothelioma; Thoracic Cancers; **Hospital:** Hosp Univ Penn - UPHS (page 68); **Address:** Hospital U Penn, Abramson Cancer Ctr, 2 PCAM, 3400 Civic Center Blvd, Philadelphia, PA 19104; **Phone:** 215-615-5121; **Board Cert:** Internal Medicine 1984; Hematology 1986; Medical Oncology 1987; **Med School:** Boston Univ 1981; **Resid:** Internal Medicine, Graduate Hosp 1984; Hematology & Oncology, Presby Hosp 1986; **Fellow:** Medical Oncology, Fox Chase Cancer Ctr 1987; **Fac Appt:** Prof Med, Univ Pennsylvania

Levine, Ellis G MD [Onc] - **Spec Exp:** Testicular Cancer; Bladder Cancer; Prostate Cancer; **Hospital:** Roswell Park Cancer Inst; **Address:** Roswell Park Cancer Inst, Elm & Carlton St, Buffalo, NY 14263-0001; **Phone:** 716-845-8547; **Board Cert:** Internal Medicine 1982; Medical Oncology 1985; **Med School:** Univ Pittsburgh 1979; **Resid:** Internal Medicine, Univ Minn Hosps 1982; **Fellow:** Medical Oncology, Univ Minn Hosps 1984; **Fac Appt:** Prof Med, SUNY Buffalo

Levy, Michael H MD/PhD [Onc] - **Spec Exp:** Pain Management; Palliative Care; Pain-Cancer; Ethics; **Hospital:** Fox Chase Cancer Ctr (page 58); **Address:** Fox Chase Cancer Ctr, Dept Med Oncology, Div Pain & Palliative Med, 333 Cottman Ave, Ste C307, Philadelphia, PA 19111; **Phone:** 215-728-3637; **Board Cert:** Internal Medicine 1979; Medical Oncology 1981; Hospice & Palliative Medicine 2008; **Med School:** Jefferson Med Coll 1976; **Resid:** Internal Medicine, Mt Sinai Med Ctr 1978; Internal Medicine, Hosp Univ Penn 1979; **Fellow:** Hematology & Oncology, Hosp Univ Penn 1981

Maki, Robert G MD/PhD [Onc] - **Spec Exp:** Sarcoma; Sarcoma-Soft Tissue; **Hospital:** Mount Sinai Med Ctr (page 63); **Address:** Mt Sinai Med Ctr, 1 Gustave Levy Pl, Box 1208, New York, NY 10029; **Phone:** 212-241-7022; **Board Cert:** Internal Medicine 2005; Medical Oncology 2007; **Med School:** Cornell Univ-Weill Med Coll 1992; **Resid:** Internal Medicine, Brigham & Womens Hosp 1995; **Fellow:** Medical Oncology, Dana-Farber Cancer Inst 1995; **Fac Appt:** Assoc Prof Med, Cornell Univ-Weill Med Coll

Marshall, John L MD [Onc] - **Spec Exp:** Gastrointestinal Cancer; Drug Development; **Hospital:** Georgetown Univ Hosp; **Address:** Lombardi Cancer Ctr, Podium A, 3800 Reservoir Rd NW, Washington, DC 20007; **Phone:** 202-444-7064; **Board Cert:** Internal Medicine 2001; Medical Oncology 2003; **Med School:** Univ Louisville Sch Med 1988; **Resid:** Internal Medicine, Georgetown Univ Hosp 1991; **Fellow:** Medical Oncology, Georgetown Univ Hosp 1993; **Fac Appt:** Assoc Prof Med, Georgetown Univ

Masters, Gregory A MD [Onc] - **Spec Exp:** Lung Cancer; Esophageal Cancer; Thoracic Cancers; **Hospital:** Christiana Hospital; **Address:** Medical Oncology-Hematology Consultants, Graham Cancer Ctr, 4701 Ogletown-Stanton Rd, Ste 3400, Newark, DE 19713; **Phone:** 302-366-1200; **Board Cert:** Internal Medicine 2003; Medical Oncology 2005; **Med School:** Northwestern Univ 1990; **Resid:** Internal Medicine, Hosp Univ Penn 1993; **Fellow:** Medical Oncology, Univ Chicago Hosps 1995; **Fac Appt:** Assoc Prof Med, Thomas Jefferson Univ

McGuire III, William P MD [Onc] - **Spec Exp:** Gynecologic Cancer; Ovarian Cancer; Breast Cancer; **Hospital:** Franklin Square Hosp; **Address:** Harry & Jeanette Weinberg Cancer Inst, 9103 Franklin Square Drive, Ste 2200, Baltimore, MD 21287; **Phone:** 443-777-7826; **Board Cert:** Internal Medicine 1974; Medical Oncology 1981; **Med School:** Baylor Coll Med 1971; **Resid:** Internal Medicine, Yale-New Haven Hosp 1973; **Fac Appt:** Clin Prof Med, Univ MD Sch Med

Miller, Vincent A MD [Onc] - **Spec Exp:** Lung Cancer; Drug Development; **Hospital:** Meml Sloan-Kettering Cancer Ctr; **Address:** Memorial Sloan-Kettering Cancer Ctr, 1275 York Ave, New York, NY 10065; **Phone:** 800-525-2225; **Board Cert:** Internal Medicine 2002; Medical Oncology 2005; **Med School:** UMDNJ-NJ Med Sch, Newark 1987; **Resid:** Internal Medicine, Thos Jefferson Univ Hosp 1991; **Fellow:** Medical Oncology, Meml Sloan Kettering Cancer Ctr 1994; **Fac Appt:** Assoc Prof Med, Cornell Univ-Weill Med Coll

Mintzer, David M MD [Onc] - **Spec Exp:** Breast Cancer; Gastrointestinal Cancer; Head & Neck Cancer; Palliative Care; **Hospital:** Pennsylvania Hosp-UPHS (page 68); **Address:** 230 W Washington Square Fl 2, Philadelphia, PA 19106; **Phone:** 215-829-6088; **Board Cert:** Internal Medicine 1980; Hematology 1982; Medical Oncology 1983; Hospice & Palliative Medicine 2004; **Med School:** Jefferson Med Coll 1977; **Resid:** Internal Medicine, Pennsylvania Hosp 1980; **Fellow:** Hematology, Jefferson Med Coll 1982; Medical Oncology, Meml Sloan Kettering Cancer Ctr 1984

Moore, Anne MD [Onc] - **Spec Exp:** Breast Cancer; **Hospital:** NY-Presby/Weill Cornell Med Ctr, NY (page 65); **Address:** Weill Cornell Breast Ctr, 425 E 61st St Fl 8, New York, NY 10065; **Phone:** 212-821-0550; **Board Cert:** Internal Medicine 1973; Hematology 1976; Medical Oncology 2008; **Med School:** Columbia P&S 1969; **Resid:** Internal Medicine, Cornell Univ Med Ctr 1973; **Fellow:** Medical Oncology, Rockefeller Univ 1973; **Fac Appt:** Prof Med, Cornell Univ-Weill Med Coll

Motzer, Robert J MD [Onc] - **Spec Exp:** Kidney Cancer; Testicular Cancer; Prostate Cancer; **Hospital:** Meml Sloan-Kettering Cancer Ctr; **Address:** 1275 York Avenue, New York, NY 10065; **Phone:** 800-525-2225; **Board Cert:** Internal Medicine 1984; Medical Oncology 1987; **Med School:** Univ Mich Med Sch 1981; **Resid:** Internal Medicine, Meml Sloan Kettering Cancer Ctr 1984; **Fellow:** Medical Oncology, Meml Sloan Kettering Cancer Ctr 1987; **Fac Appt:** Assoc Prof Med, Cornell Univ-Weill Med Coll

Muggia, Franco MD [Onc] - **Spec Exp:** Gynecologic Cancer; **Hospital:** NYU Langone Med Ctr (page 66); **Address:** NYU Clinical Cancer Ctr, 160 E 34th St Fl 4, New York, NY 10016; **Phone:** 212-731-5433; **Board Cert:** Internal Medicine 1968; Medical Oncology 1973; Hematology 1974; **Med School:** Cornell Univ-Weill Med Coll 1961; **Resid:** Internal Medicine, Hartford Hosp 1964; Internal Medicine, Francis A Delafield Hosp 1966; **Fac Appt:** Prof Med, NYU Sch Med

Nanus, David M MD [Onc] - **Spec Exp:** Prostate Cancer; Bladder Cancer; Testicular Cancer; Genitourinary Cancer; **Hospital:** NY-Presby/Weill Cornell Med Ctr, NY (page 65); **Address:** NY Hosp-Cornell Med Ctr, Payson Pavilion, 525 E 68th St Fl 3 - Ste 341, New York, NY 10021; **Phone:** 646-962-2072; **Board Cert:** Internal Medicine 1985; Medical Oncology 1987; **Med School:** Univ Hlth Scis, Chicago Med Sch 1982; **Resid:** Internal Medicine, Bronx Muni Hosp 1985; **Fellow:** Medical Oncology, Meml Sloan Kettering Canc Ctr 1989; **Fac Appt:** Prof Med, Cornell Univ-Weill Med Coll

Nissenblatt, Michael MD [Onc] - **Spec Exp:** Breast Cancer; Colon Cancer; Hereditary Cancer; Lymphoma; **Hospital:** Robert Wood Johnson Univ Hosp - New Brunswick, St. Peter's Univ Hosp; **Address:** 205 Easton Ave, New Brunswick, NJ 08901-1722; **Phone:** 732-828-9570; **Board Cert:** Internal Medicine 1976; Medical Oncology 1979; **Med School:** Columbia P&S 1973; **Resid:** Internal Medicine, Johns Hopkins Hosp 1976; **Fellow:** Medical Oncology, Johns Hopkins Hosp 1978; **Fac Appt:** Clin Prof Med

Norton, Larry MD [Onc] - **Spec Exp:** Breast Cancer; **Hospital:** Meml Sloan-Kettering Cancer Ctr; **Address:** 300 E 66th St, BAIC Bldg Fl 9 - Ste 933, New York, NY 10065; **Phone:** 646-888-5319; **Board Cert:** Internal Medicine 1975; Medical Oncology 1977; **Med School:** Columbia P&S 1972; **Resid:** Internal Medicine, Bronx Muni Hosp 1974; **Fellow:** Medical Oncology, Natl Cancer Inst 1977; **Fac Appt:** Prof Med, Cornell Univ-Weill Med Coll

O'Connor, Owen A MD/PhD [Onc] - **Spec Exp:** Lymphoma-Hodgkins & Non-Hodgkins; Drug Development; Clinical Trials; **Hospital:** NYU Langone Med Ctr (page 66); **Address:** NYU Clin Canc Ctr, 160 E 34th St Fl 7, New York, NY 10016; **Phone:** 212-731-6541; **Board Cert:** Internal Medicine 2004; Medical Oncology 2005; **Med School:** UMDNJ-RW Johnson Med Sch 1994; **Resid:** Internal Medicine, NY Presby Hosp 1996; **Fellow:** Medical Oncology, Memorial Sloan-Kettering Cancer Center 2000; **Fac Appt:** Prof Med, NYU Sch Med

O'Reilly, Eileen M MD [Onc] - **Spec Exp:** Pancreatic Cancer; Liver Cancer; Biliary Cancer; Neuroendocrine Tumors; **Hospital:** Meml Sloan-Kettering Cancer Ctr; **Address:** 1275 York Avenue, Meml Sloan-Kettering Cancer Ctr, New York, NY 10065; **Phone:** 212-639-6672; **Med School:** Ireland 1990; **Resid:** Internal Medicine, St Vincent's Hosp 1994; **Fellow:** Hematology, St Vincent's Hosp 1995; Medical Oncology, Memorial-Sloan Kettering Cancer Ctr 1997; **Fac Appt:** Assoc Prof Med, Cornell Univ-Weill Med Coll

Offit, Kenneth MD [Onc] - **Spec Exp:** Cancer Genetics; Breast Cancer; Lymphoma; **Hospital:** Meml Sloan-Kettering Cancer Ctr; **Address:** 1275 York Avenue, New York, NY 10065; **Phone:** 646-888-4050; **Board Cert:** Internal Medicine 1985; Medical Oncology 1987; **Med School:** Harvard Med Sch 1982; **Resid:** Internal Medicine, Lenox Hill Hosp 1985; **Fellow:** Hematology & Oncology, Meml Sloan Kettering Cancer Ctr 1988; **Fac Appt:** Prof Med, Cornell Univ-Weill Med Coll

Oh, William K MD [Onc] - **Spec Exp:** Genitourinary Cancer; Prostate Cancer; Testicular Cancer; Adrenal Cancer; **Hospital:** Mount Sinai Med Ctr (page 63); **Address:** 1 Gustave L Levy Pl, Box 1128, New York, NY 10029; **Phone:** 212-659-5429; **Board Cert:** Medical Oncology 2009; **Med School:** NYU Sch Med 1992; **Resid:** Internal Medicine, Brigham & Womens Hosp 1995; **Fellow:** Medical Oncology, Dana-Farber Cancer Inst 1997; **Fac Appt:** Prof Med, Mount Sinai Sch Med

Oratz, Ruth MD [Onc] - **Spec Exp:** Breast Cancer; Ovarian Cancer; **Hospital:** NYU Langone Med Ctr (page 66); **Address:** 345 E 37th St, Ste 202, New York, NY 10016; **Phone:** 212-400-4904; **Board Cert:** Internal Medicine 1985; Medical Oncology 1989; **Med School:** Albert Einstein Coll Med 1982; **Resid:** Internal Medicine, NYU Med Ctr 1982; **Fellow:** Medical Oncology, NYU Med Ctr 1985; **Fac Appt:** Assoc Clin Prof Med, NYU Sch Med

Oster, Martin W MD [Onc] - **Spec Exp:** Breast Cancer; Gastrointestinal Cancer; Head & Neck Cancer; **Hospital:** NY-Presby/Columbia Univ Med Ctr, NY (page 65); **Address:** NY Presby Hosp-Columbia Presby Med Ctr, 161 Fort Washington Ave, New York, NY 10032-3713; **Phone:** 212-305-8231; **Board Cert:** Internal Medicine 1974; Medical Oncology 1975; **Med School:** Columbia P&S 1971; **Resid:** Internal Medicine, Mass Genl Hosp 1973; **Fellow:** Medical Oncology, Natl Cancer Inst/NIH 1976; **Fac Appt:** Assoc Clin Prof Med, Columbia P&S

Pasmantier, Mark W MD [Onc] - **Spec Exp:** Lung Cancer; Ovarian Cancer; Breast Cancer; Lymphoma; **Hospital:** NY-Presby/Weill Cornell Med Ctr, NY (page 65); **Address:** 407 E 70th St Fl 3, New York, NY 10021-5302; **Phone:** 212-517-5900; **Board Cert:** Internal Medicine 1972; Hematology 1974; Medical Oncology 1975; **Med School:** NYU Sch Med 1966; **Resid:** Internal Medicine, Harlem Hosp 1970; **Fellow:** Hematology, Montefiore Med Ctr 1971; Medical Oncology, NY Hosp 1972; **Fac Appt:** Clin Prof Med, Cornell Univ-Weill Med Coll

Pavlick, Anna C MD [Onc] - **Spec Exp:** Melanoma; Skin Cancer; Merkel Cell Carcinoma; **Hospital:** NYU Langone Med Ctr (page 66); **Address:** 160 E 34th St Fl 9, MS 10016, NYU Cancer Institute, New York, NY 10016; **Phone:** 212-731-5431; **Board Cert:** Medical Oncology 2008; **Med School:** UMDNJ Sch Osteo Med 1990; **Resid:** Internal Medicine, Hackensack Med Ctr 1993; **Fellow:** Hematology & Oncology, Meml Sloan Kettering Cancer Ctr 1996; **Fac Appt:** Assoc Prof Med, NYU Sch Med

Medical Oncology

Pecora, Andrew L MD [Onc] - **Spec Exp:** Stem Cell Transplant; Myelodysplastic Syndromes; Melanoma; Immunotherapy; **Hospital:** Hackensack Univ Med Ctr; **Address:** The Cancer Ctr-Hackensack Univ Med Ctr, 92 2nd St, Hackensack, NJ 07601; **Phone:** 201-996-5900; **Board Cert:** Internal Medicine 1986; Hematology 1988; Medical Oncology 1989; **Med School:** UMDNJ-NJ Med Sch, Newark 1983; **Resid:** Internal Medicine, New York Hosp 1986; **Fellow:** Hematology & Oncology, Meml Sloan Kettering Cancer Ctr 1988; **Fac Appt:** Prof Med, UMDNJ-NJ Med Sch, Newark

Perry, David J MD [Onc] - **Spec Exp:** Gastrointestinal Cancer; Lung Cancer; Genitourinary Cancer; Clinical Trials; **Hospital:** Washington Hosp Ctr; **Address:** Washington Hosp Ctr-Dept Med Oncology, 110 Irving St NW, rm C-2151, Washington, DC 20010; **Phone:** 202-877-2843; **Board Cert:** Internal Medicine 1979; Medical Oncology 1981; Hematology 1982; **Med School:** Univ Pennsylvania 1974; **Resid:** Internal Medicine, Walter Reed AMC 1979; **Fellow:** Hematology & Oncology, Walter Reed AMC 1979; **Fac Appt:** Assoc Prof Med, Eastern VA Med Sch

Petrylak, Daniel P MD [Onc] - **Spec Exp:** Testicular Cancer; Prostate Cancer; Bladder Cancer; Kidney Cancer; **Hospital:** NY-Presby/Columbia Univ Med Ctr, NY (page 65); **Address:** 161 Fort Washington Ave Fl 9, New York, NY 10032-3729; **Phone:** 212-305-1731; **Board Cert:** Internal Medicine 2001; Medical Oncology 2003; **Med School:** Case West Res Univ 1985; **Resid:** Internal Medicine, Jacobi Med Ctr 1988; **Fellow:** Oncology, Meml-Sloan Kettering Cancer Ctr 1991; **Fac Appt:** Assoc Prof Med, Columbia P&S

Pfister, David G MD [Onc] - **Spec Exp:** Head & Neck Cancer; Laryngeal Cancer; Thyroid Cancer; Skin Cancer; **Hospital:** Meml Sloan-Kettering Cancer Ctr; **Address:** 1275 York Avenue, New York, NY 10065; **Phone:** 800-525-2225; **Board Cert:** Internal Medicine 1985; Medical Oncology 1989; **Med School:** Univ Pennsylvania 1982; **Resid:** Internal Medicine, Hosp Univ Penn 1985; **Fellow:** Epidemiology, Yale-New Haven Hosp 1987; Hematology & Oncology, Meml Sloan Kettering Cancer Ctr 1989; **Fac Appt:** Prof Med, Cornell Univ-Weill Med Coll

Posner, Marshall R MD [Onc] - **Spec Exp:** Head & Neck Cancer; Skin Cancer-Head & Neck; **Hospital:** Mount Sinai Med Ctr (page 63); **Address:** Mount Sinai Med Ctr, 1 Gustave L Levy Pl, Box 1128, New York, NY 10029; **Phone:** 212-241-6756; **Board Cert:** Internal Medicine 1978; Medical Oncology 1981; **Med School:** Tufts Univ 1975; **Resid:** Internal Medicine, Boston City Hosp 1978; **Fellow:** Oncology, Dana-Farber Cancer Inst 1981; **Fac Appt:** Assoc Prof Med, Mount Sinai Sch Med

Raptis, George MD [Onc] - **Spec Exp:** Breast Cancer; **Hospital:** Mount Sinai Med Ctr (page 63); **Address:** Ruttenberg Treatment Ctr, 1190 5th Ave, Box 1129, New York, NY 10029; **Phone:** 212-241-6756; **Board Cert:** Medical Oncology 2003; **Med School:** Mount Sinai Sch Med 1987; **Resid:** Internal Medicine, Mt Sinai Med Ctr 1990; **Fellow:** Hematology & Oncology, Meml Sloan-Kettering Canc Ctr 1993; **Fac Appt:** Assoc Prof Med, Mount Sinai Sch Med

Remick, Scot C MD [Onc] - **Spec Exp:** AIDS Related Cancers; Clinical Trials; Drug Development; Thyroid Cancer; **Hospital:** Ruby Memorial - WVU Hosp; **Address:** WVU Mary Babb Randolph Cancer Ctr, MS 0, 1801 RCB Health Sciences Center S, Box 9300, Morgantown, WV 26506-9300; **Phone:** 304-598-4552; **Board Cert:** Internal Medicine 1985; Medical Oncology 1987; **Med School:** NY Med Coll 1982; **Resid:** Internal Medicine, Johns Hopkins Hosp 1985; **Fellow:** Medical Oncology, Univ Wisconsin Clin Cancer Ctr 1988; **Fac Appt:** Prof Med, W VA Univ

Ruggiero, Joseph T MD [Onc] - **Spec Exp:** Gastrointestinal Cancer; **Hospital:** NY-Presby/Weill Cornell Med Ctr, NY (page 65); **Address:** 428 E 72nd St, Ste 300, New York, NY 10021-4635; **Phone:** 212-746-2083; **Board Cert:** Internal Medicine 1980; Hematology 1982; Medical Oncology 1983; **Med School:** NYU Sch Med 1977; **Resid:** Internal Medicine, New York Hosp 1980; **Fellow:** Hematology & Oncology, New York Hosp/Cornell 1983; **Fac Appt:** Assoc Clin Prof Med, Cornell Univ-Weill Med Coll

Saif, M Wasif MD [Onc] - **Spec Exp:** Pancreatic Cancer; Colorectal Cancer; **Address:** Irving Pavilion 10, 177 Fort Washington Ave, rm 6-435, New York, NY 10032; **Phone:** 212-305-0592; **Board Cert:** Medical Oncology 2001; **Med School:** Pakistan 1992; **Resid:** Internal Medicine, UConn Sch Med 1998; **Fellow:** Medical Oncology, Nat'l Cancer Inst 2001; Hematology, Nat'l Heart Lung & Bloos Inst; **Fac Appt:** Clin Prof Med, Columbia P&S

Saltz, Leonard B MD [Onc] - **Spec Exp:** Colon & Rectal Cancer; Gastrointestinal Cancer & Rare Tumors; Neuroendocrine Tumors; **Hospital:** Meml Sloan-Kettering Cancer Ctr; **Address:** 1275 York Ave, rm H-917, New York, NY 10065; **Phone:** 646-497-9053; **Board Cert:** Internal Medicine 1986; Hematology 1988; Medical Oncology 1989; **Med School:** Yale Univ 1983; **Resid:** Internal Medicine, New Yor Hosp 1986; **Fellow:** Hematology & Oncology, New York Hosp-Cornell/Rockefeller Univ 1989; **Fac Appt:** Prof Med, Cornell Univ-Weill Med Coll

Scheinberg, David MD/PhD [Onc] - **Spec Exp:** Leukemia; Immunotherapy; Vaccine Therapy; **Hospital:** Meml Sloan-Kettering Cancer Ctr; **Address:** 1275 York Avenue, New York, NY 10065; **Phone:** 646-888-2190; **Board Cert:** Internal Medicine 1986; Medical Oncology 2005; **Med School:** Johns Hopkins Univ 1983; **Resid:** Internal Medicine, NY Hosp-Cornell Med Ctr 1985; **Fellow:** Medical Oncology, Meml Sloan Kettering Cancer Ctr 1987; **Fac Appt:** Prof Med, Cornell Univ-Weill Med Coll

Scher, Howard MD [Onc] - **Spec Exp:** Genitourinary Cancer; Prostate Cancer; Bladder Cancer; **Hospital:** Meml Sloan-Kettering Cancer Ctr; **Address:** 1275 York Avenue, New York, NY 10065; **Phone:** 800-525-2225; **Board Cert:** Internal Medicine 1979; Medical Oncology 1985; **Med School:** NYU Sch Med 1976; **Resid:** Internal Medicine, Bellevue Hosp 1980; **Fellow:** Medical Oncology, Meml Sloan Kettering Cancer Ctr 1983; **Fac Appt:** Prof Med, Cornell Univ-Weill Med Coll

Schilder, Russell J MD [Onc] - **Spec Exp:** Gynecologic Cancer; Hematologic Malignancies; Drug Development; Clinical Trials; **Hospital:** Fox Chase Cancer Ctr (page 58); **Address:** Fox Chase Cancer Ctr, 333 Cottman Ave, Philadelphia, PA 19111; **Phone:** 215-728-3545; **Board Cert:** Internal Medicine 1986; Hematology 1988; Medical Oncology 1989; **Med School:** Univ Miami Sch Med 1983; **Resid:** Internal Medicine, Temple Univ Hosp 1986; **Fellow:** Hematology & Oncology, Fox Chase Cancer Ctr 1989; **Fac Appt:** Prof Med, Temple Univ

Schuchter, Lynn M MD [Onc] - **Spec Exp:** Melanoma; Breast Cancer; Clinical Trials; **Hospital:** Hosp Univ Penn - UPHS (page 68); **Address:** Univ Penn/Abramson Cancer Ctr, 3400 Spruce St Penn Tower Bldg Fl 16, Philadelphia, PA 19104-4206; **Phone:** 215-662-7907; **Board Cert:** Internal Medicine 1985; Medical Oncology 1989; **Med School:** Ros Franklin Univ/Chicago Med Sch 1982; **Resid:** Internal Medicine, Michael Reese Hosp 1985; **Fellow:** Medical Oncology, Johns Hopkins Hosp 1989; **Fac Appt:** Prof Med, Univ Pennsylvania

Shields, Peter G MD [Onc] - **Spec Exp:** Hematologic Malignancies; **Hospital:** Georgetown Univ Hosp; **Address:** Lombardi Cancer Ctr, 3800 Reservoir Rd NW, First Floor, Washington, DC 20007; **Phone:** 202-444-2198; **Board Cert:** Medical Oncology 1989; **Med School:** Mount Sinai Sch Med 1983; **Resid:** Internal Medicine, George Washington Univ Hosp 1986; **Fellow:** Hematology & Oncology, George Washington Univ Hosp 1990; **Fac Appt:** Prof Med, Georgetown Univ

Sidransky, David MD [Onc] - **Spec Exp:** Head & Neck Cancer; **Hospital:** Johns Hopkins Hosp (page 61); **Address:** 1550 Orleans St, rm 5-N03, Baltimore, MD 21231; **Phone:** 410-502-5153; **Board Cert:** Internal Medicine 1988; **Med School:** Baylor Coll Med 1984; **Resid:** Internal Medicine, Baylor Coll Med 1988; **Fellow:** Medical Oncology, Johns Hopkins Hosp 1992; **Fac Appt:** Prof Oto, Johns Hopkins Univ

Medical Oncology

Silverman, Lewis R MD [Onc] - **Spec Exp:** Myelodysplastic Syndromes; Leukemia & Lymphoma; Multiple Myeloma; **Hospital:** Mount Sinai Med Ctr (page 63); **Address:** Ruttenberg Treatment Ctr, 1190 5th Ave, Box 1129, New York, NY 10029; **Phone:** 212-241-6756; **Board Cert:** Internal Medicine 1981; Medical Oncology 1987; **Med School:** Belgium 1978; **Resid:** Internal Medicine, Metro Hospital 1980; Internal Medicine, Montefiore Med Ctr 1981; **Fellow:** Hematology, Montefiore Med Ctr 1982; Neoplastic Diseases, Mt Sinai Med Ctr 1984; **Fac Appt:** Assoc Prof Med, Mount Sinai Sch Med

Smith, Mitchell R MD/PhD [Onc] - **Spec Exp:** Lymphoma; Leukemia; Hodgkin's Disease; Multiple Myeloma; **Hospital:** Fox Chase Cancer Ctr (page 58); **Address:** Fox Chase Cancer Ctr, 333 Cottman Ave, Ste C307, Philadelphia, PA 19111; **Phone:** 215-728-2674; **Board Cert:** Internal Medicine 1985; Medical Oncology 1987; Hematology 1988; **Med School:** Case West Res Univ 1979; **Resid:** Pathology, Barnes Jewish Hosp 1983; Internal Medicine, Barnes Jewish Hosp 1984; **Fellow:** Medical Oncology, Meml Sloan-Ketter Cancer Ctr 1988

Speyer, James MD [Onc] - **Spec Exp:** Ovarian Cancer; Breast Cancer; Cardiac Effects in Cancer Therapy; **Hospital:** NYU Langone Med Ctr (page 66); **Address:** NYU Clinical Cancer Center, 160 E 34th St Fl 8, New York, NY 10016-4750; **Phone:** 212-731-5432; **Board Cert:** Internal Medicine 1977; Hematology 1978; Medical Oncology 1979; **Med School:** Johns Hopkins Univ 1974; **Resid:** Internal Medicine, Columbia-Presby Med Ctr 1976; Hematology, Columbia-Presby Med Ctr 1977; **Fellow:** Medical Oncology, Natl Cancer Inst 1979; **Fac Appt:** Prof Med, NYU Sch Med

Spriggs, David R MD [Onc] - **Spec Exp:** Ovarian Cancer; Drug Development; Uterine Cancer; Gynecologic Cancer; **Hospital:** Meml Sloan-Kettering Cancer Ctr; **Address:** 1275 York Ave, H Bldg Fl 9 - Ste 901, New York, NY 10065; **Phone:** 800-525-2225; **Board Cert:** Internal Medicine 1981; Medical Oncology 2006; **Med School:** Univ Wisc 1977; **Resid:** Internal Medicine, Columbia-Presby Hosp 1981; **Fellow:** Medical Oncology, Dana-Farber Cancer Inst 1985; **Fac Appt:** Prof Med, Cornell Univ-Weill Med Coll

Stadtmauer, Edward A MD [Onc] - **Spec Exp:** Bone Marrow & Stem Cell Transplant; Leukemia; Multiple Myeloma; **Hospital:** Hosp Univ Penn - UPHS (page 68); **Address:** Abramson Cancer Ctr, Univ of Penn, 2 PCAM, 34th & Cancer Ctr Blvd, Philadelphia, PA 19104; **Phone:** 215-662-7910; **Board Cert:** Internal Medicine 1986; Hematology 1988; Medical Oncology 1989; **Med School:** Univ Pennsylvania 1983; **Resid:** Internal Medicine, Bronx Muni Hosp 1986; **Fellow:** Hematology & Oncology, Hosp Univ Penn 1989; **Fac Appt:** Prof Med, Univ Pennsylvania

Stoopler, Mark Benjamin MD [Onc] - **Spec Exp:** Lung Cancer; Esophageal Cancer; Unknown Primary Cancer; **Hospital:** NY-Presby/Columbia Univ Med Ctr, NY (page 65); **Address:** 161 Fort Washington Ave, Ste 936, New York, NY 10032-3713; **Phone:** 212-305-8230; **Board Cert:** Internal Medicine 1978; Medical Oncology 1981; **Med School:** Cornell Univ-Weill Med Coll 1975; **Resid:** Internal Medicine, North Shore Univ Hosp 1978; Internal Medicine, NY Meml Hosp 1978; **Fellow:** Medical Oncology, Meml-Sloan Kettering Cancer Ctr 1980; **Fac Appt:** Assoc Clin Prof Med, Columbia P&S

Straus, David J MD [Onc] - **Spec Exp:** Lymphoma; Multiple Myeloma; **Hospital:** Meml Sloan-Kettering Cancer Ctr; **Address:** 1275 York Avenue, New York, NY 10065; **Phone:** 212-639-8365; **Board Cert:** Internal Medicine 1972; Hematology 1976; Medical Oncology 1977; **Med School:** Marquette Sch Med 1969; **Resid:** Internal Medicine, Montefiore Med Ctr 1972; Medical Oncology, Meml Sloan Kettering Cancer Ctr 1977; **Fellow:** Hematology, Beth Israel Hosp 1973; **Fac Appt:** Prof Med, Cornell Univ-Weill Med Coll

Sun, Weijing MD [Onc] - **Spec Exp:** Gastrointestinal Cancer; Pancreatic Cancer; **Hospital:** Hosp Univ Penn - UPHS (page 68); **Address:** Hosp Univ Pennsylvania, Division of Hematology-Oncology, 3400 Civic Center Blvd, Ste 300W, Philadelphia, PA 19104; **Phone:** 215-662-6319; **Board Cert:** Medical Oncology 2001; **Med School:** China 1982; **Resid:** Internal Medicine, Loyola Univ Med Ctr 1998; **Fellow:** Hematology & Oncology, Hosp Univ Penn 2001; **Fac Appt:** Assoc Prof Med, Univ Pennsylvania

Swain, Sandra MD [Onc] - **Spec Exp:** Breast Cancer; **Hospital:** Washington Hosp Ctr; **Address:** Washington Cancer Inst, 110 Irving St NW, rm C-2149, Washington, DC 20010; **Phone:** 202-877-8112; **Board Cert:** Internal Medicine 1983; Medical Oncology 1985; **Med School:** Univ Fla Coll Med 1980; **Resid:** Internal Medicine, Vanderbilt Univ Affil Hosp 1983; **Fellow:** Medical Oncology, NIH- Natl Cancer Inst 1986; **Fac Appt:** Assoc Prof Med, Georgetown Univ

Tagawa, Scott T MD [Onc] - **Spec Exp:** Prostate Cancer; Bladder Cancer; Kidney Cancer; Urologic Cancer; **Hospital:** NY-Presby/Weill Cornell Med Ctr, NY (page 65); **Address:** NY Presby-Weill Cornell Med Ctr, 525 E 68th St, Box 403, New York, NY 10065; **Phone:** 646-962-2072; **Board Cert:** Internal Medicine 2001; Medical Oncology 2005; Hematology 2006; **Med School:** USC-Keck School of Medicine 1998; **Resid:** Internal Medicine, USC Med Ctr 2001; **Fellow:** Hematology & Oncology, USC Med Ctr 2005; **Fac Appt:** Asst Prof Hem & Onc, Cornell Univ-Weill Med Coll

Tester, William MD [Onc] - **Spec Exp:** Lung Cancer; Prostate Cancer; **Hospital:** Albert Einstein Med Ctr; **Address:** AEMC Cancer Center Fl 1, 5501 Old York Rd, Philadelphia, PA 19141; **Phone:** 215-456-3880; **Board Cert:** Internal Medicine 1980; Medical Oncology 1983; Hematology 1986; **Med School:** Hahnemann Univ 1977; **Resid:** Internal Medicine, Albert Einstein Med Ctr 1980; **Fellow:** Medical Oncology, NIH-Natl Cancer Inst 1982; Hematology, Georgetown Univ Affil Hosp 1983

Tkaczuk, Katherine H MD [Onc] - **Spec Exp:** Breast Cancer; **Hospital:** Univ of MD Med Ctr; **Address:** Univ MD Cancer Ctr, 22 S Greene St, rm S9D12, Baltimore, MD 21201; **Phone:** 410-328-7904; **Board Cert:** Internal Medicine 1989; Medical Oncology 2001; **Med School:** Poland 1984; **Resid:** Internal Medicine, St Agnes Hosp 1989; **Fellow:** Hematology & Oncology, Univ Maryland Cancer Ctr 1992; **Fac Appt:** Assoc Prof Med, Univ MD Sch Med

Toppmeyer, Deborah L MD [Onc] - **Spec Exp:** Breast Cancer; Hereditary Cancer; **Hospital:** Robert Wood Johnson Univ Hosp - New Brunswick; **Address:** Cancer Inst of New Jersey, 195 Little Albany St, New Brunswick, NJ 08903; **Phone:** 732-235-9692; **Board Cert:** Internal Medicine 1988; Medical Oncology 2006; **Med School:** Albany Med Coll 1985; **Resid:** Internal Medicine, Univ Pittsburgh Hlth Ctr Hosp 1988; **Fellow:** Medical Oncology, Dana Farber Cancer Inst 1993; **Fac Appt:** Assoc Prof Med

Trump, Donald L MD [Onc] - **Spec Exp:** Prostate Cancer; Genitourinary Cancer; Drug Discovery & Development; **Hospital:** Roswell Park Cancer Inst; **Address:** Roswell Park Cancer Inst, Elm and Carlton Streets, Buffalo, NY 14263; **Phone:** 716-845-3159; **Board Cert:** Internal Medicine 1973; Medical Oncology 1977; **Med School:** Johns Hopkins Univ 1970; **Resid:** Internal Medicine, Johns Hopkins Hosp 1975; **Fellow:** Medical Oncology, Johns Hopkins Hosp 1974; **Fac Appt:** Prof Med, SUNY Buffalo

Vahdat, Linda T MD [Onc] - **Spec Exp:** Breast Cancer; Breast Cancer-Novel Therapies; **Hospital:** NY-Presby/Weill Cornell Med Ctr, NY (page 65); **Address:** 425 E 61st St Fl 8, New York, NY 10065; **Phone:** 212-821-0644; **Board Cert:** Medical Oncology 2005; **Med School:** Mount Sinai Sch Med 1987; **Resid:** Internal Medicine, Mt Sinai Hosp 1990; **Fellow:** Hematology & Oncology, Meml Sloan Kettering Cancer Ctr 1994; **Fac Appt:** Prof Med, Cornell Univ-Weill Med Coll

Vaughn, David J MD [Onc] - **Spec Exp:** Testicular Cancer; Bladder Cancer; Prostate Cancer; Genitourinary Cancer; **Hospital:** Hosp Univ Penn - UPHS (page 68); **Address:** Hosp Univ of Pennsylvania-16 Penn Tower, 3400 Spruce St, Philadelphia, PA 19104; **Phone:** 215-349-8498; **Board Cert:** Medical Oncology 2003; **Med School:** Harvard Med Sch 1987; **Resid:** Internal Medicine, NY Hosp-Cornell Med Ctr 1990; **Fellow:** Hematology & Oncology, Hosp Univ Penn 1993; **Fac Appt:** Prof Med, Univ Pennsylvania

Vinciguerra, Vincent P MD [Onc] - **Spec Exp:** Breast Cancer; Gastrointestinal Cancer; Lung Cancer; Cancer Prevention; **Hospital:** N Shore Univ Hosp; **Address:** 450 Lakeville Rd, Montra Cancer Ctr, Lake Success, NY 11042; **Phone:** 516-734-8954; **Board Cert:** Internal Medicine 1971; Hematology 1974; Medical Oncology 1975; **Med School:** Georgetown Univ 1966; **Resid:** Internal Medicine, NY Hosp-Cornell 1969; Internal Medicine, N Shore Univ Hosp 1971; **Fellow:** Hematology & Oncology, NY Hosp-Cornell 1970; Hematology & Oncology, N Shore Univ Hosp 1974; **Fac Appt:** Prof Med, NYU Sch Med

von Mehren, Margaret MD [Onc] - **Spec Exp:** Sarcoma; Melanoma; Immunotherapy; Gastrointestinal Stromal Tumors; **Hospital:** Fox Chase Cancer Ctr (page 58); **Address:** Fox Chase Cancer Ctr, Dept Med Oncology, 333 Cottman Ave, Philadelphia, PA 19111-2434; **Phone:** 215-728-2814; **Board Cert:** Medical Oncology 2007; **Med School:** Albany Med Coll 1989; **Resid:** Internal Medicine, NYU Med Ctr 1993; **Fellow:** Hematology & Oncology, Fox Chase Cancer Ctr 1996; **Fac Appt:** Assoc Prof Med, Temple Univ

Waintraub, Stanley MD [Onc] - **Spec Exp:** Breast Cancer; Bleeding/Coagulation Disorders; **Hospital:** Hackensack Univ Med Ctr; **Address:** Northern NJ Cancer Associates, 92 2nd St, Hackensack, NJ 07601; **Phone:** 201-996-5900; **Board Cert:** Internal Medicine 1980; Hematology 1982; Medical Oncology 1983; **Med School:** NY Med Coll 1977; **Resid:** Internal Medicine, Metropolitan Hosp Ctr 1980; **Fellow:** Hematology, Montefiore Hosp Med Ctr 1982; Medical Oncology, Meml Sloan Kettering Cancer Ctr 1983

Weiner, Louis M MD [Onc] - **Spec Exp:** Gastrointestinal Cancer; Immunotherapy; Liver Cancer; **Hospital:** Georgetown Univ Hosp; **Address:** Lombardi Cancer Ctr, Georgetown Univ, Research Bldg, 3800 Reservoir Rd NW, Washington, DC 20007; **Phone:** 202-444-2198; **Board Cert:** Internal Medicine 1980; Medical Oncology 1985; **Med School:** Mount Sinai Sch Med 1977; **Resid:** Internal Medicine, Med Ctr Hosp Vermont 1981; **Fellow:** Hematology & Oncology, New England Med Ctr 1984; **Fac Appt:** Prof Med, Georgetown Univ

Wetzler, Meir MD [Onc] - **Spec Exp:** Leukemia; **Hospital:** Roswell Park Cancer Inst; **Address:** Roswell Park Cancer Inst, Elm and Carlton Streets, Buffalo, NY 14263; **Phone:** 716-845-8447; **Board Cert:** Internal Medicine 2001; Medical Oncology 2003; **Med School:** Israel 1980; **Resid:** Internal Medicine, Kaplan Hosp 1986; **Fellow:** Medical Oncology, MD Anderson Cancer Ctr 1992; Clinical Immunology, MD Anderson Cancer Ctr 1992; **Fac Appt:** Prof Med, SUNY Buffalo

Wilson, Wyndham MD [Onc] - **Spec Exp:** Lymphoma; **Hospital:** Natl Inst of Hlth - Clin Ctr; **Address:** National Cancer Inst, Bldg 10 - rm 4N-115, 9000 Rockville Pike, Bethesda, MD 20892; **Phone:** 301-435-2415; **Board Cert:** Internal Medicine 1985; Medical Oncology 1987; **Med School:** Stanford Univ 1981; **Resid:** Internal Medicine, Stanford Univ 1984; **Fellow:** Oncology, NCI-NIH 1987

Wolchok, Jedd D MD/PhD [Onc] - **Spec Exp:** Melanoma; Immunotherapy; Clinical Trials; Vaccine Therapy; **Hospital:** Meml Sloan-Kettering Cancer Ctr; **Address:** Meml Sloan Kettering Cancer Ctr, 1275 York Ave, New York, NY 10065; **Phone:** 646-888-2395; **Board Cert:** Medical Oncology 2000; **Med School:** NYU Sch Med 1994; **Resid:** Internal Medicine, NYU Med Ctr 1996; **Fellow:** Medical Oncology, Meml Sloan-Kettering Canc Ctr 1997

Wolff, Antonio C MD [Onc] - **Spec Exp:** Breast Cancer; Drug Development; **Hospital:** Johns Hopkins Hosp (page 61); **Address:** 1650 Orleans St, rm 189, CRB-1 Bldg, Baltimore, MD 21231; **Phone:** 410-614-4192; **Board Cert:** Internal Medicine 2000; Medical Oncology 2000; **Med School:** Brazil 1986; **Resid:** Internal Medicine, Mt Sinai Med Ctr 1991; **Fellow:** Hematology & Oncology, Washington Univ Med Ctr 1992; Medical Oncology, Johns Hopkins Hosp 1995; **Fac Appt:** Assoc Prof Med, Johns Hopkins Univ

Zelenetz, Andrew D MD/PhD [Onc] - **Spec Exp:** Lymphoma; **Hospital:** Meml Sloan-Kettering Cancer Ctr; **Address:** 1275 York Avenue, New York, NY 10065; **Phone:** 800-525-2225; **Board Cert:** Medical Oncology 2009; **Med School:** Harvard Med Sch 1984; **Resid:** Internal Medicine, Stanford Univ Med Ctr 1986; **Fellow:** Medical Oncology, Stanford Univ Med Ctr 1991; **Fac Appt:** Asst Prof Med, Cornell Univ-Weill Med Coll

Southeast

Antonia, Scott J MD/PhD [Onc] - **Spec Exp:** Kidney Cancer; Lung Cancer; **Hospital:** H Lee Moffitt Cancer Ctr & Research Inst (page 59); **Address:** H Lee Moffitt Cancer Ctr, 12902 Magnolia Drive, Tampa, FL 33612; **Phone:** 813-979-3883; **Board Cert:** Internal Medicine 2002; Medical Oncology 2006; **Med School:** Univ Conn 1989; **Resid:** Internal Medicine, Yale-New Haven Hosp 1991; **Fellow:** Medical Oncology, Yale-New Haven Hosp 1994; **Fac Appt:** Assoc Prof Med, Univ S Fla Coll Med

Arteaga, Carlos L MD [Onc] - **Spec Exp:** Breast Cancer; **Hospital:** Vanderbilt Univ Med Ctr (page 76), TN Valley Healthcare Sys-Nashville; **Address:** Vanderbilt-Ingram Cancer Ctr, 2220 Pierce Ave, 777 Preston Rsch Bldg, Nashville, TN 37232-6838; **Phone:** 615-936-3524; **Board Cert:** Internal Medicine 1984; Medical Oncology 1989; **Med School:** Ecuador 1980; **Resid:** Internal Medicine, Grady Meml Hosp 1984; **Fellow:** Hematology & Oncology, Univ Texas Hlth Sci Ctr 1987; **Fac Appt:** Prof Med, Vanderbilt Univ

Balducci, Lodovico MD [Onc] - **Spec Exp:** Genitourinary Cancer; Breast Cancer; **Hospital:** H Lee Moffitt Cancer Ctr & Research Inst (page 59), Tampa Genl Hosp; **Address:** H Lee Moffitt Cancer Ctr, 12902 Magnolia Drive, Tampa, FL 33612; **Phone:** 813-745-8658; **Board Cert:** Internal Medicine 1987; Hematology 1978; Medical Oncology 1979; **Med School:** Italy 1968; **Resid:** Internal Medicine, Univ Miss Med Ctr 1976; Hematology & Oncology, Univ Miss Med Ctr 1979; **Fellow:** Internal Medicine, A Gemelli Genl Hosp 1970; **Fac Appt:** Prof Med, Univ S Fla Coll Med

Benedetto, Pasquale W MD [Onc] - **Spec Exp:** Genitourinary Cancer; Bone Tumors; Gastrointestinal Cancer; Pancreatic Cancer; **Hospital:** Univ of Miami Hosp & Clins/Sylvester Comp Canc Ctr (page 73), Jackson Meml Hosp (page 70); **Address:** Sylvester Comp Cancer Ctr, Med Oncology, 1475 NW 12th Ave, rm 3310, Miami, FL 33136; **Phone:** 305-243-1000; **Board Cert:** Internal Medicine 1979; Medical Oncology 1981; Hematology 1982; **Med School:** Cornell Univ-Weill Med Coll 1976; **Resid:** Internal Medicine, Johns Hopkins Hosp 1979; **Fellow:** Medical Oncology, Meml Sloan Kettering Cancer Ctr 1981; **Fac Appt:** Prof Med, Univ Miami Sch Med

Berlin, Jordan D MD [Onc] - **Spec Exp:** Gastrointestinal Cancer; Pancreatic Cancer; Liver Cancer; Clinical Trials; **Hospital:** Vanderbilt Univ Med Ctr (page 76); **Address:** Vanderbilt-Ingram Cancer Ctr, 777 Preston Rsch Bldg, Nashville, TN 37232-6307; **Phone:** 615-322-6053; **Board Cert:** Internal Medicine 2002; Medical Oncology 2005; **Med School:** Univ IL Coll Med 1989; **Resid:** Internal Medicine, Univ Cincinnati Med Ctr 1992; **Fellow:** Medical Oncology, Univ Wisconsin 1995; **Fac Appt:** Assoc Prof Med, Vanderbilt Univ

Medical Oncology

Bernard, Stephen A MD [Onc] - **Spec Exp:** Gastrointestinal Cancer; Palliative Care; Clinical Trials; **Hospital:** NC Memorial Hosp - UNC; **Address:** Univ North Carolina Sch Med, 170 Manning Drive, CB 7305, Chapel Hill, NC 27599; **Phone:** 919-966-0000; **Board Cert:** Internal Medicine 1987; Medical Oncology 1979; Hospice & Palliative Medicine 2008; **Med School:** Univ NC Sch Med 1973; **Resid:** Internal Medicine, Columbia-Presby Med Ctr 1976; **Fellow:** Hematology & Oncology, Wash Univ Hosps 1978; **Fac Appt:** Prof Med, Univ NC Sch Med

Blackwell, Kimberly L MD [Onc] - **Spec Exp:** Breast Cancer; Clinical Trials; **Hospital:** Duke Univ Hosp; **Address:** Duke Univ Medical Ctr, Box 3893, Durham, NC 27710; **Phone:** 919-668-6688; **Board Cert:** Medical Oncology 2000; **Med School:** Mayo Med Sch 1994; **Resid:** Internal Medicine, Duke Univ Med Ctr 1997; **Fellow:** Medical Oncology, Duke Univ Med Ctr 2000; **Fac Appt:** Assoc Prof Med, Duke Univ

Blobe, Gerard C MD/PhD [Onc] - **Spec Exp:** Pancreatic Cancer; Colon & Rectal Cancer; Clinical Trials; **Hospital:** Duke Univ Hosp; **Address:** Dept Hematology/Oncology, Box 91004, Durham, NC 27708; **Phone:** 919-668-6688; **Board Cert:** Internal Medicine 2009; Medical Oncology 2000; **Med School:** Duke Univ 1995; **Resid:** Internal Medicine, Brigham & Women's Hosp 1997; **Fellow:** Medical Oncology, Dana-Farber Cancer Inst 2000; **Fac Appt:** Assoc Prof Med, Duke Univ

Bolger, Graeme B MD [Onc] - **Spec Exp:** Prostate Cancer; Testicular Cancer; **Hospital:** Univ of Ala Hosp at Birmingham; **Address:** 1530 3rd Ave S, Ste FOT-1105, Birmingham, AL 35294; **Phone:** 205-934-2992; **Board Cert:** Internal Medicine 1984; Medical Oncology 2000; **Med School:** McGill Univ 1981; **Resid:** Internal Medicine, Johns Hopkins Hosp 1984; **Fellow:** Medical Oncology, Fred Hutchinson Cancer Rsch 1985; Oncology, Meml Sloan-Kettering Cancer Ctr 1992; **Fac Appt:** Assoc Prof Med, Univ Alabama

Boston, Barry MD [Onc] - **Spec Exp:** Gastrointestinal Cancer; Genitourinary Cancer; Prostate Cancer; **Hospital:** St. Francis Hosp - Memphis, Methodist Univ Hosp - Memphis; **Address:** Univ of Tennessee Cancer Inst, 7945 Wolf River Blvd, Ste 300, Germantown, TN 38138; **Phone:** 901-752-6131; **Board Cert:** Internal Medicine 1974; Medical Oncology 1977; **Med School:** Louisiana State U, New Orleans 1971; **Resid:** Internal Medicine, Univ Tenn Hosp-VA Hosp 1973; Hematology, Univ Tenn Hosp-VA Hosp 1973; **Fellow:** Medical Oncology, Yale-New Haven Hosp 1975; **Fac Appt:** Assoc Prof Med, Univ Tenn Coll Med

Brenin, Christiana M MD [Onc] - **Spec Exp:** Breast Cancer; Colon & Rectal Cancer; **Hospital:** Univ of Virginia Health Sys; **Address:** Univ Virginia Med Ctr, Division of Hematology/Oncology, PO Box 800716, Charlottesville, VA 22908; **Phone:** 434-924-8552; **Board Cert:** Internal Medicine 2003; Medical Oncology 2008; **Med School:** NY Med Coll 1990; **Resid:** Internal Medicine, Northwestern Meml Hosp 1993; **Fellow:** Hematology & Oncology, Northwestern Meml Hosp 1996; **Fac Appt:** Assoc Prof Med, Univ VA Sch Med

Burris III, Howard A MD [Onc] - **Spec Exp:** Drug Development; Drug Discovery; Breast Cancer; **Hospital:** Centennial Med Ctr, Baptist Hosp - Nashville; **Address:** Tennessee Oncology, 250 25th Ave N, Ste 100, Nashville, TN 37203; **Phone:** 615-986-4300; **Board Cert:** Internal Medicine 1988; Medical Oncology 2001; **Med School:** Univ S Ala Coll Med 1985; **Resid:** Internal Medicine, Brooke Army Med Ctr 1988; **Fellow:** Medical Oncology, Brooke Army Med Ctr 1991

Butler, William M MD [Onc] - **Spec Exp:** Breast Cancer; Prostate Cancer; Lung Cancer; Clinical Trials; **Hospital:** Palmetto Health Richland Mem Hosp; **Address:** SC Oncology Associates, 166 Stoneridge Drive, Columbia, SC 29210; **Phone:** 803-461-3000; **Board Cert:** Internal Medicine 1975; Medical Oncology 1979; Hematology 1980; **Med School:** Tulane Univ 1972; **Resid:** Internal Medicine, Charity Hosp 1975; **Fellow:** Hematology & Oncology, Walter Reed AMC 1980; **Fac Appt:** Clin Prof Med, Univ SC Sch Med

Carbone, David MD/PhD [Onc] - **Spec Exp:** Lung Cancer; **Hospital:** Vanderbilt Univ Med Ctr (page 76); **Address:** Vanderbilt-Ingram Cancer Ctr, 685 Preston Rsch Bldg, 2220 Pierce Ave, Nashville, TN 37232-6838; **Phone:** 615-936-1279; **Board Cert:** Internal Medicine 1988; Medical Oncology 2001; **Med School:** Johns Hopkins Univ 1985; **Resid:** Internal Medicine, Johns Hopkins Hosp 1988; **Fellow:** Oncology, Natl Cancer Inst 1991; **Fac Appt:** Prof Med, Vanderbilt Univ

Carey, Lisa A MD [Onc] - **Spec Exp:** Breast Cancer; **Hospital:** NC Memorial Hosp - UNC; **Address:** Univ North Carolina-Div Hem/Onc, 170 Manning Drive Fl 3rd, POB Campus Box 7305, Chapel Hill, NC 27599-7300; **Phone:** 919-966-4431; **Board Cert:** Internal Medicine 2003; Medical Oncology 2007; **Med School:** Johns Hopkins Univ 1990; **Resid:** Internal Medicine, Johns Hopkins Hosp 1993; **Fellow:** Oncology, Johns Hopkins Hosp 1996; **Fac Appt:** Asst Prof Med, Univ NC Sch Med

Carpenter Jr, John T MD [Onc] - **Spec Exp:** Breast Cancer; **Hospital:** Univ of Ala Hosp at Birmingham; **Address:** Univ Alabama Birmingham, 1530 3rd Ave S, Ste FOT-510, Birmingham, AL 35294-3300; **Phone:** 205-934-2084; **Board Cert:** Internal Medicine 1972; Hematology 1981; Medical Oncology 1975; **Med School:** Tulane Univ 1968; **Resid:** Internal Medicine, Grady Meml Hosp 1971; **Fellow:** Hematology & Oncology, Emory Univ 1973; **Fac Appt:** Prof Med, Univ Alabama

Chao, Nelson J MD [Onc] - **Spec Exp:** Bone Marrow Transplant; Lymphoma; Leukemia; **Hospital:** Duke Univ Hosp; **Address:** Duke Univ Med Ctr, Box 3961, Durham, NC 27710; **Phone:** 919-668-1002; **Board Cert:** Internal Medicine 1984; Medical Oncology 1987; **Med School:** Yale Univ 1981; **Resid:** Internal Medicine, Stanford Univ Med Ctr 1984; **Fellow:** Oncology, Stanford Univ Med Ctr 1987; **Fac Appt:** Prof Med, Duke Univ

Chung, Ki Young MD [Onc] - **Spec Exp:** Gastrointestinal Cancer; **Address:** Cancer Ctrs of the Carolinas-Spartanburg, 120 Dillon Drive, Spartanburg, SC 29307; **Phone:** 864-699-5700; **Board Cert:** Medical Oncology 2004; **Med School:** Univ NC Sch Med 1995; **Resid:** Internal Medicine, Johns Hopkins Hosp/Sinai Hosp; **Fellow:** Hematology & Oncology, Meml Sloan Kettering Cancer Ctr 2003

Colon-Otero, Gerardo MD [Onc] - **Spec Exp:** Ovarian Cancer; Breast Cancer; Hematologic Malignancies; Pancreatic Cancer-Acinar Cell; **Hospital:** Mayo - Jacksonville; **Address:** Mayo Clinic, 4500 San Pablo Rd S, Jacksonville, FL 32224-1865; **Phone:** 904-953-2000; **Board Cert:** Internal Medicine 1982; Hematology 1984; Medical Oncology 1985; **Med School:** Puerto Rico 1979; **Resid:** Internal Medicine, Mayo Clinic 1982; **Fellow:** Hematology, Mayo Clinic 1984; Medical Oncology, Univ Va Med Ctr 1986; **Fac Appt:** Assoc Prof Med, Mayo Med Sch

Conry, Robert M MD [Onc] - **Spec Exp:** Melanoma; Lung Cancer; Colon & Rectal Cancer; Sarcoma; **Hospital:** Univ of Ala Hosp at Birmingham; **Address:** The Kirklin Clinic At Acton Rd, 2145 Bonner Way, Birmingham, AL 35243; **Phone:** 205-978-0250; **Board Cert:** Hematology 2001; **Med School:** Univ Alabama 1987; **Resid:** Internal Medicine, Univ Alabama Hosp 1990; **Fellow:** Medical Oncology, Univ Alabama Hosp 1993; **Fac Appt:** Assoc Prof Med, Univ Alabama

Crawford, Jeffrey MD [Onc] - **Spec Exp:** Lung Cancer; **Hospital:** Duke Univ Hosp; **Address:** Duke Univ Med Ctr, Box 3476, Durham, NC 27710; **Phone:** 919-668-6688; **Board Cert:** Internal Medicine 1977; Hematology 1980; Medical Oncology 1981; **Med School:** Ohio State Univ 1974; **Resid:** Internal Medicine, Duke Univ Med Ctr 1977; **Fellow:** Hematology & Oncology, Duke Univ Med Ctr 1981; **Fac Appt:** Prof Med, Duke Univ

Medical Oncology

De Simone, Philip MD [Onc] - **Spec Exp:** Colon Cancer; Pancreatic Cancer; **Hospital:** Univ of Kentucky Albert B. Chandler Hosp; **Address:** UKMC Markey Cancer Ctr, 800 Rose St Fl 1, Whitney-Hendrickson bldg, Lexington, KY 40536; **Phone:** 859-323-8043; **Board Cert:** Internal Medicine 1972; Hematology 1974; **Med School:** Univ VT Coll Med 1967; **Resid:** Internal Medicine, Univ Kentucky Hosp 1972; **Fellow:** Hematology & Oncology, Univ Kentucky Hosp 1974; **Fac Appt:** Prof Med, Univ KY Coll Med

Dunphy II, Frank R MD [Onc] - **Spec Exp:** Lung Cancer; Head & Neck Cancer; **Hospital:** Duke Univ Hosp; **Address:** Duke Univ Med Ctr, Box 3685, Durham, NC 27710; **Phone:** 919-668-6688; **Board Cert:** Internal Medicine 1984; Hematology 1986; Medical Oncology 1989; **Med School:** Louisiana State U, New Orleans 1979; **Resid:** Internal Medicine, Lousiana St Univ Hosp 1983; **Fellow:** Hematology & Oncology, Louisiana St Univ Hosp 1985; **Fac Appt:** Assoc Prof Med, Duke Univ

Flinn, Ian W MD/PhD [Onc] - **Spec Exp:** Leukemia; Lymphoma; Bone Marrow Transplant; Multiple Myeloma; **Hospital:** Centennial Med Ctr; **Address:** Tennessee Oncology, 250 25th Ave N, Ste 412, Nashville, TN 37203; **Phone:** 615-986-7600; **Board Cert:** Hematology 2007; Medical Oncology 2008; **Med School:** Johns Hopkins Univ 1990; **Resid:** Internal Medicine, Univ Michigan Med Ctr 1993; **Fellow:** Hematology & Oncology, Johns Hopkins 1996

Forero, Andres MD [Onc] - **Spec Exp:** Lymphoma; **Hospital:** Univ of Ala Hosp at Birmingham; **Address:** 615 18th St S, Birmingham, AL 35233; **Phone:** 205-934-9999; **Med School:** Colombia 1982; **Resid:** Internal Medicine, Javeriana Univ 1987; **Fellow:** Medical Oncology, Javeriana Univ 1991; **Fac Appt:** Assoc Prof Med, Univ Alabama

Fracasso, Paula M MD/PhD [Onc] - **Spec Exp:** Gynecologic Cancer; Breast Cancer; **Hospital:** Univ of Virginia Health Sys; **Address:** Univ Virginia- Dept Medicine, PO Box 800716, Charlottesville, VA 22908; **Phone:** 434-243-6143; **Board Cert:** Internal Medicine 1987; Medical Oncology 2003; **Med School:** Yale Univ 1984; **Resid:** Internal Medicine, Beth Israel Hosp 1987; **Fellow:** Cancer Research, Mass Inst Tech 1989; Hematology & Oncology, Tufts-New England Med Ctr 1991; **Fac Appt:** Prof Med, Univ VA Sch Med

Friedman, Henry S MD [Onc] - **Spec Exp:** Neuro-Oncology; Brain & Spinal Cord Tumors; Gliomas; **Hospital:** Duke Univ Hosp; **Address:** Preston Robert Tisch, Brain Tumor Ctr at Duke, DUMC, Box 3624, Durham, NC 27710; **Phone:** 919-684-5301; **Board Cert:** Pediatrics 1982; Pediatric Hematology-Oncology 1982; **Med School:** SUNY Upstate Med Univ 1977; **Resid:** Pediatrics, SUNY Upstate Med Ctr 1980; **Fellow:** Pediatric Hematology-Oncology, Duke Univ Med Ctr 1983; **Fac Appt:** Prof Neuro-Onc, Duke Univ

Garst, Jennifer L MD [Onc] - **Spec Exp:** Lung Cancer; Thoracic Cancers; Cancer Survivors-Late Effects of Therapy; **Hospital:** Duke Univ Hosp; **Address:** Duke Univ Hosp, Div Medical Oncology, 2301 Erwin Rd, Box 3198, Durham, NC 27710; **Phone:** 919-681-6932; **Board Cert:** Internal Medicine 2008; **Med School:** Med Coll GA 1990; **Resid:** Internal Medicine, Univ SW Texas Hosp 1993; **Fellow:** Hematology & Oncology, Duke Univ Med Ctr 1996; **Fac Appt:** Assoc Prof Med, Duke Univ

George, Daniel J MD [Onc] - **Spec Exp:** Prostate Cancer; Kidney Cancer; **Hospital:** Duke Univ Hosp; **Address:** Duke Univ Med Ctr, Box 102002, Durham, NC 27710; **Phone:** 919-668-8108; **Board Cert:** Medical Oncology 2007; **Med School:** Duke Univ 1992; **Resid:** Internal Medicine, Johns Hopkins Hosp 1995; **Fellow:** Medical Oncology, Johns Hopkins Hosp 1998; **Fac Appt:** Assoc Prof S, Duke Univ

Gockerman, Jon Paul MD [Onc] - **Spec Exp:** Leukemia; Lymphoma; **Hospital:** Duke Univ Hosp; **Address:** Duke Univ Med Ctr, 1 Trent Drive, rm 25153, Box 3872, Morris Bldg, Durham, NC 27710; **Phone:** 919-684-8964; **Board Cert:** Internal Medicine 1972; Medical Oncology 1973; Hematology 1974; **Med School:** Univ Chicago-Pritzker Sch Med 1967; **Resid:** Internal Medicine, Duke Univ Med Ctr 1969; **Fellow:** Hematology & Oncology, Duke Univ Med Ctr 1971

Godley, Paul A MD/PhD [Onc] - **Spec Exp:** Prostate Cancer (advanced); Testicular Cancer; Penile Cancer; Bladder Cancer; **Hospital:** NC Memorial Hosp - UNC; **Address:** UNC Hematology/Oncology, POB, Campus Box 7305, 3rd Floor, 170 Manning Drive, Chapel Hill, NC 27599; **Phone:** 919-966-4431; **Board Cert:** Internal Medicine 1987; Medical Oncology 2002; **Med School:** Harvard Med Sch 1984; **Resid:** Internal Medicine, Univ Hosps 1987; **Fellow:** Epidemiology, Univ NC Sch of Public Hlth 1989; Hematology & Oncology, Univ NC Hosps 1991; **Fac Appt:** Assoc Prof Med, Univ NC Sch Med

Goldberg, Richard M MD [Onc] - **Spec Exp:** Stomach Cancer; Esophageal Cancer; Pancreatic Cancer; Neuroendocrine Tumors; **Hospital:** NC Memorial Hosp - UNC; **Address:** Division of Hematology/Oncology, CB 7305, 170 Manning Drive, Chapel Hill, NC 27599-0001; **Phone:** 919-843-7711; **Board Cert:** Internal Medicine 1982; Medical Oncology 1985; **Med School:** SUNY Upstate Med Univ 1979; **Resid:** Internal Medicine, Emory Univ Med Ctr 1982; **Fellow:** Medical Oncology, Georgetown Univ Med Ctr 1984; **Fac Appt:** Prof Med, Univ NC Sch Med

Graham II, Mark L MD [Onc] - **Spec Exp:** Breast Cancer; Breast Cancer Genetics; **Hospital:** WakeMed Cary; **Address:** Waverly Hematology/Oncology, 300 Ashville Ave, Ste 310, Cary, NC 27518; **Phone:** 919-233-8585; **Board Cert:** Internal Medicine 1989; **Med School:** Mayo Med Sch 1982; **Resid:** Internal Medicine, Duke Univ Med Ctr 1985; **Fellow:** Medical Oncology, Univ CO Hlth Sci Ctr 1990; Medical Oncology, Mayo Clinic 1991; **Fac Appt:** Assoc Clin Prof Med, Univ NC Sch Med

Greco, F Anthony MD [Onc] - **Spec Exp:** Lung Cancer; Unknown Primary Cancer; **Hospital:** Centennial Med Ctr; **Address:** Sarah Cannon Research Inst, 250 25th Ave N Atrium Bldg - Ste 100, Nashville, TN 37203; **Phone:** 615-320-5090; **Board Cert:** Internal Medicine 1975; Medical Oncology 1977; **Med School:** W VA Univ 1972; **Resid:** Internal Medicine, Univ West Virginia Hosp 1974; **Fellow:** Medical Oncology, Natl Cancer Inst 1976

Grosh, William W MD [Onc] - **Spec Exp:** Melanoma; Sarcoma; Neuroendocrine Tumors; **Hospital:** Univ of Virginia Health Sys; **Address:** UVA Health System, Div Hem/Oncology, PO Box 800716, Charlottesville, VA 22908; **Phone:** 434-924-1904; **Board Cert:** Internal Medicine 1978; Medical Oncology 1985; **Med School:** Columbia P&S 1974; **Resid:** Internal Medicine, Vanderbilt Univ Med Ctr 1977; **Fellow:** Medical Oncology, Vanderbilt Univ Med Ctr 1983; **Fac Appt:** Assoc Prof Med, Univ VA Sch Med

Hande, Kenneth R MD [Onc] - **Spec Exp:** Drug Discovery; Sarcoma; Carcinoid Tumors; **Hospital:** Vanderbilt Univ Med Ctr (page 76), TN Valley Healthcare Sys-Nashville; **Address:** Vanderbilt Univ Med Ctr, 2220 Pierce Ave, Div Hematology/Oncology, 777 Preston Rsch Bldg, Nashville, TN 37232-6307; **Phone:** 615-322-4967; **Board Cert:** Internal Medicine 1975; Medical Oncology 1977; **Med School:** Johns Hopkins Univ 1972; **Resid:** Internal Medicine, Barnes Hosp 1974; **Fellow:** Medical Oncology, Natl Cancer Inst 1977; **Fac Appt:** Prof Med, Vanderbilt Univ

Hurd, David MD [Onc] - **Spec Exp:** Lymphoma; Leukemia; Bone Marrow Transplant; **Hospital:** Wake Forest Univ Baptist Med Ctr; **Address:** Wake Forest Sch Med, Comp Cancer Ctr, Medical Center Boulevard, Winston-Salem, NC 27157-1082; **Phone:** 336-713-5440; **Board Cert:** Internal Medicine 1977; Medical Oncology 1981; **Med School:** Univ IL Coll Med 1974; **Resid:** Internal Medicine, Univ Minn Hosp 1977; **Fellow:** Medical Oncology, Univ Minn Hosp 1979; **Fac Appt:** Prof Med, Wake Forest Univ

Medical Oncology

Jahanzeb, Mohammad MD [Onc] - **Spec Exp:** Breast Cancer; Lung Cancer; **Hospital:** Boca Raton Regl Hosp; **Address:** 1192 E Newport Center Drive, Ste 200, Deerfield Beach, FL 33442; **Phone:** 954-698-3665; **Board Cert:** Medical Oncology 2003; Hematology 2005; **Med School:** Pakistan 1986; **Resid:** Internal Medicine, New Britain Genl Hosp 1990; **Fellow:** Hematology & Oncology, Washington Univ 1993; **Fac Appt:** Prof Med

Jillella, Anand MD [Onc] - **Spec Exp:** Bone Marrow Transplant; Leukemia; Lymphoma; Multiple Myeloma; **Hospital:** Med Coll of GA Hosp and Clin (MCG Health Inc); **Address:** Med Coll Ga - BMT Program, 1120 15th St, BAA 5407, Augusta, GA 30912-3125; **Phone:** 706-721-2505; **Board Cert:** Medical Oncology 2007; **Med School:** India 1985; **Resid:** Internal Medicine, Med Coll Georgia 1992; **Fellow:** Medical Oncology, Yale-New Haven Hosp 1996; **Fac Appt:** Prof Med, Med Coll GA

Khuri, Fadlo MD [Onc] - **Spec Exp:** Lung Cancer; Head & Neck Cancer; Thyroid Cancer; Mesothelioma; **Hospital:** Emory Univ Hosp, Grady Hlth Sys; **Address:** 1365 Clifton Road Rd NE, C Bldg Fl 3 - Ste C300, Atlanta, GA 30322; **Phone:** 404-778-1900; **Board Cert:** Medical Oncology 2008; **Med School:** Columbia P&S 1989; **Resid:** Internal Medicine, Boston City Hosp 1992; **Fellow:** Hematology & Oncology, New England Med Ctr-Tufts 1995; **Fac Appt:** Prof Hem & Onc, Emory Univ

Kraft, Andrew S MD [Onc] - **Spec Exp:** Prostate Cancer; Sarcoma; Drug Development; Clinical Trials; **Hospital:** MUSC Med Ctr; **Address:** 86 Jonathan Lucas St, PO BOX 250955, Charleston, SC 29425; **Phone:** 843-792-8284; **Board Cert:** Internal Medicine 1980; Medical Oncology 1985; **Med School:** Univ Pennsylvania 1975; **Resid:** Internal Medicine, Mt Sinai Hosp 1979; **Fellow:** Medical Oncology, Natl Cancer Inst 1983; **Fac Appt:** Prof Med, Med Univ SC

Kucuk, Omer MD [Onc] - **Spec Exp:** Genitourinary Cancer; Nutrition in Cancer Therapy; Prostate Cancer; Nutrition & Cancer Prevention/Control; **Hospital:** Emory Univ Hosp; **Address:** Emory Winship Cancer Inst, 1365C Clifton Rd, Ste 2110, Atlanta, GA 30322; **Phone:** 404-778-1900; **Board Cert:** Internal Medicine 1978; Hematology 1984; Medical Oncology 1989; **Med School:** Turkey 1975; **Resid:** Internal Medicine, St Francis Hosp 1978; **Fellow:** Hematology & Oncology, Northwestern Univ 1981; **Fac Appt:** Prof Hem & Onc, Emory Univ

Kvols, Larry K MD [Onc] - **Spec Exp:** Gastrointestinal Cancer; Carcinoid Tumors; Neuroendocrine Tumors; **Hospital:** H Lee Moffitt Cancer Ctr & Research Inst (page 59); **Address:** H Lee Moffitt Cancer Ctr & Research Inst, 12902 Magnolia Drive, FOB-2, Tampa, FL 33612; **Phone:** 813-745-7257; **Board Cert:** Internal Medicine 1976; Medical Oncology 1977; **Med School:** Baylor Coll Med 1970; **Resid:** Internal Medicine, Johns Hopkins Hosp 1972; **Fellow:** Hematology & Oncology, Johns Hopkins Hosp 1973; **Fac Appt:** Prof Med, Mayo Med Sch

Lawson, David H MD [Onc] - **Spec Exp:** Melanoma; **Hospital:** Emory Univ Hosp; **Address:** Emory Winship Cancer Institute, 1365 Clifton Rd NE C Bldg Fl 2, Atlanta, GA 30322; **Phone:** 404-778-1900; **Board Cert:** Internal Medicine 1977; Medical Oncology 1979; **Med School:** Emory Univ 1974; **Resid:** Internal Medicine, Emory Univ Hosps 1977; **Fellow:** Medical Oncology, Emory Univ 1979; **Fac Appt:** Assoc Prof Hem & Onc, Emory Univ

Lesser, Glenn J MD [Onc] - **Spec Exp:** Neuro-Oncology; Brain Tumors; **Hospital:** Wake Forest Univ Baptist Med Ctr; **Address:** Wake Forest Univ-Div Hematolgy/Oncology, Medical Center Blvd, Winston-Salem, NC 27157-1082; **Phone:** 336-713-5440; **Board Cert:** Medical Oncology 2007; **Med School:** Penn State Coll Med 1987; **Resid:** Internal Medicine, NC Baptist Hosp/Bowman Gray Sch Med 1991; **Fellow:** Medical Oncology, Johns Hopkins Hosp 1995; **Fac Appt:** Prof Hem & Onc, Wake Forest Univ

Lilenbaum, Rogerio MD [Onc] - **Spec Exp:** Lung Cancer; **Hospital:** Mount Sinai Med Ctr - Miami; **Address:** Mount Sinai Cancer Ctr, 4306 Alton Rd, Ste 3, Miami Beach, FL 33140-2840; **Phone:** 305-535-3310; **Board Cert:** Internal Medicine 2005; Hematology 2008; Medical Oncology 2007; **Med School:** Brazil 1986; **Resid:** Internal Medicine, Univ Hosp-Rio de Janeiro 1989; **Fellow:** Hematology & Oncology, Washington Univ Sch Med 1992; Oncology, UCSD 1994; **Fac Appt:** Assoc Clin Prof Med, Univ Miami Sch Med

Limentani, Steven A MD [Onc] - **Spec Exp:** Breast Cancer; Clinical Trials; **Hospital:** Carolinas Med Ctr; **Address:** 1100 S Tryon St, Ste 400, Charlotte, NC 28203; **Phone:** 704-446-9046; **Board Cert:** Internal Medicine 1989; Medical Oncology 2001; Hematology 2002; **Med School:** Tufts Univ 1986; **Resid:** Internal Medicine, New England Deaconess Hosp 1989; **Fellow:** Hematology & Oncology, New England Med Ctr 1992

Lippman, Marc E MD [Onc] - **Spec Exp:** Breast Cancer; **Hospital:** Univ of Miami Hosp & Clins/Sylvester Comp Canc Ctr (page 73), Univ of Miami Hosp (page 72); **Address:** Leonard M Miller Sch Med, Dept Med, 1430 NW 11th Ave, rm 1001, Miami, FL 33136; **Phone:** 305-243-1000; **Board Cert:** Internal Medicine 1987; Endocrinology 1975; Medical Oncology 1977; **Med School:** Yale Univ 1968; **Resid:** Internal Medicine, Johns Hopkins Hosp 1970; **Fellow:** Medical Oncology, Natl Cancer Inst 1973; Endocrinology, Yale-New Haven Hosp 1974; **Fac Appt:** Prof Med, Univ Mich Med Sch

List, Alan F MD [Onc] - **Spec Exp:** Myelodysplastic Syndromes; Leukemia; **Hospital:** H Lee Moffitt Cancer Ctr & Research Inst (page 59); **Address:** 12902 Magnolia Drive, MCC-VP, Tampa, FL 33612-9497; **Phone:** 813-745-6086; **Board Cert:** Internal Medicine 1983; Medical Oncology 1985; Hematology 1986; **Med School:** Univ Pennsylvania 1980; **Resid:** Internal Medicine, Good Samaritan Hosp 1983; Oncology, Vanderbilt Univ Med Ctr 1985; **Fellow:** Hematology, Vanderbilt Univ Med Ctr 1986

Lossos, Izidore MD [Onc] - **Spec Exp:** Lymphoma; Hodgkin's Disease; Leukemia; Lymphomas-Rare; **Hospital:** Univ of Miami Hosp & Clins/Sylvester Comp Canc Ctr (page 73), Jackson Meml Hosp (page 70); **Address:** Univ Miami - Sylvester Comp Cancer Ctr, 1475 NW 12th Ave, D8-4, Miami, FL 33136; **Phone:** 305-243-4785; **Med School:** Israel 1987; **Resid:** Internal Medicine, Hadassah Univ Hosp 1995; **Fellow:** Hematology & Oncology, Hadassah Univ Hosp 1997; Medical Oncology, Stanford Univ 2001; **Fac Appt:** Prof Med, Univ Miami Sch Med

Lyckholm, Laurel J MD [Onc] - **Spec Exp:** Neuro-Oncology; **Hospital:** Med Coll of VA Hosp; **Address:** Med Coll of VA, Div Hem/Onc, PO Box 980292, Richmond, VA 23298; **Phone:** 804-828-7999; **Board Cert:** Internal Medicine 1989; Medical Oncology 2003; Hematology 2004; Hospice & Palliative Medicine 2008; **Med School:** Creighton Univ 1985; **Resid:** Internal Medicine, Creighton Univ 1989; **Fellow:** Hematology & Oncology, Univ IA Coll Med 1992; **Fac Appt:** Assoc Prof Med, Med Coll VA

Lyman, Gary H MD [Onc] - **Spec Exp:** Breast Cancer; **Hospital:** Duke Univ Hosp; **Address:** Duke Comprehensive Cancer Center, Hock Plaza, 2424 Erwin Rd, Ste 205, Durham, NC 27705; **Phone:** 919-668-6688; **Board Cert:** Internal Medicine 1987; Medical Oncology 1977; Hematology 1978; **Med School:** SUNY Buffalo 1972; **Resid:** Internal Medicine, Univ North Carolina Hosp 1974; **Fellow:** Medical Oncology, Roswell Park Meml Inst 1976; Biostatistics, Harvard Med Sch 1982; **Fac Appt:** Prof Med, Duke Univ

Lynch Jr, James W MD [Onc] - **Spec Exp:** Lymphoma; Immunotherapy; Lung Cancer; **Hospital:** Shands at Univ of FL; **Address:** Shands Hlthcare, Div Hematology/Oncology, PO Box 100383, Gainesville, FL 32610-0383; **Phone:** 352-265-0725; **Board Cert:** Internal Medicine 1987; Medical Oncology 2001; **Med School:** Eastern VA Med Sch 1984; **Resid:** Internal Medicine, Univ Florida 1987; **Fellow:** Medical Oncology, Natl Cancer Inst 1991; **Fac Appt:** Prof Med, Univ Fla Coll Med

Marcom, Paul K MD [Onc] - **Spec Exp:** Breast Cancer; Clinical Trials; Cancer Genetics; **Hospital:** Duke Univ Hosp; **Address:** Duke Univ Med Ctr, Box 3476, Durham, NC 27710; **Phone:** 919-668-6688; **Board Cert:** Internal Medicine 2003; Medical Oncology 2005; **Med School:** Baylor Coll Med 1989; **Resid:** Internal Medicine, Duke Univ Med Ctr 1992; Hematology & Oncology, Duke Univ Med Ctr 1995; **Fac Appt:** Assoc Prof Med, Duke Univ

Miller, Antonius A MD [Onc] - **Spec Exp:** Lung Cancer; **Hospital:** Wake Forest Univ Baptist Med Ctr; **Address:** Wake Forest University, Comprehensive Cancer Center, Medical Center Blvd, Winston-Salem, NC 27157; **Phone:** 336-713-4392; **Med School:** Germany 1977; **Resid:** Internal Medicine, Univ Essen Med Sch 1979; Internal Medicine, Univ TN Med Ctr 1987; **Fellow:** Hematology & Oncology, UT MD Anderson Cancer Ctr 1981; **Fac Appt:** Prof Med, Wake Forest Univ

Miller, Donald M MD/PhD [Onc] - **Spec Exp:** Melanoma; Lung Cancer; **Hospital:** Univ of Louisville Hosp; **Address:** 529 S Jackson St, Louisville, KY 40202; **Phone:** 502-562-4790; **Board Cert:** Internal Medicine 1979; **Med School:** Duke Univ 1973; **Resid:** Internal Medicine, Peter Bent Brigham Hosp 1975; **Fellow:** Internal Medicine, Peter Bent Brigham Hosp 1978; Medical Oncology, Natl Cancer Inst 1979; **Fac Appt:** Prof Med, Univ Louisville Sch Med

Moore, Joseph O MD [Onc] - **Spec Exp:** Leukemia; Hodgkin's Disease; Lymphoma, Non-Hodgkin's; Neuroendocrine Tumors; **Hospital:** Duke Univ Hosp; **Address:** Duke Univ Med Ctr, Box 3872, Durham, NC 27710; **Phone:** 919-684-8964; **Board Cert:** Internal Medicine 1975; Medical Oncology 1977; **Med School:** Johns Hopkins Univ 1970; **Resid:** Internal Medicine, Johns Hopkins Hosp 1975; **Fellow:** Hematology & Oncology, Duke Univ Med Ctr 1977; **Fac Appt:** Prof Med, Duke Univ

Morgan, David S MD [Onc] - **Spec Exp:** Leukemia & Lymphoma; Hodgkin's Disease; Bone Marrow Transplant; **Hospital:** Vanderbilt Univ Med Ctr (page 76); **Address:** Vanderbilt University Medical Center, 2220 Pierce Ave, 777 Preston Research Bldg, Nashville, TN 37232-6307; **Phone:** 615-936-8422; **Board Cert:** Internal Medicine 2003; Medical Oncology 2008; **Med School:** Vanderbilt Univ 1990; **Resid:** Internal Medicine, Yale-New Haven Hosp 1993; **Fellow:** Medical Oncology, Stanford Univ Med Ctr 1997; **Fac Appt:** Asst Prof Med, Vanderbilt Univ

Muss, Hyman B MD [Onc] - **Spec Exp:** Breast Cancer; **Hospital:** NC Memorial Hosp - UNC; **Address:** Div of Hem/Onc, Physicians Office Bldg, 170 Manning Drive Fl 3 - rm 3120, Box 7305, Chapel Hill, NC 27599-7305; **Phone:** 919-966-0840; **Board Cert:** Internal Medicine 1973; Hematology 1974; Medical Oncology 1975; **Med School:** SUNY Downstate 1968; **Resid:** Internal Medicine, Peter Bent Brigham Hosp 1970; **Fellow:** Hematology & Oncology, Peter Bent Brigham Hosp 1974; Hematology & Oncology, Dana-Farber Cancer Ctr 1974; **Fac Appt:** Prof Med, Univ NC Sch Med

Nabell, Lisle M MD [Onc] - **Spec Exp:** Breast Cancer; Head & Neck Cancer; **Hospital:** Univ of Ala Hosp at Birmingham; **Address:** Univ of Alabama, 1530 3rd Ave S, Ste NP2540B, Birmingham, AL 35294; **Phone:** 205-934-3061; **Board Cert:** Internal Medicine 2000; Medical Oncology 2000; **Med School:** Univ NC Sch Med 1987; **Resid:** Internal Medicine, Univ Alabama Hosp 1990; **Fellow:** Hematology & Oncology, Univ Alabama Hosp 1992; **Fac Appt:** Assoc Prof Med, Univ Alabama

O'Regan, Ruth M MD [Onc] - **Spec Exp:** Breast Cancer; Breast Cancer Risk Assessment; Cancer Prevention; Clinical Trials; **Hospital:** Emory Univ Hosp; **Address:** Emory Winship Cancer Inst, 1365C Clifton Rd NE Fl 2, Atlanta, GA 30322; **Phone:** 404-778-1900; **Board Cert:** Medical Oncology 2000; **Med School:** Ireland 1988; **Resid:** Internal Medicine, Med Coll Wisconsin 1995; Medical Oncology, Northwestern Univ Hosp 1999; **Fellow:** Medical Oncology, Northwestern Univ 1998; **Fac Appt:** Assoc Prof Hem & Onc, Emory Univ

Pao, William MD/PhD [Onc] - **Spec Exp:** Thoracic Cancers; Lung Cancer; **Hospital:** Vanderbilt Univ Med Ctr (page 76); **Address:** 2220 Pierce Ave, rm 777 PRB, Nashville, TN 37232-6307; **Phone:** 615-322-3524; **Board Cert:** Internal Medicine 2001; Medical Oncology 2003; **Med School:** Yale Univ 1998; **Resid:** Internal Medicine, New York Hosp 2000; **Fellow:** Medical Oncology, Meml Sloan Kettering Canc Ctr 2004; **Fac Appt:** Assoc Prof Med, Vanderbilt Univ

Pasche, Boris C MD/PhD [Onc] - **Spec Exp:** Colon Cancer; Gastrointestinal Cancer; **Hospital:** Univ of Ala Hosp at Birmingham; **Address:** 2000 Morris Ave, Ste 1610, Birmingham, AL 35203; **Phone:** 205-934-9591; **Board Cert:** Medical Oncology 2008; **Med School:** Sweden 1986; **Resid:** Internal Medicine, NY Hosp/Cornell Med Ctr 1994; **Fellow:** Hematology & Oncology, Meml Sloan Kettering Cancer Ctr 1996; **Fac Appt:** Prof Med, Univ Alabama

Pegram, Mark D MD [Onc] - **Spec Exp:** Breast Cancer; Breast Cancer-Novel Therapies; **Hospital:** Univ of Miami Hosp & Clins/Sylvester Comp Canc Ctr (page 73); **Address:** UMHC/Sylvester Comp Cancer Ctr, 1475 NW 12th Ave, Miami, FL 33136; **Phone:** 305-243-1000; **Board Cert:** Internal Medicine 1989; Medical Oncology 2003; **Med School:** Univ NC Sch Med 1986; **Resid:** Internal Medicine, Parkland Meml Hosp 1989; **Fellow:** Hematology & Oncology, UCLA Med Ctr 1993; **Fac Appt:** Prof Med, Univ Miami Sch Med

Perez, Edith A MD [Onc] - **Spec Exp:** Breast Cancer; Breast Cancer Risk Assessment; Clinical Trials; **Hospital:** Mayo - Jacksonville; **Address:** Mayo Clinic-Jacksonville, 4500 San Pablo Rd Davis Bldg Fl 8, Jacksonville, FL 32224; **Phone:** 904-953-7283; **Board Cert:** Internal Medicine 1983; Hematology 1986; Medical Oncology 1987; **Med School:** Univ Puerto Rico 1979; **Resid:** Internal Medicine, Loma Linda Univ Med Ctr 1982; **Fellow:** Hematology & Oncology, Martinez VA Hosp/UC Davis 1987; **Fac Appt:** Prof Med, Mayo Med Sch

Posey III, James A MD [Onc] - **Spec Exp:** Gastrointestinal Cancer; Colon Cancer; Liver Cancer; Biliary Cancer; **Hospital:** Univ of Ala Hosp at Birmingham; **Address:** 1882 6th Ave S, NP-2540U, Birmingham, AL 35294-3300; **Phone:** 205-934-0916; **Board Cert:** Medical Oncology 1997; **Med School:** Howard Univ 1991; **Resid:** Internal Medicine, Georgetown Univ Med Ctr 1994; **Fellow:** Hematology & Oncology, Georgetown Univ Med Ctr 1997; **Fac Appt:** Assoc Prof Med, Univ Alabama

Ready, Neal E MD/PhD [Onc] - **Spec Exp:** Lung Cancer; Head & Neck Cancer; Clinical Trials; **Hospital:** Duke Univ Hosp; **Address:** Duke Univ Medical Ctr, DUMC, Box 3198, Durham, NC 27710; **Phone:** 919-668-6688; **Board Cert:** Internal Medicine 1989; Hematology 2005; Medical Oncology 2005; **Med School:** Vanderbilt Univ 1986; **Resid:** Internal Medicine, Rhode Island Hosp 1989; **Fellow:** Hematology, Rhode Island Hosp 1992; Medical Oncology, New England Med Ctr 1994

Reed, Eddie MD [Onc] - **Spec Exp:** Ovarian Cancer; Prostate Cancer; **Hospital:** Univ of S AL Med Ctr; **Address:** USA Mitchell Cancer Institute, 1660 Springhill Ave, Mobile, AL 36604; **Phone:** 251-665-8000; **Board Cert:** Internal Medicine 1982; **Med School:** Yale Univ 1979; **Resid:** Internal Medicine, Stanford Univ Med Ctr 1982; **Fellow:** Medical Oncology, Natl Cancer Inst 1985; **Fac Appt:** Prof Med, Univ S Ala Coll Med

Robert, Nicholas J MD [Onc] - **Spec Exp:** Breast Cancer; **Hospital:** Inova Fairfax Hosp; **Address:** 8503 Arlington Blvd, Ste 400, Fairfax, VA 22031; **Phone:** 703-280-5390; **Board Cert:** Internal Medicine 1978; Anatomic Pathology 1979; Medical Oncology 1981; Hematology 1984; **Med School:** McGill Univ 1974; **Resid:** Internal Medicine, Royal Victoria Hosp 1976; Pathology, Mass Genl Hosp 1979; **Fellow:** Hematology, Peter Bent Brigham Hosp 1980; Medical Oncology, Dana Farber Cancer Inst 1981

Medical Oncology

Robert-Vizcarrondo, Francisco MD [Onc] - **Spec Exp:** Lung Cancer; Mesothelioma; Drug Development; Clinical Trials; **Hospital:** Univ of Ala Hosp at Birmingham; **Address:** 1802 6th Ave S, rm NP-2555D, Birmingham, AL 35294-3300; **Phone:** 205-934-5077; **Board Cert:** Internal Medicine 1973; Medical Oncology 1975; Hematology 1976; **Med School:** Puerto Rico 1969; **Resid:** Internal Medicine, Univ PR Hosp 1972; Hematology, Univ PR Hosp 1974; **Fellow:** Medical Oncology, Univ AL Hosp at Birmingham 1976; **Fac Appt:** Prof Med, Univ Alabama

Romond, Edward H MD [Onc] - **Spec Exp:** Breast Cancer; Hemophilia; **Hospital:** Univ of Kentucky Albert B. Chandler Hosp; **Address:** Univ Kentucky Med Ctr, Div Hematology/Oncology, CC413 Markey Cancer Center, Lexington, KY 40536; **Phone:** 859-323-8043; **Board Cert:** Internal Medicine 1980; Hematology 1984; Medical Oncology 1983; **Med School:** Univ KY Coll Med 1977; **Resid:** Internal Medicine, Michigan State Univ Hosps 1980; **Fellow:** Hematology & Oncology, Michigan State Univ 1983; **Fac Appt:** Prof Med, Univ KY Coll Med

Schwartz, Michael A MD [Onc] - **Spec Exp:** Breast Cancer; Lymphoma; Prostate Cancer; **Hospital:** Mount Sinai Med Ctr - Miami; **Address:** 4306 Alton Rd Fl 3, Miami Beach, FL 33140; **Phone:** 305-535-3310; **Board Cert:** Internal Medicine 1989; Medical Oncology 2004; Hematology 2004; **Med School:** UMDNJ-RW Johnson Med Sch 1986; **Resid:** Internal Medicine, Mt Sinai Medical Ctr 1989; **Fellow:** Hematology & Oncology, Meml Sloan Kettering Cancer Ctr 1992; **Fac Appt:** Asst Clin Prof Med, Univ Miami Sch Med

Serody, Jonathan S MD [Onc] - **Spec Exp:** Breast Cancer Vaccine Therapy; Clinical Trials; Lymphoma; **Hospital:** NC Memorial Hosp - UNC; **Address:** Lineberger Comprehensive Cancer Ctr, 450 West Drive, CB 7295, Chapel Hill, NC 27599-7295; **Phone:** 919-966-8644; **Board Cert:** Internal Medicine 1989; Hematology 2007; **Med School:** Univ VA Sch Med 1986; **Resid:** Internal Medicine, Univ NC Med Ctr 1989; **Fellow:** Hematology, Univ NC Med Ctr 1992; Bone Marrow Transplant, Fred Hutchinson Transplant Program 1993; **Fac Appt:** Assoc Prof Med, Univ NC Sch Med

Shea, Thomas MD [Onc] - **Spec Exp:** Bone Marrow Transplant; Lymphoma; Leukemia; **Hospital:** NC Memorial Hosp - UNC; **Address:** Univ N Carolina, Dept Medicine, 170 Manning Drive, CB 7305, Chapel Hill, NC 27599; **Phone:** 919-966-7746; **Board Cert:** Internal Medicine 1982; Hematology 1984; Medical Oncology 1985; **Med School:** Univ NC Sch Med 1978; **Resid:** Internal Medicine, Beth Israel Deaconess Med Ctr 1982; **Fellow:** Hematology & Oncology, Beth Israel Deaconess Med Ctr 1985; Bone Marrow Transplant, Dana Farber Cancer Inst 1988; **Fac Appt:** Prof Med, Univ NC Sch Med

Sherman, Carol A MD [Onc] - **Spec Exp:** Lung Cancer; Thoracic Cancers; **Hospital:** MUSC Med Ctr; **Address:** 96 Jonathan Lucas St, Ste CSB-903, Charleston, SC 29425; **Phone:** 843-792-9621; **Board Cert:** Internal Medicine 1987; Medical Oncology 1989; **Med School:** Univ Mass Sch Med 1984; **Resid:** Internal Medicine, Univ Mass Med Ctr 1987; **Fellow:** Hematology & Oncology, Univ Mass Med Ctr 1989; **Fac Appt:** Assoc Prof Med, Med Univ SC

Shin, Dong Moon MD [Onc] - **Spec Exp:** Head & Neck Cancer; Mesothelioma; Thymoma; Lung Cancer; **Hospital:** Emory Univ Hosp; **Address:** Emory Winship Cancer Inst, 1365 C Clifton Rd NE, Ste 3094, Atlanta, GA 30322; **Phone:** 404-778-5990; **Board Cert:** Internal Medicine 1985; Medical Oncology 1989; **Med School:** South Korea 1975; **Resid:** Internal Medicine, Cook Co Hosp 1985; **Fellow:** Medical Oncology, UT- MD Anderson Cancer Ctr 1988; **Fac Appt:** Prof Med, Emory Univ

Simon, George R MD [Onc] - **Spec Exp:** Mesothelioma; Lung Cancer; Thymoma; **Hospital:** MUSC Med Ctr; **Address:** 96 Jonathan Lucas St, CSB Bldg, Ste 903, Charleston, SC 29425-6350; **Phone:** 843-792-8584; **Board Cert:** Internal Medicine 2007; Medical Oncology 2007; **Med School:** India 1986; **Resid:** Internal Medicine, St Joseph's Hosp 1995; **Fellow:** Hematology & Oncology, Univ Colorado Hlth Sciences Ctr 1997; **Fac Appt:** Assoc Prof Med, Med Univ SC

Smith, Thomas Joseph MD [Onc] - **Spec Exp:** Breast Cancer; Palliative Care; **Hospital:** VCU Med Ctr; **Address:** Massey Cancer Ctr, 9000 Stony Point Pkwy, Richmond, VA 23235; **Phone:** 804-327-8806; **Board Cert:** Internal Medicine 1982; Medical Oncology 1987; Hospice & Palliative Medicine 2008; **Med School:** Yale Univ 1979; **Resid:** Internal Medicine, Hosp Univ Penn 1982; **Fellow:** Medical Oncology, Med Coll Virginia 1987; **Fac Appt:** Prof Med, Va Commonwealth Univ Sch Med

Socinski, Mark A MD [Onc] - **Spec Exp:** Lung Cancer; **Hospital:** NC Memorial Hosp - UNC; **Address:** UNC Chapel Hill, Div Hem/Onc, 170 Manning Drive, Physicians Bldg, CB 7305, Chapel Hill, NC 27599-7305; **Phone:** 919-966-0000; **Board Cert:** Internal Medicine 1988; Medical Oncology 2002; **Med School:** Univ VT Coll Med 1984; **Resid:** Internal Medicine, Beth Israel Hosp 1986; **Fellow:** Medical Oncology, Dana-Farber Cancer Inst 1989; **Fac Appt:** Assoc Prof Med, Univ NC Sch Med

Sosman, Jeffrey MD [Onc] - **Spec Exp:** Melanoma; Skin Cancer; Immunotherapy; Drug Discovery; **Hospital:** Vanderbilt Univ Med Ctr (page 76); **Address:** Vanderbilt-Ingram Cancer Ctr, 777 Preston Rsch Bldg, Nashville, TN 37232-6307; **Phone:** 615-322-6053; **Board Cert:** Anatomic Pathology 1985; Internal Medicine 1987; Medical Oncology 1989; **Med School:** Albert Einstein Coll Med 1981; **Resid:** Anatomic Pathology, Univ Chicago Hosps 1985; Internal Medicine, Univ Wisconsin Hosp 1986; **Fellow:** Medical Oncology, Univ Wisconsin 1989; **Fac Appt:** Prof Med, Vanderbilt Univ

Sotomayor, Eduardo M MD [Onc] - **Spec Exp:** Lymphoma; Gene Therapy; Vaccine Therapy; Clinical Trials; **Hospital:** H Lee Moffitt Cancer Ctr & Research Inst (page 59); **Address:** H Lee Moffitt Cancer Inst, 12902 Magnolia Drive, FOB 3, rm 5.3125, Tampa, FL 33612; **Phone:** 813-745-1387; **Board Cert:** Medical Oncology 2009; **Med School:** Peru 1988; **Resid:** Internal Medicine, Univ Miami Sch Med 1995; **Fellow:** Immunology, Univ Miami Sch Med 1989; Oncology, Johns Hopkins Hosp 1998; **Fac Appt:** Assoc Prof Med, Univ S Fla Coll Med

Stone, Joel A MD [Onc] - **Spec Exp:** Lung Cancer; Breast Cancer; **Hospital:** St. Vincent's Med Ctr - Jacksonville; **Address:** N Florida Hematology/Oncology Assocs, 2 Shircliff Way, Ste 800, Jacksonville, FL 32204; **Phone:** 904-388-2619; **Board Cert:** Internal Medicine 1977; Medical Oncology 1979; **Med School:** Univ VA Sch Med 1974; **Resid:** Internal Medicine, Univ KY Med Ctr 1977; **Fellow:** Hematology & Oncology, Emory Univ Hosp 1979

Sutton, Linda Marie MD [Onc] - **Spec Exp:** Breast Cancer; Palliative Care; **Hospital:** Duke Univ Hosp; **Address:** University Tower, 3100 Tower Blvd, Ste 600, Durham, NC 27707; **Phone:** 919-419-5005; **Board Cert:** Internal Medicine 2002; Medical Oncology 2003; **Med School:** Univ Mass Sch Med 1987; **Resid:** Internal Medicine, Montefiore Med Ctr 1990; **Fellow:** Hematology & Oncology, Duke Univ Med Ctr 1993

Thigpen, James T MD [Onc] - **Spec Exp:** Gynecologic Cancer; Breast Cancer; Lung Cancer; **Hospital:** Univ Mississippi Med Ctr; **Address:** Univ Mississippi Med Ctr, Div Med Onc, 2500 N State St, Jackson, MS 39216; **Phone:** 601-984-5590; **Board Cert:** Internal Medicine 1972; Hematology 1974; Medical Oncology 1975; **Med School:** Univ Miss 1969; **Resid:** Internal Medicine, Univ Miss Med Ctr 1971; **Fellow:** Hematology & Oncology, Univ Miss Med Ctr 1973; **Fac Appt:** Prof Med, Univ Miss

Torti, Frank M MD [Onc] - **Spec Exp:** Prostate Cancer; Urologic Cancer; **Hospital:** Wake Forest Univ Baptist Med Ctr; **Address:** Wake Forest Med Ctr-Comp Cancer Ctr, Medical Center Blvd, Winston-Salem, NC 27157-1082; **Phone:** 336-716-7971; **Board Cert:** Internal Medicine 1978; Medical Oncology 1979; **Med School:** Harvard Med Sch 1974; **Resid:** Internal Medicine, Beth Israel Hosp 1976; **Fellow:** Medical Oncology, Stanford Univ Med Ctr 1979; **Fac Appt:** Prof Med, Wake Forest Univ

Troner, Michael MD [Onc] - **Spec Exp:** Head & Neck Cancer; Urologic Cancer; **Hospital:** Baptist Hosp of Miami; **Address:** 8940 N Kendall Drive, Ste 300, East Tower, Miami, FL 33176; **Phone:** 305-595-2141; **Board Cert:** Internal Medicine 1972; Medical Oncology 1973; **Med School:** SUNY Downstate 1968; **Resid:** Internal Medicine, Univ Maryland Hosp 1971; **Fellow:** Medical Oncology, Univ Miami Med Ctr 1973; **Fac Appt:** Assoc Clin Prof Med, Univ Miami Sch Med

Vance, Ralph MD [Onc] - **Spec Exp:** Lung Cancer; **Hospital:** Univ Mississippi Med Ctr; **Address:** Univ Mississippi Med Ctr, Div Med Onc, 2500 N State St, Jackson, MS 39216; **Phone:** 601-984-5590; **Med School:** Univ Miss 1972; **Resid:** Internal Medicine, Univ Hosp; **Fellow:** Hematology & Oncology, Univ Hosp; **Fac Appt:** Prof Med, Univ Miss

Vaughan, William P MD [Onc] - **Spec Exp:** Bone Marrow Transplant; Breast Cancer; **Hospital:** Univ of Ala Hosp at Birmingham; **Address:** Tinsley Harrison Twr, 1530 3rd Ave S, Birmingham, AL 35294; **Phone:** 205-934-1908; **Board Cert:** Internal Medicine 1975; Medical Oncology 1979; **Med School:** Univ Conn 1972; **Resid:** Internal Medicine, Univ Chicago Hosps 1975; **Fellow:** Oncology, Johns Hopkins Hosp 1977; **Fac Appt:** Prof Med, Univ Alabama

Vredenburgh, James J MD [Onc] - **Spec Exp:** Brain Tumors; Gliomas; Brain Tumors-Metastatic; **Hospital:** Duke Univ Hosp; **Address:** Duke Univ Medical Ctr, Brain Tumor Ctr, Box 3624, Durham, NC 27710; **Phone:** 919-668-2993; **Board Cert:** Internal Medicine 1986; Hematology 1988; Medical Oncology 1989; **Med School:** Univ VT Coll Med 1983; **Resid:** Internal Medicine, St Francis Med Ctr 1986; **Fellow:** Hematology & Oncology, Dartmouth-Hitchcock Med Ctr 1989; **Fac Appt:** Prof Med, Duke Univ

Waller, Edmund K MD [Onc] - **Spec Exp:** Bone Marrow & Stem Cell Transplant; **Hospital:** Emory Univ Hosp; **Address:** 1365 Clifton Rd NE, C Bldg, Atlanta, GA 30322; **Phone:** 404-778-4342; **Board Cert:** Internal Medicine 1988; Medical Oncology 2006; **Med School:** Cornell Univ-Weill Med Coll 1985; **Resid:** Internal Medicine, Stanford Univ Med Ctr 1988; **Fellow:** Oncology, Stanford Univ Med Ctr 1992; **Fac Appt:** Prof Hem & Onc, Emory Univ

Weber, Jeffrey S MD/PhD [Onc] - **Spec Exp:** Melanoma; **Hospital:** H Lee Moffitt Cancer Ctr & Research Inst (page 59); **Address:** H Lee Moffitt Cancer Ctr, 12902 Magnolia Ave, MS SRB-2, Tampa, FL 33612; **Phone:** 813-745-2691; **Board Cert:** Internal Medicine 1983; Medical Oncology 1987; **Med School:** NYU Sch Med 1980; **Resid:** Internal Medicine, UCSD Med Ctr 1983; **Fellow:** Medical Oncology, Natl Cancer Inst 1990; **Fac Appt:** Assoc Prof Med, USC Sch Med

Weiss, Geoffrey R MD [Onc] - **Spec Exp:** Gastrointestinal Cancer; Genitourinary Cancer; Melanoma; **Hospital:** Univ of Virginia Health Sys; **Address:** Univ Virginia Hlth System, Div Hem/Onc, PO Box 800716, Charlottesville, VA 22908-0716; **Phone:** 434-243-0066; **Board Cert:** Internal Medicine 1977; Medical Oncology 1981; **Med School:** St Louis Univ 1974; **Resid:** Internal Medicine, Temple Univ Hosp 1978; **Fellow:** Medical Oncology, Dana Farber Cancer Inst 1982; **Fac Appt:** Prof Med, Univ VA Sch Med

Wingard, John R MD [Onc] - **Spec Exp:** Bone Marrow Transplant; Leukemia; Multiple Myeloma; Lymphoma; **Hospital:** Shands at Univ of FL; **Address:** Gainsville Clin, PO Box 100278, Gainesville, FL 32610; **Phone:** 352-265-0111 x29452; **Board Cert:** Internal Medicine 1977; Medical Oncology 1983; **Med School:** Johns Hopkins Univ 1973; **Resid:** Internal Medicine, Memphis City Hosps 1976; Internal Medicine, VA Hosp 1977; **Fellow:** Medical Oncology, Johns Hopkins Hosp 1979; **Fac Appt:** Prof Med, Univ Fla Coll Med

Yunus, Furhan MD [Onc] - **Spec Exp:** Multiple Myeloma; Lymphoma; **Hospital:** Methodist Univ Hosp - Memphis, Regional Med Ctr - Memphis; **Address:** Univ TN Cancer Inst, 1331 Union Ave, Ste 800, Memphis, TN 38104; **Phone:** 901-725-1785; **Board Cert:** Medical Oncology 2008; **Med School:** Pakistan 1986; **Resid:** Internal Medicine, Methodist Hosp 1993; **Fellow:** Hematology & Oncology, Univ Ariz Coll Med Affil Hosp 1995; **Fac Appt:** Asst Prof Med, Univ Tenn Coll Med

Midwest

Adelstein, David J MD [Onc] - **Spec Exp:** Head & Neck Cancer; Esophageal Cancer; Lung Cancer; **Hospital:** Cleveland Clin (page 56); **Address:** Cleveland Clinic, Taussig Cancer Inst, 9500 Euclid Ave, R35, Cleveland, OH 44195; **Phone:** 216-444-9310; **Board Cert:** Internal Medicine 1978; Medical Oncology 1981; Hematology 1982; **Med School:** NYU Sch Med 1975; **Resid:** Internal Medicine, Univ Hosps Cleveland 1978; **Fellow:** Hematology & Oncology, Univ Hosps Cleveland 1981; **Fac Appt:** Prof Med, Cleveland Cl Coll Med/Case West Res

Albain, Kathy S MD [Onc] - **Spec Exp:** Breast Cancer; Lung Cancer; Cancer Survivors-Late Effects of Therapy; **Hospital:** Loyola Univ Med Ctr; **Address:** Loyola-Bernardin Cancer Ctr, 2160 S First Ave, Bldg 112 - Ste 109, Maywood, IL 60153-5590; **Phone:** 708-327-3214; **Board Cert:** Internal Medicine 1981; Medical Oncology 1983; **Med School:** Univ Mich Med Sch 1978; **Resid:** Internal Medicine, Univ Illinois Med Ctr 1981; **Fellow:** Hematology & Oncology, Univ Chicago 1984; **Fac Appt:** Prof Med, Loyola Univ-Stritch Sch Med

Albertini, Mark R MD [Onc] - **Spec Exp:** Melanoma; Melanoma-Advanced; **Hospital:** Univ WI Hosp & Clins; **Address:** Univ Wisconsin-Medical Oncology, 600 Highland Ave, Ste H4/534, Madison, WI 53792; **Phone:** 608-265-1700; **Board Cert:** Internal Medicine 1987; Medical Oncology 2002; **Med School:** Univ VT Coll Med 1984; **Resid:** Internal Medicine, Univ Wisc Hosps Clins 1987; **Fellow:** Medical Oncology, Univ Wisconsin 1991; **Fac Appt:** Assoc Prof Med, Univ Wisc

Anderson, Joseph M MD [Onc] - **Spec Exp:** Breast Cancer; Palliative Care; Neuro-Oncology; **Hospital:** Henry Ford Hosp; **Address:** 2799 W Grand Blvd, Ste K13, Detroit, MI 48202; **Phone:** 313-916-1854; **Board Cert:** Internal Medicine 1985; Medical Oncology 1989; **Med School:** Univ Mich Med Sch 1982; **Resid:** Internal Medicine, Henry Ford Hosp 1986; **Fellow:** Medical Oncology, Henry Ford Hosp 1988

Benson III, Al B MD [Onc] - **Spec Exp:** Colon Cancer; Gastrointestinal Cancer; Liver Cancer; Pancreatic Cancer; **Hospital:** Northwestern Meml Hosp, Jesse Brown VA Med Ctr; **Address:** Northwestern Div Hematology/Oncology, 676 N St Clair St, Ste 850, Chicago, IL 60611; **Phone:** 312-695-0990; **Board Cert:** Internal Medicine 1979; Medical Oncology 1983; **Med School:** SUNY Buffalo 1976; **Resid:** Internal Medicine, Univ Wisc Hosps 1979; **Fellow:** Medical Oncology, Univ Wisc Hosps 1984; **Fac Appt:** Prof Med, Northwestern Univ

Bitran, Jacob D MD [Onc] - **Spec Exp:** Breast Cancer; Bone Marrow Transplant; Lung Cancer; **Hospital:** Adv Luth Genl Hosp; **Address:** Lutheran Genl Cancer Care Specialists, 1700 Luther Lane, Park Ridge, IL 60068-1270; **Phone:** 866-611-1991; **Board Cert:** Internal Medicine 1974; Medical Oncology 1977; Hematology 1986; **Med School:** Univ IL Coll Med 1971; **Resid:** Pathology, Rush Presby St Lukes Hosp 1973; Internal Medicine, Michael Reese Hosp 1975; **Fellow:** Hematology & Oncology, Univ Chicago Hosps 1977; **Fac Appt:** Prof Med, Ros Franklin Univ/Chicago Med Sch

Bolwell, Brian J MD [Onc] - **Spec Exp:** Bone Marrow Transplant; Hematologic Malignancies; **Hospital:** Cleveland Clin (page 56); **Address:** 9500 Euclid Ave, Desk R32, Cleveland, OH 44195; **Phone:** 216-444-6922; **Board Cert:** Internal Medicine 1985; Medical Oncology 1987; **Med School:** Case West Res Univ 1981; **Resid:** Internal Medicine, Univ Hosp 1984; **Fellow:** Hematology & Oncology, Hosp Univ Penn 1987; **Fac Appt:** Prof Med, Cleveland Cl Coll Med/Case West Res

Bonomi, Philip D MD [Onc] - **Spec Exp:** Lung Cancer; Thymoma; Mesothelioma; **Hospital:** Rush Univ Med Ctr; **Address:** Rush University Medical Center, 1725 W Harrison St, Ste 824, Chicago, IL 60612; **Phone:** 312-942-5904; **Board Cert:** Internal Medicine 1975; Medical Oncology 1977; **Med School:** Univ IL Coll Med 1970; **Resid:** Internal Medicine, Geisinger Med Ctr 1972; Internal Medicine, Geisinger Med Ctr 1975; **Fellow:** Medical Oncology, Rush Presby-St Luke's Med Ctr 1977; **Fac Appt:** Prof Med, Rush Med Coll

Medical Oncology

Borden, Ernest C MD [Onc] - **Spec Exp:** Melanoma; Immunotherapy; Sarcoma; Vaccine Therapy; **Hospital:** Cleveland Clin (page 56); **Address:** 9500 Euclid Ave, Desk R40, Cleveland, OH 44195; **Phone:** 216-444-8183; **Board Cert:** Internal Medicine 1973; Medical Oncology 1975; **Med School:** Duke Univ 1966; **Resid:** Internal Medicine, Hosp Univ Penn 1968; **Fellow:** Medical Oncology, Johns Hopkins Hosp 1973; **Fac Appt:** Prof Med, Cleveland Cl Coll Med/Case West Res

Brockstein, Bruce E MD [Onc] - **Spec Exp:** Head & Neck Cancer; Sarcoma; Melanoma; **Hospital:** Evanston/North Shore Univ Hlth Sys, Highland Park/North Shore Univ Hlth Syst; **Address:** North Shore Univ Hlth Sys, Div Hematology/Oncology, 2650 Ridge Ave, rm 4816, Evanston, IL 60201; **Phone:** 847-570-2515; **Board Cert:** Internal Medicine 2003; Medical Oncology 2005; **Med School:** Univ Chicago-Pritzker Sch Med 1990; **Resid:** Internal Medicine, Hosp Univ Penn 1993; **Fellow:** Hematology & Oncology, Univ Chicago Hosps 1996; **Fac Appt:** Assoc Clin Prof Med, Northwestern Univ

Buckner, Jan Craig MD [Onc] - **Spec Exp:** Brain Tumors; Neuro-Oncology; **Hospital:** Mayo Med Ctr & Clin - Rochester; **Address:** Mayo Clinic, 200 First St SW, Rochester, MN 55905; **Phone:** 507-284-4320; **Board Cert:** Internal Medicine 1983; Medical Oncology 1985; **Med School:** Univ NC Sch Med 1980; **Resid:** Internal Medicine, Butterworth Hosp 1983; **Fellow:** Medical Oncology, Mayo Clinic 1985; **Fac Appt:** Prof Med, Mayo Med Sch

Budd, George T MD [Onc] - **Spec Exp:** Breast Cancer; **Hospital:** Cleveland Clin (page 56); **Address:** Cleveland Clinic, Taussig Cancer Ctr, 9500 Euclid Ave, Desk R35, Cleveland, OH 44195; **Phone:** 216-444-6480; **Board Cert:** Internal Medicine 1980; Medical Oncology 1983; **Med School:** Univ Kansas 1977; **Resid:** Internal Medicine, Cleveland Clinic 1980; **Fellow:** Hematology & Oncology, Cleveland Clinic 1982

Chapman, Robert A MD [Onc] - **Spec Exp:** Lung Cancer; **Hospital:** Henry Ford Hosp; **Address:** 2799 W Grand Blvd, K13, Detroit, MI 48202; **Phone:** 313-916-1841; **Board Cert:** Internal Medicine 1985; Medical Oncology 1989; **Med School:** Cornell Univ-Weill Med Coll 1976; **Resid:** Internal Medicine, Henry Ford Hosp 1979; **Fellow:** Medical Oncology, Meml Sloan Kettering Cancer Ctr 1981

Chitambar, Christopher R MD [Onc] - **Spec Exp:** Lymphoma; Leukemia; Breast Cancer; **Hospital:** Froedtert and Med Ctr of WI; **Address:** Div Neoplastic Disease, 9200 W Wisconsin Ave, Milwaukee, WI 53226-3522; **Phone:** 414-805-4600; **Board Cert:** Internal Medicine 1980; Hematology 1982; Medical Oncology 1983; **Med School:** India 1977; **Resid:** Internal Medicine, Brackenridge Hosp 1980; **Fellow:** Hematology & Oncology, Univ CO Hlth Sci Ctr 1983; **Fac Appt:** Prof Med, Med Coll Wisc

Clamon, Gerald H MD [Onc] - **Spec Exp:** Lung Cancer; Palliative Care; **Hospital:** Univ Iowa Hosp & Clinics; **Address:** Holden Comprehensive Cancer Ctr, 200 Hawkins Drive, Ste C32GH, Iowa City, IA 52242; **Phone:** 319-384-8442; **Board Cert:** Internal Medicine 1976; Medical Oncology 1979; **Med School:** Washington Univ, St Louis 1971; **Resid:** Internal Medicine, Barnes Hosp 1976; **Fellow:** Research, Natl Cancer Inst 1974; Medical Oncology, Univ Iowa Hosp & Clinics 1977; **Fac Appt:** Prof Med, Univ Iowa Coll Med

Clark, Joseph I MD [Onc] - **Spec Exp:** Kidney Cancer; Melanoma; Head & Neck Cancer; **Hospital:** Loyola Univ Med Ctr, Edward Hines, Jr. VA Hosp; **Address:** Cardinal Bernardin Cancer Ctr, Loyola Univ Med Ctr, 2160 S 1st Ave, rm 346, Maywood, IL 60153-5500; **Phone:** 708-327-3217; **Board Cert:** Internal Medicine 2002; Medical Oncology 2006; **Med School:** Loyola Univ-Stritch Sch Med 1989; **Resid:** Internal Medicine, Loyola Univ Med Ctr/Hines VA Hosp 1992; **Fellow:** Hematology & Oncology, Fox Chase Cancer Ctr/Temple Univ Hosp 1995; **Fac Appt:** Prof Med, Loyola Univ-Stritch Sch Med

Cleary, James F MD [Onc] - **Spec Exp:** Palliative Care; Head & Neck Cancer; **Hospital:** Univ WI Hosp & Clins; **Address:** 600 Highland Ave CSC Bldg - rm k6/546, Madison, WI 53792; **Phone:** 608-263-8624; **Board Cert:** Hospice & Palliative Medicine 2011; **Med School:** Australia 1984; **Resid:** Internal Medicine, Royal Adelaide Hosp 1987; **Fellow:** Medical Oncology, Royal Adelaide Hosp 1990; **Fac Appt:** Assoc Prof Med, Univ Wisc

Clinton, Steven K MD/PhD [Onc] - **Spec Exp:** Genitourinary Cancer; Prostate Cancer; Nutrition & Cancer Prevention/Control; **Hospital:** Ohio St Univ Med Ctr; **Address:** 320 W 10th Ave, rm 456 SL, Columbus, OH 43210; **Phone:** 614-293-7560; **Board Cert:** Internal Medicine 1987; **Med School:** Univ IL Coll Med 1984; **Resid:** Internal Medicine, Univ Chicago Hosps 1987; **Fellow:** Medical Oncology, Dana Farber Cancer Inst/Harvard 1991; **Fac Appt:** Assoc Prof Med, Ohio State Univ

Cobleigh, Melody A MD [Onc] - **Spec Exp:** Breast Cancer; **Hospital:** Rush Univ Med Ctr; **Address:** Rush Univ Med Ctr, 1725 W Harrison St, Ste 821, Chicago, IL 60612-3828; **Phone:** 312-942-5904; **Board Cert:** Internal Medicine 1979; Medical Oncology 1981; **Med School:** Rush Med Coll 1976; **Resid:** Internal Medicine, Rush Presby-St Lukes Med Ctr 1979; **Fellow:** Medical Oncology, Indiana Univ 1981; **Fac Appt:** Prof Med, Rush Med Coll

Davis, Mellar P MD [Onc] - **Spec Exp:** Palliative Care; Lung Cancer (advanced); Amyloidosis; **Hospital:** Cleveland Clin (page 56); **Address:** Cleveland Clin Fdn, 9500 Euclid Ave, Desk R35, Cleveland, OH 44195; **Phone:** 216-445-4622; **Board Cert:** Internal Medicine 1980; Hematology 1982; Medical Oncology 1983; Hospice & Palliative Medicine 2004; **Med School:** Ohio State Univ 1977; **Resid:** Internal Medicine, Riverside Methodist Hosp 1979; **Fellow:** Hematology, Mayo Clinic 1981; Medical Oncology, Mayo Clinic 1982; **Fac Appt:** Prof Med, Cleveland Cl Coll Med/Case West Res

Dowlati, Afshin MD [Onc] - **Spec Exp:** Lung Cancer; Thoracic Cancers; **Hospital:** Univ Hosps Case Med Ctr (page 74); **Address:** UH Seidman Cancer Center, 11100 Euclid Ave, Cleveland, OH 44106; **Phone:** 216-844-1228; **Board Cert:** Internal Medicine 2000; Medical Oncology 2001; **Med School:** Belgium 1992; **Resid:** Internal Medicine, U Liege 1996; **Fellow:** Hematology & Oncology, Case Western/Univ Hosps 1998; **Fac Appt:** Assoc Prof Med, Case West Res Univ

Dreicer, Robert MD [Onc] - **Spec Exp:** Prostate Cancer; Kidney Cancer; Bladder Cancer; Testicular Cancer; **Hospital:** Cleveland Clin (page 56); **Address:** 9500 Euclid Ave, Desk R35, Cleveland, OH 44195; **Phone:** 216-445-4623; **Board Cert:** Internal Medicine 1986; Medical Oncology 1989; **Med School:** Univ Tex, Houston 1983; **Resid:** Internal Medicine, Ind Univ Med Ctr 1986; **Fellow:** Medical Oncology, Univ Wisconsin Hosp 1989; **Fac Appt:** Prof Med, Cleveland Cl Coll Med/Case West Res

Einhorn, Lawrence H MD [Onc] - **Spec Exp:** Testicular Cancer; Lung Cancer; Urologic Cancer; **Hospital:** IU Health University Hosp; **Address:** IU Simon Cancer Center, 535 Barnhill Drive, RT 473, Indianapolis, IN 46202; **Phone:** 317-944-0920; **Board Cert:** Internal Medicine 1972; Medical Oncology 1975; **Med School:** UCLA 1967; **Resid:** Internal Medicine, Indiana Univ Hosp 1969; **Fellow:** Hematology & Oncology, Indiana Univ 1972; Hematology & Oncology, MD Anderson Cancer Ctr 1973; **Fac Appt:** Prof Med, Indiana Univ

Ellis, Matthew J MD/PhD [Onc] - **Spec Exp:** Breast Cancer; **Hospital:** Barnes-Jewish Hosp; **Address:** Washington University, 660 S Euclid Ave, Box 8056, St Louis, MO 63110; **Phone:** 314-747-1171; **Board Cert:** Internal Medicine 2004; Medical Oncology 2005; **Med School:** England, UK 1984; **Resid:** Internal Medicine, Hammersmith Hosp 1988; **Fellow:** Research, Georgetown Univ Med Ctr 1992; Medical Oncology, Georgetwon Univ Med Ctr 1994; **Fac Appt:** Prof Med, Washington Univ, St Louis

Medical Oncology

Ensminger, William D MD/PhD [Onc] - **Spec Exp:** Gastrointestinal Cancer; Liver Cancer; Clinical Trials; **Hospital:** Univ of Michigan Hosp; **Address:** 1150 W Med Ctr Drive, Med Sci II Rm #4742, Ann Arbor, MI 48109-5633; **Phone:** 734-647-8902; **Board Cert:** Internal Medicine 1976; Medical Oncology 1979; **Med School:** Harvard Med Sch 1973; **Resid:** Internal Medicine, Beth Israel Hosp 1975; **Fellow:** Medical Oncology, Dana Farber Cancer Inst 1977; **Fac Appt:** Prof Med, Univ Mich Med Sch

Fleming, Gini F MD [Onc] - **Spec Exp:** Breast Cancer-Novel Therapies; Gynecologic Cancer; Ovarian Cancer; **Hospital:** Univ of Chicago Med Ctr; **Address:** Univ Chicago Hosps, 5841 S Maryland MC2115, Chicago, IL 60637-1470; **Phone:** 773-702-6149; **Board Cert:** Internal Medicine 1988; Medical Oncology 2001; Hematology 2002; **Med School:** Univ IL Coll Med 1985; **Resid:** Internal Medicine, Univ Chicago Hosps 1988; **Fellow:** Hematology & Oncology, Univ Chicago Hosps 1992; **Fac Appt:** Prof Med, Univ Chicago-Pritzker Sch Med

Gaynor, Ellen MD [Onc] - **Spec Exp:** Breast Cancer; Gastrointestinal Cancer; Prostate Cancer; **Hospital:** Loyola Univ Med Ctr; **Address:** Loyola Bernardin Cancer Center, 2160 S First Ave Bldg 112 - rm 108, Maywood, IL 60153-3328; **Phone:** 708-327-3214; **Board Cert:** Internal Medicine 1982; Hematology 1986; Medical Oncology 1985; **Med School:** Univ Wisc 1978; **Resid:** Internal Medicine, Loyola Univ Med Ctr 1982; **Fellow:** Medical Oncology, Loyola Univ Med Ctr 1981; Hematology & Oncology, Univ Chicago 1984; **Fac Appt:** Prof Med, Loyola Univ-Stritch Sch Med

Gerson, Stanton MD [Onc] - **Spec Exp:** Leukemia; Lymphoma, Non-Hodgkin's; Stem Cell Transplant; Multiple Myeloma; **Hospital:** Univ Hosps Case Med Ctr (page 74); **Address:** Ireland Cancer Ctr, 11000 Euclid Ave, 1 WEARN 151, Cleveland, OH 44106-5065; **Phone:** 216-844-1232; **Board Cert:** Internal Medicine 1980; Hematology 1982; Medical Oncology 1983; **Med School:** Harvard Med Sch 1977; **Resid:** Internal Medicine, Hosp Univ Penn 1980; **Fellow:** Hematology & Oncology, Hosp Univ Penn 1983; **Fac Appt:** Prof Med, Case West Res Univ

Golomb, Harvey M MD [Onc] - **Spec Exp:** Lung Cancer; Leukemia; Lymphoma; **Hospital:** Univ of Chicago Med Ctr; **Address:** Univ Chicago Medical Ctr, 5841 S Maryland Ave, MC 2115, Chicago, IL 60637-1463; **Phone:** 773-702-6149; **Board Cert:** Internal Medicine 1975; Medical Oncology 1979; **Med School:** Univ Pittsburgh 1968; **Resid:** Internal Medicine, Johns Hopkins Hosp 1972; Clinical Genetics, Johns Hopkins Hosp 1973; **Fellow:** Hematology & Oncology, Univ Chicago Hosps 1975; **Fac Appt:** Prof Med, Univ Chicago-Pritzker Sch Med

Gradishar, William J MD [Onc] - **Spec Exp:** Breast Cancer; **Hospital:** Northwestern Meml Hosp; **Address:** 250 E Superior St, Ste 420, Chicago, IL 60611; **Phone:** 312-695-4125; **Board Cert:** Internal Medicine 1985; Medical Oncology 1989; **Med School:** Univ IL Coll Med 1982; **Resid:** Internal Medicine, Michael Reese Hosp 1985; **Fellow:** Hematology & Oncology, Univ Chicago Hosps 1990; **Fac Appt:** Prof Med, Northwestern Univ

Gruber, Stephen B MD/PhD [Onc] - **Spec Exp:** Cancer Genetics; Colon & Rectal Cancer; Melanoma; **Hospital:** Univ of Michigan Hosp; **Address:** 109 Zina Pitcher Pl, Ann Arbor, MI 48109-2200; **Phone:** 734-615-9712; **Board Cert:** Medical Oncology 2009; **Med School:** Univ Pennsylvania 1992; **Resid:** Internal Medicine, Hosp Univ Penn 1994; **Fellow:** Medical Oncology, Johns Hopkins Hosp 1997; Clinical Genetics, Univ Michigan Hlth Sys 1999; **Fac Appt:** Assoc Prof Med, Univ Mich Med Sch

Hartmann, Lynn Carol MD [Onc] - **Spec Exp:** Ovarian Cancer; **Hospital:** Mayo Med Ctr & Clin - Rochester; **Address:** Mayo Clinic Gonda 10 South, 200 First St SW, Rochester, MN 55905; **Phone:** 507-284-3903; **Board Cert:** Internal Medicine 1986; Medical Oncology 1989; **Med School:** Northwestern Univ 1983; **Resid:** Internal Medicine, Univ Ia Hosps/Clinics 1986; **Fellow:** Medical Oncology, Mayo Clinic 1989; **Fac Appt:** Prof Med, Mayo Med Sch

Hayes, Daniel F MD [Onc] - **Spec Exp:** Breast Cancer; **Hospital:** Univ of Michigan Hosp; **Address:** Univ Michigan Comprehensive Cancer Ctr, 6312 CCC SPC, 5942, 1500 E Medical Center Drive, Ann Arbor, MI 48109-5942; **Phone:** 734-615-6725; **Board Cert:** Internal Medicine 1982; Medical Oncology 1985; **Med School:** Indiana Univ 1979; **Resid:** Internal Medicine, Parkland Meml Hosp 1982; **Fellow:** Medical Oncology, Dana Farber Cancer Inst 1985; **Fac Appt:** Prof Med, Univ Mich Med Sch

Hoffman, Philip C MD [Onc] - **Spec Exp:** Lung Cancer; Breast Cancer; **Hospital:** Univ of Chicago Med Ctr, Little Company of Mary Hosp & Hlth Care Ctrs; **Address:** 5841 S Maryland Ave, MC 2115, Chicago, IL 60637-1447; **Phone:** 773-834-7424; **Board Cert:** Internal Medicine 1975; Hematology 1980; Medical Oncology 1981; **Med School:** Jefferson Med Coll 1972; **Resid:** Internal Medicine, Hosp Univ Penn 1975; **Fellow:** Hematology & Oncology, Univ Chicago Hosps 1980; **Fac Appt:** Prof Med, Univ Chicago-Pritzker Sch Med

Hussain, Maha H MD [Onc] - **Spec Exp:** Prostate Cancer; Bladder Cancer; Testicular Cancer; Genitourinary Cancer; **Hospital:** Univ of Michigan Hosp; **Address:** Univ Michigan Cancer Ctr, 1500 E Medical Ctr Drive, rm 7310, Ann Arbor, MI 48109; **Phone:** 734-936-8906; **Board Cert:** Internal Medicine 1986; Medical Oncology 1989; **Med School:** Iraq 1980; **Resid:** Internal Medicine, Wayne State Univ Affil Hosps 1986; **Fellow:** Medical Oncology, Wayne State Univ Affil Hosps 1989; **Fac Appt:** Prof Med, Univ Mich Med Sch

Ingle, James N MD [Onc] - **Spec Exp:** Breast Cancer; **Hospital:** Rochester Methodist Hosp, Mayo Med Ctr & Clin - Rochester; **Address:** Mayo Clinic, 200 First St SW, Gonda Bldg Fl 10, Rochester, MN 55905-0001; **Phone:** 507-284-8432; **Board Cert:** Internal Medicine 1974; Medical Oncology 1975; **Med School:** Johns Hopkins Univ 1971; **Resid:** Internal Medicine, Johns Hopkins Hosp 1976; Medical Oncology, Natl Cancer Inst 1975; **Fac Appt:** Prof Hem & Onc, Mayo Med Sch

Kalaycio, Matt E MD [Onc] - **Spec Exp:** Leukemia; Bone Marrow Transplant; **Hospital:** Cleveland Clin (page 56); **Address:** Taussig Cancer Ctr, 9500 Euclid Ave, Desk R35, Cleveland, OH 44195; **Phone:** 216-444-3705; **Board Cert:** Internal Medicine 2002; Hematology 2004; Medical Oncology 2005; **Med School:** W VA Univ 1988; **Resid:** Internal Medicine, Mercy Hosp 1991; **Fellow:** Hematology & Oncology, Cleveland Clinic 1994; **Fac Appt:** Prof Med, Cleveland Cl Coll Med/Case West Res

Kalemkerian, Gregory P MD [Onc] - **Spec Exp:** Lung Cancer; Mesothelioma; Thymoma; **Hospital:** Univ of Michigan Hosp; **Address:** 1500 E Med Ctr Drive, C350 Med Inn-SPC 5848, MS 5848, Ann Arbor, MI 48109-0848; **Phone:** 734-232-6046; **Board Cert:** Internal Medicine 1988; Medical Oncology 2001; **Med School:** Northwestern Univ 1985; **Resid:** Internal Medicine, Northwestern Meml Hosp 1988; **Fellow:** Medical Oncology, Johns Hopkins Hosp 1993; **Fac Appt:** Prof Hem & Onc, Univ Mich Med Sch

Kaminski, Mark S MD [Onc] - **Spec Exp:** Lymphoma; Bone Marrow Transplant; Drug Development; Clinical Trials; **Hospital:** Univ of Michigan Hosp; **Address:** Univ Michigan Cancer Ctr, 1500 E Medical Ctr Drive, rm 4316, Ann Arbor, MI 48109; **Phone:** 734-647-8901; **Board Cert:** Internal Medicine 1981; Medical Oncology 1983; **Med School:** Stanford Univ 1978; **Resid:** Internal Medicine, Barnes Hosp 1981; **Fellow:** Medical Oncology, Stanford Univ Med Ctr 1985; **Fac Appt:** Prof Med, Univ Mich Med Sch

Kindler, Hedy Lee MD [Onc] - **Spec Exp:** Pancreatic Cancer; Mesothelioma; Colon & Rectal Cancer; **Hospital:** Univ of Chicago Med Ctr; **Address:** Univ of Chicago Medical Ctr, 5841 S Maryland Ave, MC 2115, Chicago, IL 60637-1470; **Phone:** 773-702-6149; **Board Cert:** Internal Medicine 2002; Medical Oncology 2005; **Med School:** SUNY Buffalo 1985; **Resid:** Internal Medicine, UCLA Med Ctr 1992; **Fellow:** Medical Oncology, Meml Sloan Kettering Cancer Ctr 1995; **Fac Appt:** Assoc Prof Med, Univ Chicago-Pritzker Sch Med

Medical Oncology

Krishnamurthi, Smitha S MD [Onc] - **Spec Exp:** Gastrointestinal Cancer; Colon & Rectal Cancer; **Hospital:** Univ Hosps Case Med Ctr (page 74); **Address:** UH Case Medical Center, Seidman Cancer Center, 11100 Euclid Ave, Cleveland, OH 44106; **Phone:** 216-844-1006; **Board Cert:** Internal Medicine 2006; Medical Oncology 2008; **Med School:** Univ Pennsylvania 1993; **Resid:** Internal Medicine, Univ Penn Affil Hosps 1996; **Fellow:** Medical Oncology, Johns Hopkins Hosp 1996; **Fac Appt:** Asst Prof Med, Case West Res Univ

Kuzel, Timothy M MD [Onc] - **Spec Exp:** Kidney Cancer; Melanoma; Cutaneous Lymphoma; **Hospital:** Northwestern Meml Hosp; **Address:** Northwestern Meml Hosp, 675 N St Clair, Ste 21-100, Chicago, IL 60611; **Phone:** 312-695-0990; **Board Cert:** Internal Medicine 1987; Hematology 2000; Medical Oncology 1989; **Med School:** Univ Mich Med Sch 1984; **Resid:** Internal Medicine, McGraw MC-Northwestern Univ 1987; **Fellow:** Hematology & Oncology, McGraw MC-Northwestern Univ 1990; **Fac Appt:** Prof Med, Northwestern Univ

Loehrer, Patrick J MD [Onc] - **Spec Exp:** Thymoma; Genitourinary Cancer; Pancreatic Cancer; Esophageal Cancer; **Hospital:** IU Health University Hosp; **Address:** IU Simon Cancer Center, 535 Barnhill Drive, rm 473, Indianapolis, IN 46202-5112; **Phone:** 317-944-0920; **Board Cert:** Internal Medicine 1981; Medical Oncology 2006; **Med School:** Rush Med Coll 1978; **Resid:** Internal Medicine, Rush-Presby-St Lukes Hosp 1981; **Fellow:** Medical Oncology, Indiana Univ 1983; **Fac Appt:** Prof Med, Indiana Univ

Loprinzi, Charles L MD [Onc] - **Spec Exp:** Breast Cancer; **Hospital:** Mayo Med Ctr & Clin - Rochester; **Address:** Mayo Clinic, Dept Med Oncology, 200 First St SW, Rochester, MN 55905-0001; **Phone:** 507-284-4849; **Board Cert:** Internal Medicine 1982; Medical Oncology 1985; **Med School:** Oregon Hlth & Sci Univ 1979; **Resid:** Internal Medicine, Maricopa Co Hosp 1982; **Fellow:** Medical Oncology, Univ Wisconsin Med Ctr 1984; **Fac Appt:** Prof Med, Mayo Med Sch

Markowitz, Sanford D MD [Onc] - **Spec Exp:** Colon & Rectal Cancer; Hereditary Cancer; **Hospital:** Univ Hosps Case Med Ctr (page 74); **Address:** Ireland Cancer Ctr, 11100 Euclid Ave Fl 6, Cleveland, OH 44106; **Phone:** 216-844-3951; **Board Cert:** Internal Medicine 1984; Medical Oncology 1987; **Med School:** Yale Univ 1980; **Resid:** Internal Medicine, Univ Chicago Hosp 1984; **Fellow:** Medical Oncology, Natl Cancer Inst 1986; **Fac Appt:** Prof Med, Case West Res Univ

Meropol, Neal J MD [Onc] - **Spec Exp:** Gastrointestinal Cancer; Colon Cancer; Pancreatic Cancer; **Hospital:** Univ Hosps Case Med Ctr (page 74); **Address:** 11100 Euclid Ave, Cleveland, OH 44106; **Phone:** 216-844-5220; **Board Cert:** Internal Medicine 1988; Medical Oncology 2001; **Med School:** Vanderbilt Univ 1985; **Resid:** Internal Medicine, Univ Hosps/Case West Res 1988; **Fellow:** Hematology & Oncology, Hosp Univ Penn 1992; **Fac Appt:** Prof Med, Case West Res Univ

O'Brien, Timothy E MD [Onc] - **Spec Exp:** Gastrointestinal Cancer; Colon & Rectal Cancer; Multiple Myeloma; Lung Cancer; **Hospital:** MetroHealth Med Ctr; **Address:** MetroHealth Cancer Care Ctr, 2500 MetroHealth Drive, rm C-2100, Cleveland, OH 44109; **Phone:** 216-778-5802; **Board Cert:** Medical Oncology 1997; Hematology 1998; **Med School:** Univ Rochester 1989; **Resid:** Internal Medicine, Univ Hosps Cleveland 1992; **Fellow:** Hematology & Oncology, Univ Hosps Cleveland 1997; **Fac Appt:** Assoc Prof Med, Case West Res Univ

Olopade, Olufunmilayo I MD [Onc] - **Spec Exp:** Breast Cancer; Hereditary Cancer; Breast Cancer Genetics; Cancer Risk Assessment; **Hospital:** Univ of Chicago Med Ctr; **Address:** Univ Chicago Med Ctr, 5841 S Maryland Ave, MC 2115, Chicago, IL 60637-1470; **Phone:** 773-702-6149; **Board Cert:** Internal Medicine 1986; Hematology 2001; Medical Oncology 1989; **Med School:** Nigeria 1980; **Resid:** Internal Medicine, Cook Co Hosp 1986; **Fellow:** Hematology & Oncology, Univ Chicago Hosps 1991; **Fac Appt:** Prof Med, Univ Chicago-Pritzker Sch Med

Ozer, Howard MD [Onc] - **Spec Exp:** Lymphoma; **Hospital:** Univ of IL Med Ctr at Chicago; **Address:** UIC Hematology/Oncology, Clinical Sciences Bldg, 840 S Wood St, Ste 820E, Chicago, IL 60612; **Phone:** 312-355-1625; **Board Cert:** Internal Medicine 1979; **Med School:** Yale Univ 1975; **Resid:** Internal Medicine, Mass Genl Hosp 1977; **Fellow:** Hematology & Oncology, PB Brigham/Dana Farber Cancer Inst 1979; **Fac Appt:** Prof Med, Univ IL Coll Med

Peace, David J MD [Onc] - **Spec Exp:** Prostate Cancer; Vaccine Therapy; Leukemia & Lymphoma; Immunotherapy; **Hospital:** Univ of IL Med Ctr at Chicago, MacNeal Hosp; **Address:** 840 S Wood St CSB Bldg - Ste 820, MS 713, Chicago, IL 60607; **Phone:** 312-413-1507; **Board Cert:** Internal Medicine 1983; Medical Oncology 1987; **Med School:** Univ Pittsburgh 1980; **Resid:** Internal Medicine, Univ Pittsburgh Med Ctr 1983; **Fellow:** Hematology & Oncology, Univ Washington Med Ctr 1988

Peereboom, David M MD [Onc] - **Spec Exp:** Neuro-Oncology; Brain Tumors; Drug Development; **Hospital:** Cleveland Clin (page 56); **Address:** Cleveland Clinic Taussig Cancer Inst, 9500 Euclid Ave, MC R35, Cleveland, OH 44195; **Phone:** 216-445-6068; **Board Cert:** Internal Medicine 1989; Medical Oncology 2004; **Med School:** Med Coll VA 1986; **Resid:** Internal Medicine, Univ Hosp of Cleveland 1990; **Fellow:** Medical Oncology, Johns Hopkins Hosp 1993

Perry, Michael C MD [Onc] - **Spec Exp:** Lung Cancer; Breast Cancer; **Hospital:** Univ of Missouri Hosp; **Address:** Ellis Fischel Cancer Ctr, 115 Business Loop 70 W, DC 116.71, rm 524, Columbia, MO 65203-3299; **Phone:** 573-882-4979; **Board Cert:** Internal Medicine 1987; Hematology 1974; Medical Oncology 1975; **Med School:** Wayne State Univ 1970; **Resid:** Internal Medicine, Mayo Grad Sch 1972; **Fellow:** Hematology, Mayo Grad Sch 1974; Medical Oncology, Mayo Grad Sch 1975; **Fac Appt:** Prof Med, Univ MO-Columbia Sch Med

Peterson, Bruce MD [Onc] - **Spec Exp:** Lymphoma; Leukemia; **Address:** Univ of Minnesota, 420 Delaware St SE, MMC 480, Minneapolis, MN 55455; **Phone:** 612-625-5411; **Board Cert:** Internal Medicine 1974; Medical Oncology 1977; **Med School:** Univ Minn 1971; **Resid:** Internal Medicine, Fletcher Allen Hlthcare 1973; Internal Medicine, Fairview-Univ Med Ctr 1974; **Fellow:** Medical Oncology, Fairview-Univ Med Ctr 1977; **Fac Appt:** Prof Med, Univ Minn

Petruska, Paul J MD [Onc] - **Spec Exp:** Leukemia & Lymphoma; Solid Tumors; **Hospital:** St. Louis Univ Hosp; **Address:** SLU, Dept Hem/Onc, 3655 Vista Ave, St Louis, MO 63110; **Phone:** 314-577-6057; **Board Cert:** Internal Medicine 1972; Hematology 1974; Medical Oncology 1979; **Med School:** St Louis Univ 1967; **Resid:** Internal Medicine, St. Louis Hosp 1969; Internal Medicine, St. Louis Hosp 1972; **Fellow:** Hematology & Oncology, St. Louis Hosp 1974; **Fac Appt:** Prof Med, St Louis Univ

Pienta, Kenneth J MD [Onc] - **Spec Exp:** Prostate Cancer; **Hospital:** Univ of Michigan Hosp; **Address:** 1500 E Med Ctr Drive, rm 7303 CCC, Ann Arbor, MI 48109-5946; **Phone:** 734-647-3421; **Board Cert:** Internal Medicine 2001; Medical Oncology 2001; **Med School:** Johns Hopkins Univ 1986; **Resid:** Internal Medicine, Univ Chicago Hosps 1988; **Fellow:** Medical Oncology, Johns Hopkins Hosp 1991; **Fac Appt:** Prof Med, Univ Mich Med Sch

Pohlman, Brad L MD [Onc] - **Spec Exp:** Lymphoma; Lymphoma, Non-Hodgkin's; Bone Marrow Transplant; **Hospital:** Cleveland Clin (page 56); **Address:** Cleveland Clinic Fdn, 9500 Euclid Ave, Desk R35, Cleveland, OH 44195; **Phone:** 216-444-6070; **Board Cert:** Internal Medicine 1988; **Med School:** Indiana Univ 1985; **Resid:** Internal Medicine, Univ Wisconsin Hosp 1988; **Fellow:** Hematology, Univ Minnesota Hosp 1992

Medical Oncology

Ratain, Mark J MD [Onc] - **Spec Exp:** Solid Tumors; Drug Discovery & Development; **Hospital:** Univ of Chicago Med Ctr; **Address:** Univ Chicago Med Ctr, 5841 S Maryland Ave, MC 2115, Chicago, IL 60637; **Phone:** 773-702-6149; **Board Cert:** Internal Medicine 1983; Hematology 1986; Medical Oncology 1985; **Med School:** Yale Univ 1980; **Resid:** Internal Medicine, Johns Hopkins Hosp 1983; **Fellow:** Hematology & Oncology, Univ Chicago 1986; **Fac Appt:** Prof Med, Univ Chicago-Pritzker Sch Med

Richards, Jon M MD/PhD [Onc] - **Spec Exp:** Melanoma; **Hospital:** Adv Luth Genl Hosp, Skokie/North Shore Univ Htlh Syst; **Address:** Center for Advanced Care, 1700 Luther Ln Fl 2, Park Ridge, IL 60068; **Phone:** 847-268-8200; **Board Cert:** Medical Oncology 2007; **Med School:** Cornell Univ 1983; **Resid:** Internal Medicine, Univ Chicago Hosps 1985; **Fellow:** Hematology & Oncology, Univ Chicago Hosps 1988; **Fac Appt:** Assoc Prof Med, Univ IL Coll Med

Rosen, Steven T MD [Onc] - **Spec Exp:** Hematologic Malignancies; Breast Cancer; Leukemia & Lymphoma; **Hospital:** Northwestern Meml Hosp; **Address:** Northwestern Univ, 303 E Chicago Ave, Lurie 3-125, Chicago, IL 60611-3013; **Phone:** 312-695-0990; **Board Cert:** Internal Medicine 1979; Medical Oncology 1981; Hematology 1984; **Med School:** Northwestern Univ 1976; **Resid:** Internal Medicine, Northwestern Univ Hosp 1979; **Fellow:** Medical Oncology, Natl Cancer Inst 1981; **Fac Appt:** Prof Med, Northwestern Univ

Roth, Bruce J MD [Onc] - **Spec Exp:** Prostate Cancer; Bladder Cancer; Testicular Cancer; **Hospital:** Barnes-Jewish Hosp; **Address:** Washington University, 660 S Euclid Ave, Campus Box 8056, St Louis, MO 63110; **Phone:** 314-747-1171; **Board Cert:** Internal Medicine 1983; Medical Oncology 1985; **Med School:** St Louis Univ 1980; **Resid:** Internal Medicine, Indiana Univ Med Ctr 1983; **Fellow:** Hematology & Oncology, Indiana Univ Med Ctr 1986; **Fac Appt:** Prof Med, Washington Univ, St Louis

Salgia, Ravi MD/PhD [Onc] - **Spec Exp:** Lung Cancer; Mesothelioma; Thoracic Cancers; **Hospital:** Univ of Chicago Med Ctr; **Address:** Univ Chicago Medical Ctr, 5841 S Maryland Ave, MC 2115, Chicago, IL 60637; **Phone:** 773-702-6149; **Board Cert:** Medical Oncology 2006; **Med School:** Loyola Univ-Stritch Sch Med 1987; **Resid:** Internal Medicine, Johns Hopkins Hosp 1990; **Fellow:** Medical Oncology, Dana-Farber Cancer Inst 1993; **Fac Appt:** Prof Med, Univ Chicago-Pritzker Sch Med

Schiffer, Charles A MD [Onc] - **Spec Exp:** Leukemia; Lymphoma; Multiple Myeloma; **Hospital:** Barbara Ann Karmanos Cancer Inst, Harper Univ Hosp; **Address:** Karmanos Cancer Inst, Cancer Research Ctr, 4100 John R, HW04HO, Detroit, MI 48201; **Phone:** 313-576-8737; **Board Cert:** Internal Medicine 1972; Medical Oncology 1973; **Med School:** NYU Sch Med 1968; **Resid:** Internal Medicine, Bellevue-NY VA Hosp-NYU 1972; **Fellow:** Medical Oncology, Natl Cancer Inst 1974; **Fac Appt:** Prof Med, Wayne State Univ

Schilsky, Richard L MD [Onc] - **Spec Exp:** Gastrointestinal Cancer; Pancreatic Cancer; Drug Development; **Hospital:** Univ of Chicago Med Ctr; **Address:** Univ Chicago- Bio Sciences Div, 5841 S Maryland Ave, Chicago, IL 60637; **Phone:** 773-834-3914; **Board Cert:** Internal Medicine 1978; Medical Oncology 1979; **Med School:** Univ Chicago-Pritzker Sch Med 1975; **Resid:** Internal Medicine, Univ Texas 1977; **Fellow:** Medical Oncology, Natl Cancer Inst 1980; **Fac Appt:** Prof Med, Univ Chicago-Pritzker Sch Med

Schwartz, Burton S MD [Onc] - **Spec Exp:** Lymphoma; Breast Cancer; **Hospital:** Abbott - Northwestern Hosp; **Address:** 910 E 26th St, Ste 200, Minneapolis, MN 55404; **Phone:** 612-884-6300; **Board Cert:** Internal Medicine 1980; Hematology 1976; Medical Oncology 1977; **Med School:** Meharry Med Coll 1968; **Resid:** Internal Medicine, Michael Reese Hosp 1971; **Fellow:** Hematology, Univ Minn Hosp 1976; **Fac Appt:** Clin Prof Med, Univ Minn

Shapiro, Charles L MD [Onc] - **Spec Exp:** Breast Cancer; **Hospital:** Arthur G James Cancer Hosp & Research Inst; **Address:** 320 W 10th Ave, Starling-Loving Hall, rm B405, Columbus, OH 43210; **Phone:** 614-293-0066; **Board Cert:** Internal Medicine 1987; Medical Oncology 2005; **Med School:** SUNY Buffalo 1984; **Resid:** Internal Medicine, Temple Univ Hosp 1987; **Fellow:** Medical Oncology, Dana Farber Cancer Inst 1991; **Fac Appt:** Assoc Prof Med, Ohio State Univ

Silver, Samuel M MD/PhD [Onc] - **Spec Exp:** Hematologic Malignancies; Bleeding/Coagulation Disorders; Myelodysplastic Syndromes; Porphyria; **Hospital:** Univ of Michigan Hosp; **Address:** Univ Michigan Med Ctr, 4101 Med Sci I C- Wing, 1301 Catherine St, Ann Arbor, MI 48109-5624; **Phone:** 734-615-1332; **Board Cert:** Internal Medicine 1982; Medical Oncology 1985; Hematology 1984; **Med School:** Cornell Univ-Weill Med Coll 1978; **Resid:** Internal Medicine, UCSF-Moffit Hosp 1982; **Fellow:** Hematology & Oncology, Hosp Univ Penn 1985; **Fac Appt:** Clin Prof Med, Univ Mich Med Sch

Silverman, Paula MD [Onc] - **Spec Exp:** Breast Cancer; **Hospital:** Univ Hosps Case Med Ctr (page 74); **Address:** Univ Hosp Cleveland, Ireland Cancer Ctr, 11100 Euclid Ave Bolwell Bldg Fl 6, Cleveland, OH 44106; **Phone:** 216-844-8510; **Board Cert:** Internal Medicine 1984; Medical Oncology 1989; **Med School:** Case West Res Univ 1981; **Resid:** Internal Medicine, Univ Hosps 1984; **Fellow:** Hematology & Oncology, Case Western Reserve Univ 1987; **Fac Appt:** Assoc Prof Med, Case West Res Univ

Sledge Jr, George W MD [Onc] - **Spec Exp:** Breast Cancer; **Hospital:** IU Health University Hosp, IU Health North Hosp; **Address:** 535 Barnhill Drive, rm 473, Indianapolis, IN 46202; **Phone:** 317-274-0920; **Board Cert:** Internal Medicine 1980; Medical Oncology 1983; **Med School:** Tulane Univ 1977; **Resid:** Internal Medicine, St Louis Univ Med Ctr 1980; **Fellow:** Medical Oncology, Univ Texas SA 1983; **Fac Appt:** Prof Med, Indiana Univ

Stadler, Walter M MD [Onc] - **Spec Exp:** Kidney Cancer; Bladder Cancer; Prostate Cancer; Testicular Cancer; **Hospital:** Univ of Chicago Med Ctr; **Address:** Univ Chicago Medical Center, 5841 S Maryland Ave, MC 2115, Chicago, IL 60637; **Phone:** 773-834-7424; **Board Cert:** Internal Medicine 2002; Medical Oncology 2003; **Med School:** Yale Univ 1988; **Resid:** Internal Medicine, Michael Reese Hosp 1991; **Fellow:** Medical Oncology, Univ Chicago Hosps 1994; **Fac Appt:** Prof Med, Univ Chicago-Pritzker Sch Med

Sweetenham, John W MD [Onc] - **Spec Exp:** Lymphoma; Stem Cell Transplant; Castleman's Disease; **Hospital:** Cleveland Clin (page 56); **Address:** Cleveland Clin, Taussig Cancer Inst, 9500 Euclid Ave, Cleveland, OH 44195; **Phone:** 216-445-6707; **Med School:** England, UK 1980; **Resid:** Internal Medicine, Royal United Hosp 1984; **Fellow:** Hematology & Oncology, Univ Southampton 1989; **Fac Appt:** Prof Med, Cleveland Cl Coll Med/Case West Res

Triozzi, Pierre L MD [Onc] - **Spec Exp:** Melanoma; Vaccine Therapy; Clinical Trials; **Hospital:** Cleveland Clin (page 56); **Address:** Cleveland Clinic Fdn, 9500 Euclid Ave, MC R40, Cleveland, OH 44195; **Phone:** 216-445-5141; **Board Cert:** Internal Medicine 1983; Medical Oncology 1987; Hematology 1988; **Med School:** Ohio State Univ 1980; **Resid:** Internal Medicine, Duke Univ Med Ctr 1983; **Fellow:** Hematology & Oncology, Duke Univ Med Ctr 1987; **Fac Appt:** Prof Med, Case West Res Univ

Urba, Susan G MD [Onc] - **Spec Exp:** Head & Neck Cancer; **Hospital:** Univ of Michigan Hosp; **Address:** Level B1363, Reception C, 1500 E Med Ctr Drive, Ann Arbor, MI 48109-0922; **Phone:** 734-647-8902; **Board Cert:** Internal Medicine 1986; Medical Oncology 2002; **Med School:** Univ Mich Med Sch 1983; **Resid:** Internal Medicine, Univ Mich Med Ctr 1986; **Fellow:** Hematology & Oncology, Univ Mich Med Ctr 1988; **Fac Appt:** Assoc Prof Med, Univ Mich Med Sch

Medical Oncology

Vokes, Everett E MD [Onc] - **Spec Exp:** Lung Cancer; Head & Neck Cancer; Esophageal Cancer; **Hospital:** Univ of Chicago Med Ctr; **Address:** Univ Chicago Hosps, 5841 S Maryland Ave, MC 2115, Chicago, IL 60637-1470; **Phone:** 773-834-3093; **Board Cert:** Internal Medicine 1983; Medical Oncology 1985; **Med School:** Germany 1980; **Resid:** Internal Medicine, Ravenswood Hosp-Univ Illinois 1982; Internal Medicine, USC Med Ctr 1983; **Fellow:** Medical Oncology, Univ Chicago 1986; **Fac Appt:** Prof Med, Univ Chicago-Pritzker Sch Med

Von Roenn, Jamie H MD [Onc] - **Spec Exp:** Palliative Care; AIDS Related Cancers; Breast Cancer; **Hospital:** Northwestern Meml Hosp; **Address:** Northwestern Medical Faculty Foundation, 676 N St Clair St, Ste 850, Chicago, IL 60611; **Phone:** 312-695-6180; **Board Cert:** Internal Medicine 1983; Medical Oncology 2009; Hospice & Palliative Medicine 2008; **Med School:** Rush Med Coll 1980; **Resid:** Internal Medicine, Rush-Presby-St Lukes Hosp 1983; **Fellow:** Medical Oncology, Rush-Presby-St Lukes Hosp 1985; **Fac Appt:** Prof Med, Northwestern Univ

Weiner, George J MD [Onc] - **Spec Exp:** Lymphoma; Leukemia; Immunotherapy; **Hospital:** Univ Iowa Hosp & Clinics; **Address:** Holden Comprehensive Cancer Center, 200 Hawkins Drive, Ste 5970HJPP, Iowa City, IA 52242; **Phone:** 319-356-4422; **Board Cert:** Internal Medicine 1985; Hematology 1988; Medical Oncology 1987; **Med School:** Ohio State Univ 1981; **Resid:** Medical Oncology, Med Coll Ohio Affil Hosp 1984; **Fellow:** Hematology & Oncology, Univ Mich Med Ctr 1987; **Fac Appt:** Prof Med, Univ Iowa Coll Med

Wicha, Max S MD [Onc] - **Spec Exp:** Breast Cancer; Stem Cell Transplant; **Hospital:** Univ of Michigan Hosp; **Address:** Comp Cancer Ctr & Geriatrics Ctr, 1500 E Med Ctr Dr, rm 6302 CC, SPC 5942, Ann Arbor, MI 48109-5942; **Phone:** 734-936-1831; **Board Cert:** Internal Medicine 1977; Medical Oncology 1983; **Med School:** Stanford Univ 1974; **Resid:** Internal Medicine, Univ Chicago Hosp 1977; **Fellow:** Medical Oncology, Natl Inst Hlth 1980; **Fac Appt:** Prof Med, Univ Mich Med Sch

Wilding, George MD [Onc] - **Spec Exp:** Prostate Cancer; Kidney Cancer; Genitourinary Cancer; Drug Discovery & Development; **Hospital:** Univ WI Hosp & Clins; **Address:** 1111 Highland Ave, Ste 7057WIMR, Madison, WI 53705; **Phone:** 608-263-8610; **Board Cert:** Internal Medicine 1983; Medical Oncology 1985; **Med School:** Univ Mass Sch Med 1980; **Resid:** Internal Medicine, Univ Mass Med Ctr 1983; **Fellow:** Medical Oncology, Natl Cancer Inst 1985; **Fac Appt:** Prof Med, Univ Wisc

Worden, Francis P MD [Onc] - **Spec Exp:** Head & Neck Cancer; Palliative Care; Clinical Trials; **Hospital:** Univ of Michigan Hosp; **Address:** Level B1363, Reception C, 1500 E Medical Center Drive, Ann Arbor, MI 48109; **Phone:** 734-647-8902; **Board Cert:** Medical Oncology 2000; **Med School:** Indiana Univ 1993; **Resid:** Internal Medicine & Pediatrics, Detroit Med Ctr 1997; **Fellow:** Medical Oncology, Detroit Med Ctr 2000; **Fac Appt:** Asst Clin Prof Med, Univ Mich Med Sch

Yee, Douglas MD [Onc] - **Spec Exp:** Breast Cancer; **Address:** Masonic Cancer Ctr-Breast Ctr, 420 Delaware St SE, MMC 160, Minneapolis, MN 55455; **Phone:** 612-273-9685; **Board Cert:** Internal Medicine 1984; Medical Oncology 1987; **Med School:** Univ Chicago-Pritzker Sch Med 1981; **Resid:** Internal Medicine, Univ NC Med Ctr 1984; **Fellow:** Medical Oncology, NIH-Clin Ctr 1987; **Fac Appt:** Prof Med, Univ Minn

Great Plains and Mountains

Akerley III, Wallace L MD [Onc] - **Spec Exp:** Lung Cancer; Clinical Trials; **Hospital:** Univ Utah Hlth Care; **Address:** Huntsman Cancer Inst, 2000 Circle of Hope, rm 2165, Salt Lake City, UT 84112; **Phone:** 801-585-0100; **Board Cert:** Internal Medicine 1984; Medical Oncology 1987; Hematology 1988; **Med School:** Brown Univ 1981; **Resid:** Internal Medicine, USC Medical Ctr 1985; **Fellow:** Medical Oncology, USC Medical Ctr 1986; Hematology, Norris Cotton Cancer Ctr/Dartmouth 1988; **Fac Appt:** Prof Med, Univ Utah

Armitage, James MD [Onc] - **Spec Exp:** Lymphoma; Bone Marrow Transplant; **Hospital:** Nebraska Med Ctr; **Address:** 987630 Nebraska Medical Center, Emile @ 42nd St, Omaha, NE 68198-7630; **Phone:** 402-559-5600; **Board Cert:** Internal Medicine 1976; Medical Oncology 1977; Hematology 1984; **Med School:** Univ Nebr Coll Med 1973; **Resid:** Internal Medicine, Univ Nebraska Med Ctr 1975; **Fellow:** Hematology & Oncology, Univ Iowa Hosp 1977; **Fac Appt:** Prof Med, Univ Nebr Coll Med

Beatty, Patrick G MD/PhD [Onc] - **Spec Exp:** Hematologic Malignancies; Lymphoma; **Hospital:** St. Patrick Hospital - Missoula; **Address:** 500 W Broadway, PO Box 7877, Missoula, MT 59807; **Phone:** 406-728-2539; **Board Cert:** Internal Medicine 1980; Medical Oncology 1985; **Med School:** Univ Chicago-Pritzker Sch Med 1976; **Resid:** Internal Medicine, Vanderbilt Univ Med Ctr 1979; **Fellow:** Oncology, Univ Washington Hosps 1982

Bierman, Philip J MD [Onc] - **Spec Exp:** Lymphoma; Bone Marrow Transplant; **Hospital:** Nebraska Med Ctr; **Address:** Nebraska Medical Ctr, Dept Hem/Oncology, 987630 Nebraska Medical Ctr, Emile @ 42nd St, Omaha, NE 68198-7630; **Phone:** 402-559-5600; **Board Cert:** Internal Medicine 1982; Medical Oncology 1985; Hematology 1986; **Med School:** Univ MO-Kansas City 1979; **Resid:** Internal Medicine, Univ Nebraska Med Ctr 1983; **Fellow:** Medical Oncology, Univ Nebraska Med Ctr 1985; Hematology, City of Hope Natl Med Ctr 1986; **Fac Appt:** Prof Med, Univ Nebr Coll Med

Bunn Jr, Paul A MD [Onc] - **Spec Exp:** Lung Cancer; Clinical Trials; Thymoma; Mesothelioma; **Hospital:** Univ of CO Hosp - Anschutz Inpatient Pav; **Address:** Univ Colorado Hosp Cancer Ctr, 128001 E 17th Ave, Box 8117, Aurora, CO 80045; **Phone:** 720-848-0300; **Board Cert:** Internal Medicine 1974; Medical Oncology 1975; **Med School:** Cornell Univ-Weill Med Coll 1971; **Resid:** Internal Medicine, Moffitt Hosp/ UCSF Med Ctr 1973; **Fellow:** Medical Oncology, Natl Cancer Inst 1976; **Fac Appt:** Prof Med, Univ Colorado

Buys, Saundra S MD [Onc] - **Spec Exp:** Breast Cancer; Breast Cancer Risk Assessment; Breast Cancer Genetics; **Hospital:** Univ Utah Hlth Care; **Address:** Huntsman Cancer Inst, 2000 Circle of Hope, Salt Lake City, UT 84112; **Phone:** 801-585-0100; **Board Cert:** Internal Medicine 1982; Medical Oncology 1985; Hematology 1984; **Med School:** Tufts Univ 1979; **Resid:** Internal Medicine, Univ Utah Hosps 1982; **Fellow:** Hematology & Oncology, Univ Utah Hosps 1985; **Fac Appt:** Prof Med, Univ Utah

Cowan, Kenneth H MD/PhD [Onc] - **Spec Exp:** Breast Cancer; **Hospital:** Nebraska Med Ctr; **Address:** Eppley Cancer Center, 987630 Nebraska Medical Ctr, Emile @ 42nd St, Omaha, NE 68198-7630; **Phone:** 402-559-5600; **Board Cert:** Internal Medicine 1978; Medical Oncology 1981; **Med School:** Case West Res Univ 1975; **Resid:** Internal Medicine, Parkland Meml Hosp 1977

Dakhil, Shaker MD [Onc] - **Spec Exp:** Leukemia; Mesothelioma; Lymphoma; **Hospital:** Univ of Kansas Hosp; **Address:** Cancer Center Kansas, 818 N Emporia, Ste 403, Wichita, KS 67214; **Phone:** 316-262-4467; **Board Cert:** Internal Medicine 1978; Medical Oncology 1981; **Med School:** Lebanon 1976; **Resid:** Internal Medicine, Wayne State Univ Hosp 1978; **Fellow:** Hematology & Oncology, Univ Michigan Sch Med 1981; **Fac Appt:** Assoc Clin Prof Med, Univ Kansas

Medical Oncology

Eckhardt, S Gail MD [Onc] - **Spec Exp:** Gastrointestinal Cancer; Drug Development; **Hospital:** Univ of CO Hosp - Anschutz Inpatient Pav; **Address:** Univ Colorado Hosp Cancer Ctr, PO Box 6510, MS F-704, 1665 Aurora Court, Aurora, CO 80045-0510; **Phone:** 720-848-0300; **Board Cert:** Internal Medicine 1988; Medical Oncology 2006; **Med School:** Univ Tex Med Br, Galveston 1985; **Resid:** Internal Medicine, Univ Virginia Med Ctr 1988; **Fellow:** Research, Scripps Clinic 1989; Medical Oncology, UCSD Med Ctr 1992; **Fac Appt:** Prof Med, Univ Colorado

Elias, Anthony D MD [Onc] - **Spec Exp:** Breast Cancer; **Hospital:** Univ of CO Hosp - Anschutz Inpatient Pav; **Address:** UCH Breast Ctr, Anschutz OPD Pavillion, 1635 Aurora Ct, MS F724, Aurora, CO 80045; **Phone:** 720-848-1030; **Board Cert:** Internal Medicine 1983; Medical Oncology 1985; **Med School:** NYU Sch Med 1980; **Resid:** Internal Medicine, Johns Hopkins Hsop 1983; **Fellow:** Medical Oncology, Dana-Farber Cancer Inst 1983; **Fac Appt:** Assoc Prof Med, Univ Colorado

Fabian, Carol J MD [Onc] - **Spec Exp:** Breast Cancer; Breast Cancer Risk Assessment; **Hospital:** Univ of Kansas Hosp; **Address:** Westwood Med Pavilion, 2330 Shawnee Mission Pkwy, Ste 1102, MS 5015, Westwood, KS 66205; **Phone:** 913-588-7791; **Board Cert:** Internal Medicine 1976; Medical Oncology 1977; **Med School:** Univ Kansas 1972; **Resid:** Internal Medicine, Wesley Med Ctr 1975; **Fellow:** Medical Oncology, Univ Kansas Med Ctr 1977; **Fac Appt:** Prof Med, Univ Kansas

Glode, L Michael MD [Onc] - **Spec Exp:** Prostate Cancer; Genitourinary Cancer; **Hospital:** Univ of CO Hosp - Anschutz Inpatient Pav; **Address:** Univ Colorado Anschutz Cancer Pavilion, 1665 Aurora Court, CP 1004, MS F-710, Aurora, CO 80045; **Phone:** 720-848-0170; **Board Cert:** Internal Medicine 1975; Medical Oncology 1981; **Med School:** Washington Univ, St Louis 1972; **Resid:** Internal Medicine, Univ Texas SW Med Ctr 1973; Immunology, Natl Inst Hlth 1976; **Fellow:** Medical Oncology, Dana Farber Cancer Inst 1978; **Fac Appt:** Prof Med, Univ Colorado

Grem, Jean L MD [Onc] - **Spec Exp:** Colon & Rectal Cancer; Pancreatic Cancer; Stomach Cancer; Esophageal Cancer; **Hospital:** Nebraska Med Ctr; **Address:** 987630 Nebraska Medical Ctr, Emile @ 42nd St, Omaha, NE 68198-7630; **Phone:** 402-559-6210; **Board Cert:** Internal Medicine 1983; Medical Oncology 1985; **Med School:** Jefferson Med Coll 1980; **Resid:** Internal Medicine, Univ Iowa Hosps & Clinics 1983; **Fellow:** Medical Oncology, Univ Wisc Clin Cancer Ctr 1986; **Fac Appt:** Prof Med, Univ Nebr Coll Med

Hauke, Ralph J MD [Onc] - **Spec Exp:** Urologic Cancer; Clinical Trials; Testicular Cancer; Prostate Cancer; **Hospital:** Methodist Hosp - Omaha, Alegent Hlth - Bergan Mercy Med Ctr; **Address:** 8303 Dodge St, Ste 250, Omaha, NE 68114; **Phone:** 402-354-8124; **Board Cert:** Medical Oncology 2001; **Med School:** Panama 1990; **Resid:** Internal Medicine, Univ Nebraska Med Ctr 1996; **Fellow:** Medical Oncology, Univ Nebraska Med Ctr 2001; **Fac Appt:** Assoc Prof Med, Univ Nebr Coll Med

Kane, Madeleine A MD/PhD [Onc] - **Spec Exp:** Head & Neck Cancer; Gastrointestinal Cancer; Neuroendocrine Tumors; **Hospital:** Univ of CO Hosp - Anschutz Inpatient Pav, VA Eastern CO Health Care Sys-Denver; **Address:** Univ Colorado Hosp Cancer Ctr, PO Box 6510, MS F-704, 1665 Aurora Court, Aurora, CO 80045; **Phone:** 720-848-0300; **Board Cert:** Internal Medicine 1981; Medical Oncology 1983; Hematology 1986; **Med School:** Univ Miami Sch Med 1978; **Resid:** Internal Medicine, Stanford Univ Med Ctr 1981; **Fellow:** Hematology & Oncology, Univ Colo Hlth Sci Ctr 1984; **Fac Appt:** Prof Med, Univ Colorado

Messersmith, Wells A MD [Onc] - **Spec Exp:** Gastrointestinal Cancer; Colon & Rectal Cancer; **Hospital:** Univ of CO Hosp - Anschutz Inpatient Pav; **Address:** University of Colorado Hosp, 12605 E 16th Ave, Aurora, CO 80045; **Phone:** 720-848-0300; **Board Cert:** Internal Medicine 2001; Medical Oncology 2003; **Med School:** Harvard Med Sch 1998; **Resid:** Medical Oncology, Mass Genl Hosp 2000; **Fellow:** Medical Oncology, Johns Hopkins Hosp 2004; **Fac Appt:** Asst Prof Med, Univ Colorado

Samuels, Brian L MD [Onc] - **Spec Exp:** Sarcoma; **Hospital:** Kootenai Med Ctr; **Address:** 1440 Mullan Ave, Post Falls, ID 83854; **Phone:** 208-619-4100; **Board Cert:** Internal Medicine 1984; Medical Oncology 1987; **Med School:** Zimbabwe 1976; **Resid:** Internal Medicine, Albert Einstein Med Ctr 1981; Internal Medicine, Albert Einstein Med Ctr 1984; **Fellow:** Hematology & Oncology, Univ Chicago Hosps 1988

Steen, Preston D MD [Onc] - **Spec Exp:** Lymphoma; Lung Cancer; Breast Cancer; Palliative Care; **Hospital:** Sanford Med Ctr Fargo; **Address:** Sanford Health Roger Maris Cancer Ctr, 820 4th St N, Fargo, ND 58102; **Phone:** 701-234-6161; **Board Cert:** Internal Medicine 1987; Medical Oncology 2001; Hospice & Palliative Medicine ; **Med School:** Univ Minn 1984; **Resid:** Internal Medicine, Maricopa Med Ctr 1987; **Fellow:** Hematology & Oncology, Univ Utah 1990; **Fac Appt:** Clin Prof Med, Univ ND Sch Med

Ward, John H MD [Onc] - **Spec Exp:** Breast Cancer; Gastrointestinal Cancer; Brain Tumors; Unknown Primary Cancer; **Hospital:** Univ Utah Hlth Care, St. John's Med Ctr; **Address:** 2000 Circle of Hope, Ste 2100, rm 2141, Salt Lake City, UT 84112-5550; **Phone:** 801-585-0255; **Board Cert:** Internal Medicine 1979; Medical Oncology 1981; Hematology 1982; **Med School:** Univ Utah 1976; **Resid:** Internal Medicine, Duke Univ Med Ctr 1979; **Fellow:** Hematology & Oncology, Univ Utah Med Ctr 1982; **Fac Appt:** Prof Med, Univ Utah

Southwest

Abbruzzese, James L MD [Onc] - **Spec Exp:** Gastrointestinal Cancer; Pancreatic Cancer; Clinical Trials; **Hospital:** UT MD Anderson Cancer Ctr; **Address:** Univ Tex MD Anderson Cancer Ctr, 1515 Holcombe Blvd, Unit 426, Houston, TX 77030; **Phone:** 713-792-2828; **Board Cert:** Internal Medicine 1981; Medical Oncology 1983; **Med School:** Univ Chicago-Pritzker Sch Med 1978; **Resid:** Internal Medicine, Johns Hopkins Hosp 1981; **Fellow:** Medical Oncology, Dana-Farber Cancer Inst 1983; **Fac Appt:** Prof Med, Univ Tex, Houston

Ahmann, Frederick R MD [Onc] - **Spec Exp:** Prostate Cancer; Testicular Cancer; Bladder Cancer; **Hospital:** Univ Med Ctr - Tucson; **Address:** Arizona Cancer Ctr, 3838 N Campbell Ave, Tucson, AZ 85719; **Phone:** 520-694-2873; **Board Cert:** Internal Medicine 1977; Medical Oncology 1981; **Med School:** Univ MO-Columbia Sch Med 1974; **Resid:** Internal Medicine, Georgetown Univ Med Ctr 1977; **Fellow:** Medical Oncology, Univ Med Ctr 1980; **Fac Appt:** Prof Med, Univ Ariz Coll Med

Ajani, Jaffer A MD [Onc] - **Spec Exp:** Gastrointestinal Cancer; Esophageal Cancer; Stomach Cancer; Neuroendocrine Tumors; **Hospital:** UT MD Anderson Cancer Ctr; **Address:** Univ Tex MD Anderson Cancer Ctr, 1515 Holcombe Blvd, Unit 426, Houston, TX 77230; **Phone:** 713-792-2828; **Board Cert:** Internal Medicine 1979; Medical Oncology 1983; **Med School:** India 1971; **Resid:** Family Medicine, Penn Stae Univ-Altoona 1977; Internal Medicine, Tulane Univ Sch Med 1980; **Fellow:** Medical Oncology, MD Anderson Cancer Ctr 1983; **Fac Appt:** Prof Med, Univ Tex, Houston

Medical Oncology

Alberts, David S MD [Onc] - **Spec Exp:** Cancer Prevention; Ovarian Cancer; **Hospital:** Univ Med Ctr - Tucson; **Address:** Arizona Cancer Center, 1515N Campbell Ave, PO Box 245024, Tucson, AZ 85724; **Phone:** 520-626-7685; **Board Cert:** Internal Medicine 1973; Medical Oncology 1973; **Med School:** Univ VA Sch Med 1966; **Resid:** Medical Oncology, Natl Cancer Inst-NIH 1969; Internal Medicine, Univ Minn Hosps 1971; **Fellow:** Clinical Pharmacology, UC San Francisco 1974; **Fac Appt:** Prof Med, Univ Ariz Coll Med

Anthony, Lowell B MD [Onc] - **Spec Exp:** Gastrointestinal Cancer; Carcinoid Tumors; Neuroendocrine Tumors; **Hospital:** LSU Interim Public Hosp; **Address:** 200 W Esplanade, Ste 200, Kenner, LA 70065; **Phone:** 504-464-8500; **Board Cert:** Internal Medicine 1983; Medical Oncology 1989; **Med School:** Vanderbilt Univ 1979; **Resid:** Internal Medicine, Vanderbilt Univ Med Ctr 1982; **Fellow:** Medical Oncology, Vanderbilt Univ Med Ctr 1985; **Fac Appt:** Assoc Prof Med, Louisiana State U, New Orleans

Arun, Banu K MD [Onc] - **Spec Exp:** Breast Cancer; Cancer Prevention; Clinical Trials; **Hospital:** UT MD Anderson Cancer Ctr; **Address:** 1515 Holcombe Blvd, Unit 1354, Houston, TX 77030; **Phone:** 713-792-2817; **Med School:** Turkey 1990; **Resid:** Internal Medicine, Univ Istanbul 1994; **Fellow:** Hematology & Oncology, Lombardi Cancer Ctr-Georgetown Univ 1997; **Fac Appt:** Assoc Prof Med, Univ Tex, Houston

Benjamin, Robert S MD [Onc] - **Spec Exp:** Sarcoma; **Hospital:** UT MD Anderson Cancer Ctr; **Address:** UT MD Anderson Cancer Ctr, 1515 Holcombe Blvd, Unit 450, Houston, TX 77030; **Phone:** 713-792-3626; **Board Cert:** Internal Medicine 1973; Medical Oncology 1973; **Med School:** NYU Sch Med 1968; **Resid:** Internal Medicine, Bellevue Hosp Ctr-NYU 1970; **Fellow:** Medical Oncology, Baltimore Cancer Rsch Ctr 1972; **Fac Appt:** Prof Med, Univ Tex, Houston

Bergsagel, Peter Leif MD [Onc] - **Spec Exp:** Multiple Myeloma; Hematologic Malignancies; **Hospital:** Mayo Clinic - Scottsdale; **Address:** 13400 E Shea Blvd Fl 3, Scottsdale, AZ 85259; **Phone:** 480-301-8335; **Board Cert:** Internal Medicine 1987; Medical Oncology 1989; **Med School:** Univ Toronto 1984; **Resid:** Internal Medicine, Stanford Univ Med Ctr 1986; Internal Medicine, Sunnybrook Med Ctr 1987; **Fellow:** Medical Oncology, NIH Natl Cancer Inst 1990; **Fac Appt:** Prof Med, Mayo Med Sch

Bruera, Eduardo MD [Onc] - **Spec Exp:** Palliative Care; **Hospital:** UT MD Anderson Cancer Ctr; **Address:** 1515 Holcombe Blvd, Unit 1414, Houston, TX 77030; **Phone:** 713-792-6085; **Med School:** Argentina 1979; **Resid:** Internal Medicine, Hospital Privado; **Fellow:** Medical Oncology, Cross Cancer Inst; **Fac Appt:** Prof Med, Univ Tex, Houston

Buzdar, Aman U MD [Onc] - **Spec Exp:** Breast Cancer; **Hospital:** UT MD Anderson Cancer Ctr; **Address:** UT MD Anderson Canc Ctr, 1515 Holcome Blvd, Unit 1354, Houston, TX 77030; **Phone:** 713-792-2817; **Board Cert:** Internal Medicine 1975; Medical Oncology 1979; **Med School:** Pakistan 1967; **Resid:** Internal Medicine, Norwalk Hosp 1973; Internal Medicine, Lakewood Hosp 1971; **Fellow:** Hematology, Norwalk Hosp 1974; Oncology, MD Anderson Cancer Ctr 1975; **Fac Appt:** Prof Med, Univ Tex, Houston

Camoriano, John MD [Onc] - **Spec Exp:** Lymphoma; Breast Cancer; Bone Marrow Transplant; Castleman's Disease; **Hospital:** Mayo Clinic - Scottsdale; **Address:** Mayo Clinic - Scottsdale, 13400 E Shea Blvd Fl 3, Scottsdale, AZ 85259; **Phone:** 480-301-8335; **Board Cert:** Internal Medicine 1985; Hematology 1988; Medical Oncology 1989; **Med School:** Univ Nebr Coll Med 1982; **Resid:** Internal Medicine, Univ OK 1985; **Fellow:** Hematology & Oncology, Mayo Grad Sch Med 1989; **Fac Appt:** Asst Prof Med, Mayo Med Sch

Chang, Jenny C N MD [Onc] - **Spec Exp:** Breast Cancer; Clinical Trials; **Hospital:** Methodist Hosp - Houston; **Address:** 6445 Main St Fl 21, Outpatient Ctr, Houston, TX 77030; **Phone:** 713-441-9948; **Board Cert:** Internal Medicine 2004; **Med School:** England, UK 1989; **Resid:** Internal Medicine 1993; **Fellow:** Medical Oncology, Royal Marsden Hosp 1997; **Fac Appt:** Assoc Prof Med, Baylor Coll Med

Fay, Joseph W MD [Onc] - **Spec Exp:** Bone Marrow Transplant; Melanoma; Leukemia & Lymphoma; **Hospital:** Baylor Univ Medical Ctr-Dallas; **Address:** 3410 Worth St, Ste 300, Sammons Cancer Ctr, Dallas, TX 75246; **Phone:** 214-370-1500; **Board Cert:** Internal Medicine 1975; Medical Oncology 1977; Hematology 1978; **Med School:** Ohio State Univ 1972; **Resid:** Internal Medicine, Duke Med Ctr 1974; Oncology, Natl Cancer Institute 1976; **Fellow:** Hematology, Duke Med Ctr 1977; **Fac Appt:** Clin Prof Med, Univ Tex SW, Dallas

Fitch, Tom R MD [Onc] - **Spec Exp:** Breast Cancer; Sarcoma; Cancer Prevention; Palliative Care; **Hospital:** Mayo Clinic - Scottsdale; **Address:** Mayo Clinic - Scottsdale, 13400 E Shea Blvd Fl 3, Scottsdale, AZ 85259; **Phone:** 480-301-8335; **Board Cert:** Internal Medicine 1985; Medical Oncology 1987; Hematology 1988; **Med School:** Univ Kansas 1982; **Resid:** Internal Medicine, Univ Michigan Med Ctr 1985; **Fellow:** Hematology & Oncology, Mayo Clinic 1988; **Fac Appt:** Asst Prof Med, Mayo Med Sch

Fossella, Frank V MD [Onc] - **Spec Exp:** Lung Cancer; **Hospital:** UT MD Anderson Cancer Ctr; **Address:** Dept Thoracic Head/Neck Med Oncol, 1400 Holcombe Blvd, Unit 432, Houston, TX 77030; **Phone:** 713-792-6363; **Board Cert:** Internal Medicine 1985; Medical Oncology 1987; **Med School:** Baylor Coll Med 1982; **Resid:** Internal Medicine, Baylor Coll Med 1985; **Fellow:** Medical Oncology, Baylor Coll Med 1987; **Fac Appt:** Prof Med, Univ Tex, Houston

Glisson, Bonnie S MD [Onc] - **Spec Exp:** Head & Neck Cancer; Lung Cancer; **Hospital:** UT MD Anderson Cancer Ctr; **Address:** UTMDACC- Unit 432, PO Box 301402, Houston, TX 77230-1402; **Phone:** 713-792-6363; **Board Cert:** Internal Medicine 1982; Medical Oncology 1985; **Med School:** Ohio State Univ 1979; **Resid:** Internal Medicine, Univ VA Med Ctr 1982; **Fellow:** Medical Oncology, Univ Fla Health Sci Ctr 1985; **Fac Appt:** Prof Med, Univ Tex, Houston

Haley, Barbara MD [Onc] - **Spec Exp:** Breast Cancer; **Hospital:** UT Southwestern Med Ctr at Dallas; **Address:** 5323 Harry Hines Blvd, Suite-NB2102, Dallas, TX 75390-8852; **Phone:** 214-648-4180; **Board Cert:** Internal Medicine 1979; Hematology 1984; **Med School:** Univ Tex SW, Dallas 1976; **Resid:** Internal Medicine, Parkland Meml Hosp 1979; **Fellow:** Hematology & Oncology, Parkland Meml Hosp 1981; **Fac Appt:** Prof Med, Univ Tex SW, Dallas

Hong, Waun Ki MD [Onc] - **Spec Exp:** Lung Cancer; Head & Neck Cancer; Thoracic Cancers; **Hospital:** UT MD Anderson Cancer Ctr; **Address:** Dept Thoracic Head/Neck, 1400 Holcombe Blvd, Unit 421, Houston, TX 77030; **Phone:** 713-792-6363; **Board Cert:** Internal Medicine 1976; Medical Oncology 1979; **Med School:** South Korea 1967; **Resid:** Internal Medicine, Boston VA Hosp 1973; **Fellow:** Medical Oncology, Meml Sloan-Kettering Cancer Ctr 1975; **Fac Appt:** Prof Med, Univ Tex, Houston

Hortobagyi, Gabriel N MD [Onc] - **Spec Exp:** Breast Cancer-Male; Clinical Trials; Gene Therapy; **Hospital:** UT MD Anderson Cancer Ctr; **Address:** 1515 Holcombe Blvd, ACB Bldg - Fl 5th, MS 1354, Dept Breast Oncology, PO Box 301429, Unit 1354, Houston, TX 77030-1439; **Phone:** 713-792-2817; **Board Cert:** Internal Medicine 1975; Medical Oncology 1977; **Med School:** Colombia 1970; **Resid:** Internal Medicine, St Lukes Hosp 1974; **Fellow:** Medical Oncology, MD Anderson Cancer Ctr 1976; **Fac Appt:** Prof Med, Univ Tex, Houston

Medical Oncology

Hutchins, Laura F MD [Onc] - **Spec Exp:** Breast Cancer; Melanoma; **Hospital:** UAMS Med Ctr; **Address:** Univ Arkansas Med Scis, Dept Hem/Onc, 4301 W Markham St, Slot 508, Little Rock, AR 72205; **Phone:** 501-686-8511; **Board Cert:** Internal Medicine 1980; Hematology 1984; Medical Oncology 1987; **Med School:** Univ Ark 1977; **Resid:** Internal Medicine, Univ Ark Affil Hosp 1980; **Fellow:** Hematology & Oncology, Univ Arkansas 1983; **Fac Appt:** Prof Med, Univ Ark

Hwu, Patrick MD [Onc] - **Spec Exp:** Melanoma; Immunotherapy; Clinical Trials; **Hospital:** UT MD Anderson Cancer Ctr; **Address:** UT MD Anderson Cancer Center, Melanoma & Skin Center, 1515 Holcombe Blvd, Unit 347, Houston, TX 77030; **Phone:** 713-792-6800; **Board Cert:** Medical Oncology 2008; **Med School:** Med Coll PA 1987; **Resid:** Internal Medicine, Johns Hopkins Hosp 1989; **Fellow:** Medical Oncology, Natl Cancer Inst 1993

Johnson, David H MD [Onc] - **Spec Exp:** Lung Cancer; Drug Discovery & Development; **Hospital:** UT Southwestern Med Ctr at Dallas; **Address:** UT Southwestern Med Ctr, 5323 Harry Hines Blvd, Dallas, TX 75390-9030; **Phone:** 214-648-3486; **Board Cert:** Internal Medicine 1979; Medical Oncology 2008; **Med School:** Med Coll GA 1976; **Resid:** Internal Medicine, Univ South Alabama Med Ctr 1979; Internal Medicine, Med Coll Georgia Hosp 1980; **Fellow:** Medical Oncology, Vanderbilt Univ Med Ctr 1983; **Fac Appt:** Prof Med, Univ Tex SW, Dallas

Jonasch, Eric MD [Onc] - **Spec Exp:** Kidney Cancer; Testicular Cancer; Bladder Cancer; Genitourinary Cancer; **Hospital:** UT MD Anderson Cancer Ctr; **Address:** Dept of GU Med/Onc, 1155 Herman P Pressler, Ste 1374, Houston, TX 77030; **Phone:** 713-792-2830; **Board Cert:** Internal Medicine 2005; Hematology 2009; Medical Oncology 2010; **Med School:** Canada 1992; **Resid:** Internal Medicine, Royal Victoria Hosp 1995; **Fellow:** Hematology & Oncology, New England Med Ctr 1997; Research, Beth Israel Deaconess Med Ctr 1999; **Fac Appt:** Assoc Prof Med, Univ Tex, Houston

Karp, Daniel D MD [Onc] - **Spec Exp:** Lung Cancer; **Hospital:** UT MD Anderson Cancer Ctr; **Address:** UTMDACC- Unit 432, PO Box 301402, Houston, TX 77230-1402; **Phone:** 713-792-6363; **Board Cert:** Internal Medicine 1976; Hematology 1980; Medical Oncology 1981; **Med School:** Duke Univ 1973; **Resid:** Internal Medicine, Dartmouth-Hitchcock Med Ctr 1976; **Fellow:** Hematology, Dartmouth-Hitchcock Med Ctr 1978; Medical Oncology, Dana Farber Cancer Inst 1979; **Fac Appt:** Prof Med, Univ Tex, Houston

Kies, Merrill S MD [Onc] - **Spec Exp:** Head & Neck Cancer; Lung Cancer; **Hospital:** UT MD Anderson Cancer Ctr; **Address:** Div Cancer Med, Thoracic/Head & Neck Med Oncology, 1515 Holcombe Blvd, Unit 421, Houston, TX 77030; **Phone:** 713-792-7770; **Board Cert:** Internal Medicine 1976; Medical Oncology 1979; **Med School:** Loyola Univ-Stritch Sch Med 1973; **Resid:** Internal Medicine, Walter Reed AMC 1976; **Fellow:** Medical Oncology, Brooke AMC 1978; **Fac Appt:** Prof Med, Univ Tex, Houston

Kwak, Larry W MD/PhD [Onc] - **Spec Exp:** Lymphoma; Multiple Myeloma; Vaccine Therapy; Immunotherapy; **Hospital:** UT MD Anderson Cancer Ctr; **Address:** MD Anderson Cancer Ctr, Dept Lymphoma/Myeloma, 1515 Holcombe Blvd, Unit 429, Houston, TX 77030; **Phone:** 713-792-2860; **Board Cert:** Internal Medicine 1987; Medical Oncology 1989; **Med School:** Northwestern Univ 1982; **Resid:** Internal Medicine, Stanford Univ Hosp 1987; **Fellow:** Oncology, Stanford Univ Hosp 1989

Lippman, Scott M MD [Onc] - **Spec Exp:** Cancer Prevention; Lung Cancer; Head & Neck Cancer; **Hospital:** UT MD Anderson Cancer Ctr; **Address:** UT MD Anderson Cancer Ctr, 1515 Holcombe Blvd, Unit 432, Houston, TX 77030; **Phone:** 713-745-5439; **Board Cert:** Internal Medicine 1987; Hematology 1988; Medical Oncology 1989; **Med School:** Johns Hopkins Univ 1981; **Resid:** Internal Medicine, Harbor-UCLA Med Ctr 1983; **Fellow:** Hematology, Stanford Univ Med Ctr 1985; Hematology & Oncology, Univ Ariz Hlth Scis Ctr 1987; **Fac Appt:** Prof Med, Univ Tex, Houston

Livingston, Robert B MD [Onc] - **Spec Exp:** Bone Marrow Transplant; Breast Cancer; Lung Cancer; **Hospital:** Univ Med Ctr - Tucson; **Address:** Arizona Cancer Ctr, 3838 N Campbell Ave, Tucson, AZ 85719; **Phone:** 520-694-2873; **Board Cert:** Internal Medicine 1972; Medical Oncology 1973; **Med School:** Univ Okla Coll Med 1965; **Resid:** Internal Medicine, Univ Oklahoma Med Ctr 1971; **Fellow:** Medical Oncology, Univ Texas Cancer Ctr 1973; **Fac Appt:** Prof Med, Univ Wash

Logothetis, Christopher J MD [Onc] - **Spec Exp:** Prostate Cancer; Bladder Cancer; **Hospital:** UT MD Anderson Cancer Ctr; **Address:** UT MD Anderson Cancer Ctr, Dept GU Onc, Unit 1274, Box 301439, Houston, TX 77230; **Phone:** 713-563-7210; **Board Cert:** Internal Medicine 1978; Medical Oncology 1981; **Med School:** Greece 1974; **Resid:** Internal Medicine, Univ Texas 1979; **Fellow:** Hematology & Oncology, Univ Tex-MD Anderson Cancer Ctr 1981; **Fac Appt:** Prof Med, Univ Tex, Houston

Makhoul, Issam MD [Onc] - **Spec Exp:** Gastrointestinal Cancer; Breast Cancer; Colon Cancer; **Hospital:** UAMS Med Ctr; **Address:** 4301 W Markham St, Slot# 721-5, Little Rock, AR 72205; **Phone:** 501-686-8530; **Board Cert:** Medical Oncology 2002; Hematology 2003; **Med School:** Syria 1980; **Resid:** Internal Medicine, Genl Hosp 1984; Internal Medicine, Penn State Affil Hosp 1999; **Fellow:** Hematology & Oncology, Hershey Med Ctr 2002; **Fac Appt:** Asst Prof Med, Univ Ark

Miller, Thomas P MD [Onc] - **Spec Exp:** Lymphoma; **Hospital:** Univ Med Ctr - Tucson; **Address:** Arizona Cancer Ctr, 3838 N Campbell Ave, Tucson, AZ 85719; **Phone:** 520-694-2873; **Board Cert:** Internal Medicine 1977; Medical Oncology 1981; **Med School:** Univ IL Coll Med 1972; **Resid:** Internal Medicine, Univ Illinois Hosps 1977; **Fellow:** Hematology & Oncology, Univ Med Ctr 1980; **Fac Appt:** Prof Med, Univ Ariz Coll Med

Northfelt, Donald W MD [Onc] - **Spec Exp:** Breast Cancer; Colon & Rectal Cancer; Lung Cancer; **Hospital:** Mayo Clinic - Scottsdale; **Address:** Mayo Clinic Scottsdale, 13400 E Shea Blvd Fl 3, Scottsdale, AZ 85259; **Phone:** 480-301-8335; **Board Cert:** Internal Medicine 1988; Medical Oncology 2001; **Med School:** Univ Minn 1985; **Resid:** Internal Medicine, UCLA Med Ctr 1988; **Fellow:** Hematology & Oncology, UCSF Med Ctr 1991; **Fac Appt:** Assoc Prof Med, Mayo Med Sch

O'Brien, Susan M MD [Onc] - **Spec Exp:** Leukemia; Lymphoma; **Hospital:** UT MD Anderson Cancer Ctr; **Address:** Univ Texas MD Anderson Cancer Ctr, Dept Leukemia, Unit 428, PO Box 301402, Houston, TX 77230; **Phone:** 713-792-7305; **Board Cert:** Internal Medicine 1983; Medical Oncology 1987; **Med School:** UMDNJ-NJ Med Sch, Newark 1980; **Resid:** Internal Medicine, UMDNJ Med Ctr 1983; **Fellow:** Medical Oncology, Univ TX MD Anderson Med Ctr 1987; **Fac Appt:** Prof Med, Univ Tex, Houston

O'Shaughnessy, Joyce A MD [Onc] - **Spec Exp:** Breast Cancer; **Hospital:** Baylor Univ Medical Ctr-Dallas; **Address:** Texas Oncology, 3410 Worth St, Dallas, TX 75246; **Phone:** 214-370-1000; **Board Cert:** Internal Medicine 1985; Medical Oncology 1987; **Med School:** Yale Univ 1982; **Resid:** Internal Medicine, Mass Genl Hosp 1985; **Fellow:** Medical Oncology, National Cancer Inst 1988

Orlowski, Robert Z MD/PhD [Onc] - **Spec Exp:** Multiple Myeloma; Lymphoma, Non-Hodgkin's; Leukemia; Clinical Trials; **Hospital:** UT MD Anderson Cancer Ctr; **Address:** MD Anderson Cancer Ctr, Lymphoma & Myeloma Clinic, 1515 Holcombe Blvd, Box 429, Houston, TX 77030; **Phone:** 713-792-3510; **Med School:** Yale Univ 1991; **Resid:** Internal Medicine, Barnes Hosp/Wash Univ 1994; **Fellow:** Hematology & Oncology, Johns Hopkins Hosp 1998; **Fac Appt:** Assoc Prof Med, Univ Tex, Houston

Medical Oncology

Osborne, C Kent MD [Onc] - **Spec Exp:** Breast Cancer; **Hospital:** Methodist Hosp - Houston; **Address:** 1 Baylor Plaza, MS BCM600, Houston, TX 77030; **Phone:** 713-798-1641; **Board Cert:** Internal Medicine 1975; Medical Oncology 1977; **Med School:** Univ MO-Columbia Sch Med 1972; **Resid:** Internal Medicine, Johns Hopkins Hosp 1974; **Fellow:** Medical Oncology, Natl Cancer Inst 1977; **Fac Appt:** Prof Med, Baylor Coll Med

Papadopoulos, Nicholas E MD [Onc] - **Spec Exp:** Melanoma; **Hospital:** UT MD Anderson Cancer Ctr; **Address:** 1515 Holcombe Blvd, Unit 430, Houston, TX 77030; **Phone:** 713-792-2921; **Med School:** Greece 1966; **Resid:** Internal Medicine, Baylor Coll Med 1976; **Fellow:** Medical Oncology, MD Anderson Cancer Ctr 1978; **Fac Appt:** Assoc Prof Med, Univ Tex, Houston

Patel, Shreyaskumar MD [Onc] - **Spec Exp:** Sarcoma; **Hospital:** UT MD Anderson Cancer Ctr; **Address:** 1515 Holcombe Blvd, Box 450, Houston, TX 77030; **Phone:** 713-792-3626; **Board Cert:** Internal Medicine 1987; Medical Oncology 2000; **Med School:** India 1983; **Resid:** Internal Medicine, Wayne State Univ 1987; **Fellow:** Medical Oncology, Mayo Clinic 1990

Patt, Yehuda Z MD [Onc] - **Spec Exp:** Liver Cancer; Biliary Cancer; Colon & Rectal Cancer; Gastrointestinal Cancer; **Hospital:** Univ Hosp - New Mexico; **Address:** Univ New Mexico CRTC, Div Hem/Onc, 1201 Camino de Salud NE, Albuquerque, NM 87131; **Phone:** 505-272-4946; **Board Cert:** Internal Medicine 1982; Medical Oncology 1987; **Med School:** Israel 1967; **Resid:** Internal Medicine, Tel Aviv-Sheba Med Ctr 1974; **Fellow:** Medical Oncology, UT MD Anderson Cancer Ctr 1977; **Fac Appt:** Prof Med, Univ New Mexico

Pisters, Katherine M W MD [Onc] - **Spec Exp:** Lung Cancer; **Hospital:** UT MD Anderson Cancer Ctr; **Address:** UT MD Anderson Cancer Ctr, PO Box 301402, Unit 432, Houston, TX 77230-1402; **Phone:** 713-792-6363; **Board Cert:** Internal Medicine 1988; Medical Oncology 2002; **Med School:** Univ Western Ontario 1985; **Resid:** Internal Medicine, N Shore Univ Hosp 1988; **Fellow:** Medical Oncology, Meml Sloan Kettering Cancer Ctr 1991; **Fac Appt:** Prof Med, Univ Tex, Houston

Romaguera, Jorge MD [Onc] - **Spec Exp:** Lymphoma; **Hospital:** UT MD Anderson Cancer Ctr; **Address:** 1515 Holcombe Blvd, Box 429, Lymphoma & Myeloma Clinic, Houston, TX 77030; **Phone:** 713-792-3510; **Board Cert:** Internal Medicine 1988; Medical Oncology 1989; **Med School:** Univ Puerto Rico 1982; **Resid:** Internal Medicine, Univ Hosp 1985; **Fellow:** Hematology & Oncology, Univ Hosp 1987

Ross, Helen J MD [Onc] - **Spec Exp:** Lung Cancer; Mesothelioma; Esophageal Cancer; **Hospital:** Mayo Clinic - Scottsdale; **Address:** Mayo Clinic, 13400 E Shea Blvd, Scottsdale, AZ 85259; **Phone:** 480-301-8335; **Board Cert:** Internal Medicine 1987; Medical Oncology 1989; **Med School:** UCLA 1984; **Resid:** Internal Medicine, Cedars Sinai Med Ctr 1987; **Fellow:** Medical Oncology, UCLA Med Ctr 1989; **Fac Appt:** Assoc Prof Med, Mayo Med Sch

Saiki, John H MD [Onc] - **Hospital:** Univ Hosp - New Mexico; **Address:** University of New Mexico Cancer Center, 1201 Camino de Salud NE, Albuquerque, NM 87106; **Phone:** 505-925-0423; **Board Cert:** Internal Medicine 1970; Medical Oncology 1973; **Med School:** McGill Univ 1961; **Resid:** Internal Medicine, Univ New Mexico 1968; Hematology, Univ New Mexico 1969; **Fellow:** Medical Oncology, MD Anderson Hosp 1970; **Fac Appt:** Prof Emeritus Med, Univ New Mexico

Schiller, Joan H MD [Onc] - **Spec Exp:** Lung Cancer; **Hospital:** UT Southwestern Med Ctr at Dallas; **Address:** Univ Texas Southwestern, 5323 Harry Hines Blvd, Dallas, TX 75390-8852; **Phone:** 214-648-4180; **Board Cert:** Internal Medicine 1983; Medical Oncology 1987; **Med School:** Univ IL Coll Med 1980; **Resid:** Internal Medicine, Northwestern Meml Hosp 1983; **Fellow:** Medical Oncology, Univ Wisconsin Hosp 1985; **Fac Appt:** Prof Med, Univ Wisc

Stopeck, Alison T MD [Onc] - **Spec Exp:** Breast Cancer; Breast Cancer Risk Assessment; Hemophilia; **Hospital:** Univ Med Ctr - Tucson; **Address:** Arizona Cancer Ctr, 1515 N Campbell Ave, PO Box 245024, Tucson, AZ 85724; **Phone:** 520-626-2816; **Board Cert:** Internal Medicine 1988; Medical Oncology 2002; Hematology 2002; **Med School:** Columbia P&S 1985; **Resid:** Internal Medicine, Columbia-Presby Med Ctr 1988; **Fellow:** Hematology & Oncology, New York Hosp 1991; **Fac Appt:** Assoc Prof Med, Univ Ariz Coll Med

Taetle, Raymond MD [Onc] - **Hospital:** St. Joseph's Hosp - Tucson; **Address:** Arizona Oncology Assoc, 6565 Carondolet St, Ste 155, Tucson, AZ 85710; **Phone:** 520-886-0206; **Board Cert:** Internal Medicine 1976; Hematology 1978; Medical Oncology 1979; **Med School:** Northwestern Univ 1973; **Resid:** Internal Medicine, Univ California Med Ctr 1976; **Fellow:** Hematology & Oncology, Univ California Med Ctr 1978; **Fac Appt:** Clin Prof Med, Univ Ariz Coll Med

Valero, Vicente MD [Onc] - **Spec Exp:** Breast Cancer; **Hospital:** UT MD Anderson Cancer Ctr; **Address:** Univ Texas MD Anderson Cancer Ctr, 1515 Holcombe Blvd, Unit 1354, Houston, TX 77030; **Phone:** 713-792-2817; **Board Cert:** Internal Medicine 1985; Medical Oncology 1987; Hematology 1988; **Med School:** Mexico 1980; **Resid:** Internal Medicine, Univ Cincinnati Med Ctr 1985; Hematology & Oncology, Univ Cincinnati Med Ctr 1987; **Fellow:** Hematology & Oncology, Univ Texas Med Br 1988; **Fac Appt:** Prof Med, Univ Tex, Houston

Varadhachary, Gauri MD [Onc] - **Spec Exp:** Unknown Primary Cancer; Pancreatic Cancer; **Hospital:** UT MD Anderson Cancer Ctr; **Address:** 1515 Holcombe Blvd, Box 426, Houston, TX 77030; **Phone:** 713-792-2828; **Board Cert:** Internal Medicine 2004; Medical Oncology 2008; **Med School:** India 1991; **Resid:** Internal Medicine, Greater Baltimore Med Ctr 1995; **Fellow:** Hematology & Oncology, Baylor Univ Affil Hosp 1998

Von Burton, Gary MD [Onc] - **Spec Exp:** Breast Cancer; Sarcoma; Brain Tumors; **Hospital:** Louisiana State Univ Hosp; **Address:** LSUHSC-Shreveport, Feist-Weiller Cancer Ctr, 1501 Kings Hwy, PO Box 33932, Shreveport, LA 71130; **Phone:** 318-675-5972; **Board Cert:** Internal Medicine 1981; Medical Oncology 1983; **Med School:** Univ Utah 1978; **Resid:** Internal Medicine, Duke Univ Med Ctr 1981; **Fellow:** Hematology & Oncology, Duke Univ Med Ctr 1983; **Fac Appt:** Prof Med, Louisiana State U, Shrevport

Von Hoff, Daniel D MD [Onc] - **Spec Exp:** Pancreatic Cancer; Breast Cancer; Drug Discovery; **Hospital:** Scottsdale Hlthcare - Shea; **Address:** Translational Genomics Rsch Inst, 445 N 5th St, Ste 600, Phoenix, AZ 85004; **Phone:** 602-343-8492; **Board Cert:** Internal Medicine 1976; Medical Oncology 1979; **Med School:** Columbia P&S 1973; **Resid:** Internal Medicine, UCSF Med Ctr 1975; **Fac Appt:** Prof Med, Univ Ariz Coll Med

Willson, James KV MD [Onc] - **Spec Exp:** Gastrointestinal Cancer; Colon Cancer; Pancreatic Cancer; **Hospital:** UT Southwestern Med Ctr at Dallas; **Address:** 5323 Harry Hines Blvd, Dallas, TX 75390-8590; **Phone:** 214-645-4673; **Board Cert:** Internal Medicine 1980; Medical Oncology 1981; **Med School:** Univ Alabama 1976; **Resid:** Internal Medicine, Johns Hopkins Hosp 1978; **Fellow:** Medical Oncology, Natl Cancer Inst-NIH 1980; **Fac Appt:** Prof Med, Univ Tex SW, Dallas

Wolff, Robert A MD [Onc] - **Spec Exp:** Gastrointestinal Cancer; Pancreatic Cancer; Colon & Rectal Cancer; Clinical Trials; **Hospital:** UT MD Anderson Cancer Ctr; **Address:** 1515 Holcombe Blvd, Unit 421, Houston, TX 77030; **Phone:** 713-745-5476; **Board Cert:** Internal Medicine 1989; Medical Oncology 2008; **Med School:** Albany Med Coll 1986; **Resid:** Internal Medicine, Duke Univ Med Ctr 1989; **Fellow:** Hematology & Oncology, Duke Univ Med Ctr 1992

Medical Oncology

West Coast and Pacific

Aboulafia, David M MD [Onc] - **Spec Exp:** AIDS Related Cancers; Leukemia; Lymphoma; Multiple Myeloma; **Hospital:** Virginia Mason Med Ctr; **Address:** Virginia Mason Med Ctr, Sect of Hematology/Oncology, 1100 Ninth Ave, Seattle, WA 98101; **Phone:** 206-223-6193; **Board Cert:** Internal Medicine 1986; Medical Oncology 1989; Hematology 2003; **Med School:** Univ Mich Med Sch 1983; **Resid:** Internal Medicine, UCLA Med Ctr 1986; **Fellow:** Hematology & Oncology, UCLA Med Ctr 1989; **Fac Appt:** Clin Prof Med, Univ Wash

Abrams, Donald I MD [Onc] - **Spec Exp:** AIDS Related Cancers; Complementary Medicine; **Hospital:** San Francisco Genl Hosp; **Address:** Positive Hlth Program-SF Genl Hosp, 995 Potrero Ave, Bldg 80, Ward 84, San Francisco, CA 94110; **Phone:** 415-476-4082 x444; **Board Cert:** Internal Medicine 1980; Medical Oncology 1983; **Med School:** Stanford Univ 1977; **Resid:** Internal Medicine, Kaiser Fdn Hosp 1980; **Fellow:** Medical Oncology, UCSF Cancer Rsch 1982; **Fac Appt:** Clin Prof Med, UCSF

Advani, Ranjana H MD [Onc] - **Spec Exp:** Lymphoma; Hematologic Malignancies; Clinical Trials; **Hospital:** Stanford Univ Hosp & Clinics; **Address:** Lymphoma Clinic, 875 Blake Wilbur Drive, Clinic C, Stanford, CA 94305; **Phone:** 650-498-6000; **Board Cert:** Internal Medicine 2001; Medical Oncology 2009; **Med School:** India 1982; **Resid:** Internal Medicine, Santa Clara Vly Med Ctr 1987; Internal Medicine, Stanford Univ 1991; **Fellow:** Hematology, Stanford Univ Med Ctr 1990; **Fac Appt:** Asst Prof Med, Stanford Univ

Appelbaum, Frederick R MD [Onc] - **Spec Exp:** Bone Marrow Transplant; Leukemia-Myeloid; Graft vs Host Disease; **Hospital:** Univ Wash Med Ctr; **Address:** 1100 Fairview Ave N, rm D5-310, PO Box 19024, Seattle, WA 98109; **Phone:** 206-288-1024; **Board Cert:** Internal Medicine 1975; Medical Oncology 1977; **Med School:** Tufts Univ 1972; **Resid:** Internal Medicine, Univ Michigan Med Ctr 1974; **Fellow:** Medical Oncology, Natl Cancer Inst 1976; **Fac Appt:** Prof Med, Univ Wash

Back, Anthony MD [Onc] - **Spec Exp:** Palliative Care; Gastrointestinal Cancer; **Hospital:** Univ Wash Med Ctr; **Address:** Seattle Cancer Care Alliance, 825 Eastlake Ave E, Box G4100, Seattle, WA 98109; **Phone:** 206-288-6478; **Board Cert:** Internal Medicine 1987; Medical Oncology 2001; Hospice & Palliative Medicine 2008; **Med School:** Harvard Med Sch 1984; **Resid:** Internal Medicine, Univ Washington Med Ctr 1988; **Fellow:** Oncology, Univ Washington Med Ctr 1991; **Fac Appt:** Prof Med, Univ Wash

Ball, Edward D MD [Onc] - **Spec Exp:** Bone Marrow & Stem Cell Transplant; Leukemia & Lymphoma; Multiple Myeloma; Immunotherapy; **Hospital:** UCSD Med Ctr; **Address:** 3855 Health Sciences Dr, #0960, La Jolla, CA 92093-0960; **Phone:** 858-822-6600; **Board Cert:** Internal Medicine 1979; Medical Oncology 1983; Hematology 2011; **Med School:** Case West Res Univ 1976; **Resid:** Internal Medicine, Hartford Hosp 1979; **Fellow:** Hematology & Oncology, Univ Hosps Cleveland 1981; Hematology & Oncology, Dartmouth-Hitchcock Hosp 1982; **Fac Appt:** Prof Med, UCSD

Beer, Tomasz M MD [Onc] - **Spec Exp:** Prostate Cancer; **Hospital:** OR Hlth & Sci Univ, VA Medical Center - Portland; **Address:** 3303 SW Bond Ave, CH14R, Portland, OR 97239; **Phone:** 503-494-6594; **Board Cert:** Medical Oncology 2000; **Med School:** Johns Hopkins Univ 1991; **Resid:** Internal Medicine, Oreg Hlth Scis Univ 1994; Internal Medicine, Oreg Hlth Scis Univ 1996; **Fellow:** Hematology & Oncology, Oreg Hlth Scis Univ 1999; **Fac Appt:** Prof Med, Oregon Hlth & Sci Univ

Bensinger, William I MD [Onc] - **Spec Exp:** Multiple Myeloma; Stem Cell Transplant; **Hospital:** Univ Wash Med Ctr; **Address:** Fred Hutchinson Cancer Research Ctr, 1100 Fairview Ave N, MS DS-390, PO BOX 19024, Seattle, WA 98109-1024; **Phone:** 206-288-1024; **Board Cert:** Internal Medicine 1978; Medical Oncology 1979; **Med School:** Northwestern Univ 1973; **Resid:** Internal Medicine, Univ Wash Hosps 1978; **Fellow:** Medical Oncology, Univ Wash Hosps 1979; **Fac Appt:** Assoc Prof Med, Univ Wash

Berry, J Michael MD [Onc] - **Spec Exp:** Anal Cancer; HPV-Human Papilloma Virus; **Hospital:** UCSF - Mt Zion Med Ctr; **Address:** UCSF, Dysplasia Clinic, 1600 Divisadero St Fl 4th, Box 1705, San Francisco, CA 94143; **Phone:** 415-353-7100; **Board Cert:** Internal Medicine 1985; Medical Oncology 1989; **Med School:** Univ Miami Sch Med 1982; **Resid:** Internal Medicine, UCSF Med Ctr 1985; **Fellow:** Medical Oncology, Stanford Univ 1989; **Fac Appt:** Asst Clin Prof Med, UCSF

Carlson, Robert W MD [Onc] - **Spec Exp:** Breast Cancer; **Hospital:** Stanford Univ Hosp & Clinics; **Address:** Stanford Comprehensive Cancer Ctr, 875 Blake Wilbur Drive, rm CC-2236, Stanford, CA 94305; **Phone:** 650-498-6000; **Board Cert:** Internal Medicine 1981; Medical Oncology 1983; **Med School:** Stanford Univ 1978; **Resid:** Internal Medicine, Barnes Hosp 1980; Internal Medicine, Stanford Univ Hosp 1981; **Fellow:** Medical Oncology, Stanford Univ Hosp 1983; **Fac Appt:** Prof Med, Stanford Univ

Chang, Susan M MD [Onc] - **Spec Exp:** Brain Tumors; Spinal Cord Tumors; Pituitary Tumors; Acromegaly; **Hospital:** UCSF Med Ctr; **Address:** UCSF, Dept Neurological Surgery, 400 Parnassus Ave Fl 8 - rm A808, San Francisco, CA 94143; **Phone:** 415-353-2966; **Med School:** Univ British Columbia Fac Med 1985; **Resid:** Internal Medicine, Plains Hlth Ctr 1987; Internal Medicine, Toronto Genl Hosp 1989; **Fellow:** Medical Oncology, Princess Margaret Hosp 1991; Neuro-Oncology, UCSF Med Ctr 1995; **Fac Appt:** Prof Med, UCSF

Chap, Linnea MD [Onc] - **Spec Exp:** Breast Cancer; **Hospital:** St. John's Hlth Ctr, Santa Monica; **Address:** Beverly Hills Cancer Center, 8900 Wilshire Blvd Fl 2, Beverly Hills, CA 90211; **Phone:** 310-432-8900; **Board Cert:** Medical Oncology 2005; **Med School:** Univ Chicago-Pritzker Sch Med 1988; **Resid:** Internal Medicine, Northwestern Meml Hosp 1991; **Fellow:** Hematology & Oncology, UCLA Med Ctr 1992

Chew, Helen MD [Onc] - **Spec Exp:** Breast Cancer; **Hospital:** UC Davis Med Ctr; **Address:** UC Davis Cancer Ctr, 4501 X St Fl 3, Sacramento, CA 95817; **Phone:** 916-734-3700; **Board Cert:** Medical Oncology 2007; **Med School:** Univ Tex, San Antonio 1991; **Resid:** Internal Medicine, UT Hlth Sci Ctr 1994; **Fellow:** Medical Oncology, UT Hlth Sci Ctr 1997

Chlebowski, Rowan T MD/PhD [Onc] - **Spec Exp:** Breast Cancer; Women's Health; **Hospital:** LAC - Harbor - UCLA Med Ctr; **Address:** 1124 W Carson St J3 Bldg, Torrance, CA 90502; **Phone:** 310-222-2218; **Board Cert:** Internal Medicine 1980; Medical Oncology 1981; **Med School:** Case West Res Univ 1974; **Resid:** Internal Medicine, MetroHealth Med Ctr 1976; Medical Oncology, LAC-USC Med Ctr 1979; **Fac Appt:** Prof Med, UCLA

Chow, Warren A MD [Onc] - **Spec Exp:** Sarcoma-Soft Tissue; Sarcoma; Melanoma; **Hospital:** City of Hope Natl Med Ctr; **Address:** 1500 E Duarte Rd, Duarte, CA 91010; **Phone:** 626-256-4673 x63712; **Board Cert:** Internal Medicine 1989; Medical Oncology 2003; Hematology 2004; **Med School:** Ros Franklin Univ/Chicago Med Sch 1986; **Resid:** Internal Medicine, Cedars-Sinai Med Ctr 1990; **Fellow:** Hematology & Oncology, City of Hope Med Ctr 1992; Molecular Genetics, City of Hope Med Ctr 1994; **Fac Appt:** Assoc Prof Med

Crocenzi, Todd MD [Onc] - Spec Exp: Gastrointestinal Cancer; **Hospital:** Providence Portland Med Ctr; **Address:** Providence Cancer Ctr, 4805 NE Glisan St, Ste 6N40, Portland, OR 97213; **Phone:** 503-215-5696; **Board Cert:** Medical Oncology 2004; **Med School:** Jefferson Med Coll 1994; **Resid:** Internal Medicine, Univ MD Med Ctr 1997; **Fellow:** Hematology & Oncology, Dartmouth Hitchcock Med Ctr 2004; Immunology, Dartmouth Hitchcock Med Ctr 2005

Daud, Adil I MD [Onc] - Spec Exp: Melanoma; Skin Cancer; Drug Development; **Hospital:** UCSF Med Ctr; **Address:** 1600 Divisadero St Fl 4, Box 1706, San Francisco, CA 94115; **Phone:** 415-353-9900; **Board Cert:** Hematology 2000; Medical Oncology 2000; **Med School:** India 1987; **Resid:** Internal Medicine, Indiana Univ Affil Hosp; **Fellow:** Hematology & Oncology, Meml Sloan Kettering Cancer Ctr

Deeg, H Joachim MD [Onc] - Spec Exp: Myelodysplastic Syndromes; Bone Marrow Failure Disorders; Hematologic Malignancies; Graft vs Host Disease; **Hospital:** Univ Wash Med Ctr; **Address:** Fred Hutchinson Cancer Research Center, 1100 Fairview Avenue N, D1-100, Box 19024, Seattle, WA 98109-1024; **Phone:** 206-667-5985; **Board Cert:** Internal Medicine 1976; Medical Oncology 1979; **Med School:** Germany 1972; **Resid:** Internal Medicine, Gennessee Hosp 1976; **Fellow:** Medical Oncology, Univ Wash Med Ctr 1978; **Fac Appt:** Prof Med, Univ Wash

Disis, Mary Lenora MD [Onc] - Spec Exp: Breast Cancer; Ovarian Cancer; Clinical Trials; **Hospital:** Univ Wash Med Ctr; **Address:** Univ Washington, Tumor Vaccine Group, 815 Mercer St, Box 358050, Seattle, WA 98109; **Phone:** 206-543-8557; **Board Cert:** Internal Medicine 1989; Medical Oncology 2008; **Med School:** Univ Nebr Coll Med 1986; **Resid:** Internal Medicine, Univ Illinois Med Ctr 1990; **Fellow:** Medical Oncology, Fred Hutchinson Cancer Ctr 1993; **Fac Appt:** Assoc Prof Med, Univ Wash

Druker, Brian J MD [Onc] - Spec Exp: Leukemia; Leukemia-Chronic Myeloid; Hematologic Malignancies; **Hospital:** OR Hlth & Sci Univ; **Address:** OHSU Ctr Hematologic Malignancies, 3181 Sam Jackson Park Rd, Multnomah Pavilion, Ste 2502, MC L592, Portland, OR 97239-3098; **Phone:** 503-494-5058; **Board Cert:** Internal Medicine 1984; Medical Oncology 1987; **Med School:** UCSD 1981; **Resid:** Internal Medicine, Barnes Jewish Hosp 1984; **Fellow:** Medical Oncology, Dana-Farber Cancer Inst 1987; **Fac Appt:** Prof Med, Oregon Hlth & Sci Univ

Ellis, Georgiana K MD [Onc] - Spec Exp: Breast Cancer; Clinical Trials; **Hospital:** Univ Wash Med Ctr; **Address:** Seattle Cancer Care Alliance, 825 Eastlake Ave E, Box 358081, MS G3-630, Seattle, WA 98109-1023; **Phone:** 206-288-1000; **Board Cert:** Internal Medicine 1985; Medical Oncology 1987; **Med School:** Univ Wash 1982; **Resid:** Internal Medicine, Univ Washington Med Ctr 1985; **Fellow:** Medical Oncology, Univ Washington Med Ctr 1988; **Fac Appt:** Assoc Prof Med, Univ Wash

Estey, Elihu H MD [Onc] - Spec Exp: Leukemia; Leukemia-Myeloid; Clinical Trials; Myelodysplastic Syndromes; **Hospital:** Univ Wash Med Ctr; **Address:** Seattle Cancer Care Alliance, 825 Eastlake Ave E, UW Box 3587710, Seattle, WA 98109; **Phone:** 206-288-7176; **Board Cert:** Internal Medicine 1975; Medical Oncology 1981; **Med School:** Johns Hopkins Univ 1972; **Resid:** Internal Medicine, Bellevue Hosp Ctr 1975; **Fellow:** Medical Oncology, MD Anderson Cancer Ctr 1978

Figlin, Robert A MD [Onc] - Spec Exp: Urologic Cancer; Kidney Cancer; Immunotherapy; **Hospital:** Cedars-Sinai Med Ctr; **Address:** Cedars-Sinai Med Ctr, Division of Hematology & Oncology, 8700 Beverly Blvd, Ste AC-1085, Los Angeles, CA 90048; **Phone:** 310-423-1331; **Board Cert:** Internal Medicine 1979; Medical Oncology 1983; **Med School:** Med Coll PA Hahnemann 1976; **Resid:** Internal Medicine, Cedars Sinai Med Ctr 1980; **Fellow:** Hematology & Oncology, UCLA Ctr Hlth Sci 1982; **Fac Appt:** Prof Med, UCLA

Fisher Jr, George A MD/PhD [Onc] - **Spec Exp:** Gastrointestinal Cancer; Pancreatic Cancer; **Hospital:** Stanford Univ Hosp & Clinics; **Address:** Stanford Comp Cancer Ctr, GI Onc, 875 Blake Wilbur Drive, MC 5826, Stanford, CA 94305; **Phone:** 650-498-6000; **Board Cert:** Medical Oncology 1997; **Med School:** Stanford Univ 1987; **Resid:** Internal Medicine, Stanford Univ Med Ctr 1991; **Fellow:** Medical Oncology, Stanford Univ Med Ctr 1993; **Fac Appt:** Assoc Prof Med, Stanford Univ

Ford, James M MD [Onc] - **Spec Exp:** Gastrointestinal Cancer; Colon & Rectal Cancer; Cancer Genetics; **Hospital:** Stanford Univ Hosp & Clinics; **Address:** Stanford Comp Cancer Ctr, 875 Blake Wilbur Drive, Clinic A, Stanford, CA 94305; **Phone:** 650-723-7621; **Board Cert:** Medical Oncology 2005; **Med School:** Yale Univ 1989; **Resid:** Internal Medicine, Stanford Univ Med Ctr 1991; **Fellow:** Medical Oncology, Stanford Univ Med Ctr 1994; **Fac Appt:** Assoc Prof Med, Stanford Univ

Forscher, Charles A MD [Onc] - **Spec Exp:** Bone Tumors; Sarcoma-Soft Tissue; **Hospital:** Cedars-Sinai Med Ctr, UCLA Ronald Reagan Med Ctr; **Address:** Outpatient Cancer Ctr, Lower Level, 8700 Beverly Blvd, Ste AC1042D, Los Angeles, CA 90048; **Phone:** 310-423-8045; **Board Cert:** Internal Medicine 1981; Hematology 1986; Medical Oncology 1987; **Med School:** Albert Einstein Coll Med 1978; **Resid:** Internal Medicine, Montefiore Med Ctr 1981; **Fellow:** Hematology, Montefiore Med Ctr 1983; Neoplastic Diseases, Mt Sinai Med Ctr 1985; **Fac Appt:** Clin Prof Med, UCLA

Gandara, David R MD [Onc] - **Spec Exp:** Lung Cancer; **Hospital:** UC Davis Med Ctr; **Address:** UC Davis Cancer Ctr, 4501 X St Fl 3, Sacramento, CA 95817; **Phone:** 916-734-5959; **Board Cert:** Internal Medicine 1976; Medical Oncology 1979; **Med School:** Univ Tex Med Br, Galveston 1973; **Resid:** Internal Medicine, Madigan Med Ctr 1976; **Fellow:** Hematology & Oncology, Letterman AMC 1978; **Fac Appt:** Prof Med, UC Davis

Ganz, Patricia A MD [Onc] - **Spec Exp:** Breast Cancer; Cancer Survivors-Late Effects of Therapy; **Hospital:** UCLA Ronald Reagan Med Ctr; **Address:** UCLA, Cancer Prev/Control Rsch, A2-125 CHS, 650 Charles Young Drive S, Box 956900, Los Angeles, CA 90095-6900; **Phone:** 310-206-1404; **Board Cert:** Internal Medicine 1976; Medical Oncology 1979; **Med School:** UCLA 1973; **Resid:** Internal Medicine, UCLA Med Ctr 1976; **Fellow:** Hematology, UCLA Med Ctr 1978; **Fac Appt:** Prof Med, UCLA

Glaspy, John A MD [Onc] - **Spec Exp:** Breast Cancer; Melanoma; Lymphoma; Gastrointestinal Cancer; **Hospital:** UCLA Ronald Reagan Med Ctr, Santa Monica - UCLA Med Ctr & Ortho Hosp; **Address:** 100 UCLA Medical Plaza, Ste 550, Los Angeles, CA 90095; **Phone:** 310-794-4955; **Board Cert:** Internal Medicine 1982; Medical Oncology 1985; Hematology 1986; **Med School:** UCLA 1979; **Resid:** Internal Medicine, UCLA Med Ctr 1982; **Fellow:** Hematology & Oncology, UCLA Med Ctr 1984; **Fac Appt:** Prof Med, UCLA

Gold, Philip J MD [Onc] - **Spec Exp:** Gastrointestinal Cancer; **Hospital:** Swedish Med Ctr-First Hill-Seattle; **Address:** Swedish Cancer Inst, 1221 Madison St Fl 2 - Ste 200, Seattle, WA 98104; **Phone:** 206-386-2121; **Board Cert:** Internal Medicine 2005; Medical Oncology 2007; **Med School:** Univ Miami Sch Med 1991; **Resid:** Internal Medicine, Univ of Washington Med Ctr 1994; **Fellow:** Medical Oncology, Fred Hutchinson Cancer Rsch Ctr 1997

Gralow, Julie MD [Onc] - **Spec Exp:** Breast Cancer; **Hospital:** Univ Wash Med Ctr; **Address:** Seattle Cancer Care Alliance, 825 Eastlake Ave E, MS G3-630, Seattle, WA 98109; **Phone:** 206-288-7222; **Board Cert:** Medical Oncology 2005; **Med School:** USC Sch Med 1988; **Resid:** Internal Medicine, Brigham & Women's Hosp 1991; **Fellow:** Oncology, Univ Wash Med Ctr 1994; **Fac Appt:** Assoc Prof Med, Univ Wash

Medical Oncology

Higano, Celestia MD [Onc] - **Spec Exp:** Genitourinary Cancer; Prostate Cancer; Testicular Cancer; **Hospital:** Univ Wash Med Ctr; **Address:** Seattle Cancer Care Alliance, 825 Eastlake Ave E, PO Box 19024, Seattle, WA 98109; **Phone:** 206-288-1152; **Board Cert:** Internal Medicine 1982; Medical Oncology 1985; **Med School:** Univ Mass Sch Med 1979; **Resid:** Internal Medicine, Mayo Clin 1982; **Fellow:** Oncology, Univ Washington Med Ctr 1985; **Fac Appt:** Prof Med, Univ Wash

Jacobs, Charlotte D MD [Onc] - **Spec Exp:** Sarcoma; Unknown Primary Cancer; **Hospital:** Stanford Univ Hosp & Clinics; **Address:** 875 Blake Wilbur Drive, Clinic B, Stanford, CA 94305; **Phone:** 650-498-6000; **Board Cert:** Internal Medicine 1975; Medical Oncology 1977; **Med School:** Washington Univ, St Louis 1972; **Resid:** Internal Medicine, Barnes Hosp 1974; Internal Medicine, UCSF Med Ctr 1975; **Fellow:** Medical Oncology, Stanford Univ 1977; **Fac Appt:** Prof Med, Stanford Univ

Kaplan, Lawrence D MD [Onc] - **Spec Exp:** AIDS Related Cancers; Lymphoma; **Hospital:** UCSF Med Ctr; **Address:** UCSF Medical Center, 400 Parnassus Ave, rm 502, Box 0324, San Francisco, CA 94143-0324; **Phone:** 415-353-2421; **Board Cert:** Internal Medicine 1983; Medical Oncology 1985; **Med School:** UCLA 1980; **Resid:** Internal Medicine, Boston City Hosp 1983; **Fellow:** Hematology & Oncology, UCSF Med Ctr 1985; **Fac Appt:** Clin Prof Med, UCSF

Kelly, Karen Lee MD [Onc] - **Spec Exp:** Lung Cancer; **Hospital:** UC Davis Med Ctr; **Address:** 4501 X St, Ste 3016, Sacramento, CA 95817; **Phone:** 916-734-3735; **Board Cert:** Internal Medicine 1987; Medical Oncology 2003; **Med School:** Univ Kansas 1984; **Resid:** Internal Medicine, Univ Colo Hlth Sci Ctr 1987; **Fellow:** Medical Oncology, Univ Colo Hlth Sci Ctr 1990; **Fac Appt:** Prof Med, UCSD

Kesari, Santosh MD/PhD [Onc] - **Spec Exp:** Neuro-Oncology; Stem Cell Therapy; Leukoencephalopathy; **Hospital:** John M & Sally B Thornton Hosp, UCSD Med Ctr; **Address:** UCSD Moores Cancer Center, 3855 Health Sciences Drive, La Jolla, CA 92093; **Phone:** 858-822-7524; **Board Cert:** Neurology 2005; **Med School:** Univ Pennsylvania 1999; **Resid:** Neurology, Mass Genl Hosp 2003; **Fellow:** Neuro-Oncology, Dana Farber Cancer Inst 2004

Koczywas, Marianna MD [Onc] - **Spec Exp:** Lung Cancer; **Hospital:** City of Hope Natl Med Ctr; **Address:** City of Hope Med Ctr, Dept Med Onc, 1500 E Duarte Rd, Duarte, CA 91010; **Phone:** 626-471-9200; **Board Cert:** Hematology 2000; Medical Oncology 2001; **Med School:** Poland 1984; **Resid:** Internal Medicine, Troczewski City Hosp 1988; Internal Medicine, St Francis Med Ctr 1997; **Fellow:** Hematology & Oncology, City of Hope Natl Med Ctr 2000

Lim, Dean Wee MD [Onc] - **Hospital:** City of Hope Natl Med Ctr; **Address:** City of Hope Med Ctr, Dept Med Onc, 1500 E Duarte Rd, Duarte, CA 91010; **Phone:** 626-471-9200; **Board Cert:** Internal Medicine 1985; Medical Oncology 1989; **Med School:** Philippines 1980; **Resid:** Internal Medicine, Cabrini Med Ctr 1985; **Fellow:** Hematology & Oncology, St Lukes Roosevelt Hosp 1987; **Fac Appt:** Asst Clin Prof Med, USC-Keck School of Medicine

Maloney, David G MD/PhD [Onc] - **Spec Exp:** Lymphoma; Bone Marrow & Stem Cell Transplant; Vaccine Therapy; **Hospital:** Univ Wash Med Ctr; **Address:** Fred Hutchinson Cancer Rsch Ctr, 1100 Fairview Ave N, D1-100, Box 19024, Seattle, WA 98109-1024; **Phone:** 206-667-5616; **Board Cert:** Internal Medicine 1988; Medical Oncology 2005; **Med School:** Stanford Univ 1985; **Resid:** Internal Medicine, Brigham & Women's Hosp 1988; **Fellow:** Medical Oncology, Stanford Univ Med Ctr 1994; **Fac Appt:** Prof Med, Univ Wash

Margolin, Kim A MD [Onc] - **Spec Exp:** Melanoma; Kidney Cancer; Germ Cell Tumors; **Hospital:** Univ Wash Med Ctr; **Address:** 825 Eastlake Ave E, PO Box 19024, Seattle, WA 98109; **Phone:** 206-288-7222; **Board Cert:** Internal Medicine 1982; Medical Oncology 2006; Hematology 1986; **Med School:** Stanford Univ 1979; **Resid:** Internal Medicine, Yale-New Haven Hosp 1982; **Fellow:** Hematology & Oncology, UC San Diego Med Ctr 1983; Hematology & Oncology, City of Hope Med Ctr 1985; **Fac Appt:** Prof Med, Univ Wash

Martins, Renato G MD [Onc] - **Spec Exp:** Head & Neck Cancer; Lung Cancer; Mesothelioma; Salivary Gland Tumors; **Hospital:** Univ Wash Med Ctr; **Address:** Seattle Cancer Care Alliance, 825 Eastlake Ave E, MS G4-940, Seattle, WA 98109; **Phone:** 206-288-2048; **Board Cert:** Internal Medicine 2005; Medical Oncology 2008; **Med School:** Brazil 1992; **Resid:** Internal Medicine, Gunderson Clinic 1995; **Fellow:** Medical Oncology, Mass Genl Hosp 1998; **Fac Appt:** Assoc Prof Med, Univ Wash

Meyskens Jr, Frank MD [Onc] - **Spec Exp:** Cancer Prevention; Melanoma; Sarcoma; **Hospital:** UC Irvine Med Ctr; **Address:** UC Irvine Cancer Ctr, 101 The City Drive, Bldg 56, rm 215, Orange, CA 92868; **Phone:** 714-456-6310; **Board Cert:** Internal Medicine 1975; Medical Oncology 1981; **Med School:** UCSF 1972; **Resid:** Internal Medicine, Moffit-Calif Hosps 1974; **Fellow:** Hematology & Oncology, Natl Cancer Inst 1977; **Fac Appt:** Prof Med, UC Irvine

Mitsuyasu, Ronald T MD [Onc] - **Spec Exp:** AIDS Related Cancers; Hematologic Malignancies; **Hospital:** UCLA Ronald Reagan Med Ctr, Santa Monica - UCLA Med Ctr & Ortho Hosp; **Address:** 1399 S Roxbury Drive, Ste 100, 9911 W Pico Blvd, Ste 980, Los Angeles, CA 90035; **Phone:** 310-557-2273; **Board Cert:** Internal Medicine 1981; **Med School:** UCLA 1978; **Resid:** Internal Medicine, Rush Presby St Lukes Hosp 1981; **Fellow:** Hematology & Oncology, UCLA Med Ctr 1984; **Fac Appt:** Prof Hem & Onc, UCLA

Mortimer, Joanne MD [Onc] - **Spec Exp:** Breast Cancer; Clinical Trials; **Hospital:** City of Hope Natl Med Ctr; **Address:** 1500 E Duarte Rd, Duarte, CA 91010; **Phone:** 626-471-9200; **Board Cert:** Internal Medicine 1980; Medical Oncology 1983; **Med School:** Loyola Univ-Stritch Sch Med 1977; **Resid:** Internal Medicine, Cleveland Clinic 1980; **Fellow:** Medical Oncology, Cleveland Clinic 1982; **Fac Appt:** Prof Hem & Onc, Loyola Univ-Stritch Sch Med

Natale, Ronald B MD [Onc] - **Spec Exp:** Lung Cancer; **Hospital:** Cedars-Sinai Med Ctr; **Address:** Cedars-Sinai Outpatient Comp Cancer Ctr, 8700 Beverly Blvd, Ste MS-33, Los Angeles, CA 90048; **Phone:** 310-423-1101; **Board Cert:** Internal Medicine 1977; Medical Oncology 1979; **Med School:** Wayne State Univ 1974; **Resid:** Internal Medicine, Wayne State Univ 1977; **Fellow:** Hematology & Oncology, Meml Sloan Kettering 1980; **Fac Appt:** Prof Med, Univ Mich Med Sch

O'Day, Steven J MD [Onc] - **Spec Exp:** Melanoma; Melanoma-Advanced; **Hospital:** St. John's Hlth Ctr, Santa Monica; **Address:** 11818 Wilshire Blvd, Ste 200, Los Angeles, CA 90025; **Phone:** 310-231-2121; **Med School:** Johns Hopkins Univ 1988; **Resid:** Internal Medicine, Johns Hopkins Hosp 1991; **Fellow:** Medical Oncology, Dana Farber Cancer Inst 1992; **Fac Appt:** Assoc Clin Prof Med, USC-Keck School of Medicine

Parker, Barbara A MD [Onc] - **Spec Exp:** Breast Cancer; Nutrition in Cancer Therapy; **Hospital:** UCSD Med Ctr; **Address:** Moores UCSD Cancer Ctr, Hem/Onc Dept, 3855 Health Sciences Drive, MC 0987, La Jolla, CA 92093; **Phone:** 858-822-6195; **Board Cert:** Internal Medicine 1984; Medical Oncology 1987; **Med School:** Stanford Univ 1981; **Resid:** Internal Medicine, UCSD Med Ctr 1985; **Fellow:** Medical Oncology, UCSD Med Ctr 1987; **Fac Appt:** Prof Med, UCSD

Medical Oncology

Petersdorf, Stephen MD [Onc] - **Spec Exp:** Lymphoma; Myelodysplastic Syndromes; Leukemia; **Hospital:** Univ Wash Med Ctr; **Address:** Seattle Cancer Care Alliance, 825 Eastlake Ave E, MS E2102, Seattle, WA 98109-1023; **Phone:** 206-288-6202; **Board Cert:** Internal Medicine 1986; Hematology 2001; Medical Oncology 2001; **Med School:** Brown Univ 1983; **Resid:** Internal Medicine, Univ Washington Med Ctr 1986; **Fellow:** Hematology & Oncology, Univ Washington Med Ctr 1989; **Fac Appt:** Assoc Prof Med, Univ Wash

Picozzi Jr, Vincent J MD [Onc] - **Spec Exp:** Gastrointestinal Cancer; Pancreatic Cancer; Genitourinary Cancer; Myelodysplastic Syndromes; **Hospital:** Virginia Mason Med Ctr; **Address:** Virginia Mason Med Ctr, Div Hem/Onc, 1100 Nineth Ave, MS C2-Hem, Seattle, WA 98111; **Phone:** 206-223-6193; **Board Cert:** Internal Medicine 1981; Hematology 1986; Medical Oncology 1987; **Med School:** Stanford Univ 1978; **Resid:** Internal Medicine, Peter Bent Brigham Med Ctr 1981; **Fellow:** Hematology, Stanford Univ Med Ctr 1983; Medical Oncology, Stanford Univ MEd Ctr 1983; **Fac Appt:** Clin Prof Med, Univ Wash

Pinto, Harlan A MD [Onc] - **Spec Exp:** Head & Neck Cancer; Clinical Trials; **Hospital:** Stanford Univ Hosp & Clinics, VA Hlth Care Sys - Palo Alto; **Address:** Stanford Comp Cancer Ctr, 875 Blake Wilbur Drive, Clinic C, Stanford, CA 94305; **Phone:** 650-723-7621; **Board Cert:** Internal Medicine 1986; Medical Oncology 2002; **Med School:** Yale Univ 1983; **Resid:** Internal Medicine, Mass Genl Hosp 1986; **Fellow:** Medical Oncology, Stanford Univ Med Sch 1991; **Fac Appt:** Assoc Prof Med, Stanford Univ

Prados, Michael MD [Onc] - **Spec Exp:** Neuro-Oncology; Brain Tumors; **Hospital:** UCSF Med Ctr; **Address:** UCSF Med Ctr, Div Neuro-Oncology, 400 Parnassus Ave, rm A-808, San Francisco, CA 94143; **Phone:** 415-353-2966; **Board Cert:** Internal Medicine 1977; **Med School:** Louisiana State U, New Orleans 1974; **Resid:** Internal Medicine, Earl K Long Hosp 1977; **Fac Appt:** Prof NS, UCSF

Press, Oliver W MD/PhD [Onc] - **Spec Exp:** Lymphoma; Bone Marrow Transplant; **Hospital:** Univ Wash Med Ctr; **Address:** 1100 Fairview Ave N, MS D3-190, Seattle, WA 98109; **Phone:** 206-667-1864; **Board Cert:** Internal Medicine 1982; Medical Oncology 1985; **Med School:** Univ Wash 1979; **Resid:** Internal Medicine, Mass Genl Hosp 1982; Internal Medicine, Univ Washington Med Ctr 1983; **Fellow:** Medical Oncology, Univ Washington Med Ctr 1985; **Fac Appt:** Prof Med, Univ Wash

Quinn, David MD/PhD [Onc] - **Spec Exp:** Testicular Cancer; Kidney Cancer; Bladder Cancer; Adrenal Cancer; **Hospital:** USC Norris Cancer Hosp (page 75); **Address:** 1441 Eastlake Ave, Ste 3440, Los Angeles, CA 90033; **Phone:** 323-865-3956; **Med School:** Australia 1987; **Resid:** Internal Medicine, St Vincents Hosp 1992; **Fellow:** Medical Oncology, St Vincents Hosp 1995; **Fac Appt:** Assoc Prof Med, USC Sch Med

Reid, Tony R MD [Onc] - **Spec Exp:** Gastrointestinal Cancer; Pancreatic Cancer; Esophageal Cancer; Liver Cancer; **Hospital:** UCSD Med Ctr; **Address:** 3855 Health Sciences Drive, Ste 1102, MC 0987, La Jolla, CA 92093; **Phone:** 858-822-6100; **Board Cert:** Medical Oncology 1999; **Med School:** Stanford Univ 1991; **Resid:** Internal Medicine, Stanford Univ Med Ctr 1997; **Fellow:** Oncology, Stanford Univ Med Ctr 1999; Cancer Research, Stanford Univ Med Ctr 2000; **Fac Appt:** Assoc Prof Med, UCSD

Rosove, Michael H MD [Onc] - **Spec Exp:** Bleeding/Coagulation Disorders; Myeloproliferative Disorders; Myelodysplastic Syndromes; Hematologic Malignancies; **Hospital:** UCLA Ronald Reagan Med Ctr; **Address:** 100 UCLA Med Plaza, Ste 550, Los Angeles, CA 90024-6970; **Phone:** 310-794-4955; **Board Cert:** Internal Medicine 1976; Hematology 1982; Medical Oncology 1981; **Med School:** UCLA 1973; **Resid:** Internal Medicine, UCLA Med Ctr 1976; **Fellow:** Hematology & Oncology, UCLA Med Ctr 1979; Hematology & Oncology, Columbia Presby Med Ctr 1978; **Fac Appt:** Clin Prof Med, UCLA-David Geffen Sch Med

Rugo, Hope S MD [Onc] - **Spec Exp:** Breast Cancer; Complementary Medicine; Breast Cancer-Novel Therapies; **Hospital:** UCSF Med Ctr; **Address:** UCSF Comp Cancer Ctr-Breast Care Ctr, 1600 Divisadero St Fl 2, San Francisco, CA 94115; **Phone:** 415-353-7070; **Board Cert:** Internal Medicine 1987; Medical Oncology 1989; **Med School:** Univ Pennsylvania 1984; **Resid:** Internal Medicine, UCSF Med Ctr 1987; **Fellow:** Hematology & Oncology, UCSF Med Ctr 1989; **Fac Appt:** Clin Prof Med, UCSF

Russell, Christy A MD [Onc] - **Spec Exp:** Breast Cancer; **Hospital:** Keck Med Ctr of USC (page 75); **Address:** Norris Cancer Ctr, The Breast Ctr, 1441 Eastlake Ave, Ste 3448, Los Angeles, CA 90033; **Phone:** 323-865-3371; **Board Cert:** Internal Medicine 1983; Medical Oncology 1985; **Med School:** Med Coll PA Hahnemann 1980; **Resid:** Internal Medicine, Good Sam Med Ctr 1983; **Fellow:** Hematology & Oncology, LAC-USC Med Ctr 1986; **Fac Appt:** Assoc Prof Med, USC Sch Med

Samlowski, Wolfram E MD [Onc] - **Spec Exp:** Kidney Cancer; Melanoma; Immunotherapy; **Hospital:** St. Rose Dom Hosp-San Martin; **Address:** Nevada Cancer Institute, One Breakthrough Way, Las Vegas, NV 89135; **Phone:** 702-822-5433; **Board Cert:** Internal Medicine 1981; Medical Oncology 1985; **Med School:** Ohio State Univ 1978; **Resid:** Internal Medicine, Wayne State Univ Affil Hosp 1981; **Fellow:** Hematology & Oncology, Univ Utah Affil Hosp 1984; **Fac Appt:** Prof Hem & Onc, Univ Nevada

Sandler, Alan MD [Onc] - **Spec Exp:** Lung Cancer; Sarcoma; **Hospital:** OR Hlth & Sci Univ; **Address:** 3181 SW Sam Jackson Park Rd, MC L586, Portland, OR 97239; **Phone:** 503-494-5586; **Board Cert:** Medical Oncology 2006; **Med School:** Rush Med Coll 1987; **Resid:** Internal Medicine, Yale-New Haven Hosp 1989; **Fellow:** Medical Oncology, Yale Univ 1993; **Fac Appt:** Prof Med, Oregon Hlth & Sci Univ

Scudder, Sidney MD [Onc] - **Spec Exp:** Ovarian Cancer; Cervical Cancer; **Hospital:** UC Davis Med Ctr; **Address:** 4501 X St, Ste 3016, Sacramento, CA 95817; **Phone:** 916-734-3700; **Board Cert:** Internal Medicine 1983; Medical Oncology 1985; **Med School:** Univ Fla Coll Med 1980; **Resid:** Internal Medicine, Barnes Hosp-Washington Univ 1983; **Fellow:** Medical Oncology, Stanford Univ 1985; **Fac Appt:** Prof Med, UC Davis

Shibata, Stephen I MD [Onc] - **Spec Exp:** Gastrointestinal Cancer; Clinical Trials; **Hospital:** City of Hope Natl Med Ctr; **Address:** City of Hope Cancer Ctr, 1500 E Duarte Rd, Duarte, CA 91010; **Phone:** 626-471-9200; **Board Cert:** Internal Medicine 1988; Medical Oncology 2004; **Med School:** UC Irvine 1985; **Resid:** Internal Medicine, St Mary Med Ctr 1988; **Fellow:** Medical Oncology, City of Hope Cancer Ctr 1990; Bone Marrow Transplant, City of Hope Cancer Ctr 1991; **Fac Appt:** Assoc Prof Med

Sikic, Branimir I MD [Onc] - **Spec Exp:** Unknown Primary Cancer; Clinical Trials; **Hospital:** Stanford Univ Hosp & Clinics; **Address:** Stanford Comp Cancer Ctr, 875 Blake Wilbur Drive, Clinic C, Palo Alto, CA 94305; **Phone:** 650-723-7621; **Board Cert:** Internal Medicine 1975; Medical Oncology 1979; **Med School:** Ros Franklin Univ/Chicago Med Sch 1972; **Resid:** Internal Medicine, Georgetown Univ Hosp 1975; **Fellow:** Medical Oncology, Natl Cancer Inst 1978; Medical Oncology, Georgetown Univ Hosp 1979; **Fac Appt:** Prof Med, Stanford Univ

Small, Eric J MD [Onc] - **Spec Exp:** Prostate Cancer; Vaccine Therapy; Genitourinary Cancer; **Hospital:** UCSF Med Ctr; **Address:** UCSF Urologic Oncology Practice, 1600 Divisadero St Fl 3, San Francisco, CA 94115; **Phone:** 415-353-7171; **Board Cert:** Internal Medicine 1988; Medical Oncology 2001; **Med School:** Case West Res Univ 1985; **Resid:** Internal Medicine, Beth Israel Hosp 1988; **Fellow:** Hematology & Oncology, Cancer Research Inst/UCSF 1991; **Fac Appt:** Prof Med, UCSF

Medical Oncology

Stewart, Forrest M MD [Onc] - **Spec Exp:** Unknown Primary Cancer; Sarcoma; **Hospital:** Univ Wash Med Ctr; **Address:** Seattle Cancer Care Alliance, 825 Eastlake Ave E, Box 19023, Seattle, WA 98109; **Phone:** 206-288-7222; **Board Cert:** Internal Medicine 1980; Hematology 1982; Medical Oncology 1985; **Med School:** Indiana Univ 1977; **Resid:** Internal Medicine, Indiana Univ Med Ctr 1980; Medical Oncology, Indiana Univ Med Ctr 1981; **Fellow:** Hematology, Univ Virginia Med Ctr 1983; **Fac Appt:** Prof Med, Univ Wash

Stockdale, Frank E MD/PhD [Onc] - **Spec Exp:** Breast Cancer; Tuberous Breasts; Sarcoma-Soft Tissue; **Hospital:** Stanford Univ Hosp & Clinics; **Address:** Stanford Univ Medical Ctr, 875 Blake Wilbur Drive, Stanford, CA 94305-5826; **Phone:** 650-498-6000; **Med School:** Univ Pennsylvania 1963; **Resid:** Internal Medicine, Stanford Univ Med Ctr 1967; Medical Oncology, Stanford Univ Med Ctr; **Fac Appt:** Prof Emeritus Med, Stanford Univ

Tempero, Margaret A MD [Onc] - **Spec Exp:** Pancreatic Cancer; Gastrointestinal Cancer; **Hospital:** UCSF Med Ctr, VA Med Ctr - San Francisco; **Address:** UCSF Medical Ctr, 1600 Divisadero St Fl 4, San Francisco, CA 94115; **Phone:** 415-353-9888; **Board Cert:** Internal Medicine 1980; Medical Oncology 1983; Hematology 1984; **Med School:** Univ Nebr Coll Med 1977; **Resid:** Internal Medicine, Univ Nebraska Hosp 1980; **Fellow:** Medical Oncology, Univ Nebraska Hosp 1982; **Fac Appt:** Prof Med, UCSF

Thompson, John Ainslie MD [Onc] - **Spec Exp:** Melanoma; Kidney Cancer; **Hospital:** Univ Wash Med Ctr; **Address:** Seattle Cancer Care Alliance, 825 Eastlake Ave E, MS G4-200, Seattle, WA 98109-1023; **Phone:** 206-288-2015; **Board Cert:** Internal Medicine 1982; Medical Oncology 1985; **Med School:** Univ Alabama 1979; **Resid:** Internal Medicine, Univ Wash Med Ctr 1982; **Fellow:** Medical Oncology, Univ Washington 1985

Tripathy, Debasish MD [Onc] - **Spec Exp:** Breast Cancer; Clinical Trials; **Hospital:** USC Norris Cancer Hosp (page 75); **Address:** 1441 Eastlake Ave, rm #3429, Los Angeles, CA 90033; **Phone:** 323-865-3900; **Board Cert:** Internal Medicine 1988; Medical Oncology 2001; **Med School:** Duke Univ 1985; **Resid:** Internal Medicine, Duke Univ Med Ctr 1988; **Fellow:** Hematology & Oncology, USCF Med Ctr 1991; **Fac Appt:** Prof Med, Univ SC Sch Med

Twardowski, Przemyslaw W MD [Onc] - **Spec Exp:** Genitourinary Cancer; **Hospital:** City of Hope Natl Med Ctr; **Address:** 1500 E Duarte Rd, Duarte, CA 91010; **Phone:** 626-256-4673; **Board Cert:** Medical Oncology 2009; **Med School:** Univ MO-Columbia Sch Med 1990; **Resid:** Internal Medicine, Northwestern Meml Hosp 1994; **Fellow:** Hematology & Oncology, Northwestern Meml Hosp 1996; **Fac Appt:** Asst Prof Med, UCLA

Urba, Walter J MD/PhD [Onc] - **Spec Exp:** Breast Cancer; **Hospital:** Providence Portland Med Ctr; **Address:** Providence Oncology, 4805 NE Glisan Rd, Portland, OR 97213; **Phone:** 503-215-5696; **Board Cert:** Internal Medicine 1985; Medical Oncology 1987; **Med School:** Univ Miami Sch Med 1981; **Resid:** Internal Medicine, Morristown Meml Hosp 1983; **Fellow:** Medical Oncology, Natl Cancer Inst 1986; **Fac Appt:** Assoc Clin Prof Med, Oregon Hlth & Sci Univ

Venook, Alan P MD [Onc] - **Spec Exp:** Gastrointestinal Cancer; Colon & Rectal Cancer; Liver Cancer; **Hospital:** UCSF Med Ctr; **Address:** UCSF Comprehensive Cancer Ctr, Multi Disciplinary Practice, 1600 Divisadero St Fl 4 - rm 4202, San Francisco, CA 94115; **Phone:** 415-353-9888; **Board Cert:** Internal Medicine 1985; Medical Oncology 1987; Hematology 1988; **Med School:** UCSF 1980; **Resid:** Internal Medicine, UC Davis Med Ctr 1985; **Fellow:** Hematology & Oncology, UCSF Med Ctr 1987; **Fac Appt:** Prof Med

Vescio, Robert A MD [Onc] - **Spec Exp:** Multiple Myeloma; Amyloidosis; **Hospital:** Cedars-Sinai Med Ctr; **Address:** Cedars Sinai Med Ctr, Dept Hem/Oncology, 8700 Beverly Blvd, Ste AC1049, Los Angeles, CA 90048; **Phone:** 310-423-1825; **Board Cert:** Internal Medicine 1989; Hematology 2004; Medical Oncology 2003; **Med School:** UCSD 1986; **Resid:** Internal Medicine, UCSD Med Ctr 1989; **Fellow:** Hematology & Oncology, UCLA Med Ctr 1993; **Fac Appt:** Assoc Prof Med, UCLA

Vogelzang, Nicholas J MD [Onc] - **Spec Exp:** Prostate Cancer; Mesothelioma; Kidney Cancer; Genitourinary Cancer; **Hospital:** Sunrise Hosp & Med Ctr, Desert Springs Hosp Med Ctr - Las Vegas; **Address:** Comprehensive Cancer Ctr of Nevada, 3730 S Eastern Ave, Las Vegas, NV 89169; **Phone:** 702-952-3452; **Board Cert:** Internal Medicine 1977; Medical Oncology 1981; **Med School:** Univ IL Coll Med 1974; **Resid:** Internal Medicine, Rush-Presby St Luke's Med Ctr 1977; **Fellow:** Medical Oncology, Univ Minn Med Ctr 1980; **Fac Appt:** Prof Med, Univ Nevada

Volberding, Paul Arthur MD [Onc] - **Spec Exp:** AIDS Related Cancers; **Hospital:** UCSF Med Ctr, VA Med Ctr - San Francisco; **Address:** 4150 Clement St, VAMC 111, San Francisco, CA 94121; **Phone:** 415-750-2203; **Board Cert:** Internal Medicine 1978; Medical Oncology 1981; **Med School:** Univ Minn 1975; **Resid:** Internal Medicine, Univ Utah Med Ctr 1978; **Fellow:** Medical Oncology, UCSF Med Ctr 1981; **Fac Appt:** Prof Med, UCSF

von Gunten, Charles MD/PhD [Onc] - **Spec Exp:** Palliative Care; **Hospital:** San Diego Hospice; **Address:** San Diego Hospice, 4311 Third Ave, San Diego, CA 92103; **Phone:** 619-688-1600; **Board Cert:** Internal Medicine 2002; Medical Oncology 2003; Hospice & Palliative Medicine 2001; **Med School:** Univ Colorado 1988; **Resid:** Internal Medicine, Northwestern Univ 1991; **Fellow:** Medical Oncology, Northwestern Univ 1993; **Fac Appt:** Assoc Clin Prof Med, UCSD

Wierman, Ann MD [Onc] - **Spec Exp:** Breast Cancer; Lymphoma; Lung Cancer; **Hospital:** Mountainview Hosp - Las Vegas, Summerlin Hosp Med Ctr; **Address:** 7445 Peak Drive, Las Vegas, NV 89128; **Phone:** 702-952-2140; **Board Cert:** Internal Medicine 2002; Medical Oncology 2007; **Med School:** Baylor Coll Med 1989; **Resid:** Internal Medicine, Baylor Hosps 1992; Internal Medicine, Ben Taub Genl Hosp 1993; **Fellow:** Hematology & Oncology, Univ CO Hlth Sci Ctr 1996; **Fac Appt:** Assoc Clin Prof Med, Univ Nevada

Yen, Yun MD/PhD [Onc] - **Spec Exp:** Liver Cancer; Biliary Cancer; **Hospital:** City of Hope Natl Med Ctr; **Address:** City of Hope Comprehensive Cancer Ctr, 1500 E Duarte Rd, Duarte, CA 91010; **Phone:** 626-471-9200 x62307; **Board Cert:** Medical Oncology 2003; **Med School:** Taiwan 1982; **Resid:** Internal Medicine, St Luke's Hosp 1990; **Fellow:** Hematology & Oncology, Yale-New Haven Hosp 1993; **Fac Appt:** Prof Med, USC Sch Med

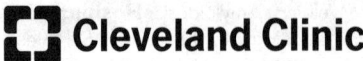
Cleveland Clinic
Every life deserves world class care.

Cleveland Clinic
Taussig Cancer Institute
9500 Euclid Avenue
Cleveland, OH 44195

clevelandclinic.org/
oncologytopdocs

Offering Same-Day Appointments
Call 800.274.2009.

Hematology/Medical Oncology

At Cleveland Clinic Taussig Cancer Institute, more than 250 top cancer specialists, researchers, nurses and technicians are dedicated to delivering the most effective medical treatments and offering access to the latest clinical trials for more than 13,000 new cancer patients every year. Our doctors are nationally and internationally known for their contributions to cancer breakthroughs and their ability to deliver superior outcomes for our patients. In recognition of these and other achievements, *U.S.News & World Report* has ranked Cleveland Clinic as one of the top cancer centers in the nation.

National Treatment Leader in Blood Cancers

The Taussig Cancer Institute is a national leader in caring for and treating patients with leukemia, lymphoma, myeloma and myelodysplastic syndromes. For example, our Bone Marrow Transplant (BMT) program has unsurpassed national outcomes. We have one of the most experienced teams in the nation, having performed more than 3,600 bone marrow transplant procedures since 1977.

Our teams of nurses, social workers, pharmacists and internationally recognized physicians work together to develop personalized treatment plans for each patient. We have a state-of-the-art, dedicated hospital floor with individual rooms for leukemia and BMT patients. We offer the most current treatments through clinical trials, many of which have been developed at Cleveland Clinic. Our goal is to promote the highest quality of care for people who have hematologic cancers.

Treatment Guides

Cleveland Clinic has developed comprehensive treatment guides for many diseases and conditions. To download our free treatment guides, visit clevelandclinic.org/treatmentguides.

Online Medical Second Opinion

Cleveland Clinic's My**Consult** Online Medical Second Opinion program securely connects patients to our physician specialists for more than 1,000 life-changing or life-threatening diagnoses all by the click of a mouse. To learn more, log onto eclevelandclinic.org/myconsult or call 800.223.2273, ext. 43223.

Special Assistance for Out-of-State Patients

Cleveland Clinic Global Patient Services offers a complimentary Medical Concierge service for patients who travel from outside of Ohio. Call 800.223.2273, ext. 55580 or email medicalconcierge@ccf.org.

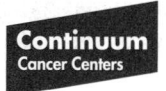

Beth Israel Medical Center
St. Luke's Hospital
Roosevelt Hospital
NY Eye & Ear Infirmary

Continuum Cancer Centers of New York

Continuum Cancer Centers of New York

(212) 844-6027

The hospitals of Continuum – Beth Israel Medical Center, St. Luke's Hospital, Roosevelt Hospital and the New York Eye and Ear Infirmary – are leading providers of cancer care through Continuum Cancer Centers of New York (CCCNY). As part of a major expansion of our cancer care services, Beth Israel Medical Center recently opened the Beth Israel Comprehensive Cancer Center-West Side Campus, a state-of-the-art facility comprising 88,000 square feet located in Manhattan.

We are dedicated to delivering care in ways that are more efficient, more attractive and more convenient for patients. Our cancer patients benefit from system-wide cancer expertise, facilities and resources. Continuum Cancer Centers feature world-renowned cancer specialists, including top-rated surgeons, medical oncologists, radiation oncologists, radiologists, pathologists, and oncology nurses.

Comprehensive diagnostic and treatment services are available for breast cancer, prostate cancer, head and neck and thyroid cancers, skin cancer, lung cancer, colorectal and other gastrointestinal cancers, lymphoma/Hodgkin's Disease, gynecological cancers, and cancers of the brain and central nervous system. Delivered efficiently in a friendly and supportive environment, our services include prevention programs – such as community education, screenings and early detection – expert diagnosis, outpatient treatment, inpatient services and home care. In addition, our Research Program offers patients access to investigational protocols through a wide number of clinical trials. Our physicians are leaders in both non-invasive and minimally invasive cancer treatments that focus on maximizing both the cure rate and the quality of life.

Support Services also play an important role at Continuum Cancer Centers. Our nurses, social workers, psychiatrists, chaplains, pharmacists, rehabilitation therapists and nutritionists all have specialized knowledge and expertise in the field of oncology.

In June 2011, CCCNY received a full three-year network accreditation from the American College of Surgeons Commission on Cancer (CoC), with commendation. Continuum first received a full, three-year accreditation in 2007, and was the only hospital system in New York State to receive such designation.

Continuum Health Partners, Inc.

Beth Israel   **Roosevelt Hospital**   **St. Luke's Hospital**   **NY Eye & Ear Infirmary**

www.chpnyc.org

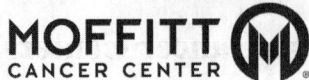

Overview

Moffitt Cancer Center & Research Institute is a National Cancer Institute (NCI) Comprehensive Cancer Center. Both private and not-for-profit the Center includes a 206 bed-hospital, a 36-bed blood and marrow transplant unit, an outpatient clinic with a complete digital imaging center, a state-of-the-art radiation therapy department, infusion center, 14 operating rooms, the Moffitt Research Institute, and off site locations including a screening center for high risk patients and a 50,000 square foot outpatient center that enables further growth and service to cancer patients. Moffitt has also created a network of strategic partners composed of 17 affiliate hospitals within the state of Florida and beyond, along with practice affiliations represented by more than 400 oncologists.

Moffitt is accredited by JCAHO, the American College of Surgeons Commission on Cancer, the American College of Radiology and the National Accreditation Program for Breast Centers.

Academic/Clinical Affiliations

Moffitt collaborates or partners with the University of South Florida, University of Florida, FAMU, Burnham Institute, Florida Atlantic University, Florida State University, Florida Institute for Human and Machine Cognition, Scripps Florida, Translational Genomics Research Institute/Arizona, University of Central Florida.

Medical Staff

The Center has more than 300 physicians known as the Moffitt Medical group, most of whom are fellowship trained. The Center's clinical services are organized into disease-oriented interdisciplinary programs, along with diagnostic imaging, interventional radiology, pathology, and anesthesiology.

Pioneering Comprehensive Medical Care

Moffitt is at the forefront of personalized medicine with Total Cancer Care™ - a system of care that encompasses prevention, genetic predisposition, the impact of lifestyle, survivorship and the uses of integrative medicine during treatment.

At the core of Total Cancer Care™ is a longitudinal research study that maintains a repository of human tissue specimens and clinical data which will further the discovery of tumor biomarkers that can be used to identify those at high risk, facilitate early detection, improve prognoses, allow drug targeting and toxicity predictions, and match individuals to the best treatment and to the right clinical trials.

International Services

Moffitt has affiliations at Ponce School of Medicine in Puerto Rico and Tianjin Medical University Cancer Institute and Hospital in China. Our international referral services oversees all necessary steps for patients who come from abroad including assistance with visas, medical records, translation, travel, lodging, transportation, language services, etc.

Moffitt has Comprehensive Research Centers (CRC) that further the Center's goal to be a leader in personalized care. Programs identified for the CRCs are Melanoma, Drug Discovery and Lung Cancer. All of the CRCs serve as a catalyst to engage collaborative research efforts with other institutions and as a training opportunity for a cadre of young investigators who will become the future leaders in the field. Additionally, the CRCs share a common mission to:

Discover: Create a milieu for discovery by fostering interdisciplinary laboratory research that generates new knowledge and understanding.

Translate: Foster the translation of new scientific discoveries, both those made at Moffitt and elsewhere into early phase clinical trials and ultimately into standard patient care.

Deliver: Support the efforts of Moffitt clinicians to deliver state-of-the-art personalized cancer care and support the training and education in prevention, research and treatment.

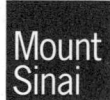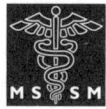

MOUNT SINAI
SCHOOL OF
MEDICINE

THE TISCH CANCER INSTITUTE
AT THE MOUNT SINAI MEDICAL CENTER
One Gustave L. Levy Place
Fifth Avenue and 100th Street
New York, NY 10029-6574
Physician Referral: 1-800-MD-SINAI (637-4624)
www.tischcancerinstitute.org

THE TISCH CANCER INSTITUTE is embedded within a renowned medical center that has world-class research facilities, one of the nation's top-ranked hospitals, and an outstanding medical school. Patients have access to the best possible cancer care across a variety of disciplines, including medical, surgical, and radiation treatments; palliative care; behavioral medicine; physical therapy; psychosocial services—and cutting-edge cancer research. For fully integrated, multidisciplinary care, our patients are also treated by the best specialists in every field at Mount Sinai and can receive seamless referrals.

Services and Programs – The Tisch Cancer Institute employs a multidisciplinary treatment approach, providing access to clinical breakthroughs, innovative techniques, leading-edge technologies, and a wide range of diagnostic, therapeutic, and support services for all types of cancer. The Institute treats: breast cancer; hematological malignancies (including multiple myeloma, myelodysplastic syndrome, and myeloproliferative disorders); genitourinary cancers (including prostate, bladder, and kidney); head and neck cancers; thoracic cancer (including lung and esophagus); gynecologic cancers; brain tumors; and other diagnoses. In addition to surgical treatment, the Institute provides radiation and medical oncology therapies, as well as bone marrow transplantation. The Dubin Breast Center, consisting of 15,000 square feet, is a newly constructed facility that opened in April 2011 and significantly expands the treatment space for breast cancer patients.

THE RUTTENBERG TREATMENT CENTER
The Derald H. Ruttenberg Treatment Center houses the ambulatory cancer program of The Tisch Cancer Institute and is operated by The Mount Sinai Hospital.

THE DUBIN BREAST CENTER
The Dubin Breast Center offers the latest, most innovative approaches available for breast health and the treatment of breast cancer.

The Tisch Cancer Institute encourages collaboration with colleagues across the Medical Center, drawing upon the knowledge of a vast network of specialists who are outstanding in their fields. These experts consist of award-winning physicians and surgeons specializing in cardiac care, neurology, urology, pediatrics, digestive diseases, obstetrics and gynecology, and other therapeutic areas. Oncologists, surgeons, radiation oncologists, and specialists from across the medical spectrum work together to provide the highest quality care to all cancer patients. Furthermore, Mount Sinai's nursing staff is an important part of the Medical Center's focus on delivering exceptional patient care, and it has received the prestigious Magnet Award for nursing excellence. Mount Sinai is also renowned for its palliative care program, which provides the highest level of care, focusing on the relief of pain, symptoms, and stress in cancer patients in both an inpatient and outpatient setting.

A Heritage of Breakthroughs – Teams of physicians and scientists at The Tisch Cancer Institute at Mount Sinai work together to rapidly translate laboratory research into new patient treatments. Among the advances pioneered at Mount Sinai are the first successful treatment of tumors of the bladder by transurethral electrocoagulation, the first demonstration of how asbestos can cause cancerous changes in the DNA of cells, and the first development of an ultrasound-guided technique to insert radioactive seeds into the prostate to treat prostate cancer.

NewYork-Presbyterian
The University Hospital of Columbia and Cornell

Affiliated with Columbia University College of Physicians and Surgeons and Weill Cornell Medical College

Herbert Irving Comprehensive Cancer Center
NewYork-Presbyterian Hospital
Columbia University Medical Center
161 Fort Washington Avenue
New York, NY 10032

Weill Cornell Cancer Center
NewYork-Presbyterian Hospital
Weill Cornell Medical Center
525 East 68th Street
New York, NY 10065

1-877-NYP-WELL (1-877-697-9355)   www.nyp.org/cancer

NewYork-Presbyterian Cancer Centers

Innovative cancer treatments. Personalized, compassionate care. Evidence-based medicine. These are the hallmarks of the cancer care available at NewYork-Presbyterian Hospital, where cutting-edge treatment goes beyond state-of-the-art. We treat more than 7,000 people who are newly diagnosed with cancer each year.

NewYork-Presbyterian features two of the country's top cancer centers: the National Cancer Institute-designated Herbert Irving Comprehensive Cancer Center (one of only three comprehensive NCI-designated cancer centers in New York State) and the Weill Cornell Cancer Center. Through a multidisciplinary team approach, we combine the expertise and talents of all of the individuals responsible for a patient's care—surgical, medical, and radiation oncologists, specialized oncology nurses, social workers, and nutritionists—to deliver seamless care in a supportive and healing environment.

Our team cares for patients with the following cancers:
- AIDS-related cancers
- Bladder cancer
- Brain and other nervous system cancers
- Breast cancer
- Colorectal, pancreatic, and other digestive cancers
- Eye cancer
- Gynecologic cancers (ovarian, cervical, endometrial)
- Head and neck cancers (oral, oropharyngeal, laryngeal)
- Kidney cancer
- Lymphomas (Hodgkin's and non-Hodgkin's)
- Leukemia and myelodysplastic syndromes
- Liver cancer
- Mesothelioma
- Myeloma
- Pediatric cancers
- Prostate cancer
- Sarcoma
- Thoracic cancers (lung, esophageal, chest wall)

Research underlies everything we do, and sets academic medical centers such as ours apart from other cancer treatment centers. Our scientists and clinical investigators are leading more than 500 clinical trials assessing new cancer management approaches in thousands of patients.

Specialized Cancer Care Includes:

- Surgical procedures for breast cancer that result in superior cosmetic outcomes, and evaluation of novel anticancer drugs for women with advanced disease

- Robotic surgery for prostate and gynecologic cancers

- Video-assisted thoracoscopy and lung-sparing surgery for some lung cancers

- Interventional endoscopy and laparoscopic surgery for colorectal and other cancers

- Targeted approaches to brain cancer treatment, including convection-enhanced chemotherapy and stereotactic radiosurgery

- Bone marrow and stem cell transplantation for hematologic cancers

- Renowned Mesothelioma Center

- Combination chemotherapy, targeted anticancer agents, novel drugs available through clinical trials, and highly targeted radiation therapy

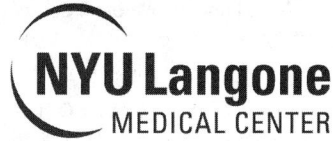

NYU Langone Medical Center
550 First Avenue , New York, NY 10016
www.NYULMC.org

NYU Clinical Cancer Center
160 East 34th Street, New York, NY 10016
www.NYUCI.org

**The Stephen D. Hassenfeld Children's Center
for Cancer and Blood Disorders**
160 East 32nd Street, New York, NY 10016
www.NYUMC.org/Hassenfeld

NYU CANCER INSTITUTE

The NYU Cancer Institute is an NCI-designated cancer center providing personalized patient care that is compassionate and state-of-the-art. The doctors and researchers work together to develop innovative therapies for patients. The Cancer Institute is world-renowned for excellence in cancer-focused research, personalized care, education and community outreach. Its mission is to discover the origins of human cancer and to use that knowledge to eradicate the personal and societal burden of cancer in our community, the nation and the world. For more information about our expert physicians, call 212-731-5000.

Patient-Focused Setting
The NYU Clinical Cancer Center is the principal outpatient facility of The Cancer Institute. The Center and its multidisciplinary team of experts provide access to the latest treatment options and clinical trials, along with a variety of programs in cancer risk reduction/prevention, screening, diagnostics, genetic counseling and supportive services. In addition, the Center emphasizes the importance of a holistic approach involving complementary medicine, psychosocial support, survivorship and palliative care. Radiology and infusion services are available in Rego Park, NY, as well.

Renowned Expertise
The NYU Cancer Institute brings together experts from a variety of disciplines to create collaborative research endeavors and clinical care teams. It offers a continuum of personalized care, from prevention through diagnosis, treatment and post-treatment support. Additionally, we have created special programs to treat diseases such as breast cancer, melanoma, GI cancer, prostate cancer, hematologic malignancies and lung cancer, as well as translational programs in cancer healthcare disparities, molecularly targeted therapy, and the cell signaling pathways involved in cancer.

A Translational Approach
Our scientists and researchers excel in uncovering how cancer develops at the molecular level, and how we can harness that knowledge to reduce the risk of cancer and treat the disease.

Stephen D. Hassenfeld Children's Center for Cancer and Blood Disorders
The center is a leading pediatric outpatient facility for the treatment of childhood cancers and blood diseases. Its unique interdisciplinary and family-centered approach combines the most advanced medical treatments with psychosocial and emotional support services for young patients and their families.

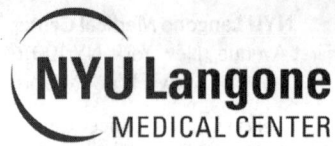

NYU Langone Medical Center
550 First Avenue , New York, NY 10016
www.NYULMC.org

NYU Clinical Cancer Center
160 East 34th Street, New York, NY 10016
www.NYUCI.org

**The Stephen D. Hassenfeld Children's Center
for Cancer and Blood Disorders**
160 East 32nd Street, New York, NY 10016
www.NYUMC.org/Hassenfeld

NYU CANCER INSTITUTE

The NYU Cancer Institute is an NCI-designated cancer center providing personalized patient care that is compassionate and state-of-the-art. The doctors and researchers work together to develop innovative therapies for patients. The Cancer Institute is world-renowned for excellence in cancer-focused research, personalized care, education and community outreach. Its mission is to discover the origins of human cancer and to use that knowledge to eradicate the personal and societal burden of cancer in our community, the nation and the world. For more information about our expert physicians, call 212-731-5000.

Patient-Focused Setting
The NYU Clinical Cancer Center is the principal outpatient facility of The Cancer Institute. The Center and its multidisciplinary team of experts provide access to the latest treatment options and clinical trials, along with a variety of programs in cancer risk reduction/prevention, screening, diagnostics, genetic counseling and supportive services. In addition, the Center emphasizes the importance of a holistic approach involving complementary medicine, psychosocial support, survivorship and palliative care. Radiology and infusion services are available in Rego Park, NY, as well.

Renowned Expertise
The NYU Cancer Institute brings together experts from a variety of disciplines to create collaborative research endeavors and clinical care teams. It offers a continuum of personalized care, from prevention through diagnosis, treatment and post-treatment support. Additionally, we have created special programs to treat diseases such as breast cancer, melanoma, GI cancer, prostate cancer, hematologic malignancies and lung cancer, as well as translational programs in cancer healthcare disparities, molecularly targeted therapy, and the cell signaling pathways involved in cancer.

A Translational Approach
Our scientists and researchers excel in uncovering how cancer develops at the molecular level, and how we can harness that knowledge to reduce the risk of cancer and treat the disease.

Stephen D. Hassenfeld Children's Center for Cancer and Blood Disorders
The center is a leading pediatric outpatient facility for the treatment of childhood cancers and blood diseases. Its unique interdisciplinary and family-centered approach combines the most advanced medical treatments with psychosocial and emotional support services for young patients and their families.

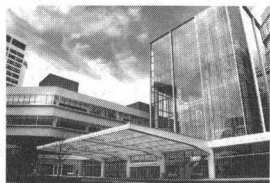

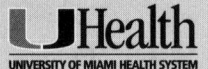
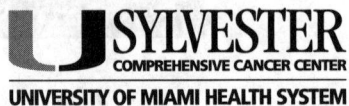

USC Norris Cancer Hospital

Part of the Keck Medical Center of USC

1441 Eastlake Ave.
Los Angeles, CA 90033
800-700-3956
KeckMedicalCenterofUSC.org

USC NORRIS CANCER HOSPITAL

USC Norris Cancer Hospital is one of only a few facilities in Southern California built exclusively for cancer research and patient care. It is part of the USC Norris Comprehensive Cancer Center, one of the original eight comprehensive cancer centers designated by the National Cancer Institute. As such, it is home to some of the most experienced, progressive doctors and cancer treatments available.

The Norris Inpatient Tower at Keck Hospital of USC includes two floors dedicated to hematology and medical oncology care. The tower features 11 operating rooms and 150 inpatient rooms and is equipped and designed to meet the medical and surgical needs of USC Norris cancer patients.

STATE-OF-THE-ART PATIENT CARE

USC hospitals are equipped with cutting-edge technology, providing the most up-to-date treatment for our patients. These features include:

+ Two surgical robots, including the newest da Vinci® Si™ Surgical System
+ Polestar® Intraoperative MRI Navigation System
+ Cyberknife® and Varian Trilogy Linear Accelerator for stereotactic radiosurgery, intensity modulated radiation therapy and image guided radiation therapy
+ Leksell Gamma Knife® PERFEXION™, a highly advanced radiation tool to treat brain tumors
+ Four endoscopy suites and two interventional radiology suites for endoscopic procedures for outpatients, as well as two fully equipped endoscopy suites for inpatient procedures

CLINICAL TRIALS

In the battle against devastating diseases such as cancer, a major USC effort is aimed at the development and testing of new treatments — surgeries, drugs, radiation therapies, preventive therapies — that might lead to a cure. USC clinical trials contribute to finding new and better ways of treating diseases. Hundreds of clinical trials take place at USC each year, giving select patients access to therapies not available elsewhere.

SPECIALTIES & RESEARCH

USC Norris Cancer Hospital is known throughout the region for expertise and excellence in:

+ Breast cancer surgery, including clinical trials for intra-operative radiotherapy for early breast cancer

+ Prostate cancer, including nerve-sparing robotic prostatectomy

+ Head and neck oncology

+ Kidney cancer and nephron sparing surgery

+ Lung cancer

+ Neuro-oncology

+ Orthopaedic oncology

+ Radiation oncology

+ Bone marrow transplant

+ GI/GU oncology

+ Adolescents and young adults

Vanderbilt-Ingram Cancer Center

2220 Pierce Ave. | Nashville, TN 37232 | Toll-free: 1 (877) 936-8422 ; Clinical Trials: 1 (800) 811-8480 | VICC.org

Overview

Vanderbilt-Ingram Cancer Center is one of only 40 in the U.S. to be named a Comprehensive Cancer Center, the National Cancer Institute's highest designation. Vanderbilt-Ingram is also a leading cancer research center, ranked in the nation's top 10 in competitive grant support from the NCI. It's also a member of the National Comprehensive Cancer Network, a nonprofit alliance working to improve care for all cancer patients.

Vanderbilt-Ingram is the only center in Tennessee ranked among the nation's Best Hospitals for cancer care by *U.S. News & World Report.*

A Specialized Approach

Cancer is not a single disease that can be treated with a generic approach. At Vanderbilt-Ingram, we provide a high level of specialization through teams of experts with the knowledge and experience to treat unique cases of all kinds.

Unlike other centers that may have a general cancer team, we have teams focused on cancers of the breast, lung, colon and other gastrointestinal organs; head and neck cancers; brain and other neurologic cancers; gynecologic cancers; bone and tissue cancers; leukemias, lymphomas and myelomas; melanoma; and pediatric cancers. We also offer expertise on rare cancers.

Personalized Cancer Medicine

We've known for some time that changes in the DNA of cancer cells can affect how they respond to treatment. Our Personalized Cancer Medicine Initiative tests patients for changes in tumor DNA known to affect treatment. The results of those tests help guide our oncologists to choose the right therapy for the patient at the right time. This approach is now used for lung cancers, melanoma and breast cancers, with other cancers to be included soon.

Clinical Trials

Studies of promising new therapies are an important option that every cancer patient should consider. Vanderbilt-Ingram offers a wide range of clinical trials. Learn more.

Survivorship and Wellness

Living through cancer can leave lasting marks. Vanderbilt-Ingram is the only cancer center in the country to offer a dedicated program for all cancer survivors once treatment ends. It includes patients regardless of age, type of cancer or where treatment took place. Learn more.

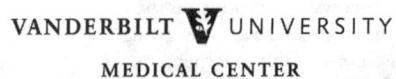

VANDERBILT ⅤUNIVERSITY
MEDICAL CENTER

Infectious Disease
a subspecialty of Internal Medicine

An internist who deals with infectious diseases of all types and in all organs. Conditions requiring selective use of antibiotics call for this special skill. This physician often diagnoses and treats AIDS patients and patients with fevers which have not been explained. Infectious disease specialists may also have expertise in preventive medicine and conditions associated with travel.

Training Required: Three years in internal medicine *plus* additional training and examination for certification in infectious disease.

INFECTIOUS DISEASE

New England

Craven, Donald Edward MD [Inf] - **Spec Exp:** AIDS/HIV; Hepatitis C; Hospital Acquired Infections; Pneumonia; **Hospital:** Lahey Clin; **Address:** Lahey Clin Med Ctr, Infectious Diseases, 41 Mall Rd, Burlington, MA 01805; **Phone:** 781-744-8608; **Board Cert:** Internal Medicine 1973; Infectious Disease 1982; **Med School:** Albany Med Coll 1970; **Resid:** Internal Medicine, Royal Victoria Hosp-McGill 1973; Internal Medicine, Royal Victoria Hosp 1974; **Fellow:** Infectious Disease, Boston Univ Hosp 1976; NIH/Bureau of Biologics 1979; **Fac Appt:** Prof Med, Tufts Univ

Flanigan, Timothy P MD [Inf] - **Spec Exp:** AIDS/HIV; **Hospital:** Miriam Hosp, Rhode Island Hosp; **Address:** 1125 N Main St, Providence, RI 02904; **Phone:** 401-793-2928; **Board Cert:** Internal Medicine 1986; Infectious Disease 1988; **Med School:** Cornell Univ-Weill Med Coll 1983; **Resid:** Internal Medicine, Hosp Univ Penn 1986; **Fellow:** Infectious Disease, Case West Res Univ 1987; **Fac Appt:** Prof Med, Brown Univ

Quagliarello, Vincent MD [Inf] - **Spec Exp:** Meningitis; Pneumonia; Endocarditis; **Hospital:** Yale-New Haven Hosp, Yale Med Group; **Address:** Yale Univ Sch Med, TAC S169A, 300 Cedar St, New Haven, CT 06520-8022; **Phone:** 203-785-3561; **Board Cert:** Internal Medicine 1984; Infectious Disease 1988; **Med School:** Washington Univ, St Louis 1980; **Resid:** Internal Medicine, Yale-New Haven Hosp 1984; **Fellow:** Infectious Disease, Univ VA Hlth Sci Ctr 1987; **Fac Appt:** Prof Med, Yale Univ

Sax, Paul E MD [Inf] - **Spec Exp:** AIDS/HIV; **Hospital:** Brigham and Women's Hosp (page 57); **Address:** Brigham & Women's Hosp, Div Infectious Disease, 15 Francis St Fl 4, Boston, MA 02115; **Phone:** 617-732-8881; **Board Cert:** Internal Medicine 2000; Infectious Disease 2000; **Med School:** Harvard Med Sch 1987; **Resid:** Internal Medicine, Brigham & Womens Hosp 1990; **Fellow:** Infectious Disease, Mass Genl Hosp 1992

Mid Atlantic

Auwaerter, Paul MD [Inf] - **Spec Exp:** Lyme Disease; Ehrlichiosis; Tick-borne Diseases; Fevers of Unknown Origin; **Hospital:** Johns Hopkins Hosp (page 61); **Address:** 10751 Falls Rd, Ste 412, Lutherville, MD 21093; **Phone:** 410-583-2900; **Board Cert:** Internal Medicine 2002; Infectious Disease 2004; **Med School:** Columbia P&S 1988; **Resid:** Internal Medicine, Johns Hopkins Med Ctr 1992; **Fellow:** Infectious Disease, Johns Hopkins Med Ctr 1996; **Fac Appt:** Assoc Prof Med, Johns Hopkins Univ

Bartlett, John G MD [Inf] - **Spec Exp:** AIDS/HIV; Fevers of Unknown Origin; Pseudomembranous Colitis; **Hospital:** Johns Hopkins Hosp (page 61); **Address:** 1830 E Monument St, Ste 447, Baltimore, MD 21287; **Phone:** 410-955-7634; **Board Cert:** Internal Medicine 1972; **Med School:** SUNY Upstate Med Univ 1963; **Resid:** Internal Medicine, Peter Bent Brigham Hosp 1965; Internal Medicine, Univ Hosp Birmingham 1968; **Fellow:** Infectious Disease, Wadsworth VA Hosp 1970

Berkowitz, Leonard B MD [Inf] - **Spec Exp:** AIDS/HIV; **Hospital:** Brooklyn Hosp Ctr-Downtown; **Address:** 121 DeKalb Ave, rm 5H, Brooklyn, NY 11201-5425; **Phone:** 718-250-6922; **Board Cert:** Internal Medicine 1980; Infectious Disease 1984; **Med School:** SUNY Downstate 1977; **Resid:** Internal Medicine, Kings Co Med Ctr 1981; **Fellow:** Infectious Disease, Kings Co Med Ctr 1983; **Fac Appt:** Asst Clin Prof Med, SUNY Hlth Sci Ctr

Brause, Barry MD [Inf] - **Spec Exp:** Bone/Joint Infections; Skin/Soft Tissue Infections; Infections in Prosthetic Devices; **Hospital:** Hosp For Special Surgery (page 60), NY-Presby/Weill Cornell Med Ctr, NY (page 65); **Address:** 535 E 70th St, New York, NY 10021-5718; **Phone:** 212-774-7411; **Board Cert:** Internal Medicine 1973; Infectious Disease 1976; **Med School:** Univ Pittsburgh 1970; **Resid:** Internal Medicine, NY Hosp 1973; **Fellow:** Infectious Disease, NY Hosp 1975; **Fac Appt:** Clin Prof Med, Cornell Univ-Weill Med Coll

Chaisson, Richard E MD [Inf] - **Spec Exp:** AIDS/HIV; Tuberculosis; **Hospital:** Johns Hopkins Hosp (page 61); **Address:** 1550 Orleans St, 1M-08, Baltimore, MD 21231; **Phone:** 410-955-1755; **Board Cert:** Internal Medicine 1985; **Med School:** Univ Mass Sch Med 1982; **Resid:** Internal Medicine, UCSF Med Ctr 1985; **Fellow:** Infectious Disease, UCSF Med Ctr 1987; **Fac Appt:** Prof Med, Johns Hopkins Univ

Cunha, Burke A MD [Inf] - **Spec Exp:** Infections in Immunocompromised Patients; Fevers of Unknown Origin; Pneumonia; Chronic Fatigue Syndrome; **Hospital:** Winthrop Univ Hosp; **Address:** 222 Station Plz N, Ste 432, Mineola, NY 11501; **Phone:** 516-663-2507; **Board Cert:** Internal Medicine 1977; Infectious Disease 1978; **Med School:** Penn State Coll Med 1972; **Resid:** Internal Medicine, Hartford Hosp 1975; **Fellow:** Infectious Disease, Hartford Hosp 1977; **Fac Appt:** Prof Med, SUNY Stony Brook

Fauci, Anthony S MD [Inf] - **Spec Exp:** AIDS/HIV; Immunotherapy; **Hospital:** Natl Inst of Hlth - Clin Ctr; **Address:** NIAID Bldg 31 - rm 7A03, 31 Center Drive, MSC 2520, Bethesda, MD 20892-2520; **Phone:** 301-496-2263; **Board Cert:** Internal Medicine 1972; Allergy & Immunology 1974; Infectious Disease 1974; **Med School:** Cornell Univ-Weill Med Coll 1966; **Resid:** Internal Medicine, New York Hosp Cornell Med Ctr 1972; **Fellow:** Infectious Disease, Natl Inst Infectious Disease NIH 1971

Frank, Ian MD [Inf] - **Spec Exp:** AIDS/HIV; **Hospital:** Hosp Univ Penn - UPHS (page 68); **Address:** Hosp U Penn, Div Infectious Disease, 3400 Spruce St, Sliverstein Bldg, Fl 3 - Ste D, Philadelphia, PA 19104; **Phone:** 215-662-6932; **Board Cert:** Internal Medicine 1983; Infectious Disease 2006; **Med School:** Dartmouth Med Sch 1980; **Resid:** Internal Medicine, Graduate Hosp 1983; **Fellow:** Infectious Disease, Hosp Univ Penn 1984; **Fac Appt:** Prof Med, Univ Pennsylvania

Gumprecht, Jeffrey P MD [Inf] - **Spec Exp:** AIDS/HIV; Travel Medicine; Infections-Surgical; **Hospital:** Mount Sinai Med Ctr (page 63); **Address:** 1100 Park Ave, New York, NY 10128; **Phone:** 212-427-9550; **Board Cert:** Internal Medicine 1987; Infectious Disease 2003; **Med School:** Albany Med Coll 1983; **Resid:** Internal Medicine, Mt Sinai Hosp 1987; **Fellow:** Infectious Disease, Montefiore Med Ctr 1990; **Fac Appt:** Asst Clin Prof Med, Mount Sinai Sch Med

Hammer, Glenn MD [Inf] - **Spec Exp:** AIDS/HIV; Hospital Acquired Infections; Infections-Surgical; **Hospital:** Mount Sinai Med Ctr (page 63); **Address:** 1100 Park Ave, New York, NY 10128-1202; **Phone:** 212-427-9550; **Board Cert:** Infectious Disease 1974; Internal Medicine 1973; **Med School:** NYU Sch Med 1969; **Resid:** Internal Medicine, Mount Sinai Hosp 1972; **Fellow:** Infectious Disease, Mount Sinai Hosp 1974; **Fac Appt:** Asst Clin Prof Med, Mount Sinai Sch Med

Hammer, Scott M MD [Inf] - **Spec Exp:** AIDS/HIV; **Hospital:** NY-Presby/Columbia Univ Med Ctr, NY (page 65); **Address:** 630 W 168th St, P&S Box 82, New York, NY 10032; **Phone:** 212-305-8039; **Board Cert:** Internal Medicine 1975; Infectious Disease 1980; **Med School:** Columbia P&S 1972; **Resid:** Internal Medicine, Columbia-Presby Hosp 1975; Internal Medicine, Stanford Univ Hosp 1975; **Fellow:** Infectious Disease, Mass Genl Hosp 1981; **Fac Appt:** Prof Med, Columbia P&S

Infectious Disease

Hartman, Barry Jay MD [Inf] - **Spec Exp:** Endocarditis; Infections-Surgical; Parasitic Infections; **Hospital:** NY-Presby/Weill Cornell Med Ctr, NY (page 65); **Address:** 407 E 70th St, Fl 4, New York, NY 10021-5302; **Phone:** 212-744-4882; **Board Cert:** Internal Medicine 1976; Infectious Disease 1980; **Med School:** Penn State Coll Med 1973; **Resid:** Internal Medicine, NY Hosp/Cornell Med Ctr 1976; **Fellow:** Infectious Disease, NY Hosp/Cornell Med Ctr 1981; **Fac Appt:** Clin Prof Med, Cornell Univ-Weill Med Coll

Lorber, Bennett MD [Inf] - **Spec Exp:** Foodborne illnesses; **Hospital:** Temple Univ Hosp; **Address:** Temple Univ Hosp - Inf Diseases, 3401 N Broad St, Parkinson Pavilion, Ste 500, Philadelphia, PA 19140; **Phone:** 215-707-3807; **Board Cert:** Internal Medicine 1974; Infectious Disease 1976; **Med School:** Univ Pennsylvania 1968; **Resid:** Internal Medicine, Temple Univ Hosp 1971; **Fellow:** Infectious Disease, Temple Univ Hosp 1973; **Fac Appt:** Prof Med, Temple Univ

Louie, Eddie MD [Inf] - **Spec Exp:** Lyme Disease; AIDS/HIV; Hospital Acquired Infections; **Hospital:** NYU Langone Med Ctr (page 66); **Address:** 345 E 37th St, Ste 207, New York, NY 10016; **Phone:** 212-682-9202; **Board Cert:** Internal Medicine 1982; Infectious Disease 1986; **Med School:** NYU Sch Med 1979; **Resid:** Internal Medicine, Kings County Hosp 1983; **Fellow:** Infectious Disease, NYU Med Ctr 1985; **Fac Appt:** Assoc Clin Prof Med, NYU Sch Med

Masur, Henry MD [Inf] - **Spec Exp:** Critical Care; AIDS/HIV; **Hospital:** Natl Inst of Hlth - Clin Ctr; **Address:** National Inst Hlth, 10 Center Drive, Clinical Ctr 7D43, Bethesda, MD 20892; **Phone:** 301-496-9320; **Board Cert:** Internal Medicine 1975; Infectious Disease 1978; **Med School:** Cornell Univ-Weill Med Coll 1972; **Resid:** Internal Medicine, New York Hosp 1974; Internal Medicine, Johns Hopkins Hosp 1975; **Fellow:** Infectious Disease, New York Hosp-Cornell 1977

McGowan, Joseph MD [Inf] - **Spec Exp:** AIDS/HIV; HIV in Pregnancy; HIV/Hepatitis Co-Infection; AIDS/HIV in Elderly; **Hospital:** NS-LIJ Hlth Sys; **Address:** 400 Community Drive, Manhasset, NY 11030; **Phone:** 516-562-4280; **Board Cert:** Internal Medicine 2002; Infectious Disease 2002; **Med School:** Mount Sinai Sch Med 1987; **Resid:** Internal Medicine, Montefiore Med Ctr 1990; **Fellow:** Infectious Disease, Montefiore Med Ctr 1993

Mildvan, Donna MD [Inf] - **Spec Exp:** AIDS/HIV; Clinical Trials; Infectious Disease; **Hospital:** Beth Israel Med Ctr - Petrie Division (page 55); **Address:** Beth Israel Med Ctr, Div Infectious Dis, 1st Ave at 16th St, 19BH17, New York, NY 10003; **Phone:** 212-420-4005; **Board Cert:** Internal Medicine 1972; Infectious Disease 1972; **Med School:** Johns Hopkins Univ 1967; **Resid:** Internal Medicine, Mt Sinai Hosp 1970; **Fellow:** Infectious Disease, Mt Sinai Hosp 1972; **Fac Appt:** Prof Med, Albert Einstein Coll Med

Nahass, Ronald MD [Inf] - **Spec Exp:** Hepatitis B & C; Lyme Disease; Wound Healing/Care; Bone Infections; **Hospital:** Robert Wood Johnson Univ Hosp - New Brunswick, Univ Med Ctr - Princeton; **Address:** 105 Raider Blvd, Ste 101, Hillsborough, NJ 08844-4254; **Phone:** 908-281-0221; **Board Cert:** Internal Medicine 1985; Infectious Disease 1988; **Med School:** UMDNJ-RW Johnson Med Sch 1982; **Resid:** Internal Medicine, RWJ Univ Hosp 1986; **Fellow:** Infectious Disease, RWJ Univ Hosp 1988; **Fac Appt:** Clin Prof Med, UMDNJ-RW Johnson Med Sch

Perlman, David MD [Inf] - **Spec Exp:** AIDS/HIV; Lyme Disease; Travel Medicine; Infectious Disease; **Hospital:** Beth Israel Med Ctr - Petrie Division (page 55), Lenox Hill Hosp; **Address:** Beth Israel Med Ctr, 120 E 16th St, Ste 12, New York, NY 10003; **Phone:** 212-844-8549; **Board Cert:** Internal Medicine 1986; Infectious Disease 1988; **Med School:** Albert Einstein Coll Med 1983; **Resid:** Internal Medicine, New York Hosp/Meml Sloan Kettering 1986; **Fellow:** Infectious Disease, Montefiore Hosp 1988; **Fac Appt:** Prof Med, Albert Einstein Coll Med

Polsky, Bruce W MD [Inf] - **Spec Exp:** AIDS/HIV; Viral Infections; Infections in Cancer Patients; AIDS Related Cancers; **Hospital:** St. Luke's - Roosevelt Hosp Ctr - Roosevelt Div (page 55); **Address:** 1111 Amsterdam Ave, New York, NY 10025-1716; **Phone:** 212-523-7335; **Board Cert:** Internal Medicine 1983; Infectious Disease 1986; **Med School:** Wayne State Univ 1980; **Resid:** Internal Medicine, Montefiore Hosp 1983; **Fellow:** Infectious Disease, Meml Sloan Kettering Cancer Ctr 1986; **Fac Appt:** Prof Med, Columbia P&S

Rao, Nalini G MD [Inf] - **Spec Exp:** Bone/Joint Infections; Tropical Diseases; Travel Medicine; **Hospital:** UPMC Presby, Pittsburgh, UPMC Shadyside; **Address:** Centre Commons, Suite 510, 5750 Centre Ave, Pittsburgh, PA 15206-3721; **Phone:** 412-661-1633; **Board Cert:** Internal Medicine 1975; Infectious Disease 1980; **Med School:** India 1970; **Resid:** Internal Medicine, Geo Wash Univ Hosp 1974; **Fellow:** Infectious Disease, Baylor Coll Med 1975; Infectious Disease, Univ Pittsburgh Sch Med 1977; **Fac Appt:** Clin Prof Med, Univ Pittsburgh

Romagnoli, Mario MD [Inf] - **Spec Exp:** AIDS/HIV; Bone/Joint Infections; **Hospital:** Lenox Hill Hosp; **Address:** 903 Park Ave, New York, NY 10075; **Phone:** 212-396-3390; **Board Cert:** Internal Medicine 1979; Infectious Disease 1982; **Med School:** Columbia P&S 1976; **Resid:** Internal Medicine, Columbia-Presby Med Ctr 1979; **Fellow:** Infectious Disease, Beth Israel Med Ctr 1981; **Fac Appt:** Assoc Prof Med, Columbia P&S

Segal, Brahm H MD [Inf] - **Spec Exp:** Infections in Cancer Patients; Immune Deficiencies-Primary; **Hospital:** Roswell Park Cancer Inst; **Address:** Roswell Park Cancer Inst, Elm & Carlton Streets, Buffalo, NY 14263; **Phone:** 716-845-5721; **Board Cert:** Infectious Disease 2009; **Med School:** Albert Einstein Coll Med 1992; **Resid:** Internal Medicine, New England Med Ctr 1995; **Fellow:** Infectious Disease, Natl Inst Allergy/Inf Dis 1997; **Fac Appt:** Prof Med, SUNY Buffalo

Sepkowitz, Kent MD [Inf] - **Spec Exp:** Tuberculosis; Infections in Cancer Patients; Fungal Infections; **Hospital:** Meml Sloan-Kettering Cancer Ctr; **Address:** 1275 York Ave, New York, NY 10065; **Phone:** 800-525-2225; **Board Cert:** Internal Medicine 1983; Infectious Disease 2010; **Med School:** Univ Okla Coll Med 1980; **Resid:** Internal Medicine, Roosevelt Hosp 1984; **Fellow:** Infectious Disease, Meml Sloan Kettering Cancer Ctr 1991; **Fac Appt:** Prof Med, Cornell Univ-Weill Med Coll

Wallach, Frances MD [Inf] - **Spec Exp:** AIDS/HIV; Infection Control; HIV & Blood Transfusions; **Hospital:** Mount Sinai Med Ctr (page 63); **Address:** Mount Sinai Medical Ctr, One Gustave L Levy Pl, Box 1090, New York, NY 10029; **Phone:** 212-241-7968; **Board Cert:** Internal Medicine 1989; Infectious Disease 2002; **Med School:** Albany Med Coll 1985; **Resid:** Internal Medicine, Montefiore Med Ctr 1989; **Fellow:** Nuclear Medicine, Montefiore Med Ctr 1990; Infectious Disease, NY Hosp-Cornell Med Ctr 1992; **Fac Appt:** Asst Prof Med, Mount Sinai Sch Med

Wormser, Gary P MD [Inf] - **Spec Exp:** Lyme Disease; AIDS/HIV; Diagnostic Problems; **Hospital:** Westchester Med Ctr; **Address:** New York Medical College, Munger Pavilion, rm 245, Valhalla, NY 10595; **Phone:** 914-493-8865; **Board Cert:** Internal Medicine 1978; Infectious Disease 1982; **Med School:** Johns Hopkins Univ 1972; **Resid:** Internal Medicine, Mt Sinai Hosp 1975; **Fellow:** Infectious Disease, Mt Sinai Hosp 1977; **Fac Appt:** Prof Med, NY Med Coll

Yancovitz, Stanley MD [Inf] - **Spec Exp:** Lyme Disease; AIDS/HIV; **Hospital:** Beth Israel Med Ctr - Petrie Division (page 55); **Address:** 1st Ave at 16th St, Ste 17 BH10, New York, NY 10003; **Phone:** 212-420-2600; **Board Cert:** Internal Medicine 1973; Infectious Disease 1976; **Med School:** SUNY Downstate 1967; **Resid:** Internal Medicine, Metropolitan Hosp 1969; Internal Medicine, Beth Israel Med Ctr 1972; **Fellow:** Infectious Disease, Mt Sinai Hosp 1975; **Fac Appt:** Clin Prof Med, Albert Einstein Coll Med

Infectious Disease

Yu, Victor L MD [Inf] - **Spec Exp:** Legionnaire's Disease; Pneumonia; Staphylococcal Infections; Skin/Soft Tissue Infections; **Hospital:** UPMC Presby, Pittsburgh; **Address:** University of Pittsburgh, 1401 Forbes Ave, Ste 209, Pittsburgh, PA 15219; **Phone:** 412-901-7707; **Board Cert:** Internal Medicine 1978; Infectious Disease 1982; **Med School:** Univ Minn 1970; **Resid:** Internal Medicine, Univ Colo Med Ctr 1972; Internal Medicine, Stanford Univ Med Ctr 1975; **Fellow:** Infectious Disease, Stanford Univ Med Ctr 1977; **Fac Appt:** Prof Med, Univ Pittsburgh

Southeast

Alvarez-Elcoro, Salvador MD [Inf] - **Spec Exp:** Tuberculosis; Travel Medicine; Infections-Transplant; **Hospital:** Mayo - Jacksonville; **Address:** Mayo Clinic, Div Infectious Disease, 4500 San Pablo Rd, Jacksonville, FL 32224; **Phone:** 904-953-2272; **Board Cert:** Internal Medicine 1977; Infectious Disease 1982; **Med School:** Mexico 1972; **Resid:** Internal Medicine, Charity Hosp 1977; **Fellow:** Infectious Disease, Boston City Hosp 1979; **Fac Appt:** Prof Med, Univ Fla Coll Med

Blumberg, Henry M MD [Inf] - **Spec Exp:** Tuberculosis; **Hospital:** Grady Hlth Sys, Emory Univ Hosp; **Address:** Emory Univ, Div Infectious Diseases, 49 Jesse Hill Jr Drive, Atlanta, GA 30303; **Phone:** 404-616-6145; **Board Cert:** Internal Medicine 1986; Infectious Disease 2010; **Med School:** Vanderbilt Univ 1983; **Resid:** Internal Medicine, Emory Univ Affil Hosps 1986; Internal Medicine, Crawford-Long Hosp 1988; **Fellow:** Infectious Disease, Emory Univ Affil Hosps 1992; **Fac Appt:** Prof Med, Emory Univ

Cancio, Margarita MD [Inf] - **Spec Exp:** AIDS/HIV; **Hospital:** Tampa Genl Hosp; **Address:** 4729 N Habana Ave, Tampa, FL 33614; **Phone:** 813-251-8444; **Board Cert:** Internal Medicine 1985; Infectious Disease 1988; **Med School:** Univ S Fla Coll Med 1982; **Resid:** Internal Medicine, Univ S Florida Affil Hosps 1985; **Fellow:** Infectious Disease, Univ S Florida Affil Hosps 1988; **Fac Appt:** Assoc Prof Med, Univ S Fla Coll Med

Cohen, Myron S MD [Inf] - **Spec Exp:** Infections in Immunocompromised Patients; **Hospital:** NC Memorial Hosp - UNC; **Address:** UNC-Chapel Hill, Div Infectious Disease, 130 Mason Farm Rd, Ste 2115, Box CB 7030, Chapel Hill, NC 27599-7030; **Phone:** 919-966-7199; **Board Cert:** Internal Medicine 1977; Infectious Disease 1982; **Med School:** Rush Med Coll 1974; **Resid:** Internal Medicine, Univ Michigan Hlth Ctr 1977; **Fellow:** Infectious Disease, Yale-New Haven Hosp 1979; **Fac Appt:** Prof Med, Univ NC Sch Med

Corey, G Ralph MD [Inf] - **Spec Exp:** Tropical Diseases; Travel Medicine; Endocarditis; Staphylococcal Infections; **Hospital:** Duke Univ Hosp; **Address:** Duke Univ Med Ctr, Box 90519, Durham, NC 27708; **Phone:** 919-668-7174; **Board Cert:** Internal Medicine 1977; Infectious Disease 1980; **Med School:** Baylor Coll Med 1973; **Resid:** Internal Medicine, Duke Univ Med Ctr 1978; **Fellow:** Infectious Disease, Duke Univ Med Ctr 1980; **Fac Appt:** Prof Med, Duke Univ

Edmond, Michael B MD [Inf] - **Spec Exp:** Bone/Joint Infections; Skin/Soft Tissue Infections; Antibiotic Resistance; Hospital Acquired Infections; **Hospital:** Med Coll of VA Hosp; **Address:** VCU/Med College Virginia, Box 980019, Richmond, VA 23298-0019; **Phone:** 804-828-2121; **Board Cert:** Internal Medicine 1989; Infectious Disease 2002; **Med School:** W VA Univ 1986; **Resid:** Internal Medicine, W Virginia Univ Hosps 1989; **Fellow:** Infectious Disease, Univ Pittsburgh 1992; Epidemiology, Univ Iowa; **Fac Appt:** Prof Med, Med Coll VA

Gorensek, Margaret J MD [Inf] - **Spec Exp:** AIDS/HIV; Infections-Transplant; Chronic Fatigue Syndrome; Pediatric Infectious Disease; **Hospital:** Holy Cross Hosp - Fort Lauderdale, Broward General Med Ctr; **Address:** Holy Cross Medical Group, 1930 NE 47th St, Ste 104, Fort Lauderdale, FL 33308; **Phone:** 954-493-9752; **Board Cert:** Internal Medicine 1985; Pediatrics 1986; Infectious Disease 1988; Pediatric Infectious Disease 2009; **Med School:** Case West Res Univ 1981; **Resid:** Internal Medicine & Pediatrics, Cleveland Clin Fdn 1985; **Fellow:** Infectious Disease, Cleveland Clin Fdn 1987; Pediatric Infectious Disease, Chldns Med Ctr 1988; **Fac Appt:** Asst Clin Prof Med, Univ Miami Sch Med

High, Kevin P MD [Inf] - **Hospital:** Wake Forest Univ Baptist Med Ctr; **Address:** Wake Forest Univ School Of Med, Section Of Infectious Disease, Winston-Salem, NC 27157; **Phone:** 336-716-4584; **Board Cert:** Internal Medicine 2009; Infectious Disease 2002; **Med School:** Univ VA Sch Med 1986; **Resid:** Internal Medicine, Univ VA Hlth Sys 1989; **Fellow:** Infectious Disease, Yale-New Haven Hosp 1993; **Fac Appt:** Prof Med, Wake Forest Univ

Katner, Harold P MD [Inf] - **Spec Exp:** AIDS/HIV; **Hospital:** Med Ctr of Central GA; **Address:** Mercer Univ Sch Med, Dept Internal Med, 707 Pine St, Macon, GA 31201; **Phone:** 478-301-5809; **Board Cert:** Internal Medicine 1983; Infectious Disease 1986; **Med School:** Louisiana State U, New Orleans 1980; **Resid:** Internal Medicine, Univ Med Ctr 1983; **Fellow:** Infectious Disease, Ochsner Fdn Hosp 1986; **Fac Appt:** Prof Med, Mercer Univ Sch Med

Pearson, Richard D MD [Inf] - **Spec Exp:** Tropical Diseases; Travel Medicine; Infectious Disease; Parasitic Infections; **Hospital:** Univ of Virginia Health Sys; **Address:** Univ VA Sch Med, Dept Internal Med, Box 800739, Charlottesville, VA 22908-0001; **Phone:** 434-924-5579; **Board Cert:** Internal Medicine 1976; Infectious Disease 1980; **Med School:** Univ Mich Med Sch 1973; **Resid:** Internal Medicine, Strong Meml Hosp 1976; **Fellow:** Infectious Disease, Strong Meml Hosp 1979; **Fac Appt:** Prof Med, Univ VA Sch Med

Ratzan, Kenneth MD [Inf] - **Spec Exp:** AIDS/HIV; **Hospital:** Mount Sinai Med Ctr - Miami, Miami Heart Inst; **Address:** Mount Sinai Med Ctr, 4300 Alton Rd, Ste 450, Miami Beach, FL 33140-2800; **Phone:** 305-673-5490; **Board Cert:** Internal Medicine 1977; Infectious Disease 1974; **Med School:** Harvard Med Sch 1965; **Resid:** Internal Medicine, Columbia Presby Med Ctr 1967; Infectious Disease, Tufts New England Med Ctr 1972; **Fellow:** Infectious Disease, Tufts New England Med Ctr 1971; **Fac Appt:** Prof Med, Univ Miami Sch Med

Saag, Michael S MD [Inf] - **Spec Exp:** AIDS/HIV; Clinical Trials; **Hospital:** Univ of Ala Hosp at Birmingham; **Address:** UAB Div Infectious Diseases, 1530 3rd Ave S, BBRB 256, Birmingham, AL 35294; **Phone:** 205-934-7349; **Board Cert:** Internal Medicine 1985; Infectious Disease 1988; **Med School:** Univ Louisville Sch Med 1981; **Resid:** Internal Medicine, Univ Ala Hosp 1984; **Fellow:** Infectious Disease, Univ Alabama 1987; **Fac Appt:** Prof Med, Univ Alabama

Scheld, W Michael MD [Inf] - **Spec Exp:** Meningitis; Septic Shock; AIDS/HIV; Antibiotic Resistance; **Hospital:** Univ of Virginia Health Sys; **Address:** Univ VA Hlth Sci Ctr, PO Box 801342, Charlottesville, VA 22908; **Phone:** 434-924-5991; **Board Cert:** Internal Medicine 1976; Infectious Disease 1978; **Med School:** Cornell Univ-Weill Med Coll 1973; **Resid:** Internal Medicine, Univ VA Med Ctr 1976; **Fellow:** Infectious Disease, Univ VA Med Ctr 1979; **Fac Appt:** Prof Med, Univ VA Sch Med

Van Der Horst, Charles M MD [Inf] - **Spec Exp:** AIDS/HIV; Fungal Infections; Viral Infections; Immune Deficiency; **Hospital:** NC Memorial Hosp - UNC; **Address:** Univ NC-Dept Med, 101 Manning Drive, Box CB 7030, Chapel Hill, NC 27514; **Phone:** 919-966-7199; **Board Cert:** Internal Medicine 1982; Infectious Disease 1986; **Med School:** Harvard Med Sch 1979; **Resid:** Internal Medicine, Montefiore Med Ctr 1982; **Fellow:** Infectious Disease, NC Meml Hosp 1985; **Fac Appt:** Prof Med, Univ NC Sch Med

Infectious Disease

Wallace, Mark R MD [Inf] - **Spec Exp:** Fever in Returning Travelers; Travel Medicine; Valley Fever; HIV; **Hospital:** Orlando Regl Med Ctr; **Address:** 77 W Underwood Fl 4 - Ste 4B, Orlando, FL 32806; **Phone:** 321-841-7750; **Board Cert:** Internal Medicine 1984; Infectious Disease 2010; **Med School:** St Louis Univ 1981; **Resid:** Internal Medicine, Univ Washington Hosp 1984; **Fellow:** Infectious Disease, Naval Hosp 1989; **Fac Appt:** Clin Prof Med, FSU College Medicine

Midwest

Bakken, Johan S MD/PhD [Inf] - **Spec Exp:** Human Granulocytic Anaplasmosis; Tick-borne Diseases; Diarrheal Diseases; Ehrlichiosis; **Hospital:** St. Luke's Hosp - Duluth, St. Mary's Med Ctr - Duluth; **Address:** 1001 E Superior St, Ste L201, Duluth, MN 55802; **Phone:** 218-249-7990; **Board Cert:** Internal Medicine 2008; **Med School:** Univ Wash 1972; **Resid:** Internal Medicine, Univ Wash Hosps 1978; Internal Medicine, Lillehammer Fylkessykehus 1981; **Fellow:** Infectious Disease, Ulleval Hosp 1985; Microbiology, Creighton Univ 1987; **Fac Appt:** Assoc Clin Prof FMed, Univ Minn

Campbell, J William MD [Inf] - **Spec Exp:** AIDS/HIV; **Hospital:** St. Luke's Hosp - Chesterfield, MO, Barnes-Jewish Hosp; **Address:** 222 S Woodsmill Rd, Ste 750N, Chesterfield, MO 63017; **Phone:** 314-205-6600; **Board Cert:** Internal Medicine 1980; Infectious Disease 1982; **Med School:** Washington Univ, St Louis 1977; **Resid:** Internal Medicine, Barnes Hosp-Wash Univ 1980; **Fellow:** Infectious Disease, Univ Tex Hlth Sci Ctr 1981; Infectious Disease, Wash Univ 1982; **Fac Appt:** Clin Prof Med, Washington Univ, St Louis

Cohn, Susan E MD [Inf] - **Spec Exp:** AIDS/HIV; AIDS/HIV in Women; Women's Health; HIV in Pregnancy; **Hospital:** Northwestern Meml Hosp; **Address:** 676 N St Clair, Ste 940, Chicago, IL 60611; **Phone:** 312-926-8358; **Board Cert:** Internal Medicine 1987; Infectious Disease 2005; **Med School:** Cornell Univ 1984; **Resid:** Internal Medicine, Boston City Hosp 1987; **Fellow:** Infectious Disease, Univ NC Affil Hosp 1992; **Fac Appt:** Prof Med, Northwestern Univ-Feinberg Sch Med

Fichtenbaum, Carl J MD [Inf] - **Spec Exp:** AIDS/HIV; **Hospital:** Univ Hosp - Cincinnati; **Address:** 231 Albert Sabin Way, ML 0560, Cincinnati, OH 45267; **Phone:** 513-584-6977; **Board Cert:** Infectious Disease 2004; Internal Medicine 2004; **Med School:** Univ MO-Kansas City 1985; **Resid:** Internal Medicine, Bridgeport Hosp 1989; Pediatrics, Bridgeport Hosp 1989; **Fellow:** Infectious Disease, Yale-New Haven Hosp 1991; Infectious Disease, Washington Univ Med Ctr 1992; **Fac Appt:** Prof Med, Univ Cincinnati

Flaherty, John P MD [Inf] - **Spec Exp:** AIDS/HIV; Travel Medicine; Orthopaedic Infectious Disease; **Hospital:** Northwestern Meml Hosp; **Address:** 676 N St Clair St, Ste 940, Chicago, IL 60611; **Phone:** 312-926-8358; **Board Cert:** Internal Medicine 1986; Infectious Disease 1988; **Med School:** Univ IL Coll Med 1983; **Resid:** Internal Medicine, Univ Iowa Hosp 1986; **Fellow:** Infectious Disease, Univ Chicago Hosps 1988; **Fac Appt:** Prof Med, Northwestern Univ

Longworth, David L MD [Inf] - **Spec Exp:** HIV; **Hospital:** Cleveland Clin (page 56); **Address:** Clevelan Clin, 9500 Euclid Ave, MC G10, Cleveland, OH 44195; **Phone:** 216-444-5665; **Board Cert:** Internal Medicine 1981; Infectious Disease 1984; **Med School:** Cornell Univ-Weill Med Coll 1978; **Resid:** Internal Medicine, UCSF-HC Moffitt Hosp 1981; **Fellow:** Infectious Disease, Brigham & Womens Hosp 1983; Research, Harvard Med School 1985; **Fac Appt:** Prof Med, Tufts Univ

Maki, Dennis G MD [Inf] - **Spec Exp:** Urinary Tract Infections; Critical Care; **Hospital:** Univ WI Hosp & Clins; **Address:** 600 Highland Ave, MC B6/242, Madison, WI 53792-2442; **Phone:** 608-263-0946; **Board Cert:** Internal Medicine 1972; Infectious Disease 1974; **Med School:** Univ Wisc 1967; **Resid:** Infectious Disease, Mass Genl Hosp 1972; Internal Medicine, Harvard-Boston City Hosp 1973; **Fellow:** Infectious Disease, Mass Genl Hosp 1974; **Fac Appt:** Prof Med, Univ Wisc

O'Keefe, J Paul MD [Inf] - **Spec Exp:** AIDS/HIV; Fungal Infections; Infections-Surgical; Travel Medicine; **Hospital:** Loyola Univ Med Ctr; **Address:** 2160 S 1st Ave, Maywood, IL 60153-3304; **Phone:** 708-216-0160; **Board Cert:** Internal Medicine 1974; Infectious Disease 1978; **Med School:** Loyola Univ-Stritch Sch Med 1971; **Resid:** Internal Medicine, Loyola Univ Med Ctr 1974; **Fellow:** Infectious Disease, VA Hosp 1975; Infectious Disease, Tufts New England Med Ctr 1977; **Fac Appt:** Prof Med, Loyola Univ-Stritch Sch Med

Salata, Robert A MD [Inf] - **Spec Exp:** AIDS/HIV; **Hospital:** Univ Hosps Case Med Ctr (page 74); **Address:** UH Case Medical Center, Infectious Disease-Foley Bldg 411, 11100 Euclid Ave, Cleveland, OH 44106; **Phone:** 216-844-1709; **Board Cert:** Internal Medicine 1982; Infectious Disease 1986; **Med School:** Case West Res Univ 1979; **Resid:** Internal Medicine, Case Med Ctr 1982; **Fellow:** Infectious Disease, Univ VA Med Ctr 1985; **Fac Appt:** Prof Med, Case West Res Univ

Schmitt, Steven K MD [Inf] - **Spec Exp:** Bone/Joint Infections; **Hospital:** Cleveland Clin (page 56); **Address:** Cleveland Clinc Main Campus, MC G21, 9500 Euclid Ave, Cleveland, OH 44195; **Phone:** 216-444-8845; **Board Cert:** Internal Medicine 2002; **Med School:** Univ Cincinnati 1988; **Resid:** Internal Medicine, Cleveland Clin 1991; **Fellow:** Infectious Disease, Cleveland Clin 1994

Sha, Beverly MD [Inf] - **Spec Exp:** AIDS/HIV in Women; **Hospital:** Rush Univ Med Ctr; **Address:** 600 S Paulina St, Ste 140-143, Chicago, IL 60612-3806; **Phone:** 312-942-5865; **Board Cert:** Internal Medicine 1989; Infectious Disease 2002; **Med School:** Johns Hopkins Univ 1986; **Resid:** Internal Medicine, Rush-Presby St Lukes Med Ctr 1989; **Fellow:** Infectious Disease, Rush-Presby St Lukes Med Ctr 1991; **Fac Appt:** Assoc Prof Med, Rush Med Coll

Slama, Thomas G MD [Inf] - **Spec Exp:** Hematologic Infections; Bone Infections; Infective Endocarditis; Infections in Prosthetic Devices; **Hospital:** St. Vincent Indianapolis Hosp; **Address:** 8240 Naab Rd, Ste 300, Indianapolis, IN 46260; **Phone:** 317-870-1970; **Board Cert:** Internal Medicine 1976; Infectious Disease 1978; **Med School:** Indiana Univ 1973; **Resid:** Internal Medicine, Indianapolis Meth Hosp 1976; **Fellow:** Infectious Disease, Ohio State Univ Hosps 1978; **Fac Appt:** Clin Prof Med, Indiana Univ

Sobel, Jack MD [Inf] - **Spec Exp:** Vaginitis; Fungal Infections; Urinary Tract Infections; **Hospital:** Harper Univ Hosp, Detroit Receiving Hospital; **Address:** 3750 Woodward Ave, Ste 200, Detroit, MI 48201; **Phone:** 313-745-9035; **Board Cert:** Internal Medicine 1978; Infectious Disease 1982; **Med School:** South Africa 1965; **Resid:** Internal Medicine 1970; **Fellow:** Infectious Disease, Univ Penn Hosps 1977; Research, Natl Inst Hlth 1978; **Fac Appt:** Prof Med, Wayne State Univ

Tomford, J Walton MD [Inf] - **Hospital:** Cleveland Clin (page 56); **Address:** Cleveland Clinic, Dept Infectious Diseases, 9500 Euclid Ave, Desk G21, Cleveland, OH 44195; **Phone:** 216-444-2764; **Board Cert:** Internal Medicine 1978; Infectious Disease 1980; **Med School:** Johns Hopkins Univ 1975; **Resid:** Internal Medicine, Johns Hopkins Hosp 1978; Internal Medicine, Univ Hosps 1981; **Fellow:** Infectious Disease, Cleveland Univ Hosp 1980; **Fac Appt:** Assoc Prof Med, Cleveland Cl Coll Med/Case West Res

Trenholme, Gordon M MD [Inf] - **Spec Exp:** Fevers of Unknown Origin; Malaria; Tropical Diseases; **Hospital:** Rush Univ Med Ctr; **Address:** Rush Univ Med Ctr, Infectious Disease, 600 S Paulina St, Ste 143, Chicago, IL 60612-3809; **Phone:** 312-942-3665; **Board Cert:** Internal Medicine 1972; Infectious Disease 1976; **Med School:** Med Coll Wisc 1970; **Resid:** Internal Medicine, Univ Chicago Hosp 1973; **Fellow:** Infectious Disease, Rush/Presby-St Luke's Med Ctr 1975; **Fac Appt:** Prof Med, Rush Med Coll

Infectious Disease

Wilson, Walter Ray MD [Inf] - **Spec Exp:** Musculoskeletal Infections; **Hospital:** Mayo Med Ctr & Clin - Rochester; **Address:** Mayo Clin, Div Infectious Disease, 200 First St SW, Rochester, MN 55905; **Phone:** 507-255-7761; **Board Cert:** Internal Medicine 1973; Infectious Disease 1974; Medical Microbiology 1975; **Med School:** Baylor Coll Med 1967; **Resid:** Internal Medicine, Methodist Hosp 1968; Internal Medicine, Mayo Clin 1973; **Fellow:** Infectious Disease, Mayo Clin 1974; Microbiology, Mayo Clin 1975; **Fac Appt:** Prof Med, Mayo Med Sch

Great Plains and Mountains

Freifeld, Alison G MD [Inf] - **Spec Exp:** Infectious Disease during Chemotherapy; Infections in Cancer Patients; **Hospital:** Nebraska Med Ctr; **Address:** Univ Nebraska Med Ctr, 985400 Nebraska Medical Center, Omaha, NE 68198-5400; **Phone:** 402-559-8650; **Board Cert:** Internal Medicine 1985; Infectious Disease 1988; **Med School:** Johns Hopkins Univ 1982; **Resid:** Internal Medicine, Johns Hopkins Univ Med Ctr 1985

Huitt, Gwen A MD [Inf] - **Spec Exp:** Tuberculosis; Cystic Fibrosis; Mycobacterial Infections; **Hospital:** Natl Jewish Med & Rsch Ctr; **Address:** National Jewish Health, 1400 Jackson St, rm J222, Denver, CO 80206; **Phone:** 303-398-1667; **Board Cert:** Internal Medicine 2003; Infectious Disease 2004; **Med School:** Univ Colorado 1988; **Resid:** Internal Medicine, Univ Colorado Hlth Sci Ctr 1991; **Fellow:** Infectious Disease, Univ Colorado Hlth Sci Ctr 1993; **Fac Appt:** Assoc Prof Med, Univ Colorado

Southwest

DuPont, Herbert L MD [Inf] - **Spec Exp:** Tropical Diseases; Diarrheal Diseases; Travel Medicine; **Hospital:** St. Luke's Episcopal Hosp-Houston; **Address:** 6720 Bertner Ave, MC 1-164, Houston, TX 77030-1602; **Phone:** 832-355-4122; **Board Cert:** Internal Medicine 1972; **Med School:** Emory Univ 1965; **Resid:** Internal Medicine, Univ Minn Hosps 1967; **Fellow:** Infectious Disease, Univ Maryland Hosp 1969; **Fac Appt:** Prof Med, Baylor Coll Med

Keiser, Philip MD [Inf] - **Spec Exp:** AIDS/HIV; **Hospital:** UT Med Br at Galveston; **Address:** 301 Harborside Drive, Mail Route 1326, Galveston, TX 77555; **Phone:** 409-722-2222; **Board Cert:** Internal Medicine 1989; **Med School:** Univ MD Sch Med 1986; **Resid:** Internal Medicine, Francis Scott Key Med Ctr 1989; **Fellow:** Infectious Disease, Univ Md 1989; **Fac Appt:** Assoc Prof Med, Univ Tex SW, Dallas

Luby, James P MD [Inf] - **Spec Exp:** Viral Infections; **Hospital:** Parkland Hlth & Hosp Sys, UT Southwestern Med Ctr at Dallas; **Address:** Univ Tex SW Med Ctr, Div Inf Dis, 5323 Harry Hines Blvd, Dallas, TX 75390-9113; **Phone:** 214-648-3480; **Board Cert:** Internal Medicine 1968; Infectious Disease 1972; **Med School:** Northwestern Univ 1961; **Resid:** Internal Medicine, Northwestern Univ 1964; **Fac Appt:** Prof Med, Univ Tex SW, Dallas

Patterson, Jan E Evans MD [Inf] - **Spec Exp:** Hospital Acquired Infections; Antibiotic Resistance; **Hospital:** Univ Hlth Syst-San Antonio; **Address:** 7400 Merton Minter Blvd, MC 111, San Antonio, TX 78229-3900; **Phone:** 210-617-5120; **Board Cert:** Internal Medicine 1985; Infectious Disease 1988; **Med School:** Univ Tex, Houston 1982; **Resid:** Internal Medicine, Vanderbilt Univ Hosp 1985; **Fellow:** Infectious Disease, Yale-New Haven Hosp 1988; **Fac Appt:** Prof Med, Univ Tex, San Antonio

Patterson, Thomas F MD [Inf] - **Spec Exp:** Fungal Infections; **Hospital:** Univ Hlth Syst-San Antonio, Rio Grande State Ctr/S TX Hlthcare Sys; **Address:** Univ Texas HSC, Dept Medicine, Div Infectious Dis, 7703 Floyd Curl Drive, MC 7881, San Antonio, TX 78229-3900; **Phone:** 210-567-4823; **Board Cert:** Internal Medicine 1986; Infectious Disease 2009; **Med School:** Univ Tex, Houston 1983; **Resid:** Internal Medicine, Vanderbilt Univ Hosp 1985; Internal Medicine, Yale-New Haven Hosp 1986; **Fellow:** Infectious Disease, Yale-New Haven Hosp 1989; **Fac Appt:** Prof Med, Univ Tex, San Antonio

Wallace Jr, Richard James MD [Inf] - **Spec Exp:** Non Tuberculous Mycobacteria; Nocardia Infection; **Hospital:** Univ of Texas Hlth Sci Ctr at Tyler; **Address:** 11937 US Hwy 271, Tyler, TX 75708; **Phone:** 903-877-5122; **Board Cert:** Internal Medicine 1975; Infectious Disease 1976; **Med School:** Baylor Coll Med 1972; **Resid:** Internal Medicine, Boston City Hosp 1974; **Fellow:** Infectious Disease, Boston City Hosp 1975; Infectious Disease, Baylor Coll Med 1977

West Coast and Pacific

Ballon-Landa, Gonzalo MD [Inf] - **Spec Exp:** Hospital Acquired Infections; AIDS/HIV; Travel Medicine; **Hospital:** Scripps Mercy Hosp & Med Ctr; **Address:** 4136 Bachman Pl, San Diego, CA 92103; **Phone:** 619-298-1443; **Board Cert:** Internal Medicine 1980; Infectious Disease 1984; **Med School:** Northwestern Univ 1977; **Resid:** Internal Medicine, Evanston Hosp 1981; **Fellow:** Infectious Disease, UCSD Med Ctr 1983

Bayer, Arnold MD [Inf] - **Spec Exp:** Infective Endocarditis; Arthritis-Septic; Coccidioidomycosis; **Hospital:** LAC - Harbor - UCLA Med Ctr, UCLA Ronald Reagan Med Ctr; **Address:** 1124 W Carson St, RB2 Fl 2, Torrance, CA 90502; **Phone:** 310-222-3813; **Board Cert:** Internal Medicine 1973; Infectious Disease 1978; **Med School:** Temple Univ 1970; **Resid:** Internal Medicine, Thomas Jefferson Univ Hosp 1972; Internal Medicine, LAC-Harbor UCLA Med Ctr 1974; **Fellow:** Infectious Disease, VA Med Ctr 1976; Infectious Disease, LAC-Harbor UCLA Med Ctr 1977; **Fac Appt:** Prof Med, UCLA

Daar, Eric S MD [Inf] - **Spec Exp:** AIDS/HIV; **Hospital:** LAC - Harbor - UCLA Med Ctr; **Address:** 1000 W Carson St, Box 449, Torrance, CA 90502; **Phone:** 310-222-2467; **Board Cert:** Internal Medicine 1988; **Med School:** Georgetown Univ 1985; **Resid:** Internal Medicine, Cedars-Sinai Med Ctr 1988; **Fellow:** Infectious Disease, Cedars-Sinai Med Ctr 1991; **Fac Appt:** Prof Med, UCLA-David Geffen Sch Med

Edwards Jr, John Ellis MD [Inf] - **Spec Exp:** Fungal Infections; Infections in Immunocompromised Patients; **Hospital:** LAC - Harbor - UCLA Med Ctr; **Address:** 1124 W Carson St, RB2 Fl 2, Torrance, CA 90502; **Phone:** 310-222-3813; **Board Cert:** Internal Medicine 1980; Infectious Disease 1974; **Med School:** UC Irvine 1968; **Resid:** Internal Medicine, Harbor-UCLA Med Ctr 1971; **Fellow:** Infectious Disease, Harbor-UCLA Med Ctr 1973; **Fac Appt:** Prof Med, UCLA

Palefsky, Joel M MD [Inf] - **Spec Exp:** AIDS Related Cancers; **Hospital:** UCSF - Mt Zion Med Ctr; **Address:** UCSF Med Ctr, Div Infectious Disease, 513 Parnassus Ave, Box 0654, San Francisco, CA 94143; **Phone:** 415-353-7100; **Board Cert:** Internal Medicine 1984; Infectious Disease 1988; **Med School:** McGill Univ 1980; **Resid:** Internal Medicine, Royal Victoria Hosp 1984; **Fellow:** Infectious Disease, Stanford Univ 1989

Richman, Douglas D MD [Inf] - **Spec Exp:** AIDS/HIV; **Hospital:** VA San Diego Hlthcre Sys, UCSD Med Ctr; **Address:** UCSD-Stein Clin Rsch Bldg, 9500 Gilman Drive, MC 0679, La Jolla, CA 92093-0679; **Phone:** 858-552-8585 x7439; **Board Cert:** Internal Medicine 1973; Infectious Disease 1976; **Med School:** Stanford Univ 1970; **Resid:** Internal Medicine, Stanford Univ Hosp 1972; **Fellow:** Infectious Disease, NIAID/NIH 1975; Infectious Disease, Beth Israel/Chldns Hosp 1976; **Fac Appt:** Prof Med, UCSD

Infectious Disease

Schooley, Robert T MD [Inf] - **Spec Exp:** AIDS/HIV; Infectious Disease; **Hospital:** UCSD Med Ctr; **Address:** UCSD - Stein Rsch Bldg, 9500 Gilman Drive, MC 0711, La Jolla, CA 92023-0665; **Phone:** 858-822-0216; **Board Cert:** Internal Medicine 1977; **Med School:** Johns Hopkins Univ 1974; **Resid:** Internal Medicine, Johns Hopkins Hosp 1976; **Fellow:** Infectious Disease, Natl Inst Hlth 1979; Infectious Disease, Mass Genl Hosp 1981; **Fac Appt:** Prof Med, UCSD

Siegel, Martin MD [Inf] - **Spec Exp:** AIDS/HIV; Infections in Cancer Patients; Orthopaedic Infectious Disease; Travel Medicine; **Hospital:** Swedish Med Ctr-First Hill-Seattle; **Address:** The Polyclinic, 1101 Madison St, Ste 900, Seattle, WA 98104; **Phone:** 206-860-4531; **Board Cert:** Internal Medicine 1976; Infectious Disease 1980; **Med School:** Case West Res Univ 1972; **Resid:** Internal Medicine, Univ N Carolina Hosp 1976; **Fellow:** Infectious Disease, Univ Washington Med Ctr 1980; **Fac Appt:** Assoc Clin Prof Med, Univ Wash

Wiviott, Lory David MD [Inf] - **Spec Exp:** AIDS/HIV; **Hospital:** CA Pacific Med Ctr-Pacific Campus, CA Pacific Med Ctr - Davies Campus; **Address:** 2100 Webster St, Ste 400, San Francisco, CA 94115; **Phone:** 415-923-3883; **Board Cert:** Internal Medicine 1986; Infectious Disease 2010; **Med School:** Albert Einstein Coll Med 1982; **Resid:** Internal Medicine, Columbia Presby Med Ctr 1985; **Fellow:** Infectious Disease, UCSF Med Ctr 1989; **Fac Appt:** Asst Clin Prof Med, UCSF

Cleveland Clinic

Every life deserves world class care.

Cleveland Clinic
Infectious Disease
9500 Euclid Avenue
Cleveland, OH 44195

clevelandclinic.org/
infectiousdiseasetopdocs

Infectious Disease

The Department of Infectious Disease, part of the Medicine Institute at Cleveland Clinic, provides patients with technologically advanced, compassionate medical care. We provide inpatient care, including general infectious disease consultation services and sub-specialty service lines including solid organ transplant, bone marrow transplant, bone and joint infections, neuroinfections, cardiothoracic and medical/surgical ICU services. We also provide transition of care to outpatient for all patients discharged on parenteral antimicrobials via our Community Outpatient Parenteral Antimicrobial Therapy Program (CoPAT). Staff members participate in the CoPAT program, which has one of the highest volumes by a single center in the country, and continues to grow.

Our outpatient sub-specialty clinics include:

Bone and Joint Infection Clinic works closely with the Orthopedic & Rheumatic Institute to treat complex infections of the musculoskeletal system.

Endocarditis Clinic evaluates and treats patients with infected heart valves, pacemakers, defibrillators and left ventricular assist devices.

Granuloma Clinic is dedicated to the care of patients with mycobacterial and fungal infections.

HIV/AIDS Clinic provides comprehensive care for HIV-infected patients.

International Travelers' Health Clinic is a full-service travel clinic that provides pre-travel health and safety advice to persons traveling abroad.

MRSA Clinic evaluates and treats patients with recurrent skin infections caused by methicillin-resistant staphylococcus aureus.

Neuroinfection Clinic is staffed with providers to treat infections of the brain, spinal cord and its linings.

Transplant Infectious Disease Clinic provides a vital role in caring for patients who are transplant candidates and recipients.

Offering Same-Day Appointments
Call 800.274.2009.

Treatment Guides

Cleveland Clinic has developed comprehensive treatment guides for many diseases and conditions. To download our free treatment guides, visit clevelandclinic.org/treatmentguides.

Online Medical Second Opinion

Cleveland Clinic's My**Consult** Online Medical Second Opinion program securely connects patients to our physician specialists for more than 1,000 life-changing or life-threatening diagnoses all by the click of a mouse. To learn more, log onto eclevelandclinic.org/myconsult or call 800.223.2273, ext. 43223.

Special Assistance for Out-of-State Patients

Cleveland Clinic Global Patient Services offers a complimentary Medical Concierge service for patients who travel from outside of Ohio. Call 800.223.2273, ext. 55580 or email medicalconcierge@ccf.org.

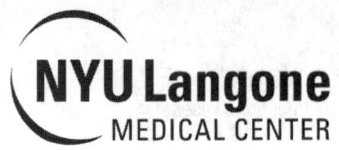

INFECTIOUS DISEASES

About the Division of Infectious Diseases and Immunology

NYU Langone Medical Center has extensive expertise in the diagnosis, treatment and prevention of rare and common acute and chronic infectious diseases. Physicians and fellows within the Division of Infectious Diseases and Immunology are actively involved in the management of complicated bone and joint infections, prevention of infection in cancer and transplant patients and developing strategies for managing hepatitis B and C. They also offer the opportunity for patients with HIV to enroll in clinical trials of new drugs that are not yet widely available. We specialize in the following areas:

HIV Prevention

The Division of Infectious Diseases and Immunology has developed a unique program in HIV prevention that has gained wide recognition and has extended the hospital's expertise from New York City to West and East Africa.

AIDS Clinical Trials

The AIDS Clinical Trials Unit is one of 35 units designated and supported by the National Institute of Allergy and Infectious Diseases, and is a dedicated resource for healthcare providers, researchers and scientists working in the field of HIV/AIDS research. It is one of the most active units in the nation in enrolling adult and pediatric patients in clinical trials supported by the NIH. Data generated by the unit has supported the licensing of several drugs and plays an essential role in defining optimal therapies and preventing complications.

Population Biology of Infectious Diseases

This novel program combines laboratory and clinical studies with epidemiology and genetics to optimize patient outcomes. Researchers in the Division of Infectious Diseases and Immunology are extensively involved in local and international studies into the early diagnosis, treatment and prevention of chronic infections such as tuberculosis and Helicobacter (bacteria associated with stomach ulcers).

Medical and Molecular Parasitology

The Division of Infectious Diseases and Immunology works alongside NYU Langone Medical Center's Department of Medical Parasitology to bring malaria and other parasitic diseases under control.

Internal Medicine

A personal physician who provides long-term, comprehensive care in the office and the hospital, managing both common and complex illness of adolescents, adults and the elderly. Internists are trained in the diagnosis and treatment of cancer, infections and diseases affecting the heart, blood, kidneys, joints and digestive, respiratory and vascular systems. They are also trained in the essentials of primary care internal medicine which incorporates an understanding of disease prevention, wellness, substance abuse, mental health and effective treatment of common problems of the eyes, ears, skin, nervous system and reproductive organs.

Note: *Internal Medicine normally includes many primary care physicians. However, for purposes of this directory, no primary care physicians are included.*

Training Required: Three years

INTERNAL MEDICINE

New England

Gillman, Matthew MD [IM] - **Spec Exp:** Obesity; Nutrition & Disease Prevention/Control; Diabetes in Pregnancy; Clinical Trials Only; **Hospital:** Children's Hospital - Boston, Brigham and Women's Hosp (page 57); **Address:** Harvard Pilgrim's Hlth Care, Dept of Population Medicine, 133 Brookline Ave Fl 6, Boston, MA 02215; **Phone:** 617-509-9968; **Board Cert:** Internal Medicine 1985; Pediatrics 1986; **Med School:** Duke Univ 1981; **Resid:** Internal Medicine, N Carolina Meml Hosp 1984; Pediatrics, N Carolina Meml Hosp 1985; **Fellow:** Research, Harvard Univ 1990; **Fac Appt:** Prof Med, Harvard Med Sch

Jackson, Vicki MD [IM] - **Spec Exp:** Palliative Care; **Hospital:** Mass Genl Hosp; **Address:** Palliative Care Service, 55 Fruit St, FND 600, Boston, MA 02114; **Phone:** 617-724-9197; **Board Cert:** Internal Medicine 2008; Hospice & Palliative Medicine 2002; **Med School:** Univ Wisc 1995; **Resid:** Internal Medicine, Cambridge Hlth Alliance 1998

Mid Atlantic

Arnold, Robert M MD [IM] - **Spec Exp:** Palliative Care; Ethics; Pain-HIV patients; **Hospital:** UPMC Montefiore, UPMC Presby, Pittsburgh; **Address:** UPMC Montefiore, Div Internal Medicine, Section of Palliative Care & Ethics, 3459 Fifth Ave, Ste 932W, Pittsburgh, PA 15213; **Phone:** 412-647-7228; **Board Cert:** Internal Medicine 1986; Hospice & Palliative Medicine 2009; **Med School:** Univ MO-Kansas City 1983; **Resid:** Internal Medicine, Rhode Island Hosp 1986; Internal Medicine, Hosp Univ Penn 1988; **Fellow:** Public Health, Robert Wood Johnson Univ Affil Hosp 1998; **Fac Appt:** Prof Med, Univ Pittsburgh

Barley, Christopher L MD [IM] - **Hospital:** NY-Presby/Weill Cornell Med Ctr, NY (page 65); **Address:** 110 E 55th St Fl 9, New York, NY 10022; **Phone:** 212-758-3590; **Board Cert:** Internal Medicine 2006; **Med School:** Geo Wash Univ 1993; **Resid:** Internal Medicine, NY Hosp Cornell Med Ctr 1996; **Fac Appt:** Asst Clin Prof Med, Cornell Univ-Weill Med Coll

Braunstein, Seth N MD/PhD [IM] - **Spec Exp:** Diabetes; **Hospital:** Hosp Univ Penn - UPHS (page 68); **Address:** Hosp of Univ Penn, Diabetes Ctr, 3400 Civic Ctr Blvd, Perelman Ctr, West Pavillion Fl 4, Philadelphia, PA 19104-4219; **Phone:** 215-662-2468; **Board Cert:** Internal Medicine 1975; **Med School:** NYU Sch Med 1972; **Resid:** Internal Medicine, Hosp Univ Penn 1975; **Fac Appt:** Assoc Prof Med, Univ Pennsylvania

Cirigliano, Michael D MD [IM] - **Spec Exp:** Complementary Medicine; Preventive Medicine; **Hospital:** Hosp Univ Penn - UPHS (page 68); **Address:** Clin Practices Michael D Cirigliano, 3701 Market St, Ste 370, Philadelphia, PA 19104; **Phone:** 215-615-3232; **Board Cert:** Internal Medicine 2005; **Med School:** Univ Pennsylvania 1990; **Resid:** Internal Medicine, Hosp U Penn 1993; **Fac Appt:** Assoc Prof Med, Univ Pennsylvania

Galland, Leo MD [IM] - **Spec Exp:** Nutrition; Chronic Illness; Complementary Medicine; **Address:** 156 5th Ave, Ste 519, New York, NY 10010; **Phone:** 212-989-6733; **Board Cert:** Internal Medicine 1972; **Med School:** NYU Sch Med 1968; **Resid:** Internal Medicine, Bellevue Hosp 1972; **Fellow:** Behavioral Medicine, Univ Conn Hlth Ctr 1981

Lewin, Neal A MD [IM] - **Spec Exp:** Preventive Medicine; Headache; Complex Diagnosis; **Hospital:** NYU Langone Med Ctr (page 66); **Address:** 120 E 36th St, Ste 1B, New York, NY 10016-3426; **Phone:** 212-889-2813; **Board Cert:** Internal Medicine 1977; Emergency Medicine 2002; Medical Toxicology 1983; **Med School:** SUNY Downstate 1974; **Resid:** Internal Medicine, NYU-Bellevue Hosp 1977; **Fac Appt:** Prof Med, NYU Sch Med

Quill, Timothy E MD [IM] - **Spec Exp:** Palliative Care; Chronic Illness; **Hospital:** Univ of Rochester Strong Meml Hosp; **Address:** University of Rochester Medical Ctr, 601 Elmwood Ave, Box 687, Rochester, NY 14642; **Phone:** 585-273-1154; **Board Cert:** Internal Medicine 1979; Hospice & Palliative Medicine 2008; **Med School:** Univ Rochester 1976; **Resid:** Internal Medicine, Univ Rochester/Strong Meml Hosp 1980; **Fellow:** Liaison Psychiatry, Univ Rochester Med Psych Liason Program 1981; **Fac Appt:** Prof Med, Univ Rochester

Rader, Daniel J MD [IM] - **Spec Exp:** Cholesterol/Lipid Disorders; Preventive Cardiology; Metabolic Disorders; **Hospital:** Hosp Univ Penn - UPHS (page 68), Penn Presby Med Ctr - UPHS (page 68); **Address:** U Penn Preventive Cardiology, Perelman Ctr for Advanced Medicine, 3400 Civic Ctr Blvd Fl 2- East, Philadelphia, PA 19104; **Phone:** 215-615-4949; **Board Cert:** Internal Medicine 1987; **Med School:** Med Coll PA Hahnemann 1984; **Resid:** Internal Medicine, Yale-New Haven Hosp 1987; **Fellow:** Research, Natl Inst Hlth 1992; **Fac Appt:** Prof Med, Univ Pennsylvania

Rivlin, Richard S MD [IM] - **Spec Exp:** Nutrition & Cancer Prevention/Control; Breast Cancer; Prostate Cancer; Colon Cancer; **Hospital:** NY-Presby/Weill Cornell Med Ctr, NY (page 65); **Address:** 1167 York Ave, New York, NY 10065; **Phone:** 646-898-2749; **Board Cert:** Internal Medicine 1969; **Med School:** Harvard Med Sch 1959; **Resid:** Internal Medicine, Johns Hopkins Hosp 1961; Internal Medicine, Johns Hopkins Hosp 1964; **Fellow:** Endocrinology, Diabetes & Metabolism, Natl Inst Hlth 1963; Biochemistry, Johns Hopkins Hosp 1966; **Fac Appt:** Prof Med, Cornell Univ-Weill Med Coll

Selwyn, Peter MD [IM] - **Spec Exp:** AIDS/HIV; Palliative Care; Addiction/Substance Abuse; **Hospital:** Montefiore Med Ctr - Div. Moses; **Address:** Montfiore Family Health Ctr, 360 E 193rd St, Bronx, NY 10458; **Phone:** 718-933-2400; **Board Cert:** Family Medicine 2005; Hospice & Palliative Medicine 2006; **Med School:** Harvard Med Sch 1981; **Resid:** Family Medicine, Montefiore Med Ctr 1984; **Fac Appt:** Prof Med, Albert Einstein Coll Med

Yaffe, Bruce MD [IM] - **Spec Exp:** Gastroscopy; Colonoscopy; **Hospital:** Lenox Hill Hosp; **Address:** 201 E 65th St, New York, NY 10065; **Phone:** 212-879-4700; **Board Cert:** Internal Medicine 1979; Gastroenterology 1981; **Med School:** Geo Wash Univ 1976; **Resid:** Internal Medicine, Mount Sinai Hosp 1979; Hepatology, Mount Sinai Hosp 1980; **Fellow:** Gastroenterology, Lenox Hill Hosp 1982

Southeast

Cushman, William C MD [IM] - **Spec Exp:** Hypertension; Preventive Cardiology; Cholesterol/Lipid Disorders; **Hospital:** VA Med Ctr - Memphis; **Address:** VA Medical Ctr, 1030 Jefferson Ave, Memphis, TN 38104-2127; **Phone:** 901-523-8990 x7357; **Board Cert:** Internal Medicine 1977; **Med School:** Univ Miss 1974; **Resid:** Internal Medicine, Univ Mississippi Med Ctr 1977; **Fac Appt:** Prof Med, Univ Tenn Coll Med

Fischl, Margaret A MD [IM] - **Spec Exp:** Immunotherapy; Infectious Disease; AIDS/HIV; Clinical Trials; **Hospital:** Univ of Miami Hosp (page 72), Univ of Miami Hosp & Clins/Sylvester Comp Canc Ctr (page 73); **Address:** 1800 NW 10th Ave, Miami, FL 33136; **Phone:** 305-243-3847; **Board Cert:** Internal Medicine 1979; **Med School:** Univ Miami Sch Med 1976; **Resid:** Internal Medicine, Univ Miami Affil Hosps 1979; **Fellow:** Infectious Disease, Univ Miami Affil Hosps 1980; **Fac Appt:** Prof Med, Univ Miami Sch Med

Internal Medicine

Tucker, Rodney O MD [IM] - **Spec Exp:** Palliative Care; **Hospital:** Univ of Ala Hosp at Birmingham; **Address:** UAB Ctr for Palliative Care, Ch19, Ste 219, 1530 3rd Ave S, Birmingham, AL 35294-2041; **Phone:** 205-975-8197; **Board Cert:** Internal Medicine 2002; **Med School:** Univ Alabama 1989; **Resid:** Internal Medicine, Carraway Methodist Med Ctr 1993; **Fac Appt:** Asst Prof Med, Univ Alabama

Tulsky, James A MD [IM] - **Spec Exp:** Palliative Care; **Hospital:** Duke Univ Hosp; **Address:** Ctr for Palliative Care, Hock Plaza, 2424 Erwin Rd, Ste 1105, Durham, NC 27705; **Phone:** 919-668-7215; **Board Cert:** Internal Medicine 2000; Hospice & Palliative Medicine 2006; **Med School:** Univ IL Coll Med 1987; **Resid:** Internal Medicine, UCSF Med Ctr 1990; **Fellow:** Pain & Palliative Care, UCSF Med Ctr 1993; **Fac Appt:** Prof Med, Duke Univ

Midwest

Burt, Richard K MD [IM] - **Spec Exp:** Stem Cell Transplant in Lupus/Crohn's; Stem Cell Transplant in MS; Autoimmune Disease; **Hospital:** Northwestern Meml Hosp; **Address:** Northwestern - Div Immunotherapy, 750 N Lakeshore Drive, rm 649, Chicago, IL 60611; **Phone:** 312-908-0059; **Board Cert:** Internal Medicine 1989; **Med School:** St Louis Univ 1984; **Resid:** Internal Medicine, Baylor Coll Med 1988; **Fellow:** Hematology & Oncology, NIH Clin Ctr 1993; **Fac Appt:** Assoc Prof Med, Northwestern Univ

Fischbein, Lewis C MD [IM] - **Spec Exp:** Rheumatoid Arthritis; Hypertension; Preventive Medicine; **Hospital:** Barnes-Jewish Hosp; **Address:** 4921 Parkview Pl, Ste 5G, St Louis, MO 63110; **Phone:** 314-747-1970; **Board Cert:** Internal Medicine 1977; Rheumatology 1980; **Med School:** Washington Univ, St Louis 1974; **Resid:** Internal Medicine, Barnes Jewish Hosp 1977; **Fellow:** Rheumatology, Washington Univ 1979; **Fac Appt:** Assoc Prof Med, Washington Univ, St Louis

Santa-Emma, Philip H MD [IM] - **Spec Exp:** Palliative Care; **Hospital:** Mt Carmel W Hosp; **Address:** 1144 Dublin Rd, Columbus, OH 43215; **Phone:** 614-234-5000; **Board Cert:** Family Medicine 2010; Hospice & Palliative Medicine 2008; **Med School:** Ohio State Univ 1988; **Resid:** Family Medicine, Mt Carmel Med Ctr 1991

Weder, Alan B MD [IM] - **Spec Exp:** Hypertension; Renovascular Disease; Peripheral Vascular Disease; Carotid Artery Disease; **Hospital:** Univ of Michigan Hosp; **Address:** Univ Mich, CVC Clinic, 1500 E Med Ctr Drive, SPC5856 Fl 3 - rm 3146, Ann Arbor, MI 48109-5856; **Phone:** 734-647-7321; **Board Cert:** Internal Medicine 1978; **Med School:** Hahnemann Univ 1975; **Resid:** Internal Medicine, Univ Chicago Hosps 1978; **Fac Appt:** Prof Med, Univ Mich Med Sch

Wright Jr, Jackson T MD/PhD [IM] - **Spec Exp:** Hypertension; **Hospital:** Univ Hosps Case Med Ctr (page 74); **Address:** CWRU Div Hypertension, 11100 Euclid Ave, Bolwell Bldg - rm 2200, Cleveland, OH 44106-6053; **Phone:** 216-844-5174; **Board Cert:** Internal Medicine 1980; **Med School:** Univ Pittsburgh 1976; **Resid:** Internal Medicine, Univ Michigan Hosps 1979; **Fellow:** Pharmacology, Univ Health Ctr 1980; **Fac Appt:** Prof Med, Case West Res Univ

Great Plains and Mountains

Mehler, Philip S MD [IM] - **Spec Exp:** Eating Disorders; Substance Abuse; Hypertension; Anorexia Nervosa-Severe; **Hospital:** Denver Health Med Ctr; **Address:** Denver Health Med Ctr, 777 Bannock St, MC 0278, Denver, CO 80204; **Phone:** 303-436-3234; **Board Cert:** Internal Medicine 1989; Addiction Medicine 1993; **Med School:** Univ Colorado 1983; **Resid:** Internal Medicine, Univ Colorado Affil Hosp 1987; **Fac Appt:** Prof Med, Univ Colorado

Southwest

Fine, Robert L MD [IM] - **Spec Exp:** Palliative Care; **Hospital:** Baylor Univ Medical Ctr-Dallas; **Address:** 3434 Swiss Ave, Ste 205, Dallas, TX 75204; **Phone:** 214-828-5090; **Board Cert:** Internal Medicine 1981; Hospice & Palliative Medicine 1993; **Med School:** Univ Tex SW, Dallas 1978; **Resid:** Internal Medicine, Baylor Univ Med Ctr 1981

West Coast and Pacific

Bissell Jr, Dwight M MD [IM] - **Spec Exp:** Porphyria; **Hospital:** UCSF Med Ctr; **Address:** UCSF Med Ctr, Dept Gastroenterology, 350 Parnassus Ave, rm 410, San Francisco, CA 94117; **Phone:** 415-353-2318; **Board Cert:** Internal Medicine 1974; **Med School:** Harvard Med Sch 1967; **Resid:** Internal Medicine, Boston City Hosp-Harvard 1970; **Fellow:** Gastroenterology, UCSF Med Ctr 1973; **Fac Appt:** Prof Med, UCSF

Cope, Dennis W MD [IM] - **Spec Exp:** Diagnostic Problems; Complex Diagnosis; **Hospital:** Olive View-UCLA Med Ctr; **Address:** Olive View Medical Ctr, 14445 Olive View Drive, Sylmar, CA 91342; **Phone:** 818-364-3205; **Board Cert:** Internal Medicine 1973; Endocrinology 1975; **Med School:** Univ Kansas 1970; **Resid:** Internal Medicine, UCLA Med Ctr 1973; **Fellow:** Endocrinology, UCLA Med Ctr 1975

Ferris, Frank D MD [IM] - **Spec Exp:** Palliative Care; **Hospital:** San Diego Hospice; **Address:** 4311 3rd Ave, San Diego, CA 92103-1407; **Phone:** 619-688-1600; **Board Cert:** Hospice & Palliative Medicine 1998; **Med School:** Canada 1981; **Resid:** Internal Medicine, Univ Toronto; Radiation Oncology, Univ Toronto; **Fellow:** Pain Management, Toronto-Sunnybrook Reg Cancer Ctr

Pantilat, Steven MD [IM] - **Spec Exp:** Palliative Care; **Hospital:** UCSF Med Ctr; **Address:** 521 Parnassus Ave, Box 0903, San Francisco, CA 94143-0903; **Phone:** 415-476-9019; **Board Cert:** Internal Medicine 2003; Hospice & Palliative Medicine 2001; **Med School:** UCSF 1989; **Resid:** Internal Medicine, UCSF Med Ctr 1992; **Fac Appt:** Asst Clin Prof Med, UCSF

Rabow, Michael W MD [IM] - **Spec Exp:** Palliative Care; **Hospital:** UCSF - Mt Zion Med Ctr; **Address:** 1545 Divisadero St, UCSF Gen Internal Med Practice, San Francisco, CA 94115; **Phone:** 415-353-7300; **Board Cert:** Internal Medicine 2006; Hospice & Palliative Medicine 2002; **Med School:** UCSF 1993; **Resid:** Internal Medicine, UCSF Med Ctr 1996; **Fellow:** Gastroenterology, UCSF Med Ctr 1997; **Fac Appt:** Assoc Clin Prof Med, UCSF

White, Jocelyn C MD [IM] - **Spec Exp:** Palliative Care; **Hospital:** Legacy Good Samaritan Med Ctr; **Address:** 1015 NW 22nd Ave, Portland, OR 97210; **Phone:** 503-413-8423; **Board Cert:** Internal Medicine 2000; Hospice & Palliative Medicine 2008; **Med School:** NYU Sch Med 1987; **Resid:** Internal Medicine, Good Samaritan Hosp 1991

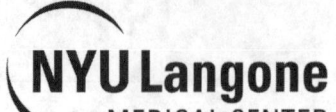
INTERNAL MEDICINE

About the Division of General Internal Medicine, Department of Medicine

Internal medicine physicians at NYU Langone Medical Center are dedicated to treating the whole patient, and not just their disease. Bound by the highest standards of their profession, they address both the physical and psychological aspects of health and disease through clear communication and a fully integrated regimen of care. We specialize in the following areas:

Primary and Specialized Healthcare

The Division of General Internal Medicine offers a multidisciplinary medical approach to treating illnesses involving the heart, lungs, gastrointestinal tract, joints, bones, muscles, endocrine organs and kidneys. A wide range of laboratory, imaging and advanced diagnostic testing, ranging from throat cultures to the complex mapping of the electrical surface of the heart, is available on-site or by referral. Comprehensive women's healthcare, including cancer screening and osteoporosis prevention and treatment, is also available.

Geriatrics

Our geriatric specialists provide comprehensive and multidisciplinary care, consultation and follow-up for elderly patients ranging from prevention and healthy aging to the treatment and care of chronic conditions including dementia, functional impairment and degenerative disorders.

Center for Healthful Behavior Change

The Center for Healthful Behavior Change (CHBC) focuses on developing evidence-based behavioral interventions aimed at improving patient health. CHBC originates, tests and spreads innovative evidence-based behavioral interventions into everyday clinical practice and community settings for patients with high blood pressure and other conditions associated with cardiovascular risk, including obesity and high cholesterol.

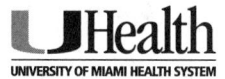

UNIVERSITY OF MIAMI
MILLER SCHOOL
of MEDICINE

305-243-4000 • 1-877-243-4340
www.uhealthsystem.com

UHEALTH

For almost 60 years, the University of Miami has been a vital part of South Florida's health care landscape. Now, known by the name UHealth – University of Miami Health System, we continue our leading role as South Florida's source for breakthrough medicine and the region's unequivocal health care leader. Backed by up-to-the-minute research, award-winning community service, and top-ranked physicians practicing in more than 100 medical specialties and subspecialties, UHealth provides health care for the 21st Century.

LEONARD M. MILLER SCHOOL OF MEDICINE

The University of Miami's Leonard M. Miller School of Medicine serves as the "engine" driving UHealth. Driven by the vision of University President Donna Shalala, (the former U.S. Secretary of Health and Human Services,) and Dean Pascal J. Goldschmidt, the Miller School of Medicine has attracted international leaders from dozens of fields. Moreover, this renowned team is transforming thousands of lives by helping our patients – and the beneficiaries of our research – live longer and live healthier.

TOP DOCTORS

UHealth doctors are among the nation's most respected. Our more than 1,500 physicians have been recognized by their peers as among the best in South Florida and the nation. In fact, more than 400 are listed as "best doctors" in regional and national rankings.* Providing care to one of the most diverse patient populations in the world and delivering services in five counties stretching from the Palm Beaches to the Florida Keys, UHealth physicians keep Florida healthy.

*Based on listings provided by Best Doctors®, Castle Connolly Medical Ltd., and Florida Super Doctors.

INNOVATIVE RESEARCH

Currently, UHealth physicians and scientists are involved in more than 1,500 ongoing studies, many of which lead to clinical trials that directly change the standard for care. They work every day to uncover new information, build better understanding, and develop new cures. It's what sets us apart, and it's why patients from all over the world choose UHealth.

UHealth's physicians and health care professionals provide care and conduct research at more than 30 facilities, including:

- University of Miami Hospital
- Sylvester Comprehensive Cancer Center
- Bascom Palmer Eye Institute
- Diabetes Research Institute
- The Miami Project to Cure Paralysis
- Mailman Center for Child Development
- John P. Hussman Institute for Human Genetics
- Interdisciplinary Stem Cell Institute

In affiliation with:

- Jackson Memorial Hospital
- Holtz Children's Hospital
- Miami VA Medical Center

UHealth: Top-ranked doctors and hospitals providing the finest health care at more than 30 convenient South Florida locations, including our hospitals: University of Miami Hospital, Bascom Palmer Eye Institute, and Sylvester Comprehensive Cancer Center. UHealth is powered by the research and education of the University of Miami Miller School of Medicine.

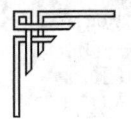
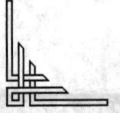
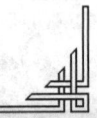

The Best in American Medicine
www.CastleConnolly.com

Maternal & Fetal Medicine
a subspecialty of Obstetrics & Gynecology

An obstetrician/gynecologist possesses special knowledge, skills and professional capability in the medical and surgical care of the female reproductive system and associated disorders. This physician serves as a consultant to other physicians and as a primary physician for women.

Training Required: Four years *plus* two years in clinical practice before certification in obstetrics and gynecology is complete *plus* additional training and examination in maternal-fetal medicine.

MATERNAL & FETAL MEDICINE

New England

Acker, David B MD [MF] - **Spec Exp:** Multiple Gestation; Pregnancy-High Risk; **Hospital:** Brigham and Women's Hosp (page 57); **Address:** Brigham & Womens Hosp, Dept Ob/Gyn, 75 Francis St, ASB1-3, Boston, MA 02115; **Phone:** 617-732-5445; **Board Cert:** Obstetrics & Gynecology 2010; Maternal & Fetal Medicine 2010; **Med School:** NYU Sch Med 1968; **Resid:** Obstetrics & Gynecology, Albert Einstein Affil Hosp 1971; Obstetrics & Gynecology, Vanderbilt Univ Affil Hosp 1974; **Fellow:** Maternal & Fetal Medicine, Boston Lying-In Hosp 1979; **Fac Appt:** Assoc Prof ObG, Harvard Med Sch

Baker, Emily MD [MF] - **Spec Exp:** Ultrasound; Pregnancy-High Risk; **Hospital:** Dartmouth - Hitchcock Med Ctr; **Address:** Dartmouth-Hitchcock Med Ctr, Dept Ob/Gyn, 1 Med Ctr Drive, Lebanon, NH 03756; **Phone:** 603-653-9306; **Board Cert:** Obstetrics & Gynecology 2007; Maternal & Fetal Medicine 2007; **Med School:** Stanford Univ 1986; **Resid:** Obstetrics & Gynecology, Univ Chicago Hosps 1990; Maternal & Fetal Medicine, Univ Washington Med Ctr 1991; **Fellow:** Maternal & Fetal Medicine, St Margaret's Hosp-Tufts Univ 1992; **Fac Appt:** Assoc Prof ObG, Dartmouth Med Sch

Carr, Stephen R MD [MF] - **Spec Exp:** Twin to Twin Transfusion Syndrome (TTTS); Multiple Gestation; Fetal Surgery; **Hospital:** Women & Infants Hosp of RI; **Address:** Women & Infants Hosp, 101 Dudley St, Providence, RI 02905; **Phone:** 401-274-1122; **Board Cert:** Obstetrics & Gynecology 2009; Maternal & Fetal Medicine 1997; **Med School:** Univ Hawaii JA Burns Sch Med 1982; **Resid:** Obstetrics & Gynecology, Univ Illinois Med Ctr 1986; **Fellow:** Maternal & Fetal Medicine, Brown Univ 1988; **Fac Appt:** Assoc Prof ObG, Brown Univ

Copel, Joshua A MD [MF] - **Spec Exp:** Prenatal Diagnosis; Fetal Echocardiography; Pregnancy-High Risk; Fetal Diagnosis & Therapy; **Hospital:** Yale-New Haven Hosp, Yale Med Group; **Address:** Yale Maternal/Fetal Medicine, 150 Sargent Drive, New Haven, CT 06511; **Phone:** 203-785-5682; **Board Cert:** Obstetrics & Gynecology 2008; Maternal & Fetal Medicine 2008; **Med School:** Tufts Univ 1979; **Resid:** Obstetrics & Gynecology, Pennsylvania Hosp 1983; **Fellow:** Maternal & Fetal Medicine, Yale-New Haven Hosp 1985; **Fac Appt:** Prof ObG, Yale Univ

Greene, Michael F MD [MF] - **Spec Exp:** Pregnancy-High Risk; Multiple Gestation; Seizure Disorders & Pregnancy; **Hospital:** Mass Genl Hosp; **Address:** Mass Genl Hosp, Dept Ob/Gyn, 55 Fruit St Yawkey Bldg - rm 4F, Boston, MA 02114; **Phone:** 617-724-2229; **Board Cert:** Obstetrics & Gynecology 2010; Maternal & Fetal Medicine 2010; **Med School:** SUNY Downstate 1976; **Resid:** Obstetrics & Gynecology, Boston Hosp Women 1980; **Fellow:** Maternal & Fetal Medicine, Brigham Hosp Women 1982; **Fac Appt:** Prof ObG, Harvard Med Sch

Heffner, Linda MD/PhD [MF] - **Spec Exp:** Pregnancy-Advanced Maternal Age; Pregnancy-High Risk; **Hospital:** Boston Med Ctr; **Address:** 85 E Concord St Fl 6, Boston, MA 02118; **Phone:** 617-414-5175; **Board Cert:** Obstetrics & Gynecology 2010; Maternal & Fetal Medicine 2010; **Med School:** Johns Hopkins Univ 1977; **Resid:** Obstetrics & Gynecology, Hosp Univ Penn 1983; **Fellow:** Maternal & Fetal Medicine, Brigham-Womens Hosp 1987; **Fac Appt:** Prof ObG, Boston Univ

Lockwood, Charles MD [MF] - **Spec Exp:** Prematurity Prevention; Miscarriage-Recurrent; Multiple Gestation; Bleeding/Coagulation Disorders; **Hospital:** Yale-New Haven Hosp, Yale Med Group; **Address:** Yale Maternal/Fetal Medicine, 150 Sargent Drive, New Haven, CT 06511; **Phone:** 203-785-5682; **Board Cert:** Obstetrics & Gynecology 2007; Maternal & Fetal Medicine 2007; **Med School:** Univ Pennsylvania 1981; **Resid:** Obstetrics & Gynecology, Penn Hosp 1985; **Fellow:** Maternal & Fetal Medicine, Yale-New Haven Hosp 1987; Thrombosis, Mt Sinai Med Ctr 1991; **Fac Appt:** Prof ObG, Yale Univ

Norwitz, Errol R MD/PhD [MF] - **Spec Exp:** Diabetes in Pregnancy; Critical Care; Prematurity Prevention; **Hospital:** Tufts Med Ctr; **Address:** Tufts Medical Center, 800 Washington St, Mailbox 324, Boston, MA 02111; **Phone:** 617-636-2382; **Board Cert:** Obstetrics & Gynecology 2010; Maternal & Fetal Medicine 2010; **Med School:** South Africa 1986; **Resid:** Obstetrics & Gynecology, Brigham & Women's Hosp 1996; **Fellow:** Maternal & Fetal Medicine, Brigham & Women's Hosp 1998; **Fac Appt:** Prof ObG, Tufts Univ

Paidas, Michael J MD [MF] - **Spec Exp:** Pregnancy-High Risk; Clotting Disorders in Pregnancy; Miscarriage-Recurrent; **Hospital:** Yale-New Haven Hosp, Yale Med Group; **Address:** Yale Maternal/Fetal Medicine, 150 Sargent Drive, New Haven, CT 06511; **Phone:** 203-785-5682; **Board Cert:** Obstetrics & Gynecology 2010; Maternal & Fetal Medicine 2010; **Med School:** Tufts Univ 1987; **Resid:** Obstetrics & Gynecology, Pennsylvania Hosp 1991; **Fellow:** Maternal & Fetal Medicine, Mount Sinai Med Ctr 1993; **Fac Appt:** Assoc Prof ObG, Yale Univ

Riley, Laura E MD [MF] - **Spec Exp:** AIDS/HIV in Pregnancy; Infectious Disease in Pregnancy; Pregnancy-High Risk; **Hospital:** Mass Genl Hosp; **Address:** Mass Genl Hosp, Dept Ob/Gyn, 55 Fruit St Yawkey Bldg - rm 4F, Boston, MA 02114; **Phone:** 617-724-2229; **Board Cert:** Obstetrics & Gynecology 2010; Maternal & Fetal Medicine 2008; **Med School:** Univ Pittsburgh 1985; **Resid:** Obstetrics & Gynecology, Univ Pittsburgh Med Ctr 1988; **Fellow:** Maternal & Fetal Medicine, Brigham & Womens Hosp 1991; Infectious Disease, Boston Univ Med Ctr 1993; **Fac Appt:** Assoc Prof ObG, Harvard Med Sch

Robinson, Julian N MD [MF] - **Spec Exp:** Prenatal Diagnosis; Fetal Echocardiography; Amniocentesis; Ultrasound; **Hospital:** Newton - Wellesley Hosp, Brigham and Women's Hosp (page 57); **Address:** Newton-Wellesley Hosp, 2014 Washington St Fl 2 West, Newton, MA 02462; **Phone:** 617-243-5909; **Board Cert:** Obstetrics & Gynecology 2010; Maternal & Fetal Medicine 2010; **Med School:** England, UK 1986; **Resid:** Obstetrics & Gynecology, Eastern VA Med Sch 1997; **Fellow:** Maternal & Fetal Medicine, Brigham & Women's Hosp 1998

Wenstrom, Katharine D MD [MF] - **Spec Exp:** Reproductive Genetics; Pregnancy-High Risk; **Hospital:** Women & Infants Hosp of RI; **Address:** Women's & Infants Hosp RI, Maternal Fetal Medicine Div, 101 Dudley St Fl 3, Providence, RI 02905; **Phone:** 401-274-1122 x1120; **Board Cert:** Obstetrics & Gynecology 2006; Maternal & Fetal Medicine 2006; Clinical Genetics 1990; **Med School:** Case West Res Univ 1983; **Resid:** Obstetrics & Gynecology, Univ Illinois Hosp 1987; **Fellow:** Maternal & Fetal Medicine, Univ Illinois Hosp 1989; Clinical Genetics, Univ Iowa Med Ctr 1990; **Fac Appt:** Prof ObG, Vanderbilt Univ

Wilkins-Haug, Louise E MD/PhD [MF] - **Spec Exp:** Fetal Diagnosis & Therapy; Pregnancy-High Risk; Genetic Disorders; Fetal Surgery; **Hospital:** Brigham and Women's Hosp (page 57); **Address:** Brigham & Womens Hosp, Div Maternal Fetal Medicine, 75 Francis St, Ste 305, Boston, MA 02115; **Phone:** 617-732-4840; **Board Cert:** Obstetrics & Gynecology 2009; Maternal & Fetal Medicine 2009; **Med School:** Stanford Univ 1985; **Resid:** Obstetrics & Gynecology, Univ Colorado Med Ctr 1989; **Fellow:** Maternal & Fetal Medicine, Brigham & Women's Hosp 1992; **Fac Appt:** Assoc Prof ObG, Harvard Med Sch

Maternal & Fetal Medicine

Mid Atlantic

Berkowitz, Richard L MD [MF] - **Spec Exp:** Fetal Therapy; Multiple Gestation; Pregnancy & Hematologic Abnormalities; **Hospital:** NY-Presby/Columbia Univ Med Ctr, NY (page 65); **Address:** 16 E 60th St, Fl 4, New York, NY 10022; **Phone:** 212-326-8951; **Board Cert:** Obstetrics & Gynecology 2005; Maternal & Fetal Medicine 2005; **Med School:** NYU Sch Med 1965; **Resid:** Obstetrics & Gynecology, NY Hosp-Cornell Med Ctr 1972; **Fac Appt:** Prof ObG, Columbia P&S

Blakemore, Karin J MD [MF] - **Spec Exp:** Fetal Diagnosis & Therapy; Pregnancy-High Risk; Ultrasound; **Hospital:** Johns Hopkins Hosp (page 61); **Address:** Johns Hopkins Hosp, Dept Maternal/Fetal Med, 600 N Wolfe St Phipps Bldg - rm 228, Baltimore, MD 21287-1228; **Phone:** 410-955-7456; **Board Cert:** Clinical Genetics 1984; Obstetrics & Gynecology 2010; Maternal & Fetal Medicine 2010; **Med School:** Med Coll OH 1978; **Resid:** Obstetrics & Gynecology, NYU Med Ctr 1982; Clinical Genetics, Yale Univ Sch Med 1985; **Fellow:** Maternal & Fetal Medicine, Washington Univ 1987; **Fac Appt:** Assoc Prof ObG, Johns Hopkins Univ

Caritis, Steve N MD [MF] - **Spec Exp:** Pregnancy-High Risk; **Hospital:** Magee-Womens Hosp - UPMC; **Address:** Dept Maternal/Fetal Medicine, 300 Halket St, Ste 0610, Pittsburgh, PA 15213-3180; **Phone:** 412-641-6361; **Board Cert:** Obstetrics & Gynecology 1999; Maternal & Fetal Medicine 1999; **Med School:** W VA Univ 1969; **Resid:** Obstetrics & Gynecology, Univ Pittsburgh Med Ctr 1973; **Fellow:** Maternal & Fetal Medicine, Columbia-Presby Med Ctr 1975; **Fac Appt:** Prof ObG, Univ Pittsburgh

Cohen, Arnold MD [MF] - **Spec Exp:** Pregnancy-High Risk; Diabetes in Pregnancy; **Hospital:** Albert Einstein Med Ctr; **Address:** AEMC 5501 Old York Rd, Lifter Bldg Fl 2, Philadelphia, PA 19141; **Phone:** 215-456-6993; **Board Cert:** Obstetrics & Gynecology 1994; Maternal & Fetal Medicine 1982; **Med School:** Cornell Univ 1971; **Resid:** Internal Medicine, Hosp Univ Pennsylvania 1973; Obstetrics & Gynecology, Hosp Univ Pennsylvania 1976; **Fellow:** Maternal & Fetal Medicine, Hosp Univ Pennsylvania 1980; **Fac Appt:** Prof ObG, Thomas Jefferson Univ

D'Alton, Mary E MD [MF] - **Spec Exp:** Pregnancy-High Risk; Multiple Gestation; Prenatal Diagnosis; **Hospital:** NY-Presby/Columbia Univ Med Ctr, NY (page 65); **Address:** 16 E 60th St, Ste 480, New York, NY 10022; **Phone:** 212-326-8951; **Board Cert:** Obstetrics & Gynecology 2010; Maternal & Fetal Medicine 2010; **Med School:** Ireland 1976; **Resid:** Obstetrics & Gynecology, Ottowa Genl Hosp 1982; **Fellow:** Maternal & Fetal Medicine, Tufts-New Eng Med Ctr 1984; **Fac Appt:** Clin Prof ObG, Columbia P&S

Eddleman, Keith A MD [MF] - **Spec Exp:** Obstetric Ultrasound; Pregnancy-High Risk; Fetal Therapy; Reproductive Genetics; **Hospital:** Mount Sinai Med Ctr (page 63); **Address:** Mount Sinai Medical Ctr, 5 E 98th St, Box 1170, New York, NY 10029; **Phone:** 212-241-5681; **Board Cert:** Obstetrics & Gynecology 2010; Maternal & Fetal Medicine 2010; Clinical Genetics 2010; **Med School:** Wake Forest Univ 1985; **Resid:** Obstetrics & Gynecology, George Washington Univ Med Ctr 1989; **Fellow:** Maternal & Fetal Medicine, Mt Sinai Med Ctr 1991; Genetics, NY-Cornell Med Ctr 1996; **Fac Appt:** Prof ObG, Mount Sinai Sch Med

Fox, Harold E MD [MF] - **Spec Exp:** Pregnancy-High Risk; Prematurity Prevention; Multiple Gestation; **Hospital:** Johns Hopkins Hosp (page 61); **Address:** Johns Hopkins Hosp, Dept Maternal/Fetal Medicine, 600 N Wolfe St Phipps Bldg - rm 264, Baltimore, MD 21287; **Phone:** 410-614-0178; **Board Cert:** Obstetrics & Gynecology 2010; Maternal & Fetal Medicine 2010; **Med School:** Univ Rochester 1972; **Resid:** Obstetrics & Gynecology, Strong Meml Hosp 1975; **Fellow:** Maternal & Fetal Medicine, Univ Rochester Hosps 1977; **Fac Appt:** Prof ObG, Johns Hopkins Univ

Grunebaum, Amos MD [MF] - **Spec Exp:** Pregnancy-High Risk; Amniocentesis; **Hospital:** NY-Presby/Weill Cornell Med Ctr, NY (page 65); **Address:** Dept Obstetrics & Gynecology, 525 E 68th St, Ste J-130, New York, NY 10065; **Phone:** 212-746-0714; **Board Cert:** Obstetrics & Gynecology 2008; Maternal & Fetal Medicine 2008; **Med School:** Germany 1974; **Resid:** Anesthesiology, Maimonides Med Ctr 1978; Obstetrics & Gynecology, Downstate Med Ctr 1982; **Fellow:** Maternal & Fetal Medicine, Downstate Med Ctr 1984; **Fac Appt:** Assoc Prof ObG, Columbia P&S

Landy, Helain J MD [MF] - **Spec Exp:** Pregnancy-High Risk; Miscarriage-Recurrent; Multiple Gestation; Diabetes in Pregnancy; **Hospital:** Georgetown Univ Hosp, Sibley Mem Hosp; **Address:** Georgetown Univ Dept Ob/Gyn, 3800 Reservoir Rd NW, 3PHC, Washington, DC 20007-2113; **Phone:** 202-444-8531; **Board Cert:** Obstetrics & Gynecology 2009; Maternal & Fetal Medicine 2009; **Med School:** Northwestern Univ 1982; **Resid:** Obstetrics & Gynecology, Penn Hosp 1986; **Fellow:** Maternal & Fetal Medicine, Geo Washington Univ Med Ctr 1988; **Fac Appt:** Prof ObG, Georgetown Univ

Parry, Samuel I MD [MF] - **Spec Exp:** Premature Labor; **Hospital:** Hosp Univ Penn - UPHS (page 68); **Address:** Univ Penn, Dept Maternal & Fetal Med, 3400 Spruce St, 2000 Court Yard, Philadelphia, PA 19104; **Phone:** 215-662-2982; **Board Cert:** Obstetrics & Gynecology 2009; **Med School:** Cornell Univ-Weill Med Coll 1990; **Resid:** Obstetrics & Gynecology, SUNY Buffalo Med Ctr 1994; **Fellow:** Maternal & Fetal Medicine, Hosp Univ Penn 1996; **Fac Appt:** Assoc Prof ObG, Univ Pennsylvania

Pinckert, Thomas L MD [MF] - **Spec Exp:** Pregnancy-High Risk; **Hospital:** Shady Grove Adven Hosp, Holy Cross Hospital - Silver Spring; **Address:** Greater Washington Maternal-Fetal Medicine, 9707 Med Ctr Drive, Ste 230, Rockville, MD 20850; **Phone:** 301-279-6060; **Board Cert:** Obstetrics & Gynecology 2009; Clinical Genetics 1990; Maternal & Fetal Medicine 2009; **Med School:** Oregon Hlth & Sci Univ 1979; **Resid:** Obstetrics & Gynecology, David Grant Med Ctr 1983; **Fellow:** Maternal & Fetal Medicine, UCSF Med Ctr 1989; Clinical Genetics, UCSF Med Ctr 1990

Plante, Lauren A MD [MF] - **Spec Exp:** Pregnancy-High Risk; **Hospital:** Hahnemann Univ Hosp; **Address:** Hahnemann Univ Hospital, Dept Ob/Gyn, Broad & Vine St, Philadelphia, PA 19102; **Phone:** 215-762-4000; **Board Cert:** Anesthesiology 2004; Critical Care Medicine 1993; Obstetrics & Gynecology 2009; Maternal & Fetal Medicine 2008; **Med School:** Albert Einstein Coll Med 1984; **Resid:** Anesthesiology, Montefiore Med Ctr 1989; Obstetrics & Gynecology, Hahnemann Univ Hosp 1994; **Fellow:** Critical Care Medicine, Montefiore Med Ctr 1990; Maternal & Fetal Medicine, Temple Univ Med Ctr 1998; **Fac Appt:** Assoc Prof ObG, Hahnemann Univ

Repke, John T MD [MF] - **Spec Exp:** Pregnancy-High Risk; Hypertension in Pregnancy; Women's Health; **Hospital:** Penn State Milton S Hershey Med Ctr; **Address:** MS Hershey Med Ctr Maternal Fetal Med, 500 University Drive, MC H103, Hershey, PA 17033; **Phone:** 717-531-3503 x4; **Board Cert:** Obstetrics & Gynecology 2010; Maternal & Fetal Medicine 2010; **Med School:** NY Med Coll 1978; **Resid:** Obstetrics & Gynecology, Johns Hopkins Hosp 1982; **Fellow:** Maternal & Fetal Medicine, Johns Hopkins Hosp 1984; **Fac Appt:** Prof ObG

Thomas, Ronald L MD [MF] - **Hospital:** Western Penn Hosp; **Address:** Federal North Bldg, 1307 Federal St, Ste B100, Pittsburgh, PA 15212; **Phone:** 412-359-3437; **Board Cert:** Obstetrics & Gynecology 2008; Maternal & Fetal Medicine 2008; **Med School:** Univ Pittsburgh 1981; **Resid:** Obstetrics & Gynecology, Natl Naval Ctr 1985; **Fellow:** Maternal & Fetal Medicine, Johns Hopkins Hosp 1988; **Fac Appt:** Assoc Prof ObG, Drexel Univ Coll Med

Maternal & Fetal Medicine

Wapner, Ronald J MD [MF] - **Spec Exp:** Perinatal Medicine; Genetic Disorders; Multiple Gestation; Vomiting-Cyclic; **Hospital:** NY-Presby/Columbia Univ Med Ctr, NY (page 65); **Address:** Div Maternal/Fetal Medicine, 16 E 60th St, rm 480, New York, NY 10022; **Phone:** 212-326-8951; **Board Cert:** Obstetrics & Gynecology 2000; Maternal & Fetal Medicine 2000; Clinical Genetics 2010; **Med School:** Jefferson Med Coll 1972; **Resid:** Obstetrics & Gynecology, Jefferson Univ Hosp 1976; **Fellow:** Maternal & Fetal Medicine, Jefferson Med Coll 1978; **Fac Appt:** Prof ObG, Columbia P&S

Southeast

Abuhamad, Alfred Z MD [MF] - **Spec Exp:** Twin to Twin Transfusion Syndrome (TTTS); Prenatal Diagnosis; Prenatal Ultrasound; Multiple Gestation; **Hospital:** Sentara Norfolk Genl Hosp; **Address:** E VA Med Sch, Div Mat Fetal Med, 825 Fairfax Ave, Ste 310, Norfolk, VA 23507; **Phone:** 757-446-7900; **Board Cert:** Obstetrics & Gynecology 2009; Maternal & Fetal Medicine 2009; **Med School:** Amer Univ Beirut 1985; **Resid:** Obstetrics & Gynecology, Jackson Meml Hosp 1989; **Fellow:** Maternal & Fetal Medicine, Jackson Meml Hosp-Univ Miami 1991; Ultrasound, Yale Univ 1991; **Fac Appt:** Prof ObG, Eastern VA Med Sch

Andrews, William W MD/PhD [MF] - **Spec Exp:** Infectious Disease; Prematurity/Low Birth Weight Infants; **Hospital:** Univ of Ala Hosp at Birmingham; **Address:** UAB Dept Obstetrics & Gynecology, 619 19th St S, 176F, rm 10360, Birmingham, AL 35233; **Phone:** 205-934-1911; **Board Cert:** Obstetrics & Gynecology 2010; **Med School:** Univ Alabama 1984; **Resid:** Obstetrics & Gynecology, Univ Alabama Hosp 1988; **Fellow:** Maternal & Fetal Medicine, Univ Texas SW Med Ctr 1990

Duff, William P MD [MF] - **Spec Exp:** Pregnancy-High Risk; Infections in Pregnancy; **Hospital:** Shands at Univ of FL; **Address:** Women's Health Magnolia Parke, 3951 NW 48th Terr, Ste 101, Gainesville, FL 32606; **Phone:** 352-265-6200; **Board Cert:** Obstetrics & Gynecology 2003; Maternal & Fetal Medicine 2003; **Med School:** Georgetown Univ 1974; **Resid:** Obstetrics & Gynecology, Walter Reed Med Ctr 1978; **Fellow:** Maternal & Fetal Medicine, UT - San Antonio 1983; **Fac Appt:** Prof ObG, Univ S Fla Coll Med

Ferguson II, James E MD [MF] - **Spec Exp:** Pregnancy-High Risk; Ultrasound; Premature Labor; **Hospital:** Univ of Virginia Health Sys; **Address:** Dept Ob/Gyn, Univ Virginia Sch Med, Box 800712, Charlottesville, VA 22908-0712; **Phone:** 434-924-9937; **Board Cert:** Obstetrics & Gynecology 2009; Maternal & Fetal Medicine 2009; **Med School:** Wake Forest Univ 1977; **Resid:** Obstetrics & Gynecology, Stanford Univ Med Ctr 1980; Obstetrics & Gynecology, Wake Forest Univ Med Ctr 1981; **Fellow:** Maternal & Fetal Medicine, Stanford Univ Med Ctr 1984; **Fac Appt:** Prof ObG, Univ VA Sch Med

Grandis, Arnold MD/PhD [MF] - **Spec Exp:** Pregnancy-High Risk; **Hospital:** Wake Forest Univ Baptist Med Ctr; **Address:** Dept Maternal & Fetal Med, Medical Center Blvd, Winston-Salem, NC 27157; **Phone:** 336-716-1025; **Board Cert:** Obstetrics & Gynecology 1980; Maternal & Fetal Medicine 1982; **Med School:** Univ Pennsylvania 1974; **Resid:** Obstetrics & Gynecology, Duke Univ Med Ctr 1978; **Fellow:** Maternal & Fetal Medicine, Duke Univ Sch Med 1980; **Fac Appt:** Assoc Prof ObG, Wake Forest Univ

Heyl, Peter S MD [MF] - **Spec Exp:** Pregnancy-High Risk; **Hospital:** Emory Univ Hosp, Emory Univ Hosp Midtown; **Address:** Emory Perinatal Center, 550 Peachtree St NE Fl 9, Atlanta, GA 30308; **Phone:** 404-778-3401; **Board Cert:** Obstetrics & Gynecology 2010; Maternal & Fetal Medicine 2010; **Med School:** Wake Forest Univ 1976; **Resid:** Obstetrics & Gynecology, Boston Hosp Women 1981; **Fellow:** Maternal & Fetal Medicine, Brigham-Womens Hosp 1983; **Fac Appt:** Prof ObG, Emory Univ

Kuller, Jeffrey MD [MF] - **Spec Exp:** Prenatal Diagnosis; **Hospital:** Duke Univ Hosp; **Address:** 2406 Blue Ridge Rd, Ste 200, Raleigh, NC 27607; **Phone:** 919-783-4299; **Board Cert:** Obstetrics & Gynecology 2009; Clinical Genetics 2010; Maternal & Fetal Medicine 2009; **Med School:** Univ Cincinnati 1984; **Resid:** Obstetrics & Gynecology, Johns Hopkins Hosp 1988; **Fellow:** Maternal & Fetal Medicine, UPMC 1990; Medical Genetics, UCSF Med Ctr 1992

Mari, Giancarlo MD [MF] - **Spec Exp:** Fetal Therapy; Obstetric Ultrasound; Twin to Twin Transfusion Syndrome (TTTS); **Hospital:** Regional Med Ctr - Memphis; **Address:** Dept OB/GYN, 853 Jefferson Ave, Ste E102, Memphis, TN 38103; **Phone:** 901-448-3700; **Board Cert:** Obstetrics & Gynecology 2009; Maternal & Fetal Medicine 2009; **Med School:** Italy 1982; **Resid:** Obstetrics & Gynecology, Yale New Haven Hosp 1994; **Fellow:** Maternal & Fetal Medicine, Yale New Haven Hosp 1996; **Fac Appt:** Prof

McLaren, Rodney A MD [MF] - **Spec Exp:** Prenatal Diagnosis; Amniocentesis; Pregnancy-High Risk; **Address:** 4001 Fair Ridge Drive, Ste 304, Fairfax, VA 22033; **Phone:** 703-359-2466; **Board Cert:** Obstetrics & Gynecology 2009; Maternal & Fetal Medicine 2009; **Med School:** Tufts Univ 1983; **Resid:** Obstetrics & Gynecology, LI Coll Hosp 1987; **Fellow:** Maternal & Fetal Medicine, Georgetown Univ 1989; **Fac Appt:** Assoc Prof ObG, Georgetown Univ

Nies, Barbara MD [MF] - **Spec Exp:** Pregnancy-High Risk; Amniocentesis; **Hospital:** Inova Fairfax Hosp, Inova Fair Oaks Hosp; **Address:** 3020 Hamaker Ct, Ste 501, Fairfax, VA 22031; **Phone:** 703-698-5350; **Board Cert:** Obstetrics & Gynecology 2009; Maternal & Fetal Medicine 2009; **Med School:** Mich State Univ 1984; **Resid:** Obstetrics & Gynecology, Univ Conn Med Ctr 1988; **Fellow:** Maternal & Fetal Medicine, George Washington Univ Med Ctr 1990

Thorp Jr, John M MD [MF] - **Spec Exp:** Multiple Gestation; Premature Labor; **Hospital:** NC Memorial Hosp - UNC; **Address:** UNC-Chapel Hill, 101 Manning Drive, Box 7600, Chapel Hill, NC 27514; **Phone:** 919-966-2131; **Board Cert:** Obstetrics & Gynecology 2009; Maternal & Fetal Medicine 2008; **Med School:** E Carolina Univ 1983; **Resid:** Obstetrics & Gynecology, Univ NC Hosp 1987; **Fellow:** Maternal & Fetal Medicine, Univ NC Hosp 1989; **Fac Appt:** Prof ObG, Univ NC Sch Med

Van Dorsten, J Peter MD [MF] - **Spec Exp:** Pregnancy-High Risk; **Hospital:** MUSC Med Ctr, McLeod Reg Med Ctr; **Address:** MUSC Med Ctr, Dept ObGyn, 96 Jonathan Lucas St, Ste 634, MS C619, Charleston, SC 29425; **Phone:** 843-792-4509; **Board Cert:** Obstetrics & Gynecology 2009; Maternal & Fetal Medicine 2009; **Med School:** Univ NC Sch Med 1971; **Resid:** Obstetrics & Gynecology, Med Univ SC Hosp 1976; **Fellow:** Maternal & Fetal Medicine, USC-LAC Hosp 1981; **Fac Appt:** Prof ObG, Med Univ SC

Midwest

Bahado-Singh, Ray O MD [MF] - **Spec Exp:** Pregnancy-High Risk; Genetic Disorders; Obstetric Ultrasound; Twin to Twin Transfusion Syndrome (TTTS); **Hospital:** Hutzel Hosp - Detroit; **Address:** 3990 John R St, 4 Webber N, Detroit, MI 48201; **Phone:** 313-993-1379; **Board Cert:** Obstetrics & Gynecology 2007; Maternal & Fetal Medicine 2007; Clinical Genetics 2006; **Med School:** Jamaica 1979; **Resid:** Obstetrics & Gynecology, Metropolitan Hosp 1985; **Fellow:** Perinatal Medicine, UC-Irvine 1987; Clinical Genetics, Yale Univ 1993

Bartelsmeyer, James MD [MF] - **Spec Exp:** Pregnancy-High Risk; Multiple Gestation; **Hospital:** St. John's Mercy Med Ctr - St Louis; **Address:** 621 S New Ballas Rd, Ste 2007B, St Louis, MO 63141; **Phone:** 314-991-5000; **Board Cert:** Obstetrics & Gynecology 2010; Maternal & Fetal Medicine 2010; **Med School:** Univ IL Coll Med 1985; **Resid:** Obstetrics & Gynecology, Univ Ill Coll Med Hosps 1989; **Fellow:** Maternal & Fetal Medicine, Barnes Hosp-Univ Wash 1991; **Fac Appt:** Assoc Prof ObG, Washington Univ, St Louis

Maternal & Fetal Medicine

Besinger, Richard MD [MF] - **Spec Exp:** Prenatal Diagnosis; Premature Labor; Critical Care; **Hospital:** Loyola Univ Med Ctr; **Address:** Loyola Univ Med Ctr, 2160 S First Ave, Outpatient Ctr, Maywood, IL 60153-5590; **Phone:** 708-216-6444; **Board Cert:** Obstetrics & Gynecology 2010; Maternal & Fetal Medicine 2010; **Med School:** Loyola Univ-Stritch Sch Med 1982; **Resid:** Obstetrics & Gynecology, Univ Mich Med Ctr 1986; **Fellow:** Maternal & Fetal Medicine, Johns Hopkins Hosp 1988; **Fac Appt:** Prof ObG, Loyola Univ-Stritch Sch Med

Dooley, Sharon L MD [MF] - **Spec Exp:** Fetal Abnormalities; Pregnancy-High Risk; Multiple Gestation; **Hospital:** Northwestern Meml Hosp; **Address:** 675 N St Clair Fl 14 - Ste 200, Chicago, IL 60611; **Phone:** 312-695-7542; **Board Cert:** Obstetrics & Gynecology 2005; Maternal & Fetal Medicine 2005; **Med School:** Univ VA Sch Med 1973; **Resid:** Obstetrics & Gynecology, Northwestern Meml Hosp 1977; **Fac Appt:** Prof ObG, Northwestern Univ

Hibbard, Judith MD [MF] - **Spec Exp:** Pregnancy-High Risk; Heart Disease in Pregnancy; Prenatal Diagnosis; Ultrasound; **Hospital:** Univ of IL Med Ctr at Chicago; **Address:** Univ Illinois at Chicago, Dept OB-GYN, 1801 W Taylor St, Chicago, IL 60612; **Phone:** 312-413-7500; **Board Cert:** Obstetrics & Gynecology 2010; Maternal & Fetal Medicine 2010; **Med School:** Loyola Univ-Stritch Sch Med 1982; **Resid:** Obstetrics & Gynecology, Univ Chicago Hosps 1986; **Fellow:** Maternal & Fetal Medicine, Univ Chicago Hosps 1988; **Fac Appt:** Prof ObG, Univ IL Coll Med

Hussey, Michael J MD [MF] - **Spec Exp:** Perinatal Medicine; Congenital Anomalies; Multiple Gestation; **Hospital:** Rush Univ Med Ctr; **Address:** 1725 W Harrison St, Ste 408, Chicago, IL 60612; **Phone:** 312-997-2229; **Board Cert:** Obstetrics & Gynecology 2010; **Med School:** Univ IL Coll Med 1986; **Resid:** Obstetrics & Gynecology, Loyola Univ Med Ctr 1993; **Fellow:** Maternal & Fetal Medicine, Rush-Presby-St Lukes Hosp 1995; Ultrasound, Univ Col Hlth Sci Ctr 1996; **Fac Appt:** Asst Prof ObG, Rush Med Coll

Ismail, Mahmoud A MD [MF] - **Spec Exp:** Pregnancy-High Risk; Perinatal Medicine; Infections-Neonatal; Infections in Pregnancy; **Hospital:** Univ of Chicago Med Ctr; **Address:** Dept Ob/Gyn, 5841 S Maryland Ave, MC 2050, Chicago, IL 60637-1463; **Phone:** 773-702-5200; **Board Cert:** Obstetrics & Gynecology 2010; Maternal & Fetal Medicine 2010; **Med School:** Egypt 1970; **Resid:** Obstetrics & Gynecology, Wayne St Univ Affil Hosps 1977; **Fellow:** Maternal & Fetal Medicine, Univ Chicago Hosps 1982; **Fac Appt:** Prof ObG, Univ Chicago-Pritzker Sch Med

Johnson, Timothy R B MD [MF] - **Spec Exp:** Prenatal Diagnosis; **Hospital:** Univ of Michigan Hosp; **Address:** Univ Mich, Dept Ob/Gyn, 1500 E Med Ctr Drive, rm L4000, Box 5276, Ann Arbor, MI 48109; **Phone:** 734-764-8123; **Board Cert:** Obstetrics & Gynecology 2001; Maternal & Fetal Medicine 2001; **Med School:** Univ VA Sch Med 1975; **Resid:** Obstetrics & Gynecology, Univ Michigan Med Ctr 1979; **Fellow:** Maternal & Fetal Medicine, Johns Hopkins Hosp 1981; **Fac Appt:** Prof ObG, Univ Mich Med Sch

Landers, Daniel V MD [MF] - **Spec Exp:** Infectious Disease; **Hospital:** Univ Minn Med Ctr, Fairview - Riverside Campus; **Address:** 606 24th Ave S, Professional Bldg Fl 4, Minneapolis, MN 55454; **Phone:** 612-273-2223; **Board Cert:** Obstetrics & Gynecology 2009; Maternal & Fetal Medicine 2009; **Med School:** UCSF 1980; **Resid:** Obstetrics & Gynecology, UCSF Med Ctr 1984; **Fellow:** Maternal & Fetal Medicine, UCSF Med Ctr 1986; Infectious Disease, UCSF Med Ctr 1988; **Fac Appt:** Prof ObG, Univ Minn

Landon, Mark B MD [MF] - **Spec Exp:** Diabetes in Pregnancy; **Hospital:** Ohio St Univ Med Ctr; **Address:** 2050 Kenny Rd Fl 5, Columbus, OH 43221; **Phone:** 614-293-2222; **Board Cert:** Obstetrics & Gynecology 2010; Maternal & Fetal Medicine 2010; **Med School:** Cornell Univ-Weill Med Coll 1980; **Resid:** Obstetrics & Gynecology, Hosp Univ Penn 1984; **Fellow:** Maternal & Fetal Medicine, Hosp Univ Penn 1986; **Fac Appt:** Assoc Prof ObG, Ohio State Univ

Leslie, Kimberly K MD [MF] - **Spec Exp:** Uterine Cancer; **Hospital:** Univ Iowa Hosp & Clinics; **Address:** 200 Hawkins Drive, Iowa City, IA 52242; **Phone:** 319-356-1976; **Board Cert:** Obstetrics & Gynecology 2011; Maternal & Fetal Medicine 2011; **Med School:** Univ Tex SW, Dallas 1981; **Resid:** Obstetrics & Gynecology, Georgetown Univ 1983; **Fellow:** Maternal & Fetal Medicine, Georgetown Univ 1987; **Fac Appt:** Prof ObG, Univ Iowa Coll Med

Macones, George A MD [MF] - **Spec Exp:** Pregnancy-High Risk; Premature Labor; **Hospital:** Barnes-Jewish Hosp, St. Louis Chldns Hosp; **Address:** Washington Univ Dept Ob/Gyn, 660 S Euclid Ave, Box 8064, St Louis, MO 63110; **Phone:** 314-454-8181; **Board Cert:** Obstetrics & Gynecology 2007; Maternal & Fetal Medicine 2007; **Med School:** Jefferson Med Coll 1988; **Resid:** Obstetrics & Gynecology, Pennsylvania Hosp 1992; **Fellow:** Maternal & Fetal Medicine, Jefferson Univ Hosp 1994; **Fac Appt:** Prof ObG, Washington Univ, St Louis

Philipson, Elliot MD [MF] - **Spec Exp:** Pregnancy-High Risk; Amniocentesis; **Hospital:** Cleveland Clin (page 56), Hillcrest Hosp-Mayfield Hts; **Address:** Hillcrest Hosp, Dept OB/Gyn, 6770 Mayfield Rd, Ste 336, Mayfield Heights, OH 44124; **Phone:** 440-312-7774; **Board Cert:** Obstetrics & Gynecology 2009; **Med School:** Italy 1975; **Resid:** Obstetrics & Gynecology, Albany Med Ctr 1980; **Fellow:** Maternal & Fetal Medicine, Metro Genl Hosp 1982; **Fac Appt:** Assoc Prof ObG, Cleveland Cl Coll Med/Case West Res

Samuels, Philip MD [MF] - **Spec Exp:** Epilepsy in Pregnancy; Hypertension in Pregnancy; Pregnancy & Hematologic Abnormalities; **Hospital:** Ohio St Univ Med Ctr; **Address:** 2050 Kenny Rd Fl 5, Columbus, OH 43221; **Phone:** 614-293-2222; **Board Cert:** Obstetrics & Gynecology 2009; Maternal & Fetal Medicine 2009; **Med School:** Texas Tech Univ 1980; **Resid:** Obstetrics & Gynecology, E VA Grad Sch Med 1984; **Fellow:** Maternal & Fetal Medicine, Hosp Univ Penn 1986; **Fac Appt:** Assoc Prof ObG, Ohio State Univ

Socol, Michael MD [MF] - **Spec Exp:** Diabetes in Pregnancy; Multiple Gestation; Premature Labor; **Hospital:** Northwestern Meml Hosp; **Address:** Prentice Womens Hosp, 250 E Superior St, Ste 3-2307, Chicago, IL 60611-3056; **Phone:** 312-472-3970; **Board Cert:** Obstetrics & Gynecology 1989; Maternal & Fetal Medicine 1981; **Med School:** Univ IL Coll Med 1974; **Resid:** Obstetrics & Gynecology, Univ Illinois Med Ctr 1977; **Fellow:** Maternal & Fetal Medicine, USC Med Ctr 1979; **Fac Appt:** Prof ObG, Northwestern Univ

Strassner, Howard T MD [MF] - **Spec Exp:** Pregnancy-High Risk; Amniocentesis; Obstetric Ultrasound; **Hospital:** Rush Univ Med Ctr, Resurrection Hlth Care St Joseph Hosp; **Address:** Women's Hlth Consultants, 1725 W Harrison St, Ste 408, Chicago, IL 60612; **Phone:** 312-997-2229; **Board Cert:** Obstetrics & Gynecology 2010; Maternal & Fetal Medicine 2010; **Med School:** Univ Chicago-Pritzker Sch Med 1974; **Resid:** Obstetrics & Gynecology, Columbia Presby Med Ctr 1978; **Fellow:** Maternal & Fetal Medicine, LA Co-USC Med Ctr 1980; **Fac Appt:** Prof ObG, Rush Med Coll

Treadwell, Marjorie C MD [MF] - **Spec Exp:** Ultrasound; Pregnancy-High Risk; Fetal Diagnosis & Therapy; **Hospital:** Univ of Michigan Hosp; **Address:** 1500 E Med Ctr Drive, F4806 MOTT Bldg, Ann Arbor, MI 48109-0264; **Phone:** 734-763-4264; **Board Cert:** Obstetrics & Gynecology 2000; Maternal & Fetal Medicine 2000; **Med School:** Univ Mich Med Sch 1984; **Resid:** Obstetrics & Gynecology, Wayne State Univ 1988; **Fellow:** Maternal & Fetal Medicine, Wayne State Univ 1990; **Fac Appt:** Prof ObG, Univ Mich Med Sch

Watson, William J MD [MF] - **Spec Exp:** Ultrasound; Prenatal Diagnosis; Clinical Genetics; Pregnancy-High Risk; **Hospital:** Mayo Med Ctr & Clin - Rochester; **Address:** 200 First St SW, Rochester, MN 55905; **Phone:** 507-284-2511; **Board Cert:** Obstetrics & Gynecology 2009; Maternal & Fetal Medicine 2009; **Med School:** Univ Wash 1980; **Resid:** Obstetrics & Gynecology, Madigan AMC 1984; **Fellow:** Maternal & Fetal Medicine, Univ NC 1990; **Fac Appt:** Prof ObG, Mayo Med Sch

Maternal & Fetal Medicine

Wilkins, Isabelle MD [MF] - **Spec Exp:** Multiple Gestation; Prenatal Ultrasound; Premature Labor; Prematurity/Low Birth Weight Infants; **Hospital:** Univ of IL Med Ctr at Chicago; **Address:** Univ Illinois Med Ctr at Chicago, Center for Womens Health, 1801 W Taylor, MS 650, Chicago, IL 60612; **Phone:** 312-413-7500; **Board Cert:** Obstetrics & Gynecology 2010; Maternal & Fetal Medicine 2010; **Med School:** Duke Univ 1980; **Resid:** Obstetrics & Gynecology, Mt Sinai Med Ctr 1984; **Fellow:** Maternal & Fetal Medicine, Mt Sinai Med Ctr 1986; **Fac Appt:** Prof ObG, Univ IL Coll Med

Winn, Hung MD [MF] - **Spec Exp:** Multiple Gestation; Pregnancy-High Risk; **Hospital:** Univ of Missouri Hosp; **Address:** 500 N Keene St, Ste 405-5, Columbia, MO 65201; **Phone:** 573-499-6041; **Board Cert:** Obstetrics & Gynecology 2000; Maternal & Fetal Medicine 2000; **Med School:** Univ IL Coll Med 1982; **Resid:** Obstetrics & Gynecology, Univ Ill Hosp 1986; **Fellow:** Maternal & Fetal Medicine, Yale-New Haven Hosp 1988; **Fac Appt:** Prof ObG, Univ MO-Columbia Sch Med

Great Plains and Mountains

Dugoff, Lorraine MD [MF] - **Spec Exp:** Pregnancy-High Risk; Prenatal Diagnosis; Ultrasound; **Hospital:** Univ of CO Hosp - Anschutz Inpatient Pav; **Address:** Univ Colorado Womens Services, 1635 Aurora Court, MS F-711, Aurora, CO 80045; **Phone:** 720-848-1060; **Board Cert:** Obstetrics & Gynecology 2010; Maternal & Fetal Medicine 2010; Clinical Genetics 2010; **Med School:** Georgetown Univ 1989; **Resid:** Obstetrics & Gynecology, Philadelphia Hosp 1990; Obstetrics & Gynecology, Univ Colorado Hlth Sci Ctr 1993; **Fellow:** Maternal & Fetal Medicine, Univ Colorado Hlth Sci Ctr 1995; Clinical Genetics, Univ Colorado Hlth Sci Ctr 1996; **Fac Appt:** Assoc Prof ObG, Univ Colorado

Gibbs, Ronald S MD [MF] - **Spec Exp:** Infectious Disease; **Hospital:** Univ of CO Hosp - Anschutz Inpatient Pav; **Address:** Univ Colorado Womens Services, 1635 Aurora Court, MS F711, Aurora, CO 80045; **Phone:** 720-848-1060; **Board Cert:** Obstetrics & Gynecology 1989; Maternal & Fetal Medicine 1981; **Med School:** Univ Pennsylvania 1969; **Resid:** Obstetrics & Gynecology, Hosp Univ Penn 1974; **Fellow:** Maternal & Fetal Medicine, Univ Tex Hlth Sci Ctr 1978; **Fac Appt:** Prof ObG, Univ Colorado

Tomich, Paul MD [MF] - **Spec Exp:** Pregnancy-High Risk; Prenatal Ultrasound; **Hospital:** Nebraska Med Ctr; **Address:** 983255 Nebraska Med Ctr, Omaha, NE 68198-3255; **Phone:** 402-559-6150; **Board Cert:** Obstetrics & Gynecology 2008; Maternal & Fetal Medicine 2008; **Med School:** Loyola Univ-Stritch Sch Med 1973; **Resid:** Obstetrics & Gynecology, Mayo Clinic 1978; **Fellow:** Maternal & Fetal Medicine, Barnes Hosp-Wash Univ 1980; **Fac Appt:** Prof ObG, Univ Nebr Coll Med

Southwest

Adam, Karolina MD [MF] - **Spec Exp:** Pregnancy-High Risk; Heart Disease in Pregnancy; **Hospital:** Methodist Hosp - Houston, St. Luke's Episcopal Hosp-Houston; **Address:** 7900 Fannin, Ste 2600, Houston, TX 77054; **Phone:** 713-791-9700; **Board Cert:** Obstetrics & Gynecology 2010; Maternal & Fetal Medicine 2010; **Med School:** Med Coll PA 1983; **Resid:** Obstetrics & Gynecology, Baylor Coll Med Ctr 1987; **Fellow:** Maternal & Fetal Medicine, Baylor Coll Med Ctr 1989

Hankins, Gary D V MD [MF] - **Spec Exp:** Pregnancy-High Risk; Hypertension in Pregnancy; **Hospital:** UT Med Br at Galveston; **Address:** 301 University Blvd, 3.400 JSA, Galveston, TX 77555-0587; **Phone:** 409-772-1957; **Board Cert:** Obstetrics & Gynecology 2000; Maternal & Fetal Medicine 2000; **Med School:** Med Coll VA 1977; **Resid:** Obstetrics & Gynecology, Wilford Hall Med Ctr 1981; **Fellow:** Critical Care Medicine, Wilford Hall Med Ctr 1982; Maternal & Fetal Medicine, Parkland Hosp 1984; **Fac Appt:** Prof ObG, Univ Tex Med Br, Galveston

Horsager, Robyn Boehrer MD [MF] - **Hospital:** UT Southwestern Med Ctr at Dallas; **Address:** 5939 Harry Hines Blvd, Ste 300, MC 9102, Dallas, TX 75390-9102; **Phone:** 214-645-3837; **Board Cert:** Obstetrics & Gynecology 2010; Maternal & Fetal Medicine 2010; **Med School:** Univ IL Coll Med 1987; **Resid:** Obstetrics & Gynecology, Parkland Meml Hosp 1991; **Fellow:** Maternal & Fetal Medicine, Univ Texas SW Med Ctr 1993; **Fac Appt:** Assoc Prof ObG, Univ Tex SW, Dallas

Mastrobattista, Joan MD [MF] - **Spec Exp:** Pregnancy-High Risk; **Hospital:** Meml Hermann Hosp - Texas Med Ctr; **Address:** 6410 Fannin St Fl 2 - Ste 250, Houston, TX 77030; **Phone:** 832-325-7133; **Board Cert:** Obstetrics & Gynecology 2010; Maternal & Fetal Medicine 2010; **Med School:** UMDNJ-NJ Med Sch, Newark 1988; **Resid:** Obstetrics & Gynecology, Cornell Univ Hosp 1992; **Fellow:** Maternal & Fetal Medicine, UT Med Ctr 1994

Pridjian, Gabriella C MD [MF] - **Spec Exp:** Pregnancy-High Risk; Prenatal Diagnosis; Genetic Disorders; Prenatal Ultrasound; **Hospital:** Tulane-Lakeside Hosp, Tulane Med Ctr; **Address:** Womens Health Center, 4720 S I-10 Service Road, Ste 302, Metairie, LA 70001; **Phone:** 504-988-8070; **Board Cert:** Obstetrics & Gynecology 2007; Maternal & Fetal Medicine 2007; Clinical Genetics 2010; **Med School:** Med Coll Wisc 1982; **Resid:** Obstetrics & Gynecology, Univ Chicago Affil Hosp 1986; **Fellow:** Maternal & Fetal Medicine, Univ Chicago Affil Hosp 1989; Clinical Genetics, Hayward Gentics Ctr/Tulane Univ 1994; **Fac Appt:** Prof ObG, Tulane Univ

Reed, Kathryn L MD [MF] - **Spec Exp:** Prenatal Diagnosis; Ultrasound; Fetal Echocardiography; **Hospital:** Univ Med Ctr - Tucson; **Address:** Univ AZ Dept Ob/Gyn-Womens Resource Ctr, 1501 N Campbell Ave Fl 8, PO Box 245078, Tucson, AZ 85724; **Phone:** 520-694-6010; **Board Cert:** Obstetrics & Gynecology 2010; Maternal & Fetal Medicine 2010; **Med School:** Univ Ariz Coll Med 1977; **Resid:** Obstetrics & Gynecology, Univ Med Ctr 1981; **Fellow:** Maternal & Fetal Medicine, Univ Arizona 1983; **Fac Appt:** Prof ObG, Univ Ariz Coll Med

Robichaux III, Alfred G MD [MF] - **Spec Exp:** Fetal Surgery; Fetal Abnormalities; Pregnancy-High Risk; **Hospital:** Ochsner Med Ctr-New Orleans; **Address:** Ochsner Clinic, Maternal-Fetal Medicine, 1514 Jefferson Hwy, New Orleans, LA 70121; **Phone:** 504-842-4151; **Board Cert:** Obstetrics & Gynecology 2010; Maternal & Fetal Medicine 2010; **Med School:** Louisiana State U, New Orleans 1978; **Resid:** Obstetrics & Gynecology, Ochsner Clinic Fdn 1982; **Fellow:** Maternal & Fetal Medicine, George Washington Univ 1984

West Coast and Pacific

Adashek, Joseph MD [MF] - **Spec Exp:** Pregnancy-High Risk; Prematurity Prevention; Prenatal Diagnosis; **Hospital:** Southern Hills Hosp & Med Ctr, Summerlin Hosp Med Ctr; **Address:** Desert Perinatal Associates, 5761 S Fort Apache, Las Vegas, NV 89144; **Phone:** 702-341-6610; **Board Cert:** Obstetrics & Gynecology 2009; Maternal & Fetal Medicine 2009; **Med School:** Penn State Coll Med 1989; **Resid:** Obstetrics & Gynecology, Northwestern Meml Hosp 1993; **Fellow:** Maternal & Fetal Medicine, UC Irvine Med Ctr 1995

Benedetti, Thomas J MD [MF] - **Spec Exp:** Prematurity Prevention; Fetal Macrosomia; **Hospital:** Univ Wash Med Ctr, Yakima Valley Mem Hosp; **Address:** Univ Washington Dept. OB/GYN, 1959 NE Pacific St, Box 356460, Health Sci Bldg, Seattle, WA 98195-6460; **Phone:** 206-543-3729; **Board Cert:** Obstetrics & Gynecology 1980; Maternal & Fetal Medicine 1981; **Med School:** Univ Wash 1973; **Resid:** Obstetrics & Gynecology, LAC-USC Med Ctr 1977; **Fellow:** Maternal & Fetal Medicine, LAC-USC Med Ctr 1979; **Fac Appt:** Prof ObG, Univ Wash

Caughey, Aaron B MD/PhD [MF] - **Spec Exp:** Pregnancy-High Risk; Diabetes in Pregnancy; Prenatal Diagnosis; **Hospital:** OR Hlth & Sci Univ; **Address:** OHSU, Dept of Perinatology, 3181 SW Sam Jackson Park Rd, MC PV420, Portland, OR 97239; **Phone:** 503-418-4200; **Board Cert:** Obstetrics & Gynecology 2007; Maternal & Fetal Medicine 2007; **Med School:** Harvard Med Sch 1995; **Resid:** Obstetrics & Gynecology, Brigham & Women's Hosp 1999; **Fellow:** Radiology, UCSF Med Ctr 2000; Maternal & Fetal Medicine, UCSF Med Ctr 2002

Cheng, Edith Y MD [MF] - **Spec Exp:** Genetic Disorders; Prenatal Diagnosis; Fetal Therapy; **Hospital:** Univ Wash Med Ctr, Seattle Chldns Hosp; **Address:** Univ Washington- Dept of Ob/Gyn, 1959 NE Pacific St, Box 356460, Seattle, WA 98195; **Phone:** 206-598-4070; **Board Cert:** Clinical Genetics 2006; Obstetrics & Gynecology 2008; Maternal & Fetal Medicine 2008; **Med School:** Univ Wash 1987; **Resid:** Obstetrics & Gynecology, Univ Washington Med Ctr 1991; **Fellow:** Clinical Genetics, Univ Washington Med Ctr 1993; Maternal & Fetal Medicine, Univ Washington Med Ctr 1995; **Fac Appt:** Assoc Prof ObG, Univ Wash

Chmait, Ramen H MD [MF] - **Spec Exp:** Fetal Surgery; Twin to Twin Transfusion Syndrome (TTTS); **Hospital:** Hollywood Presby Med Ctr; **Address:** Hollywood Presbyterian Med Ctr, 1300 N Vermont Ave, Ste 710, Los Angles, CA 90027; **Phone:** 323-361-6074; **Board Cert:** Obstetrics & Gynecology 2007; Maternal & Fetal Medicine 2007; **Med School:** UCLA 1996; **Resid:** Obstetrics & Gynecology, LAC/USC Med Ctr 2001; **Fellow:** Maternal & Fetal Medicine, UCSD Med Ctr 2003

Druzin, Maurice L MD [MF] - **Spec Exp:** Lupus/SLE in Pregnancy; Miscarriage-Recurrent; **Hospital:** Lucile Packard Chldn's Hosp; **Address:** 770 Welch Rd, Ste 201, Palo Alto, CA 94304; **Phone:** 650-498-4069; **Board Cert:** Obstetrics & Gynecology 2010; Maternal & Fetal Medicine 2008; **Med School:** South Africa 1970; **Resid:** Obstetrics & Gynecology, Rose Med Ctr-Univ Colo 1977; **Fellow:** Maternal & Fetal Medicine, LAC-USC Med Ctr 1979; **Fac Appt:** Prof ObG, Stanford Univ

Elliott, John P MD [MF] - **Spec Exp:** Twin to Twin Transfusion Syndrome (TTTS); Multiple Gestation; Premature Labor; **Hospital:** Saddleback Mem Med Ctr; **Address:** 24411 Health Center Drive, Ste 300, Laguna Hills, CA 92653; **Phone:** 949-452-7199; **Board Cert:** Obstetrics & Gynecology 1980; Maternal & Fetal Medicine 1982; **Med School:** Univ Colorado 1972; **Resid:** Obstetrics & Gynecology, Fitzsimmons Army Med Ctr 1976; **Fellow:** Maternal & Fetal Medicine, Long Beach Meml Hosp/UC Irvine 1980

Goldberg, James D MD [MF] - **Spec Exp:** Prenatal Diagnosis; Fetal Diagnosis & Therapy; **Hospital:** CA Pacific Med Ctr-Pacific Campus; **Address:** San Francisco Perinatal Assoc, One Daniel Burnham Ct, Ste 230C, San Francisco, CA 94109; **Phone:** 415-202-1200; **Board Cert:** Obstetrics & Gynecology 2010; Clinical Genetics 1987; Maternal & Fetal Medicine 2010; **Med School:** Univ Minn 1979; **Resid:** Obstetrics & Gynecology, UCSF Med Ctr 1983; **Fellow:** Maternal & Fetal Medicine, Mt Sinai Hosp 1985; Clinical Genetics, Mt Sinai Hosp 1985

Gravett, Michael G MD [MF] - **Spec Exp:** Infectious Disease-Perinatal; **Hospital:** Univ Wash Med Ctr; **Address:** Univ Washington, Dept OB/GYN, 1959 NE Pacific St, Box 356460, Hlth Sci Bldg, Seattle, WA 98195-6460; **Phone:** 206-598-4070; **Board Cert:** Obstetrics & Gynecology 1985; Maternal & Fetal Medicine 1987; **Med School:** UCLA 1977; **Resid:** Obstetrics & Gynecology, Univ Wash Med Ctr 1981; **Fellow:** Maternal & Fetal Medicine, Univ Wash Med Ctr 1983; **Fac Appt:** Prof ObG, Univ Wash

Kelly, Thomas F MD [MF] - **Spec Exp:** Pregnancy-High Risk; **Hospital:** UCSD Med Ctr; **Address:** UCSD Med Ctr, Dept Reproductive Med, 200 W Arbor Drive, MC 8433, San Diego, CA 92103; **Phone:** 619-543-2384; **Board Cert:** Obstetrics & Gynecology 2009; Maternal & Fetal Medicine 2009; **Med School:** Univ Nevada 1986; **Resid:** Obstetrics & Gynecology, USCD Med Ctr 1990; **Fellow:** Maternal & Fetal Medicine, USCD Med Ctr 1992; **Fac Appt:** Prof ObG, UCSD

Koos, Brian J MD [MF] - **Spec Exp:** Pregnancy-High Risk; Fetal Diagnosis & Therapy; Heart Disease in Pregnancy; **Hospital:** UCLA Ronald Reagan Med Ctr; **Address:** UCLA Rhonda Fleming Ob/Gyn, 200 UCLA Medical Plaza, Ste 430, Box 956928, Los Angeles, CA 90095; **Phone:** 310-794-7852; **Board Cert:** Obstetrics & Gynecology 1999; Maternal & Fetal Medicine 1999; **Med School:** Loma Linda Univ 1974; **Resid:** Obstetrics & Gynecology, Brigham & Womens Hosp 1979; **Fellow:** Maternal & Fetal Medicine, Womens Hosp 1983; **Fac Appt:** Prof ObG, UCLA

Moore, Thomas R MD [MF] - **Spec Exp:** Diabetes in Pregnancy; Fetal Diagnosis & Therapy; **Hospital:** UCSD Med Ctr, Scripps Meml Hosp - La Jolla; **Address:** 200 W Arbor Drive, MC 8433, San Diego, CA 92103; **Phone:** 619-543-7900; **Board Cert:** Obstetrics & Gynecology 2006; Maternal & Fetal Medicine 2006; **Med School:** Yale Univ 1979; **Resid:** Obstetrics & Gynecology, Naval Hosp 1983; **Fellow:** Maternal & Fetal Medicine, UCSD 1985; **Fac Appt:** Prof ObG, UCSD

Platt, Lawrence D MD [MF] - **Spec Exp:** Ultrasound; Prenatal Diagnosis; **Hospital:** Cedars-Sinai Med Ctr, St. John's Hlth Ctr, Santa Monica; **Address:** 6310 W San Vincente Blvd, Ste 520, Los Angeles, CA 90048; **Phone:** 323-857-1952; **Board Cert:** Obstetrics & Gynecology 1979; Maternal & Fetal Medicine 1981; **Med School:** Wayne State Univ 1972; **Resid:** Obstetrics & Gynecology, Sinai Hosp 1976; **Fellow:** Maternal & Fetal Medicine, USC Med Ctr 1978; **Fac Appt:** Prof ObG, UCLA

Robertson, Patricia A MD [MF] - **Spec Exp:** Pregnancy-High Risk; **Hospital:** UCSF Med Ctr; **Address:** 400 Parnassus Ave, Box 0346, San Francisco, CA 94143; **Phone:** 415-353-2566; **Board Cert:** Obstetrics & Gynecology 2009; Maternal & Fetal Medicine 2009; **Med School:** Univ Tex, San Antonio 1976; **Resid:** Obstetrics & Gynecology, UCSF Med Ctr 1980; **Fellow:** Maternal & Fetal Medicine, UCSF Med Ctr 1990; **Fac Appt:** Prof ObG, UCSF

Tabsh, Khalil M A MD [MF] - **Spec Exp:** Pregnancy-High Risk; **Hospital:** UCLA Ronald Reagan Med Ctr, Santa Monica - UCLA Med Ctr & Ortho Hosp; **Address:** 200 Med Plaza, Ste 430, Los Angeles, CA 90095; **Phone:** 310-208-4492; **Board Cert:** Obstetrics & Gynecology 1981; Maternal & Fetal Medicine 1982; **Med School:** Lebanon 1974; **Resid:** Obstetrics & Gynecology, American Univ Beirut Med Ctr 1976; Obstetrics & Gynecology, Yale-New Haven Hosp 1978; **Fellow:** Maternal & Fetal Medicine, UCLA Med Ctr 1979; **Fac Appt:** Clin Prof ObG, UCLA-David Geffen Sch Med

Zalud, Ivica MD/PhD [MF] - **Spec Exp:** Obstetric Ultrasound; Pregnancy-High Risk; **Hospital:** Kapiolani Med Ctr for Women & Chldn; **Address:** Kapliolani Med Ctr for Women & Children, 1319 Punahou St, Ste 540, Hololulu, HI 96826; **Phone:** 808-203-6546; **Board Cert:** Obstetrics & Gynecology 2005; Maternal & Fetal Medicine 2005; **Med School:** Croatia 1986; **Resid:** Obstetrics & Gynecology, Winthrop Univ Hosp 1997; **Fellow:** Maternal & Fetal Medicine, Georgetown Univ Med Ctr 2000; **Fac Appt:** Assoc Prof ObG, Univ Hawaii JA Burns Sch Med

▪▪ Cleveland Clinic

Every life deserves world class care.

Maternal & Fetal Medicine

Cleveland Clinic Ob/Gyn & Women's Health Institute is designed to meet the unique and changing medical needs of women from adolescence to mature adulthood. Our team offers coordinated and supportive care. *U.S. News & World Report* has ranked our gynecology program No. 4 in the country. Our physicians are nationally and internally known and many serve on leadership boards for professional physician societies.

Physicians and certified nurse-midwives in the Maternal-Fetal Medicine/Obstetrics Section provide three levels of obstetrical care: midwives offer a family-centered approach to low-risk prenatal care and delivery; general obstetricians provide care for low- and medium-risk pregnancies; and maternal/fetal medicine specialists provide diagnosis and treatment for more complicated high-risk pregnancies. Available services include genetic counseling, ultrasound, chorionic villus sampling and amniocentesis.

Cleveland Clinic Fetal Care Center, launched in 2005, is a multidisciplinary team of perinatologists, neonatologists and pediatric surgeons whose goal is to achieve the best possible outcome in pregnancies complicated by complex congenital anomalies. Through collaboration and communication, we provide accurate prenatal diagnosis using state-of-the-art techniques such as high-resolution ultrasound, fetal MRI and fetoscopy, then interpret and apply that information in developing a management plan for pregnancy, delivery and newborn care.

Our Fetal Care Center is staffed by pediatric specialists and maternal-fetal medicine specialists who diagnose fetal problems and can treat them immediately after birth or in the womb. Our new Special Delivery Unit and adjoining Pediatric Cardiac Catheterization Laboratory are key components of the Fetal Care Center.

Cleveland Clinic
Women's Health Institute
9500 Euclid Avenue
Cleveland, OH 44195

clevelandclinic.org/
fetalmedicinetopdocs

Offering Same-Day Appointments
Call 800.274.2009.

Treatment Guides

Cleveland Clinic has developed comprehensive treatment guides for many diseases and conditions. To download our free treatment guides, visit clevelandclinic.org/treatmentguides.

Online Medical Second Opinion

Cleveland Clinic's My**Consult** Online Medical Second Opinion program securely connects patients to our physician specialists for more than 1,000 life-changing or life-threatening diagnoses all by the click of a mouse. To learn more, log onto eclevelandclinic.org/myconsult or call 800.223.2273, ext. 43223.

Special Assistance for Out-of-State Patients

Cleveland Clinic Global Patient Services offers a complimentary Medical Concierge service for patients who travel from outside of Ohio. Call 800.223.2273, ext. 55580 or email medicalconcierge@ccf.org.

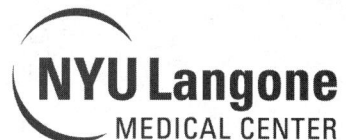
MATERNAL-FETAL MEDICINE

About the Division of Maternal-Fetal Medicine
The Division of Maternal-Fetal Medicine at NYU Langone Medical Center is committed to ensuring that both mother and fetus receive the highly specialized care they need. The Division focuses on multifetal pregnancies, genetic counseling, women who have miscarried, preterm deliveries and other medical complications that can occur during pregnancy. We also specialize in helping women who have other medical conditions that may complicate a pregnancy, such as diabetes, heart problems, high blood pressure, and lupus, among others. The Division offers the latest techniques for in-utero diagnosis and treatment as well as advanced care of complex obstetrical patients. We specialize in the following areas:

Patient Care
The Division of Maternal-Fetal Medicine focuses on ensuring that each patient delivers a healthy baby. Using minimally invasive techniques, doctors at NYU Langone Medical Center are able to repair a number of life-threatening conditions in a child before it is even born, reducing the risks of preterm labor and the need for Cesarean births. Our physicians have developed numerous new treatment protocols for high-risk obstetrics that have been adopted around the world.

Research
The Division of Maternal-Fetal Medicine has generated new treatments for high-risk obstetrics patients and introduced effective new methods of diagnosis and treatment for the fetus.

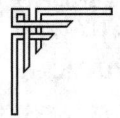

The Best in American Medicine
www.CastleConnolly.com

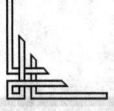
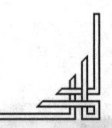

Neonatal-Perinatal Medicine
a subspecialty of Pediatrics

A subspecialist in neonatal-perinatal medicine is a pediatrician who is the principal care provider for sick newborn infants. Clinical expertise is used for direct patient care and for consulting with obstetrical colleagues to plan for the care of mothers who have high-risk pregnancies.

Training Required: Three years in pediatrics *plus* additional training and examination.

NEONATAL-PERINATAL MEDICINE

New England

Cloherty, John MD [NP] - **Spec Exp:** Neonatology; **Hospital:** Children's Hospital - Boston, Brigham and Women's Hosp (page 57); **Address:** 319 Longwood Ave, Fl 4, Boston, MA 02115; **Phone:** 617-277-7320; **Board Cert:** Pediatrics 1986; Neonatal-Perinatal Medicine 1986; **Med School:** Boston Univ 1962; **Resid:** Pediatrics, Mass Genl Hosp 1969; **Fellow:** Neonatal-Perinatal Medicine, Chldns Hosp; **Fac Appt:** Assoc Clin Prof Ped, Harvard Med Sch

Davis, Jonathan M MD [NP] - **Spec Exp:** Lung Disease in Newborns; Brain Injury; Infections-Neonatal; **Hospital:** Tufts Med Ctr; **Address:** Tufts Med Ctr, 800 Washington St, Box 44, Boston, MA 02111; **Phone:** 617-636-5322; **Board Cert:** Pediatrics 1985; Neonatal-Perinatal Medicine 1987; **Med School:** McGill Univ 1981; **Resid:** Pediatrics, Chldns Hosp 1984; **Fellow:** Neonatal-Perinatal Medicine, Chldns Hosp 1986; **Fac Appt:** Prof Ped, Tufts Univ

Ehrenkranz, Richard MD [NP] - **Spec Exp:** Nutrition; Lung Disease in Newborns; **Hospital:** Yale-New Haven Hosp, Yale Med Group; **Address:** Yale Univ-Dept Ped, PO Box 208064, New Haven, CT 06510; **Phone:** 203-688-2320; **Board Cert:** Pediatrics 1977; Neonatal-Perinatal Medicine 1979; **Med School:** SUNY Downstate 1972; **Resid:** Pediatrics, Yale-New Haven Hosp 1974; **Fellow:** Neonatal-Perinatal Medicine, Yale-New Haven Hosp 1978; **Fac Appt:** Prof Ped, Yale Univ

Frantz, Ivan MD [NP] - **Spec Exp:** Lung Disease in Newborns; Pulmonary Hypertension of Newborn (PPHN); **Hospital:** Floating Hosp for Children at Tufts Med Ce; **Address:** Tufts Med Ctr, Newborn Med, 800 Washington St, Box 44, Boston, MA 02111; **Phone:** 617-636-5322; **Board Cert:** Pediatrics 1976; Neonatal-Perinatal Medicine 2009; **Med School:** Univ Minn 1971; **Resid:** Pediatrics, Univ Minn Hosp 1973; **Fellow:** Neonatal-Perinatal Medicine, McGill Royal Victoria Hosp 1974; Neonatal-Perinatal Medicine, Mass Genl Hosp 1975; **Fac Appt:** Prof Ped, Tufts Univ

Gross, Ian MD [NP] - **Spec Exp:** Breathing Disorders; Critical Care; **Hospital:** Yale-New Haven Hosp, Yale Med Group; **Address:** Yale Sch Med, Dept Pediatrics, 333 Cedar St, PO Box 208064, New Haven, CT 06520-8064; **Phone:** 203-688-2320; **Board Cert:** Pediatrics 1974; Neonatal-Perinatal Medicine 1977; **Med School:** South Africa 1967; **Resid:** Pediatrics, Univ Witwatersrand Affil Hosps 1971; Pediatrics, Chldns Hosp Med Ctr 1973; **Fellow:** Neonatal-Perinatal Medicine, Yale-New Haven Hosp 1974; **Fac Appt:** Prof Ped, Yale Univ

Van Marter, Linda J MD [NP] - **Spec Exp:** Neonatal Chronic Lung Disease (CLD); Lung Disease in Newborns; Pulmonary Hypertension of Newborn (PPHN); **Hospital:** Brigham and Women's Hosp (page 57), Children's Hospital - Boston; **Address:** 300 Longwood Ave, Hunnewell 430 - Newborn Med, Boston, MA 02115; **Phone:** 617-355-6027; **Board Cert:** Pediatrics 1985; Neonatal-Perinatal Medicine 2009; **Med School:** Univ Pittsburgh 1980; **Resid:** Pediatrics, Childrens Hosp Med Ctr 1983; **Fellow:** Neonatology, Harvard Med Sch 1986; **Fac Appt:** Assoc Prof Ped, Harvard Med Sch

Mid Atlantic

Davidson, Dennis MD [NP] - **Spec Exp:** Lung Disease in Newborns; **Hospital:** Steven & Alexandra Cohen Chldn's Med Ctr of NY; **Address:** Steven & Alexander Cohen Chldn's Med Ctr, 269-01 76th Ave, Ste 344, Div Neonatology, New Hyde Park, NY 11040; **Phone:** 718-470-3440; **Board Cert:** Pediatrics 1980; Neonatal-Perinatal Medicine 2009; **Med School:** Loyola Univ-Stritch Sch Med 1974; **Resid:** Pediatrics, Babies Hosp-Columbia Univ 1978; **Fellow:** Neonatal-Perinatal Medicine, Babies Hosp-Columbia Univ 1981; **Fac Appt:** Clin Prof Ped, Albert Einstein Coll Med

Delivoria-Papadopoulos, Maria MD [NP] - **Spec Exp:** Neonatology; Prematurity/Low Birth Weight Infants; Breathing Disorders; Brain Injury; **Hospital:** St. Christopher's Hosp for Chldn, Hahnemann Univ Hosp; **Address:** St Christopher's Hosp for Children, 3601 A St, Ste 2212, Neonatology, Philadelphia, PA 19134; **Phone:** 215-427-5202; **Board Cert:** Pediatrics 1971; Neonatal-Perinatal Medicine 1975; **Med School:** Greece 1957; **Resid:** Pediatrics, Chldns Hosp 1959; Psychiatry, Colo State Hosp 1962; **Fellow:** Neonatology, Hosp Sick Chldn 1964; **Fac Appt:** Prof Ped

Dennery, Phyllis Armelle MD [NP] - **Spec Exp:** Lung Disease in Newborns; **Hospital:** Chldns Hosp of Philadelphia; **Address:** CHOP Div Neonatology, 34th St and Civic Ctr Blvd, rm 415, Philadelphia, PA 19104; **Phone:** 215-590-1653; **Board Cert:** Neonatal-Perinatal Medicine 2004; **Med School:** Howard Univ 1984; **Resid:** Pediatrics, Chldns Hosp Natl Med Ctr 1988; **Fellow:** Neonatal-Perinatal Medicine, Case Western Reserve Affil Hosp 1989; **Fac Appt:** Prof Ped, Univ Pennsylvania

Hendricks-Munoz, Karen MD [NP] - **Spec Exp:** Breathing Disorders; Neonatal Neurology; Retinopathy of Prematurity; **Hospital:** NYU Langone Med Ctr (page 66), Bellevue Hosp Ctr; **Address:** NYU Med Ctr, Dept Neonatology, 530 1st Ave, Ste HCC-7A, New York, NY 10016-6402; **Phone:** 212-263-7477; **Board Cert:** Pediatrics 1985; Neonatal-Perinatal Medicine 2009; **Med School:** Yale Univ 1978; **Resid:** Pediatrics, Yale-New Haven Hosp 1981; **Fellow:** Neonatology, Strong Meml Hosp 1984; **Fac Appt:** Assoc Prof Ped, NYU Sch Med

Holzman, Ian R MD [NP] - **Spec Exp:** Neonatal Nutrition; Necrotizing Enterocolitis; Ethics; Prematurity/Low Birth Weight Infants; **Hospital:** Mount Sinai Med Ctr (page 63), Elmhurst Hosp Ctr; **Address:** Newborn Assocs, One Gustave L Levy Pl, Box 1508, New York, NY 10029-6500; **Phone:** 212-241-5446; **Board Cert:** Pediatrics 1974; Neonatal-Perinatal Medicine 1977; **Med School:** Univ Pittsburgh 1971; **Resid:** Pediatrics, Chldns Hosp 1975; **Fellow:** Neonatal-Perinatal Medicine, Univ Colorado Hosp 1977; **Fac Appt:** Prof Ped, Mount Sinai Sch Med

Hurt, Hallam MD [NP] - **Spec Exp:** Neonatology; **Hospital:** Chldns Hosp of Philadelphia, Hosp Univ Penn - UPHS (page 68); **Address:** Chldns Hosp of Philadelphia, 3535 Market St Fl 14, Philadelphia, PA 19104; **Phone:** 215-590-0560; **Board Cert:** Pediatrics 1976; Neonatal-Perinatal Medicine 2002; **Med School:** Univ VA Sch Med 1971; **Resid:** Pediatrics, Univ Virginia Hosp 1974; **Fellow:** Neonatal-Perinatal Medicine, Univ Virginia Hosp 1976; **Fac Appt:** Prof Ped, Univ Pennsylvania

La Gamma, Edmund F MD [NP] - **Spec Exp:** Neonatal Infections; Prematurity/Low Birth Weight Infants; Necrotizing Enterocolitis; **Hospital:** Westchester Med Ctr, Children's & Women's Phys.of Westchester; **Address:** Maria Fareri Chldns Hosp, 100 Woods Rd, rm 2215, Valhalla, NY 10595; **Phone:** 914-493-8558; **Board Cert:** Pediatrics 1981; Neonatal-Perinatal Medicine 1981; **Med School:** NY Med Coll 1976; **Resid:** Pediatrics, NY Hosp-Cornell Med Ctr 1978; **Fellow:** Neonatal-Perinatal Medicine, NY Hosp-Cornell Med Ctr 1980; Cardiovascular Disease, UCSF Med Ctr 1981; **Fac Appt:** Prof Ped, NY Med Coll

Lawson, Edward E MD [NP] - **Spec Exp:** Prematurity/Low Birth Weight Infants; Respiratory Distress Syndrome (RDS); Neonatal Critical Care; Breathing Disorders; **Hospital:** Johns Hopkins Hosp (page 61), Johns Hopkins Bayview Med Ctr (page 61); **Address:** Johns Hopkins Chldns Ctr, 600 N Wolfe St, Nelson 2-133, Baltimore, MD 21287; **Phone:** 410-955-5259; **Board Cert:** Pediatrics 1990; Neonatal-Perinatal Medicine 1997; **Med School:** Northwestern Univ 1972; **Resid:** Pediatrics, Chldns Hosp Med Ctr 1975; **Fellow:** Neonatal-Perinatal Medicine, Harvard Med Sch 1977; **Fac Appt:** Prof Ped, Johns Hopkins Univ

Neonatal-Perinatal Medicine

Nogee, Lawrence M MD [NP] - **Spec Exp:** Lung Disease in Newborns-Genetic; **Hospital:** Johns Hopkins Hosp (page 61); **Address:** Johns Hopkins Hosp, Div Neonatolgy, 600 N Wolfe St, CMSC 6-104A, Baltimore, MD 21287-3200; **Phone:** 410-955-5259; **Board Cert:** Pediatrics 1986; Neonatal-Perinatal Medicine 1987; **Med School:** Johns Hopkins Univ 1981; **Resid:** Pediatrics, Johns Hopkins Hosp 1984; **Fellow:** Neonatal-Perinatal Medicine, Chldns Hosp Med Ctr 1986; **Fac Appt:** Prof Ped, Johns Hopkins Univ

Perlman, Jeffrey M MD [NP] - **Spec Exp:** Neonatal Critical Care; Prematurity/Low Birth Weight Infants; Neonatal Neurology; Lung Disease in Newborns; **Hospital:** NY-Presby/Weill Cornell Med Ctr, NY (page 65); **Address:** 525 E 68th St, Ste N 506, New York, NY 10065; **Phone:** 212-746-3530; **Board Cert:** Pediatrics 1983; Neonatal-Perinatal Medicine 1983; **Med School:** South Africa 1974; **Resid:** Pediatrics, Johannesburg Chldns Hosp 1979; Pediatrics, St Louis Chldns Hosp 1981; **Fellow:** Neonatology, St Louis Chldns Hosp 1983; **Fac Appt:** Prof Ped, Cornell Univ-Weill Med Coll

Polin, Richard A MD [NP] - **Spec Exp:** Neonatal Infections; **Hospital:** Morgan Stanley Children's Hosp of NY-Presby, NY (page 65); **Address:** Morgan Stanley Chlds Hosp, 3959 Broadway, CHC 115, New York, NY 10032; **Phone:** 212-305-5827; **Board Cert:** Pediatrics 1975; Neonatal-Perinatal Medicine 1977; **Med School:** Temple Univ 1970; **Resid:** Pediatrics, Chldns Meml Hosp 1972; Pediatrics, Babies Hosp 1975; **Fellow:** Neonatal-Perinatal Medicine, Babies Hosp-Columbia 1974; **Fac Appt:** Prof Ped, Columbia P&S

Short, Billie Lou MD [NP] - **Hospital:** Chldns Natl Med Ctr; **Address:** Div Neonatology, 111 Michigan Ave NW, Washington, DC 20010; **Phone:** 202-476-3314; **Board Cert:** Pediatrics 1979; Neonatal-Perinatal Medicine 1979; **Med School:** Univ Okla Coll Med 1974; **Resid:** Pediatrics, Chldn's Hosp-Oklahoma 1977; **Fellow:** Neonatal-Perinatal Medicine, Chldn's Hosp Med Ctr 1979; **Fac Appt:** Prof Ped, Geo Wash Univ

Silverman, Gary A MD/PhD [NP] - **Hospital:** Chldns Hosp of Pittsburgh - UPMC, Magee-Womens Hosp - UPMC; **Address:** Children's Hosp of Pittsburgh, 1 Children's Hospital Drive, 4401 Penn Ave, rm 7130, Pittsburgh, PA 15224; **Phone:** 412-692-9448; **Board Cert:** Neonatal-Perinatal Medicine 2011; **Med School:** Univ Chicago-Pritzker Sch Med 1984; **Resid:** Pediatrics, Children's Hosp 1087; **Fellow:** Neonatology, St Louis Chldns Hosp 1989; Research, Washington U Sch Med 1991; **Fac Appt:** Prof Ped, Univ Pittsburgh

Watchko, Jon F MD [NP] - **Hospital:** Magee-Womens Hosp - UPMC, Chldns Hosp of Pittsburgh - UPMC; **Address:** Magee-Women's Hosp, Newborn Medicine, 300 Halket St, Pittsburgh, PA 15213; **Phone:** 412-641-1834; **Board Cert:** Pediatrics 1985; Neonatal-Perinatal Medicine 1985; **Med School:** Univ Pittsburgh 1980; **Resid:** Pediatrics, Upstate Med Ctr 1983; **Fellow:** Neonatology, Univ Washington Med Ctr 1986; **Fac Appt:** Prof Ped, Univ Pittsburgh

Zubrow, Alan B MD [NP] - **Spec Exp:** Neonatology; **Hospital:** St. Christopher's Hosp for Chldn, Hahnemann Univ Hosp; **Address:** St Christopher's Hosp for Chldn, 3601 A St, Philadelphia, PA 19134; **Phone:** 215-427-5202; **Board Cert:** Pediatrics 1980; Neonatal-Perinatal Medicine 2009; **Med School:** Univ Pennsylvania 1976; **Resid:** Pediatrics, Chldns Hosp 1979; **Fellow:** Neonatology, Columbia-Presby Med Ctr 1981; **Fac Appt:** Prof Ped, Drexel Univ Coll Med

Southeast

Bancalari, Eduardo MD [NP] - **Spec Exp:** Neonatology; **Hospital:** Jackson Meml Hosp (page 70); **Address:** Dept Pediatrics (R-131), PO Box 016960, Miami, FL 33101; **Phone:** 305-585-2328; **Board Cert:** Neonatal-Perinatal Medicine 1993; Pediatrics 1993; **Med School:** Chile 1966; **Resid:** Pediatrics, Hosp Luis Calvo Mackenna 1969; **Fellow:** Pediatric Cardiology, Univ Miami Med Ctr; **Fac Appt:** Prof Ped, Univ Miami Sch Med

Boyle, Robert J MD [NP] - **Spec Exp:** Neonatology; Ethics; **Hospital:** Univ of Virginia Health Sys; **Address:** UVA Hlth Sci Ctr, Dept Peds, PO Box 800386, Charlottesville, VA 22908; **Phone:** 434-924-5429; **Board Cert:** Pediatrics 1978; Neonatal-Perinatal Medicine 1979; **Med School:** Johns Hopkins Univ 1973; **Resid:** Pediatrics, Rainbow Babies Chldns Hosp 1976; **Fellow:** Neonatal-Perinatal Medicine, Women & Infants Hosp 1978; **Fac Appt:** Prof Ped, Univ VA Sch Med

Bucciarelli, Richard L MD [NP] - **Spec Exp:** Neonatal Cardiology; **Hospital:** Shands at Univ of FL; **Address:** Shands Healthcare, 1600 SW Archer Rd, rm R1-118, PO Box 100296, Gainesville, FL 32610; **Phone:** 352-273-9001; **Board Cert:** Pediatrics 1977; Neonatal-Perinatal Medicine 1977; Pediatric Cardiology 1977; **Med School:** Univ Mich Med Sch 1972; **Resid:** Pediatrics, Shands Hosp-Univ Fla 1975; **Fellow:** Neonatal-Perinatal Medicine, Shands Hosp-Univ Fla 1977; Pediatric Cardiology, Shands Hosp-Univ Fla 1977; **Fac Appt:** Prof Ped, Univ Fla Coll Med

Dhanireddy, Ramasubbareddy MD [NP] - **Spec Exp:** Neonatology; Prematurity/Low Birth Weight Infants; **Hospital:** Regional Med Ctr - Memphis, Le Bonheur Chldns Med Ctr; **Address:** Univ Tennessee, Div Neonatology, 853 Jefferson Ave, Ste 201, Memphis, TN 38163; **Phone:** 901-448-5950; **Board Cert:** Pediatrics 1980; Neonatal-Perinatal Medicine 1997; **Med School:** India 1974; **Resid:** Pediatrics, Lousiana State Univ Med Ctr 1978; **Fellow:** Neonatology, Georgetown Univ Med Ctr 1980; **Fac Appt:** Prof Ped, Univ Tenn Coll Med

Holtzman, Ronald B MD [NP] - **Spec Exp:** Neonatology; Lung Disease in Newborns; **Hospital:** Gaston Meml Hosp; **Address:** Gaston Meml Hosp, NICU Office, 2525 Court Drive, Gastonia, NC 28056; **Phone:** 704-834-3390; **Board Cert:** Pediatrics 1987; Neonatal-Perinatal Medicine 2004; **Med School:** Rush Med Coll 1983; **Resid:** Pediatrics, Chldns Meml Hosp 1986; **Fellow:** Neonatal-Perinatal Medicine, Chldns Meml Hosp 1989

Kattwinkel, John MD [NP] - **Spec Exp:** Lung Disease in Newborns; Sudden Infant Death Syndrome (SIDS); **Hospital:** Univ of Virginia Health Sys; **Address:** Univ Va Hosp, Div Neonatology, Dept Peds, PO Box 800386, Charlottesville, VA 22908-0386; **Phone:** 434-924-5428; **Board Cert:** Pediatrics 1986; Neonatal-Perinatal Medicine 1986; **Med School:** Harvard Med Sch 1968; **Resid:** Pediatrics, Duke Univ Med Ctr 1970; **Fellow:** Neonatology, Case-West Res Univ 1974; **Fac Appt:** Prof Ped, Univ VA Sch Med

Stiles, Alan D MD [NP] - **Spec Exp:** Neonatology; **Hospital:** NC Memorial Hosp - UNC; **Address:** Dept of Pediatrics CB # 7220, Chapel Hill, NC 27599-7220; **Phone:** 919-966-4427; **Board Cert:** Pediatrics 1984; Neonatal-Perinatal Medicine 1985; **Med School:** Univ NC Sch Med 1977; **Resid:** Pediatrics, North Carolina Meml Hosp 1982; **Fellow:** Neonatal-Perinatal Medicine, Chldns Hosp/Brigham Hosp 1985; **Fac Appt:** Prof Ped, Univ NC Sch Med

Midwest

Bell, Edward F MD [NP] - **Spec Exp:** Prematurity/Low Birth Weight Infants; Neonatal Critical Care; Neonatal Hemochromatosis; **Hospital:** Univ Iowa Hosp & Clinics; **Address:** Univ Iowa Hosps, Dept Pediatrics, 200 Hawkins Drive, rm 8811 JPP, Iowa City, IA 52242; **Phone:** 319-356-4006; **Board Cert:** Pediatrics 1978; Neonatal-Perinatal Medicine 1995; **Med School:** Columbia P&S 1973; **Resid:** Pediatrics, Babies Hosp-Columbia Presby 1976; **Fellow:** Neonatology, McMaster Univ Med Ctr 1977; Neonatology, Women & Infants Hosp-Brown Univ 1979; **Fac Appt:** Prof Ped, Univ Iowa Coll Med

Cole, Francis Sessions MD [NP] - **Spec Exp:** Neonatal Chronic Lung Disease (CLD); Respiratory Distress Syndrome (RDS); Surfactant Biology; Prematurity/Low Birth Weight Infants; **Hospital:** St. Louis Chldns Hosp, Barnes-Jewish Hosp; **Address:** St Louis Chldns Hosp, 660 S Euclid Ave, Box 8116, St Louis, MO 63110; **Phone:** 314-454-6148; **Board Cert:** Pediatrics 1980; Neonatal-Perinatal Medicine 1983; **Med School:** Yale Univ 1973; **Resid:** Pediatrics, Chldns Hosp Med Ctr 1978; **Fellow:** Neonatology, Brigham & Womens Hosp 1981; **Fac Appt:** Prof Ped, Washington Univ, St Louis

Donn, Steven M MD [NP] - **Spec Exp:** Breathing Disorders; Respiratory Distress Syndrome (RDS); Pulmonary Hypertension of Newborn (PPHN); Surfactant Biology; **Hospital:** Mott Chldns Hosp, Univ of Michigan Hosp; **Address:** F5790 Mott Hosp/5254, 1500 E Med Ctr Drive, Ann Arbor, MI 48109-5254; **Phone:** 734-763-4109; **Board Cert:** Pediatrics 1981; Neonatal-Perinatal Medicine 1981; **Med School:** Tulane Univ 1974; **Resid:** Pediatrics, Univ Vermont Med Ctr 1978; **Fellow:** Neonatology, Univ Michigan 1980; **Fac Appt:** Prof Ped, Univ Mich Med Sch

Gewolb, Ira MD [NP] - **Spec Exp:** Breathing Disorders; Gastroesophageal Reflux Disease (GERD); **Hospital:** Mich State Univ-Sparrow Hos; **Address:** Sparrow Hosp, Div Neonatology Michigan State Univ., 1215 E Michigan Ave Fl 3, Lansing, MI 48912; **Phone:** 517-364-2670; **Board Cert:** Pediatrics 1980; Neonatal-Perinatal Medicine 1981; **Med School:** Yale Univ 1976; **Resid:** Pediatrics, Chldns Hosp Med Ctr 1979; **Fellow:** Neonatology, Yale Univ 1982; **Fac Appt:** Prof Ped, Mich State Univ

Hamvas, Aaron MD [NP] - **Spec Exp:** Lung Disease in Newborns-Genetic; **Hospital:** St. Louis Chldns Hosp, Barnes-Jewish Hosp; **Address:** Wash Univ-Div Newborn Med, 660 S Euclid Ave, Box 8116, St Louis, MO 63110; **Phone:** 314-454-6148; **Board Cert:** Neonatal-Perinatal Medicine 2006; **Med School:** Washington Univ, St Louis 1981; **Resid:** Pediatrics, St Louis Chldns Hosp 1984; **Fellow:** Neonatology, St Louis Chldns Hosp 1990; **Fac Appt:** Prof Ped, Washington Univ, St Louis

Lemons, James A MD [NP] - **Spec Exp:** Nutrition; Ethics; **Hospital:** Riley Hosp for Children, IU Health Methodist Hosp; **Address:** 699 Riley Hosp Drive, RR-208, Indianapolis, IN 46202-5119; **Phone:** 317-274-4716; **Board Cert:** Pediatrics 1993; Neonatal-Perinatal Medicine 1993; **Med School:** Northwestern Univ 1969; **Resid:** Pediatrics, Univ Mich Med Ctr 1972; **Fellow:** Neonatal-Perinatal Medicine, Univ Colo Med Ctr 1975; **Fac Appt:** Prof Ped, Indiana Univ

Martin, Richard John MD [NP] - **Spec Exp:** Breathing Disorders; **Hospital:** UH Rainbow Babies & Chldns Hosp (page 74); **Address:** 11100 Euclid Ave, Div Neonatology, Cleveland, OH 44106-6010; **Phone:** 216-844-3387; **Board Cert:** Pediatrics 1976; Neonatal-Perinatal Medicine 2005; **Med School:** Australia 1970; **Resid:** Pediatrics, Univ Missouri 1973; **Fellow:** Neonatal-Perinatal Medicine, Case West Res Univ 1975; **Fac Appt:** Prof Ped, Case West Res Univ

Meadow, William Lee MD/PhD [NP] - **Spec Exp:** Neonatal Infections; Ethics; **Hospital:** Univ of Chicago Med Ctr; **Address:** 5841 S Maryland Ave, MC-6060, Chicago, IL 60637; **Phone:** 773-702-6210; **Board Cert:** Pediatrics 1979; Neonatal-Perinatal Medicine 1981; **Med School:** Univ Pennsylvania 1974; **Resid:** Pediatrics, Chldns Meml Hosp 1978; **Fellow:** Neonatology, Wyler Chldns Hosp 1981; Infectious Disease, Wyler Chldns Hosp 1981; **Fac Appt:** Prof Ped, Univ Chicago-Pritzker Sch Med

Muraskas, Jonathan MD [NP] - **Spec Exp:** Prematurity/Low Birth Weight Infants; Multiple Gestation; Conjoined Twins; Ethics; **Hospital:** Loyola Univ Med Ctr; **Address:** Loyola University Medical Ctr, Bldg 107, 2160 S First Ave Fl 5 - rm 5811, Maywood, IL 60153-5500; **Phone:** 708-216-1067; **Board Cert:** Pediatrics 1987; Neonatal-Perinatal Medicine 1987; **Med School:** Loyola Univ-Stritch Sch Med 1982; **Resid:** Pediatrics, Loyola Univ Med Ctr 1985; **Fellow:** Neonatal-Perinatal Medicine, Loyola Univ Med Ctr 1987; **Fac Appt:** Prof Ped, Loyola Univ-Stritch Sch Med

Steinhorn, Robin H MD [NP] - **Spec Exp:** Pulmonary Hypertension; **Hospital:** Children's Mem Hosp -Chicago, Northwestern Meml Hosp; **Address:** 2300 Children's Plaza, Box 45, Chicago, IL 60614; **Phone:** 773-880-4142; **Board Cert:** Neonatal-Perinatal Medicine 2011; **Med School:** Washington Univ, St Louis 1980; **Resid:** Obstetrics & Gynecology, Barnes Hosp 1983; Pediatrics, Univ Minn Affil Hosp 1986; **Fellow:** Neonatal-Perinatal Medicine, Univ Minn Affil Hosp 1988; **Fac Appt:** Prof Ped, Northwestern Univ

Whitsett, Jeffrey A MD [NP] - **Spec Exp:** Lung Disease in Newborns-Genetic; **Hospital:** Cincinnati Chldns Hosp Med Ctr, Good Samaritan Hosp - Cincinnati; **Address:** Cincinnati Chldns Hosp, Div Neonatalogy, 3333 Burnet Ave, Cincinnati, OH 45229-3039; **Phone:** 513-636-4830; **Board Cert:** Pediatrics 1979; Neonatal-Perinatal Medicine 1979; **Med School:** Columbia P&S 1973; **Resid:** Pediatrics, Mt Sinai Hosp 1976; **Fellow:** Neonatology, Chldns Hosp Med Ctr 1977; **Fac Appt:** Prof Ped, Univ Cincinnati

Great Plains and Mountains

Milley, J Ross MD/PhD [NP] - **Spec Exp:** Nutrition; **Hospital:** Primary Children's Med Ctr, Univ Utah Hlth Care; **Address:** Univ Utah - Dept Pediatrics/Neonatology, Williams Bldg, PO Box 581289, Salt Lake City, UT 84158; **Phone:** 801-581-7085; **Board Cert:** Pediatrics 1980; Neonatal-Perinatal Medicine 1981; **Med School:** Univ Chicago-Pritzker Sch Med 1975; **Resid:** Pediatrics, Johns Hopkins Hosp 1978; **Fellow:** Neonatology, Johns Hopkins Hosp 1980; **Fac Appt:** Prof Ped, Univ Utah

Zach, Terence MD [NP] - **Spec Exp:** Neonatal Critical Care; **Hospital:** Creighton Univ Med Ctr; **Address:** PO Box 981205, Nebraska Med Ctr, Omaha, NE 68198-1205; **Phone:** 402-559-6750; **Board Cert:** Pediatrics 1987; Neonatal-Perinatal Medicine 2004; **Med School:** Univ Nebr Coll Med 1983; **Resid:** Pediatrics, Univ Nebr Med Ctr 1986; **Fellow:** Neonatology, Univ Minnesota 1986; **Fac Appt:** Prof Ped, Creighton Univ

Southwest

Adams, James M MD [NP] - **Spec Exp:** Lung Disease in Newborns; **Hospital:** Texas Chldns Hosp; **Address:** 6621 Fannin St, MC WT-6104, Houston, TX 77030; **Phone:** 832-826-1380; **Board Cert:** Pediatrics 1975; Neonatal-Perinatal Medicine 1975; **Med School:** Baylor Coll Med 1970; **Resid:** Pediatrics, Baylor Affil Hosps 1973; **Fellow:** Neonatal-Perinatal Medicine, Baylor Affil Hosps 1975; **Fac Appt:** Prof Ped, Baylor Coll Med

Escobedo, Marilyn B MD [NP] - **Spec Exp:** Neonatology; Nutrition; **Hospital:** Chldns Hosp OU Med Ctr; **Address:** 1200 Everett Drive, North Pavilion Fl 7 - rm 7504, Oklahoma City, OK 73104; **Phone:** 405-271-5215; **Board Cert:** Pediatrics 1986; Neonatal-Perinatal Medicine 2004; **Med School:** Washington Univ, St Louis 1970; **Resid:** Pediatrics, Chldns Hosp 1972; Neonatal-Perinatal Medicine, Chldns Hosp 1973; **Fellow:** Neonatal-Perinatal Medicine, Vanderbilt Univ 1976; **Fac Appt:** Prof Ped, Univ Okla Coll Med

Garcia-Prats, Joseph MD [NP] - **Spec Exp:** Lung Disease in Newborns; **Hospital:** Texas Chldns Hosp, Ben Taub Genl Hosp; **Address:** 6621 Fannin St, Ste W6104, Houston, TX 77030-1608; **Phone:** 713-873-3515; **Board Cert:** Pediatrics 1977; Neonatal-Perinatal Medicine 2009; **Med School:** Tulane Univ 1972; **Resid:** Pediatrics, Baylor Affil Hosp 1975; **Fellow:** Neonatal-Perinatal Medicine, Baylor Affil Hosp 1977; **Fac Appt:** Prof Ped, Baylor Coll Med

Neonatal-Perinatal Medicine

Odom, Michael W MD [NP] - **Spec Exp:** Neonatology; **Hospital:** Univ Hlth Syst-San Antonio; **Address:** Dept Peds, 7703 Floyd Curl Drive, MC 7812, San Antonio, TX 78229-3900; **Phone:** 210-567-5225; **Board Cert:** Pediatrics 1987; Neonatal-Perinatal Medicine 2011; **Med School:** Univ Tex SW, Dallas 1983; **Resid:** Pediatrics, Vanderbilt Univ Affil Hosps 1986; **Fellow:** Neonatal-Perinatal Medicine, Mt Zion Med Ctr-UCSF 1989; **Fac Appt:** Assoc Prof Ped, Univ Tex, San Antonio

Seidner, Steven R MD [NP] - **Spec Exp:** Neonatal Chronic Lung Disease (CLD); Respiratory Distress Syndrome (RDS); Pulmonary Hypertension of Newborn (PPHN); **Hospital:** Univ Hlth Syst-San Antonio; **Address:** Dept Peds, 7703 Floyd Curl Drive, MC 7812, San Antonio, TX 78229-3901; **Phone:** 210-567-5225; **Board Cert:** Pediatrics 1987; Neonatal-Perinatal Medicine 1987; **Med School:** Univ Ariz Coll Med 1982; **Resid:** Pediatrics, Harbor-UCLA Med Ctr 1985; **Fellow:** Neonatal-Perinatal Medicine, Harbor-UCLA Med Ctr 1988; **Fac Appt:** Prof Ped, Univ Tex, San Antonio

Tyson, Jon E MD [NP] - **Spec Exp:** Neonatology; **Hospital:** Meml Hermann Hosp - Texas Med Ctr; **Address:** Univ Tex, Ctr Clin Rsch, 6431 Fannin St, MSB 2.106, Houston, TX 77030; **Phone:** 713-500-5651; **Board Cert:** Pediatrics 1973; Neonatal-Perinatal Medicine 1975; **Med School:** Tulane Univ 1968; **Resid:** Pediatrics, Univ Tenn/Memphis Hosp 1971; **Fellow:** Neonatology, McMaster Univ 1975; **Fac Appt:** Prof Ped, Univ Tex, Houston

West Coast and Pacific

Ariagno, Ronald L MD [NP] - **Spec Exp:** Prematurity/Low Birth Weight Infants; Neonatal Critical Care; Sudden Infant Death Syndrome (SIDS); **Hospital:** Stanford Univ Hosp & Clinics; **Address:** Stanford Univ, Div Neonatology, 750 Welch Rd, Ste 315, Palo Alto, CA 94304; **Phone:** 650-723-5711; **Board Cert:** Pediatrics 1973; Neonatal-Perinatal Medicine 1975; **Med School:** Univ IL Coll Med 1968; **Resid:** Pediatrics, Presby-St Lukes Hosp 1971; **Fellow:** Neonatology, Chldns Hosp/UCSF 1975; **Fac Appt:** Prof Emeritus Ped, Stanford Univ

Simmons Jr, Charles F MD [NP] - **Hospital:** Cedars-Sinai Med Ctr; **Address:** Cedars-Sinai Medical Center, Maxine Dunitz Children's Health Center, 8700 Beverly Blvd, NT 4226, Los Angeles, CA 90048; **Phone:** 310-423-4416; **Board Cert:** Pediatrics 1986; Neonatal-Perinatal Medicine 1987; **Med School:** Harvard Med Sch 1980; **Resid:** Pediatrics, Children's Hosp 1983; **Fellow:** Neonatal-Perinatal Medicine, Children's Hosp 1986; **Fac Appt:** Prof Ped, UCLA-David Geffen Sch Med

Stevenson, David K MD [NP] - **Spec Exp:** Neonatology; **Hospital:** Lucile Packard Chldn's Hosp; **Address:** 750 Welch Rd, Ste 315, Palo Alto, CA 94304-1510; **Phone:** 650-723-5711; **Board Cert:** Pediatrics 1979; Neonatal-Perinatal Medicine 2004; **Med School:** Univ Wash 1975; **Resid:** Pediatrics, Univ Washington 1977; **Fellow:** Neonatal-Perinatal Medicine, Stanford Univ 1979; **Fac Appt:** Prof Ped, Stanford Univ

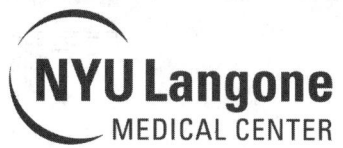
NEONATAL PERINATAL MEDICINE

Neonatal Perinatal Medicine is part of the Hassenfeld Pediatric Center, a full service specialty Children's Hospital, which supports the array of children's health services across the Medical Center where newborns, children, adolescents and young adults receive the most comprehensive and advanced care by a team of pediatricians and pediatric specialists.

The Neonatology Program at NYU Langone Medical Center addresses the unique emotional and developmental needs of infants with a program that combines family-centered care and state-of-the-art technology. We specialize in the following areas:

Neonatal Intensive Care

The Neonatal Intensive Care Unit (NICU) provides the most advanced care in New York City for neonates requiring intensive care and works closely with pediatric general and cardiac surgery, neurosurgery and craniofacial surgery. As a Regional Perinatal Center, the program additionally offers early intervention evaluation services and comprehensive family support and education.

Continuing Care

Because many premature babies may be at an increased risk for problems in growth and development, the Neonatal Comprehensive Continuing Care Program (NCCCP) follows these infants from birth through pre-school, providing evaluation and assessment of problems as soon as they arise.

Hypothermia Program

The Hypothermia Program at NYU Langone Medical Center is a full multidisciplinary service with neonatal transport and inpatient and outpatient follow-up services. The program provides rapid response treatment and assessment of infants who have birth asphyxia.

Infant Apnea and SIDS

The Infant Apnea and SIDS Program at the Bellevue Hospital Center, an affiliate of NYU Langone Medical Center, provides treatment to critically ill infants through its Neonatal Intensive Care Unit, and to other children at risk for apnea, sudden infant death syndrome (SIDS) and other life-threatening events.

Neonatal Transport

As a designated New York State Regional Perinatal Center, the Division of Neonatology cares for over one-fifth of New York City's mothers and infants. As part of that massive effort, it offers an active transport program to bring mothers and/or their newborns to NYU Langone Medical Center's Tisch Hospital for specialized intensive care.

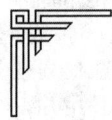

The Best in American Medicine
www.CastleConnolly.com

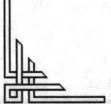
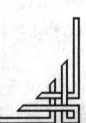

Nephrology
a subspecialty of Internal Medicine

An internist who treats disorders of the kidney, high blood pressure, fluid and mineral balance and dialysis of body wastes when the kidneys do not function. This specialist consults with surgeons about kidney transplantation.

Training Required: Three years in internal medicine *plus* additional training and examination for certification in nephrology.

NEPHROLOGY

New England

Bazari, Hasan MD [Nep] - **Spec Exp:** Kidney Failure-Acute; Nephrotic Syndrome; Hypertension; **Hospital:** Mass Genl Hosp; **Address:** Renal Assocs, Mass Genl Hosp, 55 Fruit St Gray Bldg - Ste 1003, Boston, MA 02114; **Phone:** 617-726-5050; **Board Cert:** Internal Medicine 1986; Nephrology 1988; **Med School:** Albert Einstein Coll Med 1983; **Resid:** Internal Medicine, Mass Genl Hosp 1986; **Fellow:** Nephrology, Mass Genl Hosp 1988

Brenner, Barry M MD [Nep] - **Spec Exp:** Hypertension; Diabetic Kidney Disease; Kidney Failure-Acute; Kidney Failure-Chronic; **Hospital:** Brigham and Women's Hosp (page 57); **Address:** Brigham & Women's Hosp, Renal Div, 75 Francis St, Boston, MA 02115; **Phone:** 617-732-5850; **Med School:** Univ Pittsburgh 1962; **Resid:** Internal Medicine, Albert Einstein Coll Med 1966; **Fellow:** Nephrology, Nat Inst Health 1969; **Fac Appt:** Prof Med, Harvard Med Sch

Coggins, Cecil MD [Nep] - **Spec Exp:** Kidney Disease; Hypertension; **Hospital:** Mass Genl Hosp; **Address:** 165 Cambridge St, Ste 501, Charles River Plaza, Boston, MA 02114-2712; **Phone:** 617-726-4900; **Board Cert:** Internal Medicine 1965; Nephrology 1974; **Med School:** Harvard Med Sch 1958; **Resid:** Internal Medicine, Stanford Univ Med Ctr 1965; Internal Medicine; **Fellow:** Nephrology, Stanford Univ Med Ctr 1963; Nephrology, Mass Genl Hosp 1967; **Fac Appt:** Assoc Prof Med, Harvard Med Sch

Dember, Laura MD [Nep] - **Spec Exp:** Kidney Failure-Chronic; Nephrotic Syndrome; Amyloidosis; **Hospital:** Boston Med Ctr; **Address:** 650 Albany St, EBRC 504, Renal Section, Boston, MA 02118; **Phone:** 617-638-4317; **Board Cert:** Internal Medicine 2000; Nephrology 2000; **Med School:** Yale Univ 1988; **Resid:** Internal Medicine, Hosp Univ Penn 1991; **Fellow:** Nephrology, Hosp Univ Penn 1992; Nephrology, Brigham & Womens Hosp 1995; **Fac Appt:** Assoc Prof Med, Boston Univ

Kliger, Alan MD [Nep] - **Spec Exp:** Kidney Disease; Kidney Disease-Metabolic; **Hospital:** Hosp of St Raphael; **Address:** 136 Sherman Ave, Ste 405, New Haven, CT 06511; **Phone:** 203-787-0117 x307; **Board Cert:** Internal Medicine 1973; Nephrology 1976; **Med School:** SUNY Upstate Med Univ 1970; **Resid:** Internal Medicine, SUNY Upstate Med Ctr 1973; **Fellow:** Nephrology, Georgetown Univ Hosp 1975; **Fac Appt:** Clin Prof Med, Yale Univ

Perrone, Ronald MD [Nep] - **Spec Exp:** Kidney Disease-Chronic; Kidney Failure-Acute; Polycystic Kidney Disease; Hypertension; **Hospital:** Tufts Med Ctr; **Address:** Tufts-New Eng Med Ctr, Div Nephrology, 750 Washington St, Box 391, Boston, MA 02111; **Phone:** 617-636-5866; **Board Cert:** Internal Medicine 1979; Nephrology 1982; **Med School:** Hahnemann Univ 1975; **Resid:** Internal Medicine, Grady Meml Hosp 1978; **Fellow:** Nephrology, Boston Med Ctr 1982; **Fac Appt:** Prof Med, Tufts Univ

Salant, David MD [Nep] - **Spec Exp:** Kidney Disease-Glomerular; Kidney Disease-Autoimmune; Lupus Nephritis; Vasculitis; **Hospital:** Boston Med Ctr; **Address:** 650 Albany St, Ste X504, Boston, MA 02118; **Phone:** 617-638-7330; **Board Cert:** Internal Medicine 1978; Nephrology 1980; **Med School:** South Africa 1969; **Resid:** Internal Medicine, Johannesburg Genl Hosp 1973; **Fellow:** Nephrology, Boston Univ Med Ctr 1978; **Fac Appt:** Prof Med, Boston Univ

Seifter, Julian L MD [Nep] - **Spec Exp:** Diabetic Kidney Disease; Kidney Failure-Chronic; Kidney Stones; **Hospital:** Brigham and Women's Hosp (page 57); **Address:** Brigham & Women's Hosp, Div Renal Med, 45 Francis St Fl 2, Boston, MA 02115; **Phone:** 617-732-6383; **Board Cert:** Internal Medicine 1978; Nephrology 1980; **Med School:** Albert Einstein Coll Med 1975; **Resid:** Internal Medicine, Bronx Muni Hosp Ctr 1981; **Fellow:** Nephrology, Yale-New Haven Hosp 1982; **Fac Appt:** Prof Med, Harvard Med Sch

Tolkoff-Rubin, Nina MD [Nep] - **Spec Exp:** Transplant Medicine-Kidney; Hypertension; Kidney Failure-Acute; **Hospital:** Mass Genl Hosp; **Address:** 55 Fruit St, GRB 103J, Boston, MA 02114; **Phone:** 617-726-3706; **Board Cert:** Nephrology 1974; Internal Medicine 1972; **Med School:** Harvard Med Sch 1968; **Resid:** Internal Medicine, Mass Genl Hosp 1970; Internal Medicine, Mass Genl Hosp 1972; **Fellow:** Nephrology, Mass Genl Hosp 1971; **Fac Appt:** Assoc Prof Med, Harvard Med Sch

Mid Atlantic

Appel, Gerald MD [Nep] - **Spec Exp:** Glomerulonephritis; Lupus Nephritis; Nephrotic Syndrome; **Hospital:** NY-Presby/Columbia Univ Med Ctr, NY (page 65); **Address:** 622 W 168th St, Ste PH4-124, New York, NY 10032-3720; **Phone:** 212-305-0320; **Board Cert:** Internal Medicine 1975; Nephrology 1978; **Med School:** Albert Einstein Coll Med 1972; **Resid:** Internal Medicine, Columbia Presby Hosp 1975; **Fellow:** Nephrology, Columbia Presby Hosp 1976; Nephrology, Yale-New Haven Hosp 1978; **Fac Appt:** Clin Prof Med, Columbia P&S

August, Phyllis MD [Nep] - **Spec Exp:** Hypertension; Hypertension in Pregnancy; **Hospital:** NY-Presby/Weill Cornell Med Ctr, NY (page 65); **Address:** 450 E 69th St, Hypertension Center, New York, NY 10021-4870; **Phone:** 212-746-2210; **Board Cert:** Internal Medicine 1980; Nephrology 1982; **Med School:** Yale Univ 1977; **Resid:** Internal Medicine, NY Hosp-Cornell Med Ctr 1980; **Fellow:** Nephrology, NY Hosp-Cornell Med Ctr 1983; **Fac Appt:** Prof Med, Cornell Univ-Weill Med Coll

Bernardo, Jose F MD [Nep] - **Spec Exp:** Kidney Disease; Dialysis Care; **Hospital:** UPMC Mercy, Pittsburgh; **Address:** UPMC Kidney Clin, 120 Lytton Ave, Ste 300, Pittsburgh, PA 15213; **Phone:** 412-802-3043; **Board Cert:** Internal Medicine 2009; Nephrology 2001; **Med School:** Peru 1984; **Resid:** Internal Medicine, Universidad Peruana 1989; Internal Medicine, UPMC 2000; **Fellow:** Nephrology, UPMC 2002; **Fac Appt:** Asst Prof Med, Univ Pittsburgh

Berns, Jeffrey S MD [Nep] - **Spec Exp:** Kidney Disease; Glomerulonephritis; Hypertension; **Hospital:** Hosp Univ Penn - UPHS (page 68); **Address:** Hosp Univ Penn, 3400 Spruce St Fl 1 - Ste 300S, Philadelphia, PA 19104; **Phone:** 215-662-2638; **Board Cert:** Internal Medicine 1984; Nephrology 1986; **Med School:** Case West Res Univ 1981; **Resid:** Internal Medicine, Univ Hosp 1984; **Fellow:** Nephrology, Yale-New Haven Hosp 1987; **Fac Appt:** Prof Med, Univ Pennsylvania

Blumenfeld, Jon D MD [Nep] - **Spec Exp:** Hypertension; Polycystic Kidney Disease; Adrenal Disorders; **Hospital:** NY-Presby/Weill Cornell Med Ctr, NY (page 65), Rockefeller Univ; **Address:** The Rogosin Institute, 505 E 70th St Fl 2, New York, NY 10021; **Phone:** 212-746-1495; **Board Cert:** Internal Medicine 1984; Nephrology 1986; **Med School:** Yale Univ 1981; **Resid:** Internal Medicine, New York Hosp 1984; **Fellow:** Nephrology, Brigham & Womens Hosp 1988; **Fac Appt:** Prof Med, Cornell Univ-Weill Med Coll

Cohen, David J MD [Nep] - **Spec Exp:** Transplant Medicine-Kidney; Glomerulonephritis; **Hospital:** NY-Presby/Columbia Univ Med Ctr, NY (page 65); **Address:** Columbia Univ Med Ctr, 622 W 168th St, rm PH 4-124, New York, NY 10032-3720; **Phone:** 212-305-0320; **Board Cert:** Internal Medicine 1980; Nephrology 1984; **Med School:** Albert Einstein Coll Med 1977; **Resid:** Internal Medicine, Mount Sinai Hosp 1980; **Fellow:** Nephrology, Columbia-Presby Hosp 1981; Transplant Immunobiology, Brigham & Womens Hosp 1983; **Fac Appt:** Clin Prof Med, Columbia P&S

Holzman, Lawrence B MD [Nep] - **Spec Exp:** Glomerulonephritis; **Hospital:** Hosp Univ Penn - UPHS (page 68); **Address:** Hospital Univ Penn, 3400 Spruce St Fl 1 - Ste 300, Philadelphia, PA 19104; **Phone:** 215-662-2638; **Board Cert:** Nephrology 1987; **Med School:** UMDNJ-NJ Med Sch, Newark 1984; **Resid:** Internal Medicine, Med Coll Penn 1987; **Fellow:** Nephrology, Univ Michigan 1989; **Fac Appt:** Prof Med, Univ Pennsylvania

Johnston, James R MD [Nep] - **Spec Exp:** Diabetic Kidney Disease; Hypertension; **Hospital:** UPMC Presby, Pittsburgh; **Address:** UPMC Kidney Clinic, 120 Winton Ave, Ste 300, Pittsburgh, PA 15213; **Phone:** 412-802-3043; **Board Cert:** Internal Medicine 1982; Nephrology 1984; **Med School:** Univ Pittsburgh 1979; **Resid:** Internal Medicine, Montefiore Hosp 1982; **Fellow:** Nephrology, Univ Pittsburgh Med Ctr 1983; Nephrology, Brigham & Women's Hosp 1986; **Fac Appt:** Prof Med, Univ Pittsburgh

Kelepouris, Ellie MD [Nep] - **Spec Exp:** Kidney Stones; Hypertension; **Hospital:** Hahnemann Univ Hosp; **Address:** 219 N Broad St Fl 9, Philadelphia, PA 19107; **Phone:** 215-762-2688; **Board Cert:** Nephrology 2008; **Med School:** Greece 1976; **Resid:** Internal Medicine, Mercy Cath Med Ctr 1979; **Fellow:** Nephrology, Hosp U Penn 1982; **Fac Appt:** Prof Med, Drexel Univ Coll Med

Kobrin, Sidney M MD [Nep] - **Spec Exp:** Diabetic Kidney Disease; Kidney Failure; Hypertension; **Hospital:** Hosp Univ Penn - UPHS (page 68); **Address:** Hosp U Penn, Div Nephrology, 3400 Civic Center Blvd, Fl 1 - Ste 300 South, Philadelphia, PA 19104; **Phone:** 215-662-2638; **Board Cert:** Nephrology 2002; **Med School:** South Africa 1978; **Resid:** Internal Medicine, Johannesburg Tchg Hosp 1984; **Fellow:** Nephrology, Einstein Med Ctr 1988; **Fac Appt:** Assoc Prof Med, Univ Pennsylvania

Murphy, Barbara MD [Nep] - **Spec Exp:** Transplant Medicine-Kidney; **Hospital:** Mount Sinai Med Ctr (page 63); **Address:** 5 E 98th St Fl 12, New York, NY 10029; **Phone:** 212-659-8086; **Med School:** Ireland 1989; **Resid:** Internal Medicine, Beaumont Hosp 1992; **Fellow:** Nephrology, Beaumont Hosp 1993; Nephrology, Brigham & Women's Hosp 1997; **Fac Appt:** Prof Med, Mount Sinai Sch Med

Piraino, Beth Marie MD [Nep] - **Spec Exp:** Kidney Failure; Hypertension; **Hospital:** UPMC Presby, Pittsburgh; **Address:** 3504 Fifth Ave, Ste 200, Pittsburgh, PA 15213; **Phone:** 412-383-4899; **Board Cert:** Internal Medicine 1980; Nephrology 1982; **Med School:** Med Coll PA Hahnemann 1977; **Resid:** Internal Medicine, Presby Univ Hosp 1980; **Fellow:** Nephrology, Presby Univ Hosp 1982; **Fac Appt:** Prof Med, Univ Pittsburgh

Rudnick, Michael R MD [Nep] - **Spec Exp:** Hypertension; Kidney Disease; **Hospital:** Penn Presby Med Ctr - UPHS (page 68); **Address:** Presbyterian Med Ctr, Medical Office Bldg, 39th and Market Sts, Ste 240, Philadelphia, PA 19104; **Phone:** 215-662-8730; **Board Cert:** Internal Medicine 1975; Nephrology 1976; **Med School:** Hahnemann Univ 1972; **Resid:** Internal Medicine, Hahnemann Univ Med Ctr 1974; **Fellow:** Nephrology, Hosp Univ Penn 1976; **Fac Appt:** Assoc Prof Med, Univ Pennsylvania

Stern, Leonard MD [Nep] - **Spec Exp:** Kidney Failure-Chronic; Transplant Medicine-Kidney; Bone Disorders-Metabolic; Dialysis Care; **Hospital:** NY-Presby/Columbia Univ Med Ctr, NY (page 65); **Address:** 622 W 168th St, rm PH4-124, New York, NY 10032-3702; **Phone:** 212-305-0559; **Board Cert:** Internal Medicine 1978; Nephrology 1980; **Med School:** NY Med Coll 1975; **Resid:** Internal Medicine, Jacobi Med Ctr 1978; **Fellow:** Nephrology, Montefiore Med Ctr 1979; Nephrology, Yale-New Haven Hosp 1981; **Fac Appt:** Assoc Clin Prof Med, Columbia P&S

Townsend, Raymond R MD [Nep] - **Spec Exp:** Hypertension-Complex; Renal Artery Stenosis; **Hospital:** Hosp Univ Penn - UPHS (page 68); **Address:** Hosp U Penn, Div Nephrology, 3400 Civic Center Blvd, Fl 1 - Ste 300 South, Philadelphia, PA 19104; **Phone:** 215-662-2638; **Board Cert:** Internal Medicine 1982; Nephrology 1984; **Med School:** Hahnemann Univ 1979; **Resid:** Internal Medicine, Allegheny Genl Hosp 1982; **Fellow:** Nephrology, Temple Univ Hosp 1984; **Fac Appt:** Prof Med, Univ Pennsylvania

Wilcox, Christopher S MD/PhD [Nep] - **Spec Exp:** Hypertension-Renovascular; Hypertension-Drug Resistent; **Hospital:** Georgetown Univ Hosp; **Address:** Georgetown Univ Med Ctr, 3800 Reservoir Rd NW, PHC Fl 6th, Washington, DC 20007-2113; **Phone:** 202-444-9183; **Board Cert:** Internal Medicine 1983; Nephrology 1986; **Med School:** England, UK 1968; **Resid:** Internal Medicine, Middlesex Hosp 1971; Nephrology, Middlesex Hosp 1972; **Fellow:** Nephrology, Middlesex Hosp 1975; **Fac Appt:** Prof Med, Georgetown Univ

Winston, Jonathan MD [Nep] - **Spec Exp:** Kidney Disease-Chronic; Kidney Failure; HIV Related Kidney Disease; Glomerulonephritis; **Hospital:** Mount Sinai Med Ctr (page 63); **Address:** 5 E 98th St Fl 11, New York, NY 10029-6501; **Phone:** 212-241-4060; **Board Cert:** Internal Medicine 1980; Nephrology 1984; **Med School:** Geo Wash Univ 1977; **Resid:** Internal Medicine, LI Jewish Med Ctr 1980; **Fellow:** Nephrology, Mt Sinai Hosp 1982; **Fac Appt:** Assoc Prof Med, Mount Sinai Sch Med

Southeast

Allon, Michael MD [Nep] - **Spec Exp:** Dialysis Care; **Hospital:** Univ of Ala Hosp at Birmingham; **Address:** UAB Nephrology, 1530 3rd Ave S, PB 226, Birmingham, AL 35294; **Phone:** 205-975-9676; **Board Cert:** Internal Medicine 1985; Nephrology 1988; **Med School:** Univ Mich Med Sch 1982; **Resid:** Internal Medicine, Emory Univ Hosp 1985; **Fellow:** Nephrology, Emory Univ 1987; **Fac Appt:** Prof Med, Univ Alabama

Bolton, W Kline MD [Nep] - **Spec Exp:** Kidney Disease-Glomerular; Kidney Disease-Chronic; Glomerulonephritis; **Hospital:** Univ of Virginia Health Sys; **Address:** Univ VA Hlth Scis Ctr, Dept Nephrology, Box 800133, Charlottesville, VA 22908-0001; **Phone:** 434-924-5125; **Board Cert:** Internal Medicine 1972; Nephrology 1974; **Med School:** Univ VA Sch Med 1969; **Resid:** Internal Medicine, Boston City Hosp 1971; **Fellow:** Nephrology, Univ Chicago 1973; **Fac Appt:** Prof Med, Univ VA Sch Med

Butterly, David W MD [Nep] - **Spec Exp:** Transplant Medicine-Kidney; Kidney Disease; **Hospital:** Duke Univ Hosp; **Address:** Duke Univ Med Ctr, Box 3014, Durham, NC 27710; **Phone:** 919-668-7630; **Board Cert:** Internal Medicine 2000; Nephrology 2000; **Med School:** Duke Univ 1987; **Resid:** Internal Medicine, Duke Univ Med Ctr 1990; **Fellow:** Nephrology, Duke Univ Med Ctr 1992

Coffman, Thomas M MD [Nep] - **Spec Exp:** Transplant Medicine-Kidney; Hypertension; **Hospital:** Durham VA Med Ctr, Duke Univ Hosp; **Address:** Duke Univ Med Center, Box 103015, Durham, NC 27710; **Phone:** 919-684-9788; **Board Cert:** Internal Medicine 1983; Nephrology 1988; **Med School:** Ohio State Univ 1980; **Resid:** Internal Medicine, Duke Univ Med Ctr 1983; **Fellow:** Nephrology, Duke Univ Med Ctr 1985; **Fac Appt:** Prof Med, Duke Univ

Falk, Ronald J MD [Nep] - **Spec Exp:** Glomerulonephritis; Lupus Nephritis; Wegener's Granulomatosis; Vasculitis; **Hospital:** NC Memorial Hosp - UNC; **Address:** Univ North Carolina Kidney Ctr, 7024 Burnett Womack Bldg CB #7155, Chapel Hill, NC 27599-7155; **Phone:** 919-966-2561; **Board Cert:** Internal Medicine 1980; Nephrology 1982; **Med School:** Univ NC Sch Med 1977; **Resid:** Internal Medicine, Univ North Carolina Hosps 1980; Nephrology, Univ NC 1981; **Fellow:** Research, Univ Minn 1983; **Fac Appt:** Prof Med, Univ NC Sch Med

Freedman, Barry I MD [Nep] - **Spec Exp:** Hypertension; Inherited Metabolic Disorders; Diabetes; Kidney Failure; **Hospital:** Wake Forest Univ Baptist Med Ctr; **Address:** Wake Forest Univ, Nephrology Dept, Medical Ctr Blvd, Winston-Salem, NC 27157; **Phone:** 336-716-8817; **Board Cert:** Internal Medicine 1987; Nephrology 1999; **Med School:** SUNY Downstate 1984; **Resid:** Internal Medicine, E Virgina Univ Affil Hosp 1987; **Fellow:** Nephrology, NC Baptist Hosp 1989; **Fac Appt:** Prof Med, Wake Forest Univ

Gaston, Robert S MD [Nep] - **Spec Exp:** Transplant Medicine-Kidney; Kidney Disease; Dialysis Care; **Hospital:** Univ of Ala Hosp at Birmingham; **Address:** Univ Alabama Hosp, Div Nephrology, 1530 3rd Ave S, THT 625, 625 THT, Birmingham, AL 35294; **Phone:** 205-934-7220; **Board Cert:** Internal Medicine 1982; Nephrology 1986; **Med School:** St Louis Univ 1979; **Resid:** Internal Medicine, Univ Hosp Arkansas 1982; **Fellow:** Nephrology, Univ Hosp Arkansas 1986; Transplant Medicine, Univ Alabama Med Ctr 1988; **Fac Appt:** Prof Med, Univ Alabama

Helderman, J Harold MD [Nep] - **Spec Exp:** Transplant Medicine-Kidney; Kidney Disease-Glomerular; Kidney Disease-Autoimmune; **Hospital:** Vanderbilt Univ Med Ctr (page 76); **Address:** Vanderbilt-Div Nephrology & Hypertension, 1301 Med Ctr Drive, Ste 2501, Nashville, TN 37232; **Phone:** 615-343-7592; **Board Cert:** Internal Medicine 1974; **Med School:** SUNY Downstate 1971; **Resid:** Internal Medicine, Johns Hopkins Hosp 1973; **Fellow:** Nephrology, Harvard Univ 1976; **Fac Appt:** Prof Med, Vanderbilt Univ

Lea, Janice I MD [Nep] - **Spec Exp:** Hypertension-Complex; Kidney Disease-Chronic; Diabetic Kidney Disease; Dialysis Care; **Hospital:** Emory Univ Hosp Midtown; **Address:** Emory Midtown-Div Nephrology, 550 Peachtree St NE, Medical Office Tower, Fl 8, Atlanta, GA 30308; **Phone:** 404-686-5038; **Board Cert:** Nephrology 2005; **Med School:** Univ Tex Med Br, Galveston 1988; **Resid:** Internal Medicine, Emory Univ Affil Hosps 1991; **Fellow:** Nephrology, Emory Univ Affil Hosps 1994; **Fac Appt:** Assoc Prof Med, Emory Univ

Okusa, Mark D MD [Nep] - **Spec Exp:** Kidney Failure-Chronic; Nephrotic Syndrome; Kidney Failure-Acute; **Hospital:** Univ of Virginia Health Sys; **Address:** Univ VA Hlth Sci Ctr, Div Nephrology, Lee St, Box 800-133, Charlottesville, VA 22908-0001; **Phone:** 434-924-2187; **Board Cert:** Internal Medicine 1985; Nephrology 1988; **Med School:** Med Coll VA 1982; **Resid:** Internal Medicine, Med Coll Virginia 1985; **Fellow:** Nephrology, Yale Univ Sch Med 1988; **Fac Appt:** Prof Med, Univ VA Sch Med

Rakowski, Thomas A MD [Nep] - **Spec Exp:** Polycystic Kidney Disease; Kidney Disease-Glomerular; **Hospital:** Virginia Hosp Ctr - Arlington, Inova Fairfax Hosp; **Address:** Virginia Nephrology Group, 1635 N George Mason Drive, Ste 215, Arlington, VA 22205; **Phone:** 703-841-0707; **Board Cert:** Internal Medicine 1972; Nephrology 1974; **Med School:** Hahnemann Univ 1969; **Resid:** Internal Medicine, Georgetown Univ 1971; **Fellow:** Nephrology, Georgetown Univ 1973; **Fac Appt:** Assoc Prof Med, Georgetown Univ

Roth, David MD [Nep] - **Spec Exp:** Transplant Medicine-Kidney; Kidney Failure-Chronic; **Hospital:** Jackson Meml Hosp (page 70), Univ of Miami Hosp & Clins/Sylvester Comp Canc Ctr (page 73); **Address:** Univ Miami, Div Nephrology, PO Box 016960 (R-126), Miami, FL 33101; **Phone:** 305-243-6251; **Board Cert:** Internal Medicine 1980; Nephrology 1982; **Med School:** SUNY Downstate 1977; **Resid:** Internal Medicine, Jackson Meml Hosp 1980; **Fellow:** Nephrology, Jackson Meml Hosp 1982; **Fac Appt:** Prof Med, Univ Miami Sch Med

Sands, Jeff M MD [Nep] - **Spec Exp:** Hypertension; **Hospital:** Emory Univ Hosp, Grady Hlth Sys; **Address:** The Emory Clin, 1365 Clifton Rd NE, A Bldg Fl 4, Atlanta, GA 30322; **Phone:** 404-778-5380; **Board Cert:** Internal Medicine 1984; Nephrology 2000; **Med School:** Boston Univ 1981; **Resid:** Internal Medicine, Univ Chicago Hosp Clin 1983; Internal Medicine, Natl Inst Hlth 1984; **Fellow:** Nephrology, Natl Inst Hlth 1988; Nephrology, Emory Univ Hosp 1989; **Fac Appt:** Prof Med, Emory Univ

Warnock, David G MD [Nep] - **Spec Exp:** Liddle's Syndrome; Kidney Stones; Nephrotic Syndrome; **Hospital:** Univ of Ala Hosp at Birmingham; **Address:** UAB Nephrology, 1530 3rd Ave S, ZRB 636, Birmingham, AL 35294-0006; **Phone:** 205-934-9509; **Board Cert:** Internal Medicine 1973; Nephrology 2000; **Med School:** UCSF 1970; **Resid:** Internal Medicine, UCSF Med Ctr 1973; **Fellow:** Nephrology, Natl Inst Hlth 1975; **Fac Appt:** Prof Med, Univ Alabama

Weiner, I David MD [Nep] - **Spec Exp:** Kidney Disease; Fluid/Electrolyte Balance; Kidney Stones; Adrenal Disorders; **Hospital:** Shands at Univ of FL; **Address:** Shands at Univ Florida, Dept Nephrology, PO Box 100224, Gainesville, FL 32610-0224; **Phone:** 352-273-8821; **Board Cert:** Internal Medicine 1987; Nephrology 2000; **Med School:** Vanderbilt Univ 1984; **Resid:** Internal Medicine, Univ Texas Hlth Sci Ctr 1987; **Fellow:** Nephrology, Wash Univ 1990; **Fac Appt:** Prof Med, Univ Fla Coll Med

Midwest

Brennan, Daniel C MD [Nep] - **Spec Exp:** Transplant Medicine-Kidney; **Hospital:** Barnes-Jewish Hosp; **Address:** Wash Univ School Med, Div Renal Diseases, 660 S Euclid Ave, Box 8126, St Louis, MO 63110; **Phone:** 314-362-8351; **Board Cert:** Internal Medicine 1988; Nephrology 2002; **Med School:** Univ Iowa Coll Med 1985; **Resid:** Internal Medicine, Univ Iowa Hosps 1988; **Fellow:** Nephrology, Brigham & Womens Hosp 1992; **Fac Appt:** Assoc Prof Med, Washington Univ, St Louis

Coe, Fredric MD [Nep] - **Spec Exp:** Kidney Stones; Fluid/Electrolyte Balance; **Hospital:** Univ of Chicago Med Ctr; **Address:** 5841 S Maryland Ave, MC 5100, Chicago, IL 60637; **Phone:** 773-702-1475; **Board Cert:** Internal Medicine 1968; **Med School:** Univ Chicago-Pritzker Sch Med 1961; **Resid:** Internal Medicine, Michael Reese Hosp 1965; **Fellow:** Renal Disease, Univ Texas SW 1969; **Fac Appt:** Prof Med, Univ Chicago-Pritzker Sch Med

Delmez, James MD [Nep] - **Spec Exp:** Kidney Disease; **Hospital:** Barnes-Jewish Hosp, Washington Univ Physicians; **Address:** Wash Univ Sch Med, Div Renal Disease, 660 S Euclid Ave, Box 8126, St Louis, MO 63110; **Phone:** 314-362-7603; **Board Cert:** Internal Medicine 1976; Nephrology 1982; **Med School:** Univ Rochester 1973; **Resid:** Internal Medicine, Barnes Hosp 1976; **Fellow:** Nephrology, Barnes Hosp 1978; **Fac Appt:** Prof Med, Washington Univ, St Louis

Hruska, Keith MD [Nep] - **Spec Exp:** Kidney Disease-Pediatric & Adult; Kidney Stones; Bone Disorders-Metabolic; Inherited Metabolic Disorders; **Hospital:** St. Louis Chldns Hosp, Barnes-Jewish Hosp; **Address:** St Louis Chldns Hosp, Dept Peds, 660 S Euclid Ave Fl 5MPRB, Box 8208, St Louis, MO 63110-1010; **Phone:** 314-286-2772; **Board Cert:** Internal Medicine 1972; Nephrology 1976; **Med School:** Creighton Univ 1969; **Resid:** Internal Medicine, New York Hosp-Cornell 1971; Internal Medicine, Barnes Hosp-Wash Univ 1972; **Fellow:** Nephrology, Barnes Hosp-Wash Univ 1974; **Fac Appt:** Prof Ped, Washington Univ, St Louis

Nephrology

Josephson, Michelle A MD [Nep] - **Spec Exp:** Transplant Medicine-Kidney; Hypertension; **Hospital:** Univ of Chicago Med Ctr; **Address:** Div Nephrology, 5841 S Maryland Ave, MC 5100, Chicago, IL 60637; **Phone:** 773-702-6134; **Board Cert:** Internal Medicine 1986; Nephrology 2010; **Med School:** Univ Pennsylvania 1983; **Resid:** Internal Medicine, Univ Chicago Hosps 1986; **Fellow:** Nephrology, Univ Chicago Hosps 1991; **Fac Appt:** Assoc Clin Prof Med, Univ Chicago-Pritzker Sch Med

Kasiske, Bertram MD [Nep] - **Spec Exp:** Transplant Medicine-Kidney; Kidney Disease-Geriatric; **Hospital:** Hennepin Cnty Med Ctr; **Address:** Div Nephrology, Hennepin County Med Ctr, 701 Park Ave, Minneapolis, MN 55415; **Phone:** 612-347-6088; **Board Cert:** Internal Medicine 1980; Nephrology 1982; **Med School:** Univ Iowa Coll Med 1976; **Resid:** Internal Medicine, Hennepin Co Med Ctr 1980; **Fellow:** Nephrology, Hennepin Co Med Ctr 1983; **Fac Appt:** Prof Med, Univ Minn

Kraus, Michael A MD [Nep] - **Spec Exp:** Kidney Disease-Chronic; Kidney Failure-Acute; Dialysis Care; **Hospital:** IU Health University Hosp, IU Health North Hosp; **Address:** Indiana Univ Div Nephrology, 535 Barnhill Drive, RT 150, Indianapolis, IN 46202; **Phone:** 317-963-6875; **Board Cert:** Internal Medicine 1988; Nephrology 2002; **Med School:** Indiana Univ 1985; **Resid:** Internal Medicine, Indiana Univ Med Ctr 1988; **Fellow:** Nephrology, Univ Iowa 1991; **Fac Appt:** Clin Prof Med, Indiana Univ

McCarthy, James T MD [Nep] - **Spec Exp:** Kidney Failure-Chronic; Dialysis Care; **Hospital:** Mayo Med Ctr & Clin - Rochester; **Address:** Mayo Clinic, 200 1st St SW, Rochester, MN 55905; **Phone:** 507-266-6711; **Board Cert:** Internal Medicine 1980; Nephrology 1982; **Med School:** Univ Kansas 1977; **Resid:** Internal Medicine, Mayo Clin 1980; **Fellow:** Nephrology, Mayo Clin 1983; **Fac Appt:** Prof Med, Mayo Med Sch

Miller, Brent W MD [Nep] - **Spec Exp:** Kidney Failure-Chronic; Transplant Medicine-Kidney; Dialysis Care; **Hospital:** Barnes-Jewish Hosp; **Address:** Washington Univ School Med, 660 S Euclid Ave, Campus Box 8126, St Louis, MO 63110; **Phone:** 314-362-7603; **Board Cert:** Internal Medicine 2003; Nephrology 2007; **Med School:** Washington Univ, St Louis 1990; **Resid:** Internal Medicine, Washington Univ Sch Med 1994; **Fellow:** Nephrology, Washington Univ Sch Med 1998; **Fac Appt:** Assoc Prof Med, Univ Wash

Pohl, Marc MD [Nep] - **Spec Exp:** Hypertension; Kidney Disease; Diabetes; **Hospital:** Cleveland Clin (page 56); **Address:** Dept Nephrology & Hypertension, 9500 Euclid Ave, Desk Q7, Cleveland, OH 44195; **Phone:** 216-444-6776; **Board Cert:** Internal Medicine 1972; Nephrology 1978; **Med School:** Case West Res Univ 1966; **Resid:** Internal Medicine, Univ Hosps 1968; Internal Medicine, Mass Genl Hosp 1971; **Fellow:** Nephrology, Boston City Hosp-Boston Univ 1972; Nephrology, Mass Genl Hosp 1973

Rodby, Roger A MD [Nep] - **Spec Exp:** Diabetic Kidney Disease; Glomerulonephritis; Lupus Nephritis; **Hospital:** Rush Univ Med Ctr; **Address:** 1426 W Washington Blvd, Chicago, IL 60607; **Phone:** 312-850-8434; **Board Cert:** Internal Medicine 1985; Nephrology 1988; **Med School:** Univ IL Coll Med 1982; **Resid:** Internal Medicine, UMDNJ-Rutgers 1985; **Fellow:** Nephrology, Rush/Presby-St Lukes 1987; **Fac Appt:** Assoc Prof Med, Rush Med Coll

Schreiber, Martin J MD [Nep] - **Spec Exp:** Dialysis Care; Diabetic Kidney Disease; Heart Failure in Kidney Disease; **Hospital:** Cleveland Clin (page 56); **Address:** Cleveland Clinic-Nephrology, 9500 Euclid Ave, MC Q7, Cleveland, OH 44195; **Phone:** 216-444-6365; **Board Cert:** Internal Medicine 1984; Nephrology 2003; **Med School:** Wake Forest Univ 1976; **Resid:** Internal Medicine, Cleveland Clin 1979; **Fellow:** Nephrology, Mass Genl Hosp 1980; Nephrology, Cleveland Clin 1982

Schwartz, Gary Lee MD [Nep] - **Spec Exp:** Hypertension; Kidney Disease-Chronic; Diabetic Kidney Disease; **Hospital:** St. Mary's Hosp - Rochester MN (Mayo), Rochester Methodist Hosp; **Address:** Mayo Clinic, 200 1st St SW, Rochester, MN 55905-0002; **Phone:** 507-284-4083; **Board Cert:** Internal Medicine 1980; Nephrology 1982; **Med School:** Univ Wisc 1977; **Resid:** Internal Medicine, Mayo Clinic 1980; **Fellow:** Nephrology, Mayo Clinic 1982; **Fac Appt:** Assoc Clin Prof Med, Mayo Med Sch

Somerville, James H MD [Nep] - **Hospital:** Fairview Southdale Hosp, Fairview Ridges Hosp; **Address:** 6363 France Ave S, Ste 400, Edina, MN 55435; **Phone:** 952-920-2070; **Board Cert:** Internal Medicine 1978; Nephrology 1982; **Med School:** Univ MD Sch Med 1975; **Resid:** Internal Medicine, Hennepin Co Med Ctr 1978; **Fellow:** Nephrology, Hennepin Co Med Ctr 1980

Swartz, Richard D MD [Nep] - **Spec Exp:** Kidney Failure; Dialysis Care; **Hospital:** Univ of Michigan Hosp; **Address:** Univ Mich, Div Nephrology, 1500 E Med Ctr Drive, 3914 Taubman Ctr, Ann Arbor, MI 48109-0364; **Phone:** 734-647-9342; **Board Cert:** Internal Medicine 1975; Nephrology 1978; **Med School:** Univ Mich Med Sch 1970; **Resid:** Internal Medicine, Boston City Hosp 1975; Nephrology, Beth Israel Hosp-Harvard 1977; **Fac Appt:** Prof Med, Univ Mich Med Sch

Textor, Stephen C MD [Nep] - **Spec Exp:** Transplant Medicine-Kidney; Hypertension; Renal Artery Stenosis; **Hospital:** Mayo Med Ctr & Clin - Rochester; **Address:** Mayo Clinic, Div Nephrology/Hypertension, 200 First St SW, Rochester, MN 55905; **Phone:** 507-284-4083; **Board Cert:** Internal Medicine 1977; Nephrology 1980; **Med School:** UCLA 1973; **Resid:** Internal Medicine, Boston City Hosp 1977; **Fellow:** Nephrology, Boston Univ 1978; Hypertension, Fogarty Inst 1980; **Fac Appt:** Prof Med, Mayo Med Sch

Thomas, Christie P MD [Nep] - **Spec Exp:** Transplant Medicine-Kidney; Fabry's Disease; **Hospital:** Univ Iowa Hosp & Clinics; **Address:** UIHC Nephrology Dept, 200 Hawkins Drive, SE 419 GH, Iowa City, IA 52242; **Phone:** 319-356-4216; **Board Cert:** Internal Medicine 2007; Nephrology 2008; **Med School:** India 1982; **Resid:** Internal Medicine, MMM Hosp Kolenchery 1983; Internal Medicine, Genl Hosp 1986; **Fellow:** Nephrology, Univ Sheffield Hosp 1988; Nephrology, Case Western Res Univ Hosp 1991; **Fac Appt:** Prof Med, Univ Iowa Coll Med

Torres, Vicente E MD [Nep] - **Spec Exp:** Polycystic Kidney Disease; **Hospital:** Mayo Med Ctr & Clin - Rochester; **Address:** Mayo Clinic, Div Nephrology/Hypertension, Mayo E 19, 200 First St SW, Rochester, MN 55905; **Phone:** 507-266-7093; **Board Cert:** Internal Medicine 1977; Nephrology 1980; **Med School:** Spain 1969; **Resid:** Internal Medicine, Mayo Grad Sch Med 1977; **Fellow:** Nephrology, Mayo Grad Sch Med 1979; **Fac Appt:** Prof Med, Mayo Med Sch

Venkat, K K MD [Nep] - **Spec Exp:** Transplant Medicine-Kidney; Kidney Disease; **Hospital:** Henry Ford Hosp; **Address:** Henry Ford Hosp, Div Nephrology, 2799 W Grand Blvd, Ste K16, Detroit, MI 48202-2689; **Phone:** 313-916-2702; **Board Cert:** Internal Medicine 1977; Nephrology 1978; **Med School:** India 1970; **Resid:** Internal Medicine, Henry Ford Hosp 1976; **Fellow:** Nephrology, Henry Ford Hosp 1978

Yee, Jerry MD [Nep] - **Spec Exp:** Kidney Disease-Chronic; Hypertension; Diabetic Kidney Disease; **Hospital:** Henry Ford Hosp; **Address:** Henry Ford Hospital, 2799 W Grand Blvd, CFP-5, Detroit, MI 48202; **Phone:** 313-916-9405; **Board Cert:** Internal Medicine 1985; Nephrology 2002; **Med School:** Jefferson Med Coll 1982; **Resid:** Internal Medicine, Brooke AMC-Fort Sam 1985; **Fellow:** Nephrology, Temple Univ Hosp 1986; Hypertension, Hosp U Penn 1987; **Fac Appt:** Assoc Prof Med, Wayne State Univ

Nephrology

Great Plains and Mountains

Berl, Tomas MD [Nep] - **Spec Exp:** Fluid/Electrolyte Balance; Kidney Failure-Chronic; Diabetic Kidney Disease; **Hospital:** Univ of CO Hosp - Anschutz Inpatient Pav; **Address:** Univ Colorado-Renal Disease/Hypertension, 1635 Aurora Court, MS F747, Aurora, CO 80045; **Phone:** 720-848-0749; **Board Cert:** Internal Medicine 1972; Nephrology 1976; **Med School:** NYU Sch Med 1968; **Resid:** Internal Medicine, Bronx Municipal Hosp 1970; **Fellow:** Renal Disease, Moffit Hosp-UCSF 1971; **Fac Appt:** Prof Med, Univ Colorado

Southwest

Brennan, Stephen T MD [Nep] - **Spec Exp:** Transplant Medicine-Kidney; Kidney Stones; Kidney Failure-Chronic; **Hospital:** Methodist Hosp - Houston, St. Luke's Episcopal Hosp-Houston; **Address:** 1415 La Concha Ln, Houston, TX 77054; **Phone:** 713-790-9080; **Board Cert:** Internal Medicine 1983; Nephrology 1988; **Med School:** Loyola Univ-Stritch Sch Med 1979; **Resid:** Internal Medicine, Loyola Univ Med Ctr 1983; **Fellow:** Nephrology, Univ Wash-Barnes Hosp 1986; **Fac Appt:** Assoc Clin Prof Med, Baylor Coll Med

Fadem, Stephen Z MD [Nep] - **Spec Exp:** Kidney Disease-Chronic; Kidney Failure; Hypertension; **Hospital:** Methodist Hosp - Houston, St. Luke's Episcopal Hosp-Houston; **Address:** Kidney Assocs, 6624 Fannin St, Ste 1400, Houston, TX 77030; **Phone:** 713-795-5511; **Board Cert:** Internal Medicine 1976; Nephrology 1978; **Med School:** Univ Okla Coll Med 1973; **Resid:** Internal Medicine, UT MD Anderson Hosp 1976; **Fellow:** Renal Disease, UT Hlth Sci Ctr 1978; **Fac Appt:** Clin Prof Med, Baylor Coll Med

Kasinath, Balakuntalam S MD [Nep] - **Spec Exp:** Glomerulonephritis; Diabetic Kidney Disease; **Hospital:** Univ Hlth Syst-San Antonio, Audie L Murphy Meml Vets Hosp - San Antonio; **Address:** Univ Tex Hlth Sci Ctr, Dept Med/Div Neph, 7703 Floyd Curl Drive, MC 7882, San Antonio, TX 78229-3901; **Phone:** 210-567-4707; **Board Cert:** Internal Medicine 1980; Nephrology 1982; **Med School:** India 1975; **Resid:** Internal Medicine, Ill Masonic Med Ctr 1980; **Fellow:** Nephrology, Univ Chicago Hosp 1983; **Fac Appt:** Prof Med, Univ Tex, San Antonio

Mitch, William MD [Nep] - **Spec Exp:** Nutrition; Hypertension; Kidney Failure; **Hospital:** Baylor Clinic & Hosp-Houston, Ben Taub Genl Hosp; **Address:** Baylor Clin, 6620 Main St, Ste 1375, Houston, TX 77030; **Phone:** 713-798-2500; **Board Cert:** Internal Medicine 1972; Nephrology 1978; **Med School:** Harvard Med Sch 1967; **Resid:** Internal Medicine, Brigham & Women's Hosp 1974; Nat Cancer Inst-NIH 1972; **Fellow:** Nephrology, Johns Hopkins Hosp 1973; **Fac Appt:** Prof Med, Baylor Coll Med

Olivero, Juan J MD [Nep] - **Spec Exp:** Kidney Failure-Acute; Kidney Failure-Chronic; Fluid/Electrolyte Balance; Hypertension; **Hospital:** Methodist Hosp - Houston, St. Luke's Episcopal Hosp-Houston; **Address:** 6560 Fannin St, Scurlock Twr, Ste 2206, Houston, TX 77030; **Phone:** 713-790-4615; **Board Cert:** Internal Medicine 1974; Nephrology 1976; **Med School:** Guatemala 1970; **Resid:** Internal Medicine, Baylor Affil Hosps 1973; Internal Medicine, Ben Taub Genl Hosp 1974; **Fellow:** Nephrology, Baylor Affil Hosps 1975; **Fac Appt:** Clin Prof Med, Baylor Coll Med

Suki, Wadi N MD [Nep] - **Spec Exp:** Transplant Medicine-Kidney; Hypertension; Lupus Nephritis; **Hospital:** Methodist Hosp - Houston, St. Luke's Episcopal Hosp-Houston; **Address:** 1415 La Concha Ln, Houston, TX 77054; **Phone:** 713-790-9080; **Board Cert:** Internal Medicine 1967; Nephrology 1972; **Med School:** Sudan 1959; **Resid:** Internal Medicine, Parkland Meml Hosp 1963; **Fellow:** Nephrology, Univ Tex SW Med Ctr 1961; Nephrology, Univ Tex SW Med Ctr 1965; **Fac Appt:** Clin Prof Med, Baylor Coll Med

Toto, Robert D MD [Nep] - **Spec Exp:** Hypertension/Kidney Disease; Dialysis Care; Diabetic Kidney Disease; Kidney Failure-Acute; **Hospital:** UT Southwestern Med Ctr at Dallas; **Address:** Transplant Prgm-Kidney & Liver, Professional Office Bldg 2, 5939 Harry Hines Blvd Fl 7 - Ste 700, Dallas, TX 75390; **Phone:** 214-645-1919; **Board Cert:** Internal Medicine 1980; Nephrology 1982; **Med School:** Univ IL Coll Med 1977; **Resid:** Internal Medicine, Univ Michigan Med Ctr 1979; Internal Medicine, Baylor Univ Med Ctr 1980; **Fellow:** Nephrology, US Public Hlth Svce Hosp 1981; Nephrology, UTSW Med Ctr 1983; **Fac Appt:** Prof Med, Univ Tex SW, Dallas

West Coast and Pacific

Ahmad, Suhail MD [Nep] - **Spec Exp:** Hypertension; Kidney Failure-Chronic; Kidney Stones; **Hospital:** Univ Wash Med Ctr; **Address:** Scribner Kidney Ctr, 2150 N 107th St, Ste 160, Seattle, WA 98133; **Phone:** 206-598-6430; **Med School:** India 1968; **Resid:** Internal Medicine, Univ Allahabad 1971; **Fellow:** Nephrology, Univ Washington Med Ctr 1978; **Fac Appt:** Assoc Prof Med, Univ Wash

Bennett, William M MD [Nep] - **Spec Exp:** Transplant Medicine-Kidney; **Hospital:** Legacy Good Samaritan Med Ctr; **Address:** Legacy Good Samaritan Hosp, Transplant Svcs, 1040 NW 22nd Ave, Ste 480, Portland, OR 97210; **Phone:** 503-413-6555; **Board Cert:** Internal Medicine 2002; Nephrology 2002; **Med School:** Northwestern Univ 1963; **Resid:** Internal Medicine, Chicago VA Rsch Hosp 1966; Internal Medicine, OR Hlth Sci Univ 1967; **Fellow:** Nephrology, Mass Genl Hosp 1970

Cho, Kerry C MD [Nep] - **Spec Exp:** Kidney Disease; Glomerulonephritis; **Hospital:** UCSF Med Ctr; **Address:** UCSF, Dept Nephrology, 521 Parnassus Ave, Ste C443, Box 0532, San Francisco, CA 94143-0532; **Phone:** 415-476-2173; **Board Cert:** Internal Medicine 2000; Nephrology 2003; **Med School:** Cornell Univ-Weill Med Coll 1996; **Resid:** Internal Medicine, Univ Michigan Med Ctr 1999; **Fellow:** Nephrology, USCF Med Ctr 2002; **Fac Appt:** Asst Prof Med, UCSF

Ellison, David H MD [Nep] - **Spec Exp:** Bartter's Syndrome; Gitelman's Syndrome; Hypertension; **Hospital:** OR Hlth & Sci Univ, VA Medical Center - Portland; **Address:** OHSU-Div Nephrology, 3303 SW Bond Ave, MC CH12R, Portland, OR 97239-3098; **Phone:** 503-494-3442; **Board Cert:** Internal Medicine 1981; Nephrology 1986; **Med School:** Rush Med Coll 1978; **Resid:** Internal Medicine, Oregon Hlth Scis Univ 1981; **Fellow:** Research, Oregon Hlth Scis Univ 1982; Nephrology, Yale Univ 1985; **Fac Appt:** Prof Med, Oregon Hlth & Sci Univ

Gluck, Stephen L MD [Nep] - **Spec Exp:** Kidney Disease; Fluid/Electrolyte Balance; Hypertension; Kidney Stones; **Hospital:** UCSF Med Ctr; **Address:** UCSF, Div Nephrology, 521 Parnassus Ave, rm C443, Box 0532, San Francisco, CA 94143-0532; **Phone:** 415-476-2173; **Board Cert:** Internal Medicine 1980; Nephrology 1984; **Med School:** UCLA 1977; **Resid:** Internal Medicine, Columbia Presby Med Ctr 1980; **Fellow:** Nephrology, Columbia Presby Med Ctr 1983; **Fac Appt:** Prof Med, UCSF

Kaysen, George Alan MD/PhD [Nep] - **Spec Exp:** Kidney Disease-Metabolic; Kidney Failure-Chronic; **Hospital:** UC Davis Med Ctr; **Address:** UC Davis Med Ctr, Div Nephr, One Shields Ave, GBSF 6310, Davis, CA 95616; **Phone:** 530-752-4010; **Board Cert:** Internal Medicine 1975; Nephrology 1980; **Med School:** Albert Einstein Coll Med 1972; **Resid:** Internal Medicine, Bronx Muni Hosp 1975; **Fellow:** Renal Disease, Bronx Muni Hosp 1977; **Fac Appt:** Prof Med, UC Davis

King, Andrew J MD [Nep] - **Spec Exp:** Kidney Disease-Chronic; Hypertension; Dialysis Care; **Hospital:** Scripps Green Hosp; **Address:** Scripps Clinic Torrey Pines, 10666 N Torrey Pines Rd, Mail Drop N239, La Jolla, CA 92037-1027; **Phone:** 858-554-9765; **Board Cert:** Internal Medicine 1986; Nephrology 1988; **Med School:** Northwestern Univ 1983; **Resid:** Internal Medicine, Northwestern Meml Hosp 1986; **Fellow:** Nephrology, Brigham & Womens Hosp 1990; **Fac Appt:** Clin Prof Med, UCSD

Ott, Susan M MD [Nep] - **Spec Exp:** Bone Disorders-Metabolic; Osteoporosis; **Hospital:** Univ Wash Med Ctr; **Address:** Bone & Joint Center, UWMC- Roosevelt, 4245 Roosevelt Way NE, Box 354740, Seattle, WA 98105-6920; **Phone:** 206-598-4288; **Board Cert:** Internal Medicine 1978; Nephrology 1982; **Med School:** Univ Wash 1974; **Resid:** Family Medicine, UC Davis Med Ctr 1978; **Fellow:** Nephrology, Univ Wash Med Ctr 1982; **Fac Appt:** Assoc Prof Med, Univ Wash

Riordan, John W MD [Nep] - **Hospital:** CA Pacific Med Ctr-Pacific Campus; **Address:** 2100 Webster St, Ste 412, San Francisco, CA 94115; **Phone:** 415-923-3815; **Board Cert:** Nephrology 2005; **Med School:** Univ Tex Med Br, Galveston 1987; **Resid:** Internal Medicine, Univ Texas Hlth Sci Ctr 1990; **Fellow:** Nephrology, UCSF Med Ctr 1995

Scandling Jr, John D MD [Nep] - **Spec Exp:** Transplant Medicine-Kidney; Transplant Medicine-Pancreas; **Hospital:** Stanford Univ Hosp & Clinics; **Address:** Stanford Nephrology/Transplant, 750 Welsh Rd, Ste 200, Palo Alto, CA 94304-1509; **Phone:** 650-725-9891; **Board Cert:** Internal Medicine 1981; Nephrology 1984; **Med School:** Med Coll VA 1978; **Resid:** Internal Medicine, West Virginia Univ Hosp 1981; **Fellow:** Nephrology, Univ Rochester 1983; **Fac Appt:** Prof Med, Stanford Univ

▄▟ Cleveland Clinic

Every life deserves world class care.

Nephrology

The Glickman Urological & Kidney Institute's Department of Nephrology & Hypertension provides comprehensive diagnostic and therapeutic services for patients with kidney disease and hypertension. The department participates in an active kidney transplant program, all modalities of dialysis care and clinical research studies of diabetic and other glomerular diseases. In addition to unique and proven diagnostic capabilities, the department is renowned for its expertise in the areas of renovascular hypertension, primary aldosteronism and pheochromocytoma.

Intensive Care Nephrology Services

The Department of Nephrology & Hypertension is a major participant in the intensive care setting. Our nephrologists are leaders in research into the risk factors for acute renal failure after surgeries and in evaluations and diagnosis of different techniques for treatment of acute renal failure such as slow continuous ultrafiltration, continuous arteriovenous hemofiltration and venovenous hemofiltration.

Hypertension

Utilizing the latest technology for accurate measurement of blood pressure and detailed risk assessment, specialists tailor treatment to the individual needs of each patient.

Chronic Kidney Disease (CKD)

Our CKD clinic provides health evaluation, screenings and treatment for patients. This innovative model of health management focuses on educating and involving the patient in his or her care.

Polycystic Kidney Disease (PKD)

Polycystic kidney disease can cause other health problems such as high blood pressure, frequent urination, low back pain and fatigue. Our nephrologists can help PKD patients create a health management plan for dealing with the disease.

Cleveland Clinic
Gickman Urological &
Kidney Institute
9500 Euclid Avenue
Cleveland, OH 44195

clevelandclinic.org/
nephrologytopdocs

Offering Same-Day Appointments
Call 800.274.2009.

Treatment Guides

Cleveland Clinic has developed comprehensive treatment guides for many diseases and conditions. To download our free treatment guides, visit clevelandclinic.org/treatmentguides.

Online Medical Second Opinion

Cleveland Clinic's My**Consult** Online Medical Second Opinion program securely connects patients to our physician specialists for more than 1,000 life-changing or life-threatening diagnoses all by the click of a mouse. To learn more, log onto eclevelandclinic.org/myconsult or call 800.223.2273, ext. 43223.

Special Assistance for Out-of-State Patients

Cleveland Clinic Global Patient Services offers a complimentary Medical Concierge service for patients who travel from outside of Ohio. Call 800.223.2273, ext. 55580 or email medicalconcierge@ccf.org.

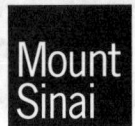
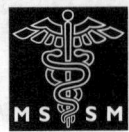

**MOUNT SINAI
SCHOOL OF
MEDICINE**

THE MOUNT SINAI MEDICAL CENTER
NEPHROLOGY
One Gustave L. Levy Place
Fifth Avenue and 100th Street
New York, NY 10029-6574
Physician Referral: 1-800-MD-SINAI (637-4624)
www.mountsinai.org/kidney

Mount Sinai's Department of Nephrology ranks among the best in the nation, according to the 2011-2012 issue of *U.S. News & World Report's "Americas Best Hospitals."* Our kidney disease program ranks in the top 25 of nearly 5,000 hospitals evaluated by the publication.

We have been an international leader in the treatment of kidney disease since we performed the first hemodialysis in the United States in the 1950s. We established New York State's first dialysis center in 1957. We currently operate the largest home dialysis program in New York City, and our **Geriatric Nephrology Program** is the only one of its kind in the country.

Under the direction of Barbara Murphy, M.D., Division Chief, we are continuing our leadership in patient care, research and education. Proof of our clinical excellence is evident daily in our practice and hospital. Our physicians care for patients referred to us by other nephrologists who recognize the need for our expertise in their most challenging and complex cases.

Our expertise spans numerous kidney diseases and treatments, including:

- Chronic kidney disease
- Polycystic kidney disease
- Geriatric kidney disease
- Diabetes-related kidney disease
- Glomerular disease
- Hypertensive kidney disease
- HIV-associated nephropathy
- Kidney transplantation
- Hemodialysis
- Peritoneal Dialysis

EXPERT PHYSICIANS

Building on the talent and expertise of our physicians, including Jonathan Winston, M.D., Tonia Kim, M.D., Mark Swidler, M.D., Joseph Vassalotti, M.D, Brian Radbill, M.D., and Richard Stein, M.D., along with transplantation specialists, Bernd Schroppel, M.D. and Vinay Nair, M.D., we provide patients with the most advanced and appropriate approach to care. With so much research taking place, we can also offer patients access to experimental treatments often unavailable elsewhere.

Initiated in 1967, our **kidney transplant program** is now one of the largest and most successful in the country, with our physician-scientists actively investigating new and innovative ways to detect, prevent, and treat rejection.

A Strong Focus on Research
With one of the largest National Institutes of Health research budgets of any nephrology division in the country, we conduct and support numerous clinical trials, and our faculty members have achieved international recognition as authorities on the causes and treatments of all forms of kidney diseases and disorders.

Neurological Surgery

A neurological surgeon provides the operative and non-operative management (i.e., prevention, diagnosis, evaluation, treatment, critical care and rehabilitation) of disorders of the central, peripheral and autonomic nervous systems, including their supporting structures and vascular supply; the evaluation and treatment of pathological processes which modify function or activity of the nervous system; and the operative and non-operative management of pain. A neurological surgeon treats patients with disorders of the nervous system; disorders of the brain, meninges, skull and their blood supply, including the extracranial carotid and vertebral arteries; disorders of the pituitary gland; disorders of the spinal cord, meninges and vertebral column, including those which may require treatment by spinal fusion or instrumentation; and disorders of the cranial and spinal nerves throughout their distribution.

Training Required: Seven years (including general surgery)

The American Board of Pediatric Neurological Surgery (ABPNS) is not a recognized ABMS subspecialty. However, this designation has been included because the certification process is meaningful and rigorous. It is awarded to those doctors who hold a current ABMS certification in Neurological Surgery, have completed a fully accredited one year, post-graduate fellowship in pediatric neurological surgery, and have submitted surgical logs indicating a practice of pediatric neurological surgery for one year, followed by a written examination.

NEUROLOGICAL SURGERY

New England

Al-Mefty, Ossama MD [NS] - **Spec Exp:** Skull Base Surgery; Brain Tumors; Cerebrovascular Surgery; **Hospital:** Brigham and Women's Hosp (page 57); **Address:** Brigham & Women's Hosp, Dept Neurosurgery, 75 Francis St, Boston, MA 02115; **Phone:** 617-525-9451; **Board Cert:** Neurological Surgery 1980; **Med School:** Syria 1972; **Resid:** Surgery, Med Coll Ohio 1974; Neurological Surgery, West Va Med Ctr 1978; **Fac Appt:** Prof NS, Harvard Med Sch

Borges, Lawrence F MD [NS] - **Spec Exp:** Spinal Surgery; Spinal Tumors; **Hospital:** Mass Genl Hosp; **Address:** Mass General Hosp, 55 Fruit St, White 1205, Boston, MA 02114; **Phone:** 617-726-6156; **Board Cert:** Neurological Surgery 1986; **Med School:** Johns Hopkins Univ 1977; **Resid:** Neurological Surgery, Mass Genl Hosp 1983; **Fac Appt:** Assoc Prof S, Harvard Med Sch

Cosgrove, G Rees MD [NS] - **Spec Exp:** Epilepsy/Seizure Disorders; Brain Tumors; **Hospital:** Rhode Island Hosp, Miriam Hosp; **Address:** 55 Claverick St, Providence, RI 02903; **Phone:** 401-490-4176; **Board Cert:** Neurological Surgery 1989; **Med School:** Queens Univ 1980; **Resid:** Neurological Surgery, Montreal Neur Inst 1986; **Fac Appt:** Prof NS, Brown Univ

David, Carlos A MD [NS] - **Spec Exp:** Cerebrovascular Surgery; Brain Tumors; Pituitary Tumors; Carotid Artery Surgery; **Hospital:** Lahey Clin, Emerson Hosp; **Address:** Lahey Clinic, Dept Neurosurgery, 41 Mall Rd, Burlington, MA 01805; **Phone:** 781-744-8643; **Board Cert:** Neurological Surgery 2001; **Med School:** Univ Miami Sch Med 1990; **Resid:** Neurological Surgery, Jackson Memorial Hosp 1995; **Fellow:** Cerebrovascular & Skull Base Surgery, Barrow Neuro Inst 1997; **Fac Appt:** Assoc Clin Prof NS, Tufts Univ

Duhaime, Ann Christine MD [NS] - **Spec Exp:** Pediatric Neurosurgery; Brain Tumors; Epilepsy; Craniofacial Surgery; **Hospital:** Mass Genl Hosp; **Address:** Mass Geneneral Hospital for Children, 15 Parkman St, WACC 331, Boston, MA 02114; **Phone:** 617-643-9175; **Board Cert:** Neurological Surgery 1990; Pediatric Neurological Surgery 2005; **Med School:** Univ Pennsylvania 1981; **Resid:** Neurological Surgery, Hosp Univ Penn 1987; **Fellow:** Pediatric Neurological Surgery, Chldns Hosp 1987

Goumnerova, Liliana MD [NS] - **Spec Exp:** Pediatric Neurosurgery; Brain Tumors; Endoscopic Surgery/Ventriculoscopy; **Hospital:** Children's Hospital - Boston, Dana-Farber Cancer Inst (page 57); **Address:** 300 Longwood Ave Hunnewell Bldg Fl 2, Boston, MA 02115; **Phone:** 617-355-6364; **Board Cert:** Neurological Surgery 1992; Pediatric Neurological Surgery 2006; **Med School:** Canada 1980; **Resid:** Neurological Surgery, Univ Ottawa 1986; **Fellow:** Pediatric Neurological Surgery, Hosp for Sick Chldn 1988; Neurological Science, Univ Hosp Penn 1990; **Fac Appt:** Assoc Prof S, Harvard Med Sch

Heilman, Carl B MD [NS] - **Spec Exp:** Skull Base Surgery; Pediatric Neurosurgery; **Hospital:** Tufts Med Ctr; **Address:** Tufts-NE Med Ctr, Dept Neurosurgery, 800 Washington St, Box 178, Bsoton, MA 02111; **Phone:** 617-636-5860; **Board Cert:** Neurological Surgery 1996; **Med School:** Univ Pennsylvania 1986; **Resid:** Neurological Surgery, Tufts New England Med Ctr 1993; **Fellow:** Skull Base Surgery, Baptist Meml Hosp 1993; **Fac Appt:** Assoc Prof NS, Tufts Univ

Madsen, Joseph R MD [NS] - **Spec Exp:** Pediatric Neurosurgery; Epilepsy/Seizure Disorders; **Hospital:** Children's Hospital - Boston; **Address:** 300 Longwood Ave, Honeywell 2, Boston, MA 02115; **Phone:** 617-355-6005; **Board Cert:** Neurological Surgery 1994; Pediatric Neurological Surgery 1997; **Med School:** Harvard Med Sch 1981; **Resid:** Neurological Surgery, Mass Genl Hosp 1989; **Fellow:** Research, Beth Israel Hosp 1983; **Fac Appt:** Assoc Prof NS, Harvard Med Sch

Martuza, Robert L MD [NS] - **Spec Exp:** Brain Tumors; Acoustic Neuroma; Skull Base Surgery; **Hospital:** Mass Genl Hosp; **Address:** Mass General Hosp, Dept Neurosurgery, 55 Fruit St, White 502, Boston, MA 02114; **Phone:** 617-726-8581; **Board Cert:** Neurological Surgery 1983; **Med School:** Harvard Med Sch 1973; **Resid:** Neurological Surgery, Mass Genl Hosp 1980; **Fac Appt:** Prof NS, Harvard Med Sch

Penar, Paul L MD [NS] - **Spec Exp:** Brain & Spinal Tumors; Epilepsy/Seizure Disorders; Movement Disorders; Stereotactic Radiosurgery; **Hospital:** Fletcher Allen Health Care- Med Ctr Campus; **Address:** Fletcher Allen Health Care, 111 Colchester Ave, Burlington, VT 05401; **Phone:** 802-847-4590; **Board Cert:** Neurological Surgery 1989; **Med School:** Univ Mich Med Sch 1981; **Resid:** Neurological Surgery, Yale-New Haven Hosp 1987

Piepmeier, Joseph MD [NS] - **Spec Exp:** Neuro-Oncology; Brain & Spinal Cord Tumors; **Hospital:** Yale-New Haven Hosp, Yale Med Group; **Address:** Yale Sch Med, Dept Neurosurgery, 333 Cedar St Fl TMP-410, New Haven, CT 06520; **Phone:** 203-785-2791; **Board Cert:** Neurological Surgery 1984; **Med School:** Univ Tenn Coll Med 1975; **Resid:** Neurological Surgery, Yale-New Haven Hosp 1982; **Fac Appt:** Prof NS, Yale Univ

Spencer, Dennis D MD [NS] - **Spec Exp:** Epilepsy/Seizure Disorders; Brain Tumors; **Hospital:** Yale-New Haven Hosp, Yale Med Group; **Address:** Yale Univ Sch Med, Dept Neurosurgery, 333 Cedar St, TMP-4, New Haven, CT 06520; **Phone:** 203-785-4891; **Board Cert:** Neurological Surgery 1980; **Med School:** Washington Univ, St Louis 1971; **Resid:** Surgery, Barnes Hosp 1972; Neurological Surgery, Yale-New Haven Hosp 1976; **Fac Appt:** Prof NS, Yale Univ

Swearingen, Brooke MD [NS] - **Spec Exp:** Pituitary Tumors; Brain & Spinal Tumors; Neuroendocrine Tumors; Spinal Surgery; **Hospital:** Mass Genl Hosp; **Address:** 15 Parkman St, WACC 331, Boston, MA 02114-3117; **Phone:** 617-726-3910; **Board Cert:** Neurological Surgery 1993; **Med School:** Harvard Med Sch 1981; **Resid:** Neurological Surgery, Mass Genl Hosp 1987; **Fac Appt:** Assoc Prof NS, Harvard Med Sch

Mid Atlantic

Andrews, David MD [NS] - **Spec Exp:** Brain Tumors; Stereotactic Radiosurgery; **Hospital:** Thomas Jefferson Univ Hosp; **Address:** Thom Jefferson Univ Hosp, Dept Neurosurg, 909 Walnut St Fl 2, Philadelphia, PA 19107-5109; **Phone:** 215-503-7005; **Board Cert:** Neurological Surgery 1992; **Med School:** Univ Colorado 1983; **Resid:** Neurological Surgery, NY Presby Hosp-Cornell Med Ctr 1989; **Fellow:** Neuro-Oncology, Meml Sloan Kettering Cancer Ctr 1987; **Fac Appt:** Prof NS, Thomas Jefferson Univ

Bailes, Julian E MD [NS] - **Spec Exp:** Neuro-Oncology; Cancer Surgery; Spinal Surgery; Cerebrovascular Surgery; **Hospital:** Ruby Memorial - WVU Hosp; **Address:** W Virgina Univ Eye Inst, PO Box 9193, Morgantown, WV 26506; **Phone:** 304-598-6127; **Board Cert:** Neurological Surgery 1992; **Med School:** Louisiana State U, New Orleans 1982; **Resid:** Surgery, Northwestern Meml Hosp 1987; **Fellow:** Neurological Surgery, Barrow Neurological Inst 1988; **Fac Appt:** Prof NS

Baltuch, Gordon MD/PhD [NS] - **Spec Exp:** Movement Disorders; Parkinson's Disease; Epilepsy/Seizure Disorders; Dystonia; **Hospital:** Hosp Univ Penn - UPHS (page 68), Pennsylvania Hosp-UPHS (page 68); **Address:** Penn Neurological Institute, 3400 Spruce St, Silverstein Bldg Fl 3, Philadelphia, PA 19104; **Phone:** 215-829-6700; **Board Cert:** Neurological Surgery 1998; **Med School:** McGill Univ 1986; **Resid:** Surgery, Montreal Genl Hosp 1988; Neurological Surgery, Montreal Neuro Inst 1994; **Fellow:** Neurological Surgery, Centre Hospitalier Univ Vaudois 1995; **Fac Appt:** Prof NS, Univ Pennsylvania

Neurological Surgery

Bederson, Joshua B MD [NS] - **Spec Exp:** Brain & Spinal Cord Tumors; Aneurysm-Cerebral; Meningioma; Pituitary Tumors; **Hospital:** Mount Sinai Med Ctr (page 63); **Address:** Mount Sinai Med Ctr, 1 Gustave Levy Pl, Box 1136, New York, NY 10029; **Phone:** 212-241-2377; **Board Cert:** Neurological Surgery 1993; **Med School:** UCSF 1984; **Resid:** Neurological Surgery, UCSF Med Ctr 1990; **Fellow:** Neurological Vascular Surgery, Barrow Neur Inst 1990; Neurological Vascular Surgery, Univ Hosp Zurich 1990; **Fac Appt:** Prof NS, Mount Sinai Sch Med

Belzberg, Allan J MD [NS] - **Spec Exp:** Peripheral Nerve Disorders; Nerve Surgery & Transplantation; Nerve Tumors; Spinal Surgery; **Hospital:** Johns Hopkins Hosp (page 61); **Address:** Johns Hopkins Dept Neurosurgery, 600 N Wolfe St, Meyer 5-109, Baltimore, MD 21287; **Phone:** 410-955-5810; **Board Cert:** Neurological Surgery 1997; **Med School:** Univ Calgary 1982; **Resid:** Neurological Surgery, Univ Calgary Affil Hosps 1990; **Fellow:** Neurological Surgery, Johns Hopkins Hosp 1992; **Fac Appt:** Assoc Prof NS, Johns Hopkins Univ

Bilsky, Mark H MD [NS] - **Spec Exp:** Brain & Spinal Tumors; Skull Base Tumors; Spinal Reconstructive Surgery; Spinal Cord Tumors; **Hospital:** Meml Sloan-Kettering Cancer Ctr, NY-Presby/Weill Cornell Med Ctr, NY (page 65); **Address:** 1275 York Ave MSKCC Bldg Fl c705, New York, NY 10065; **Phone:** 212-639-8526; **Board Cert:** Neurological Surgery 2010; **Med School:** Emory Univ 1988; **Resid:** Neurological Surgery, NY Hosp-Cornell Med Ctr 1994; **Fellow:** Neuro-Oncology, Louisville Univ Med Ctr 1995; **Fac Appt:** Prof NS, Cornell Univ-Weill Med Coll

Brem, Henry MD [NS] - **Spec Exp:** Brain & Spinal Cord Tumors; Skull Base Tumors; Pituitary Tumors; **Hospital:** Johns Hopkins Hosp (page 61), Johns Hopkins Bayview Med Ctr (page 61); **Address:** Johns Hopkins Hosp, 600 N Wolfe St Meyer 7 Bldg - rm 113, Baltimore, MD 21287; **Phone:** 410-955-2248; **Board Cert:** Neurological Surgery 1986; **Med School:** Harvard Med Sch 1978; **Resid:** Neurological Surgery, Columbia-Presby Med Ctr 1984; **Fellow:** Neurological Surgery, Johns Hopkins Hosp 1980; **Fac Appt:** Prof NS, Johns Hopkins Univ

Bruce, Jeffrey MD [NS] - **Spec Exp:** Brain Tumors; Pituitary Tumors; Skull Base Surgery; Meningioma; **Hospital:** NY-Presby/Columbia Univ Med Ctr, NY (page 65); **Address:** NY Presby Hosp, Dept Neurosurgery, 710 W 168th St N1 Bldg Fl 4 - rm 434, New York, NY 10032; **Phone:** 212-305-7346; **Board Cert:** Neurological Surgery 1993; **Med School:** UMDNJ-RW Johnson Med Sch 1983; **Resid:** Neurological Surgery, Columbia-Presby Med Ctr 1990; **Fellow:** Neurological Surgery, Nat Inst Hlth 1985; **Fac Appt:** Prof NS, Columbia P&S

Caputy, Anthony J MD [NS] - **Spec Exp:** Epilepsy/Seizure Disorders; Spinal Surgery; Brain & Spinal Tumors; Minimally Invasive Surgery; **Hospital:** G Washington Univ Hosp, Suburban Hosp; **Address:** Geo Wash Univ, Dept Neurosurgery, 2150 Pennsylvania Ave NW, Ste 7-420, Washington, DC 20037; **Phone:** 202-741-2735; **Board Cert:** Neurological Surgery 1989; **Med School:** Univ VA Sch Med 1980; **Resid:** Neurological Surgery, Georgetown Univ Hosp 1986; **Fac Appt:** Prof NS, Geo Wash Univ

Carson, Benjamin S MD [NS] - **Spec Exp:** Brain Injury; Brain & Spinal Cord Tumors; Pediatric Neurosurgery; Rasmussen's Syndrome; **Hospital:** Johns Hopkins Hosp (page 61); **Address:** 600 N Wolfe St, Harvey 811, Baltimore, MD 21287-8811; **Phone:** 410-355-4259; **Board Cert:** Neurological Surgery 1988; Pediatric Neurological Surgery 1997; **Med School:** Univ Mich Med Sch 1977; **Resid:** Neurological Surgery, Johns Hopkins Hosp 1983; **Fellow:** Pediatric Neurological Surgery, Queen Elizabeth II Med Ctr 1984; **Fac Appt:** Assoc Prof NS, Johns Hopkins Univ

Chen, Chun Siang MD [NS] - **Spec Exp:** Skull Base Tumors; Skull Base Surgery; Microsurgery; Brain & Spinal Tumors; **Hospital:** Mount Sinai Med Ctr (page 63); **Address:** Mount Sinai Med Ctr, Annenberg Bldg, One Gustave L Levy Pl Fl 8 - rm 10, New York, NY 10029; **Phone:** 212-241-8480; **Med School:** Brazil 1978; **Resid:** Neurological Surgery, Santa Casa de Misericordia of Sao Paulo Med Sch 1983; Neurological Surgery, Mt Sinai Med Ctr 2005; **Fellow:** Skull Base Surgery, St Lukes Roosevelt Hosp 2006; **Fac Appt:** Asst Prof NS, Mount Sinai Sch Med

Di Giacinto, George V MD [NS] - **Spec Exp:** Spinal Surgery; Pain Management; **Hospital:** St. Luke's - Roosevelt Hosp Ctr - Roosevelt Div (page 55); **Address:** 425 W 59th St, Ste 4E, New York, NY 10019; **Phone:** 212-523-8500; **Board Cert:** Neurological Surgery 1981; **Med School:** Harvard Med Sch 1970; **Resid:** Neurological Surgery, Columbia-Presby Hosp 1978

Dias, Mark S MD [NS] - **Spec Exp:** Pediatric Neurosurgery; Spina Bifida; Hydrocephalus; Craniosynostosis; **Hospital:** Penn State Milton S Hershey Med Ctr; **Address:** Penn State-Hersey Med Ctr, Dept Neurosurgery, 30 Hope Drive, MC EC110, Hersey, PA 17033; **Phone:** 717-531-8807; **Board Cert:** Neurological Surgery 1995; Pediatric Neurological Surgery 2006; **Med School:** Johns Hopkins Univ 1982; **Resid:** Neurological Surgery, Univ Pittsburgh Med Ctr 1989; **Fellow:** Pediatric Neurological Surgery, Univ Utah-Primary Chldns Hosp 1991; **Fac Appt:** Prof NS, Penn State Coll Med

Eisenberg, Howard M MD [NS] - **Spec Exp:** Acoustic Neuroma; Skull Base Surgery; Deep Brain Stimulation; Epilepsy/Seizure Disorders; **Hospital:** Univ of MD Med Ctr; **Address:** Univ MD Sch Med, Dept Neurosurg, 22 S Greene St, Ste S-12-D, Baltimore, MD 21201-1544; **Phone:** 410-328-3514; **Board Cert:** Neurological Surgery 1973; **Med School:** SUNY Downstate 1964; **Resid:** Surgery, New York Hosp 1966; Neurological Surgery, Peter Bent Brigham Hosp/Chldns Hosp 1970; **Fellow:** Harvard Univ 1970; **Fac Appt:** Prof NS, Univ MD Sch Med

Evans, James J MD [NS] - **Spec Exp:** Skull Base Surgery; Neuro-Oncology; Brain Tumors; Epilepsy; **Hospital:** Thomas Jefferson Univ Hosp; **Address:** 909 Walnut St Fl 2, Philadelphia, PA 19107; **Phone:** 215-955-7000; **Board Cert:** Neurological Surgery 2006; **Med School:** Univ Mass Sch Med 1995; **Resid:** Neurological Surgery, Cleveland Clinic 1999; **Fellow:** Cranial Base Surgery, Inova Fairfax Hospital 2001; **Fac Appt:** Assoc Prof NS, Thomas Jefferson Univ

Feldstein, Neil A MD [NS] - **Spec Exp:** Pediatric Neurosurgery; Chiari's Deformity; Brain Tumors-Pediatric; Spinal Cord Surgery-Pediatric; **Hospital:** Morgan Stanley Children's Hosp of NY-Presby, NY (page 65); **Address:** Neurological Inst, 710 W 168th St Fl 2 - rm 213, New York, NY 10032; **Phone:** 212-305-1396; **Board Cert:** Neurological Surgery 1995; Pediatric Neurological Surgery 2007; **Med School:** NYU Sch Med 1984; **Resid:** Neurological Surgery, Baylor Coll Med 1989; **Fellow:** Pediatric Neurological Surgery, NYU Med Ctr 1991; **Fac Appt:** Assoc Prof NS, Columbia P&S

Fenstermaker, Robert A MD [NS] - **Spec Exp:** Brain Tumors; Pituitary Tumors; Stereotactic Radiosurgery; Skull Base Surgery; **Hospital:** Roswell Park Cancer Inst; **Address:** Roswell Park Cancer Inst, Elm & Carlton Sts, Buffalo, NY 14263; **Phone:** 716-845-3154; **Board Cert:** Neurological Surgery 1991; **Med School:** NE Ohio Univ 1981; **Resid:** Neurological Surgery, Univ Hosps Cleveland 1987; **Fellow:** Pharmacology, Case Western Reserve 1989; **Fac Appt:** Prof NS, SUNY Buffalo

Gokaslan, Ziya L MD [NS] - **Spec Exp:** Spinal Tumors; Spinal Surgery-Complex; Spinal Reconstructive Surgery; **Hospital:** Johns Hopkins Hosp (page 61), Johns Hopkins Bayview Med Ctr (page 61); **Address:** Johns Hopkins Uinv, Dept Neurosurgery Spine Ctr, 600 N Wolfe St, Meyer 7-109, Baltimore, MD 21287; **Phone:** 443-287-4934; **Board Cert:** Neurological Surgery 1997; **Med School:** Turkey 1983; **Resid:** Neurological Surgery, Baylor Coll Med 1993; **Fellow:** Neurological Trauma, Baylor Coll Med 1988; Spinal Surgery, NYU Med Ctr 1994; **Fac Appt:** Prof NS, Johns Hopkins Univ

Golfinos, John G MD [NS] - **Spec Exp:** Brain Tumors; Acoustic Neuroma; Stereotactic Radiosurgery; Skull Base Surgery; **Hospital:** NYU Langone Med Ctr (page 66), Bellevue Hosp Ctr; **Address:** 530 First Ave, Ste 8R, New York, NY 10016; **Phone:** 212-263-2950; **Board Cert:** Neurological Surgery 1998; **Med School:** Columbia P&S 1988; **Resid:** Neurological Surgery, Barrow Neuro Inst 1995; **Fac Appt:** Assoc Prof NS, NYU Sch Med

Goodman, Robert R MD/PhD [NS] - **Spec Exp:** Parkinson's Disease/Movement Disorders; Epilepsy; Trigeminal Neuralgia; Hydrocephalus-Adult; **Hospital:** St. Luke's - Roosevelt Hosp Ctr - Roosevelt Div (page 55); **Address:** 1000 Tenth Ave, Ste 5G-80, New York, NY 10019; **Phone:** 212-636-3666; **Board Cert:** Neurological Surgery 1993; **Med School:** Johns Hopkins Univ 1982; **Resid:** Neurological Surgery, Columbia-Presby Med Ctr 1989; **Fac Appt:** Assoc Prof NS, Columbia P&S

Grady, M Sean MD [NS] - **Spec Exp:** Cerebrovascular Surgery; Aneurysm-Cerebral; Arteriovenous Malformations; **Hospital:** Hosp Univ Penn - UPHS (page 68), Pennsylvania Hosp-UPHS (page 68); **Address:** Dept Neurosurgery, 3400 Spruce St, Silverstein Bldg Fl 3, Philadelphia, PA 19104; **Phone:** 215-662-3483; **Board Cert:** Neurological Surgery 1990; **Med School:** Georgetown Univ 1981; **Resid:** Neurological Surgery, Univ Virginia Hosp 1987; **Fac Appt:** Prof NS, Univ Pennsylvania

Gutin, Philip H MD [NS] - **Spec Exp:** Brain Tumors; Meningioma; Acoustic Neuroma; **Hospital:** Meml Sloan-Kettering Cancer Ctr, NY-Presby/Weill Cornell Med Ctr, NY (page 65); **Address:** 1275 York Ave, rm C 703, New York, NY 10065; **Phone:** 212-639-8556; **Board Cert:** Neurological Surgery 1981; **Med School:** Univ Pennsylvania 1971; **Resid:** Neurological Surgery, UCSF Med Ctr 1979; **Fellow:** Neurological Surgery, Natl Cancer Inst 1976; **Fac Appt:** Prof NS, Cornell Univ-Weill Med Coll

Harbaugh, Robert E MD [NS] - **Spec Exp:** Carotid Artery Surgery; Aneurysm-Cerebral; Arteriovenous Malformations; **Hospital:** Penn State Milton S Hershey Med Ctr; **Address:** Penn State Hershey Med Ctr, Dept Neurosurgery, 30 Hope Drive, Hershey, PA 17033-0850; **Phone:** 717-531-4383; **Board Cert:** Neurological Surgery 1989; **Med School:** Penn State Coll Med 1978; **Resid:** Surgery, Dartmouth-Hitchcock Med Ctr 1980; Neurological Surgery, Dartmouth-Hitchcock Med Ctr 1985; **Fac Appt:** Prof NS, Penn State Coll Med

Harrop, James S MD [NS] - **Spec Exp:** Spinal Cord Injury; Spinal Trauma; Spinal Tumors; **Hospital:** Thomas Jefferson Univ Hosp; **Address:** 909 Walnut St Fl 2, Philadelphia, PA 19107; **Phone:** 215-955-7000; **Board Cert:** Neurological Surgery 2006; **Med School:** Jefferson Med Coll 1995; **Resid:** Neurological Surgery, Thomas Jefferson Univ Hosp 2001; **Fellow:** Neurological Surgery, Cleveland Clinic 2002; Spinal Surgery, Cleveland Clinic 2002; **Fac Appt:** Assoc Prof NS, Jefferson Med Coll

Hartl, Roger MD [NS] - **Spec Exp:** Spinal Surgery-Complex; Minimally Invasive Spinal Surgery; Spinal Disc Replacement; **Hospital:** NY-Presby/Weill Cornell Med Ctr, NY (page 65); **Address:** Cornell Neurosurgery, 525 E 68th St, Starr 651, New York, NY 10065; **Phone:** 212-746-2152; **Board Cert:** Neurological Surgery 2008; **Med School:** Germany 1993; **Resid:** Neurological Surgery, NY Presby-Cornell Med Ctr 2003; **Fellow:** Spinal Surgery, Barrow Neurological Inst

Hopkins, L Nelson MD [NS] - **Spec Exp:** Cerebrovascular Disease; Endovascular Surgery; **Hospital:** Millard Fillmore Gates Cir Hosp; **Address:** Univ Buffalo Neurosurgery, 3 Gates Circle, Buffalo, NY 14209; **Phone:** 716-887-5200; **Board Cert:** Neurological Surgery 1977; **Med School:** Albany Med Coll 1969; **Resid:** Neurological Surgery, SUNY Buffalo Med Ctr 1975; **Fac Appt:** Prof NS, SUNY Buffalo

Huang, Judy MD [NS] - **Spec Exp:** Brain Tumors; Spinal Disorders; Aneurysm-Cerebral; Cerebrovascular Surgery; **Hospital:** Johns Hopkins Hosp (page 61), Johns Hopkins Bayview Med Ctr (page 61); **Address:** Johns Hopkins Hosp, 600 N Wolfe St, Baltimore, MD 21287; **Phone:** 410-502-5767; **Board Cert:** Neurological Surgery 2006; **Med School:** Columbia P&S 1995; **Resid:** Neurological Surgery, NY Presby-Columbia Med Ctr 2002; **Fellow:** Vascular Neurology, NY Presby-Columbia Med Ctr 1998; Research, NY Presby-Columbia Med Ctr 1998; **Fac Appt:** Assoc Prof NS, Johns Hopkins Univ

Jallo, George I MD [NS] - **Spec Exp:** Pediatric Neurosurgery; Chiari's Deformity; Brain & Spinal Cord Tumors; Epilepsy; **Hospital:** Johns Hopkins Hosp (page 61), Johns Hopkins Bayview Med Ctr (page 61); **Address:** Johns Hopkins Hosp, Dept of Neurosurgery, 600 N Wolfe St, Ste Harvey 811, Baltimore, MD 21287; **Phone:** 410-955-7851; **Board Cert:** Neurological Surgery 2002; Pediatric Neurological Surgery 2004; **Med School:** Univ VA Sch Med 1991; **Resid:** Neurological Surgery, NYU Med Ctr 1998; **Fellow:** Pediatric Neurological Surgery, Beth Israel Med Ctr 1999; **Fac Appt:** Prof NS, Johns Hopkins Univ

Jho, Hae-Dong MD/PhD [NS] - **Spec Exp:** Minimally Invasive Surgery; Spinal Surgery; Endoscopic Surgery; **Hospital:** Allegheny General Hosp; **Address:** Jho Inst for Min Invasive Neurosurgery, 320 E North Ave, Allegheny Genl Hosp, Pittsburgh, PA 15212-4746; **Phone:** 412-359-6110; **Board Cert:** Neurological Surgery 1991; **Med School:** Korea 1971; **Resid:** Neurological Surgery, Hanyang Univ Hosp 1979; Neurological Surgery, Univ Pittsburgh 1989; **Fellow:** Microsurgery, Univ Pittsburgh 1983; **Fac Appt:** Prof NS, Drexel Univ Coll Med

Judy, Kevin MD [NS] - **Spec Exp:** Brain Tumors; Acoustic Neuroma; Skull Base Tumors; **Hospital:** Thomas Jefferson Univ Hosp; **Address:** Jefferson Neurosurgical Assocs, 909 Walnut St, Philadelphia, PA 19107; **Phone:** 215-503-7005; **Board Cert:** Neurological Surgery 1997; **Med School:** Univ Pittsburgh 1984; **Resid:** Surgery, Mercy Hosp 1986; Neurological Surgery, Johns Hopkins Hosp 1992; **Fellow:** Neurological Surgery, Johns Hopkins Hosp 1991; **Fac Appt:** Prof NS, Jefferson Med Coll

Kaiser, Michael G MD [NS] - **Spec Exp:** Spinal Surgery-Complex; Minimally Invasive Spinal Surgery; Spinal Disc Replacement; **Hospital:** NY-Presby/Columbia Univ Med Ctr, NY (page 65); **Address:** Neurological Institute, Dept Neurological Surgery, 710 W 168th St, New York, NY 10032; **Phone:** 212-305-0378; **Board Cert:** Neurological Surgery 2004; **Med School:** Yale Univ 1994; **Resid:** Neurological Surgery, Columbia Neuro Inst 2000; **Fellow:** Spinal Surgery, Emory Univ 2001; **Fac Appt:** Asst Prof NS, Columbia P&S

Kaplitt, Michael G MD/PhD [NS] - **Spec Exp:** Parkinson's Disease/Movement Disorders; Deep Brain Stimulation; Trigeminal Neuralgia; Hydrocephalus; **Hospital:** NY-Presby/Weill Cornell Med Ctr, NY (page 65); **Address:** 525 E 68th St, Box 99, New York, NY 10065; **Phone:** 212-746-4966; **Board Cert:** Neurological Surgery 2005; **Med School:** Cornell Univ-Weill Med Coll 1995; **Resid:** Neurological Surgery, New York Hosp 2000; **Fellow:** Stereo Neurological Surgery, Toronto Western Hosp 2001; **Fac Appt:** Assoc Prof NS, Cornell Univ-Weill Med Coll

Khan, Agha S MD [NS] - **Spec Exp:** Skull Base Surgery; Spinal Surgery; **Hospital:** Sinai Hosp - Baltimore, Maryland Genl Hosp; **Address:** 2411 W Belvedere Ave, Ste 402, Baltimore, MD 21215; **Phone:** 410-601-8314; **Board Cert:** Neurological Surgery 1995; **Med School:** Pakistan 1979; **Resid:** Neurological Surgery, Univ Wisconsin Hosp 1990; **Fellow:** Surgical Oncology, Roswell Park Meml Inst 1982; Neurological Surgery, Allegheny Genl Hosp 1991

Kobrine, Arthur MD/PhD [NS] - **Spec Exp:** Spinal Cord Surgery; Brain & Spinal Cord Tumors; Spinal Surgery; **Hospital:** Sibley Mem Hosp, Georgetown Univ Hosp; **Address:** 2440 M St NW, Ste 315, Washington, DC 20037-1404; **Phone:** 202-293-7136; **Board Cert:** Neurological Surgery 1976; **Med School:** Northwestern Univ 1968; **Resid:** Neurological Surgery, Northwestern Univ Hosp 1970; Neurological Surgery, Walter Reed Army Hosp 1973; **Fellow:** Physiology, Geo Wash Univ 1979; **Fac Appt:** Clin Prof NS, Georgetown Univ

Neurological Surgery

Kondziolka, Douglas MD [NS] - **Spec Exp:** Brain Tumors-Adult & Pediatric; Brain Tumors-Metastatic; Stereotactic Radiosurgery; Movement Disorders; **Hospital:** UPMC Presby, Pittsburgh, Chldns Hosp of Pittsburgh - UPMC; **Address:** Univ Pittsburgh Med Ctr, Dept Neurological Surgery, 200 Lothrop St, Ste B400, Pittsburgh, PA 15213; **Phone:** 412-647-9990; **Board Cert:** Neurological Surgery 1994; **Med School:** Univ Toronto 1985; **Resid:** Neurological Surgery, Univ Toronto 1991; **Fellow:** Stereo Neurological Surgery, UPMC Presby Med Ctr 1991; **Fac Appt:** Prof NS, Univ Pittsburgh

Kotapka, Mark J MD [NS] - **Spec Exp:** Pituitary Tumors; Skull Base Surgery; Spinal Surgery; **Hospital:** Albert Einstein Med Ctr; **Address:** Albert Einstein Medical Ctr, Klein Bldg - Ste 400, 5401 Old York Rd, Philadelphia, PA 19141; **Phone:** 215-456-6127; **Board Cert:** Neurological Surgery 1997; **Med School:** Univ MD Sch Med 1985; **Resid:** Neurological Surgery, Hosp Univ Penn 1991; **Fellow:** Pediatric Neurological Surgery, Children's Hosp Philadelphia 1992; Skull Base Surgery, Univ Pittsburgh Med Ctr 1992; **Fac Appt:** Prof NS, Albert Einstein Coll Med

Laske, Douglas W MD [NS] - **Spec Exp:** Brain & Spinal Cord Tumors; Stereotactic Radiosurgery; Brain Tumors-Metastatic; Pituitary Tumors; **Hospital:** Temple Univ Hosp, Fox Chase Cancer Ctr (page 58); **Address:** Temple University Hospital, 3401 N Broad St, Ste C540, Phildelphia, PA 19140; **Phone:** 215-707-7200; **Board Cert:** Neurological Surgery 1996; **Med School:** Columbia P&S 1985; **Resid:** Neurological Surgery, Med Coll Virginia 1991; **Fellow:** Neurosurgical Oncology, Natl Inst Hlth 1995; **Fac Appt:** Assoc Prof NS, Temple Univ

Lavyne, Michael H MD [NS] - **Spec Exp:** Spinal Surgery; Spinal Tumors; Spinal Disorders; **Hospital:** NY-Presby/Weill Cornell Med Ctr, NY (page 65), Hosp For Special Surgery (page 60); **Address:** 110 E 55th St Fl 9, New York, NY 10022; **Phone:** 212-486-9100; **Board Cert:** Neurological Surgery 1982; **Med School:** Cornell Univ-Weill Med Coll 1972; **Resid:** Neurological Surgery, Mass Genl Hosp 1979; **Fellow:** Neurology, Beth Israel Hosp 1974; **Fac Appt:** Clin Prof NS, Cornell Univ-Weill Med Coll

Loftus, Christopher M MD [NS] - **Spec Exp:** Carotid Artery Surgery; Aneurysm-Cerebral; Arteriovenous Malformations; Cerebrovascular Surgery; **Hospital:** Temple Univ Hosp; **Address:** Temple Univ School Med, 3401 N Broad St, Parkinson Pavilion, Ste C540, Philadelphia, PA 19140; **Phone:** 215-707-4109; **Board Cert:** Neurological Surgery 1987; **Med School:** SUNY Downstate 1979; **Resid:** Neurological Surgery, Columbia-Presby Med Ctr 1985; **Fac Appt:** Prof NS, Temple Univ

Lunsford, L Dade MD [NS] - **Spec Exp:** Brain Tumors; Stereotactic Radiosurgery; Movement Disorders; Vascular Malformations; **Hospital:** UPMC Presby, Pittsburgh, Chldns Hosp of Pittsburgh - UPMC; **Address:** UPMC Presbyterian Hosp; Dept Neuro Surg, 200 Lothrop St, Ste B-400, Pittsburgh, PA 15213-2536; **Phone:** 412-647-0953; **Board Cert:** Neurological Surgery 1983; **Med School:** Columbia P&S 1974; **Resid:** Neurological Surgery, Univ Pittsburgh Med Ctr 1980; **Fellow:** Stereo Neurological Surgery, Karolinska Hospital 1981; **Fac Appt:** Prof NS, Univ Pittsburgh

Maroon, Joseph C MD [NS] - **Spec Exp:** Minimally Invasive Spinal Surgery; Microdiscectomy; Brain Injury-Traumatic; Pituitary Tumors; **Hospital:** UPMC Presby, Pittsburgh, UPMC Passavant-McCandless; **Address:** UPMC Presbyterian, Dept Neuro Surg, 200 Lothrop St, Ste 5-C, Pittsburgh, PA 15213; **Phone:** 412-647-3604; **Board Cert:** Neurological Surgery 1973; **Med School:** Indiana Univ 1965; **Resid:** Surgery, Georgetown Univ Hosp 1967; Neurological Surgery, Indiana Univ Med Ctr 1971; **Fellow:** Neurological Surgery, Radcliffe Infirmary 1969; Microsurgery, Univ Vermont Affil Hosp 1972; **Fac Appt:** Prof NS, Univ Pittsburgh

McCormick, Paul C MD [NS] - **Spec Exp:** Spinal Surgery; Spinal Tumors; **Hospital:** NY-Presby/Columbia Univ Med Ctr, NY (page 65); **Address:** 710 W 168th St, Ste 506, New York, NY 10032-2603; **Phone:** 212-305-7976; **Board Cert:** Neurological Surgery 1993; **Med School:** Columbia P&S 1982; **Resid:** Neurological Surgery, Columbia Presby Med Ctr 1989; **Fellow:** Neurological Surgery, Natl Inst Hlth 1984; Spinal Surgery, Med Coll Wisconsin 1990; **Fac Appt:** Prof NS, Columbia P&S

Moore, Frank M MD [NS] - **Spec Exp:** Aneurysm-Cerebral; Brain Tumors; Spinal Cord Tumors; Spinal Surgery; **Hospital:** Englewood Hosp & Med Ctr, Mount Sinai Med Ctr (page 63); **Address:** 1158 5th Ave, New York, NY 10029-6917; **Phone:** 212-410-6990; **Board Cert:** Neurological Surgery 1992; **Med School:** France 1983; **Resid:** Neurological Surgery, Mt Sinai Hosp 1988; **Fac Appt:** Assoc Prof NS, Mount Sinai Sch Med

Murali, Raj MD [NS] - **Spec Exp:** Trigeminal Neuralgia; Skull Base Surgery; Aneurysm-Cerebral; Pituitary Tumors; **Hospital:** Westchester Med Ctr; **Address:** Westchester Med Ctr, Dept Neurosurgery, Munger Pavilion, Ste 329, Valhalla, NY 10595; **Phone:** 914-493-8392; **Board Cert:** Neurological Surgery 1982; **Med School:** India 1968; **Resid:** Neurological Surgery, Royal Infirm-Univ Edinburgh 1974; Neurological Surgery, NYU Med Ctr 1979; **Fac Appt:** Prof NS, NY Med Coll

Naff, Neal J MD [NS] - **Spec Exp:** Brain & Spinal Cord Tumors; Stereotactic Radiosurgery; Minimally Invasive Spinal Surgery; Epilepsy/Seizure Disorders; **Hospital:** St. Joseph Med Ctr, Sinai Hosp - Baltimore; **Address:** Chesapeake Neurosurgery, 2700 Quarry Lake Drive, Ste 360, Baltimore, MD 21209; **Phone:** 410-486-0090; **Board Cert:** Neurological Surgery 2000; **Med School:** Johns Hopkins Univ 1991; **Resid:** Neurological Surgery, Johns Hopkins Hosp 1998

O'Rourke, Donald M MD [NS] - **Spec Exp:** Neuro-Oncology; Brain Tumors; Spinal Surgery-Cervical; **Hospital:** Hosp Univ Penn - UPHS (page 68); **Address:** Hosp Univ Penn-Dept Neurosurgery, 3400 Spruce St, 3 Silverstein, Philadelphia, PA 19104; **Phone:** 215-662-3490; **Board Cert:** Neurological Surgery 1998; **Med School:** Univ Pennsylvania 1987; **Resid:** Neurological Surgery, Hosp Univ Penn 1994; **Fac Appt:** Assoc Prof NS, Univ Pennsylvania

Olivi, Alessandro MD [NS] - **Spec Exp:** Brain & Spinal Cord Tumors; Skull Base Tumors; Brain Tumors-Metastatic; Meningioma; **Hospital:** Johns Hopkins Hosp (page 61); **Address:** 600 N Wolfe St, Phipps Bldg - Ste 1-100, Baltimore, MD 21287-0001; **Phone:** 410-955-0703; **Board Cert:** Neurological Surgery 1994; **Med School:** Italy 1979; **Resid:** Neurological Surgery, Univ of Padova; Neurological Surgery, Mayfield Neur Inst 1998; **Fellow:** Neuro-Oncology, Johns Hopkins Hosp 1991; **Fac Appt:** Prof NS, Johns Hopkins Univ

Piatt, Joseph H MD [NS] - **Spec Exp:** Brachial Plexus Palsy-Pediatric; Spasticity & Movement Disorders; Chiari's Deformity; Syringomyelia & Spinal Cord Diseases; **Hospital:** Nemours Chldns Clinic - Wilmington; **Address:** 1600 Rockland Rd, Wilmington, DE 19803; **Phone:** 302-651-5993; **Board Cert:** Neurological Surgery 1989; Pediatric Neurological Surgery 2006; **Med School:** Univ Pennsylvania 1979; **Resid:** Neurological Surgery, Duke Univ Med Ctr 1986; **Fellow:** Pediatric Neurological Surgery, Hosp Sick Chldn 1987

Pollack, Ian F MD [NS] - **Spec Exp:** Pediatric Neurosurgery; Brain Tumors; Craniofacial Surgery; Neuro-Oncology; **Hospital:** Chldns Hosp of Pittsburgh - UPMC, UPMC Presby, Pittsburgh; **Address:** Chldns Hosp Pittsburgh, Div Neurosurgery, 4401 Penn Ave, Ste FP4129, Pittsburgh, PA 15224; **Phone:** 412-692-5881; **Board Cert:** Neurological Surgery 1996; Pediatric Neurological Surgery 2006; **Med School:** Johns Hopkins Univ 1984; **Resid:** Neurological Surgery, Univ Pittsburgh Med Ctr 1991; **Fellow:** Pediatric Neurological Surgery, Hosp Sick Chldn 1992; **Fac Appt:** Prof NS, Univ Pittsburgh

Quigley, Matthew R MD [NS] - **Spec Exp:** Brain Tumors; Spinal Cord Tumors; Neuro-Oncology; **Hospital:** Allegheny General Hosp; **Address:** Allegeny General Hosp, Neurosurgery, 420 E North Ave, Ste 302, Pittsburgh, PA 15212; **Phone:** 412-359-4764; **Board Cert:** Neurological Surgery 1991; **Med School:** Northwestern Univ-Feinberg Sch Med 1981; **Resid:** Neurological Surgery, Northwestern Univ 1987; **Fac Appt:** Assoc Prof NS, Univ Pennsylvania

Rigamonti, Daniele MD [NS] - **Spec Exp:** Hydrocephalus-Adult; Brain Tumors; Spinal Disorders; Vascular Neurosurgery; **Hospital:** Johns Hopkins Hosp (page 61); **Address:** Johns Hopkins Hosp, Dept Neurosurgery, 600 N Wolfe St, Phipps 126, Baltimore, MD 21287; **Phone:** 410-955-2259; **Board Cert:** Neurological Surgery 1988; **Med School:** Italy 1976; **Resid:** Neurological Surgery, Mt Sinai Hosp Med Ctr 1984; **Fellow:** Neurological Vascular Surgery, Barrow Neuro Inst 1987; **Fac Appt:** Prof NS, Johns Hopkins Univ

Riina, Howard A MD [NS] - **Spec Exp:** Neuroradiology; Aneurysm-Cerebral; Cerebrovascular Malformations; Stroke; **Hospital:** NYU Langone Med Ctr (page 66); **Address:** NYU Langone Med Ctr, 530 First Ave, SK1, Ste 8R, New York, NY 10016; **Phone:** 212-263-5382; **Board Cert:** Neurological Surgery 2004; **Med School:** Temple Univ 1993; **Resid:** Neurological Surgery, Hosp Univ Penn 2000; **Fellow:** Interventional Neuroradiology, Beth Israel Med Ctr 1997; Skull Base Surgery, Barrow Neuro Inst 2001; **Fac Appt:** Prof NS, NYU Sch Med

Rosenwasser, Robert H MD [NS] - **Spec Exp:** Aneurysm-Cerebral; Cerebrovascular Surgery; Arteriovenous Malformations; **Hospital:** Thomas Jefferson Univ Hosp; **Address:** Thomas Jefferson Univ Hosp, 909 Walnut St Fl 2, Philadelphia, PA 19107; **Phone:** 215-955-7000; **Board Cert:** Neurological Surgery 1987; **Med School:** Louisiana State U, New Orleans 1979; **Resid:** Neurological Surgery, Temple Univ Hosp 1984; **Fellow:** Neurological Vascular Surgery, Univ West Ontarion 1985; Interventional Neuroradiology, NYU Med Ctr 1993; **Fac Appt:** Prof NS, Thomas Jefferson Univ

Schwartz, Theodore H MD [NS] - **Spec Exp:** Brain Tumors; Pituitary Tumors; Epilepsy; Endoscopic Surgery; **Hospital:** NY-Presby/Weill Cornell Med Ctr, NY (page 65); **Address:** Cornell Neurosurgery, 525 E 68th St, Starr Pavilion, rm 651, New York, NY 10021; **Phone:** 212-746-5620; **Board Cert:** Neurological Surgery 2002; **Med School:** Harvard Med Sch 1993; **Resid:** Neurological Surgery, Columbia-Presby Med Ctr 1999; **Fellow:** Neurological Surgery, Yale-New Haven Med Ctr 2000; **Fac Appt:** Prof NS, Cornell Univ-Weill Med Coll

Sen, Chandranath MD [NS] - **Spec Exp:** Brain Tumors; Skull Base Tumors; Trigeminal Neuralgia; Hemifacial Spasm; **Hospital:** NYU Langone Med Ctr (page 66); **Address:** NYU Langone Med Ctr, Dept Neurosurgery, 550 First Ave, Ste HCC-3F, New York, NY 10016; **Phone:** 212-263-5333; **Board Cert:** Neurological Surgery 1989; **Med School:** India 1976; **Resid:** Surgery, Univ Wisconsin Hosps 1980; Neurological Surgery, Univ Wisconsin Hosps 1985; **Fellow:** Microsurgery, Univ Pittsburgh Med Ctr 1986

Sisti, Michael B MD [NS] - **Spec Exp:** Acoustic Neuroma; Brain Tumors; Stereotactic Radiosurgery; Meningioma; **Hospital:** NY-Presby/Columbia Univ Med Ctr, NY (page 65); **Address:** 710 W 168th St, New York, NY 10032-2603; **Phone:** 212-305-1728; **Board Cert:** Neurological Surgery 1991; **Med School:** Columbia P&S 1981; **Resid:** Neurological Surgery, Neuro Inst-Columbia-Presby Med Ctr 1988; **Fellow:** Neurological Surgery, Natl Inst Hlth 1983; **Fac Appt:** Assoc Prof NS, Columbia P&S

Solomon, Robert A MD [NS] - **Spec Exp:** Aneurysm-Cerebral; Arteriovenous Malformations; **Hospital:** NY-Presby/Columbia Univ Med Ctr, NY (page 65); **Address:** 710 W 168th St, Ste 439, New York, NY 10032; **Phone:** 212-305-4118; **Board Cert:** Neurological Surgery 1988; **Med School:** Johns Hopkins Univ 1980; **Resid:** Neurological Surgery, Neuro Inst-Columbia 1986; **Fac Appt:** Prof NS, Columbia P&S

Souweidane, Mark M MD [NS] - **Spec Exp:** Pediatric Neurosurgery; Minimally Invasive Surgery; Endoscopic Surgery; Brain Tumors-Pediatric; **Hospital:** NY-Presby/Weill Cornell Med Ctr, NY (page 65), Meml Sloan-Kettering Cancer Ctr; **Address:** 525 E 68th St, Box 99, New York, NY 10065-4870; **Phone:** 212-746-2363; **Board Cert:** Neurological Surgery 1999; Pediatric Neurological Surgery 2000; **Med School:** Wayne State Univ 1988; **Resid:** Neurological Surgery, NYU Med Ctr 1994; **Fellow:** Pediatric Neurological Surgery, Hosp Sick Chldn 1995; **Fac Appt:** Prof NS, Cornell Univ-Weill Med Coll

Stieg, Philip E MD/PhD [NS] - **Spec Exp:** Cerebrovascular Surgery; Acoustic Neuroma; Skull Base Surgery; Brain Tumors; **Hospital:** NY-Presby/Weill Cornell Med Ctr, NY (page 65), Hosp For Special Surgery (page 60); **Address:** 525 E 68th St, STARR 651, New York, NY 10021-9800; **Phone:** 212-746-4684; **Board Cert:** Neurological Surgery 1992; **Med School:** Med Coll Wisc 1983; **Resid:** Neurological Surgery, Dallas Chldns Hosp/Parkland Meml Hosp 1988; **Fellow:** Neurological Biology, Karolinska Inst 1988; **Fac Appt:** Prof NS, Cornell Univ-Weill Med Coll

Sundaresan, Narayan MD [NS] - **Spec Exp:** Spinal Surgery; Brain Tumors; Neuro-Oncology; Spinal Disorders-Degenerative; **Hospital:** Mount Sinai Med Ctr (page 63), Lincoln Med & Mental Hlth Ctr; **Address:** Central Park Neurosurgery, 1148 5th Ave, New York, NY 10128; **Phone:** 212-876-7575; **Board Cert:** Neurological Surgery 1980; **Med School:** India 1969; **Resid:** Neurological Surgery, Northwestern Meml Hosp 1975; **Fellow:** Neuro-Oncology, Meml Sloan Kettering Cancer Ctr 1977; **Fac Appt:** Prof NS, Mount Sinai Sch Med

Sutton, Leslie N MD [NS] - **Spec Exp:** Brain Tumors-Pediatric; Fetal Neurosurgery; Hydrocephalus; **Hospital:** Chldns Hosp of Philadelphia; **Address:** Childrens Hosp of Philadelphia, Div, Neurosurgery, 34h & Civic Ctr Blvd Wood Bldg Fl 6, Philadelphia, PA 19104; **Phone:** 215-590-2780; **Board Cert:** Neurological Surgery 1984; Pediatric Neurological Surgery 1996; **Med School:** Univ Pennsylvania 1975; **Resid:** Neurological Surgery, Hosp Univ Penn 1981; **Fac Appt:** Prof NS, Univ Pennsylvania

Tamargo, Rafael J MD [NS] - **Spec Exp:** Vascular Neurosurgery; Skull Base Surgery; **Hospital:** Johns Hopkins Hosp (page 61), Johns Hopkins Bayview Med Ctr (page 61); **Address:** Johns Hopkins Hosp, Dept Neurosurgery, 600 N Wolfe St, Meyer 8-181, Baltimore, MD 21287; **Phone:** 410-614-1533; **Board Cert:** Neurological Surgery 1995; **Med School:** Columbia P&S 1984; **Resid:** Neurological Surgery, Johns Hopkins Hosp 1992; **Fac Appt:** Prof NS, Johns Hopkins Univ

Turtz, Alan R MD [NS] - **Spec Exp:** Brain Tumors; Pituitary Tumors; Spinal Surgery; Neuro-Endoscopy; **Hospital:** Cooper Univ Hosp; **Address:** 3 Cooper Plaza, Ste 104, Camden, NJ 08103; **Phone:** 856-968-7965; **Board Cert:** Neurological Surgery 1995; **Med School:** Med Coll PA 1986; **Resid:** Neurological Surgery, Med Coll Penn 1992; **Fac Appt:** Assoc Prof NS, UMDNJ-RW Johnson Med Sch

Weiner, Howard L MD [NS] - **Spec Exp:** Pediatric Neurosurgery; Epilepsy; Brain Tumors; Tuberous Sclerosis; **Hospital:** NYU Langone Med Ctr (page 66); **Address:** NYU Med Ctr, Div Pediatric Neurosurgery, 317 E 34th St, Ste 1002, New York, NY 10016; **Phone:** 212-263-6419; **Board Cert:** Neurological Surgery 2001; **Med School:** Cornell Univ 1989; **Resid:** Neurological Surgery, NYU Med Ctr 1996; **Fellow:** Pediatric Neurological Surgery, NYU Med Ctr 1997; **Fac Appt:** Prof NS, NYU Sch Med

Weingart, Jon D MD [NS] - **Spec Exp:** Brain Tumors; Spinal Disorders; Gliomas; Chiari's Deformity; **Hospital:** Johns Hopkins Hosp (page 61); **Address:** Johns Hopkins Hosp, Dept Neurosurgery, 600 N Wolfe St Phipps Bldg - rm 101, Baltimore, MD 21287; **Phone:** 410-614-3052; **Board Cert:** Neurological Surgery 1998; **Med School:** Duke Univ 1987; **Resid:** Neurological Surgery, John Hopkins Hosp 1993; **Fellow:** Neurosurgical Oncology, Johns Hopkins Hosp; **Fac Appt:** Prof NS, Johns Hopkins Univ

Neurological Surgery

Welch, William C MD [NS] - **Spec Exp:** Spinal Surgery; **Hospital:** Pennsylvania Hosp-UPHS (page 68); **Address:** Pennsylvania Hosp, Dept Neurosurgery, 235 S 8th St, Philadelphia, PA 19106; **Phone:** 215-829-6700; **Board Cert:** Neurological Surgery 1995; **Med School:** SUNY Downstate 1985; **Resid:** Neurological Surgery, Strong Meml Hosp 1991; **Fellow:** Neuro-Oncology, Montefiore Med Ctr 1992; Spinal Surgery, Weiler/Montefiore Med Ctr 1993; **Fac Appt:** Prof NS, Univ Pennsylvania

Whiting, Donald M MD [NS] - **Spec Exp:** Movement Disorders; Pain & Spasticity; Deep Brain Stimulation; Spinal Reconstructive Surgery; **Hospital:** Allegheny General Hosp, Washington Hosp, The; **Address:** 380 West Chestnut St, Washington, PA 15301-4657; **Phone:** 724-228-1414; **Board Cert:** Neurological Surgery 1995; **Med School:** Jefferson Med Coll 1985; **Resid:** Surgery, Geisinger Med Ctr 1986; Neurological Surgery, Cleveland Clinic 1991; **Fellow:** Neurological Trauma, Allegheny Genl Hosp 1990; **Fac Appt:** Assoc Prof NS, Drexel Univ Coll Med

Wilberger Jr, James E MD [NS] - **Spec Exp:** Epilepsy; Brain Injury; Brain Tumors-Benign; **Hospital:** Allegheny General Hosp; **Address:** Allegheny General Hosp, Neorosurgery, 420 E North Ave, Ste 302, Pittsburgh, PA 15212; **Phone:** 412-359-4764; **Board Cert:** Neurological Surgery 1986; **Med School:** Med Coll VA 1978; **Resid:** Neurological Surgery, Univ Pittsburgh Med Ctr 1984; **Fac Appt:** Prof NS, Drexel Univ Coll Med

Wisoff, Jeffrey H MD [NS] - **Spec Exp:** Pediatric Neurosurgery; Brain Tumors-Pediatric; Hydrocephalus; Chiari's Deformity; **Hospital:** NYU Langone Med Ctr (page 66), Maimonides Med Ctr (page 62); **Address:** 317 E 34th St, Ste 1002, New York, NY 10016-4974; **Phone:** 212-263-6419; **Board Cert:** Neurological Surgery 1990; Pediatric Neurological Surgery 2008; **Med School:** Geo Wash Univ 1978; **Resid:** Neurological Surgery, NYU/Bellevue Hosp 1984; **Fellow:** Pediatric Neurological Surgery, NYU Med Ctr 1985; **Fac Appt:** Assoc Prof NS, NYU Sch Med

Zager, Eric L MD [NS] - **Spec Exp:** Peripheral Nerve Disorders; Carpal Tunnel Syndrome; Pediatric Neurosurgery; **Hospital:** Hosp Univ Penn - UPHS (page 68), Chldns Hosp of Philadelphia; **Address:** Hosp Univ Penn, Neurosurgery, 3400 Spruce St, 3 Silverstein, Philadelphia, PA 19104; **Phone:** 215-662-3497; **Board Cert:** Neurological Surgery 1992; **Med School:** Stanford Univ 1982; **Resid:** Neurological Surgery, Mass Genl Hosp 1988; **Fellow:** Peripheral Nerve Surgery, Univ Toronto 1989; Peripheral Nerve Surgery, LSU Med Ctr 1989; **Fac Appt:** Prof NS, Univ Pennsylvania

Southeast

Asher, Anthony MD [NS] - **Spec Exp:** Brain Tumors; Stereotactic Radiosurgery; Epilepsy; **Hospital:** Carolinas Med Ctr, Presby Hosp - Charlotte; **Address:** 225 Baldwin Ave, Charlotte, NC 28204; **Phone:** 704-376-1605; **Board Cert:** Neurological Surgery 1998; **Med School:** Wayne State Univ 1987; **Resid:** Neurological Surgery, Univ Mich Med Ctr 1995; **Fellow:** Surgical Oncology, Natl Cancer Inst 1991

Barrow, Daniel L MD [NS] - **Spec Exp:** Cerebrovascular Disease; Stroke; Aneurysm-Cerebral; Microsurgery; **Hospital:** Emory Univ Hosp; **Address:** Emory Univ Dept Neurosurgery, 1365 Clifton Rd NE B Bldg - Ste 2200, Atlanta, GA 30322; **Phone:** 404-778-5770; **Board Cert:** Neurological Surgery 1988; **Med School:** Southern IL Univ 1979; **Resid:** Neurological Surgery, Emory Univ Affil Hosps 1985; **Fellow:** Cerebrovascular Neurosurgery, Mayo Clinic 1986; **Fac Appt:** Prof NS, Emory Univ

Boop, Frederick A MD [NS] - **Spec Exp:** Pediatric Neurosurgery; Epilepsy; Brain Tumors; **Hospital:** Le Bonheur Chldns Med Ctr, Methodist Univ Hosp - Memphis; **Address:** 6325 Humphreys Blvd, Memphis, TN 38120; **Phone:** 901-259-5340; **Board Cert:** Neurological Surgery 1993; Pediatric Neurological Surgery 2005; **Med School:** Univ Ark 1983; **Resid:** Neurological Surgery, Univ Tex Hlth Sci Ctr 1989; Neurological Surgery, Inst Neur/Hosp Sick Chldn 1987; **Fellow:** Epilepsy, Univ Minn 1989; Pediatric Neurological Surgery, Ark Chldns Hosp 1990; **Fac Appt:** Assoc Prof NS, Univ Tenn Coll Med

Branch Jr, Charles L MD [NS] - **Spec Exp:** Spinal Reconstructive Surgery; Minimally Invasive Spinal Surgery; Stereotactic Radiosurgery; **Hospital:** Wake Forest Univ Baptist Med Ctr, Forsyth Med Ctr; **Address:** Wake Forest Univ Baptist Med Ctr, Medical Center Blvd, Winston-Salem, NC 27157-1029; **Phone:** 336-716-4083; **Board Cert:** Neurological Surgery 1991; **Med School:** Univ Tex SW, Dallas 1981; **Resid:** Neurological Surgery, NC Baptist Hosp 1987; **Fellow:** Neurological Surgery, UCSF Med Ctr 1987; **Fac Appt:** Prof NS, Wake Forest Univ

Brem, Steven MD [NS] - **Spec Exp:** Brain Tumors; Pituitary Tumors; Clinical Trials; Neuro-Oncology; **Hospital:** H Lee Moffitt Cancer Ctr & Research Inst (page 59); **Address:** H Lee Moffitt Cancer Ctr/Neurosurgery, 12902 Magnolia Drive, Neuro Program, Tampa, FL 33612-9497; **Phone:** 813-745-3056; **Board Cert:** Neurological Surgery 1983; **Med School:** Harvard Med Sch 1972; **Resid:** Neurological Surgery, Massachusetts Genl Hosp 1981; **Fellow:** Oncology, Natl Cancer Inst 1976; **Fac Appt:** Prof NS, Univ S Fla Coll Med

Ewend, Matthew MD [NS] - **Spec Exp:** Brain Tumors; Pituitary Tumors; Pediatric Neurosurgery; Epilepsy; **Hospital:** NC Memorial Hosp - UNC; **Address:** Univ North Carolina Neurosurgery, 170 Manning Drive, MC 7060, 2151 Physicians Office Bldg, Chapel Hill, NC 27599; **Phone:** 919-966-1374; **Board Cert:** Neurological Surgery 2001; **Med School:** Johns Hopkins Univ 1990; **Resid:** Neurological Surgery, Johns Hopkins Hospital 1994; **Fellow:** Neuro-Oncology, National Institutes of Health 1996; **Fac Appt:** Asst Prof NS, Univ NC Sch Med

Foley, Kevin T MD [NS] - **Spec Exp:** Spinal Surgery; Minimally Invasive Spinal Surgery; **Hospital:** Methodist Univ Hosp - Memphis, Baptist Memorial Hospital-Memphis; **Address:** Semmes-Murphy Clinic, 6325 Humphreys Blvd, Memphis, TN 38120; **Phone:** 901-522-7700; **Board Cert:** Neurological Surgery 1987; **Med School:** UCLA 1979; **Resid:** Neurological Surgery, UCLA Med Ctr 1985; **Fac Appt:** Prof NS, Univ Tenn Coll Med

Freeman, Thomas B MD [NS] - **Spec Exp:** Parkinson's Disease; Nerve Surgery & Transplantation; Spinal Surgery; **Hospital:** Tampa Genl Hosp; **Address:** 2 Tampa Genl Cir Fl 7, Tampa, FL 33606; **Phone:** 813-259-0889; **Board Cert:** Neurological Surgery 1993; **Med School:** Johns Hopkins Univ 1981; **Resid:** Neurological Surgery, NYU Med Ctr 1988; **Fac Appt:** Prof NS, Univ S Fla Coll Med

Friedman, Allan H MD [NS] - **Spec Exp:** Brain Tumors; Skull Base Tumors; Gliomas; **Hospital:** Duke Univ Hosp; **Address:** Duke Univ Med Ctr, DUMC 3807, Dept of Neurosurgery, Durham, NC 27710; **Phone:** 919-681-6421; **Board Cert:** Neurological Surgery 1983; **Med School:** Univ IL Coll Med 1974; **Resid:** Neurological Surgery, Duke Univ Med Ctr 1980; **Fellow:** Vascular Surgery, Univ Western Ontario 1981; **Fac Appt:** Prof S, Duke Univ

Green, Barth A MD [NS] - **Spec Exp:** Spinal Surgery; **Hospital:** Jackson Meml Hosp (page 70), Univ of Miami Hosp & Clins/Sylvester Comp Canc Ctr (page 73); **Address:** Univ Miami Dept Neurosurgery, 1095 NW 14th Terrace, Ste D4-6, Miami, FL 33136; **Phone:** 305-243-6946; **Board Cert:** Neurological Surgery 1978; **Med School:** Indiana Univ 1969; **Resid:** Neurological Surgery, Northwestern Univ Hosp 1975; **Fac Appt:** Prof NS, Univ Miami Sch Med

Guthrie, Barton L MD [NS] - **Spec Exp:** Brain Tumors; Stereotactic Radiosurgery; Parkinson's Disease/Movement Disorders; **Hospital:** Univ of Ala Hosp at Birmingham; **Address:** Univ Alabama, Div Neurosurg, 510 20th St S, Ste FOT 1038, Birmingham, AL 35294-3410; **Phone:** 205-934-8136; **Board Cert:** Neurological Surgery 1992; **Med School:** Univ Alabama 1980; **Resid:** Neurological Surgery, Mayo Clinic 1988; **Fellow:** Neurological Surgery, Stanford Univ Med Ctr 1988; **Fac Appt:** Assoc Prof NS, Univ Alabama

Hadley, Mark N MD [NS] - **Spec Exp:** Spinal Surgery-Complex; Spinal Disorders-Degenerative; **Hospital:** Univ of Ala Hosp at Birmingham; **Address:** UAB Div Neurosurgery, 1530 3rd Ave S, FOT 1030, Birmingham, AL 35294-3410; **Phone:** 205-934-1439; **Board Cert:** Neurological Surgery 1992; **Med School:** Albany Med Coll 1982; **Resid:** Neurological Surgery, St Josephs Hosp Med Ctr 1988; **Fac Appt:** Prof NS, Univ Alabama

Haid Jr, Regis W MD [NS] - **Spec Exp:** Spinal Surgery; Minimally Invasive Spinal Surgery; Spinal Disc Replacement; Microdiscectomy; **Hospital:** Piedmont Hosp; **Address:** Atlanta Brain & Spine Care, 2001 Peachtree Rd NE, Ste 575, Atlanta, GA 30309; **Phone:** 404-350-0106; **Board Cert:** Neurological Surgery 2011; **Med School:** W VA Univ 1982; **Resid:** Neurological Surgery, W Va Univ Hosps 1988; **Fellow:** Spinal Surgery, Univ Florida 1989; **Fac Appt:** Prof NS, Emory Univ

Heros, Roberto MD [NS] - **Spec Exp:** Cerebrovascular Surgery; Skull Base Surgery; Brain Tumors; **Hospital:** Jackson Meml Hosp (page 70), Univ of Miami Hosp & Clins/Sylvester Comp Canc Ctr (page 73); **Address:** Univ Miami, Dept Neurosurgery, 1095 NW 14th Terrace, Miami, FL 33136; **Phone:** 305-243-4572; **Board Cert:** Neurological Surgery 1979; **Med School:** Univ Tenn Coll Med 1968; **Resid:** Surgery, Mass Genl Hosp 1970; Neurological Surgery, Mass Genl Hosp 1976; **Fac Appt:** Prof NS, Univ Miami Sch Med

Hodes, Jonathan MD [NS] - **Spec Exp:** Spinal Cord Injury-Epidural Stimulation; Spinal Cord Injury; Movement Disorders; Brain Tumors; **Hospital:** Frazier Rehab Inst, Univ of Louisville Hosp; **Address:** Univ Louisville Hlth Care Outpt Ctr, Dept Neurosurgery, 3900 Kresge Way, Ste 41, Louisville, KY 40202; **Phone:** 502-899-3623; **Board Cert:** Internal Medicine 1986; Neurological Surgery 1984; **Med School:** Indiana Univ 1980; **Resid:** Internal Medicine, Indiana Univ Hosp 1982; Neurological Surgery, UCSF Med Ctr 1989; **Fellow:** Geriatric Medicine, NIH 1984; Neurological Radiology, Lariboisiere Hosp 1991

Landy, Howard J MD [NS] - **Spec Exp:** Stereotactic Radiosurgery; **Hospital:** Jackson Meml Hosp (page 70); **Address:** Univ Miami, Dept Neurosurgery, 1095 NW 14th Terrace Fl 2, Miami, FL 33136; **Phone:** 305-243-4675; **Board Cert:** Neurological Surgery 1991; **Med School:** Univ Miami Sch Med 1980; **Resid:** Neurological Surgery, Jackson Meml Hosp 1987; **Fac Appt:** Prof NS, Univ Miami Sch Med

Levi, Allan MD/PhD [NS] - **Spec Exp:** Spinal Surgery; Peripheral Nerve Disorders; Minimally Invasive Spinal Surgery; Spinal Cord Injury; **Hospital:** Jackson Meml Hosp (page 70), Univ of Miami Hosp (page 72); **Address:** 1095 NW 14th Terrace, Miami, FL 33136; **Phone:** 305-243-2088; **Board Cert:** Neurological Surgery 1999; **Med School:** Univ Ottawa 1986; **Resid:** Neurological Surgery, Univ Toronto Affil Hosp 1991; **Fellow:** Spinal Surgery, Barrow Neuro Inst 1995; **Fac Appt:** Prof NS, Univ Miami Sch Med

Markert Jr, James M MD [NS] - **Spec Exp:** Brain Tumors; Stereotactic Radiosurgery; Clinical Trials; **Hospital:** Univ of Ala Hosp at Birmingham; **Address:** Univ Alabama, Div Neurosurgery, 510 20th St S, FOT, rm 1060, Birmingham, AL 35294; **Phone:** 205-975-6985; **Board Cert:** Neurological Surgery 1999; **Med School:** Columbia P&S 1988; **Resid:** Neurological Surgery, Univ Mich Med Ctr 1995; **Fellow:** Neuro-Oncology, Mass Genl Hosp; **Fac Appt:** Prof NS, Univ Alabama

Morcos, Jacques J MD [NS] - **Spec Exp:** Cerebrovascular Surgery; Brain Tumors; Skull Base Tumors & Surgery; Arteriovenous Malformations; **Hospital:** Jackson Meml Hosp (page 70); **Address:** University of Miami, Dept Neurosurgery, 1095 NW 14th Terr Fl 2, Miami, FL 33136; **Phone:** 305-243-4675; **Board Cert:** Neurological Surgery 1985; **Med School:** Lebanon 1985; **Resid:** Neurological Surgery, Natl Hosp for Nervous Diseases 1990; Neurological Surgery, Univ Minnesota 1993; **Fellow:** Cerebrovascular Neurosurgery, Univ Florida/Shands Med Ctr 1994; Skull Base Surgery, Barrow Neurolical Inst 1995; **Fac Appt:** Assoc Prof NS, Univ Miami Sch Med

Myseros, John S MD [NS] - **Spec Exp:** Pediatric Neurosurgery; Brain Tumors; Congenital Nervous System Malformations; **Hospital:** Inova Fairfax Hosp for Chldn; **Address:** 8501 Arlington Blvd, Ste 450, Fairfax, VA 22031; **Phone:** 571-226-8330; **Board Cert:** Neurological Surgery 2000; Pediatric Neurological Surgery 2000; **Med School:** Johns Hopkins Univ 1990; **Resid:** Neurological Surgery, Med Coll Virginia 1996; **Fellow:** Pediatric Neurological Surgery, Hosp for Sick Children 1997; **Fac Appt:** Assoc Prof NS, Geo Wash Univ

Oakes, W Jerry MD [NS] - **Spec Exp:** Pediatric Neurosurgery; Chiari's Deformity; Occult Spinal Dysraphism (OSD); **Hospital:** Children's Hospital - Birmingham; **Address:** Children's Hosp Alabama, 1600 7th Ave S, ACC 400, Birmingham, AL 35233; **Phone:** 205-939-9653; **Board Cert:** Neurological Surgery 1981; Pediatric Neurological Surgery 2005; **Med School:** Duke Univ 1972; **Resid:** Neurological Surgery, Duke Univ Hosp 1978; **Fellow:** Neurological Surgery, Hosp for Sick Chldn 1975; Neurological Surgery, Great Ormond St Hosp 1979; **Fac Appt:** Prof NS, Univ Alabama

Olson, Jeffrey J MD [NS] - **Spec Exp:** Neuro-Oncology; Brain Tumors; Skull Base Tumors; Von Hippel-Lindau Disease; **Hospital:** Emory Univ Hosp, Emory Univ Hosp Midtown; **Address:** Emory Univ, Dept Neurosurgery, 1365B Clifton Rd NE, B Bldg - Fl 2 - Ste 2200, Atlanta, GA 30322; **Phone:** 404-778-5770; **Board Cert:** Neurological Surgery 1989; **Med School:** Univ Minn 1981; **Resid:** Neurological Surgery, Univ Iowa Hosps & Clinics 1987; **Fellow:** Neurological Surgery, Natl Inst Hlth 1990; **Fac Appt:** Prof NS, Emory Univ

Parent, Andrew D MD [NS] - **Spec Exp:** Pediatric Neurosurgery; Neuroendocrine Tumors; Pituitary Tumors; **Hospital:** Univ Mississippi Med Ctr; **Address:** Univ Miss Med Ctr-Dept Neurosurgery, 2500 N State St, Jackson, MS 39216-4500; **Phone:** 601-984-5702; **Board Cert:** Neurological Surgery 1981; Pediatric Neurological Surgery 2005; **Med School:** Univ VT Coll Med 1970; **Resid:** Neurological Surgery, Emory Univ 1978; **Fellow:** Neurological Surgery, Univ Tex Med Br 1974; **Fac Appt:** Prof NS, Univ Miss

Patel, Sunil J MD [NS] - **Spec Exp:** Brain Tumors; Skull Base Surgery; Pain-Facial; Trigeminal Neuralgia; **Hospital:** MUSC Med Ctr, R H Johnson VA Med Ctr - charleston; **Address:** MUSC-Adult Neurological Surgery, CSB, Ste 428, Charleston, SC 29425; **Phone:** 843-792-7700; **Board Cert:** Neurological Surgery 1996; **Med School:** Med Univ SC 1985; **Resid:** Neurological Surgery, Univ South Carolina 1991; **Fellow:** Neurological Surgery, Nagoya Univ Med School 1991; Skull Base Surgery, Univ Pittsburgh 1993; **Fac Appt:** Prof NS, Med Univ SC

Ragheb, John MD [NS] - **Spec Exp:** Pediatric Neurosurgery; Spinal Cord Tumors-Pediatric; Brain Injury-Pediatric; Epilepsy; **Hospital:** Miami Children's Hosp; **Address:** Miami Children's Hospital, Dept Neurosurgery, 3100 SW 62nd Ave, Ste 3109, Miami, FL 33155; **Phone:** 305-662-8386; **Board Cert:** Neurological Surgery 1996; Pediatric Neurological Surgery 1998; **Med School:** Univ Mich Med Sch 1985; **Resid:** Neurological Surgery, Univ Maryland Med Ctr 1991; **Fellow:** Pediatric Neurological Surgery, NYU Med Ctr 1992; **Fac Appt:** Prof NS, Univ Miami Sch Med

Reid, William S MD [NS] - **Spec Exp:** Spinal Surgery; Spinal Cord Surgery; Brain & Spinal Cord Tumors; **Hospital:** Univ of Tennessee Med Ctr; **Address:** 1932 Alcoa Hwy, Bldg C, Ste 280, Knoxville, TN 37920; **Phone:** 865-329-4003; **Board Cert:** Neurological Surgery 1980; **Med School:** Univ Ariz Coll Med 1971; **Resid:** Neurological Surgery, Univ Texas Hlth Sci Ctr 1975; **Fac Appt:** Assoc Clin Prof NS, Univ Tex SW, Dallas

Robertson, Jon H MD [NS] - **Spec Exp:** Brain & Spinal Cord Tumors; Skull Base Surgery; Stereotactic Radiosurgery; **Hospital:** Methodist Univ Hosp - Memphis; **Address:** Univ Tennessee, Dept Neurosurgery, 6325 Humphreys Blvd, Memphis, TN 38120; **Phone:** 901-259-5340; **Board Cert:** Neurological Surgery 1982; **Med School:** Univ Tenn Coll Med 1971; **Resid:** Surgery, City Memphis Hosp 1974; Neurological Surgery, Univ TN Med Ctr 1979; **Fac Appt:** Prof NS, Univ Tenn Coll Med

Rodts Jr, Gerald E MD [NS] - **Spec Exp:** Spinal Surgery; Spinal Trauma; Spinal Tumors; **Hospital:** Emory Univ Hosp, Emory Univ Hosp Midtown; **Address:** Emory Spine Center, 59 Executive Park South, Ste 3000, Atlanta, GA 30329; **Phone:** 404-778-7000; **Board Cert:** Neurological Surgery 1998; **Med School:** Columbia P&S 1987; **Resid:** Neurological Surgery, UCLA Med Ctr 1994; **Fellow:** Spinal Surgery, Emory Univ 1995; **Fac Appt:** Prof NS, Emory Univ

Sampson, John H MD/PhD [NS] - **Spec Exp:** Brain Tumors; Clinical Trials; **Hospital:** Duke Univ Hosp; **Address:** Duke Univ Med Ctr, Box 3050, Durham, NC 27710; **Phone:** 919-684-9041; **Board Cert:** Neurological Surgery 2002; **Med School:** Univ Manitoba 1990; **Resid:** Neurological Surgery, Duke Univ Med Ctr 1998; **Fellow:** Neurological Intensive Care, Duke Univ Med Ctr 1999; **Fac Appt:** Assoc Prof S, Duke Univ

Sandberg, David MD [NS] - **Spec Exp:** Pediatric Neurosurgery; Brain Tumors-Pediatric; Spinal Surgery; Minimally Invasive Spinal Surgery; **Hospital:** Miami Children's Hosp; **Address:** Miami Children's Hospital, Dept Neurosurgery, 3100 SW 62nd Ave, Ste 3109, Miami, FL 33135; **Phone:** 305-662-8386; **Board Cert:** Neurological Surgery 2007; **Med School:** Johns Hopkins Univ 1997; **Resid:** Surgery, NY Presby-Cornell Med Ctr 1998; Neurological Surgery, NY Presby-Cornell Med Ctr 2002; **Fellow:** Neurosurgical Oncology, Meml Sloan Kettering Cancer Ctr 2003; Pediatric Neurological Surgery, Children's Hosp 2004; **Fac Appt:** Assoc Prof NS, Univ Miami Sch Med

Sanford, Robert A MD [NS] - **Spec Exp:** Pediatric Neurosurgery; Brain Tumors-Pediatric; **Hospital:** Le Bonheur Chldns Med Ctr, St. Jude Children's Research Hosp; **Address:** 6325 Humphreys Blvd, Memphis, TN 38120; **Phone:** 901-259-5340; **Board Cert:** Neurological Surgery 1976; Pediatric Neurological Surgery 2005; **Med School:** Univ Ark 1967; **Resid:** Neurological Surgery, Univ Minneapolis Med Ctr 1973; **Fac Appt:** Prof NS, Univ Tenn Coll Med

Shaffrey, Christopher I MD [NS] - **Spec Exp:** Spinal Surgery; Spinal Surgery-Pediatric; **Hospital:** Univ of Virginia Health Sys; **Address:** Univ Virg, Dept Neurosurg, Hosp Drive, Private Clinic 3rd Fl, Rm 3508, Charlottesville, VA 22908; **Phone:** 434-243-7026; **Board Cert:** Neurological Surgery 1997; Orthopaedic Surgery 2008; **Med School:** Univ VA Sch Med 1986; **Resid:** Neurological Surgery, Univ Virginia Med Ctr 1992; Orthopaedic Surgery, Univ Virginia Med Ctr 1995; **Fellow:** Spinal Surgery, Univ Virginia Med Ctr 1996; **Fac Appt:** Prof NS, Univ VA Sch Med

Shaffrey, Mark E MD [NS] - **Spec Exp:** Brain Tumors; Clinical Trials; Spinal Cord Tumors; Spinal Tumors; **Hospital:** Univ of Virginia Health Sys; **Address:** UVA Hlth Sys, Dept Neurosurgery, PO Box 800212, Charlottesville, VA 22908; **Phone:** 434-924-1843; **Board Cert:** Neurological Surgery 2000; **Med School:** Univ VA Sch Med 1987; **Resid:** Neurological Surgery, Univ Virginia Med Ctr 1991; **Fellow:** Microvascular Physiology, NIH 1992; Neurological Pathology, Univ Virginia Med Ctr 1993; **Fac Appt:** Prof NS, Univ VA Sch Med

Sills Jr, Allen MD [NS] - **Spec Exp:** Brain & Spinal Tumors; Stereotactic Radiosurgery; Cerebrovascular Disease; **Hospital:** Vanderbilt Univ Med Ctr (page 76); **Address:** 2009 Mallory Ln, Ste 230, Franklin, TN 37067; **Phone:** 615-778-2265; **Board Cert:** Neurological Surgery 2002; **Med School:** Johns Hopkins Univ 1990; **Resid:** Neurological Surgery, Johns Hopkins Hosp 1994; **Fellow:** Neuro-Oncology, Hunterian Neurosurg Lab/Johns Hopkins 1996; **Fac Appt:** Assoc Prof NS, Vanderbilt Univ

Swaid, Swaid N MD [NS] - **Spec Exp:** Stereotactic Radiosurgery; Acoustic Neuroma; Pituitary Tumors; Brain Tumors; **Hospital:** Brookwood Med Ctr; **Address:** Neurological Surgery Assocs, 513 Brookwood Blvd, Ste 372, Birmingham, AL 35209; **Phone:** 205-802-6844; **Board Cert:** Neurological Surgery 1983; **Med School:** Univ Alabama 1976; **Resid:** Neurological Surgery, UAB Med Ctr 1981; **Fac Appt:** Assoc Prof NS, Univ Alabama

Tatter, Stephen MD/PhD [NS] - **Spec Exp:** Brain Tumors; Pituitary Tumors; Stereotactic Radiosurgery; **Hospital:** Wake Forest Univ Baptist Med Ctr; **Address:** Wake Forest Baptist Hlth, Dept Neurosurg, Medical Center Blvd, Winston-Salem, NC 27157-1029; **Phone:** 336-716-4047; **Board Cert:** Neurological Surgery 2004; **Med School:** Cornell Univ-Weill Med Coll 1990; **Resid:** Neurological Surgery, Mass Genl Hosp 1996; **Fellow:** Neurological Surgery, Mass Genl Hosp 1997; **Fac Appt:** Assoc Prof NS, Wake Forest Univ

Thompson, Reid C MD [NS] - **Spec Exp:** Neuro-Oncology; Brain & Spinal Cord Tumors; Neurovascular Surgery; Skull Base Tumors; **Hospital:** Vanderbilt Univ Med Ctr (page 76); **Address:** Vanderbilt Univ Med Ctr, Dept Neurosurg, 1500 21st Ave S, Ste 1506, Nashville, TN 37212; **Phone:** 615-322-7417; **Board Cert:** Neurological Surgery 2001; **Med School:** Johns Hopkins Univ 1989; **Resid:** Neurological Surgery, Johns Hopkins Hosp 1995; **Fellow:** Neuro-Oncology, Rsch-Johns Hopkins Hosp 1996; Cerebrovascular Neurosurgery, Stanford Univ Med Ctr 1997; **Fac Appt:** Prof NS, Vanderbilt Univ

Van Loveren, Harry R MD [NS] - **Spec Exp:** Trigeminal Neuralgia; Skull Base Surgery; **Hospital:** Tampa Genl Hosp; **Address:** Harbourside Medical Tower, 2 Tampa Genl Cir, Tampa, FL 33606; **Phone:** 813-259-0965; **Board Cert:** Neurological Surgery 1988; **Med School:** Univ Cincinnati 1979; **Resid:** Neurological Surgery, Good Samaritan Hosp 1984; **Fellow:** Neurological Surgery, Universitatspital 1985; **Fac Appt:** Prof NS, Univ S Fla Coll Med

Wharen Jr, Robert E MD [NS] - **Spec Exp:** Parkinson's Disease; Brain Tumors; Epilepsy; **Hospital:** Mayo - Jacksonville; **Address:** Mayo Clinic, Dept Neurosurgery, 4500 San Pablo Rd, Jacksonville, FL 32224-1865; **Phone:** 904-953-2103; **Board Cert:** Neurological Surgery 1988; **Med School:** Penn State Coll Med 1979; **Resid:** Neurological Surgery, Mayo Clinic 1985; **Fac Appt:** Prof NS, Mayo Med Sch

Wilson, John A MD [NS] - **Spec Exp:** Cerebrovascular Surgery; Skull Base Surgery; Spinal Surgery; **Hospital:** Wake Forest Univ Baptist Med Ctr; **Address:** Wake Forest Univ Medical Ctr, Medical Center Blvd, Winston-Salem, NC 27157-1029; **Phone:** 336-716-4020; **Board Cert:** Neurological Surgery 1996; **Med School:** Jefferson Med Coll 1982; **Resid:** Surgery, Allegheny Gen Hosp 1985; Neurological Surgery, NYU Med Ctr 1986; **Fellow:** Neurological Surgery, New England Med Ctr 1990; **Fac Appt:** Assoc Prof NS, Wake Forest Univ

Midwest

Albright, A Leland MD [NS] - **Spec Exp:** Pediatric Neurosurgery; Spasticity & Movement Disorders; Brain Tumors; **Hospital:** Univ WI Hosp & Clins; **Address:** Dept Neurosurgery, 600 Highland Ave, rm K4/836, Madison, WI 53792; **Phone:** 608-263-9651; **Board Cert:** Neurological Surgery 1981; Pediatric Neurological Surgery 2005; **Med School:** Louisiana State U, New Orleans 1969; **Resid:** Surgery, Wash Hosps 1971; Neurological Surgery, Univ Pittsburgh Med Ctr 1978; **Fellow:** Neurological Surgery, Natl Inst Hlth 1974; Immunopathology, Univ Pittsburgh Med Ctr 1978; **Fac Appt:** Prof NS, Univ Wisc

Neurological Surgery

Atkinson, John L MD [NS] - **Spec Exp:** Pituitary Surgery; Stroke; Cerebrovascular Disease; **Hospital:** Mayo Med Ctr & Clin - Rochester; **Address:** Mayo Clin, Dept Neurosurgery, 200 First St SW, Rochester, MN 55905; **Phone:** 507-284-2376; **Board Cert:** Neurological Surgery 1992; **Med School:** Univ Alabama 1984; **Resid:** Neurological Surgery, Mayo Clinic 1990; **Fac Appt:** Assoc Prof NS, Mayo Med Sch

Bakay, Roy AE MD [NS] - **Spec Exp:** Parkinson's Disease/Movement Disorders; Epilepsy; Stereotactic Radiosurgery; **Hospital:** Rush Univ Med Ctr; **Address:** University Neurosurgery, 1725 W Harrison St, Ste 970, Chicago, IL 60612; **Phone:** 312-942-6644; **Board Cert:** Neurological Surgery 1985; **Med School:** Northwestern Univ 1975; **Resid:** Neurological Surgery, Univ Washington Med Ctr 1981; **Fellow:** Neuronal Plasticity, Natl Inst Hlth 1982; **Fac Appt:** Prof NS, Rush Med Coll

Barnett, Gene H MD [NS] - **Spec Exp:** Brain Tumors; Stereotactic Radiosurgery; **Hospital:** Cleveland Clin (page 56); **Address:** Cleveland Clinic Brain Tumor Inst, 9500 Euclid Ave, MC S73, Cleveland, OH 44195; **Phone:** 216-444-5381; **Board Cert:** Neurological Surgery 1990; **Med School:** Case West Res Univ 1980; **Resid:** Neurological Surgery, Cleveland Clinic 1986; **Fellow:** Neurology, Cleveland Clinic 1982; Research, Mass Genl Hosp-Harvard 1987; **Fac Appt:** Prof NS, Cleveland Cl Coll Med/Case West Res

Batjer, Hunt Henry MD [NS] - **Spec Exp:** Aneurysm-Cerebral; Arteriovenous Malformations; Stroke; **Hospital:** Northwestern Meml Hosp; **Address:** 675 N St Clair, Galter Pavilion Fl 20 - Ste 250, Chicago, IL 60611; **Phone:** 312-695-8143; **Board Cert:** Neurological Surgery 1986; **Med School:** Univ Tex SW, Dallas 1977; **Resid:** Neurological Surgery, Parkland Meml Hosp 1981; **Fellow:** Neurological Surgery, Univ W Ontario Med Ctr 1982; **Fac Appt:** Prof NS, Northwestern Univ

Bauer, Jerry MD [NS] - **Spec Exp:** Pain-Back; Minimally Invasive Surgery; Spinal Surgery; **Hospital:** Adv Luth Genl Hosp; **Address:** Ctr Brain & Spine Surg-Parkside Ctr, 1875 Dempster St, Ste 605, Park Ridge, IL 60068-1168; **Phone:** 847-698-1088; **Board Cert:** Neurological Surgery 1982; **Med School:** Univ IL Coll Med 1974; **Resid:** Neurological Surgery, Univ Illinois Med Ctr 1979; **Fac Appt:** Asst Clin Prof NS, Univ IL Coll Med

Benzel, Edward C MD [NS] - **Spec Exp:** Spinal Surgery; **Hospital:** Cleveland Clin (page 56); **Address:** 9500 Euclid Ave, Desk S80, Cleveland, OH 44195; **Phone:** 216-445-5514; **Board Cert:** Neurological Surgery 1986; **Med School:** Univ Wisc 1975; **Resid:** Neurological Surgery, Med Coll Wisc Clins 1980; **Fellow:** Spinal Cord Injury Medicine, Wood VA Med Ctr 1981; **Fac Appt:** Prof NS, Case West Res Univ

Bierbrauer, Karin S MD [NS] - **Spec Exp:** Pediatric Neurosurgery; Spina Bifida; Craniosynostosis; Hydrocephalus; **Hospital:** Cincinnati Chldns Hosp Med Ctr; **Address:** Cincinnati Childrens Hospital, 3333 Burnet Ave, MC 2016, Cincinnati, OH 45229; **Phone:** 513-636-7124; **Board Cert:** Neurological Surgery 1994; Pediatric Neurological Surgery 2007; **Med School:** Med Univ SC 1984; **Resid:** Neurological Surgery, Emory Univ Hosp 1990; **Fellow:** Pediatric Neurological Surgery, Chldns Meml Hosp 1991; **Fac Appt:** Assoc Clin Prof NS, Ohio State Univ

Brown, Frederick D MD [NS] - **Spec Exp:** Minimally Invasive Spinal Surgery; Spinal Surgery; Pain-Chronic; **Hospital:** Univ of Chicago Med Ctr; **Address:** Univ Chicago Hosp, Dept Neurosurgery, 5841 S Maryland Ave, MC 3026, Chicago, IL 60637; **Phone:** 773-702-2123; **Board Cert:** Neurological Surgery 1982; **Med School:** Ohio State Univ 1972; **Resid:** Neurological Surgery, Univ Chicago Hosps 1978; **Fac Appt:** Assoc Prof NS, Univ Chicago-Pritzker Sch Med

Bucholz, Richard D MD [NS] - **Spec Exp:** Epilepsy/Seizure Disorders; Stereotactic Radiosurgery; **Hospital:** St. Louis Univ Hosp; **Address:** 1320 S Grand Ave, O'Donnell Hall Fl 1, St Louis, MO 63110; **Phone:** 314-977-4750; **Board Cert:** Neurological Surgery 1985; **Med School:** Yale Univ 1977; **Resid:** Neurological Surgery, Yale New Haven Hosp 1983; **Fac Appt:** Prof NS, St Louis Univ

Chandler, James P MD [NS] - **Spec Exp:** Skull Base Surgery; Neuro-Oncology; Brain Tumors; Spinal Disorders; **Hospital:** Northwestern Meml Hosp; **Address:** 675 N St Clair St, Galter Pavilion, Ste 20-250, Chicago, IL 60611; **Phone:** 312-695-8143; **Board Cert:** Neurological Surgery 2002; **Med School:** Univ MD Sch Med 1990; **Resid:** Neurological Surgery, Northwestern Meml Hosp 1996; **Fellow:** Microvascular Surgery, Inst Neurologico De S„o Paulo 1996; Cranial Base Surgery, George Washington Univ Hosp 1997; **Fac Appt:** Asst Prof NS, Northwestern Univ

Chandler, William F MD [NS] - **Spec Exp:** Pituitary Surgery; Brain Tumors; **Hospital:** Univ of Michigan Hosp; **Address:** 1500 E Med Center Drive, Ste 3552, Tauban Center, Ann Arbor, MI 48109; **Phone:** 734-936-5020; **Board Cert:** Neurological Surgery 1980; **Med School:** Univ Mich Med Sch 1971; **Resid:** Neurological Surgery, Michigan Hosp 1977; **Fac Appt:** Prof NS, Univ Mich Med Sch

Chiocca, E Antonio MD [NS] - **Spec Exp:** Brain Tumors; Spinal Cord Tumors; Peripheral Nerve Surgery; **Hospital:** Arthur G James Cancer Hosp & Research Inst, Ohio St Univ Med Ctr; **Address:** OSU Med Ctr, Dept Neurosurgery, 410 W 10th Ave, 1021-N Doan Hall, Columbus, OH 43210; **Phone:** 614-293-9312; **Board Cert:** Neurological Surgery 2000; **Med School:** Univ Tex, Houston 1988; **Resid:** Neurological Surgery, Mass Genl Hosp 1995; **Fac Appt:** Prof NS, Ohio State Univ

Cohen, Alan R MD [NS] - **Spec Exp:** Pediatric Neurosurgery; Brain & Spinal Tumors-Pediatric; Minimally Invasive Surgery; **Hospital:** UH Rainbow Babies & Chldns Hosp (page 74), Univ Hosps Case Med Ctr (page 74); **Address:** 11100 Euclid Ave, Ste B501, Cleveland, OH 44106; **Phone:** 216-844-5741; **Board Cert:** Neurological Surgery 1991; Pediatric Neurological Surgery 2007; **Med School:** Cornell Univ-Weill Med Coll 1978; **Resid:** Surgery, NYU Medical Ctr 1980; Neurological Surgery, NYU Medical Ctr 1987; **Fellow:** Neurology, Natl Hosp Queen's Square 1982; **Fac Appt:** Prof NS, Case West Res Univ

Dacey Jr, Ralph G MD [NS] - **Spec Exp:** Cerebrovascular Surgery; Aneurysm-Cerebral; Brain Tumors; **Hospital:** Barnes-Jewish Hosp, Barnes-Jewish West County Hosp; **Address:** Wash Univ Dept Neurosurgery, 660 S Euclid Ave, Box 8057, St Louis, MO 63110; **Phone:** 314-362-3577; **Board Cert:** Internal Medicine 1978; Neurological Surgery 1985; **Med School:** Univ VA Sch Med 1974; **Resid:** Internal Medicine, Strong Meml Hosp 1977; Neurological Surgery, Univ Virginia Med Ctr 1983; **Fac Appt:** Prof NS, Washington Univ, St Louis

Dempsey, Robert J MD [NS] - **Spec Exp:** Vascular Neurosurgery; Aneurysm-Cerebral; Stroke; **Hospital:** Univ WI Hosp & Clins; **Address:** Dept Neurosurgery, 600 Highland Ave, rm K4-822, Madison, WI 53792; **Phone:** 608-265-5967; **Board Cert:** Neurological Surgery 1985; **Med School:** Univ Chicago-Pritzker Sch Med 1977; **Resid:** Neurological Surgery, Univ Mich Hosps 1983; **Fac Appt:** Prof NS, Univ Wisc

Diaz, Fernando G MD/PhD [NS] - **Spec Exp:** Arteriovenous Malformations; Spinal Surgery; **Hospital:** Providence Hosp - Southfield, Beaumont Hosp-Royal Oak; **Address:** Michigan Head & Spine Inst, 29275 Northwestern Hwy, Ste 100, Southfield, MI 48034; **Phone:** 877-784-3667; **Board Cert:** Neurological Surgery 1980; **Med School:** Mexico 1968; **Resid:** Surgery, Univ Kansas Med Ctr 1973; Neurological Surgery, Univ Minn Med Ctr 1978; **Fellow:** Cerebrovascular Disease, Univ Minn Med Ctr 1979; **Fac Appt:** Prof NS, Wayne State Univ

Fessler, Richard G MD/PhD [NS] - **Spec Exp:** Skull Base Surgery; Spinal Surgery; Minimally Invasive Spinal Surgery; **Hospital:** Northwestern Meml Hosp; **Address:** 676 N St Clair St, Galter Pavillion 20-250, Chicago, IL 60611; **Phone:** 312-695-8143; **Board Cert:** Neurological Surgery 1992; **Med School:** Univ Chicago-Pritzker Sch Med 1983; **Resid:** Neurological Surgery, Univ Chicago Hosp 1989; **Fac Appt:** Prof NS, Northwestern Univ

Neurological Surgery

Frim, David M MD/PhD [NS] - Spec Exp: Pediatric Neurosurgery; Hydrocephalus; Brain & Spinal Tumors; Brain & Spinal Malformations; **Hospital:** Univ of Chicago Med Ctr; **Address:** Univ of Chicago Medical Ctr, Pediatric Neurosurgery, 5841 S Maryland Ave, MC 3026, Chicago, IL 60637-1463; **Phone:** 773-702-2475; **Board Cert:** Neurological Surgery 1998; Pediatric Neurological Surgery 1998; **Med School:** Harvard Med Sch 1988; **Resid:** Neurological Surgery, Mass Genl Hosp 1995; **Fellow:** Pediatric Neurological Surgery, Chldns Hosp 1996; **Fac Appt:** Assoc Prof S, Univ Chicago-Pritzker Sch Med

Grubb Jr, Robert L MD [NS] - Spec Exp: Brain Tumors; Acoustic Neuroma; Trigeminal Neuralgia; Skull Base Tumors; **Hospital:** Barnes-Jewish Hosp, St. Louis Chldns Hosp; **Address:** Wash Univ Sch Med, Dept Neurosurgery, 660 S Euclid Ave, Box 8057, St Louis, MO 63110; **Phone:** 314-362-3577; **Board Cert:** Neurological Surgery 1976; **Med School:** Univ NC Sch Med 1965; **Resid:** Surgery, Barnes Jewish Hosp 1967; Neurological Surgery, Barnes Jewish Hosp 1973; **Fellow:** Neurological Surgery, National Inst Health 1969; **Fac Appt:** Prof NS, Washington Univ, St Louis

Guthikonda, Murali MD [NS] - Spec Exp: Skull Base Tumors; Pituitary Tumors; Aneurysm-Cerebral; Spinal Tumors; **Hospital:** Harper Univ Hosp, Beaumont Hosp-Royal Oak; **Address:** Wayne St U Physicians Grp-Neurosurgery, 4160 John R, Ste 930, Detroit, MI 48201; **Phone:** 313-831-0777; **Board Cert:** Neurological Surgery 1982; **Med School:** India 1971; **Resid:** Surgery, St Elizabeth Hosp 1976; Neurological Surgery, Med Ctr Hosp VT 1980; **Fellow:** Skull Base Surgery, Univ Cincinnati 1993; **Fac Appt:** Prof NS, Wayne State Univ

Kaufman, Bruce A MD [NS] - Spec Exp: Pediatric Neurosurgery; Brain & Spinal Cord Tumors; Spasticity & Movement Disorders; **Hospital:** Chldns Hosp - Wisconsin; **Address:** Chldns Corporate Ctr, Dept Neurosurg, 999 N 92nd St, Ste 310, Milwaukee, WI 53226; **Phone:** 414-266-6435; **Board Cert:** Neurological Surgery 1992; Pediatric Neurological Surgery 2006; **Med School:** Case West Res Univ 1982; **Resid:** Neurological Surgery, Univ Hosp Cleveland/Case West Res 1988; **Fellow:** Pediatric Neurological Surgery, Chldns Meml Hosp/Northwestern Univ 1989; **Fac Appt:** Prof NS, Med Coll Wisc

Kuntz IV, Charles MD [NS] - Spec Exp: Spinal Surgery; Peripheral Nerve Surgery; Spinal Disorders; **Hospital:** Univ Hosp - Cincinnati; **Address:** 222 Piedmont Ave, Ste 3100, Cincinnati, OH 45219; **Phone:** 513-475-8667; **Board Cert:** Neurological Surgery 2004; **Med School:** Case West Res Univ 1991; **Resid:** Surgery, Univ Wash Med Ctr 1993; Neurological Surgery, Univ Wash Med Ctr 1999; **Fellow:** Neurological Surgery, Atkinson Morley's Hosp 1996; Neurological Surgery, Univ Wash Med Ctr 2000; **Fac Appt:** Asst Prof NS, Univ Cincinnati

Link, Michael J MD [NS] - Spec Exp: Skull Base Tumors; Brain Tumors; Cerebrovascular Surgery; **Hospital:** Mayo Med Ctr & Clin - Rochester; **Address:** Mayo Clinic, Dept Neurosurgery, 200 First St SW, Rochester, MN 55905; **Phone:** 507-284-8008; **Board Cert:** Neurological Surgery 2000; **Med School:** Mayo Med Sch 1990; **Resid:** Neurological Surgery, Mayo Clinic 1996; **Fellow:** Cerebrovascular & Skull Base Surgery, Univ Cincinnati/Mayfield Clinic 1998; **Fac Appt:** Assoc Prof NS, Mayo Med Sch

Luken, Martin MD [NS] - Spec Exp: Brain Tumors; Spinal Surgery; Chiari's Deformity; **Hospital:** Ingalls Meml Hosp, Rush Univ Med Ctr; **Address:** Ingalls Professional Office Bldg, 71 W 156th St, Ste 205, Harvey, IL 60426; **Phone:** 708-596-3344; **Board Cert:** Neurological Surgery 1983; **Med School:** Columbia P&S 1973; **Resid:** Surgery, Univ Illinois Med Ctr 1976; Neurological Surgery, Neurological Inst-Columbia Presby 1980; **Fac Appt:** Asst Prof NS, Rush Med Coll

Malik, Ghaus M MD [NS] - Spec Exp: Trigeminal Neuralgia; Cerebrovascular Surgery; Brain & Spinal Cord Tumors; **Hospital:** Henry Ford- W Bloomfield Hosp, Beaumont Hosp-Royal Oak; **Address:** Henry Ford Hosp, Dept Neurosurg, 6777 W Maple Rd, West Bloomfield, MI 48322; **Phone:** 248-661-6417; **Board Cert:** Neurological Surgery 1978; **Med School:** Pakistan 1968; **Resid:** Surgery, Henry Ford Hosp 1971; Neurological Surgery, Henry Ford Hosp 1975

Menezes, Arnold MD [NS] - **Spec Exp:** Pediatric Neurosurgery; Craniocervical Disorders; Spinal Surgery-Pediatric; **Hospital:** Univ Iowa Hosp & Clinics; **Address:** Univ Iowa Hosp, Dept Neurosurgery, 200 Hawkins Drive, Iowa City, IA 52242; **Phone:** 319-356-2768; **Board Cert:** Neurological Surgery 1976; Pediatric Neurological Surgery 2009; **Med School:** India 1967; **Resid:** Surgery, Univ Iowa Hosps 1970; Neurological Surgery, Univ Iowa Hosps 1974; **Fellow:** Child Neurology, Univ Iowa Hosps; **Fac Appt:** Prof NS, Univ Iowa Coll Med

Meyer, Fredric B MD [NS] - **Spec Exp:** Cerebrovascular Disease; Brain Tumors; Epilepsy; Pituitary Tumors; **Hospital:** Mayo Med Ctr & Clin - Rochester; **Address:** Mayo Clinic Dept Neurosurgery, 200 First St SW, Rochester, MN 55905; **Phone:** 507-284-5317; **Board Cert:** Neurological Surgery 1990; **Med School:** Boston Univ 1981; **Resid:** Neurological Surgery, Mayo Clinic 1987; **Fellow:** Neurological Surgery, Mayo Clinic 1988; **Fac Appt:** Prof NS, Mayo Med Sch

Nagib, Mahmoud MD [NS] - **Spec Exp:** Pediatric Neurosurgery; Skull Base Surgery; **Hospital:** Chldns Hosp and Clinics - Minneapolis, Abbott - Northwestern Hosp; **Address:** 913 E 26th St Piper Bldg - Ste 305, Minneapolis, MN 55404; **Phone:** 612-871-7278; **Board Cert:** Neurological Surgery 1985; **Med School:** Egypt 1973; **Resid:** Neurological Surgery, Univ Minn Hosps 1982; **Fellow:** Neurological Physiology, Univ Oslo 1976; **Fac Appt:** Clin Prof NS, Univ Minn

Park, Tae Sung MD [NS] - **Spec Exp:** Pediatric Neurosurgery; Cerebral Palsy-Select Dorsal Rhizotomy; Brachial Plexus Palsy-Pediatric; Neuro-Oncology; **Hospital:** St. Louis Chldns Hosp; **Address:** St Louis Children's Hospital, 1 Children's Place, Ste 4S20, St Louis, MO 63110; **Phone:** 314-454-2810; **Board Cert:** Neurological Surgery 1985; Pediatric Neurological Surgery 2006; **Med School:** Korea 1971; **Resid:** Neurological Surgery, Univ Virginia Hosp 1981; **Fellow:** Pediatric Neurological Surgery, Hosp for Sick Chldn 1983; **Fac Appt:** Prof NS, Washington Univ, St Louis

Raffel, Corey MD/PhD [NS] - **Spec Exp:** Pediatric Neurosurgery; Brain Tumors; Medulloblastoma; **Hospital:** Nationwide Chldn's Hosp; **Address:** Nationwide Chldn's Hosp, Dept Neurosurgery, 700 Children's Drive, Columbus, OH 43205; **Phone:** 614-722-2014; **Board Cert:** Neurological Surgery 1990; Pediatric Neurological Surgery 2006; **Med School:** UCSD 1980; **Resid:** Neurological Surgery, UCSF Med Ctr 1986; **Fellow:** Pediatric Neurological Surgery, Hosp Sick Chldn 1988

Rezai, Ali R MD [NS] - **Spec Exp:** Parkinson's Disease; Pain-Chronic; Deep Brain Stimulation; Alzheimer's Disease; **Hospital:** Ohio St Univ Med Ctr; **Address:** OSU Med Ctr, 410 W 10th Ave, rm N1047, Doan Hall, Columbus, OH 43210; **Phone:** 614-366-2420; **Board Cert:** Neurological Surgery 2003; **Med School:** USC Sch Med 1990; **Resid:** Neurological Surgery, NYU Med Ctr 1997; **Fellow:** Stereo Neurological Surgery, Univ Toronto Med Ctr 1998; Neurological Surgery, Karolinska Inst; **Fac Appt:** Assoc Prof NS, Cleveland Cl Coll Med/Case West Res

Rich, Keith M MD [NS] - **Spec Exp:** Brain Tumors; Neurovascular Surgery; Stereotactic Radiosurgery; **Hospital:** Barnes-Jewish Hosp; **Address:** Wash Univ Dept Neurosurgery, 660 S Euclid Ave, Box 8057, St Louis, MO 63110; **Phone:** 314-362-3577; **Board Cert:** Neurological Surgery 1987; **Med School:** Indiana Univ 1977; **Resid:** Neurological Surgery, Barnes Jewish Hosp 1982; **Fellow:** Neurological Pharmacology, Barnes Jewish Hosp 1984; **Fac Appt:** Assoc Prof NS, Washington Univ, St Louis

Rock, Jack P MD [NS] - **Spec Exp:** Neuro-Oncology; Pituitary Surgery; Skull Base Surgery; Brain Tumors; **Hospital:** Henry Ford Hosp; **Address:** Henry Ford Hosp, Dept Neurosurg, 2799 W Grand Blvd, Detroit, MI 48202; **Phone:** 313-916-2241; **Board Cert:** Neurological Surgery 1989; **Med School:** Univ Miami Sch Med 1979; **Resid:** Neurological Surgery, New York Hosp-Cornell 1985; **Fellow:** Univ Maryland 1986

Neurological Surgery

Rosenblum, Mark L MD [NS] - **Spec Exp:** Brain Tumors; Spinal Surgery; Infections-Neurologic; Neuro-Oncology; **Hospital:** Henry Ford Hosp; **Address:** Henry Ford Hospital, K11, 2799 W Grand Blvd, Detroit, MI 48202; **Phone:** 313-916-1340; **Board Cert:** Neurological Surgery 1982; **Med School:** NY Med Coll 1969; **Resid:** Surgery, UCLA Med Ctr 1973; Neurological Surgery, UCSF Med Ctr 1979; **Fellow:** Neuro-Oncology, NIH/Natl Cancer Inst 1972

Ruge, John R MD [NS] - **Spec Exp:** Pediatric Neurosurgery; Brain Tumors; Hydrocephalus; **Hospital:** Adv Luth Genl Hosp; **Address:** Ctr Brain & Spine Surg-Parkside Ctr, 1875 Dempster St, Ste 605, Park Ridge, IL 60068; **Phone:** 847-698-1088; **Board Cert:** Neurological Surgery 1993; **Med School:** Northwestern Univ 1983; **Resid:** Neurological Surgery, Northwestern Meml Hosp 1989; **Fellow:** Pediatric Neurological Surgery, Childrens Hosp 1990; **Fac Appt:** Asst Prof S, Rush Med Coll

Ryken, Timothy C MD [NS] - **Spec Exp:** Brain Tumors; Spinal Surgery; **Hospital:** Covenant Med Ctr; **Address:** Iowa Spine & Brain Institute, 2710 St Francis Drive, Ste 110, Waterloo, IA 50702; **Phone:** 319-272-6700; **Board Cert:** Neurological Surgery 1998; **Med School:** Univ Iowa Coll Med 1988; **Resid:** Neurological Surgery, Univ Iowa 1995; **Fellow:** Research, Cambridge Univ 1996; **Fac Appt:** Assoc Prof NS, Univ Iowa Coll Med

Selman, Warren R MD [NS] - **Spec Exp:** Stroke; Pituitary Surgery; Aneurysm-Cerebral; Microsurgery; **Hospital:** Univ Hosps Case Med Ctr (page 74); **Address:** Dept Neurosurgery, 11100 Euclid Ave, 5th Fl Hanna House, Cleveland, OH 44106; **Phone:** 216-844-5745; **Board Cert:** Neurological Surgery 1986; **Med School:** Case West Res Univ 1977; **Resid:** Neurological Surgery, Univ Hosps 1984; **Fellow:** Research, Univ Hosps 1980; Neurological Surgery, Mayo Clinic 1984; **Fac Appt:** Prof NS, Case West Res Univ

Shapiro, Scott A MD [NS] - **Spec Exp:** Brain Tumors; Aneurysm-Cerebral; Spinal Cord Injury; Pituitary Tumors; **Hospital:** IU Health Methodist Hosp, Wishard Hlth Srvs; **Address:** Indiana Univ Health Methodist Hosp, 1801 N Senate Blvd, Ste 610, Indianapolis, IN 46202; **Phone:** 317-396-1300; **Board Cert:** Neurological Surgery 1990; **Med School:** Indiana Univ 1981; **Resid:** Neurological Surgery, Indiana Univ Med Ctr 1987; **Fac Appt:** Prof NS, Indiana Univ

Spinner, Robert J MD [NS] - **Spec Exp:** Peripheral Nerve Surgery; Brachial Plexus Palsy; Brain Tumors; **Hospital:** Mayo Med Ctr & Clin - Rochester; **Address:** Mayo Clinic: Dept of Neurosurgery, 200 First St SW, Rochester, MN 55905; **Phone:** 507-284-2511; **Board Cert:** Orthopaedic Surgery 2003; Neurological Surgery 2006; **Med School:** Mayo Med Sch 1989; **Resid:** Orthopaedic Surgery, Duke Univ Med Ctr 1996; Neurological Surgery, Mayo Clinic 2000; **Fellow:** Peripheral Nerve Surgery, LSU Med Ctr 2000; **Fac Appt:** Prof NS, Mayo Med Sch

Thompson, B Gregory MD [NS] - **Spec Exp:** Acoustic Neuroma; Neurovascular Surgery; Skull Base Tumors & Surgery; Aneurysm-Cerebral; **Hospital:** Univ of Michigan Hosp; **Address:** Dept Neurosurgery, 3552 Taubman Ctr, 1500 E Medical Center Drive, Ann Arbor, MI 48109-5338; **Phone:** 734-936-7493; **Board Cert:** Neurological Surgery 1998; **Med School:** Univ Kansas 1986; **Resid:** Neurological Surgery, Univ Pittsburgh 1993; Research, Natl Inst Hlth 1992; **Fellow:** Neurological Surgery, Barrow Neuro Inst 1994; Interventional Radiology, Thomas Jefferson Univ 2005

Tomita, Tadanori MD [NS] - **Spec Exp:** Pediatric Neurosurgery; Brain Tumors-Pediatric; Hydrocephalus; **Hospital:** Children's Mem Hosp -Chicago, Northwestern Meml Hosp; **Address:** Chldns Meml Hosp, Div Ped Neurosurg, 2300 Children's Plaza, Box 28, Chicago, IL 60614-3363; **Phone:** 773-880-4373; **Board Cert:** Neurological Surgery 1984; Pediatric Neurological Surgery 1996; **Med School:** Japan 1970; **Resid:** Neurological Surgery, Kobe Univ 1974; Neurological Surgery, Northwestern Meml Hosp 1980; **Fellow:** Surgery, Meml Sloan Kettering Canc Ctr 1981; **Fac Appt:** Prof NS, Northwestern Univ

Traynelis, Vincent C MD [NS] - **Spec Exp:** Spinal Surgery; **Hospital:** Rush Univ Med Ctr; **Address:** Rush Univ Med Ctr, Dept Neurosurgery, 1725 W Harrison St, Ste 970, Chicago, IL 60612; **Phone:** 312-942-6644; **Board Cert:** Neurological Surgery 1992; **Med School:** W VA Univ 1983; **Resid:** Neurological Surgery, Univ West Virginia Med Ctr 1989; **Fac Appt:** Prof NS, Rush Med Coll

Warnick, Ronald E MD [NS] - **Spec Exp:** Neuro-Oncology; Brain Tumors; **Hospital:** Univ Hosp - Cincinnati, Good Samaritan Hosp - Cincinnati; **Address:** 222 Piedmont Ave, Ste 3100, Cincinnati, OH 45219; **Phone:** 513-475-8629; **Board Cert:** Neurological Surgery 1995; **Med School:** Univ Rochester 1982; **Resid:** Neurological Surgery, NYU Med Ctr 1989; **Fellow:** Neuro-Oncology, UCSF Med Ctr 1991; **Fac Appt:** Prof NS, Univ Cincinnati

Great Plains and Mountains

Cherny, W Bruce MD [NS] - **Spec Exp:** Pediatric Neurosurgery; Brain Tumors; Spina Bifida; **Hospital:** St. Luke's Boise Med Ctr; **Address:** Childrens Specialty Ctr, 100 E Idaho St, Ste 202, Boise, ID 83712; **Phone:** 208-381-7360; **Board Cert:** Neurological Surgery 2000; **Med School:** Univ Ariz Coll Med 1987; **Resid:** Neurological Surgery, Barrow Neuro Inst/St Joseph's Med Ctr 1994; **Fellow:** Pediatric Neurological Surgery, Primary Chldns Hosp 1995

Couldwell, William T MD/PhD [NS] - **Spec Exp:** Brain Tumors; Epilepsy; Parkinson's Disease; Skull Base Tumors; **Hospital:** Univ Utah Hlth Care; **Address:** Univ Utah, Dept Neurological Surgery, 175 N Medical Drive E, Salt Lake City, UT 84132-2303; **Phone:** 801-581-6908; **Board Cert:** Neurological Surgery 1994; **Med School:** McGill Univ 1984; **Resid:** Neurological Surgery, LAC/USC Med Ctr 1989; **Fellow:** Neurological Immunology, Montreal Neur Inst/McGill Univ 1990; Neurological Surgery, CHUV 1991; **Fac Appt:** Prof NS, Univ Utah

Johnson, Stephen D MD [NS] - **Spec Exp:** Skull Base Tumors & Surgery; **Hospital:** Presby - St Luke's Med Ctr; **Address:** Western Neurological Group, 1601 E 19th Ave, Ste 4400, Denver, CO 80218; **Phone:** 303-861-2266; **Board Cert:** Neurological Surgery 1988; **Med School:** Univ Tenn Coll Med 1974; **Resid:** Neurological Surgery, Virginia Mason Med Ctr; Neurological Surgery, New York Hosp; **Fellow:** Neurological Surgery, Univ Tennessee; **Fac Appt:** Assoc Prof NS, Univ Colorado

Kestle, John RW MD [NS] - **Spec Exp:** Pediatric Neurosurgery; Epilepsy/Seizure Disorders; **Hospital:** Primary Children's Med Ctr; **Address:** 100 N Mario Drive, Ste 1475, Salt Lake City, UT 84113; **Phone:** 801-662-5340; **Board Cert:** Neurological Surgery 2002; **Med School:** Canada 1984; **Resid:** Neurological Surgery, Univ Toronto 1990; **Fellow:** Pediatric Neurological Surgery, Hosp Sick Chldn 1992; **Fac Appt:** Prof NS, Univ Utah

Lillehei, Kevin O MD [NS] - **Spec Exp:** Neuro-Oncology; Pituitary Tumors; Peripheral Nerve Surgery; **Hospital:** Univ of CO Hosp - Anschutz Inpatient Pav; **Address:** Univ Colorado Hosp, Dept Neurosurgery, 12631 E 17th Ave, rm 501, MS C307, Aurora, CO 80045; **Phone:** 303-724-2280; **Board Cert:** Neurological Surgery 1989; **Med School:** Univ Minn 1979; **Resid:** Neurological Surgery, Univ Mich Med Ctr 1985; **Fac Appt:** Prof NS, Univ Colorado

Nazzaro, Jules M MD [NS] - **Spec Exp:** Parkinson's Disease; Movement Disorders; Stereotactic Radiosurgery; **Hospital:** Univ of Kansas Hosp; **Address:** Kansas University Medical Ctr, 3901 Rainbow Blvd, MS 3021, Kansas City, KS 66160; **Phone:** 913-588-5129; **Board Cert:** Neurological Surgery 1996; **Med School:** Albert Einstein Coll Med 1984; **Resid:** Neurological Surgery, NYU Med Ctr 1991; **Fellow:** Neurosurgical Oncology, Meml Sloan-Kettering Cancer Ctr 1992; **Fac Appt:** Assoc Prof NS, Univ Kansas

Neurological Surgery

Origitano, Thomas C MD/PhD [NS] - **Spec Exp:** Skull Base Tumors & Surgery; Brain Tumors; Pituitary Tumors; Craniofacial Surgery; **Hospital:** Kalispell Regl Med Ctr; **Address:** Northern Rockies Neurosurgical Assocs, 350 Heritage Way, Ste 1300, Kalispell, MT 59901; **Phone:** 406-752-5170; **Board Cert:** Neurological Surgery 1995; **Med School:** Loyola Univ-Stritch Sch Med 1984; **Resid:** Neurological Surgery, Loyola Univ Med Ctr 1990

Taylon, Charles MD [NS] - **Spec Exp:** Spinal Surgery-Cervical; Spinal Surgery-Low Back; Carpal Tunnel Syndrome; Trauma; **Hospital:** Creighton Univ Med Ctr; **Address:** Creighton Univ, Dept Surg, 601 N 30th St, Ste 3700, Omaha, NE 68131; **Phone:** 402-280-4497; **Board Cert:** Neurological Surgery 1984; **Med School:** Creighton Univ 1975; **Resid:** Neurological Surgery, Univ Wisc Hosps 1981; **Fac Appt:** Assoc Prof NS, Creighton Univ

Walker, Marion L MD [NS] - **Spec Exp:** Pediatric Neurosurgery; Spasticity & Movement Disorders; Hydrocephalus; Brain Tumors; **Hospital:** Primary Children's Med Ctr, Univ Utah Hlth Care; **Address:** Primary Chldns Med Ctr, Div Ped Neurosurgery, 100 N Mario Capecchi Drive, Ste 1475, Salt Lake City, UT 84113-1103; **Phone:** 801-662-5340; **Board Cert:** Neurological Surgery 1979; Pediatric Neurological Surgery 2006; **Med School:** Univ Tenn Coll Med 1969; **Resid:** Surgery, St Joseph's Hosp 1971; Neurological Surgery, St Joseph's Hosp-Barrow Neuro Inst 1976; **Fellow:** Pediatric Neurological Surgery, Hosp for Sick Chldn 1973; **Fac Appt:** Prof NS, Univ Utah

Zimmerman, Christian G MD [NS] - **Spec Exp:** Spinal Surgery-Complex; Head Injury; Trauma; **Hospital:** St. Alphonsus Regl Med Ctr; **Address:** 1075 N Curtis Rd, Ste 102, Boise, ID 83706; **Phone:** 208-367-4000; **Board Cert:** Neurological Surgery 1996; Pain Medicine 1998; **Med School:** Univ MD Sch Med 1985; **Resid:** Surgery, Univ Md Hosp-Prince Georges Med Ctr 1987; Neurological Surgery, Oreg Hlth Sci Univ 1992; **Fellow:** Spinal Surgery, Barrow Neur Inst 1993

Southwest

Adelson, P David MD [NS] - **Spec Exp:** Pediatric Neurosurgery; Brain Injury; Epilepsy/Seizure Disorders; Spinal Cord Injury; **Hospital:** Phoenix Children's Hosp; **Address:** Phoenix Childrens Hosp, Dept Neurosurgery, 1919 E Thomas Rd, B Bldg-4th Fl, Phoenix, AZ 85016; **Phone:** 602-933-0975; **Board Cert:** Neurological Surgery 1997; Pediatric Neurological Surgery 2009; **Med School:** Columbia P&S 1986; **Resid:** Neurological Surgery, UCLA Med Ctr 1992; **Fellow:** Pediatric Neurological Surgery, Children's Hosp 1994; **Fac Appt:** Prof NS, Univ Ariz Coll Med

Day, Arthur L MD [NS] - **Spec Exp:** Cerebrovascular Surgery; Carotid Artery Surgery; Skull Base Tumors; Arteriovenous Malformations; **Hospital:** Meml Hermann Hosp - Texas Med Ctr; **Address:** 6400 Fannin St, Ste 2800, Houston, TX 77030; **Phone:** 713-704-7100; **Board Cert:** Neurological Surgery 1980; **Med School:** Louisiana State U, New Orleans 1972; **Resid:** Neurological Surgery, Shands-Univ Florida Hosp 1977; **Fellow:** Neurological Pathology, Shands-Univ Florida Hosp 1978; **Fac Appt:** Prof NS, Univ Tex, Houston

De Monte, Franco MD [NS] - **Spec Exp:** Skull Base Tumors & Surgery; Neuro-Oncology; **Hospital:** UT MD Anderson Cancer Ctr; **Address:** UT MD Anderson Cancer Ctr, Dept Neurosurgery, 1515 Holcombe Blvd, Unit 442, Houston, TX 77030; **Phone:** 713-792-2400; **Board Cert:** Neurological Surgery 1995; **Med School:** Canada 1985; **Resid:** Neurological Surgery, Univ Western Ontario 1991; **Fellow:** Skull Base Surgery, Loyola Univ-Stritch Sch Med 1992; **Fac Appt:** Prof NS, Baylor Coll Med

Greene Jr, Clarence S MD [NS] - **Spec Exp:** Pediatric Neurosurgery; Congenital Nervous System Malformations; Brain Tumors; **Hospital:** Children's Hospital - New Orleans; **Address:** 200 Henry Clay Ave, Ste 210, New Orleans, LA 70118; **Phone:** 504-896-9458; **Board Cert:** Neurological Surgery 1984; Pediatric Neurological Surgery 2007; **Med School:** Howard Univ 1974; **Resid:** Neurological Surgery, Chldns Hosp 1981; Neurological Surgery, Peter Bent Brigham Hosp 1981; **Fellow:** Pediatric Neurological Surgery, Chldns Hosp 1985; **Fac Appt:** Assoc Clin Prof NS, UC Irvine

Hankinson, Hal L MD [NS] - **Spec Exp:** Brain Tumors; **Hospital:** Christus St Vincent Reg Med Ctr-Santa Fe; **Address:** 465 St Michael's Drive, Ste 107, Sante Fe, NM 87505; **Phone:** 505-988-3233; **Board Cert:** Neurological Surgery 1977; **Med School:** Tulane Univ 1967; **Resid:** Neurological Surgery, UCSF Med Ctr 1975; **Fac Appt:** Clin Prof NS, Univ New Mexico

Harper, Richard L MD [NS] - **Spec Exp:** Spinal Surgery; Brain Tumors & Hemifacial Spasms; **Hospital:** Methodist Hosp - Houston; **Address:** 6560 Fannin St, Ste 1200, Scurlock Tower, Houston, TX 77030; **Phone:** 713-790-1211; **Board Cert:** Neurological Surgery 1983; **Med School:** Baylor Coll Med 1971; **Resid:** Neurological Surgery, Baylor Hosps 1978; **Fac Appt:** Asst Clin Prof NS, Baylor Coll Med

Jimenez, David F MD [NS] - **Spec Exp:** Pediatric Neurosurgery; Craniosynostosis; Endoscopic Strip Craniectomy; Spinal Surgery; **Hospital:** Univ Hlth Syst-San Antonio, St. Luke's Baptist Hosp; **Address:** Dept of Neurosurgery, 7703 Floyd Curl Drive, MC 7843, San Antonio, TX 78229-3900; **Phone:** 210-567-5625; **Board Cert:** Neurological Surgery 1995; Pediatric Neurological Surgery 2007; **Med School:** Temple Univ 1985; **Resid:** Neurological Surgery, Temple Univ Hosp 1991; **Fellow:** Pediatric Neurological Surgery, Montefiore Med Ctr 1992; **Fac Appt:** Prof NS, Univ Tex, San Antonio

Kim, Daniel H MD [NS] - **Spec Exp:** Spinal Surgery; Peripheral Nerve Surgery; **Hospital:** St. Luke's Episcopal Hosp-Houston; **Address:** Baylor Dept Neurosurgery, 1709 Dryden Rd, Ste 750, Houston, TX 77030; **Phone:** 713-798-4696; **Board Cert:** Neurological Surgery 1998; **Med School:** Tulane Univ 1989; **Resid:** Neurological Surgery, LSU Med Ctr 1995; **Fellow:** Spinal Surgery, Univ Fla 1998; **Fac Appt:** Prof NS, Baylor Coll Med

Kim, Dong H MD [NS] - **Spec Exp:** Cerebrovascular Surgery; Aneurysm-Cerebral; Brain Tumors; Arteriovenous Malformations; **Hospital:** Meml Hermann Hosp - Texas Med Ctr; **Address:** UT Neurosurgery, 6400 Fannin St, Ste 2800, Houston, TX 77030; **Phone:** 713-704-7100; **Board Cert:** Neurological Surgery 2001; **Med School:** UCSF 1990; **Resid:** Neurological Surgery, UCSF Med Ctr 1996; **Fellow:** Cerebrovascular & Skull Base Surgery, Univ Florida 1997; **Fac Appt:** Prof NS, Univ Tex, Houston

Krisht, Ali F MD [NS] - **Spec Exp:** Skull Base Surgery; Meningioma; Vascular Neurosurgery; **Hospital:** St. Vincent Health System; **Address:** Arkansas Neuroscience Inst, 5 St Vincent Circle, Ste 503, Little Rock, AR 72205; **Phone:** 501-552-6412; **Board Cert:** Neurological Surgery 2010; **Med School:** Amer Univ Beirut 1985; **Resid:** Neurological Surgery, Emory Univ Affil Hosp 1994; **Fac Appt:** Prof NS, Univ Ark

Lang Jr, Frederick F MD [NS] - **Spec Exp:** Brain & Spinal Tumors; Gliomas; Brain Tumors-Complex; Pediatric Neurosurgery; **Hospital:** UT MD Anderson Cancer Ctr; **Address:** Univ Texas MD Anderson Cancer Ctr, 1515 Holcombe Blvd, Unit 442, Houston, TX 77030; **Phone:** 713-792-6600; **Board Cert:** Neurological Surgery 2000; **Med School:** Yale Univ 1988; **Resid:** Neurological Surgery, NYU Med Ctr 1995; **Fellow:** Neurosurgical Oncology, MD Anderson Cancer Ctr 1996; **Fac Appt:** Prof NS, Univ Tex, Houston

Neurological Surgery

Lemole, G Michael MD [NS] - **Spec Exp:** Skull Base Surgery; Stereotactic Radiosurgery; Cerebrovascular Surgery; Minimally Invasive Surgery; **Hospital:** Univ Med Ctr - Tucson; **Address:** Univ Arizona Medical Ctr, Neurosurgery PO Box 245070, 1501 N Campbell Ave, Tucson, AZ 85724-5070; **Phone:** 520-694-6144; **Board Cert:** Neurological Surgery 2007; **Med School:** Univ Pennsylvania 1995; **Resid:** Neurological Surgery, St Josephs Hosp Med Ctr 2002; **Fellow:** Cerebrovascular & Skull Base Surgery, Barrow Neuro Inst 2000; **Fac Appt:** Assoc Prof S, Univ Ariz Coll Med

Luerssen, Thomas G MD [NS] - **Spec Exp:** Pediatric Neurosurgery; Brain Injury-Traumatic; **Hospital:** Texas Chldns Hosp; **Address:** Texas Children's Hosp, Ped Neurosurgery, Clinical Care Center, Ste 1230, 6621 Fannin St, MC CC 1230.01, Houston, TX 77030-2399; **Phone:** 832-822-3950; **Board Cert:** Neurological Surgery 1985; Pediatric Neurological Surgery 2005; **Med School:** Indiana Univ 1976; **Resid:** Neurological Surgery, Indiana Univ Hosp 1981; **Fellow:** Pediatric Neurological Surgery, Chldns Hosp 1984; **Fac Appt:** Prof NS, Baylor Coll Med

Mapstone, Timothy B MD [NS] - **Spec Exp:** Brain Tumors-Adult & Pediatric; Pediatric Neurosurgery; Congenital Anomalies; **Hospital:** OU Med Ctr, Chldns Hosp OU Med Ctr; **Address:** Univ OK Hlth Sci Ctr, Dept Neurosurgery, 1000 N Lincoln Blvd, Ste 400, Oklahoma City, OK 73104; **Phone:** 405-271-4912; **Board Cert:** Neurological Surgery 1985; Pediatric Neurological Surgery 2005; **Med School:** Case West Res Univ 1977; **Resid:** Neurological Surgery, Univ Hosps 1983; **Fellow:** Research, Case West Reserve Univ; **Fac Appt:** Prof NS, Univ Okla Coll Med

Mickey, Bruce E MD [NS] - **Spec Exp:** Brain Tumors; Skull Base Surgery; Pituitary Tumors; **Hospital:** UT Southwestern Med Ctr at Dallas, Parkland Hlth & Hosp Sys; **Address:** UTSW Med Ctr, Dept Neurosurgery, 5323 Harry Hines Blvd, Dallas, TX 75390-8855; **Phone:** 214-645-2300; **Board Cert:** Neurological Surgery 1987; **Med School:** Univ Tex SW, Dallas 1978; **Resid:** Neurological Surgery, Parkland Meml Hosp 1984; **Fellow:** Research, Righospitalet 1983; **Fac Appt:** Prof NS, Univ Tex SW, Dallas

Samson, Duke S MD [NS] - **Spec Exp:** Vascular Neurosurgery; Cerebrovascular Disease; Arteriovenous Malformations; **Hospital:** UT Southwestern Med Ctr at Dallas, Parkland Hlth & Hosp Sys; **Address:** Univ Tex SW Med Ctr, Dept Neuro Surg, 5323 Harry Hines Blvd, Dallas, TX 75390-8855; **Phone:** 214-645-2300; **Board Cert:** Neurological Surgery 1978; **Med School:** Washington Univ, St Louis 1969; **Resid:** Neurological Surgery, Univ Texas SW Med Ctr 1975; **Fellow:** Neurological Surgery, Ctr Medico-Chirurgical Fech 1973; Neurological Surgery, Univ Zurich 1973; **Fac Appt:** Prof NS, Univ Tex SW, Dallas

Sawaya, Raymond MD [NS] - **Spec Exp:** Brain Tumors; **Hospital:** UT MD Anderson Cancer Ctr, Baylor Clinic & Hosp-Houston; **Address:** MD Anderson Cancer Ctr, 1515 Holcombe Blvd, Unit 442, Houston, TX 77030; **Phone:** 713-792-2400; **Board Cert:** Neurological Surgery 1985; **Med School:** Lebanon 1974; **Resid:** Neurological Surgery, Univ Cincinnati Med Ctr 1980; Neurological Surgery, Johns Hopkins Med Ctr 1981; **Fellow:** Neuro-Oncology, Natl Inst Hlth 1982; **Fac Appt:** Prof NS, Univ Tex, Houston

Sklar, Frederick H MD [NS] - **Spec Exp:** Pediatric Neurosurgery; Craniofacial Surgery; Hydrocephalus; **Hospital:** Chldns Med Ctr of Dallas, Texas Scottish Rite Hosp for Chldn; **Address:** Neurosurgeons for Chldn, 1935 Med District Drive, Dallas, TX 75235; **Phone:** 214-456-6660; **Board Cert:** Neurological Surgery 1978; **Med School:** Johns Hopkins Univ 1970; **Resid:** Neurological Surgery, Johns Hopkins Hosp 1976; **Fac Appt:** Assoc Clin Prof NS, Univ Tex SW, Dallas

Spetzler, Robert F MD [NS] - **Spec Exp:** Skull Base Tumors & Surgery; Cerebrovascular Surgery; **Hospital:** St. Joseph's Hosp & Med Ctr - Phoenix; **Address:** Barrow Neurosurgical Assocs, 2910 N Third Ave, Phoenix, AZ 85013; **Phone:** 602-406-3489; **Board Cert:** Neurological Surgery 1979; **Med School:** Northwestern Univ 1971; **Resid:** Neurological Surgery, UCSF Med Ctr 1976; **Fac Appt:** Prof S, Univ Ariz Coll Med

Walsh, John W MD/PhD [NS] - **Spec Exp:** Pediatric Neurosurgery; Epilepsy; Craniofacial Surgery/Reconstruction; Vascular Malformations; **Hospital:** Tulane Med Ctr; **Address:** Pediatric Specialties, 1415 Tulane Ave Fl 4, New Orleans, LA 70112; **Phone:** 504-988-8000; **Board Cert:** Neurological Surgery 1976; Pediatric Neurological Surgery ; **Med School:** UCLA 1969; **Resid:** Neurological Surgery, Childrens Hosp/Brigham Hosp 1974; **Fellow:** Neurological Surgery, Lahey Clin Fdn 1975; **Fac Appt:** Prof NS, Tulane Univ

Yonas, Howard MD [NS] - **Spec Exp:** Vascular Neurosurgery; Stroke; Skull Base Surgery; Trigeminal Neuralgia; **Hospital:** Univ Hosp - New Mexico; **Address:** 1 Univ of New Mexico, Dept Neurological Surgery, MSC10-5615, Albuquerque, NM 87131-0001; **Phone:** 505-272-9494; **Board Cert:** Neurological Surgery 1981; **Med School:** Ohio State Univ 1970; **Resid:** Neurological Surgery, Case West Res 1976; **Fellow:** Univ Pittsburgh 1978; **Fac Appt:** Prof NS, Univ New Mexico

West Coast and Pacific

Adler Jr, John R MD [NS] - **Spec Exp:** Stereotactic Radiosurgery; Brain Tumors; Acoustic Neuroma; **Hospital:** Stanford Univ Hosp & Clinics; **Address:** Stanford Univ Med Ctr, Dept Neurosurg, 300 Pasteur Drive R Bldg - rm 205, Stanford, CA 94305-5327; **Phone:** 650-723-5573; **Board Cert:** Neurological Surgery 1990; **Med School:** Harvard Med Sch 1980; **Resid:** Neurological Surgery, Chldns Hosp 1987; Neurological Surgery, Mass Genl Hosp 1985; **Fellow:** Cerebrovascular Disease, Karolinska Inst 1986; **Fac Appt:** Prof NS, Stanford Univ

Amar, Arun P MD/PhD [NS] - **Spec Exp:** Interventional Neuroradiology; Stroke; Stroke Prevention; **Hospital:** Keck Med Ctr of USC (page 75); **Address:** 1200 N State St, Ste 3300, Los Angeles, CA 90033; **Phone:** 323-442-5720; **Board Cert:** Neurological Surgery 2005; **Med School:** UCSF 1993; **Resid:** Neurological Surgery, USC Univ Hosp 2000; **Fellow:** Interventional Neuroradiology, USC Univ Hosp 2003; **Fac Appt:** Assoc Prof NS, USC-Keck School of Medicine

Ames, Christopher P MD [NS] - **Spec Exp:** Spinal Trauma; Spinal Cord Tumors; Spinal Reconstructive Surgery; **Hospital:** UCSF Med Ctr; **Address:** Spine Center, 400 Parnassus Ave, rm A311, San Francisco, CA 94143-0332; **Phone:** 866-817-7463; **Board Cert:** Neurological Surgery 2006; **Med School:** UCLA-David Geffen Sch Med 1994; **Resid:** Neurological Surgery, UCSD Med Ctr 2000; **Fellow:** Spinal Surgery, Barrow Neurological Inst 2002; **Fac Appt:** Assoc Clin Prof NS, UCLA-David Geffen Sch Med

Apuzzo, Michael L J MD [NS] - **Spec Exp:** Brain Tumors; Epilepsy/Seizure Disorders; Stereotactic Radiosurgery; **Hospital:** LAC & USC Med Ctr, USC Norris Cancer Hosp (page 75); **Address:** 1420 San Pablo Street, PMBA106, Los Angeles, CA 90033-1029; **Phone:** 323-226-7421; **Board Cert:** Neurological Surgery 1975; **Med School:** Boston Univ 1965; **Resid:** Neurological Surgery, Hartford Hosp 1970; Neurological Surgery, Hartford Hosp 1973; **Fellow:** Neurological Physiology, Yale Univ Hosp 1972; **Fac Appt:** Prof NS, USC Sch Med

Badie, Behnam MD [NS] - **Spec Exp:** Brain Tumors; **Hospital:** City of Hope Natl Med Ctr; **Address:** City of Hope Med Ctr, Dept Neurosurgery, 1500 E Duarte Rd, Duarte, CA 91010; **Phone:** 626-471-7100; **Board Cert:** Neurological Surgery 1998; **Med School:** UCLA 1989; **Resid:** Neurological Surgery, UCLA Med Ctr 1996; **Fac Appt:** Assoc Prof NS, UCLA

Berger, Mitchel S MD [NS] - **Spec Exp:** Brain & Spinal Cord Tumors; Pituitary Tumors; Neuro-Oncology; Pain Management; **Hospital:** UCSF Med Ctr; **Address:** UCSF Med Ctr, Dept Neurosurgery, 505 Parnassus Avenue, M-786, San Francisco, CA 94143-0112; **Phone:** 415-353-3933; **Board Cert:** Neurological Surgery 1991; **Med School:** Univ Miami Sch Med 1979; **Resid:** Neurological Surgery, UCSF Med Ctr 1984; **Fellow:** Neuro-Oncology, UCSF Med Ctr 1985; Pediatric Neurological Surgery, Hosp Sick Chldn 1986; **Fac Appt:** Prof NS, UCSF

Neurological Surgery

Black, Keith L MD [NS] - **Spec Exp:** Brain Tumors; Pineal Tumors; Spinal Tumors; Acoustic Neuroma; **Hospital:** Cedars-Sinai Med Ctr; **Address:** Cedars-Sinai Med Ctr, Dept Neurosugery, 8631 W Third St, Ste 800 East, Los Angeles, CA 90048; **Phone:** 310-423-7900; **Board Cert:** Neurological Surgery 1990; **Med School:** Univ Mich Med Sch 1981; **Resid:** Neurological Surgery, Univ Michigan Med Ctr 1987; **Fac Appt:** Prof NS

Boggan, James E MD [NS] - **Spec Exp:** Skull Base Tumors & Surgery; Pediatric Neurosurgery; **Hospital:** UC Davis Med Ctr; **Address:** Dept Neurological Surgery, 4860 Y St, Ste 3740, Sacramento, CA 95817-2307; **Phone:** 916-734-2371; **Board Cert:** Neurological Surgery 1985; **Med School:** Univ Chicago-Pritzker Sch Med 1976; **Resid:** Neurological Surgery, UCSF Med Ctr 1982; **Fac Appt:** Prof NS, UC Davis

Bray Jr, Robert S MD [NS] - **Spec Exp:** Minimally Invasive Spinal Surgery; **Address:** DISC Sports & Spine Center, 13160 Mindanao Way, Ste 300, Marina del Rey, CA 90292; **Phone:** 310-574-0400; **Board Cert:** Neurological Surgery 1991; **Med School:** Baylor Coll Med 1980; **Resid:** Neurological Surgery, Baylor Affil Hosp 1986

Burchiel, Kim J MD [NS] - **Spec Exp:** Pain Management; Stereotactic Radiosurgery; Epilepsy; Movement Disorders; **Hospital:** OR Hlth & Sci Univ; **Address:** OHSU, Dept Neurosurgery, 3303 SW Bond Ave, MC CH8N, Portland, OR 97239; **Phone:** 503-494-4314; **Board Cert:** Neurological Surgery 1984; **Med School:** UCSD 1976; **Resid:** Neurological Surgery, Univ Wash Med Ctr 1982; **Fac Appt:** Prof NS, Oregon Hlth & Sci Univ

Chen, Thomas C MD [NS] - **Spec Exp:** Brain & Spinal Tumors; Brain Tumors-Metastatic; Gliomas; Microdiscectomy; **Hospital:** USC Norris Cancer Hosp (page 75), Keck Med Ctr of USC (page 75); **Address:** USC Health Consultation Clinic 2, 1520 San Pablo St, rm 3800, MC 9197, Los Angeles, CA 90033; **Phone:** 323-442-5720; **Board Cert:** Neurological Surgery 2000; **Med School:** UCSF 1988; **Resid:** Neurological Surgery, USC Univ Hosp 1995; **Fellow:** Spinal Surgery, Med Coll Wisconsin 1997; **Fac Appt:** Assoc Prof NS, USC-Keck School of Medicine

Danielpour, Moise MD [NS] - **Spec Exp:** Pediatric Neurosurgery; Brain Tumors; Epilepsy; Craniofacial Surgery; **Hospital:** Cedars-Sinai Med Ctr; **Address:** Cedars-Sinai Medical Center, Maxine Dunitz Neurosurgical Institute, 8631 W Third St, Ste 800 E, Los Angeles, CA 90048; **Phone:** 310-423-7900; **Board Cert:** Neurological Surgery 2004; **Med School:** Albert Einstein Coll Med 1992; **Resid:** Neurological Surgery, Northwestern Univ Hosp 1999; **Fellow:** Pediatric Neurological Surgery, UCSF Med Ctr 2000

Edwards, Michael S MD [NS] - **Spec Exp:** Brain Tumors-Pediatric; Pediatric Neurosurgery; Stereotactic Radiosurgery; **Hospital:** Lucile Packard Chldn's Hosp; **Address:** Pediatric Neurosurgery, 300 Pasteur Drive, Ste R211, MC 5327, Stanford, CA 94305; **Phone:** 650-497-8775; **Board Cert:** Neurological Surgery 1980; Pediatric Neurological Surgery 2006; **Med School:** Tulane Univ 1970; **Resid:** Neurological Surgery, Oschner Fdn Hosp/Charity Hosp 1977; **Fellow:** Pediatric Neuro-Oncology, UCSF Med Ctr 1978; **Fac Appt:** Prof NS, Stanford Univ

Ellenbogen, Richard MD [NS] - **Spec Exp:** Pediatric Neurosurgery; Chiari's Deformity; Brain Tumors; **Hospital:** Seattle Chldns Hosp, Univ Wash Med Ctr; **Address:** 4800 Sand Point Way NE, MS W-7729, Seattle, WA 98145; **Phone:** 206-987-2544; **Board Cert:** Neurological Surgery 1992; Pediatric Neurological Surgery 2009; **Med School:** Brown Univ 1983; **Resid:** Neurological Surgery, Brigham Womens Hosp/Childrens Hosp 1989; **Fac Appt:** Prof NS, Univ Wash

Frazee, John G MD [NS] - **Spec Exp:** Vascular Neurosurgery; Spinal Surgery; Neuro-Endoscopy; Chiari's Deformity; **Hospital:** UCLA Ronald Reagan Med Ctr, VA Greater Los Angeles Hthecare Sys; **Address:** UCLA Neurosurgery, 750 Charles E Young Drive, Los Angeles, CA 90095-7039; **Phone:** 310-206-1231; **Board Cert:** Neurological Surgery 1984; **Med School:** Univ Rochester 1975; **Resid:** Neurological Surgery, UCLA Med Ctr 1982; **Fac Appt:** Clin Prof NS, UCLA

Giannotta, Steven L MD [NS] - **Spec Exp:** Aneurysm-Cerebral; Skull Base Tumors; Acoustic Neuroma; **Hospital:** Keck Med Ctr of USC (page 75), LAC & USC Med Ctr; **Address:** 1520 San Pablo St, Ste 3800, Los Angeles, CA 90033; **Phone:** 323-442-5720; **Board Cert:** Neurological Surgery 1980; **Med School:** Univ Mich Med Sch 1972; **Resid:** Neurological Surgery, Univ Michigan Med Ctr 1978; **Fac Appt:** Prof NS, USC Sch Med

Gupta, Nalin MD/PhD [NS] - **Spec Exp:** Pediatric Neurosurgery; **Hospital:** UCSF Med Ctr; **Address:** 400 Parnassus Ave, rm A808, San Francisco, CA 94143; **Phone:** 415-353-7500; **Board Cert:** Neurological Surgery 2002; Pediatric Neurological Surgery 2003; **Med School:** Univ Toronto 1987; **Resid:** Neurological Surgery, Univ Ottawa 1989; Neurological Surgery, Univ Toronto 1997; **Fellow:** Pediatric Neurological Surgery, Hosp for Sick Chldn 1998; **Fac Appt:** Asst Prof NS, UCSF

Harsh IV, Griffith R MD [NS] - **Spec Exp:** Brain & Spinal Cord Tumors; Skull Base Tumors; Pituitary Tumors; Acoustic Neuroma; **Hospital:** Stanford Univ Hosp & Clinics; **Address:** Stanford Center for Advanced Medicine, 875 Blake Wilbur Drive, MC 5826, Stanford, CA 94305; **Phone:** 650-723-7093; **Board Cert:** Neurological Surgery 1989; **Med School:** Harvard Med Sch 1980; **Resid:** Neurological Surgery, UCSF Med Ctr 1986; **Fellow:** Neuro-Oncology, UCSF Med Ctr 1987; **Fac Appt:** Prof NS, Stanford Univ

Kassam, Amin MD [NS] - **Spec Exp:** Skull Base Tumors & Surgery; Cranial Nerve Disorders; Cerebrovascular Surgery; Endoscopic Surgery; **Hospital:** St. John's Hlth Ctr, Santa Monica; **Address:** John Wayne Cancer Inst, 2200 Santa Monica Blvd, Santa Monica, CA 90404; **Phone:** 310-582-7450; **Med School:** Univ Toronto 1991; **Resid:** Neurological Surgery, Univ Ottawa Med Ctr 1997

Levy, Michael L MD/PhD [NS] - **Spec Exp:** Pediatric Neurosurgery; **Hospital:** Rady Children's Hosp - San Diego, UCSD Med Ctr; **Address:** 8010 Frost St, Ste 502, San Diego, CA 92123; **Phone:** 858-966-8574; **Board Cert:** Neurological Surgery 1997; Pediatric Neurological Surgery 1998; **Med School:** UCSF 1986; **Resid:** Neurological Surgery, USC Med Ctr 1993; **Fellow:** Pediatric Neurological Surgery, Chldns Hosp 1995; Physiology; **Fac Appt:** Prof NS, USC Sch Med

Liau, Linda M MD/PhD [NS] - **Spec Exp:** Brain Tumors; Neuro-Oncology; **Hospital:** UCLA Ronald Reagan Med Ctr; **Address:** CHS 74-145, Box 956901, 10833 Le Conte Ave, Los Angeles, CA 90095-6901; **Phone:** 310-267-2621; **Board Cert:** Neurological Surgery 2002; **Med School:** Stanford Univ 1991; **Resid:** Neurological Surgery, UCLA Med Ctr 1998; **Fellow:** Neuro-Oncology, UCLA Med Ctr 1998; **Fac Appt:** Prof NS, UCLA

Liker, Mark A MD [NS] - **Spec Exp:** Spinal Surgery; Deep Brain Stimulation; **Hospital:** Henry Mayo Newhall Memorial Hosp, Keck Med Ctr of USC (page 75); **Address:** 25751 McBean Pkwy, Ste 305, Valencia, CA 91355; **Phone:** 661-799-2542; **Board Cert:** Neurological Surgery 2005; **Med School:** SUNY Downstate 1995; **Resid:** Neurological Surgery, USC Med Ctr 2001; **Fellow:** Spinal Surgery, USC Med Ctr 1999; **Fac Appt:** Asst Prof NS, USC-Keck School of Medicine

Linskey, Mark E MD [NS] - **Spec Exp:** Brain Tumors; Stereotactic Radiosurgery; Skull Base Surgery; Trigeminal Neuralgia; **Hospital:** UC Irvine Med Ctr; **Address:** UCI Med Ctr, Dept Neurosurgery-Route 81, 101 The City Drive S Bldg 56 - Ste 400, Orange, CA 92868-3298; **Phone:** 714-456-6392; **Board Cert:** Neurological Surgery 1996; **Med School:** Columbia P&S 1986; **Resid:** Neurological Surgery, Univ Pittsburgh Hlth Ctrs 1993; **Fellow:** Neuro-Oncology, Ludwig Inst Cancer Rsch/Univ Coll London 1994; Neuro-Oncology, Pittsburgh Cancer Inst/Univ Pittsburgh 1992; **Fac Appt:** Assoc Prof NS, UC Irvine

Neurological Surgery

Liu, Charles Y MD [NS] - **Spec Exp:** Epilepsy; Skull Base Tumors & Surgery; Stereotactic Radio-surgery; Meningioma; **Hospital:** Keck Med Ctr of USC (page 75); **Address:** USC Dept Neuro-surgery, 1200 N State St, Ste 3300, Los Angeles, CA 90033; **Phone:** 323-442-5720; **Board Cert:** Neurological Surgery 2007; **Med School:** Yale Univ 1996; **Resid:** Neurological Surgery, LAC/USC Med Ctr 2001; **Fellow:** Spinal Surgery, LAC/USC Med Ctr 2003; **Fac Appt:** Assoc Prof NS, USC-Keck School of Medicine

Mamelak, Adam N MD [NS] - **Spec Exp:** Brain Tumors; Epilepsy; Spinal Tumors; **Hospital:** Cedars-Sinai Med Ctr; **Address:** Maxine Dunitz Neurosurgical Institute, 8631 W Third St, Ste 800-East, Los Angeles, CA 90048; **Phone:** 310-423-7900; **Board Cert:** Neurological Surgery 2000; **Med School:** Harvard Med Sch 1990; **Resid:** Neurological Surgery, UCSF Med Ctr 1994; **Fellow:** Epilepsy, UCSF Epilepsy Research Lab 1996

Martin, Neil A MD [NS] - **Spec Exp:** Vascular Neurosurgery; Aneurysm-Cerebral; Endoscopic Surgery; Microvascular Surgery; **Hospital:** UCLA Ronald Reagan Med Ctr; **Address:** UCLA Dept Neurosurgery, Box 957039, Los Angeles, CA 90095-7039; **Phone:** 310-825-5482; **Board Cert:** Neurological Surgery 1989; **Med School:** Med Coll VA 1978; **Resid:** Neurological Surgery, UCSF Med Ctr 1984; **Fellow:** Neurological Vascular Surgery, Barrow Neuro Inst 1985; **Fac Appt:** Prof NS, UCLA

Mayberg, Marc R MD [NS] - **Spec Exp:** Pituitary Surgery; Stroke/Cerebrovascular Disease; Skull Base Tumors; Acoustic Neuroma; **Hospital:** Swedish Med Ctr-First Hill-Seattle; **Address:** Seattle Neuroscience Inst, 550 17th Ave, Ste 500, James Tower, Seattle, WA 98122; **Phone:** 206-320-2800; **Board Cert:** Neurological Surgery 1988; **Med School:** Mayo Med Sch 1978; **Resid:** Neurological Surgery, Mass Genl Hosp 1984; **Fellow:** Neurological Surgery, Natl Hosp for Nervous Dis 1985

McDermott, Michael W MD [NS] - **Spec Exp:** Brain Tumors; Meningioma; Stereotactic Radio-surgery; Skull Base Tumors; **Hospital:** UCSF Med Ctr; **Address:** UCSF Dept Neurosurgery, 400 Par-nassus Ave, rm A808, San Francisco, CA 94143; **Phone:** 415-353-7500; **Board Cert:** Neurological Surgery 2003; **Med School:** Univ Toronto 1982; **Resid:** Neurological Surgery, Univ British Columbia 1988; **Fellow:** Neuro-Oncology, UCSF Med Ctr 1990; **Fac Appt:** Prof NS, UCSF

Neuwelt, Edward A MD [NS] - **Spec Exp:** Neuro-Oncology; Brain Tumors; **Hospital:** OR Hlth & Sci Univ; **Address:** Oregon Hlth Sci Univ, Dept Neurosurgery, 3181 SW Sam Jackson Pk Rd, MC-L603, Portland, OR 97239; **Phone:** 503-494-5626; **Board Cert:** Neurological Surgery 1980; **Med School:** Univ Colorado 1972; **Resid:** Neurological Surgery, Univ Tex SW Med Sch 1978; **Fellow:** Neuro-Oncology, Natl Canc Inst/NIH 1976; **Fac Appt:** Prof NS, Oregon Hlth & Sci Univ

Ojemann, Jeffrey G MD [NS] - **Spec Exp:** Pediatric Neurosurgery; Brain Tumors; Hydro-cephalus; Epilepsy; **Hospital:** Seattle Chldns Hosp, Univ Wash Med Ctr; **Address:** 4800 Sand Point Way NE, Ste W7729, Seattle, WA 98145; **Phone:** 206-987-2544; **Board Cert:** Neurological Surgery 2002; **Med School:** Washington Univ, St Louis 1992; **Resid:** Neurological Surgery, Barnes Jewish Hosp 1998; **Fellow:** Pediatric Neurological Surgery, Chldn's Hosp 2000; Neurological Surgery, Univ Wash Med Ctr 2002; **Fac Appt:** Assoc Prof NS, Univ Wash

Ott, Kenneth H MD [NS] - **Spec Exp:** Brain Tumors; Stereotactic Radiosurgery; **Hospital:** Scripps Meml Hosp - La Jolla; **Address:** Neurosurgical Med Clin, 2100 Fifth Ave, Ste 200, San Diego, CA 92101; **Phone:** 619-297-4481 x102; **Board Cert:** Neurological Surgery 1980; **Med School:** UCSF 1970; **Resid:** Surgery, Mass Genl Hosp 1972; Neurological Surgery, Mass Genl Hosp 1976; **Fac Appt:** Assoc Clin Prof S, UCSD

Sekhar, Laligam N MD [NS] - **Spec Exp:** Aneurysm-Cerebral; Arteriovenous Malformations; Brain Tumors; Skull Base Tumors; **Hospital:** Harborview Med Ctr, Univ Wash Med Ctr; **Address:** HMC-Neurosurgery, 9th & Jeff Bldg Fl 5, 908 Jefferson St, Seattle, WA 98104-2499; **Phone:** 206-744-9300; **Board Cert:** Neurological Surgery 1986; **Med School:** India 1973; **Resid:** Neurology, Univ Cincinnati Med Ctr 1977; Neurology, Univ Pittsburgh Med Ctr 1982; **Fellow:** Skull Base Surgery, Norstadt Krankenhaus 1983; Cerebrovascular Neurosurgery, Univ Zurich Hospital; **Fac Appt:** Prof NS, Univ Wash

Sekhon, Lali MD/PhD [NS] - **Spec Exp:** Spinal Surgery; Spinal Disorders-Degenerative; Spinal Disc Replacement; Minimally Invasive Spinal Surgery; **Hospital:** Renown Reg Med Ctr, St. Mary's Reg Med Ctr; **Address:** Nevada Neurosurgery, 75 Pringle Way, Ste 1007, Reno, NV 89502; **Phone:** 775-657-8844; **Med School:** Australia 1994; **Resid:** Neurological Surgery, Univ Sidney Med Ctr 1997; **Fellow:** Neurological Surgery, Mayo Clinic 1999; Neurological Orthopaedic Surgery, Toronto Western Hosp 2000

Selden, Nathan R MD/PhD [NS] - **Spec Exp:** Pediatric Neurosurgery; Brain Tumors-Pediatric; Stem Cell Transplantation; Chiari's Deformity; **Hospital:** Doernbecher Chldns Hosp/OHSU, OR Hlth & Sci Univ; **Address:** 3303 SW Bond Ave, MC CH8N, Portland, OR 97239; **Phone:** 503-494-4314; **Board Cert:** Neurological Surgery 2004; **Med School:** Harvard Med Sch 1993; **Resid:** Neurological Surgery, Univ Michigan Med Ctr 1999; **Fellow:** Pediatric Neurological Surgery, Northwestern Meml Hosp 2000; **Fac Appt:** Prof NS, Oregon Hlth & Sci Univ

Shuer, Lawrence M MD [NS] - **Spec Exp:** Pediatric Neurosurgery; Craniosynostosis; Epilepsy; Chiari's Deformity; **Hospital:** Stanford Univ Hosp & Clinics, Lucile Packard Chldn's Hosp; **Address:** Stanford Univ Dept Neurosurgery, 300 Pasteur Drive, rm R229, MC 5327, Stanford, CA 94305-5327; **Phone:** 650-723-5574; **Board Cert:** Neurological Surgery 1986; **Med School:** Univ Mich Med Sch 1978; **Resid:** Neurological Surgery, Stanford Univ Med Ctr 1984; **Fac Appt:** Prof NS, Stanford Univ

Silbergeld, Daniel MD [NS] - **Spec Exp:** Brain Tumors; Brain Tumors-Metastatic; Brain Mapping; **Hospital:** Univ Wash Med Ctr; **Address:** Univ Wash Med Ctr, Dept Neurosurg, 1959 NE Pacific, Box 356470, Seattle, WA 98195; **Phone:** 206-598-5637; **Board Cert:** Neurological Surgery 1995; **Med School:** Univ Cincinnati 1984; **Resid:** Neurological Surgery, Univ Wash Med Ctr 1990; Research, Univ Wash Med Ctr 1988; **Fellow:** Neuro-Oncology, Univ Wash Med Ctr 1991; Epilepsy, Univ Wash Med Ctr 1991; **Fac Appt:** Assoc Prof NS, Univ Wash

Steinberg, Gary K MD/PhD [NS] - **Spec Exp:** Aneurysm-Cerebral; Moya Moya Disease; Arteriovenous Malformations; Cerebrovascular Surgery; **Hospital:** Stanford Univ Hosp & Clinics; **Address:** Stanford Univ Dept Neurosurgery, 300 Pasteur Drive, rm R281, Stanford, CA 94305-5327; **Phone:** 650-725-5562; **Board Cert:** Neurological Surgery 1989; **Med School:** Stanford Univ 1980; **Resid:** Neuropathology, Stanford Univ Med Ctr 1982; Neurological Surgery, Stanford Univ Med Ctr 1987; **Fellow:** Cerebrovascular Neurosurgery, Univ West Ontario 1985; **Fac Appt:** Prof NS, Stanford Univ

Sun, Peter P MD [NS] - **Spec Exp:** Pediatric Neurosurgery; Congenital Cranial Deformities; Brain Tumors; **Hospital:** Chldns Hosp - Oakland; **Address:** 744 52nd St, Ste 5203, Oakland, CA 94609; **Phone:** 510-428-3319; **Board Cert:** Neurological Surgery 2002; Pediatric Neurological Surgery 2006; **Med School:** Columbia P&S 1991; **Resid:** Neurological Surgery, UC Davis Med Ctr 1994; Neurological Surgery, Yale-New Haven Hosp 1996; **Fellow:** Neurological Surgery, NYU Med Ctr 1997; Pediatric Neurological Surgery, Childrens Hosp 1998; **Fac Appt:** Asst Clin Prof NS, UCSF

Neurological Surgery

Yu, John S MD [NS] - **Spec Exp:** Brain Tumors; Spinal Tumors; Clinical Trials; Spinal Surgery; **Hospital:** Cedars-Sinai Med Ctr; **Address:** Maxine Dunitz Neurosurgical Institute, 8631 W 3rd St, Ste 800-East, Los Angeles, CA 90048; **Phone:** 310-423-7900; **Board Cert:** Neurological Surgery 2002; **Med School:** Harvard Med Sch 1990; **Resid:** Neurological Surgery, Mass General Hosp 1997

Cleveland Clinic

Every life deserves world class care.

Cleveland Clinic
Neurological Institute
9500 Euclid Avenue
Cleveland, OH 44195

Neurological Surgery

Cleveland Clinic Neurological Institute employs a multidisciplinary disease-specific focus, combining more than 300 medical, surgical and research specialists who treat children and adults with neurological and neurobehavioral disorders. Our clinical expertise, academic achievement and innovative research has earned the Neurological Institute an international reputation for excellence. *U.S.News & World Report* consistently ranks our neurology and neurosurgery and pediatric neurology/neurosurgery programs among the top 10 in the nation.

Our unique and collaborative clinical structure allows us to deliver coordinated, comprehensive and multidisciplinary care to our patients through more efficient treatment decision-making and consultation for complex cases. Major advances in the treatment of brain tumors, epilepsy, mood disorders, stroke, movement disorders, pain and spinal disorders are improving quality of life and survival for thousands of our patients. For those diseases resistant to available treatments, we are confident our innovative model of medicine will speed research and advances in treatment, resulting in better clinical care and more rapid breakthroughs in the full range of neurological and behavioral disorders.

Comprehensive Neurological Care

Cleveland Clinic offers expert diagnostic and treatment options for all neurologic conditions affecting children and adults, including Alzheimer's disease, aneurysms, arteriovenous malformations, back and neck disorders, brain and spine tumors, epilepsy, hydrocephalus, metastatic tumors, mild cognitive impairment, multiple sclerosis, movement disorders, neurofibromatosis, Parkinson's disease, pediatric and congential neurological disorders, pituitary disorders, sleep disorders and stroke.

clevelandclinic.org/
neurosurgerytopdocs

Offering Same-Day Appointments
Call 800.274.2009.

Treatment Guides

Cleveland Clinic has developed comprehensive treatment guides for many diseases and conditions. To download our free treatment guides, visit clevelandclinic.org/treatmentguides.

Online Medical Second Opinion

Cleveland Clinic's My**Consult** Online Medical Second Opinion program securely connects patients to our physician specialists for more than 1,000 life-changing or life-threatening diagnoses all by the click of a mouse. To learn more, log onto eclevelandclinic.org/myconsult or call 800.223.2273, ext. 43223.

Special Assistance for Out-of-State Patients

Cleveland Clinic Global Patient Services offers a complimentary Medical Concierge service for patients who travel from outside of Ohio. Call 800.223.2273, ext. 55580 or email medicalconcierge@ccf.org.

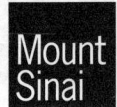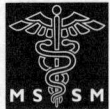

**MOUNT SINAI
SCHOOL OF
MEDICINE**

**THE MOUNT SINAI MEDICAL CENTER
NEUROSURGERY**
One Gustave L. Levy Place
Fifth Avenue and 100th Street
New York, NY 10029-6574
Physician Referral: 1-800-MD-SINAI (637-4624)
www.mountsinai.org/neurosurgery

THE DEPARTMENT OF NEUROSURGERY at Mount Sinai, established in 1920, has earned a distinguished international reputation. Areas of clinical expertise include the treatment of skull base tumors, primary and metastatic brain tumors, pituitary adenomas and acoustic neuromas, and deep brain stimulation for movement disorders. The department also provides advanced endovascular and microsurgical treatment of aneurysms, treatments for arteriovenous malformations and stroke, microvascular decompression for trigeminal neuralgia and hemifacial spasm, and advanced minimally invasive resection of spine and spinal cord tumors and degenerative spine disease.

The Comprehensive Brain Tumor Program collaborates with The Tisch Cancer Institute and the Departments of Neurology, Radiation Oncology, Radiology, and Pathology to provide comprehensive therapies for primary and metastatic brain tumors. We have pioneered minimally invasive approaches using imaging technology, frameless stereotaxy, and skull base endoscopy, awake and asleep brain mapping, and advanced microneurosurgery. Stereotactic radiosurgery, a minimally invasive treatment that does not require open surgery, gene therapy, and clinical trials are also possible options.

The Neuroendocrine Program sees more than 200 new pituitary tumor patients each year and more then 300 follow-up patients annually, and has performed more than 2,500 transphenoidal pituitary operations.

The Minimally Invasive and Endoscopic Skull Base Surgery Program provides comprehensive, highly advanced treatment for lesions located near the complex structures at the base of the skull. This multidisciplinary program unites surgical specialists in neurosurgery, otolaryngology, head and neck cancer, craniofacial surgery, oral and maxillofacial surgery, and microvascular and reconstructive procedures. We have pioneered the development of minimally invasive techniques, including transnasal endoscopic tumor resection and stereotactic radiosurgery for complex skull base lesions. This program offers renowned treatment of pituitary adenomas, acoustic neuromas, meningiomas, chordomas, craniopharyngiomas, cholesterol granulomas, chondrosarcomas, and all the pathologies of the skull base.

The Cerebrovascular Program has a highly experienced team that provides a complete range of services for the diagnosis and treatment of patients with neurovascular disorders of the brain and spinal cord, including aneurysms, arteriovenous malformations (AVMs), carotid and intracranial stenoses, and other conditions. Our team includes physicians specializing in microsurgical techniques, endovascular techniques, stereotactic radiosurgery, and neurocritical care, all working together to prevent or minimize the neurological impact of neurovascular disorders and to maximize recovery. Some current treatments include microsurgical treatment of aneurysms and AVMs with clipping and resection, endovascular treatment of aneurysms with coils and/or stents, endovascular treatment of AVMs with liquid acrylics, stereotactic radiosurgical treatment of AVMs, endovascular treatment of stenoses with stents and angioplasty and microsurgical treatment of stenoses and occlusions with bypass. We treat a high volume of patients using endovascular methods, and have the largest experience in the stent-assisted embolization of cerebral aneurysms and stent treatment of carotid artery disease amongst neurovascular centers in New York.

The Functional and Restorative Neurosurgery Program uses the latest technology to precisely target areas of abnormal activity in the brain and spinal cord. Our physicians are focused on developing minimally invasive neurosurgical techniques that either modulate neural function, replace lost neuronal populations, or halt the neurodegenerative process altogether. Currently, deep brain stimulation dominates this field, but many technologies with great potential are on the horizon. Our physicians have been honored by the Dystonia Medical Research Foundation for their pioneering work treating dystonia with deep brain stimulation. We also use gene therapy for the treatment of patients with Parkinson's disease, epilepsy, essential tremor, facial nerve disorders, and chronic pain syndromes.

The Neurosurgery Spinal Disorders Program offers treatment for all disorders of the spinal column and spinal cord, including degenerative disorders (disc herniations, spinal stenosis, spinal instability), trauma, infections, congenital disorders (including scoliosis), and tumors. Our neurosurgeons have pioneered endoscopic, minimally invasive approaches for tumors resection and treatment of degenerative diseases. These approaches reduce pain, and hospital stays, and facilitate an early return to normal activity.

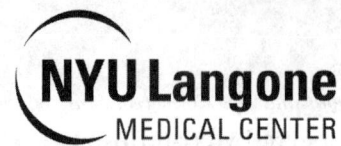

550 First Avenue *(at 31st Street)*
New York, NY 10016
www.NYULMC.org
Physician Referral: **888-7-NYU-MED** *(888-769-8633)*

NEUROLOGY

NYU Langone Medical Center evaluates and treats adults and children with a broad spectrum of neurological diseases, including stroke, epilepsy, cerebrovascular diseases, behavioral disorders and dementia, brain tumors, genetic and degenerative diseases, nerve and muscle problems, headache and pain syndromes and movement disorders. We are home to the largest multiple sclerosis (MS) program in New York and were first primary Stroke Center in NYC.

Autonomic Diseases

Our specialized Center evaluates and treats children and adults with familial dysautonomia and other inherited or acquired autonomic nervous system diseases, including orthostatic hypotension and rare forms of hereditary sensory neuropathy.

Epilepsy

The Comprehensive Epilepsy Center offers the most advanced medical and surgical options. Complementary management approaches complete the comprehensive management plan.

Multiple Sclerosis

The Comprehensive MS Care Center provides state-of-the-art diagnostic evaluations and follow-up care as part of a comprehensive program.

Neurogenetics

We focus on inherited diseases of the nervous system. Services include diagnosis and management of inherited diseases, biochemical and molecular testing and genetic counseling.

Neuro-oncology

NYU Cancer Institute includes one of the nation's leading brain and spinal cord tumor programs, with physicians highly experienced in neuro-oncology, neurosurgery and neuroradiology.

Neuromuscular Diseases

We offer multidisciplinary programs for neuromuscular diseases, including acquired peripheral neuropathy, Charcot Marie Tooth neuropathy, myasthenia gravis, amyotrophic lateral sclerosis, spinal muscular atrophy, post-polio syndrome, muscular dystrophy and Lyme neuroborreliosis.

Parkinson's Disease and Movement Disorders

The Parkinson's disease and Movement Disorders Center helps individuals and families achieve the highest possible quality of life.

Stroke Care

The multidisciplinary Comprehensive Stroke Care Center provides rapid diagnosis, effective intervention and early rehabilitation from debilitating stroke.

Penn Medicine

PENN COMPREHENSIVE NEUROSCIENCE CENTER

Philadelphia, PA 19104

800.789.PENN

PennMedicine.org

PENN NEUROLOGY

The University of Pennsylvania's history of excellence in the treatment of neurological diseases dates back to the establishment of the Department of Neurology in 1874. *The Best Doctors in America®* lists more neurologists and neurosurgeons from the Hospital of the University of Pennsylvania than from any other hospital or medical center in the Philadelphia region. Penn Neurology and Neurosurgery at the Hospital of the University of Pennsylvania (HUP) are ranked 14th in the nation by *U.S.News & World Report,* the only neuroscience programs in the region to be recognized.

The Department of Neurology is a component of the Penn Comprehensive Neuroscience Center, which is dedicated to facilitating and strengthening the integration of Penn's world-class neuroscience programs within the areas of clinical care, research and education.

Excellence and Expertise

Recognized by the National Parkinson Foundation as one of its worldwide Centers of Excellence, the **Parkinson's Disease and Movement Disorders Center** is committed to providing exceptional patient care, education, and social support services. Research is an important and ongoing mission of the Center, which actively pursues the investigation of the disease as well as exploration of new medications.

The **Multiple Sclerosis Center Program** provides comprehensive evaluation, diagnosis and treatment for patients with MS and other demyelinating disorders of the central nervous system. In addition to maintaining the highest standards for clinical service, the Penn MS program is a leader in MS training and in clinical and laboratory-based research.

The Penn **Neuro-Ophthalmology Program** bridges the fields of ophthalmology and neurology through the diagnosis and management of patients with neurological disorders that affect vision and eye movements. The program is part of Penn's **Comprehensive Neuroscience Center** and the **Scheie Eye Institute.** With five full-time faculty members and active clinical and research components, it is one of the largest neuro-ophthalmology groups in the country. Within the areas of multiple sclerosis vision research, pediatric neuro-ophthalmology, and vision-based testing for sports-related concussion, the Penn Neuro-Ophthalmology group is a world leader.

The **Penn Epilepsy Center** provides the highest standard of care to patients with epilepsy and related problems. The Center offers a comprehensive, full continuum of care including state-of-the-art diagnostic techniques, cutting-edge research, medical treatments, surgery, and support services to patients with epilepsy. Both outpatient evaluation and inpatient care are available via this multidisciplinary, full-service facility.

The **Penn Stroke Center** provides emergent care to stroke patients 24 hours a day, 365 days per year. The Center employs state-of-the-art approaches to the diagnosis, treatment and prevention of stroke and critical neurologic conditions. Inpatients are cared for by physicians and nurses with specialty training in neurological diseases in different settings, depending on their needs including the Neuroscience floor with telemetry and the Intermediate Neurological Care Unit. The Neurological Intensive Care Unit is among the most technologically advanced and sophisticated neurocritical care units in the nation, and is the only dedicated academic facility of its kind in the region.

Penn's Cognitive Neurology Program provides comprehensive, state-of-the-art assessment and treatment for patients with disorders of memory, language, attention, vision and cognition. Each patient is evaluated and treated by an experienced team of specialists and an individualized plan is developed for their ongoing care. The Center offers the latest treatment approaches available, including approved medications as well as access to numerous clinical trials of emerging treatments.

Programs

- Cognitive Neurology Program
- Center for Brain Injury and Repair
- Interventional Neuro Center
- Memory Disorders Clinic
- Multiple Sclerosis Center
- Neurological Intensive Care
- Neurogenetics Center
- Neuromuscular Disorders Program
- Neuro-Oncology Program
- Neuro-Ophthalmology Service
- Neuropsychology Service
- Parkinson's Disease and Movement Disorders Center
- Penn Epilepsy Center
- Penn Center for Sleep Disorders
- Penn Memory Center
- Stroke Center

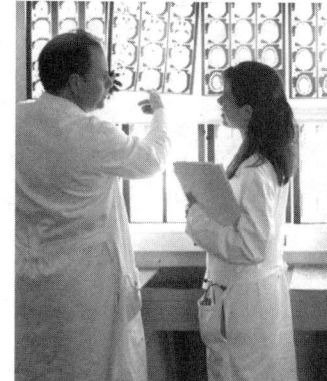

Hospital of the University of Pennsylvania | Penn Presbyterian Medical Center | Pennsylvania Hospital

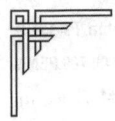

The Best in American Medicine
www.CastleConnolly.com

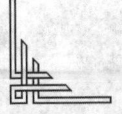
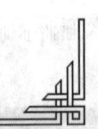

Neurology

A neurologist specializes in the diagnosis and treatment of all types of disease or impaired function of the brain, spinal cord, peripheral nerves, muscles and autonomic nervous system, as well as the blood vessels that relate to these structures. A child neurologist has special skills in the diagnosis and management of neurologic disorders of the neonatal period, infancy, early childhood and adolescence.

Training Required: Four years

NEUROLOGY

New England

Amato, Anthony A MD [N] - **Spec Exp:** Peripheral Neuropathy; Neuromuscular Disorders; Muscular Dystrophy; **Hospital:** Brigham and Women's Hosp (page 57); **Address:** Brigham & Women's Hosp, Dept Neurology, 75 Francis St, Boston, MA 02115; **Phone:** 617-732-8046; **Board Cert:** Neurology 1991; **Med School:** Univ Cincinnati 1986; **Resid:** Neurology, Wilford Hall USAF Med Ctr 1990; **Fellow:** Neuromuscular Medicine, Ohio State Med Ctr 1992; **Fac Appt:** Prof N, Harvard Med Sch

Armon, Carmel MD [N] - **Spec Exp:** Amyotrophic Lateral Sclerosis (ALS); Epilepsy/Seizure Disorders; Vascular Neurology; Sleep Medicine; **Hospital:** Baystate Med Ctr; **Address:** Baystate Neurology, 3000 Main St Fl 3 - Ste 3C, Springfield, MA 01199; **Phone:** 413-794-7192; **Board Cert:** Neurology 1990; Clinical Neurophysiology 2002; Vascular Neurology 2005; Sleep Medicine 2007; **Med School:** Israel 1980; **Resid:** Neurology, Mayo Clinic 1988; **Fellow:** Neurology, Mayo Clinic 1989; Clinical Neurophysiology, Duke Univ Med Ctr 1991; **Fac Appt:** Prof N, Tufts Univ

Batchelor, Tracy T MD [N] - **Spec Exp:** Brain Tumors; Gliomas; **Hospital:** Mass Genl Hosp; **Address:** Mass Genl Hosp Cancer Ctr - Neuro-Oncology, 55 Fruit St, Yawkey Ctr, Ste 9E, Boston, MA 02114; **Phone:** 617-724-8770; **Board Cert:** Neurology 2005; **Med School:** Emory Univ 1990; **Resid:** Neurology, Mass Genl Hosp 1994; **Fellow:** Neuro-Oncology, Meml Sloan Kettering Cancer Ctr 1995; **Fac Appt:** Prof N, Harvard Med Sch

Blum, Andrew S MD [N] - **Spec Exp:** Epilepsy; **Hospital:** Rhode Island Hosp; **Address:** Neurology Foundation Inc., 2 Dudley St, Ste 555, Providence, RI 02905; **Phone:** 401-444-3032; **Resid:** Neurology, Johns Hopkins Hosp 1994; **Fellow:** Clinical Neurophysiology, Beth Israel Deaconess Med Ctr 1995

Blumenfeld, Hal MD/PhD [N] - **Spec Exp:** Epilepsy/Seizure Disorders; **Hospital:** Yale-New Haven Hosp, Yale Med Group; **Address:** Yale Dept of Neurology, PO Box 208018, New Haven, CT 06520-8018; **Phone:** 203-785-4085; **Board Cert:** Neurology 2008; **Med School:** Columbia P&S 1992; **Resid:** Neurology, Mass Genl Hosp 1996; **Fellow:** Epilepsy, Yale-New Haven Hosp 1998; **Fac Appt:** Assoc Prof N, Yale Univ

Caplan, Louis R MD [N] - **Spec Exp:** Stroke; **Hospital:** Beth Israel Deaconess Med Ctr - Boston; **Address:** Palmer 127 West Campus BIDMC, 330 Brookline Ave, Boston, MA 02215; **Phone:** 617-632-8911; **Board Cert:** Internal Medicine 1969; Neurology 1972; Vascular Neurology 2005; **Med School:** Univ MD Sch Med 1962; **Resid:** Neurology, Boston City Hosp 1969; **Fellow:** Neurology, Harvard Univ Affil Hosp 1970; **Fac Appt:** Prof N, Harvard Med Sch

Cohen, Jeffrey Allen MD [N] - **Spec Exp:** Neuromuscular Disorders; Peripheral Neuropathy; **Hospital:** Dartmouth - Hitchcock Med Ctr; **Address:** Department of Neurology, 1 Medical Center Drive, Lebanon, NH 03756; **Phone:** 603-650-8589; **Board Cert:** Neurology 1982; Clinical Neurophysiology 1992; Neuromuscular Medicine 2008; **Med School:** Univ Okla Coll Med 1977; **Resid:** Neurology, Mt Sinai Hosp 1981; **Fellow:** Neuromuscular Disease, Mass Genl Hosp 1982; Peripheral Nerve Surgery, Mayo Clin 1986; **Fac Appt:** Prof Med, Dartmouth Med Sch

Cole, Andrew J MD [N] - **Spec Exp:** Epilepsy/Seizure Disorders; Rasmussen's Syndrome; **Hospital:** Mass Genl Hosp; **Address:** Mass Genl Hosp-Epilepsy Svc, 55 Fruit St, Wang Ambulatary Ctr, Ste 735, Boston, MA 02214; **Phone:** 617-726-3311; **Board Cert:** Neurology 1987; **Med School:** Dartmouth Med Sch 1982; **Resid:** Neurology, Neuro Inst-McGill 1986; **Fellow:** Electroencephalography, Neuro Inst-McGill 1987; Neurological Surgery, Johns Hopkins Hosp 1988; **Fac Appt:** Asst Prof N, Harvard Med Sch

Cudkowicz, Merit MD [N] - **Spec Exp:** Amyotrophic Lateral Sclerosis(ALS); Neuromuscular Disorders; **Hospital:** Beth Israel Deaconess Med Ctr - Boston; **Address:** Neurology Associates, 15 Parkman St, WAC 835, Boston, MA 02114-3117; **Phone:** 617-724-3914; **Board Cert:** Neurology 2005; **Med School:** Harvard Med Sch 1990; **Resid:** Neurology, Mass Genl Hosp 1994; **Fellow:** Neurology, Mass Genl Hosp 1996; **Fac Appt:** Prof N, Harvard Med Sch

Feldmann, Edward MD [N] - **Spec Exp:** Cerebrovascular Disease; Stroke; **Hospital:** Tufts Med Ctr; **Address:** 800 Washington St, Box 314, Boston, MA 02111; **Phone:** 617-636-5848; **Board Cert:** Neurology 1988; Vascular Neurology 2005; **Med School:** Harvard Med Sch 1983; **Resid:** Neurology, New York Hosp 1987; **Fellow:** Cerebrovascular Disease, Tufts New Eng Med Ctr 1988; **Fac Appt:** Prof N, Brown Univ

Flaherty, Alice W MD/PhD [N] - **Spec Exp:** Parkinson's Disease; Movement Disorders; Deep Brain Stimulation; Tourette's Syndrome; **Hospital:** Mass Genl Hosp, McLean Hosp; **Address:** Neurology Assocs, 15 Parkman St, WACC 715, Boston, MA 02114; **Phone:** 617-724-9234; **Board Cert:** Neurology 2009; **Med School:** Harvard Med Sch 1994; **Resid:** Neurology, Mass Genl Hosp 1998

Furie, Karen L MD [N] - **Spec Exp:** Stroke; Cerebrovascular Disease; **Hospital:** Mass Genl Hosp; **Address:** MGH Neurology Stroke Svc, 15 Parkman St, WAC 733, Boston, MA 02114; **Phone:** 617-726-8459; **Board Cert:** Neurology 2006; Vascular Neurology 2008; **Med School:** Brown Univ 1990; **Resid:** Neurology, Rhode Island Hosp 1994; **Fellow:** Cerebrovascular Disease, Brown Univ 1995

Greer, David M MD [N] - **Spec Exp:** Stroke; Cerebrovascular Disease; **Hospital:** Yale-New Haven Hosp, Yale Med Group; **Address:** Yale Univ Sch Medicine, Dept Neurology, 333 Cedar St, PO Box 208018, New Haven, CT 06520-8018; **Phone:** 203-737-1057; **Board Cert:** Neurology 2000; Vascular Neurology 2008; **Med School:** Univ Fla Coll Med 1995; **Resid:** Neurology, Mass General Hosp 1999; **Fellow:** Vascular Neurology, Mass General Hosp 2001

Gross, Paul T MD [N] - **Spec Exp:** Epilepsy; Sleep Disorders; **Hospital:** Lahey Clin; **Address:** Lahey Clinic, 41 Mall Rd, Burlington, MA 01805; **Phone:** 781-744-3263; **Board Cert:** Neurology 1981; Sleep Medicine 1992; **Med School:** Hahnemann Univ 1976; **Resid:** Neurology, Univ Wisc Hosp 1980; **Fellow:** Clinical Neurophysiology, Boston Chldn's Hosp 1981; **Fac Appt:** Clin Prof N, Tufts Univ

Jobst, Barbara C MD [N] - **Spec Exp:** Epilepsy/Seizure Disorders; Epilepsy in Women; **Hospital:** Dartmouth - Hitchcock Med Ctr; **Address:** One Medical Center Drive, Lebanon, NH 03756-1000; **Phone:** 603-653-6118; **Board Cert:** Neurology 2002; Clinical Neurophysiology 2005; **Med School:** Germany 1993; **Resid:** Neurology, Krankenhaus Barmherzigen Bruder 1996; Neurology, Dartmouth-Hitchcock Med Ctr 2000; **Fellow:** Epilepsy, Dartmouth-Hitchcock Med Ctr 2001; **Fac Appt:** Assoc Prof N, Dartmouth Med Sch

Jones Jr, H Royden MD [N] - **Spec Exp:** Neuromuscular Disorders; Amyotrophic Lateral Sclerosis (ALS); Myasthenia Gravis; Peripheral Neuropathy; **Hospital:** Lahey Clin; **Address:** Lahey Clinic, 41 Mall Rd, Burlington, MA 01805; **Phone:** 781-744-5126; **Board Cert:** Neurology 2004; Clinical Neurophysiology 2000; Neuromuscular Medicine 2006; **Med School:** Northwestern Univ 1962; **Resid:** Internal Medicine, Mayo Clinic 1965; Neurology, Mayo Clinic 1969; **Fellow:** Neurological Physiology, Mayo Clinic 1972; **Fac Appt:** Clin Prof N, Harvard Med Sch

Kase, Carlos S MD [N] - **Spec Exp:** Stroke; **Hospital:** Boston Med Ctr; **Address:** Boston Med Ctr, Shapiro Ctr, 725 Albany St Fl 7th - Ste 7B, Boston, MA 02118; **Phone:** 617-638-8456; **Board Cert:** Neurology 1980; Vascular Neurology 2005; **Med School:** Chile 1967; **Resid:** Neurology, Mass Genl Hosp 1973; Neurology, Mass Genl Hosp 1978; **Fac Appt:** Prof N, Boston Univ

Oaklander, Anne Louise MD/PhD [N] - **Spec Exp:** Nerve Injury; Peripheral Neuropathy; Pain-Neuropathic; Complex Regional Pain Syndromes; **Hospital:** Mass Genl Hosp; **Address:** Mass General Hosp, Dept Neurology, 55 Fruit St, Wayne Bldg Fl 8, Boston, MA 02114; **Phone:** 617-643-0601; **Board Cert:** Neurology 1992; Pain Medicine 2000; **Med School:** Albert Einstein Coll Med 1987; **Resid:** Neurology, UMDNJ Univ Med Ctr 1991; **Fellow:** Johns Hopkins Hosp; **Fac Appt:** Assoc Prof N, Harvard Med Sch

Pennell, Page B MD [N] - **Spec Exp:** Epilepsy in Women; Epilepsy in Pregnancy; Clinical Trials; **Hospital:** Brigham and Women's Hosp (page 57); **Address:** Brigham & Womens Hosp, Div Epilepsy, EEG & Sleep Neurology, 75 Francis St, Boston, MA 02115; **Phone:** 617-732-7547; **Board Cert:** Neurology 2004; **Med School:** Univ Fla Coll Med 1989; **Resid:** Neurology, Univ Michigan Med Ctr 1993; **Fellow:** Clinical Neurophysiology, Univ Michigan 1995; **Fac Appt:** Assoc Clin Prof N, Emory Univ

Ropper, Allan MD [N] - **Spec Exp:** Guillain-Barre Syndrome; Parkinson's Disease; **Hospital:** Brigham and Women's Hosp (page 57); **Address:** Brigham & Women's Hosp, Dept Neurology, 75 Francis St, Box BB204, Boston, MA 02115; **Phone:** 617-732-8047; **Board Cert:** Internal Medicine 1977; Neurology 1980; **Med School:** Harvard Med Sch 1974; **Resid:** Internal Medicine, UCSF Med Ctr 1976; Neurology, Mass Genl Hosp 1979; **Fac Appt:** Prof N, Tufts Univ

Rutkove, Seward B MD [N] - **Spec Exp:** Neuromuscular Disorders; Amyotrophic Lateral Sclerosis(ALS); **Hospital:** Beth Israel Deaconess Med Ctr - Boston; **Address:** 330 Brookline Ave, Ste TCC-810, Boston, MA 02215; **Phone:** 617-667-8130; **Board Cert:** Neurology 2006; Clinical Neurophysiology 2007; **Med School:** Columbia P&S 1989; **Resid:** Internal Medicine, St Joseph Mercy Hosp 1991; Neurology, Harvard-Longwood Neuro Prgm 1994; **Fellow:** Clinical Neurophysiology, Brigham & Women's Hosp 1995; **Fac Appt:** Assoc Prof N, Harvard Med Sch

Samuels, Martin A MD [N] - **Spec Exp:** Neurologic Aspects of Systemic Disease; **Hospital:** Brigham and Women's Hosp (page 57), Mass Genl Hosp; **Address:** Brigham & Women's Hosp, Dept Neurology, 75 Francis St Fl 2, Boston, MA 02115; **Phone:** 617-732-7432; **Board Cert:** Internal Medicine 1974; Neurology 1978; **Med School:** Univ Cincinnati 1971; **Resid:** Internal Medicine, Boston City Hosp 1975; Neurology, Mass Genl Hosp 1977; **Fellow:** Neurological Pathology, Mass Genl Hosp 1976; **Fac Appt:** Prof N, Harvard Med Sch

Saper, Clifford MD/PhD [N] - **Spec Exp:** Sleep Disorders/Apnea; **Hospital:** Beth Israel Deaconess Med Ctr - Boston; **Address:** 330 Brookline Ave, Dept Neurology KS 406 Bldg, Boston, MA 02215; **Phone:** 617-667-2622; **Board Cert:** Neurology 1982; **Med School:** Washington Univ, St Louis 1977; **Resid:** Neurology, NY Hosp 1981; **Fac Appt:** Prof N, Harvard Med Sch

Wen, Patrick Y MD [N] - **Spec Exp:** Neuro-Oncology; Brain Tumors; **Hospital:** Dana-Farber Cancer Inst (page 57), Brigham and Women's Hosp (page 57); **Address:** Dana-Farber Cancer Inst, 450 Brookline Ave, Ste SW430B, Boston, MA 02115; **Phone:** 617-632-2166; **Board Cert:** Neurology 1989; **Med School:** England, UK 1981; **Resid:** Internal Medicine, London Chest Hosp 1984; Internal Medicine, Nat'l Hosp for Nervous Disease 1984; **Fellow:** Harvard-Longwood Neurology 1988; **Fac Appt:** Prof N, Harvard Med Sch

Young, Anne MD/PhD [N] - **Spec Exp:** Huntington's Disease; Parkinson's Disease; Movement Disorders; **Hospital:** Mass Genl Hosp; **Address:** Mass Genl Hosp, Dept Neurology, 15 Parkman St Fl 7, Boston, MA 02114; **Phone:** 617-726-2385; **Board Cert:** Neurology 1981; **Med School:** Johns Hopkins Univ 1973; **Resid:** Neurology, UCSF Med Ctr 1978; **Fac Appt:** Prof N, Harvard Med Sch

Mid Atlantic

Apatoff, Brian R MD/PhD [N] - **Spec Exp:** Multiple Sclerosis; Neuro-Immunology; **Hospital:** NY-Presby/Weill Cornell Med Ctr, NY (page 65); **Address:** Multiple Sclerosis Inst, Ctr for Neurologic Disease, 401 E 55th St, New York, NY 10022; **Phone:** 212-593-6262; **Board Cert:** Neurology 1991; **Med School:** Univ Chicago-Pritzker Sch Med 1984; **Resid:** Neurology, Columbia Presby Med Ctr 1990; **Fellow:** Multiple Sclerosis, Neuro Inst-Columbia Univ 1992; **Fac Appt:** Assoc Prof N, Cornell Univ-Weill Med Coll

Azizi, Sayed Ausim MD/PhD [N] - **Spec Exp:** Movement Disorders; Parkinson's Disease; Stroke; **Hospital:** Temple Univ Hosp, Hahnemann Univ Hosp; **Address:** Temple Univ Sch Med, Dept of Neurology, 3401 N Broad St, Ste C525, Philadelphia, PA 19140; **Phone:** 215-707-5953; **Board Cert:** Neurology 2008; **Med School:** Univ Tex SW, Dallas 1990; **Resid:** Neurology, Yale-New Haven Hosp 1994; **Fac Appt:** Prof N, Temple Univ

Balcer, Laura J MD [N] - **Spec Exp:** Neuro-Ophthalmology; Multiple Sclerosis/Visual Disorders; Parkinson's Disease/Visual Disorders; **Hospital:** Hosp Univ Penn - UPHS (page 68); **Address:** Hosp Univ Penn, Dept Neurology, 3400 Spruce St, Philadelphia, PA 19104; **Phone:** 215-349-8072; **Board Cert:** Neurology 2006; **Med School:** Johns Hopkins Univ 1991; **Resid:** Neurology, Hosp Univ Penn 1995; **Fellow:** Neuro-Ophthalmology, Hosp Univ Penn/Scheie Inst 1995; **Fac Appt:** Prof N, Univ Pennsylvania

Baser, Susan M MD [N] - **Spec Exp:** Parkinson's Disease; Huntington's Disease; Dystonia; Movement Disorders; **Hospital:** Allegheny General Hosp; **Address:** Allegheny Neurology Assocs, 490 E North Ave Prof Bldg - rm 500, Pittsburgh, PA 15212; **Phone:** 412-359-8860; **Board Cert:** Neurology 1990; **Med School:** Loyola Univ-Stritch Sch Med 1983; **Resid:** Neurology, Univ Pittsburgh 1987; **Fellow:** Neuropharmacology, Natl Inst Hlth 1990; **Fac Appt:** Assoc Prof N, Thomas Jefferson Univ

Bell, Rodney D MD [N] - **Spec Exp:** Stroke; **Hospital:** Thomas Jefferson Univ Hosp; **Address:** Thomas Jefferson Univ Dept Neurology, 900 Walnut St, Ste 200, Philadelphia, PA 19107; **Phone:** 215-955-6488; **Board Cert:** Internal Medicine 1975; Neurotology 1981; Vascular Neurology 2005; **Med School:** Oregon Hlth & Sci Univ 1971; **Resid:** Internal Medicine, Parkland Meml Hosp 1975; Neurology, Parkland Meml Hosp 1978; **Fac Appt:** Prof N, Thomas Jefferson Univ

Bergey, Gregory K MD [N] - **Spec Exp:** Epilepsy/Seizure Disorders; Epilepsy in Women; Epilepsy in Pregnancy; **Hospital:** Johns Hopkins Hosp (page 61); **Address:** Johns Hopkins Epilepsy Ctr, 601 N Caroline St, Meyer 2-147, Baltimore, MD 21287; **Phone:** 410-955-7338; **Board Cert:** Internal Medicine 1978; Neurology 1984; **Med School:** Univ Pennsylvania 1975; **Resid:** Internal Medicine, Yale-New Haven Hosp 1977; Neurology, Johns Hopkins Hosp 1981; **Fellow:** Neurological Physiology, Natl Inst Health 1983; **Fac Appt:** Prof N, Johns Hopkins Univ

Bressman, Susan MD [N] - **Spec Exp:** Parkinson's Disease; Movement Disorders; Dystonia; **Hospital:** Beth Israel Med Ctr - Petrie Division (page 55); **Address:** 10 Union Square East, Ste 5J, New York, NY 10003-3314; **Phone:** 212-844-8379; **Board Cert:** Neurology 1983; **Med School:** Columbia P&S 1977; **Resid:** Neurology, Columbia-Presby Med Ctr 1981; **Fellow:** Movement Disorders, Columbia-Presby Med Ctr 1983; **Fac Appt:** Prof N, Albert Einstein Coll Med

Brick, John MD [N] - **Spec Exp:** Epilepsy; **Hospital:** Ruby Memorial - WVU Hosp; **Address:** WV Univ-Dept Neurology, rm 7500 HSC, PO Box 9180, Morgantown, WV 26506-9180; **Phone:** 304-598-6127; **Board Cert:** Neurology 1982; **Med School:** W VA Univ 1977; **Resid:** Neurology, W Va Univ Hosp 1981; **Fellow:** Electroencephalography, Mayo Clinic 1983; **Fac Appt:** Prof N, W VA Univ

Buchholz, David W MD [N] - **Spec Exp:** Migraine; Headache; **Hospital:** Johns Hopkins Hosp (page 61); **Address:** Johns Hopkins at Green Spring Station, 10753 Falls Rd, Ste 315, Lutherville, MD 21093; **Phone:** 410-583-2830; **Board Cert:** Neurology 1984; **Med School:** Univ Pennsylvania 1979; **Resid:** Neurology, Johns Hopkins Hosp 1983; **Fac Appt:** Assoc Prof N, Johns Hopkins Univ

Busis, Neil A MD [N] - **Spec Exp:** Electromyography; Neuromuscular Disorders; Movement Disorders; Muscle Disorders; **Hospital:** UPMC Shadyside; **Address:** Pittsburgh Neurological Associates, 532 S Aiken Ave, Ste 507, Pittsburgh, PA 15232-1326; **Phone:** 412-681-2000; **Board Cert:** Neurology 1985; **Med School:** Univ Pennsylvania 1977; **Resid:** Internal Medicine, Johns Hopkins Hosp 1979; Neurology, Mass Genl Hosp 1984; **Fellow:** Electromyography, Mass Genl Hosp 1985; **Fac Appt:** Asst Clin Prof N, Univ Pittsburgh

Calabresi, Peter A MD [N] - **Spec Exp:** Multiple Sclerosis; **Hospital:** Johns Hopkins Hosp (page 61); **Address:** Johns Hopkins, dept Neuro-Immunology, 600 Wolfe St, Pathology 627, Baltimore, MD 21287; **Phone:** 410-614-1522; **Board Cert:** Neurology 2005; **Med School:** Brown Univ 1988; **Resid:** Neurology, Strong Meml Hosp 1993; **Fellow:** Neurological Immunology, Natl Inst Hlth 1996; **Fac Appt:** Prof N, Johns Hopkins Univ

Charney, Jonathan Z MD [N] - **Spec Exp:** Headache; Stroke; **Hospital:** Mount Sinai Med Ctr (page 63); **Address:** 1111 Park Ave, Ste 1H, New York, NY 10128-1234; **Phone:** 212-831-2886; **Board Cert:** Neurology 1977; **Med School:** NY Med Coll 1969; **Resid:** Neurology, Methodist Hosp-Baylor 1971; Neurology, Columbia-Presby Med Ctr 1973; **Fac Appt:** Asst Prof N, Mount Sinai Sch Med

Cook, Stuart D MD [N] - **Spec Exp:** Multiple Sclerosis; Infectious & Demyelinating Diseases; **Hospital:** Univ Hosp-UMDNJ—Newark; **Address:** 65 Bergen St, rm 1435, Newark, NJ 07101-1709; **Phone:** 973-972-9181; **Board Cert:** Neurology 1970; **Med School:** Univ VT Coll Med 1962; **Resid:** Neurology, Albert Einstein Coll Med 1968; **Fac Appt:** Prof N, UMDNJ-NJ Med Sch, Newark

Cornblath, David R MD [N] - **Spec Exp:** Peripheral Neuropathy; **Hospital:** Johns Hopkins Hosp (page 61); **Address:** 600 N Wolfe St Meyer 6-181A, Baltimore, MD 21287-6965; **Phone:** 410-955-2229; **Board Cert:** Neurology 1982; **Med School:** Case West Res Univ 1977; **Resid:** Neurology, Hosp Univ Penn 1981; **Fellow:** Neurology, Hosp Univ Penn 1982; **Fac Appt:** Prof N, Johns Hopkins Univ

Coyle, Patricia K MD [N] - **Spec Exp:** Multiple Sclerosis; Neuro-Immunology; Lyme Disease; Infections-Neurologic; **Hospital:** Stony Brook Univ Med Ctr; **Address:** Dept Neurology, HSC T-12, rm 020, Stonybrook Univ Med Ctr, Stony Brook, NY 11794-8121; **Phone:** 631-444-2599; **Board Cert:** Neurology 2004; **Med School:** Johns Hopkins Univ 1974; **Resid:** Neurology, Johns Hopkins Hosp 1978; **Fellow:** Neurological Immunology, Johns Hopkins Hosp 1980; **Fac Appt:** Prof N, SUNY Stony Brook

Dalmau, Josep O MD/PhD [N] - **Spec Exp:** Brain Tumors; **Hospital:** Hosp Univ Penn - UPHS (page 68); **Address:** Hosp Univ Penn, Dept Neuro-Oncology, 3 W Gates Bldg, 3400 Spruce St, Phildelphia, PA 19104; **Phone:** 215-746-4707; **Med School:** Spain 1971; **Resid:** Neurology, Univ Hosp de la Sta Cruz y San Pablo 1983; **Fellow:** Neurology, NY Hosp-Cornell Med Ctr 1992; Neuro-Oncology, Meml Sloan Kettering Cancer Ctr 1993

De Angelis, Lisa M MD [N] - **Spec Exp:** Neuro-Oncology; **Hospital:** Meml Sloan-Kettering Cancer Ctr; **Address:** 1275 York Avenue, New York, NY 10065; **Phone:** 212-639-7123; **Board Cert:** Neurology 1986; **Med School:** Columbia P&S 1980; **Resid:** Neurology, Neuro Inst-Presby Hosp 1984; **Fellow:** Neuro-Oncology, Neuro Inst-Presby Hosp 1985; Neuro-Oncology, Meml Sloan-Kettering Cancer Ctr 1986; **Fac Appt:** Prof N, Cornell Univ-Weill Med Coll

Devinsky, Orrin MD [N] - **Spec Exp:** Epilepsy; Tuberous Sclerosis; Behavioral Neurology; **Hospital:** NYU Langone Med Ctr (page 66), Saint Barnabas Med Ctr; **Address:** 223 E 34th St Fl Ground, New York, NY 10016-4972; **Phone:** 646-558-0803; **Board Cert:** Neurology 1987; Clinical Neurophysiology 1990; **Med School:** Harvard Med Sch 1982; **Resid:** Neurology, NY Hosp-Cornell Med Ctr 1986; **Fellow:** Epilepsy, Natl Inst Health 1988; **Fac Appt:** Prof N, NYU Sch Med

Dewberry, Robert G MD [N] - **Hospital:** Maryland Genl Hosp; **Address:** 827 Linden Ave, Armory Bldg - Fl 2 - Ste 2A, Baltimore, MD 21201; **Phone:** 410-225-8290; **Board Cert:** Neurology 1992; **Med School:** Univ MD Sch Med 1987; **Resid:** Neurology, Barnes Hosp 1991; **Fellow:** Neuromuscular Disease, Univ Virginia Hosp 1993

Dichter, Marc A MD/PhD [N] - **Spec Exp:** Epilepsy/Seizure Disorders; **Hospital:** Hosp Univ Penn - UPHS (page 68); **Address:** Dept Neurology, 3W Gates Bldg, 3400 Spruce St, Philadelphia, PA 19104; **Phone:** 215-349-5166; **Board Cert:** Neurology 1978; **Med School:** NYU Sch Med 1969; **Resid:** Neurology, Beth Israel Hosp/Chldns Hosp/ Brigham Hosp 1975; **Fac Appt:** Prof N, Univ Pennsylvania

Fahn, Stanley MD [N] - **Spec Exp:** Movement Disorders; Parkinson's Disease; **Hospital:** NY-Presby/Columbia Univ Med Ctr, NY (page 65); **Address:** Neurological Institute, 710 W 168th St Fl 3 - rm 350, New York, NY 10032; **Phone:** 212-305-5277; **Board Cert:** Neurology 1968; **Med School:** UCSF 1958; **Resid:** Neurology, Neuro Inst-Columbia 1962; **Fellow:** Neurological Chemistry, Natl Inst Hlth 1968; **Fac Appt:** Prof N, Columbia P&S

Feinberg, Todd E MD [N] - **Spec Exp:** Alzheimer's Disease; Dementia; **Hospital:** Beth Israel Med Ctr - Petrie Division (page 55); **Address:** Beth Israel Med Ctr, Yarmon Neurobehavioral Ctr, First Ave at 16th St, New York, NY 10003; **Phone:** 212-420-4111; **Board Cert:** Psychiatry 1984; Neurology 1987; **Med School:** Mount Sinai Sch Med 1978; **Resid:** Psychiatry, Mt Sinai Med Ctr 1982; Neurology, Mt Sinai Med Ctr 1984; **Fellow:** Behavioral Neurology, Univ Florida 1986; **Fac Appt:** Clin Prof N, Albert Einstein Coll Med

Fellus, Jonathan L MD [N] - **Spec Exp:** Brain Injury; Neuro-Rehabilitation; Stroke; Dementia; **Hospital:** Meadowlands Hosp Med Ctr; **Address:** Meadowlands Hospital, 55 Meadowlands Pkwy, Secaucus, NJ 07094; **Phone:** 201-392-3524; **Board Cert:** Neurology 2009; **Med School:** UMDNJ-RW Johnson Med Sch 1992; **Resid:** Neurology, Penn Hosp 1996; **Fellow:** Neurological Rehabilitation, Kernan Hosp-Univ Md Med Ctr 1997; **Fac Appt:** Asst Clin Prof N, UMDNJ-NJ Med Sch, Newark

Fink, Matthew E MD [N] - **Spec Exp:** Cerebrovascular Disease; Stroke; **Hospital:** NY-Presby/Weill Cornell Med Ctr, NY (page 65); **Address:** NY Cornell Med Ctr Dept Neurology, 525 E 68th St, rm F610, New York, NY 10065; **Phone:** 212-746-4564; **Board Cert:** Internal Medicine 1980; Neurology 1983; Vascular Neurology 2005; **Med School:** Univ Pittsburgh 1976; **Resid:** Internal Medicine, Boston Med Ctr 1980; Neurology, Columbia-Presby Hosp 1982; **Fac Appt:** Prof N, Cornell Univ

Foo, Sun-Hoo MD [N] - **Spec Exp:** Stroke; Headache; Parkinson's Disease; Dementia; **Hospital:** NYU Langone Med Ctr (page 66), NY Downtown Hosp; **Address:** 650 1st Ave Fl 4, New York, NY 10016-3240; **Phone:** 212-213-0270; **Board Cert:** Internal Medicine 1976; Neurology 1980; **Med School:** Taiwan 1972; **Resid:** Internal Medicine, St Vincent's Hosp 1976; Neurology, NYU Med Ctr 1979; **Fac Appt:** Prof N, NYU Sch Med

Neurology

French, Jacqueline MD [N] - **Spec Exp:** Epilepsy/Seizure Disorders; **Hospital:** NYU Langone Med Ctr (page 66); **Address:** 223 E 34th St, New York, NY 10016; **Phone:** 646-558-0805; **Board Cert:** Neurology 1987; **Med School:** Brown Univ 1982; **Resid:** Neurology, Mount Sinai Hosp 1986; **Fellow:** Epilepsy, Mount Sinai Hosp 1988; Epilepsy, Yale-New Haven Hosp 1989; **Fac Appt:** Prof N, NYU Sch Med

Galetta, Steven MD [N] - **Spec Exp:** Neuro-Ophthalmology; Optic Nerve Disorders; Multiple Sclerosis; **Hospital:** Hosp Univ Penn - UPHS (page 68); **Address:** Hosp Univ Penn, Dept Neurology, 3W Gates Bldg, 3400 Spruce St, Philadelphia, PA 19104; **Phone:** 215-662-3381; **Board Cert:** Neurology 1988; **Med School:** Cornell Univ-Weill Med Coll 1983; **Resid:** Neurology, Hosp Univ Penn 1987; **Fellow:** Neuro-Ophthalmology, Bascom Palmer Eye Inst 1988; **Fac Appt:** Prof N, Univ Pennsylvania

Gendelman, Seymour MD [N] - **Spec Exp:** Parkinson's Disease; Dementia; Headache; **Hospital:** Mount Sinai Med Ctr (page 63); **Address:** 5 E 98th St Fl 7, Box 1139, New York, NY 10029-6501; **Phone:** 212-241-8172; **Board Cert:** Neurology 1971; **Med School:** Geo Wash Univ 1964; **Resid:** Neurology, Mt Sinai Hosp 1968; **Fac Appt:** Clin Prof N, Mount Sinai Sch Med

Gizzi, Martin S MD/PhD [N] - **Spec Exp:** Neuro-Ophthalmology; Stroke; Progressive Supranuclear Palsy (PSP); Stroke; **Hospital:** JFK Med Ctr - Edison; **Address:** NJ Neuroscience Insitute, 65 James St, Edison, NJ 08820-3947; **Phone:** 732-321-7010; **Board Cert:** Neurology 1990; Vascular Neurology 2008; **Med School:** Univ Miami Sch Med 1985; **Resid:** Neurology, Mount Sinai Hosp 1989; **Fellow:** Neuro-Ophthalmology, Mount Sinai Hosp 1991

Glass, Jon MD [N] - **Spec Exp:** Neuro-Oncology; Brain Tumors; Spinal Tumors; **Hospital:** Thomas Jefferson Univ Hosp; **Address:** 909 Walnut St Fl 2, Philadelphia, PA 19107; **Phone:** 215-503-7005; **Board Cert:** Neurology 1993; **Med School:** SUNY Downstate 1986; **Resid:** Neurology, Boston Univ 1990; **Fellow:** Neuro-Oncology, Mass Genl Hosp 1992; **Fac Appt:** Asst Prof N, NYU Sch Med

Golbe, Lawrence I MD [N] - **Spec Exp:** Parkinson's Disease; Progressive Supranuclear Palsy (PSP); Movement Disorders; **Hospital:** Robert Wood Johnson Univ Hosp - New Brunswick; **Address:** 125 Paterson St Fl 6 - rm 6200, New Brunswick, NJ 08901-2160; **Phone:** 732-235-7733; **Board Cert:** Neurology 1984; **Med School:** NYU Sch Med 1978; **Resid:** Internal Medicine, Hahnemann Univ Hosp 1980; Neurology, Bellevue Hosp 1983; **Fac Appt:** Prof N, UMDNJ-RW Johnson Med Sch

Goodgold, Albert MD [N] - **Spec Exp:** Parkinson's Disease; Spinal Cord Disorders; Multiple Sclerosis; Movement Disorders; **Hospital:** NYU Langone Med Ctr (page 66); **Address:** 530 First Ave Fl 5 - Ste 5A, New York, NY 10016; **Phone:** 212-263-7205; **Med School:** Switzerland 1955; **Resid:** Neurology, Bellevue Hosp 1960; **Fac Appt:** Prof N, NYU Sch Med

Hiesiger, Emile MD [N] - **Spec Exp:** Pain-Spine; Pain-Cancer, Spine; Pain-Back; **Hospital:** NYU Langone Med Ctr (page 66), VA NY Harbor Hlthcare Sys-Manhattan Campus; **Address:** 530 1st Ave, Ste 5A, New York, NY 10016-6402; **Phone:** 212-263-6123; **Board Cert:** Neurology 1983; **Med School:** NY Med Coll 1978; **Resid:** Neurology, NYU Med Ctr 1982; **Fellow:** Neurology, Meml Sloan-Kettering Cancer Ctr 1984; **Fac Appt:** Assoc Clin Prof N, NYU Sch Med

Hurtig, Howard MD [N] - **Spec Exp:** Parkinson's Disease; Movement Disorders; **Hospital:** Pennsylvania Hosp-UPHS (page 68); **Address:** Pennsylvania Hosp Neurological Inst, 330 S 9th St Fl 3, Philadelphia, PA 19107; **Phone:** 215-829-6500; **Board Cert:** Neurology 1976; **Med School:** Tulane Univ 1966; **Resid:** Internal Medicine, New York Hosp 1968; Neurology, Hosp Univ Penn 1973; **Fac Appt:** Prof N, Univ Pennsylvania

Jordan, Barry D MD [N] - **Spec Exp:** Brain Injury; Sports Neurology; Concussion; Memory Disorders; **Hospital:** Burke Rehab Hosp; **Address:** Burke Rehabilitation Hosp, 785 Mamaroneck Ave, White Plains, NY 10605; **Phone:** 914-597-2332; **Board Cert:** Neurology 1989; **Med School:** Harvard Med Sch 1981; **Resid:** Neurology, New York Hosp 1986; **Fellow:** Hosp Spec Surgery 1987; UCLA Med Ctr 1998; **Fac Appt:** Assoc Prof N, Cornell Univ-Weill Med Coll

Kasner, Scott E MD [N] - **Spec Exp:** Cerebrovascular Disease; Stroke; **Hospital:** Hosp Univ Penn - UPHS (page 68); **Address:** Hosp Univ Penn - Neurology 3W-Gates, 3400 Spruce St, Philadelphia, PA 19104; **Phone:** 215-662-3564; **Board Cert:** Neurology 2007; Vascular Neurology 2006; **Med School:** Yale Univ 1992; **Resid:** Neurology, Hosp Univ Penn 1996; **Fellow:** Stroke, Univ Texas Affil Hosp 1997; Neurocritical Care, Univ Texas Affil Hosp 1997; **Fac Appt:** Prof N, Univ Pennsylvania

Klein, Patricia MD [N] - **Spec Exp:** Headache; Dizziness; **Hospital:** Holy Name Med Ctr, Hackensack Univ Med Ctr; **Address:** 680 Kinderkamack Rd, Oradell, NJ 07649; **Phone:** 201-261-6222; **Board Cert:** Neurology 1980; **Med School:** UMDNJ-NJ Med Sch, Newark 1976; **Resid:** Neurology, UMDNJ 1979; **Fac Appt:** Asst Clin Prof N, UMDNJ-NJ Med Sch, Newark

Kolodny, Edwin H MD [N] - **Spec Exp:** Pediatric Neurology; Inherited Disorders of Nervous System; Gaucher Disease; Fabry's Disease; **Hospital:** NYU Langone Med Ctr (page 66), Bellevue Hosp Ctr; **Address:** 403 E 34 St Fl 2, New York, NY 10016-6402; **Phone:** 212-263-8344; **Board Cert:** Neurology 1971; Clinical Genetics 1984; Clinical Biochemical Genetics 1987; **Med School:** NYU Sch Med 1962; **Resid:** Internal Medicine, Bellevue Hosp 1964; Neurology, Mass Genl Hosp 1967; **Fellow:** Neurological Pathology, Mass Genl Hosp 1966; Neurology, Nat Inst Neurol Dis & Stroke 1970; **Fac Appt:** Prof N, NYU Sch Med

Krauss, Gregory L MD [N] - **Spec Exp:** Epilepsy/Seizure Disorders; **Hospital:** Johns Hopkins Hosp (page 61); **Address:** Johns Hopkins Hosp, Dept Neurology, 600 N Wolfe St, Meyer 2-147, Baltimore, MD 21287; **Phone:** 410-955-2822; **Board Cert:** Neurology 1990; **Med School:** Oregon Hlth & Sci Univ 1985; **Resid:** Neurology, Johns Hopkins Hosp 1989; **Fellow:** Epilepsy, Johns Hopkins Hosp 1991; **Fac Appt:** Assoc Prof N, Johns Hopkins Univ

Krumholz, Allan MD [N] - **Spec Exp:** Epilepsy/Seizure Disorders; Sleep Disorders/Apnea; **Hospital:** Univ of MD Med Ctr; **Address:** Univ Maryland Med System, Dept Neurology, 22 S Greene St, rm S12C09, Baltimore, MD 21201-1544; **Phone:** 410-328-6266; **Board Cert:** Neurology 1977; Clinical Neurophysiology 2006; **Med School:** Ros Franklin Univ/Chicago Med Sch 1970; **Resid:** Internal Medicine, Baltimore City Hosp 1972; Neurology, Johns Hopkins Hosp 1975; **Fellow:** Electroencephalography, Johns Hopkins Hosp 1980; **Fac Appt:** Prof N, Univ MD Sch Med

Kula, Roger W MD [N] - **Spec Exp:** Neuromuscular Disorders; Myasthenia Gravis; Syringomyelia & Spinal Cord Diseases; Chiari's Deformity; **Hospital:** N Shore Univ Hosp, Steven & Alexandra Cohen Chldn's Med Ctr of NY; **Address:** 865 Northern Blvd, Ste 302, Great Neck, NY 11021; **Phone:** 516-570-4400; **Board Cert:** Internal Medicine 1975; Neurology 1977; Neuromuscular Medicine 2008; **Med School:** Johns Hopkins Univ 1970; **Resid:** Internal Medicine, New York Hosp 1972; Neurology, UCSF Med Ctr 1974; **Fellow:** Neuromuscular Medicine, Natl Inst Hlth 1977; **Fac Appt:** Assoc Prof N, SUNY Hlth Sci Ctr

Kunschner, Lara MD [N] - **Spec Exp:** Neuro-Oncology; Brain Tumors; **Hospital:** Allegheny General Hosp; **Address:** 420 E North Ave, Ste 206, Ste 206, Pittsburgh, PA 15212; **Phone:** 412-359-8850; **Board Cert:** Neurology 1999; **Med School:** Univ Pittsburgh 1994; **Resid:** Neurology, Univ Michigan Hosps 1999; **Fellow:** Neuro-Oncology, MD Anderson Cancer Ctr 2000

Neurology

Kuzniecky, Ruben MD [N] - **Spec Exp:** Epilepsy/Seizure Disorders; MRI; Developmental Disorders; **Hospital:** NYU Langone Med Ctr (page 66); **Address:** 223 E 34th St Fl Ground, New York, NY 10016; **Phone:** 646-558-0802; **Board Cert:** Neurology 1990; **Med School:** Argentina 1980; **Resid:** Neurology, McGill Univ 1986; **Fellow:** Epilepsy, McGill Univ 1988; **Fac Appt:** Prof N, NYU Sch Med

Labar, Douglas R MD/PhD [N] - **Spec Exp:** Epilepsy/Seizure Disorders; **Hospital:** NY-Presby/Weill Cornell Med Ctr, NY (page 65); **Address:** NY Weill Cornell Med Ctr, 525 E 68th St, New York, NY 10065; **Phone:** 212-746-2359; **Board Cert:** Neurology 1987; **Med School:** Med Coll PA 1982; **Resid:** Neurology, Columbia Presby Med Ctr 1986; **Fellow:** Epilepsy, Columbia Presby Med Ctr 1988; **Fac Appt:** Prof N, Cornell Univ-Weill Med Coll

Lacomis, David MD [N] - **Spec Exp:** Amyotrophic Lateral Sclerosis (ALS); Muscle Disorders; Myasthenia Gravis; Neuromuscular Disorders; **Hospital:** UPMC Presby, Pittsburgh; **Address:** Dept Neurology-Kaufmann Med Bldg, 3471 Fifth Ave, Ste 810, Pittsburgh, PA 15213; **Phone:** 412-692-4917; **Board Cert:** Neurology 1992; Clinical Neurophysiology 2004; Neuromuscular Medicine 2009; **Med School:** Penn State Coll Med 1987; **Resid:** Neurology, Harvard Affil Hosp 1991; **Fellow:** Neuromuscular Disease, Univ Mass Med Ctr 1993; **Fac Appt:** Prof N, Univ Pittsburgh

Laterra, John J MD/PhD [N] - **Spec Exp:** Neuro-Oncology; Brain Tumors; **Hospital:** Johns Hopkins Hosp (page 61), Kennedy Krieger Inst; **Address:** Phipps 115, 600 N Wolfe St, Baltimore, MD 21287; **Phone:** 410-614-3853; **Board Cert:** Neurology 1990; **Med School:** Case West Res Univ 1984; **Resid:** Neurology, Univ Mich Hosps 1988; **Fellow:** Research, Johns Hopkins Hosp 1989; **Fac Appt:** Prof N, Johns Hopkins Univ

Latov, Norman MD/PhD [N] - **Spec Exp:** Peripheral Neuropathy; Neuro-Immunology; **Hospital:** NY-Presby/Weill Cornell Med Ctr, NY (page 65); **Address:** 1305 York Ave Fl 2 - Ste 217, New York, NY 10021; **Phone:** 646-962-3202; **Board Cert:** Neurology 1989; **Med School:** Univ Pennsylvania 1975; **Resid:** Internal Medicine, Boston City Hosp 1976; Neurology, Columbia-Presby Med Ctr 1979; **Fellow:** Immunology, Columbia-Presby Med Ctr 1981; **Fac Appt:** Prof N, Cornell Univ-Weill Med Coll

Levine, David N MD [N] - **Spec Exp:** Dementia; Stroke; Spinal Cord Disorders; **Hospital:** NYU Langone Med Ctr (page 66); **Address:** 400 E 34th St, Ste RIR-311, New York, NY 10016-4901; **Phone:** 212-263-7744; **Board Cert:** Neurology 1976; **Med School:** Harvard Med Sch 1968; **Resid:** Neurology, Mass Genl Hosp 1974; **Fellow:** Neurology, Mass Genl Hosp 1976; **Fac Appt:** Prof N, NYU Sch Med

Levine, Steven R MD [N] - **Spec Exp:** Stroke; Cerebrovascular Disease; **Hospital:** SUNY Downstate Med Ctr; **Address:** SUNY Downstate Medical Center, 450 Clarkson Ave, Box 1213, Brooklyn, NY 11203; **Phone:** 718-221-5188; **Board Cert:** Neurology 1986; Vascular Neurology 2005; **Med School:** Med Coll Wisc 1981; **Resid:** Neurology, Univ Mich Hosps 1985; **Fellow:** Cerebrovascular Disease, Henry Ford Hosp 1987; **Fac Appt:** Prof N, Mount Sinai Sch Med

Liporace, Joyce D MD [N] - **Spec Exp:** Epilepsy in Women; Women's Health; Epilepsy in Pregnancy; **Hospital:** Riddle Meml Hosp; **Address:** Riddle Healthcare 2, 1088 Baltimore Pike, Ste 2205, Media, PA 19063; **Phone:** 610-744-2960; **Board Cert:** Neurological Surgery 1993; **Med School:** Johns Hopkins Univ 1988; **Resid:** Neurology, Hosp U Penn 1992; **Fellow:** Clinical Neurophysiology, Hosp U Penn 1994; **Fac Appt:** Assoc Prof Med, Thomas Jefferson Univ

Lipton, Richard MD [N] - **Spec Exp:** Headache; Clinical Trials; **Hospital:** Montefiore Med Ctr - Div. Weiler; **Address:** Montefiore Headache Center, 1575 Blondell Ave, Ste 225, Bronx, NY 10461-2662; **Phone:** 718-405-8360; **Board Cert:** Neurology 1985; **Med School:** Univ Chicago-Pritzker Sch Med 1980; **Resid:** Neurology, Montefiore Med Ctr 1984; **Fellow:** Neurological Physiology, Montefiore Med Ctr 1985; NeuroEpidemiology, Columbia Univ 1990; **Fac Appt:** Prof N, Albert Einstein Coll Med

Liu, Grant T MD [N] - **Spec Exp:** Pediatric Neuro-Ophthalmology; Neuro-Ophthalmology; **Hospital:** Hosp Univ Penn - UPHS (page 68), Chldns Hosp of Philadelphia; **Address:** Hosp Univ Penn, Dept Neurology, 3W Gates Bldg, 3400 Spruce St, Philadelphia, PA 19104; **Phone:** 215-349-8460; **Board Cert:** Neurology 1993; **Med School:** Columbia P&S 1988; **Resid:** Neurology, Harvard-Nolgwood Neurology Program 1992; **Fellow:** Neuro-Ophthalmology, Bascom Palmer Eye Inst 1993; **Fac Appt:** Prof N, Univ Pennsylvania

Logigian, Eric L MD [N] - **Spec Exp:** Neuromuscular Disorders; Electromyography; Lyme Disease; Peripheral Neuropathy; **Hospital:** Univ of Rochester Strong Meml Hosp, Highland Hosp of Rochester; **Address:** Univ Rochester, Dept of Neurology, 601 Elmwood Ave, Box 673, Rochester, NY 14642; **Phone:** 585-275-4568; **Board Cert:** Internal Medicine 1981; Neurology 1985; Clinical Neurophysiology 2009; **Med School:** Boston Univ 1978; **Resid:** Internal Medicine, Beth Israel Hosp 1981; Neurology, Mass Genl Hosp 1984; **Fellow:** Clinical Neurophysiology, Mass Genl Hosp 1985; **Fac Appt:** Prof N, Univ Rochester

Lublin, Fred D MD [N] - **Spec Exp:** Multiple Sclerosis; **Hospital:** Mount Sinai Med Ctr (page 63); **Address:** Dickinson Ctr for Multiple Sclerosis, 5 E 98th St, Box 1138, New York, NY 10029-6574; **Phone:** 212-241-6854; **Board Cert:** Neurology 1977; **Med School:** Jefferson Med Coll 1972; **Resid:** Neurology, New York Hosp/Cornell 1976; **Fac Appt:** Prof N, Mount Sinai Sch Med

McArthur, Justin C MD [N] - **Spec Exp:** AIDS/HIV; Multiple Sclerosis; **Hospital:** Johns Hopkins Hosp (page 61); **Address:** Johns Hopkins Hosp, Dept Neurology, 600 N Wolfe St, Meyer 6-113, Baltimore, MD 21287; **Phone:** 410-955-3730; **Board Cert:** Internal Medicine 1984; Neurology 1986; **Med School:** England, UK 1979; **Resid:** Internal Medicine, Johns Hopkins Hosp 1982; Neurology, Johns Hopkins Hosp 1985; **Fac Appt:** Prof N, Johns Hopkins Univ

McCluskey, Leo MD [N] - **Spec Exp:** Amyotrophic Lateral Sclerosis (ALS); **Hospital:** Pennsylvania Hosp-UPHS (page 68); **Address:** 330 S 9th St, Philadelphia, PA 19107; **Phone:** 215-829-3053; **Board Cert:** Neurology 1986; **Med School:** Columbia P&S 1980; **Resid:** Internal Medicine, Univ Mich 1982; Neurology, Hosp Univ Penn 1985; **Fellow:** Neuromuscular Disease, Hosp Univ Penn 1986; **Fac Appt:** Assoc Prof N, Univ Pennsylvania

Miller, Aaron MD [N] - **Spec Exp:** Multiple Sclerosis; Alzheimer's Disease; Autoimmune Disease; **Hospital:** Mount Sinai Med Ctr (page 63), Maimonides Med Ctr (page 62); **Address:** Corinne Goldsmith Dickinson Ctr for MS, 5 E 98th St, Box 1138, New York, NY 10029; **Phone:** 212-241-6854; **Board Cert:** Internal Medicine 1972; Neurology 1977; **Med School:** NYU Sch Med 1968; **Resid:** Internal Medicine, Jacobi Med Ctr 1970; Neurology, Montefiore Med Ctr 1975; **Fellow:** Neurovirology, Johns Hopkins Hosp 1977; **Fac Appt:** Prof N, Mount Sinai Sch Med

Mitsumoto, Hiroshi MD [N] - **Spec Exp:** Amyotrophic Lateral Sclerosis (ALS); Neuromuscular Disorders; Clinical Trials; **Hospital:** NY-Presby/Columbia Univ Med Ctr, NY (page 65); **Address:** Neurological Inst, 710 W 168th St Fl 9, New York, NY 10032; **Phone:** 212-305-1319; **Board Cert:** Neurology 1978; **Med School:** Japan 1968; **Resid:** Internal Medicine, Toho Univ Hosps 1972; Neurology, Univ Hosps 1976; **Fellow:** Neurological Pathology, Cleveland Clinic 1978; Neuromuscular Medicine, New England Med Ctr 1981; **Fac Appt:** Prof N, Columbia P&S

Neurology

Mohr, JP MD [N] - **Spec Exp:** Aphasia; Stroke; Arteriovenous Malformations; Moya Moya; **Hospital:** NY-Presby/Columbia Univ Med Ctr, NY (page 65); **Address:** Neurological Inst-Dept Neurology, 710 W 168 St, Ste 615, Box 141, New York, NY 10032-2603; **Phone:** 212-305-8033; **Board Cert:** Neurology 1971; Vascular Neurology 2005; **Med School:** Univ VA Sch Med 1963; **Resid:** Neurology, Columbia Presby Med Ctr 1966; Neurology, Mass Genl Hosp 1968; **Fellow:** Neurology, Mass Genl Hosp 1969; **Fac Appt:** Clin Prof N, Columbia P&S

Newman, Lawrence C MD [N] - **Spec Exp:** Headache; Pain-Facial; **Hospital:** St. Luke's - Roosevelt Hosp Ctr - Roosevelt Div (page 55); **Address:** St Luke's-Roosevelt Hosp-Headache Inst, 425 W 59th St Fl 4 - Ste A, New York, NY 10019; **Phone:** 212-523-5869; **Board Cert:** Neurology 2005; Headache Medicine 2006; **Med School:** Mexico 1983; **Resid:** Internal Medicine, Elmhurst Hosp 1986; Neurology, Montefiore Med Ctr 1989; **Fellow:** Headache, Montefiore Med Ctr 1990; **Fac Appt:** Prof N, Albert Einstein Coll Med

Olanow, C Warren MD [N] - **Spec Exp:** Parkinson's Disease; Movement Disorders; **Hospital:** Mount Sinai Med Ctr (page 63); **Address:** 1468 Madison Ave, Box 1137, New York, NY 10029; **Phone:** 212-241-8435; **Med School:** Univ Toronto 1965; **Resid:** Neurology, Toronto Genl Hosp 1968; Neurology, Columbia Presby Hosp 1970; **Fellow:** Neurological Anatomy, Columbia Presby Hosp 1971; **Fac Appt:** Prof N, Mount Sinai Sch Med

Pedley, Timothy A MD [N] - **Spec Exp:** Epilepsy/Seizure Disorders; **Hospital:** NY-Presby/Columbia Univ Med Ctr, NY (page 65); **Address:** The Neurological Inst, 710 W 168th St, rm 1406, New York, NY 10032; **Phone:** 212-305-6489; **Board Cert:** Neurology 1975; **Med School:** Yale Univ 1969; **Resid:** Neurology, Stanford Univ Hosp 1973; **Fellow:** Clinical Neurophysiology, Stanford Univ Hosp 1975; **Fac Appt:** Prof N, Columbia P&S

Petito, Frank A MD [N] - **Spec Exp:** Multiple Sclerosis; Headache; Lyme Disease; **Hospital:** NY-Presby/Weill Cornell Med Ctr, NY (page 65); **Address:** 525 E 68th St, Ste 607, New York, NY 10065; **Phone:** 212-746-2309; **Board Cert:** Neurology 1974; **Med School:** Columbia P&S 1967; **Resid:** Neurology, New York Hosp 1971; **Fac Appt:** Prof N, Cornell Univ-Weill Med Coll

Posner, Jerome B MD [N] - **Spec Exp:** Neuro-Oncology; Brain Tumors; Paraneoplastic Syndromes; **Hospital:** Meml Sloan-Kettering Cancer Ctr; **Address:** 1275 York Ave, rm C731, New York, NY 10065; **Phone:** 212-639-7047; **Board Cert:** Neurology 1962; **Med School:** Univ Wash 1955; **Resid:** Neurology, Univ WA Affil Hosp 1959; **Fellow:** Biochemistry, Univ WA Affil Hosp 1963; **Fac Appt:** Prof N, Cornell Univ-Weill Med Coll

Pula, Thaddeus MD [N] - **Spec Exp:** Neurophysiology; Electromyography; **Hospital:** Maryland Genl Hosp; **Address:** Maryland Genl Hosp, Div Neurology, 827 Linden Ave Fl 2, Baltimore, MD 21201-4606; **Phone:** 410-225-8290; **Board Cert:** Neurology 1981; **Med School:** Univ MD Sch Med 1976; **Resid:** Internal Medicine, Mercy Hosp Med Ctr; **Fellow:** Neurology, Univ Maryland

Reich, Stephen G MD [N] - **Spec Exp:** Movement Disorders; Parkinson's Disease; Ataxia; Dystonia-Botox Therapy; **Hospital:** Univ of MD Med Ctr; **Address:** Univ Maryland Med System, Frenkil Bldg, 16 S Eutaw St Fl 3, Baltimore, MD 21201; **Phone:** 410-328-5858; **Board Cert:** Neurology 1989; **Med School:** Tulane Univ 1983; **Resid:** Neurology, Case West Res Univ Hosp 1987; **Fellow:** Movement Disorders, Johns Hopkins Hosp 1988; **Fac Appt:** Assoc Prof N, Univ MD Sch Med

Relkin, Norman R MD/PhD [N] - **Spec Exp:** Alzheimer's Disease; Dementia; Memory Disorders; **Hospital:** NY-Presby/Weill Cornell Med Ctr, NY (page 65); **Address:** Weill Cornell Memory Disorders Program, 428 E 72nd St, Ste 500, New York, NY 10021; **Phone:** 212-746-2441; **Board Cert:** Neurology 1992; **Med School:** Albert Einstein Coll Med 1987; **Resid:** Neurology, New York Hosp 1991; **Fellow:** Behavioral Neurology, New York Hosp-Cornell 1992; **Fac Appt:** Asst Prof N, Cornell Univ-Weill Med Coll

Rosenfeld, Myrna MD/PhD [N] - **Spec Exp:** Neuro-Oncology; Brain Tumors; **Hospital:** Hosp Univ Penn - UPHS (page 68); **Address:** Hosp Univ Penn, Dept Neurology, 3 West Gates Bldg, 3400 Spruce St, Philadelphia, PA 19104; **Phone:** 215-746-4707; **Board Cert:** Neurology 2004; **Med School:** Northwestern Univ 1985; **Resid:** Neurology, Northwestern Univ Hosp 1987; Neurology, Univ Hosp Cleveland 1989; **Fellow:** Neuro-Oncology, Meml Sloan Kettering Cancer Ctr

Sage, Jacob MD [N] - **Spec Exp:** Parkinson's Disease; **Hospital:** Robert Wood Johnson Univ Hosp - New Brunswick; **Address:** UMDNJ, Dept Neurology, 125 Paterson St, Ste 6200, New Brunswick, NJ 08901-2160; **Phone:** 732-235-7733; **Board Cert:** Neurology 1979; **Med School:** Univ Pittsburgh 1972; **Resid:** Neurology, Univ Pittsburgh Hosps 1978; **Fellow:** Neurological Chemistry, NY Hosp-Cornell 1980; **Fac Appt:** Prof N, UMDNJ-RW Johnson Med Sch

Schwartzman, Robert J MD [N] - **Spec Exp:** Reflex Sympathetic Dystrophy (RSD); Pain Management; **Hospital:** Hahnemann Univ Hosp; **Address:** Drexel Neurological Assocs, 219 N Broad St Fl 7, Philadelphia, PA 19107; **Phone:** 215-762-6915; **Board Cert:** Internal Medicine 1971; Neurology 1974; **Med School:** Univ Pennsylvania 1965; **Resid:** Internal Medicine, Duke Univ Hosp 1967; Neurology, Hosp Univ Penn 1969; **Fellow:** Neurology, NIH-Med Neur Br 1971; **Fac Appt:** Prof N, Drexel Univ Coll Med

Shefner, Jeremy M MD/PhD [N] - **Spec Exp:** Amyotrophic Lateral Sclerosis (ALS); Neuromuscular Disorders; **Hospital:** SUNY Upstate Med Univ Shos; **Address:** 750 E Adams St, Syracuse, NY 13210-1834; **Phone:** 315-464-4243; **Board Cert:** Neurology 1989; Clinical Neurophysiology 2004; **Med School:** Northwestern Univ 1983; **Resid:** Neurology, Harvard-Longwood Neur Trng 1988; **Fellow:** Neuromuscular Disease, Brigham & Womens Hosp 1990; **Fac Appt:** Prof N, SUNY Upstate Med Univ

Shulman, Lisa M MD [N] - **Spec Exp:** Movement Disorders; Movement Disorders-Botox Therapy; Parkinson's Disease; **Hospital:** Univ of MD Med Ctr; **Address:** 110 S Paca St Fl 3, Baltimore, MD 21201; **Phone:** 410-328-2164; **Board Cert:** Neurology 1994; **Med School:** Univ Miami Sch Med 1988; **Resid:** Neurology, Jackson Meml Hosp 1992; **Fellow:** Movement Disorders, Jackson Meml Hosp 1994; **Fac Appt:** Assoc Prof N, Univ MD Sch Med

Silberstein, Stephen D MD [N] - **Spec Exp:** Headache; Migraine; **Hospital:** Thomas Jefferson Univ Hosp; **Address:** Jefferson Headache Center, 111 S 11th St, Gibbon Bldg, Ste 8130, Philadelphia, PA 19107; **Phone:** 215-955-2243; **Board Cert:** Neurology 1975; Headache Medicine 2006; **Med School:** Univ Pennsylvania 1967; **Resid:** Internal Medicine, Hosp Univ Penn 1969; Neurology, Hosp Univ Penn 1975; **Fac Appt:** Clin Prof N, Temple Univ

Simpson, David M MD [N] - **Spec Exp:** Infections-CNS; AIDS-Neurologic Complications; Peripheral Neuropathy; Neuromuscular Disorders; **Hospital:** Mount Sinai Med Ctr (page 63); **Address:** Mt Sinai Med Ctr, Dept Neurology, 1 Gustave L Levy Pl, Box 1052, Annenberg, 2nd Flr, New York, NY 10029; **Phone:** 212-241-8748; **Board Cert:** Neurology 1984; Clinical Neurophysiology 2005; Neuromuscular Medicine 2008; **Med School:** SUNY Buffalo 1979; **Resid:** Neurology, New York Hosp-Cornell Med Ctr 1983; **Fellow:** Clinical Neurophysiology, Mass Genl Hosp 1984; **Fac Appt:** Prof N, Mount Sinai Sch Med

Sirdofsky, Michael D MD [N] - **Spec Exp:** Neuromuscular Disorders; Electrodiagnosis; **Hospital:** Georgetown Univ Hosp; **Address:** Entrance 1 PHC Bldg Fl 7, 3800 Resevoir Rd NW, Washington, DC 20007; **Phone:** 202-444-8525; **Board Cert:** Neurology 1981; **Med School:** Georgetown Univ 1976; **Resid:** Neurology, Georgetown Univ Hosp 1980; **Fac Appt:** Assoc Prof N, Georgetown Univ

Sperling, Michael R MD [N] - **Spec Exp:** Epilepsy; **Hospital:** Thomas Jefferson Univ Hosp; **Address:** Thomas Jefferson Univ Hosp, Dept Neurology, 900 Walnut St, Ste 200, Philadelphia, PA 19107; **Phone:** 215-955-1222; **Board Cert:** Neurology 1984; Clinical Neurophysiology 2009; **Med School:** Temple Univ 1978; **Resid:** Neurology, Mt Sinai Hosp 1982; **Fellow:** Epilepsy, UCLA Med Ctr 1984; **Fac Appt:** Prof N, Thomas Jefferson Univ

Stern, Matthew B MD [N] - **Spec Exp:** Parkinson's Disease; Movement Disorders; Botox Therapy; **Hospital:** Pennsylvania Hosp-UPHS (page 68), Hosp Univ Penn - UPHS (page 68); **Address:** Pennsylvania Hosp, Dept Neurology, 330 S 9th St Fl 3, Philadelphia, PA 19107; **Phone:** 215-829-6500; **Board Cert:** Neurology 1983; **Med School:** Duke Univ 1978; **Resid:** Neurology, Hosp Univ Penn 1982; **Fac Appt:** Prof N, Univ Pennsylvania

Swerdlow, Michael L MD [N] - **Spec Exp:** Myasthenia Gravis; Spinal Disorders; Multiple Sclerosis; **Hospital:** Montefiore Med Ctr - Div. Moses; **Address:** 3400 Bainbridge Ave, Bronx, NY 10467-2401; **Phone:** 718-920-4178; **Board Cert:** Neurology 1975; **Med School:** Univ Pennsylvania 1967; **Resid:** Internal Medicine, Mount Sinai Hosp 1969; Neurology, Montefiore Med Ctr 1972; **Fellow:** Neurology, Natl Inst Hlth 1974; **Fac Appt:** Prof N, Albert Einstein Coll Med

Tayal, Ashis H MD [N] - **Spec Exp:** Stroke; Vascular Neurology; **Hospital:** Allegheny General Hosp; **Address:** Allegheny Neurology Assocs, 420 E North Ave, Ste 206, E Wing Professional Bldg, Pittsburgh, PA 15212; **Phone:** 412-359-8850; **Board Cert:** Internal Medicine 2007; Neurology 2006; Vascular Neurology 2008; **Med School:** Tufts Univ 1994; **Resid:** Internal Medicine, Mount Sinai Med Ctr 1997; Neurology, Univ Pittsburgh Med Ctr 2001; **Fellow:** Vascular Neurology, Univ Pittsburgh Med Ctr 2006

Vas, George A MD [N] - **Spec Exp:** Stroke; Multiple Sclerosis; **Hospital:** SUNY Downstate Med Ctr, Kings County Hosp Ctr; **Address:** 450 Clarkson Ave, Ste A, Brooklyn, NY 11203-2056; **Phone:** 718-270-2502; **Board Cert:** Internal Medicine 1973; Neurology 1977; Clinical Neurophysiology 2002; **Med School:** Univ Pittsburgh 1970; **Resid:** Internal Medicine, New York Hosp 1972; Neurology, New York Hosp 1975; **Fac Appt:** Prof N, SUNY Downstate

Waters, Cheryl H MD [N] - **Spec Exp:** Parkinson's Disease; Movement Disorders; **Hospital:** NY-Presby/Columbia Univ Med Ctr, NY (page 65); **Address:** 710 W 168th St Fl 3, New York, NY 10032; **Phone:** 212-305-3665; **Board Cert:** Neurology 1986; **Med School:** Univ Toronto 1980; **Resid:** Internal Medicine, Univ Toronto Med Ctr 1982; Neurology, Univ Toronto Med Ctr 1985; **Fellow:** Neurological Pharmacology, Univ Toronto Med Ctr 1987; **Fac Appt:** Prof N, Columbia P&S

Wechsler, Lawrence R MD [N] - **Spec Exp:** Cerebrovascular Disease; Stroke; **Hospital:** UPMC Presby, Pittsburgh, UPMC Shadyside; **Address:** UPMC Stroke Institute, 3471 Fifth Ave, Ste 810, Pittsburgh, PA 15213; **Phone:** 412-692-4920; **Board Cert:** Internal Medicine 1983; Neurology 1984; Vascular Neurology 2005; **Med School:** Univ Pennsylvania 1978; **Resid:** Internal Medicine, Presby-Univ Hosp 1980; Neurology, Mass Genl Hosp 1983; **Fellow:** Clinical Neurophysiology, Mass Genl Hosp 1984; Cerebrovascular Disease, Mass Genl Hosp 1985; **Fac Appt:** Prof N, Univ Pittsburgh

Weinberg, Harold J MD [N] - **Spec Exp:** Stroke; Spinal Disorders; Neuromuscular Disorders; Memory Disorders; **Hospital:** NYU Langone Med Ctr (page 66); **Address:** 650 1st Ave Fl 4, New York, NY 10016-3240; **Phone:** 212-213-9339; **Board Cert:** Neurology 1983; Electrodiagnostic Medicine 1989; **Med School:** Albert Einstein Coll Med 1978; **Resid:** Neurology, Columbia-Presby Med Ctr 1982; **Fellow:** Neuromuscular Medicine, Columbia-Presby Med Ctr 1982; **Fac Appt:** Clin Prof N, NYU Sch Med

Weiner, William J MD [N] - **Spec Exp:** Movement Disorders; Parkinson's Disease; Huntington's Disease; Progressive Supranuclear Palsy (PSP); **Hospital:** Univ of MD Med Ctr; **Address:** Univ Maryland Med System, Dept Neurology, 110 S Paca St, rm S124, Baltimore, MD 21201; **Phone:** 410-328-2172; **Board Cert:** Neurology 1975; **Med School:** Univ IL Coll Med 1969; **Resid:** Neurology, Univ Minn 1971; Neurology, Rush-Presby Med Ctr 1973; **Fac Appt:** Prof N, Univ MD Sch Med

Wityk, Robert J MD [N] - **Spec Exp:** Stroke; Cerebrovascular Disease; **Hospital:** Johns Hopkins Hosp (page 61); **Address:** Johns Hopkins Outpatient Ctr, 601 N Caroline St, Ste 5073A, Baltimore, MD 21287; **Phone:** 410-955-2228; **Board Cert:** Internal Medicine 1988; Neurology 1992; **Med School:** Case West Res Univ 1985; **Resid:** Internal Medicine, UCSD Med Ctr 1988; Neurology, Mass Genl Hosp 1991; **Fellow:** Cardiovascular Disease, Tufts U-New Eng MC 1992; **Fac Appt:** Assoc Prof N, Johns Hopkins Univ

Zimmerman, Earl A MD [N] - **Spec Exp:** Memory Disorders; Alzheimer's Disease; Dementia; **Hospital:** Albany Med Ctr; **Address:** Albany Med Ctr-Neurology, 47 New Scotland Ave, MC 65, Albany, NY 12208; **Phone:** 518-262-0800; **Board Cert:** Neurology 1970; Internal Medicine 1970; **Med School:** Univ Pennsylvania 1963; **Resid:** Internal Medicine, Presbyterian Hosp 1965; Neurology, Neurological Inst 1968; **Fellow:** Endocrinology, Presbyterian Hosp 1972; **Fac Appt:** Prof N, Albany Med Coll

Southeast

Abou-Khalil, Bassel MD [N] - **Spec Exp:** Epilepsy; Neurophysiology; **Hospital:** Vanderbilt Univ Med Ctr (page 76); **Address:** Vanderbilt Univ-Dept Neurology, 1161 21st Ave S, rm A-0118 MCN, Nashville, TN 37232-2551; **Phone:** 615-936-0060; **Board Cert:** Neurology 1986; Clinical Neurophysiology 2002; **Med School:** Amer Univ Beirut 1978; **Resid:** Neurology, Strong Meml Hosp 1980; Neurology, Univ Mich Hosps 1982; **Fellow:** Epilepsy, Univ Mich Hosps 1985; Electroencephalography, Univ Mich Hosps 1985; **Fac Appt:** Prof N, Vanderbilt Univ

Adams, David J MD [N] - **Spec Exp:** Diagnostic Problems; Hydrocephalus-normal pressure; Pseudotumor Cerebri; Autoimmune Disease; **Hospital:** Univ of Miami Hosp (page 72), Jackson Meml Hosp (page 70); **Address:** Univ Miami Dept Neurology, 1150 NW 14th St, Ste 609, Miami, FL 33136; **Phone:** 305-243-6732; **Board Cert:** Neurology 1977; **Med School:** Columbia P&S 1969; **Resid:** Neurology, Neurological Inst 1975; **Fac Appt:** Clin Prof N, Univ Miami Sch Med

Adams, Robert J MD [N] - **Spec Exp:** Stroke; **Hospital:** MUSC Med Ctr; **Address:** MUSC Stroke Center, 19 Hagood Ave, Ste 501, Charleston, SC 29425; **Phone:** 843-792-7058; **Board Cert:** Neurology 1987; Vascular Neurology 2008; **Med School:** Univ Ark 1980; **Resid:** Neurology, Med Coll Georgia 1985; **Fac Appt:** Assoc Prof N, Med Coll GA

Alexandrov, Andrei MD [N] - **Spec Exp:** Stroke; Cerebrovascular Disease; **Hospital:** Univ of Ala Hosp at Birmingham; **Address:** 2000 6th Ave S, Birmingham, AL 35253; **Phone:** 205-801-8986; **Med School:** Russia 1989; **Resid:** Child Neurology, Russian Academy of Med Sciences 1991; **Fellow:** Neuroimaging, Univ Texas Affil Hosp 1998; **Fac Appt:** Prof N, Univ Alabama

Ashizawa, Tetsuo MD [N] - **Spec Exp:** Movement Disorders; Myasthenia Gravis; Parkinson's Disease; Huntington's Disease; **Hospital:** Shands at Univ of FL; **Address:** Neurology at Shands Med Plaza, 2000 SW Archer Rd Fl 3, PO Box 100236, Gainesville, FL 32608-0236; **Phone:** 352-265-8408; **Board Cert:** Neurology 1980; **Med School:** Japan 1973; **Resid:** Neurology, Baylor Coll of Med Affil Hosp 1978; **Fellow:** Neuromuscular Disease, Baylor Coll of Med Affil Hosp 1978; **Fac Appt:** Prof N, Univ Fla Coll Med

Bebin, E Martina MD [N] - **Spec Exp:** Epilepsy; Child Neurology; Tuberous Sclerosis; **Hospital:** Univ of Ala Hosp at Birmingham; **Address:** 1719 6th Ave S, Birmingham, AL 35294; **Phone:** 205-801-8986; **Board Cert:** Child Neurology 2003; **Med School:** Univ Miss 1986; **Resid:** Neurology, Mayo Clnic 1991; **Fac Appt:** Assoc Prof N, Univ Alabama

Berger, Joseph MD [N] - **Spec Exp:** Multiple Sclerosis; AIDS/HIV; Infectious & Demyelinating Diseases; **Hospital:** Univ of Kentucky Albert B. Chandler Hosp; **Address:** Kentucky Neuroscience Clinic, 740 S Limestone St, Lexington, KY 40536; **Phone:** 859-323-5661; **Board Cert:** Internal Medicine 1977; Neurology 1983; **Med School:** Jefferson Med Coll 1974; **Resid:** Internal Medicine, Georgetown Univ Hosp 1977; Neurology, Jackson Meml Hosp 1981; **Fac Appt:** Prof N, Univ KY Coll Med

Bertorini, Tulio E MD [N] - **Spec Exp:** Clinical Neurophysiology; Neuromuscular Disorders; Electromyography; **Hospital:** Methodist Univ Hosp - Memphis; **Address:** 1211 Union Ave, Ste 400, Memphis, TN 38104; **Phone:** 901-725-8920; **Board Cert:** Neurology 1977; **Med School:** Peru 1970; **Resid:** Neurology, Georgetown Univ Sch Med 1973; Neurology, VA Hosp/Armed Forces Inst Path 1974; **Fellow:** Electrodiagnosis, Mass Genl Hosp 1975; Clinical Neurophysiology, Natl Inst Neuro Comm Dis & Stroke/NIH 1977; **Fac Appt:** Prof N, Univ Tenn Coll Med

Brooks, Benjamin R MD [N] - **Spec Exp:** Neuromuscular Disorders; Multiple Sclerosis; Neurotoxicology; **Hospital:** Carolinas Med Ctr, Levine Chldns Hosp; **Address:** CMC Dept Neurology, 1010 Edgehill Rd N, Charlotte, NC 28207-1885; **Phone:** 704-446-1900; **Board Cert:** Internal Medicine 1974; Neurology 1978; **Med School:** Harvard Med Sch 1970; **Resid:** Neurology, Mass Genl Hosp 1974; Neurology, Natl Inst Neuro Disorders & Stroke-NIH 1976; **Fellow:** Neurovirology, Johns Hopkins Hosp 1978

Corbett, James MD [N] - **Spec Exp:** Neuro-Ophthalmology; Pseudotumor Cerebri; Neurosarcoidosis; Headache; **Hospital:** Univ Mississippi Med Ctr; **Address:** Univ Mississippi Med Ctr, Dept Neurology, 2500 N State St, Jackson, MS 39216-4505; **Phone:** 601-984-5501; **Board Cert:** Neurology 2004; **Med School:** Ros Franklin Univ/Chicago Med Sch 1966; **Resid:** Internal Medicine, Rhode Island Hosp 1968; Neurology, Univ Hosp-Case Western Reserve 1971; **Fac Appt:** Prof N, Univ Miss

DeKosky, Steven T MD [N] - **Spec Exp:** Alzheimer's Disease; Dementia; Behavioral Neurology; Geriatric Neurology; **Hospital:** Univ of Virginia Health Sys; **Address:** Univ Virgina School of Med, Box 800973, Charlottesville, VA 22908; **Phone:** 434-924-5118; **Board Cert:** Neurology 2004; **Med School:** Univ Fla Coll Med 1974; **Resid:** Internal Medicine, Johns Hopkins Hosp 1975; Neurology, Univ Florida 1978; **Fellow:** Neurological Chemistry, Univ Virginia Hosp 1979; **Fac Appt:** Prof N, Univ VA Sch Med

DeLong, Mahlon R MD [N] - **Spec Exp:** Parkinson's Disease; Movement Disorders; **Hospital:** Emory Univ Hosp, Wesley Woods Ger Hosp; **Address:** Wesley Woods Health Ctr, 1841 Clifton Rd NE, Atlanta, GA 30329; **Phone:** 404-778-3444; **Board Cert:** Neurology 1980; **Med School:** Harvard Med Sch 1966; **Resid:** Internal Medicine, Boston City Hosp 1968; Neurology, Johns Hopkins Hosp 1976; **Fellow:** Neurology, NIMH 1973; **Fac Appt:** Prof N, Emory Univ

Finkel, Alan G MD [N] - **Spec Exp:** Headache; Pain-Facial; Migraine; **Hospital:** NC Memorial Hosp - UNC; **Address:** Carolina Headache Inst, 103 Market St, Chapel Hill, NC 27516; **Phone:** 919-942-4424; **Board Cert:** Neurology 1991; Pain Medicine 2003; Headache Medicine 2006; **Med School:** SUNY Buffalo 1985; **Resid:** Neurology, NC Meml Hosp 1989; **Fellow:** Pain & Headache Medicine, Univ NC Hosp; **Fac Appt:** Prof N, Univ NC Sch Med

Finkel, Michael F MD [N] - **Spec Exp:** Movement Disorders-Lower Limb; ADD/ADHD; Headache in Women; Trauma Neurology; **Hospital:** Physicians Regl Hlthcare Med Ctr-Pine Ridge; **Address:** Physicians Regl Med Grp, 6101 Pine Ridge Rd, Naples, FL 34119; **Phone:** 239-348-4093; **Board Cert:** Neurology 1979; **Med School:** Washington Univ, St Louis 1973; **Resid:** Neurology, Strong Meml Hosp 1977

Glass, Jonathan D MD [N] - **Spec Exp:** Neuro-Pathology; Amyotrophic Lateral Sclerosis (ALS); Peripheral Neuropathy; Neuromuscular Disorders; **Hospital:** Emory Univ Hosp, Grady Hlth Sys; **Address:** 1365 Clifton Rd NE, A Bldg Fl 3 - Ste A3100, Atlanta, GA 30322; **Phone:** 404-778-3444; **Board Cert:** Neurology 1990; Neuropathology 1997; **Med School:** Univ VT Coll Med 1985; **Resid:** Neurology, Johns Hopkins Hosp 1989; **Fellow:** Neuropathology, Johns Hopkins Univ 1991; **Fac Appt:** Prof N, Emory Univ

Goldstein, Larry B MD [N] - **Spec Exp:** Stroke; Carotid Artery Disease; **Hospital:** Duke Univ Hosp, Durham VA Med Ctr; **Address:** Duke Univ Med Ctr, 200 Trent Dr, Clinic 1-L, Durham, NC 27710; **Phone:** 919-684-3801; **Board Cert:** Neurology 1987; Vascular Neurology 2005; **Med School:** Mount Sinai Sch Med 1981; **Resid:** Neurology, Mt Sinai Hosp 1985; **Fellow:** Cerebrovascular Disease, Duke Univ Med Ctr 1986; **Fac Appt:** Prof N, Duke Univ

Gress, Daryl Ray MD [N] - **Spec Exp:** Critical Care; Stroke; **Hospital:** Univ of Virginia Health Sys; **Address:** Univ of VA Health Sys, Dept Neurology, Box 800394, Charlottesville, VA 22908; **Phone:** 434-924-8371; **Board Cert:** Neurology 1989; **Med School:** Washington Univ, St Louis 1982; **Resid:** Internal Medicine, Johns Hopkins Hosp 1984; Neurology, Mass Genl Hosp 1987; **Fellow:** Stroke, Mass Genl Hosp 1988

Haley Jr, Elliott C MD [N] - **Spec Exp:** Stroke; **Hospital:** Univ of Virginia Health Sys; **Address:** Univ VA Hlth Sys, Dept Neurology, Box 800394, Charlottesville, VA 22908; **Phone:** 434-982-6952; **Board Cert:** Internal Medicine 1978; Neurology 1985; Vascular Neurology 2008; **Med School:** Tulane Univ 1974; **Resid:** Internal Medicine, Univ Va Hosp 1978; Neurology, Univ Va Hosp 1982; **Fellow:** Cerebrovascular Disease, Mass Genl Hosp 1984; **Fac Appt:** Prof N, Univ VA Sch Med

Hauser, Robert A MD [N] - **Spec Exp:** Movement Disorders; Parkinson's Disease; **Hospital:** Tampa Genl Hosp; **Address:** Parkinsons Disease & Movement Ctr, 5 Tampa Genl Cir, Ste 410, Tampa, FL 33606-3500; **Phone:** 813-844-4077; **Board Cert:** Neurology 1989; **Med School:** Temple Univ 1982; **Resid:** Neurological Surgery, Eastern VA Med Ctr 1985; Neurology, Eastern VA Med Ctr 1988; **Fellow:** Movement Disorders, Univ S Florida Affil Hosp 1990; **Fac Appt:** Prof N, Univ S Fla Coll Med

Heilman, Kenneth M MD [N] - **Spec Exp:** Behavioral Neurology; Memory Disorders; Aphasia; Speech Disorders; **Hospital:** Shands at Univ of FL, Malcolm Randall VA Med Ctr; **Address:** Hlth Ctr Univ Fla Coll Med, Dept Neur, PO Box 100236, Gainesville, FL 32610-0236; **Phone:** 352-273-5550; **Board Cert:** Neurology 1973; **Med School:** Univ VA Sch Med 1963; **Resid:** Internal Medicine, Bellevue Hosp Ctr 1965; Neurology, Boston City Hosp 1970; **Fac Appt:** Prof N, Univ Fla Coll Med

Hess, David C MD [N] - **Spec Exp:** Stroke; Antiphospholipid Syndrome (APS); **Hospital:** Med Coll of GA Hosp and Clin (MCG Health Inc); **Address:** Med Coll Ga Dept Neurology, 1120 15th St, rm Bl-3080, Augusta, GA 30912; **Phone:** 706-721-1691; **Board Cert:** Internal Medicine 1986; Neurology 1990; Vascular Surgery 2008; **Med School:** Univ MD Sch Med 1983; **Resid:** Internal Medicine, Allegheny Genl Hosp 1985; Neurology, Med Coll Ga 1989; **Fellow:** Cerebrovascular Disease, Med Coll Ga 1990; **Fac Appt:** Prof N, Med Coll GA

Janss, Anna J MD/PhD [N] - **Spec Exp:** Brain Tumors-Pediatric; Clinical Trials; Cancer Survivors-Late Effects of Therapy; **Hospital:** Chldns Hlthcare Atlanta @ Egleston, Chldns Hlthcare Atlanta @ Scottish Rite; **Address:** Aflac Cancer & Blood Disorders Ctr, Outpatient Clin, Tower 1 Fl 4, 1405 Clifton Rd NE, Atlanta, GA 30322; **Phone:** 404-785-1200; **Board Cert:** Neurology 1993; **Med School:** Univ Iowa Coll Med 1988; **Resid:** Neurology, Hosp Univ Penn 1992; **Fellow:** Pediatric Neuro-Oncology, Chldns Hosp 1996; **Fac Appt:** Assoc Prof N, Emory Univ

Kirshner, Howard S MD [N] - **Spec Exp:** Stroke; Aphasia; Neuro-Rehabilitation; Behavioral Neurology; **Hospital:** Vanderbilt Univ Med Ctr (page 76), Vanderbilt Stallworth Rehab Hosp (page 76); **Address:** Vanderbilt Univ Med Ctr, Dept Neurology, A-0118 Medical Center North, Nashville, TN 37232-2551; **Phone:** 615-936-1354; **Board Cert:** Neurology 1980; Vascular Neurology 2005; **Med School:** Harvard Med Sch 1972; **Resid:** Neurology, Mass Genl Hosp 1978; **Fellow:** Neurological Science, Natl Inst Hlth 1975; **Fac Appt:** Prof N, Vanderbilt Univ

Kurtzke, Robert N MD [N] - **Spec Exp:** Electromyography; Nerve/Muscle Disorders; **Hospital:** Inova Fairfax Hosp, Reston Hosp Ctr; **Address:** Neurology Ctr of Fairfax, 3020 Hamaker Ct, Ste 400, Fairfax, VA 22031-2220; **Phone:** 703-876-0800; **Board Cert:** Neurology 1990; Clinical Neurophysiology 2004; **Med School:** Georgetown Univ 1985; **Resid:** Neurology, Neurology Inst-Columbia Presby 1989; **Fellow:** Neuromuscular Disease, Duke Univ Med Ctr 1990

Lavin, Patrick J MD [N] - **Spec Exp:** Neuro-Ophthalmology; Eye Movement Disorders; Headache; Neuro-Otology; **Hospital:** Vanderbilt Univ Med Ctr (page 76); **Address:** Vanderbilt Univ Dept Neurology, 1161 21st Ave S, A-0118 MCN, Nashville, TN 37232-2551; **Phone:** 615-936-0060; **Board Cert:** Neurology 1985; **Med School:** Ireland 1970; **Resid:** Internal Medicine, St Vincent Hosp Elm Pk 1973; Internal Medicine, Genl Hosp-Royal Infirm 1976; **Fellow:** Neurology, Case Western Reserve Univ 1981; Neuro-Ophthalmology, Case Western Reserve Univ 1983; **Fac Appt:** Prof N, Vanderbilt Univ

Montgomery Jr, Erwin B MD [N] - **Spec Exp:** Parkinson's Disease; Movement Disorders; **Hospital:** Univ of Ala Hosp at Birmingham; **Address:** UAB Dept Neurology, 1720 7th Ave S, SC 350, Birmingham, AL 35233; **Phone:** 205-934-0683; **Board Cert:** Neurology 1982; **Med School:** SUNY Buffalo 1976; **Resid:** Neurology, Barnes Jewish Hosp 1980; **Fellow:** Neurological Physiology, Washington Univ 1981; **Fac Appt:** Prof N, Univ Alabama

Moots, Paul L MD [N] - **Spec Exp:** Neuro-Oncology; Brain Tumors; Neurologic Complications of Cancer; Pain-Neuropathic; **Hospital:** Vanderbilt Univ Med Ctr (page 76), TN Valley Healthcare Sys-Nashville; **Address:** Vanderbilt Dept Neurology, 1161 21st Ave S, A-0118 Med Ctr North, Nashville, TN 37232; **Phone:** 615-322-6053; **Board Cert:** Neurology 1989; **Med School:** Ohio State Univ 1980; **Resid:** Neurology, Univ Va Med Ctr 1984; **Fellow:** Neuropathology, Univ Virginia 1986; Neuro-Oncology, Meml Sloan Kettering Canc 1989; **Fac Appt:** Assoc Prof N, Vanderbilt Univ

Morgenlander, Joel C MD [N] - **Spec Exp:** Nerve/Muscle Disorders; Stroke; Multiple Sclerosis; **Hospital:** Duke Univ Hosp; **Address:** Duke Univ Med Ctr, 200 Trent Dr, Clinic 1-L, Durham, NC 27710; **Phone:** 919-684-6887; **Board Cert:** Neurology 1992; **Med School:** Univ Pittsburgh 1986; **Resid:** Neurology, Duke Univ Med Ctr 1990; **Fellow:** Neuromuscular Disease, Duke Univ Med Ctr 1991; **Fac Appt:** Prof N, Duke Univ

Nabors III, L Burt MD [N] - **Spec Exp:** Neuro-Oncology; Brain Tumors; **Hospital:** Univ of Ala Hosp at Birmingham; **Address:** UAB, FOT 1020, 510 20th St S, Birmingham, AL 35294-0001; **Phone:** 205-934-1432; **Board Cert:** Neurology 2009; **Med School:** Univ Tenn Coll Med 1991; **Resid:** Neurology, Univ Alabama Med Ctr; **Fellow:** Neuro-Oncology, Univ Alabama; **Fac Appt:** Prof N, Univ Alabama

Newman, Nancy J MD [N] - **Spec Exp:** Neuro-Ophthalmology; **Hospital:** Emory Univ Hosp, Chldns Hlthcare Atlanta @ Egleston; **Address:** Emory Eye Center, 1365 Clifton Rd NE B Bldg - Ste 4500, Atlanta, GA 30322; **Phone:** 404-778-5360; **Board Cert:** Neurology 1989; **Med School:** Harvard Med Sch 1984; **Resid:** Neurology, Mass Genl Hosp 1988; **Fellow:** Neuro-Ophthalmology, Mass EE Infirmary 1989; **Fac Appt:** Prof N, Emory Univ

Nolan, Bruce A MD [N] - **Spec Exp:** Sleep Disorders/Apnea; **Hospital:** Jackson Meml Hosp (page 70); **Address:** Univ Miami Dept Neurology, 1501 NW 9th Ave, Miami, FL 33136; **Phone:** 305-243-5195; **Board Cert:** Neurology 1974; **Med School:** Wayne State Univ 1966; **Resid:** Neurology, Univ Miami Affil Hosp 1970; **Fac Appt:** Assoc Prof N, Univ Miami Sch Med

Oh, Shin Joong MD [N] - **Spec Exp:** Neuromuscular Disorders; Electromyography; Myasthenia Gravis; **Hospital:** Univ of Ala Hosp at Birmingham; **Address:** UAB Dept Neurology, 1530 3rd Ave S, SC 200, Birmingham, AL 35294-0017; **Phone:** 205-934-2120; **Board Cert:** Neurology 1973; Clinical Neurophysiology 2001; Neuromuscular Medicine 2009; **Med School:** Korea 1960; **Resid:** Internal Medicine, Seoul National Univ Hosp 1964; Neurology, Georgetown Univ Hosp 1967; **Fellow:** NeuroEpidemiology, Univ Minnesota Hosps 1968; **Fac Appt:** Prof N, Univ Alabama

Rothrock, John F MD [N] - **Spec Exp:** Headache; Stroke; **Hospital:** Univ of Ala Hosp at Birmingham; **Address:** UAB, Dept Neurology, 1530 3rd Ave S, SC 426, Birmingham, AL 35294-0017; **Phone:** 205-996-7945; **Board Cert:** Neurology 1984; Vascular Neurology 2009; Headache Medicine 2009; **Med School:** Univ VA Sch Med 1977; **Resid:** Neurology, Univ Ariz Med Ctr 1981; **Fac Appt:** Prof N, Univ Alabama

Sacco, Ralph L MD [N] - **Spec Exp:** Stroke; Stroke Prevention; **Hospital:** Jackson Meml Hosp (page 70), Univ of Miami Hosp & Clins/Sylvester Comp Canc Ctr (page 73); **Address:** Univ of Miami-Dept of Neurology, 1120 NW 14th St Fl 13 - Ste 1352, Miami, FL 33136; **Phone:** 305-243-7519; **Board Cert:** Neurology 1989; **Med School:** Boston Univ 1983; **Resid:** Neurology, Columbia-Presby Med Ctr 1987; **Fellow:** Cerebrovascular Disease, Columbia-Presby Med Ctr 1989; **Fac Appt:** Prof N, Univ Miami Sch Med

Sadowsky, Carl H MD [N] - **Spec Exp:** Memory Disorders; Alzheimer's Disease; **Hospital:** Columbia Hosp - W Palm Beach; **Address:** 4631 N Congress Ave, Ste 200, West Palm Beach, FL 33407-2234; **Phone:** 561-845-0500 x129; **Board Cert:** Neurology 1977; **Med School:** Cornell Univ 1971; **Resid:** Internal Medicine, Dartmouth-Hitchcock Med Ctr 1973; Neurology, Dartmouth-Hitchcock Med Ctr 1976; **Fac Appt:** Assoc Clin Prof N, Nova SE Univ, Coll Osteo Med

Schatz, Norman J MD [N] - **Spec Exp:** Neuro-Ophthalmology; Multiple Sclerosis & Visual Loss; Vision-Unexplained Loss; **Hospital:** Bascom Palmer Eye Inst (page 71), Univ of Miami Hosp (page 72); **Address:** 4701 N Meridian Ave, Adams Bldg - Ste 500A, Miami Beach, FL 33140; **Phone:** 305-532-2885; **Board Cert:** Neurology 1969; **Med School:** Hahnemann Univ 1961; **Resid:** Neurology, Jefferson Hosp 1965; **Fellow:** Neuro-Ophthalmology, Bascom Palmer Eye Inst 1966; **Fac Appt:** Clin Prof N, Univ Pennsylvania

Schiff, David MD [N] - **Spec Exp:** Brain Tumors; Spinal Cord Tumors; Neurologic Complications of Cancer; Neuro-Oncology; **Hospital:** Univ of Virginia Health Sys; **Address:** Univ VA, Div of Neuro-Oncology, PO Box 800432, Charlottesville, VA 22908; **Phone:** 434-982-4415; **Board Cert:** Neurology 1994; **Med School:** Harvard Med Sch 1988; **Resid:** Neurology, Harvard Longwood 1992; **Fellow:** Neuro-Oncology, Meml Sloan Kettering Cancer Ctr 1993; Mayo Clinic 1994; **Fac Appt:** Assoc Prof NS, Univ VA Sch Med

Neurology

Sethi, Kapil D MD [N] - **Spec Exp:** Parkinson's Disease; Restless Legs Syndrome; Movement Disorders; Botox Therapy; **Hospital:** Med Coll of GA Hosp and Clin (MCG Health Inc); **Address:** Med Coll Georgia, Dept Neurology, 1459 Harper St, Augusta, GA 30912-0004; **Phone:** 706-721-2798; **Board Cert:** Neurology 1987; **Med School:** India 1976; **Resid:** Neurology, Pgimer 1981; Neurology, Med Coll Georgia 1985; **Fac Appt:** Prof N, Med Coll GA

Singer, Carlos MD [N] - **Spec Exp:** Parkinson's Disease; Movement Disorders; Botox Therapy; **Hospital:** Jackson Meml Hosp (page 70); **Address:** Univ Miami Dept Neurology, 1501 NW 9th Ave, Miami, FL 33136; **Phone:** 305-243-3876; **Board Cert:** Internal Medicine 1976; Neurology 1981; **Med School:** Venezuela 1972; **Resid:** Internal Medicine, Montefiore Hosp 1976; Neurology, Albert Einstein Affil Hosp 1979; **Fellow:** Electromyography, Jackson Meml Hosp 1981; Movement Disorders, Univ Miami 1989; **Fac Appt:** Prof N, Univ Miami Sch Med

Watts, Ray L MD [N] - **Spec Exp:** Parkinson's Disease; Movement Disorders; **Hospital:** Univ of Ala Hosp at Birmingham; **Address:** 510 20th St S, FOT 1203, Birmingham, AL 35294; **Phone:** 205-934-0683; **Board Cert:** Neurology 1985; **Med School:** Washington Univ, St Louis 1980; **Resid:** Neurology, Mass Genl Hosp 1984; **Fellow:** Electromyography, Mass Genl Hosp 1983; **Fac Appt:** Prof N, Univ Alabama

Wooten Jr, George F MD [N] - **Spec Exp:** Movement Disorders; Parkinson's Disease; Tremor & Dystonia; **Hospital:** Univ of Virginia Health Sys; **Address:** Univ VA Hlth Sys, Dept Neuro-McKim Hall, Box 800394, Charlottesville, VA 22908; **Phone:** 434-924-2706; **Board Cert:** Neurology 1977; **Med School:** Cornell Univ-Weill Med Coll 1970; **Resid:** Neurology, NY Hosp-Cornell 1977; **Fellow:** Pharmacology, Natl Inst Hlth-NIMH 1974; **Fac Appt:** Prof N, Univ VA Sch Med

Midwest

Adams Jr, Harold P MD [N] - **Spec Exp:** Stroke; Cerebrovascular Disease; **Hospital:** Univ Iowa Hosp & Clinics; **Address:** Univ Iowa Hosp, Dept Neurology, 200 Hawkins Drive, rm 2148-RCP, Iowa City, IA 52242; **Phone:** 319-356-4110; **Board Cert:** Neurology 2004; Vascular & Interventional Radiology 2005; **Med School:** Northwestern Univ 1970; **Resid:** Neurology, Univ Iowa Hosp 1974; **Fac Appt:** Prof N, Univ Iowa Coll Med

Ahlskog, J Eric MD/PhD [N] - **Spec Exp:** Parkinson's Disease; Movement Disorders; **Hospital:** Mayo Med Ctr & Clin - Rochester, St. Mary's Hosp - Rochester MN (Mayo); **Address:** Mayo Clinic, Dept Neurology, 200 First St SW, Rochester, MN 55905; **Phone:** 507-538-1038; **Board Cert:** Neurology 1984; **Med School:** Dartmouth Med Sch 1976; **Resid:** Internal Medicine, Univ Chicago Hosps Clins 1978; Neurology, Mayo Grad Sch Med 1981; **Fac Appt:** Prof N, Mayo Med Sch

Alberts, Mark J MD [N] - **Spec Exp:** Stroke/Cerebrovascular Disease; **Hospital:** Northwestern Meml Hosp; **Address:** 675 N St Clair, Galter Bldg Fl 20 - Ste 100, Chicago, IL 60611; **Phone:** 312-695-7950; **Board Cert:** Neurology 1987; Vascular Neurology 2005; **Med School:** Tufts Univ 1982; **Resid:** Neurology, Duke Univ Med Ctr 1986; **Fellow:** Cerebrovascular Disease, Duke Univ Med Ctr 1987; **Fac Appt:** Prof N, Northwestern Univ

Arnason, Barry G W MD [N] - **Spec Exp:** Multiple Sclerosis; Guillain-Barre Syndrome; Myasthenia Gravis; **Hospital:** Univ of Chicago Med Ctr; **Address:** 5841 S Maryland Ave, MC 2030, Chicago, IL 60637; **Phone:** 773-702-6222; **Board Cert:** Neurology 1971; **Med School:** Univ Manitoba 1957; **Resid:** Neurology, Mass Genl Hosp 1959; Neurology, Mass Genl Hosp 1962; **Fac Appt:** Prof N, Univ Chicago-Pritzker Sch Med

Barger, Geoffrey R MD [N] - **Spec Exp:** Neuro-Oncology; Brain Tumors; **Hospital:** Harper Univ Hosp, Barbara Ann Karmanos Cancer Inst; **Address:** Wayne State Univ Hlth Ctr, 4201 St Antoine, Ste 8D-UHC, Detroit, MI 48201; **Phone:** 313-745-4275; **Board Cert:** Neurology 1981; **Med School:** Jefferson Med Coll 1975; **Resid:** Neurology, Penn Hosp 1979; **Fellow:** Neuro-Oncology, Moffitt Hosp & Brain Tumor Ctr/UCSF 1982; **Fac Appt:** Assoc Prof N, Wayne State Univ

Barkley, Gregory L MD [N] - **Spec Exp:** Epilepsy/Seizure Disorders; **Hospital:** Henry Ford Hosp; **Address:** Henry Ford Hosp, Dept Neurology, 2799 W Grand Blvd, Detroit, MI 48202; **Phone:** 313-916-3922; **Board Cert:** Neurology 1988; Clinical Neurophysiology 2001; **Med School:** Mich State Univ 1981; **Resid:** Neurology, Henry Ford Hosp 1985; **Fellow:** Clinical Neurophysiology, Henry Ford Hosp 1986; **Fac Appt:** Assoc Prof N, Wayne State Univ

Bernstein, Richard A MD/PhD [N] - **Spec Exp:** Stroke/Cerebrovascular Disease; **Hospital:** Northwestern Meml Hosp; **Address:** 675 N St Claire, Ste 20-100, Chicago, IL 60026; **Phone:** 312-695-7950; **Board Cert:** Neurology 2001; Vascular Neurology 2005; **Med School:** Cornell Univ-Weill Med Coll 1996; **Resid:** Neurology, Columbia-Presby Med Ctr 2000; **Fellow:** Vascular Neurology, UCSF Med Ctr 2001; Stroke, Stanford Med Ctr 2002; **Fac Appt:** Assoc Prof N, Northwestern Univ-Feinberg Sch Med

Broderick, Joseph P MD [N] - **Spec Exp:** Stroke; **Hospital:** Univ Hosp - Cincinnati; **Address:** Univ Cincinnati, Dept Neurology, 222 Piedmont Ave, Ste 3200, Cincinnati, OH 45219; **Phone:** 513-475-8730; **Board Cert:** Neurology 1988; Vascular Neurology 2005; **Med School:** Univ Cincinnati 1982; **Resid:** Neurology, Mayo Clinic 1986; **Fellow:** Cerebrovascular Disease, Mayo Clinic 1987; **Fac Appt:** Clin Prof N, Univ Cincinnati

Brown, Robert D MD [N] - **Spec Exp:** Stroke; Cerebrovascular Disease; **Hospital:** Mayo Med Ctr & Clin - Rochester; **Address:** Mayo Clinic, Dept Neurology, 200 First St SW, Rochester, MN 55905; **Phone:** 507-266-4143; **Board Cert:** Neurology 1994; Vascular Surgery 2008; **Med School:** Mayo Med Sch 1987; **Resid:** Neurology, Mayo Clin 1991; **Fellow:** Cerebrovascular Disease, Mayo Clin 1992; **Fac Appt:** Prof N, Mayo Med Sch

Burke, Allan M MD [N] - **Spec Exp:** Cerebrovascular Disease; Neurologic Imaging; **Hospital:** Northwestern Meml Hosp; **Address:** 233 E Erie St, Ste 500, Chicago, IL 60611-2912; **Phone:** 312-944-0063; **Board Cert:** Neurology 1982; Neuroimaging 2002; **Med School:** Columbia P&S 1976; **Resid:** Internal Medicine, NY Hosp 1978; Neurology, Columbia-Presby Med Ctr 1981; **Fellow:** Cerebrovascular Disease, Hosp Univ Penn 1983; **Fac Appt:** Clin Prof N, Northwestern Univ

Cascino, Terrence L MD [N] - **Spec Exp:** Neuro-Oncology; **Hospital:** Mayo Med Ctr & Clin - Rochester; **Address:** Mayo Clinic, Dept Neurology, 200 1st St SW, Rochester, MN 55905; **Phone:** 507-284-2576; **Board Cert:** Neurology 1984; **Med School:** Loyola Univ-Stritch Sch Med 1972; **Resid:** Neurology, Mayo Clinic 1980; **Fellow:** Neuro-Oncology, Meml Sloan Kettering Cancer Ctr; **Fac Appt:** Assoc Prof N, Mayo Med Sch

Chelimsky, Thomas C MD [N] - **Hospital:** Univ Hosps Case Med Ctr (page 74); **Address:** UH Neurological Institute, 11100 Euclid Ave, Ste 5, Cleveland, OH 44106; **Phone:** 216-844-3495; **Board Cert:** Internal Medicine 1986; Neurology 1992; Pain Medicine 2000; **Med School:** Washington Univ, St Louis 1983; **Resid:** Internal Medicine, Mayo Clinic 1986; Neurology, Mayo Clinic 1989; **Fellow:** Physiology, Mayo Clinic 1987; **Fac Appt:** Prof N, Case West Res Univ

Cohen, Jeffrey Alan MD [N] - **Spec Exp:** Multiple Sclerosis; Neuro-Immunology; **Hospital:** Cleveland Clin (page 56); **Address:** Cleveland Clinic, 9500 Euclid Ave, Desk U10, Cleveland, OH 44195; **Phone:** 216-445-8110; **Board Cert:** Neurology 1985; **Med School:** Univ Chicago-Pritzker Sch Med 1980; **Resid:** Neurology, Hosp Univ Penn 1984; **Fellow:** Neurological Immunology, Hosp Univ Penn 1987

Neurology

Cutrer, F Michael MD [N] - **Spec Exp:** Headache; Pain-Facial; Migraine; **Hospital:** Mayo Med Ctr & Clin - Rochester, Rochester Methodist Hosp; **Address:** Mayo Clinic, Dept Neurology, 200 First St SW, Rochester, MN 55905-0001; **Phone:** 507-284-4409; **Board Cert:** Neurology 1993; **Med School:** Univ Miss 1988; **Resid:** Neurology, UCLA Med Ctr 1992; **Fellow:** Neurology, Mass Genl Hosp-Harvard 1994; **Fac Appt:** Assoc Prof N, Mayo Med Sch

Elias, Stanton B MD [N] - **Spec Exp:** Multiple Sclerosis; Myasthenia Gravis; **Hospital:** Henry Ford Hosp; **Address:** Henry Ford Hosp, Dept Neurology, 2799 W Grand Blvd, Fl K-11, Detroit, MI 48202-2689; **Phone:** 313-916-7207; **Board Cert:** Neurology 1979; **Med School:** Univ Pittsburgh 1972; **Resid:** Neurology, Duke Univ Med Ctr 1976; **Fellow:** Neurology, Duke Univ Med Ctr 1977

Farlow, Martin R MD [N] - **Spec Exp:** Alzheimer's Disease; Neurodegenerative Disorders; Multiple Sclerosis; Prion Diseases; **Hospital:** IU Health University Hosp, Wishard Hlth Srvs; **Address:** IU Health - Neurology, 541 Clinical Drive, Ste 292, Indianapolis, IN 46202; **Phone:** 317-948-5450; **Board Cert:** Neurology 1988; **Med School:** Indiana Univ 1979; **Resid:** Neurology, Indiana Univ Hosp 1983; **Fac Appt:** Prof N, Indiana Univ

Feldman, Eva L MD/PhD [N] - **Spec Exp:** Neuromuscular Disorders; Amyotrophic Lateral Sclerosis (ALS); Peripheral Neuropathy; **Hospital:** Univ of Michigan Hosp; **Address:** Univ Mich, Dept Neurology, 1500 E Med Ctr Drive, Taubman 1324 SPC 5322, Ann Arbor, MI 48109; **Phone:** 734-936-9020; **Board Cert:** Neurology 1988; **Med School:** Univ Mich Med Sch 1983; **Resid:** Neurology, Johns Hopkins Hosp 1987; **Fellow:** Neuromuscular Medicine, Univ Mich Hosps 1988; **Fac Appt:** Prof N, Univ Mich Med Sch

Furlan, Anthony J MD [N] - **Spec Exp:** Stroke; Thrombolytic Therapy; **Hospital:** Univ Hosps Case Med Ctr (page 74); **Address:** Dept Neurology, 11100 Euclid Ave, Fl 5, Hanna House, Cleveland, OH 44106; **Phone:** 216-844-3193; **Board Cert:** Neurology 1979; Vascular Neurology 2005; **Med School:** Loyola Univ-Stritch Sch Med 1973; **Resid:** Neurology, Cleveland Clinic 1977; **Fellow:** Cerebrovascular Disease, Mayo Clinic 1978; **Fac Appt:** Assoc Prof N, Ohio State Univ

Gilman, Sid MD [N] - **Spec Exp:** Parkinson's Disease/Movement Disorders; Alzheimer's Disease; Multiple Sclerosis; Ataxia; **Hospital:** Univ of Michigan Hosp; **Address:** Univ Mich, Dept Neurology, 300 N Ingalls 3D15, Ann Arbor, MI 48109-0489; **Phone:** 734-936-1808; **Board Cert:** Neurology 1966; **Med School:** UCLA 1957; **Resid:** Neurology, Boston City Hosp-Harvard 1963; **Fellow:** Neurological Physiology, Boston City Hosp-Harvard 1965; **Fac Appt:** Prof N, Univ Mich Med Sch

Goetz, Christopher G MD [N] - **Spec Exp:** Movement Disorders; Parkinson's Disease; Dyskinesias; **Hospital:** Rush Univ Med Ctr; **Address:** 1725 W Harrison St, Ste 755, Chicago, IL 60612-3835; **Phone:** 312-563-2030; **Board Cert:** Neurology 1982; **Med School:** Rush Med Coll 1975; **Resid:** Neurology, Michael Reese Med Ctr 1977; Neurology, Rush-Presby-St Luke's Med Ctr 1979; **Fac Appt:** Prof N, Rush Med Coll

Goodwin, James MD [N] - **Spec Exp:** Neuro-Ophthalmology; Optic Nerve Disorders; Neuromuscular Disorder & Vision Problems; **Hospital:** Univ of IL Med Ctr at Chicago; **Address:** Univ Illinois Eye & Ear Infirm, 1855 W Taylor St, rm 3.158, MC 64, Chicago, IL 60612; **Phone:** 312-996-9120; **Board Cert:** Neurology 1975; **Med School:** Univ IL Coll Med 1969; **Resid:** Neurology, Univ Minnesota Hosps 1973; **Fellow:** Neuro-Ophthalmology, Bascom Palmer Eye Inst 1976; **Fac Appt:** Prof Oph, Univ IL Coll Med

Hain, Timothy C MD [N] - **Spec Exp:** Neuro-Otology; Balance Disorders; Motion Sickness; **Hospital:** Northwestern Meml Hosp; **Address:** 645 N Michigan Ave, Ste 410, Chicago, IL 60611; **Phone:** 312-274-0197; **Board Cert:** Neurology 1983; **Med School:** Univ IL Coll Med 1978; **Resid:** Neurology, Univ Illinois Affil Hosp 1982; **Fellow:** Neurology, Johns Hopkins Hosp 1984; Ophthalmology, Johns Hopkins Hosp 1984; **Fac Appt:** Prof N, Northwestern Univ

Hecox, Kurt E MD [N] - **Spec Exp:** Pediatric Neurology; Epilepsy/Seizure Disorders; Hearing Loss; **Hospital:** Chldns Hosp - Wisconsin; **Address:** Dept Neurology, 9000 W Wisconsin Ave, rm CCC-540, PO Box 1997, Milwaukee, WI 53226; **Phone:** 414-266-3464; **Board Cert:** Clinical Neurophysiology 1977; **Med School:** UCSD 1971; **Resid:** Neurology, Univ Texas Southwestern Med Ctr 1975; **Fellow:** Pediatric Neurology, Children's Med Ctr/Parkland Hosp 1978; **Fac Appt:** Prof N, Med Coll Wisc

Homer, Daniel MD [N] - **Spec Exp:** Stroke; **Hospital:** Evanston/North Shore Univ Hlth Sys, Highland Park/North Shore Univ Hlth Syst; **Address:** Evanston Hosp, Dept Neurology, 1000 Central St, Ste 615, Evanston, IL 60201; **Phone:** 847-570-2570; **Board Cert:** Neurology 1990; Vascular Neurology 2008; **Med School:** Northwestern Univ 1979; **Resid:** Neurology, Stanford Univ Hosp 1983; **Fellow:** Stroke, Mayo Clinic 1984; **Fac Appt:** Asst Prof N, Northwestern Univ

Josephson, David A MD [N] - **Spec Exp:** Electromyography; Epilepsy; Stroke; **Hospital:** St. Vincent Indianapolis Hosp, Comm Hosp N - Indianapolis; **Address:** 8402 Harcourt Rd, Ste 615, Indianapolis, IN 46260; **Phone:** 317-806-6991; **Board Cert:** Neurology 2004; **Med School:** Indiana Univ 1971; **Resid:** Neurology, Univ Mich Med Ctr 1973; Neurology, Indiana Univ Med Ctr 1975; **Fac Appt:** Assoc Clin Prof N, Indiana Univ

Katirji, Bashar MD [N] - **Spec Exp:** Neuromuscular Disorders; **Hospital:** Univ Hosps Case Med Ctr (page 74); **Address:** UH Neurological Institute, 11100 Euclid Ave, Cleveland, OH 44106; **Phone:** 216-844-4854; **Board Cert:** Neurology 1985; Clinical Neurophysiology 2002; Neuromuscular Medicine 2008; **Med School:** Syria 1977; **Resid:** Internal Medicine, King Faisal Spec Hosp 1980; Neurology, Univ Pittsburgh Med Ctr 1983; **Fellow:** Electromyography, Cleveland Clinic 1984; **Fac Appt:** Prof N, Case West Res Univ

Kincaid, John C MD [N] - **Spec Exp:** Neuromuscular Disorders; Electromyography; Pain-Facial; Peripheral Neuropathy; **Hospital:** IU Health University Hosp; **Address:** IU Health Physicians-Neurology, 550 N University Blvd, Ste 1710, Indianapolis, IN 46202; **Phone:** 317-944-0311; **Board Cert:** Neurology 2010; Clinical Neurophysiology 2000; **Med School:** Indiana Univ 1975; **Resid:** Neurology, Indiana Univ Affil Hosp 1979; **Fellow:** Electromyography, Mayo Clinic 1980; **Fac Appt:** Prof N, Indiana Univ

Lewis, Richard A MD [N] - **Spec Exp:** Neuromuscular Disorders; **Hospital:** Harper Univ Hosp; **Address:** 4201 St Aintoine, Univ Health Center, Ste 8A, Detroit, MI 48201; **Phone:** 313-745-4275; **Board Cert:** Neurology 1980; **Med School:** Med Coll VA 1974; **Resid:** Neurology, Hosp Univ Penn 1978

Lisak, Robert P MD [N] - **Spec Exp:** Multiple Sclerosis; Myasthenia Gravis; Vasculitis; Demyelinating Neuropathy; **Hospital:** Harper Univ Hosp, Detroit Receiving Hospital; **Address:** Wayne State Univ Sch Med, 4201 St Antoine, Hlth Ctr 8D, Detroit, MI 48201; **Phone:** 313-745-4240; **Board Cert:** Neurology 1975; **Med School:** Columbia P&S 1965; **Resid:** Internal Medicine, Bronx Municipal Hosp-Einstein 1969; Neurology, Hosp Univ Penn 1972; **Fac Appt:** Prof N, Wayne State Univ

Logan, William R MD [N] - **Spec Exp:** Stroke; Cerebrovascular Disease; **Hospital:** St. John's Mercy Med Ctr - St Louis; **Address:** St Johns Mercy Med Ctr, Tower B, 621 New Ballas Rd, Ste 5003, St Louis, MO 63141; **Phone:** 314-227-2020; **Board Cert:** Internal Medicine 1981; Neurology 1986; Vascular Neurology 2009; **Med School:** Univ Okla Coll Med 1978; **Resid:** Internal Medicine, Univ Missouri Hosps 1982; Neurology, Unix Texas Hlth Sci Ctr 1984

Luders, Hans MD/PhD [N] - **Spec Exp:** Epilepsy; **Hospital:** Univ Hosps Case Med Ctr (page 74); **Address:** University Hosps-Case Med Ctr, 11100 Euclid Ave, Dept Neurology, Lakeside Bldg - Ste 3200, Cleveland, OH 44106; **Phone:** 216-844-3650; **Board Cert:** Neurology 1985; **Med School:** Chile 1965; **Resid:** Neurology, Neur Inst-Kyushu Univ 1971; **Fellow:** Neurological Physiology, Mayo Grad Sch Med 1975; **Fac Appt:** Prof N, Ohio State Univ

Mahowald, Mark W MD [N] - **Spec Exp:** Sleep Disorders/Apnea; **Hospital:** Hennepin Cnty Med Ctr; **Address:** Minn Regional Sleep Disorders Ctr, 701 Park Ave Green Bldg Fl 8 - Ste 220, Minneapolis, MN 55415; **Phone:** 612-873-6201; **Board Cert:** Neurology 1976; **Med School:** Univ Minn 1968; **Resid:** Neurology, Fairview Univ Med Ctr 1974; **Fac Appt:** Prof N, Univ Minn

Maraganore, Demetrius MD [N] - **Spec Exp:** Movement Disorders; Parkinson's Disease; **Hospital:** Evanston/North Shore Univ Hlth Sys, Glenbrook Hosp-NorthShore Univ Hlth Syst; **Address:** 2150 Pfingsten Rd, Ste 3000, Glenview, IL 60026; **Phone:** 847-570-2570; **Board Cert:** Neurology 1990; **Med School:** Northwestern Univ-Feinberg Sch Med 1985; **Resid:** Neurology, Mayo Clinic 1989; **Fellow:** Movement Disorders, Natl Hosp for Nervous Disorders 1990

Mesulam, Marsel MD [N] - **Spec Exp:** Alzheimer's Disease; Tourette's Syndrome; Dementia; **Hospital:** Northwestern Meml Hosp; **Address:** 320 E Superior St Fl 11 - rm 453, Chicago, IL 60611; **Phone:** 312-908-9339; **Board Cert:** Neurology 1977; **Med School:** Harvard Med Sch 1972; **Resid:** Neurology, Boston City Hosp 1976; **Fac Appt:** Prof N, Northwestern Univ

Mikkelsen, Tommy MD [N] - **Spec Exp:** Brain Tumors; Gliomas; **Hospital:** Henry Ford Hosp; **Address:** Henry Ford Hospital, ER 3096, 2799 W Grand Blvd, Detroit, MI 48202; **Phone:** 313-916-8641; **Board Cert:** Neurology 2008; **Med School:** Univ Calgary 1983; **Resid:** Internal Medicine, Calgary General Hosp 1985; Neurology, Montreal Neuro Inst 1988; **Fellow:** Neuro-Oncology, Royal Victoria Hosp 1990; Neuro-Oncology, Ludwig Inst for Cancer Rsch 1992; **Fac Appt:** Assoc Prof N, Case West Res Univ

Mohammad, Yousef M MD [N] - **Spec Exp:** Headache; Migraine; Stroke; **Hospital:** Rush Univ Med Ctr; **Address:** Rush Professional Office Bldg, 1725 W Harrison St, Ste 1118, Chicago, IL 60612; **Phone:** 312-942-4500; **Board Cert:** Neurology 2004; Vascular Neurology 2008; **Med School:** Amer Univ Beirut 1989; **Resid:** Neurology, Wayne State Univ Affil Hosps 1996; **Fellow:** Stroke, Emory Univ Hosp 1999

Morris, John C MD [N] - **Spec Exp:** Alzheimer's Disease; **Hospital:** Barnes-Jewish Hosp; **Address:** Memory Diagnostic Ctr, 4488 Forest Park, Ste 160, St Louis, MO 63108-2215; **Phone:** 314-286-1967; **Board Cert:** Internal Medicine 1979; Neurology 1985; **Med School:** Univ Rochester 1974; **Resid:** Internal Medicine, Akron Genl Med Ctr 1979; Neurology, Cleveland Metro Genl Hosp 1982; **Fellow:** Neuropharmacology, Washington Univ 1985; **Fac Appt:** Prof N, Washington Univ, St Louis

Newman, Daniel S MD [N] - **Spec Exp:** Amyotrophic Lateral Sclerosis (ALS); Nerve/Muscle Disorders; **Hospital:** Henry Ford Hosp; **Address:** Henry Ford Hospital, 2799 W Grand Blvd Fl K11, Detroit, MI 48202; **Phone:** 313-916-2594; **Board Cert:** Neurology 1992; Neuromuscular Medicine 2008; **Med School:** Univ Mich Med Sch 1983; **Resid:** Neurology, Henry Ford Hosp 1988; **Fellow:** Electromyography, Mayo Clinic 1989; **Fac Appt:** Assoc Prof N, Wayne State Univ

Newton, Herbert B MD [N] - **Spec Exp:** Neuro-Oncology; Brain & Spinal Tumors; Clinical Trials; **Hospital:** Ohio St Univ Med Ctr, Arthur G James Cancer Hosp & Research Inst; **Address:** 320 W 10th Ave, Starling Loving Bldg, rm M410, Columbus, OH 43210; **Phone:** 614-293-8930; **Board Cert:** Neurology 1989; **Med School:** SUNY Buffalo 1984; **Resid:** Neurology, Univ Michigan Med Ctr 1988; **Fellow:** Neuro-Oncology, Meml Sloan-Kettering Cancer Ctr 1990; **Fac Appt:** Prof N, Ohio State Univ

Pascuzzi, Robert M MD [N] - **Spec Exp:** Neuromuscular Disorders; Amyotrophic Lateral Sclerosis (ALS); Myasthenia Gravis; Post Polio Syndrome; **Hospital:** IU Health University Hosp, Wishard Hlth Srvs; **Address:** Indiana Univ Dept Neurology, 545 Barnhill Drive, EH 125, Indianapolis, IN 46202; **Phone:** 317-274-4455; **Board Cert:** Neurology 2004; **Med School:** Indiana Univ 1979; **Resid:** Neurology, Univ Va Med Ctr 1983; **Fellow:** Neuromuscular Medicine, Univ Virginia 1985; **Fac Appt:** Prof N, Indiana Univ

Perlmutter, Joel S MD [N] - **Spec Exp:** Parkinson's Disease; Movement Disorders; Huntington's Disease; **Hospital:** Barnes-Jewish Hosp; **Address:** Wash Univ Sch Med, Dept Neurology, 660 S Euclid Ave, Box 8111, St Louis, MO 63110; **Phone:** 314-362-6908; **Board Cert:** Neurology 1985; **Med School:** Univ MO-Columbia Sch Med 1979; **Resid:** Neurology, Barnes Hosp-Wash Univ 1983; **Fellow:** Movement Disorders, Barnes Hosp-Wash Univ 1984; **Fac Appt:** Prof N, Washington Univ, St Louis

Pestronk, Alan MD [N] - **Spec Exp:** Neuromuscular Disorders; Peripheral Neuropathy; **Hospital:** Barnes-Jewish Hosp; **Address:** Washington Univ Sch Med, Dept Neurology, Dept Neuro, Div Neuromuscular Disorders, 660 S Euclid Ave, Box 8111, St Louis, MO 63110; **Phone:** 314-362-6981; **Board Cert:** Neurology 1978; Neuromuscular Medicine 2008; **Med School:** Johns Hopkins Univ 1970; **Resid:** Neurology, Johns Hopkins Hosp 1974; **Fellow:** Neuromuscular Medicine, Johns Hopkins Hosp 1977; **Fac Appt:** Prof NPath, Washington Univ, St Louis

Petersen, Ronald C MD/PhD [N] - **Spec Exp:** Alzheimer's Disease; Cognitive Impairment/Mild; **Hospital:** Mayo Med Ctr & Clin - Rochester; **Address:** Mayo Clinic, Dept Neurology, 200 1st St SW, Rochester, MN 55905; **Phone:** 507-538-1038; **Board Cert:** Neurology 1986; **Med School:** Mayo Med Sch 1980; **Resid:** Neurology, Mayo Clinic 1984; **Fellow:** Behavioral Neurology, Beth Israel Med Ctr 1986; **Fac Appt:** Prof N, Mayo Med Sch

Reder, Anthony T MD [N] - **Spec Exp:** Multiple Sclerosis; Tetanus; Myasthenia Gravis; Reflex Sympathetic Dystrophy (RSD); **Hospital:** Univ of Chicago Med Ctr; **Address:** Univ Chicago- Dept Neurology, 5841 S Maryland Ave, MC 2030, Chicago, IL 60637; **Phone:** 773-702-6222; **Board Cert:** Neurology 1984; **Med School:** Univ Mich Med Sch 1978; **Resid:** Neurology, Univ Minn Hosps 1982; **Fellow:** Neurological Immunology, Univ Chicago Med Ctr 1984; **Fac Appt:** Assoc Prof N, Univ Chicago-Pritzker Sch Med

Reed, Robert L MD [N] - **Spec Exp:** Multiple Sclerosis; Stroke; **Hospital:** Good Samaritan Hosp - Cincinnati; **Address:** 111 Wellington Pl, Cincinnati, OH 45219; **Phone:** 513-241-2370; **Board Cert:** Neurology 1975; **Med School:** Univ Cincinnati 1966; **Resid:** Internal Medicine, Mayo Grad Sch Med 1970; Neurology, Mayo Grad Sch Med 1973

Richerson, George B MD/PhD [N] - **Hospital:** Univ Iowa Hosp & Clinics, Iowa City VA Hlth Care Sys; **Address:** UIHC Neurology Dept, 200 Hawkins Drive, Iowa City, IA 52242; **Phone:** 319-356-4296; **Board Cert:** Neurology 1993; **Med School:** Univ Iowa Coll Med 1984; **Resid:** Neurology, Yale-New Haven Hosp 1990; **Fac Appt:** Prof N, Univ Iowa Coll Med

Rogers, Lisa R DO [N] - **Spec Exp:** Neuro-Oncology; Brain Tumors; Brain Radiation Toxicity; **Hospital:** Univ Hosps Case Med Ctr (page 74); **Address:** Univ Hosps-Case Med Ctr, Dept Neuro, Hanna House 506, MS HAN 5040, 11100 Euclid Ave, Cleveland, OH 44106-5040; **Phone:** 216-844-5160; **Board Cert:** Neurology 1982; **Med School:** Kirksville Coll Osteo Med 1976; **Resid:** Neurology, Cleveland Clin Fdn 1980; **Fellow:** Neuro-Oncology, Meml-Sloan Kettering Cancer Ctr 1982; **Fac Appt:** Prof N, Case West Res Univ

Roos, Karen L MD [N] - **Spec Exp:** Infections-Neurologic; Encephalitis; Vascular Disease; Neurofibromatosis; **Hospital:** IU Health University Hosp, Wishard Hlth Srvs; **Address:** Indiana Univ Med Ctr, 550 N University Blvd, rm 1710, Indianapolis, IN 46202-5149; **Phone:** 317-948-5450; **Board Cert:** Neurology 1986; **Med School:** Hahnemann Univ 1981; **Resid:** Neurology, Univ Virginia Med Ctr 1985; **Fac Appt:** Prof N, Indiana Univ

Neurology

Roos, Raymond MD [N] - **Spec Exp:** Amyotrophic Lateral Sclerosis (ALS); Multiple Sclerosis; Neuromuscular Disorders; **Hospital:** Univ of Chicago Med Ctr; **Address:** Univ Chicago, Dept Neurology, 5841 S Maryland Ave, MC-2030, Chicago, IL 60637; **Phone:** 773-702-7852; **Board Cert:** Neurology 1976; **Med School:** SUNY Downstate 1968; **Resid:** Neurology, Johns Hopkins Hosp 1974; **Fellow:** Neurology, Natl Inst Neur Dis & Stroke 1971; Neurological Viral Immunology, Johns Hopkins Hosp 1976; **Fac Appt:** Prof N, Univ Chicago-Pritzker Sch Med

Rosenfeld, Steven S MD [N] - **Spec Exp:** Brain Tumors; Gliomas; Neuro-Oncology; **Hospital:** Cleveland Clin (page 56); **Address:** Cleveland Clinic, 9500 Euclid Ave, S-73, Cleveland, OH 44195; **Phone:** 216-444-4461; **Board Cert:** Neurology 1994; **Med School:** Northwestern Univ 1985; **Resid:** Neurology, Duke Univ Med Ctr 1989; **Fellow:** Neuro-Oncology, Duke Univ Med Ctr 1990; **Fac Appt:** Prof N, Cleveland Cl Coll Med/Case West Res

Rubin, Susan M MD [N] - **Spec Exp:** Multiple Sclerosis in Women; Epilepsy in Pregnancy; Headache in Women; Migraine in Women; **Hospital:** Glenbrook Hosp-NorthShore Univ Hlth Syst, Evanston/North Shore Univ Hlth Sys; **Address:** Glenbrook Hosp, Dept Neurology, 2150 Pfingsten Rd, Ste 3000, Glenview, IL 60026; **Phone:** 847-657-5875; **Board Cert:** Neurology 2006; **Med School:** Univ IL Coll Med 1988; **Resid:** Neurology, Northwestern Meml Hosp 1993; **Fellow:** Neurological Physiology, Northwestern Meml Hosp 1994; **Fac Appt:** Asst Clin Prof N, Univ Chicago-Pritzker Sch Med

Saper, Joel R MD [N] - **Spec Exp:** Headache; Pain-Chronic after Head Injury; **Hospital:** Chelsea Comm Hosp; **Address:** Michigan Head Pain & Neurological Inst, 3120 Professional Drive, Ann Arbor, MI 48104; **Phone:** 734-677-6000; **Board Cert:** Neurology 1975; Pain Medicine 1996; Headache Medicine 2006; **Med School:** Univ IL Coll Med 1969; **Resid:** Neurology, Univ Mich Med Ctr 1973; **Fac Appt:** Clin Prof N, Mich State Univ

Siddique, Teepu MD [N] - **Spec Exp:** Amyotrophic Lateral Sclerosis (ALS); Muscular Dystrophy; Neurogenetics; Spasticity Management; **Hospital:** Northwestern Meml Hosp; **Address:** 675 N St Clair St Fl 20 - Ste 100, Chicago, IL 60611; **Phone:** 312-695-7950; **Board Cert:** Neurology 1980; **Med School:** Pakistan 1973; **Resid:** Neurology, UMDNJ Affil Hosp 1979; **Fellow:** Electromyography, Hosp Special Surg 1980; Neuromuscular Disease, Natl Inst Hlth 1981; **Fac Appt:** Prof N, Northwestern Univ

Sila, Cathy A MD [N] - **Spec Exp:** Cerebrovascular Disease; Stroke-Young Adults; **Hospital:** Univ Hosps Case Med Ctr (page 74); **Address:** University Hospitals - Case Me Ctr, Dept of Neurology, 11100 Euclid Ave, Cleveland, OH 44106-5040; **Phone:** 216-844-8334; **Board Cert:** Neurology 1986; Vascular Neurology 2005; **Med School:** Case West Res Univ 1981; **Resid:** Neurology, Cleveland Clin 1983; Neurology, Mayo Clin 1985; **Fellow:** Research, Cleveland Clin 1986; Vascular Neurology, Cleveland Clin 1986; **Fac Appt:** Prof N, Case West Res Univ

Swanson, Jerry W MD [N] - **Spec Exp:** Headache; Migraine; **Hospital:** Mayo Med Ctr & Clin - Rochester; **Address:** Mayo Clinic, Dept Neurology, 200 First St SW, Rochester, MN 55905-0001; **Phone:** 507-538-1036; **Board Cert:** Neurology 1984; Headache Medicine 2006; **Med School:** Northwestern Univ 1977; **Resid:** Neurology, Mayo Clinic 1982; **Fellow:** Electroencephalography, Mayo Clinic 1983; **Fac Appt:** Prof N, Mayo Med Sch

Taylor, Frederick R MD [N] - **Spec Exp:** Headache; Pain-Facial; Migraine; **Hospital:** Park Nicollet Methodist Hosp - Minnesota; **Address:** Park Nicollet Clinic, 3931 Louisiana Ave S, Ste W505, Minneapolis, MN 55426; **Phone:** 952-993-3432; **Board Cert:** Pediatrics 1982; Neurology 1985; Headache Medicine 2006; **Med School:** Univ New Mexico 1977; **Resid:** Pediatrics, Univ Wisc Hlth Sci Ctr 1980; Neurology, Univ Wisc Hlth Sci Ctr 1983; **Fellow:** Neurological Physiology, Univ Wisc Hlth Sci Ctr 1984

Vick, Nicholas A MD [N] - **Spec Exp:** Brain Tumors; Neuro-Oncology; **Hospital:** Evanston/North Shore Univ Hlth Sys; **Address:** Evanston Kellog Cancer Ctr, 2650 Ridge Ave, Evanston, IL 60201; **Phone:** 847-570-1808; **Board Cert:** Neurology 1971; **Med School:** Univ Chicago-Pritzker Sch Med 1965; **Resid:** Neurology, Univ Chicago Hosps 1968; **Fellow:** Neurology, Natl Inst Hlth 1970; **Fac Appt:** Prof N, Northwestern Univ

Vitek, Jerrold Lee MD/PhD [N] - **Spec Exp:** Parkinson's Disease/Movement Disorders; Tremor & Dystonia; Deep Brain Stimulation; **Address:** Univ Minn, Dept Neurology, MMC 295 420 Delaware St SE, Minneapolis, MN 55455; **Phone:** 612-625-9900; **Board Cert:** Neurology 1992; **Med School:** Univ Minn 1984; **Resid:** Neurology, Johns Hopkins Hosp 1988; **Fac Appt:** Prof N, Univ Minn

Windebank, Anthony J MD [N] - **Spec Exp:** Peripheral Neuropathy; Amyotrophic Lateral Sclerosis (ALS); Multiple Sclerosis; **Hospital:** Mayo Med Ctr & Clin - Rochester; **Address:** Mayo Clin, Dept Neurology, 200 First St SW, Rochester, MN 55905; **Phone:** 507-284-1588; **Board Cert:** Neurology 1982; **Med School:** England, UK 1974; **Resid:** Internal Medicine, Radcliffe Infirm 1977; Neurology, Mayo Clin 1981; **Fellow:** Neurology, Mayo Clin 1982; **Fac Appt:** Prof N, Mayo Med Sch

Wright, Robert B MD [N] - **Spec Exp:** Myasthenia Gravis; Migraine; **Hospital:** Rush Univ Med Ctr; **Address:** 1725 W Harrison St, Ste 1118, Chicago, IL 60612-3841; **Phone:** 312-942-5936; **Board Cert:** Neurology 1988; **Med School:** Univ IL Coll Med 1982; **Resid:** Neurology, Rush Presby-St Luke's Med Ctr 1986; **Fellow:** Neuromuscular Medicine, Rush Presby-St Luke's Med Ctr 1987; **Fac Appt:** Asst Prof N, Rush Med Coll

Great Plains and Mountains

Barohn, Richard J MD [N] - **Spec Exp:** Peripheral Neuropathy; Myasthenia Gravis; Amyotrophic Lateral Sclerosis (ALS); Guillain-Barre Syndrome; **Hospital:** Univ of Kansas Hosp; **Address:** Univ Kansas Medical Ctr, Dept Neurology, 3599 Rainbow Blvd, MS 2012, Kansas City, KS 66160; **Phone:** 913-588-6970; **Board Cert:** Neurology 1987; Clinical Neurophysiology 2004; Neuromuscular Medicine 2008; **Med School:** Univ MO-Kansas City 1980; **Resid:** Neurology, Lackland AFB 1985

Bromberg, Mark B MD/PhD [N] - **Spec Exp:** Peripheral Neuropathy; Neuromuscular Disorders; **Hospital:** Univ Utah Hlth Care; **Address:** 175 N Medical Drive, Clinical Neurosciences Ctr, Salt Lake City, UT 84132; **Phone:** 801-585-7575; **Board Cert:** Neurology 1988; Clinical Neurophysiology 2000; **Med School:** Univ Mich Med Sch 1982; **Resid:** Neurology, Univ Mich Med Ctr 1986; **Fellow:** Electromyography, Univ Mich Med Ctr 1987; Neuromuscular Disease, Univ Mich Med Ctr 1987; **Fac Appt:** Prof N, Univ Utah

Filley, Christopher M MD [N] - **Spec Exp:** Leukoencephalopathy; Alzheimer's Disease; Brain Injury-Traumatic; Multiple Sclerosis; **Hospital:** Univ of CO Hosp - Anschutz Inpatient Pav, VA Eastern CO Health Care Sys-Denver; **Address:** Univ CO, Neurology Dept, Behavioral Neurology Sect, 12631 E 17th Ave, MS B185, Aurora, CO 80045; **Phone:** 303-724-2187; **Board Cert:** Neurology 1984; Behavioral Neurology & Neuropsychiatry 2006; **Med School:** Johns Hopkins Univ 1979; **Resid:** Neurology, Univ Colorado Hosp 1983; **Fellow:** Behavioral Neurology, Boston VA Hosp 1984; **Fac Appt:** Prof N, Univ Colorado

Neurology

Kelly, James P MD [N] - **Spec Exp:** Brain Injury; Memory Disorders; Neurologic Rehabilitation; Brain Injury-Traumatic; **Hospital:** Univ of CO Hosp - Anschutz Inpatient Pav; **Address:** Univ Co Hosp, Outpt Neurology, PO Box 6510, MS F727, Aurora, CO 80045; **Phone:** 720-848-2080; **Board Cert:** Neurology 1991; **Med School:** Northwestern Univ 1983; **Resid:** Neurology, Univ Colorado Med Ctr 1988; **Fellow:** Behavioral Neurology, Univ Colorado Med Ctr 1989; **Fac Appt:** Prof NS, Univ Colorado

Ringel, Steven P MD [N] - **Spec Exp:** Neuromuscular Disorders; **Hospital:** Univ of CO Hosp - Anschutz Inpatient Pav; **Address:** Univ Colorado Hosp, Neuromuscular Dept, 12631 E 17th Ave, Box B185, Aurora, CO 80045; **Phone:** 303-724-2209; **Board Cert:** Neurology 1974; **Med School:** Univ Mich Med Sch 1968; **Resid:** Neurology, Rush-Presby-St Lukes Med Ctr 1972; **Fellow:** Neurology, Natl Inst Neuro Dis-NIH 1976; **Fac Appt:** Prof N, Univ Colorado

Vollmer, Timothy L MD [N] - **Spec Exp:** Multiple Sclerosis; Myasthenia Gravis; Vasculitis of the Nervous System; Stroke; **Hospital:** Univ of CO Hosp - Anschutz Inpatient Pav; **Address:** Univ Colorado Dept Neurology, MS B-185, 12631 E 17th Ave, Aurora, CO 80045; **Phone:** 720-848-2080; **Board Cert:** Neurology 1991; **Med School:** Stanford Univ 1983; **Resid:** Neurology, Stanford Univ Hosp 1987; **Fellow:** Neurological Immunology, Stanford Univ 1986; **Fac Appt:** Prof N, Univ Colorado

Southwest

Ahern, Geoffrey L MD/PhD [N] - **Spec Exp:** Behavioral Neurology; Dementia; Alzheimer's Disease; **Hospital:** Univ Med Ctr - Tucson; **Address:** Univ Arizona, Dept Neurology, 1501 N Campbell Ave, PO Box 245023, Tucson, AZ 85724; **Phone:** 520-626-6524; **Board Cert:** Neurology 1992; Behavioral Neurology & Neuropsychiatry 2006; **Med School:** Yale Univ 1984; **Resid:** Neurology, Boston Univ Affil Hosps 1988; **Fellow:** Behavioral Neurology, Beth Israel Hosp 1990; **Fac Appt:** Prof N, Univ Ariz Coll Med

Burns, Richard S MD [N] - **Spec Exp:** Movement Disorders; Ataxia; Neurodegenerative Disorders; **Hospital:** St. Joseph's Hosp & Med Ctr - Phoenix; **Address:** Barrow Neurological Institute, 500 W Thomas Rd, Ste 300, Phoenix, AZ 85013; **Phone:** 602-406-6262; **Board Cert:** Neurology 1985; **Med School:** Univ Minn 1969; **Resid:** Internal Medicine, Huntington Meml Hosp 1971; Neurology, UC Irvine Med Ctr 1978; **Fellow:** Clinical Pharmacology, Natl Inst Genl Med Sci 1980

Couch Jr, James R MD/PhD [N] - **Spec Exp:** Headache; Stroke; Neuro-Rehabilitation; Tourette's Syndrome; **Hospital:** OU Med Ctr, VA Med Ctr - Oklahoma City; **Address:** 711 Stanton L Young Blvd, Ste 210, Oklahoma City, OK 73104-5021; **Phone:** 405-271-3635; **Board Cert:** Neurology 1974; Clinical Neurophysiology 2002; Headache Medicine 2006; **Med School:** Baylor Coll Med 1965; **Resid:** Neurology, Washington Univ Med Ctr 1972; **Fellow:** Neuropharmacology, Natl Inst Hlth 1969; **Fac Appt:** Prof N, Univ Okla Coll Med

Coull, Bruce M MD [N] - **Spec Exp:** Stroke; Cerebrovascular Disease; **Hospital:** University Physicians Hosp at Kino; **Address:** Univ Physicians Dept Neurology, UPH Clinic Bldg, 2800 E Ajo Way, Tucson, AZ 85713; **Phone:** 520-874-2700; **Board Cert:** Neurology 1979; Vascular Neurology 2005; **Med School:** Univ Pittsburgh 1972; **Resid:** Neurology, Stanford Univ Med Ctr 1976; **Fellow:** Developmental Neurology, Stanford Univ 1978; **Fac Appt:** Prof N, Univ Ariz Coll Med

Diaz-Arrastia, Ramon R MD/PhD [N] - **Spec Exp:** Brain Injury-Traumatic; MRI; Epilepsy/Seizure Disorders; **Hospital:** UT Southwestern Med Ctr at Dallas; **Address:** 5323 Harry Hines Blvd, Dallas, TX 75390-7208; **Phone:** 214-645-8800; **Board Cert:** Neurology 1993; **Med School:** Baylor Coll Med 1988; **Resid:** Neurology, Columbia Univ Med Ctr 1992; **Fellow:** Neurology, UT SW Med Ctr 1993; **Fac Appt:** Prof N, Univ Tex SW, Dallas

Dodick, David W MD [N] - **Spec Exp:** Headache; Migraine; **Hospital:** Mayo Clinic - Scottsdale, Mayo Clinic - Phoenix; **Address:** Mayo Clinic, Dept of Neurology, 5777 E Mayo Blvd, 5 East Neurology, Phoenix, AZ 85054; **Phone:** 480-342-3078; **Board Cert:** Neurology 2006; Vascular Neurology 2005; Headache Medicine 2006; **Med School:** Dalhousie Univ 1990; **Resid:** Neurology, Mayo Clinic 1994; **Fellow:** Headache, Univ Toronto 1996; **Fac Appt:** Prof N, Mayo Med Sch

Doody, Rachelle Smith MD/PhD [N] - **Spec Exp:** Alzheimer's Disease; Memory Disorders; **Hospital:** Methodist Hosp - Houston; **Address:** Alzheimer's & Memory Disorder Ctr, Dept of Neurology, 1977 Butler Blvd, Ste E5.101, Houston, TX 77030; **Phone:** 713-798-4734; **Board Cert:** Neurology 1988; **Med School:** Baylor Coll Med 1983; **Resid:** Neurology, Baylor Coll of Med Affil Hosp 1987; **Fac Appt:** Prof N, Baylor Coll Med

Ferrendelli, James A MD [N] - **Spec Exp:** Epilepsy/Seizure Disorders; Geriatric Neurology; **Hospital:** Meml Hermann Hosp - Texas Med Ctr; **Address:** UT Houston Sch Med, Dept Neurology, 6431 Fannin ST, MSB 7109, Houston, TX 77030; **Phone:** 713-500-7080; **Board Cert:** Neurology 1973; **Med School:** Univ Colorado 1962; **Resid:** Neurology, Cleveland Metro Genl Hosp 1968; **Fellow:** Neuropharmacology, Washington Univ Med Sch 1971; **Fac Appt:** Prof N, Univ Tex, Houston

Frohman, Elliot M MD [N] - **Spec Exp:** Multiple Sclerosis; Neuro-Ophthalmology; **Hospital:** UT Southwestern Med Ctr at Dallas, Parkland Hlth & Hosp Sys; **Address:** MS Clinic, 5323 Harry Hines Blvd, MC 8829, Dallas, TX 75390-8829; **Phone:** 214-645-8800; **Board Cert:** Neurology 2005; **Med School:** UC Irvine 1990; **Resid:** Neurology, Johns Hopkins Hosp 1994; **Fellow:** Neuro-Ophthalmology, Johns Hopkins Hosp 1995; **Fac Appt:** Assoc Prof N, Univ Tex SW, Dallas

Gilbert, Mark R MD [N] - **Spec Exp:** Brain Tumors; Neuro-Oncology; **Hospital:** UT MD Anderson Cancer Ctr; **Address:** Univ Tex MD Anderson Cancer Ctr, 1515 Holcombe Blvd, Unit 431, Houston, TX 77030; **Phone:** 713-792-4008; **Board Cert:** Internal Medicine 1985; Neurology 1990; **Med School:** Johns Hopkins Univ 1982; **Resid:** Internal Medicine, Johns Hopkins Hosp 1985; Neurology, Johns Hopkins Hosp 1988; **Fellow:** Neuro-Oncology, Johns Hopkins Hosp 1988; **Fac Appt:** Assoc Prof N, Univ Tex, Houston

Grotta, James C MD [N] - **Spec Exp:** Stroke; **Hospital:** Meml Hermann Hosp - Texas Med Ctr; **Address:** UT Houston Med Sch, Dept Neur, 6410 Fannin St, Ste 1014, Houston, TX 77030; **Phone:** 832-325-7080; **Board Cert:** Neurology 1978; Vascular Neurology 2005; **Med School:** Univ VA Sch Med 1971; **Resid:** Neurology, Univ Colorado Hlth Sci Ctr 1977; **Fellow:** Diagnostic Radiology, Mass Genl Hosp 1979; **Fac Appt:** Prof N, Univ Tex, Houston

Harati, Yadollah MD [N] - **Spec Exp:** Neuromuscular Disorders; Amyotrophic Lateral Sclerosis (ALS); Myasthenia Gravis; Nerve/Muscle Disorders; **Hospital:** St. Luke's Episcopal Hosp-Houston; **Address:** Baylor Neurology, Smith Tower, 6550 Fannin, Ste 1801, Houston, TX 77030; **Phone:** 713-798-7411; **Board Cert:** Neurology 1978; **Med School:** Iran 1970; **Resid:** Neurology, Univ Nebraska Affil Hosp 1974; Neurology, Baylor Coll of Med Affil Hosp 1975; **Fellow:** Neuromuscular Disease, Baylor Coll of Med Affil Hosp 1976; **Fac Appt:** Prof N, Baylor Coll Med

Infante, Ernesto MD [N] - **Spec Exp:** Neuromuscular Disorders; Movement Disorders; Headache; **Hospital:** Meml Hermann Hosp - Texas Med Ctr, LBJ General Hosp; **Address:** 6410 Fannin St, Ste 1014, UT Professional Building Fl 10, Houston, TX 77030; **Phone:** 832-325-7080; **Board Cert:** Neurology 1973; Electrodiagnostic Medicine 1989; **Med School:** Spain 1964; **Resid:** Neurology, Univ Minn Hosps 1969; **Fellow:** Electromyography, Mayo Clinic 1970; **Fac Appt:** Assoc Clin Prof N, Univ Tex, Houston

Jankovic, Joseph MD [N] - **Spec Exp:** Movement Disorders; Parkinson's Disease; Tourette's Syndrome; **Hospital:** Methodist Hosp - Houston, St. Luke's Episcopal Hosp-Houston; **Address:** Parkinson's Dis Ctr & Movement Disorders Clin, 6550 Fannin St, Smith Twr, Ste 1801, Houston, TX 77030; **Phone:** 713-798-5998; **Board Cert:** Neurology 1979; **Med School:** Univ Ariz Coll Med 1973; **Resid:** Neurology, Columbia-Presby Med Ctr 1977; **Fac Appt:** Prof N, Baylor Coll Med

Kent, Thomas Andrew MD [N] - **Spec Exp:** Stroke; Neuro-Psychiatry; **Hospital:** DeBakey VA Med·Ctr-Houston; **Address:** 2002 Holcombe Blvd, MC 127, Neurology Care Line, Houston, TX 77030; **Phone:** 713-794-7393; **Board Cert:** Psychiatry 1993; Neurology 2006; **Med School:** Univ Kansas 1979; **Resid:** Psychiatry, Univ Kansas Affil Hosp 1983; Neurology, Univ Texas Affil Hosp 1985; **Fellow:** Psychopharmacology, Univ Kansas Affil Hosp 1983; **Fac Appt:** Prof N, Baylor Coll Med

Labiner, David M MD [N] - **Spec Exp:** Epilepsy; Seizure Disorders; **Hospital:** Univ Med Ctr - Tucson; **Address:** Univ Arizona HSC, Dept Neurology, 1501 N Campbell Ave, PO Box 245023, Tucson, AZ 85724-5023; **Phone:** 520-626-2006; **Board Cert:** Neurology 1992; **Med School:** Med Coll GA 1984; **Resid:** Neurology, Neuro Inst/Columbia 1988; **Fellow:** Epilepsy, Duke Univ Med Ctr 1989; **Fac Appt:** Prof N, Univ Ariz Coll Med

Nicholl, Jeffrey S MD [N] - **Spec Exp:** Seizure Disorders; Epilepsy; **Hospital:** Tulane Med Ctr; **Address:** Tulane Dept Neurology, 1430 Tulane Ave, #8065, New Orleans, LA 70112; **Phone:** 504-988-2241; **Board Cert:** Neurology 2009; Psychiatry 1981; Clinical Neurophysiology 2001; Emergency Medicine 2004; **Med School:** Georgetown Univ 1974; **Resid:** Psychiatry, UCLA Neuro Psyc Inst 1979; Neurology, Tulane Univ 1997; **Fellow:** Clinical Neurophysiology, Tulane Univ 1998; Epilepsy, UCLA 2000; **Fac Appt:** Assoc Prof N, Tulane Univ

Oommen, Kalarickal J MD [N] - **Spec Exp:** Epilepsy; **Hospital:** Univ Med Ctr-Lubbock, Covenant Med Ctr; **Address:** 3506 21st St, Ste 400, Lubbock, TX 79410; **Phone:** 806-725-4115; **Board Cert:** Neurology 1983; **Med School:** India 1973; **Resid:** Psychiatry, Arizona Hlth Sci Ctr 1979; Neurology, Arizona Hlth Sci Ctr 1982; **Fellow:** Electroencephalography, Med Coll Georgia 1983; **Fac Appt:** Prof N, Texas Tech Univ

Patchell, Roy Andrew MD [N] - **Spec Exp:** Neuro-Oncology; Brain Tumors; Spinal Tumors; **Hospital:** St. Joseph's Hosp & Med Ctr - Phoenix; **Address:** Barrow Neurology Clinics, 350 W Thomas·Rd, Ste 300, Phoenix, AZ 85013-4409; **Phone:** 602-406-2616; **Board Cert:** Neurology 1984; **Med School:** Univ KY Coll Med 1979; **Resid:** Neurology, Johns Hopkins Hosp 1983; **Fellow:** Neuro-Oncology, Meml Sloan-Kettering Canc Ctr 1985; **Fac Appt:** Prof N, Univ KY Coll Med

Shapiro, William R MD [N] - **Spec Exp:** Neuro-Oncology; **Hospital:** St. Joseph's Hosp & Med Ctr - Phoenix; **Address:** Barrow Neurology Clins, 500 W Thomas Rd, Ste 300, Phoenix, AZ 85013; **Phone:** 602-406-6262; **Board Cert:** Neurology 1969; **Med School:** UCSF 1961; **Resid:** Internal Medicine, Univ Wash Hosp 1963; Neurology, NY Hosp-Cornell Med Ctr 1966; **Fellow:** Neuro-Oncology, Natl Inst Hlth 1969; **Fac Appt:** Prof N, Univ Ariz Coll Med

Suarez, Jose MD [N] - **Spec Exp:** Stroke; Critical Care; **Hospital:** St. Luke's Episcopal Hosp-Houston; **Address:** Neurology Associates, Smith Tower, 6550 Fannin St Fl 18 - Ste 1801, Houston, TX 77030; **Phone:** 713-798-7411; **Board Cert:** Neurology 2008; Vascular Neurology 2005; **Med School:** Colombia 1988; **Resid:** Neurology, Case Western Reserve Univ Hosp 1996; **Fellow:** Neurocritical Care, Johns Hopkins Univ Hosp 1998; **Fac Appt:** Assoc Prof N, Baylor Coll Med

Wolinsky, Jerry S MD [N] - **Spec Exp:** Multiple Sclerosis; Clinical Trials; MRI; **Hospital:** Meml Hermann Hosp - Texas Med Ctr; **Address:** Univ Texas Med Sch, 6431 Fannin St, MSMB 7.044, Houston, TX 77030-1503; **Phone:** 713-500-7135; **Board Cert:** Neurology 1975; **Med School:** Univ IL Coll Med 1969; **Resid:** Neurology, UCSF Med Ctr 1973; **Fellow:** Neuropathology, VA Hosp 1975; **Fac Appt:** Prof N, Univ Tex, Houston

Yung, WK Alfred MD [N] - **Spec Exp:** Neuro-Oncology; Brain Tumors; **Hospital:** UT MD Anderson Cancer Ctr; **Address:** 1515 Holcombe Blvd, Unit 431, Houston, TX 77030-4017; **Phone:** 713-794-1285; **Board Cert:** Neurology 1980; **Med School:** Univ Chicago-Pritzker Sch Med 1975; **Resid:** Neurology, UCSD Med Ctr 1978; **Fellow:** Neuro-Oncology, Meml Sloan Kettering Cancer Ctr 1981; **Fac Appt:** Prof N, Univ Tex, Houston

West Coast and Pacific

Adornato, Bruce T MD [N] - **Spec Exp:** Stroke; Peripheral Neuropathy; Sleep Disorders/Apnea; **Hospital:** Stanford Univ Hosp & Clinics, VA Hlth Care Sys - Palo Alto; **Address:** 326 Bryant St, Palo Alto, CA 94301; **Phone:** 650-324-4300; **Board Cert:** Internal Medicine 1975; Neurology 1978; **Med School:** UCSD 1972; **Resid:** Internal Medicine, UCSF-Moffitt Hosp 1974; Neurology, UCSF-Moffitt Hosp 1976; **Fellow:** Neurology, Natl Inst Hlth 1978; **Fac Appt:** Clin Prof N, Stanford Univ

Albers, Gregory W MD [N] - **Spec Exp:** Cerebrovascular Disease; Stroke; Clinical Trials; **Hospital:** Stanford Univ Hosp & Clinics; **Address:** Stanford Univ Med Ctr, Dept Neurology, 780 Welch Rd, Ste 205, Palo Alto, CA 94304; **Phone:** 650-723-4448; **Board Cert:** Neurology 1990; Vascular Neurology 2008; **Med School:** UCSD 1984; **Resid:** Neurology, Stanford Univ Med Ctr 1988; **Fellow:** Stroke, Stanford Univ Med Ctr 1989; **Fac Appt:** Prof N, Stanford Univ

Aminoff, Michael J MD [N] - **Spec Exp:** Movement Disorders; Parkinson's Disease; **Hospital:** UCSF Med Ctr; **Address:** 400 Parnassus Ave Fl 8, Box 0348, San Francisco, CA 94143-0216; **Phone:** 415-353-2273; **Board Cert:** Neurology 2004; Clinical Neurophysiology 2000; **Med School:** England, UK 1965; **Resid:** Internal Medicine, Univ London Hosps 1970; Neurology, Middlesex Hosp/Natl Hosp Queen Sq 1972; **Fac Appt:** Prof N, UCSF

Aurora, Sheena K MD [N] - **Spec Exp:** Headache; Migraine; Electromyography; Movement Disorders; **Hospital:** Swedish Med Ctr-First Hill-Seattle; **Address:** Swedish Headache Ctr, 1101 Madison St, Ste 200, Seattle, WA 98104; **Phone:** 206-215-2243; **Board Cert:** Neurology 2006; Electrodiagnostic Medicine 1998; Headache Medicine 2006; **Med School:** India 1990; **Resid:** Neurology, Henry Ford Hosp 1997

Becker, Kyra J MD [N] - **Spec Exp:** Stroke/Cerebrovascular Disease; Neuro-Immunology; Stroke-Young Adults; Critical Care; **Hospital:** Harborview Med Ctr; **Address:** Harborview Medical Ctr, Dept Neurology, 325 9th Ave, Box 359859, Seattle, WA 98104; **Phone:** 206-744-6285; **Board Cert:** Neurology 2006; Vascular Neurology 2005; **Med School:** Duke Univ 1989; **Resid:** Neurology, Johns Hopkins Hosp 1993; **Fellow:** Critical Care Neurology, Johns Hopkins Hosp 1995; Research, NIH-NINDS 1996; **Fac Appt:** Assoc Prof N, Univ Wash

Bourdette, Dennis MD [N] - **Spec Exp:** Multiple Sclerosis; Guillain-Barre Syndrome; Myasthenia Gravis; **Hospital:** OR Hlth & Sci Univ; **Address:** OHSU, Dept Neurology, 3181 SW Sam Jackson Park Rd, MC L226, Portland, OR 97239; **Phone:** 503-494-5759; **Board Cert:** Neurology 1985; **Med School:** UC Davis 1978; **Resid:** Neurology, Oregon Hlth Sci Univ Hosp 1982; **Fellow:** Neurological Immunology, VA Med Ctr 1985; **Fac Appt:** Prof N, Oregon Hlth & Sci Univ

Bruno, Michiko K MD [N] - **Spec Exp:** Movement Disorders; Parkinson's Disease; Tourette's Syndrome; **Hospital:** Queen's Med Ctr - Honolulu; **Address:** Queens Physicians Office, 1380 Lusitana St, Ste 705, Honolulu, HI 96813; **Phone:** 808-537-9105; **Board Cert:** Neurology 2003; **Med School:** Japan 1996; **Resid:** Neurology, NY Presby-Cornell Med Ctr 2002; **Fellow:** Movement Disorders, NIH 2004

Neurology

Chamberlain, Marc C MD [N] - **Spec Exp:** Brain Tumors; Neuro-Oncology; Clinical Trials; **Hospital:** Univ Wash Med Ctr; **Address:** Seattle Cancer Care Alliance, 825 Eastlake Ave E, POB 10923, MS G4940, Seattle, WA 98109-1023; **Phone:** 206-288-8280; **Board Cert:** Pediatrics 1985; Child Neurology 1989; **Med School:** Columbia P&S 1977; **Resid:** Pediatrics, Montefiore Med Ctr 1981; Neurology, UCLA Med Ctr 1983; **Fellow:** Neuro-Oncology, UCSF Med Ctr 1986; **Fac Appt:** Prof N, Univ Wash

Charles, Andrew C MD [N] - **Spec Exp:** Headache; Migraine; **Hospital:** UCLA Ronald Reagan Med Ctr; **Address:** UCLA Neurological Svcs, 300 UCLA Medical Plaza, Ste B200, Los Angeles, CA 90095; **Phone:** 310-794-1195; **Board Cert:** Neurology 1992; **Med School:** UCLA 1986; **Resid:** Neurology, UCLA Med Ctr 1990; **Fellow:** Neurology, UCLA 1992; **Fac Appt:** Prof N, UCLA

Chui, Helena C MD [N] - **Spec Exp:** Stroke; Dementia; Alzheimer's Disease; **Hospital:** Keck Med Ctr of USC (page 75), Rancho Los Amigos Natl Rehab Ctr; **Address:** USC Dept Neurology, 1510 San Pablo St, Ste 618, Los Angeles, CA 90033; **Phone:** 323-442-7591; **Board Cert:** Neurology 1984; **Med School:** Johns Hopkins Univ 1977; **Resid:** Neurology, Univ Iowa Med Ctr 1981; **Fellow:** Behavioral Neurology, Univ Iowa Med Ctr 1979; **Fac Appt:** Prof N, USC Sch Med

Cloughesy, Timothy F MD [N] - **Spec Exp:** Neuro-Oncology; Seizure Disorders; Brain Tumors; **Hospital:** UCLA Ronald Reagan Med Ctr; **Address:** UCLA Neurological Services, 710 Westwood Plaza, Ste 1230, Los Angeles, CA 90095; **Phone:** 310-825-5321; **Board Cert:** Neurology 1993; **Med School:** Tulane Univ 1987; **Resid:** Neurology, UCLA Med Ctr 1991; **Fellow:** Neuro-Oncology, Meml Sloan-Kettering Canc Ctr; **Fac Appt:** Clin Prof N, UCLA

Corey-Bloom, Jody MD/PhD [N] - **Spec Exp:** Multiple Sclerosis; **Hospital:** UCSD Med Ctr; **Address:** 8950 Via La Jolla Drive, Ste C129, La Jolla, CA 92037-0973; **Phone:** 858-657-8540; **Board Cert:** Neurology 1993; **Med School:** UCSD 1986; **Resid:** Neurology, UCSD Med Ctr 1990; **Fellow:** Neurology, UCSD Med Ctr 1992; **Fac Appt:** Prof N, UCSD

Cummings, Jeffrey Lee MD [N] - **Spec Exp:** Neuro-Psychiatry; Alzheimer's Disease; Parkinson's Disease; **Address:** Cleveland Clinic Nevada, Lou Ruvo Ctr for Brain Health, 888 W Bonneville Ave, Las Vegas, NV 89106; **Phone:** 702-483-6000; **Board Cert:** Neurology 1979; **Med School:** Univ Wash 1974; **Resid:** Neurology, Boston Univ Sch Med 1978; **Fellow:** Behavioral Neurology and Psychiatry, Boston Univ Sch Med 1979; Neurological Pathology, The Natl Hosp 1980; **Fac Appt:** Assoc Prof N, UCLA

DeGiorgio, Christopher M MD [N] - **Spec Exp:** Epilepsy; Seizure Disorders; **Hospital:** UCLA Ronald Reagan Med Ctr; **Address:** UCLA Neurological Svcs, 300 UCLA Medical Plaza, rm B200, Los Angeles, CA 90095; **Phone:** 310-794-1195; **Board Cert:** Neurology 1987; **Med School:** Loyola Univ-Stritch Sch Med 1981; **Resid:** Neurology, Wadsworth VA Hosp 1985; **Fellow:** Epilepsy, UCLA 1987; **Fac Appt:** Prof N, UCLA

Engel, William King MD [N] - **Spec Exp:** Neuromuscular Disorders; Peripheral Neuropathy; Amyotrophic Lateral Sclerosis (ALS); Myasthenia Gravis; **Hospital:** Good Samaritan Hosp - LA, Keck Med Ctr of USC (page 75); **Address:** 637 S Lucas Ave Fl 3, Los Angeles, CA 90017; **Phone:** 213-975-9950; **Board Cert:** Neurology 1962; **Med School:** McGill Univ 1955; **Resid:** Neurology, Natl Inst Hlth 1959; Neurology, Natl Hosp 1960; **Fellow:** Neuromuscular Medicine, Natl Inst Hlth 1961; **Fac Appt:** Prof N, USC Sch Med

Engstrom, John W MD [N] - **Spec Exp:** Peripheral Neuropathy; Spinal Cord Disorders; **Hospital:** UCSF Med Ctr; **Address:** UCSF Med Ctr, Dept Neurology, 400 Parnassus Ave Fl 8, Box 0348, San Francisco, CA 94143; **Phone:** 415-353-2273; **Board Cert:** Internal Medicine 1984; Neurology 1991; Clinical Neurophysiology 2002; **Med School:** Stanford Univ 1981; **Resid:** Internal Medicine, Johns Hopkins Hosp 1984; Neurology, UCSF Med Ctr 1988; **Fellow:** Neurology, UCSF Med Ctr 1989; **Fac Appt:** Prof N, UCSF

Fisher, Mark Jay MD [N] - **Spec Exp:** Stroke; Cerebrovascular Disease; **Hospital:** UC Irvine Med Ctr, VA Long Beach Hlthcare Sys; **Address:** UC Irvine Med Ctr, Dept Neurology, 101 The City Drive S, Shanbrom Hall Bldg 55 - rm 121, Orange, CA 92868; **Phone:** 714-456-6856; **Board Cert:** Neurology 1981; Vascular Neurology 2005; **Med School:** Univ Cincinnati 1975; **Resid:** Neurology, UCLA-Wadsworth VA Hosp 1980; **Fac Appt:** Prof N, UC Irvine

Fisher, Robert S MD [N] - **Spec Exp:** Epilepsy; Seizure Disorders; **Hospital:** Stanford Univ Hosp & Clinics; **Address:** Stanford Univ Dept Neurology, 300 Pasteur Drive, rm A-343, Stanford, CA 94305-5235; **Phone:** 650-498-3056; **Board Cert:** Neurology 1983; Clinical Neurophysiology 2002; **Med School:** Stanford Univ 1977; **Resid:** Internal Medicine, Stanford Univ 1979; **Fellow:** Neurology, Johns Hopkins Univ 1982; **Fac Appt:** Prof N, Stanford Univ

Goodin, Douglas S MD [N] - **Spec Exp:** Multiple Sclerosis; **Hospital:** UCSF Med Ctr, VA Med Ctr - San Francisco; **Address:** UCSF Multiple Sclerosis Ctr, 400 Parnassus Ave Fl 8, San Francisco, CA 94143; **Phone:** 415-353-2069; **Board Cert:** Neurology 1985; **Med School:** UC Irvine 1978; **Resid:** Neurology, UCSF Med Ctr 1981; **Fac Appt:** Clin Prof N, UCSF

Graves, Michael C MD [N] - **Spec Exp:** Amyotrophic Lateral Sclerosis (ALS); Electromyography; Guillain-Barre Syndrome; Muscular Dystrophy; **Hospital:** UCLA Ronald Reagan Med Ctr; **Address:** UCLA Neurological Svcs, 300 Medical Plaza, Ste B200, Box 956975, Los Angeles, CA 90095-6975; **Phone:** 310-794-1195; **Board Cert:** Neurology 1977; **Med School:** Stanford Univ 1970; **Resid:** Internal Medicine, UCSD Med Ctr 1972; Neurology, Johns Hopkins Hosp 1975; **Fellow:** Rockefeller Univ; **Fac Appt:** Assoc Prof N, UCLA

Guilleminault, Christian MD [N] - **Spec Exp:** Sleep Disorders/Apnea; **Hospital:** Stanford Univ Hosp & Clinics; **Address:** Stanford Sleep Medicine Center, 450 Broadway St, Pavilion B, Redwood City, CA 94063-5704; **Phone:** 650-723-6601; **Med School:** France 1962; **Resid:** Neurology, Hospital Foch 1966; Hosp de la Salpetriere 1968; **Fellow:** Univ Geneva 1967; **Fac Appt:** Prof Psyc, Stanford Univ

Hauser, Stephen L MD [N] - **Spec Exp:** Multiple Sclerosis; **Hospital:** UCSF Med Ctr; **Address:** UCSF Multiple Sclerosis Center, 400 Parnassus Ave, 8th Fl, San Francisco, CA 94143; **Phone:** 415-353-2069; **Board Cert:** Internal Medicine 1978; Neurology 1981; **Med School:** Harvard Med Sch 1975; **Resid:** Internal Medicine, NY Presby-Cornell 1977; Neurology, Mass Genl Hosp 1980; **Fellow:** Neurology, Harvard Univ 1980; **Fac Appt:** Prof N, UCSF

Heck, Christianne N MD [N] - **Spec Exp:** Epilepsy; **Hospital:** Keck Med Ctr of USC (page 75); **Address:** Neurologic Care & Research Ctr, 1520 San Pablo St, Ste 3000, Los Angeles, CA 90033; **Phone:** 323-442-5710; **Board Cert:** Neurology 2001; **Med School:** USC-Keck School of Medicine 1991; **Resid:** Neurology, LAC/USC Med Ctr 1995; **Fellow:** Epilepsy, USC Med Ctr 1996; **Fac Appt:** Assoc Prof N, USC-Keck School of Medicine

Henderson, Victor W MD [N] - **Spec Exp:** Alzheimer's Disease; Dementia; Memory Disorders; **Hospital:** Stanford Univ Hosp & Clinics; **Address:** Stanford Univ Dept Health Rsch & Policy, 150 Governors Lane, Rredwood Bldg, rm T 152, Stanford, CA 94305-5405; **Phone:** 650-723-6469; **Board Cert:** Neurology 1981; **Med School:** Johns Hopkins Univ 1976; **Resid:** Internal Medicine, Duke Univ Med Ctr 1977; Neurology, Barnes Hosp- Wash Univ 1980; **Fellow:** Behavioral Neurology, Aphasia Rsch Ctr-Boston Univ 1981; **Fac Appt:** Prof N, Stanford Univ

Langston, J William MD [N] - **Spec Exp:** Parkinson's Disease; Movement Disorders; Tremor; **Hospital:** Parkinson's Inst/Movement Disorders Trmt Ctr, The; **Address:** The Parkinsons Inst, 675 Almanor Ave, Sunnyvale, CA 94085; **Phone:** 408-542-5633; **Board Cert:** Neurology 1986; **Med School:** Univ MO-Columbia Sch Med 1967; **Resid:** Neurology, Stanford Univ 1974; **Fellow:** Electroencephalography, Stanford Univ

Lew, Mark F MD [N] - **Spec Exp:** Movement Disorders; Parkinson's Disease; Dystonia; **Hospital:** Keck Med Ctr of USC (page 75); **Address:** USC Consultation Center 2, 1520 San Pablo St, Ste 3000, Los Angeles, CA 90033; **Phone:** 323-442-5817; **Board Cert:** Neurology 1993; **Med School:** Geo Wash Univ 1987; **Resid:** Neurology, USC-LAC Med Ctr 1991; **Fellow:** Movement Disorders, USC-LAC Med Ctr 1992; **Fac Appt:** Prof N, USC Sch Med

Longo, Frank M MD/PhD [N] - **Spec Exp:** Alzheimer's Disease; Huntington's Disease; **Hospital:** Stanford Univ Hosp & Clinics, UCSF Med Ctr; **Address:** Stanford Univ Med Ctr, Neurology, 300 Pasteur Drive, MC 5235, H3160, Stanford, CA 94305; **Phone:** 650-723-6469; **Board Cert:** Neurology 1981; **Med School:** UCSD 1981; **Resid:** Neurology, UCSF Med Ctr 1987; **Fellow:** Neurology, UCSF Med Ctr 1989; **Fac Appt:** Prof N, Stanford Univ

Lutsep, Helmi L MD [N] - **Spec Exp:** Stroke/Cerebrovascular Disease; Stroke Prevention; **Hospital:** OR Hlth & Sci Univ; **Address:** Oregon Stroke Ctr, OHSU, 3181 SW Sam Jackson Park Rd, CR-131, Portland, OR 97239; **Phone:** 503-494-7225; **Board Cert:** Neurology 1994; Vascular Neurology 2005; **Med School:** Mayo Med Sch 1988; **Resid:** Neurology, Mayo Clinic 1992; **Fellow:** Behavioral Neurology, UC Davis Med Ctr 1995; Stroke, Stanford Univ Med Ctr 1996; **Fac Appt:** Prof N, Oregon Hlth & Sci Univ

Morrell, Martha J MD [N] - **Spec Exp:** Epilepsy; Epilepsy in Women; **Hospital:** Stanford Univ Hosp & Clinics; **Address:** Stanford Univ Dept Neurology, 300 Pasteur Drive, rm A-343, Stanford, CA 94305-5235; **Phone:** 650-725-6648; **Board Cert:** Neurology 1989; Clinical Neurophysiology 2003; **Med School:** Stanford Univ 1984; **Resid:** Neurology, Hosp Univ Penn 1988; **Fellow:** Epilepsy, Graduate Hosp-Univ Penn 1990; **Fac Appt:** Clin Prof N, Stanford Univ

Nutt Jr, John G MD [N] - **Spec Exp:** Parkinson's Disease; Movement Disorders; **Hospital:** OR Hlth & Sci Univ; **Address:** Parkinson's Ctr of Oregon, 3181 SW Sam Jackson Park Rd, MC OP32, Portland, OR 97239; **Phone:** 503-494-7230; **Board Cert:** Neurology 1978; **Med School:** Baylor Coll Med 1970; **Resid:** Neurology, Univ Wash Med Ctr 1976; **Fellow:** Pharmacology, Natl Inst Neuro Disorders /Stroke 1978; **Fac Appt:** Prof N, Oregon Hlth & Sci Univ

Phuphanich, Surasak MD [N] - **Spec Exp:** Brain Tumors-Metastatic; Stem Cell Therapy; Spinal Tumors; Neurologic Complications of Cancer; **Hospital:** Cedars-Sinai Med Ctr; **Address:** 8631 W 3rd St, Ste 410E, Los Angeles, CA 90048; **Phone:** 310-423-4413; **Board Cert:** Neurology 1983; **Med School:** Thailand 1975; **Resid:** Neurology, Univ Illinois Med Ctr 1981; **Fellow:** Neuro-Oncology, UCSF Med Ctr 1984; **Fac Appt:** Prof Neuro-Onc

Raskin, Neil H MD [N] - **Spec Exp:** Headache; Migraine; **Hospital:** UCSF Med Ctr; **Address:** UCSF Neurology Faculty Practice, 400 Parnassus Ave Fl 8, Box 0348, San Francisco, CA 94143-0348; **Phone:** 415-353-2273; **Board Cert:** Neurology 1969; **Med School:** Harvard Med Sch 1959; **Resid:** Internal Medicine, Bellevue Hosp Ctr 1961; Neurology, Neuro Inst/Columbia 1964; **Fellow:** Neurology, Neuro Inst/Columbia 1965; **Fac Appt:** Prof N, UCSF

Rosenbaum, Richard B MD [N] - **Spec Exp:** Neuromuscular Disorders; Parkinson's Disease; **Hospital:** OR Hlth & Sci Univ, Providence Portland Med Ctr; **Address:** Oregon Clinic Neurology Department, 5050 NE Hoyt St, Ste 315, Portland, OR 97213-2975; **Phone:** 503-963-3100; **Board Cert:** Internal Medicine 1975; Neurology 1979; **Med School:** Harvard Med Sch 1971; **Resid:** Internal Medicine, Stanford Med Ctr 1973; Neurology, UCSF Med Ctr 1977; **Fac Appt:** Clin Prof N, Oregon Hlth & Sci Univ

Samii, Ali MD [N] - **Spec Exp:** Movement Disorders; Parkinson's Disease; Tremor & Dystonia; **Hospital:** Univ Wash Med Ctr; **Address:** UW Medical Center, Dept Neurology, 1959 NE Pacific St, Box 356169, Seattle, WA 98195; **Phone:** 206-598-7688; **Board Cert:** Neurology 2007; **Med School:** McGill Univ 1989; **Resid:** Neurology, UC Davis Med Ctr 1993; **Fellow:** Movement Disorders, NIH/Motor Control Sect 1996; Movement Disorders, Univ BC 1997; **Fac Appt:** Assoc Prof N, Univ Wash

Saver, Jeffrey L MD [N] - **Spec Exp:** Stroke; Stroke Prevention; **Hospital:** UCLA Ronald Reagan Med Ctr; **Address:** UCLA Stroke Ctr, 710 Westwood Plaza, rm 4126, Los Angeles, CA 90095; **Phone:** 310-794-6379; **Board Cert:** Neurology 1991; Vascular Neurology 2005; **Med School:** Harvard Med Sch 1986; **Resid:** Neurological Surgery, Brigham & Womens Hosp 1990; **Fellow:** Behavioral Neurology, Univ Iowa Hosps 1991; Cerebrovascular Disease, Rhode Island Hosp 1992; **Fac Appt:** Prof N, UCLA

Smith, Wade S MD/PhD [N] - **Spec Exp:** Stroke; Pain-Back & Shoulder; **Hospital:** UCSF Med Ctr; **Address:** UCSF Vascular Neurology, 400 Parnassus Ave, Box 0114, San Francisco, CA 94143-0114; **Phone:** 415-353-1489; **Board Cert:** Neurology 2006; Vascular Neurology 2008; **Med School:** Univ Wash 1989; **Resid:** Neurology, UCSF-Moffitt Hosp 1993; **Fellow:** Critical Care Medicine, UCSF Med Ctr 1994; **Fac Appt:** Prof N, UCSF

Starr, Arnold MD [N] - **Spec Exp:** Hearing Disorders; Neurophysiology-Aging; Neurophysiology-Dementia; Hearing Disorders; **Hospital:** UC Irvine Med Ctr; **Address:** Dept Neurology, Gottschalk Medical Plaza, 1 Medical Plaza Drive, Irvine, CA 92697; **Phone:** 714-456-7239; **Board Cert:** Neurology 1970; **Med School:** NYU Sch Med 1957; **Resid:** Neurology, Boston City Hosp 1959; **Fellow:** Neurology, Natl Inst Hlth 1962; Clinical Neurophysiology, Inst Neurophysiology 1963; **Fac Appt:** Prof N, UC Irvine

Tanner, Caroline M MD/PhD [N] - **Spec Exp:** Parkinson's Disease; Movement Disorders; Dystonia; **Hospital:** Parkinson's Inst/Movement Disorders Trmt Ctr, The; **Address:** The Parkinson's Inst, 675 Almanor Ave, Sunnyvale, CA 94085; **Phone:** 408-734-2800; **Board Cert:** Neurology 1982; **Med School:** Loyola Univ-Stritch Sch Med 1976; **Resid:** Neurology, Rush-Presby-St Luke's Med Ctr 1980; **Fellow:** Neurological Pharmacology, Rush-Presby-St Luke's Med Ctr 1982

Taylor, Lynne P MD [N] - **Spec Exp:** Brain Tumors; Gliomas; **Hospital:** Virginia Mason Med Ctr; **Address:** Virginia Mason Medical Ctr, Neurology, 1100 9th Ave, Fl 7, Seattle, WA 98101; **Phone:** 206-341-0420; **Board Cert:** Neurology 1987; Hospice & Palliative Medicine 2010; **Med School:** Washington Univ, St Louis 1982; **Resid:** Neurology, Hosp Univ Penn 1986; **Fellow:** Neuro-Oncology, Meml Sloan Kettering Cancer Ctr 1988; **Fac Appt:** Assoc Clin Prof N, Univ Wash

Tetrud, James W MD [N] - **Spec Exp:** Movement Disorders; Parkinson's Disease; Tremor; **Hospital:** Parkinson's Inst/Movement Disorders Trmt Ctr, The; **Address:** The Parkinson's Inst, 675 Almanor Ave, Sunnyvale, CA 94085; **Phone:** 408-734-2800; **Board Cert:** Neurology 1981; **Med School:** NYU Sch Med 1973; **Resid:** Internal Medicine, VA Med Ctr-West Los Angeles 1974; Neurology, VA Med Ctr-West Los Angeles 1978

Weiner, Leslie P MD [N] - **Spec Exp:** Multiple Sclerosis; Amyotrophic Lateral Sclerosis (ALS); **Hospital:** Keck Med Ctr of USC (page 75), LAC & USC Med Ctr; **Address:** USC Dept Neurology, 1520 San Pablo St, Ste 3000, Los Angeles, CA 90033; **Phone:** 323-442-5710; **Board Cert:** Neurology 1969; **Med School:** Univ Cincinnati 1961; **Resid:** Neurology, Baltimore City Hosp 1963; Neurology, Johns Hopkins Hosp 1965; **Fellow:** Neurology, Johns Hopkins Hosp 1969; **Fac Appt:** Prof N, USC Sch Med

Cleveland Clinic

Every life deserves world class care.

Cleveland Clinic
Neurological Institute
9500 Euclid Avenue
Cleveland, OH 44195

clevelandclinic.org/
neurotopdocs

Offering Same-Day Appointments
Call 800.274.2009.

Neurology

Cleveland Clinic Neurological Institute employs a multidisciplinary disease-specific focus, combining more than 300 medical, surgical and research specialists who treat children and adults with neurological and neurobehavioral disorders. Our clinical expertise, academic achievement and innovative research has earned the Neurological Institute an international reputation for excellence. *U.S.News & World Report* consistently ranks our neurology and neurosurgery and pediatric neurology/neurosurgery programs among the top 10 in the nation.

Our unique and collaborative clinical structure allows us to deliver coordinated, comprehensive and multidisciplinary care to our patients through more efficient treatment decision-making and consultation for complex cases. Major advances in the treatment of brain tumors, epilepsy, mood disorders, stroke, movement disorders, pain and spinal disorders are improving quality of life and survival for thousands of our patients. For those diseases resistant to available treatments, we are confident our innovative model of medicine will speed research and advances in treatment, resulting in better clinical care and more rapid breakthroughs in the full range of neurological and behavioral disorders.

Comprehensive Neurological Care

Cleveland Clinic offers expert diagnostic and treatment options for all neurologic conditions affecting children and adults, including Alzheimer's disease, aneurysms, arteriovenous malformations, back and neck disorders, brain and spine tumors, epilepsy, hydrocephalus, metastatic tumors, mild cognitive impairment, multiple sclerosis, movement disorders, neurofibromatosis, Parkinson's disease, pediatric and congential neurological disorders, pituitary disorders, sleep disorders and stroke.

Treatment Guides

Cleveland Clinic has developed comprehensive treatment guides for many diseases and conditions. To download our free treatment guides, visit clevelandclinic.org/ treatmentguides.

Online Medical Second Opinion

Cleveland Clinic's My**Consult** Online Medical Second Opinion program securely connects patients to our physician specialists for more than 1,000 life-changing or life-threatening diagnoses all by the click of a mouse. To learn more, log onto eclevelandclinic.org/myconsult or call 800.223.2273, ext. 43223.

Special Assistance for Out-of-State Patients

Cleveland Clinic Global Patient Services offers a complimentary Medical Concierge service for patients who travel from outside of Ohio. Call 800.223.2273, ext. 55580 or email medicalconcierge@ccf.org.

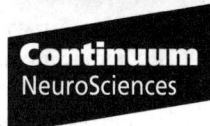

Neurology and Neurosurgery Expertise
(800) 420-4004

The member hospitals of the Continuum Neurosciences consortium—St. Luke's and Roosevelt Hospitals and Beth Israel Medical Center—are home to many international leaders in neurology, neurosurgery, neuro-radiology and endovascular neurosurgery. Each of the hospitals has clinicians who are nationally and internationally recognized for their accomplishments and attract patients from throughout the United States and other countries who are looking for innovative treatment programs delivered by physicians specializing in both clinical care and research. Our expertise includes treatments for:

- Complex brain tumors, spine and spinal cord; chordomas, meningiomas, acoustic neuromas, trigeminal neuralgia and hemifacial spasms
- Headaches
- Disorders of the brain, spinal cord, peripheral nerves and muscles
- Stroke/cerebrovascular diseases
- Epilepsy and seizures
- Movement disorders (Parkinson's disease, dystonia and essential tremor)
- Neuro-ophthalmologic conditions
- Neuro-oncology-related illnesses
- Neuro-psychiatry/psychology-based conditions
- Many adult and pediatric neurologic conditions

A few of our Centers of Excellence include:

St. Luke's and Roosevelt Hospitals

- The Hyman-Newman Institute for Neurology and Neurosurgery
- Center for Endovascular Surgery
- The Vascular Birthmarks Institute
- Vascular Malformations Center of NY
- New York Brain Tumor Center
- The Headache Institute
- The Stroke Center

Beth Israel Medical Center

- The Alan and Barbara Mirken Department of Neurology
- Bachmann-Strauss Dystonia Center of Excellence
- National Parkinson Foundation Center of Excellence
- The Betty and Morton Yarmon Stroke Center
- Internationally respected divisions of adult and pediatric epilepsy
- ALS (Lou Gehrig's disease) Center sponsored by the ALS Association
- Neurosurgery
- Peripheral Nerve Center

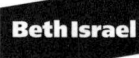 **Beth Israel**   **Roosevelt Hospital**   **St. Luke's Hospital**   **NY Eye & Ear Infirmary**

www.chpnyc.org

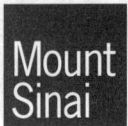
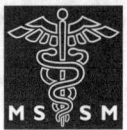

MOUNT SINAI
SCHOOL OF
MEDICINE

THE MOUNT SINAI MEDICAL CENTER
NEUROLOGY

One Gustave L. Levy Place
Fifth Avenue and 100th Street
New York, NY 10029-6574
Physician Referral: 1-800-MD-SINAI (637-4624)
www.mountsinai.org/neurology

THE ESTELLE AND DANIEL MAGGIN DEPARTMENT OF NEUROLOGY at Mount Sinai provides compassionate, state-of-the-art, interdisciplinary care for disorders of the brain and nervous system.

The Robert and John M. Bendheim Parkinson and Movement Disorders Center is one of the world's leading multidisciplinary centers for clinical care and translational research aimed at Parkinson's disease, dystonia, tremor, and a variety of movement disorders. The Center incorporates a world-renowned deep-brain stimulation program, and is at the forefront in clinical trials and experimental therapeutics for movement disorders.

The Corinne Goldsmith Dickinson Center for Multiple Sclerosis is an internationally recognized comprehensive center, uniting the efforts of leading physicians and scientists from many disciplines to understand the causes and consequences of MS. The Center provides services in all aspects of diagnosis, disease management, rehabilitation, and patient support, and the opportunity for patients to participate in potentially groundbreaking clinical trials.

The Clinical Program for Cerebrovascular Disorders comprises an outstanding team of medical experts who specialize in the most advanced approaches in the evaluation, treatment, and rehabilitation of patients with cerebrovascular diseases. Services include the early diagnosis of stroke, a specialized Neurointensive Care Unit, and an advanced inpatient stroke unit. Physicians are available at all times for emergency consultation with referring physicians. The Stroke Center was the first JCAHO-certified primary stroke center in Manhattan.

The NeuroAIDS Program provides diagnosis and treatment for neurological disorders associated with HIV disease. This program is one of the few in the world to treat the various complications of the disease that affect the central and peripheral nervous systems in as many as 70 percent of patients.

THE ESTELLE AND DANIEL MAGGIN DEPARTMENT OF NEUROLOGY is renowned for its unique integration of outstanding patient care and cutting-edge research in neurological disease, and can bring the latest advances in treatment to our patients. Our physicians and neuroscientists have made enormous strides in basic and translational research, bringing medical breakthroughs that will change the course of neurological treatment. The department is led by some of the most prominent figures in American neurology, is #3 nationally in the number of academic neurologists trained in our residency program, and receives annual research grants of more than $20 million.

The Epilepsy Center provides specific expertise in the diagnosis and treatment of epilepsy and related disorders. The Center encompasses outstanding epileptologists, a new modern inpatient epilepsy monitoring unit, and full outpatient EEG and diagnostic capabilities.

The Center for Headache and Pain Medicine is a multidisciplinary center for the diagnosis and treatment of chronic and acute headaches and other painful disorders of the skull, brain, or face in both adults and children. Specialists in neurology, pain medicine, ENT, ophthalmology, psychiatry, and rehabilitation medicine are available to evaluate and treat individuals with painful disorders.

The Division of Neuromuscular Diseases provides diagnosis, treatment, and compassionate care for patients with disorders in neuromuscular transmission, muscle diseases, peripheral nerve problems, and spasticity resulting from stroke or damage to the central nervous system.

Mount Sinai's Neurological Tumor Program is world-acclaimed for the treatment of pituitary adenomas, acoustic neuromas, meningiomas, and cancerous brain tumors. The program's multispecialty group of physicians works together to provide outstanding care through state-of-the-art surgical procedures, radiation therapy, chemotherapy, and supportive therapy. Our physicians have pioneered the treatment of tumors with stereotactic radiosurgery, as well as developed a number of experimental treatment protocols to improve patients' lives.

The Eye Movement and Vestibular Disorder Program provides outstanding diagnosis and treatment for visual problems, balance problems, and motion sickness. Our physicians participate in NASA programs, employing technology used to assess these disorders in space, and studying possible treatment applications on earth.

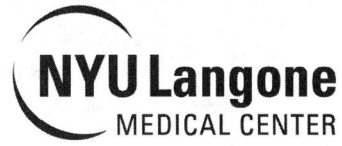

550 First Avenue *(at 31st Street)*
New York, NY 10016
www.NYULMC.org
Physician Referral: **888-7-NYU-MED** *(888-769-8633)*

NEUROSURGERY

The Department of Neurosurgery at NYU Langone Medical Center offers some of the medical field's most skilled and experienced surgeons in advanced, minimally invasive procedures. Patients also benefit from cutting-edge research and fully integrated approach to medical care.

Brain Tumor
The Department of Neurosurgery specializes in both malignant and benign brain tumors, including skull base tumors. Expertise includes glioblastoma, ependymoma, hemangioblastoma, other gliomas, meningiomas and vestibular schwannomas (acoustic neuromas).

Cerebrovascular Surgery
The Division of Cerebrovascular Surgery is a premier center for brain aneurysms, giant intracranial aneurysms, brain vascular malformations and cavernomas, and stroke.

Epilepsy
The Comprehensive Epilepsy Center is the largest epilepsy center in the U.S. offering patients an array of advanced surgical and medical options.

Spinal Neurosurgery
The Division of Spine Surgery provides treatment for degenerative spinal diseases, spinal tumors, spinal trauma and spinal infections.

Hyperhidrosis
The Department offers expertise in the surgical treatment of primary hyperhidrosis (excessive sweating) including Endoscopic Thoracic Sympathectomy.

Neurosurgical Technology
Our neurosurgeons remove deep-seated tumors, vascular malformations and other disease sites using a highly advanced Leksell Gamma Knife. Aided by 3-D MRI technology, the Gamma Knife bombards its target with precise doses of radiation, while preserving healthy tissue.

We also provide state-of-the-art care and research through the following divisions:
- Facial Pain: provides patients a thorough examination and, if required, nerve injections and minimally invasive surgery.
- Functional Neurosurgery: offers diagnosis and treatment of Parkinson's disease and conditions that involve involuntary muscle contractions.
- Pediatric Neurosurgery: provides treatment to children with brain and spinal cord tumors, congenital and development disorders.
- Peripheral Nerve Surgery: focuses on the diagnosis and treatment of nerve compressions, nerve tremors, Brachial Plexus (nerve fiber) and nerve injuries.

Neuro-Critical Care
Intensive care and treatment of critical neurosurgical illnesses is provided.

![Penn Medicine]
Penn Medicine
PENN COMPREHENSIVE NEUROSCIENCE CENTER

Philadelphia, PA 19104
800.789.PENN
PennMedicine.org

PENN NEUROLOGY

The University of Pennsylvania's history of excellence in the treatment of neurological diseases dates back to the establishment of the Department of Neurology in 1874. *The Best Doctors in America*® lists more neurologists and neurosurgeons from the Hospital of the University of Pennsylvania than from any other hospital or medical center in the Philadelphia region. Penn Neurology and Neurosurgery at the Hospital of the University of Pennsylvania (HUP) are ranked 14th in the nation by *U.S.News & World Report,* the only neuroscience programs in the region to be recognized.

The Department of Neurology is a component of the Penn Comprehensive Neuroscience Center, which is dedicated to facilitating and strengthening the integration of Penn's world-class neuroscience programs within the areas of clinical care, research and education.

Excellence and Expertise

Recognized by the National Parkinson Foundation as one of its worldwide Centers of Excellence, the **Parkinson's Disease and Movement Disorders Center** is committed to providing exceptional patient care, education, and social support services. Research is an important and ongoing mission of the Center, which actively pursues the investigation of the disease as well as exploration of new medications.

The **Multiple Sclerosis Center Program** provides comprehensive evaluation, diagnosis and treatment for patients with MS and other demyelinating disorders of the central nervous system. In addition to maintaining the highest standards for clinical service, the Penn MS program is a leader in MS training and in clinical and laboratory-based research.

The **Penn Neuro-Ophthalmology Program** bridges the fields of ophthalmology and neurology through the diagnosis and management of patients with neurological disorders that affect vision and eye movements. The program is part of Penn's **Comprehensive Neuroscience Center** and the **Scheie Eye Institute**. With five full-time faculty members and active clinical and research components, it is one of the largest neuro-ophthalmology groups in the country. Within the areas of multiple sclerosis vision research, pediatric neuro-ophthalmology, and vision-based testing for sports-related concussion, the Penn Neuro-Ophthalmology group is a world leader.

The **Penn Epilepsy Center** provides the highest standard of care to patients with epilepsy and related problems. The Center offers a comprehensive, full continuum of care including state-of-the-art diagnostic techniques, cutting-edge research, medical treatments, surgery, and support services to patients with epilepsy. Both outpatient evaluation and inpatient care are available via this multidisciplinary, full-service facility.

The **Penn Stroke Center** provides emergent care to stroke patients 24 hours a day, 365 days per year. The Center employs state-of-the-art approaches to the diagnosis, treatment and prevention of stroke and critical neurologic conditions. Inpatients are cared for by physicians and nurses with specialty training in neurological diseases in different settings, depending on their needs including the Neuroscience floor with telemetry and the Intermediate Neurological Care Unit. The Neurological Intensive Care Unit is among the most technologically advanced and sophisticated neurocritical care units in the nation, and is the only dedicated academic facility of its kind in the region.

Penn's **Cognitive Neurology Program** provides comprehensive, state-of-the-art assessment and treatment for patients with disorders of memory, language, attention, vision and cognition. Each patient is evaluated and treated by an experienced team of specialists and an individualized plan is developed for their ongoing care. The Center offers the latest treatment approaches available, including approved medications as well as access to numerous clinical trials of emerging treatments.

Programs

- Cognitive Neurology Program
- Center for Brain Injury and Repair
- Interventional Neuro Center
- Memory Disorders Clinic
- Multiple Sclerosis Center
- Neurological Intensive Care
- Neurogenetics Center
- Neuromuscular Disorders Program
- Neuro-Oncology Program
- Neuro-Ophthalmology Service
- Neuropsychology Service
- Parkinson's Disease and Movement Disorders Center
- Penn Epilepsy Center
- Penn Center for Sleep Disorders
- Penn Memory Center
- Stroke Center

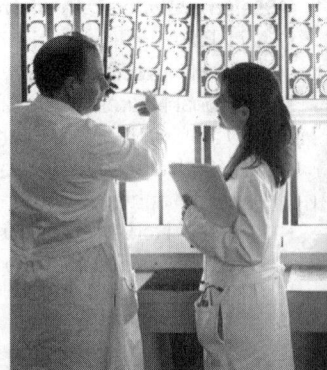

Nuclear Medicine

A nuclear medicine specialist employs the properties of radioactive atoms and molecules in the diagnosis and treatment of disease, and in research. Radiation detection and imaging instrument systems are used to detect disease as it changes the function and metabolism of normal cells, tissues and organs. A wide variety of diseases can be found in this way, usually before the structure of the organ involved by the disease can be seen to be abnormal by any other techniques. Early detection of coronary artery disease (including acute heart attack); early cancer detection and evaluation of the effect of tumor treatment; diagnosis of infection and inflammation anywhere in the body; and early detection of blood clot in the lungs, are all possible with these techniques. Unique forms of radioactive molecules can attack and kill cancer cells (e.g., lymphoma, thyroid cancer) or can relieve the severe pain of cancer that has spread to bone.

The nuclear medicine specialist has special knowledge in the biologic effects of radiation exposure, the fundamentals of the physical sciences and the principles and operation of radiation detection and imaging instrumentation systems.

Training required: Three years

NUCLEAR MEDICINE

Mid Atlantic

Agress Jr, Harry MD [NuM] - **Spec Exp:** PET Imaging; Cancer Detection & Staging; Nuclear Oncology; CT Scan; **Hospital:** Hackensack Univ Med Ctr; **Address:** Hackensack Univ Med Ctr, 30 Prospect Ave, Hackensack, NJ 07601; **Phone:** 201-996-2196; **Board Cert:** Nuclear Medicine 1976; Diagnostic Radiology 1978; **Med School:** Tufts Univ 1972; **Resid:** Radiology, Columbia-Presby Med Ctr 1978; **Fellow:** Nuclear Medicine, Natl Inst Hlth 1975; **Fac Appt:** Clin Prof Rad, Columbia P&S

Alavi, Abass MD [NuM] - **Spec Exp:** Brain Tumors; Neurologic Imaging; PET Imaging-Brain; Brain Infections; **Hospital:** Hosp Univ Penn - UPHS (page 68), Chldns Hosp of Philadelphia; **Address:** Hosp Univ Penn, Div Nuclear Med, 3400 Spruce St, Donner Bldg rm 110, Philadelphia, PA 19104; **Phone:** 215-662-3069; **Board Cert:** Internal Medicine 1972; Nuclear Medicine 1973; **Med School:** Iran 1964; **Resid:** Internal Medicine, Albert Einstein Med Ctr/Phila VA Hosp 1969; Hematology, Hosp Univ Penn 1970; **Fellow:** Nuclear Medicine, Hosp Univ Penn 1973; **Fac Appt:** Prof Rad, Univ Pennsylvania

Carrasquillo, Jorge A MD [NuM] - **Spec Exp:** Radioimmunotherapy of Cancer; PET Imaging; **Hospital:** Meml Sloan-Kettering Cancer Ctr; **Address:** 1275 York Avenue, Nuclear Medicine Svc, Box 77, New York, NY 10065; **Phone:** 212-639-2459; **Board Cert:** Internal Medicine 1977; Nuclear Medicine 1982; **Med School:** Univ Puerto Rico 1974; **Resid:** Internal Medicine, Univ Dist Hosp 1977; Nuclear Medicine, Univ Wash Hosp 1982

Freeman, Leonard M MD [NuM] - **Spec Exp:** Nuclear Oncology; Gastrointestinal Disorders; PET Imaging; CT Scan; **Hospital:** Montefiore Med Ctr - Div. Moses; **Address:** 111 E 210th St, Bronx, NY 10467-2401; **Phone:** 718-920-6060; **Board Cert:** Diagnostic Radiology 1966; Nuclear Medicine 1972; Nuclear Radiology 1974; **Med School:** Ros Franklin Univ/Chicago Med Sch 1961; **Resid:** Diagnostic Radiology, Bronx Municipal Hosp 1965; **Fac Appt:** Prof NuM, Albert Einstein Coll Med

Goldsmith, Stanley J MD [NuM] - **Spec Exp:** Thyroid Cancer; PET Imaging; Neuroendocrine Tumors; **Hospital:** NY-Presby/Weill Cornell Med Ctr, NY (page 65); **Address:** 525 E 68th St Starr Bldg - rm 2-21, New York, NY 10021-9800; **Phone:** 212-746-4588; **Board Cert:** Internal Medicine 1969; Nuclear Medicine 1972; Endocrinology 1972; **Med School:** SUNY Downstate 1962; **Resid:** Internal Medicine, Kings Co Hosp 1967; **Fellow:** Endocrinology, Diabetes & Metabolism, Mt Sinai Hosp 1968; Nuclear Medicine, Bronx VA Hosp 1969; **Fac Appt:** Prof Rad, Cornell Univ-Weill Med Coll

Lamonica, Dominick M MD [NuM] - **Spec Exp:** Thyroid Cancer; Lymphoma, Non-Hodgkin's; **Hospital:** Roswell Park Cancer Inst; **Address:** Roswell Park Cancer Inst, Elm & Carlton St, Dept of Nuclear Medicine, Buffalo, NY 14263; **Phone:** 716-845-3282; **Board Cert:** Internal Medicine 2005; Nuclear Medicine 2006; **Med School:** Mount Sinai Sch Med 1987; **Resid:** Internal Medicine, Univ Hosp-SUNY Stony Brook 1991; Diagnostic Radiology, Nassau City Med Ctr 1992; **Fellow:** Nuclear Medicine, DVAMC North Port-SUNY Stony Brook 1994; Nuclear Medicine, SUNY Buffalo-RPCI 1995; **Fac Appt:** Asst Prof, SUNY Buffalo

Larson, Steven M MD [NuM] - **Spec Exp:** Thyroid Cancer; PET Imaging; **Hospital:** Meml Sloan-Kettering Cancer Ctr; **Address:** 1275 York Ave, New York, NY 10065; **Phone:** 800-525-2225; **Board Cert:** Nuclear Medicine 1972; Internal Medicine 1973; **Med School:** Univ Wash 1965; **Resid:** Internal Medicine, Virginia Mason Hosp 1970; Nuclear Medicine, Natl Inst Hlth 1972; **Fac Appt:** Prof NuM, Cornell Univ-Weill Med Coll

Majd, Massoud MD [NuM] - **Spec Exp:** Pediatric Nuclear Medicine; **Hospital:** Chldns Natl Med Ctr; **Address:** 111 Michigan Ave NW, Washington, DC 20010-2978; **Phone:** 202-476-3698; **Board Cert:** Radiology 1972; Nuclear Medicine 1973; **Med School:** Iran 1960; **Resid:** Diagnostic Radiology, Georgetown Univ Hosp 1966; **Fac Appt:** Prof Rad, Geo Wash Univ

Mountz, James M MD/PhD [NuM] - **Spec Exp:** Neurologic Imaging; Brain Imaging; **Hospital:** UPMC Presby, Pittsburgh; **Address:** UPMC Hlth Sys, Presby Univ Hosp, 200 Lothrop St, PET Facility, rm B 932, Pittsburgh, PA 15213; **Phone:** 412-647-0104; **Board Cert:** Diagnostic Radiology 1985; Nuclear Medicine 1986; **Med School:** Case West Res Univ 1981; **Resid:** Diagnostic Radiology, Univ Michigan Hosps 1985; **Fellow:** Nuclear Medicine, Univ Michigan Hosps 1986; **Fac Appt:** Prof Rad, Univ Pittsburgh

Neumann, Ronald D MD [NuM] - **Hospital:** Natl Inst of Hlth - Clin Ctr; **Address:** NIH, Bldg 10, 1C-401, 9000 Rockville Drive, MSC 1180, Bethesda, MD 20892-1180; **Phone:** 301-496-6455; **Board Cert:** Nuclear Medicine 1979; **Med School:** Yale Univ 1974; **Resid:** Pathology, Yale-New Haven Hosp 1977; Nuclear Medicine, Yale-New Haven Hosp 1979

Sanger, Joseph J MD [NuM] - **Spec Exp:** Nuclear Cardiology; Nuclear Oncology; **Hospital:** NYU Langone Med Ctr (page 66), Bellevue Hosp Ctr; **Address:** Old Bellevue C & D Bldg, 1st Floor, rm 7, 462 First Ave, New York, NY 10016-6402; **Phone:** 212-731-5001; **Board Cert:** Nuclear Medicine 1981; **Med School:** NYU Sch Med 1977; **Resid:** Diagnostic Radiology, NYU Med Ctr 1979; **Fellow:** Nuclear Medicine, NYU Med Ctr 1981; **Fac Appt:** Assoc Prof Rad, NYU Sch Med

Strashun, Arnold M MD [NuM] - **Spec Exp:** Neurologic Imaging; Nuclear Cardiology; Thyroid Disorders; PET Imaging-Brain; **Hospital:** SUNY Downstate Med Ctr, Kings County Hosp Ctr; **Address:** SUNY Downstate Med Ctr, Dept Radiology, 450 Clarkson Ave, Box 1198, Brooklyn, NY 11203; **Phone:** 718-270-1603; **Board Cert:** Internal Medicine 1977; Nuclear Medicine 1979; **Med School:** Baylor Coll Med 1974; **Resid:** Internal Medicine, Baylor Med Ctr 1975; Internal Medicine, Texas Med Ctr 1977; **Fellow:** Nuclear Medicine, VA Med Ctr 1978; Nuclear Medicine, Mount Sinai Hosp 1979; **Fac Appt:** Prof NuM, SUNY Downstate

Strauss, H William MD [NuM] - **Spec Exp:** Cardiac Imaging in Cancer Therapy; Thyroid Cancer; Cardiac Imaging; **Hospital:** Meml Sloan-Kettering Cancer Ctr; **Address:** 1275 York Avenue, New York, NY 10065; **Phone:** 212-639-7238; **Board Cert:** Nuclear Medicine 1988; **Med School:** SUNY Downstate 1965; **Resid:** Internal Medicine, Downstate Med Ctr 1967; Internal Medicine, Bellevue Hosp 1968; **Fellow:** Nuclear Medicine, Johns Hopkins Hosp 1970; **Fac Appt:** Prof NuM, Cornell Univ-Weill Med Coll

Wahl, Richard L MD [NuM] - **Spec Exp:** Radioimmunotherapy of Cancer; PET Imaging; PET Imaging-Breast; **Hospital:** Johns Hopkins Hosp (page 61); **Address:** Johns Hopkins Hosp, Radiology Dept, Nuclear Medicine Fl 3, 601 N Caroline St, JHOC-3223, Baltimore, MD 21287; **Phone:** 410-955-5465; **Board Cert:** Diagnostic Radiology 1982; Nuclear Radiology 1983; Nuclear Medicine 1985; **Med School:** Washington Univ, St Louis 1978; **Resid:** Diagnostic Radiology, Mallinckrodt Inst 1982; **Fellow:** Nuclear Radiology, Mallinckrodt Inst 1983; **Fac Appt:** Prof Rad, Johns Hopkins Univ

Southeast

Alazraki, Naomi P MD [NuM] - **Spec Exp:** Nuclear Oncology; **Hospital:** Atlanta VA Med Ctr, Emory Univ Hosp; **Address:** VA Medical Ctr - Atlanta, 1670 Clairmont Rd, MC 115, Decatur, GA 30033; **Phone:** 404-321-6111; **Board Cert:** Nuclear Medicine 1972; Diagnostic Radiology 1972; **Med School:** Albert Einstein Coll Med 1966; **Resid:** Diagnostic Radiology, Univ Hospital 1971; **Fac Appt:** Prof Rad, Emory Univ

Nuclear Medicine

Coleman, R Edward MD [NuM] - **Spec Exp:** PET Imaging; SPECT Imaging; Tumor Imaging; **Hospital:** Duke Univ Hosp; **Address:** Duke Univ Med Ctr, Erwin Rd, Box 3949, Durham, NC 27710-0001; **Phone:** 919-684-7244; **Board Cert:** Internal Medicine 1973; Nuclear Medicine 1974; **Med School:** Washington Univ, St Louis 1968; **Resid:** Internal Medicine, Royal Victoria Hosp 1970; **Fellow:** Nuclear Medicine, Mallinckrodt Inst Radiology 1974; **Fac Appt:** Prof Rad, Duke Univ

Sandler, Martin P MD [NuM] - **Spec Exp:** Nuclear Endocrinology; Cardiac Imaging; PET Imaging; **Hospital:** Vanderbilt Univ Med Ctr (page 76); **Address:** Vanderbilt Univ Med Ctr, CCC 1121 MCN, 1161 21st Ave S, Nashville, TN 37232-2675; **Phone:** 615-322-0860; **Board Cert:** Nuclear Medicine 1983; **Med School:** South Africa 1972; **Resid:** Internal Medicine, Groote Schur Hosp; **Fellow:** Endocrinology, Diabetes & Metabolism, Vanderbilt Univ Med Ctr 1980; Nuclear Medicine, Vanderbilt Univ Med Ctr 1982; **Fac Appt:** Prof Rad, Vanderbilt Univ

Ziffer, Jack A MD/PhD [NuM] - **Spec Exp:** Nuclear Cardiology; Cardiac CT Angiography; Thyroid Disease; Thyroid Cancer; **Hospital:** Baptist Hosp of Miami; **Address:** Baptist Hosp of Miami, Dept Radiology, 8900 N Kendall Drive, Miami, FL 33176; **Phone:** 786-596-5917; **Board Cert:** Nuclear Medicine 1988; Nuclear Radiology 1988; Diagnostic Radiology 1987; Nuclear Cardiology 1996; **Med School:** Univ Miami Sch Med 1983; **Resid:** Diagnostic Radiology, Emory Univ Affil Hosps 1987; **Fellow:** Nuclear Medicine, Emory Univ 1988; **Fac Appt:** Prof Rad, Univ Miami Sch Med

Midwest

Dillehay, Gary L MD [NuM] - **Spec Exp:** Lymphoma; Bone Densitometry; PET Imaging; Thyroid Cancer; **Hospital:** Northwestern Meml Hosp; **Address:** Northwestern Meml Hosp, Dept Nuclear Medicine, 675 N St Clair St, Galter 8-110, Chicago, IL 60611; **Phone:** 312-926-5119; **Board Cert:** Nuclear Medicine 1985; Nuclear Radiology 1987; **Med School:** Mayo Med Sch 1979; **Resid:** Diagnostic Radiology, Northwestern Meml Hosp 1983; Nuclear Medicine, Northwestern Meml Hosp 1984; **Fac Appt:** Prof Rad, Northwestern Univ-Feinberg Sch Med

Neumann, Donald R MD [NuM] - **Spec Exp:** Nuclear Oncology; Nuclear Cardiology; Parathyroid Disease; Pheochromocytoma; **Hospital:** Cleveland Clin (page 56); **Address:** 9500 Euclid Ave, MS Jb3, Cleveland, OH 44195; **Phone:** 216-444-2193; **Board Cert:** Diagnostic Radiology 1987; Nuclear Radiology 1990; **Med School:** Wright State Univ 1980; **Resid:** Diagnostic Radiology, Mount Sinai Med Ctr 1987; **Fellow:** Magnetic Resonance Imaging, Mount Sinai Med Ctr 1988

Siegel, Barry A MD [NuM] - **Spec Exp:** Cancer Detection & Staging; PET Imaging; Thyroid Disorders; **Hospital:** Barnes-Jewish Hosp, St. Louis Chldns Hosp; **Address:** 510 S Kingshighway Blvd, St Louis, MO 63110-1016; **Phone:** 314-362-2809; **Board Cert:** Nuclear Medicine 1973; Diagnostic Radiology 1977; Nuclear Radiology 1981; **Med School:** Washington Univ, St Louis 1969; **Resid:** Diagnostic Radiology, Mallinckrodt Inst Radiology 1973; **Fellow:** Nuclear Medicine, Mallinckrodt Inst Radiology 1973; **Fac Appt:** Prof Rad, Washington Univ, St Louis

Wiseman, Gregory MD [NuM] - **Spec Exp:** Lymphoma, Non-Hodgkin's; Multiple Myeloma; Radioimmunotherapy of Cancer; **Hospital:** Mayo Med Ctr & Clin - Rochester; **Address:** Mayo Clinic, Dept Nuc Med, 200 First St SW, Charlton Bldg, Rochester, MN 55905; **Phone:** 507-284-9599; **Board Cert:** Internal Medicine 1986; Hematology 1988; Nuclear Medicine 2002; **Med School:** Univ Utah 1983; **Resid:** Internal Medicine, Mayo Clinic 1986; Nuclear Medicine, Univ Washington Med Ctr 1992; **Fellow:** Hematology, Mayo Clinic 1989; Medical Oncology, Univ Washington 1991; **Fac Appt:** Asst Prof, Mayo Med Sch

Southwest

Podoloff, Donald A MD [NuM] - **Spec Exp:** Prostate Cancer; Breast Cancer; **Hospital:** UT MD Anderson Cancer Ctr; **Address:** UT MD Anderson Cancer Ctr, 1515 Holcombe Blvd, Box 57, Houston, TX 77030; **Phone:** 713-745-1160; **Board Cert:** Diagnostic Radiology 1973; Nuclear Medicine 1975; Nuclear Radiology 1975; **Med School:** SUNY Downstate 1964; **Resid:** Internal Medicine, Beth Israel Med Ctr 1968; Diagnostic Radiology, Wilford Hall USAF Med Ctr 1973; **Fac Appt:** Prof Rad, Univ Tex, Houston

West Coast and Pacific

Dae, Michael W MD [NuM] - **Spec Exp:** Nuclear Cardiology; Pediatric Nuclear Medicine; **Hospital:** UCSF Med Ctr; **Address:** UCSF, Dept Nuclear Medicine, 505 Parnassus Ave, Box 0252, San Francisco, CA 94143-0252; **Phone:** 415-353-1521; **Board Cert:** Pediatrics 1983; Nuclear Medicine 1984; **Med School:** Duke Univ 1976; **Resid:** Pediatrics, Chldns Hosp 1978; **Fellow:** Pediatric Cardiology, UCSF Med Ctr 1982; Nuclear Cardiology, UCSF Med Ctr 1983; **Fac Appt:** Prof, UCSF

Klaas, Virginia E MD [NuM] - **Spec Exp:** Nuclear Radiology; **Hospital:** Valley Med Ctr-Renton, WA, Auburn Reg Med Ctr; **Address:** Valley Radiologists, PO BOX 26730, Federal Way, WA 98093-3730; **Phone:** 253-661-1700; **Board Cert:** Diagnostic Radiology 1994; Nuclear Radiology 1995; Nuclear Medicine 2004; **Med School:** UC Irvine 1989; **Resid:** Diagnostic Radiology, Stanford Univ Med Ctr 1994; **Fellow:** Nuclear Medicine, Mallinckrodt Inst of Radiology 1995

Scheff, Alice M MD [NuM] - **Spec Exp:** PET Imaging; Thyroid Disorders; Neurologic Imaging; Cardiac Imaging; **Hospital:** Santa Clara Vly Med Ctr; **Address:** 751 S Bascom Ave, Nuclear Med, San Jose, CA 95128; **Phone:** 408-885-6970; **Board Cert:** Nuclear Medicine 1982; Nuclear Radiology 1983; **Med School:** Penn State Coll Med 1978; **Resid:** Diagnostic Radiology, Penn State-Hershey Med Ctr 1982; Nuclear Medicine, Penn State-Hershey Med Ctr 1982; **Fellow:** Magnetic Resonance Imaging, Long Beach Meml Med Ctr 1993

Schelbert, Heinrich R MD/PhD [NuM] - **Spec Exp:** Nuclear Cardiology; Coronary Artery Disease; **Hospital:** UCLA Ronald Reagan Med Ctr, Santa Monica - UCLA Med Ctr & Ortho Hosp; **Address:** UCLA Dept Molecular & Med Pharmacology, B2-085J CHS, Box 95648, Los Angeles, CA 90095-6948; **Phone:** 310-825-3076; **Board Cert:** Nuclear Medicine 1976; **Med School:** Germany 1964; **Resid:** Internal Medicine, Mercy Med Ctr 1968; Cardiovascular Disease, Univ Duesseldorf 1972; **Fellow:** Cardiovascular Disease, UCSD Med Ctr 1975; Nuclear Medicine, UCSD Med Ctr 1976; **Fac Appt:** Prof Pharm, UCLA-David Geffen Sch Med

Waxman, Alan D MD [NuM] - **Spec Exp:** PET Imaging-Brain; Thyroid Cancer; Cancer Detection & Staging; **Hospital:** Cedars-Sinai Med Ctr, Keck Med Ctr of USC (page 75); **Address:** Cedars-Sinai Med Ctr, Taper Imaging, 8700 Beverly Blvd, rm 1258, Los Angeles, CA 90048-1804; **Phone:** 310-423-4216; **Board Cert:** Nuclear Medicine 1972; **Med School:** USC Sch Med 1963; **Resid:** Nuclear Medicine, Wadsworth VA Hosp 1965; **Fellow:** Internal Medicine, Natl Inst Hlth 1967; **Fac Appt:** Clin Prof, USC Sch Med

Cleveland Clinic

Every life deserves world class care.

Cleveland Clinic
Imaging Institute
9500 Euclid Avenue
Cleveland, OH 44195

clevelandclinic.org/
nuclearmedicinetopdocs

Offering Same-Day Appointments
Call 800.274.2009.

Nuclear Medicine

Cleveland Clinic Imaging Institute is one of the leading academic imaging centers in the world and one of the busiest clinical departments in the country. Each year, Cleveland Clinic imagers perform and interpret more than 1.8 million examinations, for which all images are acquired digitally.

Cleveland Clinic's Department of Nuclear Medicine's advanced imaging capabilities can identify both anatomic and physiologic changes in organ function. A Cyclotron enables on-site production of customized PET tracers for both clinical and research needs. Cleveland Clinic has 12 gamma cameras — three PET/CT scanners, three SPECT/CT scanners and six traditional gamma cameras. Our mobile PET/CT system brings main campus capabilities to Cleveland Clinic community hospitals.

Our unique expertise and unsurpassed technology are available to individualize patient diagnosis and management and treatment with the highest degree possible of accuracy and timeliness. Hybrid SPECT/CT and PET/CT fusion imaging is performed on specialized scanners that directly map the abnormal tissue depicted on the nuclear images to the affected area displayed on the high-resolution CT images.

The department possesses an abundant depth of expertise in both imaging and clinical medicine. Physicians are board-certified and clinically experienced in a broad array of specialties, including cardiology, neurology and radiology.

Patient therapy is a significant component of nuclear medicine. Treatments, and sometimes pain relief, are offered for conditions such as Graves' disease, thyroid cancer, liver cancer, cancer that has spread to the bone and refractory lymphomas. PET/CT scans also assist radiation oncologists in planning treatment with external sources of radiation.

Treatment Guides
Cleveland Clinic has developed comprehensive treatment guides for many diseases and conditions. To download our free treatment guides, visit clevelandclinic.org/treatmentguides.

Online Medical Second Opinion
Cleveland Clinic's My**Consult** Online Medical Second Opinion program securely connects patients to our physician specialists for more than 1,000 life-changing or life-threatening diagnoses all by the click of a mouse. To learn more, log onto eclevelandclinic.org/myconsult or call 800.223.2273, ext. 43223.

Special Assistance for Out-of-State Patients
Cleveland Clinic Global Patient Services offers a complimentary Medical Concierge service for patients who travel from outside of Ohio. Call 800.223.2273, ext. 55580 or email medicalconcierge@ccf.org.

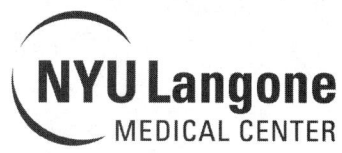
NUCLEAR MEDICINE

About the Division of Nuclear Medicine, Department of Radiology

Nuclear medicine at NYU Langone Medical Center spans all medical specialties to deliver safe techniques that image body physiology for the diagnosis, monitoring and prevention of disease. In addition to cutting-edge imaging, the Medical Center offers a full spectrum of radioiodine therapy protocols for the treatment of hyperthyroidism and thyroid cancer. Our nuclear medicine physicians are also experts in the field of radioimmunotherapy for lymphoma. We specialize in the following areas:

Advanced Imaging Equipment

NYU Langone Medical Center houses some of the most advanced nuclear medicine equipment in the world, including best-of-breed SPECT, SPECT and PET/CT scanners. Cameras are linked by advanced data management systems to allow rapid, accurate reading and digital report generation. Image data is available to referring physicians over a digital network that allows for timely patient management.

Nuclear Medicine

NYU Langone Medical Center's Tisch Hospital offers a wide range of nuclear medicine services, specializing in a full complement of non-invasive nuclear imaging techniques designed to diagnose and monitor disease of the neurological, cardiovascular, endocrine, gastrointestinal, pulmonary, genitourinary and hepatobiliary systems. Specialized blood volume and lymphedema evaluation protocols are also offered. Advanced dosimetry protocols are used to optimize therapy for patients with thyroid cancer and lymphoma.

PET/CT Scans

PET/CT scans allow for simultaneous imaging of metabolic processes as well as anatomic structures in the body. These advanced scanners have revolutionized the care of cancer patients and are making great strides in the diagnosis and management of neurological and cardiac diseases. NYU Langone Medical Center's nuclear medicine physicians are fellowship-trained experts in the field of PET/CT.

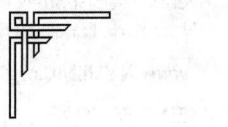

The Best in American Medicine
www.CastleConnolly.com

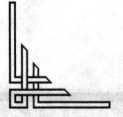
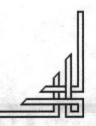

Obstetrics & Gynecology

An obstetrician/gynecologist possesses special knowledge, skills and professional capability in the medical and surgical care of the female reproductive system and associated disorders. This physician serves as a consultant to other physicians and as a primary physician for women.

Training Required: Four years *plus* two years in clinical practice before certification is complete.

OBSTETRICS & GYNECOLOGY

New England

Cramer, Daniel W MD [ObG] - **Spec Exp:** Ovarian Cancer; Ovarian Cancer-High Risk; **Hospital:** Dana-Farber Cancer Inst (page 57), Brigham and Women's Hosp (page 57); **Address:** Brigham & Women's Hosp, Ob/Gyn Epidemiology Ctr, 221 Longwood Ave, RFB 366, Boston, MA 02115; **Phone:** 617-732-4895; **Board Cert:** Obstetrics & Gynecology 1979; **Med School:** Univ Colorado 1970; **Resid:** Obstetrics & Gynecology, Boston Womens Hosp 1976; **Fellow:** Public Health, Harvard Med Sch 1982; **Fac Appt:** Prof ObG, Harvard Med Sch

Eckler, Kristen MD [ObG] - **Spec Exp:** Pelvic Reconstruction; Uro-Gynecology; **Hospital:** Mass Genl Hosp; **Address:** 55 Fruit St, MGH-Founders 468, Boston, MA 02114; **Phone:** 617-724-9019; **Board Cert:** Obstetrics & Gynecology 2001; **Med School:** Tufts Univ 1994; **Resid:** Obstetrics & Gynecology, Brigham & Women's Hosp 1998

Einarsson, Jon I MD [ObG] - **Spec Exp:** Minimally Invasive Surgery; Endometriosis; Pelvic Organ Prolapse Repair; Incontinence-Female; **Hospital:** Brigham and Women's Hosp (page 57); **Address:** Brigham & Womens Hosp, Dept Obstetrics & Gynecology, 75 Francis St, Boston, MA 02115; **Phone:** 617-525-8582; **Board Cert:** Obstetrics & Gynecology 2005; **Med School:** Iceland 1995; **Resid:** Obstetrics & Gynecology, Baylor Affil Hosp 2002; **Fellow:** Minimally Invasive Surgery, Baylor Affil Hosp 2004; **Fac Appt:** Asst Prof ObG, Harvard Med Sch

Laufer, Marc MD [ObG] - **Spec Exp:** Adolescent Gynecology; Endometriosis-Adolescent; Congenital Anomalies-Gynecologic; Pediatric Gynecology; **Hospital:** Children's Hospital - Boston, Brigham and Women's Hosp (page 57); **Address:** Chldns Hosp, Dept of Ped Gynecology, 300 Longwood Ave, Boston, MA 02115; **Phone:** 617-355-5785; **Board Cert:** Obstetrics & Gynecology 2010; **Med School:** Univ Pennsylvania 1986; **Resid:** Obstetrics & Gynecology, Brigham & Womens Hosp/Mass Genl Hosp 1990; **Fellow:** Reproductive Endocrinology, Brigham & Womens Hosp/Chldns Hosp 1992; Gynecology, Chldns Hosp 1992; **Fac Appt:** Assoc Prof ObG, Harvard Med Sch

Myers, Deborah L MD [ObG] - **Spec Exp:** Uro-Gynecology; **Hospital:** Women & Infants Hosp of RI; **Address:** Women & Infants Hosp, 695 Eddy St, Providence, RI 02905; **Phone:** 401-453-7560; **Board Cert:** Obstetrics & Gynecology 2008; **Med School:** SUNY Stony Brook 1981; **Resid:** Obstetrics & Gynecology, Women & Infants Hosp 1985; **Fac Appt:** Asst Prof ObG, Brown Univ

Nour, Nawal M MD [ObG] - **Spec Exp:** Female Genital Cutting (FGC) Education; Gynecology-African women only; Pregnancy-African women only; **Hospital:** Brigham and Women's Hosp (page 57); **Address:** Brigham & Women's Hosp, Dept Ob/Gyn, 75 Francis St CWN-3 Bldg - Ste 340, Boston, MA 02115; **Phone:** 617-732-4740; **Board Cert:** Obstetrics & Gynecology 2010; **Med School:** Harvard Med Sch 1994; **Resid:** Obstetrics & Gynecology, Brgham & Women's Hosp 1998

Mid Atlantic

Bader, Thomas J MD [ObG] - **Spec Exp:** Pregnancy-High Risk; **Hospital:** Crozer - Chester Med Ctr; **Address:** 1 Medical Center Blvd, Upland, PA 19013; **Phone:** 610-872-7660; **Board Cert:** Obstetrics & Gynecology 2006; **Med School:** Georgetown Univ 1989; **Resid:** Obstetrics & Gynecology, Hosp Univ Penn 1993

Brodman, Michael L MD [ObG] - **Spec Exp:** Incontinence-Female; Laparoscopic Surgery; Pelvic Organ Prolapse Repair; Uro-Gynecology; **Hospital:** Mount Sinai Med Ctr (page 63); **Address:** Dept Gynecology/Urogynecology, 5 E 98th St Fl 2, New York, NY 10029; **Phone:** 212-241-7952; **Board Cert:** Obstetrics & Gynecology 2010; **Med School:** Mount Sinai Sch Med 1982; **Resid:** Obstetrics & Gynecology, Mt Sinai Hosp 1986; **Fellow:** Pelvic Surgery, Mt Sinai Hosp 1987; **Fac Appt:** Assoc Prof ObG, Mount Sinai Sch Med

Carson, Donald G MD [ObG] - **Spec Exp:** Gynecology Only; **Hospital:** Magee-Womens Hosp - UPMC; **Address:** Ob/Gyn Assocs of Pittsburgh, 3380 Boulevard of the Allies, Ste 1, Pittsburgh, PA 15213; **Phone:** 412-621-7575; **Board Cert:** Obstetrics & Gynecology 2010; **Med School:** Univ Pittsburgh 1977; **Resid:** Obstetrics & Gynecology, Magee-Women's Hosp 1981; **Fac Appt:** Assoc Clin Prof ObG, Univ Pittsburgh

De Cherney, Alan H MD [ObG] - **Spec Exp:** Infertility-Female; Reproductive Endocrinology; Gynecologic Surgery; **Hospital:** Natl Inst of Hlth - Clin Ctr, Unif Serv Univ of the Hlth Sci; **Address:** NICHD, NIH, Bldg 10, CRC, 1 East, 10 Center Drive, rm 1-3140, MS 1109, Bethesda, MD 20892-5800; **Phone:** 301-496-5800; **Board Cert:** Obstetrics & Gynecology 1989; Reproductive Endocrinology 1979; **Med School:** Temple Univ 1967; **Resid:** Obstetrics & Gynecology, Hosp Univ Penn 1972; **Fac Appt:** Prof ObG, Uniformed Srvs Univ, Bethesda

Evans, Mark I MD [ObG] - **Spec Exp:** Reproductive Genetics; Fetal Diagnosis & Therapy; Multiple Gestation; Ultrasound; **Hospital:** Mount Sinai Med Ctr (page 63); **Address:** Comprehensive Genetics, 131 E 65th St, New York, NY 10065; **Phone:** 212-288-1422; **Board Cert:** Obstetrics & Gynecology 2010; Clinical Genetics 1984; **Med School:** SUNY Downstate 1978; **Resid:** Obstetrics & Gynecology, Lying-In Hosp 1982; **Fellow:** Clinical Genetics, Natl Inst Hlth 1984; **Fac Appt:** Prof ObG, Mount Sinai Sch Med

Goldstein, Martin S MD [ObG] - **Spec Exp:** Uterine Fibroids; Laparoscopic Surgery; Pelvic Organ Prolapse Repair; Endometriosis; **Hospital:** Mount Sinai Med Ctr (page 63); **Address:** 40 E 84th St, New York, NY 10028-1314; **Phone:** 212-472-6500; **Board Cert:** Obstetrics & Gynecology 1980; **Med School:** SUNY Hlth Sci Ctr 1966; **Resid:** Obstetrics & Gynecology, Mount Sinai Hosp 1971; **Fac Appt:** Assoc Clin Prof ObG, Mount Sinai Sch Med

Hockstein, Steven MD [ObG] - **Spec Exp:** Uterine Fibroids; **Hospital:** NY-Presby/Weill Cornell Med Ctr, NY (page 65); **Address:** 425 E 61st St Fl 11, New York, NY 10021; **Phone:** 212-821-0810; **Board Cert:** Obstetrics & Gynecology 2010; **Med School:** Univ MD Sch Med 1993; **Resid:** Obstetrics & Gynecology, McGaw Med Ctr 1997; **Fac Appt:** Asst Clin Prof ObG, Cornell Univ-Weill Med Coll

Iglesia, Cheryl MD [ObG] - **Spec Exp:** Uro-Gynecology; **Hospital:** Washington Hosp Ctr; **Address:** Washington Hosp Ctr, 106 Irving St NW, Ste 405-S, Washington, DC 20010; **Phone:** 202-877-6526; **Board Cert:** Obstetrics & Gynecology 2007; **Med School:** Univ MD Sch Med 1991; **Resid:** Obstetrics & Gynecology, Univ FL Hlth Sci Ctr 1995; **Fellow:** Uro-Gynecology, Rush Med Coll 1997

Lucente, Vincent R MD [ObG] - **Spec Exp:** Uro-Gynecology; Pelvic Floor Reconstruction; Incontinence-Female; Pelvic Organ Prolapse Repair; **Hospital:** St. Luke's Hosp - Allentown, Abington Mem Hosp; **Address:** Hamilton Court Professional Ctr, 3050 Hamilton Blvd, Ste 200, Allentown, PA 18103; **Phone:** 610-435-9575; **Board Cert:** Obstetrics & Gynecology 2010; **Med School:** SUNY Stony Brook 1985; **Resid:** Obstetrics & Gynecology, N Shore Univ Hosp 1989; **Fellow:** Uro-Gynecology, Methodist Hosp 1990; **Fac Appt:** Clin Prof ObG, Temple Univ

Obstetrics & Gynecology

Maynard, Steven MD [ObG] - **Spec Exp:** Minimally Invasive Surgery; Incontinence; **Hospital:** Georgetown Univ Hosp; **Address:** 3800 Resovoir Rd NW, Pasquerilla Health Center Fl 3, Washington, DC 20007; **Phone:** 202-444-8531; **Board Cert:** Obstetrics & Gynecology 2009; **Med School:** McGill Univ 1986; **Resid:** Obstetrics & Gynecology, Women & Infants Hosp 1993; **Fac Appt:** Asst Prof ObG, Georgetown Univ

Ordorica, Steven A MD [ObG] - **Spec Exp:** Pregnancy-High Risk; Miscarriage-Recurrent; Maternal & Fetal Medicine; **Hospital:** NYU Langone Med Ctr (page 66); **Address:** NYU Med Ctr, Dept OB/GYN, 530 1st Ave, Ste 10Q, New York, NY 10016-6402; **Phone:** 212-263-5982; **Board Cert:** Obstetrics & Gynecology 2010; **Med School:** SUNY Stony Brook 1983; **Resid:** Obstetrics & Gynecology, NYU Med Ctr 1987; **Fellow:** Maternal & Fetal Medicine, NYU Med Ctr 1989; **Fac Appt:** Assoc Prof ObG, NYU Sch Med

Pfeifer, Samantha MD [ObG] - **Spec Exp:** Infertility-Female; Endometriosis; Laparoscopic Surgery; Congenital Anomalies-Gynecologic; **Hospital:** Hosp Univ Penn - UPHS (page 68); **Address:** Penn Health for Women, 250 King of Prussia Rd, Radnor, PA 19087; **Phone:** 610-902-2500; **Board Cert:** Obstetrics & Gynecology 2010; Reproductive Endocrinology 2010; **Med School:** Univ Pennsylvania 1986; **Resid:** Obstetrics & Gynecology, Hosp Univ Penn 1990; **Fellow:** Reproductive Endocrinology, Hosp Univ Penn 1993; **Fac Appt:** Assoc Prof ObG, Univ Pennsylvania

Scher, Jonathan MD [ObG] - **Spec Exp:** Miscarriage-Recurrent; Pregnancy-High Risk; Infertility-IVF Failure; **Hospital:** Mount Sinai Med Ctr (page 63); **Address:** 1126 Park Ave, New York, NY 10128-1203; **Phone:** 212-427-7400; **Board Cert:** Obstetrics & Gynecology 1981; **Med School:** South Africa 1964; **Resid:** Obstetrics & Gynecology, Groote Schuur Hosp 1970; Obstetrics & Gynecology, Kings College Hosp 1972; **Fac Appt:** Asst Clin Prof ObG, Mount Sinai Sch Med

Sewell, Catherine A MD [ObG] - **Spec Exp:** Uterine Fibroids; Minimally Invasive Surgery; **Hospital:** Johns Hopkins Hosp (page 61); **Address:** Johns Hopkins Fibroid Ctr, 600 N Wolfe St Phipps Bldg - Ste 249, Baltimore, MD 21287; **Phone:** 410-614-4496; **Board Cert:** Obstetrics & Gynecology 2010; **Med School:** Univ Pennsylvania 1994; **Resid:** Obstetrics & Gynecology, Johns Hopkins Hosp 1998; **Fac Appt:** Asst Prof ObG, Johns Hopkins Univ

Simon, James A MD [ObG] - **Spec Exp:** Infertility; Menopause Problems; Osteoporosis; Sexual Dysfunction; **Hospital:** G Washington Univ Hosp, Sibley Mem Hosp; **Address:** 1850 M St NW, Ste 450, Washington, DC 20036; **Phone:** 202-293-1000; **Board Cert:** Obstetrics & Gynecology 2009; Reproductive Endocrinology 2009; **Med School:** Rush Med Coll 1978; **Resid:** Obstetrics & Gynecology, George Washington Univ Hosp 1982; **Fellow:** Reproductive Endocrinology, Harbor-UCLA Medical Ctr 1984; **Fac Appt:** Clin Prof ObG, Geo Wash Univ

Wiesenfeld, Harold C MD [ObG] - **Spec Exp:** Infectious Diseases-Gynecologic; Sexually Transmitted Diseases; **Hospital:** Magee-Womens Hosp - UPMC; **Address:** Dept Ob/Gyn, 300 Halket St, Ste 0610, Pittsburgh, PA 15213; **Phone:** 412-641-6412; **Board Cert:** Obstetrics & Gynecology 2010; **Med School:** McGill Univ 1987; **Resid:** Obstetrics & Gynecology, McGill Univ 1990; **Fac Appt:** Assoc Prof ObG, Univ Pittsburgh

Witter, Frank R MD [ObG] - **Spec Exp:** Pregnancy-High Risk; Multiple Gestation; Lupus/SLE in Pregnancy; **Hospital:** Johns Hopkins Hosp (page 61), Johns Hopkins Bayview Med Ctr (page 61); **Address:** 600 N Wolfe St, Nelson 2170, Baltimore, MD 21287; **Phone:** 410-502-3200; **Board Cert:** Obstetrics & Gynecology 2010; Maternal & Fetal Medicine 2010; **Med School:** Univ Chicago-Pritzker Sch Med 1976; **Resid:** Obstetrics & Gynecology, Johns Hopkins Hosp 1980; **Fellow:** Maternal & Fetal Medicine, Johns Hopkins Hosp 1982; Clinical Pharmacology, Johns Hopkins Hosp 1984; **Fac Appt:** Prof ObG, Johns Hopkins Univ

Young, Bruce MD [ObG] - **Spec Exp:** Infertility; Minimally Invasive Surgery; Twin to Twin Transfusion Syndrome (TTTS); Miscarriage-Recurrent; **Hospital:** NYU Langone Med Ctr (page 66), Bellevue Hosp Ctr; **Address:** 530 1st Ave, HCC-5th Fl, Ste 5G, New York, NY 10016; **Phone:** 212-263-6359; **Board Cert:** Obstetrics & Gynecology 1970; Maternal & Fetal Medicine 1975; **Med School:** NYU Sch Med 1963; **Resid:** Obstetrics & Gynecology, NYU Med Ctr 1968; **Fellow:** Reproductive Endocrinology, NYU Med Ctr 1968; **Fac Appt:** Prof ObG, NYU Sch Med

Southeast

Andersen, Glenna R MD [ObG] - **Hospital:** Inova Fairfax Hosp; **Address:** 8501 Arlington Blvd, Ste 300, Fairfax, VA 22031; **Phone:** 703-560-1611; **Board Cert:** Obstetrics & Gynecology 2009; **Med School:** Univ VA Sch Med 1981; **Resid:** Obstetrics & Gynecology, SUNY Buffalo Affil Hosps 1985

Berga, Sarah L MD [ObG] - **Spec Exp:** Menstrual Disorders; Hormonal Disorders; Reproductive Endocrinology; **Hospital:** Emory Univ Hosp, Emory Univ Hosp Midtown; **Address:** Dept Gynecology & Obstetrics, 1365 Clifton Rd A Bldg Fl 4 - Ste 4100, Atlanta, GA 30322; **Phone:** 404-778-3401; **Board Cert:** Obstetrics & Gynecology 2010; Reproductive Endocrinology 2010; **Med School:** Univ VA Sch Med 1980; **Resid:** Obstetrics & Gynecology, Mass Genl Hosp 1984; **Fellow:** Reproductive Endocrinology, UCSD Med Ctr 1986; **Fac Appt:** Prof ObG, Emory Univ

Filip, Stanley J MD [ObG] - **Spec Exp:** Uterine Fibroids; Menopause Problems; Hysterectomy Alternatives; Endometriosis; **Hospital:** Duke Univ Hosp, Durham Regional Hosp; **Address:** Duke Univ Med Ctr, Box 3267, Durham, NC 27704; **Phone:** 919-684-9699; **Board Cert:** Obstetrics & Gynecology 1985; **Med School:** Mount Sinai Sch Med 1979; **Resid:** Obstetrics & Gynecology, Univ Colo Affil Hosp 1983

Hager, W David MD [ObG] - **Spec Exp:** Infectious Diseases-Gynecologic; Sexually Transmitted Diseases; HPV-Human Papilloma Virus; Laparoscopic Surgery; **Hospital:** Central Baptist Hosp, St. Joseph Hosp; **Address:** Womens Care Ctr, 1720 Nicholasville Rd, Ste 506, Lexington, KY 40503; **Phone:** 859-278-0363; **Board Cert:** Obstetrics & Gynecology 1993; **Med School:** Univ KY Coll Med 1972; **Resid:** Obstetrics & Gynecology, Univ Kentucky Med Ctr 1976; **Fac Appt:** Prof ObG, Univ KY Coll Med

Hullfish, Kathie L MD [ObG] - **Spec Exp:** Uro-Gynecology; Pelvic Reconstruction; Pelvic Organ Prolapse Repair; Incontinence; **Hospital:** Univ of Virginia Health Sys; **Address:** Univ Virginia Med Ctr, Div Urogynecology, Pelvic Reconst Med, P.O. Box 801305, Charlottesville, VA 22908-0712; **Phone:** 434-924-2103; **Board Cert:** Obstetrics & Gynecology 2009; **Med School:** Univ VA Sch Med 1992; **Resid:** Obstetrics & Gynecology, Univ Virginia Med Ctr 1996; **Fellow:** Uro-Gynecology, Rush Med Ctr 1998; **Fac Appt:** Assoc Prof ObG, Univ VA Sch Med

Jenkins, Todd MD [ObG] - **Spec Exp:** Minimally Invasive Surgery; Hysteroscopic Surgery; Endometriosis; Uterine Fibroids; **Hospital:** Univ of Ala Hosp at Birmingham; **Address:** UAB Dept Obstetrics/Gynecology, 619 19th St S, 176F 1026, Birmingham, AL 35249-7333; **Phone:** 205-801-8000; **Board Cert:** Obstetrics & Gynecology 2010; **Med School:** Univ Alabama 1994; **Resid:** Obstetrics & Gynecology, Univ Alabama Hosp 1998; **Fac Appt:** Assoc Prof ObG, Univ Alabama

Morgan, Linda S MD [ObG] - **Spec Exp:** Gynecologic Cancer; Women's Health; **Hospital:** Shands at Univ of FL; **Address:** 2000 SW Archer Rd, Gainesville, FL 32610; **Phone:** 352-265-8200; **Board Cert:** Obstetrics & Gynecology 2008; Gynecologic Oncology 2008; **Med School:** Med Coll PA Hahnemann 1975; **Resid:** Obstetrics & Gynecology, Shands Hosp 1979; **Fellow:** Gynecologic Oncology, Mass Genl Hosp 1981; **Fac Appt:** Prof ObG, Univ Fla Coll Med

Obstetrics & Gynecology

Sanz, Luis E MD [ObG] - **Spec Exp:** Uro-Gynecology; Hysteroscopic Surgery; Vaginal Reconstruction; Pelvic Reconstruction; **Hospital:** Virginia Hosp Ctr - Arlington; **Address:** 1625 N George Mason Drive, Ste 475, Arlington, VA 22205; **Phone:** 703-717-4000; **Board Cert:** Obstetrics & Gynecology 1982; **Med School:** Georgetown Univ 1976; **Resid:** Obstetrics & Gynecology, Georgetown Univ Hosp 1980; **Fellow:** Advanced Pelvic Surgery, Georgetown Univ 1982; **Fac Appt:** Prof ObG, Georgetown Univ

Simpson, Joe L MD [ObG] - **Spec Exp:** Prenatal Diagnosis; Ovarian Failure; Infertility/Genetics; **Hospital:** Jackson N Med Ctr; **Address:** Florida International University, University Park AHC 693, 11200 SW 8 St, Miami, FL 33199; **Phone:** 305-348-0613; **Board Cert:** Obstetrics & Gynecology 2010; Clinical Genetics 1982; **Med School:** Duke Univ 1968; **Resid:** Obstetrics & Gynecology, NY Hosp-Cornell Med Ctr 1973; **Fac Appt:** Prof ObG, FIU Coll Med

Steege, John F MD [ObG] - **Spec Exp:** Laparoscopic Surgery; Endometriosis; Pain-Pelvic & Perineal; Gynecologic Surgery; **Hospital:** NC Memorial Hosp - UNC; **Address:** Univ NC-Dept OB/GYN, CB 7570, Chapel Hill, NC 27599-7570; **Phone:** 919-966-7764; **Board Cert:** Obstetrics & Gynecology 1978; **Med School:** Yale Univ 1972; **Resid:** Obstetrics & Gynecology, Yale - New Haven Hosp 1976; **Fac Appt:** Prof ObG, Univ NC Sch Med

Visco, Anthony G MD [ObG] - **Spec Exp:** Uro-Gynecology; Pelvic Organ Prolapse Repair; Robotic Hysterectomy; Minimally Invasive Surgery; **Hospital:** Duke Univ Hosp; **Address:** Duke Univ Medical Ctr, 5324 McFarland Drive, Durham, NC 27707; **Phone:** 919-401-1000; **Board Cert:** Obstetrics & Gynecology 2008; **Med School:** SUNY Upstate Med Univ 1993; **Resid:** Obstetrics & Gynecology, Univ Rochester Med Ctr 1997; **Fellow:** Uro-Gynecology, Duke Univ Med Ctr 2000; Reconstructive Pelvic Surgery, Duke Univ Med Ctr 2000; **Fac Appt:** Assoc Prof ObG, Duke Univ

Midwest

Argenta, Peter A MD [ObG] - **Spec Exp:** Laparoscopic Surgery; Women's Health; Cervical Cancer; Ovarian Cancer; **Address:** Womens Health Clin, 516 Delaware St SE, Clinic 1C Fl 1, Minneapolis, MN 55455; **Phone:** 612-626-3444; **Board Cert:** Obstetrics & Gynecology 2005; Gynecologic Oncology 2005; **Med School:** Duke Univ 1995; **Resid:** Obstetrics & Gynecology, Hosp U Penn 1999; **Fellow:** Gynecologic Oncology, Mt Sinai Med Ctr 2002; **Fac Appt:** Assoc Prof ObG, Univ Minn

Bartholomew, Deborah A MD [ObG] - **Spec Exp:** Gynecologic Pathology; Robotic Surgery; Minimally Invasive Surgery; **Hospital:** Ohio St Univ Med Ctr; **Address:** 4053 W Dublin Granville Rd, Dublin, OH 43017; **Phone:** 614-764-2262; **Board Cert:** Anatomic Pathology 1990; Obstetrics & Gynecology 2010; **Med School:** Med Coll VA 1983; **Resid:** Obstetrics & Gynecology, David Grant USAF Med Ctr 1987; Anatomic Pathology, UC Davis Med Ctr 1987; **Fellow:** Gynecologic Pathology, UC Davis Med Ctr 1989; **Fac Appt:** Assoc Prof ObG

Bradley, Linda D MD [ObG] - **Spec Exp:** Hysteroscopic Surgery; Menstrual Disorders; Endoscopy; Uterine Fibroids; **Hospital:** Cleveland Clin (page 56); **Address:** Cleveland Clinic Fdn, Dept Ob/Gyn, 9500 Euclid Ave, Desk A81, Cleveland, OH 44195; **Phone:** 216-444-6601; **Board Cert:** Obstetrics & Gynecology 2004; **Med School:** Univ Cincinnati 1981; **Resid:** Obstetrics & Gynecology, Cleveland Metro Genl Hosp 1985

Corteville, Jane E MD [ObG] - **Spec Exp:** Fetal Diagnosis & Therapy; Maternal & Fetal Medicine; Prenatal Genetic Diagnosis; Obstetric Ultrasound; **Hospital:** Univ Hosps Case Med Ctr (page 74); **Address:** UH MacDonald Women's Hospital, 11100 Euclid Ave, Cleveland, OH 44106; **Phone:** 216-844-8545; **Board Cert:** Obstetrics & Gynecology 2009; Clinical Genetics 2010; **Med School:** Washington Univ, St Louis 1992; **Resid:** Obstetrics & Gynecology, Barnes-Jewish Hosp 1987; **Fellow:** Ultrasound/CT, Barnes-Jewish Hosp 1989; Medical Genetics, Chldns Hosp 1992; **Fac Appt:** Asst Prof ObG, Case West Res Univ

De Lancey, John O MD [ObG] - **Spec Exp:** Uro-Gynecology; Incontinence; Pelvic Organ Prolapse Repair; **Hospital:** Univ of Michigan Hosp; **Address:** Univ Mich Med Ctr, Dept ObGyn, 1500 E Med Ctr Drive, rm L4000, Box 5276, Ann Arbor, MI 48109-0276; **Phone:** 734-764-8429; **Board Cert:** Obstetrics & Gynecology 1997; **Med School:** Univ Mich Med Sch 1977; **Resid:** Obstetrics & Gynecology, Univ Mich Med Ctr 1981; **Fac Appt:** Prof ObG, Univ Mich Med Sch

De Lia, Julian E MD [ObG] - **Spec Exp:** Fetal Surgery; Twin to Twin Transfusion Syndrome (TTTS); **Hospital:** Wheaton Franciscan Hlthcare-St Joseph-Milwaukee; **Address:** TTTS Inst, WFHC-St Joseph, 5000 W Chambers St, Milwaukee, WI 53210-1688; **Phone:** 414-447-3535; **Board Cert:** Obstetrics & Gynecology 1993; **Med School:** UMDNJ-NJ Med Sch, Newark 1972; **Resid:** Obstetrics & Gynecology, St Barnabas Med Ctar 1976; **Fac Appt:** Assoc Prof ObG, Med Coll Wisc

Famuyide, Abimbola MD [ObG] - **Spec Exp:** Minimally Invasive Surgery; Uterine Fibroids; **Hospital:** Mayo Med Ctr & Clin - Rochester; **Address:** Mayo Clinic, Dept Ob/Gyn, 200 First St SW, 4A Eisenberg, Rochester, MN 55905; **Phone:** 507-284-2511; **Board Cert:** Obstetrics & Gynecology 2004; **Med School:** Nigeria 1985; **Resid:** Obstetrics & Gynecology, Barnsley District Hosp/Central Sheffield Hosp; **Fellow:** Obstetrics & Gynecology, Mayo Grad Sch; **Fac Appt:** Asst Prof ObG, Mayo Med Sch

Gonik, Bernard MD [ObG] - **Spec Exp:** Infectious Disease in Pregnancy; Prenatal Diagnosis; Vaccinations in Pregnancy; **Hospital:** Sinai-Grace Hosp; **Address:** Womens Diagnostic Unit, 6071 W Outer Drive Fl 2 - rm 284, Detroit, MI 48235-2624; **Phone:** 313-966-1880; **Board Cert:** Obstetrics & Gynecology 2009; Maternal & Fetal Medicine 2009; **Med School:** Mich State Univ 1978; **Resid:** Obstetrics & Gynecology, Univ Texas Med Sch 1982; **Fellow:** Maternal & Fetal Medicine, Univ Texas Med Sch 1985; **Fac Appt:** Prof ObG, Wayne State Univ

Greenfield, Marjorie L MD [ObG] - **Spec Exp:** Adolescent Gynecology; **Hospital:** Univ Hosps Case Med Ctr (page 74); **Address:** UH MacDonald Women's Hosp, Obstetrics & Gynecology, 11100 Euclid Ave, Ste 1200, Cleveland, OH 44106; **Phone:** 216-844-3941; **Board Cert:** Obstetrics & Gynecology 2009; **Med School:** Case West Res Univ 1983; **Resid:** Obstetrics & Gynecology, Univ Hosp 1987; **Fac Appt:** Assoc Prof ObG, Case West Res Univ

Hale, Douglass S MD [ObG] - **Spec Exp:** Uro-Gynecology; Pelvic Floor Reconstruction; Reconstructive Surgery; Robotic Surgery; **Hospital:** IU Health Methodist Hosp; **Address:** Urogynecology Assocs, 1633 N Capital Ave, Ste 436, Indianapolis, IN 46202; **Phone:** 317-962-6600; **Board Cert:** Obstetrics & Gynecology 2010; **Med School:** Med Coll OH 1989; **Resid:** Obstetrics & Gynecology, T Jefferson Univ Hosp 1993; **Fellow:** Uro-Gynecology, Methodist Hosp 1995; Reconstructive Surgery, Methodist Hosp 1995; **Fac Appt:** Assoc Clin Prof ObG, Indiana Univ

Karram, Mickey M MD [ObG] - **Spec Exp:** Uro-Gynecology; Pelvic Floor Reconstruction; Incontinence-Female; **Hospital:** Christ Hosp, The - Cincinnati; **Address:** 7759 University Drive, Ste G, Westchester, OH 45069; **Phone:** 513-463-2500; **Board Cert:** Obstetrics & Gynecology 2009; **Med School:** Egypt 1982; **Resid:** Obstetrics & Gynecology, Good Samaritan Hosp 1985; **Fellow:** Gynecologic Urology, Harbor Hosp-UCLA 1986; **Fac Appt:** Prof ObG, Univ Cincinnati

Lengyel, Ernst MD/PhD [ObG] - **Spec Exp:** Ovarian Cancer; Cervical Cancer; **Hospital:** Univ of Chicago Med Ctr; **Address:** 5841 S Maryland Ave, rm L250, MC 2050, Chicago, IL 60637; **Phone:** 773-702-6722; **Board Cert:** Obstetrics & Gynecology 2010; **Med School:** Germany ; **Resid:** Obstetrics & Gynecology, Univ Munich; **Fellow:** Gynecologic Oncology, UCSF Med Ctr; **Fac Appt:** Prof ObG, Univ Chicago-Pritzker Sch Med

Levine, Elliot MD [ObG] - **Spec Exp:** Sexually Transmitted Diseases; Sexual Dysfunction; Vulvar & Vaginal Disorders; Vulvar Pain; **Hospital:** Adv Illinois Masonic Med Ctr, Weiss Meml Hosp; **Address:** 3000 N Halsted St, Ste 625, Chicago, IL 60657; **Phone:** 773-296-3450; **Board Cert:** Obstetrics & Gynecology 1984; **Med School:** Ros Franklin Univ/Chicago Med Sch 1978; **Resid:** Obstetrics & Gynecology, Illinois Masonic Med Ctr 1982; **Fac Appt:** Asst Prof ObG, Rush Med Coll

Merritt, Diane F MD [ObG] - **Spec Exp:** Adolescent Gynecology; Pediatric Gynecology; Endometriosis; Congenital Anomalies-Gynecologic; **Hospital:** Barnes-Jewish Hosp, St. Louis Chldns Hosp; **Address:** Washington Univ Sch Medicine, 660 S Euclid Ave, St Louis, MO 63110; **Phone:** 314-362-4211; **Board Cert:** Obstetrics & Gynecology 1984; **Med School:** NYU Sch Med 1975; **Resid:** Surgery, Barnes Hosp-Wash Univ 1977; Obstetrics & Gynecology, Barnes Hosp-Wash Univ 1980; **Fac Appt:** Prof ObG, Washington Univ, St Louis

Niebyl, Jennifer R MD [ObG] - **Spec Exp:** Nutrition; **Hospital:** Univ Iowa Hosp & Clinics; **Address:** Univ Iowa Hosps & Clins, 200 Hawkins Drive, Dept Ob/Gyn, Iowa City, IA 52242; **Phone:** 319-356-2294; **Board Cert:** Obstetrics & Gynecology 1998; Maternal & Fetal Medicine 1998; **Med School:** Yale Univ 1967; **Resid:** Obstetrics & Gynecology, NY Hosp-Cornell Med Ctr 1970; Obstetrics & Gynecology, Johns Hopkins Hosp 1973; **Fellow:** Maternal & Fetal Medicine, Johns Hopkins Hosp 1978; **Fac Appt:** Prof ObG, Univ Iowa Coll Med

Valaitis, Sandra MD [ObG] - **Spec Exp:** Pelvic Organ Prolapse Repair; Incontinence; **Hospital:** Univ of Chicago Med Ctr; **Address:** Univ Chicago Med Ctr, Dept Ob/Gyn, 5841 S Maryland Ave, MC 2050, Chicago, IL 60637; **Phone:** 773-834-8622; **Board Cert:** Obstetrics & Gynecology 2010; **Med School:** Univ Chicago-Pritzker Sch Med 1989; **Resid:** Obstetrics & Gynecology, Univ Chicago Med Ctr 1993; **Fellow:** Uro-Gynecology, St Georges Hosp; **Fac Appt:** Assoc Prof ObG, Univ Chicago-Pritzker Sch Med

Walters, Mark D MD [ObG] - **Spec Exp:** Uro-Gynecology; Vaginal Reconstruction; Incontinence-Female; Pelvic Organ Prolapse Repair; **Hospital:** Cleveland Clin (page 56); **Address:** 9500 Euclid Ave, MC A81, Cleveland, OH 44195; **Phone:** 216-445-6586; **Board Cert:** Obstetrics & Gynecology 1996; **Med School:** Ohio State Univ 1980; **Resid:** Obstetrics & Gynecology, New England Med Ctr 1984; **Fac Appt:** Prof ObG, Cleveland Cl Coll Med/Case West Res

Great Plains and Mountains

Byrne, Janice LB MD [ObG] - **Spec Exp:** Prenatal Diagnosis; Ultrasound; Reproductive Genetics; **Hospital:** Univ Utah Hlth Care; **Address:** 50 N Medical Drive, Ste 2B200, Salt Lake City, UT 84132; **Phone:** 801-585-5156; **Board Cert:** Obstetrics & Gynecology 2010; Clinical Genetics 2010; Maternal & Fetal Medicine 2010; **Med School:** Univ Tex SW, Dallas 1987; **Resid:** Obstetrics & Gynecology, Univ Utah Hosps & Clins 1991; **Fellow:** Clinical Genetics, Univ Utah Hosps & Clins 1993; Maternal & Fetal Medicine, Univ Utah Hosps & Clins 1994; **Fac Appt:** Assoc Prof ObG, Univ Utah

King, Aileen MD [ObG] - **Spec Exp:** Women's Health; **Hospital:** St. Luke's Boise Med Ctr; **Address:** 333 N First St, Ste 240, Boise, ID 83702; **Phone:** 208-338-8900; **Board Cert:** Obstetrics & Gynecology 2010; **Med School:** UC Irvine 1996; **Resid:** Obstetrics & Gynecology, Univ CO Hlth Sci Ctr 2000

Southwest

Berens, Pamela D MD [ObG] - **Hospital:** Meml Hermann Hosp - Texas Med Ctr; **Address:** 6140 Fannin St, Ste 250, Houston, TX 77030; **Phone:** 713-572-8122; **Board Cert:** Obstetrics & Gynecology 2010; **Med School:** Univ Minn 1989; **Resid:** Obstetrics & Gynecology, UT Hlth Sci-Meml Hermann 1993; **Fac Appt:** Assoc Prof ObG, Univ Tex, Houston

Bradshaw, Karen D MD [ObG] - **Spec Exp:** Women's Health; Preventive Medicine; Pediatric & Adolescent Gynecology; Menstrual Disorders; **Hospital:** UT Southwestern Med Ctr at Dallas; **Address:** Lowe Ctr for Womens Preventive Health, 5939 Harry Hines Blvd, Dallas, TX 75390-8865; **Phone:** 214-645-3888; **Board Cert:** Obstetrics & Gynecology 2010; Reproductive Endocrinology 2010; **Med School:** Univ Tex SW, Dallas 1981; **Resid:** Obstetrics & Gynecology, Parkland Hosp 1985; **Fellow:** Reproductive Endocrinology, UT-Southwestern Med Ctr 1987; **Fac Appt:** Prof ObG, Univ Tex SW, Dallas

Cornella, Jeffrey L MD [ObG] - **Spec Exp:** Pelvic Reconstruction; Robotic Surgery; Uro-Gynecology; Vaginal Reconstruction; **Hospital:** Mayo Clinic - Phoenix; **Address:** Mayo Clinic Gynecology, 5779 E Mayo Blvd, Phoenix, AZ 85054; **Phone:** 480-301-8484; **Board Cert:** Obstetrics & Gynecology 2010; **Med School:** Washington Univ, St Louis 1981; **Resid:** Obstetrics & Gynecology, Mayo Clinic 1986; **Fellow:** Uro-Gynecology, UC Irvine 1987; **Fac Appt:** Prof ObG, Mayo Med Sch

Emerson, S Cameron MD [ObG] - **Spec Exp:** Uro-Gynecology; Incontinence; Urodynamics; **Hospital:** Ochsner Med Ctr-New Orleans; **Address:** Oschner Clinic, Dept Ob/Gyn, 1514 Jefferson Hwy, New Orleans, LA 70121; **Phone:** 504-842-4155; **Board Cert:** Obstetrics & Gynecology 2010; **Med School:** Univ Wash 1979; **Resid:** Obstetrics & Gynecology, Tulane Univ Med Ctr 1983; **Fellow:** Advanced Pelvic Surgery, Mayo Clinic 1984

Faro, Sebastian MD/PhD [ObG] - **Spec Exp:** Infectious Diseases-Gynecologic; Sexually Transmitted Diseases; Pelvic Reconstruction; **Hospital:** Woman's Hosp TX, St. Luke's Episcopal Hosp-Houston; **Address:** 7400 Fannin St, Ste 840, Houston, TX 77054; **Phone:** 713-799-9091; **Board Cert:** Obstetrics & Gynecology 2009; **Med School:** Creighton Univ 1975; **Resid:** Obstetrics & Gynecology, Creighton Univ 1978; **Fac Appt:** Clin Prof ObG, Univ Tex, Houston

Putterman, Bart D MD [ObG] - **Spec Exp:** Diabetes in Pregnancy; **Hospital:** Methodist Hosp - Houston; **Address:** 6560 Fannin St, Scurlock Tower, Ste 1980, Houston, TX 77030-2727; **Phone:** 713-335-0335; **Board Cert:** Obstetrics & Gynecology 2010; **Med School:** Baylor Coll Med 1984; **Resid:** Obstetrics & Gynecology, Baylor Affil Hosps 1988

West Coast and Pacific

Eschenbach, David A MD [ObG] - **Spec Exp:** Gynecologic Surgery-Complex; Vulvar & Vaginal Disorders; **Hospital:** Univ Wash Med Ctr; **Address:** Univ Washington Women's Health Care, 4245 Roosevelt Way NE, Box 354765, Seattle, WA 98105; **Phone:** 206-598-5500; **Board Cert:** Obstetrics & Gynecology 1975; **Med School:** Univ Wisc 1968; **Resid:** Obstetrics & Gynecology, Univ Wash Hosp 1973; **Fellow:** Infectious Disease, Univ Wash Hosp 1974; **Fac Appt:** Prof ObG, Univ Wash

Goldman, Mindy E MD [ObG] - **Spec Exp:** Breast Cancer; **Hospital:** UCSF Med Ctr; **Address:** 2356 Sutter St, San Francisco, CA 94115; **Phone:** 415-885-7788; **Board Cert:** Obstetrics & Gynecology 2007; **Med School:** Univ VT Coll Med 1989; **Resid:** Obstetrics & Gynecology, UCSF Med Ctr 1993

Obstetrics & Gynecology

Parker, William H MD [ObG] - **Spec Exp:** Gynecologic Surgery; Hysteroscopic Surgery; Laparoscopic Surgery; Uterine Fibroids; **Hospital:** St. John's Hlth Ctr, Santa Monica; **Address:** 1450 10th St, Ste 404, Santa Monica, CA 90401-2804; **Phone:** 310-451-8144; **Board Cert:** Obstetrics & Gynecology 1981; **Med School:** SUNY Downstate 1974; **Resid:** Obstetrics & Gynecology, UC San Diego 1978; **Fac Appt:** Clin Prof ObG, UCLA

Sweet, Richard L MD [ObG] - **Spec Exp:** Sexually Transmitted Diseases; Infectious Diseases-Gynecologic; Women's Health; Infections in Pregnancy; **Hospital:** UC Davis Med Ctr; **Address:** UC Davis Women's Center for Health, 4860 Y St, Ste 2500, Sacramento, CA 95817; **Phone:** 916-734-6670; **Board Cert:** Obstetrics & Gynecology 1975; **Med School:** Univ Mich Med Sch 1966; **Resid:** Obstetrics & Gynecology, Univ Mich Med Ctr 1973; **Fac Appt:** Prof ObG, UC Davis

Cleveland Clinic

Every life deserves world class care.

Obstetrics & Gynecology

Cleveland Clinic Ob/Gyn & Women's Health Institute is designed to meet the unique and changing medical needs of women from adolescence to mature adulthood. *U.S. News & World Report* has ranked our gynecology program No.4 in the country.

Reproductive Endocrinology and Infertility: This team involves close collaboration between male and female infertility specialists, andrologists and embryologists. We offer all available treatment options including medications, artificial insemination, in vitro fertilization (IVF) and reproductive surgery.

Urogynecology and Reconstructive Pelvic Surgery: This center offers cutting-edge and traditional surgery for urinary incontinence and pelvic organ prolapse, along with medical and behavioral therapy.

Center for Female Pelvic Medicine & Reconstructive Surgery: Urogynecologist, urologists and colorectal surgeons in this center treat incontinence and prolapse via the abdominal, vaginal and laparoscopic routes. Pelvic floor subspecialists collaborate to advance research, education and to improve patient outcomes.

Maternal-Fetal Medicine/Obstetrics: Specialists provide management for high-risk pregnancies. Services include genetic counseling, ultrasound, antepartum fetal surveillance, prenatal diagnostic testing and consultation.

Fetal Care Center: The team of perinatologists, neonatologists, pediatric subspecialists and surgeons provides prenatal diagnosis for complex fetal abnormalities.

Center for Menstrual Disorders, Fibroids and Hysteroscopic Services: This center offers individualized evaluation of abnormal menstrual bleeding, post-menopausal bleeding and uterine fibroids. Clinicians utilize in-office, minimally invasive technology.

Center for Specialized Women's Health: This center offers a full range of specialized women's health services in one location.

Cleveland Clinic
Women's Health Institute
9500 Euclid Avenue
Cleveland, OH 44195

clevelandclinic.org/
obgyntopdocs

Offering Same-Day Appointments
Call 800.274.2009.

Treatment Guides
Cleveland Clinic has developed comprehensive treatment guides for many diseases and conditions. To download our free treatment guides, visit clevelandclinic.org/treatmentguides.

Online Medical Second Opinion
Cleveland Clinic's My**Consult** Online Medical Second Opinion program securely connects patients to our physician specialists for more than 1,000 life-changing or life-threatening diagnoses all by the click of a mouse. To learn more, log onto eclevelandclinic.org/myconsult or call 800.223.2273, ext. 43223.

Special Assistance for Out-of-State Patients
Cleveland Clinic Global Patient Services offers a complimentary Medical Concierge service for patients who travel from outside of Ohio. Call 800.223.2273, ext. 55580 or email medicalconcierge@ccf.org.

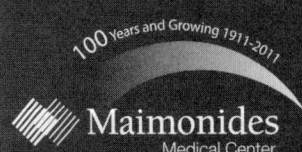

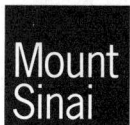 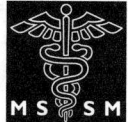

**MOUNT SINAI
SCHOOL OF
MEDICINE**

THE MOUNT SINAI MEDICAL CENTER
OBSTETRICS, GYNECOLOGY,
AND REPRODUCTIVE SCIENCE

One Gustave L. Levy Place
Fifth Avenue and 100th Street
New York, NY 10029-6574
Physician Referral: 1-800-MD-SINAI (637-4624)
www.mountsinai.org/obgyn

Building on more than a century of leadership in providing health care to women, the **DEPARTMENT OF OBSTETRICS, GYNECOLOGY, AND REPRODUCTIVE SCIENCE** at The Mount Sinai Medical Center offers special expertise in:

General obstetrics – Genetic counseling, prenatal care, labor and delivery management, and postpartum care. In addition to our talented physicians, other health care professionals are integrated into our practice, including genetic counselors, nutritionists, social workers, nurse midwives, childbirth educators, and lactation/breastfeeding specialists.

High-risk obstetrics – Advanced techniques in prenatal diagnosis and consultations in the management of complicated pregnancies. Our ultrasound unit is recognized for its expertise in fetal anatomy ultrasound assessments. The latest technology, including 4D imaging, is employed. Antepartum testing, including amniocentesis, chorionic villus sampling, and fetal blood sampling, are all routinely performed at Mount Sinai.

Reproductive endocrinology and infertility – Diagnosis and treatment of both female and male factor infertility. Treatment options for women include fertility medications, intrauterine insemination, in vitro fertilization, intracytoplasmic sperm injection, and ovum donation.

General gynecology – Cancer screening, management of abnormal Pap smears, family planning, and surgical management of fibroids, endometriosis, and other benign gynecologic conditions.

Gynecologic infectious diseases – Treatment and prevention of sexually transmitted infections and consultations on obstetrical and gynecological infections.

Gynecologic oncology – Care for women with cancers of the ovary, uterus, cervix, vulva, and vagina.

Minimally invasive surgery – For many conditions.

Urogynecology and reconstructive pelvic surgery – Lower urinary tract disorders.

INNOVATIVE APPROACHES TO PRENATAL CARE AND THE TREATMENT OF GYNECOLOGIC CANCERS
Known worldwide for excellence and innovative approaches to prenatal diagnosis and fetal therapy, Mount Sinai's Department of Obstetrics, Gynecology, and Reproductive Science has a long tradition of advancing clinical practice through patient-oriented research. Faculty members are pioneering work in diverse areas, including first- and second-trimester screening for fetal chromosomal abnormalities, vaccines for the prevention of sexually transmitted infections, minimally invasive surgical techniques, and new approaches to the diagnosis and treatment of gender-specific cancers.

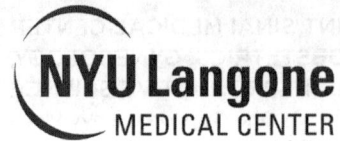
OBSTETRICS AND GYNECOLOGY

About the Department of Obstetrics and Gynecology
NYU Langone Medical Center provides comprehensive programs and services designed specifically for women, from primary care to highly specialized programs that are supported by sophisticated research and advanced training. We specialize in the following areas:

Fertility-Related Services
NYU Langone offers state-of-the-art programs in egg donation, egg freezing and wellness (acupuncture, mind/body, psychology and yoga). Diagnosis and treatment include ovulation induction, assisted reproductive technologies and surgical options that incorporate the latest endoscopic techniques. The Center also tests for genetic abnormalities, as well as for immunity and infectious diseases.

Gynecologic Oncology
The NCI-designated NYU Cancer Institute's Women's Cancer Program specializes in the treatment of cervical cancer, endometrial cancer, ovarian cancer, uterine cancer, vaginal cancer and vulvar cancer.

Maternal Fetal Medicine
Prenatal care for high-risk pregnancies and detailed consultations before, during and after pregnancy are offered. Special attention is given to multifetal pregnancies and to women who have other medical conditions that may complicate a pregnancy, such as diabetes, heart problems, high blood pressure and lupus.

Obstetrics
We offer a broad range of obstetrical services, including prenatal care that gives equal emphasis to the well-being of the mother and the fetus; fetal monitoring through ultrasound and other techniques; childbirth preparedness and breastfeeding classes; consultation for high-risk pregnancies, including treatment for women who have experienced recurrent pregnancy loss.

Specialty Services
In addition to routine gynecological care, we offer pelvic ultrasound; aspiration of breast cysts; evaluation of infertility (including the special needs of same-sex couples); colposcopy (a diagnostic evaluation of abnormal pap smears); LEEP (a loop electrosurgical procedure used to diagnose and treat cervical cancer); cryotherapy for vaginal warts; and bone density testing.

Urogynecology and Reconstructive Pelvic Surgery
Our urogynecologists treat all forms of incontinence and pelvic disorders; malformations of the reproductive tract found at birth, during childhood or in young adults; and conditions such as overactive bladder, urinary and/or fecal incontinence and pelvic organ prolapse.

Sponsored Page

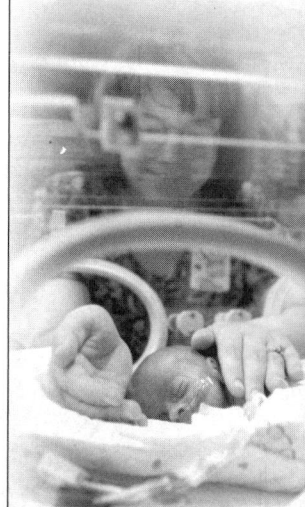

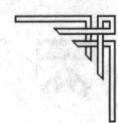

The Best in American Medicine
www.CastleConnolly.com

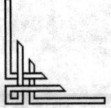
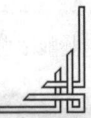

Ophthalmology

An ophthalmologist has the knowledge and professional skills needed to provide comprehensive eye and vision care. Ophthalmologists are medically trained to diagnose, monitor and medically or surgically treat all ocular and visual disorders. This includes problems affecting the eye and its component structures, the eyelids, the orbit and the visual pathways. In so doing, an ophthalmologist prescribes vision services, including glasses and contact lenses.

Training Required: Four years

OPHTHALMOLOGY

New England

Dana, Reza MD [Oph] - **Spec Exp:** Corneal Disease & Transplant; Dry Eye Syndrome; Uveitis; **Hospital:** Mass Eye & Ear Infirmary; **Address:** Mass Eye & Ear Infirmary, 243 Charles St, Boston, MA 02114; **Phone:** 617-573-4331; **Board Cert:** Ophthalmology 2006; **Med School:** Johns Hopkins Univ 1989; **Resid:** Ophthalmology, Illinois Eye & Ear Infirm 1993; **Fellow:** Cornea & Ext Eye Disease, Wills Eye Hosp 1994; Uveitis, Mass Eye & Ear Infirm 1995; **Fac Appt:** Prof Oph, Harvard Med Sch

Duker, Jay S MD [Oph] - **Spec Exp:** Retinal Disorders; Retinal Disorders-Pediatric; Diabetic Eye Disease/Retinopathy; **Hospital:** Tufts Med Ctr; **Address:** New England Eye Ctr, 800 Washington St, Box 450, Boston, MA 02111; **Phone:** 617-636-4600; **Board Cert:** Ophthalmology 1989; **Med School:** Jefferson Med Coll 1984; **Resid:** Ophthalmology, Wills Eye Hosp 1988; **Fellow:** Vitreoretinal Surgery & Disease, Wills Eye Hosp 1990; **Fac Appt:** Assoc Prof Oph, Tufts Univ

Foster, C Stephen MD [Oph] - **Spec Exp:** Uveitis; Corneal Disease; Cataract Surgery; **Hospital:** Mass Eye & Ear Infirmary, Mount Auburn Hosp; **Address:** 5 Cambridge Ctr, Fl 8, Cambridge, MA 02142; **Phone:** 866-353-6377; **Board Cert:** Ophthalmology 1976; **Med School:** Duke Univ 1969; **Resid:** Ophthalmology, Barnes Hosp 1975; **Fellow:** Cornea, Mass EE Infirm-Harvard 1976; Ocular Immunology, Mass EE Infirm-Harvard 1977; **Fac Appt:** Prof Oph, Harvard Med Sch

Hedges, Thomas R MD [Oph] - **Spec Exp:** Neuro-Ophthalmology; **Hospital:** Tufts Med Ctr; **Address:** New England Med Ctr, 800 Washington St, Box 450, Boston, MA 02111; **Phone:** 617-636-5488; **Board Cert:** Ophthalmology 1980; **Med School:** Tufts Univ 1975; **Resid:** Ophthalmology, Mass EE Infirm 1980; **Fellow:** Neuro-Ophthalmology, UCSF Med Ctr 1981; **Fac Appt:** Prof Oph, Tufts Univ

Hunter, David G MD/PhD [Oph] - **Spec Exp:** Pediatric Ophthalmology; Eye Muscle Disorders; Strabismus; Congenital Fibrosis-Extraocular Muscles; **Hospital:** Children's Hospital - Boston; **Address:** Chlds Hosp Boston, Dept Ophthalmology, 300 Longwood Ave, Fegan 4 Bldg, Boston, MA 02115; **Phone:** 617-355-6766; **Board Cert:** Ophthalmology 2003; **Med School:** Baylor Coll Med 1987; **Resid:** Ophthalmology, Mass EE Infirm 1991; **Fellow:** Pediatric Ophthalmology, Wilmer Ophthalmic Inst/Johns Hopkins 1992; **Fac Appt:** Assoc Prof Oph, Harvard Med Sch

Kornmehl, Ernest W MD [Oph] - **Spec Exp:** LASIK-Refractive Surgery; PRK-Refractive Surgery; Cataract Surgery; Dry Eye Syndrome; **Hospital:** Mass Eye & Ear Infirmary, Brigham and Women's Hosp (page 57); **Address:** Kornmehl Laser Eye Assoc, 44 Washington St, Brookline, MA 02445; **Phone:** 877-870-2010; **Board Cert:** Ophthalmology 1989; **Med School:** SUNY Downstate 1984; **Resid:** Ophthalmology, Yale-New Haven Hosp 1988; **Fellow:** Cornea & Ext Eye Disease, Mass E&E Infirm 1990; **Fac Appt:** Assoc Clin Prof Oph, Harvard Med Sch

Miller, Joan W MD [Oph] - **Spec Exp:** Macular Degeneration; Retinal Disorders; **Hospital:** Mass Eye & Ear Infirmary; **Address:** Mass Eye & Ear Infirm, Ophthalmology, 243 Charles St, Boston, MA 02114; **Phone:** 617-573-3915; **Board Cert:** Ophthalmology 1991; **Med School:** Harvard Med Sch 1985; **Resid:** Ophthalmology, Mass Eye & Ear Infirm 1989; **Fellow:** Retina, Mass Eye & Ear Infirm 1991; **Fac Appt:** Prof Oph, Harvard Med Sch

Mitchell, Paul R MD [Oph] - **Spec Exp:** Pediatric Ophthalmology; Nystagmus; Strabismus; **Hospital:** CT Chldns Med Ctr, Hartford Hosp; **Address:** 366 Colt Hwy, Route 6, Farmington, CT 06032; **Phone:** 860-409-0449; **Board Cert:** Ophthalmology 1977; **Med School:** Geo Wash Univ 1970; **Resid:** Ophthalmology, Wills Eye Hosp 1976; **Fellow:** Pediatric Ophthalmology, Chldns Hosp MC/Geo Wash 1977; **Fac Appt:** Asst Clin Prof Oph, Univ Conn

Rizzo III, Joseph F MD [Oph] - **Spec Exp:** Neuro-Ophthalmology; **Hospital:** Mass Eye & Ear Infirmary; **Address:** Mass Eye & Ear Infirmary, 243 Charles St Fl 9, Boston, MA 02114; **Phone:** 617-573-3412; **Board Cert:** Neurology 1984; Ophthalmology 1987; **Med School:** Louisiana State U, New Orleans 1978; **Resid:** Neurology, Tufts-New Engl Med Ctr 1982; Ophthalmology, Boston Univ 1985; **Fellow:** Neuro-Ophthalmology, Harvard Univ 1986; **Fac Appt:** Assoc Prof Oph, Harvard Med Sch

Rubin, Peter A D MD [Oph] - **Spec Exp:** Oculoplastic Surgery; Orbital & Eyelid Tumors/Cancer; Eyelid Cancer & Reconstruction; Eyelid Cosmetic & Reconstructive Surgery; **Hospital:** Beth Israel Deaconess Med Ctr - Boston; **Address:** 44 Washington St, Brookline, MA 02445; **Phone:** 617-232-9600; **Board Cert:** Ophthalmology 1991; **Med School:** Yale Univ 1985; **Resid:** Ophthalmology, Manhattan EET Hosp 1989; **Fellow:** Oculoplastic Surgery, Mass EE Infirmary 1990; **Fac Appt:** Assoc Clin Prof Oph, Univ Tenn Coll Med

Shingleton, Bradford J MD [Oph] - **Spec Exp:** Cataract Surgery; Glaucoma; **Hospital:** Mass Eye & Ear Infirmary; **Address:** Ophthalmic Cons Boston, 50 Staniford St, Ste 600, Boston, MA 02114; **Phone:** 617-314-2614; **Board Cert:** Ophthalmology 1982; **Med School:** Univ Mich Med Sch 1977; **Resid:** Ophthalmology, Mass E&E Infirm 1981; **Fellow:** Refractive Surgery, Mass E&E Infirm 1982; **Fac Appt:** Asst Clin Prof Oph, Harvard Med Sch

Tsai, James C MD [Oph] - **Spec Exp:** Glaucoma; **Hospital:** Yale-New Haven Hosp, Yale Med Group; **Address:** Yale Eye Center, 40 Temple St, New Haven, CT 06520-8061; **Phone:** 203-785-2020; **Board Cert:** Ophthalmology 2006; **Med School:** Stanford Univ 1989; **Resid:** Ophthalmology, Doheny Eye Inst/USC 1993; **Fellow:** Glaucoma, Bascom Palmer Eye Inst 1994; Glaucoma, Moorfields Eye Hosp 1995; **Fac Appt:** Prof Oph, Yale Univ

Walton, David S MD [Oph] - **Spec Exp:** Glaucoma-Pediatric; Cataract-Pediatric; Neuro-Ophthalmology; **Hospital:** Mass Eye & Ear Infirmary, Mass Genl Hosp; **Address:** 2 Longfellow Pl, Ste 201, Boston, MA 02114; **Phone:** 617-227-3011; **Board Cert:** Ophthalmology 1969; Pediatrics 1983; **Med School:** Duke Univ 1961; **Resid:** Ophthalmology, Mass EE Infirm 1967; **Fellow:** Glaucoma, Mass EE Infirm 1968; **Fac Appt:** Prof Oph, Harvard Med Sch

Mid Atlantic

Abramson, David H MD [Oph] - **Spec Exp:** Eye Tumors/Cancer; Orbital Tumors/Cancer; Retinoblastoma; Melanoma-Choroidal (eye); **Hospital:** Meml Sloan-Kettering Cancer Ctr, NY-Presby/Weill Cornell Med Ctr, NY (page 65); **Address:** 70 E 66th St, New York, NY 10065; **Phone:** 212-744-1700; **Board Cert:** Ophthalmology 1975; **Med School:** Albert Einstein Coll Med 1969; **Resid:** Ophthalmology, Harkness Eye Inst 1974; **Fellow:** Ocular Oncology, Columbia-Presby Med Ctr 1975; **Fac Appt:** Prof Oph, Cornell Univ-Weill Med Coll

Behrens, Myles MD [Oph] - **Spec Exp:** Neuro-Ophthalmology; **Hospital:** NY-Presby/Columbia Univ Med Ctr, NY (page 65); **Address:** 635 W 165th St, New York, NY 10032-3701; **Phone:** 212-305-5415; **Board Cert:** Ophthalmology 1971; **Med School:** Columbia P&S 1962; **Resid:** Internal Medicine, Columbia Presby Hosp 1964; Ophthalmology, Columbia Presby Hosp 1970; **Fellow:** Neuro-Ophthalmology, UCSF Med Ctr 1971; **Fac Appt:** Clin Prof Oph, Columbia P&S

Bressler, Neil M MD [Oph] - **Spec Exp:** Retinal Disorders; **Hospital:** Johns Hopkins Hosp (page 61); **Address:** Wilmer Eye Institute, 600 N Wolfe St, Maumenee Bldg-752, Baltimore, MD 21287; **Phone:** 410-955-8342; **Board Cert:** Ophthalmology 1987; **Med School:** Johns Hopkins Univ 1982; **Resid:** Internal Medicine, Johns Hopkins Hosp 1983; Ophthalmology, Mass Eye & Ear Infirm 1986; **Fellow:** Retina, Wilmer Inst/Johns Hopkins Hosp 1987; **Fac Appt:** Assoc Prof Oph, Johns Hopkins Univ

Bressler, Susan B MD [Oph] - **Spec Exp:** Diabetic Eye Disease/Retinopathy; Retinal Disorders; Macular Degeneration; **Hospital:** Johns Hopkins Hosp (page 61); **Address:** The Johns Hopkins Hospital, Wilmer Eye Institute-Maumenee 706, 600 N Wolfe St, Baltimore, MD 21287; **Phone:** 410-955-3618; **Board Cert:** Ophthalmology 1987; **Med School:** Johns Hopkins Univ 1982; **Resid:** Ophthalmology, Mass Eye & Ear Infirmary 1986; **Fellow:** Ophthalmology, Wilmer Eye Inst 1987; Retinal Surgery, Mass Eye & Ear Infirmary 1988; **Fac Appt:** Prof Oph, Johns Hopkins Univ

Brown, Gary C MD [Oph] - **Spec Exp:** Retinal Disorders; Retinal Vascular Diseases; Macular Degeneration; **Hospital:** Wills Eye Hosp, Thomas Jefferson Univ Hosp; **Address:** Mid-Atlantic Retina, 910 E Willow Grove Ave, Wyndmoor, PA 19038; **Phone:** 215-233-4300; **Board Cert:** Ophthalmology 2003; **Med School:** SUNY Upstate Med Univ 1975; **Resid:** Ophthalmology, Wills Eye Hosp 1979; **Fellow:** Vitreoretinal Disease, Wills Eye Hosp 1981; **Fac Appt:** Prof Oph, Jefferson Med Coll

Brucker, Alexander J MD [Oph] - **Spec Exp:** Retinal Disorders; Retina/Vitreous Surgery; Macular Degeneration; **Hospital:** Penn Presby Med Ctr - UPHS (page 68); **Address:** Univ Penn, Scheie Eye Inst, 51 N 39th St, rm 517, Philadelphia, PA 19104; **Phone:** 215-662-9702; **Board Cert:** Ophthalmology 1977; **Med School:** NY Med Coll 1972; **Resid:** Ophthalmology, Friedenwald Inst 1976; **Fellow:** Retina/Vitreous, Johns Hopkins Hosp 1977; **Fac Appt:** Prof Oph, Univ Pennsylvania

Campochiaro, Peter MD [Oph] - **Spec Exp:** Retina/Vitreous Surgery; **Hospital:** Johns Hopkins Hosp (page 61); **Address:** Wilmer Ophthalmological Inst, 600 N Wolfe St, 747 Maumenee, Baltimore, MD 21287-9277; **Phone:** 410-955-5106; **Board Cert:** Ophthalmology 1983; **Med School:** Johns Hopkins Univ 1978; **Resid:** Ophthalmology, Univ Virginia 1982; **Fellow:** Retina/Vitreous, John Hopkins Univ 1984; **Fac Appt:** Prof Oph, Johns Hopkins Univ

Caputo, Anthony R MD [Oph] - **Spec Exp:** Pediatric Ophthalmology; Strabismus; **Hospital:** Clara Maass Med Ctr; **Address:** 556 Eagle Rock Ave, Ste 203, Roseland, NJ 07068-1500; **Phone:** 973-228-3111; **Board Cert:** Ophthalmology 1976; **Med School:** Italy 1969; **Resid:** Ophthalmology, UMDNJ-Univ Hosp 1974; **Fellow:** Ophthalmology, Wills Eye Hosp 1975; **Fac Appt:** Prof Oph, UMDNJ-NJ Med Sch, Newark

Chang, Stanley MD [Oph] - **Spec Exp:** Diabetic Eye Disease/Retinopathy; Macular Disease/Degeneration; Retina/Vitreous Surgery; Retinal Disorders; **Hospital:** NY-Presby/Columbia Univ Med Ctr, NY (page 65); **Address:** 635 W 165th St, New York, NY 10032; **Phone:** 212-305-9535; **Board Cert:** Ophthalmology 1979; **Med School:** Columbia P&S 1974; **Resid:** Ophthalmology, Mass Eye & Ear Infirm 1978; **Fellow:** Vitreoretinal Surgery, Bascom Palmer Eye Inst 1979; **Fac Appt:** Prof Oph, Columbia P&S

D'Amico, Donald J MD [Oph] - **Spec Exp:** Diabetic Eye Disease/Retinopathy; Retinal Detachment; Retinal Disorders; **Hospital:** NY-Presby/Weill Cornell Med Ctr, NY (page 65); **Address:** Weill Cornell Medical College, Dept of Ophthalmology, 1305 York Ave Fl 11th, New York, NY 10021; **Phone:** 646-962-2020; **Board Cert:** Ophthalmology 1982; **Med School:** Univ IL Coll Med 1977; **Resid:** Ophthalmology, Mass Eye & Ear Infirm 1981; **Fellow:** Vitreoretinal Surgery, Bascom Palmer Eye Inst 1982; **Fac Appt:** Prof Oph, Cornell Univ-Weill Med Coll

Del Priore, Lucian MD/PhD [Oph] - **Spec Exp:** Diabetic Eye Disease/Retinopathy; Macular Degeneration; Retinal Detachment; Retina-Artificial; **Hospital:** NY-Presby/Columbia Univ Med Ctr, NY (page 65), Lenox Hill Hosp (Manh Eye, Ear & Throat Hosp); **Address:** Harkness Eye Inst, 635 W 165th St, New York, NY 10032; **Phone:** 212-305-9535; **Board Cert:** Ophthalmology 1989; **Med School:** Univ Rochester 1982; **Resid:** Ophthalmology, Wilmer Eye Inst/Johns HopkinsHosp 1987; **Fellow:** Glaucoma, Wilmer Eye Inst/Johns Hopkins Hosp 1988; Vitreoretinal Surgery, Wilmer Eye Inst/Johns Hopkins Hosp 1989; **Fac Appt:** Prof Oph, Columbia P&S

Della Rocca, Robert C MD [Oph] - **Spec Exp:** Orbital Tumors/Cancer; Eyelid Tumors/Cancer; Thyroid Eye Disease; Oculoplastic Surgery; **Hospital:** New York Eye & Ear Infirm (page 64), Sound Shore Med Ctr - Westchester; **Address:** 310 E 14th St, South Bldg, rm 319, New York, NY 10003; **Phone:** 212-979-4575; **Board Cert:** Ophthalmology 1975; **Med School:** Creighton Univ 1967; **Resid:** Ophthalmology, NY Eye & Ear Infirm 1973; **Fellow:** Oculoplastic Surgery, Albany Med Ctr

Dhaliwal, Deepinder K MD [Oph] - **Spec Exp:** Refractive Surgery; Corneal & External Eye Disease; Anterior Segment Surgery; **Hospital:** UPMC Presby, Pittsburgh; **Address:** UPMC Eye Center, 203 Lothrop St, Pittsburgh, PA 15213; **Phone:** 412-647-2200; **Board Cert:** Ophthalmology 2007; **Med School:** Northwestern Univ-Feinberg Sch Med 1990; **Resid:** Ophthalmology, Univ Pitt Eye & Ear Inst 1994; **Fellow:** Refractive Surgery, Univ Utah 1995; **Fac Appt:** Assoc Prof Oph, Univ Pittsburgh

Dodick, Jack M MD [Oph] - **Spec Exp:** Cataract Surgery-Lens Implant; Laser Vision Surgery; **Hospital:** NYU Langone Med Ctr (page 66), Lenox Hill Hosp (Manh Eye, Ear & Throat Hosp); **Address:** 535 Park Ave, New York, NY 10065; **Phone:** 212-288-7638; **Board Cert:** Ophthalmology 1969; **Med School:** Univ Toronto 1963; **Resid:** Ophthalmology, Manhattan EE&T Hosp 1967; **Fellow:** Anterior Segment - External Disease, Westchester Co Med Ctr 1968; **Fac Appt:** Prof Oph, NYU Sch Med

Eagle, Ralph C MD [Oph] - **Spec Exp:** Ophthalmic Pathology; **Hospital:** Wills Eye Hosp; **Address:** Wills Eye Hosp, Dept Pathology, 840 Walnut St, Ste 1410, Philadelphia, PA 19107; **Phone:** 215-928-3280; **Board Cert:** Ophthalmology 1976; **Med School:** Univ Pennsylvania 1970; **Resid:** Ophthalmology, Scheie Eye Inst 1975; **Fellow:** Ophthalmic Pathology, Armed Forces Inst Path 1978; **Fac Appt:** Prof Oph, Jefferson Med Coll

Eggers, Howard M MD [Oph] - **Spec Exp:** Pediatric Ophthalmology; Strabismus-Adult & Pediatric; **Hospital:** NY-Presby/Columbia Univ Med Ctr, NY (page 65); **Address:** Harkness Eye Institute, 635 W 165th St, New York, NY 10032-3724; **Phone:** 212-305-5409; **Board Cert:** Ophthalmology 1978; **Med School:** Columbia P&S 1971; **Resid:** Ophthalmology, Harkness Inst-Presby Hosp 1975; **Fac Appt:** Prof Oph, Columbia P&S

Feldon, Steven E MD [Oph] - **Spec Exp:** Neuro-Ophthalmology; Orbital Surgery; Strabismus; Thyroid Eye Disease; **Hospital:** Univ of Rochester Strong Meml Hosp, Rochester Genl Hosp; **Address:** 601 Elmwood Ave, Box 659, Rochester, NY 14642; **Phone:** 585-275-1126; **Board Cert:** Ophthalmology 1979; **Med School:** Albert Einstein Coll Med 1973; **Resid:** Ophthalmology, Mass Eye & Ear Infirmary 1978; **Fellow:** Neuro-Ophthalmology, UCSF Med Ctr 1979; **Fac Appt:** Prof Oph, Univ Rochester

Finger, Paul T MD [Oph] - **Spec Exp:** Eye Tumors/Cancer; Melanoma-Choroidal (eye); Retinoblastoma; Orbital Tumors/Cancer; **Hospital:** New York Eye & Ear Infirm (page 64), NYU Langone Med Ctr (page 66); **Address:** 115 E 61 St Fl 5 - Ste B, New York, NY 10065; **Phone:** 212-832-8170; **Board Cert:** Ophthalmology 1990; **Med School:** Tulane Univ 1982; **Resid:** Ophthalmology, Manhattan EET Hosp 1986; **Fellow:** Ocular Oncology, N Shore Univ Hosp 1987; **Fac Appt:** Clin Prof Oph, NYU Sch Med

Ophthalmology

Florakis, George J MD [Oph] - **Spec Exp:** Cornea Transplant; Corneal Disease; Keratoconus; Anterior Segment Trauma/Reconstruction; **Hospital:** NY-Presby/Columbia Univ Med Ctr, NY (page 65), White Plains Hosp Ctr; **Address:** Harkness Eye Institute, 635 W 165th St, Ste 303, New York, NY 10032; **Phone:** 212-927-2394; **Board Cert:** Ophthalmology 1989; **Med School:** Columbia P&S 1983; **Resid:** Ophthalmology, Harkness Eye Inst 1987; **Fellow:** Cornea & Ext Eye Disease, Univ Iowa Hosps & Clins 1988; **Fac Appt:** Clin Prof Oph, Columbia P&S

Friberg, Thomas R MD [Oph] - **Spec Exp:** Retinal Disorders; Diabetic Eye Disease/Retinopathy; Macular Degeneration; **Hospital:** UPMC Presby, Pittsburgh; **Address:** UPMC Eye Center, 203 Lothrop St, rm 824, Pittsburgh, PA 15213-2548; **Phone:** 412-647-2200; **Board Cert:** Ophthalmology 1979; **Med School:** Univ Minn 1973; **Resid:** Ophthalmology, Stanford Univ Med Ctr 1977; **Fellow:** Retina, Mass EE Infirmary 1978; Vitreoretinal Surgery, Duke Univ Med Ctr 1979; **Fac Appt:** Prof Oph, Univ Pittsburgh

Fuchs, Wayne MD [Oph] - **Spec Exp:** Diabetic Eye Disease/Retinopathy; Macular Disease/Degeneration; Retinal Disorders; Pseudoxanthoma Elasticum; **Hospital:** Mount Sinai Med Ctr (page 63), Lenox Hill Hosp (Manh Eye, Ear & Throat Hosp); **Address:** 121 E 60th St, Ste 5B, New York, NY 10022-1186; **Phone:** 212-319-8205; **Board Cert:** Ophthalmology 1985; **Med School:** Mount Sinai Sch Med 1979; **Resid:** Ophthalmology, Mt Sinai Hosp 1983; **Fellow:** Vitreoretinal Surgery & Disease, NY Hosp-Cornell Med Ctr 1984; **Fac Appt:** Clin Prof Oph, Mount Sinai Sch Med

Gaasterland, Douglas E MD [Oph] - **Spec Exp:** Glaucoma; Laser Surgery; Anterior Segment Surgery; **Hospital:** Georgetown Univ Hosp; **Address:** 2 Wisconsin Circle, Ste 200, Chevy Chase, MD 20815; **Phone:** 301-215-7100; **Board Cert:** Ophthalmology 1971; **Med School:** Johns Hopkins Univ 1965; **Resid:** Ophthalmology, Yale-New Haven Hosp 1970; **Fellow:** Glaucoma, National Eye Inst-NIH 1971; **Fac Appt:** Clin Prof Oph, Georgetown Univ

Gallin, Pamela F MD [Oph] - **Spec Exp:** Pediatric Ophthalmology; Amblyopia; Strabismus; Lacrimal Gland Disorders; **Hospital:** NY-Presby/Columbia Univ Med Ctr, NY (page 65), Lenox Hill Hosp (Manh Eye, Ear & Throat Hosp); **Address:** NY Presby/Columbia Univ, 635 W 165th St, Ste 224, New York, NY 10032-3701; **Phone:** 212-305-5407; **Board Cert:** Ophthalmology 1983; **Med School:** Washington Univ, St Louis 1978; **Resid:** Ophthalmology, Mount Sinai Med Ctr 1982; **Fellow:** Pediatric Ophthalmology, Chldns Natl Med Ctr 1983; Strabismus, Columbia-Presby Med Ctr 1983; **Fac Appt:** Clin Prof Oph, Columbia P&S

Gentile, Ronald MD [Oph] - **Spec Exp:** Retina/Vitreous Surgery; Diabetic Eye Disease/Retinopathy; Macular Degeneration; Retinal Disorders; **Hospital:** New York Eye & Ear Infirm (page 64); **Address:** 310 E 14th St, Ste 310 South, New York, NY 10003-4201; **Phone:** 212-979-4120; **Board Cert:** Ophthalmology 2008; **Med School:** SUNY Downstate 1991; **Resid:** Ophthalmology, NY Eye & Ear Infirm 1995; **Fellow:** Vitreoretinal Surgery & Disease, Kresge Eye Inst 1998; **Fac Appt:** Prof Oph, NY Med Coll

Gibralter, Richard P MD [Oph] - **Spec Exp:** Cataract Surgery; Laser Vision Surgery; Cornea Transplant; Corneal Disease & Surgery; **Hospital:** Lenox Hill Hosp (Manh Eye, Ear & Throat Hosp), New York Eye & Ear Infirm (page 64); **Address:** 154 E 71st St, New York, NY 10021-5123; **Phone:** 212-628-2202; **Board Cert:** Ophthalmology 1981; **Med School:** Mount Sinai Sch Med 1976; **Resid:** Ophthalmology, Manhattan EE&T Hosp 1980; **Fellow:** Cornea, Manhattan EE&T Hosp 1981; **Fac Appt:** Assoc Clin Prof Oph, NYU Sch Med

Goldberg, Daniel MD [Oph] - **Spec Exp:** LASIK-Refractive Surgery; Cornea Transplant; Cataract Surgery; Lens Implants; **Address:** Atlantic Laser Vision Center, 180 White Rd, Ste 202, Little Silver, NJ 07739-1166; **Phone:** 732-219-9220; **Board Cert:** Ophthalmology 1979; **Med School:** SUNY Downstate 1974; **Resid:** Ophthalmology, SUNY Downstate 1978; **Fellow:** Cornea, Eye & Ear Hosp 1979; **Fac Appt:** Assoc Clin Prof Oph, Drexel Univ Coll Med

Goldberg, Morton MD [Oph] - **Spec Exp:** Macular Disease/Degeneration; Diabetic Eye Disease/Retinopathy; Retinal Disorders; **Hospital:** Johns Hopkins Hosp (page 61); **Address:** Johns Hopkins Hosp, 600 N Wolfe St, Maumenee 713, Baltimore, MD 21287-9128; **Phone:** 410-955-6846; **Board Cert:** Ophthalmology 1968; **Med School:** Harvard Med Sch 1962; **Resid:** Ophthalmology, Wilmer Ophth Inst 1966; **Fellow:** Ophthalmology, Wilmer Ophth Inst 1967; Research, Johns Hopkins Hosp 1967; **Fac Appt:** Prof Oph, Johns Hopkins Univ

Guyton, David MD [Oph] - **Spec Exp:** Strabismus; Pediatric Ophthalmology; **Hospital:** Johns Hopkins Hosp (page 61); **Address:** Johns Hopkins Hosp, 600 N Wolfe, Wilmer 233, Baltimore, MD 21282-9028; **Phone:** 410-955-8314; **Board Cert:** Ophthalmology 1977; **Med School:** Harvard Med Sch 1969; **Resid:** Ophthalmology, Johns Hopkins Hosp 1976; **Fellow:** Pediatric Ophthalmology, Baylor Coll Med 1977; **Fac Appt:** Prof Oph, Johns Hopkins Univ

Hall, Lisabeth S MD [Oph] - **Spec Exp:** Pediatric Ophthalmology; Strabismus-Adult & Pediatric; Eye Muscle Disorders; Cataract-Pediatric; **Hospital:** New York Eye & Ear Infirm (page 64), NYU Langone Med Ctr (page 66); **Address:** 40 W 72nd St, New York, NY 10023; **Phone:** 212-979-4614; **Board Cert:** Ophthalmology 2009; **Med School:** SUNY Stony Brook 1992; **Resid:** Ophthalmology, Manhattan Eye & Ear Infirm 1996; **Fellow:** Pediatric Ophthalmology, Jules Stein Eye Inst 1997; **Fac Appt:** Assoc Prof Oph, NY Med Coll

Haller, Julia Allison MD [Oph] - **Spec Exp:** Retina/Vitreous Surgery; Retinal Disorders; **Hospital:** Wills Eye Hosp, Thomas Jefferson Univ Hosp; **Address:** 840 Walnut St, Ste 1510, Philadelphia, PA 19107; **Phone:** 215-928-3073; **Board Cert:** Ophthalmology 1987; **Med School:** Harvard Med Sch 1980; **Resid:** Ophthalmology, Wilmer Eye Inst/Johns Hopkins 1985; **Fellow:** Retina/Vitreous, Wilmer Eye Inst/Johns Hopkins 1986; **Fac Appt:** Prof Oph, Jefferson Med Coll

Handa, James T MD [Oph] - **Spec Exp:** Macular Degeneration; Melanoma-Choroidal (eye); Retinoblastoma; **Hospital:** Johns Hopkins Hosp (page 61); **Address:** 600 N Wolfe St, Maumenee Building 710, Baltimore, MD 21287; **Phone:** 410-955-3518; **Board Cert:** Ophthalmology 1991; **Med School:** Univ Pennsylvania 1986; **Resid:** Ophthalmology, Wills Eye Hosp 1990; **Fellow:** Retina/Vitreous, Duke Eye Ctr 1992; Ophthalmic Oncololgy, USC Sch Med 1993; **Fac Appt:** Assoc Prof Oph, Johns Hopkins Univ

Hersh, Peter MD [Oph] - **Spec Exp:** LASIK-Refractive Surgery; Cornea Transplant; Keratoconus; **Hospital:** Univ Hosp-UMDNJ—Newark; **Address:** Glenpointe Center East, 300 Frank W Burr Blvd, Ste 71, Teaneck, NJ 07666-6704; **Phone:** 201-883-0505; **Board Cert:** Ophthalmology 1987; **Med School:** Johns Hopkins Univ 1982; **Resid:** Internal Medicine, Lenox Hill Hosp 1983; Ophthalmology, Mass Eye & Ear Infirm 1986; **Fellow:** Cornea & Ext Eye Disease, Mass Eye & Ear Infirm 1987; **Fac Appt:** Prof Oph, UMDNJ-NJ Med Sch, Newark

Ho, Allen C MD [Oph] - **Spec Exp:** Retina/Vitreous Surgery; Macular Degeneration; Diabetic Eye Disease/Retinopathy; **Hospital:** Wills Eye Hosp, Abington Mem Hosp; **Address:** 910 E Willow Grove Ave, Mid Atlantic Retina, Wyndmoor, PA 19038; **Phone:** 215-233-4300; **Board Cert:** Ophthalmology 2004; **Med School:** Columbia P&S 1988; **Resid:** Ophthalmology, Wills Eye Hosp 1992; **Fellow:** Retina/Vitreous, Manhattan E&E Hosp 1994; **Fac Appt:** Prof Oph, Jefferson Med Coll

Iliff, Nicholas T MD [Oph] - **Spec Exp:** Oculoplastic Surgery; Orbital & Eyelid Tumors/Cancer; **Hospital:** Johns Hopkins Hosp (page 61); **Address:** Wilmer at Bayview Med Ctr, 4940 Eastern Ave, Baltimore, MD 21224; **Phone:** 410-550-2360; **Board Cert:** Ophthalmology 1978; **Med School:** Johns Hopkins Univ 1972; **Resid:** Ophthalmology, Johns Hopkins-Wilmer Inst 1977; **Fellow:** Retinal Surgery, Johns Hopkins-Wilmer Inst 1978; Oculoplastic & Reconstructive Surgery, Johns Hopkins-Wilmer Inst 1980; **Fac Appt:** Prof Oph, Johns Hopkins Univ

Ophthalmology

Jaafar, Mohamad S MD [Oph] - **Spec Exp:** Pediatric Ophthalmology; Strabismus-Adult & Pediatric; Glaucoma-Pediatric; **Hospital:** Chldns Natl Med Ctr, G Washington Univ Hosp; **Address:** Dept Ophthalmology, 111 Michigan Ave NW, Washington, DC 20010-2970; **Phone:** 202-476-3045; **Board Cert:** Ophthalmology 2008; **Med School:** Amer Univ Beirut 1978; **Resid:** Ophthalmology, Am Univ Beirut Med Ctr 1981; Ophthalmology, Washington Hosp Ctr 1994; **Fellow:** Pediatric Ophthalmology, Chldn's Hosp 1982; Pediatric Ophthalmology, Baylor Coll Med 1983; **Fac Appt:** Prof Oph, Geo Wash Univ

Jabs, Douglas MD [Oph] - **Spec Exp:** Uveitis; **Hospital:** Mount Sinai Med Ctr (page 63); **Address:** One Gustave L Levy Pl, Box 1183, New York, NY 10029; **Phone:** 212-241-6752; **Board Cert:** Ophthalmology 1982; Internal Medicine 1983; **Med School:** Johns Hopkins Univ 1977; **Resid:** Ophthalmology, Wilmer Eye Inst 1981; Internal Medicine, Johns Hopkins Hosp 1983; **Fellow:** Rheumatology, Johns Hopkins Hosp 1984; **Fac Appt:** Prof Oph, Mount Sinai Sch Med

Katowitz, James A MD [Oph] - **Spec Exp:** Oculoplastic & Orbital Surgery; Pediatric Ophthalmology; Corneal Disease & Surgery; **Hospital:** Chldns Hosp of Philadelphia, Hosp Univ Penn - UPHS (page 68); **Address:** Childrens Hosp, Div Ophthalmology, 3400 Civic Center Blvd, Wood Bldg Fl 1, Philadelphia, PA 19104; **Phone:** 215-590-2791; **Board Cert:** Ophthalmology 1969; **Med School:** Univ Pennsylvania 1963; **Resid:** Ophthalmology, Hosp Univ Penn 1967; **Fellow:** Oculoplastic Surgery, Queen Victoria Hosp 1968; Oculoplastic Surgery, Moorfield Eye Hosp 1968; **Fac Appt:** Prof Emeritus Oph, Univ Pennsylvania

Kidwell, Earl MD [Oph] - **Spec Exp:** Oculoplastic Surgery; **Hospital:** Howard Univ Hosp; **Address:** Ophthalmology Associates, 2041 Georgia Ave NW, Ste 2000, Washington, DC 20060; **Phone:** 202-865-4601; **Board Cert:** Ophthalmology 1978; **Med School:** Johns Hopkins Univ 1973; **Resid:** Ophthalmology, Johns Hopkins Hosp 1977; **Fellow:** Oculoplastic Surgery, Univ Miami Hosps 1978

Koller, Harold Paul MD [Oph] - **Spec Exp:** Pediatric Ophthalmology; Eye Muscle Surgery; Visual Perception & Learning Disorders; Strabismus; **Hospital:** Wills Eye Hosp, Abington Mem Hosp; **Address:** 1650 Huntington Pike, Ste 150, Meadowbrook, PA 19046-8001; **Phone:** 215-947-6660; **Board Cert:** Ophthalmology 1971; **Med School:** Tulane Univ 1964; **Resid:** Ophthalmology, Tulane Hosp Med Ctr 1968; **Fellow:** Pediatric Ophthalmology, Washington Chldn's Hosp 1970; **Fac Appt:** Clin Prof Oph, Thomas Jefferson Univ

Kupersmith, Mark J MD [Oph] - **Spec Exp:** Neuro-Ophthalmology; **Hospital:** St. Luke's - Roosevelt Hosp Ctr - Roosevelt Div (page 55); **Address:** Roosevelt Hosp, 1000 10th Ave, 10th Fl - INN, New York, NY 10019; **Phone:** 212-870-9418; **Board Cert:** Ophthalmology 1981; Neurology 1981; **Med School:** Northwestern Univ 1974; **Resid:** Neurology, NYU Med Ctr 1978; Ophthalmology, NYU Med Ctr 1980; **Fac Appt:** Prof Oph, Albert Einstein Coll Med

Liebmann, Jeffrey M MD [Oph] - **Spec Exp:** Glaucoma; Cataract Surgery; **Hospital:** New York Eye & Ear Infirm (page 64), Lenox Hill Hosp (Manh Eye, Ear & Throat Hosp); **Address:** 121 E 60th St Fl 8, New York, NY 10022; **Phone:** 212-477-7540; **Board Cert:** Ophthalmology 1989; **Med School:** Boston Univ 1983; **Resid:** Ophthalmology, SUNY Downstate Med Ctr 1987; **Fellow:** Glaucoma, New York EE Infirmary 1988; **Fac Appt:** Clin Prof Oph, NYU Sch Med

Lisman, Richard D MD [Oph] - **Spec Exp:** Oculoplastic Surgery; Eyelid/Tear Duct Reconstruction; Eyelid Cosmetic & Reconstructive Surgery; Orbital & Eyelid Tumors/Cancer; **Hospital:** NYU Langone Med Ctr (page 66), Lenox Hill Hosp (Manh Eye, Ear & Throat Hosp); **Address:** 635 Park Ave, New York, NY 10021-6546; **Phone:** 212-585-1405; **Board Cert:** Ophthalmology 1981; **Med School:** NYU Sch Med 1976; **Resid:** Ophthalmology, Manhattan EE Hosp 1980; **Fellow:** Ophthalmic Plastic Surgery, NY Eye & Ear Infirmary 1981; Plastic Surgery, Manhattan EE&T Hosp 1982; **Fac Appt:** Clin Prof Oph, NYU Sch Med

Mackool, Richard J MD [Oph] - **Spec Exp:** Cataract Surgery; LASIK-Refractive Surgery; Lens Implants-Multifocal; Corneal Disease & Surgery; **Hospital:** New York Eye & Ear Infirm (page 64), NYU Langone Med Ctr (page 66); **Address:** 31-27 41st St, Astoria, NY 11103; **Phone:** 718-728-3400; **Board Cert:** Ophthalmology 1975; **Med School:** Boston Univ 1968; **Resid:** Ophthalmology, New York EE Infirm 1973; **Fac Appt:** Clin Prof Oph, NYU Sch Med

Magramm, Irene MD [Oph] - **Spec Exp:** Pediatric Ophthalmology; Strabismus; Cataract Surgery; Diplopia; **Hospital:** Lenox Hill Hosp (Manh Eye, Ear & Throat Hosp), New York Eye & Ear Infirm (page 64); **Address:** 220 E 63rd St, Ste LM, New York, NY 10055; **Phone:** 212-644-5100; **Board Cert:** Ophthalmology 1987; **Med School:** Cornell Univ-Weill Med Coll 1981; **Resid:** Ophthalmology, North Shore Univ Hosp 1985; **Fellow:** Pediatric Ophthalmology, Manhattan EE&T Hosp 1986; **Fac Appt:** Asst Clin Prof Oph, Cornell Univ-Weill Med Coll

Maguire, Joseph I MD [Oph] - **Spec Exp:** Retinal Disorders; **Hospital:** Wills Eye Hosp, Lankenau Hosp; **Address:** 840 Walnut St, Ste 1020, Philadelphia, PA 19107; **Phone:** 215-928-3300; **Board Cert:** Ophthalmology 1989; **Med School:** Jefferson Med Coll 1983; **Resid:** Ophthalmology, Wills Eye Hosp 1987; **Fellow:** Retina/Vitreous, Wills Eye Hosp 1989; Retina, Moorfields Hosp 1990; **Fac Appt:** Assoc Prof Oph, Thomas Jefferson Univ

Mandel, Eric R MD [Oph] - **Spec Exp:** LASIK-Refractive Surgery; Corneal Disease; PRK-Refractive Surgery; **Hospital:** Lenox Hill Hosp; **Address:** 211 E 70th St, New York, NY 10021; **Phone:** 212-734-0111; **Board Cert:** Ophthalmology 1988; **Med School:** SUNY Stony Brook 1982; **Resid:** Ophthalmology, Lenox Hill Hosp 1986; **Fellow:** Cornea & Ext Eye Disease, Mass EE Infirm 1987

McDonnell, Peter J MD [Oph] - **Spec Exp:** Cornea Transplant; Corneal Disease; Refractive Surgery; **Hospital:** Johns Hopkins Hosp (page 61); **Address:** Johns Hopkins Hospital, Wilmer Eye Institute, 727 Maumenee, 600 N Wolfe St, Baltimore, MD 21287; **Phone:** 443-287-1511; **Board Cert:** Ophthalmology 1988; **Med School:** Johns Hopkins Univ 1982; **Resid:** Ophthalmology, Wilmer Eye Inst 1986; **Fellow:** Cornea & Ext Eye Disease, Doheny Eye Inst 1987; **Fac Appt:** Prof Oph, USC Sch Med

Medow, Norman MD [Oph] - **Spec Exp:** Cataract-Pediatric; Glaucoma-Pediatric; Corneal Disease-Pediatric; **Hospital:** Montefiore Med Ctr - Div. Moses; **Address:** Montefiore Hosp Ctr, Dept Ophthalmology, 3332 Rochambeau Ave, rm 306, Bronx, NY 10467; **Phone:** 718-920-6178; **Board Cert:** Ophthalmology 1975; **Med School:** SUNY Hlth Sci Ctr 1966; **Resid:** Ophthalmology, Manhattan EE&T Hosp 1972; **Fellow:** Cataract/Lens Implant Surgery, Charles Kelman, MD 1973; **Fac Appt:** Assoc Clin Prof Oph, Cornell Univ-Weill Med Coll

Miller, Neil MD [Oph] - **Spec Exp:** Neuro-Ophthalmology; Orbital Diseases; Thyroid Eye Disease; **Hospital:** Johns Hopkins Hosp (page 61); **Address:** Johns Hopkins - Wilmer Eye Inst, 600 N Wolfe St Wilmer Bldg - rm 233, Baltimore, MD 21287-0001; **Phone:** 410-955-8679; **Board Cert:** Ophthalmology 1976; **Med School:** Johns Hopkins Univ 1971; **Resid:** Ophthalmology, Johns Hopkins Hosp 1975; **Fellow:** Neuro-Ophthalmology, UCSF Med Ctr 1975; **Fac Appt:** Prof Oph, Johns Hopkins Univ

Mills, Monte D MD [Oph] - **Spec Exp:** Pediatric Ophthalmology; Eye Muscle Disorders; Strabismus; **Hospital:** Chldns Hosp of Philadelphia; **Address:** Chldns Hosp, Dept Ophthalmology, 3400 Civic Center Blvd, Wood Bldg Fl 1, Philadelphia, PA 19104; **Phone:** 215-590-2791; **Board Cert:** Ophthalmology 2004; **Med School:** Baylor Coll Med 1988; **Resid:** Ophthalmology, Mass Eye & Ear Infirm 1992; **Fellow:** Pediatric Ophthalmology, Chldns Hosp 1993; **Fac Appt:** Assoc Clin Prof Oph, Univ Pennsylvania

Muldoon, Thomas O MD [Oph] - **Spec Exp:** Retina/Vitreous Surgery; Macular Disease/Degeneration; Diabetic Eye Disease/Retinopathy; **Hospital:** New York Eye & Ear Infirm (page 64); **Address:** 310 E 14th St, Ste 402, New York, NY 10003-4201; **Phone:** 212-979-4595; **Board Cert:** Ophthalmology 1971; **Med School:** Univ Rochester 1962; **Resid:** Surgery, St Lukes Hosp 1966; Ophthalmology, NY EE Infirm 1969; **Fellow:** Retinal Surgery, NY EE Infirm 1970; **Fac Appt:** Assoc Clin Prof Oph, NY Med Coll

Myers, Jonathan S MD [Oph] - **Spec Exp:** Glaucoma; **Hospital:** Wills Eye Hosp; **Address:** Wills Eye Inst, 840 Walnut St, Ste 1110, Philadelphia, PA 19107; **Phone:** 215-928-3197; **Board Cert:** Ophthalmology 2008; **Med School:** Univ Pennsylvania 1992; **Resid:** Ophthalmology, Wills Eye Hosp 1996; **Fellow:** Glaucoma, Duke Univ Med Ctr 1997; **Fac Appt:** Asst Prof Oph, Thomas Jefferson Univ

Nelson, Leonard B MD [Oph] - **Spec Exp:** Pediatric Ophthalmology; Strabismus; Eye Muscle Disorders; **Hospital:** Wills Eye Hosp; **Address:** Wills Eye Hospital, 840 Walnut St, Ste 1210, Philadelphia, PA 19107; **Phone:** 215-928-3244; **Board Cert:** Ophthalmology 1981; **Med School:** Harvard Med Sch 1976; **Resid:** Ophthalmology, Bellevue Hosp Ctr-NYU 1980; **Fellow:** Pediatric Ophthalmology, Chldns Hosp Med Ctr 1981; Ocular Disease, Johns Hopkins Hosp 1982; **Fac Appt:** Assoc Prof Oph, Jefferson Med Coll

O'Brien, Joan M MD [Oph] - **Spec Exp:** Eye Tumors/Cancer; Retinoblastoma; **Hospital:** Hosp Univ Penn - UPHS (page 68); **Address:** Penn Presbyterian Med Ctr, Scheie Eye Inst, 51 N 39th St, Philadelphia, PA 19104; **Phone:** 215-662-8100; **Board Cert:** Ophthalmology 2007; **Med School:** Dartmouth Med Sch 1986; **Resid:** Ophthalmology, Mass Eye & Ear Infirm 1992; **Fellow:** Ophthalmic Pathology, Mass Eye & Ear Infirm 1989; Ophthalmological Pathology, UCSF Med Ctr 1993; **Fac Appt:** Prof Oph, Univ Pennsylvania

Odel, Jeffrey G MD [Oph] - **Spec Exp:** Neuro-Ophthalmology; Retinal Disorders; Optic Nerve Disorders; **Hospital:** NY-Presby/Columbia Univ Med Ctr, NY (page 65); **Address:** Harkness Eye Institute, 635 W 165th St, rm 316, New York, NY 10032-3701; **Phone:** 212-305-5415; **Board Cert:** Ophthalmology 1981; **Med School:** Univ Rochester 1975; **Resid:** Ophthalmology, Mt Sinai Hosp 1981; **Fellow:** Ophthalmology, Bascom-Palmer Eye Inst 1977; Ophthalmology, Columbia Presby Med Ctr 1982; **Fac Appt:** Assoc Clin Prof Oph, Columbia P&S

Orlin, Stephen E MD [Oph] - **Spec Exp:** Cataract Surgery; Corneal Disease & Surgery; Refractive Surgery; **Hospital:** Penn Presby Med Ctr - UPHS (page 68), Hosp Univ Penn - UPHS (page 68); **Address:** Univ Penn Scheie Eye Inst, 51 N 39th St, Philadelphia, PA 19104; **Phone:** 215-662-8022; **Board Cert:** Ophthalmology 1987; **Med School:** South Africa 1977; **Resid:** Ophthalmology, Scheie Eye Inst 1985; **Fellow:** Cornea & Ext Eye Disease, Scheiev Eye Inst 1986; **Fac Appt:** Assoc Prof Oph, Univ Pennsylvania

Quigley, Harry A MD [Oph] - **Spec Exp:** Glaucoma; **Hospital:** Johns Hopkins Hosp (page 61); **Address:** 600 N Wolfe St, Maumenee B-110, Baltimore, MD 21287-9205; **Phone:** 410-955-6052; **Board Cert:** Ophthalmology 1976; **Med School:** Johns Hopkins Univ 1971; **Resid:** Ophthalmology, Wilmer Inst-Johns Hopkins Hosp 1975; **Fellow:** Ophthalmology, Bascom Palmer Eye Inst 1977; **Fac Appt:** Prof Oph, Johns Hopkins Univ

Quinn, Graham E MD [Oph] - **Spec Exp:** Pediatric Ophthalmology; Eye Growth/Development; **Hospital:** Chldns Hosp of Philadelphia; **Address:** Chldns Hosp of Philadelphia, Div Ophthalmology, 3400 Civic Center Blvd, Wood Bldg Fl 1, Philadelphia, PA 19104-4399; **Phone:** 215-590-2791; **Board Cert:** Ophthalmology 1979; **Med School:** Duke Univ 1973; **Resid:** Pathology, Metro Genl Hosp 1975; Ophthalmology, Hosp Univ Penn 1978; **Fellow:** Pediatric Ophthalmology, Childrens Hosp 1979; **Fac Appt:** Prof Oph, Univ Pennsylvania

Regillo, Carl D MD [Oph] - **Spec Exp:** Retinal Disorders; **Hospital:** Wills Eye Hosp, Thomas Jefferson Univ Hosp; **Address:** Mid Atlantic Retina, 910 E Willow Grove Ave, Wyndmoor, PA 19038; **Phone:** 800-331-6634; **Board Cert:** Ophthalmology 2004; **Med School:** Harvard Med Sch 1988; **Resid:** Ophthalmology, Wills Eye Hosp 1992; **Fellow:** Retinal Surgery, Wills Eye Hosp 1994; **Fac Appt:** Prof Oph, Jefferson Med Coll

Reynolds, James D MD [Oph] - **Spec Exp:** Pediatric Ophthalmology; Strabismus; Retinopathy of Prematurity; **Hospital:** Women's & Chldn's Hosp of Buffalo, The; **Address:** Ross Eye Institute, 1176 Main St, Buffalo, NY 14209; **Phone:** 716-881-7900; **Board Cert:** Ophthalmology 1982; **Med School:** SUNY Buffalo 1978; **Resid:** Ophthalmology, Erie Co Med Ctr 1981; **Fellow:** Pediatric Ophthalmology, Pittsburgh EE Hospital 1982; **Fac Appt:** Prof Oph, SUNY Buffalo

Ritch, Robert MD [Oph] - **Spec Exp:** Glaucoma; **Hospital:** New York Eye & Ear Infirm (page 64); **Address:** 310 E 14th St, rm 304S, New York, NY 10003-4201; **Phone:** 212-477-7540; **Board Cert:** Ophthalmology 1977; **Med School:** Albert Einstein Coll Med 1972; **Resid:** Ophthalmology, Mt Sinai Hosp 1976; **Fellow:** Glaucoma, Mt Sinai Hosp 1978; **Fac Appt:** Clin Prof Oph, NY Med Coll

Schein, Oliver D MD [Oph] - **Spec Exp:** Cataract Surgery; Corneal Disease & Surgery; **Hospital:** Johns Hopkins Hosp (page 61); **Address:** Johns Hopkins Hosp, 600 N Wolfe St, Maumenee 317, Baltimore, MD 21287; **Phone:** 410-955-7677; **Board Cert:** Internal Medicine 1984; Ophthalmology 1990; **Med School:** Johns Hopkins Univ 1981; **Resid:** Internal Medicine, Johns Hopkins Hosp 1984; Ophthalmology, Mass Eye & Ear Infirm 1987; **Fellow:** Cornea & Ext Eye Disease, Mass Eye & Ear Infirm 1988; **Fac Appt:** Prof Oph, Johns Hopkins Univ

Schiff, William M MD [Oph] - **Spec Exp:** Macular Disease/Degeneration; Diabetic Eye Disease/Retinopathy; Retinal Detachment; Macular Disease/Degeneration; **Hospital:** NY-Presby/Columbia Univ Med Ctr, NY (page 65), St. Luke's - Roosevelt Hosp Ctr - Roosevelt Div (page 55); **Address:** Columbia Ophthalmic Consultants, 635 W 165th St, New York, NY 10032; **Phone:** 212-305-9535; **Board Cert:** Ophthalmology 2006; **Med School:** NYU Sch Med 1988; **Resid:** Ophthalmology, New York Eye & Ear Infirm 1994; **Fellow:** Retina/Vitreous, NY Hosp-Harkness Eye Inst 1996; **Fac Appt:** Prof Oph, Columbia P&S

Schuman, Joel S MD [Oph] - **Spec Exp:** Glaucoma; Cataract Surgery; **Hospital:** UPMC Presby, Pittsburgh, UPMC Shadyside; **Address:** Eye & Ear Institute, Ste 816, 203 Lothrop St, Pittsburgh, PA 15213; **Phone:** 412-647-2200; **Board Cert:** Ophthalmology 1990; **Med School:** Mount Sinai Sch Med 1984; **Resid:** Ophthalmology, Med Coll Virginia Hosps 1988; **Fellow:** Glaucoma, Mass EE Infirmary 1990; **Fac Appt:** Prof Oph, Univ Pittsburgh

Sergott, Robert C MD [Oph] - **Spec Exp:** Neuro-Ophthalmology; Optic Nerve Disorders; Glaucoma; Thyroid Eye Disease; **Hospital:** Thomas Jefferson Univ Hosp, Wills Eye Hosp; **Address:** Wills Eye Hosp, Dept Neuro-Opthalmology, 840 Walnut St Fl 9 - Ste 930, Philadelphia, PA 19107; **Phone:** 215-928-3130; **Board Cert:** Ophthalmology 1982; **Med School:** Johns Hopkins Univ 1975; **Resid:** Internal Medicine, Mary Imogene Bassett Hosp 1976; Ophthalmology, Jackson Meml Hosp 1980; **Fellow:** Ophthalmology, Jackson Meml Hosp 1980

Shabto, Uri MD [Oph] - **Spec Exp:** Retinopathy of Prematurity; Macular Disease/Degeneration; Diabetic Eye Disease/Retinopathy; **Hospital:** New York Eye & Ear Infirm (page 64); **Address:** 310 E 14th St South Bldg - Ste 419, New York, NY 10003-4201; **Phone:** 212-677-2000; **Board Cert:** Ophthalmology 1991; **Med School:** Harvard Med Sch 1986; **Resid:** Ophthalmology, NY Eye & Ear Infirm 1990; **Fellow:** Vitreoretinal Surgery, Montefiore Hosp 1991; **Fac Appt:** Asst Prof Oph, NYU Sch Med

Ophthalmology

Shields, Carol L MD [Oph] - **Spec Exp:** Orbital Tumors/Cancer; Melanoma-Choroidal (eye); Retinoblastoma; Pediatric Ophthalmology; **Hospital:** Wills Eye Hosp, Jefferson Reg Med Ctr - Pittsburgh; **Address:** Wills Eye Inst, Ocular Oncology Service, 840 Walnut St, Ste 1440, Phildelphia, PA 19107; **Phone:** 215-928-3105; **Board Cert:** Ophthalmology 1989; **Med School:** Univ Pittsburgh 1983; **Resid:** Ophthalmology, Willis Eye Hosp 1988; **Fellow:** Ophthalmic Pathology, Willis Eye Hosp 1988; Ophthalmic Oncololgy, Willis Eye Hosp 1989; **Fac Appt:** Prof Oph, Jefferson Med Coll

Shields, Jerry MD [Oph] - **Spec Exp:** Eye Tumors/Cancer; Pediatric Ophthalmology; Retinoblastoma; Melanoma-Choroidal (eye); **Hospital:** Wills Eye Hosp, Thomas Jefferson Univ Hosp; **Address:** Wills Eye Hosp, Ocular Oncology Svce, 840 Walnut St, Ste 1440, Philadelphia, PA 19107; **Phone:** 215-928-3105; **Board Cert:** Ophthalmology 1972; **Med School:** Univ Mich Med Sch 1964; **Resid:** Ophthalmology, Wills Eye Hosp 1970; **Fellow:** Ophthalmology, Wills Eye Hosp 1972; **Fac Appt:** Prof Oph, Thomas Jefferson Univ

Simon, John W MD [Oph] - **Spec Exp:** Pediatric Ophthalmology; Strabismus; **Hospital:** Albany Med Ctr, St. Peter's Hosp - Albany; **Address:** 1220 New Scotland Rd, Ste 202, Slingerlands, NY 12159; **Phone:** 518-533-6502; **Board Cert:** Ophthalmology 1981; **Med School:** Mount Sinai Sch Med 1976; **Resid:** Ophthalmology, Mt Sinai Hosp 1980; **Fellow:** Pediatric Ophthalmology, Wills Eye Hosp 1981; **Fac Appt:** Prof Oph, Albany Med Coll

Smith, Scott D MD [Oph] - **Spec Exp:** Glaucoma; **Hospital:** NY-Presby/Columbia Univ Med Ctr, NY (page 65); **Address:** Edward Harkness Eye Inst, 635 W 165th St, New York, NY 10030; **Phone:** 212-305-9535; **Board Cert:** Ophthalmology 2006; **Med School:** Yale Univ 1990; **Resid:** Ophthalmology, Mass Eye & Ear Infirm 1994; **Fellow:** Glaucoma, Wilmer Eye Inst 1996; **Fac Appt:** Assoc Prof Oph, Columbia P&S

Stark, Walter J MD [Oph] - **Spec Exp:** Corneal Disease & Transplant; Cataract Surgery; Refractive Surgery; **Hospital:** Johns Hopkins Hosp (page 61); **Address:** Wilmer Eye Inst, 600 N Wolfe St Maumenee Bldg - rm 327, Baltimore, MD 21287-9238; **Phone:** 410-955-5490; **Board Cert:** Ophthalmology 1973; **Med School:** Univ Okla Coll Med 1967; **Resid:** Ophthalmology, Wilmer Inst-Johns Hopkins 1971; **Fac Appt:** Prof Oph, Johns Hopkins Univ

Stefanyszyn, Mary MD [Oph] - **Spec Exp:** Cosmetic Surgery-Eyes; Oculoplastic & Orbital Surgery; Eyelid Surgery; **Hospital:** Wills Eye Hosp; **Address:** Wills Eye Hosp, 840 Walnut St, Ste 912, Philadelphia, PA 19107; **Phone:** 215-928-3171; **Board Cert:** Ophthalmology 1983; **Med School:** Harvard Med Sch 1978; **Resid:** Ophthalmology, Wills Eye Hosp 1982; Ophthalmic Pathology, Armed Forces Inst of Pathology 1982; **Fellow:** Oculoplastic & Reconstructive Surgery, Wills Eye Hosp 1983; Orbital Surgery, Moorfields Eye Hosp 1985

Sterns, Gwen K MD [Oph] - **Spec Exp:** Geriatric Ophthalmology; Low Vision; **Hospital:** Rochester Genl Hosp, Univ of Rochester Strong Meml Hosp; **Address:** 1425 Portland Ave, Box 224, Ophthalmology Dept, Rochester, NY 14621; **Phone:** 585-922-4794; **Board Cert:** Ophthalmology 1976; **Med School:** Med Coll PA 1970; **Resid:** Ophthalmology, Nassau Co Med Ctr 1974; **Fellow:** Ophthalmology, Colum-Presby Eye Inst 1975; **Fac Appt:** Assoc Prof Oph, Univ Rochester

Vander, James F MD [Oph] - **Spec Exp:** Diabetic Eye Disease/Retinopathy; Retinal Disorders; Macular Degeneration; **Hospital:** Wills Eye Hosp; **Address:** Mid Atlantic Retina, 910 E Willow Grove Ave, Wyndmoor, PA 19038-7910; **Phone:** 215-233-4300; **Board Cert:** Ophthalmology 1989; **Med School:** Univ Mich Med Sch 1984; **Resid:** Ophthalmology, Univ Michigan Med Ctr 1988; **Fellow:** Retina/Vitreous, Wills Eye Hosp 1990; **Fac Appt:** Prof Oph, Thomas Jefferson Univ

Walsh, Joseph B MD [Oph] - **Spec Exp:** Diabetic Eye Disease/Retinopathy; Macular Degeneration; Retinal Disorders; **Hospital:** New York Eye & Ear Infirm (page 64), Beth Israel Med Ctr - Petrie Division (page 55); **Address:** 310 E 14th St Bldg S Fl 3, New York, NY 10003-4201; **Phone:** 212-979-4500; **Board Cert:** Ophthalmology 2005; **Med School:** Georgetown Univ 1966; **Resid:** Internal Medicine, Univ Hosp 1968; Ophthalmology, NY Eye & Ear Infirm 1973; **Fellow:** Retina, Montefiore Med Ctr 1974; **Fac Appt:** Prof Oph, NY Med Coll

Wang, Frederick MD [Oph] - **Spec Exp:** Pediatric Ophthalmology; Strabismus; Eye Muscle Disorders; **Hospital:** New York Eye & Ear Infirm (page 64), Montefiore Med Ctr - Div. Moses; **Address:** 30 E 40th St, Ste 405, New York, NY 10016-1201; **Phone:** 212-684-3980; **Board Cert:** Pediatrics 1978; Ophthalmology 1980; **Med School:** Albert Einstein Coll Med 1972; **Resid:** Pediatrics, Jacobi Med Ctr 1974; Ophthalmology, Albert Einstein 1979; **Fellow:** Pediatric Ophthalmology, Children's Hosp Natl Med Ctr 1980; **Fac Appt:** Clin Prof Oph, Albert Einstein Coll Med

Yannuzzi, Lawrence MD [Oph] - **Spec Exp:** Retina/Vitreous Surgery; Macular Disease/Degeneration; Diabetic Eye Disease/Retinopathy; **Hospital:** NY-Presby/Columbia Univ Med Ctr, NY (page 65), Lenox Hill Hosp (Manh Eye, Ear & Throat Hosp); **Address:** 460 Park Ave Fl 5, New York, NY 10022; **Phone:** 212-861-9797; **Board Cert:** Ophthalmology 1970; **Med School:** Boston Univ 1964; **Resid:** Ophthalmology, Manhattan EE&T Hosp 1968; **Fellow:** Ophthalmology, Manhattan EE&T Hosp 1971; **Fac Appt:** Clin Prof Oph, Columbia P&S

Zaidman, Gerald MD [Oph] - **Spec Exp:** Laser Vision Surgery; Cornea Transplant; Cataract Surgery; Corneal Disease-Pediatric; **Hospital:** Westchester Med Ctr, Montefiore Med Ctr - Div. North; **Address:** Westchester Med Ctr, Macy Pavilion, Dept Ophthalmology, rm 1100, Valhalla, NY 10595; **Phone:** 914-493-1599; **Board Cert:** Ophthalmology 1981; **Med School:** Albert Einstein Coll Med 1975; **Resid:** Ophthalmology, Beth Abraham Hosp 1977; Ophthalmology, Lenox Hill Hosp 1980; **Fellow:** Cornea & Ext Eye Disease, Univ Pittsburgh 1982; **Fac Appt:** Assoc Prof Oph, NY Med Coll

Southeast

Afshari, Natalie A MD [Oph] - **Spec Exp:** Cataract Surgery; Cornea Transplant; LASIK-Refractive Surgery; PRK-Refractive Surgery; **Hospital:** Duke Univ Hosp; **Address:** Duke Eye Center at DUMC, 2351 Erwin Rd, Box 3802, Durham, NC 27710; **Phone:** 919-684-3799; **Board Cert:** Ophthalmology 2011; **Med School:** Stanford Univ 1995; **Resid:** Ophthalmology, Mass Eye & Ear Infirmary 1999; **Fellow:** Cornea & Refractive Surgery, Mass Eye & Ear Infirmary 2001

Alfonso, Eduardo MD [Oph] - **Spec Exp:** Corneal Disease & Surgery; Cornea Transplant & Artificial Cornea; **Hospital:** Bascom Palmer Eye Inst (page 71), Jackson Meml Hosp (page 70); **Address:** Bascom Palmer Eye Institute, 900 NW 17th St, Miami, FL 33136-1119; **Phone:** 305-243-2020; **Board Cert:** Ophthalmology 1985; **Med School:** Yale Univ 1980; **Resid:** Ophthalmology, Bascom Palmer Eye Inst 1984; **Fellow:** Cornea, Mass Eye & Ear Hosp 1986; Ophthalmological Pathology, Mass Eye & Ear Hosp 1986; **Fac Appt:** Prof Oph, Univ Miami Sch Med

Biousse, Valerie MD [Oph] - **Spec Exp:** Neuro-Ophthalmology; Optic Nerve Disorders; **Hospital:** Emory Univ Hosp; **Address:** Emory Eye Center, 1365 Clifton Rd NE B Bldg - Ste 4500, Atlanta, GA 30322; **Phone:** 404-778-2020; **Board Cert:** Ophthalmology 2004; **Med School:** France 1988; **Resid:** Neurology, Univ Paris VI Affil Hosp 1994; Ophthalmology, Emory Univ Med Ctr 2002; **Fellow:** Stroke, Univ Paris VI 1996; Neuro-Ophthalmology, Emory Univ 1996; **Fac Appt:** Prof Oph, Emory Univ

Ophthalmology

Buckley, Edward G MD [Oph] - **Spec Exp:** Pediatric Ophthalmology; Strabismus; Cataract-Pediatric; Neuro-Ophthalmology; **Hospital:** Duke Univ Hosp; **Address:** Duke Eye Center, 2352 Erwin Rd, Box 3802, Durham, NC 27710; **Phone:** 919-681-3937; **Board Cert:** Ophthalmology 2007; **Med School:** Duke Univ 1977; **Resid:** Ophthalmology, Duke Univ Eye Ctr 1981; **Fellow:** Pediatric Ophthalmology, Bascom Palmer Eye Inst 1983; Neuro-Ophthalmology, Bascom Palmer Eye Inst 1983; **Fac Appt:** Prof Oph, Duke Univ

Budenz, Donald L MD [Oph] - **Spec Exp:** Glaucoma; **Hospital:** Bascom Palmer Eye Inst (page 71); **Address:** Bascom Palmer Eye Inst, 900 NW 17th St, Ste 341, Miami, FL 33136; **Phone:** 305-543-2020; **Board Cert:** Ophthalmology 2003; **Med School:** Harvard Med Sch 1987; **Resid:** Ophthalmology, Scheie Eye Inst 1991; **Fellow:** Glaucoma, Bascom Palmer Eye Inst 1992; **Fac Appt:** Assoc Prof Oph, Univ Miami Sch Med

Capo, Hilda MD [Oph] - **Spec Exp:** Pediatric Ophthalmology; Strabismus; Neuro-Ophthalmology; **Hospital:** Bascom Palmer Eye Inst (page 71); **Address:** Bascom Palmer Eye Institute, 900 NW 17th St, Miami, FL 33136; **Phone:** 305-243-2020; **Board Cert:** Ophthalmology 1989; **Med School:** Puerto Rico 1982; **Resid:** Ophthalmology, Univ Puerto Rico Affil Hosp 1987; **Fellow:** Neuro-Ophthalmology, NYU Med Ctr 1989; Pediatric Ophthalmology, Johns Hopkins Hosp 1988; **Fac Appt:** Clin Prof Oph, Univ Miami Sch Med

Carlson, Alan N MD [Oph] - **Spec Exp:** Cornea & External Eye Disease; Cornea Transplant; LASIK-Refractive Surgery; **Hospital:** Duke Univ Hosp; **Address:** Duke Univ Eye Center, Box 3802, Durham, NC 27710; **Phone:** 919-684-5769; **Board Cert:** Ophthalmology 1988; **Med School:** Duke Univ 1982; **Resid:** Ophthalmology, Baylor Med Ctr 1986; **Fellow:** Cornea & Ext Eye Disease, Baylor Med Ctr 1987; Cornea & Ext Eye Disease, Duke Univ Med Ctr 1988; **Fac Appt:** Prof Oph, Duke Univ

Culbertson, William MD [Oph] - **Spec Exp:** LASIK-Refractive Surgery; Corneal Disease & Surgery; Cataract Surgery; **Hospital:** Bascom Palmer Eye Inst (page 71); **Address:** Bascom Palmer Eye Institute, 900 NW 17th St, Miami, FL 33136-1119; **Phone:** 305-243-2020; **Board Cert:** Ophthalmology 1976; **Med School:** Emory Univ 1970; **Resid:** Ophthalmology, Vanderbilt Univ Hosp 1974; **Fellow:** Cornea & Ext Eye Disease, Bascom Palmer Eye Inst 1979; **Fac Appt:** Prof Oph, Univ Miami Sch Med

Davis, Janet L MD [Oph] - **Spec Exp:** Uveitis; Retina/Vitreous Surgery; Macular Degeneration; Diabetic Eye Disease/Retinopathy; **Hospital:** Bascom Palmer Eye Inst (page 71); **Address:** Bascom Palmer Eye Inst, 900 NW 17th St, Miami, FL 33136-1119; **Phone:** 305-243-2020; **Board Cert:** Ophthalmology 2006; **Med School:** Baylor Coll Med 1981; **Resid:** Ophthalmology, Baylor Affil Hosp 1986; **Fellow:** Vitreoretinal Surgery, Bascom Palmer Eye Inst 1987; Ocular Immunology, NIH-Natl Eye Inst 1989; **Fac Appt:** Prof Oph, Univ Miami Sch Med

Dutton, Jonathan J MD/PhD [Oph] - **Spec Exp:** Oculoplastic Surgery; Eye Tumors/Cancer; Melanoma-Choroidal (eye); **Hospital:** NC Memorial Hosp - UNC; **Address:** Univ North Carolina - Dept Ophthalmology, 130 Mason Farm Rd, 5156 Bioinformatics, CB 7040, Chapel Hill, NC 27599; **Phone:** 919-966-5296; **Board Cert:** Ophthalmology 1983; **Med School:** Washington Univ, St Louis 1977; **Resid:** Ophthalmology, Washington Univ Med Ctr 1982; **Fellow:** Oculoplastic Surgery, Univ Iowa Med Ctr 1983; **Fac Appt:** Prof Oph, Univ NC Sch Med

Flynn Jr, Harry W MD [Oph] - **Spec Exp:** Retina/Vitreous Surgery; Diabetic Eye Disease/Retinopathy; **Hospital:** Bascom Palmer Eye Inst (page 71), Univ of Miami Hosp & Clins/Sylvester Comp Canc Ctr (page 73); **Address:** Bascom Palmer Eye Institute, 900 NW 17th St, Miami, FL 33136-1119; **Phone:** 305-243-2020; **Board Cert:** Ophthalmology 1976; **Med School:** Univ VA Sch Med 1971; **Resid:** Ophthalmology, Univ Virginia Hosp 1975; **Fellow:** Retina, Pacific Med Ctr 1976; **Fac Appt:** Prof Oph, Univ Miami Sch Med

Forster, Richard K MD [Oph] - **Spec Exp:** Cornea Transplant; Cataract Surgery; **Hospital:** Bascom Palmer Eye Inst (page 71); **Address:** Bascom Palmer Eye Institute, 900 NW 17th St, Miami, FL 33136; **Phone:** 305-243-2020; **Board Cert:** Ophthalmology 1971; **Med School:** Boston Univ 1963; **Resid:** Ophthalmology, Bascom Palmer Eye Inst 1969; **Fellow:** Ophthalmology, Fl Proctor Fdn/UCSF 1970; **Fac Appt:** Prof Oph, Univ Miami Sch Med

Freedman, Sharon F MD [Oph] - **Spec Exp:** Pediatric Ophthalmology; Glaucoma-Pediatric; Strabismus; Retinopathy of Prematurity; **Hospital:** Duke Univ Hosp; **Address:** Duke Eye Center, 2352 Erwin Rd, Box 3802, Durham, NC 27710; **Phone:** 919-681-3937; **Board Cert:** Ophthalmology 1991; **Med School:** Harvard Med Sch 1985; **Resid:** Ophthalmology, Mass Eye & Ear Infirm 1989; **Fellow:** Pediatric Ophthalmology, Childns Hosp 1990; Glaucoma, Duke Eye Ctr 1992; **Fac Appt:** Prof Oph, Duke Univ

Gorovoy, Mark S MD [Oph] - **Spec Exp:** Corneal Disease & Transplant; Cataract Surgery; Glaucoma; LASIK-Refractive Surgery; **Hospital:** Lee Memorial Hlth Systems; **Address:** 12381 S Cleveland Ave, Ste 300, Fort Myers, FL 33907; **Phone:** 239-939-1444; **Board Cert:** Ophthalmology 1982; **Med School:** Geo Wash Univ 1973; **Resid:** Ophthalmology, Geo Washington Univ Hosp 1980; **Fellow:** Cornea & Ext Eye Disease, Univ Florida 1982

Greenfield, David S MD [Oph] - **Spec Exp:** Glaucoma; Cataract Surgery-Lens Implant; **Hospital:** Bascom Palmer Eye Inst (page 71); **Address:** Bascom Palmer Eye Inst, 7101 Fairway Drive, Palm Beach Gardens, FL 33418; **Phone:** 561-515-1500; **Board Cert:** Ophthalmology 2007; **Med School:** NYU Sch Med 1990; **Resid:** Ophthalmology, New England Eye Center 1994; **Fellow:** Glaucoma, Bascom Palmer Eye Inst 1995; Neuro-Ophthalmology, Bascom Palmer Eye Inst 1995; **Fac Appt:** Prof Oph, Univ Miami Sch Med

Grossniklaus, Hans E MD [Oph] - **Spec Exp:** Ophthalmic Pathology; Melanoma-Choroidal (eye); Macular Disease/Degeneration; Retinal Disorders; **Hospital:** Emory Univ Hosp; **Address:** Emory Clinic - LF Montgomery Lab, 1365-B Clifton Rd NE, rm BT428, Atlanta, GA 30322; **Phone:** 404-778-4611; **Board Cert:** Ophthalmology 1985; Anatomic Pathology 1987; **Med School:** Ohio State Univ 1980; **Resid:** Ophthalmology, Case West Res Univ Hosp 1984; Pathology, Case West Res Univ Hosp 1987; **Fellow:** Ophthalmological Pathology, Johns Hopkins Hosp 1985; **Fac Appt:** Prof Oph, Emory Univ

Guy, John R MD [Oph] - **Spec Exp:** Neuro-Ophthalmology; **Hospital:** Bascom Palmer Eye Inst (page 71); **Address:** Bascom Palmer Eye Inst, 900 NW 17th St Fl 4, Miami, FL 33136; **Phone:** 305-243-2020; **Board Cert:** Ophthalmology 1983; **Med School:** Univ Miami Sch Med 1977; **Resid:** Neurology, Temple Univ Hosp 1979; Ophthalmology, Georgetown Univ Med Ctr 1988; **Fellow:** Neuro-Ophthalmology, Willis Eye Hosp 1983; **Fac Appt:** Assoc Prof Oph, Univ Miami Sch Med

Haik, Barrett MD [Oph] - **Spec Exp:** Eye Tumors/Cancer; Orbital Diseases; **Hospital:** St. Jude Children's Research Hosp; **Address:** Univ Tenn Med Group, Ophthamology, 930 Madison Ave, Ste 400, Memphis, TN 38103-3452; **Phone:** 901-448-6650; **Board Cert:** Ophthalmology 1981; **Med School:** Louisiana State U, New Orleans 1976; **Resid:** Ophthalmology, Columbia-Presby/Harkness Eye Inst 1980; **Fac Appt:** Prof Oph, Univ Tenn Coll Med

Hess, J Bruce MD [Oph] - **Spec Exp:** Pediatric Ophthalmology; Strabismus; **Hospital:** All Children's Hosp, Bayfront Med Ctr; **Address:** 601 5th St S, Ste 601, St Petersburg, FL 33701; **Phone:** 727-767-4393; **Board Cert:** Ophthalmology 1978; **Med School:** Baylor Coll Med 1971; **Resid:** Ophthalmology, Geisinger Med Ctr 1977; **Fellow:** Ophthalmology, Wills Eye Hosp 1978; **Fac Appt:** Assoc Prof Oph, Univ S Fla Coll Med

Ophthalmology

Hodapp, Elizabeth A MD [Oph] - **Spec Exp:** Pediatric Glaucoma; **Hospital:** Bascom Palmer Eye Inst (page 71); **Address:** Bascom Palmer Eye Inst, 900 NW 17th St, Miami, FL 33136; **Phone:** 305-243-2020; **Board Cert:** Ophthalmology 1980; **Med School:** Harvard Med Sch 1975; **Resid:** Ophthalmology, Wash Univ Affil Hosp 1979; **Fellow:** Glaucoma, Washington Univ 1981

Kerr, Natalie C MD [Oph] - **Spec Exp:** Pediatric Ophthalmology; Strabismus; Cataract-Pediatric; Genetic Disorders-Eye; **Hospital:** Le Bonheur Chldns Med Ctr, St. Jude Children's Research Hosp; **Address:** Hamilton Eye Inst, 930 Madison Ave, Ste 400, Memphis, TN 38103; **Phone:** 901-448-6650; **Board Cert:** Ophthalmology 2003; **Med School:** Univ Fla Coll Med 1987; **Resid:** Ophthalmology, Univ FL Affil Hosp 1991; **Fellow:** Pediatric Ophthalmology, Univ TN Affil Hosp 1992; **Fac Appt:** Prof Oph, Univ Tenn Coll Med

Lambert, Scott R MD [Oph] - **Spec Exp:** Pediatric Ophthalmology; Strabismus; Cataract-Pediatric; **Hospital:** Chldns Hlthcare Atlanta @ Egleston, Emory Univ Hosp; **Address:** Emory Eye Center, Pediatric Ophthalmology Clinic, 1365B Clifton Rd NE, Ste 4513, Atlanta, GA 30322; **Phone:** 404-778-3431; **Board Cert:** Ophthalmology 1989; **Med School:** Yale Univ 1983; **Resid:** Ophthalmology, UCSF Med Ctr 1987; **Fellow:** Pediatric Ophthalmology, Hosp for Sick Chldn 1988; Strabismus, Smith Kuttlewell 1988; **Fac Appt:** Prof Oph, Emory Univ

Lee, Paul P MD [Oph] - **Spec Exp:** Glaucoma; **Hospital:** Duke Univ Hosp; **Address:** Duke Univ Med Ctr, 2352 Erwin Rd, Box 3802, Durham, NC 27710; **Phone:** 919-681-3937; **Board Cert:** Ophthalmology 1991; **Med School:** Univ Mich Med Sch 1986; **Resid:** Ophthalmology, Wilmer Eye Inst/Johns Hopkins 1990; **Fellow:** Glaucoma, Mass EE Infirm 1991; **Fac Appt:** Prof Oph, Duke Univ

Mawn, Louise MD [Oph] - **Spec Exp:** Orbital Surgery; Reconstructive Surgery; Neuro-Ophthalmology; Eyelid/Tear Duct Reconstruction; **Hospital:** Vanderbilt Univ Med Ctr (page 76); **Address:** Vanderbilt Eye Institute, 2311 Pierce Ave, Nashville, TN 37232; **Phone:** 615-936-2020; **Board Cert:** Ophthalmology 2008; **Med School:** Wake Forest Univ 1990; **Resid:** Ophthalmology, Univ Iowa Hosps & Clin 1995; **Fellow:** Neuro-Ophthalmology, New England Med Ctr 1996; Ophthalmic Plastic & Reconstructive Surgery, Univ Ottawa Eye Inst 1997; **Fac Appt:** Assoc Prof Oph, Vanderbilt Univ

McKeown, Craig A MD [Oph] - **Spec Exp:** Pediatric Ophthalmology; Strabismus-Adult & Pediatric; Eye Muscle Disorders; **Hospital:** Bascom Palmer Eye Inst (page 71); **Address:** Bascom Palmer Eye Inst, 900 NW 17th St, Miami, FL 33136; **Phone:** 305-243-2020; **Board Cert:** Ophthalmology 1982; **Med School:** Northwestern Univ 1971; **Resid:** Ophthalmology, Walter Reed Med Ctr 1980; **Fellow:** Pediatric Ophthalmology, Chldns Hosp Natl Med Ctr 1984; Pediatric Ophthalmology, Wilmer Inst-Johns Hospkins 1985; **Fac Appt:** Assoc Clin Prof Oph, Univ Miami Sch Med

Meredith, Travis A MD [Oph] - **Spec Exp:** Retina/Vitreous Surgery; Macular Degeneration; Diabetic Eye Disease/Retinopathy; **Hospital:** NC Memorial Hosp - UNC; **Address:** 5151 Bioinformatics, CB#7040, Chapel Hill, NC 27599-7040; **Phone:** 919-966-5296; **Board Cert:** Ophthalmology 1976; **Med School:** Johns Hopkins Univ 1969; **Resid:** Ophthalmology, Wilmer Inst-Johns Hopkins 1971; Ophthalmology, Wilmer Inst-Johns Hopkins 1975; **Fellow:** Vitreoretinal Surgery, Med Coll Wisconsin 1976; **Fac Appt:** Prof Oph, Univ NC Sch Med

Murray, Timothy G MD [Oph] - **Spec Exp:** Retinal Disorders; Eye Tumors/Cancer; **Hospital:** Bascom Palmer Eye Inst (page 71); **Address:** Bascom Palmer Eye Inst, 900 NW 17th St, rm 254, Miami, FL 33136-1119; **Phone:** 305-326-6166; **Board Cert:** Ophthalmology 1990; **Med School:** Johns Hopkins Univ 1985; **Resid:** Ophthalmology, UCSF Med Ctr 1989; **Fellow:** Ophthalmology, UCSF 1999; Ophthalmology, Med Coll Wisconsin 1991; **Fac Appt:** Prof Oph, Univ Miami Sch Med

Nunery, William R MD [Oph] - **Spec Exp:** Orbital Surgery; Oculoplastic Surgery; Thyroid Eye Disease; **Hospital:** Univ of Louisville Hosp; **Address:** Kentucky Lions Eye Ctr, 301 E Muhammad Ali Blvd, Louisville, KY 40202; **Phone:** 502-889-1000; **Board Cert:** Ophthalmology 1980; **Med School:** Case West Res Univ 1975; **Resid:** Ophthalmology, Indiana Univ Hosp 1979; **Fellow:** Ophthalmic Plastic Surgery, Emory Univ 1980

Nussbaum, Julian MD [Oph] - **Spec Exp:** Diabetic Eye Disease/Retinopathy; Macular Degeneration; Retinopathy of Prematurity; **Hospital:** Med Coll of GA Hosp and Clin (MCG Health Inc); **Address:** 1120 15th St BA Bldg Fl 2 - rm 2331, Augusta, GA 30912; **Phone:** 706-721-1148; **Board Cert:** Ophthalmology 1981; **Med School:** Univ Miami Sch Med 1976; **Resid:** Internal Medicine, Jackson Memorial Hosp 1977; Ophthalmology, Med Coll Georgia 1980; **Fellow:** Vitreoretinal Surgery, Mass Eye & Ear Infirmary 1982; **Fac Appt:** Prof Oph, Med Coll GA

O'Brien, Terrence P MD [Oph] - **Spec Exp:** Cataract Surgery-Lens Implant; Laser Vision Surgery; Corneal & External Eye Disease; Eye Infections; **Hospital:** Bascom Palmer Eye Inst (page 71); **Address:** Bascom Palmer Eye Inst, 7101 Fairway Drive, Palm Beach Gardens, FL 33418; **Phone:** 561-515-1544; **Board Cert:** Ophthalmology 2004; **Med School:** Univ Mich Med Sch 1985; **Resid:** Ophthalmology, Wilmer Eye Inst 1989; **Fellow:** Cornea & Ext Eye Disease, Cullen Eye Inst-Baylor 1990; **Fac Appt:** Prof Oph, Univ Miami Sch Med

Olsen, Timothy W MD [Oph] - **Spec Exp:** Macular Degeneration; Diabetic Eye Disease/Retinopathy; Retinal Detachment; Retinal Disorders-Pediatric; **Hospital:** Emory Univ Hosp; **Address:** Emory Eye Center, 1365B Clifton Rd NE, Ste 3500, Atlanta, GA 30322; **Phone:** 404-778-2020; **Board Cert:** Ophthalmology 2007; **Med School:** Univ Kansas 1989; **Resid:** Ophthalmology, Univ Minn Affil Hosps 1993; **Fellow:** Vitreoretinal Surgery & Disease, Emory Univ 1996; **Fac Appt:** Prof Oph, Emory Univ

Parrish, Richard K MD [Oph] - **Spec Exp:** Glaucoma; Cataract Surgery; Anterior Segment Surgery; **Hospital:** Bascom Palmer Eye Inst (page 71), Jackson Meml Hosp (page 70); **Address:** Bascom Palmer Eye Institute, 900 NW 17th St, rm 4501, Miami, FL 33136; **Phone:** 305-243-2020; **Board Cert:** Ophthalmology 1981; **Med School:** Indiana Univ 1976; **Resid:** Ophthalmology, Wills Eye Hosp 1980; **Fellow:** Glaucoma, Bascom Palmer Eye Inst 1982; **Fac Appt:** Prof Oph, Univ Miami Sch Med

Patrinely, James R MD [Oph] - **Spec Exp:** Ophthalmic Plastic Surgery; Eyelid Surgery; Orbital Surgery; **Hospital:** Methodist Hosp - Houston, St. Luke's Episcopal Hosp-Houston; **Address:** 17 E Main St, Ste 100, Morgan Stanley Bldg, Pensacola, FL 32504; **Phone:** 850-473-0990; **Board Cert:** Ophthalmology 2002; **Med School:** Vanderbilt Univ 1980; **Resid:** Ophthalmology, Bayloy College Med 1984; **Fellow:** Ophthalmological Pathology, Johns Hopkins Hosp 1985; Ophthalmic Plastic & Reconstructive Surgery, Univ Utah Med Ctr 1986; **Fac Appt:** Clin Prof Oph, Baylor Coll Med

Perez, Victor L MD [Oph] - **Spec Exp:** Cornea & External Eye Disease; Cornea Transplant; Cataract Surgery-Lens Implant; Uveitis; **Hospital:** Bascom Palmer Eye Inst (page 71); **Address:** 900 NW 17 St, Miami, FL 33136; **Phone:** 305-243-2020; **Board Cert:** Ophthalmology 2001; **Med School:** Univ Puerto Rico 1991; **Resid:** Ophthalmology, Mass Eye & Ear Infirmary 2000; **Fellow:** Immunology, Brigham & Women's Hosp 1996; Cornea, Mass Eye & Ear Infirmary 2002; **Fac Appt:** Assoc Prof Oph, Univ Miami Sch Med

Pollard, Zane F MD [Oph] - **Spec Exp:** Pediatric Ophthalmology; Strabismus; Tear Duct Problems; **Hospital:** Chldns Hlthcare Atlanta @ Scottish Rite, Piedmont Hosp; **Address:** 5445 Meridian Mark Rd, Ste 220, Atlanta, GA 30342-4722; **Phone:** 404-255-2419; **Board Cert:** Ophthalmology 1975; **Med School:** Tulane Univ 1966; **Resid:** Surgery, UCSF Med Ctr 1968; Ophthalmology, USC Med Ctr 1973; **Fellow:** Pediatric Ophthalmology, Wills Eye Hosp 1975

Ophthalmology

Rosenfeld, Philip J MD/PhD [Oph] - **Spec Exp:** Macular Disease/Degeneration; Diabetic Eye Disease/Retinopathy; Retinal Detachment; Retina/Vitreous Surgery; **Hospital:** Bascom Palmer Eye Inst (page 71); **Address:** Bascom Palmer Eye Inst, 900 NW 17th St, Miami, FL 33136; **Phone:** 305-243-2020; **Board Cert:** Ophthalmology 2008; **Med School:** Johns Hopkins Univ 1988; **Resid:** Ophthalmology, Mass Eye & Ear Infirm 1995; **Fellow:** Retina, Bascom Palmer Eye Inst 1996; **Fac Appt:** Prof Oph, Univ Fla Coll Med

Sherwood, Mark B MD [Oph] - **Spec Exp:** Glaucoma; **Hospital:** Shands at Univ of FL; **Address:** Shands at Univ Florida, Dept Ophthalmology, 1600 SW Archer Rd, Box 100284, Gainesville, FL 32610; **Phone:** 352-273-8708; **Med School:** England, UK 1976; **Resid:** Ophthalmology, Moorefield's Eye Hosp 1980; **Fellow:** Glaucoma, Wills Eye Hosp 1982; Glaucoma, Moorefield's Eye Hosp 1983; **Fac Appt:** Prof Oph, Univ Fla Coll Med

Sternberg Jr, Paul MD [Oph] - **Spec Exp:** Retina/Vitreous Surgery; Macular Degeneration; Eye Tumors/Cancer; **Hospital:** Vanderbilt Univ Med Ctr (page 76), Vanderbilt Monroe Carrell Jr. Chldn's Hosp (page 76); **Address:** Vanderbilt Eye Institute, 2311 Pierce Ave, Nashville, TN 37232-8808; **Phone:** 615-936-1453; **Board Cert:** Ophthalmology 1985; **Med School:** Univ Chicago-Pritzker Sch Med 1979; **Resid:** Ophthalmology, Johns Hopkins Hosp 1983; **Fellow:** Vitreoretinal Surgery, Duke Univ Med Ctr 1984; **Fac Appt:** Prof Oph, Vanderbilt Univ

Stulting, R Doyle MD/PhD [Oph] - **Spec Exp:** Corneal Disease & Transplant; Laser Vision Surgery; Cataract Surgery; Keratoconus; **Address:** Woolfson Eye Institute, 800 Mount Vernon Highway NE, Ste 125, Atlanta, GA 30328; **Phone:** 404-256-1125; **Board Cert:** Ophthalmology 1982; **Med School:** Duke Univ 1976; **Resid:** Internal Medicine, Barnes Hosp 1978; Ophthalmology, Bascom Palmer Eye Inst 1981; **Fellow:** Cornea, Emory Univ 1982

Tse, David MD [Oph] - **Spec Exp:** Oculoplastic Surgery; Orbital Tumors/Cancer; Lacrimal Gland Disorders; Anophthalmia; **Hospital:** Bascom Palmer Eye Inst (page 71), Jackson Meml Hosp (page 70); **Address:** Bascom Palmer Eye Inst, 900 NW 17th St, Miami, FL 33136; **Phone:** 305-326-6086; **Board Cert:** Ophthalmology 2002; **Med School:** Univ Miami Sch Med 1976; **Resid:** Ophthalmology, LAC/USC Med Ctr 1981; **Fellow:** Oculoplastic Surgery, Univ Iowa Hosps 1982; **Fac Appt:** Prof Oph, Univ Miami Sch Med

Updegraff, Stephen A MD [Oph] - **Spec Exp:** LASIK-Refractive Surgery; Corneal Disease & Surgery; Refractive Surgery; **Address:** Updegraff Vision, 1601 38th Ave N, Saint Petersburg, FL 33713; **Phone:** 727-822-4287; **Board Cert:** Ophthalmology 2008; **Med School:** Penn State Coll Med 1989; **Resid:** Ophthalmology, LSU Eye Ctr 1994; **Fellow:** Cornea, Univ Texas 1995

Wang, Ming X MD/PhD [Oph] - **Spec Exp:** Laser Vision Surgery; Corneal Disease; Cataract Surgery; **Address:** 1801 West End Ave, Ste 1150, Nashville, TN 37203; **Phone:** 615-321-8881; **Board Cert:** Ophthalmology 2009; **Med School:** Harvard Med Sch 1991; **Resid:** Ophthalmology, Wills Eye Hosp 1996; **Fellow:** Refractive Surgery, Bascom Palmer Eye Inst 1997; **Fac Appt:** Assoc Clin Prof Oph, Univ Tenn Coll Med

Waring III, George O MD [Oph] - **Spec Exp:** LASIK-Refractive Surgery; Cataract Surgery; Lens Implants; **Hospital:** Northside Hosp; **Address:** 5505 Peachtree Dunwoody Rd, Ste 220, Atlanta, GA 30342; **Phone:** 404-442-9577; **Board Cert:** Ophthalmology 1975; **Med School:** Baylor Coll Med 1967; **Resid:** Ophthalmology, Wills Eye Hosp 1973; **Fellow:** Cornea & Ext Eye Disease, Wills Eye Hosp 1974

Wilson Jr, Marion E MD [Oph] - **Spec Exp:** Cataract-Pediatric; Strabismus; Lens Implants-Pediatric; Pediatric Ophthalmology; **Hospital:** MUSC Chldns Hosp; **Address:** MUSC Storm Eye Inst, 167 Ashley Ave, PO Box 250676, Charleston, SC 29425; **Phone:** 843-792-7622; **Board Cert:** Ophthalmology 1987; **Med School:** Med Univ SC 1980; **Resid:** Ophthalmology, Natl Naval Med Ctr 1986; **Fellow:** Pediatric Ophthalmology, Chldns Hosp - Naval Med Ctr 1987; **Fac Appt:** Prof Oph, Med Univ SC

Wilson, Matthew W MD [Oph] - **Spec Exp:** Eye Tumors/Cancer; Retinoblastoma; Melanoma-Choroidal (eye); **Hospital:** St. Jude Children's Research Hosp, Methodist Univ Hosp - Memphis; **Address:** Univ Tenn Med Grp, Ophthalmology, 930 Madison Ave, Ste 200, Memphis, TN 38103; **Phone:** 901-448-6650; **Board Cert:** Ophthalmology 2007; **Med School:** Emory Univ 1990; **Resid:** Ophthalmology, Emory Univ Med Ctr 1994; Ophthalmic Pathology, Emory Univ Med Ctr 1995; **Fellow:** Ocular Oncology, Moorfields Eye Hosp 1996; Ophthalmic Plastic & Reconstructive Surgery, Casey Eye Inst 1998; **Fac Appt:** Assoc Prof Oph, Univ Tenn Coll Med

Yeatts, R Patrick MD [Oph] - **Spec Exp:** Oculoplastic Surgery; Orbital Tumors/Cancer; Eyelid Tumors/Cancer; Orbital Diseases; **Hospital:** Wake Forest Univ Baptist Med Ctr; **Address:** Wake Forest Univ Eye Ctr, Janeway Clinical Sciences Bldg Fl 6, Medical Ctr Blvd, Winston-Salem, NC 27157; **Phone:** 336-716-4091; **Board Cert:** Ophthalmology 1983; **Med School:** Wake Forest Univ 1978; **Resid:** Ophthalmology, Mayo Clin 1982; **Fellow:** Oculoplastic & Reconstructive Surgery, Mass Eye & Ear Infirmary 1983; **Fac Appt:** Prof Oph, Wake Forest Univ

Midwest

Abrams, Gary W MD [Oph] - **Spec Exp:** Retina/Vitreous Surgery; **Hospital:** Hutzel Hosp - Detroit; **Address:** Kresge Eye Inst, 4717 St Antoine St, Detroit, MI 48201; **Phone:** 313-577-8900; **Board Cert:** Ophthalmology 1977; **Med School:** Univ Okla Coll Med 1968; **Resid:** Ophthalmology, Med Coll Wisc Affil Hosps 1976; **Fellow:** Vitreoretinal Surgery, Bascom Palmer Eye Inst 1978; **Fac Appt:** Prof Oph, Wayne State Univ

Ahmad, Amjad Z MD [Oph] - **Spec Exp:** Oculoplastic & Orbital Surgery; Cosmetic & Reconstructive Surgery; Eyelid Cosmetic & Reconstructive Surgery; Tear Duct Problems; **Hospital:** Univ of IL Med Ctr at Chicago; **Address:** Univ Ill at Chicago, Dept, Ophthalmology & Visual Scis, 1855 W Taylor St Fl 3 - rm 3.158, Chicago, IL 60612; **Phone:** 312-996-9120; **Board Cert:** Ophthalmology 2011; **Med School:** Univ Mich Med Sch 1994; **Resid:** Ophthalmology, Univ Michigan Affil Hosp 1998; **Fellow:** Oculoplastic & Reconstructive Surgery, Univ Michigan Affil Hosp 2000; **Fac Appt:** Asst Prof Oph, Univ IL Coll Med

Albert, Daniel M MD [Oph] - **Spec Exp:** Eye Tumors/Cancer; Ophthalmic Pathology; **Hospital:** Univ WI Hosp & Clins; **Address:** 600 Highland Ave CSC Bldg - rm K6/412, Madison, WI 53792-3284; **Phone:** 608-263-9798; **Board Cert:** Ophthalmology 1969; **Med School:** Univ Pennsylvania 1962; **Resid:** Ophthalmology, Hosp Univ Penn 1966; **Fellow:** Neuro-Ophthalmology, Natl Inst Hlth 1968; Pathology, Armed Forces Inst Path 1969; **Fac Appt:** Prof Oph, Univ Wisc

Alward, Wallace MD [Oph] - **Spec Exp:** Glaucoma; **Hospital:** Univ Iowa Hosp & Clinics; **Address:** 200 Hawkins Drive, Iowa City, IA 52242-1009; **Phone:** 319-356-3938; **Board Cert:** Ophthalmology 2006; **Med School:** Ohio State Univ 1976; **Resid:** Ophthalmology, Univ Louisville 1986; **Fellow:** Glaucoma, Univ Miami-Bascom Palmer Eye Inst 1987; **Fac Appt:** Prof Oph, Univ Iowa Coll Med

Ophthalmology

Archer, Steven M MD [Oph] - **Spec Exp:** Pediatric Ophthalmology; **Hospital:** Univ of Michigan Hosp; **Address:** Kellogg Eye Ctr, 1000 Wall St, Ann Arbor, MI 48105-1912; **Phone:** 734-764-7558; **Board Cert:** Ophthalmology 1986; **Med School:** Univ Chicago-Pritzker Sch Med 1978; **Resid:** Ophthalmology, Univ Chicago 1984; **Fellow:** Pediatric Ophthalmology, Indiana Univ 1986; **Fac Appt:** Asst Prof Oph, Univ Mich Med Sch

Augsburger, James MD [Oph] - **Spec Exp:** Eye Tumors/Cancer; Melanoma-Choroidal (eye); Retinoblastoma; **Hospital:** Univ Hosp - Cincinnati, Cincinnati Chldns Hosp Med Ctr; **Address:** Medical Arts Bldg, Ste 1500, 222 Piedmont Ave, ML 665-E, Cincinnati, OH 45267-0665; **Phone:** 513-475-7300; **Board Cert:** Ophthalmology 1979; **Med School:** Univ Cincinnati 1974; **Resid:** Ophthalmology, Univ Hosp-Cincinnati 1978; **Fellow:** Ocular Oncology, Wills Eye Hosp 1980; **Fac Appt:** Prof Oph, Univ Cincinnati

Azar, Dimitri T MD [Oph] - **Spec Exp:** LASIK-Refractive Surgery; **Hospital:** Univ of IL at Chicago Eye & Ear Infirm, Univ of IL Med Ctr at Chicago; **Address:** Illinois Eye & Ear Infirmary, 30 N Michigan, Ste 410, Chicago, IL 60602; **Phone:** 312-996-2020; **Board Cert:** Ophthalmology 1991; **Med School:** Lebanon 1983; **Resid:** Ophthalmology, American Univ Med Ctr 1986; Ophthalmology, Mass E&E Infirm 1991; **Fellow:** Cornea & Ext Eye Disease, Mass E&E Infirm 1988; Cornea Research, Harvard Med Sch 1991; **Fac Appt:** Prof Oph, Univ IL Coll Med

Azar, Nathalie F MD [Oph] - **Spec Exp:** Pediatric Ophthalmology; Strabismus; **Hospital:** Univ of IL at Chicago Eye & Ear Infirm; **Address:** Illinois Eye & Ear Infirmary, 30 N Michigan Ave, Ste 410, Chicago, IL 60602; **Phone:** 312-996-2020; **Board Cert:** Ophthalmology 1996; **Med School:** Boston Univ 1990; **Resid:** Ophthalmology, George Washington U Med Ctr 1994; **Fellow:** Pediatric Ophthalmology, Wilmer Eye Inst 1995; **Fac Appt:** Assoc Clin Prof Oph, Univ IL Coll Med

Baker, John D MD [Oph] - **Spec Exp:** Pediatric Ophthalmology; **Hospital:** Chldns Hosp of Michigan; **Address:** 2355 Monroe Blvd, Dearborn, MI 48124-3009; **Phone:** 313-561-1777; **Board Cert:** Ophthalmology 1974; **Med School:** Wayne State Univ 1967; **Resid:** Ophthalmology, Detroit Genl Hosp 1971; **Fellow:** Pediatric Ophthalmology, Chldns Natl Med Ctr 1972; **Fac Appt:** Clin Prof Oph, Wayne State Univ

Burke, Miles J MD [Oph] - **Spec Exp:** Pediatric Ophthalmology; Eye Muscle Surgery; Amblyopia & Vision Development; Optic Nerve Disorders; **Hospital:** Cincinnati Chldns Hosp Med Ctr, Jewish Hosp - Kenwood - Cincinnati; **Address:** 10475 Montgomery Rd, Ste 4F, Cincinnati, OH 45242-5200; **Phone:** 513-984-4949; **Board Cert:** Ophthalmology 1979; **Med School:** Univ Ariz Coll Med 1974; **Resid:** Ophthalmology, Univ Michigan Med Ctr 1978; **Fellow:** Pediatric Ophthalmology, Wills Eye Hosp 1979

Cahill, Kenneth V MD [Oph] - **Spec Exp:** Eyelid Surgery; Eyelid/Tear Duct Reconstruction; Orbital Surgery; Oculoplastic Surgery; **Hospital:** Nationwide Chldn's Hosp; **Address:** The Eye Center, 262 Neil Ave, Ste 430, Columbus, OH 43215; **Phone:** 614-221-7464; **Board Cert:** Ophthalmology 1984; **Med School:** Ohio State Univ 1979; **Resid:** Ophthalmology, Univ of Pittsburgh 1983; **Fellow:** Oculoplastic Surgery, OSU Med Ctr 1984; Oculoplastic Surgery, Chldns Hosp Philadelphia 1984; **Fac Appt:** Clin Prof Oph, Ohio State Univ

Carter, Keith D MD [Oph] - **Spec Exp:** Oculoplastic & Orbital Surgery; Eyelid Surgery; Botox Therapy; **Hospital:** Univ Iowa Hosp & Clinics; **Address:** Univ Iowa, Dept Ophthalmology, 200 Hawkins Dr, PFP 11136-F, Iowa City, IA 52242; **Phone:** 319-356-2852; **Board Cert:** Ophthalmology 1988; **Med School:** Indiana Univ 1983; **Resid:** Ophthalmology, Univ Michigan Med Ctr 1987; **Fellow:** Oculoplastic Surgery, Univ Iowa 1988; **Fac Appt:** Prof Oph, Univ Iowa Coll Med

Del Monte, Monte A MD [Oph] - **Spec Exp:** Pediatric Ophthalmology; Strabismus-Adult & Pediatric; Glaucoma-Pediatric; Cataract-Pediatric; **Hospital:** Univ of Michigan Hosp; **Address:** Kellogg Eye Center, 1000 Wall St, Ann Arbor, MI 48105-1912; **Phone:** 734-764-3111; **Board Cert:** Ophthalmology 1982; **Med School:** Johns Hopkins Univ 1974; **Resid:** Pediatrics, Chldns Hosp Med Ctr 1977; Ophthalmology, Wilmer Eye Inst 1981; **Fellow:** Ophthalmology, Wilmer Eye Inst 1978; Pediatric Ophthalmology, Chldns Hosp 1981; **Fac Appt:** Prof Oph, Univ Mich Med Sch

Drack, Arlene V MD [Oph] - **Spec Exp:** Eye Diseases-Hereditary; Eye Tumors/Cancer; Pediatric Ophthalmology; Strabismus; **Hospital:** Univ Iowa Hosp & Clinics; **Address:** UIHC Dept of Ophth and Vis Science, 200 Hawkins Drive, Iowa City, IA 52242; **Phone:** 319-356-2859; **Board Cert:** Ophthalmology 1994; **Med School:** Penn State Coll Med 1986; **Resid:** Ophthalmology, Georgetown Univ Med Ctr 1990; **Fellow:** Pediatric Ophthalmology, Univ IA Hosps & Clin 1991; Molecular Genetics, Univ IA Hosps & Clin 1992; **Fac Appt:** Assoc Prof Oph, Univ Iowa Coll Med

Edwards, Paul A MD [Oph] - **Spec Exp:** Retinal Disorders; Macular Degeneration; Diabetic Eye Disease/Retinopathy; Ophthalmic Genetics; **Hospital:** Henry Ford Hosp, Henry Ford- W Bloomfield Hosp; **Address:** Henry Ford Hosp, Dept Ophthalmology, 2799 W Grand Blvd, K-10, Detroit, MI 48202; **Phone:** 313-916-3245; **Board Cert:** Ophthalmology 2005; **Med School:** West Indies 1979; **Resid:** Surgery, Washington Hosp Ctr 1984; Ophthalmology, Henry Ford Hosp 1989; **Fellow:** Research, Natl Eye Inst 1991; Retina/Vitreous, Henry Ford Hosp 1993; **Fac Appt:** Prof Oph, Wayne State Univ

Elner, Victor H MD/PhD [Oph] - **Spec Exp:** Eyelid Tumors/Cancer; Orbital Tumors/Cancer; **Hospital:** Univ of Michigan Hosp; **Address:** Kellogg Eye Ctr, 1000 Wall St, Ann Arbor, MI 48105; **Phone:** 734-763-9142; **Board Cert:** Ophthalmology 1983; Pathology 1988; **Med School:** Univ Chicago-Pritzker Sch Med 1979; **Resid:** Ophthalmology, Univ Chicago 1982; Pathology, Univ Chicago 1984; **Fellow:** Ophthalmological Pathology, Armed Forces Inst 1985; Ophthalmic Plastic & Reconstructive Surgery, Univ Wisconsin 1987; **Fac Appt:** Prof Oph, Univ Mich Med Sch

Feder, Robert S MD [Oph] - **Spec Exp:** Corneal Disease; LASIK-Refractive Surgery; Cataract Surgery; **Hospital:** Northwestern Meml Hosp; **Address:** 675 N St Clair St, Galter Pavilion Fl 15, Chicago, IL 60611-5975; **Phone:** 312-695-8150; **Board Cert:** Ophthalmology 1983; **Med School:** Northwestern Univ 1978; **Resid:** Ophthalmology, Barnes Hosp 1982; **Fellow:** Cornea & Ext Eye Disease, Univ Iowa Med Ctr 1983; **Fac Appt:** Assoc Prof Oph, Northwestern Univ

Fishman, Gerald MD [Oph] - **Spec Exp:** Retinitis Pigmentosa; Retinal Disorders-Inherited; **Address:** Chicago Lighthouse, 1850 W Roosevelt Rd, Chicago, IL 60608; **Phone:** 312-997-3666; **Board Cert:** Ophthalmology 1975; **Med School:** Ohio State Univ 1969; **Resid:** Ophthalmology, Univ Illinois EE Infirmary 1973; **Fellow:** Ocular Pathology, Univ Illinois EE Infirmary 1974; **Fac Appt:** Prof Oph, Univ IL Coll Med

Greenwald, Mark MD [Oph] - **Spec Exp:** Pediatric Ophthalmology; **Hospital:** Univ of Chicago Med Ctr; **Address:** Dept Ophthalmology, 5758 S Maryland Ave, Chicago, IL 60637; **Phone:** 773-834-5685; **Board Cert:** Ophthalmology 1981; **Med School:** Harvard Med Sch 1976; **Resid:** Ophthalmology, Univ Illinois Hosp 1980; **Fellow:** Pediatric Ophthalmology, Chldns Hosp 1981; **Fac Appt:** Assoc Prof Oph, Univ Wash

Harbour, J William MD [Oph] - **Spec Exp:** Eye Tumors/Cancer; Melanoma-Choroidal (eye); Retinoblastoma; **Hospital:** Barnes-Jewish Hosp, St. Louis Chldns Hosp; **Address:** 1600 S Brentwood, Ste 800, St Louis, MO 63144; **Phone:** 314-367-1278 x2156; **Board Cert:** Ophthalmology 2007; **Med School:** Johns Hopkins Univ 1990; **Resid:** Ophthalmology, Wills Eye Hosp 1994; **Fellow:** Retina/Vitreous, Bascom Palmer Eye Inst 1995; Ocular Oncology, UCSF Med Ctr 1996; **Fac Appt:** Prof Oph, Washington Univ, St Louis

Ophthalmology

Heckenlively, John R MD [Oph] - **Spec Exp:** Eye Diseases-Hereditary; Retinal Disorders; Opthalmic Genetics; **Hospital:** Univ of Michigan Hosp; **Address:** MI Kellogg Eye Ctr, 1000 Wall St, Ann Arbor, MI 48105; **Phone:** 734-763-2280; **Board Cert:** Ophthalmology 1977; **Med School:** Univ Colorado 1972; **Resid:** Ophthalmology, Univ KY 1976; **Fellow:** Vitreoretinal Disease, Jules Stein Eye Inst 1977; Johns Hopkins Hosp 1978; **Fac Appt:** Prof Oph, Univ Mich Med Sch

Heuer, Dale K MD [Oph] - **Spec Exp:** Glaucoma; **Hospital:** Froedtert and Med Ctr of WI; **Address:** The Eye Institute, 925 N 87th St, Milwaukee, WI 53226; **Phone:** 414-456-2020; **Board Cert:** Ophthalmology 1983; **Med School:** Northwestern Univ 1978; **Resid:** Ophthalmology, Med Coll Wisc Affil Hosp 1982; **Fellow:** Glaucoma, Bascom Palmer Eye Inst 1984; **Fac Appt:** Prof Oph, Med Coll Wisc

Holland, Edward J MD [Oph] - **Spec Exp:** Corneal Disease; Refractive Surgery; Cataract Surgery; **Hospital:** St. Elizabeth Hlthcare-Edgewood; **Address:** Cincinnati Eye Institute, 1945 CEI Drive, Edgewood, OH 45242; **Phone:** 513-984-5133; **Board Cert:** Ophthalmology 1986; **Med School:** Loyola Univ-Stritch Sch Med 1981; **Resid:** Ophthalmology, Univ Minn Med Ctr 1985; **Fellow:** Cornea & Ext Eye Disease, Univ Iowa Affil Hosp 1986; Ocular Immunology, Natl Eye Inst 1987; **Fac Appt:** Clin Prof Oph, Univ Cincinnati

John, Thomas MD [Oph] - **Spec Exp:** Cornea Transplant & Artificial Cornea; Amniotic Membrane Transplant; Cataract Surgery; Refractive Surgery; **Hospital:** Loyola Univ Med Ctr, Adv S Suburban Hosp; **Address:** 16532 S Oak Park Ave, Tinley Park, IL 60477; **Phone:** 708-429-2223; **Board Cert:** Ophthalmology 1987; **Med School:** India 1977; **Resid:** Ophthalmology, Hosp Univ Penn 1984; **Fellow:** Cornea & Ext Eye Disease, Univ Rochester Sch Med & Dentistry 1985; Cornea & Ext Eye Disease, Mass Eye & Ear Infirmary 1987; **Fac Appt:** Assoc Clin Prof Oph, Loyola Univ-Stritch Sch Med

Kaufman, Paul L MD [Oph] - **Spec Exp:** Glaucoma; **Hospital:** Univ WI Hosp & Clins; **Address:** Univ Wisconsin Hosp, Dept Ophthalmology, 2880 University Ave, MC 9030, Madison, WI 53705; **Phone:** 608-263-7171; **Board Cert:** Ophthalmology 1976; **Med School:** NYU Sch Med 1967; **Resid:** Ophthalmology, Washington Univ-Barnes Hosp 1973; **Fellow:** Ocular Pharmacology, Univ Uppsala 1975; **Fac Appt:** Prof Oph, Univ Wisc

Krueger, Ronald MD [Oph] - **Spec Exp:** Corneal Disease; Refractive Surgery; **Hospital:** Cleveland Clin (page 56); **Address:** Cleveland Clinic Fdn - Cole Eye Inst, 9500 Euclid Ave, Desk I32, Cleveland, OH 44195; **Phone:** 216-444-8158; **Board Cert:** Ophthalmology 2003; **Med School:** UMDNJ-NJ Med Sch, Newark 1987; **Resid:** Ophthalmology, Columbia Presby Med Ctr 1991; **Fellow:** Refractive Surgery, Univ Okla Hlth Sci Ctr-McGee Eye Inst 1992; Cornea, USC-Doheny Eye Inst 1993

Kushner, Burton J MD [Oph] - **Spec Exp:** Pediatric Ophthalmology; Strabismus-Adult & Pediatric; **Hospital:** Univ WI Hosp & Clins; **Address:** Pediatric Eye Clinic, 2880 University Ave, MC 9030, Madison, WI 53709; **Phone:** 608-263-7171; **Board Cert:** Ophthalmology 1975; **Med School:** Northwestern Univ 1969; **Resid:** Ophthalmology, Univ Wisc Hosp 1973; **Fellow:** Pediatric Ophthalmology, Bascom Palmer Eye Inst 1974; **Fac Appt:** Prof Oph, Univ Wisc

Kwon, Young H MD/PhD [Oph] - **Spec Exp:** Glaucoma; **Hospital:** Univ Iowa Hosp & Clinics; **Address:** UIHC Dept of Ophthalmology, 200 Hawkins Drive, 11190-B PFP, Iowa City, IA 52242; **Phone:** 319-356-3933; **Board Cert:** Ophthalmology 2008; **Med School:** Yale Univ 1991; **Resid:** Ophthalmology, Mass Eye & Ear Infirmary 1995; **Fellow:** Glaucoma, Yale Univ Affil Hosp 1996; **Fac Appt:** Prof Oph, Univ Iowa Coll Med

Lane, Stephen S MD [Oph] - **Spec Exp:** Laser Vision Surgery; Cataract Surgery; **Hospital:** United Hosp; **Address:** Associated Eye Care, 2950 Curve Crest Blvd, Stillwater, MN 55082; **Phone:** 651-275-3000; **Board Cert:** Ophthalmology 1986; **Med School:** Univ Minn 1980; **Resid:** Ophthalmology, MS Hershey Med Ctr 1984; **Fellow:** Cornea & Ext Eye Disease, Univ Minn 1984; **Fac Appt:** Clin Prof Oph, Univ Minn

Lass, Jonathan H MD [Oph] - **Spec Exp:** Cataract Surgery-Lens Implant; Corneal & External Eye Disease; **Hospital:** Univ Hosps Case Med Ctr (page 74); **Address:** UH Case Medical Center, Ophthalmology, 11100 Euclid Ave, MS WRN-5068, Cleveland, OH 44106; **Phone:** 216-844-8590; **Board Cert:** Ophthalmology 1978; **Med School:** Boston Univ 1973; **Resid:** Ophthalmology, Boston Univ Med Ctr 1977; **Fellow:** Ophthalmology, Mass Eye & Ear Infirmary 1979; **Fac Appt:** Prof Oph, Case West Res Univ

Lichter, Paul R MD [Oph] - **Spec Exp:** Cataract Surgery; Glaucoma; **Hospital:** Univ of Michigan Hosp; **Address:** 1000 Wall St, WK Kellogg Eye Ctr, Ann Arbor, MI 48105; **Phone:** 734-763-5874; **Board Cert:** Ophthalmology 1970; **Med School:** Univ Mich Med Sch 1964; **Resid:** Ophthalmology, Univ Mich Med Ctr 1968; **Fellow:** Ophthalmology, UCSF Med Ctr 1969; **Fac Appt:** Prof Oph, Univ Mich Med Sch

Lindstrom, Richard L MD [Oph] - **Spec Exp:** Corneal Disease; Cataract Surgery; Refractive Surgery; **Hospital:** Abbott - Northwestern Hosp, Phillips Eye Inst; **Address:** 9801 DuPont Ave S, Ste 200, Bloomington, MN 55431; **Phone:** 612-813-3600; **Board Cert:** Ophthalmology 1978; **Med School:** Univ Minn 1972; **Resid:** Ophthalmology, Univ Minn 1979; Ophthalmology, Univ Minn 1980; **Fellow:** Anterior Segment - External Disease, Mary Shields Eye Hosp; Glaucoma, Univ Hosps; **Fac Appt:** Prof Oph, Univ Minn

Lucarelli, Mark J MD [Oph] - **Spec Exp:** Ophthalmic Plastic Surgery; Reconstructive Plastic Surgery; Oculoplastic & Orbital Surgery; Thyroid Eye Disease; **Hospital:** Univ WI Hosp & Clins; **Address:** Univ Wisconsin Hosp & Clinics, 2880 University Ave, MC 9030, Madison, WI 53792; **Phone:** 608-263-7171; **Board Cert:** Ophthalmology 2008; **Med School:** Washington Univ, St Louis 1991; **Resid:** Ophthalmology, Mass Eye & Ear Infirm 1995; **Fellow:** Ophthalmic Plastic & Reconstructive Surgery, Univ Wisconsin Hosp & Clins 1997; **Fac Appt:** Prof Oph, Univ Wisc

Lueder, Gregg T MD [Oph] - **Spec Exp:** Retinoblastoma; Eye Tumors-Pediatric; Pediatric Ophthalmology; **Hospital:** St. Louis Chldns Hosp; **Address:** St Louis Children's Hospital, One Children's Pl, Ste 2 South 89, St Louis, MO 63110; **Phone:** 314-454-6026; **Board Cert:** Ophthalmology 2003; **Med School:** Univ Iowa Coll Med 1985; **Resid:** Pediatrics, St Louis Children's Hosp 1988; Ophthalmology, Univ Iowa Med Ctr 1991; **Fellow:** Pediatric Ophthalmology, Hosp for Sick Children 1993; **Fac Appt:** Assoc Prof Oph, Washington Univ, St Louis

Maguire, Leo J MD [Oph] - **Spec Exp:** Cornea Transplant; Refractive Surgery; **Hospital:** Mayo Med Ctr & Clin - Rochester; **Address:** Mayo Clinic-Ophthalmology, 200 First St SW, Rochester, MN 55905; **Phone:** 507-284-4152; **Board Cert:** Ophthalmology 1986; **Med School:** Jefferson Med Coll 1980; **Resid:** Ophthalmology, Univ Michigan Med Ctr 1984; **Fellow:** Cornea & Ext Eye Disease, LSU Eye Ctr 1986; **Fac Appt:** Assoc Prof Oph, Mayo Med Sch

Mets, Marilyn MD [Oph] - **Spec Exp:** Pediatric Ophthalmology; Ophthalmic Genetics; Strabismus; Retinal Disorders; **Hospital:** Children's Mem Hosp -Chicago; **Address:** 2300 Children's Plaza, Box 70, Chicago, IL 60614; **Phone:** 773-880-4020; **Board Cert:** Ophthalmology 2005; **Med School:** Geo Wash Univ 1976; **Resid:** Ophthalmology, Cleveland Clinic Fdn 1980; **Fellow:** Pediatric Ophthalmology, Natl Chldns Hosp 1981; **Fac Appt:** Prof Oph, Northwestern Univ

Mieler, William F MD [Oph] - **Spec Exp:** Retina/Vitreous Surgery; Eye Tumors/Cancer; Macular Disease/Degeneration; Trauma; **Hospital:** Univ of IL Med Ctr at Chicago, Weiss Meml Hosp; **Address:** Univ IL Chicago, Dept Ophthalmology, 1855 W Taylor St, MS 648, Chicago, IL 60637; **Phone:** 773-996-6660; **Board Cert:** Ophthalmology 1984; **Med School:** Univ Wisc 1979; **Resid:** Ophthalmology, Bascom-Palmer Eye Inst 1983; **Fellow:** Vitreoretinal Surgery & Disease, Med Ctr Wisconsin Eye Inst 1984; Oculoplastic Surgery, Wills Eye Hosp 1986; **Fac Appt:** Prof Oph, Univ IL Coll Med

Mizen, Thomas R MD [Oph] - **Spec Exp:** Neuro-Ophthalmology; Optic Nerve Disorders; **Hospital:** Rush Univ Med Ctr; **Address:** 1725 W Harrison St, Ste 928, Chicago, IL 60612-3862; **Phone:** 312-942-3500; **Board Cert:** Ophthalmology 1986; **Med School:** Finch/Chicago Med Sch 1980; **Resid:** Ophthalmology, Rush-Presby-St Lukes Med Ctr 1984; **Fellow:** Neuro-Ophthalmology, Barnes Hosp/Wash Univ 1985; **Fac Appt:** Asst Prof Oph, Rush Med Coll

Nerad, Jeffrey MD [Oph] - **Spec Exp:** Orbital Tumors/Cancer; Eyelid Cancer & Reconstruction; Oculoplastic Surgery; **Address:** Cincinnati Eye Institute, 1945 CEI Drive, Cincinnati, OH 45242; **Phone:** 513-984-5133; **Board Cert:** Ophthalmology 1984; **Med School:** St Louis Univ 1979; **Resid:** Ophthalmology, St Louis Univ Med Ctr 1983; **Fellow:** Oculoplastic & Reconstructive Surgery, Univ Iowa 1984; **Fac Appt:** Prof Oph, Univ Iowa Coll Med

Olitsky, Scott E MD [Oph] - **Spec Exp:** Pediatric Ophthalmology; Strabismus; **Hospital:** Chldns Mercy Hosps & Clinics; **Address:** Chldns Mercy Hosp, Dept Oph, 2401 Gillham Rd, Kansas City, MO 64108; **Phone:** 816-234-3046; **Board Cert:** Ophthalmology 2004; **Med School:** Jefferson Med Coll 1988; **Resid:** Ophthalmology, SUNY Buffalo Med Ctr 1992; **Fellow:** Pediatric Ophthalmology, Wills Eye Hosp 1993; **Fac Appt:** Prof Oph, Univ MO-Kansas City

Osher, Robert H MD [Oph] - **Spec Exp:** Cataract Surgery-Lens Implant; **Address:** Cincinnati Eye Inst, 1945 CEI Drive, Cincinnati, OH 45242; **Phone:** 513-984-5133; **Board Cert:** Ophthalmology 1981; **Med School:** Univ Rochester 1976; **Resid:** Ophthalmology, Bascom Palmer Eye Inst 1980; **Fellow:** Ophthalmology, Wills Eye Hosp 1977; Ophthalmology, Bascom Palmer Eye Inst 1981; **Fac Appt:** Prof Oph, Univ Cincinnati

Pepose, Jay MD [Oph] - **Spec Exp:** LASIK-Refractive Surgery; Cataract Surgery; Corneal & External Eye Disease; **Hospital:** Barnes-Jewish Hosp, St. John's Mercy Med Ctr - St Louis; **Address:** 1815 Clarkson Rd, Chesterfield, MO 63017; **Phone:** 636-728-0111; **Board Cert:** Ophthalmology 1989; **Med School:** UCLA 1982; **Resid:** Ophthalmology, Johns Hopkins Hosp 1987; **Fellow:** Cornea & Ext Eye Disease, Georgetown Univ Med Ctr 1988; **Fac Appt:** Prof Oph, Washington Univ, St Louis

Petersen, Michael R MD/PhD [Oph] - **Spec Exp:** Diabetic Eye Disease/Retinopathy; Macular Degeneration; Retinal Detachment; Uveitis; **Hospital:** Bethesda North Hosp; **Address:** Cincinnati Eye Institute, 1945 CEI Drive, Blue Ash, OH 45242-5664; **Phone:** 513-984-5133; **Board Cert:** Ophthalmology 1991; **Med School:** Univ Mich Med Sch 1986; **Resid:** Ophthalmology, Kellogg Eye Ctr 1990; **Fellow:** Vitreoretinal Surgery, Univ Wash Affil Hosp 1992

Plager, David A MD [Oph] - **Spec Exp:** Pediatric Ophthalmology; Strabismus; Cataract-Pediatric; Glaucoma-Pediatric; **Hospital:** Riley Hosp for Children; **Address:** IU Pediatric Ophthalmology, 702 Rotary Circle Fl 2, Indianapolis, IN 46202; **Phone:** 317-944-8103; **Board Cert:** Ophthalmology 2006; **Med School:** Indiana Univ 1983; **Resid:** Ophthalmology, Indiana Univ Hosps 1987; **Fellow:** Pediatric Ophthalmology, Chldns Hosp Natl Med Ctr 1988; Strabismus, Chldns Hosp Natl Med Ctr 1988; **Fac Appt:** Prof Oph, Indiana Univ

Pulido, Jose S MD [Oph] - **Spec Exp:** Retina/Vitreous Surgery; Eye Tumors/Cancer; **Hospital:** Mayo Med Ctr & Clin - Rochester; **Address:** 200 1st St SW, Rochester, MN 55905; **Phone:** 507-284-3721; **Board Cert:** Ophthalmology 1986; **Med School:** Tulane Univ 1981; **Resid:** Ophthalmology, Illinois Eye & Ear Infirm 1986; **Fellow:** Vitreoretinal Surgery & Disease, Bascom-Palmer Eye Inst 1987; Ocular Oncology, Wills Eye Hosp; **Fac Appt:** Prof Oph, Mayo Med Sch

Putterman, Allen M MD [Oph] - **Spec Exp:** Oculoplastic & Orbital Surgery; Cosmetic Surgery-Face & Eyes; Thyroid Eye Disease; Eyelid Cosmetic & Reconstructive Surgery; **Hospital:** St. Joseph Hosp, Univ of IL Med Ctr at Chicago; **Address:** 111 N Wabash Ave, Ste 1722, Chicago, IL 60602-2002; **Phone:** 312-372-2256; **Board Cert:** Ophthalmology 1971; **Med School:** Univ Wisc 1963; **Resid:** Ophthalmology, Michael Reese Hosp 1969; **Fellow:** Oculoplastic Surgery, Manhattan Eye/Ear Infirm 1970; **Fac Appt:** Prof Oph, Univ IL Coll Med

Rogers, Gary L MD [Oph] - **Spec Exp:** Strabismus-Adult & Pediatric; **Hospital:** Nationwide Chldn's Hosp; **Address:** 555 S 18th St, Ste 4C, Columbus, OH 43205; **Phone:** 614-224-6222; **Board Cert:** Ophthalmology 1974; **Med School:** Ohio State Univ 1968; **Resid:** Ophthalmology, Mt Sinai Hosp 1972; **Fellow:** Pediatric Ophthalmology, Chldns Hosp Natl Med Ctr 1974; **Fac Appt:** Clin Prof Oph, Ohio State Univ

Rosenberg, Michael A MD [Oph] - **Spec Exp:** Refractive Surgery; Cataract Surgery; Eye Muscle Surgery; **Hospital:** Northwestern Meml Hosp; **Address:** Northwestern Med Fac Fdn, 675 N St Clair St, Ste 15-150, Chicago, IL 60611-5967; **Phone:** 312-695-8150; **Board Cert:** Ophthalmology 1975; **Med School:** Northwestern Univ 1967; **Resid:** Ophthalmology, Bascom Palmer Eye Inst 1973; **Fellow:** Neuro-Ophthalmology, UCSF Med Ctr 1974; Refractive Surgery, Univ Monterrey 1998; **Fac Appt:** Assoc Clin Prof Oph, Northwestern Univ

Samuelson, Thomas W MD [Oph] - **Spec Exp:** Glaucoma; Cataract Surgery; Anterior Segment Surgery; Refractive Surgery; **Hospital:** Phillips Eye Inst, Regions Hosp - St Paul; **Address:** Minnesota Eye Consultants, 710 E 24th St, Ste 100, Minneapolis, MN 55404-3810; **Phone:** 612-813-3600; **Board Cert:** Ophthalmology 1991; **Med School:** Univ Minn 1985; **Resid:** Ophthalmology, Univ S Florida 1990; **Fellow:** Glaucoma, Wills Eye Hosp 1991; **Fac Appt:** Assoc Clin Prof Oph, Univ Minn

Schachat, Andrew P MD [Oph] - **Spec Exp:** Retina/Vitreous Surgery; Diabetic Eye Disease/Retinopathy; Melanoma-Choroidal (eye); **Hospital:** Cleveland Clin (page 56); **Address:** The Cleveland Clinic Fdn, Cole Eye Inst, 9500 Euclid Ave, Desk I30, Cleveland, OH 44195; **Phone:** 216-444-7963; **Board Cert:** Ophthalmology 1983; **Med School:** Johns Hopkins Univ 1979; **Resid:** Ophthalmology, Wilmer Inst-John Hopkins Hosp 1982; **Fellow:** Vitreoretinal Surgery & Disease, Wilmer Eye Inst-Johns Hopkins Hosp 1983; **Fac Appt:** Prof Oph

Stone, Edwin MD [Oph] - **Spec Exp:** Retinal Disorders; Eye Diseases-Hereditary; **Hospital:** Univ Iowa Hosp & Clinics; **Address:** Dept Ophthalmology, 200 Hawkins Dr, PFP 11136-F, Iowa City, IA 52242; **Phone:** 319-356-2852; **Board Cert:** Ophthalmology 1990; **Med School:** Baylor Coll Med 1985; **Resid:** Ophthalmology, Univ Iowa Hosps 1989; **Fellow:** Retina, Univ Iowa Hosps 1992; **Fac Appt:** Prof Oph, Univ Iowa Coll Med

Summers, C Gail MD [Oph] - **Spec Exp:** Eye Diseases-Hereditary; Albinism; **Address:** Riverside Park Pl Bldg, 701 25th Ave S, Ste 302, Minneapolis, MN 55454; **Phone:** 612-365-8350; **Board Cert:** Ophthalmology 1984; **Med School:** Univ Minn 1979; **Resid:** Ophthalmology, Univ Minnesota Med Ctr 1983; **Fellow:** Pediatric Ophthalmology, Unin Minnesota Med Ctr 1984; **Fac Appt:** Prof Oph, Univ Minn

Ophthalmology

Traboulsi, Elias Iskandar MD [Oph] - **Spec Exp:** Pediatric Ophthalmology; Glaucoma-Pediatric; **Hospital:** Cleveland Clin (page 56); **Address:** Cleveland Clinic Fdn, Cole Eye Inst, 9500 Euclid Ave, Ste I32, Cleveland, OH 44195; **Phone:** 216-444-4363; **Board Cert:** Clinical Genetics 1987; Ophthalmology 1991; **Med School:** Amer Univ Beirut 1982; **Resid:** Ophthalmology, American Univ Beirut Hosp 1985; Ophthalmology, Georgetown Hosp 1989; **Fellow:** Ophthalmology, Johns Hopkins Hosp 1986; Pediatric Ophthalmology, Chldns Hosp Natl Med Ctr 1990; **Fac Appt:** Prof Oph, Ohio State Univ

Trese, Michael T MD [Oph] - **Spec Exp:** Retina/Vitreous Surgery; Retinal Disorders-Pediatric; **Hospital:** Beaumont Hosp-Royal Oak, Chldns Hosp of Michigan; **Address:** 3535 W 13 Mile Rd, Ste 344, Royal Oak, MI 48073-6710; **Phone:** 248-288-2280; **Board Cert:** Ophthalmology 1981; **Med School:** Georgetown Univ 1976; **Resid:** Ophthalmology, Jules Stein Eye Inst-UCLA 1980; **Fellow:** Retina, Duke Univ Med Ctr 1981; **Fac Appt:** Assoc Clin Prof Oph, Wayne State Univ

Trobe, Jonathan D MD [Oph] - **Spec Exp:** Neuro-Ophthalmology; Optic Nerve Disorders; **Hospital:** Univ of Michigan Hosp; **Address:** WK Kellogg Eye Ctr, 1000 Wall St, Ann Arbor, MI 48105-1912; **Phone:** 734-763-5114; **Board Cert:** Ophthalmology 1974; Neurology 1988; **Med School:** Harvard Med Sch 1968; **Resid:** Ophthalmology, Wills Eye Hosp 1972; Neurology, Jackson Meml Hosp/U Miami 1986; **Fellow:** Neuro-Ophthalmology, Bascom Palmer Eye Inst 1977; **Fac Appt:** Prof Oph, Univ Mich Med Sch

Tychsen, Lawrence MD [Oph] - **Spec Exp:** Pediatric Ophthalmology; Strabismus; Amblyopia; **Hospital:** St. Louis Chldns Hosp, Barnes-Jewish Hosp; **Address:** Chldns Eye Care Ctr, 1 Children's Pl, Ste 2 South 89, St Louis, MO 63110; **Phone:** 314-454-6026; **Board Cert:** Ophthalmology 1984; **Med School:** Georgetown Univ 1979; **Resid:** Ophthalmology, Univ Iowa Hosp 1983; **Fellow:** Pediatric Ophthalmology, UCSF Med Ctr 1985; **Fac Appt:** Assoc Prof Oph, Washington Univ, St Louis

Vajaranant, Thasarat S MD [Oph] - **Spec Exp:** Glaucoma; Women's Eye Health; **Hospital:** Univ of IL at Chicago Eye & Ear Infirm; **Address:** Univ of Illinois at Chicago, Glaucoma Service, 1855 W Taylor St, MC 648, Chicago, IL 60612; **Phone:** 312-996-7030; **Board Cert:** Ophthalmology 2008; **Med School:** Thailand 1996; **Resid:** Ophthalmology, Univ of Illinois 2006; **Fellow:** Glaucoma, Univ of Illinois 2007; Research, Univ of Illinois 2008; **Fac Appt:** Asst Prof Oph, Univ IL Coll Med

Volpe, Nicholas J MD [Oph] - **Spec Exp:** Neuro-Ophthalmology; Strabismus; **Hospital:** Northwestern Meml Hosp; **Address:** Sorrel Rosin Eye Ctr, 675 N St Clair, Galter Pavilion, Ste 15-150, Chicago, IL 60611; **Phone:** 312-695-8150; **Board Cert:** Ophthalmology 2003; **Med School:** SUNY Downstate 1987; **Resid:** Ophthalmology, Mass E&E Infirmary 1993; **Fellow:** Neuro-Ophthalmology, Mass E&E Infirmary 1992; **Fac Appt:** Prof Oph, Northwestern Univ-Feinberg Sch Med

Williams, George A MD [Oph] - **Spec Exp:** Retinal Disorders; Macular Degeneration; **Hospital:** Beaumont Hosp-Royal Oak; **Address:** Associated Retinal Consultants, 3535 W 13 Mile Rd, Ste 344, Royal Oak, MI 48073; **Phone:** 248-288-2280; **Board Cert:** Ophthalmology 2005; **Med School:** Northwestern Univ 1978; **Resid:** Ophthalmology, Med Coll Wisconsin 1982; **Fellow:** Retina/Vitreous, Med Coll Wisconsin 1984; **Fac Appt:** Clin Prof Oph, Univ Mich Med Sch

Wilson, Steven E MD [Oph] - **Spec Exp:** PRK-Refractive Surgery; Corneal Disease; **Hospital:** Cleveland Clin (page 56); **Address:** Cleveland Clinic Fdn - Cole Eye Inst, 9500 Euclid Ave, Ste I32, Cleveland, OH 44195; **Phone:** 216-444-5887; **Board Cert:** Ophthalmology 1990; **Med School:** UCSD 1984; **Resid:** Ophthalmology, Mayo Clinic 1988; **Fellow:** Refractive Surgery, Med Ctr Louisiana-LSU 1990; **Fac Appt:** Prof Oph, Case West Res Univ

Great Plains and Mountains

Anderson, Richard L MD [Oph] - **Spec Exp:** Orbital & Eyelid Tumors/Cancer; Eyelid Problems/Ptosis/Blepharospasm; Cosmetic Surgery-Face & Eyes; **Hospital:** Salt Lake Regional Med Ctr, Intermountain Shriners Hosp; **Address:** 1002 E South Temple, Ste 308, Salt Lake City, UT 84102-1525; **Phone:** 801-363-3355; **Board Cert:** Ophthalmology 1976; **Med School:** Univ Iowa Coll Med 1971; **Resid:** Ophthalmology, Univ Iowa Hosps-Clins 1975; **Fellow:** Oculoplastic & Reconstructive Surgery, Albany Med Ctr 1975; Oculoplastic & Reconstructive Surgery, UCSF Med Ctr 1976; **Fac Appt:** Prof PlS, Univ Utah

Cionni, Robert J MD [Oph] - **Spec Exp:** Cataract Surgery-Lens Implant; Refractive Surgery; **Hospital:** LDS Hosp, Univ Utah Hlth Care; **Address:** The Eye Inst of Utah, 755 E 3900 South, Salt Lake City, UT 84107; **Phone:** 801-266-2283; **Board Cert:** Ophthalmology 1991; **Med School:** Univ Cincinnati 1985; **Resid:** Ophthalmology, Univ Louisville Hosp 1987; **Fellow:** Cataract/Lens Implant Surgery, Cincinnati Eye Inst

Crandall, Alan S MD [Oph] - **Spec Exp:** Glaucoma; Cataract Surgery; **Hospital:** Univ Utah Hlth Care; **Address:** Moran Eye Ctr- Univ Utah Hosp, 65 N Mario Cappecchi Drive, Salt Lake City, UT 84132; **Phone:** 801-581-2352; **Board Cert:** Ophthalmology 1977; **Med School:** Univ Utah 1973; **Resid:** Ophthalmology, Hosp Univ Penn 1976; **Fellow:** Glaucoma, Scheie Eye Inst; **Fac Appt:** Clin Prof Oph, Univ Utah

Durrie, Daniel MD [Oph] - **Spec Exp:** LASIK-Refractive Surgery; Corneal Disease; **Hospital:** Univ of Kansas Hosp; **Address:** 5520 College Blvd, Ste 201, Overland Park, KS 66211; **Phone:** 913-491-3330; **Board Cert:** Ophthalmology 1979; **Med School:** Univ Nebr Coll Med 1975; **Resid:** Ophthalmology, Univ Nebr Med Coll Affil Hosp 1979; **Fellow:** Cornea, Filkins Eye Inst 1980; **Fac Appt:** Clin Prof Oph, Univ Kansas

Gigantelli, James W MD [Oph] - **Spec Exp:** Orbital Tumors/Cancer; Eyelid Cancer & Reconstruction; Lymphoma-Ocular (eye); **Hospital:** Nebraska Med Ctr; **Address:** 985540 Nebraska Medical Center, 985540 Nebraska Medical Ctr, Omaha, NE 68198-5540; **Phone:** 402-559-4276; **Board Cert:** Ophthalmology 1991; **Med School:** Vanderbilt Univ 1985; **Resid:** Ophthalmology, Baylor Coll Med 1989; **Fellow:** Ophthalmic Plastic & Reconstructive Surgery, Duke Unv Med Ctr 1990; **Fac Appt:** Prof Oph, Univ Nebr Coll Med

McCann, John D MD/PhD [Oph] - **Spec Exp:** Cosmetic Surgery-Face & Eyes; Orbital Diseases; Botox Therapy; **Hospital:** Intermountain Med Ctr; **Address:** Center for Facial Appearances, 1002 E South Temple, Ste 308, Salt Lake City, UT 84102; **Phone:** 801-363-3355; **Board Cert:** Ophthalmology 2007; **Med School:** Univ Iowa Coll Med 1991; **Resid:** Ophthalmology, Univ CA Affil Hosp 1995; **Fellow:** Oculoplastic Surgery, Univ Utah Med Ctr 1996

Southwest

Ellis Jr, George S MD [Oph] - **Spec Exp:** Pediatric Ophthalmology; Eye Muscle Disorders; **Hospital:** Children's Hospital - New Orleans, E Jefferson Genl Hosp; **Address:** Children's Hospital, 200 Henry Clay Ave, Ste 3106, New Orleans, LA 70118; **Phone:** 504-896-9426; **Board Cert:** Ophthalmology 1982; **Med School:** Tulane Univ 1977; **Resid:** Ophthalmology, LSU-Eye Center 1979; Ophthalmology, Duke Univ-Eye Ctr 1982; **Fellow:** Pediatric Ophthalmology, Hall Eye Clinic 1982; Pediatric Ophthalmology, Chldns Hosp 1982; **Fac Appt:** Assoc Clin Prof Oph, Tulane Univ

Ophthalmology

Esmaeli-Azad, Bita MD [Oph] - **Spec Exp:** Orbital & Eyelid Tumors/Cancer; Eyelid Cancer & Reconstruction; Oculoplastic Surgery; **Hospital:** UT MD Anderson Cancer Ctr; **Address:** Dept of Head & Neck Surgery, Ophthalmology Section, 1515 Holcombe Blvd, Unit 1445, Houston, TX 77030; **Phone:** 713-792-6523; **Board Cert:** Ophthalmology 2006; **Med School:** Ros Franklin Univ/Chicago Med Sch 1990; **Resid:** Ophthalmology, Univ Michigan Affil Hosp 1994; **Fellow:** Ophthalmic Plastic & Reconstructive Surgery, Univ Toronto Affil Hosp 1996; **Fac Appt:** Assoc Prof Oph, Univ Tex, Houston

Eustis, H Sprague MD [Oph] - **Spec Exp:** Pediatric Ophthalmology; Strabismus; **Hospital:** Ochsner Med Ctr-New Orleans, Children's Hospital - New Orleans; **Address:** Ochsner Clinic, Dept Ophthalmology, 1514 Jefferson Hwy Fl 10, New Orleans, LA 70121; **Phone:** 504-842-3995; **Board Cert:** Ophthalmology 1985; **Med School:** Louisiana State U, New Orleans 1980; **Resid:** Ophthalmology, LSU Eye Ctr 1984; **Fellow:** Pediatric Ophthalmology, Hosp Sick Chldn 1985; Pediatric Ophthalmology, Natl Chldns Med Ctr 1985; **Fac Appt:** Clin Prof Oph, Louisiana State U, New Orleans

Koch, Douglas D MD [Oph] - **Spec Exp:** Cataract Surgery; Refractive Surgery; **Hospital:** Methodist Hosp - Houston; **Address:** 1977 Butler Blvd, Houston, TX 77030-2704; **Phone:** 713-798-6100; **Board Cert:** Ophthalmology 1982; **Med School:** Harvard Med Sch 1977; **Resid:** Ophthalmology, Baylor Coll Med 1981; **Fellow:** Cornea, Moorfields Eye Hosp 1982; Refractive Surgery, Baylor Coll Med 1982; **Fac Appt:** Prof Oph, Baylor Coll Med

Lambert, H Michael MD [Oph] - **Spec Exp:** Retina/Vitreous Surgery; Macular Disease/Degeneration; Diabetic Eye Disease/Retinopathy; **Hospital:** Methodist Hosp - Houston, St. Luke's Episcopal Hosp-Houston; **Address:** 2727 Gramercy, Ste 200, Houston, TX 77025-1633; **Phone:** 713-799-9975; **Board Cert:** Ophthalmology 1983; **Med School:** Baylor Coll Med 1977; **Resid:** Ophthalmology, Wilford Hall USAF Med Ctr 1982; **Fellow:** Vitreoretinal Surgery, Duke Univ Eye Ctr 1983; **Fac Appt:** Assoc Clin Prof Oph, Baylor Coll Med

Lee, Andrew G MD [Oph] - **Spec Exp:** Neuro-Ophthalmology; Optic Nerve Disorders; Optic Nerve Tumors; **Hospital:** Methodist Hosp - Houston; **Address:** Methodist Hosp, Dept Ophthalmology, 6560 Fannin St, Ste 450, Houston, TX 77030; **Phone:** 713-441-8843; **Board Cert:** Ophthalmology 2006; **Med School:** Univ VA Sch Med 1989; **Resid:** Ophthalmology, Cullen Eye Inst-Baylor 1993; **Fellow:** Neuro-Ophthalmology, Wilmer Eye Inst-Johns Hopkins 1994; **Fac Appt:** Prof Oph, Cornell Univ-Weill Med Coll

Lewis, Richard Alan MD [Oph] - **Spec Exp:** Eye Diseases-Hereditary; Ophthalmic Genetics; Retinal Disorders; Macular Degeneration; **Hospital:** St. Luke's Episcopal Hosp-Houston, Texas Chldns Hosp; **Address:** Cullen Eye Inst, Baylor Coll Med, 6501 Fannin, Ste NC-206, Houston, TX 77030; **Phone:** 713-798-6100; **Board Cert:** Ophthalmology 1976; **Med School:** Univ Mich Med Sch 1969; **Resid:** Ophthalmology, Univ Michigan Hosp 1973; **Fellow:** Retina, Univ Michigan Hosp 1974; Macular Disease, Bascom Palmer Eye Inst 1975; **Fac Appt:** Prof Oph, Baylor Coll Med

Mazow, Malcolm L MD [Oph] - **Spec Exp:** Strabismus-Adult & Pediatric; Pediatric Ophthalmology; **Hospital:** Meml Hermann Hosp - Texas Med Ctr; **Address:** 2855 Gramercy St Fl 2, Houston, TX 77025; **Phone:** 713-668-6828; **Board Cert:** Ophthalmology 1967; **Med School:** Univ Tex Med Br, Galveston 1961; **Resid:** Ophthalmology, Univ Iowa Hosp 1965; **Fellow:** Strabismus, Univ Iowa Hosp 1966; **Fac Appt:** Clin Prof Oph, Univ Tex, Houston

McCulley, James P MD [Oph] - **Spec Exp:** Corneal & External Eye Disease; Laser Vision Surgery; Cataract Surgery; **Hospital:** UT Southwestern Med Ctr at Dallas; **Address:** Univ Tex SW Med Ctr, Dept Oph, 5323 Harry Hines Blvd, Dallas, TX 75390-9057; **Phone:** 214-645-2020; **Board Cert:** Ophthalmology 1974; **Med School:** Washington Univ, St Louis 1968; **Resid:** Ophthalmology, Mass EE Infirm 1973; **Fellow:** Cornea, Cornea Rsch-Retina Fdn 1974; Cornea, Mass EE Infirm 1974; **Fac Appt:** Prof Oph, Univ Tex SW, Dallas

Miller, Joseph M MD [Oph] - **Spec Exp:** Pediatric Ophthalmology; Strabismus; Amblyopia; **Hospital:** Univ Med Ctr - Tucson; **Address:** Univ Ariz, Dept Ophthalmology, 707 N Alvernon Way, Ste 301, Tucson, AZ 85711; **Phone:** 520-694-1460; **Board Cert:** Ophthalmology 1991; **Med School:** NE Ohio Univ 1985; **Resid:** Ophthalmology, Yale New Haven Hosp 1990; **Fellow:** Pediatric Ophthalmology, Johns Hopkins Hosp 1991; Refractive Surgery, Univ Arizona Hosp 2001; **Fac Appt:** Prof Oph, Univ Ariz Coll Med

Mims III, James Luther MD [Oph] - **Spec Exp:** Pediatric Ophthalmology; Strabismus-Adult & Pediatric; **Hospital:** Baptist Med Ctr - San Antonio, Methodist Chldns Hosp of South Texas; **Address:** 311 Camden St, Ste 511, San Antonio, TX 78215-2015; **Phone:** 210-225-0084; **Board Cert:** Ophthalmology 1977; **Med School:** Tulane Univ 1968; **Resid:** Ophthalmology, Wills Eye Hosp 1976; **Fellow:** Pediatric Ophthalmology, Wills Eye Hosp 1977; **Fac Appt:** Clin Prof Oph, Univ Tex, San Antonio

Pflugfelder, Stephen C MD [Oph] - **Spec Exp:** Corneal & External Eye Disease; Refractive Surgery; Cataract Surgery; Lens Implants; **Hospital:** Methodist Hosp - Houston; **Address:** 1977 Butler Blvd, Houston, TX 77030; **Phone:** 713-798-6100; **Board Cert:** Ophthalmology 1987; **Med School:** SUNY Upstate Med Univ 1981; **Resid:** Ophthalmology, Baylor Coll of Med Affil Hosp 1985; **Fellow:** Cornea & Ext Eye Disease, Bascom Palmer Eye Inst 1986; **Fac Appt:** Prof Oph, Baylor Coll Med

Richard, James M MD [Oph] - **Spec Exp:** Pediatric Ophthalmology; Eye Muscle Surgery; **Hospital:** Chldns Hosp OU Med Ctr, Integris Baptist Med Ctr - OK; **Address:** 11013 Hefner Pointe Drive, Oklahoma City, OK 73120-5050; **Phone:** 405-751-2020; **Board Cert:** Ophthalmology 1979; **Med School:** Univ Okla Coll Med 1974; **Resid:** Ophthalmology, Baylor Coll Med 1978; **Fellow:** Pediatric Ophthalmology, Chldns Hosp 1979; Ophthalmology, Johns Hopkins Hosp 1980; **Fac Appt:** Clin Prof Oph, Univ Okla Coll Med

Schiffman, Jade S MD [Oph] - **Spec Exp:** Neuro-Ophthalmology; **Hospital:** UT MD Anderson Cancer Ctr; **Address:** MD Anderson Cancer, 1515 Holcombe Blvd, Box 342, Houston, TX 77035; **Phone:** 713-792-3798; **Board Cert:** Neurology 1983; Ophthalmology 1991; **Med School:** SUNY Upstate Med Univ 1975; **Resid:** Neurology, Univ Miami Affil Hosp 1980; Ophthalmology, Univ California Affil Hosp 1989; **Fellow:** Neuro-Ophthalmology, Univ California Med Ctr 1981; **Fac Appt:** Prof Oph, Univ Tex, Houston

Siatkowski, R Michael MD [Oph] - **Spec Exp:** Pediatric Ophthalmology; Neuro-Ophthalmology; Retinopathy of Prematurity; Strabismus; **Hospital:** OU Med Ctr; **Address:** Dean Mcgee Eye Institute, 608 Stanton L Young Blvd, Oklahoma City, OK 73104; **Phone:** 405-271-1094; **Board Cert:** Ophthalmology 2009; **Med School:** Jefferson Med Coll 1987; **Resid:** Ophthalmology, St Francis Med Ctr 1991; **Fellow:** Neuro-Ophthalmology, Bascom Palmer Eye Inst 1992; Pediatric Ophthalmology, Bascom Palmer Eye Inst 1993; **Fac Appt:** Prof Oph, Univ Okla Coll Med

Soparkar, Charles MD [Oph] - **Spec Exp:** Eye Tumors/Cancer; Orbital & Eyelid Tumors/Cancer; Oculoplastic Surgery; **Hospital:** Methodist Hosp - Houston, Texas Chldns Hosp; **Address:** Plastic Eye Surg Assocs, 3730 Kirby Drive, Ste 900, Houston, TX 77098; **Phone:** 713-795-0705; **Board Cert:** Ophthalmology 2007; **Med School:** Univ Mass Sch Med 1990; **Resid:** Ophthalmology, Baylor Affil Hosps 1994; **Fellow:** Ophthalmic Oncololgy, Texas Med Ctr 1995; Ophthalmic Plastic Surgery, Texas Med Ctr 1995; **Fac Appt:** Asst Clin Prof Oph, Baylor Coll Med

Wallace III, Robert B MD [Oph] - **Spec Exp:** Refractive Surgery; Cataract Surgery; Glaucoma; **Hospital:** CHRISTUS St. Frances Cabrini Hosp; **Address:** 4110 Parliament Drive, Alexandria, LA 71303; **Phone:** 318-448-4488; **Board Cert:** Ophthalmology 1979; **Med School:** Tulane Univ 1974; **Resid:** Ophthalmology, Tulane Affil Hosp 1978; **Fac Appt:** Clin Prof Oph, Louisiana State U, New Orleans

West Coast and Pacific

Abbott, Richard L MD [Oph] - **Spec Exp:** Cornea & External Eye Disease; **Hospital:** UCSF Med Ctr; **Address:** UCSF, Dept Ophthalmology, 8 Koret Way, K301, San Francisco, CA 94143-0730; **Phone:** 415-514-8200; **Board Cert:** Ophthalmology 1978; **Med School:** Geo Wash Univ 1971; **Resid:** Ophthalmology, Presby-Pacific Med Ctr 1977; **Fellow:** Cornea & Ext Eye Disease, Bascom Palmer Eye Inst 1978; **Fac Appt:** Clin Prof Oph, UCSF

Arnold, Anthony C MD [Oph] - **Spec Exp:** Neuro-Ophthalmology; **Hospital:** UCLA Ronald Reagan Med Ctr; **Address:** 100 Stein Plaza, Box 957000, Los Angeles, CA 90095-7005; **Phone:** 310-825-4344; **Board Cert:** Ophthalmology 2008; **Med School:** UCLA 1975; **Resid:** Ophthalmology, Jules Stein Eye Inst-UCLA 1979; **Fellow:** Neuro-Ophthalmology, Jules Stein Eye Inst-UCLA 1983; **Fac Appt:** Clin Prof Oph, UCLA

Baerveldt, George MD [Oph] - **Spec Exp:** Glaucoma; **Hospital:** UC Irvine Med Ctr; **Address:** UC Irvine Med Ctr, Dept Ophthalmology, Gottschalk Med Plaza, 1 Medical Plaza Dr, Multi-Spec Ste, Irvine, CA 92697-4375; **Phone:** 949-824-2020; **Med School:** South Africa 1967; **Resid:** Ophthalmology, Univ of Witwatersrand 1975; **Fellow:** Neuro-Ophthalmology, SUNY Downstate Med Ctr 1975; **Fac Appt:** Prof Oph, UC Irvine

Baylis, Henry I MD [Oph] - **Spec Exp:** Oculoplastic Surgery; Eyelid Surgery; **Hospital:** UCLA Ronald Reagan Med Ctr, Hoag Meml Hosp Presby; **Address:** 1260 15th St, Ste 917, Santa Monica, CA 90404; **Phone:** 310-207-0300; **Board Cert:** Ophthalmology 1969; **Med School:** Univ Mich Med Sch 1960; **Resid:** Ophthalmology, UCLA Med Ctr 1966; **Fellow:** Oculoplastic Surgery, Manhattan EET Hosp 1967; **Fac Appt:** Clin Prof Oph, UCLA

Bernardino, Carlo Robert MD [Oph] - **Spec Exp:** Oculoplastic Surgery; Orbital Surgery; Thyroid Eye Disease; Anophthalmia; **Hospital:** Comm Hosp of Monterey Pen; **Address:** Vantage Eye Center, Medical Bldg B, Ste 130, 2 Upper Ragsdale Drive, Monterey, CA 93940; **Phone:** 831-647-3900; **Board Cert:** Ophthalmology 2003; **Med School:** Jefferson Med Coll 1997; **Resid:** Ophthalmology, Wills Eye Hosp 2001; **Fellow:** Oculoplastic Surgery, Mass Eye & Ear Infirm 2003; **Fac Appt:** Assoc Prof Oph, Yale Univ

Blumenkranz, Mark S MD [Oph] - **Spec Exp:** Retinal Disorders; Macular Degeneration; **Hospital:** Stanford Univ Hosp & Clinics; **Address:** The Eye Institute, 2452 Watson Court, Palo Alto, CA 94303-5353; **Phone:** 650-723-6995; **Board Cert:** Ophthalmology 1980; **Med School:** Brown Univ 1975; **Resid:** Ophthalmology, Stanford Univ Hosp 1979; **Fellow:** Vitreoretinal Surgery, Bascom Palmer Eye Inst 1980; **Fac Appt:** Prof Oph, Stanford Univ

Borchert, Mark S MD [Oph] - **Spec Exp:** Pediatric Ophthalmology; Vision-Unexplained Loss; Optic Nerve Disorders; **Hospital:** Chldns Hosp - Los Angeles; **Address:** Chldns Hosp, Div Ophthalmology, MS 88, 4650 Sunset Blvd, MS 88, Los Angeles, CA 90027-6062; **Phone:** 323-361-4510; **Board Cert:** Ophthalmology 1989; **Med School:** Baylor Coll Med 1983; **Resid:** Ophthalmology, LAC-USC Med Ctr 1987; **Fellow:** Neuro-Ophthalmology, Mass EE Infirm-Harvard 1988; **Fac Appt:** Assoc Prof Oph, USC Sch Med

Boxer Wachler, Brian S MD [Oph] - **Spec Exp:** LASIK-Refractive Surgery; Keratoconus; Corneal Disease & Surgery; Cataract Surgery; **Hospital:** Cedars-Sinai Med Ctr; **Address:** Boxer Wachler Vision Inst, 465 N Roxbury Drive, Ste 902, Beverly Hills, CA 90210; **Phone:** 310-860-1900; **Board Cert:** Ophthalmology 2010; **Med School:** Dartmouth Med Sch 1993; **Resid:** Ophthalmology, St Louis Univ Eye Inst 1997; **Fellow:** Refractive Surgery, Univ Kansas Med Ctr 1998

Boxrud, Cynthia Ann MD [Oph] - **Spec Exp:** Oculoplastic Surgery; Eye Tumors/Cancer; Orbital Diseases; **Hospital:** UCLA Ronald Reagan Med Ctr, St. John's Hlth Ctr, Santa Monica; **Address:** 2021 Santa Monica Blvd, Ste 700E, Santa Monica, CA 90404-2208; **Phone:** 310-829-9060; **Board Cert:** Ophthalmology 2008; **Med School:** Case West Res Univ 1986; **Resid:** Ophthalmology, NYU-Bellevue Hosp Ctr 1990; **Fellow:** Ophthalmic Oncololgy, New York Hosp-Cornell Med Ctr 1992; Ophthalmic Plastic Surgery, UCLA-Jules Stein Eye Inst 1993; **Fac Appt:** Asst Prof Oph, UCLA

Caprioli, Joseph MD [Oph] - **Spec Exp:** Glaucoma; Cataract Surgery; Anterior Segment Surgery; **Hospital:** UCLA Ronald Reagan Med Ctr; **Address:** UCLA-Jules Stein Eye Institute, 100 Stein Plaza Fl 2 - Ste 2-273, Los Angeles, CA 90095-7006; **Phone:** 310-794-9442; **Board Cert:** Ophthalmology 1985; **Med School:** SUNY Buffalo 1979; **Resid:** Ophthalmology, Yale-New Haven Hosp. 1983; **Fellow:** Glaucoma, Wills Eye Hosp 1984; **Fac Appt:** Prof Oph, UCLA

Caster, Andrew I MD [Oph] - **Spec Exp:** LASIK-Refractive Surgery; Laser Vision Surgery; **Hospital:** Cedars-Sinai Med Ctr; **Address:** 9100 Wilshire Blvd, Ste 265E, Beverly Hills, CA 90212; **Phone:** 310-274-1221; **Board Cert:** Ophthalmology 1986; **Med School:** Harvard Med Sch 1980; **Resid:** Ophthalmology, UCLA Jules Stein Eye Inst 1984

Char, Devron H MD [Oph] - **Spec Exp:** Eye Tumors/Cancer; Thyroid Eye Disease; Oculoplastic Surgery; **Hospital:** CA Pacific Med Ctr-Pacific Campus, UCSF Med Ctr; **Address:** 45 Castro St, Ste 309, San Francisco, CA 94114; **Phone:** 415-522-0700; **Board Cert:** Ophthalmology 1978; **Med School:** Univ Minn 1970; **Resid:** Internal Medicine, Mass Genl Hosp 1972; Ophthalmology, UCSF Med Ctr 1977; **Fellow:** Medical Oncology, Natl Cancer Inst 1974; Ophthalmology, UCSF Med Ctr 1978; **Fac Appt:** Prof Oph, Stanford Univ

Choy, Andrew MD [Oph] - **Spec Exp:** Eye Muscle Disorders; Oculoplastic & Orbital Surgery; Orbital Tumors/Cancer; **Hospital:** Long Beach Meml Med Ctr, Los Alamitos Med Ctr; **Address:** 4100 Long Beach Blvd, Ste 108, Long Beach, CA 90807-2619; **Phone:** 562-426-3925; **Board Cert:** Ophthalmology 1976; **Med School:** USC Sch Med 1969; **Resid:** Neurology, LAC-USC Med Ctr 1971; Ophthalmology, Bellevue Hosp Ctr-NYU 1974; **Fellow:** Strabismus, Columbia-Presby Med Ctr 1975; **Fac Appt:** Assoc Clin Prof Oph, UCLA

Cockerham, Kimberly P MD [Oph] - **Spec Exp:** Meningioma-Orbital (eye); Orbital Tumors/Cancer; Eyelid Cancer & Reconstruction; Neuro-Ophthalmology; **Hospital:** El Camino Hosp, Stanford Univ Hosp & Clinics; **Address:** 762 Altos Oaks Drive, Ste 2, Los Altos, CA 94024; **Phone:** 650-559-9150; **Board Cert:** Ophthalmology 2004; **Med School:** Geo Wash Univ 1987; **Resid:** Ophthalmology, Walter Reed Army Med Ctr 1992; **Fellow:** Neuro-Ophthalmology, Walter Reed Army Med Ctr 1993; Neuro-Ophthalmology, Allegheny General Hosp 1995

Day, Susan H MD [Oph] - **Spec Exp:** Pediatric Ophthalmology; Strabismus-Adult & Pediatric; **Hospital:** CA Pacific Med Ctr-Pacific Campus, Chldns Hosp - Oakland; **Address:** 2340 Clay St, Ste 100, San Francisco, CA 94115; **Phone:** 415-202-1500; **Board Cert:** Ophthalmology 2009; **Med School:** Louisiana State U, New Orleans 1975; **Resid:** Ophthalmology, California Pacific Med Ctr 1979; **Fellow:** Pediatric Ophthalmology, Hosp Sick Chldn 1980

De Juan Jr, Eugene MD [Oph] - **Spec Exp:** Retina/Vitreous Surgery; **Hospital:** UCSF Med Ctr; **Address:** UCSF Dept Ophthalmology, 10 Koret Way, San Francisco, CA 94143-0730; **Phone:** 415-353-2800; **Board Cert:** Ophthalmology 1985; **Med School:** Univ S Ala Coll Med 1979; **Resid:** Ophthalmology, Johns Hopkins Hosp 1983; **Fellow:** Vitreoretinal Surgery, Duke Univ Eye Ctr 1984; **Fac Appt:** Prof Oph, UCSF

Demer, Joseph L MD/PhD [Oph] - **Spec Exp:** Pediatric Ophthalmology; Strabismus; Nystagmus; **Hospital:** UCLA Ronald Reagan Med Ctr; **Address:** Jules Stein Eye Institute, 100 Stein Plaza, MC 7002, Los Angeles, CA 90095-7065; **Phone:** 310-825-5931; **Board Cert:** Ophthalmology 1988; **Med School:** Johns Hopkins Univ 1983; **Resid:** Ophthalmology, Baylor Coll Med 1987; **Fellow:** Pediatric Ophthalmology, Texas Chldns Hosp 1988; **Fac Appt:** Prof Oph, UCLA

Gorin, Michael B MD/PhD [Oph] - **Spec Exp:** Retinal Disorders; Macular Disease/Degeneration; Eye Diseases-Hereditary; **Hospital:** UCLA Ronald Reagan Med Ctr; **Address:** Dept Ophthalmology, Jules Stein Eye Inst, 100 Stein Plaza, Los Angeles, CA 90095-7000; **Phone:** 310-794-5400; **Board Cert:** Ophthalmology 1987; **Med School:** Univ Pennsylvania 1980; **Resid:** Ophthalmology, Jules Stein Eye Inst 1986; **Fellow:** Medical Retina, Moorfields Eye Hosp 1987; **Fac Appt:** Prof Oph, UCLA-David Geffen Sch Med

Granet, David B MD [Oph] - **Spec Exp:** Pediatric Ophthalmology; Eye Muscle Disorders; Strabismus; **Hospital:** UCSD Med Ctr, Rady Children's Hosp - San Diego; **Address:** UCSD-Shiley Eye Ctr, 9415 Campus Point Drive, La Jolla, CA 92093; **Phone:** 858-534-2020; **Board Cert:** Ophthalmology 2005; **Med School:** Yale Univ 1987; **Resid:** Ophthalmology, Bellevue Hosp-NYU 1991; **Fellow:** Pediatric Ophthalmology, Chldns Hosp & U Penn Scheie Inst 1993; **Fac Appt:** Prof Oph, UCSD

Humayun, Mark S MD/PhD [Oph] - **Spec Exp:** Retina/Vitreous Surgery; Retinal Disorders; Retinal Vascular Diseases; Diabetic Eye Disease/Retinopathy; **Hospital:** Keck Med Ctr of USC (page 75); **Address:** Doheny Eye Center, 1450 San Pablo St Fl 4, Los Angeles, CA 90033; **Phone:** 323-442-6522; **Board Cert:** Ophthalmology 2006; **Med School:** Duke Univ 1989; **Resid:** Ophthalmology, Duke Univ Hosp 1993; **Fellow:** Vitreoretinal Surgery, Wilmer Inst-Johns Hopkins 1995; **Fac Appt:** Prof Oph, USC-Keck School of Medicine

Irvine, John A MD [Oph] - **Spec Exp:** Corneal & External Eye Disease; **Hospital:** Keck Med Ctr of USC (page 75); **Address:** USC-Doheny Eye Institute, 1450 San Pablo St, Ste 5703, Los Angeles, CA 90033; **Phone:** 323-442-6335; **Board Cert:** Ophthalmology 1989; **Med School:** USC Sch Med 1982; **Resid:** Ophthalmology, Mass EE Infirm 1986; **Fellow:** Cornea & Ext Eye Disease, Mass EE Infirm 1987; **Fac Appt:** Prof Oph, USC Sch Med

Isenberg, Sherwin Jay MD [Oph] - **Spec Exp:** Strabismus; Pediatric Ophthalmology; **Hospital:** LAC - Harbor - UCLA Med Ctr, UCLA Ronald Reagan Med Ctr; **Address:** Jules Stein Eye Inst, 100 Stein Plaza, Los Angeles, CA 90095-7000; **Phone:** 310-825-8840; **Board Cert:** Ophthalmology 1978; **Med School:** UCLA 1973; **Resid:** Ophthalmology, Illinois Ear & Eye Infirm 1977; **Fellow:** Pediatric Ophthalmology, Chldns Hosp Natl Med Ctr 1978; **Fac Appt:** Prof Oph, UCLA

Iwach, Andrew G MD [Oph] - **Spec Exp:** Glaucoma; **Hospital:** UCSF Med Ctr, CA Pacific Med Ctr-Pacific Campus; **Address:** Glaucoma Ctr of San Francisco, 55 Stevenson St, San Francisco, CA 94105; **Phone:** 415-981-2020; **Board Cert:** Ophthalmology 1991; **Med School:** UCLA 1984; **Resid:** Ophthalmology, Stanford Univ Med Ctr 1988; **Fellow:** Glaucoma, UCSF Med Ctr 1989; **Fac Appt:** Assoc Prof Oph, UCSF

Kim, Jonathan W MD [Oph] - **Spec Exp:** Oculoplastic Surgery; Orbital Tumors/Cancer; **Hospital:** Stanford Univ Hosp & Clinics; **Address:** 900 Blake Wilbur Drive, rm W3002, MC 5353, Palo Alto, CA 94304; **Phone:** 650-723-6995; **Board Cert:** Ophthalmology 2000; **Med School:** Univ Iowa Coll Med 1994; **Resid:** Ophthalmology, CA Pacific Med Ctr 1998; **Fellow:** Oculoplastic Surgery, Jules Stein Eye Inst/UCLA Med Ctr 2000; Orbital Surgery, Mass Eye & Ear Infirm 2004

Maloney, Robert K MD [Oph] - **Spec Exp:** Refractive Surgery; LASIK-Refractive Surgery; Cataract Surgery; **Hospital:** UCLA Ronald Reagan Med Ctr; **Address:** Maloney Vision Inst, 10921 Wilshire Blvd, Ste 900, Los Angeles, CA 90024-4002; **Phone:** 310-208-3937; **Board Cert:** Ophthalmology 1991; **Med School:** UCSF 1985; **Resid:** Ophthalmology, Johns Hopkins Hosp 1989; **Fellow:** Refractive Surgery, Emory Univ Hosp 1991; **Fac Appt:** Clin Prof Oph, UCLA

Manche, Edward E MD [Oph] - **Spec Exp:** LASIK-Refractive Surgery; Corneal Disease & Transplant; PRK-Refractive Surgery; **Hospital:** Stanford Univ Hosp & Clinics; **Address:** The Eye Institute at Stanford, 2452 Watson Court, Palo Alto, CA 94303-5353; **Phone:** 650-723-6995; **Board Cert:** Ophthalmology 2007; **Med School:** Albert Einstein Coll Med 1990; **Resid:** Ophthalmology, UMDNJ Affil Hosp 1994; **Fellow:** Cornea & Ext Eye Disease, Jules Stein Eye Inst-UCLA 1996; **Fac Appt:** Assoc Prof Oph, Stanford Univ

Mannis, Mark J MD [Oph] - **Spec Exp:** Cornea Transplant & Artificial Cornea; Cornea & External Eye Disease; **Hospital:** UC Davis Med Ctr; **Address:** UC Davis Med Ctr, Dept Ophthalmology, 4860 Y St, Ste 2400, Sacramento, CA 95817; **Phone:** 916-734-6602; **Board Cert:** Ophthalmology 2009; **Med School:** Univ Fla Coll Med 1975; **Resid:** Ophthalmology, Washington Univ 1979; **Fellow:** Cornea & Ext Eye Disease, Univ IA Hosps & Clins 1980; **Fac Appt:** Prof Oph, UC Davis

Marmor, Michael F MD [Oph] - **Spec Exp:** Retinal Disorders; Retinal Dystrophies; Electroretinograms (ERG); Retinal Drug Toxicity; **Hospital:** Stanford Univ Hosp & Clinics; **Address:** California VitreoRetinal Ctr, 2452 Watson Ct, Palo Alto, CA 94303-5353; **Phone:** 650-723-6995; **Board Cert:** Ophthalmology 1974; **Med School:** Harvard Med Sch 1966; **Resid:** Ophthalmology, Mass EE Infirm 1973; **Fellow:** Neurological Physiology, NaTl Inst Hlth 1970; **Fac Appt:** Prof Oph, Stanford Univ

Masket, Samuel MD [Oph] - **Spec Exp:** Cataract Surgery; Cataract Surgery Revision; Congenital Eye Disorders-Rare; **Address:** 2080 Century Park E, Ste 911, Los Angeles, CA 90067; **Phone:** 310-229-1220; **Board Cert:** Ophthalmology 1974; **Med School:** NY Med Coll 1968; **Resid:** Ophthalmology, Metropolitan Hosp Ctr 1973; **Fellow:** Ophthalmology, Columbia Presby Med Ctr 1973; **Fac Appt:** Clin Prof Oph, UCLA

Mathers, William MD [Oph] - **Spec Exp:** Corneal & External Eye Disease; Refractive Surgery; Laser Surgery; **Hospital:** OR Hlth & Sci Univ; **Address:** Casey Eye Inst, 3375 SW Terwilliger Blvd, Portland, OR 97239-4197; **Phone:** 503-494-7674; **Board Cert:** Anesthesiology 1980; Ophthalmology 1987; **Med School:** Stanford Univ 1973; **Resid:** Anesthesiology, Stanford Univ Hosp 1977; Ophthalmology, Univ Wash Med Ctr 1985; **Fellow:** Cornea, Georgetown Univ Med Ctr 1986; **Fac Appt:** Prof Oph, Oregon Hlth & Sci Univ

Miller, Kevin M MD [Oph] - **Spec Exp:** Cataract Surgery-Lens Implant; Refractive Surgery; **Hospital:** UCLA Ronald Reagan Med Ctr; **Address:** Jules Stein Eye Institute, 100 Stein Plaza, UCLA, Los Angeles, CA 90095; **Phone:** 310-206-9951; **Board Cert:** Ophthalmology 2003; **Med School:** Johns Hopkins Univ 1985; **Resid:** Ophthalmology, Jules Stein Eye Inst 1991; **Fellow:** Ophthalmic Optics, Wilmer Inst/Johns Hopkins 1988; **Fac Appt:** Clin Prof Oph, UCLA

Mondino, Bartly MD [Oph] - **Spec Exp:** Cornea & External Eye Disease; **Hospital:** UCLA Ronald Reagan Med Ctr; **Address:** 100 Stein Plaza, MC 700019, Los Angeles, CA 90095-7065; **Phone:** 310-825-5053; **Board Cert:** Ophthalmology 1976; **Med School:** Stanford Univ 1971; **Resid:** Ophthalmology, NY Hosp/Cornell Univ 1975; **Fellow:** Cornea & Ext Eye Disease, Univ Pittsburgh Eye & Ear Hosp 1976; **Fac Appt:** Prof Oph, UCLA

Ophthalmology

Murphree, A Linn MD [Oph] - **Spec Exp:** Retinoblastoma; Eye Tumors/Cancer; Ophthalmic Genetics; Pediatric Ophthalmology; **Hospital:** Chldns Hosp - Los Angeles, USC Norris Cancer Hosp (page 75); **Address:** Chldns Hosp, Div Oph, 4650 Sunset Blvd, MS 88, Los Angeles, CA 90027-6016; **Phone:** 323-361-2347; **Board Cert:** Ophthalmology 1978; **Med School:** Baylor Coll Med 1972; **Resid:** Ophthalmology, Baylor Coll Med 1973; Ophthalmology, Baylor Coll Med 1976; **Fellow:** Pediatric Ophthalmology, Wilmer Inst/Johns Hopkins 1977; **Fac Appt:** Prof Oph, USC Sch Med

Ng, John MD [Oph] - **Spec Exp:** Oculoplastic & Orbital Surgery; Reconstructive Surgery; Trauma; **Hospital:** OR Hlth & Sci Univ; **Address:** Casey Eye Inst, 3375 SW Terwilliger Blvd, Portland, OR 97239; **Phone:** 503-494-3004; **Board Cert:** Ophthalmology 2007; **Med School:** Geo Wash Univ 1988; **Resid:** Ophthalmology, Letterman/Madigan Army Med Ctr 1994; Ophthalmology; **Fellow:** Oculoplastic & Reconstructive Surgery, Midwest Eye Inst 1997; **Fac Appt:** Assoc Prof Oph, Oregon Hlth & Sci Univ

Paul, T Otis MD [Oph] - **Spec Exp:** Pediatric Ophthalmology; Strabismus-Adult & Pediatric; **Hospital:** Chldns Hosp - Oakland, CA Pacific Med Ctr-Pacific Campus; **Address:** 5275 Claremont Ave Fl 1, Oakland, CA 94618; **Phone:** 510-428-3050; **Board Cert:** Ophthalmology 1974; **Med School:** UCLA 1967; **Resid:** Ophthalmology, Naval Hosp 1972; **Fellow:** Pediatric Ophthalmology, Ca Pacific Med Ctr 1974

Puliafito, Carmen A MD [Oph] - **Spec Exp:** Retinal Disorders; Macular Degeneration; **Hospital:** Keck Med Ctr of USC (page 75); **Address:** USC Dept Ophthalmology, 1975 Zonal Ave, Ste KAM 500, Los Angeles, CA 90033; **Phone:** 323-442-6335; **Board Cert:** Ophthalmology 1983; **Med School:** Harvard Med Sch 1978; **Resid:** Ophthalmology, Mass Eye & Ear Infirm 1982; **Fellow:** Vitreoretinal Surgery, Mass Eye & Ear Infirm 1983; **Fac Appt:** Prof Oph, USC-Keck School of Medicine

Rao, Narsing A MD [Oph] - **Spec Exp:** Uveitis/AIDS; Eye Pathology; **Hospital:** Keck Med Ctr of USC (page 75); **Address:** USC Doheny Eye Center, 1450 San Pablo St, Los Angeles, CA 90033-4697; **Phone:** 323-442-6522; **Board Cert:** Pathology 1974; Ophthalmology 1977; **Med School:** India 1967; **Resid:** Pathology, Georgetown Univ Hosp 1972; Ophthalmology, Georgetown Univ Hosp 1975; **Fac Appt:** Prof Oph, USC Sch Med

Sadda, SriniVas R MD [Oph] - **Spec Exp:** Macular Degeneration; Diabetic Eye Disease/Retinopathy; Retinal Disorders-Inherited; Retinal Vascular Diseases; **Hospital:** Keck Med Ctr of USC (page 75); **Address:** USC Doheny Eye Ctr, 9033 Wilshire Blvd, Ste 360, Beverly Hills, CA 90210; **Phone:** 310-601-3366; **Board Cert:** Ophthalmology 2010; **Med School:** Johns Hopkins Univ 1994; **Resid:** Ophthalmology, Wilmer Eye Inst 1997; **Fellow:** Neuro-Ophthalmology, Wilmer Eye Inst 1998; Retina, Wilmer Eye Inst 1998; **Fac Appt:** Assoc Prof Oph, USC-Keck School of Medicine

Salz, James J MD [Oph] - **Spec Exp:** LASIK-Refractive Surgery; PRK-Refractive Surgery; Cataract Surgery; **Hospital:** Cedars-Sinai Med Ctr; **Address:** 11620 Wilshire Blvd, Ste 711, Los Angeles, CA 90025; **Phone:** 310-444-1134; **Board Cert:** Ophthalmology 1971; **Med School:** Duke Univ 1965; **Resid:** Ophthalmology, LAC-USC Med Ctr 1969; **Fac Appt:** Clin Prof Oph, USC Sch Med

Savino, Peter J MD [Oph] - **Spec Exp:** Neuro-Ophthalmology; **Hospital:** UCSD Med Ctr; **Address:** Shiley Eye Ctr, 9415 Campus Point Drive, MC 0946, La Jolla, CA 92093-0946; **Phone:** 858-534-6290; **Board Cert:** Ophthalmology 1975; **Med School:** Italy 1968; **Resid:** Ophthalmology, Georgetown Med Ctr 1973; **Fellow:** Neuro-Ophthalmology, Bascom Palmer Eye Inst 1974; **Fac Appt:** Prof Oph, Thomas Jefferson Univ

Seibel, Barry S MD [Oph] - **Spec Exp:** Cataract Surgery; **Hospital:** Cedars-Sinai Med Ctr; **Address:** 11620 Wilshire Blvd, Ste 711, Los Angeles, CA 90025; **Phone:** 310-444-1134; **Board Cert:** Ophthalmology 1991; **Med School:** Univ Tex, Houston 1985; **Resid:** Ophthalmology, Hollywood Presby Med Ctr 1987; Ophthalmology, USC-Doheny Eye Clin 1989; **Fac Appt:** Asst Clin Prof Oph, UCLA

Seiff, Stuart R MD [Oph] - **Spec Exp:** Oculoplastic Surgery; Orbital Tumors/Cancer; **Hospital:** UCSF Med Ctr, CA Pacific Med Ctr-Pacific Campus; **Address:** 2100 Webster St, Ste 214, San Francisco, CA 94115; **Phone:** 415-923-3007; **Board Cert:** Ophthalmology 1986; **Med School:** UCSF 1980; **Resid:** Ophthalmology, UCSF Med Ctr 1984; **Fellow:** Ophthalmic Plastic & Reconstructive Surgery, UCLA Med Ctr 1985; Oculoplastic Surgery, Moorfield's Eye Hosp 1986; **Fac Appt:** Prof Oph, UCSF

Serafano, Donald N MD [Oph] - **Spec Exp:** LASIK-Refractive Surgery; Cataract Surgery; Lens Implants; **Hospital:** Los Alamitos Med Ctr, Long Beach Meml Med Ctr; **Address:** 10861 Cherry St, Ste 204, Box 250, Los Alamitos, CA 90720-5403; **Phone:** 562-598-3160; **Board Cert:** Ophthalmology 1978; **Med School:** Wayne State Univ 1971; **Resid:** Ophthalmology, Mayo Clinic 1978; **Fac Appt:** Assoc Clin Prof Oph, USC Sch Med

Shamie, Neda MD [Oph] - **Spec Exp:** Cornea Transplant; Cataract Surgery; Anterior Segment Surgery; Keratoconus; **Hospital:** Keck Med Ctr of USC (page 75); **Address:** USC Doheny Eye Ctr, 9033 Wilshire Blvd, Ste 360, Beverly Hills, CA 90210; **Phone:** 310-601-3366; **Board Cert:** Ophthalmology 2006; **Med School:** UCSF 1998; **Resid:** Ophthalmology, UC-Irvine Med Ctr 2002; **Fellow:** Cornea & Refractive Surgery, UC-Irvine Med Ctr 2993; **Fac Appt:** Assoc Clin Prof Oph, USC-Keck School of Medicine

Smith, Ronald Edward MD [Oph] - **Spec Exp:** Corneal Disease; Uveitis; **Hospital:** Keck Med Ctr of USC (page 75); **Address:** USC-Doheny Eye Center, 1450 San Pablo Rd, Ste 5703, Los Angeles, CA 90033; **Phone:** 323-442-6335; **Board Cert:** Ophthalmology 1974; **Med School:** Johns Hopkins Univ 1967; **Resid:** Ophthalmology, Wilmer Ophthal Inst 1973; **Fellow:** Research, UCSF 1972; **Fac Appt:** Prof Oph, USC Sch Med

Steinert, Roger F MD [Oph] - **Spec Exp:** Refractive Surgery; Cataract Surgery; Cornea Transplant; **Hospital:** UC Irvine Med Ctr; **Address:** Gottschalk Med Plaza, 1 Medical Plaza Drive Fl 2, Irvine, CA 92697; **Phone:** 949-824-2020; **Board Cert:** Ophthalmology 1982; **Med School:** Harvard Med Sch 1977; **Resid:** Ophthalmology, Mass EE Infirm 1981; **Fac Appt:** Prof Oph, UC Irvine

Stout, J Timothy MD/PhD [Oph] - **Spec Exp:** Retinal Disorders-Pediatric; Retinoblastoma; Retinopathy of Prematurity; **Hospital:** OR Hlth & Sci Univ, Providence St Vincent Med Ctr; **Address:** 3375 SW Terwilliger Blvd, Portland, OR 97239; **Phone:** 503-494-2435; **Board Cert:** Ophthalmology 2010; **Med School:** Baylor Coll Med 1989; **Resid:** Ophthalmology, Doheny Eye Inst 1993; **Fellow:** Ophthalmology, Moorfields Eye Hosp 1994; Retinal Surgery, Doheny Eye Inst 1995; **Fac Appt:** Assoc Prof Oph, Oregon Hlth & Sci Univ

Weiss, Avery H MD [Oph] - **Spec Exp:** Pediatric Ophthalmology; Strabismus; Amblyopia; **Hospital:** Seattle Chldns Hosp; **Address:** 4800 Sand Point Way NE, MS W-4753, Seattle, WA 98105; **Phone:** 206-987-2177; **Board Cert:** Ophthalmology 1981; **Med School:** Univ Miami Sch Med 1974; **Resid:** Internal Medicine, Barnes-Jewish Hosp 1976; Ophthalmology, Barnes-Jewish Hosp 1980; **Fellow:** Research, Barnes-Jewish Hosp 1977; Pediatric Ophthalmology, Chldns Hosp Natl Med Ctr 1981; **Fac Appt:** Assoc Prof Oph, Univ Wash

Ophthalmology

Wilson, David Jean MD [Oph] - **Spec Exp:** Eye Tumors/Cancer; Ophthalmic Pathology; **Hospital:** OR Hlth & Sci Univ; **Address:** 3375 SW Terwilliger Blvd, Portland, OR 97239; **Phone:** 503-494-7881; **Board Cert:** Ophthalmology 2009; **Med School:** Baylor Coll Med 1981; **Resid:** Ophthalmology, Univ Oregon 1985; **Fellow:** Ophthalmic Pathology, John Hopkins Univ Hosp 1987; Retina/Vitreous, Mass Eye & Ear Infirm 1988; **Fac Appt:** Prof Oph, Oregon Hlth & Sci Univ

Wright, Kenneth W MD [Oph] - **Spec Exp:** Cataract Surgery-Lens Implant; Strabismus-Adult & Pediatric; Pediatric Eye Surgery-Ptosis; Pediatric Ophthalmology; **Hospital:** Cedars-Sinai Med Ctr; **Address:** 520 S San Vincente Blvd, Los Angeles, CA 90048; **Phone:** 310-652-6420; **Board Cert:** Ophthalmology 1983; **Med School:** Boston Univ 1977; **Resid:** Ophthalmology, LAC-USC Med Ctr 1981; **Fellow:** Pediatric Ophthalmology, Johns Hopkins Hosp 1981; Pediatric Ophthalmology, Chldns Hosp Natl Med Ctr 1982; **Fac Appt:** Clin Prof Oph, USC Sch Med

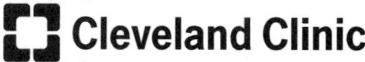
Cleveland Clinic

Every life deserves world class care.

Ophthalmology

Cleveland Clinic Cole Eye Institute is a center of excellence for highly specialized ophthalmologic care and research, with a reputation for innovation and superior outcomes. Our staff has one of the highest patient volumes in the United States, with advanced expertise in retina and vitreous surgery, cornea and external diseases, glaucoma, neuro-ophthalmology, oculoplastics and orbital surgery, ocular oncology, pediatric ophthalmology, refractive surgery and uveitis. We rank among the top ophthalmology programs in the nation according to *U.S.News & World Report* — the highest ranking in Ohio.

National Leader in Retina Conditions

Surgical procedures developed by our vitreoretinal faculty are used worldwide to treat retinal detachments, diabetic macular edema, diabetic traction detachments, macular holes and pediatric retinal surgery. The dedicated team utilizes advanced retinal imaging devices and provides access to the latest clinical trials for patients who are in the early stages of age-related macular degeneration or who have failed standard medical therapy.

Unique Provider for Pediatric Ophthalmology

Our pediatric specialists offer expert treatment for strabismus, retinopathy of prematurity and congenital cataracts, and performs about 150 surgical procedures annually for esotropia, exotropia, thyroid eye disease, cranial nerve palsies, dissociated deviations, hyper-tropia and hypotropias, Duane and Brown syndromes, nystagmus and related conditions.

Cleveland Clinic
Cole Eye Institute
9500 Euclid Avenue
Cleveland, OH 44195

clevelandclinic.org/
eyetopdocs

Offering Same-Day Appointments
Call 800.274.2009.

Treatment Guides

Cleveland Clinic has developed comprehensive treatment guides for many diseases and conditions. To download our free treatment guides, visit clevelandclinic.org/treatmentguides.

Online Medical Second Opinion

Cleveland Clinic's My**Consult** Online Medical Second Opinion program securely connects patients to our physician specialists for more than 1,000 life-changing or life-threatening diagnoses all by the click of a mouse. To learn more, log onto eclevelandclinic.org/myconsult or call 800.223.2273, ext. 43223.

Special Assistance for Out-of-State Patients

Cleveland Clinic Global Patient Services offers a complimentary Medical Concierge service for patients who travel from outside of Ohio. Call 800.223.2273, ext. 55580 or email medicalconcierge@ccf.org.

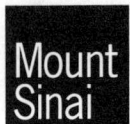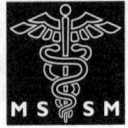

MOUNT SINAI
SCHOOL OF
MEDICINE

THE MOUNT SINAI MEDICAL CENTER
OPHTHALMOLOGY

One Gustave L. Levy Place
Fifth Avenue and 100th Street
New York, NY 10029-6574
Physician Referral: 1-800-MD-SINAI (637-4624)
www.mountsinai.org/opthalmology

Specializing in the prevention, diagnosis, and treatment of eye disorders, the **DEPARTMENT OF OPHTHALMOLOGY** at Mount Sinai features faculty with wide experience in special eye problems. The department offers the full spectrum of comprehensive eye care services, as well as a state-of-the-art optical shop.

Services include:

- Refractive errors and comprehensive ophthalmology
- Corneal and external diseases of the eye
- Refractive surgery
- Retinal disorders (diabetic retinopathy, macular degeneration, inherited retinal diseases)
- Glaucoma
- Dry eyes (Sjögren's syndrome)
- Intravitreal injections, including Lucentis and Avastin
- Pediatric eye care and strabismus
- Uveitis (inflammation of the eye)
- Neuro-ophthalmic disorders
- Oculplastic surgery, including lidand orbital tumors and thyroid-related eye problems
- Cosmetic procedures—Botox and Restalayne injections
- Trauma

A PIONEERING METHOD OF CORRECTING FARSIGHTEDNESS
Mount Sinai ophthalmologists helped pioneer a new radiofrequency method of correcting farsightedness. Known as conductive keratoplasty (CK), the brief procedure is performed in the doctor's office with only topical anesthesia (eye drops). For most farsighted patients—especially those over age 40 whose eyes are naturally aging—the CK procedure eliminates the need for glasses.

The department offers the full range of sophisticated diagnostic tests for evaluating patient conditions, including optical coherence tomography, fundus photography, fluorescein angiography, diagnostic ultrasound, electroretinography, visually evoked potentials, electro-oculography, corneal topography, and confocal microscopy, as well as state-of-the-art techniques for assessing glaucoma. These techniques include perimetry, HRT II imaging and ultrasound biomicroscopy, a noninvasive method to achieve high-resolution imaging of the inside of the eye. In certain cases of glaucoma, it is the only noninvasive way to identify the exact cause of the condition and ascertain optimal treatment. These methods allow for faster, more accurate diagnosis and help determine the best treatment plan for each individual patient.

Our highly skilled eye surgeons perform cataract surgery, corneal transplants, refractive surgery, glaucoma surgery, strabismus surgery, ophthalmic plastic and reconstructive surgery, laser surgery, and vitreoretinal surgery for complicated retinal problems. We also offer minimally invasive procedures to treat eye disease, including non-laser refractive surgeries, small-incision cataract surgery, bladeless laser procedures and Intacs for keratoconus.

LEADERS IN CLINICAL RESEARCH
Mount Sinai ophthalmologists helped pioneer and evaluate new treatments for eye diseases and problems, including glaucoma, uvetis, ocular infections and farsightedness.

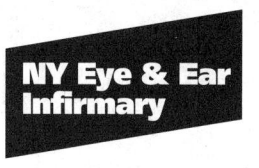

NY Eye & Ear Infirmary

Continuum Health Partners, Inc.

THE NEW YORK EYE AND EAR INFIRMARY

310 East 14th Street
New York, New York 10003
Tel. 212.979.4000   Fax. 212.228.0664
http://www.nyee.edu

PROVIDING EXCEPTIONAL EYE CARE

The Department of Ophthalmology is the region's most comprehensive center for the delivery of primary through tertiary eye care. It is also by far the largest provider of eye care in the metropolitan area—with some 155,000 outpatient visits and 22,000 surgical cases performed each year. 365 board-certified ophthalmologists located throughout New York City and its tri-state area comprise the attending Medical Staff.

IN A HIGHLY SPECIALIZED SETTING

As a specialty hospital, The New York Eye and Ear Infirmary is uniquely qualified to handle the most complicated cases. It serves as a nationwide referral center with a commitment to teaching, research, and high-technology based patient care. Cutting edge ocular imaging instrumentation provides highest resolution to diagnose diseases of the cornea, retina and optic nerve and glaucoma. Highly experienced staff in state-of-the-art facilities have made the New York Eye and Ear Infirmary's 17 operating rooms a national benchmark in efficiency in eye surgery cases.

FOR PATIENTS OF ALL AGES

The New York Eye and Ear Infirmary's Ophthalmology staff are sensitive to the specific needs of patients of all ages. Senior citizens are the vast majority of the NYEE's 12,000 cataract patients each year, as well as individuals receiving treatment for age-related macular degeneration. Young children are now 25 percent of the patient population, with conditions such as strabismus, acquired and congenital cataracts, corneal diseases and ocular trauma. For those rare cases of children who have a disease ordinarily associated with age, the Infirmary runs New York's only Pediatric Glaucoma Service. Active adults of all ages utilize the New York Metropolitan Eye Trauma Center and Oculoplastic and Orbital Surgery Services.

Ophthalmology Clinical Services

Ambulatory Care Services
Comprehensive Eye Care
Cornea & Refractive Surgery
Eye Trauma
Glaucoma
Low Vision
Neuro-Ophthalmology
Ocular Pathology
Ocular Tumor
Oculoplastic &
Orbital Surgery
Pediatric Ophthalmology
& Strabismus
Retinal-Vitreal
Uveitis/Ocular Immunology

Facilities

Ambulatory Surgery Center
Bendheim Family Retina Center
Einhorn Clinical Trials Area
*(supporting more than 100
ophthalmology studies a year)*
Jorge N. Buxton Microsurgical
Education Center
*(for residents, fellows and
attending physicians)*

About The New York Eye and Ear Infirmary

Founded in 1820, it is the nation's first and foremost, continuously operating specialty hospital. More than 10 million people have sought treatment here since its inception.

Physician Referral
1.800.449.HOPE (4673)

The Best in American Medicine
www.CastleConnolly.com

Orthopaedic Surgery

An orthopaedic surgeon is trained in the preservation, investigation and restoration of the form and function of the extremities, spine and associated structures by medical, surgical and physical means.

An orthopaedic surgeon is involved with the care of patients whose musculoskeletal problems include congenital deformities, trauma, infections, tumors, metabolic disturbances of the musculoskeletal system, deformities, injuries and degenerative diseases of the spine, hands, feet, knee, hip, shoulder and elbow in children and adults. An orthopaedic surgeon is also concerned with primary and secondary muscular problems and the effects of central or peripheral nervous system lesions of the musculoskeletal system.

Note: *There are many Orthopaedic Surgeons who are trained in Sports Medicine and prefer to be listed under that heading; some trained in Sports Medicine prefer to be listed under Orthopaedics.*

Training Required: Five years (including general surgery training) *plus* two years in clinical practice before final certification is achieved.

ORTHOPAEDIC SURGERY

New England

Abdu, William A MD [OrS] - **Spec Exp:** Spinal Surgery; Spinal Disorders; Spinal Cord Injury; **Hospital:** Dartmouth - Hitchcock Med Ctr; **Address:** Darthmouth-Hitchcock Med Ctr, Spine Ctr, 1 Med Ctr Drive, Lebanon, NH 03756; **Phone:** 603-650-2225; **Board Cert:** Orthopaedic Surgery 2004; **Med School:** Tufts Univ 1985; **Resid:** Surgery, Darthmouth-Hitchcock Med Ctr 1990; Orthopaedic Surgery, Newington Chldns Hosp 1989; **Fellow:** Spinal Surgery, Case Western Reserve Univ Hosp 1991; **Fac Appt:** Assoc Prof OrS, Dalhousie Univ

Bono, James Vincent MD [OrS] - **Spec Exp:** Hip Surgery; Knee Surgery; **Hospital:** New England Bapt Hosp; **Address:** 125 Parker Hill Ave, Ste 573, Boston, MA 02120; **Phone:** 617-731-6337; **Board Cert:** Orthopaedic Surgery 2008; **Med School:** Albany Med Coll 1987; **Resid:** Orthopaedic Surgery, Albany Med Ctr 1993; **Fellow:** Hip & Knee Surgery, Hosp for Special Surgery 1994; **Fac Appt:** Clin Prof OrS, Tufts Univ

Brick, Gregory W MD [OrS] - **Spec Exp:** Hip Replacement; Knee Replacement; Spinal Surgery; **Hospital:** Brigham and Women's Hosp (page 57); **Address:** Brigham & Womens, Dept Orth Surg, 75 Francis St, Boston, MA 02115; **Phone:** 617-732-5386; **Med School:** New Zealand 1976; **Resid:** Surgery, Greenlane Hosp 1981; Orthopaedic Surgery, Middlemore Hosp 1984; **Fellow:** Joint Replacement Surgery, Brigham & Women's Hosp 1986; Spinal Surgery, Vanderbilt Univ Med Ctr 1987; **Fac Appt:** Assoc Clin Prof OrS, Harvard Med Sch

Browner, Bruce D MD [OrS] - **Spec Exp:** Fractures-Complex; Osteomyelitis; Bone Infections; Fractures-Non Union; **Hospital:** Univ of Conn Hlth Ctr, John Dempsey Hosp, Hartford Hosp; **Address:** Med Arts & Rsch Bldg, 263 Farmington Ave Fl 3 - Ste 2, Farmington, CT 06030-4038; **Phone:** 860-679-6650; **Board Cert:** Orthopaedic Surgery 1979; **Med School:** SUNY Downstate 1973; **Resid:** Orthopaedic Surgery, Albany Med Ctr 1978; **Fellow:** Trauma, Albany Med Ctr 1975; **Fac Appt:** Prof OrS, Univ Conn

Burke, Dennis MD [OrS] - **Spec Exp:** Knee Replacement; Hip Replacement; Reconstructive Surgery; **Hospital:** Mass Genl Hosp; **Address:** Mass General Hosp, Yawkey 3B, 55 Fruit St, Boston, MA 02114; **Phone:** 617-726-3411; **Board Cert:** Orthopaedic Surgery 2009; **Med School:** Loyola Univ-Stritch Sch Med 1978; **Resid:** Surgery, Beth Israel Deaconess Med Ctr 1980; Orthopaedic Surgery, Mass Genl Hosp 1984

Cassidy, Charles MD [OrS] - **Spec Exp:** Hand & Upper Extremity Surgery; Elbow Surgery; Trauma-Upper & Lower Extremity; **Hospital:** Tufts Med Ctr; **Address:** New England Med Ctr, 800 Washington St, Box 306, Boston, MA 02111; **Phone:** 617-636-5150; **Board Cert:** Hand Surgery 2007; Orthopaedic Surgery 2007; **Med School:** Northwestern Univ 1987; **Resid:** Orthopaedic Surgery, New England Med Ctr 1993; **Fellow:** Hand Surgery, Tufts Univ Med Ctr 1995; **Fac Appt:** Assoc Prof OrS, Tufts Univ

DiGiovanni, Christopher W MD [OrS] - **Spec Exp:** Foot & Ankle Surgery; **Hospital:** Rhode Island Hosp; **Address:** University Orthopedics Inc, 100 Butler Dr, Providence, RI 02906-4862; **Phone:** 401-330-1430; **Board Cert:** Orthopaedic Surgery 2001; **Med School:** Brown Univ 1991; **Resid:** Orthopaedic Surgery, Rhode Island Hosp 1997; **Fellow:** Joint Replacement Surgery, Hosp Spec Surgery 1998; Foot & Ankle Surgery, Harborview Med Ctr 1999; **Fac Appt:** Prof OrS, Brown Univ

Einhorn, Thomas A MD [OrS] - **Spec Exp:** Hip & Knee Replacement; Bone Disorders-Metabolic; Hip & Knee Reconstruction; Osteonecrosis; **Hospital:** Boston Med Ctr; **Address:** Orthopaedic Surgical Associates, 720 Harrison Ave, Ste 805, Boston, MA 02118; **Phone:** 617-638-8435; **Board Cert:** Orthopaedic Surgery 1998; **Med School:** Cornell Univ-Weill Med Coll 1976; **Resid:** Orthopaedic Surgery, St Lukes-Roosevelt Hosp 1981; Pediatric Orthopaedic Surgery, Alfred DuPont Inst 1981; **Fellow:** Orthopaedic Surgery, Hosp Special Surgery 1982; **Fac Appt:** Prof OrS, Boston Univ

Endrizzi, Donald P MD [OrS] - **Spec Exp:** Shoulder Surgery; Rotator Cuff Surgery; Elbow Surgery; Joint Replacement; **Hospital:** Maine Med Ctr, Mercy Hosp-Portland, Maine; **Address:** Orthopaedic Associates, 33 Sewall St, Portland, ME 04102; **Phone:** 207-828-2100; **Board Cert:** Orthopaedic Surgery 2011; **Med School:** Columbia P&S 1982; **Resid:** Surgery, Columbia-Presby Med Ctr 1984; Orthopaedic Surgery, Columbia Presby Med Ctr 1987; **Fac Appt:** Assoc Clin Prof S, Univ VT Coll Med

Friedlaender, Gary E MD [OrS] - **Spec Exp:** Bone & Soft Tissue Tumors; Limb Surgery/Reconstruction; Fractures-Complex & Non Union; Tissue Banking; **Hospital:** Yale-New Haven Hosp, Yale Med Group; **Address:** 800 Howard Ave, Yale Physicians Fl 1, New Haven, CT 06519; **Phone:** 203-737-5660; **Board Cert:** Orthopaedic Surgery 1975; **Med School:** Univ Mich Med Sch 1969; **Resid:** Surgery, Michigan Med Ctr 1971; Orthopaedic Surgery, Yale-New Haven Hosp 1974; **Fellow:** Musculoskeletal Oncology, Mass Genl Hosp 1983; **Fac Appt:** Prof OrS, Yale Univ

Fulkerson, John P MD [OrS] - **Spec Exp:** Knee-Patella Problems; Arthroscopic Surgery-Knee; Sports Medicine; **Hospital:** Hartford Hosp; **Address:** 499 Farmington Ave Fl 3, Farmington, CT 06032; **Phone:** 860-549-8269; **Board Cert:** Orthopaedic Surgery 1980; **Med School:** Yale Univ 1972; **Resid:** Orthopaedic Surgery, Yale-New Haven Hosp 1978; **Fellow:** Sports Medicine, Hosp for Special Surg 1979; **Fac Appt:** Clin Prof OrS, Univ Conn

Gebhardt, Mark MD [OrS] - **Spec Exp:** Musculoskeletal Tumors; Bone Tumors; **Hospital:** Beth Israel Deaconess Med Ctr - Boston, Children's Hospital - Boston; **Address:** 330 Brookline Ave, Stoneman 10, Boston, MA 02215; **Phone:** 617-667-9598; **Board Cert:** Orthopaedic Surgery 2007; **Med School:** Univ Cincinnati 1975; **Resid:** Surgery, Univ Pittsburg Med Ctr 1977; Orthopaedic Surgery, Harvard Affil Hosps 1982; **Fellow:** Pediatric Orthopaedic Surgery, Boston Chldns Hosp 1983; Orthopaedic Oncology, Mass Genl Hosp 1983; **Fac Appt:** Prof OrS, Harvard Med Sch

Green, Andrew MD [OrS] - **Spec Exp:** Shoulder Surgery; Elbow Surgery; Rotator Cuff Surgery; Arthroscopic Surgery; **Hospital:** Rhode Island Hosp, Miriam Hosp; **Address:** Univ Orthopedics Inc, 2 Dudley St, Ste 200, Providence, RI 02905-3248; **Phone:** 401-457-1533; **Board Cert:** Orthopaedic Surgery 2006; **Med School:** Columbia P&S 1987; **Resid:** Orthopaedic Surgery, Rhode Island Hosp 1992; **Fellow:** Pacific Med Ctr 1993; **Fac Appt:** Assoc Prof OrS, Brown Univ

Hornicek, Francis J MD/PhD [OrS] - **Spec Exp:** Bone Tumors; Sarcoma; Bone Tumors-Metastatic; Soft Tissue Tumors; **Hospital:** Mass Genl Hosp; **Address:** MGH Orthpaedic Oncology, 55 Fruit St, Yawkey 3700, Boston, MA 02114; **Phone:** 617-724-3700; **Board Cert:** Orthopaedic Surgery 2010; **Med School:** Univ Pittsburgh 1991; **Resid:** Orthopaedic Surgery, Jackson Meml Hosp 1996; **Fellow:** Orthopaedic Oncology, Mass Genl Hosp/Chldns Hosp 1997; **Fac Appt:** Assoc Prof OrS, Harvard Med Sch

Jokl, Peter MD [OrS] - **Spec Exp:** Knee Surgery; Sports Medicine; Shoulder Surgery; **Hospital:** Yale-New Haven Hosp, Yale Med Group; **Address:** Yale Sports Med, Dept Orthopaedics, 800 Howard Ave, Ste 133, New Haven, CT 06519-1369; **Phone:** 203-785-2579; **Board Cert:** Orthopaedic Surgery 1974; **Med School:** Yale Univ 1968; **Resid:** Orthopaedic Surgery, Yale-New Haven Hosp 1972; **Fac Appt:** Prof OrS, Yale Univ

Orthopaedic Surgery

Jupiter, Jesse B MD [OrS] - **Spec Exp:** Upper Extremity Trauma; Hand Surgery; Fractures-Non Union; **Hospital:** Mass Genl Hosp, Newton - Wellesley Hosp; **Address:** Yawkey Center, Ste 2100, 55 Fruit St, Boston, MA 02114; **Phone:** 617-726-5100; **Board Cert:** Orthopaedic Surgery 1982; **Med School:** Yale Univ 1972; **Resid:** Surgery, Mass Genl Hosp 1976; Orthopaedic Surgery, Mass Genl Hosp 1979; **Fellow:** Hand Surgery, Univ Louisville 1981; Trauma, AO/ASIF 1980; **Fac Appt:** Prof OrS, Harvard Med Sch

Kasser, James MD [OrS] - **Spec Exp:** Pediatric Orthopaedic Surgery; **Hospital:** Children's Hospital - Boston; **Address:** Chldns Hosp, Dept Ortho Surgery, 300 Longwood Ave, Honeywell 221, Boston, MA 02115; **Phone:** 617-355-6617; **Board Cert:** Orthopaedic Surgery 2005; **Med School:** Tufts Univ 1976; **Resid:** Orthopaedic Surgery, Tufts Med Ctr 1981; **Fellow:** Pediatric Orthopaedic Surgery, Dupont Inst 1984; **Fac Appt:** Prof OrS, Harvard Med Sch

Kocher, Mininder S MD [OrS] - **Spec Exp:** Pediatric Orthopaedic Surgery; Pediatric Sports Medicine; Arthroscopic Surgery; Arthroscopic Surgery-Hip; **Hospital:** Children's Hospital - Boston, Beth Israel Deaconess Med Ctr - Boston; **Address:** Children's Hosp, Dept Orthopaedic Surg, 319 Longwood Ave Fl 6, Boston, MA 02115; **Phone:** 617-355-3501; **Board Cert:** Orthopaedic Surgery 2002; Orthopaedic Sports Medicine 2008; **Med School:** Duke Univ 1993; **Resid:** Orthopaedic Surgery, Beth Israel Deaconess Med Ctr 1999; **Fellow:** Pediatric Orthopaedic Surgery, Chldns Hosp 1999; Sports Medicine, Steadman Hawkins Clin 2000; **Fac Appt:** Asst Prof OrS, Harvard Med Sch

Laurencin, Cato T MD/PhD [OrS] - **Spec Exp:** Shoulder & Knee Surgery; Sports Medicine; **Hospital:** Univ of Conn Hlth Ctr, John Dempsey Hosp; **Address:** Univ Conn Health Ctr, 263 Farmington Ave, Farmington, CT 06030-3800; **Phone:** 860-679-8384; **Board Cert:** Orthopaedic Surgery 2007; **Med School:** Harvard Med Sch 1987; **Resid:** Orthopaedic Surgery, Harvard Combined Program 1993; **Fellow:** Sports Medicine & Shoulder Surgery, Hosp for Special Surg 1994; **Fac Appt:** Prof OrS, Univ Conn

Marsh, James S MD [OrS] - **Spec Exp:** Pediatric Orthopaedic Surgery; **Hospital:** Yale-New Haven Hosp, Hosp of St Raphael; **Address:** 800 Howard Ave, Ste 133, New Haven, CT 06519; **Phone:** 203-785-2579; **Med School:** Harvard Med Sch 1981; **Resid:** Orthopaedic Surgery, Stanford Univ 1986; **Fellow:** Pediatric Orthopaedic Surgery, Mass Genl Hosp 1987; **Fac Appt:** Assoc Prof OrS, Yale Univ

Minas, Tom MD [OrS] - **Spec Exp:** Arthroscopic Surgery; Cartilage Damage & Transplant; Joint Replacement; Pelvic & Acetabular Fractures; **Hospital:** Brigham and Women's Hosp (page 57); **Address:** Brigham & Wmns Hosp, Dept of Orthopedic Surg, 850 Boylston St, Ste 112, Chestnut Hill, MA 02467; **Phone:** 617-732-5322; **Board Cert:** Orthopaedic Surgery 2008; **Med School:** Univ Toronto 1982; **Resid:** Orthopaedic Surgery, University of Toronto 1988; **Fellow:** Orthopaedic Surgery, Sunnybrook Univ 1989; Joint Reconstruction, Brigham & Womens Hosp 1990; **Fac Appt:** Assoc Prof OrS, Harvard Med Sch

Ready, John E MD [OrS] - **Spec Exp:** Bone Cancer; Sarcoma-Soft Tissue; Hip & Knee Replacement in Bone Tumors; Hip & Knee Replacement; **Hospital:** Brigham and Women's Hosp (page 57), Dana-Farber Cancer Inst (page 57); **Address:** Brigham & Women's Hospital, Dept of Orthopedic Surgery, 75 Francis St, Boston, MA 02115; **Phone:** 617-732-5368; **Board Cert:** Orthopaedic Surgery 2002; **Med School:** Dalhousie Univ 1982; **Resid:** Orthopaedic Surgery, Dalhousie Univ Hosp 1987; **Fellow:** Orthopaedic Oncology, St Michael's Hosp 1988; Orthopaedic Oncology, Mass Genl Hosp/Childns Hosp 1989

Reilly, Donald T MD [OrS] - **Spec Exp:** Knee Replacement; Hip Replacement; **Hospital:** New England Bapt Hosp; **Address:** Pro Sports Orthopaedics, 235 Cypres St, Ste 300, Brookline, MA 02445; **Phone:** 617-738-8642; **Board Cert:** Orthopaedic Surgery 1984; **Med School:** Case West Res Univ 1975; **Resid:** Orthopaedic Surgery, Harvard Combined Ortho 1981

Richmond, John C MD [OrS] - **Spec Exp:** Shoulder Injuries; Rotator Cuff Surgery; Knee Surgery; Arthroscopic Surgery; **Hospital:** New England Bapt Hosp; **Address:** Boston Sports & Shoulder Ctr, 830 Boylston St, Ste 107, Chestnut Hill, MA 02467; **Phone:** 617-264-1100; **Board Cert:** Orthopaedic Surgery 1984; **Med School:** Tufts Univ 1976; **Resid:** Surgery, Hosp UPenn 1978; Orthopaedic Surgery, New England Med Ctr 1981; **Fac Appt:** Prof OrS, Tufts Univ

Scott, Richard D MD [OrS] - **Spec Exp:** Hip Replacement; Knee Replacement; **Hospital:** Brigham and Women's Hosp (page 57), New England Bapt Hosp; **Address:** 125 Parker Hill Ave, Boston, MA 02120; **Phone:** 617-738-9151; **Board Cert:** Orthopaedic Surgery 1975; **Med School:** Temple Univ 1968; **Resid:** Orthopaedic Surgery, Mass Genl Hosp 1974; **Fellow:** Orthopaedic Surgery, Mass Genl Hosp 1974; **Fac Appt:** Prof OrS, Harvard Med Sch

Thornhill, Thomas S MD [OrS] - **Spec Exp:** Hip & Knee Replacement; Arthritis; Shoulder & Elbow Surgery; Joint Replacement; **Hospital:** Brigham and Women's Hosp (page 57); **Address:** Brigham & Women's Hosp, Dept Orth Surg, 45 Francis St, Boston, MA 02115; **Phone:** 617-732-5322; **Board Cert:** Internal Medicine 1973; Orthopaedic Surgery 1979; **Med School:** Cornell Univ-Weill Med Coll 1970; **Resid:** Internal Medicine, Peter Brent Brigham Hosp 1972; Orthopaedic Surgery, Harvard Combined Prgm 1978; **Fellow:** Joint Replacement Surgery, Robert Breck Brigham Hosp; **Fac Appt:** Prof OrS, Harvard Med Sch

Tornetta III, Paul MD [OrS] - **Spec Exp:** Trauma; Fractures-Complex; Minimally Invasive Surgery; Fractures in the Elderly; **Hospital:** Boston Med Ctr; **Address:** Boston Med Ctr, 725 Albany St, Shapiro-Ste 4B, Boston, MA 02118; **Phone:** 617-414-4865; **Board Cert:** Orthopaedic Surgery 2006; **Med School:** SUNY Downstate 1987; **Resid:** Orthopaedic Surgery, Downstate Med Ctr 1992; **Fellow:** Trauma, Good Samaritan Hosp 1993; **Fac Appt:** Prof OrS, Boston Univ

Weinstein, James DO [OrS] - **Spec Exp:** Pain-Back; Spinal Tumors; **Hospital:** Dartmouth - Hitchcock Med Ctr; **Address:** DHMC, Dept Orthopaedic Surgery, One Medical Ctr Drive, Lebanon, NH 03756; **Phone:** 603-650-2225; **Board Cert:** Orthopaedic Surgery 2002; **Med School:** Chicago Coll Osteo Med 1973; **Resid:** Orthopaedic Surgery, Rush Presby-St Lukes Med Ctr 1983; **Fac Appt:** Prof OrS, Dartmouth Med Sch

Zarins, Bertram MD [OrS] - **Spec Exp:** Knee Injuries/ACL; Rotator Cuff Surgery; Cartilage Damage; Shoulder Injuries; **Hospital:** Mass Genl Hosp; **Address:** MGH Sports Medicine, 175 Cambridge St, Ste 400, Boston, MA 02114; **Phone:** 617-726-3421; **Board Cert:** Orthopaedic Surgery 1975; **Med School:** SUNY Upstate Med Univ 1967; **Resid:** Surgery, Johns Hopkins Hosp 1969; Orthopaedic Surgery, Harvard Ortho Prog 1973; **Fellow:** Sports Medicine, Mass Genl Hosp 1976; **Fac Appt:** Clin Prof OrS, Harvard Med Sch

Mid Atlantic

Aboulafia, Albert J MD [OrS] - **Spec Exp:** Bone Cancer; **Hospital:** Sinai Hosp - Baltimore; **Address:** Lapidus Cancer Inst, 2401 W Belvedere Ave, Baltimore, MD 21215; **Phone:** 410-601-9266; **Board Cert:** Orthopaedic Surgery 2004; **Med School:** Univ Mich Med Sch 1985; **Resid:** Orthopaedic Surgery, LAC/USC Sch Med 1990; **Fellow:** Orthopaedic Oncology, Chldn's Natl Med Ctr/NIH 1991; **Fac Appt:** Asst Clin Prof OrS, Univ MD Sch Med

Albert, Todd J MD [OrS] - **Spec Exp:** Spinal Surgery; Spinal Surgery-Cervical; Spinal Deformity; **Hospital:** Thomas Jefferson Univ Hosp; **Address:** Rothman Institute, 925 Chesnut St Fl 5, Philadelphia, PA 19107; **Phone:** 800-321-9999; **Board Cert:** Orthopaedic Surgery 2006; **Med School:** Univ VA Sch Med 1987; **Resid:** Orthopaedic Surgery, Thomas Jefferson Univ Hosp 1992; **Fellow:** Spinal Surgery, Minnesota Spine Ctr 1993; **Fac Appt:** Prof OrS, Thomas Jefferson Univ

Orthopaedic Surgery

Balderston, Richard MD [OrS] - **Spec Exp:** Scoliosis; Spinal Surgery; Spinal Disc Replacement; **Hospital:** Pennsylvania Hosp-UPHS (page 68); **Address:** Pennsylvania Hosp, 800 Spruce St, Philadelphia, PA 19107; **Phone:** 215-829-2222; **Board Cert:** Orthopaedic Surgery 1985; **Med School:** Univ Pennsylvania 1977; **Resid:** Orthopaedic Surgery, Hosp Univ Penn 1982; **Fellow:** Spinal Surgery, Univ Minn Affil Hosp 1983; **Fac Appt:** Clin Prof OrS, Univ Pennsylvania

Bartolozzi, Arthur R MD [OrS] - **Spec Exp:** Sports Medicine; Arthroscopic Surgery-Knee; Knee Ligament Reconstruction; Shoulder Surgery; **Hospital:** Pennsylvania Hosp-UPHS (page 68); **Address:** Pennsylvania Hosp, 800 Spruce St, Philadelphia, PA 19107; **Phone:** 215-829-2222; **Board Cert:** Orthopaedic Surgery 2010; **Med School:** UCSD 1981; **Resid:** Orthopaedic Surgery, Hosp Univ Penn 1986; **Fellow:** Sports Medicine, UCLA Med Ctr 1987; **Fac Appt:** Assoc Clin Prof OrS, Univ Pennsylvania

Bauman, Phillip A MD [OrS] - **Spec Exp:** Foot & Ankle Surgery; Knee Surgery; Dance/Sports Medicine; Arthroscopic Surgery; **Hospital:** St. Luke's - Roosevelt Hosp Ctr - Roosevelt Div (page 55), NY-Presby/Columbia Univ Med Ctr, NY (page 65); **Address:** Orthopaedic Associates of NY, 343 W 58th St, Ste 1, New York, NY 10019; **Phone:** 212-506-0228; **Board Cert:** Orthopaedic Surgery 2009; **Med School:** Columbia P&S 1981; **Resid:** Surgery, St Lukes-Roosevelt Hosp Ctr 1983; Orthopaedic Surgery, Columbia-Presby Med Ctr 1987; **Fac Appt:** Asst Prof OrS, Columbia P&S

Benevenia, Joseph MD [OrS] - **Spec Exp:** Limb Sparing Surgery; Bone Cancer; Sarcoma-Soft Tissue; **Hospital:** Univ Hosp-UMDNJ—Newark; **Address:** 140 Bergen St, Ste ACC1610, Newark, NJ 07103; **Phone:** 973-972-2153; **Board Cert:** Orthopaedic Surgery 2003; **Med School:** UMDNJ-NJ Med Sch, Newark 1984; **Resid:** Orthopaedic Surgery, UMDNJ-NJ Med Sch Hosp 1988; **Fellow:** Orthopaedic Oncology, Case Western Reserve Univ 1991; **Fac Appt:** Prof OrS, UMDNJ-NJ Med Sch, Newark

Betz, Randal R MD [OrS] - **Spec Exp:** Spinal Cord Injury-Pediatric; Praxis Functional Electrical Stim (FES); Scoliosis; Spinal Deformity-Pediatric; **Hospital:** Philadelphia Shriners Hosp; **Address:** Shriners Hospital for Children, 3551 N Broad St, Philadelphia, PA 19140; **Phone:** 215-430-4026; **Board Cert:** Orthopaedic Surgery 1985; Spinal Cord Injury Medicine 2008; **Med School:** Temple Univ 1977; **Resid:** Orthopaedic Surgery, Shriners Hospital 1980; Orthopaedic Surgery, Temple Univ Hospital 1982; **Fellow:** Pediatric Orthopaedic Surgery, DuPont Inst 1983; **Fac Appt:** Prof OrS, Temple Univ

Bigliani, Louis U MD [OrS] - **Spec Exp:** Shoulder Surgery; Sports Medicine; Arthroscopic Surgery; Rotator Cuff Surgery; **Hospital:** NY-Presby/Columbia Univ Med Ctr, NY (page 65); **Address:** 622 W 168th St, rm 1130, New York, NY 10032-3720; **Phone:** 212-305-0998; **Board Cert:** Orthopaedic Surgery 1994; **Med School:** Loyola Univ-Stritch Sch Med 1973; **Resid:** Surgery, Roosevelt Hosp 1974; Orthopaedic Surgery, Columbia Presby Med Ctr 1977; **Fac Appt:** Prof OrS, Columbia P&S

Bitan, Fabien D MD [OrS] - **Spec Exp:** Spinal Surgery-Pediatric & Adult; Spinal Disc Replacement; Spinal Deformity; Spinal Disorders-Degenerative; **Hospital:** Lenox Hill Hosp, Beth Israel Med Ctr - Petrie Division (page 55); **Address:** Manhattan Orthopaedics, 130 E 77th St Fl 7, New York, NY 10075; **Phone:** 212-744-8114; **Med School:** France 1981; **Resid:** Orthopaedic Surgery, Hospital Beaujon 1987; Pediatric Orthopaedic Surgery, Hosp des Enfants Malades 1990; **Fellow:** Pediatric Orthopaedic Surgery, Hosp Special Surgery 1997; Spinal Surgery, Beth Israel Med Ctr 1998

Boachie-Adjei, Oheneba MD [OrS] - **Spec Exp:** Spinal Surgery; Scoliosis; **Hospital:** Hosp For Special Surgery (page 60); **Address:** Hosp for Special Surgery, 535 E 70th St, New York, NY 10021; **Phone:** 212-606-1948; **Board Cert:** Orthopaedic Surgery 2010; **Med School:** Columbia P&S 1980; **Resid:** Surgery, St Vincents Hosp 1982; Orthopaedic Surgery, Hosp Spec Surg 1986; **Fellow:** Orthopaedic Pathology, Hosp Spec Surg 1983; Spinal Surgery, Twin Cities Scoliosis Ctr/Minn Spine Ctr 1987; **Fac Appt:** Assoc Clin Prof S, Cornell Univ-Weill Med Coll

Booth Jr, Robert E MD [OrS] - **Spec Exp:** Knee Replacement & Revision; **Hospital:** Pennsylvania Hosp-UPHS (page 68); **Address:** Pennsylvania Hosp, 800 Spruce St, Philadelphia, PA 19107; **Phone:** 215-829-2222; **Board Cert:** Orthopaedic Surgery 1978; **Med School:** Univ Pennsylvania 1971; **Resid:** Surgery, Penn Hosp 1973; Orthopaedic Surgery, Hosp Univ Penn 1977; **Fac Appt:** Clin Prof OrS, Univ Pennsylvania

Bronson, Michael J MD [OrS] - **Spec Exp:** Joint Replacement; Knee Replacement; Hip Replacement; Arthritis; **Hospital:** Mount Sinai Med Ctr (page 63); **Address:** Mt Sinai Med Ctr, Dept Orthopedic Surgery, 5 E 98th St, Box 1188, New York, NY 10029; **Phone:** 212-241-1640; **Board Cert:** Orthopaedic Surgery 1984; **Med School:** NY Med Coll 1976; **Resid:** Orthopaedic Surgery, Lenox Hill Hosp 1980; **Fellow:** Hip & Knee Surgery, Columbia-Presby Med Ctr 1981; **Fac Appt:** Assoc Prof OrS, Mount Sinai Sch Med

Buly, Robert L MD [OrS] - **Spec Exp:** Hip Replacement; Minimally Invasive Surgery; Arthritis; Knee Replacement; **Hospital:** Hosp For Special Surgery (page 60), NY-Presby/Weill Cornell Med Ctr, NY (page 65); **Address:** Hospital for Special Surgery, 535 E 70th St, New York, NY 10021; **Phone:** 212-606-1971; **Board Cert:** Orthopaedic Surgery 2004; **Med School:** Cornell Univ-Weill Med Coll 1985; **Resid:** Orthopaedic Surgery, Hosp for Special Surg 1990; **Fellow:** Hip Surgery, Mueller Fdn 1991; Joint Reconstruction, Case Western Res/ Univ Hosp 1992; **Fac Appt:** Assoc Prof OrS, Cornell Univ-Weill Med Coll

Cammisa Jr, Frank P MD [OrS] - **Spec Exp:** Spinal Surgery; Spinal Disc Replacement; Minimally Invasive Spinal Surgery; Scoliosis; **Hospital:** Hosp For Special Surgery (page 60), NY-Presby/Weill Cornell Med Ctr, NY (page 65); **Address:** 523 E 72nd St, Fl 3, New York, NY 10021; **Phone:** 212-606-1946; **Board Cert:** Orthopaedic Surgery 2011; **Med School:** Columbia P&S 1982; **Resid:** Surgery, Columbia-Presby Hosp 1983; Orthopaedic Surgery, Hosp for Special Surgery 1987; **Fellow:** Spinal Surgery, Jackson Meml Hosp 1988; **Fac Appt:** Assoc Prof OrS, Cornell Univ-Weill Med Coll

Cappuccino, Andrew MD [OrS] - **Spec Exp:** Spinal Surgery; Spinal Disc Replacement; Minimally Invasive Spinal Surgery; **Hospital:** Kenmore Mercy Hosp, Erie County Med Ctr; **Address:** Buffalo Spine Surgery, 46 Davison Ct, Lockport, NY 14094; **Phone:** 716-438-2973; **Board Cert:** Orthopaedic Surgery 2007; **Med School:** SUNY Buffalo 1988; **Resid:** Orthopaedic Surgery, Monmouth Med Ctr 1993; Pediatric Orthopaedic Surgery, Childrens Hosp 1992; **Fellow:** Spinal Surgery, Johns Hopkins/Paul McAfee, MD 1994

Chu, Constance R MD [OrS] - **Spec Exp:** Sports Medicine; Knee Injuries/ACL; Cartilage Damage; **Hospital:** UPMC Montefiore, UPMC Shadyside; **Address:** Kaufmann Bldg, 3471 5th Ave, Ste 1010, Pittsburgh, PA 15213; **Phone:** 412-687-3900; **Board Cert:** Orthopaedic Surgery 2002; **Med School:** Harvard Med Sch 1992; **Resid:** Orthopaedic Surgery, UCSD Med Ctr 1995; **Fellow:** Joint Replacement Surgery, Brigham & Women's Hosp 1999; **Fac Appt:** Assoc Prof OrS, Univ Pittsburgh

Cornell, Charles MD [OrS] - **Spec Exp:** Trauma; Joint Replacement; Hip & Knee Replacement; **Hospital:** Hosp For Special Surgery (page 60); **Address:** 535 E 70th St, New York, NY 10021; **Phone:** 212-606-1414; **Board Cert:** Orthopaedic Surgery 2009; **Med School:** Cornell Univ-Weill Med Coll 1980; **Resid:** Surgery, Presby Hosp 1982; Orthopaedic Surgery, Hosp For Special Surg/New York Hosp 1985; **Fellow:** Orthopaedic Surgery, Univ Wash Med Ctr 1986; **Fac Appt:** Clin Prof OrS, Cornell Univ-Weill Med Coll

Orthopaedic Surgery

Craig, Edward V MD [OrS] - **Spec Exp:** Shoulder Arthroscopic Surgery; Shoulder Replacement; Sports Medicine; Elbow Surgery; **Hospital:** Hosp For Special Surgery (page 60), NY-Presby/Weill Cornell Med Ctr, NY (page 65); **Address:** 535 E 70th St, New York, NY 10021-4892; **Phone:** 212-606-1966; **Board Cert:** Orthopaedic Surgery 1984; **Med School:** Columbia P&S 1973; **Resid:** Internal Medicine, Columbia-Presby Hosp 1976; Orthopaedic Surgery, Columbia-Presby Hosp 1980; **Fellow:** Shoulder Surgery, Columbia-Presby Hosp 1981; Hand Surgery, Columbia-Presby Hosp 1982; **Fac Appt:** Clin Prof OrS, Cornell Univ-Weill Med Coll

Crossett, Lawrence MD [OrS] - **Spec Exp:** Hip Surgery; Knee Surgery; **Hospital:** UPMC Shadyside, UPMC Presby, Pittsburgh; **Address:** Shadyside Med Bldg, 5200 Centre Ave, Ste 415, Pittsburgh, PA 15232; **Phone:** 412-802-4100; **Board Cert:** Orthopaedic Surgery 2010; **Med School:** Temple Univ 1981; **Resid:** Orthopaedic Surgery, Temple Univ Hosp 1986; Orthopaedic Surgery, Shriners Children's Hosp 1984; **Fac Appt:** Assoc Prof OrS, Univ Pittsburgh

Davidson, Richard S MD [OrS] - **Spec Exp:** Limb Lengthening (Ilizarov Procedure); Limb Deformities; Foot Deformities; Clubfoot; **Hospital:** Chldns Hosp of Philadelphia; **Address:** Children's Hospital, Dept Orthopaedics, 34th & Civic Ctr Blvd, Wood Center Fl 2, Philadelphia, PA 19104; **Phone:** 215-590-1527; **Board Cert:** Orthopaedic Surgery 2007; **Med School:** NYU Sch Med 1976; **Resid:** Orthopaedic Surgery, Hosp Special Surgery 1981; **Fellow:** Pediatric Orthopaedic Surgery, Hosp for Sick Children 1982; **Fac Appt:** Assoc Prof OrS, Univ Pennsylvania

Delahay, John N MD [OrS] - **Spec Exp:** Pediatric Orthopaedic Surgery; Trauma; **Hospital:** Georgetown Univ Hosp; **Address:** G-PHC 3800 Reservoir Rd NW, Washington, DC 20007; **Phone:** 202-444-1438; **Board Cert:** Orthopaedic Surgery 1975; **Med School:** Georgetown Univ 1969; **Resid:** Orthopaedic Surgery, Georgetown Univ Hosp 1974; **Fac Appt:** Prof OrS, Georgetown Univ

Deland, Jonathan T MD [OrS] - **Spec Exp:** Foot & Ankle Surgery; Sports Medicine; Arthritis; **Hospital:** Hosp For Special Surgery (page 60); **Address:** Hosp Spec Surg, Foot & Ankle Service, 535 E 70th St, New York, NY 10021-4099; **Phone:** 212-606-1665; **Board Cert:** Orthopaedic Surgery 2003; **Med School:** Columbia P&S 1980; **Resid:** Orthopaedic Surgery, St Luke's-Roosevelt Hosp Ctr 1982; Orthopaedic Surgery, Mass Genl Hosp 1987; **Fac Appt:** Asst Prof S, Cornell Univ-Weill Med Coll

Dines, David M MD [OrS] - **Spec Exp:** Shoulder Surgery; Sports Medicine; Shoulder Replacement; **Hospital:** Long Island Jewish Med Ctr, Hosp For Special Surgery (page 60); **Address:** 935 Northern Blvd, Ste 303, Great Neck, NY 11021-5309; **Phone:** 516-482-1037; **Board Cert:** Orthopaedic Surgery 1980; **Med School:** UMDNJ-NJ Med Sch, Newark 1974; **Resid:** Surgery, NY Hosp-Cornell Med Ctr 1976; Orthopaedic Surgery, Hosp Special Surg 1979; **Fac Appt:** Clin Prof OrS, Albert Einstein Coll Med

Donaldson III, William F MD [OrS] - **Spec Exp:** Spinal Surgery; **Hospital:** UPMC Presby, Pittsburgh; **Address:** Univ Pittsburgh Physicians, Orthopaedics, 3471 5th Ave, Ste 1010, Pittsburgh, PA 15213; **Phone:** 412-605-3218; **Board Cert:** Orthopaedic Surgery 2009; **Med School:** Rush Med Coll 1980; **Resid:** Surgery, Rush Presby-St Luke's Med Ctr 1981; Orthopaedic Surgery, Hosp Special Surg 1985; **Fellow:** Spinal Surgery, Hosp Special Surg 1986; **Fac Appt:** Assoc Prof OrS, Univ Pittsburgh

Dormans, John P MD [OrS] - **Spec Exp:** Bone Cancer; Spinal Surgery-Pediatric; Pediatric Orthopaedic Surgery; **Hospital:** Chldns Hosp of Philadelphia; **Address:** 34th Street & Civic Center Blvd, Wood Bldg Fl 2 - rm 2315, Philadelphia, PA 19104-4399; **Phone:** 215-590-1534; **Board Cert:** Orthopaedic Surgery 2002; **Med School:** Indiana Univ 1983; **Resid:** Orthopaedic Surgery, Michigan State Univ Hosps 1988; **Fellow:** Pediatric Orthopaedic Surgery, Hosp for Sick Children 1989; **Fac Appt:** Prof OrS, Univ Pennsylvania

Errico, Thomas J MD [OrS] - **Spec Exp:** Spinal Surgery; Spinal Disc Replacement; Scoliosis; **Hospital:** NYU Langone Med Ctr (page 66), NYU Hosp For Joint Diseases; **Address:** 530 1st Ave, Ste 8U, New York, NY 10016-6402; **Phone:** 212-263-7182; **Board Cert:** Orthopaedic Surgery 2007; **Med School:** UMDNJ-NJ Med Sch, Newark 1978; **Resid:** Orthopaedic Surgery, NYU Med Ctr 1983; **Fellow:** Spinal Surgery, Toronto Genl Hosp 1984; **Fac Appt:** Assoc Prof OrS, NYU Sch Med

Feldman, David S MD [OrS] - **Spec Exp:** Limb Deformities; Spinal Surgery; Pediatric Orthopaedic Surgery; Scoliosis; **Hospital:** NYU Hosp For Joint Diseases, NYU Langone Med Ctr (page 66); **Address:** 67 Irving Pl Fl 8, New York, NY 10003; **Phone:** 212-533-5310; **Board Cert:** Orthopaedic Surgery 2007; **Med School:** Albert Einstein Coll Med 1988; **Resid:** Orthopaedic Surgery, Hosp for Joint Diseases 1993; **Fellow:** Pediatric Surgery, Hosp For Sick Chldn 1994; **Fac Appt:** Asst Prof OrS, NYU Sch Med

Flatow, Evan MD [OrS] - **Spec Exp:** Rotator Cuff Surgery; Shoulder Injuries; Shoulder Replacement; Shoulder Arthroscopic Surgery; **Hospital:** Mount Sinai Med Ctr (page 63); **Address:** 5 E 98th St Fl 9, Box 1188, New York, NY 10029; **Phone:** 212-241-1663; **Board Cert:** Orthopaedic Surgery 2010; **Med School:** Columbia P&S 1981; **Resid:** Surgery, Roosevelt Hosp 1983; Orthopaedic Surgery, Columbia-Presby Med Ctr 1985; **Fellow:** Shoulder Surgery, Columbia-Presby Med Ctr 1987; **Fac Appt:** Prof OrS, Mount Sinai Sch Med

Frassica, Frank J MD [OrS] - **Spec Exp:** Bone Cancer; **Hospital:** Johns Hopkins Hosp (page 61), Univ of MD Med Ctr; **Address:** 601 N Caroline St, Ste 5215, Baltimore, MD 21287; **Phone:** 410-502-2698; **Board Cert:** Orthopaedic Surgery 2011; **Med School:** Univ SC Sch Med 1982; **Resid:** Orthopaedic Surgery, Mayo Clinic 1987; **Fellow:** Orthopaedic Oncology, Mayo Clinic 1988; **Fac Appt:** Prof OrS, Johns Hopkins Univ

Fu, Freddie H MD [OrS] - **Spec Exp:** Sports Medicine; Knee Injuries/ACL; Shoulder Injuries; **Hospital:** UPMC Presby, Pittsburgh, UPMC South Side-Out Pt Ctr; **Address:** Presbyterian Univ Hosp, Kaufmann Bldg, 3471 5th Ave, Ste 1011, Pittsburgh, PA 15213; **Phone:** 412-432-3611; **Board Cert:** Orthopaedic Surgery 1984; **Med School:** Univ Pittsburgh 1977; **Resid:** Orthopaedic Surgery, Univ Pittsburgh Med Ctr 1982; **Fellow:** Orthopaedic Research, Univ Pittsburgh Med Ctr 1979; **Fac Appt:** Prof OrS, Univ Pittsburgh

Gladstone, James N MD [OrS] - **Spec Exp:** Shoulder & Knee Surgery; Cartilage Damage; Knee-Patella Problems; Arthritis; **Hospital:** Mount Sinai Med Ctr (page 63); **Address:** Mt Sinai Med Ctr, 5 E 98th St Fl 9, Box 1188, New York, NY 10029; **Phone:** 212-241-1645; **Board Cert:** Orthopaedic Surgery 2009; Orthopaedic Sports Medicine 2007; **Med School:** Tufts Univ 1990; **Resid:** Orthopaedic Surgery, Columbia-Presby Med Ctr 1995; **Fellow:** Sports Medicine, American Sports Med Inst 1996; **Fac Appt:** Assoc Prof OrS, Mount Sinai Sch Med

Glashow, Jonathan L MD [OrS] - **Spec Exp:** Sports Medicine; Shoulder Surgery; Knee Surgery; Arthroscopic Surgery; **Hospital:** Mount Sinai Med Ctr (page 63), Lenox Hill Hosp; **Address:** 737 Park Ave, Ste 1C, New York, NY 10021; **Phone:** 212-794-5096; **Board Cert:** Orthopaedic Surgery 2004; **Med School:** Cornell Univ-Weill Med Coll 1984; **Resid:** Orthopaedic Surgery, Lenox Hill Hosp 1989; **Fellow:** Arthroscopic Surgery, S Calif Ortho Inst 1990; Shoulder Surgery, Univ Texas Med Ctr 1990; **Fac Appt:** Assoc Clin Prof OrS, Mount Sinai Sch Med

Goldstein, Jeffrey A MD [OrS] - **Spec Exp:** Spinal Surgery; Minimally Invasive Spinal Surgery; Spinal Disc Replacement; Scoliosis; **Hospital:** NYU Hosp For Joint Diseases, NYU Langone Med Ctr (page 66); **Address:** NYU Hosp for Joint Diseases, 19 Beekman St Fl 5, New York, NY 10038; **Phone:** 212-513-7711; **Board Cert:** Orthopaedic Surgery 2004; **Med School:** SUNY Downstate 1990; **Resid:** Orthopaedic Surgery, Case West Univ Med Ctr 1995; **Fellow:** Spinal Surgery, Maryland Spine Ctr 1996; **Fac Appt:** Assoc Clin Prof OrS, NYU Sch Med

Orthopaedic Surgery

Greisberg, Justin K MD [OrS] - **Spec Exp:** Foot & Ankle Surgery; Ankle Replacement & Revision; Reconstructive Surgery; Trauma; **Hospital:** NY-Presby/Columbia Univ Med Ctr, NY (page 65); **Address:** NY Presbyterian-Columbia Medical Ctr, 622 W 168th St, PH-11, rm 1153, New York, NY 10032; **Phone:** 212-305-5604; **Board Cert:** Orthopaedic Surgery 2004; **Med School:** Albert Einstein Coll Med 1995; **Resid:** Orthopaedic Surgery, Rhode Island Hosp 2000; **Fellow:** Orthopaedic Trauma Surgery, Rhode Island Hosp 2001; Foot & Ankle Surgery, Harbor; **Fac Appt:** Assoc Prof OrS, Columbia P&S

Grelsamer, Ronald P MD [OrS] - **Spec Exp:** Knee-Patella Problems; Sports Medicine; Knee Reconstruction; Arthritis-Hip & Knee; **Hospital:** Mount Sinai Med Ctr (page 63); **Address:** Mount Sinai Medical Ctr, Dept Orthopaedics, 5 E 98th St, Box 1188, New York, NY 10029-6574; **Phone:** 212-241-2914; **Board Cert:** Orthopaedic Surgery 2008; **Med School:** Columbia P&S 1979; **Resid:** Orthopaedic Surgery, Columbia Presby Med Ctr 1984; **Fellow:** Hip & Knee Surgery, Columbia Presby Med Ctr 1985; **Fac Appt:** Assoc Prof OrS, Mount Sinai Sch Med

Haas, Steven B MD [OrS] - **Spec Exp:** Knee Surgery; Knee Replacement; Minimally Invasive Surgery; **Hospital:** Hosp For Special Surgery (page 60); **Address:** Hospital for Special Surgery, 535 E 70th St Fl 3, New York, NY 10021; **Phone:** 212-606-1852; **Board Cert:** Orthopaedic Surgery 2004; **Med School:** Univ Rochester 1985; **Resid:** Orthopaedic Surgery, Hosp Special Surgery 1990; **Fellow:** Knee Surgery, Hosp Special Surgery 1991; **Fac Appt:** Clin Prof OrS, Cornell Univ-Weill Med Coll

Hannafin, Jo A MD/PhD [OrS] - **Spec Exp:** Sports Medicine-Women; Shoulder Arthroscopic Surgery; Knee Injuries/Ligament Surgery; Ligament Reconstruction; **Hospital:** Hosp For Special Surgery (page 60), NY-Presby/Weill Cornell Med Ctr, NY (page 65); **Address:** 535 E 70th St, New York, NY 10021-4872; **Phone:** 212-606-1469; **Board Cert:** Orthopaedic Surgery 2005; Orthopaedic Sports Medicine 2009; **Med School:** Albert Einstein Coll Med 1985; **Resid:** Orthopaedic Surgery, Montefiore Med Ctr 1990; **Fellow:** Sports Medicine, Hosp Special Surgery 1992; **Fac Appt:** Assoc Prof OrS, Cornell Univ-Weill Med Coll

Hausman, Michael R MD [OrS] - **Spec Exp:** Hand Reconstruction; Elbow Reconstruction; Reconstructive Microvascular Surgery; Arthroscopic Surgery; **Hospital:** Mount Sinai Med Ctr (page 63); **Address:** 5 E 98th St Fl 9, Box 1188, New York, NY 10029-6501; **Phone:** 212-241-1658; **Board Cert:** Orthopaedic Surgery 2010; Hand Surgery 2010; **Med School:** Yale Univ 1979; **Resid:** Surgery, Yale-New Haven Hosp 1981; Orthopaedic Surgery, Yale-New Haven Hosp 1985; **Fellow:** Hand Surgery, Roosevelt Hosp 1987; **Fac Appt:** Assoc Clin Prof OrS, Mount Sinai Sch Med

Healey, John H MD [OrS] - **Spec Exp:** Bone Tumors; Hip & Knee Replacement in Bone Tumors; Sarcoma; Sarcoma-Soft Tissue; **Hospital:** Meml Sloan-Kettering Cancer Ctr, Hosp For Special Surgery (page 60); **Address:** 1275 York Ave, New York, NY 10065; **Phone:** 212-639-7610; **Board Cert:** Orthopaedic Surgery 2007; **Med School:** Univ VT Coll Med 1978; **Resid:** Orthopaedic Surgery, Hosp Special Surg 1983; **Fellow:** Musculoskeletal Oncology, Meml Sloan Kettering Cancer Ctr 1984; Orthopaedic Surgery, Hosp Special Surgery 1984; **Fac Appt:** Prof OrS, Cornell Univ-Weill Med Coll

Hecht, Andrew MD [OrS] - **Spec Exp:** Spinal Surgery; Spinal Disc Replacement; Minimally Invasive Spinal Surgery; **Hospital:** Mount Sinai Med Ctr (page 63); **Address:** Mount Sinai Med Ctr, Dept Orthopaedic Surg, 5 E 98th St Fl 9, Box 1188, New York, NY 10029; **Phone:** 212-241-0735; **Board Cert:** Orthopaedic Surgery 2003; **Med School:** Harvard Med Sch 1994; **Resid:** Orthopaedic Surgery, Mass Genl Hosp 1999; **Fellow:** Spinal Surgery, Emory Univ Spine Ctr 2001; **Fac Appt:** Asst Prof OrS, Mount Sinai Sch Med

Helfet, David L MD [OrS] - **Spec Exp:** Fractures-Complex; Fractures-Complex & Non Union; Fractures-Stress; Deformity Reconstruction; **Hospital:** Hosp For Special Surgery (page 60), NY-Presby/Weill Cornell Med Ctr, NY (page 65); **Address:** 535 E 70th St, New York, NY 10021; **Phone:** 212-606-1888; **Board Cert:** Orthopaedic Surgery 1984; **Med School:** South Africa 1975; **Resid:** Surgery, Edendale Hosp 1977; Orthopaedic Surgery, Johns Hopkins Hosp 1981; **Fellow:** Orthopaedic Surgery, Inselspita Hosp 1981; Orthopaedic Surgery, UCLA Med Ctr 1982; **Fac Appt:** Prof OrS, Cornell Univ-Weill Med Coll

Henshaw, Robert M MD [OrS] - **Spec Exp:** Musculoskeletal Tumors; Bone Tumors; **Hospital:** Washington Hosp Ctr, Chldns Natl Med Ctr; **Address:** 110 Irving St NW, Ste C2173, Washington, DC 20010; **Phone:** 202-877-3970; **Board Cert:** Orthopaedic Surgery 2010; **Med School:** Tufts Univ 1990; **Resid:** Orthopaedic Surgery, UCLA Med Ctr 1995; **Fellow:** Orthopaedic Surgery, Washington Hosp Ctr 1997; **Fac Appt:** Assoc Prof OrS, Georgetown Univ

Herman, Martin J MD [OrS] - **Spec Exp:** Pediatric Orthopaedic Surgery; Hip Disorders-Pediatric; Scoliosis; Musculoskeletal Disorders; **Hospital:** St. Christopher's Hosp for Chldn; **Address:** St Christophers Hosp for Children, Dept Orthopaedic Surgery, 3601 A St, Philadelphia, PA 19134; **Phone:** 215-427-3131; **Board Cert:** Orthopaedic Surgery 2009; **Med School:** Columbia P&S 1990; **Resid:** Orthopaedic Surgery, RW Johnson Univ Hosp 1995; **Fellow:** Pediatric Orthopaedic Surgery, ampbell Clinic/Univ Tenn 1996; **Fac Appt:** Assoc Prof OrS, Drexel Univ Coll Med

Herzenberg, John E MD [OrS] - **Spec Exp:** Limb Lengthening (Ilizarov Procedure); Limb Deformities; Pediatric Orthopaedic Surgery; Clubfoot; **Hospital:** Sinai Hosp - Baltimore; **Address:** Rubin Inst for Advanced Orthopaedics, 2401 W Belvedere Ave, Baltimore, MD 21215; **Phone:** 410-601-8700; **Board Cert:** Orthopaedic Surgery 2009; **Med School:** Boston Univ 1979; **Resid:** Orthopaedic Surgery, Duke Univ Med Ctr 1985; **Fellow:** Pediatric Orthopaedic Surgery, Hosp for Sick Children 1986

Hilibrand, Alan S MD [OrS] - **Spec Exp:** Spinal Surgery; Spinal Trauma; Spinal Surgery-Cervical; Spinal Deformity; **Hospital:** Thomas Jefferson Univ Hosp, Atlantic City Medical Center- City Division; **Address:** Rothman Institute, 925 Chestnut St Fl 5, Philadelphia, PA 19107; **Phone:** 800-321-9999; **Board Cert:** Orthopaedic Surgery 2009; **Med School:** Yale Univ 1990; **Resid:** Orthopaedic Surgery, Univ Michigan Hlth System 1995; **Fellow:** Spinal Surgery, Cleveland Spine Inst 1996; **Fac Appt:** Prof OrS, Jefferson Med Coll

Hotchkiss, Robert N MD [OrS] - **Spec Exp:** Hand Surgery; Wrist Surgery; Elbow Reconstruction; Dupuytren's Contracture; **Hospital:** Hosp For Special Surgery (page 60), NY-Presby/Weill Cornell Med Ctr, NY (page 65); **Address:** 523 E 72nd St Fl 4, New York, NY 10021-4099; **Phone:** 212-606-1964; **Board Cert:** Orthopaedic Surgery 2010; Hand Surgery 2010; **Med School:** Johns Hopkins Univ 1980; **Resid:** Surgery, Johns Hopkins Hosp 1982; Orthopaedic Surgery, Johns Hopkins Hosp 1985; **Fellow:** Hand Surgery, Union Meml Hosp 1987; **Fac Appt:** Assoc Prof OrS, Cornell Univ-Weill Med Coll

Hozack, William J MD [OrS] - **Spec Exp:** Hip Surgery; Knee Surgery; Joint Replacement; **Hospital:** Thomas Jefferson Univ Hosp; **Address:** Rothman Institute, 925 Chesnut St Fl 5, Philadelphia, PA 19107; **Phone:** 800-321-9999; **Board Cert:** Orthopaedic Surgery 2010; **Med School:** McGill Univ 1981; **Resid:** Orthopaedic Surgery, Hosp Univ Penn 1986; **Fellow:** Joint Reconstruction, Penn Hosp/Thomas Jefferson Univ 1987; **Fac Appt:** Prof OrS, Jefferson Med Coll

Hume, Eric L MD [OrS] - **Spec Exp:** Hip Replacement; Knee Replacement; **Hospital:** Penn Presby Med Ctr - UPHS (page 68); **Address:** Penn Presbyterian Medical Center, 51 N 39th St, Cupp Bldg Fl 1, Philadelphia, PA 19104; **Phone:** 215-662-3340; **Board Cert:** Orthopaedic Surgery 2007; **Med School:** SUNY Upstate Med Univ 1978; **Resid:** Orthopaedic Surgery, Jefferson Univ Hosp 1983; **Fac Appt:** Assoc Clin Prof OrS, Univ Pennsylvania

Orthopaedic Surgery

Hungerford, Marc W MD [OrS] - **Spec Exp:** Knee Replacement & Revision; Hip Replacement & Revision; Cartilage Damage; **Hospital:** Mercy Med Ctr - Baltimore; **Address:** Mercy Medical Center, Joint Replacement & Trauma Ctr, 301 Saint Paul Pl, Baltimore, MD 21202; **Phone:** 410-539-2227; **Board Cert:** Orthopaedic Surgery 2001; **Med School:** Vanderbilt Univ 1992; **Resid:** Orthopaedic Surgery, Johns Hopkins Hosp 1997; **Fac Appt:** Asst Prof OrS, Johns Hopkins Univ

Hyman, Joshua E MD [OrS] - **Spec Exp:** Pediatric Orthopaedic Surgery; Fractures-Pediatric; Scoliosis; Clubfoot/Foot Deformities in Children; **Hospital:** Morgan Stanley Children's Hosp of NY-Presby, NY (page 65), NY-Presby/Columbia Univ Med Ctr, NY (page 65); **Address:** Children's Hosp New York, 3959 Broadway, Ste 8 North, New York, NY 10032-3784; **Phone:** 212-305-5475; **Board Cert:** Orthopaedic Surgery 2002; **Med School:** Columbia P&S 1990; **Resid:** Surgery, Beth Israel Hosp 1993; Orthopaedic Surgery, Mass Genl Hosp/Beth Israel Hosp 1998; **Fellow:** Pediatric Orthopaedic Surgery, Hosp for Sick Children 1999; **Fac Appt:** Assoc Prof OrS, Columbia P&S

Johanson, Norman A MD [OrS] - **Spec Exp:** Hip Replacement & Revision; Knee Replacement & Revision; Juvenile Arthritis; **Hospital:** Hahnemann Univ Hosp; **Address:** Drexel Orthopaedic Assocs, 216 N Broad St, Feinstein Bldg, Fl 2, Philadelphia, PA 19102; **Phone:** 215-762-2663; **Board Cert:** Orthopaedic Surgery 2007; **Med School:** Cornell Univ 1978; **Resid:** Orthopaedic Surgery, Hosp Special Surg 1984; **Fac Appt:** Prof OrS, Drexel Univ Coll Med

Johnson, Carl A MD [OrS] - **Spec Exp:** Knee Surgery; **Hospital:** Johns Hopkins Bayview Med Ctr (page 61), Johns Hopkins Hosp (page 61); **Address:** Johns Hopkins at Whitemarsh, 4924 Campbell Blvd, Ste 130, Nottingham, MD 21236; **Phone:** 443-442-2086; **Board Cert:** Orthopaedic Surgery 1983; **Med School:** Johns Hopkins Univ 1976; **Resid:** Surgery, Johns Hopkins Hosp 1978; Orthopaedic Surgery, Johns Hopkins Hosp 1981; **Fac Appt:** Assoc Prof OrS, Johns Hopkins Univ

Kaplan, Frederick S MD [OrS] - **Spec Exp:** Bone Disorders-Metabolic; Fibrodysplasia Ossificans Progressiv FOP; Progressive Osseous Heteroplasia POH; **Hospital:** Hosp Univ Penn - UPHS (page 68); **Address:** Orthopaedic Inst, 3400 Spruce St, 2 Silverstein, Philadelphia, PA 19104; **Phone:** 215-349-8727; **Med School:** Johns Hopkins Univ 1976; **Resid:** Orthopaedic Surgery, Hosp Univ Penn 1981; **Fellow:** Orthopaedic Research, Hosp Univ Penn 1982; Musculoskeletal Disorders, Dr Michael Zasloff/U Penn 1991; **Fac Appt:** Prof OrS, Univ Pennsylvania

Kenan, Samuel MD [OrS] - **Spec Exp:** Bone Tumors; **Hospital:** NYU Hosp For Joint Diseases, NYU Langone Med Ctr (page 66); **Address:** 300 Old Country Rd, Ste 221, Mineola, NY 11501; **Phone:** 516-280-3733; **Med School:** Israel 1976; **Resid:** Orthopaedic Surgery, Hadassah Univ Hosp 1984; **Fellow:** Orthopaedic Pathology, Hosp for Joint Diseases 1987; **Fac Appt:** Prof OrS, NYU Sch Med

Krackow, Kenneth A MD [OrS] - **Spec Exp:** Knee Replacement; Knee Reconstruction; Hip Replacement & Revision; **Hospital:** Buffalo General Hosp; **Address:** Bufffalo General Hosp, Dept Orthopaedic Surgery, 100 High St, Ste B276, Buffalo, NY 14203; **Phone:** 716-859-1256; **Board Cert:** Orthopaedic Surgery 1993; **Med School:** Duke Univ 1971; **Resid:** Surgery, Johns Hopkins Hosp 1973; Orthopaedic Surgery, Johns Hopkins Hosp 1976; **Fac Appt:** Prof OrS, SUNY Buffalo

Lackman, Richard D MD [OrS] - **Spec Exp:** Bone Cancer; Sarcoma; Limb Sparing Surgery; **Hospital:** Pennsylvania Hosp-UPHS (page 68), Penn Presby Med Ctr - UPHS (page 68); **Address:** Penn Orthopaedics, 301 S 8th St, Garfield Duncan Bldg, Ste 2C, Philadelphia, PA 19106; **Phone:** 215-829-5022; **Board Cert:** Orthopaedic Surgery 1985; **Med School:** Univ Pennsylvania 1977; **Resid:** Orthopaedic Surgery, Hosp Univ Penn 1982; **Fellow:** Orthopaedic Oncology, Mayo Clin 1983; **Fac Appt:** Prof OrS, Univ Pennsylvania

Lane, Joseph MD [OrS] - **Spec Exp:** Bone Disorders-Metabolic; Osteoporosis Spine-Kyphoplasty; Bone Cancer; **Hospital:** Hosp For Special Surgery (page 60), NY-Presby/Weill Cornell Med Ctr, NY (page 65); **Address:** Hosp for Special Surgery, 535 E 70th St, New York, NY 10021; **Phone:** 212-606-1172; **Board Cert:** Orthopaedic Surgery 1974; **Med School:** Harvard Med Sch 1965; **Resid:** Surgery, Hosp Univ Penn 1967; Orthopaedic Surgery, Hosp Univ Penn 1973; **Fac Appt:** Prof OrS, Cornell Univ-Weill Med Coll

Lauerman, William MD [OrS] - **Spec Exp:** Spinal Deformity-Pediatric & Adult; Spinal Surgery; Pain-Back; Scoliosis; **Hospital:** Georgetown Univ Hosp; **Address:** 3800 Reservoir Rd NW, Spine Surgery Clinic-1 Gorman, Washington, DC 20007; **Phone:** 202-444-8766 x2; **Board Cert:** Orthopaedic Surgery 2001; **Med School:** Georgetown Univ 1982; **Resid:** Orthopaedic Surgery, Georgetown Univ Med Ctr 1987; **Fellow:** Orthopaedic Surgery, Univ Minn-Twin Cities Scoliosis Ctr 1988; **Fac Appt:** Prof OrS, Georgetown Univ

Leadbetter, Wayne MD [OrS] - **Spec Exp:** Knee-Patella Problems; Arthritis-Knee; **Hospital:** Sinai Hosp - Baltimore; **Address:** Ctr Joint Preservation & Sportss Med, 11110 Med Campus Rd, Ste 103, Baltimore, MD 21742; **Phone:** 301-665-4575; **Board Cert:** Orthopaedic Surgery 1977; **Med School:** Creighton Univ 1970; **Resid:** Surgery, Johns Hopkins Hosp 1972; Orthopaedic Surgery, Johns Hopkins Hosp 1976; **Fellow:** Orthopaedic Surgery, Jonhs Hopkins Hosp 1973; **Fac Appt:** Asst Clin Prof S, Uniformed Srvs Univ, Bethesda

Lee, Francis Y MD/PhD [OrS] - **Spec Exp:** Bone Tumors; Pediatric Orthopaedic Cancers; Pediatric Orthopaedic Surgery; **Hospital:** Morgan Stanley Children's Hosp of NY-Presby, NY (page 65), NY-Presby/Columbia Univ Med Ctr, NY (page 65); **Address:** 3959 Broadway, Ste 800N, New York, NY 10032; **Phone:** 212-305-3293; **Board Cert:** Orthopaedic Surgery 2001; **Med School:** South Korea 1986; **Resid:** Orthopaedic Surgery, NJ Med Ctr 1997; **Fellow:** Orthopaedic Oncology, Harvard Med Sch 1998; Pediatric Orthopaedic Surgery, Hosp for Sick Chldn/Univ Toronto 1999; **Fac Appt:** Asst Prof OrS, Columbia P&S

Levine, David S MD [OrS] - **Spec Exp:** Foot & Ankle Surgery; Ankle Reconstruction; **Hospital:** Hosp For Special Surgery (page 60); **Address:** Hospital for Special Surgery, 535 East 70th St, New York, NY 10021; **Phone:** 212-606-1940; **Board Cert:** Orthopaedic Surgery 2011; **Med School:** Cornell Univ-Weill Med Coll 1992; **Resid:** Orthopaedic Surgery, Hosp for Special Surgery 1997; **Fellow:** Foot & Ankle Surgery, Harborview Med Ctr 1998

Macaulay, William B MD [OrS] - **Spec Exp:** Hip Replacement; Knee Replacement; Minimally Invasive Surgery; Reconstructive Surgery; **Hospital:** NY-Presby/Columbia Univ Med Ctr, NY (page 65); **Address:** Columbia Orthopaedics, 161 Fort Washington Ave, Irving Pavilion Fl 2, New York, NY 10032; **Phone:** 212-305-6959; **Board Cert:** Orthopaedic Surgery 2001; **Med School:** Columbia P&S 1992; **Resid:** Orthopaedic Surgery, Univ Pittsburgh Med Ctr 1997; **Fellow:** Adult Reconstructive Surgery, Hosp for Special Surgery 1999; **Fac Appt:** Prof OrS, Columbia P&S

Malawer, Martin M MD [OrS] - **Spec Exp:** Bone Tumors; Limb Sparing Surgery; Pediatric Orthopaedic Surgery; Sarcoma; **Hospital:** Georgetown Univ Hosp, G Washington Univ Hosp; **Address:** 7830 Old Georgetown Rd, Ste C15, Bethesda, MD 20814; **Phone:** 301-215-7940; **Board Cert:** Orthopaedic Surgery 1976; **Med School:** NYU Sch Med 1969; **Resid:** Surgery, Bronx Muni Hosp 1972; Orthopaedic Surgery, Bellevue Hosp Ctr 1975; **Fellow:** Orthopaedic Oncology, Shands Hosp-Univ Florida 1978; **Fac Appt:** Prof OrS, Geo Wash Univ

Marx, Robert G MD [OrS] - **Spec Exp:** Shoulder Surgery; Knee Injuries/Ligament Surgery; Knee Replacement; Sports Medicine; **Hospital:** Hosp For Special Surgery (page 60); **Address:** Hospital for Special Surgery, 535 E 70th St, New York, NY 10021; **Phone:** 212-606-1645; **Board Cert:** Orthopaedic Surgery 2003; **Med School:** McGill Univ 1991; **Resid:** Orthopaedic Surgery, Univ Toronto 1996; **Fellow:** Sports Medicine, Hosp Special Surgery 1998; **Fac Appt:** Prof OrS, Cornell Univ-Weill Med Coll

Orthopaedic Surgery

McAfee, Paul C MD [OrS] - **Spec Exp:** Spinal Reconstructive Surgery; Spinal Disc Replacement; Scoliosis; **Hospital:** St. Joseph Med Ctr; **Address:** Scoliosis & Spine Ctr, 7505 Osler Drive, Ste 104, Towson, MD 21204; **Phone:** 410-337-8888; **Board Cert:** Orthopaedic Surgery 2007; **Med School:** SUNY Upstate Med Univ 1979; **Resid:** Orthopaedic Surgery, SUNY Upstate Med Ctr 1984; **Fellow:** Spinal Surgery, Case West Res Univ Hosps 1986; **Fac Appt:** Assoc Prof OrS, Johns Hopkins Univ

McCann, Peter D MD [OrS] - **Spec Exp:** Shoulder Surgery; Elbow Surgery; **Hospital:** Beth Israel Med Ctr - Petrie Division (page 55); **Address:** 10 Union Square E, Ste 3M, New York, NY 10003; **Phone:** 212-844-6735; **Board Cert:** Orthopaedic Surgery 2009; **Med School:** Columbia P&S 1980; **Resid:** Surgery, St Vincent's Hosp 1982; Orthopaedic Surgery, Columbia-Presby Med Ctr 1985; **Fellow:** Shoulder Surgery, Columbia-Presby Med Ctr 1986; **Fac Appt:** Assoc Prof OrS, Albert Einstein Coll Med

McFarland, Edward G MD [OrS] - **Spec Exp:** Sports Medicine; Rotator Cuff Surgery; Shoulder Surgery; **Hospital:** Johns Hopkins Hosp (page 61); **Address:** 10753 Falls Rd, Ste 215, Lutherville, MD 21093; **Phone:** 410-583-2851; **Board Cert:** Orthopaedic Surgery 2011; Orthopaedic Sports Medicine 2010; **Med School:** Univ Louisville Sch Med 1982; **Resid:** Orthopaedic Surgery, Mayo Clinic 1987; **Fellow:** Sports Medicine, Kerlan-Jobe Orthopaedic Group 1989; **Fac Appt:** Prof OrS, Johns Hopkins Univ

Myerson, Mark MD [OrS] - **Spec Exp:** Foot & Ankle Surgery; **Hospital:** Mercy Med Ctr - Baltimore; **Address:** 301 St Paul Pl, Baltimore, MD 21202; **Phone:** 410-659-2800; **Board Cert:** Orthopaedic Surgery 2008; **Med School:** South Africa 1979; **Resid:** Surgery, Sinai Hospital 1981; Orthopaedic Surgery, Johns Hopkins Hosp 1985; **Fellow:** Foot & Ankle Surgery, Hospital Joint Disease

Neuwirth, Michael MD [OrS] - **Spec Exp:** Scoliosis; Spinal Surgery; **Hospital:** Beth Israel Med Ctr - Petrie Division (page 55); **Address:** Beth Israel Med Ctr - Spine Institute, 10 Union Square E, Ste 5P, New York, NY 10003-3314; **Phone:** 212-844-8692; **Board Cert:** Orthopaedic Surgery 1980; **Med School:** SUNY Hlth Sci Ctr 1974; **Resid:** Orthopaedic Surgery, Hosp for Joint Diseases 1978; **Fellow:** Spinal Surgery, Rush-Presby Med Ctr 1979; **Fac Appt:** Assoc Clin Prof OrS, NYU Sch Med

Nicholas, Stephen J MD [OrS] - **Spec Exp:** Sports Medicine; Shoulder & Knee Surgery; Arthroscopic Surgery; **Hospital:** Lenox Hill Hosp; **Address:** 130 E 77 St, New York, NY 10075; **Phone:** 212-737-3301; **Board Cert:** Orthopaedic Surgery 2005; **Med School:** NY Med Coll 1986; **Resid:** Orthopaedic Surgery, Hosp for Special Surgery 1991; **Fellow:** Sports Medicine, Lenox Hill Hosp 1992

O'Keefe, Regis J MD/PhD [OrS] - **Spec Exp:** Bone & Soft Tissue Tumors; Reconstructive Surgery; Bone Disorders-Metabolic; **Hospital:** Univ of Rochester Strong Meml Hosp, Highland Hosp of Rochester; **Address:** Univ Rochester, Dept Orthopaedic Surgery, 601 Elmwood Ave, Box 665, Rochester, NY 14642; **Phone:** 585-275-3100; **Board Cert:** Orthopaedic Surgery 2007; **Med School:** Harvard Med Sch 1985; **Resid:** Surgery, New Eng Deaconess Hosp/Harvard 1986; Orthopaedic Surgery, Univ Rochester 1992; **Fellow:** Orthopaedic Oncology, Mass Genl Hosp 1993; **Fac Appt:** Prof S, Univ Rochester

O'Leary, Patrick MD [OrS] - **Spec Exp:** Spinal Surgery; **Hospital:** Hosp For Special Surgery (page 60); **Address:** 1015 Madison Ave Fl 4, New York, NY 10075; **Phone:** 212-249-8100; **Board Cert:** Orthopaedic Surgery 1983; **Med School:** Ireland 1968; **Resid:** Surgery, Roosevelt Hosp 1972; Orthopaedic Surgery, Hosp Spec Surg-Cornell 1975; **Fellow:** Spinal Surgery, Univ Toronto Genl Ortho Hosp 1976; **Fac Appt:** Assoc Clin Prof OrS, Cornell Univ-Weill Med Coll

Padgett, Douglas E MD [OrS] - **Spec Exp:** Hip & Knee Replacement; Arthroscopic Surgery-Hip; Arthroscopic Surgery-Knee; Dance Medicine; **Hospital:** Hosp For Special Surgery (page 60); **Address:** Hosp for Special Surgery, 535 E 70 St, New York, NY 10021; **Phone:** 212-606-1642; **Board Cert:** Orthopaedic Surgery 2003; **Med School:** NY Med Coll 1982; **Resid:** Orthopaedic Surgery, Hosp Spec Surg 1989; **Fellow:** Orthopaedic Surgery, Rush Presby Med Ctr 1990; **Fac Appt:** Assoc Prof OrS, Cornell Univ-Weill Med Coll

Parvizi, Javad MD [OrS] - **Spec Exp:** Hip Replacement & Revision; Knee Replacement & Revision; **Hospital:** Thomas Jefferson Univ Hosp; **Address:** Rothman Institute, 925 Chestnut St Fl 5, Philadelphia, PA 19107; **Phone:** 800-321-9999; **Board Cert:** Orthopaedic Surgery 2005; **Med School:** England, UK 1991; **Resid:** Orthopaedic Surgery, Mayo Clinic; **Fellow:** Joint Arthroplasty, Univ of Berne; **Fac Appt:** Prof OrS, Thomas Jefferson Univ

Pellicci, Paul M MD [OrS] - **Spec Exp:** Hip Replacement-Young Adults; Hip Resurfacing; Knee Replacement; Joint Replacement; **Hospital:** Hosp For Special Surgery (page 60), NY-Presby/Weill Cornell Med Ctr, NY (page 65); **Address:** 535 E 70th St, Ste 354, New York, NY 10021-4872; **Phone:** 212-606-1010; **Board Cert:** Orthopaedic Surgery 1982; **Med School:** Cornell Univ-Weill Med Coll 1975; **Resid:** Surgery, NY Hosp 1977; Orthopaedic Surgery, Hosp Spec Surg 1980; **Fellow:** Joint Replacement Surgery, Brigham & Womens Hosp 1981; **Fac Appt:** Prof OrS, Cornell Univ-Weill Med Coll

Pizzutillo, Peter D MD [OrS] - **Spec Exp:** Pediatric Orthopaedic Surgery; Sports Medicine; Congenital Anomalies-Orthopaedic; **Hospital:** St. Christopher's Hosp for Chldn; **Address:** St Christophers Hosp for Children, Dept Orthopaedic Surgery, 3601 A St, Philadelphia, PA 19134; **Phone:** 215-427-3131; **Board Cert:** Orthopaedic Surgery 1976; **Med School:** Jefferson Med Coll 1970; **Resid:** Orthopaedic Surgery, Thosd Jefferson Univ Hosp 1975; Pediatric Orthopaedic Surgery, Alfred I Du Pont Inst 1974; **Fac Appt:** Prof OrS, Jefferson Med Coll

Plancher, Kevin D MD [OrS] - **Spec Exp:** Shoulder Surgery; Elbow Surgery; Cartilage Damage & Transplant; Shoulder Replacement; **Hospital:** Beth Israel Med Ctr - Petrie Division (page 55), Lenox Hill Hosp; **Address:** 1160 Park Ave, New York, NY 10128; **Phone:** 212-876-5200; **Board Cert:** Orthopaedic Surgery 2007; Hand Surgery 2008; Orthopaedic Sports Medicine 2009; **Med School:** Georgetown Univ 1986; **Resid:** Orthopaedic Surgery, Mass Genl Hosp/Brigham & Womens Hosp 1991; **Fellow:** Hand Surgery, Indiana Hand Ctr 1993; Sports Medicine, Steadman-Hawkins Clinic 1994; **Fac Appt:** Assoc Clin Prof OrS, Albert Einstein Coll Med

Ramsey, Matthew L MD [OrS] - **Spec Exp:** Shoulder Surgery; Elbow Surgery; Sports Medicine; **Hospital:** Bucks Specialty Inst, Thomas Jefferson Univ Hosp; **Address:** Rothman Institute, 925 Chestnut St, Fl 5, Philadelphia, PA 19107; **Phone:** 800-321-9999; **Board Cert:** Orthopaedic Surgery 2009; **Med School:** SUNY Hlth Sci Ctr 1990; **Resid:** Orthopaedic Surgery, Thomas Jefferson Univ Hosp 1995; **Fellow:** Shoulder Surgery, Hosp Univ Penn 1996; **Fac Appt:** Assoc Prof OrS, Thomas Jefferson Univ

Ranawat, Chitranjan MD [OrS] - **Spec Exp:** Hip Replacement; Knee Replacement; **Hospital:** Hosp For Special Surgery (page 60); **Address:** Hosp for Special Surgery, 535 E 70th St Fl 6, New York, NY 10021; **Phone:** 646-797-8700; **Board Cert:** Orthopaedic Surgery 1969; **Med School:** India 1958; **Resid:** Surgery, MY Hosp 1963; Orthopaedic Surgery, Albany Med Ctr 1965; **Fellow:** Orthopaedic Surgery, Hosp Special Surg 1969; **Fac Appt:** Prof OrS, Cornell Univ-Weill Med Coll

Orthopaedic Surgery

Rechtine, Glenn MD [OrS] - **Spec Exp:** Spinal Surgery; Spinal Disorders-Degenerative; Spinal Trauma; **Hospital:** Univ of Rochester Strong Meml Hosp; **Address:** Univ Rochester, Dept Orthopaedics, 601 Elmwood Ave, Box 665, Rochester, NY 14642; **Phone:** 585-275-2225; **Board Cert:** Orthopaedic Surgery 2010; **Med School:** Univ S Fla Coll Med 1975; **Resid:** Orthopaedic Surgery, Naval Regional Med Ctr 1980; **Fellow:** Spinal Surgery, Case West Res Univ 1981; **Fac Appt:** Prof OrS, Univ Rochester

Rodosky, Mark W MD [OrS] - **Spec Exp:** Sports Medicine; Shoulder Surgery; Rotator Cuff Surgery; **Hospital:** UPMC South Side-Out Pt Ctr; **Address:** UPMC Center for Sports Medicine, 3200 S Water St, Pittsburgh, PA 15203; **Phone:** 412-432-3621; **Board Cert:** Orthopaedic Surgery 2008; **Med School:** Mount Sinai Sch Med 1987; **Resid:** Surgery, Univ Pittsburgh Med Ctr 1993; **Fellow:** Orthopaedic Surgery, NY Presby-Columbia Presby Med Ctr 1994; **Fac Appt:** Asst Prof OrS, Univ Pittsburgh

Rothman, Richard H MD/PhD [OrS] - **Spec Exp:** Hip Replacement; Knee Replacement; Joint Replacement; **Hospital:** Thomas Jefferson Univ Hosp; **Address:** Rothman Institute, 925 Chestnut St Fl 5, Philadelphia, PA 19107; **Phone:** 800-321-9999; **Board Cert:** Orthopaedic Surgery 1970; **Med School:** Univ Pennsylvania 1962; **Resid:** Orthopaedic Surgery, Jefferson Hosp 1968; **Fac Appt:** Prof OrS, Jefferson Med Coll

Roye Jr, David P MD [OrS] - **Spec Exp:** Pediatric Orthopaedic Surgery; Scoliosis; Hip Disorders-Pediatric; Neuromuscular Disorders; **Hospital:** Morgan Stanley Children's Hosp of NY-Presby, NY (page 65), NY-Presby/Columbia Univ Med Ctr, NY (page 65); **Address:** Morgan Stanley Chlds Hosp NewYork-Presby, 3959 Broadway, 8 North, New York, NY 10032-1559; **Phone:** 212-305-5475; **Board Cert:** Orthopaedic Surgery 1981; **Med School:** Columbia P&S 1975; **Resid:** Orthopaedic Surgery, Columbia-Presby Med Ctr 1979; **Fellow:** Orthopaedic Surgery, Hosp for Sick Chldn 1980; **Fac Appt:** Prof OrS, Columbia P&S

Rozbruch, S Robert MD [OrS] - **Spec Exp:** Limb Lengthening; Limb Deformities; Limb Surgery/Reconstruction; Fractures-Complex & Non Union; **Hospital:** Hosp For Special Surgery (page 60), NY-Presby/Weill Cornell Med Ctr, NY (page 65); **Address:** 535 E 70th St, New York, NY 10021; **Phone:** 212-606-1415; **Board Cert:** Orthopaedic Surgery 2009; **Med School:** Cornell Univ-Weill Med Coll 1990; **Resid:** Orthopaedic Surgery, Hosp Special Surgery 1995; **Fellow:** Trauma, Univ Bern Hosp 1997; Limb Lengthening, Intl Ctr Limb Length/Univ MD 1999; **Fac Appt:** Assoc Clin Prof OrS, Cornell Univ-Weill Med Coll

Salvati, Eduardo A MD [OrS] - **Spec Exp:** Hip Surgery; Hip & Knee Replacement; **Hospital:** Hosp For Special Surgery (page 60); **Address:** Hosp for Spec Surg, 535 E 70th Street, New York, NY 10021; **Phone:** 212-606-1472; **Board Cert:** Orthopaedic Surgery 1972; **Med School:** Argentina 1963; **Resid:** Orthopaedic Surgery, Univ Florence Ortho Clinic 1965; Orthopaedic Surgery, Hosp Buenos Aires 1969; **Fellow:** Hip Surgery, Hosp For Spec Surg 1972; **Fac Appt:** Clin Prof OrS, Cornell Univ-Weill Med Coll

Sandhu, Harvinder S MD [OrS] - **Spec Exp:** Minimally Invasive Surgery; Spinal Disc Replacement; Spinal Surgery; **Hospital:** Hosp For Special Surgery (page 60), NY-Presby/Weill Cornell Med Ctr, NY (page 65); **Address:** 535 E 70th St, New York, NY 10021; **Phone:** 212-606-1798; **Board Cert:** Orthopaedic Surgery 2007; **Med School:** Northwestern Univ 1987; **Resid:** Orthopaedic Surgery, Univ Hosp-SUNY Hlth Sci Ctr 1992; **Fellow:** Spinal Surgery, UCLA Med Ctr 1993; **Fac Appt:** Assoc Prof OrS, Cornell Univ-Weill Med Coll

Schmidt, Richard G MD [OrS] - **Spec Exp:** Bone Tumors; Sarcoma-Soft Tissue; Limb Sparing Surgery; Bone Tumors-Metastatic; **Hospital:** Lankenau Hosp, Fox Chase Cancer Ctr (page 58); **Address:** Musculoskeletal Tumor Ctr, 15 N Presidential Blvd, Ste 300, Bala Cynwyd, PA 19004; **Phone:** 610-667-2663; **Board Cert:** Orthopaedic Surgery 2009; **Med School:** Penn State Coll Med 1980; **Resid:** Orthopaedic Surgery, Hosp Univ Penn 1985; **Fellow:** Orthopaedic Oncology, Shands Hosp 1986

Schwab, Frank J MD [OrS] - **Spec Exp:** Spinal Surgery; Pain-Back; Spinal Deformity; Scoliosis; **Hospital:** NYU Hosp For Joint Diseases, New York Methodist Hosp; **Address:** 306 E 15th St, Ste 1F, New York, NY 10003; **Phone:** 646-794-8646; **Board Cert:** Orthopaedic Surgery 2010; **Med School:** Columbia P&S 1990; **Resid:** Surgery, NY Presby-Columbia Med Ctr 1992; Orthopaedic Surgery, NY Presby-Columbia Med Ctr 1996; **Fellow:** Orthopaedic Surgery, Hospital Lariboisiere 1991; Spinal Surgery, Maimonides Med Ctr 1997; **Fac Appt:** Assoc Clin Prof OrS, NYU Sch Med

Scott, W Norman MD [OrS] - **Spec Exp:** Knee Injuries; Knee Replacement; Sports Medicine; **Hospital:** Lenox Hill Hosp, Franklin Hosp; **Address:** 210 E 64th St Fl 4, New York, NY 10065; **Phone:** 646-293-7501; **Board Cert:** Orthopaedic Surgery 1978; **Med School:** Cornell Univ-Weill Med Coll 1972; **Resid:** Surgery, St Lukes-Roosevelt Hosp Ctr 1974; Orthopaedic Surgery, Hosp Special Surg 1977; **Fac Appt:** Clin Prof OrS, Cornell Univ-Weill Med Coll

Sculco, Thomas P MD [OrS] - **Spec Exp:** Hip Replacement; Knee Replacement; Minimally Invasive Surgery; Joint Replacement; **Hospital:** Hosp For Special Surgery (page 60); **Address:** 535 E 70th St, New York, NY 10021-4872; **Phone:** 212-606-1475; **Board Cert:** Orthopaedic Surgery 1976; **Med School:** Columbia P&S 1969; **Resid:** Surgery, Roosevelt Hosp 1971; Orthopaedic Surgery, Hosp For Special Surgery 1974; **Fellow:** Orthopaedic Surgery, The London Hosp 1975; **Fac Appt:** Prof OrS, Cornell Univ-Weill Med Coll

Sharkey, Peter F MD [OrS] - **Spec Exp:** Hip Replacement; Knee Replacement; **Hospital:** Thomas Jefferson Univ Hosp, Riddle Meml Hosp; **Address:** Rothman Institute, 925 Chestnut St Fl 5, Philadelphia, PA 19107; **Phone:** 800-321-9999; **Board Cert:** Orthopaedic Surgery 2003; **Med School:** SUNY Upstate Med Univ 1984; **Resid:** Orthopaedic Surgery, Thomas Jefferson Univ Hosp 1990; **Fellow:** Hip & Knee Surgery, Rothman Inst; **Fac Appt:** Prof OrS, Thomas Jefferson Univ

Spivak, Jeffrey M MD [OrS] - **Spec Exp:** Spinal Surgery; Scoliosis; Sports Medicine Back Injuries; **Hospital:** NYU Hosp For Joint Diseases, NYU Langone Med Ctr (page 66); **Address:** Hosp for Joint Diseases, Spine Ctr, 301 E 17th St, Ste 400, New York, NY 10003-3804; **Phone:** 212-598-6696; **Board Cert:** Orthopaedic Surgery 2006; **Med School:** Cornell Univ-Weill Med Coll 1986; **Resid:** Orthopaedic Surgery, Hosp for Joint Diseases 1992; **Fellow:** Spinal Surgery, Thomas Jefferson Univ Hosp 1993; **Fac Appt:** Asst Prof OrS, NYU Sch Med

Sponseller, Paul D MD [OrS] - **Spec Exp:** Cerebral Palsy; Scoliosis; Pediatric Orthopaedic Surgery; **Hospital:** Johns Hopkins Hosp (page 61); **Address:** 601 N Caroline St, Ste 5212, Baltimore, MD 21287-0882; **Phone:** 410-955-3136; **Board Cert:** Orthopaedic Surgery 2010; **Med School:** Univ Mich Med Sch 1980; **Resid:** Orthopaedic Surgery, Univ Wisc Hosp 1985; **Fellow:** Pediatric Orthopaedic Surgery, Children's Hosp 1986; **Fac Appt:** Prof OrS, Johns Hopkins Univ

Strongwater, Allan M MD [OrS] - **Spec Exp:** Pediatric Orthopaedic Surgery; Cerebral Palsy; Deformity Reconstruction; **Hospital:** St. Joseph's Regl Med Ctr - Paterson, NYU Langone Med Ctr (page 66); **Address:** St Josephs Childrens Hospital, Dept Orthopaedic Surgery, 703 Main St - Xavier 702, Paterson, NJ 07503; **Phone:** 973-754-2414; **Board Cert:** Orthopaedic Surgery 2007; **Med School:** Rush Med Coll 1978; **Resid:** Orthopaedic Surgery, Yale-New Haven Hosp 1983; **Fellow:** Pediatric Orthopaedic Surgery, Hosp Joint Diseases 1984; **Fac Appt:** Clin Prof OrS, NYU Sch Med

Orthopaedic Surgery

Stuchin, Steven MD [OrS] - **Spec Exp:** Hand Surgery; Arthritis; Hip & Knee Replacement; Hip Resurfacing; **Hospital:** NYU Hosp For Joint Diseases, Lenox Hill Hosp; **Address:** 301 E 17th St, Ste 1402, New York, NY 10003-3804; **Phone:** 212-598-6708; **Board Cert:** Orthopaedic Surgery 1984; **Med School:** Columbia P&S 1976; **Resid:** Surgery, Roosevelt Hosp 1978; Orthopaedic Surgery, Hosp For Special Surg 1981; **Fellow:** Hand Surgery, Thomas Jefferson Univ Hosp 1982; **Fac Appt:** Assoc Prof OrS, NYU Sch Med

Vaccaro, Alexander R MD/PhD [OrS] - **Spec Exp:** Spinal Surgery; Spinal Trauma; Spinal Cord Injury; **Hospital:** Thomas Jefferson Univ Hosp; **Address:** Rothman Institute, 925 Chestnut St Fl 5, Philadelphia, PA 19107; **Phone:** 800-321-9999; **Board Cert:** Orthopaedic Surgery 2006; **Med School:** Georgetown Univ 1987; **Resid:** Orthopaedic Surgery, Thos Jefferson Univ Hosp 1992; **Fellow:** Spinal Surgery, UCSD Med Ctr 1993; **Fac Appt:** Prof OrS, Thomas Jefferson Univ

Wapner, Keith L MD [OrS] - **Spec Exp:** Foot & Ankle Surgery; Tendon Surgery; Arthritis; **Hospital:** Pennsylvania Hosp-UPHS (page 68); **Address:** 230 W Washington Square, The Farm Journal Bldg Fl 5, Philadelphia, PA 19106-3500; **Phone:** 215-829-3668; **Board Cert:** Orthopaedic Surgery 2009; **Med School:** Temple Univ 1980; **Resid:** Surgery, Hosp Univ Penn 1981; Orthopaedic Surgery, Hosp Univ Penn 1985; **Fellow:** Joint Reconstruction, Ohio St Univ Med Ctr 1986; Foot & Ankle Surgery, UCSF Med Ctr 1987

Warren, Russell MD [OrS] - **Spec Exp:** Knee Injuries/Ligament Surgery; Shoulder Surgery; Shoulder Replacement; Rotator Cuff Surgery; **Hospital:** Hosp For Special Surgery (page 60), NY-Presby/Weill Cornell Med Ctr, NY (page 65); **Address:** 535 E 70th St, New York, NY 10021-4892; **Phone:** 212-606-1178; **Board Cert:** Orthopaedic Surgery 1974; **Med School:** SUNY Upstate Med Univ 1966; **Resid:** Surgery, St Lukes Hosp 1968; Orthopaedic Surgery, Hosp For Special Surgery 1973; **Fellow:** Shoulder Surgery, Columbia-Presby Med Ctr 1977; **Fac Appt:** Prof OrS, Cornell Univ-Weill Med Coll

Weinfeld, Steven B MD [OrS] - **Spec Exp:** Foot & Ankle Surgery; Diabetic Leg/Foot; **Hospital:** Mount Sinai Med Ctr (page 63), Hackensack Univ Med Ctr; **Address:** 5 E 98th St Fl 9, Box 1188, New York, NY 10029; **Phone:** 212-241-1634; **Board Cert:** Orthopaedic Surgery 2009; **Med School:** Albany Med Coll 1990; **Resid:** Orthopaedic Surgery, Albany Med Ctr 1995; **Fellow:** Ankle and Foot Surgery, Union Meml Hosp 1996; **Fac Appt:** Assoc Prof OrS, Mount Sinai Sch Med

Westrich, Geoffrey H MD [OrS] - **Spec Exp:** Hip Replacement & Revision; Knee Replacement & Revision; Arthroscopic Surgery-Hip; Arthroscopic Surgery-Knee; **Hospital:** Hosp For Special Surgery (page 60), NY-Presby/Weill Cornell Med Ctr, NY (page 65); **Address:** Hospital for Special Surgery, 535 E 70th St, New York, NY 10021; **Phone:** 212-606-1510; **Board Cert:** Orthopaedic Surgery 2009; **Med School:** Tufts Univ 1990; **Resid:** Orthopaedic Surgery, Hosp for Special Surg 1995; **Fellow:** Trauma, Inselspital 1995; Adult Reconstructive Surgery, Hosp for Special Surg 1996; **Fac Appt:** Assoc Prof OrS, Cornell Univ-Weill Med Coll

Wetzel, F Todd MD [OrS] - **Spec Exp:** Spinal Surgery; Minimally Invasive Surgery; **Hospital:** Temple Univ Hosp, Jeanes Hosp; **Address:** Temple Univ Hosp Fl 5, 3509 N Broad St, Philadelphia, PA 19140; **Phone:** 215-707-2111; **Board Cert:** Orthopaedic Surgery 2011; **Med School:** Univ Pennsylvania 1981; **Resid:** Surgery, Yale-New Haven Hosp 1983; Orthopaedic Surgery, Yale Univ Affil Hosps 1986; **Fellow:** Spinal Surgery, Dr Henry LaRocca 1987; **Fac Appt:** Prof OrS, Temple Univ

Wickiewicz, Thomas L MD [OrS] - **Spec Exp:** Shoulder Surgery; Sports Medicine; Knee Injuries/ACL; Rotator Cuff Surgery; **Hospital:** Hosp For Special Surgery (page 60), NY-Presby/Weill Cornell Med Ctr, NY (page 65); **Address:** 535 E 70th St, New York, NY 10021; **Phone:** 212-606-1450; **Board Cert:** Orthopaedic Surgery 1984; **Med School:** UMDNJ-NJ Med Sch, Newark 1976; **Resid:** Orthopaedic Surgery, Hosp for Special Surg 1981; **Fellow:** Sports Medicine, UCLA Med Ctr 1982; **Fac Appt:** Clin Prof OrS, Cornell Univ-Weill Med Coll

Wiesel, Sam W MD [OrS] - **Spec Exp:** Spinal Surgery; **Hospital:** Georgetown Univ Hosp; **Address:** 3800 Reservoir Rd NW, PHC Bldg Fl Ground, Washington, DC 20007-2113; **Phone:** 202-444-8766 x2; **Board Cert:** Orthopaedic Surgery 1977; **Med School:** Univ Pennsylvania 1971; **Resid:** Orthopaedic Surgery, Hosp Univ Penn 1976; **Fellow:** Orthopaedic Surgery, Hosp Univ Penn 1973; **Fac Appt:** Prof OrS, Georgetown Univ

Williams, Gerald MD [OrS] - **Spec Exp:** Shoulder Reconstruction; Shoulder Cartilage Implant; Shoulder Replacement; Rotator Cuff Surgery; **Hospital:** Thomas Jefferson Univ Hosp, Methodist Hosp; **Address:** Rothman Institute, 925 Chestnut St Fl 5, Philadelphia, PA 19107; **Phone:** 800-321-9999; **Board Cert:** Orthopaedic Surgery 2003; **Med School:** Temple Univ 1984; **Resid:** Orthopaedic Surgery, Univ Texas San Antonio Affil Hosp 1989; **Fellow:** Shoulder Surgery, Univ Texas San Antonio Affil Hosp 1990; **Fac Appt:** Prof OrS, Thomas Jefferson Univ

Williams, Riley J MD [OrS] - **Spec Exp:** Cartilage Damage & Transplant; Shoulder Arthroscopic Surgery; Knee Injuries/ACL; Knee Surgery; **Hospital:** Hosp For Special Surgery (page 60), NY-Presby/Weill Cornell Med Ctr, NY (page 65); **Address:** Hosp Special Surgery, 535 E 70th St, New York, NY 10021; **Phone:** 212-606-1855; **Board Cert:** Orthopaedic Surgery 2000; **Med School:** Stanford Univ 1992; **Resid:** Orthopaedic Surgery, Hosp Special Surgery 1997; **Fellow:** Sports Medicine & Shoulder Surgery, Hosp Special Surgery 1998; **Fac Appt:** Assoc Prof OrS, Cornell Univ-Weill Med Coll

Wittig, James C MD [OrS] - **Spec Exp:** Bone Tumors; Sarcoma-Soft Tissue; Hip & Knee Replacement; Shoulder Tumors; **Hospital:** Mount Sinai Med Ctr (page 63), Hackensack Univ Med Ctr; **Address:** 5 E 98th St, Fl 9, New York, NY 10029; **Phone:** 212-241-1807 x4817; **Board Cert:** Orthopaedic Surgery 2003; **Med School:** NYU Sch Med 1994; **Resid:** Orthopaedic Surgery, Columbia Presby Med Ctr 1999; **Fellow:** Orthopaedic Oncology, Washington Cancer Inst 2001; Orthopaedic Oncology, NIH 2001; **Fac Appt:** Assoc Prof OrS, Mount Sinai Sch Med

Zuckerman, Joseph D MD [OrS] - **Spec Exp:** Shoulder Surgery; Hip Replacement; Knee Replacement; Rotator Cuff Surgery; **Hospital:** NYU Hosp For Joint Diseases, NYU Langone Med Ctr (page 66); **Address:** NYU Hosp for Joint Diseases, Dept Ortho Surg, 301 E 17th St Fl 14 - Ste 1402, New York, NY 10003; **Phone:** 212-598-6674; **Board Cert:** Orthopaedic Surgery 2007; **Med School:** Med Coll Wisc 1978; **Resid:** Orthopaedic Surgery, Univ WA Med Ctr 1983; **Fellow:** Arthritis Surgery, Brigham & Womans Hosp 1984; Shoulder Surgery, Mayo Clinic 1984; **Fac Appt:** Prof OrS, NYU Sch Med

Southeast

Beaty, James H MD [OrS] - **Spec Exp:** Pediatric Orthopaedic Surgery; Clubfoot; Fractures-Pediatric; **Hospital:** Le Bonheur Chldns Med Ctr; **Address:** Campbell Clinic, 1400 S Germantown Rd, Germantown, TN 38138; **Phone:** 901-759-3125; **Board Cert:** Orthopaedic Surgery 2007; **Med School:** Univ Tenn Coll Med 1976; **Resid:** Surgery, Baptist Meml Hosp 1979; Orthopaedic Surgery, Campbell Clin Fdn 1981; **Fellow:** Pediatric Orthopaedic Surgery, Alfred I Dupont Inst 1982; **Fac Appt:** Prof OrS, Univ Tenn Coll Med

Berrey, B Hudson MD [OrS] - **Spec Exp:** Musculoskeletal Tumors; Bone Cancer; Soft Tissue Tumors; Sarcoma; **Hospital:** Shands Jacksonville, Wolfson Chldns Hosp; **Address:** University of Florida Coll Med, Dept Orthopaedic Surgery, 655 W Eighth St ACC Bldg Fl 2, Jacksonville, FL 32209-6511; **Phone:** 904-244-5942; **Board Cert:** Orthopaedic Surgery 1982; **Med School:** Univ Tex Med Br, Galveston 1977; **Resid:** Orthopaedic Surgery, Tripler Army Med Ctr 1981; **Fellow:** Medical Oncology, Mass Genl Hosp/Harvard 1985; **Fac Appt:** Prof OrS, Univ Fla Coll Med

Orthopaedic Surgery

Boden, Scott D MD [OrS] - **Spec Exp:** Spinal Disorders; Spinal Surgery; Spinal Disc Replacement; Microdiscectomy; **Hospital:** Emory Univ Hosp; **Address:** Emory Orthopaedics & Spine Center, 59 Executive Park South, Ste 3000, Atlanta, GA 30329; **Phone:** 404-778-7143; **Board Cert:** Orthopaedic Surgery 2005; **Med School:** Univ Pennsylvania 1986; **Resid:** Orthopaedic Surgery, Geo Washington Univ Hosp 1991; **Fellow:** Spinal Surgery, Case Western Reserve Univ 1992; **Fac Appt:** Prof OrS, Emory Univ

Curl, Walton W MD [OrS] - **Spec Exp:** Sports Medicine; **Hospital:** Wake Forest Univ Baptist Med Ctr; **Address:** Wake Forest Med Ctr, Comp Rehab, 131 Miller St, Winston-Salem, NC 27103; **Phone:** 336-716-8091; **Board Cert:** Orthopaedic Surgery 1980; **Med School:** Duke Univ 1973; **Resid:** Orthopaedic Surgery, Letterman Army Med Ctr 1978; **Fellow:** Sports Medicine, Keller Army Hosp 1979; **Fac Appt:** Prof OrS, Wake Forest Univ

DeOrio, James K MD [OrS] - **Spec Exp:** Ankle Replacement & Revision; Foot & Ankle Surgery; Foot Deformities; **Hospital:** Duke Univ Hosp; **Address:** 4709 Creekstone Drive, Ste 200, Durham, NC 27703; **Phone:** 919-660-2358; **Board Cert:** Orthopaedic Surgery 1983; **Med School:** Geo Wash Univ 1977; **Resid:** Orthopaedic Surgery, Mayo Clinic 1982; **Fellow:** Orthopaedic Surgery, Chur Hosp 1983; **Fac Appt:** Assoc Prof OrS, Duke Univ

Diduch, David R MD [OrS] - **Spec Exp:** Sports Medicine; Knee Injuries/ACL; Shoulder Reconstruction; Rotator Cuff Surgery; **Hospital:** Univ of Virginia Health Sys; **Address:** Univ Virginia Dept Ortho Surg, Box 800243, Charlottesville, VA 22908; **Phone:** 434-243-0274; **Board Cert:** Orthopaedic Surgery 2008; Orthopaedic Sports Medicine 2009; **Med School:** Harvard Med Sch 1988; **Resid:** Orthopaedic Surgery, Univ Virginia Med Ctr 1994; **Fellow:** Sports Medicine, Insall-Scott-Kelly Inst 1995; **Fac Appt:** Prof OrS, Univ VA Sch Med

Eismont, Frank MD [OrS] - **Spec Exp:** Spinal Surgery; Spinal Tumors; Spinal Trauma; **Hospital:** Jackson Meml Hosp (page 70), Univ of Miami Hosp (page 72); **Address:** Univ Miami Sch Med, Dept Orth Surg, PO Box 016960 (D-27), Miami, FL 33101; **Phone:** 305-243-3000; **Board Cert:** Orthopaedic Surgery 2007; **Med School:** Univ Rochester 1973; **Resid:** Orthopaedic Surgery, Case Western Res Univ Hosp 1978; **Fellow:** Spinal Surgery, Case Western Res Univ Hosp 1979; Spinal Surgery, PA Hosp 1980; **Fac Appt:** Prof OrS, Univ Miami Sch Med

Garrett, William MD/PhD [OrS] - **Spec Exp:** Sports Medicine; Shoulder & Knee Surgery; Shoulder & Knee Reconstruction; Rotator Cuff Surgery; **Hospital:** Duke Univ Hosp; **Address:** Duke Univ Med Center, Box 3338, Durham, NC 27710; **Phone:** 919-684-5678; **Board Cert:** Orthopaedic Surgery 2007; Orthopaedic Sports Medicine 2007; **Med School:** Duke Univ 1976; **Resid:** Orthopaedic Surgery, Duke Univ Med Ctr 1982; **Fac Appt:** Prof OrS, Duke Univ

Goldner, Richard D MD [OrS] - **Spec Exp:** Hand & Wrist Surgery; Hand & Wrist Reconstrction; Arthroscopic Surgery-Wrist; **Hospital:** Duke Univ Hosp; **Address:** Duke Univ Med Center, Box 3480, Durham, NC 27710; **Phone:** 919-684-6461; **Board Cert:** Orthopaedic Surgery 1982; Hand Surgery 2000; **Med School:** Duke Univ 1974; **Resid:** Orthopaedic Surgery, Univ Virginia Med Ctr 1980; Surgery, Duke Univ Med Ctr 1976; **Fellow:** Hand Surgery, Duke Univ Med Ctr 1981; **Fac Appt:** Assoc Prof OrS, Duke Univ

Jiranek, William A MD [OrS] - **Spec Exp:** Knee Replacement; Arthritis; Minimally Invasive Surgery; Hip Replacement; **Hospital:** Med Coll of VA Hosp; **Address:** MCV Dept Orthopaedic Surgery, 9000 Stony Point Pkwy, Richmond, VA 23235; **Phone:** 804-228-4155; **Board Cert:** Orthopaedic Surgery 2005; **Med School:** Univ VA Sch Med 1985; **Resid:** Orthopaedic Surgery, Tufts Combined Program 1991; **Fellow:** Orthopaedic Surgery, Mass Genl Hosp/Harvard 1992; **Fac Appt:** Assoc Prof OrS, Med Coll VA

Johnson, Darren L MD [OrS] - **Spec Exp:** Knee Injuries; Sports Medicine; Knee Ligament Reconstruction; Arthroscopic Surgery; **Hospital:** Univ of Kentucky Albert B. Chandler Hosp; **Address:** Univ Kentucky-Orthopedic Surgery, 740 S Limestone, Ste K-401, Lexington, KY 40536-0284; **Phone:** 859-257-4969; **Board Cert:** Orthopaedic Surgery 2006; Orthopaedic Sports Medicine 2007; **Med School:** UCLA 1987; **Resid:** Orthopaedic Surgery, LAC-USC Med Ctr 1992; **Fellow:** Sports Medicine, Univ Pittsburgh 1993; **Fac Appt:** Prof OrS, Univ KY Coll Med

Karas, Spero G MD [OrS] - **Spec Exp:** Sports Medicine; Shoulder Injuries; Knee Injuries/ACL/Meniscus Tears; Cartilage Damage; **Hospital:** Emory Univ Hosp; **Address:** Emory Orthopaedics & Sports Medicine, 59 Executive Park South, Ste 1000, Atlanta, GA 30329; **Phone:** 404-778-7204; **Board Cert:** Orthopaedic Surgery 2002; Orthopaedic Sports Medicine 2008; **Med School:** Indiana Univ 1993; **Resid:** Orthopaedic Surgery, Duke Univ Med Ctr 1999; **Fellow:** Orthopaedic Surgery, Steadman Hawkins Clinic 2000; **Fac Appt:** Assoc Prof OrS, Emory Univ

Kneisl, Jeffrey S MD [OrS] - **Spec Exp:** Bone Cancer; Musculoskeletal Tumors; **Hospital:** Carolinas Med Ctr; **Address:** 1025 Morhead Medical Drive, Ste 300, Charlotte, NC 28204; **Phone:** 704-355-5982; **Board Cert:** Orthopaedic Surgery 2010; **Med School:** Northwestern Univ 1980; **Resid:** Orthopaedic Surgery, Northwestern Univ 1987; **Fellow:** Orthopaedic Oncology, Univ Chicago 1990

Kress, Kenneth J MD [OrS] - **Spec Exp:** Knee Replacement; Knee Reconstruction; Sports Medicine; **Hospital:** St. Joseph's Hosp - Atlanta; **Address:** Resergens Orthopaedics, 5671 Peachtree Dunwoody Rd NE, Ste 700, Atlanta, GA 30342; **Phone:** 404-847-9999; **Board Cert:** Orthopaedic Surgery 2004; **Med School:** Cornell Univ 1985; **Resid:** Orthopaedic Surgery, Hosp for Special Surg 1990; **Fellow:** Knee Reconstruction, Dr John C Garrett 1991

Lebwohl, Nathan MD [OrS] - **Spec Exp:** Spinal Surgery; **Hospital:** Jackson Meml Hosp (page 70); **Address:** Univ Miami, Dept Orthopaedic Surgery, PO Box 016960, Miami, FL 33101; **Phone:** 305-585-8225; **Board Cert:** Orthopaedic Surgery 2003; **Med School:** Harvard Med Sch 1983; **Resid:** Surgery, Mt Sinai Hosp 1985; Orthopaedic Surgery, New York Ortho Hosp-Columbia Univ 1988; **Fellow:** Spinal Surgery, Univ Louisville 1989; **Fac Appt:** Assoc Clin Prof OrS, Univ Miami Sch Med

Miller, Mark D MD [OrS] - **Spec Exp:** Sports Medicine; Knee Ligament Reconstruction; Knee Cartilage/Meniscus Transplants; Shoulder Arthroscopic Surgery; **Hospital:** Univ of Virginia Health Sys; **Address:** Univ Virginia Dept Ortho Surg, Box 800243, Charlottesville, VA 22908; **Phone:** 434-982-4832; **Board Cert:** Orthopaedic Surgery 2006; Orthopaedic Sports Medicine 2007; **Med School:** Uniformed Srvs Univ, Bethesda 1987; **Resid:** Orthopaedic Surgery, Wilford Hall USAF Med Ctr 1992; **Fellow:** Shoulder Surgery, Univ Pittsburgh 1993; Sports Medicine, Univ Pittsburgh 1993; **Fac Appt:** Prof OrS, Univ VA Sch Med

Nunley II, James A MD [OrS] - **Spec Exp:** Foot & Ankle Surgery; Ankle Replacement & Revision; Arthritis; Sports Injuries-Foot & Ankle; **Hospital:** Duke Univ Hosp; **Address:** Duke University Med Ctr, Box 2923, Durham, NC 27710-0001; **Phone:** 919-684-4033; **Board Cert:** Orthopaedic Surgery 1981; **Med School:** Tulane Univ 1973; **Resid:** Orthopaedic Surgery, Duke Univ Med Ctr 1979; **Fellow:** Hand Surgery, Duke Univ Med Ctr 1980; **Fac Appt:** Prof OrS, Duke Univ

Paley, Dror MD [OrS] - **Spec Exp:** Limb Lengthening (Ilizarov Procedure); Limb Deformities; Pediatric Orthopaedic Surgery; **Hospital:** St. Mary's Med Ctr - W Palm Bch; **Address:** 901 45th St, Kimmel Bldg, West Palm Beach, FL 33407; **Phone:** 561-844-5255; **Board Cert:** Orthopaedic Surgery 2010; **Med School:** Univ Toronto 1979; **Resid:** Orthopaedic Surgery, Univ Toronto Hosp 1985; **Fellow:** Hand Surgery, Sunny Brook Hosp 1986; Pediatric Orthopaedic Surgery, Hosp for Sick Children 1987

Pettrone, Frank A MD [OrS] - **Spec Exp:** Sports Medicine; Shoulder & Knee Surgery; **Hospital:** Virginia Hosp Ctr - Arlington; **Address:** Commonwealth Ortho & Rehabilitation, 1635 N George Mason Drive, Ste 310, Arlington, VA 22205-3616; **Phone:** 703-525-6100; **Board Cert:** Orthopaedic Surgery 1975; **Med School:** Georgetown Univ 1969; **Resid:** Orthopaedic Surgery, Georgetown Hosp 1974; **Fac Appt:** Clin Prof OrS, Georgetown Univ

Poehling, Gary G MD [OrS] - **Spec Exp:** Hand Surgery; Arthroscopic Surgery; Sports Medicine; **Hospital:** Wake Forest Univ Baptist Med Ctr; **Address:** Wake Forest Medical Ctr, Comp Rehab Plaza, 131 Miller St, Winston-Salem, NC 27103; **Phone:** 336-716-8091; **Board Cert:** Orthopaedic Surgery 1977; **Med School:** Marquette Sch Med 1968; **Resid:** Surgery, Duke Univ Med Ctr 1970; Orthopaedic Surgery, Duke Univ Med Ctr 1976; **Fac Appt:** Prof OrS, Wake Forest Univ

Richardson, William J MD [OrS] - **Spec Exp:** Spinal Surgery; Spinal Deformity; Spinal Disc Replacement; Spinal Trauma; **Hospital:** Duke Univ Hosp; **Address:** Duke Univ Med Center, Box 3077, Durham, NC 27710; **Phone:** 919-684-5711; **Board Cert:** Orthopaedic Surgery 2010; **Med School:** Eastern VA Med Sch 1979; **Resid:** Orthopaedic Surgery, Duke Univ Med Ctr 1986; **Fellow:** Spinal Surgery, Totonto General Hosp 1987

Scarborough, Mark T MD [OrS] - **Spec Exp:** Bone Tumors; Sarcoma; **Hospital:** Shands at Univ of FL; **Address:** Shands Healthcare Univ FL, PO Box 112-733, Gainesville, FL 32611-2733; **Phone:** 352-273-7000; **Board Cert:** Orthopaedic Surgery 2004; **Med School:** Univ Fla Coll Med 1985; **Resid:** Orthopaedic Surgery, Univ Texas Med Ctr 1990; **Fellow:** Orthopaedic Surgery, Mass Genl Hosp 1991; **Fac Appt:** Prof OrS, Univ Fla Coll Med

Schuler, Thomas C MD [OrS] - **Spec Exp:** Spinal Surgery-Cervical; Spinal Surgery-Low Back; Sports Medicine Back Injuries; **Hospital:** Reston Hosp Ctr; **Address:** Virginia Spine Inst, 1831 Wiehle Ave, rm 200, Reston, VA 20190; **Phone:** 703-709-1114; **Board Cert:** Orthopaedic Surgery 2005; **Med School:** Indiana Univ 1986; **Resid:** Surgery, William Beaumont Hosp 1987; **Fellow:** Orthopaedic Surgery, William Beaumont Hosp 1991; Spinal Surgery, Kerlan-Jobe Orth Clinic

Schwartz, Herbert S MD [OrS] - **Spec Exp:** Bone Tumors-Metastatic; Bone Tumors; Pelvic Surgery-Complex; Musculoskeletal Tumors; **Hospital:** Vanderbilt Univ Med Ctr (page 76), Baptist Hosp - Nashville; **Address:** Vanderbilt Orthopaedic Institute, Medical Center East, South Tower, Ste 4200, Nashville, TN 37232-8774; **Phone:** 615-322-0543; **Board Cert:** Orthopaedic Surgery 2007; **Med School:** Univ Chicago-Pritzker Sch Med 1981; **Resid:** Orthopaedic Surgery, Univ Chicago Hosps 1986; **Fellow:** Orthopaedic Oncology, Mayo Clinic 1987; **Fac Appt:** Prof OrS, Vanderbilt Univ

Siegel, Herrick J MD [OrS] - **Spec Exp:** Hip and Knee Replacement; Bone & Soft Tissue Tumors; Shoulder Replacement; Hip & Knee Replacement; **Hospital:** Univ of Ala Hosp at Birmingham, UAB Highlands Hosp; **Address:** 1313 13th St S, Birmingham, AL 35205; **Phone:** 205-930-8554; **Board Cert:** Orthopaedic Surgery 2005; **Med School:** NYU Sch Med 1995; **Resid:** Orthopaedic Surgery, USC Univ Hosp 2000; **Fellow:** Orthopaedic Oncology, Mayo Clinic 2002; **Fac Appt:** Assoc Prof OrS, Univ Alabama

Spengler, Dan M MD [OrS] - **Spec Exp:** Spinal Surgery; **Hospital:** Vanderbilt Univ Med Ctr (page 76); **Address:** Vanderbilt Orthopedic Inst, Medical Ctr E, S Tower Rm#4200, Nashville, TN 37232-8774; **Phone:** 615-343-6364; **Board Cert:** Orthopaedic Surgery 1988; **Med School:** Univ Mich Med Sch 1966; **Resid:** Orthopaedic Surgery, Univ Mich Med Ctr 1968; Orthopaedic Surgery, Univ Mich Med Ctr 1973; **Fellow:** Orthopaedic Surgery, Case West Res Hosps 1974; **Fac Appt:** Prof OrS, Vanderbilt Univ

Spindler, Kurt P MD [OrS] - **Spec Exp:** Sports Medicine; Ligament Reconstruction; Arthroscopic Surgery; Adolescent Sports Medicine; **Hospital:** Vanderbilt Univ Med Ctr (page 76); **Address:** Vanderbilt Orthopaedic Inst, 3200 Medical Center East, South Tower, 1215 21st Ave S, Nashville, TN 37232-8774; **Phone:** 615-322-7878; **Board Cert:** Orthopaedic Surgery 2004; Orthopaedic Sports Medicine 2007; **Med School:** Univ Pennsylvania 1985; **Resid:** Orthopaedic Surgery, Hosp Univ Penn 1990; **Fellow:** Sports Medicine, Cleveland Clinic Fdn 1991; **Fac Appt:** Prof OrS, Vanderbilt Univ

Taft, Timothy N MD [OrS] - **Spec Exp:** Sports Medicine; Knee Injuries/ACL; Shoulder Surgery; **Hospital:** NC Memorial Hosp - UNC; **Address:** UNC Orthopaedics, CB # 7055, Bioinformatics Bldg, Chapel Hill, NC 27599-7055; **Phone:** 919-962-6637; **Board Cert:** Orthopaedic Surgery 1976; **Med School:** Univ MO-Columbia Sch Med 1969; **Resid:** Orthopaedic Surgery, UNC Hosps 1974; Orthopaedic Surgery, N Carolina Ortho Hosp 1972; **Fac Appt:** Prof OrS, Univ NC Sch Med

Walling, Arthur K MD [OrS] - **Spec Exp:** Bone Tumors; Soft Tissue Tumors; Foot & Ankle Surgery; **Hospital:** Tampa Genl Hosp; **Address:** Florida Orthopaedic Inst, 13020 Telecom Pkwy N, Tampa, FL 33637; **Phone:** 813-978-9700; **Board Cert:** Orthopaedic Surgery 1982; **Med School:** Creighton Univ 1976; **Resid:** Orthopaedic Surgery, Univ South Florida Affil Hosps 1980; **Fellow:** Surgical Oncology, Univ Florida 1981; **Fac Appt:** Assoc Clin Prof OrS, Univ S Fla Coll Med

Ward Sr, William G MD [OrS] - **Spec Exp:** Bone Tumors; Soft Tissue Tumors; Reconstructive Surgery; Sarcoma; **Hospital:** Wake Forest Univ Baptist Med Ctr; **Address:** First Floor Comp Rehab, 131 Miller St, Winston-Salem, NC 27103; **Phone:** 336-716-8093; **Board Cert:** Orthopaedic Surgery 2004; **Med School:** Duke Univ 1975; **Resid:** Surgery, Duke Univ Med Ctr 1985; Orthopaedic Surgery, Duke Univ Med Ctr 1989; **Fellow:** Sports Medicine, Cleveland Clinic 1990; Orthopaedic Oncology, UCLA Med Ctr 1991; **Fac Appt:** Prof OrS, Wake Forest Univ

Webb, Lawrence MD [OrS] - **Spec Exp:** Trauma; Pelvic & Acetabular Fractures; Fractures-Complex & Non Union; Musculoskeletal Infections; **Hospital:** Med Ctr of Central GA; **Address:** 840 Pine St, Ste 500, Macon, GA 31201; **Phone:** 478-633-8682; **Board Cert:** Orthopaedic Surgery 2007; **Med School:** Temple Univ 1978; **Resid:** Orthopaedic Surgery, Bowman Gray Affil Hosp 1983; **Fellow:** Trauma, Harborview Med Ctr 1984; **Fac Appt:** Prof OrS, Mercer Univ Sch Med

Weiner, Richard L MD [OrS] - **Spec Exp:** Knee Replacement; Knee Reconstruction; Hip Replacement; Hip Reconstruction; **Hospital:** St. Mary's Med Ctr - W Palm Bch, Palm Beach Gardens Med Ctr; **Address:** 733 US Highway 1, North Palm Beach, FL 33408-4508; **Phone:** 561-840-1090; **Board Cert:** Orthopaedic Surgery 2004; **Med School:** Univ Pennsylvania 1986; **Resid:** Orthopaedic Surgery, UMDNJ-Univ Hosp 1991

Midwest

Albright, John P MD [OrS] - **Spec Exp:** Sports Medicine; **Hospital:** Univ Iowa Hosp & Clinics; **Address:** UIHC Dept of Orthopaedic Surg, 200 Hawkins Drive, Iowa City, IA 52242; **Phone:** 319-384-7070; **Board Cert:** Orthopaedic Surgery 2007; **Med School:** Loyola Univ-Stritch Sch Med 1967; **Resid:** Orthopaedic Surgery, Yale-New Haven Hosp 1971; **Fellow:** Research, Yale-New Haven Hosp 1972; **Fac Appt:** Prof OrS, Univ Iowa Coll Med

An, Howard MD [OrS] - **Spec Exp:** Spinal Surgery; Scoliosis; Spinal Microdiscectomy; **Hospital:** Rush Univ Med Ctr; **Address:** 1611 W Harrison, Ste 300, Chicago, IL 60612; **Phone:** 312-243-4244; **Board Cert:** Orthopaedic Surgery 2002; **Med School:** Med Coll OH 1982; **Resid:** Orthopaedic Surgery, Med College Ohio Hosps 1988; **Fellow:** Spinal Surgery, Jefferson Med College 1989; **Fac Appt:** Prof OrS, Rush Med Coll

Orthopaedic Surgery

Anglen, Jeffrey O MD [OrS] - **Spec Exp:** Trauma; Fractures-Complex & Non Union; Bone Infections; **Hospital:** IU Health University Hosp; **Address:** Indiana Univ Dept Ortho Surgery, 541 Clinical Drive, Ste 600, Indianapolis, IN 46202; **Phone:** 317-274-7372; **Board Cert:** Orthopaedic Surgery 2011; **Med School:** Johns Hopkins Univ 1983; **Resid:** Orthopaedic Surgery, Johns Hopkins Hosp 1988; **Fellow:** Orthopaedic Trauma Surgery, Tampa Genl Hosp 1989; **Fac Appt:** Prof OrS, Indiana Univ

Archdeacon, Michael T MD [OrS] - **Spec Exp:** Trauma; Pelvic & Acetabular Fractures; **Hospital:** Univ Hosp - Cincinnati; **Address:** 222 Piedmont Ave, Ste 2200, Cincinnati, OH 45219; **Phone:** 513-475-8690; **Board Cert:** Orthopaedic Surgery 2003; **Med School:** Ohio State Univ 1993; **Resid:** Orthopaedic Surgery, Case Western Univ Hosp 2000; **Fellow:** Orthopaedic Trauma Surgery, Tampa Gen Hosp 2001; **Fac Appt:** Prof OrS, Univ Cincinnati

Bach Jr, Bernard R MD [OrS] - **Spec Exp:** Sports Medicine; Knee Surgery; Knee Injuries/ACL; Shoulder Surgery; **Hospital:** Rush Univ Med Ctr; **Address:** Midwest Orthopaedics, 1611 W Harrison St, Ste 300, Chicago, IL 60612; **Phone:** 312-243-4244; **Board Cert:** Orthopaedic Surgery 2010; Orthopaedic Sports Medicine 2010; **Med School:** Univ Cincinnati 1979; **Resid:** Surgery, New Eng Deaconess Hosp 1981; Orthopaedic Surgery, Mass Genl Hosp 1984; **Fellow:** Sports Medicine, Hosp Special Surgery 1986; **Fac Appt:** Prof OrS, Rush Med Coll

Berry, Daniel John MD [OrS] - **Spec Exp:** Hip Replacement & Revision; Knee Replacement & Revision; **Hospital:** Mayo Med Ctr & Clin - Rochester; **Address:** Mayo Clinic, 200 1st St SW, Gonda-14, Rochester, MN 55905; **Phone:** 507-284-4204; **Board Cert:** Orthopaedic Surgery 2004; **Med School:** Harvard Med Sch 1984; **Resid:** Orthopaedic Surgery, Harvard Univ Affil Hosps 1989; **Fellow:** Adult Reconstructive Surgery, Mauric E Muller Foundation 1990; Hip Surgery, Mayo Clinic 1991; **Fac Appt:** Prof OrS, Mayo Med Sch

Biermann, J Sybil MD [OrS] - **Spec Exp:** Sarcoma; Bone Cancer; Multiple Myeloma; Limb Sparing Surgery; **Hospital:** Univ of Michigan Hosp; **Address:** Univ Michigan Cancer Ctr, 1500 E Medical Ctr Drive, SPC 5912, Ann Arbor, MI 48109; **Phone:** 734-647-8902; **Board Cert:** Orthopaedic Surgery 2006; **Med School:** Stanford Univ 1987; **Resid:** Orthopaedic Surgery, Univ Iowa Hosp 1992; **Fellow:** Orthopaedic Oncology, Univ Chicago Hosps 1993; **Fac Appt:** Assoc Prof OrS, Univ Mich Med Sch

Blaha, John D MD [OrS] - **Spec Exp:** Hip & Knee Replacement; **Hospital:** Univ of Michigan Hosp; **Address:** Univ Michigan, Dept Orthopaedic Surg, 1500 E Medical Ctr Dr, Taubman 2912, Ann Arbor, MI 48109; **Phone:** 734-647-9961; **Board Cert:** Orthopaedic Surgery 1979; **Med School:** Univ Mich Med Sch 1973; **Resid:** Surgery, Univ Mich Hosp 1975; Orthopaedic Surgery, Univ Mich Hosp 1978; **Fellow:** Joint Replacement Surgery, Univ London 1980; **Fac Appt:** Prof OrS, Univ Mich Med Sch

Bridwell, Keith MD [OrS] - **Spec Exp:** Spinal Deformity; Scoliosis; Spinal Surgery; **Hospital:** Barnes-Jewish Hosp, St. Louis Chldns Hosp; **Address:** Washington Univ School of Med, 660 S Euclid Ave, Campus Box 8233, St Louis, MO 63110; **Phone:** 314-747-2560; **Board Cert:** Orthopaedic Surgery 1985; **Med School:** Washington Univ, St Louis 1977; **Resid:** Orthopaedic Surgery, Barnes Hosp-Wash Univ 1981; **Fellow:** Spinal Surgery, Rush Presby-St Lukes Med Ctr 1982; **Fac Appt:** Prof OrS, Washington Univ, St Louis

Buckwalter IV, Joseph A MD [OrS] - **Spec Exp:** Bone Cancer; Bone Tumors-Metastatic; Fractures-Complex; **Hospital:** Univ Iowa Hosp & Clinics; **Address:** Univ Iowa Hosps, Dept Orthopaedics, 200 Hawkins Drive, Iowa City, IA 52242; **Phone:** 319-356-2595; **Board Cert:** Orthopaedic Surgery 1991; **Med School:** Univ Iowa Coll Med 1974; **Resid:** Orthopaedic Surgery, Iowa Hosp 1979; **Fac Appt:** Prof OrS, Univ Iowa Coll Med

Callaghan, John J MD [OrS] - **Spec Exp:** Hip & Knee Replacement; Sports Medicine; **Hospital:** Univ Iowa Hosp & Clinics; **Address:** Univ Iowa Hosp, Dept Orthopaedics, 200 Hawkins Drive, Iowa City, IA 52242; **Phone:** 319-356-3110; **Board Cert:** Orthopaedic Surgery 2011; **Med School:** Loyola Univ-Stritch Sch Med 1978; **Resid:** Orthopaedic Surgery, Univ Iowa Hosp 1983; **Fellow:** Orthopaedic Surgery, Hosp Special Surg 1984; **Fac Appt:** Prof OrS, Univ Iowa Coll Med

Cheng, Edward Y MD [OrS] - **Spec Exp:** Bone & Soft Tissue Tumors; Reconstructive Surgery; **Address:** Univ Minnesota, Dept Orthopaedic Surgery, 2512 S Seventh St, Ste R-200, Minneapolis, MN 55454; **Phone:** 612-273-1177; **Board Cert:** Orthopaedic Surgery 2003; **Med School:** Northwestern Univ 1983; **Resid:** Surgery, Northwestern Univ 1985; Orthopaedic Surgery, Beth Israel Hosp 1989; **Fellow:** Surgical Oncology, Mass Genl Hosp 1990; **Fac Appt:** Prof OrS, Univ Minn

Clohisy, Denis MD [OrS] - **Spec Exp:** Bone Cancer; **Address:** Univ Minn, Dept Orthopaedic Surgery, 2512 S Seveth St, Ste R200, Minneapolis, MN 55454; **Phone:** 612-273-1177; **Board Cert:** Orthopaedic Surgery 2004; **Med School:** Northwestern Univ 1983; **Resid:** Orthopaedic Surgery, Univ Minn 1990; **Fellow:** Pathology, Wash Univ Med Ctr 1987; Musculoskeletal Oncology, Mass Genl Hosp 1991; **Fac Appt:** Prof OrS, Univ Minn

Ebraheim, Nabil A MD [OrS] - **Spec Exp:** Trauma; Fractures-Complex & Non Union; Bone Infections; Reconstructive Surgery; **Hospital:** Univ of Toledo Med Ctr; **Address:** Univ Toledo Med Ctr, Dept Orthopaedics, 3065 Arlington Ave, MS 1094, Toledo, OH 43614; **Phone:** 419-383-3761; **Board Cert:** Orthopaedic Surgery 2008; **Med School:** Egypt 1975; **Resid:** Surgery, St Clare's Hosp 1980; Orthopaedic Surgery, SUNY-Downstate Med Ctr 1983; **Fellow:** Trauma, Univ Maryland Hosps 1984; Orthopaedic Surgery, Hanover Trauma Ctr 1985; **Fac Appt:** Prof OrS, Univ Toledo, Med Univ OH

Gitelis, Steven MD [OrS] - **Spec Exp:** Bone Cancer; Soft Tissue Tumors; Limb Sparing Surgery; Hip Replacement; **Hospital:** Rush Univ Med Ctr; **Address:** 1611 W Harrison St, Ste 300, Chicago, IL 60612; **Phone:** 312-432-2397; **Board Cert:** Orthopaedic Surgery 1982; **Med School:** Rush Med Coll 1975; **Resid:** Orthopaedic Surgery, Rush Presby-St Lukes Med Ctr 1980; **Fellow:** Orthopaedic Oncology, Mayo Clinic 1982; **Fac Appt:** Prof OrS, Rush Med Coll

Goitz, Henry MD [OrS] - **Spec Exp:** Sports Medicine; Knee Injuries/ACL/Meniscus Tears; Rotator Cuff Surgery; Elbow Surgery; **Hospital:** DMC Surgery Hosp, Harper Univ Hosp; **Address:** Detroit Med Ctr, Sports Medicine, 28800 Ryan Rd, Ste 220, Warren, MI 48092; **Phone:** 586-558-2860; **Board Cert:** Orthopaedic Surgery 2006; **Med School:** UMDNJ-Rutgers Med Sch 1985; **Resid:** Orthopaedic Surgery, Univ Virginia Affil Hosp 1991; **Fellow:** Sports Medicine & Hand Surgery, Univ Virginia Affil Hosp 1991; Sports Medicine, American Sports Med Inst 1992

Goldstein, Wayne MD [OrS] - **Spec Exp:** Hip Replacement; Knee Replacement; **Hospital:** Adv Luth Genl Hosp; **Address:** 9000 Waukegan Rd, Ste 200, Morton Grove, IL 60053; **Phone:** 847-375-3000; **Board Cert:** Orthopaedic Surgery 2007; **Med School:** Univ IL Coll Med 1978; **Resid:** Orthopaedic Surgery, Univ Ilinois Med Ctr 1983; **Fellow:** Arthritis Surgery, Brigham & Women's Hosp 1984; **Fac Appt:** Assoc Clin Prof OrS, Univ Chicago-Pritzker Sch Med

Graf, Ben K MD [OrS] - **Spec Exp:** Sports Medicine; **Hospital:** Univ WI Hosp & Clins; **Address:** 1685 Highland Ave, MFCB Bldg - rm 6124, Madison, WI 53792-3228; **Phone:** 608-263-8850; **Board Cert:** Orthopaedic Surgery 2008; Orthopaedic Sports Medicine 2007; **Med School:** Univ Wisc 1979; **Resid:** Orthopaedic Surgery, Univ Wisc Hosps 1984; **Fellow:** Sports Medicine, Long Beach Meml Hosp 1985; **Fac Appt:** Assoc Prof S, Univ Wisc

Orthopaedic Surgery

Grant, Richard E MD [OrS] - **Spec Exp:** Hip & Knee Replacement; Spinal Surgery-Low Back; Sickle Cell Disease-Hip Surgery; **Hospital:** Univ Hosps Case Med Ctr (page 74); **Address:** Univ Hosps Cleveland, Dept Ortho Surgery, 11100 Euclid Ave, Bolwell Bldg Fl 5, Cleveland, OH 44106; **Phone:** 216-844-1118; **Board Cert:** Orthopaedic Surgery 2007; **Med School:** Howard Univ 1976; **Resid:** Orthopaedic Surgery, Wilford Hall Med Ctr-Lackland 1984; **Fellow:** Joint Arthroplasty, Ohio State Univ Hosp 1985; Spinal Cord Injury Medicine, St Lukes/Baylor Univ 1986; **Fac Appt:** Prof OrS, Howard Univ

Hanssen, Arlen D MD [OrS] - **Spec Exp:** Hip Surgery; Knee Surgery; **Hospital:** Mayo Med Ctr & Clin - Rochester; **Address:** Mayo Clinic, Dept Orthopaedic Surgery, 200 First St SW, Rochester, MN 55905; **Phone:** 507-284-2884; **Board Cert:** Orthopaedic Surgery 2001; **Med School:** St Louis Univ 1983; **Resid:** Orthopaedic Surgery, Mayo Clin 1988; **Fac Appt:** Prof OrS, Mayo Med Sch

Hensinger, Robert N MD [OrS] - **Spec Exp:** Pediatric Orthopaedic Surgery; Spinal Surgery-Pediatric; **Hospital:** Univ of Michigan Hosp; **Address:** Univ Michigan Med Ctr, Dept Ortho Surg, 1500 E Med Ctr Drive, 2912 Taubman Ctr, Ann Arbor, MI 48109-0328; **Phone:** 734-936-5715; **Board Cert:** Orthopaedic Surgery 2007; **Med School:** Univ Mich Med Sch 1964; **Resid:** Orthopaedic Surgery, Univ Michigan 1966; Orthopaedic Surgery, Univ Michigan 1971; **Fellow:** Pediatric Orthopaedic Surgery, AI DuPont Inst 1972; **Fac Appt:** Prof OrS, Univ Mich Med Sch

Iannotti, Joseph MD/PhD [OrS] - **Spec Exp:** Shoulder Surgery; Rotator Cuff Surgery; **Hospital:** Cleveland Clin (page 56); **Address:** Cleveland Clinic, Dept Orthopaedic Surg, 9500 Euclid Ave, Desk A41, Cleveland, OH 44195-5027; **Phone:** 216-445-5151; **Board Cert:** Orthopaedic Surgery 2007; **Med School:** Northwestern Univ 1979; **Resid:** Orthopaedic Surgery, Hosp Univ Penn 1984; **Fellow:** Orthopaedic Research, Hosp Univ Penn 1985; **Fac Appt:** Prof OrS, Cleveland Cl Coll Med/Case West Res

Irwin, Ronald B MD [OrS] - **Spec Exp:** Bone Cancer; Limb Sparing Surgery; Sarcoma-Soft Tissue; **Hospital:** Mount Clemens Regional Med Ctr; **Address:** Mount Clemens Regional Med Ctr, 1080 Harrington Blvd, Ste 201, Mount Clemens, MI 48043; **Phone:** 586-493-7575; **Board Cert:** Orthopaedic Surgery 1979; **Med School:** Univ Mich Med Sch 1971; **Resid:** Orthopaedic Surgery, William Beaumont Hosp 1978; **Fellow:** Orthopaedic Oncology, Mayo Clinic 1978

Jacobs, Joshua J MD [OrS] - **Spec Exp:** Hip Replacement & Revision; Knee Replacement & Revision; **Hospital:** Rush Univ Med Ctr; **Address:** 1611 W Harrison St, Ste 300, Chicago, IL 60612; **Phone:** 312-243-4244; **Board Cert:** Orthopaedic Surgery 2011; **Med School:** Univ IL Coll Med 1981; **Resid:** Orthopaedic Surgery, Harvard Univ Affil Hosp 1987; **Fellow:** Joint Replacement Surgery, Rush Univ Med Ctr 1988; **Fac Appt:** Prof OrS, Rush Med Coll

Joyce, Michael J MD [OrS] - **Spec Exp:** Bone & Soft Tissue Tumors; Fractures-Complex & Non Union; Musculoskeletal Tissue Banking; Pelvic & Acetabular Fractures; **Hospital:** Cleveland Clin (page 56); **Address:** 9500 Euclid Ave, Desk A41, Dept Orthopaedic Surgery, Cleveland, OH 44195; **Phone:** 216-444-4282; **Board Cert:** Orthopaedic Surgery 1985; **Med School:** Univ Louisville Sch Med 1976; **Resid:** Surgery, Johns Hopkins Hosp 1978; Orthopaedic Surgery, Harvard Combined Program 1981; **Fellow:** Orthopaedic Oncology, Mass General Hosp 1982; Trauma, Univ Toronto-Sunnybrook Hosp 1983; **Fac Appt:** Assoc Clin Prof OrS, Case West Res Univ

Kaeding, Christopher C MD [OrS] - **Spec Exp:** Sports Medicine; Knee Injuries/ACL; Shoulder Injuries; Rotator Cuff Surgery; **Hospital:** Ohio St Univ Med Ctr; **Address:** OSU Sports Med Ctr, 2050 Kenny Rd, Ste 3100, Columbus, OH 43221; **Phone:** 614-293-8813; **Board Cert:** Orthopaedic Surgery 2002; Orthopaedic Sports Medicine 2007; **Med School:** Northwestern Univ 1983; **Resid:** Orthopaedic Surgery, Northwestern Univ 1988; **Fellow:** Sports Medicine, Cleveland Clinic 1989; **Fac Appt:** Clin Prof OrS, Ohio State Univ

Kenter, Keith MD [OrS] - **Spec Exp:** Sports Medicine; Shoulder Reconstruction; Knee Surgery; **Hospital:** Univ Hosp - Cincinnati; **Address:** University of Cincinnati Physicians, 222 Piedmont Ave, Ste 2200, Cincinnati, OH 45219; **Phone:** 513-475-8690; **Board Cert:** Orthopaedic Surgery 2010; Orthopaedic Sports Medicine 2007; **Med School:** Univ MO-Columbia Sch Med 1990; **Resid:** Surgery, Duke Univ Med Ctr 1992; Orthopaedic Surgery, Duke Univ Med Ctr 1996; **Fellow:** Sports Medicine & Shoulder Surgery, Hosp for Special Surgery 1997; **Fac Appt:** Asst Prof OrS, Univ Cincinnati

Kraay, Matthew J MD [OrS] - **Spec Exp:** Arthritis; Reconstructive Surgery; Joint Replacement; **Hospital:** Univ Hosps Case Med Ctr (page 74); **Address:** UH Case Medical Center, Dept of Orthopaedic Surgery, 11100 Euclid Ave, Cleveland, OH 44106; **Phone:** 216-844-8372; **Board Cert:** Orthopaedic Surgery 2004; **Med School:** Wayne State Univ 1983; **Resid:** Orthopaedic Surgery, Univ Hosps 1989; **Fellow:** Adult Reconstructive Surgery, Univ Hosps 1990; Orthopaedic Surgery, Hosp Special Surgery 1991; **Fac Appt:** Prof OrS, Case West Res Univ

Lenke, Lawrence G MD [OrS] - **Spec Exp:** Spinal Surgery; Spinal Deformity; Scoliosis; Spinal Reconstructive Surgery; **Hospital:** Barnes-Jewish Hosp, St. Louis Chldns Hosp; **Address:** Washington Univ School Med, 660 S Euclid Ave, Campus Box 8233, St Louis, MO 63110; **Phone:** 314-747-2500; **Board Cert:** Orthopaedic Surgery 2005; **Med School:** Northwestern Univ 1986; **Resid:** Orthopaedic Surgery, Barnes-Jewish Hosp 1989; **Fellow:** Spinal Surgery, Barnes-Jewish Hosp 1992; **Fac Appt:** Prof OrS, Washington Univ, St Louis

Les, Kimberly A MD [OrS] - **Spec Exp:** Bone Cancer; **Hospital:** Beaumont Hosp-Royal Oak; **Address:** Rose Cancer Treatment Ctr, 3577 W 13 Mile Rd, Ste 402, Royal Oak, MI 48073; **Phone:** 248-551-9910; **Board Cert:** Orthopaedic Surgery 2000; **Med School:** Geo Wash Univ 1992; **Resid:** Orthopaedic Surgery, Henry Ford Hosp 1997; **Fellow:** Orthopaedic Oncology, Univ Chicago Hosps 1978

Lock, Terrence Ralph MD [OrS] - **Spec Exp:** Sports Medicine; Arthroscopic Surgery; Shoulder & Knee Reconstruction; **Hospital:** Henry Ford Hosp, Henry Ford Med Ctr-Cottage; **Address:** Henry Ford Hosp, Ctr for Athletic Med, 6525 Second Ave, Detroit, MI 48202; **Phone:** 313-972-4060; **Board Cert:** Orthopaedic Surgery 2002; Orthopaedic Sports Medicine 2007; **Med School:** Wayne State Univ 1983; **Resid:** Orthopaedic Surgery, Wayne St Univ Sch Med 1988; **Fellow:** Sports Medicine, Mass Genl Hosp 1989

Manoli II, Arthur MD [OrS] - **Spec Exp:** Foot & Ankle Surgery; Reconstructive Surgery; **Hospital:** St. Joseph Mercy Oakland Hosp; **Address:** 44555 Woodward Ave, Ste 503, Pontiac, MI 48341; **Phone:** 248-858-6773; **Board Cert:** Orthopaedic Surgery 2007; **Med School:** Univ Mich Med Sch 1970; **Resid:** Surgery, Oakwood Hosp 1972; Orthopaedic Surgery, Wayne St Univ Affil Hosps 1975; **Fellow:** Ankle and Foot Surgery, Univ Wash/Vanderbilt Univ 1990

Mayerson, Joel L MD [OrS] - **Spec Exp:** Bone Tumors; Sarcoma-Soft Tissue; Limb Surgery/Reconstruction; Musculoskeletal Tumors; **Hospital:** Ohio St Univ Med Ctr; **Address:** Ohio State, Div of Musculoskeletal Onc, 410 W 10 Ave N Doan Hall Bldg - rm 1049, Columbus, OH 43210; **Phone:** 614-293-4420; **Board Cert:** Orthopaedic Surgery 2003; **Med School:** Johns Hopkins Univ 1994; **Resid:** Orthopaedic Surgery, Cleveland Clinic 1999; **Fellow:** Orthopaedic Oncology, Univ Wash Med Ctr 2000; **Fac Appt:** Assoc Prof OrS, Ohio State Univ

McCarthy, James J MD [OrS] - **Spec Exp:** Lower Limb Surgery in Children; Arthroscopic Surgery-Hip; Pediatric Orthopaedic Surgery; Hip Disorders-Pediatric; **Hospital:** Cincinnati Chldns Hosp Med Ctr; **Address:** Cincinnati Chldn's, Dept Ped Ortho Surg, 3333 Burnet Ave, Cincinnati, OH 45229; **Phone:** 513-636-4454; **Board Cert:** Orthopaedic Surgery 2010; **Med School:** Univ NC Sch Med 1991; **Resid:** Orthopaedic Surgery, Cleveland Clinic 1996; **Fellow:** Arthroscopic Surgery, Children's Hosp 1997; **Fac Appt:** Prof OrS, Univ Wisc

Orthopaedic Surgery

McDonald, Douglas J MD [OrS] - **Spec Exp:** Bone & Soft Tissue Tumors; Ewing's Sarcoma; Sarcoma; Hip & Knee Reconstruction; **Hospital:** Barnes-Jewish Hosp, St. Louis Chldns Hosp; **Address:** Ctr Advanced Med, Orthopaedic Surg Ctr, 4921 Parkview Pl Fl 6 - Ste A, Box 8605, St Louis, MO 63110; **Phone:** 314-747-2500; **Board Cert:** Orthopaedic Surgery 2011; **Med School:** Univ Minn 1982; **Resid:** Orthopaedic Surgery, Mayo Clinic 1987; **Fellow:** Orthopaedic Oncology, Mayo Clinic 1988; Orthopaedic Surgery, Rizzoli Inst 1989; **Fac Appt:** Prof OrS, Washington Univ, St Louis

Morcuende, Jose A MD/PhD [OrS] - **Spec Exp:** Clubfoot; Pediatric Orthopaedic Surgery; **Hospital:** Univ Iowa Hosp & Clinics; **Address:** UIHC Orthopaedic & Rehab Dept, 200 Hawkins Drive, Iowa City, IA 52242; **Phone:** 319-356-2223; **Board Cert:** Orthopaedic Surgery 2004; **Med School:** Spain 1981; **Resid:** Orthopaedic Surgery, Univ IA Hosp & Clin 2001; **Fellow:** Pediatric Orthopaedic Surgery, Univ IA Hosp & Clin 2002; **Fac Appt:** Assoc Prof OrS, Univ Iowa Coll Med

Mott, Michael P MD [OrS] - **Spec Exp:** Soft Tissue Tumors; Musculoskeletal Tumors; Bone Cancer; **Hospital:** Henry Ford Hosp, Henry Ford- W Bloomfield Hosp; **Address:** Henry Ford Hosp, Dept Ortho Surg, 2799 W Grand Blvd Fl 12, Detroit, MI 48202; **Phone:** 313-916-1961; **Board Cert:** Orthopaedic Surgery 2007; **Med School:** Univ Mich Med Sch 1989; **Resid:** Orthopaedic Surgery, Wayne State Univ Affil Hosp 1994; **Fellow:** Musculoskeletal Oncology, Mass Genl Hosp 1995; Orthopaedic Oncology, Wayne State Univ 1996; **Fac Appt:** Assoc Prof OrS, Wayne State Univ

Muschler, George F MD [OrS] - **Spec Exp:** Hip Replacement; Knee Replacement; Fractures-Complex & Non Union; **Hospital:** Cleveland Clin (page 56); **Address:** Cleveland Clinic, Dept Orthopaedic Surg, 9500 Euclid Ave, Desk A41, Cleveland, OH 44195-0001; **Phone:** 216-444-2601; **Board Cert:** Orthopaedic Surgery 2001; **Med School:** Northwestern Univ 1981; **Resid:** Orthopaedic Surgery, Univ Texas SW Med Ctr 1986; **Fellow:** Metabolic Bone Research, Hosp Special Surgery 1988; Musculoskeletal Oncology, Meml Sloan Kettering Cancer Ctr 1988; **Fac Appt:** Prof OrS, Cleveland Cl Coll Med/Case West Res

Nepola, James V MD [OrS] - **Spec Exp:** Trauma; Shoulder Reconstruction; **Hospital:** Univ Iowa Hosp & Clinics; **Address:** UIHC Dept Orthopedic Surgery, 200 Hawkins Drive, Iowa City, IA 52242; **Phone:** 319-356-2223; **Board Cert:** Orthopaedic Surgery 2009; **Med School:** Columbia P&S 1978; **Resid:** Surgery, Roosevelt Hosp 1980; Orthopaedic Surgery, NY-Presby Hosp/Columbia 1983; **Fellow:** Orthopaedic Trauma Surgery, NY-Presby Hosp/Columbia 1984; **Fac Appt:** Prof OrS, Univ Iowa Coll Med

Nuber, Gordon W MD [OrS] - **Spec Exp:** Shoulder Reconstruction; Rotator Cuff Surgery; Cartilage Damage; Arthroscopic Surgery-Knee; **Hospital:** Northwestern Meml Hosp; **Address:** Northwestern Orthopaedic Inst, 680 N Lake Shore, Ste 1028, Chicago, IL 60611-4451; **Phone:** 312-664-6848; **Board Cert:** Orthopaedic Surgery 2007; **Med School:** Wayne State Univ 1978; **Resid:** Orthopaedic Surgery, Northwestern Meml Hosp 1983; **Fellow:** Sports Medicine, Natl Athletic Hlth Inst 1984; **Fac Appt:** Clin Prof OrS, Northwestern Univ

O'Driscoll, Shawn MD/PhD [OrS] - **Spec Exp:** Sports Medicine; Shoulder Surgery; Elbow Surgery; Cartilage Damage; **Hospital:** Mayo Med Ctr & Clin - Rochester; **Address:** Mayo Clinic, Dept Orthopaedic Surgery, 200 1st St SW, Rochester, MN 55905; **Phone:** 507-538-1953; **Board Cert:** Orthopaedic Surgery 2003; Orthopaedic Sports Medicine 2007; **Med School:** Univ Toronto 1980; **Resid:** Orthopaedic Surgery, Univ Toronto 1987; **Fellow:** Arthroscopic Surgery, Toronto Western Hosp; Elbow & Shoulder Surgery, Mayo Clinic 1988; **Fac Appt:** Prof OrS, Mayo Med Sch

Parsons III, Theodore W MD [OrS] - **Spec Exp:** Bone & Soft Tissue Tumors; Reconstructive Surgery; **Hospital:** Henry Ford Hosp; **Address:** Henry Ford Hosp, Dept Orthopaedics, 2799 West Grand Blvd, CFP-6, Detroit, MI 48202; **Phone:** 313-916-1964; **Board Cert:** Orthopaedic Surgery 2005; **Med School:** Uniformed Srvs Univ, Bethesda 1986; **Resid:** Orthopaedic Surgery, Wilford Hall USAF Med Ctr 1991; **Fellow:** Pediatric Oncology, Boston Chldns Hosp 1992; Orthopaedic Oncology, Mass Genl Hosp 1992; **Fac Appt:** Prof OrS, Wayne State Univ

Peabody, Terrance D MD [OrS] - **Spec Exp:** Soft Tissue Tumors; Bone Tumors; Pediatric Orthopaedic Cancers; Limb Sparing Surgery; **Hospital:** Univ of Chicago Med Ctr; **Address:** Univ Chicago Medical Ctr, 5841 S Maryland Ave, MC 3079, Chicago, IL 60637; **Phone:** 773-702-3442; **Board Cert:** Orthopaedic Surgery 2004; **Med School:** UC Irvine 1985; **Resid:** Orthopaedic Surgery, UC Irvine Med Ctr 1990; **Fellow:** Orthopaedic Oncology, Univ Chicago Hosps 1991; **Fac Appt:** Prof OrS, Univ Chicago-Pritzker Sch Med

Pinzur, Michael S MD [OrS] - **Spec Exp:** Diabetes-Amputation; Foot & Ankle Surgery; Amputation Surgery; Charcot Foot; **Hospital:** Loyola Univ Med Ctr; **Address:** Loyola Univ Med Ctr, Dept Orth Surg, 2160 S 1st Ave Maguire Bldg - Ste 1700, Maywood, IL 60153-3304; **Phone:** 708-216-4993; **Board Cert:** Orthopaedic Surgery 1980; **Med School:** Rush Med Coll 1974; **Resid:** Orthopaedic Surgery, Northwestern Meml Hosp 1979; **Fac Appt:** Prof OrS, Loyola Univ-Stritch Sch Med

Polly, David W MD [OrS] - **Spec Exp:** Spinal Surgery; Scoliosis; Aging; **Address:** Univ Minnesota, Orthopaedic Dept, 2512 S 7th St, rm R-102, Minneapolis, MN 55454; **Phone:** 612-273-9400; **Board Cert:** Orthopaedic Surgery 2005; **Med School:** Uniformed Srvs Univ, Bethesda 1985; **Resid:** Orthopaedic Surgery, Walter Reed Army Med Ctr 1991; **Fellow:** Spinal Surgery, Univ Minn Affil Hosp 1992

Riew, K Daniel MD [OrS] - **Spec Exp:** Spinal Surgery-Cervical; Minimally Invasive Spinal Surgery; Spinal Microdiscectomy; **Hospital:** Barnes-Jewish Hosp; **Address:** Ctr for Advanced Med-Spine Ctr, 4921 Parkview Pl, CAM Bldg Fl 12 - Ste A, St Louis, MO 63110; **Phone:** 314-514-3500; **Board Cert:** Internal Medicine 1987; Orthopaedic Surgery 2008; **Med School:** Case West Res Univ 1984; **Resid:** Internal Medicine, NY Hosp-Cornell Med Ctr 1987; Orthopaedic Surgery, George Wash Univ Med Ctr 1994; **Fellow:** Spinal Surgery, Case West Res Univ 1995; **Fac Appt:** Prof OrS, Washington Univ, St Louis

Romeo, Anthony A MD [OrS] - **Spec Exp:** Shoulder Reconstruction; Shoulder Problems-Complex; Sports Medicine; Elbow Surgery; **Hospital:** Rush Univ Med Ctr, Rush Oak Park Hosp; **Address:** 1611 W Harrison St, Ste 300, Chicago, IL 60612; **Phone:** 312-432-2342; **Board Cert:** Orthopaedic Surgery 2008; Orthopaedic Sports Medicine 2010; **Med School:** St Louis Univ 1987; **Resid:** Orthopaedic Surgery, Cleveland Clinic 1992; **Fellow:** Shoulder Surgery, Univ Washington 1993; **Fac Appt:** Assoc Prof OrS, Rush Med Coll

Schafer, Michael F MD [OrS] - **Spec Exp:** Sports Medicine; Spinal Surgery; Scoliosis; **Hospital:** Northwestern Meml Hosp, Children's Mem Hosp -Chicago; **Address:** 675 N St Clair, Galter Pavillion Fl 17 - Ste 100, Chicago, IL 60611-5968; **Phone:** 312-695-6800; **Board Cert:** Orthopaedic Surgery 1983; **Med School:** Univ Iowa Coll Med 1967; **Resid:** Orthopaedic Surgery, Northwestern Univ Hosp 1972; **Fellow:** Spinal Surgery, Natl Fdn Traveling Fellowship 1973; **Fac Appt:** Prof OrS, Northwestern Univ

Shelbourne, K Donald MD [OrS] - **Spec Exp:** Knee Surgery; Arthroscopic Surgery; Knee Rehabilitation (Non-Surgical); Knee Ligament Reconstruction; **Hospital:** IU Health Methodist Hosp; **Address:** 1815 N Capitol Ave, Ste 600, Indianapolis, IN 46202; **Phone:** 317-924-8636; **Board Cert:** Orthopaedic Surgery 1984; **Med School:** Indiana Univ 1976; **Resid:** Orthopaedic Surgery, Indiana Univ Hosp 1981; **Fellow:** Sports Medicine, Univ Wisconsin 1982; **Fac Appt:** Assoc Clin Prof OrS, Indiana Univ

Sim, Franklin H MD [OrS] - **Spec Exp:** Sarcoma; Bone Cancer; **Hospital:** Mayo Med Ctr & Clin - Rochester; **Address:** Mayo Clinic, Orthopaedic Surg, Gonda 14, 200 1st St SW, Rochester, MN 55905; **Phone:** 507-284-2511; **Board Cert:** Orthopaedic Surgery 1971; **Med School:** Dalhousie Univ 1965; **Resid:** Orthopaedic Surgery, Mayo Clinic 1970; **Fac Appt:** Prof OrS, Mayo Med Sch

Orthopaedic Surgery

Stulberg, S David MD [OrS] - **Spec Exp:** Hip & Knee Replacement; **Hospital:** Northwestern Meml Hosp; **Address:** 680 N Lake Shore Drive, Ste 924, Chicago, IL 60611; **Phone:** 312-664-6848; **Board Cert:** Orthopaedic Surgery 1977; **Med School:** Univ Mich Med Sch 1969; **Resid:** Orthopaedic Surgery, Mass Genl Hosp 1974; **Fellow:** Research, Toronto Hosp Sick Chldn 1976; **Fac Appt:** Prof OrS, Northwestern Univ

Swiontkowski, Marc F MD [OrS] - **Spec Exp:** Osteomyelitis; Fractures-Non Union; Trauma; Bone Infections; **Address:** Tria Orthopedic Ctr, 8100 Northland Drive, Bloomington, MN 55431; **Phone:** 952-831-8742; **Board Cert:** Orthopaedic Surgery 2008; **Med School:** USC Sch Med 1979; **Resid:** Orthopaedic Surgery, Univ Washington Med Ctr 1984; **Fac Appt:** Prof OrS, Univ Minn

Thompson, George H MD [OrS] - **Spec Exp:** Orthopaedic Surgery-Pediatric; Scoliosis; Spinal Deformity-Pediatric; **Hospital:** UH Rainbow Babies & Chldns Hosp (page 74); **Address:** UH Rainbow Babies & Children's Hospital, Ped Ortho Surg, 11100 Euclid Ave, Cleveland, OH 44106; **Phone:** 216-844-5416; **Board Cert:** Orthopaedic Surgery 1994; **Med School:** Univ Okla Coll Med 1970; **Resid:** Surgery, UCLA Med Ctr 1972; Orthopaedic Surgery, UCLA Med Ctr 1977; **Fellow:** Pediatric Orthopaedic Surgery, Hosp for Sick Chldn; **Fac Appt:** Prof OrS, Case West Res Univ

Weinstein, Stuart L MD [OrS] - **Spec Exp:** Scoliosis; Hip Disorders & Dysplasia; Hip Disorders-Pediatric; Spinal Deformity; **Hospital:** Univ Iowa Hosp & Clinics; **Address:** Univ Iowa, Dept Orthopaedics, 200 Hawkins Drive, Iowa City, IA 52242-1009; **Phone:** 319-356-1872; **Board Cert:** Orthopaedic Surgery 2007; **Med School:** Univ Iowa Coll Med 1972; **Resid:** Orthopaedic Surgery, Univ Iowa Hosps 1976; **Fac Appt:** Prof OrS, Univ Iowa Coll Med

Wixson, Richard L MD [OrS] - **Spec Exp:** Hip & Knee Replacement; **Hospital:** Northwestern Meml Hosp; **Address:** 680 N Lake Shore Drive Fl 9 - rm 924, Chicago, IL 60611; **Phone:** 312-664-6848; **Board Cert:** Orthopaedic Surgery 1979; **Med School:** Univ Wisc 1972; **Resid:** Orthopaedic Surgery, Henry Ford Hosp 1977; Orthopaedic Surgery, New Eng Baptist Hosp 1979; **Fellow:** Orthopaedic Surgery, Mass Genl Hosp 1978; **Fac Appt:** Clin Prof OrS, Northwestern Univ

Wurtz, L Daniel MD [OrS] - **Spec Exp:** Bone & Soft Tissue Tumors; Limb Sparing Surgery; Sarcoma; Pediatric Orthopaedic Cancers; **Hospital:** IU Health University Hosp, Riley Hosp for Children; **Address:** University Orthopaedic Assocs, 541 Clinical Drive, Ste 600, Indianapolis, IN 46202; **Phone:** 317-274-3227; **Board Cert:** Orthopaedic Surgery 2004; **Med School:** Univ S Ala Coll Med 1985; **Resid:** Orthopaedic Surgery, Wilford Hall USAF Med Ctr 1990; **Fellow:** Musculoskeletal Oncology, Univ Chicago; **Fac Appt:** Assoc Prof OrS, Indiana Univ

Yamaguchi, Ken MD [OrS] - **Spec Exp:** Shoulder Surgery; Elbow Surgery; Rotator Cuff Surgery; **Hospital:** Barnes-Jewish Hosp; **Address:** Washington Univ School of Med, 660 S Euclid Ave, Campus Box 8233, St Louis, MO 63110; **Phone:** 314-747-2500; **Board Cert:** Orthopaedic Surgery 2008; **Med School:** Geo Wash Univ 1989; **Resid:** Orthopaedic Surgery, George Wash Univ Med Ctr 1994; **Fellow:** Shoulder Surgery, Columbia Presby Med Ctr 1995; **Fac Appt:** Prof OrS, Washington Univ, St Louis

Zdeblick, Thomas MD [OrS] - **Spec Exp:** Spinal Surgery; **Hospital:** Univ WI Hosp & Clins; **Address:** 1685 Highland Ave, Madison, WI 53705-2281; **Phone:** 608-265-3207; **Board Cert:** Orthopaedic Surgery 2002; **Med School:** Tufts Univ 1982; **Resid:** Orthopaedic Surgery, Case West Res Univ 1988; **Fellow:** Spinal Surgery, Johns Hopkins Univ 1989; **Fac Appt:** Prof OrS, Univ Wisc

Great Plains and Mountains

Coughlin, Michael J MD [OrS] - **Spec Exp:** Foot & Ankle Surgery; **Hospital:** St. Alphonsus Regl Med Ctr; **Address:** 1075 N Curtis Rd, Ste 300, Boise, ID 83706; **Phone:** 208-377-1000; **Board Cert:** Orthopaedic Surgery 1980; **Med School:** Oregon Hlth & Sci Univ 1974; **Resid:** Orthopaedic Surgery, UCSF Med Ctr 1978; **Fellow:** Foot & Ankle Surgery, Samuel Merrit Hosp 1979; **Fac Appt:** Clin Prof OrS, Oregon Hlth & Sci Univ

Garvin, Kevin L MD [OrS] - **Spec Exp:** Hip Surgery; Knee Surgery; Joint Replacement; **Hospital:** Nebraska Med Ctr; **Address:** UNMC Orthopaedic Clinic, 989265 Nebraska Medical Ctr Fl 2, Omaha, NE 68198-9265; **Phone:** 402-559-8000; **Board Cert:** Orthopaedic Surgery 2010; **Med School:** Med Coll Wisc 1982; **Resid:** Orthopaedic Surgery, Univ Arkansas Hosp 1987; **Fellow:** Hip Surgery, Hosp for Special Surgery 1988; **Fac Appt:** Prof OrS, Univ Nebr Coll Med

Heiden, Eric A MD [OrS] - **Spec Exp:** Sports Medicine; Knee Surgery; **Hospital:** Ortho Spec Hosp, The (TOSH); **Address:** 2200 Park Ave D Bldg - Ste 100, 5848 Fashion Blvd, Park City, UT 84060; **Phone:** 801-703-8397; **Board Cert:** Orthopaedic Surgery 2000; **Med School:** Stanford Univ 1991; **Resid:** Orthopaedic Surgery, UC Davis Med Ctr 1996; **Fellow:** Sports Medicine, Amer Sports Med Inst 1997

Kelly, Cynthia M MD [OrS] - **Spec Exp:** Osteonecrosis; Bone Tumors; Soft Tissue Tumors; Bone Cancer; **Hospital:** Presby - St Luke's Med Ctr; **Address:** 1601 E 19th Ave, Ste 3300, Denver, CO 80218; **Phone:** 303-837-0072; **Board Cert:** Orthopaedic Surgery 2000; **Med School:** UCLA 1989; **Resid:** Orthopaedic Surgery, Harbor-UCLA Med Ctr 1994; **Fellow:** Orthopaedic Oncology, UCLA Med Ctr 1995

Millett, Peter J MD [OrS] - **Spec Exp:** Shoulder Surgery; Sports Medicine; Arthroscopic Surgery; **Hospital:** Vail Valley Med Ctr; **Address:** Steadman-Hawkins Clinic, 181 W Meadow Drive, Ste 400, Vail, CO 81657; **Phone:** 970-476-1100; **Board Cert:** Orthopaedic Surgery 2003; **Med School:** Dartmouth Med Sch 1995; **Resid:** Orthopaedic Surgery, Hosp Special Surgery 2000; **Fellow:** Sports Medicine, Steadman Hawkins Clinic 2001

Randall, R Lawrence L MD [OrS] - **Spec Exp:** Bone Tumors; Sarcoma-Soft Tissue; Pediatric Orthopaedic Surgery; **Hospital:** Univ Utah Hlth Care, Primary Children's Med Ctr; **Address:** Ped Ortho Surg, Primary Chlds Med Ctr, 100 N Mario Capecchi Drive, Ste 4550, Salt Lake City, UT 84113; **Phone:** 801-662-5600; **Board Cert:** Orthopaedic Surgery 2001; **Med School:** Yale Univ 1992; **Resid:** Orthopaedic Surgery, UCSF Med Ctr 1997; **Fellow:** Musculoskeletal Oncology, Univ WA Med Ctr 1998; **Fac Appt:** Assoc Prof OrS, Univ Utah

Rosenberg, Thomas D MD [OrS] - **Spec Exp:** Knee Surgery; Sports Medicine; **Hospital:** Ortho Spec Hosp, The (TOSH); **Address:** 900 Round Valley Drive, Ste 100, Park City, UT 84060; **Phone:** 435-655-6600; **Board Cert:** Orthopaedic Surgery 1979; **Med School:** Univ Utah 1973; **Resid:** Orthopaedic Surgery, Univ Utah Affil Hosps 1977; **Fellow:** Sports Medicine, Univ Wisconsin Hosp 1978

Saltzman, Charles L MD [OrS] - **Spec Exp:** Foot & Ankle Surgery; **Hospital:** Univ Utah Hlth Care; **Address:** Dept Orthopaedic Surgery, 590 Wakara Way, Salt Lake City, UT 84108; **Phone:** 801-587-5404; **Board Cert:** Orthopaedic Surgery 2004; **Med School:** Univ NC Sch Med 1985; **Resid:** Orthopaedic Surgery, Univ Michigan Med Ctr; **Fellow:** Orthopaedic Surgery, Mayo Clinic; **Fac Appt:** Prof OrS, Univ Utah

Orthopaedic Surgery

Steadman, J Richard MD [OrS] - **Spec Exp:** Knee-Microfracture Surgery; Sports Medicine; **Hospital:** Vail Valley Med Ctr; **Address:** The Steadman Clinic, 181 W Meadow Drive, Ste 400, Vail, CO 81657; **Phone:** 970-476-1100; **Board Cert:** Orthopaedic Surgery 1972; **Med School:** Univ Tex SW, Dallas 1963; **Resid:** Orthopaedic Surgery, Charity Hosp 1966; Orthopaedic Surgery, Louisiana St Univ Hosp 1967

Wilkins, Ross M MD [OrS] - **Spec Exp:** Bone Cancer; Bone Infections; Fractures-Non Union; **Hospital:** Presby - St Luke's Med Ctr; **Address:** 1601 E 19th Ave, Ste 3300, Denver, CO 80218; **Phone:** 303-837-0072; **Board Cert:** Orthopaedic Surgery 2007; **Med School:** Wayne State Univ 1978; **Resid:** Orthopaedic Surgery, Univ Colorado Med Ctr 1983; **Fellow:** Orthopaedic Oncology, Mayo Clinic 1984

Southwest

Agarwal, Animesh MD [OrS] - **Spec Exp:** Trauma; Fractures-Complex; **Hospital:** Univ Hlth Syst-San Antonio; **Address:** UTHSCSA Div Orthopaedic Trauma, 7703 Floyd Curl Drive, MC 7774, San Antonio, TX 78229-3900; **Phone:** 210-567-5125; **Board Cert:** Orthopaedic Surgery 2011; **Med School:** Univ Tex, San Antonio 1992; **Resid:** Orthopaedic Surgery, Unix TX Med Ctr 1997; **Fellow:** Trauma, Grant Med Ctr 1998; **Fac Appt:** Prof OrS, Univ Tex, San Antonio

Aronson, James MD [OrS] - **Spec Exp:** Limb Lengthening (Ilizarov Procedure); Hip Disorders & Dysplasia; Clubfoot; Limb Deformities; **Hospital:** Arkansas Chldns Hosp; **Address:** Arkansas Chldns Hosp, Dept Orthopaedics, 1 Children's Way, Slot 839, Little Rock, AR 72202; **Phone:** 501-364-1468; **Board Cert:** Orthopaedic Surgery 2007; **Med School:** Univ Pittsburgh 1975; **Resid:** Surgery, Maine Med Ctr 1977; Orthopaedic Surgery, Duke Univ Med Ctr 1982; **Fellow:** Pediatric Orthopaedic Surgery, Alfred I DuPont Inst 1983; **Fac Appt:** Prof OrS, Univ Ark

Brodsky, James W MD [OrS] - **Spec Exp:** Foot & Ankle Surgery; **Hospital:** Baylor Univ Medical Ctr-Dallas; **Address:** 3900 Junius St, Ste 500, Dallas, TX 75246; **Phone:** 214-823-7090; **Board Cert:** Orthopaedic Surgery 2008; **Med School:** Case West Res Univ 1979; **Resid:** Orthopaedic Surgery, Bellevue Hosp Ctr/NYU 1981; Orthopaedic Surgery, Baylor Coll Med 1984; **Fellow:** Foot & Ankle Surgery, Rancho Los Amigos/USC/LAC Hosp 1985; **Fac Appt:** Clin Prof OrS, Univ Tex SW, Dallas

Bucholz, Robert W MD [OrS] - **Spec Exp:** Hip & Knee Replacement; **Hospital:** UT Southwestern Med Ctr at Dallas, Parkland Hlth & Hosp Sys; **Address:** Dept Ortho Surg, 1801 Inwood Rd, Dallas, TX 75390-8882; **Phone:** 214-645-3300; **Board Cert:** Orthopaedic Surgery 2005; **Med School:** Yale Univ 1973; **Resid:** Orthopaedic Surgery, Yale-New Haven Hosp 1977; **Fac Appt:** Prof OrS, Univ Tex SW, Dallas

Cooper, Daniel E MD [OrS] - **Spec Exp:** Sports Medicine; Knee Injuries/ACL; Arthroscopic Surgery; Reconstructive Surgery; **Hospital:** Baylor Univ Medical Ctr-Dallas, Mary Shiels Hosp; **Address:** WB Carrell Clin, 9301 N Central Expwy, Ste 400, Tower 1, Dallas, TX 75231; **Phone:** 214-220-2468; **Board Cert:** Orthopaedic Surgery 2003; **Med School:** Univ Tex SW, Dallas 1984; **Resid:** Orthopaedic Surgery, Univ Texas Health Scis Ctr 1989; **Fellow:** Sports Medicine, Hosp for Special Surgery 1990

Gugenheim Jr, Joseph J MD [OrS] - **Spec Exp:** Limb Lengthening (Ilizarov Procedure); Limb Deformities; **Hospital:** Texas Ortho Hosp; **Address:** Foundren Orthopaedic Group, 7401 S Main St, Houston, TX 77030; **Phone:** 713-799-2300; **Board Cert:** Orthopaedic Surgery 1978; **Med School:** Northwestern Univ 1972; **Resid:** Orthopaedic Surgery, Baylor Univ Hosp 1976; **Fellow:** Pediatric Orthopaedic Surgery, Boston Chldns Hosp 1977; **Fac Appt:** Assoc Prof S, Baylor Coll Med

Hochschuler, Stephen H MD [OrS] - **Spec Exp:** Spinal Surgery; **Hospital:** TX Hlth Presby Hosp Plano; **Address:** Texas Back Institute, 6020 W Parker Rd, Ste 200, Plano, TX 75093-7916; **Phone:** 972-608-5000; **Board Cert:** Orthopaedic Surgery 1978; **Med School:** Harvard Med Sch 1968; **Resid:** Surgery, Boston City Hosp 1971; Orthopaedic Surgery, Univ Texas SW Med Ctr 1976

Mabrey, Jay D MD [OrS] - **Spec Exp:** Knee Replacement & Revision; Hip Replacement & Revision; Arthroscopic Surgery-Hip; **Hospital:** Baylor Univ Medical Ctr-Dallas, Mary Shiels Hosp; **Address:** Baylor Univ Med Ctr, Dept Orthopaedics, 3500 Gaston Ave Bldg Hob Fl 6, Dallas, TX 75246; **Phone:** 214-820-3434; **Board Cert:** Orthopaedic Surgery 2009; **Med School:** Cornell Univ-Weill Med Coll 1981; **Resid:** Surgery, Duke Univ Med Ctr 1983; Orthopaedic Surgery, Duke Univ Med Ctr 1987; **Fellow:** Joint Replacement Surgery, Hosp Special Surg 1991; **Fac Appt:** Clin Prof OrS, Univ Tex SW, Dallas

Seltzer, Dana G MD [OrS] - **Spec Exp:** Sports Medicine; Trauma; Arthroscopic Surgery; Shoulder Problems-Complex; **Hospital:** St. Joseph's Hosp & Med Ctr - Phoenix; **Address:** 500 W Thomas Rd, Ste 850, Phoenix, AZ 85013; **Phone:** 602-406-2663; **Board Cert:** Orthopaedic Surgery 2007; **Med School:** USC Sch Med 1986; **Resid:** Orthopaedic Surgery, Univ Miami-Jackson Meml Hosp 1991; **Fellow:** Sports Medicine, Kerlan-Jobe Clinic 1992; Shoulder Surgery, UTSA 1993

Souryal, Tarek O MD [OrS] - **Spec Exp:** Sports Medicine; Knee Injuries/ACL; **Hospital:** TX Hlth Presby Hosp Dallas; **Address:** 6901 Snider Plaza, Ste 200, Dallas, TX 75205; **Phone:** 214-369-7733; **Board Cert:** Orthopaedic Surgery 2011; **Med School:** Univ Tex, San Antonio 1982; **Resid:** Orthopaedic Surgery, UTSW Med Ctr 1987; **Fellow:** Sports Medicine, Sports Med Clin N Tex 1987; Sports Medicine, Hughston Ortho Clinic 1988; **Fac Appt:** Clin Prof OrS, Univ Tex SW, Dallas

Williams, Ronald P MD [OrS] - **Spec Exp:** Bone Tumors; **Hospital:** Univ Hlth Syst-San Antonio; **Address:** Scarcoma Ctr at CTRC, 7979 Wurzbach Rd, Ste U219, MC 8226, San Antonio, TX 78229-3900; **Phone:** 210-450-1170; **Board Cert:** Orthopaedic Surgery 2003; **Med School:** Univ Tex, San Antonio 1984; **Resid:** Orthopaedic Surgery, Univ Kans Sch Med 1989; **Fellow:** Orthopaedic Oncology, Case West Res Univ 1990; **Fac Appt:** Prof OrS, Univ Tex, San Antonio

Wirth, Michael A MD [OrS] - **Spec Exp:** Shoulder Surgery; Shoulder Replacement; **Hospital:** Univ Hlth Syst-San Antonio, Methodist Hosp-San Antonio; **Address:** Univ Tex Hlth Sci Ctr, Dept Orth, 7703 Floyd Curl Drive, MC 7774, San Antonio, TX 78229-3900; **Phone:** 210-567-5135; **Board Cert:** Orthopaedic Surgery 2004; **Med School:** Oregon Hlth & Sci Univ 1985; **Resid:** Orthopaedic Surgery, Univ Texas Hlth Sci Ctr 1990; **Fellow:** Shoulder Surgery, Charles Rockwood Jr MD 1991; **Fac Appt:** Prof OrS, Univ Tex, San Antonio

West Coast and Pacific

Anderson, Lesley J MD [OrS] - **Spec Exp:** Knee Injuries/ACL; Knee Cartilage/Meniscus Transplants; Cartilage Damage; Stem Cells in Orthopedics; **Hospital:** CA Pacific Med Ctr-Pacific Campus; **Address:** 2100 Webster St, Ste 309, San Francisco, CA 94115; **Phone:** 415-923-3029; **Board Cert:** Orthopaedic Surgery 2007; **Med School:** Penn State Coll Med 1976; **Resid:** Orthopaedic Surgery, UCLA Med Ctr 1983; **Fellow:** Sports Medicine/Knee Surgery, Blazina Ortho Clinic 1984; **Fac Appt:** Asst Clin Prof OrS, UCSF

Bos, Gary D MD [OrS] - **Spec Exp:** Musculoskeletal Tumors; Sarcoma; Reconstructive Surgery; **Hospital:** Yakima Valley Mem Hosp; **Address:** 3003 TIETON Drive, Ste 350, Yakima, WA 98902; **Phone:** 509-573-3989; **Board Cert:** Orthopaedic Surgery 2008; **Med School:** Univ Chicago-Pritzker Sch Med 1978; **Resid:** Orthopaedic Surgery, Case West Reserve Univ 1984; **Fellow:** Orthopaedic Surgery, Case West Reserve Univ 1980; Orthopaedic Oncology, Mayo Clinic 1985; **Fac Appt:** Asst Clin Prof OrS

Orthopaedic Surgery

Brien, Earl Warren MD [OrS] - **Spec Exp:** Bone & Soft Tissue Tumors; **Hospital:** Cedars-Sinai Med Ctr; **Address:** 8700 Beverly Blvd, rm AC1058, Los Angeles, CA 90048; **Phone:** 310-423-9887; **Board Cert:** Orthopaedic Surgery 2006; **Med School:** Howard Univ 1986; **Resid:** Orthopaedic Surgery, LAC-King Drew Med Ctr 1992; **Fellow:** Musculoskeletal Disorders, Memorial Sloan Kettering 1993; Metabolic Bone Research, Hosp for Special Surgery 1994

Caillouette, James Thompson MD [OrS] - **Spec Exp:** Joint Replacement; Hip & Knee Reconstruction; **Hospital:** Hoag Meml Hosp Presby; **Address:** Newport Orthopaedic Institute, 22 Corporate Plaza Drive, Newport Beach, CA 92660; **Phone:** 949-722-5000; **Board Cert:** Orthopaedic Surgery 2011; **Med School:** USC Sch Med 1983; **Resid:** Orthopaedic Surgery, Univ CA Affil Hosp 1988; **Fac Appt:** Assoc Clin Prof OrS, UC Irvine

Carragee, Eugene J MD [OrS] - **Spec Exp:** Spinal Surgery; Spinal Disc Replacement; **Hospital:** Stanford Univ Hosp & Clinics, Lucile Packard Chldn's Hosp; **Address:** Orthopaedic Spine Center, 450 Broadway St, Pavilion A, 1st Fl, Redwood City, CA 94063-6110; **Phone:** 650-725-5905; **Board Cert:** Orthopaedic Surgery 2005; **Med School:** Stanford Univ 1982; **Resid:** Internal Medicine, Stanford Univ Hosp 1984; Orthopaedic Surgery, Stanford Univ Hosp 1988; **Fac Appt:** Prof OrS, Stanford Univ

Chambers, Richard Byron MD [OrS] - **Spec Exp:** Diabetes-Amputation; **Hospital:** Rancho Los Amigos Natl Rehab Ctr; **Address:** Rancho Los Amigos Natl Rehab Ctr, Dept Surgery, 7601 E Imperial Hwy, Downey, CA 90242; **Phone:** 562-401-7166; **Board Cert:** Orthopaedic Surgery 1977; **Med School:** Columbia P&S 1971; **Resid:** Surgery, NY Hosp; Orthopaedic Surgery, Hosp Special Surg

Chapman, Jens Robert MD [OrS] - **Spec Exp:** Spinal Surgery; Trauma; **Hospital:** Harborview Med Ctr; **Address:** Roosevelt Bone & Joint Surgery Ctr, 4245 Roosevelt Way NE Fl 2, Box 354740, Seattle, WA 98105; **Phone:** 206-598-4288; **Board Cert:** Orthopaedic Surgery 2004; **Med School:** Germany 1983; **Resid:** Surgery, Klinkum F.D. Isar 1985; Orthopaedic Surgery, Univ Texas Southern Med Ctr 1990; **Fellow:** Trauma, Harborview Med Ctr 1990; Spinal Surgery, Univ Washington Med School 1991; **Fac Appt:** Prof OrS, Univ Wash

Conrad, Ernest U MD [OrS] - **Spec Exp:** Pediatric Orthopaedic Surgery; Bone Tumors; Sarcoma; **Hospital:** Seattle Chldns Hosp, Univ Wash Med Ctr; **Address:** 4800 Sand Point Way NE, #W7706, Box 359300, Seattle, WA 98195-5371; **Phone:** 206-987-5678; **Board Cert:** Orthopaedic Surgery 2009; **Med School:** Univ VA Sch Med 1979; **Resid:** Orthopaedic Surgery, Hosp for Special Surgery 1984; **Fellow:** Orthopaedic Oncology, Univ Fla Coll Med 1985; Pediatric Orthopaedic Surgery, Hosp for Sick Chldn 1986; **Fac Appt:** Prof OrS, Univ Wash

Copp, Steven N MD [OrS] - **Spec Exp:** Foot & Ankle Surgery; Hip & Knee Replacement; Reconstructive Surgery-Complex; **Hospital:** Scripps Green Hosp; **Address:** Scripps Clinic Torrey Pines, 10666 N Torrey Pines Rd, MS 116, La Jolla, CA 92037; **Phone:** 858-554-8519; **Board Cert:** Orthopaedic Surgery 2002; **Med School:** UCSD 1983; **Resid:** Orthopaedic Surgery, UCSD Med Ctr 1988

Delamarter, Rick B MD [OrS] - **Spec Exp:** Spinal Surgery; Minimally Invasive Spinal Surgery; Spinal Disc Replacement; Spinal Reconstructive Surgery; **Hospital:** Cedars-Sinai Med Ctr; **Address:** Spine Institute of Santa Monica, 444 S San Vincente Blvd, Ste 901, Los Angeles, CA 90048; **Phone:** 310-248-7310; **Board Cert:** Orthopaedic Surgery 2010; **Med School:** Oregon Hlth & Sci Univ 1981; **Resid:** Orthopaedic Surgery, UCLA Med Ctr 1986; **Fac Appt:** Assoc Prof S, UCLA

Dillingham, Michael F MD [OrS] - **Spec Exp:** Sports Medicine; **Hospital:** Stanford Univ Hosp & Clinics, CA Pacific Med Ctr-Pacific Campus; **Address:** 500 Arguello St, Ste 100, Redwood City, CA 94063; **Phone:** 650-851-4900; **Board Cert:** Orthopaedic Surgery 1977; Physical Medicine & Rehabilitation 1979; **Med School:** Stanford Univ 1971; **Resid:** Orthopaedic Surgery, Standford Univ Med Ctr 1975; Physical Medicine & Rehabilitation, Santa Clara Valley Med Ctr 1977; **Fellow:** Spinal Surgery, Santa Clara Valley Med Ctr 1976; **Fac Appt:** Clin Prof OrS, Stanford Univ

Dorr, Lawrence D MD [OrS] - **Spec Exp:** Hip & Knee Replacement; **Hospital:** Good Samaritan Hosp - LA; **Address:** Dorr Arthritis Institute, 637 S Lucas Ave, Ste 101, Los Angeles, CA 90017; **Phone:** 213-977-2280; **Board Cert:** Orthopaedic Surgery 1978; **Med School:** Univ Iowa Coll Med 1967; **Resid:** Orthopaedic Surgery, LAC-USC Med Ctr 1976; **Fellow:** Joint Replacement Surgery, Hosp Special Surgery 1977

Eckardt, Jeffrey J MD [OrS] - **Spec Exp:** Bone Tumors; Soft Tissue Tumors; Limb Sparing Surgery; **Hospital:** Santa Monica - UCLA Med Ctr & Ortho Hosp, UCLA Ronald Reagan Med Ctr; **Address:** UCLA Med Ctr, Dept Ortho Surg/Oncology, 1250 16th St Tower # 713, Santa Monica, CA 90404; **Phone:** 310-319-3816; **Board Cert:** Orthopaedic Surgery 1981; **Med School:** Cornell Univ-Weill Med Coll 1971; **Resid:** Orthopaedic Surgery, UCLA Med Ctr 1979; **Fellow:** Orthopaedic Oncology, Mayo Clinic 1980; **Fac Appt:** Prof OrS, UCLA

Elattrache, Neal S MD [OrS] - **Spec Exp:** Shoulder & Elbow Surgery; Knee Surgery; Sports Medicine; **Hospital:** Keck Med Ctr of USC (page 75); **Address:** Kerlan-Jobe Orthopaedic Clin, 6801 Park Terrace Drive, Los Angeles, CA 90045; **Phone:** 310-665-7257; **Board Cert:** Orthopaedic Surgery 2004; Orthopaedic Sports Medicine 2007; **Med School:** Univ Pittsburgh 1985; **Resid:** Orthopaedic Surgery, Univ Pittsburgh Med Ctr 1990; **Fellow:** Sports Medicine, Kerlan-Jobe Orthpaedic Clin 1991; **Fac Appt:** Assoc Clin Prof OrS, USC-Keck School of Medicine

Finerman, Gerald MD [OrS] - **Spec Exp:** Sports Medicine; Hip & Knee Replacement; **Hospital:** UCLA Ronald Reagan Med Ctr, Santa Monica - UCLA Med Ctr & Ortho Hosp; **Address:** 1245 16 St, Ste 202, Santa Monica, CA 90404; **Phone:** 310-825-6019; **Board Cert:** Orthopaedic Surgery 1971; **Med School:** Johns Hopkins Univ 1962; **Resid:** Surgery, Johns Hopkins Hosp 1964; Orthopaedic Surgery, Johns Hopkins Hosp 1969; **Fac Appt:** Prof Emeritus OrS, UCLA

Garfin, Steven R MD [OrS] - **Spec Exp:** Spinal Surgery; Minimally Invasive Spinal Surgery; **Hospital:** UCSD Med Ctr; **Address:** UCSD, Dept Orthopedic Surgery, 9350 Campus Pointe Drive, Ste 1B, La Jolla, CA 92037; **Phone:** 858-657-8200; **Board Cert:** Orthopaedic Surgery 1982; **Med School:** Univ Minn 1972; **Resid:** Orthopaedic Surgery, UCSD Med Ctr 1980; **Fellow:** Spinal Surgery, Pennsylvania Hosp 1981; **Fac Appt:** Prof OrS, UCSD

Goodman, Stuart B MD/PhD [OrS] - **Spec Exp:** Arthritis; Joint Replacement; Reconstructive Surgery; **Hospital:** Stanford Univ Hosp & Clinics, Lucile Packard Chldn's Hosp; **Address:** Joint Replacement Center, 450 Broadway St, Redwood City, CA 94063-6110; **Phone:** 650-723-5643; **Board Cert:** Orthopaedic Surgery 2008; **Med School:** Univ Toronto 1978; **Resid:** Orthopaedic Surgery, Univ Toronto Affil Hosp 1984; **Fellow:** Trauma, Univ Toronto 1985; **Fac Appt:** Prof OrS, Stanford Univ

Gorab II, Robert S MD [OrS] - **Spec Exp:** Knee Replacement; Hip Replacement; Arthritis; **Hospital:** St. Joseph's Hosp - Orange; **Address:** Orthopaedic Specialty Inst, 280 Main St, Ste 200, Orange, CA 92868; **Phone:** 714-937-2136; **Board Cert:** Orthopaedic Surgery 2006; **Med School:** Univ Pittsburgh 1989; **Resid:** Orthopaedic Surgery, UC-Irvine Med Ctr 1995; **Fellow:** Joint Reconstruction, Cleveland Clinic 1996; **Fac Appt:** Assoc Prof OrS, UC Irvine

Orthopaedic Surgery

Johnson, Eric E MD [OrS] - **Spec Exp:** Pelvic & Acetabular Fractures; Trauma; Limb Lengthening; Hip Replacement; **Hospital:** UCLA Ronald Reagan Med Ctr; **Address:** UCLA Med Ctr-Dept Orthopedic Surgery, 10833 Le Conte Ave, rm 73-143 CHF, Los Angeles, CA 90095-6902; **Phone:** 310-206-1169; **Board Cert:** Orthopaedic Surgery 1985; **Med School:** Univ Utah 1976; **Resid:** Surgery, Univ Utah Med Ctr 1978; Orthopaedic Surgery, UCLA Med Ctr 1981; **Fellow:** Orthopaedic Trauma Surgery, Univ Hanover 1982; Hip Surgery, Univ Paris 1984; **Fac Appt:** Prof OrS, UCLA

Kim, Choll W MD/PhD [OrS] - **Spec Exp:** Minimally Invasive Spinal Surgery; Spinal Surgery; Scoliosis; Spinal Surgery-Cervical; **Hospital:** UCSD Med Ctr, Alvarado Hosp & Med Ctr; **Address:** Spine Institute of San Diego, Ctr for Minimally Invasive Spine Surgery, 6719 Alvarado Rd, Ste 308, San Diego, CA 92120; **Phone:** 619-265-7912; **Board Cert:** Orthopaedic Surgery 2005; **Med School:** Harvard Med Sch 1996; **Resid:** Orthopaedic Surgery, UCSD Affil Hosp 2001; **Fellow:** Spinal Surgery, Mayo Clin 2002; **Fac Appt:** Assoc Clin Prof OrS, UCSD

Lowenberg, David W MD [OrS] - **Spec Exp:** Osteomyelitis; Limb Lengthening (Ilizarov Procedure); Fractures-Complex & Non Union; Limb Deformities; **Hospital:** Stanford Univ Hosp & Clinics; **Address:** 450 Broadway, Pavilion A, Redwood City, CA 94063; **Phone:** 650-723-5643; **Board Cert:** Orthopaedic Surgery 2003; **Med School:** UCLA 1985; **Resid:** Orthopaedic Surgery, UCSF Med Ctr 1990; **Fac Appt:** Prof OrS, Stanford Univ

Luck Jr, James V MD [OrS] - **Spec Exp:** Hemophilia Related Disease; Hip & Knee Replacement; Musculoskeletal Tumors; **Hospital:** Santa Monica - UCLA Med Ctr & Ortho Hosp; **Address:** 2400 S Flower St, Fl 3, Los Angeles, CA 90007; **Phone:** 213-749-8255; **Board Cert:** Orthopaedic Surgery 2000; **Med School:** USC Sch Med 1967; **Resid:** Orthopaedic Surgery, Orthopaedic Hosp 1973; **Fellow:** Orthopaedic Oncology, Orthopaedic Hosp 1974; Reconstructive Surgery, Rancho Los Amigos 1974; **Fac Appt:** Prof OrS, UCLA

Mandelbaum, Bert R MD [OrS] - **Spec Exp:** Sports Medicine; Knee Injuries/ACL; Cartilage Damage; **Hospital:** St. John's Hlth Ctr, Santa Monica; **Address:** Santa Monica Orthopaedic Group, 2020 Santa Monica Blvd Fl 4, Santa Monica, CA 90404; **Phone:** 310-829-2663; **Board Cert:** Orthopaedic Surgery 2009; Orthopaedic Sports Medicine 2010; **Med School:** Washington Univ, St Louis 1980; **Resid:** Orthopaedic Surgery, Johns Hopkins Hosp 1985

Matsen, Frederick MD [OrS] - **Spec Exp:** Shoulder Replacement; Elbow Replacement; Rotator Cuff Surgery; **Hospital:** Univ Wash Med Ctr; **Address:** Bone & Joint Ctr, 4245 Roosevelt Way NE, Box 354740, Seattle, WA 98105; **Phone:** 206-598-4288; **Board Cert:** Orthopaedic Surgery 1978; **Med School:** Baylor Coll Med 1968; **Resid:** Orthopaedic Surgery, Univ Washington Med Ctr 1974; **Fac Appt:** Prof OrS, Univ Wash

O'Donnell, Richard John MD [OrS] - **Spec Exp:** Bone Cancer; Sarcoma-Soft Tissue; Pediatric Orthopaedic Cancers; **Hospital:** UCSF Med Ctr; **Address:** UCSF Helen Diller Cancer Ctr, 1600 Divisadero St Fl 4, San Francisco, CA 94115; **Phone:** 415-885-3800; **Board Cert:** Orthopaedic Surgery 2010; **Med School:** Harvard Med Sch 1989; **Resid:** Orthopaedic Surgery, Mass Genl Hosp 1995; **Fellow:** Musculoskeletal Oncology, Univ WA Med Ctr 1996; **Fac Appt:** Assoc Prof OrS, UCSF

Oakes, Daniel A MD [OrS] - **Spec Exp:** Hip & Knee Replacement; Hip & Knee Reconstruction; Hip Resurfacing; Osteonecrosis; **Hospital:** Keck Med Ctr of USC (page 75); **Address:** USC Univ Hospital, Dept Orthopaedics, 1520 San Pablo St, Ste 2000, Los Angeles, CA 90033; **Phone:** 323-442-5860; **Board Cert:** Orthopaedic Surgery 2006; **Med School:** Harvard Med Sch 1997; **Resid:** Orthopaedic Surgery, UCLA Med Ctr 2003; **Fellow:** Joint Reconstruction, Mayo Clinic 2004; **Fac Appt:** Assoc Prof OrS, UCLA

Oppenheim, William L MD [OrS] - **Spec Exp:** Limb Lengthening; Scoliosis; Clubfoot/Foot Deformities in Children; Pediatric Orthopaedic Surgery; **Hospital:** UCLA Ronald Reagan Med Ctr, Santa Monica - UCLA Med Ctr & Ortho Hosp; **Address:** Luskin Childrens Clinic, 1530 Arizona Ave, Santa Monica, CA 90404; **Phone:** 310-206-6345; **Board Cert:** Orthopaedic Surgery 1980; **Med School:** Georgetown Univ 1970; **Resid:** Orthopaedic Surgery, Univ Washington Hosp 1976; **Fellow:** Pediatric Orthopaedic Surgery, Orthopaedic Hosp UCLA 1979; **Fac Appt:** Prof OrS, UCLA

Patzakis, Michael J MD [OrS] - **Spec Exp:** Osteomyelitis; Fractures-Non Union; Joint Infections; **Hospital:** Keck Med Ctr of USC (page 75); **Address:** 1200 N State St GNH3900, Los Angeles, CA 90033-1029; **Phone:** 323-226-7201; **Board Cert:** Orthopaedic Surgery 1983; **Med School:** Ohio State Univ 1963; **Resid:** Orthopaedic Surgery, LAC-USC Med Ctr 1968; **Fellow:** Rheumatology, Univ CO Med Ctr 1969; **Fac Appt:** Prof OrS, USC Sch Med

Peterson, Davis C MD [OrS] - **Spec Exp:** Spinal Surgery; Scoliosis; Trauma; **Hospital:** Providence Alaska Med Ctr, Alaska Regl Hosp; **Address:** Anchorage Fracture & Orthopaedics, 3031 Piper St, Ste 220, Anchorage, AK 99508; **Phone:** 907-563-3145; **Board Cert:** Orthopaedic Surgery 2009; **Med School:** Baylor Coll Med 1980; **Resid:** Orthopaedic Surgery, Madigan Army Med Ctr 1986; **Fellow:** Spinal Surgery, St Luke's Med Ctr 1990

Rajacich, Nicholas MD [OrS] - **Spec Exp:** Pediatric Orthopaedic Surgery; **Hospital:** Mary Bridge Chldns Hosp & Hlth Ctr; **Address:** Mary Bridge Orthopaedic Clin, 311 S L St, Tacoma, WA 98405; **Phone:** 253-403-1507; **Board Cert:** Orthopaedic Surgery 2003; **Med School:** Johns Hopkins Univ 1982; **Resid:** Orthopaedic Surgery, Rhode Island Hosp 1985; Orthopaedic Surgery, San Francisco Or Res Program 1989; **Fellow:** Pediatric Orthopaedic Surgery, Hosp for Sick Chldn 1990

Sangeorzan, Bruce J MD [OrS] - **Spec Exp:** Foot & Ankle Surgery; Trauma; Ankle Replacement & Revision; **Hospital:** Harborview Med Ctr, Univ Wash Med Ctr; **Address:** 908 Jefferson St, MS 359799, Seattle, WA 98104; **Phone:** 206-744-4830; **Board Cert:** Orthopaedic Surgery 2010; **Med School:** Wayne State Univ 1981; **Resid:** Orthopaedic Surgery, Wayne State Univ 1986; **Fellow:** Trauma, Univ Wash 1986; Foot & Ankle Reconstruction, Univ Wash 1987; **Fac Appt:** Prof OrS, Univ Wash

Schmalzried, Thomas P MD [OrS] - **Spec Exp:** Hip & Knee Replacement; **Hospital:** St. Vincent's Med Ctr - Los Angeles; **Address:** The Joint Replacement Inst, 2200 W 3rd St, Ste 400, Los Angeles, CA 90057; **Phone:** 213-484-7600; **Board Cert:** Orthopaedic Surgery 2004; **Med School:** UCLA 1984; **Resid:** Orthopaedic Surgery, UCLA Med Ctr 1990; **Fellow:** Joint Replacement Surgery, UCLA 1987; Hip Surgery, Mass Genl Hosp/Harvard 1991; **Fac Appt:** Asst Prof OrS, UCLA

Singer, Daniel I MD [OrS] - **Spec Exp:** Hand Surgery; Bone Cancer; Hand & Upper Extremity Tumors; **Hospital:** Queen's Med Ctr - Honolulu; **Address:** Queen's Physicians' Office Blg 1, 1380 Lusitana St, Ste 615, Honolulu, HI 96813-2442; **Phone:** 808-521-8109; **Board Cert:** Orthopaedic Surgery 2010; Hand Surgery 2010; **Med School:** Boston Univ 1979; **Resid:** Surgery, Univ Conn Hlth Ctr 1981; Orthopaedic Surgery, Univ Hawaii Affil Hosp 1984; **Fellow:** Hand Surgery, Thomas Jefferson Univ Hosp 1985; Microvascular Surgery, St Vincent's Hosp 1986; **Fac Appt:** Assoc Prof OrS, Univ Hawaii JA Burns Sch Med

Smith, Douglas George MD [OrS] - **Spec Exp:** Amputation Surgery; Foot & Ankle Surgery; Limb Sparing Surgery; **Hospital:** Harborview Med Ctr; **Address:** Harborview Medical Center, 325 9th Ave, Box 359798, Seattle, WA 98104; **Phone:** 206-744-3466; **Board Cert:** Orthopaedic Surgery 2003; **Med School:** Univ Chicago-Pritzker Sch Med 1984; **Resid:** Orthopaedic Surgery, Loyola Univ Hosp 1989; **Fellow:** Foot & Ankle Surgery, Harborview Med Ctr 1990; **Fac Appt:** Prof OrS, Univ Wash

Orthopaedic Surgery

Song, Kit M MD [OrS] - **Spec Exp:** Spinal Deformity-Pediatric; Joint Infections; Bone Infections; Trauma; **Hospital:** Seattle Chldns Hosp; **Address:** Seattle Chldns Hosp- Ortho Div, 4800 Sand Point Way NE, MS WW7706, Seattle, WA 98105; **Phone:** 206-987-2109; **Board Cert:** Orthopaedic Surgery 2005; **Med School:** Univ Iowa Coll Med 1985; **Resid:** Orthopaedic Surgery, Univ Wash Affil Hosp 1991; **Fellow:** Pediatric Orthopaedic Surgery, Texas Scottish Rite Chldns Hosp 1992; **Fac Appt:** Asst Prof OrS, Univ Wash

Thomas, Bert J MD [OrS] - **Spec Exp:** Hip Replacement & Revision; Hip Resurfacing; Knee Replacement & Revision; Arthroscopic Surgery; **Hospital:** UCLA Ronald Reagan Med Ctr, Santa Monica - UCLA Med Ctr & Ortho Hosp; **Address:** 1250 16th St, 7th Fl Tower, #745, Santa Monica, CA 90404; **Phone:** 310-319-3828; **Board Cert:** Orthopaedic Surgery 2008; **Med School:** Univ Pennsylvania 1979; **Resid:** Orthopaedic Surgery, UCLA Med Ctr 1984; **Fellow:** Hip Replacement Surgery, Hosp Special Surg 1985; **Fac Appt:** Clin Prof OrS, UCLA-David Geffen Sch Med

Thordarson, David B MD [OrS] - **Spec Exp:** Foot & Ankle Surgery-Complex; Reconstructive Surgery; Trauma; **Hospital:** Keck Med Ctr of USC (page 75); **Address:** USC Orthopaedic Surgery Assocs, 1520 San Pablo St, Ste 2000, Los Angeles, CA 90033; **Phone:** 323-442-5860; **Board Cert:** Orthopaedic Surgery 2003; **Med School:** UCLA 1984; **Resid:** Orthopaedic Surgery, UCLA Med Ctr 1989; **Fellow:** Foot & Ankle Surgery, UCLA-Kaiser 1990; **Fac Appt:** Prof OrS, USC-Keck School of Medicine

Tolo, Vernon T MD [OrS] - **Spec Exp:** Pediatric Orthopaedic Surgery; Spinal Surgery-Pediatric; Spinal Deformity-Pediatric; Scoliosis; **Hospital:** Chldns Hosp - Los Angeles, Keck Med Ctr of USC (page 75); **Address:** Chldns Hosp LA, Orthopaedic Surgery, 4650 W Sunset Blvd, MS 69, Los Angeles, CA 90027-6062; **Phone:** 323-361-4658; **Board Cert:** Orthopaedic Surgery 1977; **Med School:** Johns Hopkins Univ 1968; **Resid:** Orthopaedic Surgery, Johns Hopkins Hosp 1975; **Fellow:** Pediatric Orthopaedic Surgery, Hosp Sick Chldn 1976; **Fac Appt:** Prof OrS, USC Sch Med

Vail, Thomas P MD [OrS] - **Spec Exp:** Hip & Knee Replacement; Hip Resurfacing; Arthritis; Osteonecrosis; **Hospital:** UCSF Med Ctr; **Address:** 1500 Owens St Fl 2, 500 Parnassus Ave, Box MU320W, San Francisco, CA 94143-0728; **Phone:** 415-502-5183; **Board Cert:** Orthopaedic Surgery 2005; **Med School:** Loyola Univ-Stritch Sch Med 1985; **Resid:** Thoracic Surgery, Duke Univ Med Ctr 1987; Orthopaedic Surgery, Duke Univ Med Ctr 1991; **Fellow:** Reconstructive Surgery, North Amer/Euro Trav Prgm 1992; **Fac Appt:** Prof OrS, UCSF

Wang, Jeffrey C MD [OrS] - **Spec Exp:** Spinal Surgery; Minimally Invasive Surgery; Spinal Trauma; **Hospital:** UCLA Ronald Reagan Med Ctr, Santa Monica - UCLA Med Ctr & Ortho Hosp; **Address:** UCLA Spine Center, 1250 16th St, Ste 745, Santa Monica, CA 90404; **Phone:** 310-319-3334; **Board Cert:** Orthopaedic Surgery 2010; **Med School:** Univ Pittsburgh 1991; **Resid:** Orthopaedic Surgery, Orthopaedic Hosp UCLA 1996; **Fellow:** Spinal Surgery, Case Western Reserve Univ 1997; **Fac Appt:** Prof OrS, UCLA

Watkins III, Robert G MD [OrS] - **Spec Exp:** Spinal Surgery; Spinal Disc Replacement; **Hospital:** Marina Del Rey Hosp; **Address:** 4640 Admiralty Way, Ste 600, Marina Del Rey, CA 90292; **Phone:** 310-448-7890; **Board Cert:** Orthopaedic Surgery 2007; **Med School:** Univ Tenn Coll Med 1969; **Resid:** Orthopaedic Surgery, LAC-USC Med Ctr 1978; **Fellow:** Spinal Surgery, Jones-Hunt Orth Hosp 1979; **Fac Appt:** Assoc Prof OrS, USC Sch Med

Yoo, Jung MD [OrS] - **Spec Exp:** Spinal Surgery; **Hospital:** OR Hlth & Sci Univ; **Address:** 3181 SW Sam Jackson Park Rd, MC OP31, Portland, OR 97239; **Phone:** 503-494-6406; **Board Cert:** Orthopaedic Surgery 2004; **Med School:** Univ Chicago-Pritzker Sch Med 1984; **Resid:** Orthopaedic Surgery, Case Western Reserve Univ 1990; **Fellow:** Orthopaedic Surgery, SUNY Hlth Sci Ctr 1991; **Fac Appt:** Prof OrS, Oregon Hlth & Sci Univ

Cleveland Clinic

Every life deserves world class care.

Cleveland Clinic
Orthopaedic Surgery
9500 Euclid Avenue
Cleveland, OH 44195

clevelandclinic.org/
orthotopdocs

Offering Same-Day Appointments
Call 800.274.2009.

Orthopaedic Surgery

The Cleveland Clinic Department of Orthopaedic Surgery has a long history of excellence and innovation in treating musculoskeletal injuries and diseases. Since 1992, *U.S.News & World Report* has consistently ranked the Department of Orthopaedic Surgery among the top five orthopaedic programs in the nation.

Foot and Ankle: All specialists and surgeons have extensive training in the diagnosis and care of foot and ankle disorders.

Joint Replacement: The Center for Adult Reconstruction performs joint replacement, resurfacing and revision surgery of the hip and knee. Our experienced surgeons offer the most advanced implants and minimally invasive techniques to restore patient mobility.

Upper Extremity: This center provide a diagnosis and treatment for problems affecting the hand, wrist, elbow and shoulder.

Pediatrics: The Center for Pediatric Orthopaedics handles more than 14,000 outpatient visits each year. Our physicians offer expertise in the management of all musculoskeletal conditions in children, and sports injuries.

Center for Spine Health: The Center for Spine Health diagnoses and treats more than 13,000 patients annually. The center brings together the expertise of specialists in neurosurgery, orthopaedic surgery and non-surgical spine care.

Trauma: Cleveland Clinic is a leader in the treatment of fractures and non-union and in the development of methods to improve outcomes through advanced bone grafting techniques.

Center for Musculoskeletal Tumors: As one of the largest multidisciplinary centers of its kind, we offer expertise in treating bone and soft tissue sarcomas and performing limb salvage.

Treatment Guides

Cleveland Clinic has developed comprehensive treatment guides for many diseases and conditions. To download our free treatment guides, visit clevelandclinic.org/treatmentguides.

Online Medical Second Opinion

Cleveland Clinic's My**Consult** Online Medical Second Opinion program securely connects patients to our physician specialists for more than 1,000 life-changing or life-threatening diagnoses all by the click of a mouse. To learn more, log onto eclevelandclinic.org/myconsult or call 800.223.2273, ext. 43223.

Special Assistance for Out-of-State Patients

Cleveland Clinic Global Patient Services offers a complimentary Medical Concierge service for patients who travel from outside of Ohio. Call 800.223.2273, ext. 55580 or email medicalconcierge@ccf.org.

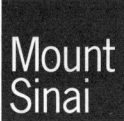 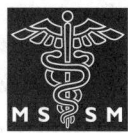

MOUNT SINAI
SCHOOL OF
MEDICINE

THE MOUNT SINAI MEDICAL CENTER
ORTHOPAEDICS

One Gustave L. Levy Place
Fifth Avenue and 100th Street
New York, NY 10029-6574
Physician Referral: 1-800-MD-SINAI (637-4624)
www.mountsinai.org/orthopaedics

Beyond its reputation for depth and breadth of expertise, **THE LENI AND PETER W. MAY DEPARTMENT OF ORTHOPAEDICS** at The Mount Sinai Medical Center is known for personalized care. The faculty and staff invest the time to get to know their patients as individuals, ensuring that they receive direct care from subspecialty-trained orthopedists. The faculty share expertise in surgery of the foot and ankle, knee, hip, hand, elbow, shoulder, and spine; total joint replacement; microvascular surgery; cancer surgery; and minimally invasive surgery. Taking a whole-patient approach to care, they work in close collaboration with specialists in geriatrics, neurology, oncology, pathology, and rehabilitation medicine.

Investigation and Innovation – Recent years have seen successive refinements in the techniques of orthopedic surgery at Mount Sinai, including joint replacement, minimally invasive fracture repair, and microvascular surgery. Faculty members have been instrumental in the design and perfection of hip and shoulder prostheses. Additionally, Mount Sinai has broadened the applications of arthroscopic surgery—the fiber optic technology that first heralded the arrival of minimally invasive surgery.

Mount Sinai orthopedic bone, spine and tendon scientists are known for their studies of diseases of the skeletal system. Researchers are currently investigating disc degeneration in the spine; rotator cuff degeneration; methods of determining bone strength; how genetic alterations change the skeleton's function; and the fundamental molecular mechanisms of arthritis.

Use of Cutting-Edge Techniques – Mount Sinai uses innovative, minimally invasive approaches for joint replacement and fracture repair. The Department's oncology service is renowned for saving limbs with both bone and joint malignancies.

The Sports Service is one of few departments in New York that provides patients with the option of arthroscopic surgery of the hip. Patients have the ability to return to activities faster and with less pain with this minimally invasive procedure. Our arthroscopists also specialize in cartilage preservation techniques, including cartilage transplantation, allowing patients to preserve their own joints and delaying the need for joint replacement surgery.

GROUNDBREAKING PROCEDURES ENHANCE QUALITY OF LIFE

Today at Mount Sinai, arthroscopy is used to repair not only the knee but virtually every joint. Converting what used to be major open surgery to outpatient procedures has dramatically shortened rehabilitation and return to work times. More significantly, it has allowed many more patients to get help for painful, function-limiting conditions. That is the case for many elderly or frail patients who are physically unable to undergo major surgery. The fact that such procedures are now more widely accessible is enhancing the quality of life for many patients and allowing them to lead more active lives.

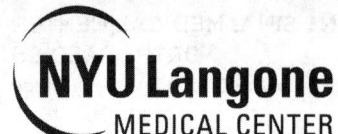
ORTHOPAEDIC SERVICES

The Department of Orthopaedic Surgery at NYU Langone Medical Center continues to be recognized as a national leader, ranked one of the top 10 in U.S. News & World Report's 2011-2012 "Best Hospitals" survey. Expert physicians combine extensive experience with cutting-edge research and technology to address bone and joint problems that affect a patient's ability to function. The department's nine specialty divisions provide care at NYU Langone's premier outpatient facility, the Center for Musculoskeletal Care, as well as at the Hospital for Joint Diseases, our internationally-renowned inpatient musculoskeletal hospital. In addition to our subspecialty divisions, the department features specialized orthopaedic patient care centers:

The Bone Healing Center evaluates and treats problem fractures and are leaders in technologies and procedures to help patients facing a long and difficult recovery from complex fracture reconstruction or fracture healing problems.

Harkness Center for Dance Injuries offers many subsidized and free services for dancers, including clinics staffed by orthopaedists and dance physical therapists. The Center also offers state-of-the-art rehabilitation technology and free injury prevention screenings and lectures.

The Diabetes Foot and Ankle Center focuses on the prevention and recurrence of foot and ankle problems associated with complications of diabetes.

The Hip Center evaluates and treats developmental, traumatic, and degenerative hip disorders and specializes in the cutting-edge, minimally invasive anterior total hip replacement technique.

The Orthopaedic Immediate Care Center ("i-Care"), New York City's only walk-in orthopaedic clinic, uses state-of-the-art diagnostic equipment to evaluate and treat hand and foot injuries, hip, arm or leg fractures, dislocation or joint injury, sprains, and bone or joint infection.

The Joint Preservation Center (JPC) is dedicated to operative and non-operative treatment of joint problems, aiming to reduce symptoms, restore function and delay the onset of degenerative arthritis and potential need for an eventual joint replacement.

Joint Replacement Center physicians are experts in knee, hip and shoulder replacements, complex joint revisions, and minimally invasive surgeries, conducting 3,000+ procedures annually.

The Occupational and Industrial Orthopaedic Center (OIOC) provides clinical, educational, research and consulting services in the prevention and treatment of musculoskeletal injuries and disorders that arise from work or the work environment.

The Spine Center specializes in spine disorders, including lower back and neck pain, scoliosis, osteoporosis and complex spine problems. The Center performs minimally invasive spinal fusions and was one of the first in the country to successfully perform artificial disc implantation.

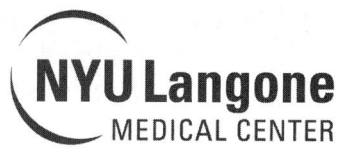

HOSPITAL FOR JOINT DISEASES

About the Hospital for Joint Diseases

The Hospital for Joint Diseases at NYU Langone Medical Center (HJD) is one of the nation's leading inpatient orthopaedic and rheumatologic specialty hospitals, and is ranked among the nation's top 10 for both orthopaedics and rheumatology in the 2011-2012 U.S. News & World Report annual survey of "Best Hospitals" in America. HJD is dedicated to the prevention and treatment of musculoskeletal diseases, providing some of the most advanced programs in the region for musculoskeletal disorders and the largest pediatric orthopaedic program in New York City. HJD also offers a number of unique and highly specialized services to provide tailored, world-class care to patients with specific musculoskeletal conditions and needs. We specialize in the following areas:

Orthopaedic Surgery

The clinical expertise of HJD's internationally-renowned surgeons represents all subspecialty areas of orthopaedic surgery, including Adult Reconstructive, Sports Medicine, Spine, Shoulder & Elbow, Foot & Ankle, Hand Surgery, Trauma & Fracture, Orthopaedic Oncology, and Pediatric Orthopaedics; additional areas of focus include minimally-invasive hip surgery and robotic-assisted joint replacement.

Rheumatology

HJD is devoted to the care of patients with clinical problems involving joints, soft tissues and the combined conditions of connective tissues. Conditions treated include osteoarthritis, rheumatoid and psoriatic arthritis, lupus, fibromyalgia and vasculitis.

Neurology – Spine & Nerve

HJD provides a broad range of diagnostic and therapeutic services to patients with neurological disorders. Its outstanding clinical staff includes specialists in pain management, spine and nerve pain, and cerebral palsy.

Radiology

HJD provides complete inpatient and outpatient diagnostic orthopaedic radiology services, including MRI, computed tomography, ultrasonography and conventional radiography, as well as a multitude of musculoskeletal interventional procedures. Neurointerventional specialists also perform the highly effective vertebroplasty (a new medical spinal repair procedure) for treatment of osteoporotic compression fractures. The medical team includes several internationally-known musculoskeletal radiologists with expertise in all aspects of osteoradiology.

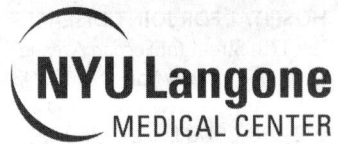

550 First Avenue *(at 31st Street)*
New York, NY 10016

www.NYULMC.org

Children's Services Access Line: **855-NYU-KIDS**

PEDIATRIC ORTHOPAEDIC SURGERY

Pediatric Orthopaedics is part of the Hassenfeld Pediatric Center, a full service specialty Children's Hospital, which supports the array of children's health services across the Medical Center where newborns, children, adolescents and young adults receive the most comprehensive and advanced care by a team of pediatricians and pediatric specialists.

From common injuries to the most complex congenital disorders, NYU Langone's pediatric orthopaedic service, based at the Hospital for Joint Diseases (HJD), is one of the most extensive orthopaedic programs for children in the country and is a renowned multidisciplinary center featuring a strong collaborative approach to care. Areas of specialization include scoliosis, limb deformities, hip dysplasia, cerebral palsy, congenital insensitivity to pain, arthrogryposis, sports injuries, anterior cruciate ligament injuries, bone tumors, juvenile idiopathic arthritis, Charcot-Marie-Tooth disease, and brachial plexus injuries.

Specialized Orthopaedic Services
The Center for Children at HJD is a full-service pediatric outpatient facility that offers multidisciplinary management of pediatric musculoskeletal and neuromuscular disorders and brings together outstanding board-certified pediatric specialists in orthopaedic surgery, rheumatology, genetics, neurology, rehabilitation and pediatrics.

The Orthopaedic Immediate Care Center (i-Care), New York City's only walk-in orthopaedic clinic, uses state-of-the-art diagnostic equipment to evaluate and treat urgent orthopaedic injuries, such as fractures, dislocation or joint injury, sprains, and bone or joint infection.

The Ambulatory Care Clinic is available for convenient, streamlined treatment of both children and adults. A team of pediatric hospitalists evaluates patients with multiple medical problems prior to surgery, and helps to manage their postoperative care.

Nationally Recognized Surgical Care
The Wallace B. Lehman, MD Center for Pediatric Orthopaedic Surgery at HJD is at the forefront of specialized surgery and personalized care for children. The Center is proud to be the largest teaching program in the country to offer a pediatric orthopaedic surgical residency, as well as fellowship training. It is also a recognized leader in surgical innovation and advanced technology, which helps ensure that patients receive the best possible care.

Convenient Satellite Sites
Satellite locations in the outlying areas of Westchester, Long Island, Rockland and New Jersey provide added convenience for parents seeking top orthopaedic care for their children within their own communities.

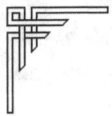

The Best in American Medicine
www.CastleConnolly.com

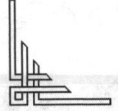
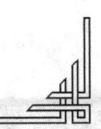

Otolaryngology

An otolaryngologist-head and neck surgeon provides comprehensive medical and surgical care for patients with diseases and disorders that affect the ears, nose, throat, the respiratory and upper alimentary systems and related structures of the head and neck.

An otolaryngologist diagnoses and provides medical and/or surgical therapy or prevention of diseases, allergies, neoplasms, deformities, disorders and/or injuries of the ears, nose, sinuses, throat, respiratory and upper alimentary systems, face, jaws and the other head and neck systems. Head and neck oncology, facial plastic and reconstructive surgery and the treatment of disorders of hearing and voice are fundamental areas of expertise.

Training Required: Five years

Certification in the following subspecialty requires additional training and examination.

Plastic Surgery within the Head and Neck: An otolaryngologist with additional training in plastic and reconstructive procedures within the head, face, neck and associated structures, including cutaneous head and neck oncology and reconstruction, management of maxillofacial trauma, soft tissue repair and neural surgery.

Facial Plastic and Reconstructive Surgery is not a recognized ABMS subspecialty. However this designation has been included because the certification process is meaningful and rigorous. It is awarded to those doctors who hold a current ABMS certification in Otolaryngology, but those board certified in Plastic Surgery, Ophthalmology, or Dermatology are also eligible. Certification requires a post-graduate fellowship in Facial Plastic and Reconstructive Surgery followed by a written examination.

This field is diverse and involves a wide age range of patients, from the newborn to the aged. While both cosmetic and reconstructive surgeries are practiced, there are many additional procedures which interface with them.

OTOLARYNGOLOGY

New England

Bhattacharyya, Neil MD [Oto] - **Spec Exp:** Head & Neck Surgery; **Hospital:** Brigham and Women's Hosp (page 57), Dana-Farber Cancer Inst (page 57); **Address:** Brigham and Women's Hosp, 45 Francis St Fl 2, Boston, MA 02115; **Phone:** 617-525-6540; **Board Cert:** Otolaryngology 1998; **Med School:** Univ IL Coll Med 1992; **Resid:** Otolaryngology, Mass Eye & Ear Infirm 1997; **Fac Appt:** Assoc Prof Oto, Harvard Med Sch

Burns, James A MD [Oto] - **Spec Exp:** Laryngeal & Vocal Cord Surgery; Laryngeal & Tracheal Disorders; Voice Disorders; **Hospital:** Mass Genl Hosp; **Address:** Ctr for Laryngeal Surgery, One Bowdoin Square Fl 11, BS01-11, Boston, MA 02114; **Phone:** 617-726-1444; **Board Cert:** Otolaryngology 1997; **Med School:** Univ VA Sch Med 1991; **Resid:** Otolaryngology, Univ Virginia Affil Hosp 1996; **Fellow:** Laryngology, Mass Eye & Ear Infirmary 2003

Couch, Marion E MD [Oto] - **Spec Exp:** Head & Neck Cancer; Thyroid & Parathyroid Cancer & Surgery; Microvascular Surgery; Airway Reconstruction; **Hospital:** Fletcher Allen Health Care- Med Ctr Campus; **Address:** 111 Colchester Ave, Div Otolaryngology, Burlington, VT 05401; **Phone:** 802-847-4537; **Board Cert:** Otolaryngology 1997; **Med School:** Rush Med Coll 1990; **Resid:** Surgery, Johns Hopkins Hosp 1991; Otolaryngology, Johns Hopkins Hosp 1995; **Fac Appt:** Assoc Prof Oto, Univ VT Coll Med

Deschler, Daniel G MD [Oto] - **Spec Exp:** Head & Neck Cancer; Head & Neck Reconstruction; Salivary Gland Tumors & Surgery; Voice after Laryngeal Cancer Surgery; **Hospital:** Mass Eye & Ear Infirmary, Mass Genl Hosp; **Address:** Mass Eye & Ear Infirmary, Head & Neck Surgery, 243 Charles St, Boston, MA 02114; **Phone:** 617-573-4100; **Board Cert:** Otolaryngology 1996; **Med School:** Harvard Med Sch 1990; **Resid:** Otolaryngology, UCSF Med Ctr 1995; **Fellow:** Head & Neck Surgical Oncology, Hahneman Univ Med Ctr 1996; **Fac Appt:** Assoc Prof Oto, Harvard Med Sch

Gliklich, Richard E MD [Oto] - **Spec Exp:** Cosmetic Surgery-Face & Neck; Rhinoplasty; Skin Laser Surgery-Resurfacing; **Hospital:** Mass Eye & Ear Infirmary; **Address:** Mass Eye & Ear Infirmary, 243 Charles St Fl 9, Boston, MA 02114; **Phone:** 617-573-4105; **Board Cert:** Otolaryngology 1994; Facial Plastic & Reconstr Surgery 1996; **Med School:** Harvard Med Sch 1988; **Resid:** Otolaryngology, Mass E&E Infirm 1993; **Fellow:** Facial Plastic Surgery, Harvard Univ 1994; **Fac Appt:** Prof Oto, Harvard Med Sch

Gosselin, Benoit J MD [Oto] - **Spec Exp:** Head & Neck Cancer; Facial Plastic & Reconstructive Surgery; Head & Neck Reconstruction; **Hospital:** Dartmouth - Hitchcock Med Ctr; **Address:** Dartmouth-Hitchcock Med Ctr, Dept Oto, 1 Med Ctr Drive, Lebanon, NH 03756; **Phone:** 603-650-8123; **Board Cert:** Otolaryngology 1994; **Med School:** Univ Ottawa 1988; **Resid:** Head and Neck Surgery, Univ Ottawa 1993; **Fellow:** Head and Neck Surgery, Univ Toronto 1994; Facial Plastic Surgery, Mercy Hosp 1995; **Fac Appt:** Assoc Clin Prof Oto, Dartmouth Med Sch

Grillone, Gregory A MD [Oto] - **Spec Exp:** Laryngeal Disorders; Laryngeal Cancer; Head & Neck Cancer; Voice Disorders; **Hospital:** Boston Med Ctr; **Address:** Boston Med Ctr, Dept Otolaryngology, 830 Harrison Ave, Moakley Bldg - Ste 1400, Boston, MA 02118; **Phone:** 617-414-4913; **Board Cert:** Otolaryngology 1988; **Med School:** Mount Sinai Sch Med 1983; **Resid:** Otolaryngology, Boston Univ Med Ctr 1988; **Fac Appt:** Assoc Prof Oto, Boston Univ

Otolaryngology

Grundfast, Kenneth M MD [Oto] - **Spec Exp:** Hearing Loss; Pediatric Otolaryngology; **Hospital:** Boston Med Ctr, VA Boston Hlthcare Sys-Jamaica Plain Div; **Address:** Boston Med Ctr, 830 Harrison Ave, Ste 1400, Boston, MA 02118; **Phone:** 617-638-8124; **Board Cert:** Otolaryngology 1977; **Med School:** SUNY Upstate Med Univ 1969; **Resid:** Surgery, Sibley Meml Hosp 1974; Otolaryngology, Boston-Affil Hosps 1977; **Fellow:** Pediatric Otolaryngology, Chldns Hosp 1978; **Fac Appt:** Prof Oto, Boston Univ

Hadlock, Theresa MD [Oto] - **Spec Exp:** Facial Paralysis; **Hospital:** Mass Eye & Ear Infirmary; **Address:** Mass Eye & Ear Infirm, Facial Plastic Surgery, 243 Charles St, Boston, MA 02114; **Phone:** 617-573-3641; **Board Cert:** Otolaryngology 2002; **Med School:** Harvard Med Sch 1994; **Resid:** Otolaryngology, Mass Eye & Ear Infirm 1998; **Fellow:** Facial Plastic Surgery, Mass Eye & Ear Infirm 1999; **Fac Appt:** Asst Prof Oto, Harvard Med Sch

Kveton, John MD [Oto] - **Spec Exp:** Ear Disorders/Surgery; Cochlear Implants; Acoustic Neuroma; Hearing Loss; **Hospital:** Yale-New Haven Hosp; **Address:** 46 Prince St, Ste 601, New Haven, CT 06519-1634; **Phone:** 203-752-1726; **Board Cert:** Otolaryngology 1982; Neurotology 2004; **Med School:** St Louis Univ 1978; **Resid:** Otolaryngology, Yale-New Haven Hosp 1982; **Fellow:** Neurotology, The Otology Group 1983; **Fac Appt:** Clin Prof Oto, Yale Univ

McKenna, Michael J MD [Oto] - **Spec Exp:** Skull Base Surgery; Otology; Neuro-Otology; **Hospital:** Mass Eye & Ear Infirmary; **Address:** Massachusetts Eye & Ear Infirm, 243 Charles St Fl 2, Boston, MA 02114-3002; **Phone:** 617-573-3672; **Board Cert:** Otolaryngology 1988; Neurotology 2004; **Med School:** USC Sch Med 1982; **Resid:** Otolaryngology, Mass Eye & Ear Infirm 1988; **Fellow:** Neurotology, Otologic Med Grp 1989; **Fac Appt:** Prof Oto, Harvard Med Sch

Metson, Ralph MD [Oto] - **Spec Exp:** Sinus Disorders/Surgery; **Hospital:** Mass Eye & Ear Infirmary; **Address:** Zero Emerson Pl, Ste 2D, Boston, MA 02114; **Phone:** 617-227-4366; **Board Cert:** Otolaryngology 1985; **Med School:** UCSD 1979; **Resid:** Otolaryngology, UCLA Med Ctr 1985; **Fac Appt:** Assoc Clin Prof Oto, Harvard Med Sch

Randolph, Gregory W MD [Oto] - **Spec Exp:** Thyroid Disorders; Thyroid Cancer; Parathyroid Disease; **Hospital:** Mass Eye & Ear Infirmary; **Address:** Mass Eye & Ear Infirmary, 243 Charles St Fl 2, Boston, MA 02114; **Phone:** 617-573-4115; **Board Cert:** Otolaryngology 1993; **Med School:** Cornell Univ-Weill Med Coll 1987; **Resid:** Otolaryngology, Mass E&E Infirmary 1992; **Fellow:** Thyroid Oncology, Mass E&E Infirmary 1993; **Fac Appt:** Asst Prof Oto, Harvard Med Sch

Rauch, Steven D MD [Oto] - **Spec Exp:** Hearing & Balance Disorders; Meniere's Disease; Neuro-Otology; **Hospital:** Mass Eye & Ear Infirmary; **Address:** Mass Eye & Ear Infirm Dept Otolary, 243 Charles St, Boston, MA 02114; **Phone:** 617-573-3644; **Board Cert:** Otolaryngology 1984; **Med School:** Univ Cincinnati 1979; **Resid:** Surgery, U Mass Med Ctr 1981; Otolaryngology, Mass Eye & Ear Infirm 1984; **Fac Appt:** Assoc Prof Oto, Harvard Med Sch

Rebeiz, Elie E MD [Oto] - **Spec Exp:** Head & Neck Surgery; Sinus Disorders/Surgery; Skull Base Surgery; **Hospital:** Tufts Med Ctr; **Address:** Tufts Med Ctr, Dept Otolaryngology, 750 Washington St, Boston, MA 02111; **Phone:** 617-636-1664; **Board Cert:** Otolaryngology 2000; **Med School:** Lebanon 1984; **Resid:** Otolaryngology, Amer Univ Med Ctr 1988; **Fellow:** Otolaryngology, Mass E&E Infirm 1990; **Fac Appt:** Prof Oto, Tufts Univ

Sasaki, Clarence T MD [Oto] - **Spec Exp:** Head & Neck Cancer; Skull Base Surgery; Voice Disorders; Zenker Diverticulum; **Hospital:** Yale-New Haven Hosp, Yale Med Group; **Address:** Yale Sch Med, Dept Otolaryngology, 333 Cedar St, Box 208041, New Haven, CT 06520-8041; **Phone:** 203-785-2592; **Board Cert:** Otolaryngology 1973; **Med School:** Yale Univ 1966; **Resid:** Surgery, Mary Hitchcock Hosp 1968; Otolaryngology, Yale-New Haven Hosp 1973; **Fellow:** Head and Neck Surgery, Univ of Milan 1978; Skull Base Surgery, Univ Zurich 1982; **Fac Appt:** Prof Oto, Yale Univ

Silverman, Damon A MD [Oto] - **Spec Exp:** Head & Neck Cancer & Surgery; Voice Disorders; Throat Disorders; **Hospital:** Fletcher Allen Health Care- Med Ctr Campus; **Address:** Fletcher Allen Otolaryngology, West Pavilion, Level 4, Med Ctr Campus, 111 Colchester Ave, MS 210WP4, Burlington, VT 05401; **Phone:** 802-847-4041; **Board Cert:** Otolaryngology 2004; **Med School:** UC Davis 1997; **Resid:** Otolaryngology, Cleveland Clinic 2003; **Fellow:** Laryngology, Vanderbilt Univ 2004; **Fac Appt:** Asst Prof Oto, Univ VT Coll Med

Vining, Eugenia M MD [Oto] - **Spec Exp:** Sinus Disorders/Surgery; Skull Base Tumors; Sinus Tumors; **Hospital:** Yale-New Haven Hosp; **Address:** 46 Prince St, Ste 601, New Haven, CT 06519; **Phone:** 203-752-1726; **Board Cert:** Otolaryngology 1993; **Med School:** Yale Univ 1987; **Resid:** Otolaryngology, Yale-New Haven Hosp 1991; Otolaryngology, Yale-New Haven Hosp 1992; **Fellow:** Sinus Surgery, Univ Penn 1993

Zeitels, Steven MD [Oto] - **Spec Exp:** Laryngeal Disorders; Voice Disorders; Laryngeal Cancer; Head & Neck Cancer & Surgery; **Hospital:** Mass Genl Hosp; **Address:** MGH Center for Laryngeal Surgery, 1 Bowdoin Square Fl 11, Boston, MA 02114; **Phone:** 617-726-0218; **Board Cert:** Otolaryngology 1988; **Med School:** Boston Univ 1982; **Resid:** Surgery, Univ Hosp-Boston City Hosp 1983; Otolaryngology, Boston Univ-Tufts Univ Affil Hosps 1987; **Fellow:** Head and Neck Surgery, Boston VA Med Ctr 1988; **Fac Appt:** Prof Oto, Harvard Med Sch

Mid Atlantic

Aviv, Jonathan MD [Oto] - **Spec Exp:** Voice Disorders; Swallowing Disorders; Cough; Endoscopy; **Hospital:** Mount Sinai Med Ctr (page 63); **Address:** 210 E 86th St Fl 9, New York, NY 10028; **Phone:** 212-722-5570; **Board Cert:** Otolaryngology 1990; **Med School:** Columbia P&S 1985; **Resid:** Surgery, Mt Sinai Med Ctr 1987; Otolaryngology, Mt Sinai Med Ctr 1990; **Fellow:** Otolaryngology, Mt Sinai Med Ctr 1991; **Fac Appt:** Prof Oto, Mount Sinai Sch Med

Blitzer, Andrew MD/DDS [Oto] - **Spec Exp:** Voice Disorders; Swallowing Disorders; Nasal & Sinus Surgery; Botox Therapy; **Hospital:** St. Luke's - Roosevelt Hosp Ctr - Roosevelt Div (page 55); **Address:** 425 W 59th St Fl 10, New York, NY 10019-1104; **Phone:** 212-262-9500; **Board Cert:** Otolaryngology 1977; **Med School:** Mount Sinai Sch Med 1973; **Resid:** Surgery, Beth Israel Med Ctr 1974; Otolaryngology, Mt Sinai Hosp 1977; **Fac Appt:** Clin Prof Oto, Columbia P&S

Califano III, Joseph A MD [Oto] - **Spec Exp:** Head & Neck Cancer; Thyroid Cancer; Skull Base Tumors; Melanoma; **Hospital:** Johns Hopkins Hosp (page 61), Greater Baltimore Med Ctr; **Address:** Johns Hopkins Hosp, 601 N Caroline St Fl 6th, Baltimore, MD 21287-0910; **Phone:** 410-502-2692; **Board Cert:** Otolaryngology 2000; **Med School:** Harvard Med Sch 1993; **Resid:** Otolaryngology, Johns Hopkins Hosp 1999; **Fellow:** Otolaryngology, Meml Sloan Kettering Cancer Ctr 2000; **Fac Appt:** Prof Oto, Johns Hopkins Univ

Carey, John P MD [Oto] - **Spec Exp:** Skull Base Surgery; Hearing Disorders; Neurotology; **Hospital:** Johns Hopkins Hosp (page 61); **Address:** John Hopkins Outpt Ctr, 601 N Caroline St, Baltimore, MD 21287; **Phone:** 410-955-1686; **Board Cert:** Otolaryngology 1999; Neurotology 2008; **Med School:** Univ Wash 1991; **Resid:** Internal Medicine, Univ Washington 1998; **Fellow:** Otolaryngology, John Hopkins Med Inst 1999; **Fac Appt:** Prof Oto, Johns Hopkins Univ

Chalian, Ara A MD [Oto] - **Spec Exp:** Head & Neck Cancer; Head & Neck Reconstruction; Thyroid Cancer; Reconstructive Surgery; **Hospital:** Hosp Univ Penn - UPHS (page 68); **Address:** Hosp Univ Penn, Dept Otolaryngology, 3400 Spruce St, 5 Silverstein Bldg, Philadelphia, PA 19104; **Phone:** 215-349-5559; **Board Cert:** Otolaryngology 1994; **Med School:** Indiana Univ 1988; **Resid:** Surgery, Indiana Univ Hosp 1990; Otolaryngology, Indiana Univ Hosp 1993; **Fellow:** Molecular Biology, Hosp U Penn 1994; Head and Neck Surgery, Hosp U Penn 1995; **Fac Appt:** Assoc Prof Oto, Univ Pennsylvania

Otolaryngology

Close, Lanny G MD [Oto] - **Spec Exp:** Skull Base Surgery; Head & Neck Cancer; Sinus Disorders/Surgery; Endoscopic Sinus Surgery; **Hospital:** NY-Presby/Columbia Univ Med Ctr, NY (page 65); **Address:** 16 E 60th St, Ste 470, New York, NY 10022; **Phone:** 212-326-8475; **Board Cert:** Otolaryngology 1977; **Med School:** Baylor Coll Med 1972; **Resid:** Surgery, Johns Hopkins Hosp 1974; Otolaryngology, Baylor Affil Hosps 1977; **Fellow:** Head and Neck Surgery, MD Anderson Cancer Ctr 1979; **Fac Appt:** Prof Oto, Columbia P&S

Costantino, Peter D MD [Oto] - **Spec Exp:** Skull Base Tumors; Head & Neck Cancer; Craniofacial Surgery/Reconstruction; **Hospital:** Lenox Hill Hosp, NY-Presby/Columbia Univ Med Ctr, NY (page 65); **Address:** New York Head & Neck Inst, 110 E 59th St, Ste 10A, New York, NY 10022; **Phone:** 212-434-4500; **Board Cert:** Otolaryngology 1990; Facial Plastic & Reconstr Surgery 2000; **Med School:** Northwestern Univ 1984; **Resid:** Surgery, Northwestern Meml Hosp 1986; Otolaryngology, Northwestern Meml Hosp 1989; **Fellow:** Head and Neck Surgery, Northwestern Meml Hosp 1990; Skull Base Surgery, Univ Pittsburgh 1991; **Fac Appt:** Prof Oto, Columbia P&S

Davidson, Bruce J MD [Oto] - **Spec Exp:** Head & Neck Cancer; Thyroid Disorders; **Hospital:** Georgetown Univ Hosp; **Address:** Georgetown Univ Med Ctr, Dept Otolaryngology-Head & Neck Surgery, 3800 Reservoir Rd NW, Gorman Bldg - Fl 1, Washington, DC 20007; **Phone:** 202-444-1351; **Board Cert:** Otolaryngology 1993; **Med School:** W VA Univ 1987; **Resid:** Otolaryngology, Georgetown Univ Med Ctr 1992; **Fellow:** Head and Neck Surgery, Memorial Sloan-Kettering Cancer Ctr 1994; **Fac Appt:** Asst Prof Oto, Georgetown Univ

Edelstein, David R MD [Oto] - **Spec Exp:** Endoscopic Sinus Surgery; Nasal Reconstruction; Rhinoplasty; Sleep Disorders/Apnea; **Hospital:** Lenox Hill Hosp (Manh Eye, Ear & Throat Hosp), Lenox Hill Hosp; **Address:** 1421 3rd Ave Fl 4, New York, NY 10028; **Phone:** 212-452-1500; **Board Cert:** Otolaryngology 1985; **Med School:** Boston Univ 1980; **Resid:** Otolaryngology, Mount Sinai Hosp 1984; **Fac Appt:** Clin Prof Oto, Cornell Univ-Weill Med Coll

Feghali, Joseph G MD [Oto] - **Spec Exp:** Ear Disorders/Surgery; Acoustic Neuroma; Hearing Disorders; Neuro-Otology; **Hospital:** Montefiore Med Ctr - Div. Moses; **Address:** 182 E 210th St, Bronx, NY 10467; **Phone:** 718-881-3277; **Board Cert:** Otolaryngology 1990; **Med School:** Lebanon 1978; **Resid:** Otolaryngology, American Univ Beirut 1982; Otolaryngology, Montefiore Med Ctr 1990; **Fellow:** Otology & Neurotology, House Ear Inst 1983; Neurological Surgery, Meml Sloan Kettering Cancer Ctr 1984; **Fac Appt:** Clin Prof Oto, Albert Einstein Coll Med

Ferris, Robert L MD/PhD [Oto] - **Spec Exp:** Head & Neck Cancer; Thyroid & Parathyroid Cancer & Surgery; **Hospital:** UPMC Presby, Pittsburgh; **Address:** 200 Lothrop St, Ste 500, Pittsburgh, PA 15213; **Phone:** 412-647-7110; **Board Cert:** Otolaryngology 2002; **Med School:** Johns Hopkins Univ 1995; **Resid:** Otolaryngology, Johns Hopkins Univ Hosp 2001; **Fac Appt:** Assoc Prof Oto, Univ Pittsburgh

Fried, Marvin P MD [Oto] - **Spec Exp:** Endoscopic Sinus Surgery; Head & Neck Tumors; Laryngeal & Voice Disorders; Sinus Disorders/Surgery; **Hospital:** Montefiore Med Ctr - Div. Moses, Montefiore Med Ctr - Div. Weiler; **Address:** 3400 Bainbridge Ave Fl 3, Bronx, NY 10467; **Phone:** 718-920-4646; **Board Cert:** Otolaryngology 1975; **Med School:** Tufts Univ 1969; **Resid:** Surgery, Jewish Hosp 1971; Otolaryngology, Barnes Hosp 1975; **Fellow:** Stroke, Washington Univ 1976; **Fac Appt:** Prof Oto, Albert Einstein Coll Med

Genden, Eric M MD [Oto] - **Spec Exp:** Head & Neck Cancer & Surgery; Head & Neck Cancer Reconstruction; Airway Reconstruction; Thyroid & Parathyroid Cancer & Surgery; **Hospital:** Mount Sinai Med Ctr (page 63); **Address:** Mt Sinai Dept Otolaryngology, 1 Gustave L Levy Pl, Box 1191, New York, NY 10029; **Phone:** 212-241-9410; **Board Cert:** Otolaryngology 1999; Facial Plastic & Reconstr Surgery 2000; **Med School:** Mount Sinai Sch Med 1992; **Resid:** Otolaryngology, Barnes Jewish Hosp 1998; **Fellow:** Head and Neck Surgery, Mt Sinai Med Ctr 1999; **Fac Appt:** Assoc Prof Oto, Mount Sinai Sch Med

Gold, Scott D MD [Oto] - **Spec Exp:** Endoscopic Sinus Surgery; Sinus Disorders/Surgery; **Hospital:** Beth Israel Med Ctr - Petrie Division (page 55), Mount Sinai Med Ctr (page 63); **Address:** 36A E 36th St, Ste 200, New York, NY 10016-3401; **Phone:** 212-889-8575; **Board Cert:** Otolaryngology 1983; **Med School:** Mount Sinai Sch Med 1979; **Resid:** Otolaryngology, Mt Sinai Med Ctr 1983; **Fac Appt:** Asst Clin Prof Oto, Mount Sinai Sch Med

Goldenberg, David MD [Oto] - **Spec Exp:** Head & Neck Cancer & Surgery; Thyroid & Parathyroid Cancer & Surgery; Salivary Gland Tumors & Surgery; **Hospital:** Penn State Milton S Hershey Med Ctr; **Address:** Otolaryngology-Head and Neck Surgery, 500 University Drive, MC H091, Hershey, PA 17033-0850; **Phone:** 717-531-8945; **Med School:** Israel 1995; **Resid:** Otolaryngology, Rambam Med Ctr; **Fellow:** Head & Neck Surgical Oncology, Johns Hopkins Med Ctr; **Fac Appt:** Assoc Prof S

Grandis, Jennifer R MD [Oto] - **Spec Exp:** Head & Neck Cancer; **Hospital:** UPMC Presby, Pittsburgh, Magee-Womens Hosp - UPMC; **Address:** Univ Pittsburgh Med Ctr EELB, 200 Lothrop St Fl 3, Ear, Nose & Throat Dept, Pittsburgh, PA 15213; **Phone:** 412-647-2100; **Board Cert:** Otolaryngology 1994; **Med School:** Univ Pittsburgh 1987; **Resid:** Otolaryngology, Univ Pittsburgh Med Ctr 1993; **Fac Appt:** Prof Oto, Univ Pittsburgh

Hammerschlag, Paul E MD [Oto] - **Spec Exp:** Cochlear Implants; Hearing Loss; Meniere's Disease; Balance Disorders; **Hospital:** NYU Langone Med Ctr (page 66), New York Eye & Ear Infirm (page 64); **Address:** 650 First Ave, New York, NY 10016-3240; **Phone:** 212-889-2600; **Board Cert:** Otolaryngology 1978; **Med School:** Albert Einstein Coll Med 1972; **Resid:** Surgery, Virginia Mason Hosp 1974; Otolaryngology, Mass Eye & Ear Infirm 1978; **Fellow:** Otolaryngology, Mass Eye & Ear Infirm 1978; **Fac Appt:** Assoc Clin Prof Oto, NYU Sch Med

Har-El, Gady MD [Oto] - **Spec Exp:** Head & Neck Cancer; Thyroid & Parathyroid Surgery; Sinus Tumors; Skull Base Tumors; **Hospital:** Lenox Hill Hosp, Lenox Hill Hosp (Manh Eye, Ear & Throat Hosp); **Address:** 186 E 76th St Fl 2, New York, NY 10021; **Phone:** 212-434-2323; **Board Cert:** Otolaryngology 1992; **Med School:** Israel 1982; **Resid:** Otolaryngology, SUNY Downstate Med Ctr 1991; **Fac Appt:** Prof Oto, SUNY Hlth Sci Ctr

Hicks Jr, Wesley L MD/DDS [Oto] - **Spec Exp:** Head & Neck Cancer & Surgery; Reconstructive Surgery; **Hospital:** Roswell Park Cancer Inst; **Address:** Roswell Park Cancer Inst, Dept Head & Neck Surgery, Elm & Carlton Sts, Buffalo, NY 14263; **Phone:** 716-845-3158; **Board Cert:** Otolaryngology 1993; **Med School:** SUNY Buffalo 1984; **Resid:** Otolaryngology, Manhattan Eye Ear & Throat Hosp 1988; Otolaryngology, New York Hosp/Meml Sloan Kettering Cancer Ctr 1989; **Fellow:** Head and Neck Surgery, Stanford Univ Med Ctr 1990; **Fac Appt:** Prof Oto, SUNY Buffalo

Hirsch, Barry MD [Oto] - **Spec Exp:** Hearing Loss; Ear Infections; Ear Tumors; Skull Base Tumors; **Hospital:** UPMC Presby, Pittsburgh, UPMC St Margaret; **Address:** 200 Lothrop St Fl 3, Ear Nose Throat Inst, Dept Otolaryngology, Pittsburgh, PA 15213; **Phone:** 412-647-2100; **Board Cert:** Otolaryngology 1982; Neurotology 2005; **Med School:** Univ Pennsylvania 1977; **Resid:** Otolaryngology, Univ Pittsburgh Med Ctr 1982; **Fellow:** Neurotology, Univ Pittsburgh 1985; Neurotology, Univ Zurich 1986; **Fac Appt:** Prof Oto, Univ Pittsburgh

Hoffman, Ronald MD [Oto] - **Spec Exp:** Cochlear Implants; Balance Disorders; Ear Disorders/Surgery; **Hospital:** New York Eye & Ear Infirm (page 64); **Address:** 380 2nd Ave Fl 9, New York, NY 10010; **Phone:** 212-614-8388; **Board Cert:** Otolaryngology 1976; **Med School:** Jefferson Med Coll 1971; **Resid:** Otolaryngology, NYU Med Ctr 1976; **Fellow:** Otology & Neurotology, Lenox Hill Hosp 1977; **Fac Appt:** Prof Oto, Albert Einstein Coll Med

Otolaryngology

Holliday, Michael J MD [Oto] - **Spec Exp:** Neuro-Otology; Skull Base Surgery; Otology; **Hospital:** Johns Hopkins Hosp (page 61), Johns Hopkins Bayview Med Ctr (page 61); **Address:** Johns Hopkins Hosp-Otology Division, 601 N Caroline St Fl 6, Baltimore, MD 21287; **Phone:** 410-955-1686; **Board Cert:** Otolaryngology 1976; **Med School:** Marquette Sch Med 1969; **Resid:** Otolaryngology, Johns Hopkins Hosp 1976; **Fellow:** Neurotology, Univ Zurich 1979; **Fac Appt:** Assoc Prof Oto, Johns Hopkins Univ

Hopping, Steven B MD [Oto] - **Spec Exp:** Cosmetic Surgery-Face; Hair Restoration/Transplant; **Hospital:** G Washington Univ Hosp; **Address:** The Center for Cosmetic Surgery, 2311 M St NW, Ste 503, Washington, DC 20037; **Phone:** 202-785-3175; **Board Cert:** Otolaryngology 1980; Facial Plastic & Reconstr Surgery 1986; Hair Restoration Surgery 1990; **Med School:** Univ Cincinnati 1975; **Resid:** Surgery, George Washington Hosp 1977; Otolaryngology, Maa E&E Infirmary 1980; **Fellow:** Plastic Surgery, Mass E&E Infirmary 1981; **Fac Appt:** Clin Prof S, Geo Wash Univ

Hurst, Michael K MD/DDS [Oto] - **Spec Exp:** Nasal Allergy; Sleep Disorders/Apnea; Thyroid Surgery; **Hospital:** Ruby Memorial - WVU Hosp, Monongalia Genl Hosp; **Address:** 1188 Pineview Drive, Morgantown, WV 26505; **Phone:** 304-599-3959; **Board Cert:** Otolaryngology 1994; **Med School:** Marshall Univ 1988; **Resid:** Otolaryngology, Univ West Virginia Hosps 1993; Head and Neck Surgery, Univ West Virginia Hosps 1993; **Fac Appt:** Assoc Prof Oto, W VA Univ

Jacobs, Joseph B MD [Oto] - **Spec Exp:** Endoscopic Sinus Surgery; Sinus Disorders/Surgery; Sinus Surgery-Revision; **Hospital:** NYU Langone Med Ctr (page 66); **Address:** NYU Med Ctr, 530 1st Ave, Ste 3C, New York, NY 10016-6402; **Phone:** 212-263-7398; **Board Cert:** Otolaryngology 1978; **Med School:** Albert Einstein Coll Med 1974; **Resid:** Otolaryngology, NYU Med Ctr 1978; **Fellow:** Plastic/Reconstructive Surgery, UCLA Med Ctr 1979; **Fac Appt:** Prof Oto, NYU Sch Med

Johnson, Jonas T MD [Oto] - **Spec Exp:** Head & Neck Surgery; Head & Neck Cancer; Sleep Disorders/Apnea/Snoring; Parotid Gland Tumors; **Hospital:** UPMC Montefiore, Magee-Womens Hosp - UPMC; **Address:** Univ Physicians UPMC, Eye & Ear Inst, 200 Lothrop St, Ste 300, Pittsburgh, PA 15213; **Phone:** 412-647-2100; **Board Cert:** Otolaryngology 1977; **Med School:** SUNY Upstate Med Univ 1972; **Resid:** Surgery, Med Coll Virginia Hosps 1974; Otolaryngology, SUNY-Univ Hosp 1977; **Fac Appt:** Prof Oto, Univ Pittsburgh

Josephson, Jordan S MD [Oto] - **Spec Exp:** Rhinoplasty Revision; Endoscopic Sinus Surgery; Nasal & Sinus Disorders; Sleep Apnea; **Hospital:** Lenox Hill Hosp (Manh Eye, Ear & Throat Hosp), Lenox Hill Hosp; **Address:** 205 E 76th St, Ste M1, New York, NY 10021; **Phone:** 212-717-1773; **Board Cert:** Otolaryngology 1988; **Med School:** SUNY Downstate 1983; **Resid:** Otolaryngology, LI Jewish Med Ctr 1988; **Fellow:** Sinus Surgery, Johns Hopkins Hosp 1989

Keane, William M MD [Oto] - **Spec Exp:** Head & Neck Cancer & Surgery; Thyroid Cancer; **Hospital:** Thomas Jefferson Univ Hosp; **Address:** Thomas Jefferson Hosp, 925 Chestnut St Fl 6, Philadelphia, PA 19107; **Phone:** 215-955-6760; **Board Cert:** Otolaryngology 1978; **Med School:** Harvard Med Sch 1970; **Resid:** Surgery, Strong Meml Hosp 1972; Otolaryngology, Univ Penn Hosp 1977; **Fac Appt:** Prof Oto, Thomas Jefferson Univ

Kennedy, David W MD [Oto] - **Spec Exp:** Sinus Disorders/Surgery; Skull Base Tumors & Surgery; Minimally Invasive Surgery; Esthesioneuroblastoma; **Hospital:** Hosp Univ Penn - UPHS (page 68), Pennsylvania Hosp-UPHS (page 68); **Address:** 3400 Spruce St, Ravdin Bldg Fl 5, Philadelphia, PA 19104-4229; **Phone:** 215-662-6971; **Board Cert:** Otolaryngology 1978; **Med School:** Ireland 1972; **Resid:** Surgery, Johns Hopkins Hosp 1974; Otolaryngology, Johns Hopkins Hosp 1978; **Fac Appt:** Prof Oto, Univ Pennsylvania

Koch, Wayne Martin MD [Oto] - **Spec Exp:** Head & Neck Cancer; Sinus Tumors; **Hospital:** Johns Hopkins Hosp (page 61); **Address:** Johns Hopkins Hosp, Dept Otolaryngology, 601 N Caroline St, rm 6221, Baltimore, MD 21287; **Phone:** 410-955-1686; **Board Cert:** Otolaryngology 1987; **Med School:** Univ Pittsburgh 1982; **Resid:** Otolaryngology, Tufts-Boston Univ Hosps 1987; **Fellow:** Surgical Oncology, Johns Hopkins Hosp 1989; **Fac Appt:** Assoc Prof Oto, Johns Hopkins Univ

Koufman, Jamie A MD [Oto] - **Spec Exp:** Voice Disorders; Laryngeal Disorders; **Hospital:** New York Eye & Ear Infirm (page 64); **Address:** 200 W 57th St, Ste 1203, New York, NY 10019; **Phone:** 212-463-8014; **Board Cert:** Otolaryngology 1978; **Med School:** Boston Univ 1973; **Resid:** Surgery, Hartford Hosp 1975; Otolaryngology, Boston Univ Med Ctr 1978

Kraus, Dennis H MD [Oto] - **Spec Exp:** Head & Neck Cancer; Skull Base Tumors; Thyroid & Parathyroid Surgery; **Hospital:** Meml Sloan-Kettering Cancer Ctr; **Address:** 1275 York Ave, Box 285, New York, NY 10065; **Phone:** 212-639-5621; **Board Cert:** Otolaryngology 1990; **Med School:** Univ Rochester 1985; **Resid:** Surgery, Cleveland Clinic 1987; Otolaryngology, Cleveland Clinic 1990; **Fellow:** Head and Neck Surgery, Meml Sloan Kettering Cancer Ctr 1991; **Fac Appt:** Prof Oto, Cornell Univ-Weill Med Coll

Krespi, Yosef P MD [Oto] - **Spec Exp:** Nasal & Sinus Cancer & Surgery; Sleep Disorders/Apnea; Head & Neck Cancer & Surgery; Snoring/Sleep Apnea; **Hospital:** Lenox Hill Hosp (Manh Eye, Ear & Throat Hosp), St. Luke's - Roosevelt Hosp Ctr - Roosevelt Div (page 55); **Address:** 425 W 59th St, Fl 10, New York, NY 10019-1128; **Phone:** 212-262-2929; **Board Cert:** Otolaryngology 1981; **Med School:** Israel 1973; **Resid:** Surgery, Mt Sinai Hosp 1976; Otolaryngology, Mt Sinai Hosp 1980; **Fellow:** Surgery, Northwestern Meml Hosp 1981; **Fac Appt:** Clin Prof Oto, Columbia P&S

Kuhel, William I MD [Oto] - **Spec Exp:** Head & Neck Cancer & Surgery; Thyroid Cancer; Parathyroid Cancer; **Hospital:** NY-Presby/Weill Cornell Med Ctr, NY (page 65); **Address:** 1305 York Ave Fl 5, New York, NY 10021; **Phone:** 646-962-6325; **Board Cert:** Otolaryngology 1988; **Med School:** Univ Mich Med Sch 1983; **Resid:** Surgery, St Vincent's Hosp 1985; Otolaryngology, Indiana Univ 1988; **Fellow:** Head and Neck Surgery, MD Anderson Cancer Ctr 1989; **Fac Appt:** Assoc Clin Prof Oto, Cornell Univ-Weill Med Coll

Lalwani, Anil K MD [Oto] - **Spec Exp:** Ear Disorders/Surgery; Facial Nerve Disorders; Pediatric Otolaryngology; Skull Base Surgery; **Hospital:** NYU Langone Med Ctr (page 66); **Address:** 550 First Ave, Ste 7Q, New York, NY 10016; **Phone:** 212-263-7167; **Board Cert:** Otolaryngology 1992; Neurotology 2010; **Med School:** Univ Mich Med Sch 1985; **Resid:** Surgery, Duke Univ Med Ctr 1987; Otolaryngology, UCSF Med Ctr 1991; **Fellow:** Skull Base Surgery, UCSF Med Ctr 1992; **Fac Appt:** Prof Oto, NYU Sch Med

Lawson, William MD [Oto] - **Spec Exp:** Nasal & Sinus Cancer & Surgery; Head & Neck Cancer; Skull Base Surgery; Head & Neck Inflammatory Disorders; **Hospital:** Mount Sinai Med Ctr (page 63); **Address:** 5 E 98th St Fl 8, Box 1191, New York, NY 10029-6501; **Phone:** 212-241-9410; **Board Cert:** Otolaryngology 1974; **Med School:** NYU Sch Med 1965; **Resid:** Surgery, Bronx VA Hosp 1967; Otolaryngology, Mt Sinai Hosp 1973; **Fellow:** Otolaryngology, Mt Sinai Hosp 1970; **Fac Appt:** Prof Oto, Mount Sinai Sch Med

Lebovics, Robert S MD [Oto] - **Spec Exp:** Head & Neck Inflammatory Disorders; Head & Neck Autoimmune Disease; Head & Neck Infectious Disease; Relapsing Polychondritis; **Hospital:** St. Luke's - Roosevelt Hosp Ctr - Roosevelt Div (page 55); **Address:** 425 W 59th St Fl 10, New York, NY 10019; **Phone:** 212-262-2002; **Board Cert:** Otolaryngology 1988; **Med School:** SUNY Downstate 1982; **Resid:** Surgery, Montefiore-Weiler Einstein Div 1983; Otolaryngology, Montefiore-Weiler Einstein Div 1987

Otolaryngology

Linstrom, Christopher MD [Oto] - **Spec Exp:** Cochlear Implants; Acoustic Neuroma; Encephalocele; Cholesteatoma; **Hospital:** New York Eye & Ear Infirm (page 64); **Address:** NY Eye & Ear Infirmary, Dept Otolaryngology, 310 E 14th St, New York, NY 10003-4201; **Phone:** 212-979-4200; **Board Cert:** Otolaryngology 1987; **Med School:** McGill Univ 1982; **Resid:** Surgery, Geo Wash Med Ctr 1984; Otolaryngology, NY Hosp 1987; **Fellow:** Otology & Neurotology, Michigan Ear Inst 1989; **Fac Appt:** Assoc Prof Oto, NY Med Coll

Newkirk, Kenneth Allen MD [Oto] - **Spec Exp:** Head & Neck Cancer; Sinus Disorders; **Hospital:** Georgetown Univ Hosp; **Address:** 3800 Reservoir Rd NW, Gorman Bldg, 1st Fl, rm G-104, Washington, DC 20007; **Phone:** 202-444-8186; **Board Cert:** Otolaryngology 2002; **Med School:** Mount Sinai Sch Med 1993; **Resid:** Otolaryngology, Lombardi Cancer Center 2000; **Fellow:** Otolaryngology, Lombardi Cancer Center 2003; Otolaryngology, MD Anderson Cancer Ctr 2005; **Fac Appt:** Asst Prof Oto, Georgetown Univ

Niparko, John MD [Oto] - **Spec Exp:** Ear Disorders/Surgery; Neuro-Otology; **Hospital:** Johns Hopkins Hosp (page 61); **Address:** Johns Hopkins Hosp, Dept Otolaryngology, 601 N Caroline St, rm 6223, Baltimore, MD 21287-0910; **Phone:** 410-955-2689; **Board Cert:** Otolaryngology 1986; Neurotology 2004; **Med School:** Univ Mich Med Sch 1980; **Resid:** Surgery, William Beaumont Hosp 1982; Otolaryngology, Univ Michigan Hosp 1986; **Fellow:** Otolaryngology, Univ Michigan Hosp; **Fac Appt:** Prof Oto, Johns Hopkins Univ

O'Malley Jr, Bert W MD [Oto] - **Spec Exp:** Head & Neck Cancer; Sinus Tumors; Skull Base Tumors; **Hospital:** Hosp Univ Penn - UPHS (page 68); **Address:** Hosp Univ Penn, Dept Otolaryngology, 3400 Spruce St, 5 Ravdin, Philadelphia, PA 19104; **Phone:** 215-615-4325; **Board Cert:** Otolaryngology 1995; **Med School:** Univ Tex SW, Dallas 1988; **Resid:** Surgery, UTSW Med Ctr/Parkland Meml Hosp 1989; Otolaryngology, Baylor Coll Med 1993; **Fellow:** Head & Neck Oncology, Univ Pittsburgh 1994; Skull Base Surgery, Univ Pittsburgh 1995; **Fac Appt:** Prof Oto, Univ Pennsylvania

Papel, Ira D MD [Oto] - **Spec Exp:** Rhinoplasty; Cosmetic Surgery-Face; Reconstructive Surgery-Face; Skin Cancer/Facial Reconstruction; **Hospital:** Greater Baltimore Med Ctr, Johns Hopkins Hosp (page 61); **Address:** 1838 Greene Tree Rd, Ste 370, Baltimore, MD 21208; **Phone:** 410-486-3400; **Board Cert:** Otolaryngology 1986; Facial Plastic & Reconstr Surgery 1991; **Med School:** Boston Univ 1981; **Resid:** Otolaryngology, Johns Hopkins Hosp 1986; **Fellow:** Facial Plastic Surgery, UCSF Med Ctr 1987; **Fac Appt:** Assoc Prof Oto, Johns Hopkins Univ

Parisier, Simon C MD [Oto] - **Spec Exp:** Cochlear Implants; Hearing Loss; Ear Disorders/Surgery; Cholesteatoma; **Hospital:** New York Eye & Ear Infirm (page 64); **Address:** NY Eye & Ear Infirmary - Otolaryngology, 380 2nd Ave Fl 9, New York, NY 10010; **Phone:** 212-979-4542; **Board Cert:** Otolaryngology 1967; **Med School:** Boston Univ 1961; **Resid:** Otolaryngology, Mount Sinai Hosp 1966; **Fac Appt:** Prof Oto, NY Med Coll

Persky, Mark S MD [Oto] - **Spec Exp:** Head & Neck Cancer; Skull Base Tumors; Thyroid Cancer; Vascular Lesions-Head & Neck; **Hospital:** Beth Israel Med Ctr - Petrie Division (page 55), New York Eye & Ear Infirm (page 64); **Address:** 10 Union Square East, Ste 4J, New York, NY 10003; **Phone:** 212-844-8648; **Board Cert:** Otolaryngology 1976; **Med School:** SUNY Upstate Med Univ 1972; **Resid:** Otolaryngology, Bellevue Hosp 1976; **Fellow:** Head and Neck Surgery, Beth Israel Med Ctr 1977; **Fac Appt:** Clin Prof Oto, Albert Einstein Coll Med

Picken, Catherine A MD [Oto] - **Spec Exp:** Head & Neck Reconstruction; Thyroid Disorders; Sinus Disorders/Surgery; **Hospital:** Georgetown Univ Hosp, Sibley Mem Hosp; **Address:** 2440 M St NW, Ste 620, Washington, DC 20037; **Phone:** 202-785-5000; **Board Cert:** Otolaryngology 1989; **Med School:** Northwestern Univ 1979; **Resid:** Surgery, Natl Heart Lung Blood Inst 1983; Otolaryngology, Georgetown Univ Hosp 1989; **Fac Appt:** Assoc Prof Oto, Georgetown Univ

Pribitkin, Edmund A MD [Oto] - **Spec Exp:** Rhinoplasty; Thyroid Disorders; Facial Plastic Surgery; **Hospital:** Thomas Jefferson Univ Hosp; **Address:** 925 Chestnut St Fl 6, Philadelphia, PA 19107; **Phone:** 215-955-6760; **Board Cert:** Otolaryngology 1992; **Med School:** Univ Pennsylvania 1986; **Resid:** Otolaryngology, Univ Penn Hosp 1991; **Fellow:** Facial Plastic & Reconstr Surgery, Stanford Univ Hosp 1992; **Fac Appt:** Assoc Prof Oto, Thomas Jefferson Univ

Quatela, Vito C MD [Oto] - **Spec Exp:** Facial Plastic Surgery; Rhinoplasty; Reconstructive Surgery; **Hospital:** Univ of Rochester Strong Meml Hosp, Rochester Genl Hosp; **Address:** 973 East Ave, Ste 100, Rochester, NY 14607; **Phone:** 585-244-1000; **Board Cert:** Otolaryngology 1985; Facial Plastic & Reconstr Surgery 1991; **Med School:** Northwestern Univ 1979; **Resid:** Surgery, Med Ctr Hosp Vermont 1981; Otolaryngology, Northwestern Univ Hosp 1985; **Fellow:** Facial Plastic Surgery, Tulane Univ 1986; Facial Plastic Surgery, Oregon Hlth Science Univ 1987; **Fac Appt:** Assoc Clin Prof Oto, Univ Rochester

Rassekh, Christopher MD [Oto] - **Spec Exp:** Laryngeal Cancer-Organ Preservation; Skull Base Tumors; Salivary Gland Tumors & Surgery; **Hospital:** Hosp Univ Penn - UPHS (page 68); **Address:** Hosp Univ Penn-Otorhinolaryngology, 5 Silverstein, Philadelphia, PA 19104; **Phone:** 215-662-2777; **Board Cert:** Otolaryngology 1993; **Med School:** Univ Iowa Coll Med 1986; **Resid:** Otolaryngology, Univ Iowa Med Ctr 1992; **Fellow:** Head and Neck Surgery, Univ Pittsburgh Med Ctr 1993; **Fac Appt:** Assoc Prof Oto, Univ Pennsylvania

Roland Sr, J Thomas MD [Oto] - **Spec Exp:** Acoustic Neuroma; Cochlear Implants; Neuro-Otology; Facial Nerve Disorders; **Hospital:** NYU Langone Med Ctr (page 66), Bellevue Hosp Ctr; **Address:** 550 First Avenue, Ste 7Q, New York, NY 10016; **Phone:** 212-263-5565; **Board Cert:** Otolaryngology 1993; Neurotology 2004; **Med School:** Temple Univ 1983; **Resid:** Otolaryngology, NYU Med Ctr 1992; **Fellow:** Neurotology, NYU Med Ctr 1993; **Fac Appt:** Assoc Prof Oto, NYU Sch Med

Rosen, Clark A MD [Oto] - **Spec Exp:** Voice Disorders; **Hospital:** UPMC Mercy, Pittsburgh, UPMC Presby, Pittsburgh; **Address:** UPMC The Voice Ctr, 1400 Locust St, D Bldg Fl 2 - Ste 2100, Pittsburgh, PA 15219; **Phone:** 412-232-7464; **Board Cert:** Otolaryngology 1995; **Med School:** Rush Med Coll 1989; **Resid:** Otolaryngology, Oregon Hlth Sci Univ 1994; **Fellow:** Otolaryngology, Univ Tenn Med Ctr 1995; **Fac Appt:** Prof Oto, Univ Pittsburgh

Sataloff, Robert T MD [Oto] - **Spec Exp:** Neuro-Otology; Voice Disorders; Laryngeal Disorders; Throat Disorders; **Hospital:** Hahnemann Univ Hosp, St. Christopher's Hosp for Chldn; **Address:** 1721 Pine Street, Philadelphia, PA 19103-6701; **Phone:** 215-545-3322; **Board Cert:** Otolaryngology 1980; **Med School:** Jefferson Med Coll 1975; **Resid:** Otolaryngology, Univ Mich Hosp 1980; **Fellow:** Neurotology, Univ Mich Hosp 1981; **Fac Appt:** Prof Oto, Drexel Univ Coll Med

Schaefer, Steven D MD [Oto] - **Spec Exp:** Sinus Disorders/Surgery; Head & Neck Surgery; Endoscopic Sinus Surgery; **Hospital:** Lenox Hill Hosp (Manh Eye, Ear & Throat Hosp), Beth Israel Med Ctr - Petrie Division (page 55); **Address:** 110 E 59th St, Ste 8C, New York, NY 10022; **Phone:** 212-434-4500; **Board Cert:** Otolaryngology 1978; **Med School:** UC Irvine 1972; **Resid:** Surgery, UCLA Med Ctr 1974; Otolaryngology, Stanford Med Ctr 1977; **Fac Appt:** Prof Oto, NY Med Coll

Schaitkin, Barry M MD [Oto] - **Spec Exp:** Sinus Disorders/Surgery; Endoscopic Sinus Surgery; Rhinosinusitis; **Hospital:** UPMC Shadyside; **Address:** Shadyside Medical Bldg, 5200 Centre Ave, Ste 211, Pittsburgh, PA 15232; **Phone:** 412-621-0123; **Board Cert:** Otolaryngology 1990; **Med School:** Penn State Coll Med 1984; **Resid:** Otolaryngology, Hershey Med Ctr 1990; **Fac Appt:** Assoc Prof Oto, Univ Pittsburgh

Otolaryngology

Schantz, Stimson P MD [Oto] - **Spec Exp:** Head & Neck Surgery; Head & Neck Cancer; Thyroid Cancer; **Hospital:** New York Eye & Ear Infirm (page 64), Beth Israel Med Ctr - Petrie Division (page 55); **Address:** 310 E 14th St Fl 6N, New YorkNew York, NY 10003; **Phone:** 212-979-4535; **Board Cert:** Surgery 2005; **Med School:** Univ Cincinnati 1975; **Resid:** Surgery, Georgetown Univ Med CtrGeorgetown Univ Med Ctr 1982; Otolaryngology, Univ Illinois Eye & Ear Infirm 1980; **Fellow:** Surgical Oncology, MD Anderson Cancer Ctr 1984; **Fac Appt:** Prof Oto, NY Med Coll

Schley, W Shain MD [Oto] - **Spec Exp:** Nasal & Sinus Disorders; Throat Disorders; Voice Disorders; Sleep Disorders; **Hospital:** NY-Presby/Weill Cornell Med Ctr, NY (page 65); **Address:** 449 E 68th St Fl 2 - Ste DS 10, New York, NY 10065; **Phone:** 212-746-2223; **Board Cert:** Otolaryngology 1973; **Med School:** Emory Univ 1966; **Resid:** Surgery, Roosevelt Hosp 1968; Otolaryngology, New York Hosp 1973; **Fac Appt:** Assoc Clin Prof Oto, Cornell Univ-Weill Med Coll

Setzen, Michael MD [Oto] - **Spec Exp:** Nasal & Sinus Surgery; Rhinoplasty; Sleep Disorders/Apnea; Snoring/Sleep Apnea; **Hospital:** N Shore Univ Hosp, St. Francis Hosp - The Heart Ctr (page 69); **Address:** 600 Northern Blvd, Ste 312, Great Neck, NY 11021-5200; **Phone:** 516-829-0045; **Board Cert:** Otolaryngology 1982; **Med School:** South Africa 1974; **Resid:** Surgery, Cleveland Clinic Fdn 1978; Otolaryngology, Barnes Jewish Hosp 1982; **Fac Appt:** Assoc Clin Prof Oto, NYU Sch Med

Shapshay, Stanley M MD [Oto] - **Spec Exp:** Laryngeal Cancer; Vocal Cord Disorders; Sleep Apnea; **Hospital:** Albany Med Ctr; **Address:** University Ear, Nose & Throat Ctr, 35 Hackett Blvd, Albany, NY 12208-3420; **Phone:** 518-262-5575; **Board Cert:** Otolaryngology 1975; **Med School:** Med Coll VA 1968; **Resid:** Surgery, New England Med Ctr 1971; Otolaryngology, Boston Med Ctr 1975; **Fellow:** Surgery, Serafimer Hosp/Karolinska Med Sch 1972; **Fac Appt:** Prof Oto, Albany Med Coll

Snyderman, Carl H MD [Oto] - **Spec Exp:** Skull Base Tumors & Surgery; Sinus Tumors; Head & Neck Cancer; Endoscopic Surgery; **Hospital:** UPMC Presby, Pittsburgh; **Address:** Eye Ear Inst, Dept of Otolaryngology, 200 Lothrop St, Ste 500, Pittsburgh, PA 15213; **Phone:** 412-647-8186; **Board Cert:** Otolaryngology 1987; **Med School:** Univ Chicago-Pritzker Sch Med 1982; **Resid:** Otolaryngology, Eye-Ear Hosp/Univ Pittsburgh 1987; **Fellow:** Skull Base Surgery, Eye-Ear Hosp/Univ Pittsburgh 1988; **Fac Appt:** Prof Oto, Univ Pittsburgh

Stewart, Michael G MD [Oto] - **Spec Exp:** Nasal & Sinus Disorders; Sleep Disorders/Apnea; Head & Neck Surgery; **Hospital:** NY-Presby/Weill Cornell Med Ctr, NY (page 65); **Address:** Weill Cornell Physicians, 1305 York Ave, New York, NY 10011; **Phone:** 646-962-6673; **Board Cert:** Otolaryngology 1995; **Med School:** Johns Hopkins Univ 1988; **Resid:** Otolaryngology, Baylor Coll Med 1994; **Fac Appt:** Prof Oto, Cornell Univ-Weill Med Coll

Strome, Marshall MD [Oto] - **Spec Exp:** Sleep Disorders/Apnea; Voice Disorders; Head & Neck Cancer; Swallowing Disorders; **Hospital:** St. Luke's - Roosevelt Hosp Ctr - St Luke's Hosp (page 55), Mount Sinai Med Ctr (page 63); **Address:** 110 E 59th St, Ste 10A, New York, NY 10022; **Phone:** 212-223-1333; **Board Cert:** Otolaryngology 1970; **Med School:** Univ Mich Med Sch 1964; **Resid:** Surgery, Harper Hosp 1966; Otolaryngology, Univ Michigan Hosp 1970; **Fac Appt:** Prof Oto

Strome, Scott E MD [Oto] - **Spec Exp:** Microsurgery; Head & Neck Cancer; Head & Neck Reconstruction; Laryngeal Cancer; **Hospital:** Univ of MD Med Ctr; **Address:** 16 S Eutaw St, Ste 500, Baltimore, MD 21201; **Phone:** 410-328-6467; **Board Cert:** Otolaryngology 1998; **Med School:** Harvard Med Sch 1991; **Resid:** Otolaryngology, Univ Michigan 1997; **Fellow:** Head and Neck Surgery, Allegheny Genl Hosp 1998; Microvascular Surgery, Allegheny Genl Hosp 1998; **Fac Appt:** Prof Oto, Univ MD Sch Med

Sulica, Radu Lucian MD [Oto] - **Spec Exp:** Laryngeal & Vocal Cord Surgery; Voice Disorders; Vocal Cord Disorders; Botox Therapy; **Hospital:** NY-Presby/Weill Cornell Med Ctr, NY (page 65); **Address:** Weill Cornell Otorhinolaryngology, 1305 York Ave Fl 5, New York, NY 10021; **Phone:** 646-962-4734; **Board Cert:** Otolaryngology 2000; **Med School:** Georgetown Univ 1993; **Resid:** Surgery, Georgetown Univ Hosp 1995; Otolaryngology, Georgetown Univ Hosp 1999; **Fellow:** Laryngology, St Lukes Roosevelt Hosp 2000; **Fac Appt:** Assoc Prof Oto, Cornell Univ-Weill Med Coll

Tufano, Ralph P MD [Oto] - **Spec Exp:** Thyroid Disorders; Parathyroid Disease; Head & Neck Cancer; **Hospital:** Johns Hopkins Hosp (page 61); **Address:** Johns Hopkins Hosp, Oto-Head & Neck Surg, 601 North Caroline St, Ste JHOC 6210, Baltimore, MD 21287; **Phone:** 410-955-3628; **Board Cert:** Otolaryngology 2001; **Med School:** SUNY Buffalo 1995; **Resid:** Otolaryngology, Univ Penn 2000; **Fellow:** Head and Neck Surgery, Johns Hopkins Hosp 2001; **Fac Appt:** Assoc Prof Oto, Johns Hopkins Univ

Urken, Mark MD [Oto] - **Spec Exp:** Head & Neck Cancer & Surgery; Head & Neck Cancer Reconstruction; Thyroid & Parathyroid Cancer & Surgery; Salivary Gland Tumors; **Hospital:** Beth Israel Med Ctr - Petrie Division (page 55); **Address:** Inst for Head, Neck & Thyroid Cancer, 10 Union Square E, Ste 5B, New York, NY 10003-3314; **Phone:** 212-844-8775; **Board Cert:** Otolaryngology 1986; **Med School:** Univ VA Sch Med 1981; **Resid:** Otolaryngology, Mt Sinai Hosp 1986; **Fellow:** Microvascular Surgery, Mercy Hosp 1987; **Fac Appt:** Prof Oto, Albert Einstein Coll Med

Waner, Milton MD [Oto] - **Spec Exp:** Pediatric Facial Plastic Surgery; Birthmarks/Hemangiomas; Vascular Malformations; **Hospital:** St. Luke's - Roosevelt Hosp Ctr - St Luke's Hosp (page 55), Beth Israel Med Ctr - Petrie Division (page 55); **Address:** Vascular Birthmark Institute, 126 W 60th St, New York, NY 10023; **Phone:** 212-636-3970; **Med School:** South Africa 1977; **Resid:** Surgery, Univ of Witwatersrand 1980; Otolaryngology, Univ of Witwatersrand 1984; **Fellow:** Otolaryngology, Univ Cincinnatti Med Ctr 1985

Weinstein, Gregory MD [Oto] - **Spec Exp:** Head & Neck Cancer; Laryngeal Cancer; **Hospital:** Hosp Univ Penn - UPHS (page 68); **Address:** Hosp Univ Penn, Dept Otolaryngology, 3400 Spruce St, 5 Ravdin, Philadelphia, PA 19104; **Phone:** 215-349-5390; **Board Cert:** Otolaryngology 1990; **Med School:** NY Med Coll 1985; **Resid:** Otolaryngology, Univ Iowa Hosp 1990; **Fellow:** Head & Neck Oncology, UC Davis Med Ctr 1991; **Fac Appt:** Prof Oto, Univ Pennsylvania

Woo, Peak MD [Oto] - **Spec Exp:** Voice Disorders; Laryngeal Disorders; Laryngeal Cancer; **Hospital:** Mount Sinai Med Ctr (page 63); **Address:** 300 Central Park West, Ste 1-H, New York, NY 10024; **Phone:** 212-580-1004; **Board Cert:** Otolaryngology 1983; **Med School:** Boston Univ 1978; **Resid:** Otolaryngology, Boston Univ Med Ctr 1983; **Fac Appt:** Clin Prof Oto, Mount Sinai Sch Med

Zalzal, George MD [Oto] - **Spec Exp:** Airway Disorders; Laryngeal & Tracheal Disorders; Ear Disorders/Surgery; **Hospital:** Chldns Natl Med Ctr; **Address:** Childrens Natl Med Ctr, Dept Otolaryngology, 111 Michigan Ave NW Fl 1 - Ste 1000, Washington, DC 20010; **Phone:** 202-476-2159; **Board Cert:** Otolaryngology 1996; **Med School:** Lebanon 1979; **Resid:** Otolaryngology, American Univ Hosp 1983; **Fellow:** Pediatric Otolaryngology, Univ Cincinnati 1985; **Fac Appt:** Prof Ped, Geo Wash Univ

Otolaryngology

Southeast

Balkany, Thomas J MD [Oto] - **Spec Exp:** Ear Disorders/Surgery; Neuro-Otology; Cochlear Implants; Hearing Loss; **Hospital:** Jackson Meml Hosp (page 70); **Address:** Univ Miami Dept Otolaryngology, PO Box 016960, Miami, FL 33101; **Phone:** 305-243-2000; **Board Cert:** Otolaryngology 1977; Neurotology 2004; **Med School:** Univ Miami Sch Med 1972; **Resid:** Surgery, St Joseph Hosp 1974; Otolaryngology, Colorado Med Ctr 1977; **Fellow:** Otology & Neurotology, House Ear Inst 1978; **Fac Appt:** Clin Prof Oto, Univ Miami Sch Med

Becker, Ferdinand F MD [Oto] - **Spec Exp:** Cosmetic Surgery-Face; **Hospital:** Indian River Med Ctr; **Address:** 5070 N A1A, Ste A, Vero Beach, FL 32963-1229; **Phone:** 772-234-3700; **Board Cert:** Otolaryngology 1972; **Med School:** Tulane Univ 1965; **Resid:** Surgery, Charity Hosp 1969; Otolaryngology, Charity Hosp 1972; **Fac Appt:** Asst Clin Prof Oto, Univ Fla Coll Med

Bolger, William E MD [Oto] - **Spec Exp:** Sinus Disorders/Surgery; **Hospital:** Mayo - Jacksonville; **Address:** Mayo Clinic, Otolaryngology Dept, 4500 San Pablo Rd, Jacksonville, FL 32224; **Phone:** 904-953-2217; **Board Cert:** Otolaryngology 1992; **Med School:** Uniformed Srvs Univ, Bethesda 1986; **Resid:** Otolaryngology, Willford Hall USAF Med Ctr 1991; **Fellow:** Rhinology, Hosp Univ Penn 1992; **Fac Appt:** Prof S, Uniformed Srvs Univ, Bethesda

Browne, J Dale MD [Oto] - **Spec Exp:** Head & Neck Cancer; Thyroid Cancer; Skull Base Surgery; Head & Neck Reconstruction; **Hospital:** Wake Forest Univ Baptist Med Ctr; **Address:** Wake Forest Baptist Med Ctr, Dept Otolaryngology, Medical Center Blvd, Winston Salem, NC 27103; **Phone:** 336-716-3854; **Board Cert:** Otolaryngology 1987; **Med School:** Med Coll GA 1982; **Resid:** Otolaryngology, NC Baptist Hosp 1987; **Fellow:** Otolaryngology, Univ Hosp 1991; **Fac Appt:** Prof Oto, Wake Forest Univ

Bumpous, Jeffrey MD [Oto] - **Spec Exp:** Head & Neck Cancer; Head & Neck Reconstruction; Thyroid & Parathyroid Cancer & Surgery; **Hospital:** Univ of Louisville Hosp, Norton Hosp; **Address:** 401 E Chestnut St, Ste 710, Louisville, KY 40202-1845; **Phone:** 502-583-8303; **Board Cert:** Otolaryngology 1994; **Med School:** Univ Louisville Sch Med 1988; **Resid:** Otolaryngology, Univ Louisville Hosp 1993; **Fellow:** Head and Neck Surgery, Univ Pittsburgh 1994; **Fac Appt:** Prof Oto, Univ Louisville Sch Med

Civantos, Francisco J MD [Oto] - **Spec Exp:** Head & Neck Cancer; Skull Base Surgery; **Hospital:** Univ of Miami Hosp & Clins/Sylvester Comp Canc Ctr (page 73); **Address:** Sylvester Cancer Ctr, Otolaryngology, 1475 NW 12th Ave, Miami, FL 33136; **Phone:** 305-243-5276; **Board Cert:** Otolaryngology 1992; **Med School:** Columbia P&S 1986; **Resid:** Otolaryngology, Univ Illinois Coll Med 1991; **Fellow:** Head & Neck Oncology, Vanderbilt Univ 1992; **Fac Appt:** Assoc Prof Oto, Univ Miami Sch Med

Day, Terrence A MD [Oto] - **Spec Exp:** Head & Neck Cancer; Reconstructive Microvascular Surgery; Skull Base Surgery; Facial Plastic & Reconstructive Surgery; **Hospital:** MUSC Med Ctr; **Address:** MUSC, Dept Otolaryngology, 135 Rutledge Ave, MSC550, Charleston, SC 29425; **Phone:** 843-792-0719; **Board Cert:** Otolaryngology 1996; **Med School:** Univ Okla Coll Med 1989; **Resid:** Otolaryngology, LSU Med Ctr 1995; **Fellow:** Head & Neck Surgical Oncology, UC Davis Med Ctr 1996; Maxillofacial Surgery, Univ Hosp 1994; **Fac Appt:** Assoc Prof Oto, Med Univ SC

DiNardo, Laurence J MD [Oto] - **Spec Exp:** Head & Neck Cancer; Endoscopic Sinus Surgery; Skull Base Surgery; Sinus Disorders/Surgery; **Hospital:** Med Coll of VA Hosp; **Address:** VCU Dept Otolaryngology, 401 N 11th St, rm 7-100, Box 980146, Richmond, VA 23298-0146; **Phone:** 804-628-4368; **Board Cert:** Otolaryngology 1992; **Med School:** Stanford Univ 1986; **Resid:** Otolaryngology, Hosp Univ Penn 1991; **Fac Appt:** Prof Oto, Va Commonwealth Univ Sch Med

Epstein, Jeffrey S MD [Oto] - **Spec Exp:** Hair Restoration/Transplant; Facial Plastic Surgery; **Hospital:** South Miami Hosp; **Address:** 6280 Sunset Drive, Ste 504, Miami, FL 33143; **Phone:** 305-666-1774; **Board Cert:** Otolaryngology 1994; Facial Plastic & Reconstr Surgery 1995; Hair Restoration Surgery 1998; **Med School:** Univ VT Coll Med 1988; **Resid:** Otolaryngology, Jackson Meml Hosp 1993; **Fellow:** Facial Plastic Surgery, Sheldon S Kabaker MD 1994; **Fac Appt:** Clin Prof Oto, Univ Miami Sch Med

Farrior, Edward H MD [Oto] - **Spec Exp:** Rhinoplasty; Ear Reshaping (Otoplasty); Facial Plastic Surgery; **Hospital:** Tampa Genl Hosp, St. Joseph's Hosp - Tampa; **Address:** 2908 W Azeele St, Tampa, FL 33609-3109; **Phone:** 813-875-3223; **Board Cert:** Otolaryngology 1987; Facial Plastic & Reconstr Surgery 1992; **Med School:** Univ VA Sch Med 1982; **Resid:** Otolaryngology, Univ Mich Hosps 1987; **Fellow:** Facial Plastic & Reconstr Surgery, Tampa Genl Hosp 1988; **Fac Appt:** Assoc Clin Prof S, Univ S Fla Coll Med

Farrior III, Joseph Brown MD [Oto] - **Spec Exp:** Otosclerosis/Stapedectomy; Hearing Loss; Meniere's Disease; Otology; **Hospital:** St. Joseph's Hosp - Tampa, Tampa Genl Hosp; **Address:** Farrior Ear Clinic, 2727 W Martin Luther King Jr Blvd, Ste 520, Tampa, FL 33607; **Phone:** 800-342-3277; **Board Cert:** Otolaryngology 1981; **Med School:** Emory Univ 1975; **Resid:** Surgery, Johns Hopkins Hosp 1977; Otolaryngology, Johns Hopkins Hosp 1981; **Fellow:** Otolaryngology, Farrior Clin/St Josephs Hosp 1980; **Fac Appt:** Assoc Clin Prof Oto, Univ S Fla Coll Med

Goodwin, W Jarrard MD [Oto] - **Spec Exp:** Head & Neck Cancer; **Hospital:** Univ of Miami Hosp & Clins/Sylvester Comp Canc Ctr (page 73), Jackson Meml Hosp (page 70); **Address:** Sylvester Comp Cancer Ctr, Dept Otolaryngology, 1475 NW 12th Ave, rm 4037, Miami, FL 33136-1015; **Phone:** 305-243-3564; **Board Cert:** Otolaryngology 1978; **Med School:** Albany Med Coll 1972; **Resid:** Surgery, Jackson Meml Hosp 1974; Otolaryngology, Jackson Meml Hosp 1977; **Fellow:** Head & Neck Surgical Oncology, MD Anderson Hosp 1980; **Fac Appt:** Prof Oto, Univ Miami Sch Med

Haynes, David S MD [Oto] - **Spec Exp:** Otology; Neurotology; Hearing Disorders; Cochlear Implants; **Hospital:** Vanderbilt Univ Med Ctr (page 76), Saint Thomas Hosp - Nashville; **Address:** Otology Group of Vanderbilt, Ste 7209, Medical Center East, 1215 21st Ave S, Nashville, TN 37232; **Phone:** 615-322-6180; **Board Cert:** Otolaryngology 1994; Neurotology 2004; **Med School:** Univ Tenn Coll Med 1987; **Resid:** Surgery, Vanderbilt Univ Med Ctr 1989; Otolaryngology, Vanderbilt Univ Med Ctr 1993; **Fellow:** Otology & Neurotology, Otology Grp/ Ear Fdn 1995; **Fac Appt:** Assoc Prof Oto, Vanderbilt Univ

Kesser, Bradley W MD [Oto] - **Spec Exp:** Aural Atresia Repair; Neuro-Otology; **Hospital:** Univ of Virginia Health Sys; **Address:** Univ VA Dept Otolaryngology, PO Box 800713, Charlottesville, VA 22908; **Phone:** 434-924-2040; **Board Cert:** Otolaryngology 1999; **Med School:** Univ VA Sch Med 1993; **Resid:** Otolaryngology, Univ Va Med Ctr 1998; **Fellow:** Otology & Neurotology, House Ear Clinic 2000; **Fac Appt:** Asst Prof Oto, Univ VA Sch Med

Kuhn, Frederick MD [Oto] - **Spec Exp:** Endoscopic Sinus Surgery; Allergic Fungal Sinusitis; Rhinoplasty Revision; **Hospital:** Meml Hlth Univ Med Ctr - Savannah, St. Joseph's-Candler Hosp; **Address:** Georgia Nasal & Sinus Inst, 4750 Waters Ave, Ste 112, Savannah, GA 31404; **Phone:** 912-355-1070; **Board Cert:** Otolaryngology 1972; **Med School:** Univ Okla Coll Med 1966; **Resid:** Surgery, St Lukes Hosp 1968; **Fellow:** Otolaryngology, Barnes Hosp/Wash Univ 1972

Lambert, Paul R MD [Oto] - **Spec Exp:** Neuro-Otology; Acoustic Neuroma; Meniere's Disease; Cholesteatoma; **Hospital:** MUSC Med Ctr; **Address:** MUSC, Dept Otolaryngology, 135 Rutledge Ave, Box 250550, Charleston, SC 29425; **Phone:** 843-792-3531; **Board Cert:** Otolaryngology 1981; Neurotology 2004; **Med School:** Duke Univ 1976; **Resid:** Surgery, UCLA Med Ctr 1978; Otolaryngology, UCLA Med Ctr 1981; **Fellow:** Neurotology, Otologic Med Group 1982; **Fac Appt:** Prof Oto, Med Univ SC

Otolaryngology

Lanza, Donald C MD [Oto] - **Spec Exp:** Skull Base Tumors; Sinus Disorders/Surgery; Rhinitis; Graves' Disease-Eye; **Hospital:** St. Anthony's Hosp - St Petersburg, All Children's Hosp; **Address:** 550 94th Ave N, St Petersburg, FL 33702; **Phone:** 727-573-0074; **Board Cert:** Otolaryngology 1990; **Med School:** SUNY Hlth Sci Ctr 1985; **Resid:** Surgery, Albany Med Ctr 1987; Otolaryngology, Albany Med Ctr 1990; **Fellow:** Rhinology, Johns Hopkins Univ 1990; Rhinology, Univ Penn 1991

Levine, Paul A MD [Oto] - **Spec Exp:** Head & Neck Cancer; Head & Neck Reconstruction; Skull Base Tumors; **Hospital:** Univ of Virginia Health Sys; **Address:** Dept Otolaryngology, PO Box 800713, Charlottesville, VA 22908; **Phone:** 434-924-5593; **Board Cert:** Otolaryngology 1978; **Med School:** Albany Med Coll 1973; **Resid:** Otolaryngology, Yale-New Haven Hosp 1977; **Fellow:** Head and Neck Surgery, Stanford Med Ctr 1978; **Fac Appt:** Prof Oto, Univ VA Sch Med

Mangat, Devinder S MD [Oto] - **Spec Exp:** Cosmetic & Reconstructive Surgery-Face; **Hospital:** St. Elizabeth Hlthcare-Edgewood; **Address:** 133 Barnwood Drive, Edgewood, KY 41017; **Phone:** 513-984-3223; **Board Cert:** Otolaryngology 1978; Facial Plastic & Reconstr Surgery 1991; **Med School:** Univ KY Coll Med 1973; **Resid:** Surgery, Univ KY Med Ctr 1975; Otolaryngology, Univ Okla Hlth Scis Ctr 1978; **Fellow:** Facial Plastic Surgery, McCullough Clinic 1979; **Fac Appt:** Assoc Prof Oto, Univ Cincinnati

Mattox, Douglas E MD [Oto] - **Spec Exp:** Neuro-Otology; Meniere's Disease; Hearing Loss; Cochlear Implants; **Hospital:** Emory Univ Hosp, Chldns Hlthcare Atlanta @ Egleston; **Address:** Emory Univ Dept Otolaryngology, 1365A Clifton Rd NE, Ste 2300, Atlanta, GA 30322; **Phone:** 404-778-3381; **Board Cert:** Otolaryngology 1977; Neurotology 2004; **Med School:** Yale Univ 1973; **Resid:** Otolaryngology, Stanford Univ Hosp 1977; **Fellow:** Neurotology, Ugo Fisch, MD 1985; **Fac Appt:** Prof Oto, Emory Univ

McCaffrey, Thomas V MD [Oto] - **Spec Exp:** Head & Neck Cancer; Thyroid Cancer; Tracheal Surgery; **Hospital:** H Lee Moffitt Cancer Ctr & Research Inst (page 59), Tampa Genl Hosp; **Address:** H Lee Moffitt Cancer Ctr, Dept Otolaryngology-HNS, 12902 Magnolia Drive, MS FOB2-HN, Tampa, FL 33612; **Phone:** 813-745-8463; **Board Cert:** Otolaryngology 1980; **Med School:** Loyola Univ-Stritch Sch Med 1974; **Resid:** Surgery, Mayo Affil Hosps 1976; Otolaryngology, Mayo Affil Hosps 1980; **Fac Appt:** Prof Oto, Univ S Fla Coll Med

Netterville, James L MD [Oto] - **Spec Exp:** Head & Neck Surgery; Head & Neck Cancer; Vocal Cord Disorders; Skull Base Tumors; **Hospital:** Vanderbilt Univ Med Ctr (page 76), Vanderbilt Monroe Carrell Jr. Chldn's Hosp (page 76); **Address:** Vanderbilt Univ Med Ctr, Dept Oto, 7209 Med Ctr East, South Twr, 1215 21st Ave S, Nashville, TN 37232-8605; **Phone:** 615-343-8840; **Board Cert:** Otolaryngology 1985; **Med School:** Univ Tenn Coll Med 1980; **Resid:** Surgery, Methodist Hosp 1982; Otolaryngology, Univ Tenn Med Ctr 1985; **Fellow:** Surgical Oncology, Univ Iowa 1986; **Fac Appt:** Prof Oto, Vanderbilt Univ

Osguthorpe, John D MD [Oto] - **Spec Exp:** Head & Neck Cancer; Thyroid & Parathyroid Cancer & Surgery; Nasal & Sinus Disorders; Salivary Gland Tumors & Surgery; **Hospital:** MUSC Med Ctr, E Cooper Med Ctr; **Address:** MUSC Med Ctr-Dept Otolaryngology, 135 Rutledge Ave, PO Box 250550, Charleston, SC 29425; **Phone:** 843-792-3533; **Board Cert:** Otolaryngology 1978; **Med School:** Univ Utah 1973; **Resid:** Surgery, UCLA Med Ctr 1975; Otolaryngology, UCLA Med Ctr 1978; **Fellow:** Skull Base Surgery, Univ Zurich 1989; **Fac Appt:** Prof Oto, Med Univ SC

Ossoff, Robert H MD [Oto] - **Spec Exp:** Voice Disorders; Laryngeal Disorders; Vocal Cord Disorders; Endoscopic Surgery; **Hospital:** Vanderbilt Univ Med Ctr (page 76); **Address:** Vanderbilt Univ Med Ctr, 1215 21st Ave S, Med Ctr E, Ste 7302, Nashville, TN 37212-8200; **Phone:** 615-343-7464; **Board Cert:** Otolaryngology 1982; **Med School:** Tufts Univ 1975; **Resid:** Otolaryngology, Northwestern Meml Hosp 1980; **Fellow:** Head and Neck Surgery, Northwestern Meml Hosp 1981; **Fac Appt:** Prof Oto, Vanderbilt Univ

Peters, Glenn E MD [Oto] - **Spec Exp:** Thyroid & Parathyroid Cancer & Surgery; **Hospital:** Univ of Ala Hosp at Birmingham; **Address:** UAB Med Ctr, Div of Head & Neck Surgery, 1530 3rd Ave S, Ste BDB 563, Birmingham, AL 35294-0012; **Phone:** 205-934-9767; **Board Cert:** Otolaryngology 1985; **Med School:** Louisiana State U, New Orleans 1980; **Resid:** Surgery, Baptist Med Ctr 1982; Otolaryngology, Univ Alabama Hosp 1984; **Fellow:** Head & Neck Surgical Oncology, Johns Hopkins Hosp 1987; **Fac Appt:** Prof S, Univ Alabama

Pillsbury, Harold C MD [Oto] - **Spec Exp:** Cochlear Implants; Neuro-Otology; Ear Disorders/Surgery; **Hospital:** NC Memorial Hosp - UNC; **Address:** 170 Manning Drive, Physicians Bldg, CB 7070, Chapel Hill, NC 27599-7070; **Phone:** 919-966-8926; **Board Cert:** Otolaryngology 1978; Neurotology 2004; **Med School:** Geo Wash Univ 1972; **Resid:** Surgery, Univ NC Hosp 1973; Otolaryngology, NC Meml Hosp 1976; **Fac Appt:** Prof Oto, Univ NC Sch Med

Pitman, Karen MD [Oto] - **Spec Exp:** Head & Neck Cancer & Surgery; Thyroid & Parathyroid Cancer & Surgery; Sentinel Node Surgery; **Hospital:** Univ Mississippi Med Ctr; **Address:** Univ Miss Med Ctr, Dept Otolaryngology, 2500 N State St, Jackson, MS 39216; **Phone:** 601-984-5160; **Board Cert:** Otolaryngology 1995; **Med School:** Uniformed Srvs Univ, Bethesda 1987; **Resid:** Otolaryngology, Naval Med Ctr 1994; **Fellow:** Head & Neck Oncology, Univ Pittsburgh 1996; **Fac Appt:** Prof Oto, Univ Miss

Poole, Michael D MD/PhD [Oto] - **Spec Exp:** Pediatric Otolaryngology; Ear Infections; Sleep Disorders/Apnea; Sinus Disorders; **Hospital:** Meml Hlth Univ Med Ctr - Savannah, St. Joseph's-Candler Hosp; **Address:** Georgia Ear Institute, 4700 Waters Ave, Savannah, GA 31404; **Phone:** 912-356-1515; **Board Cert:** Otolaryngology 1986; **Med School:** Univ NC Sch Med 1981; **Resid:** Otolaryngology, NC Meml Hosp 1986; **Fac Appt:** Prof Oto, Mercer Univ Sch Med

Postma, Gregory N MD [Oto] - **Spec Exp:** Voice Disorders; **Hospital:** Med Coll of GA Hosp and Clin (MCG Health Inc); **Address:** Med Coll Georgia, Voice & Swallowing Center, 1120 15th St, BP-4109, Augusta, GA 30912; **Phone:** 706-721-4400; **Board Cert:** Otolaryngology 1994; **Med School:** Hahnemann Univ 1984; **Resid:** Otolaryngology, Oakland Naval Hosp 1992; Otolaryngology, Univ N Carolina Hosps 1993; **Fellow:** Otolaryngology, Vanderbilt Univ 1996; **Fac Appt:** Prof Oto, Med Coll GA

Ries, W Russell MD [Oto] - **Spec Exp:** Facial Plastic & Reconstructive Surgery; Cosmetic Surgery-Face; Skin Laser Surgery; **Hospital:** Vanderbilt Univ Med Ctr (page 76); **Address:** Vanderbilt Univ Dept Otolaryngology, 7209 Medical Center East, South Tower, 1215 21st Ave S, Nashville, TN 37232; **Phone:** 615-322-6180; **Board Cert:** Otolaryngology 1985; Facial Plastic & Reconstr Surgery 1992; **Med School:** Univ Tenn Coll Med 1978; **Resid:** Surgery, Baptist Meml Hosp 1981; Otolaryngology, Northwestern Meml Hosp 1984; **Fellow:** Facial Plastic Surgery, Tulane Med Ctr 1985; **Fac Appt:** Prof Oto, Vanderbilt Univ

Rosenthal, Eben MD [Oto] - **Spec Exp:** Head & Neck Cancer; Microvascular Surgery; Reconstructive Surgery; Minimally Invasive Surgery; **Hospital:** Univ of Ala Hosp at Birmingham; **Address:** 2000 6th Ave S, Birmingham, AL 35233; **Phone:** 205-934-9766; **Board Cert:** Otolaryngology 2001; **Med School:** Univ Mich Med Sch 1994; **Resid:** Otolaryngology, Univ MI Med Ctr 2000; **Fellow:** Head and Neck Surgery, OR Hlth Sci Univ 2001; **Fac Appt:** Assoc Prof S, Univ Alabama

Samant, Sandeep MD [Oto] - **Spec Exp:** Head & Neck Cancer & Surgery; Skull Base Surgery; Endoscopic Surgery; Thyroid & Parathyroid Cancer & Surgery; **Hospital:** Methodist Univ Hosp - Memphis; **Address:** UT Med Grp-Oto-Head & Neck Surgery, 7945 Wolf River Blvd, Ste 220, Memphis, TN 38138; **Phone:** 901-347-8220; **Board Cert:** Otolaryngology 2009; **Med School:** India 1986; **Resid:** Otolaryngology, ALL-Indian Inst 1989; Otolaryngology, Royal Coll Surgeons 1994; **Fellow:** Head and Neck Surgery, Univ Miami/Sylvester Comprehensive Cancer Ctr 1995; Head & Neck Oncology, Univ TN Med Ctr 1996

Otolaryngology

Senior, Brent A MD [Oto] - **Spec Exp:** Sinus Disorders/Surgery; Nasal Allergy; Sleep Disorders; **Hospital:** NC Memorial Hosp - UNC; **Address:** Physicians Office G-120 Bldg, 17D Manning CB #7070 Drive, Chapel Hill, NC 27599-7070; **Phone:** 919-966-6483; **Board Cert:** Otolaryngology 1996; **Med School:** Univ Mich Med Sch 1990; **Resid:** Otolaryngology, Boston Univ/Tufts Univ 1995; **Fellow:** Sinus Surgery, Univ Penn 1996; **Fac Appt:** Prof Oto, Univ NC Sch Med

Shockley, William W MD [Oto] - **Spec Exp:** Facial Plastic & Reconstructive Surgery; Rhinoplasty; Salivary Gland Tumors & Surgery; Thyroid Surgery; **Hospital:** NC Memorial Hosp - UNC; **Address:** 170 Manning Drive, Physicians Bldg, CB 7070, Chapel Hill, NC 27599-7070; **Phone:** 919-966-8926; **Board Cert:** Otolaryngology 1981; Facial Plastic & Reconstr Surgery ; **Med School:** Indiana Univ 1976; **Resid:** Otolaryngology, Univ Cincinnati Hosps 1981; **Fellow:** Head and Neck Surgery, H&N Surg Assoc 1982; **Fac Appt:** Prof Oto, Univ NC Sch Med

Sillers, Michael J MD [Oto] - **Spec Exp:** Nasal & Sinus Disorders; Sinus Disorders/Surgery; **Hospital:** St. Vincent's Hosp - Birmingham; **Address:** Alabama Nasal & Sinus Ctr, 7191 Cahaba Valley Rd, Ste 301, Birmingham, AL 35242; **Phone:** 205-980-2091; **Board Cert:** Otolaryngology 1994; **Med School:** Univ Alabama 1988; **Resid:** Otolaryngology, Univ Alabama Hosp 1993; **Fellow:** Sinus Surgery, Med Coll Georgia 1994; **Fac Appt:** Asst Prof S, Univ Alabama

Silverstein, Herbert MD [Oto] - **Spec Exp:** Ear Disorders/Surgery; Meniere's Disease; **Hospital:** Sarasota Meml Hosp; **Address:** Silverstein Institute, 1901 Floyd St, Sarasota, FL 34239; **Phone:** 941-366-9222; **Board Cert:** Otolaryngology 1967; **Med School:** Temple Univ 1961; **Resid:** Surgery, Hosp Univ Penn 1963; Otolaryngology, Mass EE Infirm 1966; **Fac Appt:** Clin Prof S, Univ S Fla Coll Med

Stringer, Scott P MD [Oto] - **Spec Exp:** Rhinitis; Skull Base Surgery; **Hospital:** Univ Mississippi Med Ctr, G.V. (Sonny) Montgomery VA Med Ctr - Jackson; **Address:** Univ Miss Med Ctr, Dept Otolaryngology, 2500 N State St, Jackson, MS 39216-4505; **Phone:** 601-984-5160; **Board Cert:** Otolaryngology 1987; **Med School:** Univ Tex SW, Dallas 1982; **Resid:** Surgery, Univ Tex SW Med Ctr 1984; Otolaryngology, Univ Tex SW Med Ctr 1987; **Fac Appt:** Prof Oto, Univ Miss

Telischi, Fred F MD [Oto] - **Spec Exp:** Ear Disorders/Surgery; Hearing Loss; Cochlear Implants; Neuro-Otology; **Hospital:** Jackson Meml Hosp (page 70); **Address:** Univ Miami Sch Med, Dept Otolaryngology, 1120 NW 14th St, PO Box 016960, Miami, FL 33101; **Phone:** 305-243-2000; **Board Cert:** Otolaryngology 1990; Neurotology 2010; **Med School:** Univ Miami Sch Med 1985; **Resid:** Otolaryngology, Jackson Meml Hosp 1990; **Fellow:** Neurotology, House Ear Clinic 1992; **Fac Appt:** Prof Oto, Univ Miami Sch Med

Terris, David J MD [Oto] - **Spec Exp:** Thyroid Surgery; Thyroid Cancer; Parathyroid Disease; **Hospital:** Med Coll of GA Hosp and Clin (MCG Health Inc), Doctors Hosp; **Address:** MCG Health - Dept Otolaryngology, 1447 Harper St, Medical Office Bldg Fl 4, Augusta, GA 30912; **Phone:** 706-721-4400; **Board Cert:** Otolaryngology 1994; **Med School:** Duke Univ 1988; **Resid:** Surgery, Stanford Univ Med Ctr 1989; Otolaryngology, Stanford Univ Med Ctr 1993; **Fellow:** Head and Neck Surgery, Stanford Univ Med Ctr 1994; **Fac Appt:** Prof Oto, Med Coll GA

Tucci, Debara L MD [Oto] - **Spec Exp:** Skull Base Surgery; Middle Ear Disorders; Otology; Neurotology; **Hospital:** Duke Univ Hosp; **Address:** Duke Univ Med Center, Div Otolaryngology, Box 3805, Durham, NC 27710; **Phone:** 919-684-6968; **Board Cert:** Otolaryngology 1990; Neurotology 2004; **Med School:** Univ VA Sch Med 1985; **Resid:** Otolaryngology, Univ Va Med ctr 1990; **Fellow:** Otology & Neurotology, Univ Mich Med Ctr 1992; **Fac Appt:** Assoc Prof S, Duke Univ

Valentino, Joseph MD [Oto] - **Spec Exp:** Head & Neck Cancer; Reconstructive Microvascular Surgery; Thyroid Cancer; **Hospital:** Univ of Kentucky Albert B. Chandler Hosp; **Address:** 800 Rose St, rm C236, Lexington, KY 40536; **Phone:** 859-257-5405; **Board Cert:** Otolaryngology 1993; **Med School:** UMDNJ-RW Johnson Med Sch 1987; **Resid:** Otolaryngology, Univ Minn 1992; **Fellow:** Otolaryngology, Univ Iowa Coll Med 1993; **Fac Appt:** Assoc Prof Oto, Univ KY Coll Med

Wazen, Jack J MD [Oto] - **Spec Exp:** Skull Base Surgery; Meniere's Disease; Acoustic Neuroma; Hearing & Balance Disorders; **Hospital:** Sarasota Meml Hosp; **Address:** Silverstein Institute, 1901 Floyd St, Sarasota, FL 34239; **Phone:** 941-366-9222; **Board Cert:** Otolaryngology 1983; **Med School:** Lebanon 1978; **Resid:** Surgery, St Lukes Hosp 1980; Otolaryngology, Columbia Presby Hosp 1983; **Fellow:** Neurotology, Ear Rsch Fdn 1984

Weissler, Mark C MD [Oto] - **Spec Exp:** Head & Neck Cancer; Laryngeal & Tracheal Disorders; Voice Disorders; Salivary Gland Tumors; **Hospital:** NC Memorial Hosp - UNC; **Address:** 170 Manning Drive, G106 Physician's Office Bldg, CB#7070, Chapel Hill, NC 27599-7070; **Phone:** 919-843-4820; **Board Cert:** Otolaryngology 1985; **Med School:** Boston Univ 1980; **Resid:** Surgery, Mass Genl Hosp 1982; Otolaryngology, Mass Eye & Ear Infirm 1985; **Fellow:** Head & Neck Oncology, Univ Cincinnati 1986; **Fac Appt:** Prof Oto, Univ NC Sch Med

Yarbrough, Wendell G MD [Oto] - **Spec Exp:** Head & Neck Cancer; **Hospital:** Vanderbilt Univ Med Ctr (page 76); **Address:** Vanderbilt Otolaryngology, 1215 21st Ave S, Ste 7209, Nashville, TN 37232-8605; **Phone:** 615-322-6180; **Board Cert:** Otolaryngology 1995; **Med School:** Univ NC Sch Med 1989; **Resid:** Otolaryngology, Univ NC Hosps 1994; **Fellow:** Surgical Oncology, Univ NC Hosps 1996; **Fac Appt:** Assoc Prof Oto, Vanderbilt Univ

Midwest

Akervall, Jan A MD [Oto] - **Spec Exp:** Head & Neck Cancer; Head & Neck Reconstruction; Minimally Invasive Surgery; **Hospital:** Beaumont Hosp-Royal Oak, St. Joseph Mercy Hosp - Ann Arbor; **Address:** 28300 Orchard Lake Rd, Ste 100, Farmington Hills, MI 48334; **Phone:** 248-737-4030; **Med School:** Sweden 1990; **Resid:** Otolaryngology, Lund Univ Fac Med 1998; **Fellow:** Head & Neck Oncology, Univ MI Hosps 2002; **Fac Appt:** Clin Prof Oto, Oakland Univ-William Beaumont Med Sch

Alam, Daniel Syed MD [Oto] - **Spec Exp:** Nasal Reconstruction; Head & Neck Reconstruction; Parotid Gland Tumors; Cancer Reconstruction; **Hospital:** Cleveland Clin (page 56); **Address:** Cleveland Clin Main Campus, 9500 Euclid Ave, MC A71, Cleveland, OH 44195; **Phone:** 216-445-6594; **Board Cert:** Otolaryngology 2002; **Med School:** Johns Hopkins Univ 1996; **Resid:** Otolaryngology, Mass Genl Hosp 2001; **Fellow:** Facial Plastic & Reconstr Surgery, UCLA Med Ctr 2002

Arts, H Alexander MD [Oto] - **Spec Exp:** Skull Base Tumors & Surgery; Neuro-Otology; Hearing Loss; Cochlear Implants; **Hospital:** Univ of Michigan Hosp; **Address:** Univ Michigan Health Systems, Dept Otolaryngology, 1500 E Medical Ctr Dr, 1904 Taubman Ctr, Ann Arbor, MI 48109; **Phone:** 734-936-8006; **Board Cert:** Otolaryngology 1992; Neurotology 2004; **Med School:** Baylor Coll Med 1983; **Resid:** Surgery, Univ Washington Med Ctr 1985; Otolaryngology, Univ Washington Med Ctr 1990; **Fellow:** Neurotology, Univ Virginia 1991; **Fac Appt:** Prof Oto, Univ Mich Med Sch

Baim, Howard M MD [Oto] - **Spec Exp:** Head & Neck Surgery; Sleep Disorders/Apnea; Sinus Disorders; **Hospital:** Adv Illinois Masonic Med Ctr, Highland Park/North Shore Univ Hlth Syst; **Address:** 2532 N Lincoln Ave, Chicago, IL 60614-2468; **Phone:** 773-883-1177; **Board Cert:** Otolaryngology 1978; **Med School:** Univ IL Coll Med 1973; **Resid:** Surgery, Illinois Met Grp Hosps 1975; Otolaryngology, Illinois EE Infirmary 1978; **Fac Appt:** Asst Clin Prof Oto, Univ IL Coll Med

Otolaryngology

Baker, Shan R MD [Oto] - **Spec Exp:** Cosmetic Surgery-Face & Neck; Reconstructive Surgery; **Hospital:** Univ of Michigan Hosp; **Address:** Ctr Facial & Cosmetic Surgery, 19900 Haggerty Rd, Ste 103, Livonia, MI 48152-1054; **Phone:** 734-432-7634; **Board Cert:** Otolaryngology 1977; Facial Plastic & Reconstr Surgery 1990; **Med School:** Univ Iowa Coll Med 1971; **Resid:** Surgery, UCSD Med Ctr 1973; Otolaryngology, Univ Iowa Hosps 1977; **Fac Appt:** Prof Oto, Univ Mich Med Sch

Bastian, Robert W MD [Oto] - **Spec Exp:** Voice Disorders; Swallowing Disorders; Laryngeal Disorders; **Hospital:** Adv Good Samaritan Hosp; **Address:** Bastian Voice Inst, 3010 Highland Parkway, Ste 550, Downers Grove, IL 60515-5500; **Phone:** 630-724-1100; **Board Cert:** Otolaryngology 1983; **Med School:** Washington Univ, St Louis 1978; **Resid:** Surgery, Barnes Hosp 1979; Otolaryngology, Barnes Hosp 1983; **Fellow:** Otolaryngology, Hosp Foch 1983

Beatty, Charles W MD [Oto] - **Spec Exp:** Otology & Neuro-Otology; Acoustic Neuroma; Meniere's Disease; Cochlear Implants; **Hospital:** Mayo Med Ctr & Clin - Rochester; **Address:** Mayo Clinic-Dept of Ear, Nose and Throat, 200 First St SW, Gonda-12, Rochester, MN 55905; **Phone:** 507-284-8532; **Board Cert:** Otolaryngology 1982; **Med School:** Univ Iowa Coll Med 1977; **Resid:** Otolaryngology, Mayo Clinic 1982; **Fac Appt:** Prof Oto, Mayo Med Sch

Benninger, Michael S MD [Oto] - **Spec Exp:** Voice Disorders; Nasal & Sinus Disorders; Sinus Disorders/Surgery; Laryngeal Disorders; **Hospital:** Cleveland Clin (page 56); **Address:** Cleveland Clinic, MC A71, 9500 Euclid Ave, Cleveland, OH 44195; **Phone:** 216-444-6686; **Board Cert:** Otolaryngology 1988; **Med School:** Case West Res Univ 1983; **Resid:** Surgery, Cleveland Clin Fdn 1985; Otolaryngology, Cleveland Clin Fdn 1988; **Fac Appt:** Prof S, Cleveland Cl Coll Med/Case West Res

Blair, Elizabeth MD [Oto] - **Spec Exp:** Head & Neck Cancer & Surgery; Thyroid & Parathyroid Surgery; Salivary Gland Tumors; Skull Base Tumors; **Hospital:** Univ of Chicago Med Ctr; **Address:** 5841 S Maryland Ave, MC 1035, Chicago, IL 60637; **Phone:** 773-702-4934; **Board Cert:** Otolaryngology 1994; **Med School:** Creighton Univ 1988; **Resid:** Otolaryngology, Univ Pittsburgh Med Ctr 1993; **Fellow:** Head & Neck Surgical Oncology, MD Anderson Cancer Ctr 1994; **Fac Appt:** Assoc Prof Oto, Univ Chicago-Pritzker Sch Med

Bojrab, Dennis I MD [Oto] - **Spec Exp:** Otology & Neuro-Otology; Facial Nerve Disorders; Skull Base Tumors; **Hospital:** Providence Hosp - Southfield, Beaumont Hosp-Royal Oak; **Address:** Michigan Ear Inst, 30055 Northwestern Hwy, Ste 101, Farmington Hills, MI 48334; **Phone:** 248-865-4444; **Board Cert:** Otolaryngology 1985; Neurotology 2005; **Med School:** Indiana Univ 1979; **Resid:** Surgery, Butterworth Hosp 1981; Otolaryngology, Univ Indiana Sch Med 1984; **Fellow:** Skull Base Surgery, Vanderbilt Univ Med Ctr 1985; **Fac Appt:** Clin Prof Oto, Wayne State Univ

Bradford, Carol MD [Oto] - **Spec Exp:** Head & Neck Cancer; Melanoma-Head & Neck; Skin Cancer-Head & Neck; **Hospital:** Univ of Michigan Hosp; **Address:** University of Michigan Health System, 1500 E Medical Center Drive, rm 1904-TC, Ann Arbor, MI 48109-0312; **Phone:** 734-936-8029; **Board Cert:** Otolaryngology 1993; **Med School:** Univ Mich Med Sch 1986; **Resid:** Otolaryngology, Univ Michigan Med Ctr 1992; **Fellow:** Head and Neck Surgery, Univ Michigan Med Ctr 1988; **Fac Appt:** Prof Oto, Univ Mich Med Sch

Branham, Gregory H MD [Oto] - **Spec Exp:** Cosmetic & Reconstructive Surgery-Face; Nasal Surgery; Botox Therapy; Skin Laser Surgery-Resurfacing; **Hospital:** Washington Univ Physicians, Barnes-Jewish Hosp; **Address:** 605 Old Ballas Rd, Ste 100, St Louis, MO 63141; **Phone:** 314-432-7760; **Board Cert:** Otolaryngology 1989; Facial Plastic & Reconstr Surgery 1993; **Med School:** Washington Univ, St Louis 1983; **Resid:** Otolaryngology, St Louis Univ Hosp 1989; **Fellow:** Facial Plastic & Reconstr Surgery, Washington Univ Affil Hosp 1990; **Fac Appt:** Assoc Prof Oto, St Louis Univ

Burkey, Brian MD [Oto] - **Spec Exp:** Parotid Gland Tumors; Head & Neck Cancer; Reconstructive Microvascular Surgery; **Hospital:** Cleveland Clin (page 56); **Address:** Head & Neck Inst, Desk A71, The Cleveland Clin, 9500 Euclid Ave, Cleveland, OH 44195; **Phone:** 216-445-8838; **Board Cert:** Otolaryngology 1992; **Med School:** Univ VA Sch Med 1986; **Resid:** Otolaryngology, Univ Mich Med Ctr 1991; **Fellow:** Microsurgery, Ohio State Univ 1991; **Fac Appt:** Assoc Prof Oto, Vanderbilt Univ

Caldarelli, David D MD [Oto] - **Spec Exp:** Laryngeal & Vocal Cord Surgery; Sinus Disorders/Surgery; Ear Disorders/Surgery; Meniere's Disease; **Hospital:** Rush Univ Med Ctr; **Address:** Rush Otolaryngology, 1611 W Harrison St, Ste 550, Chicago, IL 60612; **Phone:** 312-733-4341; **Board Cert:** Otolaryngology 1970; **Med School:** Univ IL Coll Med 1965; **Resid:** Surgery, Presby-St Lukes Hosp 1967; Otolaryngology, Univ Illinois Eye/Ear Infirm 1970; **Fac Appt:** Prof Oto, Rush Med Coll

Campbell, Bruce H MD [Oto] - **Spec Exp:** Head & Neck Cancer; Thyroid Surgery; **Hospital:** Froedtert and Med Ctr of WI, Chldns Hosp - Wisconsin; **Address:** Med Coll Wisc-Dept Oto, 9200 W Wisconsin Ave, Milwaukee, WI 53226; **Phone:** 414-805-5583; **Board Cert:** Otolaryngology 1986; **Med School:** Rush Med Coll 1980; **Resid:** Otolaryngology, Med Coll Wisconsin 1985; **Fellow:** Head and Neck Surgery, MD Anderson Cancer Ctr 1987; **Fac Appt:** Prof Oto, Med Coll Wisc

Corey, Jacquelynne P MD [Oto] - **Spec Exp:** Nasal & Sinus Disorders; Allergy; Voice Disorders; **Hospital:** Univ of Chicago Med Ctr; **Address:** 57841 S Maryland Ave, MC 1035, Chicago, IL 60637; **Phone:** 773-702-1865; **Board Cert:** Otolaryngology 1985; **Med School:** Univ IL Coll Med 1979; **Resid:** Otolaryngology, Rush Presby-St Lukes Med Ctr 1984; **Fac Appt:** Assoc Prof Oto, Univ Chicago-Pritzker Sch Med

Driscoll, Colin L W MD [Oto] - **Spec Exp:** Acoustic Neuroma; Cochlear Implants; Skull Base Tumors; **Hospital:** Mayo Med Ctr & Clin - Rochester; **Address:** Mayo Clinic, Dept of Ear, Nose and Throat, 200 First St SW, Rochester, MN 55905; **Phone:** 507-284-4065; **Board Cert:** Otolaryngology 1998; Neurology 2006; **Med School:** Univ New Mexico 1992; **Resid:** Otolaryngology, Mayo Clinic 1997; **Fellow:** Neurotology, UCSF Med Ctr 1998; Skull Base Surgery, UCSF Med Ctr 1999; **Fac Appt:** Assoc Prof Oto, Mayo Med Sch

Ford, Charles N MD [Oto] - **Spec Exp:** Voice Disorders; Laryngeal Disorders; **Hospital:** Univ WI Hosp & Clins; **Address:** Univ of WI Hosp & Clinics, 600 Highland Ave, G3/225 Otolaryngology, MC 2400, Madison, WI 53792-3284; **Phone:** 608-263-6190; **Board Cert:** Otolaryngology 1971; **Med School:** Univ Louisville Sch Med 1965; **Resid:** Otolaryngology, Henry Ford Hosp 1970; **Fac Appt:** Prof Oto, Univ Wisc

Friedman, Michael MD [Oto] - **Spec Exp:** Sleep Disorders/Apnea/Snoring; Thyroid & Parathyroid Surgery; Sinus Disorders/Surgery; **Hospital:** Adv Illinois Masonic Med Ctr, Rush Univ Med Ctr; **Address:** 3000 N Halsted St, Ste 400, Chicago, IL 60657; **Phone:** 312-236-3642; **Board Cert:** Otolaryngology 1977; **Med School:** Univ IL Coll Med 1972; **Resid:** Surgery, Illinois Masonic Hosp 1974; Otolaryngology, Univ Illinois Med Ctr 1977; **Fac Appt:** Prof Oto, Rush Med Coll

Funk, Gerry F MD [Oto] - **Spec Exp:** Head & Neck Cancer; Head & Neck Reconstruction; Head & Neck Trauma; **Hospital:** Univ Iowa Hosp & Clinics; **Address:** UIHC, Dept Otolaryngology, 200 Hawkins Drive, Iowa City, IA 52242-1007; **Phone:** 319-356-2165; **Board Cert:** Otolaryngology 1992; **Med School:** Univ Chicago-Pritzker Sch Med 1986; **Resid:** Surgery, LAC-USC Med Ctr 1987; Otolaryngology, LAC-USC Med Ctr 1991; **Fellow:** Head and Neck Surgery, Univ Iowa Hosp 1992; **Fac Appt:** Prof Oto, Univ Iowa Coll Med

Otolaryngology

Gantz, Bruce J MD [Oto] - **Spec Exp:** Cochlear Implants; Neuro-Otology; Skull Base Surgery; **Hospital:** Univ Iowa Hosp & Clinics; **Address:** Univ Hosp & Clins, Dept Otolaryngology, 200 Hawkins Drive, rm 21201PFP, Iowa City, IA 52242-1078; **Phone:** 319-356-2173; **Board Cert:** Otolaryngology 1980; Neurotology 2004; **Med School:** Univ Iowa Coll Med 1974; **Resid:** Otolaryngology, Univ Iowa Hosps 1980; **Fellow:** Neurotology, Univ Zurich 1982; **Fac Appt:** Prof Oto, Univ Iowa Coll Med

Goebel, Joel Alan MD [Oto] - **Spec Exp:** Dizziness; Hearing Disorders; Otology & Neuro-Otology; **Hospital:** Barnes-Jewish Hosp, St. Louis Chldns Hosp; **Address:** Barnes Jewish Hosp South, Campus Box 8115, St Louis, MO 63110; **Phone:** 314-362-7509; **Board Cert:** Otolaryngology 1985; **Med School:** Washington Univ, St Louis 1980; **Resid:** Otolaryngology, Barnes Hosp/Wash Univ 1985; **Fac Appt:** Prof Oto, Washington Univ, St Louis

Hartig, Gregory K MD [Oto] - **Spec Exp:** Head & Neck Cancer; Skull Base Tumors; **Hospital:** Univ WI Hosp & Clins; **Address:** 600 Highland Ave, rm K4/720, Madison, WI 53792-7375; **Phone:** 608-263-6190; **Board Cert:** Otolaryngology 1994; **Med School:** Univ Mich Med Sch 1988; **Resid:** Otolaryngology, Univ Mich Med Ctr 1993; **Fellow:** Otolaryngology, Univ Penn Med Ctr 1994; **Fac Appt:** Prof Oto, Univ Mich Med Sch

Haughey, Bruce H MD [Oto] - **Spec Exp:** Reconstructive Surgery-Face; Head & Neck Cancer; Head & Neck Reconstruction; **Hospital:** Barnes-Jewish Hosp, St. Louis Chldns Hosp; **Address:** Barnes Jewish Hosp South, 660 S Euclid Ave, Box 8115, St Louis, MO 63110; **Phone:** 314-362-7509; **Board Cert:** Otolaryngology 1984; **Med School:** New Zealand 1976; **Resid:** Surgery, Univ Auckland 1981; Otolaryngology, Univ Iowa Med Ctr 1984; **Fellow:** Otolaryngology, Univ Iowa Med Ctr 1985; **Fac Appt:** Prof Oto, Washington Univ, St Louis

Hilger, Peter A MD [Oto] - **Spec Exp:** Head & Neck Surgery; Facial Plastic Surgery; **Hospital:** Regions Hosp - St Paul, Fairview Southdale Hosp; **Address:** Centennial Lakes Med Bldg, 7373 France Ave S, Ste 410, Edina, MN 55435; **Phone:** 952-844-0404; **Board Cert:** Otolaryngology 1979; **Med School:** Univ Minn 1974; **Resid:** Surgery, Univ Minn Hosp 1975; Otolaryngology, Univ Minn Hosp 1979; **Fellow:** Plastic Surgery, Mass Eye & Ear Infirm 1980; **Fac Appt:** Asst Prof Oto, Univ Minn

Hoffman, Henry T MD [Oto] - **Spec Exp:** Voice Disorders; Head & Neck Cancer; Salivary Gland Tumors & Surgery; **Hospital:** Univ Iowa Hosp & Clinics; **Address:** Univ Iowa Hosp & Clins-Dept Oto, 200 Hawkins Drive, Iowa City, IA 52242; **Phone:** 319-356-2201; **Board Cert:** Otolaryngology 1985; **Med School:** UCSD 1980; **Resid:** Otolaryngology, Univ Iowa Hosp & Clinics 1985; **Fellow:** Head & Neck Oncology, Univ Michigan Hosp 1989; **Fac Appt:** Clin Prof Oto, Univ Iowa Coll Med

Hogikyan, Norman D MD [Oto] - **Spec Exp:** Voice Disorders; Vocal Cord Disorders; Swallowing Disorders; Airway Disorders; **Hospital:** Univ of Michigan Hosp; **Address:** Univ Michigan Hlth Sys, Taubman Ctr, rm 1904, 1500 E Medical Ctr Drive, Ann Arbor, MI 48109; **Phone:** 734-936-8051; **Board Cert:** Otolaryngology 1995; **Med School:** Univ Mich Med Sch 1988; **Resid:** Otolaryngology, Barnes Jewish Med Ctr 1994; **Fellow:** Otolaryngology, Loyola Univ Med Ctr 1995; **Fac Appt:** Assoc Prof Oto, Univ Mich Med Sch

Hotaling, Andrew J MD [Oto] - **Spec Exp:** Pediatric Otolaryngology; Sleep Disorders/Apnea; Neck Masses; Ear Infections; **Hospital:** Loyola Univ Med Ctr; **Address:** Loyola Univ Med Ctr, 2160 S 1st Ave Maguire Bldg - rm 1870, Maywood, IL 60153-5590; **Phone:** 708-216-9183; **Board Cert:** Otolaryngology 1985; **Med School:** Case West Res Univ 1979; **Resid:** Surgery, Case Western 1981; Otolaryngology, Northwestern Meml Hosp 1984; **Fellow:** Pediatric Otolaryngology, Univ Pittsburgh Med Ctr 1985; **Fac Appt:** Prof Oto, Loyola Univ-Stritch Sch Med

Jones, Paul J MD [Oto] - **Spec Exp:** Pediatric Otolaryngology; **Hospital:** Rush Univ Med Ctr; **Address:** 1611 W Harrison St, Ste 550, Chicago, IL 60612; **Phone:** 312-942-2175; **Board Cert:** Otolaryngology 1989; **Med School:** Rush Med Coll 1983; **Resid:** Otolaryngology, Rush Presby-St Lukes Med Ctr 1988; **Fac Appt:** Asst Prof Oto, Rush Med Coll

Kang, Dong-Kyoo Richard MD [Oto] - **Spec Exp:** Cochlear Implants; Ear Disorders/Surgery; **Hospital:** Nationwide Chldn's Hosp; **Address:** Nationwide Children's Hospital, 700 Children's Drive, Columbus, OH 43205; **Phone:** 614-722-6600; **Board Cert:** Otolaryngology 1986; **Med School:** Boston Univ 1980; **Resid:** Otolaryngology, Naval Med Ctr 1986; **Fellow:** Pediatric Otolaryngology, St. Louis Chldn's Hosp 1991; Pediatric Otolaryngology, San Diego Chldn's Hosp 1993; **Fac Appt:** Assoc Clin Prof Oto, Ohio State Univ

Kartush, Jack MD [Oto] - **Spec Exp:** Ear Disorders/Surgery; Balance Disorders; **Hospital:** Providence Hosp - Southfield; **Address:** Michigan Ear Inst, 30055 Northwestern Hwy, Ste 101, Farmington Hills, MI 48334; **Phone:** 248-865-4444; **Board Cert:** Otolaryngology 1984; **Med School:** Univ Mich Med Sch 1978; **Resid:** Otolaryngology, Univ Mich Med Ctr 1984; **Fellow:** Neurotology, Univ Mich Med Ctr 1985; **Fac Appt:** Assoc Clin Prof Oto, Wayne State Univ

Kern, Robert C MD [Oto] - **Spec Exp:** Sinus Disorders/Surgery; Nasal & Sinus Disorders; Snoring/Sleep Apnea; Taste & Smell Disorders; **Hospital:** Northwestern Meml Hosp, Stroger Hosp of Cook Co; **Address:** Northwestern Medical Faculty Fdn, 675 N St Clair St Bldg 15 - Ste 200, Chicago, IL 60611; **Phone:** 312-695-8182; **Board Cert:** Otolaryngology 1990; **Med School:** Jefferson Med Coll 1985; **Resid:** Otolaryngology, Wayne State Affil Hosp 1990; **Fellow:** Research, Natl Inst Hlth 1991; **Fac Appt:** Prof Oto, Northwestern Univ

Lavertu, Pierre MD [Oto] - **Spec Exp:** Thyroid Cancer; Head & Neck Cancer; Skull Base Tumors; **Hospital:** Univ Hosps Case Med Ctr (page 74); **Address:** Univ Hosps, Dept Oto-Head & Neck Surg, 11100 Euclid Ave, Cleveland, OH 44106-5045; **Phone:** 216-844-4773; **Board Cert:** Otolaryngology 1981; **Med School:** Univ Montreal 1976; **Resid:** Otolaryngology, Univ Montreal Med Ctr 1981; **Fellow:** Head and Neck Surgery, Univ Montreal Med Ctr 1982; Head and Neck Surgery, Cleveland Clinic 1983; **Fac Appt:** Prof Oto, Case West Res Univ

Leonetti, John P MD [Oto] - **Spec Exp:** Skull Base Tumors & Surgery; Neuro-Otology; Head & Neck Cancer; Facial Paralysis; **Hospital:** Loyola Univ Med Ctr; **Address:** Loyola University Medical Ctr, Dept Otolaryngology, 2160 S First Ave Bldg 105 - rm 1870, Maywood, IL 60153; **Phone:** 708-216-4804; **Board Cert:** Otolaryngology 1987; **Med School:** Loyola Univ-Stritch Sch Med 1982; **Resid:** Otolaryngology, Loyola Univ Med Ctr 1987; Research, House Ear Inst 1987; **Fellow:** Neurotology, Barnes Jewish Hosp 1988; **Fac Appt:** Prof Oto, Loyola Univ-Stritch Sch Med

Marentette, Lawrence J MD [Oto] - **Spec Exp:** Skull Base Tumors & Surgery; Facial Plastic & Reconstructive Surgery; **Hospital:** Univ of Michigan Hosp; **Address:** Univ Michigan Hlth Sys, Dept Oto, 1500 E Med Ctr Drive, 1904 Taubman Ctr, Ann Arbor, MI 48109; **Phone:** 734-936-8051; **Board Cert:** Otolaryngology 1981; Facial Plastic & Reconstr Surgery 1995; **Med School:** Wayne State Univ 1976; **Resid:** Otolaryngology, Wayne State Univ 1980; **Fellow:** Maxillofacial Surgery, Univ of Zurich 1985; **Fac Appt:** Prof Oto, Univ Mich Med Sch

Miyamoto, Richard T MD [Oto] - **Spec Exp:** Neurotology; Acoustic Neuroma; Middle Ear Disorders; Cochlear Implants; **Hospital:** IU Health University Hosp, Riley Hosp for Children; **Address:** 702 Barnhill Drive, RI 0860, Indianapolis, IN 46202; **Phone:** 317-274-3556; **Board Cert:** Otolaryngology 1975; Neurotology 2004; **Med School:** Univ Mich Med Sch 1970; **Resid:** Surgery, Butterworth Hosp 1972; Otolaryngology, Indiana Univ Hosps 1975; **Fellow:** Otology & Neurotology, Otologic Med Grp 1978; **Fac Appt:** Prof Oto, Indiana Univ

Otolaryngology

Naclerio, Robert M MD [Oto] - **Spec Exp:** Head & Neck Surgery; Pediatric Otolaryngology; Sinus Disorders/Surgery; **Hospital:** Univ of Chicago Med Ctr; **Address:** Univ Chicago Med Ctr, 5841 S Maryland Ave, MC 1035, Chicago, IL 60637; **Phone:** 773-702-0080; **Board Cert:** Otolaryngology 1983; **Med School:** Baylor Coll Med 1976; **Resid:** Surgery, Johns Hopkins Hosp 1978; Otolaryngology, Baylor Coll Med 1980; **Fellow:** Clinical Immunology, Johns Hopkins Hosp 1982; **Fac Appt:** Prof Oto, Univ Chicago-Pritzker Sch Med

Olsen, Kerry D MD [Oto] - **Spec Exp:** Head & Neck Cancer & Surgery; Esthesioneuroblastoma; Salivary Gland Tumors & Surgery; Skull Base Tumors; **Hospital:** Mayo Med Ctr & Clin - Rochester; **Address:** Mayo Clinic, Dept Otolaryngology, 200 1st St SW, Rochester, MN 55905-0001; **Phone:** 507-284-3542; **Board Cert:** Otolaryngology 1981; **Med School:** Mayo Med Sch 1976; **Resid:** Otolaryngology, Mayo Clinic 1981; **Fac Appt:** Prof Oto, Mayo Med Sch

Ozer, Enver MD [Oto] - **Spec Exp:** Head & Neck Cancer; Head & Neck Surgery; **Hospital:** Ohio St Univ Med Ctr; **Address:** 456 W 10th Ave, Ste 4A, Columbus, OH 43210; **Phone:** 614-293-8074; **Med School:** Turkey 1994; **Resid:** Otolaryngology, Marmara Univ Med Sch 1996; Head and Neck Surgery, Marmara Univ Med Sch 2000; **Fellow:** Head & Neck Oncology, Ohio St Univ Med Ctr 2005; **Fac Appt:** Asst Prof Oto, Ohio State Univ

Paparella, Michael M MD [Oto] - **Spec Exp:** Hearing Disorders; Neuro-Otology; Meniere's Disease; **Hospital:** Univ Minn Med Ctr, Fairview - Riverside Campus; **Address:** 701 25th Ave S, Ste 200, Minneapolis, MN 55454-1443; **Phone:** 612-339-2836; **Board Cert:** Otolaryngology 1963; **Med School:** Univ Mich Med Sch 1957; **Resid:** Otolaryngology, Henry Ford Hosp 1961; **Fac Appt:** Clin Prof Oto, Univ Minn

Pelzer, Harold J MD/DDS [Oto] - **Spec Exp:** Head & Neck Cancer; Swallowing Disorders; **Hospital:** Northwestern Meml Hosp; **Address:** Northwestern Dept Otolaryngology, 675 N St Clair St, Ste 15-200, Chicago, IL 60611; **Phone:** 312-695-8182; **Board Cert:** Otolaryngology 1985; **Med School:** Northwestern Univ 1979; **Resid:** Surgery, Northwestern Meml Hosp 1983; **Fellow:** Head and Neck Surgery, Northwestern Meml Hosp 1985; **Fac Appt:** Assoc Prof Oto, Northwestern Univ

Pensak, Myles L MD [Oto] - **Spec Exp:** Skull Base Tumors; Facial Paralysis; Hearing & Balance Disorders; **Hospital:** Univ Hosp - Cincinnati, Good Samaritan Hosp - Cincinnati; **Address:** Univ Medical Arts Building, 222 Piedmont Ave, Ste 5200, Cincinnati, OH 45219; **Phone:** 513-475-8400; **Board Cert:** Otolaryngology 1983; Neurotology 2004; **Med School:** NY Med Coll 1978; **Resid:** Surgery, Upstate Med Ctr 1980; Otolaryngology, Yale Univ 1983; **Fellow:** Otology & Neurotology, The Otology Group 1984; **Fac Appt:** Prof Oto, Univ Cincinnati

Petruzzelli, Guy MD/PhD [Oto] - **Spec Exp:** Head & Neck Cancer & Surgery; Skull Base Tumors; Thyroid Cancer; Pituitary Tumors; **Hospital:** Rush Univ Med Ctr; **Address:** Rush Otolaryngology Head & Neck Surgery, 1611 W Harrison St, Ste 550, Chicago, IL 60612; **Phone:** 312-942-6100; **Board Cert:** Otolaryngology 1993; **Med School:** Rush Med Coll 1987; **Resid:** Otolaryngology, Univ Pittsburgh Med Ctr 1992; **Fellow:** Head & Neck Oncology, Univ Pittsburgh Med Ctr 1993; Skull Base Surgery, Univ Pittsburgh Ctr Cranial Base Surg 1993; **Fac Appt:** Prof Oto, Rush Med Coll

Piccirillo, Jay MD [Oto] - **Spec Exp:** Sleep Disorders/Apnea; Sinus Disorders/Surgery; **Hospital:** Barnes-Jewish Hosp; **Address:** Barnes Jewish Hosp South, Campus Box 8115, St Louis, MO 63110; **Phone:** 314-362-7509; **Board Cert:** Otolaryngology 1990; **Med School:** Univ VT Coll Med 1985; **Resid:** Otolaryngology, Albany Med Ctr 1990; **Fellow:** Yale Univ 1992; **Fac Appt:** Asst Prof Oto, Washington Univ, St Louis

Siegel, Gordon J MD [Oto] - **Spec Exp:** Head & Neck Cancer; Nasal & Sinus Disorders; **Hospital:** Northwestern Meml Hosp; **Address:** 3 E Huron St Fl 1, Chicago, IL 60611-2705; **Phone:** 312-988-7777; **Board Cert:** Otolaryngology 1984; **Med School:** Ros Franklin Univ/Chicago Med Sch 1978; **Resid:** Otolaryngology, Northwestern Univ Affil Hosp 1982; **Fac Appt:** Asst Clin Prof Oto, Northwestern Univ

Stankiewicz, James MD [Oto] - **Spec Exp:** Endoscopic Sinus Surgery; Rhinosinusitis; Nasal & Sinus Disorders; **Hospital:** Loyola Univ Med Ctr; **Address:** Loyola Univ Med Ctr, Dept Oto, 2160 S First Ave, Maywood, IL 60153-5590; **Phone:** 708-216-9183; **Board Cert:** Otolaryngology 1978; **Med School:** Univ Chicago-Pritzker Sch Med 1974; **Resid:** Otolaryngology, Univ Chicago Hosp 1978; **Fac Appt:** Prof Oto, Loyola Univ-Stritch Sch Med

Stenson, Kerstin M MD [Oto] - **Spec Exp:** Head & Neck Cancer & Surgery; Head & Neck Cancer Reconstruction; Trauma; Vocal Cord Disorders; **Hospital:** Univ of Chicago Med Ctr; **Address:** 5741 S Maryland Ave, MC 1035, Chicago, IL 60637-1463; **Phone:** 773-702-1865; **Board Cert:** Otolaryngology 1994; **Med School:** Ros Franklin Univ/Chicago Med Sch 1988; **Resid:** Otolaryngology, Univ Illinois Affil Hosp 1993; **Fellow:** Head & Neck Oncology, Univ Michigan Hosp 1994; Microvascular Surgery, Univ Michigan Hosp 1994; **Fac Appt:** Prof S, Univ Chicago-Pritzker Sch Med

Szachowicz II, Edward H MD [Oto] - **Spec Exp:** Cosmetic Surgery-Face; Rhinoplasty; **Hospital:** Abbott - Northwestern Hosp; **Address:** Centennial Lakes Med Bldg, 7373 France Ave S, Ste 508, Edina, MN 55435-4538; **Phone:** 952-835-5665; **Board Cert:** Otolaryngology 1984; **Med School:** Univ IL Coll Med 1979; **Resid:** Surgery, Fairview Univ Med Ctr 1980; Otolaryngology, Fairview Univ Med Ctr 1984; **Fellow:** Facial Plastic Surgery, Fairview Univ Med Ctr 1986; **Fac Appt:** Asst Clin Prof Oto, Univ Minn

Teknos, Theodoros N MD [Oto] - **Spec Exp:** Head & Neck Cancer; Thyroid Cancer; Facial Plastic & Reconstructive Surgery; Reconstructive Microvascular Surgery; **Hospital:** Ohio St Univ Med Ctr; **Address:** 456 W 10th Ave, Ste 4A, Columbus, OH 43210; **Phone:** 614-293-8074; **Board Cert:** Otolaryngology 1997; **Med School:** Harvard Med Sch 1991; **Resid:** Otolaryngology, Mass Eye & Ear Hosp 1996; **Fellow:** Head and Neck Surgery, Vanderbilt Univ Med Ctr 1997; Microvascular Surgery, Vanderbilt Univ Med Ctr 1997; **Fac Appt:** Prof Oto, Ohio State Univ

Telian, Steven A MD [Oto] - **Spec Exp:** Cochlear Implants; Ear Disorders/Surgery; Acoustic Neuroma; **Hospital:** Univ of Michigan Hosp; **Address:** Univ Mich Med Ctr, Dept Otolaryngology-Head & Neck Surgery, 1500 E Med Ctr Drive, 1904 Taubman Ctr, Ann Arbor, MI 48109-0312; **Phone:** 734-936-8006; **Board Cert:** Otolaryngology 1985; Neurotology 2004; **Med School:** Univ Pennsylvania 1980; **Resid:** Otolaryngology, Hosp Univ Penn 1985; **Fellow:** Neurotology, Univ Mich Med Ctr 1986; **Fac Appt:** Prof Oto, Univ Mich Med Sch

Toriumi, Dean MD [Oto] - **Spec Exp:** Rhinoplasty; Cosmetic Surgery-Face; Reconstructive Plastic Surgery; **Hospital:** Univ of IL Med Ctr at Chicago; **Address:** 60 E Delaware Pl, Ste 1460, Chicago, IL 60611; **Phone:** 312-255-8812; **Board Cert:** Otolaryngology 1988; **Med School:** Rush Med Coll 1981; **Resid:** Surgery, Univ Illinois Med Ctr 1985; Otolaryngology, Northwestern Univ Med Sch 1987; **Fellow:** Facial Plastic Surgery, Tulane Med Sch 1988; Facial Plastic Surgery, Virginia Mason Med Ctr 1989; **Fac Appt:** Assoc Prof Oto, Univ IL Coll Med

Wiet, Richard J MD [Oto] - **Spec Exp:** Acoustic Neuroma; Hearing Loss; Otosclerosis/Stapedectomy; Cochlear Implants; **Hospital:** Adventist Hinsdale Hosp, Northwestern Meml Hosp; **Address:** Ear Institute of Chicago, 11 Salt Creek Ln, Ste 101, Hinsdale, IL 60521; **Phone:** 630-789-3110; **Board Cert:** Otolaryngology 1976; Neurotology 2004; **Med School:** Loyola Univ-Stritch Sch Med 1971; **Resid:** Otolaryngology, Cincinnati Med Ctr 1976; **Fellow:** Neurotology, Univ Zurich/Ear Fdn 1979; **Fac Appt:** Clin Prof Oto, Northwestern Univ

Otolaryngology

Wilson, Keith M MD [Oto] - **Spec Exp:** Head & Neck Cancer & Surgery; Voice Disorders; **Hospital:** Univ Hosp - Cincinnati; **Address:** Univ Cincinnati Medical Ctr, 222 Piedmont Ave, Ste 5200, Cincinnati, OH 45219-4222; **Phone:** 513-475-8400; **Board Cert:** Otolaryngology 1992; **Med School:** Cornell Univ-Weill Med Coll 1986; **Resid:** Otolaryngology, St Louis Univ Med Ctr 1991; **Fellow:** Head & Neck Surgical Oncology, Ohio State Med Ctr 1992; **Fac Appt:** Assoc Prof Oto, Univ Cincinnati

Wolf, Gregory T MD [Oto] - **Spec Exp:** Head & Neck Cancer; Laryngeal Cancer; **Hospital:** Univ of Michigan Hosp; **Address:** Univ Mich Med Ctr, Dept Oto-HNS, 1500 E Med Ctr, Taubman Ctr, rm 1904, Ann Arbor, MI 48109-0312; **Phone:** 734-936-8029; **Board Cert:** Otolaryngology 1978; **Med School:** Univ Mich Med Sch 1973; **Resid:** Surgery, Georgetown Univ Hosp 1975; Otolaryngology, SUNY Upstate Med Ctr 1977; **Fellow:** Immunology, NIH 1980; **Fac Appt:** Prof Oto, Univ Mich Med Sch

Woodson, B Tucker MD [Oto] - **Spec Exp:** Sleep Disorders/Apnea; **Hospital:** Froedtert and Med Ctr of WI, Chldns Hosp - Wisconsin; **Address:** Froedtert West ENT Clinic, 9200 W Wisconsin Ave, Milwaukee, WI 53226-3522; **Phone:** 414-805-7667; **Board Cert:** Otolaryngology 1988; **Med School:** Univ MO-Columbia Sch Med 1983; **Resid:** Surgery, Henry Ford Hosp 1984; Otolaryngology, Henry Ford Hosp 1988; **Fac Appt:** Assoc Prof Oto, Med Coll Wisc

Woodson, Gayle Ellen MD [Oto] - **Spec Exp:** Voice Disorders; Swallowing Disorders; **Hospital:** St. John's Hosp - Springfield, Memorial Med Ctr-Springfield; **Address:** Div Otolaryngology, PO Box 19662, Springfield, IL 62794-9662; **Phone:** 217-545-6099; **Board Cert:** Otolaryngology 1981; **Med School:** Baylor Coll Med 1975; **Resid:** Surgery, Johns Hopkins Hosp 1978; Otolaryngology, Baylor Coll Med 1981; **Fellow:** Laryngology, Inst Laryngology and Otology 1982; **Fac Appt:** Prof Oto, Southern IL Univ

Young, Nancy MD [Oto] - **Spec Exp:** Cochlear Implants; Cholesteatoma; Hearing Loss; Baha Implant; **Hospital:** Children's Mem Hosp -Chicago, Glenbrook Hosp-NorthShore Univ Hlth Syst; **Address:** Children's Memorial, Div Otolaryngology, 2300 Children's Plaza, Box 265, Chicago, IL 60614; **Phone:** 773-880-3020; **Board Cert:** Otolaryngology 1987; **Med School:** NYU Sch Med 1982; **Resid:** Surgery, Montefiore Med Ctr 1984; Otolaryngology, Northwestern Univ Hosp 1987; **Fellow:** Neurotology, Hinsdale Hosp 1988; **Fac Appt:** Assoc Prof Oto, Northwestern Univ

Yueh, Bevan MD [Oto] - **Spec Exp:** Head & Neck Cancer; Hearing Loss; **Address:** Univ Minn Med Ctr, Dept Otolaryngology/Head & Neck Surgery, 420 Delaware St SE, MMC 396, Minneapolis, MN 55455-0932; **Phone:** 612-625-2410; **Board Cert:** Otolaryngology 1995; **Med School:** Stanford Univ 1989; **Resid:** Otolaryngology, Johns Hopkins Hosp 1994; **Fellow:** Otolaryngology, Johns Hopkins Hosp 1995; **Fac Appt:** Assoc Prof Oto, Univ Minn

Great Plains and Mountains

Abaza, Mona M MD [Oto] - **Spec Exp:** Voice Disorders; Swallowing Disorders; **Hospital:** Univ of CO Hosp - Anschutz Inpatient Pav; **Address:** Univ Colorado Dept ENT, 1635 Aurora Court, MS F737, Aurora, CO 80045; **Phone:** 720-848-2820; **Board Cert:** Otolaryngology 1999; **Med School:** Med Coll PA Hahnemann 1991; **Resid:** Otolaryngology, Univ Texas Affil Hosps 1998; **Fellow:** Research, Natl Insts of Deafness & Communicative Disorders 1994; Laryngology, Jefferson Univ Hosp 1999; **Fac Appt:** Assoc Prof Oto, Univ Colorado

Chowdhury, Khalid MD [Oto] - **Spec Exp:** Skull Base Tumors & Surgery; Craniofacial Surgery; Maxillofacial Surgery; Head & Neck Cancer; **Hospital:** Porter Adventist Hosp, Denver Health Med Ctr; **Address:** Center for Craniofacial Surgery, 1601 E 19th Ave, Ste 3000, Denver, CO 80218; **Phone:** 303-839-5155; **Board Cert:** Otolaryngology 1990; Facial Plastic & Reconstr Surgery 1995; **Med School:** Univ Saskatchewan 1982; **Resid:** Surgery, Univ Saskatchewan Hosp 1985; Otolaryngology, McGill Univ Hosps 1989; **Fellow:** Craniofacial Surgery, Univ Bern Hosp 1990; Facial Plastic & Reconstr Surgery, Univ Bern Hosp 1990; **Fac Appt:** Assoc Prof Oto, Univ Colorado

Denenberg, Steven M MD [Oto] - **Spec Exp:** Cosmetic Surgery-Face; Rhinoplasty; **Hospital:** Nebraska Meth Hosp, Alegent Hlth - Bergan Mercy Med Ctr; **Address:** 7640 Pacific St, Omaha, NE 68114-5421; **Phone:** 402-391-7640; **Board Cert:** Otolaryngology 1984; Facial Plastic & Reconstr Surgery 1992; **Med School:** Univ Nebr Coll Med 1980; **Resid:** Otolaryngology, Stanford Univ Med Ctr 1984; **Fellow:** Facial Plastic Surgery, McCollough Ctr 1985; **Fac Appt:** Asst Clin Prof Oto, Univ Nebr Coll Med

Jenkins, Herman A MD [Oto] - **Spec Exp:** Ear Disorders/Surgery; Neuro-Otology; Acoustic Neuroma; Cochlear Implants; **Hospital:** Univ of CO Hosp - Anschutz Inpatient Pav, Chldn's Hosp - Aurora (CO); **Address:** Univ Colorado Hosp, Dept Otolaryngology, 1635 Aurora Court, MC F737, Aurora, CO 80045; **Phone:** 720-848-2820; **Board Cert:** Otolaryngology 1977; Neurotology 2004; **Med School:** Vanderbilt Univ 1970; **Resid:** Surgery, UCLA Med Ctr 1972; Otolaryngology, UCLA Med Ctr 1977; **Fellow:** Neurotology, Univ Hosp 1980; **Fac Appt:** Prof Oto, Univ Colorado

Kingdom, Todd T MD [Oto] - **Spec Exp:** Nasal & Sinus Disorders; Endoscopic Sinus Surgery; Skull Base Surgery; **Hospital:** Univ of CO Hosp - Anschutz Inpatient Pav, Natl Jewish Med & Rsch Ctr; **Address:** Univ Colorado Hospital, 1635 Aurora Court, MS F737, Aurora, CO 80045; **Phone:** 720-848-2820; **Board Cert:** Otolaryngology 1997; **Med School:** Emory Univ 1991; **Resid:** Otolaryngology, UCSF Med Ctr 1996; **Fac Appt:** Assoc Prof Oto, Univ Colorado

Lydiatt, Daniel D MD/DDS [Oto] - **Spec Exp:** Head & Neck Cancer; **Hospital:** Nebraska Med Ctr, Methodist Hosp - Omaha; **Address:** Nebraska Med Ctr, Dept Otolaryngology, 981225 Nebraska Medical Ctr, Omaha, NE 68198-1225; **Phone:** 402-559-6500; **Board Cert:** Otolaryngology 1992; **Med School:** Univ Nebr Coll Med 1983; **Resid:** Otolaryngology, Univ Nebraska Med Ctr 1990; **Fellow:** Head and Neck Surgery, MD Anderson Med Ctr 1991; **Fac Appt:** Assoc Prof Oto, Univ Nebr Coll Med

Lydiatt, William M MD [Oto] - **Spec Exp:** Head & Neck Cancer; Thyroid Cancer; Salivary Gland Tumors & Surgery; **Hospital:** Nebraska Med Ctr, Nebraska Meth Hosp; **Address:** 981225 Nebraska Medical Ctr, Omaha, NE 68198-7630; **Phone:** 402-559-6500; **Board Cert:** Otolaryngology 1994; **Med School:** Univ Nebr Coll Med 1988; **Resid:** Otolaryngology, Univ Nebraska Med Ctr 1993; **Fellow:** Head and Neck Surgery, Meml Sloan Kettering Cancer Ctr 1995; **Fac Appt:** Prof Oto, Univ Nebr Coll Med

Shelton, Clough MD [Oto] - **Spec Exp:** Facial Nerve Disorders; Acoustic Neuroma; Hearing & Balance Disorders; Cochlear Implants; **Hospital:** Univ Utah Hlth Care; **Address:** Univi Utah Sch Med, 50 N Med Drive, 1900 East, Ste 3C120, Salt Lake City, UT 84132; **Phone:** 801-585-5450; **Board Cert:** Otolaryngology 1986; Neurotology 2004; **Med School:** Univ Tex SW, Dallas 1981; **Resid:** Otolaryngology, Stanford Univ Med Ctr 1986; **Fellow:** Neurotology, Otologic Med Group 1987; **Fac Appt:** Prof Oto, Univ Utah

Otolaryngology

Smith, Russell B MD [Oto] - **Spec Exp:** Head & Neck Cancer; Thyroid Cancer; Skull Base Tumors; **Hospital:** Nebraska Med Ctr, Nebraska Meth Hosp; **Address:** 981225 Nebraska Medical Center, Omaha, NE 68198-1225; **Phone:** 402-559-6500; **Board Cert:** Otolaryngology 2001; **Med School:** Univ MO-Columbia Sch Med 1995; **Resid:** Otolaryngology, Univ Missouri Med Ctr 2000; **Fellow:** Head & Neck Surgical Oncology, Univ Iowa Hosps & Clins 2001; **Fac Appt:** Assoc Prof Oto, Univ Nebr Coll Med

Song, John I MD [Oto] - **Spec Exp:** Head & Neck Cancer; Skull Base Tumors; Swallowing Disorders; **Hospital:** Univ of CO Hosp - Anschutz Inpatient Pav; **Address:** Univ Colorado Hosp, Otolaryngology, 1635 Aurora Ct, MS F737, Aurora, CO 80045; **Phone:** 720-848-2820; **Board Cert:** Otolaryngology 1998; **Med School:** NYU Sch Med 1991; **Resid:** Otolaryngology, UCLA Med Ctr 1997; **Fellow:** Head and Neck Surgery, Univ Pittsburgh Med Ctr 1998; **Fac Appt:** Asst Prof Oto, Univ Colorado

Southwest

Amedee, Ronald G MD [Oto] - **Spec Exp:** Otology & Neuro-Otology; Skull Base Surgery; Sinus Disorders/Surgery; Hearing & Balance Disorders; **Hospital:** Ochsner Med Ctr-New Orleans, Tulane Med Ctr; **Address:** Ochsner Medical Ctr-Otolaryngology, 1514 Jefferson Hwy, New Orleans, LA 70121; **Phone:** 504-842-3640; **Board Cert:** Otolaryngology 1987; **Med School:** Louisiana State U, New Orleans 1981; **Resid:** Surgery, Charity Hosp 1983; Otolaryngology, Charity Hosp 1986; **Fellow:** Skull Base Surgery, Klinikum der Albert Ludwigs 1988; **Fac Appt:** Prof Oto, Tulane Univ

Arriaga, Moises A MD [Oto] - **Spec Exp:** Meniere's Disease; Skull Base Surgery; Acoustic Neuroma; Cochlear Implants; **Hospital:** Our Lady of the Lake Regl Med Ctr, Children's Hospital - New Orleans; **Address:** Hearing & Balance Ctr, 7777 Hennessy Blvd, Ste 709, Baton Rouge, LA 70808; **Phone:** 225-765-7735; **Board Cert:** Otolaryngology 1990; Neurotology 2004; **Med School:** Brown Univ 1985; **Resid:** Otolaryngology, Univ Pittsburgh Med Ctr 1990; **Fellow:** Neurotology, House Ear Clinic 1991; **Fac Appt:** Prof Oto, Louisiana State U, New Orleans

Clark, Keith F MD/PhD [Oto] - **Spec Exp:** Pediatric Otolaryngology; Airway Reconstruction; Voice Disorders; Vocal Cord Disorders-Botox Therapy; **Hospital:** St. Anthony Hosp -Oklahoma City; **Address:** 535 NW 9th St, Ste 300, Oklahoma City, OK 73102; **Phone:** 405-272-6027; **Board Cert:** Otolaryngology 1983; **Med School:** Univ Mich Med Sch 1978; **Resid:** Otolaryngology, Univ Iowa Med Ctr 1983

Clayman, Gary Lee MD/DMD [Oto] - **Spec Exp:** Thyroid Cancer & Surgery; Salivary Gland Tumors & Surgery; Head & Neck Cancer; Thyroid & Parathyroid Surgery; **Hospital:** UT MD Anderson Cancer Ctr; **Address:** Univ TX/MD Anderson Cancer Center, 1515 Holcombe Blvd, Unit 1445, Houston, TX 77030-4009; **Phone:** 713-792-8837; **Board Cert:** Otolaryngology 1992; **Med School:** NE Ohio Univ 1986; **Resid:** Surgery, Hennepin Co Med Ctr 1987; Otolaryngology, Univ Minn Med Ctr 1991; **Fellow:** Head and Neck Surgery, MD Anderson Cancer Ctr 1993; **Fac Appt:** Prof Oto, Univ Tex, Houston

Diaz, Eduardo M MD [Oto] - **Spec Exp:** Head & Neck Cancer; Laryngeal Cancer; Laryngeal Cancer-Organ Preservation; Tongue Cancer; **Hospital:** UT MD Anderson Cancer Ctr; **Address:** UT MD Anderson Cancer Center, Head & Neck Center, 1515 Holcombe Blvd, Unit 460, Houston, TX 77030; **Phone:** 713-792-6920; **Board Cert:** Otolaryngology 1995; **Med School:** Baylor Coll Med 1989; **Resid:** Surgery, Univ Tex Hlth Sci Ctr 1991; Ophthalmology, Univ Tex Hlth Sci Ctr 1994; **Fellow:** Head & Neck Surgical Oncology, UT MD Anderson Cancer Ctr 1995; **Fac Appt:** Prof Oto, Univ Tex, Houston

Donovan, Donald T MD [Oto] - **Spec Exp:** Head & Neck Cancer; Voice Disorders; Vocal Cord Disorders; Thyroid Disorders; **Hospital:** Methodist Hosp - Houston, St. Luke's Episcopal Hosp-Houston; **Address:** 6550 Fannin St, Ste 1701, Smith Tower, Houston, TX 77030; **Phone:** 713-798-5900; **Board Cert:** Otolaryngology 1981; **Med School:** Baylor Coll Med 1976; **Resid:** Surgery, Baylor Affil Hosps 1978; Otolaryngology, Baylor Affil Hosps 1981; **Fellow:** Head and Neck Surgery, Columbia-Presby Med Ctr 1982; **Fac Appt:** Prof Oto, Baylor Coll Med

Dornhoffer, John L MD [Oto] - **Spec Exp:** Hearing & Balance Disorders; Neuro-Otology; Hearing Loss; **Hospital:** UAMS Med Ctr; **Address:** UAMS, Dept Otolaryngology, Head & Neck Surgery, 4301 W Markham St, Ste 547-05, Little Rock, AR 72205; **Phone:** 501-686-5878; **Board Cert:** Otolaryngology 1994; **Med School:** Univ Kansas 1988; **Resid:** Otolaryngology, UAMS Med Ctr 1992; **Fellow:** Otology, Univ of Zurich Affil Hosp 1994; Otology, Univ of Wuzburg Affil Hosp 1994; **Fac Appt:** Prof Oto, Univ Ark

Gianoli, Gerard MD [Oto] - **Spec Exp:** Dizziness; Hearing Loss; Ear Disorders/Surgery; Balance Disorders; **Hospital:** North Oaks Med Ctr; **Address:** 17050 Medical Center Drive, Ste 315, The Ear & Balance Institute, Baton Rouge, LA 70816-3249; **Phone:** 225-293-6973; **Board Cert:** Otolaryngology 1993; Neurotology 2004; **Med School:** Tulane Univ 1986; **Resid:** Pediatrics, Tulane Univ 1988; Otolaryngology, Tulane Univ 1992; **Fellow:** Otology & Neurotology, Michigan Ear Inst; **Fac Appt:** Assoc Clin Prof Oto, Tulane Univ

Graham III, H Devon MD [Oto] - **Spec Exp:** Cosmetic & Reconstructive Surgery-Face; Snoring/Sleep Apnea; Nasal Reconstruction; Facial Rejuvenation; **Hospital:** Ochsner Med Ctr-New Orleans; **Address:** 1514 Jefferson Hwy, 4th Fl, New Orleans, LA 70121; **Phone:** 504-842-3950; **Board Cert:** Otolaryngology 1989; Facial Plastic & Reconstr Surgery 1993; **Med School:** Louisiana State U, New Orleans 1984; **Resid:** Surgery, Ochsner Foundation Hosp 1986; Otolaryngology, Tulane Univ Med Ctr 1989; **Fellow:** Facial Plastic Surgery, Baptist Hosp 1990; Facial Plastic Surgery, St Joseph Hosp 1990; **Fac Appt:** Asst Clin Prof Oto, Tulane Univ

Hanna, Ehab YN MD [Oto] - **Spec Exp:** Skull Base Tumors & Surgery; Head & Neck Cancer & Surgery; **Hospital:** UT MD Anderson Cancer Ctr; **Address:** Univ Tex MD Anderson Cancer Ctr, 1515 Holcolmbe Blvd, Unit 1445, Houston, TX 77030; **Phone:** 713-745-1815; **Board Cert:** Otolaryngology 1994; **Med School:** Egypt 1982; **Resid:** Otolaryngology, Cleveland Clinic 1989; Otolaryngology, Cleveland Clinic 1993; **Fellow:** Otolaryngology, Univ Pittsburgh Med Ctr 1994; **Fac Appt:** Prof Oto, Univ Tex, Houston

Hayden, Richard E MD [Oto] - **Spec Exp:** Head & Neck Surgery; Thyroid & Parathyroid Surgery; Facial Plastic & Reconstructive Surgery; Microvascular Surgery; **Hospital:** Mayo Clinic - Phoenix; **Address:** Mayo Clinic, Dept Otolaryngology, 5777 E Mayo Blvd, Phoenix, AZ 85054; **Phone:** 480-342-2912; **Board Cert:** Otolaryngology 1978; **Med School:** McGill Univ 1974; **Resid:** Otolaryngology, Univ Toronto Affil Hosp 1978; **Fellow:** Head & Neck Oncology, MD Anderson Hosp 1979; Radiation Oncology, Princess Margaret Hosp 1980; **Fac Appt:** Prof Oto, Mayo Med Sch

Johnson Jr, Calvin M MD [Oto] - **Spec Exp:** Ear Disorders/Surgery; Nasal Surgery; Cosmetic Surgery-Face; **Address:** Hedgewood Surgical Ctr, 2427 St Charles Ave, New Orleans, LA 70130; **Phone:** 504-895-7642; **Board Cert:** Otolaryngology 1974; Facial Plastic & Reconstr Surgery 1989; **Med School:** Tulane Univ 1967; **Resid:** Surgery, Tulane Univ Sch Med 1971; Otolaryngology, Tulane Univ Sch Med 1974; **Fellow:** Facial Plastic Surgery, Amer Academy Facial Plastic & Recon Surg 1975

Otolaryngology

Macias, John D MD [Oto] - **Spec Exp:** Otology; Neuro-Otology; Cochlear Implants; Hearing Loss; **Hospital:** Banner Good Samaritan Regl Med Ctr - Phoenix, Phoenix Children's Hosp; **Address:** 1515 N 9th St, Ste B, Phoenix, AZ 85006-2523; **Phone:** 602-257-4228; **Board Cert:** Otolaryngology 1994; Neurotology 2005; **Med School:** Stanford Univ 1988; **Resid:** Otolaryngology, Univ Iowa Hosps & Clins 1993; **Fellow:** Otology & Neurotology, Ear Fdn/Otology Grp 1994

Medina, Jesus E MD [Oto] - **Spec Exp:** Head & Neck Cancer & Surgery; **Hospital:** OU Med Ctr; **Address:** 825 NE 10th St Fl 4 - Ste 4200, Oklahoma City, OK 73104; **Phone:** 405-271-7559; **Board Cert:** Otolaryngology 1980; **Med School:** Peru 1974; **Resid:** Surgery, Wayne St Univ Affil Hosp 1977; Otolaryngology, Wayne St Univ Affil Hosp 1980; **Fellow:** Head and Neck Surgery, MD Anderson Hosp 1981; **Fac Appt:** Prof Oto, Univ Okla Coll Med

Myers, Jeffrey N MD/PhD [Oto] - **Spec Exp:** Head & Neck Cancer; Melanoma-Head & Neck; Tongue Cancer; **Hospital:** UT MD Anderson Cancer Ctr; **Address:** Univ Texas MD Anderson Cancer Ctr, 1515 Holcombe Blvd, Box 441, Houston, TX 77030; **Phone:** 713-745-2667; **Board Cert:** Otolaryngology 1997; **Med School:** Univ Pennsylvania 1991; **Resid:** Otolaryngology, Univ Pittsburgh Med Ctr 1996; **Fellow:** Head & Neck Surgical Oncology, MD Anderson Cancer Ctr 1997; **Fac Appt:** Assoc Prof Oto, Univ Tex, Houston

Nuss, Daniel W MD [Oto] - **Spec Exp:** Head & Neck Cancer; Skull Base Tumors & Surgery; **Hospital:** Our Lady of the Lake Regl Med Ctr; **Address:** Our Lady of the Lake Regl Med Ctr, 7777 Hennessy Blvd, Ste 409, Baton Rouge, LA 70808; **Phone:** 225-765-1765; **Board Cert:** Otolaryngology 1987; **Med School:** Louisiana State U, New Orleans 1981; **Resid:** Surgery, Charity Hosp 1983; Otolaryngology, LSU Med Ctr 1987; **Fellow:** Surgical Oncology, MD Anderson Hosp & Tumor Inst 1984; Head and Neck Surgery, Ctr Cranial Base Surg-Univ Pittsburgh 1991; **Fac Appt:** Prof Oto, Louisiana State U, New Orleans

Otto, Randal A MD [Oto] - **Spec Exp:** Head & Neck Cancer; Thyroid & Parathyroid Cancer & Surgery; Sinus Disorders/Surgery; **Hospital:** Univ Hlth Syst-San Antonio, Audie L Murphy Meml Vets Hosp - San Antonio; **Address:** 8300 Floyd Curl Drive, MSC 7777, San Antonio, TX 78229-3900; **Phone:** 210-450-0700; **Board Cert:** Otolaryngology 1987; **Med School:** Univ MO-Columbia Sch Med 1981; **Resid:** Pathology, Queens Med Ctr 1982; Otolaryngology, Univ of Missouri 1987; **Fac Appt:** Prof Oto, Univ Tex, San Antonio

Stasney, C Richard MD [Oto] - **Spec Exp:** Voice Disorders; Vocal Cord Disorders; Laryngeal Disorders; **Hospital:** Methodist Hosp - Houston; **Address:** Texas Voice Center, 6550 Fannin St, Ste 2025, Houston, TX 77030; **Phone:** 713-796-2001; **Board Cert:** Otolaryngology 1974; **Med School:** Baylor Coll Med 1969; **Resid:** Surgery, Baylor Affil Hosps 1971; Otolaryngology, Baylor Affil Hosps 1974; **Fac Appt:** Clin Prof Oto, Cornell Univ-Weill Med Coll

Suen, James Y MD [Oto] - **Spec Exp:** Head & Neck Cancer; Vascular Lesions-Head & Neck; Laryngeal Disorders; Thyroid Cancer; **Hospital:** UAMS Med Ctr, Arkansas Chldns Hosp; **Address:** Univ Hosp Arkansas Med Scis, 4301 W Markham St, Slot 543, Little Rock, AR 72205; **Phone:** 501-686-8224; **Board Cert:** Otolaryngology 1973; **Med School:** Univ Ark 1966; **Resid:** Surgery, Univ Arkansas Med Ctr 1970; Otolaryngology, Univ Arkansas Med Ctr 1973; **Fellow:** Head and Neck Surgery, MD Anderson Cancer Ctr 1974; **Fac Appt:** Prof Oto, Univ Ark

Weber, Randal S MD [Oto] - **Spec Exp:** Skin Cancer; Thyroid & Parathyroid Cancer & Surgery; Salivary Gland Tumors & Surgery; Head & Neck Cancer; **Hospital:** UT MD Anderson Cancer Ctr; **Address:** 1515 Holcombe Blvd, Unit 1445, Houston, TX 77030-4009; **Phone:** 713-745-0497; **Board Cert:** Otolaryngology 1985; **Med School:** Univ Tenn Coll Med 1976; **Resid:** Surgery, Baylor Coll Med 1982; Otolaryngology, Baylor Coll Med 1985; **Fellow:** Head and Neck Surgery, MD Anderson Cancer Ctr 1986; **Fac Appt:** Prof Oto, Univ Tex, Houston

Weber, Samuel C MD [Oto] - **Spec Exp:** Thyroid Cancer; Parathyroid Cancer; Nasal & Sinus Surgery; Head & Neck Surgery; **Hospital:** St. Luke's Episcopal Hosp-Houston, Methodist Hosp - Houston; **Address:** 6624 Fannin St, Ste 1480, Houston, TX 77030-2385; **Phone:** 713-795-5343; **Board Cert:** Otolaryngology 1972; **Med School:** Univ Tenn Coll Med 1965; **Resid:** Surgery, Baylor Coll Med 1971; Otolaryngology, Baylor Coll Med 1972; **Fac Appt:** Clin Prof Oto, Baylor Coll Med

West Coast and Pacific

Andersen, Peter MD [Oto] - **Spec Exp:** Laryngeal Cancer; Nasal & Sinus Cancer & Surgery; Head & Neck Cancer & Surgery; Neck Masses; **Hospital:** OR Hlth & Sci Univ; **Address:** Dept of Otolaryngology, 3181 SW Sam Jackson Park Rd, MC PV-01, Portland, OR 97239; **Phone:** 503-494-5355; **Board Cert:** Otolaryngology 1994; **Med School:** Washington Univ, St Louis 1988; **Resid:** Otolaryngology, Oregon Hlth & Science Univ 1993; **Fellow:** Head & Neck Surgical Oncology, Meml Sloan Kettering Cancer Ctr 1995; **Fac Appt:** Prof Oto, Oregon Hlth & Sci Univ

Berke, Gerald S MD [Oto] - **Spec Exp:** Head & Neck Surgery; Head & Neck Cancer; Voice Disorders; Laryngeal Disorders; **Hospital:** UCLA Ronald Reagan Med Ctr; **Address:** 200 UCLA Med Plaza, Ste 550, Los Angeles, CA 90095; **Phone:** 310-825-5179; **Board Cert:** Otolaryngology 1984; **Med School:** USC Sch Med 1978; **Resid:** Otolaryngology, LAC-USC Med Ctr 1979; **Fellow:** Head and Neck Surgery, UCLA Med Ctr 1984; **Fac Appt:** Prof Oto, UCLA

Blackwell, Keith Edward MD [Oto] - **Spec Exp:** Head & Neck Reconstruction; Head & Neck Cancer & Surgery; Microvascular Surgery; **Hospital:** UCLA Ronald Reagan Med Ctr; **Address:** UCLA Medical Center, Ste 550, Box 951624, Los Angeles, CA 90095; **Phone:** 310-206-6688; **Board Cert:** Otolaryngology 1995; **Med School:** Northwestern Univ 1988; **Resid:** Otolaryngology, UCLA Med Ctr1 1994; **Fellow:** Otolaryngology, Mt Sinai Med Ctr 1995; **Fac Appt:** Prof Oto, UCLA

Brackmann, Derald E MD [Oto] - **Spec Exp:** Ear Disorders/Surgery; Facial Nerve Disorders; Acoustic Neuroma; Otosclerosis/Stapedectomy; **Hospital:** St. Vincent's Med Ctr - Los Angeles; **Address:** House Clinic, 2100 W 3rd St, 1st Fl, Los Angeles, CA 90057-1902; **Phone:** 213-483-9930; **Board Cert:** Otolaryngology 1971; Neurotology 2005; **Med School:** Univ IL Coll Med 1962; **Resid:** Otolaryngology, LAC/USC Med Ctr 1970; **Fellow:** Otology & Neurotology, House Ear Clinic 1971; **Fac Appt:** Clin Prof Oto, USC-Keck School of Medicine

Courey, Mark S MD [Oto] - **Spec Exp:** Laryngeal Disorders; Swallowing Disorders; Laryngeal Cancer; **Hospital:** UCSF - Mt Zion Med Ctr, UCSF Med Ctr; **Address:** UCSF Voice & Swallowing Ctr, 2330 Post St Fl 5 - Ste 526, San Francisco, CA 94115; **Phone:** 415-885-7700; **Board Cert:** Otolaryngology 1993; **Med School:** SUNY Buffalo 1987; **Resid:** Otolaryngology, SUNY-Buffalo Med Ctr 1992; **Fellow:** Laryngology, Vanderbilt Univ 1993; **Fac Appt:** Prof Oto, UCSF

Donald, Paul J MD [Oto] - **Spec Exp:** Skull Base Tumors & Surgery; Head & Neck Cancer; **Hospital:** UC Davis Med Ctr; **Address:** 2521 Stockton Blvd, rm 7200, Sacramento, CA 95817; **Phone:** 916-734-2832; **Board Cert:** Otolaryngology 1973; **Med School:** Univ British Columbia Fac Med 1964; **Resid:** Surgery, St Pauls Hosp 1969; Otolaryngology, Univ Iowa Hosp 1973; **Fac Appt:** Prof Oto, UC Davis

Duckert, Larry G MD/PhD [Oto] - **Spec Exp:** Otology & Neuro-Otology; Otosclerosis/Stapedectomy; Acoustic Neuroma; Skull Base Surgery; **Hospital:** Univ Wash Med Ctr; **Address:** 1959 NE Pacific St, Box 356161, Seattle, WA 98195; **Phone:** 206-598-4022; **Board Cert:** Otolaryngology 1978; **Med School:** Univ Minn 1972; **Resid:** Otolaryngology, Univ Minnesota Hosp 1978; **Fellow:** Research, Ohio State Univ Coll of Med 1972; Otology & Neurotology, Univ Wuzburg Affil Hosp 1990; **Fac Appt:** Prof Oto, Univ Wash

Eisele, David W MD [Oto] - **Spec Exp:** Salivary Gland Tumors & Surgery; Head & Neck Cancer; Thyroid Cancer; Neck Masses; **Hospital:** UCSF Med Ctr; **Address:** UCSF, Dept Head & Neck Surgery, 2380 Sutter St Fl 2, Box 1703, San Francisco, CA 94115-1703; **Phone:** 415-885-7528; **Board Cert:** Otolaryngology 1988; **Med School:** Cornell Univ-Weill Med Coll 1982; **Resid:** Surgery, Univ Wash Med Ctr 1984; Otolaryngology, Univ Wash Med Ctr 1988; **Fac Appt:** Prof Oto, UCSF

Fee Jr, Willard E MD [Oto] - **Spec Exp:** Head & Neck Cancer; Parotid Gland Tumors; Thyroid Cancer; **Hospital:** Stanford Univ Hosp & Clinics; **Address:** Stanford Cancer Ctr, 875 Blake Lake Wilbur Dr, CC-2227, Stanford, CA 94305-5826; **Phone:** 650-498-6000; **Board Cert:** Otolaryngology 1974; **Med School:** Univ Colorado 1969; **Resid:** Surgery, Wadsworth VA Hosp 1971; Otolaryngology, UCLA Med Ctr 1974; **Fac Appt:** Prof Oto, Stanford Univ

Flint, Paul W MD [Oto] - **Spec Exp:** Voice Disorders; Laryngeal Disorders; **Hospital:** OR Hlth & Sci Univ; **Address:** Oregon Health & Science Univ, 3181 SW Sam Jackson Park Rd, MC PV01, Portland, OR 97239; **Phone:** 503-494-8510; **Board Cert:** Otolaryngology 1989; **Med School:** Baylor Coll Med 1983; **Resid:** Surgery, Univ Washington 1985; Otolaryngology, Univ Washington 1989; **Fellow:** Otolaryngology, Guys Hosp 1989; **Fac Appt:** Prof Oto, Oregon Hlth & Sci Univ

Futran, Neal D MD/DMD [Oto] - **Spec Exp:** Head & Neck Cancer & Surgery; Head & Neck Cancer Reconstruction; Skull Base Tumors & Surgery; **Hospital:** Univ Wash Med Ctr, Harborview Med Ctr; **Address:** Univ Wash Med Ctr, Oto Office, 1959 NE Pacific St, Box 356161, Seattle, WA 98195-6515; **Phone:** 206-543-3060; **Board Cert:** Otolaryngology 1993; **Med School:** SUNY Downstate 1987; **Resid:** Surgery, Kings Co-SUNY Downstate 1985; Otolaryngology, Univ Rochester Med Ctr 1992; **Fellow:** Microvascular Surgery, Mt Sinai Hosp 1993; **Fac Appt:** Prof Oto, Univ Wash

Harris, Jeffrey P MD/PhD [Oto] - **Spec Exp:** Neuro-Otology; Hearing & Balance Disorders; Skull Base Surgery; Meniere's Disease; **Hospital:** UCSD Med Ctr, VA San Diego Hlthcre Sys; **Address:** UCSD Med Ctr, 9350 Campus Point Drive, La Jolla, CA 92037; **Phone:** 858-657-8590; **Board Cert:** Otolaryngology 1979; Neurotology 2004; **Med School:** Univ Pennsylvania 1974; **Resid:** Otolaryngology, Mass EE Infirmary 1979; **Fellow:** Neurological Surgery, Univ Zurich Med Ctr 1983; **Fac Appt:** Prof S, UCSD

Jackler, Robert K MD [Oto] - **Spec Exp:** Neuro-Otology; Skull Base Surgery; Ear Tumors; **Hospital:** Stanford Univ Hosp & Clinics; **Address:** Stanford Univ Med Ctr, Dept Head & Neck Surg, 801 Welch Rd Fl 2, Stanford, CA 94305-5739; **Phone:** 650-725-6500; **Board Cert:** Otolaryngology 1984; Neurotology 2004; **Med School:** Boston Univ 1979; **Resid:** Otolaryngology, UCSF Med Ctr 1984; **Fellow:** Otolaryngology, Oto Med Grp 1985; **Fac Appt:** Prof Oto, Stanford Univ

Kaplan, Michael J MD [Oto] - **Spec Exp:** Head & Neck Surgery; Skull Base Surgery; Head & Neck Cancer; **Hospital:** Stanford Univ Hosp & Clinics; **Address:** 875 Blake Wilbur Drive, Fl 1st, Ste Clinic B, MS 5820, 801 Welch Rd, Fl 2, MS 5739, Stanford, CA 94305-5739; **Phone:** 650-498-6000; **Board Cert:** Otolaryngology 1982; **Med School:** Harvard Med Sch 1977; **Resid:** Surgery, Beth Israel-Chldns Hosps 1979; Otolaryngology, Mass EE Infirm 1982; **Fellow:** Head and Neck Surgery, Univ Virginia 1984; **Fac Appt:** Prof Oto, Stanford Univ

Keller, Gregory S MD [Oto] - **Spec Exp:** Cosmetic Surgery-Face; **Hospital:** Santa Barbara Cottage Hosp, UCLA Ronald Reagan Med Ctr; **Address:** 221 W Pueblo St, Ste A, Santa Barbara, CA 93105; **Phone:** 805-687-6408; **Board Cert:** Otolaryngology 1976; **Med School:** Univ IL Coll Med 1971; **Resid:** Surgery, Cottage Hosp 1973; Otolaryngology, Univ Illinois Affil Hosp 1976; **Fac Appt:** Assoc Clin Prof S, UCLA

Larrabee Jr, Wayne F MD [Oto] - **Spec Exp:** Cosmetic Surgery-Face; Eyelid Surgery; Rhinoplasty; Nasal Surgery; **Hospital:** Swedish Med Ctr-First Hill-Seattle; **Address:** Facial Plastic Surgery Ctr, 600 Broadway Ste 280, Seattle, WA 98122-5371; **Phone:** 206-386-3550; **Board Cert:** Otolaryngology 1979; Facial Plastic & Reconstr Surgery 1999; **Med School:** Tulane Univ 1971; **Resid:** Surgery, Charity Hosp 1976; Otolaryngology, Tulane Univ Med Ctr 1979; **Fac Appt:** Clin Prof Oto, Univ Wash

Lustig, Lawrence R MD [Oto] - **Spec Exp:** Cochlear Implants; Hearing Loss; **Hospital:** UCSF Med Ctr; **Address:** Cochlear Implant Center, 2380 Sutter St Fl 1, San Francisco, CA 94115; **Phone:** 415-353-2464; **Board Cert:** Otolaryngology 1998; Neurotology 2006; **Med School:** UCSF 1992; **Resid:** Otolaryngology, UCSF Med Ctr 1997; **Fellow:** Neurotology, John Hopkins Hosp 1999

McMenomey, Sean O MD [Oto] - **Spec Exp:** Otology & Neuro-Otology; Skull Base Tumors & Surgery; Head & Neck Surgery; Stereotactic Radiosurgery; **Hospital:** OR Hlth & Sci Univ, Providence St Vincent Med Ctr; **Address:** Oregon Hlth & Sci Univ, Dept Otolaryngology, 3181 SW Sam Jackson Park Rd, MC PV-01, Portland, OR 97239; **Phone:** 503-494-8135; **Board Cert:** Otolaryngology 1993; Neurotology 2004; **Med School:** St Louis Univ 1987; **Resid:** Otolaryngology, Oregon Hlth Sci Ctr 1992; **Fellow:** Otology & Neurotology, Baptist Hosp 1993; **Fac Appt:** Prof Oto, Oregon Hlth & Sci Univ

Oghalai, John S MD [Oto] - **Spec Exp:** Neuro-Otology; **Hospital:** Stanford Univ Hosp & Clinics, Lucile Packard Chldn's Hosp; **Address:** Stanford Univ, 801 Welch Rd, Stanford, CA 94305; **Phone:** 650-723-5281; **Board Cert:** Otolaryngology 2002; Neurotology 2010; **Med School:** Univ Wisc 1994; **Resid:** Otolaryngology, Baylor Coll Med Ctr 2001; **Fellow:** Otolaryngology, UCSF Med Ctr 2003; Neurological Surgery, UCSF Med Ctr 2003; **Fac Appt:** Assoc Prof Oto, Baylor Coll Med

Orloff, Lisa MD [Oto] - **Spec Exp:** Thyroid & Parathyroid Cancer & Surgery; Minimally Invasive Surgery; Head & Neck Surgery; **Hospital:** UCSF Med Ctr; **Address:** Head & Neck Surg Canc Clin, 2380 Sutter St Fl 2, San Francisco, CA 94115; **Phone:** 415-885-7528; **Board Cert:** Otolaryngology 1993; **Med School:** UCLA 1986; **Resid:** Surgery, Univ Washington 1988; Otolaryngology, Univ Washington 1992; **Fellow:** Microvascular Surgery, Mt Sinai Med Ctr; **Fac Appt:** Assoc Prof S, UCSD

Powell, Nelson B MD/DDS [Oto] - **Spec Exp:** Sleep Disorders/Apnea; Maxillofacial Surgery; **Hospital:** Stanford Univ Hosp & Clinics; **Address:** California Sleep Institute, 1900 University Ave, Ste 101, East Palo Alto, CA 94303; **Phone:** 650-328-0511; **Board Cert:** Otolaryngology 1984; **Med School:** Univ Wash 1979; **Resid:** Surgery, Stanford Univ Hosp 1980; Otolaryngology, Stanford Univ Hosp 1983; **Fac Appt:** Clin Prof S, Stanford Univ

Rice, Dale H MD [Oto] - **Spec Exp:** Head & Neck Cancer; Sinus Disorders/Surgery; **Hospital:** Keck Med Ctr of USC (page 75), USC Norris Cancer Hosp (page 75); **Address:** 1520 San Pablo St, Ste 4600, Los Angeles, CA 90033-1029; **Phone:** 323-442-5790; **Board Cert:** Otolaryngology 1976; **Med School:** Univ Mich Med Sch 1968; **Resid:** Surgery, Univ Mich Med Ctr 1970; Otolaryngology, Univ Mich Med Ctr 1976; **Fac Appt:** Prof Oto, USC Sch Med

Rubinstein, Jay T MD/PhD [Oto] - **Spec Exp:** Cochlear Implants; Acoustic Neuroma; Hearing Loss; Skull Base Surgery; **Hospital:** Univ Wash Med Ctr; **Address:** Univ Washington Med Ctr, 1959 NE Pacific St, Box 356161, Seattle, WA 98195; **Phone:** 206-598-4022; **Board Cert:** Otolaryngology 1995; Neurotology 2005; **Med School:** Univ Wash 1987; **Resid:** Otolaryngology, Mass Eye & Ear Infirmary 1994; **Fellow:** Laryngology, Mass Eye & Ear Infirmary 1990; Otology & Neurotology, Univ Iowa Affil Hosp 1995; **Fac Appt:** Prof Oto, Univ Wash

Otolaryngology

Senders, Craig W MD [Oto] - **Spec Exp:** Pediatric Otolaryngology; Cleft Palate/Lip; Endoscopic Sinus Surgery; Sleep Disorders/Apnea; **Hospital:** UC Davis Med Ctr; **Address:** UC Davis, Dept Otolaryngology, 2521 Stockton Blvd, Ste 7200, Sacramento, CA 95817; **Phone:** 916-734-5400; **Board Cert:** Otolaryngology 1984; **Med School:** Oregon Hlth & Sci Univ 1979; **Resid:** Otolaryngology, Univ Iowa Hosps & Clins 1983; **Fellow:** Maxillofacial Surgery, Univ Iowa Hosps & Clins 1984; **Fac Appt:** Prof Oto, UC Davis

Shindo, Maisie L MD [Oto] - **Spec Exp:** Head & Neck Cancer & Surgery; Thyroid Cancer; Parathyroid Surgery; Parathyroid Cancer; **Hospital:** OR Hlth & Sci Univ; **Address:** Thyroid & Parathyroid Clinic, 3181 SW Sam Jackson Park Rd, MC PV-01, Portland, OR 97239-3098; **Phone:** 503-494-2544; **Board Cert:** Otolaryngology 1989; **Med School:** Univ Saskatchewan 1984; **Resid:** Otolaryngology, LAC-USC Med Ctr 1989; **Fellow:** Head and Neck Surgery, Northwestern Meml Hosp 1991; **Fac Appt:** Prof Oto, Oregon Hlth & Sci Univ

Singer, Mark I MD [Oto] - **Spec Exp:** Head & Neck Surgery; Head & Neck Cancer; Melanoma; **Hospital:** CA Pacific Med Ctr-Pacific Campus; **Address:** 2340 Clay St Fl 2, San Francisco, CA 94115; **Phone:** 415-600-3800; **Board Cert:** Otolaryngology 1976; **Med School:** Columbia P&S 1970; **Resid:** Surgery, Northwestern Meml Hosp 1973; Otolaryngology, Northwestern Meml Hosp 1976; **Fellow:** Oncology, Northwestern Meml Hosp 1976

Sinha, Uttam K MD [Oto] - **Spec Exp:** Head & Neck Cancer; Voice Disorders; Thyroid Cancer; Swallowing Disorders; **Hospital:** Keck Med Ctr of USC (page 75), House Ear Inst; **Address:** 1200 N State St, rm 4136, Los Angeles, CA 90033; **Phone:** 323-226-7315; **Board Cert:** Otolaryngology 1998; **Med School:** India 1985; **Resid:** Otolaryngology, LAC-USC Med Ctr 1995; **Fellow:** Microvascular Surgery, Mount Sinai Med Ctr 1996; Laryngology 1997; **Fac Appt:** Assoc Prof Oto, USC Sch Med

Wackym, P Ashley MD [Oto] - **Spec Exp:** Cochlear Implants; Acoustic Neuroma; Head & Neck Surgery; **Hospital:** Legacy Good Samaritan Med Ctr, Legacy Emanuel Chldn's Hosp; **Address:** Ear and Skull Base Ctr, 1225 NE 2nd Ave, Ste 305, Portland, OR 97232; **Phone:** 503-233-6068; **Board Cert:** Otolaryngology 1992; Neurotology 2004; **Med School:** Vanderbilt Univ 1985; **Resid:** Neurological Surgery, UCLA Med Ctr 1987; Head and Neck Surgery, UCLA Med Ctr 1991; **Fellow:** Otology & Neurotology, Univ Iowa 1992; Neurological Science, UCLA Med Ctr 1989; **Fac Appt:** Prof Oto

Wang, Steven J MD [Oto] - **Spec Exp:** Head & Neck Cancer & Surgery; **Hospital:** UCSF Med Ctr; **Address:** 2380 Sutter St Fl Second, San Francisco, CA 94115; **Phone:** 415-885-7528; **Board Cert:** Otolaryngology 2002; **Med School:** Harvard Med Sch 1995; **Resid:** Otolaryngology, UCLA Med Ctr 2001; Head and Neck Surgery, UCLA Med Ctr 2001; **Fellow:** Head & Neck Surgical Oncology, Univ Michigan 2003; **Fac Appt:** Assoc Prof Oto, UCSF

Wax, Mark K MD [Oto] - **Spec Exp:** Facial Nerve Disorders; Skull Base Tumors & Surgery; Facial Plastic & Reconstructive Surgery; Microvascular Surgery; **Hospital:** OR Hlth & Sci Univ; **Address:** Oregon Hlth Scis Univ, Dept Ototlaryngology, 3181 SW Sam Jackson Park Rd, MC PV-01, Portland, OR 97201; **Phone:** 503-494-5355; **Board Cert:** Otolaryngology 1985; Facial Plastic & Reconstr Surgery 2000; **Med School:** Univ Toronto 1980; **Resid:** Otolaryngology, Univ Toronto 1985; Surgery, Cedars-Sinai Med Ctr 1983; **Fellow:** Head and Neck Surgery, St Michaels Hosp 1991; **Fac Appt:** Prof Oto, Oregon Hlth & Sci Univ

Weisman, Robert A MD [Oto] - **Spec Exp:** Head & Neck Cancer; Clinical Trials; Thyroid & Parathyroid Cancer & Surgery; Head & Neck Cancer Reconstruction; **Hospital:** UCSD Med Ctr; **Address:** Moores-UCSD Cancer Center, 3855 Hlth Sci Drive, MC 0987, La Jolla, CA 92093-0987; **Phone:** 858-822-6197; **Board Cert:** Otolaryngology 1978; **Med School:** Washington Univ, St Louis 1973; **Resid:** Head and Neck Surgery, UCLA Med Ctr 1978; **Fac Appt:** Prof S, UCSD

Weymuller Jr, Ernest MD [Oto] - **Spec Exp:** Head & Neck Cancer; Sinus Disorders/Surgery; **Hospital:** Univ Wash Med Ctr; **Address:** 1959 NE Pacific St, Box 356161, Seattle, WA 98159; **Phone:** 206-598-4022; **Board Cert:** Otolaryngology 1973; **Med School:** Harvard Med Sch 1966; **Resid:** Surgery, Vanderbilt Univ Hosp 1968; Otolaryngology, Mass Eye and Ear Infirm 1973; **Fac Appt:** Prof Oto, Univ Wash

Wong, Brian JF MD [Oto] - **Spec Exp:** Facial Plastic & Reconstructive Surgery; Head & Neck Surgery; Vascular Malformations; **Hospital:** UC Irvine Med Ctr; **Address:** UC Irvine, Dept Head & Neck Surgery, 101 The City Drive, Pavillion II, 1st Fl, Orange, CA 92868; **Phone:** 714-456-7017; **Board Cert:** Otolaryngology 1998; Facial Plastic & Reconstr Surgery 2007; **Med School:** Johns Hopkins Univ 1990; **Resid:** Otolaryngology, UC Irvine Med Ctr 1996; **Fellow:** Facial Plastic & Reconstr Surgery, UC Irvine Med Ctr 1998; **Fac Appt:** Prof Oto, UC Irvine

Cleveland Clinic

Every life deserves world class care.

Otolaryngology

Cleveland Clinic's Head & Neck Institute is recognized nationally and internationally in this multidisciplinary field, and is consistently ranked as a top program by *U.S.News & World Report.* The Institute is comprised of extensively trained specialists in these areas:

Audiology: comprehensive evaluation and treatment through assistive listening devices, hearing aids, bone anchored auditory implants and cochlear implants.

Facial Plastic and Reconstructive Surgery: Treatments range from office-based injectables to rhinoplasty, face-lifts and major facial reconstructive surgery, including the world's first near-total face transplant.

Head and Neck Surgery: Evaluation and treatment of benign and malignant tumors.

Laryngotracheal Reconstruction: Laryngeal airway obstruction, esophageal reflux, tracheal aspiration, voice preservation/rehabilitation and removal of respiratory foreign bodies.

Nasal and Sinus Disorders: Sinusitis, polyps, septal deviation, nasal obstruction and allergies. Minimally invasive, computer-aided techniques for sinus and skull base surgery.

Otology-Neurotology: Middle and posterior cranial fossa surgery for cerebellopontine and skull base tumors, immune-mediated inner ear disease (deafness), Meniere's disease and cochlear implantation are handled here.

Pediatric Otolaryngology: Treatment of all forms of pediatric disorders.

Speech-Language Pathology: Evaluation and treatment for pediatric through geriatric patients with speech, language, voice, cognitive and swallowing disorders.

Vestibular and Balance Disorders: Diagnosis and vestibular rehabilitation for dizziness and disequilibrium.

Voice Center: Voice therapies and effective management options for all conditions related to the voice.

Cleveland Clinic
Head & Neck Institute
9500 Euclid Avenue
Cleveland, OH 44195

clevelandclinic.org/
headandnecktopdocs

Offering Same-Day Appointments
Call 800.274.2009.

Treatment Guides
Cleveland Clinic has developed comprehensive treatment guides for many diseases and conditions. To download our free treatment guides, visit clevelandclinic.org/ treatmentguides.

Online Medical Second Opinion
Cleveland Clinic's My**Consult** Online Medical Second Opinion program securely connects patients to our physician specialists for more than 1,000 life-changing or life-threatening diagnoses all by the click of a mouse. To learn more, log onto eclevelandclinic.org/myconsult or call 800.223.2273, ext. 43223.

Special Assistance for Out-of-State Patients
Cleveland Clinic Global Patient Services offers a complimentary Medical Concierge service for patients who travel from outside of Ohio. Call 800.223.2273, ext. 55580 or email medicalconcierge@ccf.org.

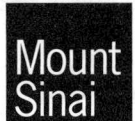 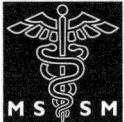

**MOUNT SINAI
SCHOOL OF
MEDICINE**

**THE MOUNT SINAI MEDICAL CENTER
OTOLARYNGOLOGY – EAR, NOSE, AND THROAT**
One Gustave L. Levy Place
Fifth Avenue and 100th Street
New York, NY 10029-6574
Physician Referral: 1-800-MD-SINAI (637-4624)
www.mountsinai.org/ENT

Mount Sinai's **DEPARTMENT OF OTOLARYNGOLOGY – HEAD AND NECK SURGERY** is recognized as one of the finest head and neck surgery programs in the nation. In 2011, *U.S. News & World Report* ranked our otolaryngology specialty in the top 20 in the United States and #2 in New York, Mount Sinai's department of Otolaryngology-Head and Neck Surgery is one of the oldest in the country. Since the early nineteenth century, Mount Sinai faculty have pioneered surgical advances in endoscopy, otology, skull-base surgery, laryngology, rhinology, facial plastic surgery, and head and neck oncology and reconstruction. Over the past decade, the department has expanded to include cutting-dge technology in robotic and endoscopic surgery, basic science research, and translational science programs.

Robotic Head and Neck Surgery – The Department of Otolaryngology-Head and Neck Surgery is a world leader in robotic head and neck surgery using the da Vinci® Surgical Robotic System. Mount Sinai surgeons and researchers have published new techniques in robotic surgery that have changed the paradigm for management of head and neck cancer. These techniques allow for endoscopic surgery without external incisions shortening hospital stay and improving quality-of-life outcomes.

Endoscopic Laser Surgery of the Larynx and Trachea – Surgeons and researchers at the Mount Sinai School of Medicine have introduced new techniques in laryngeal and tracheal surgery including endoscopic laser surgery, tracheal transplantation, and reconstructive surgery that allows for removal of malignant disease with voice and swallowing preservation.

The Grabsheid Voice Center – For more than a century, Mount Sinai has provided professional singers and patients in need with cutting-edge technology using endoscopic laser surgery and minimally invasive surgical techniques. Surgeons at the Grabsheid Voice Center have pioneered office-based surgical techniques that offer patients the opportunity to undergo therapy without the need for general anesthesia.

Cranial Base Surgery – Techniques in endoscopic trans-nasal surgery have revolutionized the management of skull base tumors and cerebrospinal leaks. Surgeons at Mount Sinai have developed procedures for accessing the cranial base and frontal lobes of the brain through the nose. Outcomes using these methods have demonstrated that patients have excellent outcomes with lower complications rates.

Thyroid and Parathyroid Surgery – The Mount Sinai Thyroid and Parathyroid Center is nationally recognized for excellence in clinical care and clinical outcomes research. Minimally invasive and robotic surgical techniques have provided patients the opportunity for surgery to be performed through an minimally invasive incision. Cure rates for thyroid cancer using these techniques are higher than 95 percent. Parathyroid surgery is performed using similar techniques and intraoperative parathyroid hormone monitoring.

Otology and Neurotology – The multidisciplinary team has long been recognized as one of the best in the nation. Outcomes for acoustic tumors and hearing restoration procedures are among the best in the country. Otologic surgeons at Mount Sinai have pioneered surgical techniques for the management of chronic ear disease and cochlear implantation that have resulted is excellent outcomes.

THE MULTIDISCIPLINARY HEAD AND NECK ONCOLOGY TEAM Recognized as one of the finest programs in the country, members of the multidisciplinary team include 35 physicians, surgeons, and ancillary staff from 12 different departments focused on the care of patients. The head and neck oncology program offers world-renown courses, training fellowships, and research fellowships that are respected as the finest in the country. Mount Sinai's multi-disciplinary head and neck cancer team has gained national recognition for its expertise and innovation in the management of head, neck, and skull-base cancer. The Mount Sinai team of experts in minimally invasive and endoscopic head and neck surgery comprises a group of surgeons and oncologists focused on curative treatment for head and neck malignancies. The expert team works to treat tumors of the oral cavity, jaw, and larynx, and preserve each patient's quality of life. Speech and swallowing rehabilitation therapists work with patients to help them recover. Mount Sinai is on the cutting edge of head and neck cancer therapy, reconstruction, and rehabilitation.

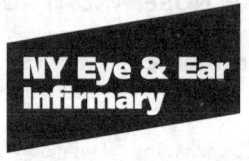

NY Eye & Ear Infirmary

Continuum Health Partners, Inc.

THE NEW YORK EYE AND EAR INFIRMARY

310 East 14th Street
New York, New York 10003
Tel. 212.979.4000   Fax. 212.228.0664
http://www.nyee.edu

PROVIDING EXCEPTIONAL CARE OF THE EAR, NOSE, THROAT, AND HEAD & NECK

Established in 1820 the Department of Otolaryngology/Head & Neck Surgery is the first training program in this specialty in the Western Hemisphere. Over nearly two centuries the department has evolved to be an international referral center for the medical and surgical treatment of diseases of the ear, nose, throat and face.

OUTSTANDING SERVICES:

Ear Institute (Otology – Neuro-otology): Specializing in the care of acute and chronic ear disease including hearing loss, cochlear implantation, dizziness, tinnitus, intra cranial tumors and facial nerve disorders. Our advanced otologic and vestibular diagnostic labs assist physicians in treatment.

Facial Plastic Surgery: Highly specialized and renowned surgeons perform in-office or ambulatory procedures utilizing state-of-the-art technology and techniques to produce outstanding results with minimal incisions, rapid recovery and a natural, youthful appearance.

Facial Paralysis: Comprehensive center treating all causes and offering reconstruction of the paralyzed face.

Head & Neck Oncology: A multi-disciplinary team including board-certified surgeons, medical & radiation oncologists, nutritionists and rehabilitation specialists insure rapid recovery from complex, life-saving surgical procedures and return to daily activities.

Pediatric Otolaryngology: Treating children has long been a priority at the Infirmary. Pediatric care ranges from middle ear infection, tonsil and adenoid disease, and neck masses to complex sinus and airway diseases.

Rhinology and Sinus Surgery: Internationally known specialists utilize minimally invasive techniques to treat disorders from sinusitis to intra cranial tumors.

Thyroid Center: A comprehensive program to streamline the diagnosis and treatment of thyroid diseases and cancers. A highly skilled team of surgeons, endocrinologists and radiologists manage the patient's care.

Voice & Swallowing Institute: Combining the expertise of physicians, speech pathologists and a voice physiologist to diagnose and treat voice problems – not only for performing artists but also for teachers, stockbrokers, receptionists, salespeople – anyone for whom voice is an important part of life.

Otolaryngology Clinical Services

General Otolaryngology *plus*

Facial Plastic & Reconstructive Surgery

Cochlear Implantation

Voice & Vocal Dynamics

Head & Neck Oncology

Laryngology

Otology & Neuro-otology

Pediatric Otolaryngology

Rhinology & Sinus Surgery

Swallowing Disorders

Thyroid Center

Facilities

Academic Faculty Practice,
including multiple locations throughout metropolitan NY

Hearing Aid Dispensary

Vestibular Rehabilitation

Ambulatory Care Services

About The New York Eye and Ear Infirmary

The New York Eye and Ear Infirmary is the nation's first specialty hospital and one of the most experienced in terms of the number of patients it treats and complexity of its cases. Each year the otolaryngology department performs more than 6,000 surgeries and sees more than 70,000 visits from outpatients

Physician Referral
1.800.449.HOPE (4673)

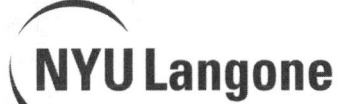
OTOLARYNGOLOGY

About the Department of Otolaryngology

The Department of Otolaryngology at NYU Langone Medical Center provides the highest quality treatment for ear, nose, throat, head and neck disorders, including one of the premier head and neck surgery programs in the country. We specialize in the following areas:

Cochlear Implants

Patients are provided with extensive evaluation, device programming and speech rehabilitation both pre- and post-operatively.

Facial Plastic and Reconstructive Surgery

Care is provided to patients requiring facial reconstructive surgery for a wide variety of facial deformities, and to those seeking facial cosmetic surgery. Specialties include functional and aesthetic rhinoplasty, facial rejuvenation surgery, injectable fillers, Botulinum Toxin (Botox) for facial spasm or wrinkles, and chemical peels and microdermabrasion.

General Otolaryngology and Sleep Surgery

Care is provided to adult patients with voice, sleep, allergy and nasal breathing disorders. Additionally, services for children are provided through our pediatric otolaryngologists.

Head and Neck Surgery and Oncology

Care is provided to patients with cancer of the head and neck, including cancer of the larynx, oral cavity, throat, nasal cavity and sinuses, salivary glands and lymph nodes in the neck.

Neutology/Skull Base Program

The Otolaryngology team provides expert care to patients with hearing loss, facial nerve palsy, vertigo and tinnitus, and treats lesions such as acoustic neuromas and skull base meningiomas. Featured services include facial palsy rehabilitation, auditory brainstem Implants, cochlear implants, laser surgery and endoscopic anterior and lateral skull base surgery.

Voice and Swallowing Disorders

We treat voice and swallowing disorders, including sore throat, chronic cough, hoarseness, voice loss, swallowing dysfunction, benign growths and cancerous tumors, vocal cord paralysis, the aging voice, recurrent or chronic laryngitis, gastroesophageal reflux, and injuries from overuse and misuse of the voice.

Audiology treats patients suffering with hearing or balance disorders; Head and Neck Speech Pathology treats voice, speech or swallowing problems; Rhinology treats all diseases of the paranasal sinuses, nose and related structures; Skull Base Surgery offers a minimally invasive and advanced surgical approach to tumors of the anterior and posterior skull base.

The Best in American Medicine
www.CastleConnolly.com

Pain Medicine

subspecialty of Anesthesiology, Neurology, and in Physical Medicine and Rehabilitation or Psychiatry

Some physicians who have their primary board certification in anesthesiology, neurology, physical medicine and rehabilitation, or psychiatry have completed additional training and passed an examination in the subspecialty called pain management. These doctors provide a high level of care, either as a primary physician or consultant, for patients experiencing problems with acute, chronic and/or cancer pain in both hospital and ambulatory settings.

For more information about the main specialties of these physicians, see **Anesthesiology, Neurology, Physical Medicine** and **Rehabilitation** or **Psychiatry** section(s).

Training Required: Number of years required for primary specialty *plus* additional training and examination

PAIN MEDICINE

New England

Abrahm, Janet L MD [PM] - **Spec Exp:** Palliative Care; Pain-Cancer; **Hospital:** Dana-Farber Cancer Inst (page 57), Brigham and Women's Hosp (page 57); **Address:** Dana-Farber Cancer Institute, 450 Brookline St, Shields-Warren 420, Boston, MA 02215; **Phone:** 617-632-6464; **Board Cert:** Internal Medicine 1976; Medical Oncology 1981; Hematology 1978; Hospice & Palliative Medicine 2008; **Med School:** UCSF 1973; **Resid:** Internal Medicine, Mass Genl Hosp 1975; Internal Medicine, Moffitt Hosp-UCSF 1977; **Fellow:** Hematology, Mass Genl Hosp 1976; Hematology & Oncology, Hosp Univ Penn 1980; **Fac Appt:** Assoc Prof Med, Harvard Med Sch

Berde, Charles Benjamin MD/PhD [PM] - **Spec Exp:** Pain Management-Pediatric; Critical Care; Reflex Sympathetic Dystrophy (RSD); **Hospital:** Children's Hospital - Boston, Spaulding Rehab Hosp; **Address:** Chldns Hosp, PTS, 333 Longwood Ave Fl 5, Boston, MA 02115; **Phone:** 617-355-7040; **Board Cert:** Pediatrics 1988; Anesthesiology 2009; Pain Medicine 2004; **Med School:** Stanford Univ 1980; **Resid:** Pediatrics, Chldns Hosp 1983; Anesthesiology, Mass Genl Hosp 1985; **Fellow:** Pediatric Anesthesiology, Chldns Hosp 1985; **Fac Appt:** Prof Ped, Harvard Med Sch

Loder, Elizabeth W MD [PM] - **Spec Exp:** Headache; Migraine; **Hospital:** Brigham and Women's Hosp (page 57), Faulkner Hosp; **Address:** 1153 Centre St, Ste 4970, Boston, MA 02130; **Phone:** 617-983-7580; **Board Cert:** Internal Medicine 2000; **Med School:** Univ ND Sch Med 1985; **Resid:** Internal Medicine, Faulkner Hosp 1989; **Fellow:** Headache, Graham Headache Ctr 1990; **Fac Appt:** Asst Prof Med, Harvard Med Sch

Peeters-Asdourian, Christine MD [PM] - **Hospital:** Beth Israel Deaconess Med Ctr - Boston; **Address:** Arnold Pain Management Ctr, One Brookline Pl, Ste 105, Brookline, MA 02445; **Phone:** 617-278-8000; **Board Cert:** Anesthesiology 1987; Pain Medicine 2004; **Med School:** Belgium 1978; **Resid:** Anesthesiology, U Mass Med Ctr 1982; **Fac Appt:** Asst Prof Anes, Univ Mass Sch Med

Ross, Edgar L MD [PM] - **Hospital:** Brigham and Women's Hosp (page 57); **Address:** Brigham & Women's Dept of Pain Medicine, 850 Boylston St Fl 3 - Ste 320, Chestnut Hill, MA 02467; **Phone:** 617-732-9056; **Board Cert:** Anesthesiology 1984; Pain Medicine 2004; **Med School:** Wayne State Univ 1980; **Resid:** Anesthesiology, Case West Univ Hosps 1983; **Fellow:** Pain Medicine, Case West Univ Hosps 1984; **Fac Appt:** Asst Prof Anes, Harvard Med Sch

Mid Atlantic

Argoff, Charles E MD [PM] - **Spec Exp:** Pain Management; Headache; Botox for Pain; Pain-Interventional Techniques; **Hospital:** Albany Med Ctr, St. Catherine's of Siena Med Ctr; **Address:** AMC Neurology Group, 47 New Scotland Ave, MC 70, Physicians Pavilion, 1st Fl, Albany, NY 12208; **Phone:** 518-262-5226; **Board Cert:** Neurology 1990; Pain Medicine 2009; **Med School:** Northwestern Univ-Feinberg Sch Med 1984; **Resid:** Neurology, Stony Brook Univ Affil Hosp 1988; **Fellow:** Neurology, Natl Inst of Hlth 1990; **Fac Appt:** Prof N, Albany Med Coll

Christo, Paul J MD [PM] - **Spec Exp:** Reflex Sympathetic Dystrophy (RSD); Spinal Cord Stimulation; Pain-Spine; Pain-Low Back; **Hospital:** Johns Hopkins Hosp (page 61); **Address:** Pain Treatment Ctr, 601 N Caroline St, Ste 3062, Baltimore, MD 21287; **Phone:** 410-955-7246; **Board Cert:** Anesthesiology 2001; Pain Medicine 2002; **Med School:** Univ Louisville Sch Med 1995; **Resid:** Anesthesiology, Mass General Hosp 2000; **Fellow:** Pain Medicine, Johns Hopkins Hosp 2001; **Fac Appt:** Assoc Prof Anes, Johns Hopkins Univ

Cope, Doris K MD [PM] - **Hospital:** UPMC St Margaret, UPMC Shadyside; **Address:** UPMC St Margaret Pain Med Ctr, 200 Delafield Rd, Ste 2070, Pittsburgh, PA 15215; **Phone:** 412-784-5119; **Board Cert:** Anesthesiology 1989; Pain Medicine 2007; **Med School:** Med Coll GA 1982; **Resid:** Anesthesiology, Univ S Alabama 1986; **Fac Appt:** Prof Anes, Univ Pittsburgh

DeLeon, Oscar A MD [PM] - **Spec Exp:** Pain-Acute; Pain-Chronic; Pain-Cancer; **Hospital:** Roswell Park Cancer Inst; **Address:** Roswell Park Cancer Inst, Dept Anesthesia/Pain Medicine, Elm & Carlton Sts, Buffalo, NY 14263; **Phone:** 716-845-4595; **Board Cert:** Anesthesiology 1991; Critical Care Medicine 1993; Pain Medicine 2005; **Med School:** Guatemala 1982; **Resid:** Surgery, SUNY-Downstate Med Ctr 1986; Anesthesiology, Univ Buffalo 1989; **Fac Appt:** Prof Anes, SUNY Buffalo

Diwan, Sudhir MD [PM] - **Spec Exp:** Pain-after Spinal Intervention; Pain-Musculoskeletal; Pain-Neuropathic; Pain-Cancer; **Hospital:** Staten Island Univ Hosp - North; **Address:** Spine & Pain Inst of New York, 1534 Victory Blvd, Staten Island, NY 10314; **Phone:** 718-667-3577; **Board Cert:** Anesthesiology 2001; Pain Medicine 2002; **Med School:** India 1983; **Resid:** Surgery, St Luke's-Roosevelt Hosp Ctr 1994; Anesthesiology, St Luke's-Roosevelt Hosp Ctr 1997; **Fellow:** Pain Medicine, NY Presby Hosp 1998

Dubois, Michel Y MD [PM] - **Spec Exp:** Pain-Back & Neck; Pain-Neuropathic; Pain-Cancer; **Hospital:** NYU Langone Med Ctr (page 66), Bellevue Hosp Ctr; **Address:** 317 E 34th St, Ste 902, New York, NY 10016-4974; **Phone:** 212-201-1004; **Board Cert:** Anesthesiology 1985; Pain Medicine 2004; **Med School:** France 1974; **Resid:** Anesthesiology, Georgetown Univ Hosp 1980; **Fellow:** Pain Medicine, Georgetown Univ Hosp 1983; **Fac Appt:** Prof Anes, NYU Sch Med

Falco, Frank J.E MD [PM] - **Spec Exp:** Spinal Disorders; Pain-Musculoskeletal-Spine; Pain-Chronic; **Hospital:** Christiana Hospital; **Address:** Mid Atlantic Spine & Pain Ctr, 100 Biddle Ave, Ste 101, Newark, DE 19702; **Phone:** 302-392-6501; **Board Cert:** Pain Medicine 2000; Physical Medicine & Rehabilitation 2003; Sports Medicine 2007; Electrodiagnostic Medicine 2004; **Med School:** Temple Univ 1988; **Resid:** Physical Medicine & Rehabilitation, Temple Univ Hosp 1992; **Fellow:** Pain Management, Georgia Spine & Sports Ctr 1994; **Fac Appt:** Asst Clin Prof PMR, Temple Univ

Gharibo, Christopher G MD [PM] - **Spec Exp:** Pain-Back & Neck; Pain-Neuropathic; Pain-Chronic; Complex Regional Pain Syndromes; **Hospital:** NYU Langone Med Ctr (page 66), NYU Hosp For Joint Diseases; **Address:** 301 E 17th St, Ste 1001, New York, NY 10003; **Phone:** 212-598-6174; **Board Cert:** Anesthesiology 1997; Pain Medicine 2009; **Med School:** UMDNJ-NJ Med Sch, Newark 1992; **Resid:** Anesthesiology, NYU Med Ctr 1995; **Fellow:** Pain Medicine, Jefferson Univ Hosp 1997; **Fac Appt:** Asst Prof Anes, NYU Sch Med

Jain, Subhash MD [PM] - **Spec Exp:** Pain-Cancer; Pain-Pelvic; Reflex Sympathetic Dystrophy; Complex Regional Pain Syndromes; **Hospital:** Beth Israel Med Ctr - Petrie Division (page 55); **Address:** 360 E 72nd St, Ste C, New York, NY 10021; **Phone:** 212-439-6100; **Board Cert:** Anesthesiology 1994; Pain Medicine 1998; **Med School:** India 1968; **Resid:** Surgery, St Vincent Med Ctr 1977; Anesthesiology, New York Hosp 1979; **Fellow:** Pain Medicine, New York Hosp/Meml Sloan Kettering Cancer Ctr 1980; **Fac Appt:** Assoc Prof Anes, Cornell Univ-Weill Med Coll

Kreitzer, Joel MD [PM] - **Spec Exp:** Pain-Back; Pain-Cancer; Pain-Neuropathic; **Hospital:** Mount Sinai Med Ctr (page 63), Mount Sinai Hosp of Queens (page 63); **Address:** Upper East Side Pain Medicine, 1540 York Ave, New York, NY 10028; **Phone:** 212-288-2180; **Board Cert:** Anesthesiology 1990; Pain Medicine 2004; **Med School:** Albert Einstein Coll Med 1985; **Resid:** Anesthesiology, Mt Sinai Hosp 1989; **Fellow:** Pain Medicine, Mt Sinai Hosp 1989; **Fac Appt:** Assoc Clin Prof Anes, Mount Sinai Sch Med

Pain Medicine

Ngeow, Jeffrey MD [PM] - **Spec Exp:** Pain-Musculoskeletal-Spine & Neck; Acupuncture; Reflex Sympathetic Dystrophy (RSD); Pain-Neuropathic; **Hospital:** Hosp For Special Surgery (page 60); **Address:** 535 E 70th St, New York, NY 10021-4872; **Phone:** 212-606-1059; **Board Cert:** Anesthesiology 1980; Pain Medicine 2005; **Med School:** England, UK 1971; **Resid:** Anesthesiology, Peter Bent Brigham Hosp 1977; **Fellow:** Pain Medicine, Tufts New England Med Ctr 1978; **Fac Appt:** Assoc Clin Prof Anes, Cornell Univ-Weill Med Coll

Portenoy, Russell MD [PM] - **Spec Exp:** Pain-Cancer; Palliative Care; **Hospital:** Beth Israel Med Ctr - Petrie Division (page 55); **Address:** Beth Israel Med Ctr, Dept Pain Medicine/Palliative Care, First Ave at 16th St, New York, NY 10003; **Phone:** 212-844-1403; **Board Cert:** Neurology 1985; Hospice & Palliative Medicine 2008; **Med School:** Univ MD Sch Med 1980; **Resid:** Neurology, Montefiore Med Ctr 1984; **Fellow:** Pain Medicine, Meml Sloan-Kettering Cancer Ctr 1985; **Fac Appt:** Prof N, Albert Einstein Coll Med

Raja, Srinivasa MD [PM] - **Spec Exp:** Pain-Neuropathic; Herpetic Neuralgia (Shingles); Reflex Sympathetic Dystrophy (RSD); **Hospital:** Johns Hopkins Hosp (page 61); **Address:** 601 N Caroline St Fl 3rd - rm 3062A, Baltimore, MD 21287; **Phone:** 410-955-7246; **Board Cert:** Anesthesiology 1982; Pain Medicine 2004; **Med School:** India 1974; **Resid:** Anesthesiology, Univ Washington Med Ctr 1979; **Fellow:** Pain Medicine, Univ Virginia Hosp 1981; **Fac Appt:** Prof Anes, Johns Hopkins Univ

Staats, Peter MD [PM] - **Spec Exp:** Pain-Cancer; Pain-Back; **Hospital:** Riverview Med Ctr, CentraState Med Ctr; **Address:** Metzger Staats Pain Mgmt, 160 Avenue at the Commons, Ste 1, Shrewsbury, NJ 07702; **Phone:** 732-380-0200; **Board Cert:** Anesthesiology 1994; Pain Medicine 2005; **Med School:** Univ Mich Med Sch 1989; **Resid:** Anesthesiology, Johns Hopkins Hosp 1993; **Fellow:** Pain Medicine, Johns Hopkins Hosp 1994

Weinberger, Michael L MD [PM] - **Spec Exp:** Pain-Cancer; Pain-Back; Palliative Care; **Hospital:** NY-Presby/Columbia Univ Med Ctr, NY (page 65); **Address:** 630 W 168th St, PH5, rm 500, New York, NY 10032-3720; **Phone:** 212-305-7114; **Board Cert:** Internal Medicine 1986; Anesthesiology 1990; Pain Medicine 2004; Hospice & Palliative Medicine 2006; **Med School:** Columbia P&S 1983; **Resid:** Internal Medicine, St Vincent's Hosp 1986; Anesthesiology, Columbia-Presby Med Ctr 1989; **Fellow:** Pain Medicine, Meml Sloan Kettering Cancer Ctr 1990; **Fac Appt:** Assoc Prof Anes, Columbia P&S

Southeast

Anghelescu, Doralina L MD [PM] - **Spec Exp:** Pain Management-Pediatric; Pain-Cancer; **Hospital:** St. Jude Children's Research Hosp; **Address:** St Jude Chldn's Rsch Hosp, Anesthesiology, 262 Danny Thomas Pl, MS 130, Memphis, TN 38105; **Phone:** 901-595-4034; **Board Cert:** Anesthesiology 1998; Pain Medicine 2001; **Med School:** Romania 1985; **Resid:** Anesthesiology, Univ N Mex Hosp 1997; **Fellow:** Pain Medicine, Chldns Natl Med Ctr 1998; Pain Medicine, Univ NMex Hosp 1999

Baumann, Patricia L MD [PM] - **Spec Exp:** Pain-Back; Pain-Neuropathic; Spinal Disorders; **Hospital:** Emory Univ Hosp Midtown, Emory Univ Hosp; **Address:** Emory Center for Pain Management, 550 Peachtree St NE, Ste 7085, Atlanta, GA 30308; **Phone:** 404-686-2410; **Board Cert:** Anesthesiology 1993; Pain Medicine 2005; **Med School:** Emory Univ 1988; **Resid:** Anesthesiology, Emory Univ Med Ctr 1992; **Fac Appt:** Asst Prof Anes, Emory Univ

Gobrial, Wagih W MD [PM] - **Hospital:** Cleveland Clin - Weston; **Address:** Cleveland Clinic Weston-Pain Management, 2950 Cleveland Clinic Blvd, Weston, FL 33331; **Phone:** 954-659-5046; **Board Cert:** Anesthesiology 1997; Pain Medicine 2009; **Med School:** Egypt 1976; **Resid:** Anesthesiology, Cleveland Clinic 1996; **Fellow:** Pain Management, Cleveland Clinic 1997; **Fac Appt:** Asst Clin Prof Anes, Nova SE Univ, Coll Osteo Med

Rauck, Richard L MD [PM] - **Spec Exp:** Pain-Cancer; Spinal Cord Stimulation; Complex Regional Pain Syndromes; **Hospital:** Forsyth Med Ctr, Wake Forest Univ Baptist Med Ctr; **Address:** Carolinas Pain Institute, 145 Kimel Park Drive, Ste 330, Winston-Salem, NC 27103; **Phone:** 336-765-6181; **Board Cert:** Anesthesiology 1987; Pain Medicine 2005; **Med School:** Bowman Gray 1982; **Resid:** Anesthesiology, Univ Cincinnati Hosp 1985; **Fellow:** Pain Medicine, Univ Cincinnati Hosp 1986; **Fac Appt:** Assoc Prof Anes, Wake Forest Univ

Vetter, Thomas R MD [PM] - **Spec Exp:** Pain Management-Pediatric; Pain-Chronic; **Hospital:** Children's Hospital - Birmingham, Univ of Ala Hosp at Birmingham; **Address:** UAB Anesthesiology/Pain Medicine, 619 19th St S, JT 865, Birmingham, AL 35249-6810; **Phone:** 205-934-6501; **Board Cert:** Anesthesiology 2009; Pain Medicine 2009; **Med School:** Ohio State Univ 1984; **Resid:** Anesthesiology, Univ Pittsburgh Med Ctr 1988; **Fellow:** Pain Management, Childrens Hosp 1989; **Fac Appt:** Prof Anes, Univ Alabama

Midwest

Abram, Stephen E MD [PM] - **Hospital:** Froedtert and Med Ctr of WI; **Address:** Pain Management Clinic/Med College WI, 1155 N Mayfair Rd, Wauwatosa, WI 53226; **Phone:** 414-456-7600; **Board Cert:** Anesthesiology 2001; Pain Medicine 2004; **Med School:** Jefferson Med Coll 1970; **Resid:** Anesthesiology, Mary Hitchcock Meml Hosp 1973; **Fac Appt:** Prof Anes, Med Coll Wisc

Amin, Sandeep D MD [PM] - **Spec Exp:** Headache-Supraorbital Stimulation; Complex Regional Pain Syndromes; Pain-Cancer; Pain-after Spinal Intervention; **Hospital:** Rush Univ Med Ctr, Rush Oak Park Hosp; **Address:** Rush Pain Ctr, 1725 W Harrison St, Ste 550, Chicago, IL 60612; **Phone:** 312-942-6631; **Board Cert:** Anesthesiology 1998; Pain Medicine 2011; **Med School:** India 1991; **Resid:** Anesthesiology, Univ Illinois Hosps 1997; **Fellow:** Pain Medicine, Univ Illinois Hosps 1998; Pain Medicine, Johns Hopkins Hosp 1999; **Fac Appt:** Prof Anes, Rush Med Coll

Benedetti, Costantino MD [PM] - **Spec Exp:** Pain-Cancer; Palliative Care; Pain-Acute; Pain-Chronic; **Hospital:** Ohio St Univ Med Ctr, Arthur G James Cancer Hosp & Research Inst; **Address:** Ohio State Univ Med Ctr, 300 W 10th Ave, Ste 410, Columbus, OH 43210; **Phone:** 614-293-8487; **Board Cert:** Hospice & Palliative Medicine 1997; **Med School:** Italy 1972; **Resid:** Anesthesiology, Univ Colorado Hosp 1975; Anesthesiology, Univ Wash Med Ctr 1976; **Fellow:** Pain Medicine, Univ Wash Med Ctr 1978; **Fac Appt:** Clin Prof Anes, Ohio State Univ

Benzon, Honorio T MD [PM] - **Spec Exp:** Pain-Back; Complex Regional Pain Syndromes; Pain-Neuropathic; Pain-Cancer; **Hospital:** Northwestern Meml Hosp; **Address:** 675 N Saint Clair St, Fl 20, Ste 100, Chicago, IL 60611-3015; **Phone:** 312-695-2500; **Board Cert:** Anesthesiology 2009; Pain Medicine 2004; **Med School:** Philippines 1971; **Resid:** Anesthesiology, Univ Cincinnati Med Ctr 1975; Anesthesiology, Northwestern Meml Hosp 1976; **Fellow:** Research, Brigham & Womens Hosp 1986; **Fac Appt:** Prof Anes, Northwestern Univ

Covington, Edward C MD [PM] - **Spec Exp:** Pain-Chronic; **Hospital:** Cleveland Clin (page 56); **Address:** 9500 Euclid Ave, Desk C21, Cleveland, OH 44195; **Phone:** 216-444-5964; **Board Cert:** Psychiatry 1978; Pain Medicine 2001; **Med School:** Univ Tenn Coll Med 1970; **Resid:** Psychiatry, Mayo Clinic 1975

Green, Carmen R MD [PM] - **Spec Exp:** Pain Care-Racial/Ethnic Disparities; **Hospital:** Univ of Michigan Hosp; **Address:** Univ Mich Hlth Sys, Dept Anesthesiology, rm 1H247, 1500 E Med Ctr Drive, SPC5048, Ann Arbor, MI 48109-5048; **Phone:** 734-936-4240; **Board Cert:** Anesthesiology 1996; Pain Medicine 2009; **Med School:** Mich State Univ 1987; **Resid:** Anesthesiology, Univ Mich Med Ctr 1989; **Fellow:** Pain Medicine, Univ Mich Med Ctr 1992; **Fac Appt:** Asst Prof Anes, Univ Mich Med Sch

Harden, R Norman MD [PM] - **Spec Exp:** Reflex Sympathetic Dystrophy (RSD); Fibromyalgia; **Hospital:** Rehab Inst of Chicago; **Address:** 980 N Michigan Ave, Ste 800, Chicago, IL 60611; **Phone:** 312-238-7800; **Med School:** Med Coll GA 1984; **Resid:** Neurology, Univ South Carolina Med Ctr 1985; **Fellow:** Pain Medicine, Rehab Inst-Georgia 1989; **Fac Appt:** Asst Prof PMR, Northwestern Univ

Huntoon, Marc MD [PM] - **Spec Exp:** Pain-Cancer; Pain-after Spinal Intervention; Palliative Care; **Hospital:** Mayo Med Ctr & Clin - Rochester; **Address:** Mayo Clinic-Pain Medicine, 200 First St SW, Rochester, MN 55905; **Phone:** 507-266-9240; **Board Cert:** Anesthesiology 2003; Pain Medicine 2004; Hospice & Palliative Medicine 2004; **Med School:** Wayne State Univ 1985; **Resid:** Anesthesiology, Naval Hosp Med Ctr 1991; **Fellow:** Pain Medicine, Naval Hosp Med Ctr 1992

Mekhail, Nagy A MD/PhD [PM] - **Spec Exp:** Pain-Back & Neck; Pain-Chronic; Pain-Neuropathic; Pain-Cancer; **Hospital:** Cleveland Clin (page 56); **Address:** Cleveland Clinic, 9500 Euclid Ave, MC C25, Cleveland, OH 44195; **Phone:** 216-445-7370; **Board Cert:** Pain Medicine 2004; **Med School:** Egypt 1975; **Resid:** Anesthesiology, Cleveland Clinic 1991; **Fellow:** Pain Medicine, Cleveland Clinic 1992; **Fac Appt:** Prof Anes, Cleveland Cl Coll Med/Case West Res

Robbins, Larry D MD [PM] - **Spec Exp:** Headache; Migraine; Psychopharmacology; Pain Management; **Address:** 60 Revere Drive, Ste 330, MS 60062, Northbrook, IL 60062; **Phone:** 847-480-9399; **Board Cert:** Anesthesiology 2005; **Med School:** Univ IL Coll Med 1981; **Resid:** Neurology, Univ Illinois Med Ctr 1985; **Fellow:** Pain Medicine, Diamond Headache Clinic 1986

Rosenquist, Richard W MD [PM] - **Spec Exp:** Complex Regional Pain Syndromes; Pain-Back; Pain-Facial; Headache; **Hospital:** Cleveland Clin (page 56); **Address:** Cleveland Clinic-Pain Management, 10524 Euclid Ave, MC C25, Cleveland, OH 44106; **Phone:** 216-445-7370; **Board Cert:** Anesthesiology 1988; Pain Medicine 2004; **Med School:** Northwestern Univ 1984; **Resid:** Anesthesiology, Northwestern Univ Med Ctr 1987; **Fellow:** Anesthesiology & Pain Management, Emory Univ Hosp 1988

Suresh, Santhanam MD [PM] - **Hospital:** Children's Mem Hosp -Chicago; **Address:** Chldns Meml Hosp, Dept Anesthesia, 2300 Children's Plaza, Box 19, Chicago, IL 60614; **Phone:** 773-880-4006; **Board Cert:** Pediatrics 2011; Anesthesiology 2012; Pain Medicine 2009; **Med School:** India 1983; **Resid:** Pediatrics, Cook Co Hosp 1988; Anesthesiology, Loyola Univ Med Ctr 1990; **Fellow:** Pediatric Anesthesiology, Northwestern Meml Hosp 1991; **Fac Appt:** Prof Anes, Northwestern Univ-Feinberg Sch Med

Swarm, Robert A MD [PM] - **Spec Exp:** Pain-Acute; Pain-Chronic; Pain-Cancer; **Hospital:** Barnes-Jewish Hosp; **Address:** Ctr for Advanced Med-Pain Mngmt Ctr, 4921 Parkview Pl, Ste 10A, MS 90-35-706, St Louis, MO 63110; **Phone:** 314-362-8820; **Board Cert:** Anesthesiology 1990; Pain Medicine 2004; **Med School:** Washington Univ, St Louis 1983; **Resid:** Surgery, Barnes Hosp 1986; Anesthesiology, Barnes Hosp 1989; **Fellow:** Pain Medicine, Univ Sydney 1991; **Fac Appt:** Assoc Prof Anes, Washington Univ, St Louis

Weisman, Steven J MD [PM] - **Spec Exp:** Pain Management-Pediatric; Palliative Care-Pediatric; Complex Regional Pain Syndromes; Pain-Cancer; **Hospital:** Chldns Hosp - Wisconsin; **Address:** Chldns Hosp Wisconsin, Chldns Pain Clin, PO Box 1997, Milwaukee, WI 53201-1997; **Phone:** 414-266-2775; **Board Cert:** Pediatrics 1982; Pediatric Hematology-Oncology 1984; Anesthesiology 1996; **Med School:** Albert Einstein Coll Med 1978; **Resid:** Pediatrics, Chldns Hosp 1981; Anesthesiology, Univ Conn Hlth Ctr 1994; **Fellow:** Pediatric Hematology-Oncology, Indiana Univ Sch Med 1984; **Fac Appt:** Prof Anes, Med Coll Wisc

Great Plains and Mountains

Fine, Perry G MD [PM] - **Spec Exp:** Pain-Cancer; Palliative Care; Pain-Chronic; **Hospital:** Univ Utah Hlth Care; **Address:** 546 S Chipeta Way, Ste 220, Salt Lake City, UT 84108; **Phone:** 801-581-7246; **Board Cert:** Anesthesiology 1985; Pain Medicine 2004; **Med School:** Med Coll VA 1981; **Resid:** Anesthesiology, Univ Utah Hlth Sci Ctr 1984; **Fellow:** Pain Medicine, Univ Toronto Affil Hosp 1985; **Fac Appt:** Prof Anes, Univ Utah

Weinstein, Sharon M MD [PM] - **Spec Exp:** Pain-Cancer; Palliative Care; **Hospital:** Univ Utah Hlth Care; **Address:** Huntsman Cancer Institute, 2000 Circle of Hope, Salt Lake City, UT 84112; **Phone:** 801-585-0112; **Board Cert:** Neurology 1993; Pain Medicine 2000; Hospice & Palliative Medicine 2008; **Med School:** Albert Einstein Coll Med 1986; **Resid:** Neurology, Montefiore Med Ctr 1990; **Fellow:** Pain Medicine, Meml Sloan Kettering Cancer Ctr 1991; **Fac Appt:** Assoc Prof Anes, Univ Utah

Southwest

Burton, Allen W MD [PM] - **Spec Exp:** Pain-Cancer; Palliative Care; **Hospital:** St. Luke's Episcopal Hosp-Houston; **Address:** 7700 Main St, Ste 400, Houston, TX 77030; **Phone:** 832-553-1336; **Board Cert:** Anesthesiology 1996; Pain Medicine 1998; **Med School:** Baylor Coll Med 1991; **Resid:** Anesthesiology, Brigham & Women's Hosp 1995; **Fellow:** Pain Medicine, U Texas Med Branch Hosp 1998; **Fac Appt:** Assoc Prof Anes, Univ Tex Med Br, Galveston

Driver, Larry C MD [PM] - **Spec Exp:** Pain-Cancer; Palliative Care; **Hospital:** UT MD Anderson Cancer Ctr; **Address:** UT MD Anderson Cancer Ctr, Dept Pain Medicine, 1400 Holcombe Blvd, Unit 409, Houston, TX 77030; **Phone:** 713-745-7246; **Board Cert:** Anesthesiology 1992; Pain Medicine 2002; **Med School:** Univ Tex, San Antonio 1980; **Resid:** Anesthesiology, Univ Colorado Hlth Sci Ctr 1984; **Fellow:** Pain Medicine, MD Anderson Cancer Ctr 1999; **Fac Appt:** Assoc Prof Anes, Univ Tex, Houston

Freitag, Frederick G DO [PM] - **Spec Exp:** Headache; Migraine-Chronic; Botox Therapy; **Hospital:** Baylor Univ Medical Ctr-Dallas; **Address:** Baylor Univ Med Ctr, Research Inst, Comprehensive Headache Ctr, 9101 N Central Expressway, Ste 400, Dallas, TX 75231; **Phone:** 214-820-9272; **Board Cert:** Family Medicine 1982; Pain Medicine 2001; **Med School:** Chicago Coll Osteo Med 1979; **Resid:** Family Medicine, Brentwood Hosp 1981; **Fellow:** Headache, Cleveland Clinic 1982; **Fac Appt:** Assoc Clin Prof FMed, Baylor Coll Med

Noe, Carl E MD [PM] - **Spec Exp:** Pain-Back & Neck; **Hospital:** UT Southwestern Med Ctr at Dallas; **Address:** 1801 Inwood Rd, Dallas, TX 75390; **Phone:** 214-645-8450; **Board Cert:** Anesthesiology 1989; Pain Medicine 2004; Critical Care Medicine 1989; **Med School:** Univ Tex, San Antonio 1984; **Resid:** Anesthesiology, TX Tech Univ Hlth Sci Ctr 1987; Anesthesiology, Stanford Univ Med Ctr 1988; **Fellow:** Critical Care Medicine, Stanford Univ Med Ctr 1988; Pain Management, TX Tech Univ Hlth Sci Ctr 1989; **Fac Appt:** Assoc Prof Anes, Univ Tex SW, Dallas

Pain Medicine

Racz, Gabor MD [PM] - **Spec Exp:** Pain-after Spinal Intervention; Reflex Sympathetic Dystrophy (RSD); Pain-Back, Head & Neck; Headache/Facial Pain; **Hospital:** Univ Med Ctr-Lubbock; **Address:** 3601 4th St, MS 8182, Lubbock, TX 79430-0002; **Phone:** 806-743-3112; **Board Cert:** Anesthesiology 1993; Pain Medicine 2004; **Med School:** England, UK 1962; **Resid:** Anesthesiology, SUNY Upstate Med Ctr 1969; **Fac Appt:** Prof Anes, Texas Tech Univ

Ramamurthy, Somayaji MD [PM] - **Spec Exp:** Pain-Back; Pain-Chronic; **Hospital:** Univ Hlth Syst-San Antonio; **Address:** UT Medicine Pain Consultants, 5282 Medical Drive, Ste 614, San Antonio, TX 78229; **Phone:** 210-450-9857; **Board Cert:** Anesthesiology 1972; Pain Medicine 2004; **Med School:** India 1965; **Resid:** Anesthesiology, Cook Co Hosp 1970; **Fac Appt:** Prof Anes, Univ Tex, San Antonio

Walsh, Nicolas E MD [PM] - **Spec Exp:** Pain-Back; Trauma Rehabilitation; Post Polio Syndrome; **Hospital:** Univ Hlth Syst-San Antonio, Audie L Murphy Meml Vets Hosp - San Antonio; **Address:** Univ Tex Hlth Sci Ctr, Rehab Med, 7703 Floyd Curl Drive, MC 7798, San Antonio, TX 78229-3901; **Phone:** 210-567-5350; **Board Cert:** Physical Medicine & Rehabilitation 2009; Pain Medicine 2000; **Med School:** Univ Colorado 1979; **Resid:** Physical Medicine & Rehabilitation, Univ Tex Hlth Sci Ctr 1982; **Fac Appt:** Prof PMR, Univ Tex, San Antonio

West Coast and Pacific

Audell, Laura G MD [PM] - **Spec Exp:** Complex Regional Pain Syndromes; Reflex Sympathetic Dystrophy (RSD); Herpetic Neuralgia (Shingles); Spinal Cord Disorders; **Hospital:** Cedars-Sinai Med Ctr; **Address:** 444 S San Vincente, Ste 1101, Los Angeles, CA 90048; **Phone:** 310-423-9600; **Board Cert:** Internal Medicine 1986; Anesthesiology 1988; Pain Medicine 2007; **Med School:** Univ Wash 1982; **Resid:** Internal Medicine, UCLA-Hosps 1985; Anesthesiology, UCLA-Hosps 1987; **Fellow:** Pain Medicine, UCLA-Hosps 1988

Ballantyne, Jane C MD [PM] - **Spec Exp:** Pain-Chronic; Pain-Cancer; **Hospital:** Harborview Med Ctr; **Address:** Univ Wash Pain Ctr, 4225 Roosevelt Way NE, Ste 401, Seattle, WA 98105; **Phone:** 206-744-7065; **Board Cert:** Anesthesiology 2007; **Med School:** England, UK 1978; **Resid:** Surgery, London & Oxford 1985; Anesthesiology, John Radcliffe Hosp 1990; **Fellow:** Anesthesiology, Mass Genl Hosp 1992; Pain Medicine, Mass Genl Hosp 1994; **Fac Appt:** Prof Anes, Univ Wash

Ferrante, F Michael MD [PM] - **Spec Exp:** Pain-Back & Neck; Reflex Sympathetic Dystrophy (RSD); Botox for Pain; Pain-Neuropathic; **Hospital:** Santa Monica - UCLA Med Ctr & Ortho Hosp, UCLA Ronald Reagan Med Ctr; **Address:** UCLA Pain Program, 1245 16th St, Ste 225, Santa Monica, CA 90404; **Phone:** 310-319-2241; **Board Cert:** Internal Medicine 1985; Anesthesiology 1987; Pain Medicine 2004; **Med School:** NY Med Coll 1980; **Resid:** Internal Medicine, Emroy Univ Affil Hosp 1983; Anesthesiology, Emroy Univ Affil Hosp 1986; **Fellow:** Infectious Disease, Barnes Hosp-Wash Univ 1984; Pain Medicine, Brigham & Womens Hosp 1987; **Fac Appt:** Prof Anes, UCLA

Fishman, Scott M MD [PM] - **Spec Exp:** Pain-Cancer; Pain-Chronic; **Hospital:** UC Davis Med Ctr; **Address:** UC Davis Med Ctr, Pain Management Clinic, 4860 Y St, Ste 2700, Sacramento, CA 95817; **Phone:** 916-734-7246; **Board Cert:** Psychiatry 1998; Pain Medicine 1995; **Med School:** Univ Mass Sch Med 1990; **Resid:** Internal Medicine, Greenwich Hosp 1993; Psychiatry, Mass Genl Hosp 1996; **Fellow:** Pain Medicine, Mass Genl Hosp 1995; **Fac Appt:** Prof Anes, UC Davis

Fitzgibbon, Dermot R MD [PM] - **Spec Exp:** Pain-Cancer; **Hospital:** Univ Wash Med Ctr; **Address:** Univ Wash Med Ctr, Dept Anesthesiology, 1959 NE Pacific St, Box 356540, Seattle, WA 98195; **Phone:** 206-598-4100; **Board Cert:** Anesthesiology 1996; Pain Medicine 2009; **Med School:** Ireland 1983; **Resid:** Anesthesiology, St Vincent's Hosp 1992; Anesthesiology, Univ Washington Med Ctr 1995; **Fellow:** Pain Medicine, Univ Wash-Pain Mngmt Clinic 1994; **Fac Appt:** Assoc Prof Anes, Univ Wash

Fuller, Nicholas S MD [PM] - **Hospital:** Cedars-Sinai Med Ctr; **Address:** 120 S Spalding Drive, Ste 301, Beverly Hills, CA 90212; **Phone:** 310-385-7755; **Board Cert:** Anesthesiology 1996; **Med School:** SUNY Buffalo 1991; **Resid:** Anesthesiology, Brigham & Women's Hosp 1995; **Fellow:** Pain Medicine, Univ Washington Med Ctr 1997

Jasmin, Luc MD/PhD [PM] - **Spec Exp:** Spinal Cord Stimulation; Spasticity & Movement Disorders; Stereotactic Radiosurgery; Pain-Cancer; **Hospital:** Cedars-Sinai Med Ctr; **Address:** Los Angeles Neurosurgical Institute, 8670 Wilshire Blvd, Ste 201, Los Angeles, CA 90211; **Phone:** 877-635-2674; **Med School:** Canada 1981; **Resid:** Neurological Surgery, Notre-Dame Hospital; **Fellow:** Research, UCSF Med Ctr; Neurosurgical Oncology, UCSF Med Ctr

Koh, Jeffrey MD [PM] - **Spec Exp:** Pain Management-Pediatric; **Hospital:** Doernbecher Chldns Hosp/OHSU, OR Hlth & Sci Univ; **Address:** 3181 SW Sam Jackson Park Rd, MC UHS-2, Portland, OR 97239; **Phone:** 503-418-5188; **Board Cert:** Pediatrics 2011; Anesthesiology 1993; Pain Medicine 2007; **Med School:** Wayne State Univ 1985; **Resid:** Pediatrics, Emory Univ Hosp 1988; Anesthesiology, Brigham & Women's Hosp 1991; **Fellow:** Pediatric Anesthesiology, Chldn's Hosp 1992; Pediatric Pain Management, UCLA Med Ctr 1993; **Fac Appt:** Prof Ped, Oregon Hlth & Sci Univ

Mackey, Sean MD/PhD [PM] - **Spec Exp:** Pain-Cancer; Pain-Chronic; **Hospital:** Stanford Univ Hosp & Clinics; **Address:** Stanford Univ Pain Management Ctr, 450 Broadway St, Pavilion A, 1st Fl, Redwood City, CA 94305-5340; **Phone:** 650-723-6238; **Board Cert:** Anesthesiology 2009; Pain Medicine 2011; **Med School:** Univ Ariz Coll Med 1994; **Resid:** Anesthesiology, Stanford Univ Med Ctr 1998; **Fellow:** Pain Medicine, Stanford Univ Med Ctr 1999; **Fac Appt:** Assoc Prof Anes, Stanford Univ

Prager, Joshua P MD [PM] - **Spec Exp:** Complex Regional Pain Syndromes; **Hospital:** UCLA Ronald Reagan Med Ctr; **Address:** California Pain Medicine Ctr, 100 UCLA Medical Plaza, Ste 760, Los Angeles, CA 90095; **Phone:** 310-794-7246 x100; **Board Cert:** Internal Medicine 1984; Anesthesiology 1987; Pain Medicine 2004; **Med School:** Stanford Univ 1981; **Resid:** Internal Medicine, UCLA Med Ctr 1984; Anesthesiology, Mass Genl Hosp 1986

Rosner, Howard L MD [PM] - **Spec Exp:** Pain-after Spinal Intervention; Pain-Back; Reflex Sympathetic Dystrophy (RSD); **Hospital:** Cedars-Sinai Med Ctr; **Address:** 444 S San Vincente Blvd, Ste 1101, Cedars-Sinai Med Ctr,Mark Goodson Bldg, Los Angeles, CA 90048; **Phone:** 310-423-9612; **Board Cert:** Anesthesiology 1989; Pain Medicine 2004; **Med School:** Univ Miami Sch Med 1980; **Resid:** Anesthesiology, Mass Genl Hosp 1983; **Fellow:** Pain Medicine, Columbia-Presby Med Ctr 1984

Slatkin, Neal E MD [PM] - **Spec Exp:** Pain-Cancer; Palliative Care; Neurology; **Hospital:** El Camino Hosp, Good Samaritan Hosp - San Jose; **Address:** 4850 Union Ave, San Jose, CA 95124-5156; **Phone:** 408-559-5600; **Board Cert:** Neurology 1982; Pain Medicine 2000; **Med School:** SUNY Stony Brook 1976; **Resid:** Neurology, Bellevue Hosp Ctr-NYU 1978; Neurology, Med Coll Va Hosps 1981; **Fellow:** Neurology, Med Coll Va 1982; Neuro-Oncology, Meml Sloan-Kettering Cancer Ctr 1984

Pain Medicine

Wallace, Mark Steven MD [PM] - **Spec Exp:** Pain-Chronic; Pain-Cancer; Palliative Care;
Hospital: UCSD Med Ctr; **Address:** 9350 Campus Point Drive, MC 7651, La Jolla, CA 92037;
Phone: 858-657-6035; **Board Cert:** Anesthesiology 1992; Pain Medicine 2005; **Med School:**
Creighton Univ 1987; **Resid:** Anesthesiology, Univ Maryland Hosp 1991; **Fellow:** Pain Medicine,
UCSD Med Ctr 1994

Cleveland Clinic

Every life deserves world class care.

Pain Management

At Cleveland Clinic's Department of Pain Management, 28 board-certified pain management physicians and researchers are dedicated to the goal of helping every patient with chronic pain return to a normal, productive lifestyle. Our committed staff uses the latest in diagnostic technology, paired with medical and interventional therapeutics, to work with patients to identify the source of the pain, eliminate or reduce the pain and teach them to manage it.

Cleveland Clinic Pain Management specialists treat chronic pain related to any type of disease, injury or accident, including:

- Back and neck pain, including herniated discs, spinal stenosis, tumors and arthritis
- Chronic abdominal pain and pelvic pain
- Complex regional pain syndrome (also known as reflex sympathetic dystrophy or RSD)
- Muscle and joint pain and arthritis
- Headache
- Sports injuries
- Disorders of the nervous system, including shingles and trigeminal, and occipital neuralgia (facial pain)
- Pain associated with AIDS
- Sickle cell anemia
- Cancer pain
- Intractable spasticity associated with multiple sclerosis or spinal cord injuries
- Pain associated with osteoporosis and vertebral compression fractures

The mission of Cleveland Clinic's Department of Pain Management is to be the leader in patient care, education and outcomes-oriented clinical and basic research in pain medicine. The department is home to one of the largest and most sought-after pain medicine fellowship programs in the world.

Cleveland Clinic
Anesthesiology Institute
9500 Euclid Avenue
Cleveland, OH 44195

clevelandclinic.org/
painmanagementtopdocs

Offering Same-Day Appointments
Call 800.274.2009.

Treatment Guides

Cleveland Clinic has developed comprehensive treatment guides for many diseases and conditions. To download our free treatment guides, visit clevelandclinic.org/treatmentguides.

Online Medical Second Opinion

Cleveland Clinic's My**Consult** Online Medical Second Opinion program securely connects patients to our physician specialists for more than 1,000 life-changing or life-threatening diagnoses all by the click of a mouse. To learn more, log onto eclevelandclinic.org/myconsult or call 800.223.2273, ext. 43223.

Special Assistance for Out-of-State Patients

Cleveland Clinic Global Patient Services offers a complimentary Medical Concierge service for patients who travel from outside of Ohio. Call 800.223.2273, ext. 55580 or email medicalconcierge@ccf.org.

The Best in American Medicine
www.CastleConnolly.com

Pathology

A pathologist deals with the causes and nature of disease and contributes to diagnosis, prognosis and treatment through knowledge gained by the laboratory application of the biologic, chemical and physical sciences.

A pathologist uses information gathered from the microscopic examination of tissue specimens, cells and body fluids, and from clinical laboratory tests on body fluids and secretions for the diagnosis, exclusion and monitoring of disease.

Training Required: Five to seven years

Certification in the following subspecialty requires additional training and examination.

Dermatopathology: A dermatopathologist has the expertise to diagnose and monitor diseases of the skin including infectious, immunologic, degenerative and neoplastic diseases. This entails the examination and interpretation of specially prepared tissue sections, cellular scrapings and smears of skin lesions by means of routine and special (electron and flourescent) microscopes.

PATHOLOGY

New England

Bhan, Atul K MD [Path] - **Spec Exp:** Immunopathology; Liver Pathology; Liver Cancer; **Hospital:** Mass Genl Hosp; **Address:** Mass Genl Hosp, Dept Pathology, 55 Fruit St, Warren 501, Boston, MA 02114-2620; **Phone:** 617-726-2588; **Board Cert:** Anatomic Pathology 1976; Immunopathology 1985; **Med School:** India 1965; **Resid:** Pathology, Boston Univ Hosp 1971; Pathology, Chldns Univ Hosp 1974; **Fac Appt:** Prof Path, Harvard Med Sch

Connolly, James L MD [Path] - **Spec Exp:** Breast Pathology; Breast Cancer; **Hospital:** Beth Israel Deaconess Med Ctr - Boston, Brigham and Women's Hosp (page 57); **Address:** Beth Israel Deaconess Med Ctr, Dept Path, Dept Pathology, 330 Brookline Ave, rm ES 112, Boston, MA 02215-5400; **Phone:** 617-667-4344; **Board Cert:** Anatomic Pathology 1980; **Med School:** Vanderbilt Univ 1974; **Resid:** Anatomic Pathology, Beth Israel Hosp 1978; **Fac Appt:** Prof Path, Harvard Med Sch

De Las Morenas, Antonio MD [Path] - **Spec Exp:** Thyroid Disorders; **Hospital:** Boston Med Ctr; **Address:** Boston Med Ctr, 670 Albany St Fl 3rd - Ste 307, Boston, MA 02118; **Phone:** 617-414-5059; **Board Cert:** Pathology 1989; Cytopathology 1990; **Med School:** Spain 1978; **Resid:** Anatomic Pathology, Mallory Inst 1987; **Fellow:** Cytopathology, Hosp UPenn 1988; **Fac Appt:** Prof Path, Boston Univ

DeLellis, Ronald A MD [Path] - **Spec Exp:** Thyroid Cancer; Endocrine Cancers; Endocrine Pathology; **Hospital:** Rhode Island Hosp, Miriam Hosp; **Address:** Rhode Island Hosp, Dept Pathology, 593 Eddy St, Providence, RI 02903-4923; **Phone:** 401-444-5154; **Board Cert:** Anatomic Pathology 1972; **Med School:** Tufts Univ 1966; **Resid:** Anatomic Pathology, Natl Inst Hlth 1971; **Fellow:** Pathology, Univ Hosp 1973; **Fac Appt:** Prof Path, Brown Univ

Fletcher, Christopher D M MD [Path] - **Spec Exp:** Soft Tissue Tumors; Sarcoma; Surgical Pathology; **Hospital:** Brigham and Women's Hosp (page 57), Dana-Farber Cancer Inst (page 57); **Address:** Brigham & Women's Hospital, Dept Pathology, 75 Francis St, Boston, MA 02115-6110; **Phone:** 617-732-8558; **Med School:** England, UK 1981; **Resid:** Pathology, St Thomas Hosp 1985; **Fellow:** Pathology, St Thomas Hosp 1986; **Fac Appt:** Prof Path, Harvard Med Sch

Harris, Nancy L MD [Path] - **Spec Exp:** Lymphoma; Hematopathology; **Hospital:** Mass Genl Hosp; **Address:** Mass Genl Hosp, Dept Pathology, 55 Fruit St, Warren 211, Boston, MA 02114; **Phone:** 617-726-5155; **Board Cert:** Anatomic Pathology 1978; Clinical Pathology 1978; **Med School:** Stanford Univ 1970; **Resid:** Pathology, Beth Israel Hosp 1978; **Fellow:** Immunopathology, Mass Genl Hosp 1980; **Fac Appt:** Prof Path, Harvard Med Sch

Kaufman, Richard Max MD [Path] - **Spec Exp:** Transfusion Medicine; **Hospital:** Brigham and Women's Hosp (page 57), Dana-Farber Cancer Inst (page 57); **Address:** Brigham & Women's Hosp, 75 Francis St, Boston, MA 02115; **Phone:** 617-732-4749; **Board Cert:** Clinical Pathology 2000; Blood Banking Transfusion Medicine 2002; **Med School:** Washington Univ, St Louis 1992; **Resid:** Pathology, Washington Univ 2000; **Fellow:** Blood Banking Transfusion Medicine, Washington Univ 2001; **Fac Appt:** Asst Prof Path, Harvard Med Sch

Mark, Eugene J MD [Path] - **Spec Exp:** Pulmonary Pathology; Forensic Pathology; Occupational Lung Disease; Lung Pathology-Rare Tumors; **Hospital:** Mass Genl Hosp; **Address:** Mass Genl Hosp, Dept Path, 55 Fruit St, Warren 246, Boston, MA 02114; **Phone:** 617-726-8891; **Board Cert:** Anatomic & Clinical Pathology 1973; Dermatopathology 1975; **Med School:** Harvard Med Sch 1967; **Resid:** Pathology, Mass Genl Hosp 1972; **Fellow:** Pathology, Kantonspital 1966; **Fac Appt:** Prof Path, Harvard Med Sch

Morrow, Jon Stanley MD/PhD [Path] - **Spec Exp:** Kidney Cancer; Colon Cancer; Breast Cancer; Hematopathology; **Hospital:** Yale-New Haven Hosp; **Address:** Yale Pathology, Bady Memorial Laboratory, 310 Cedar St, BML 140, New Haven, CT 06510; **Phone:** 203-785-3624; **Board Cert:** Pathology 1980; **Med School:** Yale Univ 1976; **Resid:** Pathology, Yale-New Haven Hosp 1978; **Fellow:** Pathology, Yale-New Haven Hosp 1980; **Fac Appt:** Prof Path, Yale Univ

Odze, Robert D MD [Path] - **Spec Exp:** Gastrointestinal Pathology; Liver Pathology; Esophageal Cancer; **Hospital:** Brigham and Women's Hosp (page 57); **Address:** Brigham & Women's Hosp, Dept Pathology, 75 Francis St, Boston, MA 02115; **Phone:** 617-732-7549; **Board Cert:** Anatomic Pathology 1990; **Med School:** McGill Univ 1984; **Resid:** Surgery, McGill Univ 1987; Pathology, McGill Univ 1990; **Fellow:** Gastrointestinal Pathology, New England Deaconess Med Ctr 1991; **Fac Appt:** Assoc Prof Path, Harvard Med Sch

Rennke, Helmut G MD [Path] - **Spec Exp:** Kidney Pathology; **Hospital:** Brigham and Women's Hosp (page 57); **Address:** Brigham & Womens Hosp, Dept Pathology, 75 Francis St Emory Bldg, Boston, MA 02115; **Phone:** 617-732-6518; **Board Cert:** Anatomic Pathology 1980; **Med School:** Chile 1971; **Resid:** Pathology, Boston City Hosp 1974; Pathology, Peter Bent Brigham Hosp 1977; **Fac Appt:** Prof Path, Harvard Med Sch

Rosenberg, Andrew E MD [Path] - **Spec Exp:** Bone & Joint Pathology; **Hospital:** Mass Genl Hosp; **Address:** Mass Genl Hosp, Dept Pathology, 55 Fruit St, Boston, MA 02114; **Phone:** 617-726-5127; **Board Cert:** Anatomic Pathology 1985; **Med School:** Temple Univ 1981; **Resid:** Anatomic Pathology, Mass Genl Hosp 1984; **Fellow:** Immunopathology, Mass Genl Hosp 1985

Schnitt, Stuart J MD [Path] - **Spec Exp:** Breast Pathology; Breast Cancer; **Hospital:** Beth Israel Deaconess Med Ctr - Boston; **Address:** Beth Israel Deaconess Med Ctr, Dept Pathology, 330 Brookline Ave, rm ES 112, Boston, MA 02215-5400; **Phone:** 617-667-4344; **Board Cert:** Anatomic & Clinical Pathology 1983; **Med School:** Albany Med Coll 1979; **Resid:** Anatomic Pathology, Beth Israel Deaconess Med Ctr 1983; **Fellow:** Surgical Pathology, Beth Israel Deaconess Med Ctr 1984; **Fac Appt:** Assoc Prof Path, Harvard Med Sch

Smith, Thomas W MD [Path] - **Spec Exp:** Neuropathology; **Hospital:** UMass Meml Med Ctr - Univ Campus; **Address:** Univ Mass Dept Pathology, Div Neuropathology, 55 Lake Ave N, Worcester, MA 01655; **Phone:** 508-856-2331; **Board Cert:** Neuropathology 1976; **Med School:** Cornell Univ 1972; **Resid:** Neuropathology, Peter Bent Brigham Hosp 1976; Radiology, Mass General Hosp 1977; **Fellow:** Anatomic Pathology, Peter Bent Brigham Hosp 1978; **Fac Appt:** Prof Path, Univ Mass Sch Med

Young, Robert H MD [Path] - **Spec Exp:** Ovarian Cancer; Gynecologic Cancer; **Hospital:** Mass Genl Hosp; **Address:** Mass General Hosp, 55 Fruit St, Dept Pathology, Warren 215, Boston, MA 02114; **Phone:** 617-726-8892; **Board Cert:** Anatomic Pathology 1980; **Med School:** Ireland 1974; **Resid:** Pathology, Mass Genl Hosp 1979; Pathology, Dublin Univ 1977; **Fac Appt:** Prof Path, Harvard Med Sch

Mid Atlantic

Bagg, Adam MD [Path] - **Spec Exp:** Hematopathology; Leukemia & Lymphoma; Myelodysplastic Syndromes; **Hospital:** Hosp Univ Penn - UPHS (page 68); **Address:** Hosp Univ Penn, Dept Pathology & Lab Med, 3400 Spruce St, Phildelphia, PA 19104; **Phone:** 215-662-4280; **Board Cert:** Clinical Pathology 1992; Hematology 1999; **Med School:** South Africa 1981; **Resid:** Internal Medicine, Univ Witwatersrand 1992; Clinical Pathology, Georgetown Univ 1992; **Fellow:** Hematopathology, Georgetown Univ 1993; **Fac Appt:** Prof Path, Univ Pennsylvania

Bastian, Boris C MD/PhD [Path] - **Spec Exp:** Melanoma; Skin Cancer; Dermatopathology; **Hospital:** Meml Sloan-Kettering Cancer Ctr; **Address:** Meml Sloan Kettering Cancer Ctr, 1275 York Ave, Dept Pathology, New York, NY 10065; **Phone:** 212-639-8410; **Med School:** Germany 1988; **Resid:** Dermatology, University of Wurzburg 1994; **Fellow:** Hematology, Ludwig-Maximilian-University 1989; UCSF Canc Ctr; **Fac Appt:** Asst Prof D, UCSF

Brooks, John S MD [Path] - **Spec Exp:** Tumor Pathology; Sarcoma; Bone & Soft Tissue Pathology; **Hospital:** Pennsylvania Hosp-UPHS (page 68), Hosp Univ Penn - UPHS (page 68); **Address:** Pennsylvania Hospital, Preston 6 FL, 800 Spruce St, Philadelphia, PA 19107; **Phone:** 215-829-3541; **Board Cert:** Anatomic Pathology 1978; Immunopathology 1983; **Med School:** Thomas Jefferson Univ 1974; **Resid:** Pathology, Hosp Univ Penn 1978; **Fellow:** Immunopathology, Hosp Univ Penn 1978; **Fac Appt:** Prof Path, Univ Pennsylvania

Burger, Peter MD [Path] - **Spec Exp:** Brain Tumors; Neuro-Pathology; **Hospital:** Johns Hopkins Hosp (page 61); **Address:** Johns Hopkins Hosp-Dept Pathology, 600 N Wolfe St, Pathology 710, Baltimore, MD 21287; **Phone:** 410-955-8378; **Board Cert:** Anatomic Pathology 1976; Neuropathology 1976; **Med School:** Northwestern Univ 1966; **Resid:** Anatomic Pathology, Duke Univ Med Ctr 1973; **Fellow:** Neuropathology, Duke Univ Med Ctr 1973

Crawford, James M MD/PhD [Path] - **Spec Exp:** Liver Pathology; Gastrointestinal Pathology; Gastrointestinal Cancer; **Hospital:** N Shore Univ Hosp, Long Island Jewish Med Ctr; **Address:** N Shore-LI Jewish Laboratories, 10 Nevada Drive, Lake Success, NY 11042-1114; **Phone:** 516-719-1060; **Board Cert:** Anatomic Pathology 1987; **Med School:** Duke Univ 1982; **Resid:** Pathology, Brigham & Women's Hosp 1984; **Fellow:** Gastrointestinal Pathology, Brigham & Women's Hosp 1987; Pathology, Royal Free hosp 1989

Demetris, Anthony J MD [Path] - **Spec Exp:** Transplant Pathology; Liver Pathology; **Hospital:** UPMC Montefiore; **Address:** UPMC - Montefiore, 3459 5th Ave, rm E741, Pittsburgh, PA 15213; **Phone:** 412-647-2067; **Board Cert:** Anatomic & Clinical Pathology 1987; **Med School:** Univ Pittsburgh 1982; **Resid:** Anatomic & Clinical Pathology, Univ Pittsburgh Med Ctr 1986; **Fac Appt:** Prof Path, Univ Pittsburgh

Ehya, Hormoz MD [Path] - **Spec Exp:** Cytopathology; Breast Pathology; Lung Pathology; **Hospital:** Fox Chase Cancer Ctr (page 58); **Address:** Fox Chase Cancer Center, 333 Cottman Ave, rm C427, Philadelphia, PA 19111-2497; **Phone:** 215-728-5389; **Board Cert:** Anatomic Pathology 1979; Cytopathology 1989; **Med School:** Iran 1974; **Resid:** Pathology, Univ Miss Med Ctr 1979; **Fellow:** Cytopathology, Meml Sloan-Kettering Cancer Ctr 1980

Epstein, Jonathan MD [Path] - **Spec Exp:** Bladder Cancer; Prostate Cancer; Urologic Pathology; **Hospital:** Johns Hopkins Hosp (page 61); **Address:** 401 N Broadway, Weinberg 2242, Baltimore, MD 21231; **Phone:** 410-955-5043; **Board Cert:** Anatomic Pathology 1986; **Med School:** Boston Univ 1981; **Resid:** Pathology, Johns Hopkins Hosp 1985; **Fellow:** Pathology, Meml Sloan Kettering Cancer Ctr 1984; **Fac Appt:** Prof Path, Johns Hopkins Univ

Fogt, Franz MD/PhD [Path] - **Spec Exp:** Gastrointestinal Pathology; **Hospital:** Penn Presby Med Ctr - UPHS (page 68); **Address:** Presbyterian Medical Ctr, Dept Pathology, 51 N 39th St, 551 Wright Saunders Bldg, Philadelphia, PA 19104; **Phone:** 215-662-8077; **Board Cert:** Anatomic & Clinical Pathology 1995; **Med School:** Germany 1988; **Resid:** Anatomic & Clinical Pathology, New England Deaconess Hosp 1995; **Fellow:** Gastrointestinal Pathology, New England Deaconess Hosp 1996; **Fac Appt:** Prof Path, Univ Pennsylvania

Gottlieb, Geoffrey J MD [Path] - **Spec Exp:** Dermatopathology; Melanoma; **Address:** Ackerman Academy Dermatopathology, 145 E 32nd St Fl 10, New York, NY 10016; **Phone:** 212-889-6225; **Board Cert:** Anatomic Pathology 1979; Dermatopathology 1982; **Med School:** Cornell Univ-Weill Med Coll 1976; **Resid:** Pathology, NY Hosp-Cornell Med Ctr 1979; **Fellow:** Dermatopathology, NYU Med Ctr 1982

Gupta, Prabodh K MD [Path] - **Spec Exp:** Lung Pathology; Cervical Cancer; Fine Needle Aspiration Biopsy; **Hospital:** Hosp Univ Penn - UPHS (page 68); **Address:** Hosp Univ Penn - Cytopathology, 3400 Spruce St, 6 Founders, Philadelphia, PA 19104; **Phone:** 215-662-3238; **Board Cert:** Anatomic Pathology 1975; Cytopathology 1989; **Med School:** India 1960; **Resid:** Pathology, All India Inst Med Scis 1967; **Fellow:** Pathology, Mass Genl Hosp 1968; Cytopathology, Johns Hopkins Hosp 1969; **Fac Appt:** Prof Path, Univ Pennsylvania

Heller, Debra S MD [Path] - **Spec Exp:** Gynecologic Pathology; Pediatric Pathology; Perinatal Pathology; **Hospital:** Univ Hosp-UMDNJ—Newark; **Address:** UMDNJ-NJ Med Sch Dept Pathology, 185 S Orange Ave, UH/E158, Newark, NJ 07101; **Phone:** 973-972-0751; **Board Cert:** Anatomic Pathology 1988; Obstetrics & Gynecology 2008; Pediatric Pathology 1999; **Med School:** NY Med Coll 1977; **Resid:** Obstetrics & Gynecology, Beth Israel Med Ctr 1981; Anatomic Pathology, Mt Sinai Med Ctr 1988; **Fellow:** Pediatric Pathology, Mt Sinai Med Ctr 1987; Gynecologic Pathology, Mt Sinai Med Ctr 1989; **Fac Appt:** Prof Path, UMDNJ-NJ Med Sch, Newark

Hoda, Syed A MD [Path] - **Spec Exp:** Breast Cancer; Surgical Pathology; **Hospital:** NY-Presby/Weill Cornell Med Ctr, NY (page 65); **Address:** 525 E 68th St, 1028 Starr, New York, NY 10021-4870; **Phone:** 212-746-2700; **Board Cert:** Anatomic & Clinical Pathology 1990; Cytopathology 1991; Pathology 2001; **Med School:** Pakistan 1984; **Resid:** Anatomic & Clinical Pathology, Tulane Univ Affil Hosps 1990; **Fellow:** Cytopathology, Meml Sloan Kettering Cancer Ctr 1991; Pathology, Meml Sloan Kettering Cancer Ctr 1992; **Fac Appt:** Clin Prof Path, Cornell Univ-Weill Med Coll

Hruban, Ralph H MD [Path] - **Spec Exp:** Gastrointestinal Pathology; Pancreatic Cancer; **Hospital:** Johns Hopkins Hosp (page 61); **Address:** Johns Hopkins Hosp, Dept Pathology, 401 N Broadway Bldg Weinberg - rm 2242, Baltimore, MD 21231; **Phone:** 410-955-2660; **Board Cert:** Anatomic Pathology 1990; **Med School:** Johns Hopkins Univ 1985; **Resid:** Pathology, Johns Hopkins Hosp 1990; **Fellow:** Anatomic Pathology, Meml Sloan Kettering Cancer Ctr 1989; **Fac Appt:** Prof Path, Johns Hopkins Univ

Jones, Robert V MD [Path] - **Spec Exp:** Neuro-Pathology; Brain Tumors; **Hospital:** G Washington Univ Hosp; **Address:** GWUMC, Dept Path, 2300 I (Eye) St NW, Ross Hall, Ste 502, Washington, DC 20037; **Phone:** 202-994-3391; **Board Cert:** Anatomic & Clinical Pathology 1981; Neuropathology 1994; **Med School:** Univ VA Sch Med 1977; **Resid:** Anatomic & Clinical Pathology, Walter Reed AMC 1981; **Fellow:** Neurological Pathology, ARmed Forces Inst Path 1990; **Fac Appt:** Assoc Prof Path, Geo Wash Univ

Kahn, Leonard B MD [Path] - **Spec Exp:** Bone Pathology; Head & Neck Pathology; Soft Tissue Tumors; Jaw Tumors; **Hospital:** Long Island Jewish Med Ctr, N Shore Univ Hosp; **Address:** 6 Ohio Drive, Ste 202 - rm 621, Lake Success, NY 10042; **Phone:** 516-304-7264; **Board Cert:** Anatomic Pathology 1980; **Med School:** South Africa 1960; **Resid:** Pathology, Univ Cape Town 1966; **Fellow:** Pathology, Washington Univ 1969; **Fac Appt:** Prof Path, Albert Einstein Coll Med

Katzenstein, Anna-Luise A MD [Path] - **Spec Exp:** Lung Cancer; Pulmonary Pathology; Interstitial Lung Disease; **Hospital:** SUNY Upstate Med Univ Shos, Crouse Hosp; **Address:** SUNY Upstate Medical Univ, 750 E Adams St UH Bldg - rm 6709, Syracuse, NY 13210; **Phone:** 315-464-7125; **Board Cert:** Anatomic Pathology 1976; **Med School:** Johns Hopkins Univ 1971; **Resid:** Pathology, Univ Hosp 1975; **Fellow:** Surgical Pathology, Barnes Hosp-Wash Univ 1976; **Fac Appt:** Prof Path, SUNY Upstate Med Univ

Pathology

Kurman, Robert J MD [Path] - **Spec Exp:** Gynecologic Pathology; Ovarian Cancer; Uterine Cancer; **Hospital:** Johns Hopkins Hosp (page 61); **Address:** Johns Hopkins Hosp, Dept Pathology, 401 N Broadway, Weinberg-2242, Baltimore, MD 21231; **Phone:** 410-955-0471; **Board Cert:** Anatomic Pathology 1972; Obstetrics & Gynecology 1980; **Med School:** SUNY Upstate Med Univ 1968; **Resid:** Pathology, Peter Bent Brigham Hosp/Mass Genl Hosp 1977; Obstetrics & Gynecology, LAC Hosp/USC 1978; **Fellow:** Obstetrics & Gynecology, Harvard Univ 1973; **Fac Appt:** Prof Path, Johns Hopkins Univ

Li Volsi, Virginia A MD [Path] - **Spec Exp:** Endocrine Cancers; Thyroid Cancer; Gynecologic Cancer; **Hospital:** Hosp Univ Penn - UPHS (page 68); **Address:** Hosp Univ Penn - Pathology, 3400 Spruce St, Founders Bldg Fl 6 - rm 6009, Philadelphia, PA 19104; **Phone:** 215-662-6545; **Board Cert:** Anatomic Pathology 1974; **Med School:** Columbia P&S 1969; **Resid:** Anatomic Pathology, Presbyterian Hosp 1974; **Fac Appt:** Prof Path, Univ Pennsylvania

Melamed, Jonathan MD [Path] - **Spec Exp:** Prostate Cancer; Tumor Banking-Prostate; **Hospital:** NYU Langone Med Ctr (page 66); **Address:** NYU Medical Ctr, Dept Pathology, TH-461, 560 First Ave, New York, NY 10016; **Phone:** 212-263-8927; **Board Cert:** Anatomic & Clinical Pathology 1992; **Med School:** South Africa 1985; **Resid:** Pathology, Lenox Hill Hosp 1991; **Fellow:** Pathology, Meml Sloan Kettering Cancer Ctr 1992; Urologic Pathology, Meml Sloan Kettering Cancer Ctr 1993; **Fac Appt:** Assoc Prof Path, NYU Sch Med

Mies, Carolyn MD [Path] - **Spec Exp:** Breast Cancer; **Hospital:** Hosp Univ Penn - UPHS (page 68); **Address:** Hosp Univ Penn-Surgical Pathology, 3400 Spruce St, Founders 6, Philadelphia, PA 19104; **Phone:** 215-662-6503; **Board Cert:** Anatomic Pathology 1984; **Med School:** Rush Med Coll 1980; **Resid:** Pathology, Tufts-New England Med Ctr 1982; Pathology, New England Deaconess Hosp 1984; **Fellow:** Surgical Pathology, Meml Sloan Kettering Cancer Ctr 1986; **Fac Appt:** Assoc Prof Path, Univ Pennsylvania

Montgomery, Elizabeth A MD [Path] - **Spec Exp:** Barrett's Esophagus; Esophageal Cancer; Gastrointestinal Pathology; **Hospital:** Johns Hopkins Hosp (page 61); **Address:** Johns Hopkins Univ, Dept Pathology, 401 N Broadway Weinberg Bldg - rm 2242, Baltimore, MD 21231; **Phone:** 410-614-2308; **Board Cert:** Anatomic Pathology 1988; Cytopathology 1994; **Med School:** Geo Wash Univ 1984; **Resid:** Pathology, Walter Reed AMC 1988; **Fac Appt:** Assoc Prof Path, Johns Hopkins Univ

Orazi, Attilio MD [Path] - **Spec Exp:** Hematopathology; Bone Marrow Pathology; Lymph Node Pathology; Spleen Pathology; **Hospital:** NY-Presby/Weill Cornell Med Ctr, NY (page 65); **Address:** NY Presby-Cornell Medical Ctr, 525 E 68th St, Starr Pavilion, rm 715, New York, NY 10021; **Phone:** 212-746-2050; **Board Cert:** Anatomic Pathology 1997; Hematology 1998; **Med School:** Italy 1979; **Resid:** Internal Medicine, Leicester Royal Infirmary 1982; Histopathology, Northampton Genl Hosp 1983; **Fellow:** Anatomic Pathology, Natl Cancer Inst 1985; **Fac Appt:** Prof Path, Cornell Univ-Weill Med Coll

Patchefsky, Arthur S MD [Path] - **Spec Exp:** Breast Cancer; Pulmonary Pathology; Sarcoma; **Hospital:** Fox Chase Cancer Ctr (page 58); **Address:** Fox Chase Cancer Center, 333 Cottman Ave, rm C4333, Philadelphia, PA 19111; **Phone:** 215-728-5390; **Board Cert:** Anatomic Pathology 1969; **Med School:** Hahnemann Univ 1963; **Resid:** Pathology, John Hopkins Hosp 1966; Pathology, Hosp Univ Penn 1967; **Fellow:** Pathology, Meml Sloan Kettering Cancer Ctr 1968; **Fac Appt:** Prof Path, Thomas Jefferson Univ

Reuter, Victor E MD [Path] - **Spec Exp:** Prostate Cancer; Genitourinary Pathology; Bladder Cancer; Testicular Cancer; **Hospital:** Meml Sloan-Kettering Cancer Ctr; **Address:** Memorial Sloan Kettering Cancer Ctr, Dept Pathology, 1275 York Ave, New York, NY 10021; **Phone:** 212-639-8225; **Board Cert:** Anatomic & Clinical Pathology 1983; **Med School:** Dominican Republic 1978; **Resid:** Anatomic Pathology, Thos Jefferson Univ Hosp 1981; Clinical Pathology, Thos Jefferson Univ Hosp 1983; **Fellow:** Surgical Pathology, Meml Sloan Kettering Cancer Ctr 1985; **Fac Appt:** Prof Path, Cornell Univ-Weill Med Coll

Rosenblum, Marc K MD [Path] - **Spec Exp:** Neuropathology; Brain Tumors; **Hospital:** Meml Sloan-Kettering Cancer Ctr; **Address:** 1275 York Ave, Meml Sloan-Kettering Cancer Ctr, New York, NY 10065; **Phone:** 212-639-3844; **Board Cert:** Anatomic Pathology 1984; Neuropathology 1988; **Med School:** Univ Miami Sch Med 1979; **Resid:** Anatomic Pathology, Mt Sinai Med Ctr 1984; **Fellow:** Pathology, Meml Sloan-Kettering Cancer Ctr 1985; Neurological Pathology, Bellevue-NYU Med Ctr 1987; **Fac Appt:** Prof Path, Cornell Univ-Weill Med Coll

Ross, Jeffrey S MD [Path] - **Spec Exp:** Urologic Cancer; Prostate Cancer; Breast Cancer; **Hospital:** Albany Med Ctr; **Address:** Albany Med Coll, Dept Path, 47 New Scotland Ave, MC 81, Albany, NY 12208; **Phone:** 518-262-5471; **Board Cert:** Anatomic & Clinical Pathology 1974; **Med School:** SUNY Buffalo 1970; **Resid:** Pathology, Mass Genl Hosp 1974; **Fellow:** Pathology, Harvard Med Sch 1974; **Fac Appt:** Prof Path, Albany Med Coll

Sanchez, Miguel A MD [Path] - **Spec Exp:** Breast Cancer; Thyroid Cancer; **Hospital:** Englewood Hosp & Med Ctr; **Address:** 350 Engle St Dean Bldg Fl LL1, Englewood, NJ 07631-1898; **Phone:** 201-894-3423; **Board Cert:** Anatomic Pathology 1975; Clinical Pathology 1979; Cytopathology 1991; **Med School:** Spain 1969; **Resid:** Pathology, Englewood Hosp 1972; Pathology, Temple Univ 1973; **Fellow:** Pathology, Meml Sloan Kettering Cancer Ctr 1974; Clinical Pathology, St Vincents Hosp 1975; **Fac Appt:** Assoc Prof Path, Mount Sinai Sch Med

Schiller, Alan L MD [Path] - **Spec Exp:** Bone & Joint Pathology; Soft Tissue Pathology; Bone Tumors; **Hospital:** Mount Sinai Med Ctr (page 63); **Address:** Mt Sinai Sch Med, Dept Pathology, 1 Gustave Levy Pl, Box 1194, New York, NY 10029-6500; **Phone:** 212-241-8014; **Board Cert:** Anatomic Pathology 1973; **Med School:** Ros Franklin Univ/Chicago Med Sch 1967; **Resid:** Pathology, Mass Genl Hosp 1972; **Fac Appt:** Prof Path, Mount Sinai Sch Med

Silverman, Jan F MD [Path] - **Spec Exp:** Fine Needle Aspiration Biopsy; Surgical Pathology; Gastrointestinal Pathology; Cytopathology; **Hospital:** Allegheny General Hosp, West Penn Hosp-Forbes Campus; **Address:** Allegheny Gen Hosp-Dept Lab Medicine, 320 E North Ave, Pittsburgh, PA 15212; **Phone:** 412-359-6886; **Board Cert:** Anatomic & Clinical Pathology 1975; Cytopathology 1989; **Med School:** Med Coll VA 1970; **Resid:** Pathology, Med Coll Virginia 1975; **Fellow:** Surgical Pathology, Med Coll Virginia 1975; **Fac Appt:** Prof Path, Drexel Univ Coll Med

Soslow, Robert A MD [Path] - **Spec Exp:** Gynecologic Pathology; **Hospital:** Meml Sloan-Kettering Cancer Ctr; **Address:** 1275 York Avenue, Pathology Department, New York, NY 10065; **Phone:** 800-525-2225; **Board Cert:** Anatomic Pathology 1995; **Med School:** Univ Pennsylvania 1991; **Resid:** Anatomic Pathology, Stanford Univ Med Ctr 1994; **Fellow:** Immunopathology, Stanford Univ Med Ctr 1995; **Fac Appt:** Assoc Prof Path, Cornell Univ

Swerdlow, Steven H MD [Path] - **Spec Exp:** Lymphoma; Hematopathology; Transplant Pathology; **Hospital:** UPMC Presby, Pittsburgh; **Address:** Div Hematopathology, 200 Lothrop St, Ste G-300, Pittsburgh, PA 15213-2536; **Phone:** 412-647-5191; **Board Cert:** Anatomic & Clinical Pathology 2005; **Med School:** Harvard Med Sch 1975; **Resid:** Pathology, Beth Israel Hosp 1979; **Fellow:** Hematopathology, Vanderbilt Univ 1981; Hematopathology, St Bartholmew's Hosp 1983; **Fac Appt:** Prof Path, Univ Pittsburgh

Pathology

Tomaszewski, John E MD [Path] - **Spec Exp:** Kidney Pathology; Lung Pathology; Uterine Cancer; Genitourinary Pathology; **Hospital:** Hosp Univ Penn - UPHS (page 68); **Address:** Hosp Univ Penn, Dept Pathology & Lab Med, 3400 Spruce St, 6 Founders Bldg, Ste 6042, Philadelphia, PA 19104; **Phone:** 215-662-6852; **Board Cert:** Anatomic Pathology 1982; Immunopathology 1983; **Med School:** Univ Pennsylvania 1977; **Resid:** Pathology, Hosp Univ Penn 1982; **Fellow:** Surgical Pathology, Hosp Univ Penn 1983; **Fac Appt:** Prof Path, Univ Pennsylvania

Tornos, Carmen MD [Path] - **Spec Exp:** Gynecologic Cancer; Breast Cancer; Ovarian Cancer; **Hospital:** Stony Brook Univ Med Ctr; **Address:** Stony Brook Univ Hosp, Dept Pathology, Level 2, rm 766, Stony Brook, NY 11794; **Phone:** 631-444-2222; **Board Cert:** Anatomic & Clinical Pathology 1989; **Med School:** Spain 1977; **Resid:** Hematology, Ciudad Sanitaria Valle de Hebron 1982; Anatomic & Clinical Pathology, Univ Texas HSC 1989; **Fellow:** Surgical Pathology, MD Anderson Cancer Ctr 1990; **Fac Appt:** Prof Path, SUNY Stony Brook

Travis, William MD [Path] - **Spec Exp:** Pulmonary Pathology; Lung Cancer; Interstitial Lung Disease; **Hospital:** Meml Sloan-Kettering Cancer Ctr; **Address:** 1275 York Ave, MSKCC Bldg, Pathology Dept, New York, NY 10065; **Phone:** 212-639-6364; **Board Cert:** Anatomic & Clinical Pathology 1985; **Med School:** Univ Fla Coll Med 1981; **Resid:** Anatomic Pathology, New England Deaconess Hosp 1983; Clinical Pathology, Mayo Clinic 1985; **Fellow:** Surgical Pathology, Mayo Clinic 1986

Wang, Beverly Y MD [Path] - **Spec Exp:** Head & Neck Pathology; **Hospital:** NYU Langone Med Ctr (page 66); **Address:** NYU Medical Ctr, Dept Pathology, 530 First Ave Fl 4 - rm 461, New York, NY 10016; **Phone:** 212-263-6032; **Board Cert:** Anatomic Pathology 1998; Cytopathology 1999; **Med School:** China 1982; **Resid:** Pathology, Mount Sinai Med Ctr 1999; **Fac Appt:** Prof Path, NYU Sch Med

Yousem, Samuel A MD [Path] - **Spec Exp:** Pulmonary Pathology; Transplant-Lung (Pathology); Lung Cancer; **Hospital:** UPMC Presby, Pittsburgh; **Address:** Dept Pathology, A-610, UPMC-Presbyterian Campus, 200 Lothrop St, Pittsburgh, PA 15213; **Phone:** 412-647-6193; **Board Cert:** Anatomic Pathology 1985; Cytopathology 1997; **Med School:** Univ MD Sch Med 1981; **Resid:** Pathology, Stanford Univ Med Ctr 1983; **Fellow:** Surgical Pathology, Stanford Univ Med Ctr 1984; **Fac Appt:** Prof Path, Univ Pittsburgh

Zagzag, David MD/PhD [Path] - **Spec Exp:** Neuropathology; Brain Tumors; Tumor Banking-Brain; **Hospital:** NYU Langone Med Ctr (page 66), Bellevue Hosp Ctr; **Address:** NYU Med Ctr, Dept Pathology, 550 First Ave, Div Neuropathology, NB-4N30, New York, NY 10016; **Phone:** 212-263-6449; **Board Cert:** Anatomic Pathology 1993; Neuropathology 1993; **Med School:** France 1984; **Resid:** Surgical Pathology, NYU Med Ctr 1990; **Fellow:** Neurological Pathology, NYU Med Ctr 1992; **Fac Appt:** Assoc Prof Path, NYU Sch Med

Southeast

Banks, Peter MD [Path] - **Spec Exp:** Hematopathology; Lymphoma; **Hospital:** Carolinas Med Ctr; **Address:** Dept Pathology, 1000 Blythe Blvd, 4th Fl Pathology Lab, Charlotte, NC 28203; **Phone:** 704-355-2251; **Board Cert:** Anatomic Pathology 2008; **Med School:** Harvard Med Sch 1971; **Resid:** Pathology, National Cancer Inst 1974; Pathology, Duke Univ Med Ctr 1975; **Fellow:** Surgical Pathology, Univ Minn Med Ctr 1976; **Fac Appt:** Prof Path, Univ NC Sch Med

Bostwick, David MD [Path] - **Spec Exp:** Urologic Pathology; Prostate Cancer; Bladder Cancer; Gastrointestinal Pathology; **Address:** 4355 Innslake Drive, Glen Allen, VA 23060; **Phone:** 804-967-9225; **Board Cert:** Anatomic Pathology 2003; **Med School:** Univ MD Sch Med 1979; **Resid:** Pathology, Stanford Univ Med Ctr 1981; **Fellow:** Surgical Pathology, Stanford Univ Med Ctr 1984

Chesney, Carolyn M MD [Path] - **Spec Exp:** Hematopathology; Bleeding/Coagulation Disorders; **Hospital:** Baptist Memorial Hospital-Memphis; **Address:** Pathology Grp of MidSouth Inc, 7550 Wolf River Blvd, Ste 200, Germantown, TN 38138; **Phone:** 901-542-6800; **Board Cert:** Internal Medicine 1972; Hematology 1999; **Med School:** Vanderbilt Univ 1968; **Resid:** Internal Medicine, Vanderbilt Univ Hosp 1970; **Fellow:** Hematology, Mass Genl Hosp 1972; **Fac Appt:** Prof Med, Univ Tenn Coll Med

Cote, Richard J MD [Path] - **Spec Exp:** Lymph Node Pathology; Bladder Cancer; Breast Cancer; **Hospital:** Univ of Miami Hosp (page 72); **Address:** 1120 NW 14th St, CRB Bldg - Fl 14 - Ste 1416 (R5), Miami, FL 33136; **Phone:** 305-243-2683; **Board Cert:** Anatomic Pathology 1987; **Med School:** Univ Chicago-Pritzker Sch Med 1980; **Resid:** Pathology, New York Hosp 1987; **Fellow:** Pathology, Meml Sloan-Kettering Cancer Ctr 1990; **Fac Appt:** Prof Path, USC-Keck School of Medicine

Faye-Petersen, Ona MD [Path] - **Spec Exp:** Perinatal Pathology; Fetal Pathology; Neonatal Pathology; Pediatric Pathology; **Hospital:** Univ of Ala Hosp at Birmingham, UAB Highlands Hosp; **Address:** UAB Dept Pathology, 619 19th St S, NP 3547, Birmingham, AL 35249; **Phone:** 205-975-8880; **Board Cert:** Anatomic & Clinical Pathology 1987; Pediatric Pathology 1991; **Med School:** Univ Colorado 1980; **Resid:** Pathology, Presby-Denver Hosp 1985; **Fellow:** Surgical Pathology, Meml Sloan Ketter Cancer Ctr 1986; Pediatric Pathology, Mt Sinai Hosp 1987; **Fac Appt:** Prof Path, Univ Alabama

Lage, Janice MD [Path] - **Spec Exp:** Obstetric Pathology; Gynecologic Pathology; Breast Pathology; **Hospital:** MUSC Med Ctr; **Address:** MUSC Med Ctr, Dept Path, 165 Ashley Ave, Ste 309, Box 250908, Charleston, SC 29425; **Phone:** 843-792-3121; **Board Cert:** Anatomic Pathology 2001; **Med School:** Washington Univ, St Louis 1980; **Resid:** Pathology, Barnes Hosp/Wash Univ 1982; Obstetrics & Gynecology, Barnes Hosp/Wash Univ 1983; **Fellow:** Surgical Pathology, Barnes Hosp/Wash Univ 1984; **Fac Appt:** Prof Path, Med Univ SC

Masood, Shahla MD [Path] - **Spec Exp:** Breast Cancer; Breast Pathology; **Hospital:** Shands Jacksonville; **Address:** Univ of Florida, Dept Pathology, 655 W 8th St, Jacksonville, FL 32209-6511; **Phone:** 904-244-4387; **Board Cert:** Anatomic & Clinical Pathology 1977; Cytopathology 1990; **Med School:** Iran 1973; **Resid:** Anatomic Pathology, Univ Hosp 1977; **Fac Appt:** Prof Path, Univ Fla Coll Med

McCurley, Thomas L MD [Path] - **Spec Exp:** Hematopathology; Immunopathology; **Hospital:** Vanderbilt Univ Med Ctr (page 76), TN Valley Healthcare Sys-Nashville; **Address:** Hematopathology Dept, 1301 Med Ctr Drive, 4601 TVC, Nashville, TN 37232-5310; **Phone:** 615-343-9167; **Board Cert:** Anatomic & Clinical Pathology 1981; Immunopathology 1986; Hematology 1999; **Med School:** Vanderbilt Univ 1974; **Resid:** Internal Medicine, UCSF Med Ctr 1976; Pathology, Vanderbilt Univ Med Ctr 1981; **Fellow:** Hematopathology, Vanderbilt Univ 1984; **Fac Appt:** Assoc Prof Path, Vanderbilt Univ

Mills, Stacey E MD [Path] - **Spec Exp:** Breast Pathology; Ear, Nose & Throat Pathology; Surgical Pathology; Bone Pathology; **Hospital:** Univ of Virginia Health Sys; **Address:** Univ VA Hlth System, Dept Pathology, PO Box 800214, Charlottesville, VA 22908-0214; **Phone:** 434-982-4406; **Board Cert:** Anatomic Pathology 2009; **Med School:** Univ VA Sch Med 1977; **Resid:** Pathology, Univ Virginia Med Ctr 1980; **Fellow:** Pathology, Univ Virginia Med Ctr 1981; **Fac Appt:** Prof Path, Univ VA Sch Med

Nicosia, Santo MD [Path] - **Spec Exp:** Ovarian Cancer; Cytopathology; **Hospital:** H Lee Moffitt Cancer Ctr & Research Inst (page 59); **Address:** 12901 Bruce B Downs Blvd, MDC Box 11, Tampa, FL 33612-4742; **Phone:** 813-974-3133; **Board Cert:** Anatomic Pathology 1978; Cytopathology 1990; **Med School:** Italy 1967; **Resid:** Anatomic Pathology, Michael Reese Hosp 1972; **Fellow:** Hosp Univ Penn 1973; **Fac Appt:** Prof Path, Univ S Fla Coll Med

Pathology

Norenberg, Michael D MD [Path] - **Spec Exp:** Liver Pathology; Parkinson's Disease; **Hospital:** Jackson Meml Hosp (page 70); **Address:** Jackson Meml Hosp, Dept Pathology, 1611 NW 12th Ave Holtz Ctr, rm 2142, Miami, FL 33136; **Phone:** 305-585-7017; **Board Cert:** Anatomic Pathology 1972; Neuropathology 1974; **Med School:** Univ Rochester 1965; **Resid:** Pathology, Strong Meml Hosp 1970; **Fellow:** Neuropathology, Strong Meml Hosp 1972; **Fac Appt:** Prof Path, Univ Miami Sch Med

Petito, Carol K MD [Path] - **Spec Exp:** Neuro-Pathology; **Hospital:** Jackson Meml Hosp (page 70); **Address:** Univ Miami Dept Pathology (R-5), 1550 NW 10th Ave, PAP Bldg, rm 417, Miami, FL 33136; **Phone:** 305-585-8970; **Board Cert:** Anatomic Pathology 1973; Neuropathology 1973; **Med School:** Columbia P&S 1967; **Resid:** Pathology, NY Hosp-Cornell Med Ctr 1970; Neuropathology, Armed Forces Inst; **Fac Appt:** Prof Path, Univ Miami Sch Med

Sewell, C Whitaker MD [Path] - **Spec Exp:** Breast Pathology; Surgical Pathology; **Hospital:** Emory Univ Hosp; **Address:** Emory Univ Hosp, Dept Pathology, 1364 Clifton Rd NE, rm H185C, Atlanta, GA 30322; **Phone:** 404-712-7003; **Board Cert:** Anatomic & Clinical Pathology 1974; **Med School:** Emory Univ 1969; **Resid:** Pathology, Emory Univ Hosp 1974; **Fac Appt:** Prof Path, Emory Univ

Weiss, Sharon A W MD [Path] - **Spec Exp:** Soft Tissue Pathology; Surgical Pathology; Sarcoma; **Hospital:** Emory Univ Hosp; **Address:** Emory Univ Hosp, Dept Pathology, 1364 Clifton Rd NE, rm H176, Atlanta, GA 30322; **Phone:** 404-712-0708; **Board Cert:** Anatomic Pathology 1974; **Med School:** Johns Hopkins Univ 1971; **Resid:** Pathology, Johns Hopkins Hosp 1975; **Fac Appt:** Prof Path, Emory Univ

Midwest

Allred, D Craig MD [Path] - **Spec Exp:** Breast Cancer; Breast Pathology; Breast Cancer Risk Assessment; **Hospital:** Barnes-Jewish Hosp; **Address:** Washington Univ Sch Med, Path & Immunology, 660 S Euclid Ave, Box 8118, St Louis, MO 63110; **Phone:** 314-362-6313; **Board Cert:** Anatomic Pathology 1984; **Med School:** Univ Utah 1979; **Resid:** Anatomic Pathology, Univ Conn Hlth Ctr 1983; **Fellow:** Immunopathology, Univ Conn Hlth Ctr 1982; **Fac Appt:** Prof Path, Baylor Coll Med

Appelman, Henry MD [Path] - **Spec Exp:** Gastrointestinal Pathology; Liver Pathology; **Hospital:** Univ of Michigan Hosp; **Address:** Univ Michigan, Dept Pathology, 1500 E Med Ctr Drive, Ann Arbor, MI 48109-0054; **Phone:** 734-936-6770; **Board Cert:** Anatomic & Clinical Pathology 1966; **Med School:** Univ Mich Med Sch 1961; **Resid:** Pathology, Univ Mich Med Ctr 1966; **Fac Appt:** Prof Path, Univ Mich Med Sch

Balla, Andre K MD/PhD [Path] - **Spec Exp:** Prostate Cancer; Gynecologic Pathology; Tumor Banking; **Hospital:** Univ of IL Med Ctr at Chicago; **Address:** Univ Illinois Chicago, Dept Path, 840 S Wood St, 130 CSN Bldg, MC 847, Chicago, IL 60612; **Phone:** 312-996-3879; **Board Cert:** Anatomic & Clinical Pathology 1988; **Med School:** Brazil 1972; **Resid:** Pathology, Hahnemann Univ Hosp 1988; **Fellow:** Clinical Immunology, Scripps Clin Rsch Fdn 1981; **Fac Appt:** Prof Path, Univ IL Coll Med

Behm, Frederick G MD [Path] - **Spec Exp:** Hematopathology; **Hospital:** Univ of IL Med Ctr at Chicago; **Address:** Univ Illinois Chicago, Dept Pathology, 840 S Wood St, 130 CSN Bldg, MC 847, Chicago, IL 60612-7335; **Phone:** 312-996-3150; **Board Cert:** Anatomic & Clinical Pathology 1980; Hematology 1983; **Med School:** Med Coll Wisc 1974; **Resid:** Pathology, Med Coll Va Hosps 1979; **Fac Appt:** Prof Path, Univ IL Coll Med

Bell, Debra A MD [Path] - **Spec Exp:** Gynecologic Pathology; Ovarian Cancer; **Hospital:** Mayo Med Ctr & Clin - Rochester; **Address:** Mayo Clinic-Pathology Dept, 200 First St SW, Rochester, MN 55905; **Phone:** 507-284-1800; **Board Cert:** Anatomic Pathology 1980; Cytopathology 1989; **Med School:** Albany Med Coll 1976; **Resid:** Pathology, NYU Med Ctr 1981; **Fellow:** Cytopathology, Meml Sloan Kettering Cancer Ctr 1982; **Fac Appt:** Assoc Prof Path, Mayo Med Sch

Cho, Kathleen R MD [Path] - **Spec Exp:** Gynecologic Pathology; Ovarian Cancer; Cervical Cancer; **Hospital:** Univ of Michigan Hosp; **Address:** Univ Michigan Med Sch, 109 Zina Pitcher Pl, rm 1506, Ann Arbor, MI 48109-2200; **Phone:** 734-764-1549; **Board Cert:** Anatomic Pathology 1990; **Med School:** Vanderbilt Univ 1984; **Resid:** Pathology, Johns Hopkins Hosp 1988; **Fellow:** Gynecologic Pathology, Johns Hopkins Hosp 1990; **Fac Appt:** Prof Path, Univ Mich Med Sch

Cohen, Michael B MD [Path] - **Spec Exp:** Urologic Cancer; Cytopathology; **Hospital:** Univ Iowa Hosp & Clinics, Iowa City VA Hlth Care Sys; **Address:** Univ Iowa - Dept Pathology, 200 Hawkins Drive, C670GH, Iowa City, IA 52242; **Phone:** 319-384-9609; **Board Cert:** Anatomic Pathology 2008; Cytopathology 1996; **Med School:** Albany Med Coll 1982; **Resid:** Pathology, UCSF Hosps & Clinics 1986; **Fellow:** Cytopathology, UCSF Hosps & Clinics 1987; **Fac Appt:** Prof Path, Univ Iowa Coll Med

Dahmoush, Laila MD [Path] - **Spec Exp:** Breast Pathology; Gynecologic Pathology; Urologic Pathology; **Hospital:** Univ Iowa Hosp & Clinics; **Address:** UIHC Dept of Pathology, 200 Hawkins Dr 5216D RCP, Iowa City, IA 52242; **Phone:** 319-356-4440; **Board Cert:** Anatomic & Clinical Pathology 1999; Cytopathology 2001; **Med School:** Egypt 1983; **Resid:** Anatomic & Clinical Pathology, Washington Univ Hosp 1997; Anatomic & Clinical Pathology, Univ MD Med Sys 1999; **Fellow:** Surgical Pathology, Univ MD Med Sys 2000; Cytopathology, Natl Inst Hlth/Natl Canc Inst 2001; **Fac Appt:** Assoc Prof Path, Univ Iowa Coll Med

Gambetti, Pierluigi MD [Path] - **Spec Exp:** Neuro-Pathology; Neurodegenerative Disorders; Creutzfeldt-Jakob Disease (CJD); **Hospital:** Univ Hosps Case Med Ctr (page 74); **Address:** Case Western Reserve Univ, Inst Path, 2085 Adelbert Rd, rm 419, Cleveland, OH 44106; **Phone:** 216-368-0587; **Board Cert:** Neuropathology 1981; **Med School:** Italy 1960; **Resid:** Neurology, Univ Bologna Med Ctr 1963; **Fellow:** Neurological Pathology, Institut Bunge 1965; Neurological Pathology, Hosp Univ Penn 1968; **Fac Appt:** Prof Path, Case West Res Univ

Goldblum, John R MD [Path] - **Spec Exp:** Soft Tissue Pathology; Esophageal Cancer; Gastrointestinal Pathology; Sarcoma; **Hospital:** Cleveland Clin (page 56); **Address:** Cleveland Clinic, Anatomic Pathology L25, 9500 Euclid Ave, Cleveland, OH 44195; **Phone:** 216-444-8238; **Board Cert:** Anatomic Pathology 1993; **Med School:** Univ Mich Med Sch 1989; **Resid:** Anatomic Pathology, Univ Michigan Hosps 1993; **Fac Appt:** Prof Path, Cleveland Cl Coll Med/Case West Res

Greenson, Joel K MD [Path] - **Spec Exp:** Liver Cancer; Gastrointestinal Pathology; Liver Pathology; **Hospital:** Univ of Michigan Hosp; **Address:** Univ Michigan Hospitals, Dept Pathology, 1301 Catherine St, Med Sci 1 Bldg - rm 5218, Ann Arbor, MI 48109-5602; **Phone:** 734-936-6770; **Board Cert:** Anatomic & Clinical Pathology 1988; **Med School:** Univ Mich Med Sch 1984; **Resid:** Pathology, Cedars-Sinai Med Ctr 1988; **Fellow:** Gastrointestinal Pathology, Johns Hopkins Hosp 1990; **Fac Appt:** Prof Path, Univ Mich Med Sch

Kurtin, Paul J MD [Path] - **Spec Exp:** Lymph Node Pathology; Bone Marrow Pathology; Lymphoma; **Hospital:** Mayo Med Ctr & Clin - Rochester; **Address:** Mayo Clinic - Div Hematopathology, 200 First St SW, Hilton 1160A, Rochester, MN 55905; **Phone:** 507-284-4939; **Board Cert:** Anatomic & Clinical Pathology 1983; Hematology 1988; **Med School:** Med Coll Wisc 1979; **Resid:** Anatomic & Clinical Pathology, Vanderbilt Univ Med Ctr 1983; **Fellow:** Hematopathology, Brigham & Women's Hosp 1984; Surgical Pathology, Brigham & Women's Hosp 1986; **Fac Appt:** Prof Path, Mayo Med Sch

Pathology

Lucas, David R MD [Path] - **Spec Exp:** Bone Tumors; Soft Tissue Tumors; Surgical Pathology; **Hospital:** Univ of Michigan Hosp; **Address:** 1500 E Medical Ctr Drive, rm 2G332-UH, Ann Arbor, MI 48109; **Phone:** 734-232-0022; **Board Cert:** Anatomic Pathology 1993; **Med School:** Wayne State Univ 1988; **Resid:** Pathology, Wayne State Univ Med Ctr 1991; **Fellow:** Surgical Pathology, Mayo Clinic 1993; **Fac Appt:** Prof Path, Univ Mich Med Sch

Mitros, Frank A MD [Path] - **Spec Exp:** Liver Pathology; Gastrointestinal Pathology; Surgical Pathology; **Hospital:** Univ Iowa Hosp & Clinics; **Address:** Univ Iowa Hosp & Clins, Dept Pathology, 200 Hawkins Dr, 5244B RCP, Iowa City, IA 52242; **Phone:** 319-356-1760; **Board Cert:** Anatomic Pathology 1979; **Med School:** UMDNJ-NJ Med Sch, Newark 1969; **Resid:** Pathology, Univ Chicago Hosps 1976; **Fac Appt:** Prof Path, Univ Iowa Coll Med

Moore, Steven A MD/PhD [Path] - **Spec Exp:** Muscular Dystrophy; Neuropathology; **Hospital:** Univ Iowa Hosp & Clinics; **Address:** UIHC Dept of Pathology, 200 Hawkins Dr 5239B RCP, Iowa City, IA 52242; **Phone:** 319-384-9084; **Board Cert:** Anatomic Pathology 1986; Neuropathology 1986; **Med School:** Indiana Univ 1982; **Resid:** Pathology, Univ IA Hosp & Clin 1984; **Fellow:** Neurological Pathology, Univ IA Hosp & Clin 1986; **Fac Appt:** Prof NPath, Univ Iowa Coll Med

Myers, Jeffrey L MD [Path] - **Spec Exp:** Lung Cancer; Lung Pathology; **Hospital:** Univ of Michigan Hosp; **Address:** 1500 E Medical Center Drive, Univ Michigan, 2G332 UH, Ann Arbor, MI 48109-5912; **Phone:** 734-936-1888; **Board Cert:** Anatomic Pathology 1986; **Med School:** Washington Univ, St Louis 1981; **Resid:** Anatomic Pathology, Barnes Jewish Hosp 1984; **Fellow:** Surgical Pathology, Univ Alabama Med Ctr 1985; **Fac Appt:** Prof Path, Univ Mich Med Sch

Petras, Robert E MD [Path] - **Spec Exp:** Gastrointestinal Pathology; **Address:** Ameripath GI Institute, 7730 First Pl, Ste A, Oakwood Village, OH 44146; **Phone:** 440-703-2100; **Board Cert:** Anatomic & Clinical Pathology 2004; **Med School:** Ohio State Univ 1978; **Resid:** Anatomic & Clinical Pathology, Cleveland Clinic 1982; **Fellow:** Gastrointestinal Pathology, St Marks Hosp; **Fac Appt:** Assoc Prof Path, NE Ohio Univ

Rubin, Brian P MD [Path] - **Spec Exp:** Bone & Soft Tissue Pathology; Sarcoma; **Hospital:** Cleveland Clin (page 56); **Address:** Cleveland Clinic, Dept Anatomic Pathology, L25, 9500 Euclid Ave, Cleveland, OH 44195; **Phone:** 216-445-5551; **Board Cert:** Anatomic Pathology 1999; **Med School:** Cornell Univ-Weill Med Coll 1995; **Resid:** Pathology, Brigham & Womens Hosp 2000; **Fac Appt:** Asst Prof Path, Univ Wash

Scheithauer, Bernd W MD [Path] - **Spec Exp:** Brain Tumors; Pituitary Tumors; Neuro-Pathology; Pituitary Disorders; **Hospital:** Mayo Med Ctr & Clin - Rochester; **Address:** Mayo Clinic, Dept Pathology, 200 First St SW, Hilton Bldg, Rochester, MN 55905; **Phone:** 507-284-8350; **Board Cert:** Anatomic Pathology 1979; Neuropathology 1979; **Med School:** Loma Linda Univ 1973; **Resid:** Anatomic Pathology, Stanford Univ Med Ctr 1976; Neuropathology, Stanford Univ Med Ctr 1978; **Fellow:** Surgical Pathology, Stanford Univ Med Ctr 1979; **Fac Appt:** Prof Path, Mayo Med Sch

Suster, Saul M MD [Path] - **Spec Exp:** Lung Cancer; Mediastinal Tumors; Surgical Pathology; **Hospital:** Froedtert and Med Ctr of WI; **Address:** Med College of Wisconsin, Dept Pathology, Dynacare Lab Bldg, rm 226, 9200 W Wisconsin Ave, Milwaukee, WI 53226; **Phone:** 414-805-6968; **Board Cert:** Anatomic & Clinical Pathology 1988; **Med School:** Ecuador 1976; **Resid:** Anatomic Pathology, Tel Aviv Univ Med Ctr 1984; Anatomic & Clinical Pathology, Mt Sinai Med Ctr 1988; **Fellow:** Surgical Pathology, Yale-New Haven Hosp 1990; **Fac Appt:** Prof Path, Med Coll Wisc

Ulbright, Thomas M MD [Path] - **Spec Exp:** Testicular Cancer; Gynecologic Pathology; **Hospital:** IU Health University Hosp; **Address:** IU Health Pathology Laboratory, 350 W 11th St, rm 4078, Indianapolis, IN 46202; **Phone:** 317-491-6498; **Board Cert:** Anatomic Pathology 1980; **Med School:** Washington Univ, St Louis 1975; **Resid:** Pathology, Barnes Jewish Hosp 1978; Surgical Pathology, Barnes Jewish Hosp 1979; **Fellow:** Gynecologic Pathology, St Johns Mercy Med Ctr 1980; **Fac Appt:** Prof Path, Indiana Univ

Wollmann, Robert MD [Path] - **Spec Exp:** Neuro-Pathology; Brain Tumors; **Hospital:** Univ of Chicago Med Ctr; **Address:** Univ Chicago Med Ctr, 5841 S Maryland Ave, MC 6101, Chicago, IL 60615-2707; **Phone:** 773-702-6166; **Board Cert:** Anatomic Pathology 1975; Neuropathology 1977; **Med School:** Univ IL Coll Med 1969; **Resid:** Anatomic Pathology, Univ Chicago Med Ctr 1972; **Fellow:** Neuropathology, Max Planck Inst 1972; **Fac Appt:** Prof Path, Univ Chicago-Pritzker Sch Med

Great Plains and Mountains

De Masters, Bette K MD [Path] - **Spec Exp:** Neuro-Pathology; Brain Tumors; **Hospital:** Univ of CO Hosp - Anschutz Inpatient Pav, Chldn's Hosp - Aurora (CO); **Address:** Univ CO Hlth Sci Ctr, Dept Pathology, 12605 East 16th Ave MS F-768, Aurora, CO 80045; **Phone:** 270-848-4421; **Board Cert:** Anatomic & Clinical Pathology 1982; Neuropathology 1985; **Med School:** Univ Wisc 1977; **Resid:** Internal Medicine, Presby Hosp 1979; Pathology, Univ Colo Med Sch 1982; **Fellow:** Neurological Pathology, Univ Colo/Univ Kansas 1984; **Fac Appt:** Prof Path, Univ Colorado

Thor, Ann D MD [Path] - **Spec Exp:** Breast Cancer; Gynecologic Cancer; **Hospital:** Univ of CO Hosp - Anschutz Inpatient Pav; **Address:** 12631 E 17th Ave, Rm 2215, Box B216, Anschutz Med Campus, Box 6511, MS B216, Aurora, CO 80045-0508; **Phone:** 303-724-3704; **Board Cert:** Anatomic Pathology 1987; Cytopathology 1989; **Med School:** Vanderbilt Univ 1981; **Resid:** Pathology, Vanderbilt Univ 1983; **Fellow:** Immunopathology, Natl Cancer Inst 1986; Gynecologic Pathology, Mass Genl Hosp 1990; **Fac Appt:** Prof Path, Univ Colorado

Weisenburger, Dennis D MD [Path] - **Spec Exp:** Hematopathology; Lymphoma; **Hospital:** Nebraska Med Ctr; **Address:** Dept Pathology and Microbiology, 983135 Nebraska Medical Center, Omaha, NE 68198-3135; **Phone:** 402-559-7688; **Board Cert:** Anatomic & Clinical Pathology 1979; **Med School:** Univ Minn 1974; **Resid:** Anatomic Pathology, Univ Iowa Hosps 1978; **Fellow:** Hematopathology, City of Hope Natl Med Ctr 1980; **Fac Appt:** Prof Path, Univ Nebr Coll Med

Southwest

Bruner, Janet M MD [Path] - **Spec Exp:** Brain Tumors; Neuro-Pathology; **Hospital:** UT MD Anderson Cancer Ctr; **Address:** MD Anderson Cancer Ctr, 1515 Holcombe Blvd, Ste 85, Houston, TX 77030; **Phone:** 713-792-6127; **Board Cert:** Anatomic Pathology 1982; Neuropathology 1984; **Med School:** Med Coll OH 1979; **Resid:** Anatomic & Clinical Pathology, Med Coll Ohio Hosp 1982; **Fellow:** Neurological Pathology, Baylor Coll Med 1984; **Fac Appt:** Prof Path, Univ Tex, Houston

Cagle, Philip MD [Path] - **Spec Exp:** Pulmonary Pathology; Lung Cancer; Mesothelioma; **Hospital:** Methodist Hosp - Houston; **Address:** Methodist Hospital, Dept Pathology, 6565 Fannin St, Ste 227, Houston, TX 77030; **Phone:** 713-441-6478; **Board Cert:** Anatomic & Clinical Pathology 1985; **Med School:** Univ Tenn Coll Med 1981; **Resid:** Pathology, Baylor Coll Med Ctr 1985; **Fellow:** Pulmonary Pathology 1987; **Fac Appt:** Prof Path, Baylor Coll Med

Foucar, M Kathryn MD [Path] - **Spec Exp:** Leukemia; Lymph Node Pathology; Bone Marrow Pathology; **Hospital:** Univ Hosp - New Mexico; **Address:** TriCore Reference Lab, Hematopathology, 1001 Woodward Pl NE, Albuquerque, NM 87102; **Phone:** 505-938-8456; **Board Cert:** Anatomic & Clinical Pathology 1978; **Med School:** Ohio State Univ 1974; **Resid:** Anatomic Pathology, Univ NM Health & Sci Ctr 1976; Anatomic Pathology, Univ Minn Med Ctr 1978; **Fellow:** Surgical Pathology, Univ Minn Med Ctr 1979; **Fac Appt:** Prof Path, Univ New Mexico

Grogan, Thomas M MD [Path] - **Spec Exp:** Immunopathology; Lymphoma; **Hospital:** Univ Med Ctr - Tucson; **Address:** AHSC, Dept Pathology, 1501 N Campbell Ave, rm 5211, Tucson, AZ 85724; **Phone:** 520-626-7477; **Board Cert:** Anatomic Pathology 1976; **Med School:** Geo Wash Univ 1971; **Resid:** Pathology, Letterman Army Med Ctr 1976; **Fellow:** Immunopathology, Stanford Univ Sch Med 1979; **Fac Appt:** Prof Path, Univ Ariz Coll Med

Hamilton, Stanley R MD [Path] - **Spec Exp:** Surgical Pathology; Gastrointestinal Pathology; Liver Pathology; **Hospital:** UT MD Anderson Cancer Ctr; **Address:** Univ Texas MD Anderson Cancer Ctr, 1515 Holcombe Blvd, Unit 085, Houston, TX 77030-4009; **Phone:** 713-792-2040; **Board Cert:** Anatomic & Clinical Pathology 1978; **Med School:** Indiana Univ 1973; **Resid:** Pathology, Johns Hopkins Hosp 1978; **Fellow:** St Marks Hosp 1979; **Fac Appt:** Prof Path, Univ Tex, Houston

Kinney, Marsha C MD [Path] - **Spec Exp:** Hematopathology; Lymphoma; Leukemia; **Hospital:** Univ Hlth Syst-San Antonio; **Address:** Univ Texas Hlth & Sci Ctr, Dept Path, 7703 Floyd Curl Drive, MC 7750, San Antonio, TX 78229-3900; **Phone:** 210-567-4072; **Board Cert:** Anatomic & Clinical Pathology 1985; Hematology 1998; **Med School:** Univ Tex SW, Dallas 1981; **Resid:** Pathology, Vanderbilt Univ Med Ctr 1985; **Fellow:** Hematopathology, Vanderbilt Univ Med Ctr 1988; **Fac Appt:** Prof Path, Univ Tex, San Antonio

Leslie, Kevin O MD [Path] - **Spec Exp:** Pulmonary Pathology; Lung Cancer; Surgical Pathology; **Hospital:** Mayo Clinic - Scottsdale; **Address:** Mayo Clinic, Scottsdale, 13400 E Shea Blvd, Dept Pathology, Scottsdale, AZ 85259; **Phone:** 480-301-8021; **Board Cert:** Anatomic & Clinical Pathology 1982; **Med School:** Albert Einstein Coll Med 1976; **Resid:** Anatomic & Clinical Pathology, Univ Colorado Health Sci Ctr 1982; **Fellow:** Surgical Pathology, Stanford Univ Med Ctr 1983; **Fac Appt:** Prof Path, Mayo Med Sch

Moran, Cesar A MD [Path] - **Spec Exp:** Lung Cancer; Mediastinal Tumors; Mesothelioma; **Hospital:** UT MD Anderson Cancer Ctr; **Address:** MD Anderson Cancer Ctr, Dept Pathology, 1515 Holcombe Blvd, rm G1-3738, Houston, TX 77030; **Phone:** 713-792-8134; **Board Cert:** Anatomic Pathology 1992; **Med School:** Guatemala 1981; **Resid:** Anatomic Pathology, Mt Sinai Med Ctr 1988; **Fellow:** Surgical Pathology, Yale-New Haven Med Ctr 1989; **Fac Appt:** Prof Path, Univ Tex, Houston

Prieto, Victor G MD/PhD [Path] - **Spec Exp:** Dermatopathology; Melanoma; Skin Cancer; **Hospital:** UT MD Anderson Cancer Ctr; **Address:** MD Anderson Cancer Ctr, Dept Pathology, 1515 Holcombe Blvd, Box 85, Houston, TX 77030-4000; **Phone:** 713-792-0918; **Board Cert:** Anatomic Pathology 1995; Dermatopathology 1997; **Med School:** Spain 1986; **Resid:** Pathology, New York Hosp-Cornell Med Ctr 1993; **Fellow:** Pathology, Meml Sloan Kettering Cancer Ctr 1995; Dermatopathology, New York Hosp-Cornell Med Ctr 1996; **Fac Appt:** Prof Path, Univ Tex, Houston

Rashid, Asif MD/PhD [Path] - **Spec Exp:** Gastrointestinal Pathology; Liver Pathology; **Hospital:** UT MD Anderson Cancer Ctr; **Address:** MD Anderson Cancer Ctr, Dept Pathology, 1515 Holcombe Blvd, Box 85, Houston, TX 77030; **Phone:** 713-745-1101; **Board Cert:** Anatomic Pathology 1994; **Med School:** Pakistan 1984; **Resid:** Anatomic Pathology, Mass Genl Hosp 1993; **Fellow:** Anatomic Pathology, Mass Genl Hosp 1994; Anatomic Pathology, Johns Hopkins 1996

Roberts, William C MD [Path] - **Spec Exp:** Cardiac Pathology; **Hospital:** Baylor Univ Medical Ctr-Dallas; **Address:** Baylor Univ Med Ctr, Heart & Vascular Inst, 3500 Gaston Ave, Ste H-030, Dallas, TX 75246-2017; **Phone:** 214-820-7911; **Board Cert:** Anatomic Pathology 1965; **Med School:** Emory Univ 1958; **Resid:** Anatomic Pathology, Natl Heart Inst-NIH 1962; Internal Medicine, Johns Hopkins Hosp 1963; **Fellow:** Cardiovascular Disease, Natl Heart Inst-NIH 1964

Sahin, Aysegul MD [Path] - **Spec Exp:** Breast Cancer; **Hospital:** UT MD Anderson Cancer Ctr; **Address:** 1515 Holcombe Blvd, Box 0085, Houston, TX 77030; **Phone:** 713-794-1500; **Board Cert:** Pathology 1987; **Med School:** Turkey 1980; **Resid:** Pathology, Oregon Hlth Sci Univ 1986; **Fellow:** Surgical Pathology, Univ Iowa Hosps & Clins 1987; **Fac Appt:** Prof Path, Univ Tex, Houston

Silva, Elvio G MD [Path] - **Spec Exp:** Gynecologic Pathology; Gynecologic Cancer; **Hospital:** UT MD Anderson Cancer Ctr, Cedars-Sinai Med Ctr; **Address:** MD Anderson Cancer Ctr, Dept Pathology, 1515 Holcombe Blvd, Unit 85, MC G1-3563B, Houston, TX 77030; **Phone:** 713-792-3154; **Board Cert:** Anatomic Pathology 2007; **Med School:** Argentina 1969; **Resid:** Pathology, National Univ Med Ctr 1975; Anatomic Pathology, Univ Toronto 1978; **Fellow:** Surgical Pathology, MD Anderson Cancer Ctr 1979; **Fac Appt:** Prof Path

Walker, David H MD [Path] - **Spec Exp:** Infections-Emerging; Tropical Diseases; Bioterrorism Preparedness; **Hospital:** UTMB - John Sealy Hospital; **Address:** UT Med Br Galveston, Dept Path, 301 University Blvd, Galveston, TX 77555-0609; **Phone:** 409-772-3989; **Board Cert:** Anatomic & Clinical Pathology 1974; **Med School:** Vanderbilt Univ 1969; **Resid:** Anatomic & Clinical Pathology, Peter Bent Brigham Hosp 1973; **Fellow:** Pathology, Harvard Univ 1973; **Fac Appt:** Prof Path, Univ Tex Med Br, Galveston

Wheeler, Thomas M MD [Path] - **Spec Exp:** Thyroid Disorders; Thyroid Cancer; Genitourinary Cancer; **Hospital:** Ben Taub Genl Hosp; **Address:** Baylor Coll Med, Dept Pathology, One Baylor Plaza, rm T203, MS 315, Houston, TX 77030; **Phone:** 713-798-4664; **Board Cert:** Anatomic & Clinical Pathology 1981; Cytopathology 1990; **Med School:** Baylor Coll Med 1977; **Resid:** Pathology, Baylor Affil Hosps 1981; **Fac Appt:** Prof Path, Baylor Coll Med

West Coast and Pacific

Amin, Mahul MD [Path] - **Spec Exp:** Genitourinary Pathology; Bladder Cancer; **Hospital:** Cedars-Sinai Med Ctr; **Address:** Cedars Sinai Med Ctr, 8700 Beverly Blvd, Ste 8728, Los Angeles, CA 90048; **Phone:** 310-423-6631; **Board Cert:** Anatomic & Clinical Pathology 1996; **Med School:** India 1983; **Resid:** Pathology, Henry Ford Hosp 1992; **Fellow:** Surgical Pathology, MD Anderson Cancer Ctr 1993; **Fac Appt:** Prof Path, UCLA-David Geffen Sch Med

Arber, Daniel A MD [Path] - **Spec Exp:** Bone Marrow Pathology; Lymph Node Pathology; Spleen Pathology; **Hospital:** Stanford Univ Hosp & Clinics, Lucile Packard Chldn's Hosp; **Address:** Clinic Laboratories, Stanford Univ Med Ctr, 300 Pasteur Drive, rm H1507, MC 5627, Stanford, CA 94305; **Phone:** 650-725-5604; **Board Cert:** Anatomic & Clinical Pathology 1991; Hematology 1993; **Med School:** Univ Tex, San Antonio 1986; **Resid:** Anatomic & Clinical Pathology, Scott & White Meml Hosp 1991; **Fellow:** Hematopathology, City of Hope Natl Med Ctr 1993; **Fac Appt:** Prof Path, Stanford Univ

Bollen, Andrew W MD [Path] - **Spec Exp:** Neuro-Pathology; Brain Tumors; Brain Infections; **Hospital:** UCSF Med Ctr, San Francisco Genl Hosp; **Address:** UCSF School of Medicine, Dept Pathology/Neuropathology, 505 Parnassus Ave, rm M553, Box 0102, San Francisco, CA 94143-0511; **Phone:** 415-476-5236; **Board Cert:** Neuropathology 1992; Anatomic Pathology 1992; Clinical Pathology 1993; **Med School:** UCSD 1985; **Resid:** Anatomic Pathology, UCSF Med Ctr 1991; **Fellow:** Neuropathology, UCSF Med Ctr 1989; **Fac Appt:** Prof Path, UCSF

Pathology

Chandrasoma, Parakrama T MD [Path] - **Spec Exp:** Gastrointestinal Pathology; Gastrointestinal Cancer; Neuro-Pathology; **Hospital:** LAC & USC Med Ctr; **Address:** LAC-USC Med Ctr, Dept Path, Clinic Tower Fl 7 - rm A7A127, 1100 N State St, Los Angeles, CA 90033; **Phone:** 323-226-4600; **Board Cert:** Anatomic Pathology 1982; **Med School:** Sri Lanka 1971; **Resid:** Anatomic Pathology, Univ Sri Lanka 1978; Anatomic Pathology, LAC-USC Med Ctr 1982; **Fac Appt:** Prof Path, USC Sch Med

Chang, Karen L MD [Path] - **Spec Exp:** Leukemia; **Hospital:** City of Hope Natl Med Ctr; **Address:** 1500 E Duarte Rd, Duarte, CA 91010-3012; **Phone:** 626-256-4673 x62456; **Board Cert:** Anatomic & Clinical Pathology 1992; **Med School:** Mount Sinai Sch Med 1985; **Resid:** Anatomic Pathology, Stanford Univ Med Ctr 1988; Clinical Pathology, Stanford Univ Med Ctr 1991; **Fellow:** Surgical Pathology, Stanford Univ Med Ctr 1989

Cochran, Alistair J MD [Path] - **Spec Exp:** Melanoma; Dermatopathology; **Hospital:** UCLA Ronald Reagan Med Ctr; **Address:** UCLA Med Ctr, Dept Path & Med, 10833 Le Conte Ave, rm 13-145CHS, MC 173216, Los Angeles, CA 90095-1732; **Phone:** 310-825-2743; **Med School:** Scotland, UK 1959; **Resid:** Dermatopathology, Western Infirmary 1968; Pathology, Western Infirmary 1968; **Fellow:** Immunology, Karolinska Inst 1970; **Fac Appt:** Prof Path, UCLA

Dubeau, Louis MD/PhD [Path] - **Spec Exp:** Ovarian Cancer; Breast Cancer; **Hospital:** USC Norris Cancer Hosp (page 75); **Address:** USC Norris Cancer Ctr, Dept Pathology, 1441 Eastlake Ave, rm 6338, Los Angeles, CA 90033-1048; **Phone:** 323-865-0720; **Board Cert:** Anatomic Pathology 1984; **Med School:** McGill Univ 1979; **Resid:** Anatomic Pathology, McGill Univ Med Ctr 1984; **Fac Appt:** Prof Path, USC Sch Med

Ferrell, Linda MD [Path] - **Spec Exp:** Liver Pathology; **Hospital:** UCSF Med Ctr; **Address:** UCSF Med Ctr, Dept Pathology, 505 Parnassus Ave, rm M590, Box 0102, San Francisco, CA 94143-0102; **Phone:** 415-353-1090; **Board Cert:** Anatomic Pathology 1982; **Med School:** Univ Kansas 1977; **Resid:** Anatomic Pathology, Univ Kansas Med Ctr 1979; Anatomic Pathology, UCSF Med Ctr 1981; **Fac Appt:** Prof Path, UCSF

Fishbein, Michael C MD [Path] - **Spec Exp:** Cardiovascular Pathology; Pulmonary Pathology; **Hospital:** UCLA Ronald Reagan Med Ctr; **Address:** UCLA Pathology & Lab Medicine, 10833 Le Conte Ave, Los Angeles, CA 90095-1732; **Phone:** 310-825-8940; **Board Cert:** Anatomic & Clinical Pathology 1975; **Med School:** Univ IL Coll Med 1971; **Resid:** Anatomic & Clinical Pathology, UCLA-Harbor General Hosp 1975; **Fellow:** Pathology, Heart Lung Inst-NIH 1975; **Fac Appt:** Prof Path, UCLA

Govindarajan, Sugantha MD [Path] - **Spec Exp:** Liver Pathology; **Hospital:** Rancho Los Amigos Natl Rehab Ctr; **Address:** Rancho Los Amigos Natl Rehab Ctr, 7601 E Imperial Hwy, Bldg JPI - rm B170, Dept Pathology, Downey, CA 90242; **Phone:** 562-401-8996; **Board Cert:** Anatomic Pathology 1976; **Med School:** India 1969; **Resid:** Pathology, St Lukes Hosp 1976; **Fellow:** Pathology, Cleveland Clinic 1977; **Fac Appt:** Prof Path, USC Sch Med

Hammar, Samuel P MD [Path] - **Spec Exp:** Lung Cancer; Pulmonary Pathology; **Hospital:** Harrison Med Ctr; **Address:** Diagnostic Specialties Laboratory, 700 Lebo Blvd, Bremerton, WA 98310; **Phone:** 360-479-7707; **Board Cert:** Anatomic & Clinical Pathology 1975; **Med School:** Univ Wash 1970

Kanel, Gary MD [Path] - **Spec Exp:** Liver Pathology; **Hospital:** Keck Med Ctr of USC (page 75); **Address:** USC Univ Hosp, Dept Pathology, 1500 San Pablo St Fl 2, Los Angeles, CA 90033; **Phone:** 323-226-7127; **Board Cert:** Anatomic & Clinical Pathology 1979; **Med School:** Tufts Univ 1974; **Resid:** Pathology, Tufts-New England Med Ctr 1976; Pathology, Univ Chicagos Hosp 1977; **Fellow:** Pathology, Tufts-New England Med Ctr 1979; **Fac Appt:** Prof Path, USC Sch Med

Koss, Michael N MD [Path] - **Spec Exp:** Pulmonary Pathology; Lung Cancer; Kidney Pathology; **Hospital:** USC Norris Cancer Hosp (page 75), Keck Med Ctr of USC (page 75); **Address:** 2222 Ocean View Ave, Ste 212, Los Angeles, CA 90057; **Phone:** 213-381-2260; **Board Cert:** Anatomic Pathology 1979; **Med School:** Stanford Univ 1970; **Resid:** Pathology, Columbia Presby Med Ctr 1974; **Fellow:** Renal Pathology, Columbia Presby Med Ctr 1975; Pulmonary Pathology, Armed Forces Inst Path 1978; **Fac Appt:** Prof Path, USC Sch Med

Le Boit, Philip E MD [Path] - **Spec Exp:** Cutaneous Lymphoma; Skin Cancer; Dermatopathology; **Hospital:** UCSF Med Ctr; **Address:** UCSF - Dermatopathology Section, 1701 Divisadero St, rm 499, San Francisco, CA 94115; **Phone:** 415-353-7546; **Board Cert:** Anatomic Pathology 1983; Dermatopathology 1983; Clinical Pathology 1986; **Med School:** Albany Med Coll 1979; **Resid:** Anatomic Pathology, UCSF Med Ctr 1981; Clinical Pathology, Mt Sinai Hosp 1982; **Fellow:** Dermatopathology, New York Hosp-Cornell Med Ctr 1983; **Fac Appt:** Prof Path, UCSF

Ljung, Britt-Marie E MD [Path] - **Spec Exp:** Breast Cancer; Cytopathology; Fine Needle Aspiration Biopsy; **Hospital:** UCSF - Mt Zion Med Ctr; **Address:** UCSF - Dept Pathology, 1600 Divisadero St, Box 1785, R-200, San Francisco, CA 94143-1785; **Phone:** 415-353-7320; **Board Cert:** Anatomic Pathology 1985; Cytopathology 1989; **Med School:** Sweden 1975; **Resid:** Pathology, Karolinska Hosp 1979; Anatomic Pathology, UCLA Med Ctr 1983; **Fac Appt:** Prof Path, UCSF

Mischel, Paul S MD [Path] - **Spec Exp:** Neuro-Pathology; Brain Tumors; **Hospital:** UCLA Ronald Reagan Med Ctr; **Address:** UCLA Med Ctr, Div Neuropathology, 10833 Le Conte Ave, rm 13-317 CHS, Los Angeles, CA 90095-1732; **Phone:** 310-825-2339; **Board Cert:** Anatomic Pathology 1997; Neuropathology 1997; **Med School:** Cornell Univ-Weill Med Coll 1991; **Resid:** Anatomic & Clinical Pathology, UCLA Med Center 1996; **Fellow:** Neurological Pathology, UCLA 1995; Research, Howard Hughes Med Inst/UCSF 1998; **Fac Appt:** Prof Path, UCLA

Nathwani, Bharat N MD [Path] - **Spec Exp:** Hematopathology; Leukemia; Lymphoma; **Hospital:** Cedars-Sinai Med Ctr; **Address:** Cedars-Sinai Dept Pathology, 8700 Beverly Blvd, South Tower, rm 7706, Los Angeles, CA 90048; **Phone:** 310-248-6659; **Board Cert:** Anatomic Pathology 1977; **Med School:** India 1969; **Resid:** Pathology, JJ Group-Grant Med Ctr 1972; Pathology, Rush-Presby-St Lukes Med Ctr 1974; **Fellow:** Hematopathology, City Hope Natl Med Ctr 1975; **Fac Appt:** Prof Path, USC Sch Med

Perry, Arie MD [Path] - **Spec Exp:** Neuro-Pathology; Brain Tumors; **Hospital:** UCSF Med Ctr; **Address:** UCSF-Dept of Neuropathology, 505 Parnassus Ave, rm M-551, San Francisco, CA 94143; **Phone:** 415-476-5236; **Board Cert:** Anatomic & Clinical Pathology 1995; Neuropathology 1997; **Med School:** Univ Tex SW, Dallas 1990; **Resid:** Pathology, Univ Tex SW 1994; **Fellow:** Surgical Pathology, Mayo Clin 1995; Neurological Pathology, Mayo Clin 1998; **Fac Appt:** Assoc Prof Path, Washington Univ, St Louis

Rutgers, Joanne MD [Path] - **Spec Exp:** Gynecologic Cancer; Cytopathology; Gastrointestinal Pathology; **Hospital:** Long Beach Meml Med Ctr; **Address:** 2801 Atlantic Ave, Dept of Pathology, Long Beach, CA 90806; **Phone:** 562-933-0717; **Board Cert:** Clinical Pathology 1992; Anatomic Pathology 1985; Cytopathology 1997; **Med School:** UCSD 1981; **Resid:** Pathology, Montefiore Med Ctr 1983; Pathology, NYU Med Ctr 1985; **Fellow:** Gynecologic Pathology, Mass Genl Hosp 1989; **Fac Appt:** Clin Prof Path, UC Irvine

Sibley, Richard K MD [Path] - **Spec Exp:** Kidney Pathology; Breast Pathology; Liver Pathology; **Hospital:** Stanford Univ Hosp & Clinics; **Address:** Stanford Univ Med Ctr, Surg Path Lab, 300 Pasteur Drive, rm H2110, MC 5324, Stanford, CA 94305; **Phone:** 650-723-7211; **Board Cert:** Anatomic Pathology 1975; **Med School:** Univ Tex SW, Dallas 1971; **Resid:** Anatomic Pathology, Univ Chicago Hosps 1974; **Fellow:** Stanford Univ Med Ctr 1975; **Fac Appt:** Prof Path, Stanford Univ

Triche, Timothy J MD/PhD [Path] - **Spec Exp:** Pediatric Pathology; Pediatric Cancers; Sarcoma; **Hospital:** Chldns Hosp - Los Angeles; **Address:** Chldns Hosp Los Angeles, Dept Patholgy, 4650 Sunset Blvd, MS 133, Los Angeles, CA 90027; **Phone:** 323-361-8898; **Board Cert:** Anatomic Pathology 1975; **Med School:** Tulane Univ 1971; **Resid:** Anatomic Pathology, Barnes Hosp-Wash Univ 1973; Surgical Pathology, Barnes Hosp 1974; **Fellow:** Pathology, Natl Cancer Inst 1975; **Fac Appt:** Prof Path, USC Sch Med

True, Lawrence D MD [Path] - **Spec Exp:** Urologic Pathology; Prostate Cancer; Bladder Cancer; **Hospital:** Univ Wash Med Ctr; **Address:** Univ Wash Med Ctr, Dept Anatomic Path, Campus Box 356100, rm NE110, 1959 NE Pacific St, Seattle, WA 98195-6100; **Phone:** 206-598-6400; **Board Cert:** Anatomic Pathology 1981; **Med School:** Tulane Univ 1971; **Resid:** Pathology, Univ Colo Hlth Sci Ctr 1980; **Fac Appt:** Prof Path, Univ Wash

Warnke, Roger A MD [Path] - **Spec Exp:** Lymphoma; Hematopathology; **Hospital:** Stanford Univ Hosp & Clinics; **Address:** Stanford Hosp, 300 Pasteur, Pathology, rm L235, Stanford, CA 94305-5324; **Phone:** 650-725-5167; **Board Cert:** Anatomic Pathology 1975; **Med School:** Washington Univ, St Louis 1971; **Resid:** Pathology, Stanford Univ Med Ctr 1974; **Fellow:** Surgical Pathology, Stanford Univ Med Ctr 1975; Immunology, Stanford Univ Med Ctr 1976; **Fac Appt:** Prof Path, Stanford Univ

Weiss, Lawrence M MD [Path] - **Spec Exp:** Lymphoma; Hematopathology; Adrenal Pathology; **Hospital:** City of Hope Natl Med Ctr; **Address:** City of Hope Natl Med Ctr, Div Pathology, 1500 E Duarte Rd, Duarte, CA 91010-0269; **Phone:** 626-256-4673 x62456; **Board Cert:** Anatomic Pathology 1985; **Med School:** Univ MD Sch Med 1981; **Resid:** Pathology, Brigham & Women's Hosp 1983; **Fellow:** Surgical Pathology, Stanford Univ Hosp 1984

Wilczynski, Sharon P MD/PhD [Path] - **Spec Exp:** Gynecologic Cancer; Breast Cancer; Ovarian Cancer; Clinical Trials; **Hospital:** City of Hope Natl Med Ctr; **Address:** City Hope Natl Med Ctr-Dept of Pathology, 1500 E Duarte Rd, Duarte, CA 91010; **Phone:** 626-256-4673 x62456; **Board Cert:** Anatomic & Clinical Pathology 1985; Cytopathology 1991; **Med School:** Med Coll PA Hahnemann 1981; **Resid:** Pathology, Hosp Univ Penn 1983; Anatomic & Clinical Pathology, Long Beach Meml Hosp 1985; **Fac Appt:** Prof Path, USC-Keck School of Medicine

Pediatrics

A pediatrician is concerned with the physical, emotional and social health of children from birth to young adulthood. Care encompasses a broad spectrum of health services ranging from preventive health-care to the diagnosis and treatment of acute and chronic diseases.

A pediatrician deals with biological, social and environmental influences on the developing child, and with the impact of disease and dysfunction on development.

Training Required: Three years

Pediatric Allergy and Immunology: An allergist-immunologist is trained in evaluation, physical and laboratory diagnosis and management of disorders involving the immune system. Selected examples of such conditions include asthma, anaphylaxis, rhinitis, eczema and adverse reactions to drugs, foods and insect stings as well as immune deficiency diseases (both acquired and congenital), defects in host defense and problems related to autoimmune disease, organ transplantation or malignancies of the immune system. As our understanding of the immune system develops, the scope of this specialty is widening.

Training Required: Prior certification in pediatrics *plus* two years in allergy/immunology. (Training programs are available at some medical centers to provide individuals with expertise in both allergy/immunology and pediatric pulmonology. Such individuals are candidates for dual certification.)

(continued on next page)

Certification in one of the following subspecialties requires additional training and examination.

Pediatric Cardiology: A pediatric cardiologist provides comprehensive care to patients with cardiovascular problems. This specialist is skilled in selecting, performing and evaluating the structural and functional assessment of the heart and blood vessels and the clinical evaluation of cardiovascular disease.

Pediatric Critical Care Medicine: A pediatrician who cares for children who are victims of life threatening disorders such as severe accidents, shock and diabetic acidosis.

Pediatric Endocrinology: A pediatrician who provides expert care to infants, children and adolescents who have diseases that result from an abnormality in the endocrine glands (glands which secrete hormones). These diseases include diabetes mellitus, growth failure, unusual size for age, early or late pubertal development, birth defects, the genital anomalies and disorders of the thyroid, the adrenal and pituitary glands.

Pediatric Gastroenterology: A pediatrician who specializes in the diagnosis and treatment of diseases of the digestive systems of infants, children and adolescents. This specialist treats conditions such as abdominal pain, ulcers, diarrhea, cancer and jaundice and performs complex diagnostic and therapeutic procedures using lighted scopes to see internal organs.

Pediatric Hematology-Oncology: A pediatrician trained in the combination of pediatrics, hematology and oncology to recognize and manage pediatric blood disorders and cancerous diseases.

Pediatric Infectious Diseases: A pediatrician trained to care for children in the diagnosis, treatment and prevention of infectious diseases. This specialist can apply specific knowledge to effect a better outcome for pediatric infections with complicated courses, underlying diseases that predispose to unusual or severe infections, unclear diagnoses, uncommon diseases and complex or investigational treatments.

Pediatric Nephrology: A pediatrician who deals with the normal and abnormal development and maturation of the kidney and urinary tract, the mechanisms by which the kidney can be damaged, the evaluation and treatment of renal diseases, fluid and electrolyte abnormalities, hypertension and renal replacement therapy.

Pediatric Otolaryngology: A pediatric otolaryngologist has special expertise in the management of infants and children with disorders that include congenital and acquired conditions involving the aerodigestive tract, nose and paranasal sinuses, the ear and other areas of the head and neck. The pediatric otolaryngologist has special skills in the diagnosis, treatment and management of childhood disorders of voice, speech, language and hearing.

Pediatric Pulmonology: A pediatrician dedicated to the prevention and treatment of all respiratory diseases affecting infants, children and young adults. This specialist is knowledgeable about the growth and development of the lung, assessment of respiratory function in infants and children and experienced in a variety of invasive and noninvasive diagnostic techniques.

Pediatric Rheumatology: A pediatrician who treats diseases of joints, muscle, bones and tendons. A pediatric rheumatologist diagnoses and treats arthritis, back pain, muscle strains, common athletic injuries and "collagen" diseases.

Pediatric Surgery: A surgeon with expertise in the management of surgical conditions in premature and newborn infants, children and adolescents.

PEDIATRICS

New England

Miller, Karen J MD [Ped] - **Spec Exp:** Developmental & Behavioral Disorders; **Hospital:** Tufts Med Ctr; **Address:** Tufts New England Med Ctr, 800 Washington St, rm 334, Boston, MA 02111; **Phone:** 617-636-7242; **Board Cert:** Internal Medicine 1982; Neurodevelopmental Disabilities 2001; Developmental-Behavioral Pediatrics 2002; **Med School:** Tulane Univ 1977; **Resid:** Pediatrics, Georgetown Univ Hosp 1980; **Fellow:** Developmental-Behavioral Pediatrics, Schneider's Chldn's Hosp 1996; **Fac Appt:** Assoc Prof Ped, Tufts Univ

Palfrey, Judith S MD [Ped] - **Spec Exp:** Special Health Care Needs (CSHCN); Developmental Disorders; **Hospital:** Children's Hospital - Boston; **Address:** Chldns Hosp, 300 Longwood Ave, Honeywell 201.3, Boston, MA 02115; **Phone:** 617-355-4662; **Board Cert:** Pediatrics 1976; Developmental-Behavioral Pediatrics 2002; **Med School:** Columbia P&S 1971; **Resid:** Pediatrics, Montefiore Med Ctr 1974; **Fac Appt:** Prof Ped, Harvard Med Sch

Rappaport, Leonard MD [Ped] - **Spec Exp:** Developmental & Behavioral Disorders; **Hospital:** Children's Hospital - Boston; **Address:** Chldns Hosp, Fegan 10, 300 Longwood Ave, Boston, MA 02115; **Phone:** 617-355-4683; **Board Cert:** Pediatrics 1983; Developmental-Behavioral Pediatrics 2002; **Med School:** Yale Univ 1977; **Resid:** Pediatrics, Chldns Hosp 1980; **Fellow:** Developmental-Behavioral Pediatrics, Chldns Hosp 1982; **Fac Appt:** Prof Ped, Harvard Med Sch

Shaywitz, Sally E MD [Ped] - **Spec Exp:** Learning Disorders; Dyslexia; **Hospital:** Yale-New Haven Hosp, Yale Med Group; **Address:** Yale Univ Dept Pediatrics, 333 Cedar St, PO Box 208064, New Haven, CT 06520-8064; **Phone:** 203-785-4641; **Board Cert:** Pediatrics 1971; **Med School:** Albert Einstein Coll Med 1966; **Resid:** Pediatrics, Albert Einstein Coll Med 1970; **Fellow:** Pediatrics, Bronx Muni Hosp Ctr 1968; Behavioral Pediatrics, Albert Einstein Coll Med 1970; **Fac Appt:** Prof Ped, Yale Univ

Mid Atlantic

Berlin Jr, Cheston M MD [Ped] - **Spec Exp:** Phenylketonuria (PKU); Tourette's Syndrome; **Hospital:** Penn State Milton S Hershey Med Ctr; **Address:** Penn State Univ Coll Med, Dept Peds, 500 University Drive, PO Box 850, Hershey, PA 17033; **Phone:** 717-531-8006; **Board Cert:** Pediatrics 1982; **Med School:** Harvard Med Sch 1962; **Resid:** Pediatrics, Childrens Hosp 1967; **Fac Appt:** Prof Ped

Burgess, David B MD [Ped] - **Spec Exp:** Developmental & Behavioral Disorders; ADD/ADHD; Autism; **Hospital:** Chldns Hosp of Philadelphia; **Address:** Children's Hosp Philadelphia, Specialty Care Ctr, 4009 Black Horse Pike, Mays Landing, NJ 08330; **Phone:** 609-677-7895; **Board Cert:** Pediatrics 1978; Developmental-Behavioral Pediatrics 2004; **Med School:** Univ Wisc 1973; **Resid:** Pediatrics, Charity Hosp 1977; **Fellow:** Child Development, JFK Child Dev Ctr, Univ Colorado 1980; **Fac Appt:** Assoc Clin Prof Ped, Univ Pennsylvania

Gartner Jr, J Carlton MD [Ped] - **Spec Exp:** Diagnostic Problems; Multisystem Disorders; **Hospital:** Alfred I duPont Hosp for Children; **Address:** Alfred I duPont Hosp for Children, 1600 Rockland Rd, rm 3B367, Wilmington, DE 19803; **Phone:** 302-651-5946; **Board Cert:** Pediatrics 2007; **Med School:** Johns Hopkins Univ 1971; **Resid:** Pediatrics, Childrens Hosp 1974; **Fac Appt:** Prof Ped, Thomas Jefferson Univ

Hofkosh, Dena MD [Ped] - **Spec Exp:** Developmental & Behavioral Disorders; Developmental Disorders; **Hospital:** Chldns Hosp of Pittsburgh - UPMC; **Address:** Childrens Hosp Pittsburgh, Chldn's Oakland Med Bldg, 3420 5th Ave, Pittsburgh, PA 15213; **Phone:** 412-692-5560; **Board Cert:** Pediatrics 2009; Neurodevelopmental Disabilities 2001; **Med School:** NYU Sch Med 1979; **Resid:** Pediatrics, Univ Pittsburgh Med Ctr 1982; **Fellow:** Ambulatory Pediatrics, Univ Pittsburgh Med Ctr 1984; **Fac Appt:** Prof Ped, Univ Pittsburgh

Morton, D Holmes MD [Ped] - **Spec Exp:** Genetic Disorders; Rare Disorders; **Hospital:** Lancaster Genl Hosp; **Address:** Clinic For Special Children, 535 Bunker Hill Rd, PO Box 128, Strasburg, PA 17579; **Phone:** 717-687-9407; **Board Cert:** Pediatrics 1987; **Med School:** Harvard Med Sch 1983; **Resid:** Pediatrics, Childrens Hosp 1986; **Fellow:** Research, Childrens Hosp 1988

Oeffinger, Kevin MD [Ped] - **Spec Exp:** Cancer Survivors-Late Effects of Therapy; **Hospital:** Meml Sloan-Kettering Cancer Ctr; **Address:** 300 E 66th St, New York, NY 10065; **Phone:** 800-525-2225; **Board Cert:** Family Medicine 2006; **Med School:** Univ Tex, San Antonio 1984; **Resid:** Family Medicine, Baylor Coll Med 1985; **Fellow:** Family Medicine, Fam Practice Faculty Dev Ctr 1999; Natl Cancer Inst 2000

Vining, Eileen P MD [Ped] - **Spec Exp:** Pediatric Neurology; Epilepsy; Rasmussen's Syndrome; **Hospital:** Johns Hopkins Hosp (page 61); **Address:** 600 N Wolfe St Meyer Bldg, 601 N Caroline St, Baltimore, MD 21227; **Phone:** 410-502-0964; **Board Cert:** Pediatrics 1977; **Med School:** Johns Hopkins Univ 1972; **Resid:** Pediatrics, Chldns Hosp 1974; **Fellow:** Developmental-Behavioral Pediatrics, JFK Inst/Johns Hopkins Hosp 1976; **Fac Appt:** Assoc Prof Ped, Johns Hopkins Univ

Zitelli, Basil MD [Ped] - **Spec Exp:** Complex Diagnosis; **Hospital:** Chldns Hosp of Pittsburgh - UPMC; **Address:** Childrens Hospital Drive, 45th St & Penn Ave, Faculty Pavilion Fl 3, Pittsburgh, PA 15201; **Phone:** 412-692-5135; **Board Cert:** Pediatrics 1976; **Med School:** Univ Pittsburgh 1971; **Resid:** Pediatrics, Johns Hopkins Hosp 1974; **Fellow:** Pediatrics, Johns Hopkins Hosp 1978; **Fac Appt:** Prof Ped, Univ Pittsburgh

Southeast

Hershorin, Eugene R MD [Ped] - **Spec Exp:** ADD/ADHD; Developmental & Mood Disorders; Learning Disorders; **Hospital:** Jackson Meml Hosp (page 70), Baptist Hosp of Miami; **Address:** 8932 SW 97th Ave, Ste D, Miami, FL 33176; **Phone:** 305-270-5050; **Board Cert:** Pediatrics 1980; Developmental-Behavioral Pediatrics 2004; **Med School:** Penn State Coll Med 1976; **Resid:** Pediatrics, Chldn's Hosp 1979; **Fac Appt:** Assoc Prof Ped, Univ Miami Sch Med

Midwest

Berman, Brian W MD [Ped] - **Spec Exp:** Sickle Cell Disease; Thrombotic Disorders; Thalassemia; Fanconi Aplastic Anemia; **Hospital:** UH Rainbow Babies & Chldns Hosp (page 74); **Address:** Rainbow Babies & Chldn's Hosp, 11100 Euclid Ave, MS RBC6019, Cleveland, OH 44106-6019; **Phone:** 216-884-3752; **Board Cert:** Pediatrics 2009; Pediatric Hematology-Oncology 1989; **Med School:** Temple Univ 1975; **Resid:** Pediatrics, St Chris Hosp for Chldn 1978; **Fellow:** Pediatric Hematology-Oncology, Yale-New Haven Hosp 1980; **Fac Appt:** Prof Ped, Case West Res Univ

Bull, Marilyn J MD [Ped] - **Spec Exp:** Developmental Disorders; Down Syndrome; Birth Defects; **Hospital:** Riley Hosp for Children; **Address:** 705 Riley Hospital Drive, rm 1601, Indianapolis, IN 46202; **Phone:** 317-944-4846; **Board Cert:** Pediatrics 1973; Clinical Genetics 1982; Neurodevelopmental Disabilities 2001; **Med School:** Univ Mich Med Sch 1968; **Resid:** Pediatrics, Childrens Meml Hosp 1972; **Fellow:** Genetics, Boston Floating Hosp 1973; **Fac Appt:** Prof Ped, Indiana Univ

Pediatrics

Fost, Norman C MD [Ped] - **Spec Exp:** Ethics; **Hospital:** Univ WI Hosp & Clins; **Address:** Dept Pediatrics 4108, 600 Highland Ave, Madison, WI 53792-4108; **Phone:** 608-265-6050; **Board Cert:** Pediatrics 1970; **Med School:** Yale Univ 1964; **Resid:** Pediatrics, Johns Hopkins Hosp 1971; **Fellow:** Pediatrics, Harvard Sch Public Hlth 1973; **Fac Appt:** Prof Ped, Univ Wisc

Jacob, Molly MD [Ped] - **Spec Exp:** Asthma; ADD/ADHD; Nutrition; **Hospital:** Children's Mem Hosp -Chicago, Adv Illinois Masonic Med Ctr; **Address:** 2742 W Montrose Ave, Chicago, IL 60610; **Phone:** 773-463-0136; **Board Cert:** Pediatrics 1980; **Med School:** India 1968; **Resid:** Pediatrics, Ill Masonic Med Ctr 1979; **Fellow:** Ambulatory Pediatrics, Ill Masonic Med Ctr 1979; **Fac Appt:** Asst Clin Prof Ped, Univ IL Coll Med

Lantos, John D MD [Ped] - **Spec Exp:** Ethics; Palliative Care; Ethics Issues in Neonatalogy; **Hospital:** Chldns Mercy Hosps & Clinics; **Address:** Childrens Mercy Bioethics Center, 2401 Gilham Rd, Kansas City, MO 64108; **Phone:** 816-701-5284; **Board Cert:** Pediatrics 2009; **Med School:** Univ Pittsburgh 1981; **Resid:** Pediatrics, Chldns Natl Med Ctr 1984; **Fellow:** Clinical Ethics, Univ Chicago Hosps 1987; **Fac Appt:** Prof Ped, Univ MO-Kansas City

Roizen, Nancy Jean M MD [Ped] - **Spec Exp:** ADD/ADHD; Autism; Developmental & Behavioral Disorders; **Hospital:** UH Rainbow Babies & Chldns Hosp (page 74), Univ Hosps Case Med Ctr (page 74); **Address:** UH Rainbow Specialty Center - Westlake, 10524 Euclid Ave, rm 3150, Cleveland, OH 44106; **Phone:** 216-844-3230; **Board Cert:** Pediatrics 1987; Neurodevelopmental Disabilities 2001; Developmental-Behavioral Pediatrics 2010; **Med School:** Tufts Univ 1972; **Resid:** Pediatrics, Johns Hopkins Hosp 1974; **Fellow:** Developmental-Behavioral Pediatrics, Johns Hopkins Hosp 1975; Behavioral Pediatrics, UCSF 1976; **Fac Appt:** Prof Psyc, Case West Res Univ

Southwest

Infante, Anthony J MD/PhD [Ped] - **Spec Exp:** Immune Deficiencies-Primary; Autoimmune Disease; Fevers-Periodic; **Hospital:** Christus Santa Rosa Children's Hosp, Univ Hlth Syst-San Antonio; **Address:** 7703 Floyd Curl Drive, MC 7811, San Antonio, TX 78229-3900; **Phone:** 210-704-2187; **Board Cert:** Pediatrics 2004; **Med School:** Indiana Univ 1978; **Resid:** Pediatrics, Mayo Clinic 1980; **Fellow:** Pediatric Immunology, Mayo Clinic 1981; Immunology, Stanford Univ Hosp 1983; **Fac Appt:** Prof Ped, Univ Tex, San Antonio

Kleinerman, Eugenie S MD [Ped] - **Spec Exp:** Ewing's Sarcoma; Cancer Survivors-Late Effects of Therapy; **Hospital:** UT MD Anderson Cancer Ctr; **Address:** MD Anderson Cancer Ctr, Dept Pediatrics, 1515 Holcombe Blvd, Unit 87, Houston, TX 77030; **Phone:** 713-792-8110; **Board Cert:** Pediatrics 1980; **Med School:** Duke Univ 1975; **Resid:** Pediatrics, Chldns Hosp-Natl Med Ctr 1978; **Fellow:** Immunology, Natl Cancer Inst 1981; **Fac Appt:** Prof Ped, Univ Tex, Houston

West Coast and Pacific

Berkowitz, Carol D MD [Ped] - **Spec Exp:** Child Abuse; **Hospital:** LAC - Harbor - UCLA Med Ctr; **Address:** LAC-Harbor-UCLA Med Ctr, 1000 W Carson St, Box 437, Torrance, CA 90509-2910; **Phone:** 310-222-3091; **Board Cert:** Pediatrics 2000; Pediatric Emergency Medicine 2006; Child Abuse Pediatrics 2009; **Med School:** Columbia P&S 1969; **Resid:** Pediatrics, Roosevelt Hosp 1972; **Fac Appt:** Clin Prof Ped, UCLA

Feldman, Kenneth W MD [Ped] - **Spec Exp:** Child Abuse; **Hospital:** Seattle Chldns Hosp; **Address:** Odessa Brown Chldns Clin, 2101 E Yesler Way, Ste 100, Seattle, WA 98122; **Phone:** 206-987-7225; **Board Cert:** Pediatrics 1975; Child Abuse Pediatrics 2009; **Med School:** Univ Wisc 1970; **Resid:** Pediatrics, Chldns Regl Med Ctr 1974; **Fac Appt:** Clin Prof Ped, Univ Wash

Jones Jr, Kenneth Lyons MD [Ped] - **Spec Exp:** Genetic Disorders; Dysmorphology; **Hospital:** UCSD Med Ctr; **Address:** 9500 Gilman Drive, MC 0828, Dept Pediatrics, La Jolla, CA 92093-0828; **Phone:** 858-246-0047; **Board Cert:** Pediatrics 1971; **Med School:** Hahnemann Univ 1966; **Resid:** Pediatrics, Chldns Ortho Hosp 1969; **Fac Appt:** Prof Ped, UCSD

Walker, William O MD [Ped] - **Spec Exp:** Developmental & Behavioral Disorders; Autism; Cerebral Palsy; Spina Bifida; **Hospital:** Seattle Chldns Hosp; **Address:** Seattle Children's, 4800 Sand Point Way NE, MS A-7938, Seattle, WA 98145-5005; **Phone:** 206-987-2210; **Board Cert:** Pediatrics 1984; Neurodevelopmental Disabilities 2001; Developmental-Behavioral Pediatrics 2010; **Med School:** Tulane Univ 1979; **Resid:** Pediatrics, W Beaumont Army Med Ctr 1982; **Fellow:** Behavioral Pediatrics, W Beaumont Army Med Ctr 1987; **Fac Appt:** Prof Ped, Univ Wash

Zeltzer, Lonnie K MD [Ped] - **Spec Exp:** Pain Management; Complementary Medicine; **Hospital:** Mattel Chldns Hosp at UCLA; **Address:** UCLA Pediatric Pain Program, 10833 Le Conte Ave, #22-464 MDCC, Los Angeles, CA 90095-1752; **Phone:** 310-825-0731; **Board Cert:** Pediatrics 1976; **Med School:** Univ Cincinnati 1970; **Resid:** Pediatrics, Univ Ariz Hosp 1973; **Fellow:** Adolescent Medicine, Chldns Hosp 1976; **Fac Appt:** Prof Ped, UCLA

PEDIATRIC ALLERGY & IMMUNOLOGY

New England

Klein, Robert B MD [PA&I] - **Spec Exp:** Asthma; **Hospital:** Rhode Island Hosp; **Address:** Rhode Island Hosp, Dept of Pediatrics, 593 Eddy St, Providence, RI 02903; **Phone:** 401-444-5648; **Board Cert:** Pediatrics 1976; Allergy & Immunology 1977; **Med School:** Switzerland 1971; **Resid:** Pediatrics, Dartmouth/Hitchcock Med Ctr 1974; **Fellow:** Allergy & Immunology, UCLA 1976; **Fac Appt:** Prof Ped, Brown Univ

Mid Atlantic

Ehrlich, Paul M MD [PA&I] - **Spec Exp:** Asthma; Food Allergy; **Hospital:** New York Eye & Ear Infirm (page 64), NYU Langone Med Ctr (page 66); **Address:** 35 E 35th St, Ste 202, New York, NY 10016-3823; **Phone:** 212-685-4225; **Board Cert:** Pediatrics 1975; Allergy & Immunology 1977; **Med School:** NYU Sch Med 1970; **Resid:** Pediatrics, Bellevue Hosp Ctr 1973; **Fellow:** Allergy & Immunology, Walter Reed Army Med Ctr 1976; **Fac Appt:** Assoc Clin Prof Ped, NYU Sch Med

Josephs, Shelby H MD [PA&I] - **Spec Exp:** Food Allergy; **Hospital:** Georgetown Univ Hosp; **Address:** 6000 Executive Blvd, Ste 615, North Bethesda, MD 20852; **Phone:** 240-747-5750; **Board Cert:** Pediatrics 1979; Allergy & Immunology 1985; **Med School:** Duke Univ 1975; **Resid:** Pediatrics, Chldns Hosp 1977; Allergy & Immunology, Duke Univ Med Ctr 1979; **Fac Appt:** Assoc Clin Prof Ped, Georgetown Univ

Kamani, Naynesh R MD [PA&I] - **Spec Exp:** Stem Cell Transplant; Immunotherapy; Bone Marrow Transplant; **Hospital:** Chldns Natl Med Ctr; **Address:** Chldns Natl Med Ctr, Div Hematology, 111 Michigan Ave NW, Washington, DC 20010; **Phone:** 202-476-2140; **Board Cert:** Pediatrics 1983; Allergy & Immunology 1983; Diagnostic Lab Immunology 1986; **Med School:** Ethiopia 1975; **Resid:** Pediatrics, Downstate Med Ctr-Kings Co Hosp 1981; **Fellow:** Pediatric Allergy & Immunology, Chldns Hosp 1983; **Fac Appt:** Prof Ped, Geo Wash Univ

Pediatric Allergy & Immunology

Schuberth, Kenneth Charles MD [PA&I] - Spec Exp: Allergy; Asthma; **Hospital:** Johns Hopkins Hosp (page 61), Greater Baltimore Med Ctr; **Address:** 10807 Falls Rd, Ste 200, Lutherville, MD 21093; **Phone:** 410-321-9393; **Board Cert:** Pediatrics 1979; Allergy & Immunology 1983; **Med School:** Johns Hopkins Univ 1973; **Resid:** Pediatrics, Johns Hopkins Hosp 1978; **Fellow:** Allergy & Immunology, Johns Hopkins Hosp 1980; **Fac Appt:** Assoc Prof Ped, Johns Hopkins Univ

Sicherer, Scott H MD [PA&I] - Spec Exp: Food Allergy; Drug Sensitivity; Eczema; **Hospital:** Mount Sinai Med Ctr (page 63); **Address:** One Gustave L Levy Pl, Box 1198, New York, NY 10029-6500; **Phone:** 212-241-5548; **Board Cert:** Pediatrics 2008; Allergy & Immunology 2007; **Med School:** Johns Hopkins Univ 1990; **Resid:** Pediatrics, Mt Sinai Hosp 1994; **Fellow:** Allergy & Immunology, Johns Hopkins Hosp 1997; **Fac Appt:** Prof Ped, Mount Sinai Sch Med

Skoner, David Peter MD [PA&I] - Spec Exp: Asthma & Allergy; Rhinitis; **Hospital:** Allegheny General Hosp; **Address:** Allegheny Genl Hosp, Div Asthma, Allergy & Immunology, 320 E North Ave, Fl 7-South Tower, Pittsburgh, PA 15212; **Phone:** 412-359-6640; **Board Cert:** Pediatrics 1985; Allergy & Immunology 1985; **Med School:** Temple Univ 1980; **Resid:** Pediatrics, Chldns Hosp Med Ctr 1983; **Fellow:** Allergy & Immunology, Chldns Hosp 1985; **Fac Appt:** Prof Ped, Drexel Univ Coll Med

Sly, R Michael MD [PA&I] - Spec Exp: Asthma; Allergy; Atopic Dermatitis; **Hospital:** Chldns Natl Med Ctr; **Address:** Children's Natl Med Ctr, Dept Allergy, Pulmonary, Sleep Med, 111 Michigan Ave NW, Ste 1030, Washington, DC 20010-2970; **Phone:** 202-476-2128; **Board Cert:** Pediatric Allergy & Immunology 1967; Pediatrics 1980; Allergy & Immunology 1987; **Med School:** Washington Univ, St Louis 1960; **Resid:** Pediatrics, St Louis Chldns Hosp 1962; Pediatrics, Univ Kentucky Med Ctr 1963; **Fellow:** Pediatric Allergy & Immunology, UCLA Med Ctr 1967; **Fac Appt:** Prof Ped, Geo Wash Univ

Spergel, Jonathan MD/PhD [PA&I] - Spec Exp: Atopic Dermatitis; Food Allergy; Asthma; **Hospital:** Chldns Hosp of Philadelphia; **Address:** 3550 Market St Fl 3, Philadelphia, PA 19104; **Phone:** 215-590-2549; **Board Cert:** Allergy & Immunology 2006; **Med School:** Mount Sinai Sch Med 1992; **Resid:** Pediatrics, Yale New Haven Hosp 1994; **Fellow:** Allergy & Immunology, Chldn's Hosp 1995; **Fac Appt:** Assoc Prof Ped, Univ Pennsylvania

Sullivan, Kathleen MD/PhD [PA&I] - Spec Exp: Immune Deficiency; **Hospital:** Chldns Hosp of Philadelphia; **Address:** Children's Hosp, Div Immunology, 34th St & Civic Ctr Blvd, Philadelphia, PA 19104; **Phone:** 215-590-2549; **Board Cert:** Pediatrics 2001; Pediatric Rheumatology 2002; Clinical & Laboratory Immunology 1997; **Med School:** UCSF 1988; **Resid:** Pediatrics, UCSF 1990; **Fellow:** Pediatric Rheumatology, Jonhs Hopkins Hosp 1993; **Fac Appt:** Prof Ped, Univ Pennsylvania

Wood, Robert A MD [PA&I] - Spec Exp: Food Allergy; Asthma; **Hospital:** Johns Hopkins Hosp (page 61); **Address:** Johns Hopkins Children's Ctr, 600 N Wolfe St, CMSC-1102, Baltimore, MD 21287; **Phone:** 410-955-5883; **Board Cert:** Pediatrics 1987; Allergy & Immunology 2010; **Med School:** Univ Rochester 1982; **Resid:** Pediatrics, Johns Hopkins Hosp 1985; **Fellow:** Allergy & Immunology, Johns Hopkins Hosp 1988; **Fac Appt:** Prof Ped, Johns Hopkins Univ

Southeast

Burks Jr, A Wesley MD [PA&I] - Spec Exp: Asthma; Allergic Rhinitis; Food Allergy; Anaphylaxis; **Hospital:** Duke Univ Hosp; **Address:** Duke Univ Med Ctr, Box 2644, Durham, NC 27710; **Phone:** 919-681-2949; **Board Cert:** Pediatrics 1985; Allergy & Immunology 1985; **Med School:** Univ Ark 1980; **Resid:** Pediatrics, Ark Chldns Hosp 1983; **Fellow:** Allergy & Immunology, Duke Univ Med Ctr 1985; **Fac Appt:** Prof Ped, Duke Univ

Kelly, Cynthia S MD [PA&I] - **Spec Exp:** Asthma; Rhinitis; Sinusitis; **Hospital:** Chldns Hosp of King's Daughters; **Address:** Chlds Hosp of The Kings Daughters, 601 Childrens Lane, Fl 4th, Norfolk, VA 23507; **Phone:** 757-668-8255; **Board Cert:** Pediatrics 2004; Allergy & Immunology 2007; **Med School:** Wayne State Univ 1985; **Resid:** Pediatrics, Univ Mich 1987; **Fellow:** Allergy & Immunology, UCLA Med Ctr 1988; Pediatric Infectious Disease, Vanderbilt Univ 1989; **Fac Appt:** Assoc Prof Ped, Eastern VA Med Sch

Ownby, Dennis R MD [PA&I] - **Spec Exp:** Food Allergy; Anaphylaxis; Latex Allergy; Asthma; **Hospital:** Med Coll of GA Hosp and Clin (MCG Health Inc); **Address:** Allergy & Immunology, 1120 15th St Bldg BG - rm 1019, Augusta, GA 30912-0004; **Phone:** 706-721-2390; **Board Cert:** Pediatrics 1977; Allergy & Immunology 2006; Clinical & Laboratory Immunology 1986; **Med School:** Med Coll OH 1972; **Resid:** Pediatrics, Duke Univ Med Ctr 1974; **Fellow:** Pediatric Allergy & Immunology, Duke Univ Med Ctr 1977; **Fac Appt:** Prof Ped, Med Coll GA

Sleasman, John W MD [PA&I] - **Spec Exp:** Infectious Disease; Immunodeficiency Disorders; Hypogammaglobulinemia; **Hospital:** All Children's Hosp; **Address:** All Childrens Hosp, Div Ped Immun/Rheumatology, 601 5th St S, St Petersburg, FL 33701; **Phone:** 727-767-4150; **Board Cert:** Pediatrics 1988; Diagnostic Lab Immunology 1990; **Med School:** Univ Tenn Coll Med 1981; **Resid:** Pediatrics, Shands Hosp 1984; **Fellow:** Pediatric Infectious Disease, Shands Hosp 1987; Immunology, Dana Farber Cancer Inst 1988

Midwest

Lemanske Jr, Robert F MD [PA&I] - **Spec Exp:** Asthma; Allergy; Immune Deficiency; **Hospital:** Univ WI Hosp & Clins; **Address:** 600 Highland Ave, K4/916 CSC, Madison, WI 53792; **Phone:** 608-265-2206; **Board Cert:** Pediatrics 1980; Allergy & Immunology 1981; **Med School:** Univ Wisc 1975; **Resid:** Pediatrics, Univ Wisc Hosp 1978; **Fellow:** Allergy & Immunology, Univ Wisc Hosp 1980; Allergy & Immunology, Natl Inst Hlth 1983; **Fac Appt:** Prof Ped, Univ Wisc

Pongracic, Jacqueline MD [PA&I] - **Spec Exp:** Latex Allergy; Asthma; Food Allergy; **Hospital:** Children's Mem Hosp -Chicago; **Address:** 2300 Children's Plaza, Box 60, Chicago, IL 60614; **Phone:** 773-327-3710; **Board Cert:** Internal Medicine 1988; Allergy & Immunology 2001; **Med School:** Northwestern Univ 1985; **Resid:** Internal Medicine, North Shore Univ Hosp 1988; **Fellow:** Allergy & Immunology, Johns Hopkins Hosp 1991; **Fac Appt:** Asst Prof Ped, Northwestern Univ

Strunk, Robert C MD [PA&I] - **Spec Exp:** Asthma; **Hospital:** St. Louis Chldns Hosp; **Address:** 660 S Euclid Ave, Box 8116, St Louis, MO 63110; **Phone:** 314-454-2694; **Board Cert:** Pediatrics 1974; Allergy & Immunology 1987; **Med School:** Northwestern Univ 1968; **Resid:** Pediatrics, Cincinnati Chldns Hosp 1970; **Fellow:** Pediatric Allergy & Immunology, Boston Chldns Hosp 1974; **Fac Appt:** Prof Ped, Washington Univ, St Louis

Wolf, Raoul MD [PA&I] - **Spec Exp:** Asthma; Allergy; Immune Deficiency; **Hospital:** Univ of Chicago Med Ctr, La Rabida Chlds Hosp; **Address:** Dept of Allergy & Immunology, E 65th St at Lake Michigan, Chicago, IL 60649; **Phone:** 773-702-6169; **Board Cert:** Pediatrics 1980; Allergy & Immunology 1983; **Med School:** South Africa 1969; **Resid:** Pediatrics, Baragwanath Hosp 1973; Pediatrics, Transvaal Meml Hosp Chldn 1976; **Fellow:** Allergy & Immunology, Chldns Hosp Med Ctr 1979; **Fac Appt:** Prof Ped, Univ Chicago-Pritzker Sch Med

Pediatric Allergy & Immunology

Great Plains and Mountains

Bock, Samuel A MD [PA&I] - **Spec Exp:** Asthma up to age 50; Allergy up to age 50; Food Allergy; **Hospital:** Boulder Community Hospital, Natl Jewish Med & Rsch Ctr; **Address:** Boulder Asthma & Allergy Clinics, 3950 Broadway, Boulder, CO 80304; **Phone:** 303-444-5991; **Board Cert:** Pediatrics 1977; Allergy & Immunology 1977; **Med School:** Univ MD Sch Med 1972; **Resid:** Pediatrics, Colo Med Ctr/Natl Jewish Med Ctr 1974; **Fellow:** Allergy & Immunology, Colo Med Ctr/Natl Jewish Med Ctr 1976; **Fac Appt:** Clin Prof Ped, Univ Colorado

Gelfand, Erwin W MD [PA&I] - **Spec Exp:** Immune Deficiency; Asthma; Allergy; **Hospital:** Natl Jewish Med & Rsch Ctr, Chldn's Hosp - Aurora (CO); **Address:** National Jewish Health, 1400 Jackson St, Denver, CO 80206; **Phone:** 303-398-1196; **Board Cert:** Pediatrics 1972; **Med School:** McGill Univ 1966; **Resid:** Pediatrics, Montreal Childrens Hosp 1968; Pediatrics, Childrens Hosp Med Ctr 1969; **Fellow:** Immunology, Childrens Hosp Med Ctr 1971; **Fac Appt:** Prof Ped, Univ Colorado

Leung, Donald YM MD/PhD [PA&I] - **Spec Exp:** Atopic Dermatitis; Asthma; Food Allergy; **Hospital:** Natl Jewish Med & Rsch Ctr, Chldn's Hosp - Aurora (CO); **Address:** National Jewish Health, 1400 Jackson St, Goodman Bldg, K926i, Denver, CO 80206; **Phone:** 303-398-1379; **Board Cert:** Pediatrics 1982; Allergy & Immunology 1983; Clinical & Laboratory Immunology 1990; **Med School:** Univ Chicago-Pritzker Sch Med 1977; **Resid:** Pediatrics, Chldn's Hosp 1979; **Fellow:** Allergy & Immunology, Chldn's Hosp 1981; **Fac Appt:** Prof Ped, Univ Colorado

Southwest

Bahna, Sami L MD [PA&I] - **Spec Exp:** Food Allergy; Asthma; Eczema; **Hospital:** Louisiana State Univ Hosp; **Address:** LSU Hlth Scis Ctr, Dept Pediatrics, 1501 Kings Hwy, rm 5-323, Shreveport, LA 71103; **Phone:** 318-675-7625; **Board Cert:** Pediatrics 1980; Allergy & Immunology 1981; **Med School:** Egypt 1964; **Resid:** Pediatrics, Univ Maryland Hosp 1975; **Fellow:** Allergy & Immunology, Harbor-UCLA Med Ctr 1978; **Fac Appt:** Prof Ped, Louisiana State U, New Orleans

Shearer, William T MD/PhD [PA&I] - **Spec Exp:** AIDS/HIV; Immune Deficiency; **Hospital:** Texas Chldns Hosp; **Address:** Dept Allergy & Immunology, 1102 Bates St, Ste 330, Houston, TX 77030-2399; **Phone:** 832-824-1319; **Board Cert:** Pediatrics 1986; Allergy & Immunology 1989; Clinical & Laboratory Immunology 1986; **Med School:** Washington Univ, St Louis 1970; **Resid:** Pediatrics, Chldns Hosp-Wash Univ 1972; **Fellow:** Allergy & Immunology, Barnes Hosp-Wash Univ 1974; **Fac Appt:** Prof Ped, Baylor Coll Med

Wasserman, Richard L MD/PhD [PA&I] - **Hospital:** Med City Dallas Hosp, Chldns Med Ctr of Dallas; **Address:** DallasAllergyImmunology, 7777 Forest Ln, B-332, Dallas, TX 75230; **Phone:** 972-566-7788; **Board Cert:** Pediatrics 1982; Allergy & Immunology 1987; **Med School:** Univ Tex SW, Dallas 1977; **Resid:** Pediatrics, Chldns Hosp of Philadelphia 1979; **Fellow:** Immunology, Chldns Hosp of Philadelphia 1980; Rheumatology, Rockefeller Univ 1982; **Fac Appt:** Clin Prof A&I, Univ Tex SW, Dallas

West Coast and Pacific

Church, Joseph A MD [PA&I] - **Spec Exp:** AIDS/HIV; Immune Deficiency; **Hospital:** Chldns Hosp - Los Angeles; **Address:** Childrens Hosp LA, MS75, Clinical Immunology & Allergy, 4650 W Sunset Blvd, MC 75, Los Angeles, CA 90027; **Phone:** 323-361-2501; **Board Cert:** Pediatrics 1977; Allergy & Immunology 1977; **Med School:** UMDNJ-NJ Med Sch, Newark 1972; **Resid:** Pediatrics, Chldns Hosp/Natl Med Ctr 1974; **Fellow:** Allergy & Immunology, Georgetown Med Ctr 1976; **Fac Appt:** Prof Ped, USC Sch Med

Cowan, Morton J MD [PA&I] - **Spec Exp:** Immunodeficiency Disorders; Stem Cell Transplant-Fetal; Bone Marrow Transplant; **Hospital:** UCSF Med Ctr; **Address:** UCSF Med Ctr, Peds BMT Program, 505 Parnassus Ave, rm M659, San Francisco, CA 94143-1278; **Phone:** 415-476-2188; **Board Cert:** Pediatrics 1981; Allergy & Immunology 1983; **Med School:** Univ Pennsylvania 1970; **Resid:** Surgery, Duke Univ Med Ctr 1972; Pediatrics, UCSF Med Ctr 1977; **Fellow:** Research, Natl Inst Hlth 1975; Immunology, UCSF Med Ctr 1979; **Fac Appt:** Prof Ped, UCSF

Epstein, Stuart MD [PA&I] - **Spec Exp:** Asthma & Allergy; Food Allergy; **Hospital:** Cedars-Sinai Med Ctr, UCLA Ronald Reagan Med Ctr; **Address:** 9735 Wilshire Blvd, Ste 121, Beverly Hills, CA 90212-2101; **Phone:** 310-274-6853; **Board Cert:** Allergy & Immunology 1999; **Med School:** Univ IL Coll Med 1978; **Resid:** Pediatrics, Cedars Sinai Med Ctr 1980; **Fellow:** Pediatrics, UC Irvine 1981; Pediatrics, USC Med Ctr 1982; **Fac Appt:** Assoc Clin Prof Ped, UCLA

Fanous, Yvonne F MD [PA&I] - **Spec Exp:** Asthma & Allergy; Cystic Fibrosis; Immune Deficiency; **Hospital:** Loma Linda Univ Med Ctr; **Address:** Loma Linda Hlth Care Pediatrics, 250 E Caroline St, Ste J, San Bernardino, CA 92408; **Phone:** 909-651-1900; **Board Cert:** Pediatrics 1983; Allergy & Immunology 1985; **Med School:** Egypt 1973; **Resid:** Pediatrics, Texas Tech Univ Hosp 1980; Pediatrics, Loma Linda Univ 1981; **Fellow:** Allergy & Immunology, UC Irvine 1984; **Fac Appt:** Assoc Prof A&I, Loma Linda Univ

PEDIATRIC CARDIOLOGY

New England

Hellenbrand, William E MD [PCd] - **Spec Exp:** Interventional Cardiology; **Hospital:** Yale-New Haven Hosp; **Address:** Yale Univ School of Med, Dept of Pediatrics, 333 Cedar St, New Haven, CT 06520-8064; **Phone:** 203-785-2110; **Board Cert:** Pediatrics 1975; Pediatric Cardiology 1977; **Med School:** SUNY Downstate 1970; **Resid:** Pediatrics, Yale-New Haven Hosp 1972; **Fellow:** Pediatric Cardiology, Yale-New Haven Hosp 1976; **Fac Appt:** Prof Ped, Columbia P&S

Lang, Peter MD [PCd] - **Spec Exp:** Interventional Cardiology; Cardiac Catheterization; **Hospital:** Children's Hospital - Boston; **Address:** Chldns Hosp, Dept Cardiology, 300 Longwood Ave, Boston, MA 02114; **Phone:** 617-355-8539; **Board Cert:** Pediatrics 1977; Pediatric Cardiology 1979; **Med School:** Mount Sinai Sch Med 1972; **Resid:** Pediatrics, Babies Hosp-Presby Med Ctr 1975; **Fellow:** Pediatric Cardiology, Chldns Hosp Med Ctr 1978; **Fac Appt:** Assoc Prof Ped, Harvard Med Sch

Lock, James E MD [PCd] - **Spec Exp:** Interventional Cardiology; Angioplasty-Pulmonary Artery; Cardiac Catheterization; Fetal Surgery; **Hospital:** Children's Hospital - Boston; **Address:** Chldns Hosp, Dept Cardiology, 300 Longwood Ave, Boston, MA 02115-5724; **Phone:** 617-355-7313; **Board Cert:** Pediatrics 1978; Pediatric Cardiology 1981; **Med School:** Stanford Univ 1973; **Resid:** Pediatrics, Univ Minn Hosp 1975; Pediatric Cardiology, Univ Minn Hosp 1977; **Fellow:** Cardiovascular Disease, Hosp Sick Chldn 1979; **Fac Appt:** Prof Ped, Harvard Med Sch

Newburger, Jane MD [PCd] - **Spec Exp:** Kawasaki Disease; Cholesterol/Lipid Disorders; Congenital Heart Disease; **Hospital:** Children's Hospital - Boston, Brigham and Women's Hosp (page 57); **Address:** Chldns Hosp, Dept Ped Cardiology, 300 Longwood Ave, Farley Bldg Fl 2, Boston, MA 02115; **Phone:** 617-355-5427; **Board Cert:** Pediatrics 1979; Pediatric Cardiology 1983; **Med School:** Harvard Med Sch 1974; **Resid:** Pediatrics, Chldns Hosp Med Ctr 1976; **Fellow:** Pediatric Cardiology, Chldns Hosp Med Ctr 1979; **Fac Appt:** Prof Ped, Harvard Med Sch

Pediatric Cardiology

Walsh, Edward P MD [PCd] - **Spec Exp:** Arrhythmias; **Hospital:** Children's Hospital - Boston; **Address:** Chldns Hosp, Dept Cardiology, 300 Longwood Ave Bader Bldg Fl 2, Boston, MA 02115; **Phone:** 617-355-6328; **Board Cert:** Pediatrics 1985; Pediatric Cardiology 1985; **Med School:** Univ Pennsylvania 1979; **Resid:** Pediatrics, Chldns Hosp 1982; **Fellow:** Pediatric Cardiology, Chldns Hosp 1985; **Fac Appt:** Assoc Prof Ped, Harvard Med Sch

Mid Atlantic

Beerman, Lee B MD [PCd] - **Spec Exp:** Congenital Heart Disease-Adult & Child; Arrhythmias; **Hospital:** Chldns Hosp of Pittsburgh - UPMC; **Address:** Chldns Hosp-Heart Ctr, 4401 Penn Ave Fl 5, Faculty Pavilion, Pittsburgh, PA 15224; **Phone:** 412-692-5540; **Board Cert:** Pediatrics 1979; Pediatric Cardiology 1979; **Med School:** Univ Pittsburgh 1974; **Resid:** Pediatrics, Chldns Hosp 1977; **Fellow:** Pediatric Cardiology, Chldns Hosp 1979; **Fac Appt:** Prof Ped, Univ Pittsburgh

Biancaniello, Thomas MD [PCd] - **Spec Exp:** Congenital Heart Disease; Fetal Echocardiography; Interventional Cardiology; Cardiac Catheterization; **Hospital:** Stony Brook Univ Med Ctr, Steven & Alexandra Cohen Chldn's Med Ctr of NY; **Address:** Stony Brook Univ Hosp, Dept Pediatrics, HSC T11, 040, Stony Brook, NY 11794-8111; **Phone:** 631-444-5437; **Board Cert:** Pediatrics 1979; Pediatric Cardiology 1981; **Med School:** NY Med Coll 1975; **Resid:** Pediatrics, North Shore Univ Hosp 1977; **Fellow:** Pediatric Cardiology, Cincinnati Chldns Hosp 1980; **Fac Appt:** Prof Ped, SUNY Stony Brook

Bierman, Fredrick MD [PCd] - **Spec Exp:** Fetal Echocardiography; Kawasaki Disease; Congenital Heart Disease; Echocardiography; **Hospital:** Westchester Med Ctr; **Address:** Westchester Med Ctr, Taylor Care Center, Taylor Pavilion, rm 219, 100 Woods Rd, Valhalla, NY 10595; **Phone:** 914-493-6753; **Board Cert:** Pediatrics 1978; Pediatric Cardiology 1981; **Med School:** SUNY Downstate 1973; **Resid:** Pediatrics, Mount Sinai Med Ctr 1976; **Fellow:** Pediatric Cardiology, Harvard Chldns Hosp 1979; **Fac Appt:** Prof Ped, Albert Einstein Coll Med

Brenner, Joel I MD [PCd] - **Spec Exp:** Congenital Heart Disease; **Hospital:** Johns Hopkins Hosp (page 61); **Address:** Johns Hopkins Hosp, Pediatric Cardiology, 600 N Wolfe St, Brady 522, Baltimore, MD 21287; **Phone:** 410-955-5987; **Board Cert:** Pediatrics 1975; Pediatric Cardiology 1977; **Med School:** NY Med Coll 1970; **Resid:** Pediatrics, NY Hosp 1972; **Fellow:** Pediatric Cardiology, Yale-New Haven Hosp 1974; **Fac Appt:** Assoc Prof Ped, Johns Hopkins Univ

Cooper, Rubin MD [PCd] - **Spec Exp:** Congenital Heart Disease; Rheumatic Heart Disease; Kawasaki Disease; **Hospital:** Steven & Alexandra Cohen Chldn's Med Ctr of NY; **Address:** Steven & Alexandra Cohen Chldns Med Ctr, 269-01 76th Ave, Ste 139, New Hyde Park, NY 11040; **Phone:** 718-470-3661; **Board Cert:** Pediatrics 1976; Pediatric Cardiology 1979; **Med School:** NY Med Coll 1971; **Resid:** Pediatrics, Strong Meml Hosp 1973; **Fellow:** Pediatric Cardiology, Strong Meml Hosp 1975; **Fac Appt:** Prof Ped, Cornell Univ-Weill Med Coll

Crosson, Jane MD [PCd] - **Spec Exp:** Congenital Heart Disease-Adult & Child; Pacemakers; Syncope; Fetal Echocardiography; **Hospital:** Johns Hopkins Hosp (page 61); **Address:** 600 N Wolfe St, Brady 502, Baltimore, MD 21287; **Phone:** 410-614-0706; **Board Cert:** Pediatrics 1987; Pediatric Cardiology 2010; **Med School:** Med Coll GA 1982; **Resid:** Pediatrics, Univ MD Hosp 1986; **Fellow:** Pediatric Cardiology, Univ Minn Hosp 1990

Gelb, Bruce D MD [PCd] - **Spec Exp:** Transplant Medicine-Heart; Marfan's Syndrome; Noonan Syndrome; **Hospital:** Mount Sinai Med Ctr (page 63); **Address:** One Gustave L Levy Pl, Box 1201, New York, NY 10029; **Phone:** 212-241-8592; **Board Cert:** Pediatric Cardiology 2006; **Med School:** Univ Rochester 1984; **Resid:** Pediatrics, NY Presby Hosp 1987; **Fellow:** Pediatric Cardiology, Baylor College Med 1991; **Fac Appt:** Prof Ped, Mount Sinai Sch Med

Gewitz, Michael MD [PCd] - **Spec Exp:** Neonatal Cardiology; Kawasaki Disease; Echocardiography; Heart Failure; **Hospital:** Westchester Med Ctr, Children's & Women's Phys.of Westchester; **Address:** Maria Fareri Children's Hospital, Rte 100, Munger Pavillion, Ste 618, Valhalla, NY 10595; **Phone:** 914-594-4370; **Board Cert:** Pediatrics 1979; Pediatric Cardiology 1981; **Med School:** Hahnemann Univ 1974; **Resid:** Pediatrics, Chldns Hosp 1976; Pediatrics, Hosp Sick Chldn 1977; **Fellow:** Pediatric Cardiology, Yale-New Haven Hosp 1979; **Fac Appt:** Prof Ped, NY Med Coll

Hsu, Daphne MD [PCd] - **Spec Exp:** Interventional Cardiology; Heart Failure; Transplant Medicine-Heart; **Hospital:** Montefiore Med Ctr - Div. Moses; **Address:** Chldn's Hosp at Montefiore, 3415 Bainbridge Ave, Bronx, NY 10467; **Phone:** 718-741-2315; **Board Cert:** Pediatrics 1988; Pediatric Cardiology 2003; **Med School:** Yale Univ 1982; **Resid:** Pediatrics, Columbia Babies & Chldn's Hosp 1985; **Fellow:** Pediatric Cardiology, Columbia Babies & Chldn's Hosp 1988; **Fac Appt:** Prof Ped, Albert Einstein Coll Med

Murphy, John D MD [PCd] - **Spec Exp:** Cardiac Catheterization; Interventional Cardiology; **Hospital:** St. Christopher's Hosp for Chldn; **Address:** St Christophers Hosp for Children, The Heart Center, 3601 A St, Philadelphia, PA 19134; **Phone:** 215-427-4820; **Board Cert:** Pediatrics 1980; Pediatric Cardiology 1981; **Med School:** Univ VT Coll Med 1975; **Resid:** Pediatrics, Chldns Hosp 1977; **Fellow:** Pediatric Cardiology, Chldns Hosp Med Ctr 1980

Parness, Ira A MD [PCd] - **Spec Exp:** Echocardiography; Congenital Heart Disease; Fetal Echocardiography; **Hospital:** Mount Sinai Med Ctr (page 63), Englewood Hosp & Med Ctr; **Address:** One Gustave L Levy Pl, Box 1201, New York, NY 10029-6500; **Phone:** 212-241-6640; **Board Cert:** Pediatrics 1984; Pediatric Cardiology 1985; **Med School:** SUNY Downstate 1979; **Resid:** Pediatrics, Brookdale Hosp 1982; **Fellow:** Pediatric Cardiology, Chldns Hosp 1985; **Fac Appt:** Prof Ped, Mount Sinai Sch Med

Radtke, Wolfgang MD [PCd] - **Spec Exp:** Interventional Cardiology; Cardiac Catheterization; Congenital Heart Disease-Adult & Child; **Hospital:** Alfred I duPont Hosp for Children; **Address:** Nemours Cardiac Ctr, 1600 Rockland Rd, Wilmington, DE 19803; **Phone:** 302-651-6600; **Board Cert:** Pediatrics 2002; Pediatric Cardiology 2004; **Med School:** Germany 1980; **Resid:** Pediatrics, Kiel Univ Chldns Hosp 1985; **Fellow:** Pediatric Cardiology, Chldns Hosp 1988; **Fac Appt:** Prof Ped, Jefferson Med Coll

Sherman, Frederick S MD [PCd] - **Hospital:** Chldns Hosp of Pittsburgh - UPMC, Magee-Womens Hosp - UPMC; **Address:** Children's Hosp Heart Ctr, 4401 Penn Ave Fl 5, Pittsburgh, PA 15224; **Phone:** 412-692-5540; **Board Cert:** Pediatrics 1980; Pediatric Cardiology 1985; **Med School:** Yale Univ 1975; **Resid:** Internal Medicine, Univ Virginia Hosp 1978; **Fellow:** Pediatric Cardiology, Boston Children's Hosp 1984; **Fac Appt:** Prof Ped, Univ Pittsburgh

Sommer, Robert J MD [PCd] - **Spec Exp:** Congenital Heart Disease; Atrial Septal Defect; Cardiac Catheterization; **Hospital:** Morgan Stanley Children's Hosp of NY-Presby, NY (page 65), St. Joseph's Regl Med Ctr - Paterson; **Address:** 173 Fort Washington Ave Fl 4, New York, NY 10032; **Phone:** 212-342-0886; **Board Cert:** Pediatric Cardiology 2006; **Med School:** NYU Sch Med 1985; **Resid:** Pediatrics, Mt Sinai Med Ctr 1988; **Fellow:** Pediatric Cardiology, Mt Sinai Med Ctr 1991; Interventional Cardiology, Childrens Hosp 1991; **Fac Appt:** Assoc Prof Ped, Columbia P&S

Steinherz, Laurel MD [PCd] - **Spec Exp:** Cardiac Effects of Cancer/Cancer Therapy; **Hospital:** Meml Sloan-Kettering Cancer Ctr, NY-Presby/Weill Cornell Med Ctr, NY (page 65); **Address:** 1275 York Avenue, New York, NY 10065; **Phone:** 212-639-8103; **Board Cert:** Pediatrics 1976; Pediatric Cardiology 1978; **Med School:** Albert Einstein Coll Med 1970; **Resid:** Pediatrics, Chldns Hosp 1972; **Fellow:** Pediatric Cardiology, NY Hosp-Cornell Med Ctr 1975; **Fac Appt:** Prof Ped, Cornell Univ-Weill Med Coll

Pediatric Cardiology

Velvis, Harm MD [PCd] - **Spec Exp:** Cardiac Catheterization; Congenital Heart Disease; Heart Disease in Down Syndrome; Interventional Cardiology; **Hospital:** Albany Med Ctr, St. Peter's Hosp - Albany; **Address:** Capital Dist Ped Cardio Assoc, 319 S Manning Blvd, Ste 203, Albany, NY 12208-1743; **Phone:** 518-489-3292; **Board Cert:** Pediatric Cardiology 2009; **Med School:** Netherlands 1980; **Resid:** Pediatrics, Albany Med Ctr 1987; **Fellow:** Pediatric Cardiology, UCSF Med Ctr 1990; **Fac Appt:** Assoc Clin Prof Ped, Albany Med Coll

Walsh, Christine A MD [PCd] - **Spec Exp:** Arrhythmias; Congenital Heart Disease; Sudden Infant Death Syndrome (SIDS); **Hospital:** Montefiore Med Ctr - Div. Moses, Montefiore Med Ctr - Div. Weiler; **Address:** 3415 Bainbridge Ave, Bronx, NY 10467-2401; **Phone:** 718-741-2343; **Board Cert:** Pediatrics 1978; Pediatric Cardiology 1983; Pediatric Critical Care Medicine 2003; **Med School:** Yale Univ 1973; **Resid:** Pediatrics, Columbia-Presby Med Ctr 1976; **Fellow:** Pediatric Cardiology, Columbia-Presby Med Ctr 1978; Cardiac Electrophysiology, Columbia P&S 1980; **Fac Appt:** Prof Ped, Albert Einstein Coll Med

Weinberg, Paul M MD [PCd] - **Spec Exp:** Cardiac MRI; **Hospital:** Chldns Hosp of Philadelphia; **Address:** Chldns Hosp, Div Cardiology, 34th St & Civic Ctr Blvd, Ste 8NW90, Philadelphia, PA 19104; **Phone:** 215-590-3274; **Board Cert:** Pediatrics 1974; Pediatric Cardiology 1975; **Med School:** Jefferson Med Coll 1969; **Resid:** Pediatrics, Chldns Hosp 1971; Cardiology & Pathology, Chldns Hosp Med Ctr 1977; **Fellow:** Pediatric Cardiology, Chldns Hosp 1973; **Fac Appt:** Prof Ped, Univ Pennsylvania

Southeast

Colvin, Edward V MD [PCd] - **Spec Exp:** Congenital Heart Disease-Adult & Child; Fetal Echocardiography; Transplant Medicine-Heart; **Hospital:** Children's Hospital - Birmingham, Univ of Ala Hosp at Birmingham; **Address:** UAB Pediatric Cardiology, 176F Ste 9100, 619 19th St S, Birmingham, AL 35249; **Phone:** 205-934-3460; **Board Cert:** Pediatrics 1982; Pediatric Cardiology 1985; **Med School:** Univ Alabama 1977; **Resid:** Pediatrics, Chldns Hosp 1980; **Fellow:** Pediatric Cardiology, Baylor Coll Med 1983; **Fac Appt:** Prof Ped, Univ Alabama

Epstein, Michael L MD [PCd] - **Spec Exp:** Congenital Heart Disease; **Hospital:** All Children's Hosp; **Address:** All Children's Hosp, 601 5th St S, St Petersburg, FL 33701; **Phone:** 727-767-3333; **Board Cert:** Pediatrics 1976; Pediatric Cardiology 1981; **Med School:** Univ Tex Med Br, Galveston 1971; **Resid:** Pediatrics, Univ Ariz Hlth Sci Ctr 1974; **Fellow:** Pediatric Cardiology, Univ Minn Hosp 1979; **Fac Appt:** Prof Ped, Univ S Fla Coll Med

Fish, Frank A MD [PCd] - **Spec Exp:** Arrhythmias-Pediatric & Adult; Congenital Heart Disease-Adult; Pacemakers; Cardiac Electrophysiology; **Hospital:** Vanderbilt Monroe Carrell Jr. Chldn's Hosp (page 76), Vanderbilt Univ Med Ctr (page 76); **Address:** Vanderbilt Chldns Hosp, Div Pediatric Cardiology, 2200 Children's Way, 5230 DOT, Nashville, TN 37232-9119; **Phone:** 615-322-7447; **Board Cert:** Pediatrics 1987; Pediatric Cardiology 2006; **Med School:** Indiana Univ 1983; **Resid:** Pediatrics, Indiana Univ Hosp 1986; **Fellow:** Pediatric Cardiology, Vanderbilt Univ Med Ctr 1989; Cardiac Electrophysiology, Chldns Meml Hosp 1990; **Fac Appt:** Assoc Prof Ped, Vanderbilt Univ

Fricker, Frederick Jay MD [PCd] - **Spec Exp:** Transplant Medicine-Heart; **Hospital:** Shands at Univ of FL; **Address:** Shands Hlthcre, Div Pediatric Cardiology, 1600 SW Archer Rd, Box 100296, Gainesville, FL 32610-0296; **Phone:** 352-273-7770; **Board Cert:** Pediatrics 1975; Pediatric Cardiology 1981; **Med School:** Loyola Univ-Stritch Sch Med 1970; **Resid:** Pediatrics, Chldns Hosp 1973; **Fellow:** Pediatric Cardiology, Chldns Hosp 1977; **Fac Appt:** Prof Ped, Univ Fla Coll Med

Gullquist, Scott D MD [PCd] - **Hospital:** VCU Med Ctr; **Address:** VCU Medical Ctr, Pediatric Cardiology, Box 980301, Richmond, VA 23298; **Phone:** 804-828-5745; **Board Cert:** Pediatric Cardiology 2009; **Med School:** Georgetown Univ 1987; **Resid:** Pediatrics, Chldns Hosp 1990; Pediatric Cardiology, Chldns Hosp 1993; **Fac Appt:** Assoc Prof Ped, Med Coll VA

Latson, Larry A MD [PCd] - **Spec Exp:** Congenital Heart Disease; Interventional Cardiology; **Hospital:** Joe DiMaggio Chldns Hosp; **Address:** 1150 N 35th Ave, Ste 575, Hollywood, FL 33021; **Phone:** 954-985-6939; **Board Cert:** Pediatrics 1981; Pediatric Cardiology 1983; Pediatric Critical Care Medicine 2010; **Med School:** Baylor Coll Med 1976; **Resid:** Pediatrics, Baylor Affil Hosp 1978; **Fellow:** Pediatric Cardiology, Baylor Coll Med 1981; **Fac Appt:** Prof Ped, Cleveland Cl Coll Med/Case West Res

Moskowitz, William B MD [PCd] - **Spec Exp:** Patent Foramen Ovale; Cardiac Catheterization; Coarctation of the Aorta; Congenital Heart Disease-Adult & Child; **Hospital:** Med Coll of VA Hosp; **Address:** Childrens Heart Ctr, Med Coll Virginia, 1200 E Broad St, PO Box 980543, Richmond, VA 23298; **Phone:** 804-828-9143; **Board Cert:** Pediatrics 1983; Pediatric Cardiology 1985; **Med School:** Univ S Fla Coll Med 1978; **Resid:** Pediatrics, Chldns Hosp 1981; **Fellow:** Pediatric Cardiology, Chldns Hosp 1984; **Fac Appt:** Prof Ped, Med Coll VA

Young, Ming-Lon MD [PCd] - **Spec Exp:** Arrhythmias; Syncope; **Hospital:** Joe DiMaggio Chldns Hosp, Jackson Meml Hosp (page 70); **Address:** Joe DiMaggio Childrens Hosp, 1150 N 35th Ave, Ste 575, Hollywood, FL 33021; **Phone:** 954-265-3437; **Board Cert:** Pediatrics 1985; Pediatric Cardiology 2009; **Med School:** Taiwan 1976; **Resid:** Preventive Medicine, Johns Hopkins Hosp 1979; Pediatrics, St Agnes Hosp 1981; **Fellow:** Pediatric Cardiology, Univ Miami Hosps 1985; **Fac Appt:** Prof Ped, Univ Miami Sch Med

Zahn, Evan M MD [PCd] - **Spec Exp:** Interventional Cardiology; Ventricular Septal Defect (Amplatzer R); Congenital Heart Disease; **Hospital:** Miami Children's Hosp, Baptist Hosp of Miami; **Address:** Miami Childrens Hosp, 3100 SW 62nd Ave, ACB Bldg Fl 2, Miami, FL 33155-5009; **Phone:** 305-662-8301 x5; **Board Cert:** Pediatric Cardiology 2007; **Med School:** NY Med Coll 1986; **Resid:** Pediatrics, Univ Colorado Hosp 1989; **Fellow:** Interventional Cardiology, Hosp for Sick Children 1992

Midwest

Ackerman, Michael J MD/PhD [PCd] - **Spec Exp:** Long QT Interval Syndrome; Sudden Infant Death Syndrome (SIDS); Hypertrophic Cardiomyopathy; Sudden Unexplained Death Syndrome (SUDS); **Hospital:** Mayo Med Ctr & Clin - Rochester; **Address:** Mayo Clin, Dept Ped Cardiology, 200 First St SW, Rochester, MN 55905; **Phone:** 507-284-0101; **Board Cert:** Pediatric Cardiology 2002; **Med School:** Mayo Med Sch 1995; **Resid:** Pediatric & Adolescent Medicine, Mayo Clin 1998; **Fellow:** Pediatric Cardiology, Mayo Clin 2000; **Fac Appt:** Prof Ped, Mayo Med Sch

Agarwala, Brojendra MD [PCd] - **Spec Exp:** Congenital Heart Disease; **Hospital:** Univ of Chicago Med Ctr; **Address:** 5841 S Maryland Ave, rm C-104, MC 4051, Chicago, IL 60637; **Phone:** 773-702-6172; **Board Cert:** Pediatrics 1970; Pediatric Cardiology 1978; **Med School:** India 1965; **Resid:** Pediatrics, St Vincent Hosp Med Ctr 1969; **Fellow:** Pediatric Cardiology, NYU Med Ctr 1972; **Fac Appt:** Prof Ped, Univ Chicago-Pritzker Sch Med

Beekman III, Robert H MD [PCd] - **Spec Exp:** Interventional Cardiology; Cardiac Catheterization; **Hospital:** Cincinnati Chldns Hosp Med Ctr; **Address:** Cincinnati Chldns Hosp Med Ctr, Div Cardiology, 3333 Burnet Ave, MC 2003, Cincinnati, OH 45229-3026; **Phone:** 513-636-7072; **Board Cert:** Pediatrics 1981; Pediatric Cardiology 1983; **Med School:** Duke Univ 1976; **Resid:** Pediatrics, UCLA Med Ctr 1979; **Fellow:** Pediatric Cardiology, Univ Mich Hosp 1981; **Fac Appt:** Prof Ped, Univ Cincinnati

Pediatric Cardiology

Caldwell, Randall L MD [PCd] - **Spec Exp:** Transplant Medicine-Heart; Echocardiography; Congenital Heart Disease; **Hospital:** Riley Hosp for Children; **Address:** 702 Barnhill Drive, RR-127, Indianapolis, IN 46202-5128; **Phone:** 317-274-8906; **Board Cert:** Pediatrics 1976; Pediatric Cardiology 1978; **Med School:** Indiana Univ 1971; **Resid:** Pediatrics, Indiana Univ Med Ctr 1974; **Fellow:** Pediatric Cardiology, Indiana Univ Med Ctr 1978; **Fac Appt:** Prof Ped, Indiana Univ

Cetta Jr, Frank MD [PCd] - **Spec Exp:** Congenital Heart Disease-Adult; Congenital Heart Disease; **Hospital:** Mayo Med Ctr & Clin - Rochester; **Address:** Mayo Clinic, Gonda 6-138 NW, 200 First St SW, Rochester, MN 55905; **Phone:** 507-266-0676; **Board Cert:** Pediatric Cardiology 2004; **Med School:** Loyola Univ-Stritch Sch Med 1987; **Resid:** Internal Medicine & Pediatrics, Loyola Med Ctr 1991; **Fac Appt:** Assoc Prof Ped, Mayo Med Sch

Cheatham, John P MD [PCd] - **Spec Exp:** Congenital Heart Disease-Adult & Child; Cardiac Catheterization; **Hospital:** Nationwide Chldn's Hosp; **Address:** The Heart Center, 700 Children's Drive, Columbus, OH 43205; **Phone:** 614-722-2459; **Board Cert:** Pediatrics 1981; Pediatric Cardiology 1983; **Med School:** Univ Okla Coll Med 1976; **Resid:** Pediatrics, Children's Hosp 1978; **Fellow:** Pediatric Cardiology, Texas Children's Hosp 1981; **Fac Appt:** Prof Ped, Ohio State Univ

Dick, Macdonald MD [PCd] - **Spec Exp:** Congenital Heart Disease; **Hospital:** Mott Chldns Hosp; **Address:** C.S. Motts Chldns Hosp, Dept Ped Cardio, 1500 E Med Ctr Drive, rm L1242, Box 0204, Ann Arbor, MI 48109; **Phone:** 734-936-7418; **Board Cert:** Pediatrics 1989; Pediatric Cardiology 2007; **Med School:** Univ VA Sch Med 1967; **Resid:** Pediatrics, Univ Va Hosp 1971; **Fellow:** Pediatric Cardiology, Chldns Hosp Med Ctr 1974; **Fac Appt:** Prof Ped, Univ Mich Med Sch

Driscoll, David J MD [PCd] - **Spec Exp:** Exercise Physiology; Klippel-Trenaunay Syndrome; Cardiomyopathy; **Hospital:** Mayo Med Ctr & Clin - Rochester; **Address:** Mayo Clinic - Pediatric Cardiology, 200 First St SW, Rochester, MN 55905; **Phone:** 507-284-3297; **Board Cert:** Pediatrics 1976; Pediatric Cardiology 2006; **Med School:** Marquette Sch Med 1970; **Resid:** Pediatrics, Milwaukee Chldns Hosp 1972; Pediatrics, Milwaukee Chldns Hosp 1975; **Fellow:** Pediatric Cardiology, Baylor Coll Med 1978; **Fac Appt:** Prof Ped, Mayo Med Sch

Feltes, Timothy F MD [PCd] - **Spec Exp:** Congenital Heart Disease; **Hospital:** Nationwide Chldn's Hosp; **Address:** 700 Children's Drive, rm ED619, Nationwide Chldn's Hosp, Columbus, OH 43205; **Phone:** 614-722-2565; **Board Cert:** Pediatrics 1985; Pediatric Cardiology 2010; **Med School:** Univ Toledo, Med Univ OH 1980; **Resid:** Pediatrics, Emory Univ Med Ctr 1983; **Fellow:** Pediatric Cardiology, Texas Children's Hosp 1986; **Fac Appt:** Clin Prof Ped, Ohio State Univ

Hardin, Joel T MD [PCd] - **Spec Exp:** Congenital Heart Disease-Adult & Child; Cardiac Intensive Care; Marfan's Syndrome; **Hospital:** Loyola Univ Med Ctr; **Address:** Loyola University Medical Center, 2160 S 1st Ave, Maguire Bldg, rm 3312, Maywood, IL 60153-3328; **Phone:** 708-327-9103; **Board Cert:** Pediatrics 2005; Pediatric Cardiology 2009; **Med School:** Univ Tenn Coll Med 1987; **Resid:** Pediatrics, St Louis Children's Hosp 1990; **Fellow:** Pediatric Cardiology, St Louis Children's Hosp 1993; **Fac Appt:** Assoc Prof Ped, Loyola Univ-Stritch Sch Med

Hijazi, Ziyad M MD [PCd] - **Spec Exp:** Interventional Cardiology; Congenital Heart Disease; Coarctation of the Aorta; **Hospital:** Rush Univ Med Ctr; **Address:** 1653 W Congress Pkwy, Ste 770 Jones, Chicago, IL 60612; **Phone:** 312-942-8941; **Board Cert:** Pediatric Cardiology 2007; **Med School:** Jordan 1982; **Resid:** Pediatrics, Yale-New Haven Hosp 1988; **Fellow:** Pediatric Cardiology, Yale-New Haven Hosp 1991; **Fac Appt:** Prof Ped, Rush Med Coll

Pahl, Elfriede MD [PCd] - **Spec Exp:** Transplant Medicine-Heart; Heart Failure; Congenital Heart Disease; Kawasaki Disease; **Hospital:** Children's Mem Hosp -Chicago; **Address:** Children's Memorial Hosp, Ped Cardiology, 2300 Children's Plaza, Box 21, Chicago, IL 60614-3394; **Phone:** 773-880-6388; **Board Cert:** Pediatrics 1987; Pediatric Cardiology 2010; **Med School:** Northwestern Univ 1983; **Resid:** Pediatrics, Chldns Meml Hosp 1986; **Fellow:** Pediatric Cardiology, Chldns Hosp of Pittsburgh 1988; **Fac Appt:** Prof Ped, Northwestern Univ

Rocchini, Albert P MD [PCd] - **Spec Exp:** Congenital Heart Disease; Interventional Cardiology; Hypertension in Obesity; **Hospital:** Univ of Michigan Hosp; **Address:** Mott Chldns Hosp, Dept Ped Cardiology, 1500 E Med Ctr Drive, rm L1242, Box 0204, Ann Arbor, MI 48109-0204; **Phone:** 734-936-8993; **Board Cert:** Pediatrics 1989; Pediatric Cardiology 1989; **Med School:** Univ Pittsburgh 1972; **Resid:** Pediatrics, Univ Minn 1974; **Fellow:** Pediatric Cardiology, Chldns Hosp 1977; **Fac Appt:** Prof Ped, Univ Mich Med Sch

Great Plains and Mountains

Minich, Lois LuAnn MD [PCd] - **Spec Exp:** Echocardiography; **Hospital:** Primary Children's Med Ctr; **Address:** Dept Ped Cardiology, 100 N Mario Capecchi Drive, Ste 1500, Salt Lake City, UT 84113; **Phone:** 801-662-5400; **Board Cert:** Pediatric Cardiology 2007; **Med School:** W VA Univ 1986; **Resid:** Pediatrics, Fletcher Allen Health Care 1989; **Fellow:** Pediatric Cardiology, Univ Michigan Hosps 1992

O'Laughlin, Martin P MD [PCd] - **Spec Exp:** Cardiac Catheterization; Congenital Heart Disease-Adult & Child; Interventional Cardiology; **Hospital:** Chldns Mercy Hosps & Clinics, St. Luke's Hosp of Kansas City; **Address:** 3901 Rainbow Blvd, Kansas City, KS 66160; **Phone:** 913-588-6311; **Board Cert:** Pediatrics 1985; Pediatric Cardiology 2003; **Med School:** Columbia P&S 1980; **Resid:** Pediatrics, Baylor Coll Med 1984; **Fellow:** Pediatric Cardiology, Texas Chldns Hosp/Baylor 1987

Southwest

Bricker, John T MD [PCd] - **Spec Exp:** Transplant Medicine-Heart; Congenital Heart Disease-Adult & Child; **Hospital:** Univ Genl Hosp-Houston; **Address:** 6410 Fannin St, rm 425, Houston, TX 77030; **Phone:** 713-500-5738; **Board Cert:** Pediatrics 1981; Pediatric Cardiology 1997; **Med School:** Ohio State Univ 1976; **Resid:** Pediatrics, Tex Chldns Hosp 1980; **Fellow:** Pediatric Cardiology, Tex Chldns Hosp 1983; **Fac Appt:** Prof Ped, Univ Tex, Houston

Dreyer, William J MD [PCd] - **Spec Exp:** Congenital Heart Disease; Transplant Medicine-Heart; **Hospital:** Texas Chldns Hosp; **Address:** Texas Chldns Hosp, 6621 Fannin St, MC 19345-C, Houston, TX 77030; **Phone:** 832-826-5659; **Board Cert:** Pediatrics 1987; Pediatric Cardiology 2006; **Med School:** Univ Fla Coll Med 1981; **Resid:** Pediatrics, UCSF Med Ctr 1984; **Fellow:** Pediatric Cardiology, Baylor Coll Med 1988; **Fac Appt:** Assoc Prof Ped, Baylor Coll Med

Gillette, Paul C MD [PCd] - **Spec Exp:** Arrhythmias; **Hospital:** Cook Chldns Med Ctr, Harris Methodist Hosp - Fort Worth; **Address:** Pediatric Cardiology, 209 N Bonnie Brae St, Ste 100, Med Bldg 3, Denton, TX 76201; **Phone:** 940-243-0104; **Board Cert:** Pediatrics 1974; Pediatric Cardiology 1975; **Med School:** Med Univ SC 1969; **Resid:** Pediatrics, Baylor Coll Med 1972; **Fellow:** Pediatric Cardiology, Baylor Coll Med 1974

Pediatric Cardiology

Mahony, Lynn MD [PCd] - **Spec Exp:** Congenital Heart Disease; Marfan's Syndrome; Congestive Heart Failure; Complex Diagnosis; **Hospital:** Chldns Med Ctr of Dallas; **Address:** 1935 Medical District Drive, Ste 3, Dept Cardiology, Dallas, TX 75235; **Phone:** 214-456-2333; **Board Cert:** Pediatrics 1979; Pediatric Cardiology 1997; **Med School:** Stanford Univ 1975; **Resid:** Pediatrics, Stanford Univ 1978; **Fellow:** Pediatric Cardiology, UCSF Med Ctr 1981; **Fac Appt:** Prof Ped, Univ Tex SW, Dallas

Moodie, Douglas S MD [PCd] - **Spec Exp:** Marfan's Syndrome; Congenital Heart Disease-Adult & Child; **Hospital:** Texas Chldns Hosp; **Address:** 6621 Fannin St, MC 19345-C, Houston, TX 77030; **Phone:** 832-826-5659; **Board Cert:** Pediatrics 1977; Pediatric Cardiology 1977; **Med School:** Med Coll Wisc 1972; **Resid:** Pediatrics, Mayo Clinic 1974; **Fellow:** Pediatric Cardiology, Mayo Clinic 1977

Rogers Jr, James H MD [PCd] - **Spec Exp:** Congenital Heart Disease; **Hospital:** Christus Santa Rosa Children's Hosp, Univ Hlth Syst-San Antonio; **Address:** Chldns Heart Network, 1901 Babcock Rd, Ste 301, San Antonio, TX 78229; **Phone:** 210-341-7722; **Board Cert:** Pediatrics 1976; Pediatric Cardiology 2009; **Med School:** Med Coll GA 1971; **Resid:** Pediatrics, Wilford Hall USAF Med Ctr 1974; **Fellow:** Pediatric Cardiology, Med Coll Georgia 1976; **Fac Appt:** Clin Prof Ped, Univ Tex, San Antonio

West Coast and Pacific

Bernstein, Daniel MD [PCd] - **Spec Exp:** Transplant Medicine-Heart; Congenital Heart Disease; Heart Failure; **Hospital:** Lucile Packard Chldn's Hosp, Stanford Univ Hosp & Clinics; **Address:** Lucile Packard Chldns Hosp, Div Ped Card, 750 Welch Rd, Ste 305, Palo Alto, CA 94304-5731; **Phone:** 650-723-7913; **Board Cert:** Pediatrics 1984; Pediatric Cardiology 1985; **Med School:** NYU Sch Med 1978; **Resid:** Pediatrics, Montefiore Hosp-Einstein 1982; **Fellow:** Pediatric Cardiology, UCSF Med Ctr 1986; **Fac Appt:** Prof Ped, Stanford Univ

Lewin, Mark MD [PCd] - **Spec Exp:** Echocardiography; Arrhythmias; Marfan's Syndrome; **Hospital:** Seattle Chldns Hosp, Univ Wash Med Ctr; **Address:** Seattle Chldn's Hosp, 4800 Sand Point Way NE, G-0035-Cardiology Admin, Seattle, WA 98105; **Phone:** 206-987-2018; **Board Cert:** Pediatric Cardiology 2006; **Med School:** USC-Keck School of Medicine 1991; **Resid:** Pediatrics, Chldns Hosp 1994; **Fellow:** Pediatric Cardiology, Texas Chldns Hosp 1998; **Fac Appt:** Assoc Prof Ped, Univ Wash

Perry, Stanton Bruce MD [PCd] - **Spec Exp:** Interventional Cardiology; **Hospital:** Lucile Packard Chldn's Hosp; **Address:** Lucile Packard Chldns Hosp, Dept Ped Cardiology, 750 Welch Rd, Ste 305, Palo Alto, CA 94304; **Phone:** 650-723-7913; **Board Cert:** Pediatrics 1986; **Med School:** Iceland 1978; **Resid:** Pediatrics, St Louis Chldn's Hosp 1983; **Fellow:** Pediatric Cardiology, Chldns Hosp 1984; **Fac Appt:** Assoc Prof Ped, Stanford Univ

Teitel, David F MD [PCd] - **Spec Exp:** Cardiac Catheterization; Congenital Heart Disease; **Hospital:** UCSF Med Ctr; **Address:** UCSF, Pediatric Heart Center, 400 Parnassus Ave, 2nd Fl, San Francisco, CA 94143-0544; **Phone:** 415-353-2008; **Board Cert:** Pediatrics 1980; Pediatric Cardiology 2004; **Med School:** Univ Toronto 1975; **Resid:** Pediatrics, Chldns Hosp 1980; **Fellow:** Pediatric Cardiology, UCSF Med Ctr 1982; **Fac Appt:** Prof Ped, UCSF

PEDIATRIC CRITICAL CARE MEDICINE

Mid Atlantic

Hinkle, Andrea S MD [PCCM] - **Hospital:** Univ of Rochester Strong Meml Hosp; **Address:** Golisano Childrens Hosp at Strong, 601 Elmwood Ave, Box 667, Rochester, NY 14642; **Phone:** 585-275-8138; **Board Cert:** Pediatrics 2006; Pediatric Hematology-Oncology 2008; **Med School:** Brown Univ 1987; **Resid:** Pediatrics, Boston City Hosp 1991; **Fellow:** Pediatric Hematology-Oncology, Chldns Natl Med Ctr 1994; **Fac Appt:** Asst Prof Ped, Univ Rochester

Thompson, Ann Ellen MD [PCCM] - **Spec Exp:** Mechanical Ventilation; Critical Care; Respiratory Failure; **Hospital:** Chldns Hosp of Pittsburgh - UPMC; **Address:** Chldns Hosp, Dept Ped Crit Care, 4401 Penn Ave, Pittsburgh, PA 15224; **Phone:** 412-692-5164; **Board Cert:** Pediatrics 1992; Anesthesiology 1980; Pediatric Critical Care Medicine 2010; **Med School:** Tufts Univ 1974; **Resid:** Pediatrics, Chldns Hosp 1977; Anesthesiology, Hosp Univ Penn 1980; **Fellow:** Pediatric Critical Care Medicine, Chldns Hosp 1979; **Fac Appt:** Prof Ped, Univ Pittsburgh

Southeast

Anand, Kanwaljeet Singh MD/PhD [PCCM] - **Spec Exp:** Pain Management; Critical Care; **Hospital:** Le Bonheur Chldns Med Ctr, St. Jude Children's Research Hosp; **Address:** 50 N Dunlap St, Memphis, TN 38103-2893; **Phone:** 901-287-6292; **Board Cert:** Pediatric Critical Care Medicine 2004; **Med School:** India 1981; **Resid:** Pediatrics, Chldns Hosp 1991; Neonatal-Perinatal Medicine, John Radcliffe Hosp 1985; **Fellow:** Pediatric Critical Care Medicine, Mass Genl Hosp 1993; **Fac Appt:** Prof Ped, Univ Tenn Coll Med

Midwest

Sarnaik, Ashok P MD [PCCM] - **Spec Exp:** Critical Care; Perinatal Medicine; **Hospital:** Chldns Hosp of Michigan; **Address:** Chldns Hosp, Div Crit Care Med, 3901 Beaubien St, Carl's Bldg - Ste 4134, Detroit, MI 48201-2119; **Phone:** 313-745-5629; **Board Cert:** Pediatrics 1975; Neonatal-Perinatal Medicine 1979; Pediatric Critical Care Medicine 2003; **Med School:** India 1969; **Resid:** Pediatrics, JJ Hosp-Bombay Univ 1971; Pediatrics, Chldns Hosp Mich 1974; **Fellow:** Neonatal-Perinatal Medicine, Chldns Hosp Mich 1975; **Fac Appt:** Prof Ped, Wayne State Univ

Sichting, Kay A MD [PCCM] - **Hospital:** Peyton Manning Children's Hosp at St. Vincent; **Address:** Peyton Manning Chldns Hosp-PICU, 2001 W 86th St, Indianapolis, IN 46260; **Phone:** 317-338-5230; **Board Cert:** Pediatric Critical Care Medicine 2006; **Med School:** Indiana Univ 1990; **Resid:** Pediatrics, Riley Hosp for Chldn 1993; **Fellow:** Pediatric Critical Care Medicine, Riley Hosp for Chldn 1994; Pediatric Critical Care Medicine, Chldns Hosp of WI 1997

Great Plains and Mountains

Dean, Jonathan M MD [PCCM] - **Hospital:** Primary Children's Med Ctr; **Address:** Pediatric Critical Care, Univ Utah, PO Box 518289, Salt Lake City, UT 84158; **Phone:** 801-587-7572; **Board Cert:** Pediatrics 1981; Pediatric Critical Care Medicine 2003; **Med School:** Northwestern Univ 1977; **Resid:** Pediatrics, Children's Hosp 1981; **Fellow:** Pediatric Critical Care Medicine, Johns Hopkins Hosp 1983; **Fac Appt:** Prof Ped, Univ Utah

Pediatric Critical Care Medicine

Southwest

Fuhrman, Bradley P MD [PCCM] - ; **Address:** Pediatrics Admin Elp, Paul L Foster School of Medicine, 4800 Alberta Ave, El Paso, TX 79905-2799; **Phone:** 915-545-6785; **Board Cert:** Pediatrics 1992; Pediatric Critical Care Medicine 2003; Neonatal-Perinatal Medicine 1979; Pediatric Cardiology 1979; **Med School:** NYU Sch Med 1971; **Resid:** Pediatrics, Univ Minnesota Med Ctr 1973; **Fellow:** Pediatric Cardiology, Univ Minnesota 1974; Neonatal-Perinatal Medicine, Univ Minnesota 1979; **Fac Appt:** Prof Ped, Texas Tech Univ

Perez Fontan, J Julio MD [PCCM] - **Spec Exp:** Respiratory Failure; **Hospital:** UT Southwestern Med Ctr at Dallas, Chldns Med Ctr of Dallas; **Address:** UT SW Med Ctr, Dept Peds, 5323 Harry Hines Blvd, Dallas, TX 75390-9063; **Phone:** 214-648-9618; **Board Cert:** Pediatrics 1987; Pediatric Critical Care Medicine 2003; **Med School:** Spain 1977; **Resid:** Pediatrics, Chldns Hosp/Univ Barcelona 1981; **Fellow:** Critical Care Medicine, UCSF Med Ctr 1984; **Fac Appt:** Prof Ped, Univ Tex SW, Dallas

Taylor, Richard P MD [PCCM] - **Hospital:** Univ Hlth Syst-San Antonio; **Address:** Dept Ped Critical Care, 7703 Floyd Curl Drive, MC 7829, San Antonio, TX 78229; **Phone:** 210-562-5816; **Board Cert:** Internal Medicine 1988; Pediatric Critical Care Medicine 2004; **Med School:** Univ Tex Med Br, Galveston 1984; **Resid:** Internal Medicine, St Joseph Mercy Hosp 1988; Pediatrics, UNiv Michigan Med Ctr 1988; **Fellow:** Pediatric Critical Care Medicine, Univ Michigan Med Ctr 1995; **Fac Appt:** Assoc Prof Ped

West Coast and Pacific

Schwarz, Adam J MD [PCCM] - **Hospital:** Chldns Hosp Orange Co; **Address:** Chldns Hosp of Orange, 455 S Main St, Orange, CA 92868; **Phone:** 714-532-8620; **Board Cert:** Pediatric Critical Care Medicine 2011; Pediatrics 2009; **Med School:** Stanford Univ 1990; **Resid:** Pediatrics, Stanford Med Ctr 1993; **Fellow:** Pediatric Critical Care Medicine, Harbor-UCLA Med Ctr 1996; **Fac Appt:** Assoc Clin Prof Ped

Zimmerman, Jerry John MD [PCCM] - **Spec Exp:** Inflammation in Critical Illness; Sepsis; Septic Shock; **Hospital:** Seattle Chldns Hosp, Harborview Med Ctr; **Address:** Seattle Chldn's Hosp, 4800 Sand Point Way NE, MS W8866, PO Box 5371/41-A, Seattle, WA 98105-0371; **Phone:** 206-987-3862; **Board Cert:** Pediatrics 1992; Pediatric Critical Care Medicine 2010; **Med School:** Univ Wisc 1979; **Resid:** Pediatrics, Univ Wisconsin Hosp 1982; **Fellow:** Pediatric Critical Care Medicine, Chldns Natl Med Ctr 1984; **Fac Appt:** Prof Ped, Univ Wash

PEDIATRIC ENDOCRINOLOGY

New England

Casella, Samuel Joseph MD [PEn] - **Spec Exp:** Thyroid Disorders; Growth/Development Disorders; **Hospital:** Dartmouth - Hitchcock Med Ctr; **Address:** Dartmouth-Hitchcock Med Ctr, Dept Ped Endo, 1 Med Ctr Drive, Lebanon, NH 03756; **Phone:** 603-653-9877; **Board Cert:** Pediatrics 1985; Pediatric Endocrinology 1986; **Med School:** SUNY Upstate Med Univ 1981; **Resid:** Pediatrics, Upstate Med Ctr 1984; **Fellow:** Pediatric Endocrinology, NC Meml Hosp-Univ NC 1986; **Fac Appt:** Assoc Prof Ped, Johns Hopkins Univ

Gordon, Catherine M MD [PEn] - **Spec Exp:** Bone Disorders-Metabolic; **Hospital:** Children's Hospital - Boston; **Address:** Chldns Hosp, Ped Endocrinology, 333 Longwood Ave Fl 6, Boston, MA 02115; **Phone:** 617-355-7476; **Board Cert:** Pediatric Endocrinology 2007; Adolescent Medicine 2001; **Med School:** Univ NC Sch Med 1991; **Resid:** Pediatrics, Chldns Hosp 1994; **Fellow:** Pediatric Endocrinology, Chldns Hosp 1996; **Fac Appt:** Assoc Prof Ped, Harvard Med Sch

Levitsky, Lynne Lipton MD [PEn] - **Spec Exp:** Diabetes; Growth/Development Disorders; Cushing's Syndrome; **Hospital:** Mass Genl Hosp; **Address:** Mass Genl Hosp, Ped Endocrinology, 55 Fruit St Yawkey Bldg Fl 6 - rm 6C, Boston, MA 02114; **Phone:** 617-726-2909; **Board Cert:** Pediatrics 1971; Pediatric Endocrinology 1978; **Med School:** Yale Univ 1966; **Resid:** Pediatrics, Chldns Hosp 1968; **Fellow:** Pediatric Endocrinology, Univ Maryland Hosp 1970; **Fac Appt:** Assoc Prof Ped, Harvard Med Sch

Ludwig, David S MD/PhD [PEn] - **Spec Exp:** Obesity; Nutrition; **Hospital:** Children's Hospital - Boston; **Address:** Chldns Hosp, Div Endocrinology, 333 Longwood Ave Fl 6 - rm 624, Boston, MA 02115; **Phone:** 617-355-7476; **Board Cert:** Pediatric Endocrinology 2003; **Med School:** Stanford Univ 1990; **Resid:** Pediatrics, Chldns Hosp 1993; **Fellow:** Pediatric Endocrinology, Chldns Hosp 1995; **Fac Appt:** Asst Prof Ped, Harvard Med Sch

Spack, Norman P MD [PEn] - **Spec Exp:** Diabetes; Growth Disorders; Transgender Issues; **Hospital:** Children's Hospital - Boston; **Address:** Chldns Hosp, Div Endocrinology, 300 Longwood Ave, Boston, MA 02115; **Phone:** 617-355-7476; **Board Cert:** Pediatrics 1975; Pediatric Endocrinology 2003; **Med School:** Univ Rochester 1969; **Resid:** Pediatrics, Boston City Hosp/Chldns Hosp 1972; **Fellow:** Adolescent Medicine, Chldns Hosp 1975; Pediatric Endocrinology, Chldns Hosp 1978; **Fac Appt:** Assoc Prof Ped, Harvard Med Sch

Tamborlane, William V MD [PEn] - **Spec Exp:** Diabetes; **Hospital:** Yale-New Haven Hosp, Yale Med Group; **Address:** Yale Pediatric Endocrinology, 333 Cedar St, rm 3091-LMP, New Haven, CT 06519; **Phone:** 203-764-6747; **Board Cert:** Pediatrics 1978; Pediatric Endocrinology 1986; **Med School:** Georgetown Univ 1972; **Resid:** Pediatrics, Georgetown Univ Hosp 1975; **Fellow:** Pediatric Endocrinology, Yale-New Haven Hosp 1977; **Fac Appt:** Prof Ped, Yale Univ

Mid Atlantic

Alter, Craig A MD [PEn] - **Spec Exp:** Diabetes; Growth Disorders; Thyroid Disorders; Pubertal Disorders; **Hospital:** Chldns Hosp of Philadelphia; **Address:** Children's Hosp of Philadelphia, Dept Pediatric Endocrinology, 34th & Civic Ctr Blvd, Philadelphia, PA 19104; **Phone:** 215-590-3174; **Board Cert:** Pediatrics 2005; Pediatric Endocrinology 2010; **Med School:** Harvard Med Sch 1987; **Resid:** Pediatrics, Boston Children's Hosp 1990; **Fellow:** Pediatric Endocrinology, Children's Hosp 1993; **Fac Appt:** Clin Prof Ped, Univ Pennsylvania

Arslanian, Silva MD [PEn] - **Spec Exp:** Diabetes; Obesity; **Hospital:** Chldns Hosp of Pittsburgh - UPMC; **Address:** 4401 Penn Ave, Pittsburgh, PA 15224; **Phone:** 412-692-6935; **Board Cert:** Pediatrics 1983; Pediatric Endocrinology 1983; **Med School:** Lebanon 1978; **Resid:** Pediatrics, American Univ Hosp 1980; **Fellow:** Pediatric Endocrinology, Chldns Hosp 1983; **Fac Appt:** Prof Ped, Univ Pittsburgh

Becker, Dorothy J MD [PEn] - **Spec Exp:** Diabetes; **Hospital:** Chldns Hosp of Pittsburgh - UPMC; **Address:** Children's Hospital Drive, Div Endocrinology, 4401 Penn Ave, Pittsburgh, PA 15224; **Phone:** 412-692-5172; **Board Cert:** Pediatrics 1978; Pediatric Endocrinology 1978; **Med School:** South Africa 1964; **Resid:** Pediatrics, Univ Capetown 1972; Endocrinology, Diabetes & Metabolism, Univ Capetown 1974; **Fellow:** Pediatric Endocrinology, Univ Pittsburgh Hosp 1976; **Fac Appt:** Prof Ped, Univ Pittsburgh

Pediatric Endocrinology

De Luca, Francesco MD [PEn] - **Spec Exp:** Growth Disorders; Metabolic Syndrome; Osteoporosis; Diabetes; **Hospital:** St. Christopher's Hosp for Chldn; **Address:** St Christophers Hosp for Children, Endocrinology Section, Ste 3303, 3601 A St, Philadelphia, PA 19134; **Phone:** 215-427-8100; **Board Cert:** Pediatric Endocrinology 2010; **Med School:** Italy 1983; **Resid:** Pediatrics, Cath Univ Sacred Heart Affil Hosp; Pediatrics, Albert Einstein Med Ctr; **Fellow:** Pediatric Endocrinology, St Christophers Hosp; Pediatric Endocrinology, Natl Inst Hlth; **Fac Appt:** Assoc Prof Ped, Drexel Univ Coll Med

Levine, Michael A MD [PEn] - **Spec Exp:** Bone Disorders-Metabolic; Osteoporosis; **Hospital:** Chldns Hosp of Philadelphia; **Address:** Childrens Hosp Philadelphia, Div Endocrinology, 34th St & Civic Center Blvd, Philadelphia, PA 19104; **Phone:** 215-590-3174; **Board Cert:** Internal Medicine 1979; Endocrinology, Diabetes & Metabolism 1981; **Med School:** Hahnemann Univ 1976; **Resid:** Internal Medicine, Johns Hopkins Hosp 1979; **Fellow:** Endocrinology, Natl Inst Hlth 1981; Genetics, Natl Inst Hlth 1981; **Fac Appt:** Prof Med, Univ Pennsylvania

Maclaren, Noel K MD [PEn] - **Spec Exp:** Diabetes; Obesity; Metabolic Syndrome; **Hospital:** Lenox Hill Hosp; **Address:** Bioseek Endocrine Clinic, 200 W 57th St, Ste 610, New York, NY 10019; **Phone:** 212-371-0658; **Board Cert:** Pediatrics 1977; Pediatric Endocrinology 1978; **Med School:** New Zealand 1963; **Resid:** Pediatrics, Wellington Public Hosp 1967; **Fellow:** Pediatric Endocrinology, Johns Hopkins Hosp 1973; **Fac Appt:** Prof Ped, Cornell Univ-Weill Med Coll

New, Maria I MD [PEn] - **Spec Exp:** Adrenal Disorders; Growth/Development Disorders; **Hospital:** Mount Sinai Med Ctr (page 63); **Address:** Mount Sinai Medical Ctr, 1 Gustave L Levy Pl, Box 1198, New York, NY 10029; **Phone:** 212-241-8210; **Board Cert:** Pediatrics 1960; **Med School:** Univ Pennsylvania 1954; **Resid:** Pediatrics, New York Hosp 1957; **Fellow:** Pediatric Endocrinology, New York Hosp 1958; Endocrinology, Diabetes & Metabolism, New York Hosp 1964; **Fac Appt:** Prof Ped, Cornell Univ-Weill Med Coll

Oberfield, Sharon E MD [PEn] - **Spec Exp:** Adrenal Disorders; Neuroendocrine Growth Disorders; Growth Disorders; **Hospital:** Morgan Stanley Children's Hosp of NY-Presby, NY (page 65); **Address:** 630 W 168th St PH East Bldg - Ste 522, New York, NY 10032; **Phone:** 212-305-6559; **Board Cert:** Pediatrics 1979; Pediatric Endocrinology 2000; **Med School:** Cornell Univ-Weill Med Coll 1974; **Resid:** Pediatrics, NY Hosp-Cornell 1976; **Fellow:** Pediatric Endocrinology, NY Hosp-Cornell 1979; **Fac Appt:** Prof Ped, Columbia P&S

Plotnick, Leslie P MD [PEn] - **Spec Exp:** Diabetes; Growth Disorders; Thyroid Disorders; Pubertal Disorders; **Hospital:** Johns Hopkins Hosp (page 61); **Address:** Johns Hopkins Hospital, 200 N Wolfe St, Dept Pediatric Endocrinology #3120, Baltimore, MD 21287; **Phone:** 410-955-6463; **Board Cert:** Pediatrics 1975; Pediatric Endocrinology 2009; **Med School:** Univ MD Sch Med 1970; **Resid:** Pediatrics, Johns Hopkins Hosp 1972; **Fellow:** Pediatric Endocrinology, Johns Hopkins Hosp 1974; **Fac Appt:** Prof Ped, Johns Hopkins Univ

Sklar, Charles A MD [PEn] - **Spec Exp:** Cancer Survivors-Late Effects of Therapy; Growth Disorders in Childhood Cancer; Pituitary Disorders; **Hospital:** Meml Sloan-Kettering Cancer Ctr; **Address:** 1275 York Avenue, New York, NY 10065; **Phone:** 800-525-2225; **Board Cert:** Pediatrics 1979; Pediatric Endocrinology 1980; **Med School:** USC Sch Med 1974; **Resid:** Pediatrics, Childrens Hosp 1976; **Fellow:** Pediatric Endocrinology, UCSF Med Ctr 1979; **Fac Appt:** Assoc Prof Ped, Cornell Univ-Weill Med Coll

Sperling, Mark A MD [PEn] - **Spec Exp:** Diabetes; Growth/Development Disorders; Hypoglycemia; Neonatal Diabetes; **Hospital:** Chldns Hosp of Pittsburgh - UPMC, UPMC Presby, Pittsburgh; **Address:** Chldns Hosp Pittsburgh, Endocrinology, 4401 Penn Ave, Faculty Pavillion, rm 8139, Pittsburgh, PA 15224; **Phone:** 412-692-5172; **Board Cert:** Pediatrics 1986; Pediatric Endocrinology 1986; **Med School:** Australia 1962; **Resid:** Internal Medicine, Prince Henry Hosp 1964; Pediatrics, Royal Chldns Hosp 1968; **Fellow:** Pediatric Endocrinology, Chldns Hosp 1970; **Fac Appt:** Prof Ped, Univ Pittsburgh

Stanley, Charles MD [PEn] - **Spec Exp:** Hyperinsulinism-Congenital; Hypoglycemia; **Hospital:** Chldns Hosp of Philadelphia; **Address:** Chldns Hosp, Div Endocrinology, 34th St & Civic Ctr Blvd, Philadelphia, PA 19104; **Phone:** 215-590-3174; **Board Cert:** Pediatrics 1976; Pediatric Endocrinology 1978; **Med School:** Univ VA Sch Med 1970; **Resid:** Pediatrics, Children's Hosp 1972; **Fellow:** Pediatric Endocrinology, Children's Hosp 1976; **Fac Appt:** Prof Emeritus Ped, Univ Pennsylvania

Southeast

Diamond, Frank B MD [PEn] - **Spec Exp:** Growth Disorders; Obesity; Calcium Disorders in Newborn; **Hospital:** All Children's Hosp, Tampa Genl Hosp; **Address:** All Chldn's Hosp, 601 5th St S, St Petersburg, FL 33701; **Phone:** 727-767-4237; **Board Cert:** Pediatrics 1979; Pediatric Endocrinology 1980; **Med School:** Penn State Coll Med 1974; **Resid:** Pediatrics, Chldns Hosp-Univ Alabama 1976; **Fellow:** Pediatric Endocrinology, Chldns Hosp-Univ Penn 1978; **Fac Appt:** Prof Ped, Univ S Fla Coll Med

Freemark, Michael S MD [PEn] - **Spec Exp:** Prader-Willi Syndrome; Growth Disorders; Pubertal Disorders; Diabetes; **Hospital:** Duke Univ Hosp, Durham Regional Hosp; **Address:** Ped Endocrinology & Diabetes, DUMC, Box 102820, Durham, NC 27710; **Phone:** 919-684-8350; **Board Cert:** Pediatrics 1980; Pediatric Endocrinology 1983; **Med School:** Duke Univ 1976; **Resid:** Pediatrics, Duke Univ Med Ctr 1979; **Fellow:** Pediatric Endocrinology, Duke Univ Med Ctr 1983; Pediatric Endocrinology, Hospital Necker Enfants Malades 1993; **Fac Appt:** Prof Ped, Duke Univ

Friedman, Nancy E MD [PEn] - **Spec Exp:** Calcium Disorders; Bone Disorders-Metabolic; Growth/Development Disorders; Cancer Survivors-Late Effects of Therapy; **Hospital:** Duke Univ Hosp; **Address:** Duke Consultative Services, 3480 Wake Forest Rd, Ste 310, Raleigh, NC 27609; **Phone:** 919-684-3772 x2; **Board Cert:** Pediatrics 1979; Pediatric Endocrinology 2003; **Med School:** Med Coll VA 1975; **Resid:** Pediatrics, Childrens Hosp Med Ctr 1977; Pediatrics, Childrens Meml Hosp 1978; **Fellow:** Endocrinology, Diabetes & Metabolism, Michael Reese Hosp 1980; **Fac Appt:** Asst Clin Prof Ped, Duke Univ

Meacham, Lillian R MD [PEn] - **Spec Exp:** Growth Disorders in Childhood Cancer; Cancer Survivors-Late Effects of Therapy; **Hospital:** Chldns Hlthcare Atlanta @ Egleston, Chldns Hlthcare Atlanta @ Scottish Rite; **Address:** Aflac Outpatient Center, 1405 Clifton Rd NE, 4th Fl, Tower 1, Atlanta, GA 30322; **Phone:** 404-785-1200; **Board Cert:** Pediatrics 2006; Pediatric Endocrinology 2006; **Med School:** Emory Univ 1984; **Resid:** Pediatrics, Emory Univ Hosp 1987; **Fellow:** Pediatric Endocrinology, Emory Univ 1990; **Fac Appt:** Prof Ped, Emory Univ

Silverstein, Janet H MD [PEn] - **Spec Exp:** Diabetes; Growth/Development Disorders; Obesity; **Hospital:** Shands at Univ of FL; **Address:** Univ Florida - Shands Hlthcare, 1701 SW Archer Rd, Gainesville, FL 32610-3003; **Phone:** 352-334-1390; **Board Cert:** Pediatrics 1975; Pediatric Endocrinology 2004; **Med School:** Univ Pennsylvania 1970; **Resid:** Pediatrics, Chldns Hosp 1972; Pediatrics, Chldns Hosp 1975; **Fellow:** Pediatric Endocrinology, Duke Univ Med Ctr 1977; **Fac Appt:** Prof Ped, Univ Fla Coll Med

Pediatric Endocrinology

Midwest

Allen, David Bruce MD [PEn] - **Spec Exp:** Growth Disorders; Pubertal Disorders; Diabetes; **Hospital:** Univ WI Hosp & Clins; **Address:** Univ Wisc American Fam Chldn's Hosp, H4/448 CSC-Pediatrics, 600 Highland Ave, Madison, WI 53792-4108; **Phone:** 608-263-5835; **Board Cert:** Pediatrics 1986; Pediatric Endocrinology 2011; **Med School:** Duke Univ 1980; **Resid:** Pediatrics, Univ Wisc Hosp 1985; **Fellow:** Pediatric Endocrinology, Univ Wisc Hosp 1988; **Fac Appt:** Prof Ped, Univ Wisc

Cuttler, Leona MD [PEn] - **Hospital:** UH Rainbow Babies & Chldns Hosp (page 74); **Address:** UH Rainbow Babies & Children's Hosp, 11100 Euclid Ave, Cleveland, OH 44106; **Phone:** 216-844-3661; **Board Cert:** Pediatrics 1980; Pediatric Endocrinology 1983; **Med School:** Univ Iowa Coll Med 1975; **Resid:** Pediatrics, Hosp for Sick Chldn 1980; **Fellow:** Pediatric Endocrinology, Hosp for Sick Chldn 1982; Pediatric Endocrinology, UCSF Med Ctr 1984; **Fac Appt:** Prof Ped, Case West Res Univ

Eugster, Erica A MD [PEn] - **Spec Exp:** Pubertal Disorders; Turner Syndrome; Growth/Development Disorders; Sex Development Disorders; **Hospital:** Riley Hosp for Children, Franciscan St. Francis Hlth-Indianapolis; **Address:** Riley Childrens Hosp, Pediatric Endocrinology, 705 Riley Hospital Drive, rm 5960, Indianapolis, IN 46202; **Phone:** 317-944-3889; **Board Cert:** Pediatric Endocrinology 2005; **Med School:** Med Coll PA 1990; **Resid:** Pediatrics, Marshfield Clin-St Josephs Hosp 1994; **Fellow:** Pediatric Endocrinology, Univ Minn 1997; **Fac Appt:** Prof Ped, Indiana Univ

Gutai, James MD [PEn] - **Hospital:** Chldns Hosp of Michigan, Marquette Genl Hosp; **Address:** Morris J Hood Comp Diabetes Ctr, 4201 St Antoine St, Univ Hlth Ctr, Box 247, Detroit, MI 48201; **Phone:** 313-577-0133; **Board Cert:** Pediatrics 1977; Pediatric Endocrinology 1980; **Med School:** Temple Univ 1970; **Resid:** Pediatrics, Johns Hopkins Hosp 1976; **Fellow:** Pediatric Endocrinology, Johns Hopkins Hosp 1976; **Fac Appt:** Prof Ped, Wayne State Univ

Levy, Richard Alshuler MD [PEn] - **Spec Exp:** Growth Disorders; Pituitary Disorders; Thyroid Disorders; **Hospital:** Rush Univ Med Ctr, Ingalls Meml Hosp; **Address:** 1725 W Harrison St, Ste 328, Chicago, IL 60612-3863; **Phone:** 312-942-8989; **Board Cert:** Internal Medicine 1976; Pediatrics 1983; Endocrinology 1985; Pediatric Endocrinology 1986; **Med School:** Louisiana State U, New Orleans 1971; **Resid:** Internal Medicine, Univ Mass Med Ctr 1977; Pediatrics, Beth Israel Hosp 1978; **Fellow:** Endocrinology, Diabetes & Metabolism, Barnes Jewish Hosp 1982; **Fac Appt:** Asst Prof Ped, Rush Med Coll

Menon, Ram K MD [PEn] - **Spec Exp:** Growth/Development Disorders; Diabetes; **Hospital:** Univ of Michigan Hosp; **Address:** Univ Mich Med Ctr, 1500 E Med Ctr Drive, D1205 MPB-SPC5718, Ann Arbor, MI 48109; **Phone:** 734-764-5175; **Board Cert:** Pediatrics 2009; Pediatric Endocrinology 2003; **Med School:** India 1979; **Resid:** Pediatrics, All India Inst of Med Sci 1984; **Fellow:** Endocrinology & Metabolism, Royal Free Hosp & Med Coll 1986; Pediatric Endocrinology, Chldn's Hosp 1989; **Fac Appt:** Assoc Prof Ped, Univ Mich Med Sch

Mirmira, Raghu G MD/PhD [PEn] - **Spec Exp:** Diabetes; **Hospital:** Riley Hosp for Children; **Address:** Riley Hosp Chldn-Endocrinology, 705 Riley Hospital Drive, rm 5960, Indianapolis, IN 46202; **Phone:** 317-274-3889; **Board Cert:** Endocrinology, Diabetes & Metabolism 2008; **Med School:** Univ Chicago-Pritzker Sch Med 1993; **Resid:** Internal Medicine, UCSF Med Ctr 1995; **Fellow:** Endocrinology, Diabetes & Metabolism, UCSF 1998; **Fac Appt:** Assoc Prof Ped, Indiana Univ

Norris, Andrew W MD/PhD [PEn] - **Spec Exp:** Diabetes; **Hospital:** Univ Iowa Hosp & Clinics; **Address:** UIHC Pediatric Endocrinology, 200 Hawkins Dr 2857 JPP, Iowa City, IA 52242; **Phone:** 319-356-2229; **Board Cert:** Pediatric Endocrinology 2003; **Med School:** Washington Univ, St Louis 1997; **Resid:** Pediatrics, Univ IA Hosp & Clin 2000; **Fellow:** Pediatric Endocrinology, Chldns Hosp 2003; **Fac Appt:** Asst Prof Ped, Univ Wash

Rogers, Douglas G MD [PEn] - **Spec Exp:** Diabetes; Growth/Development Disorders; Thyroid Disorders; **Hospital:** Cleveland Clin (page 56); **Address:** Div Pediatric Endocrinology, 9500 Euclid Ave, Box A120, Cleveland, OH 44195-0001; **Phone:** 216-444-5515; **Board Cert:** Pediatrics 1984; Pediatric Endocrinology 1986; **Med School:** Ros Franklin Univ/Chicago Med Sch 1978; **Resid:** Pediatrics, Cardinal Glennon Chldns Hosp 1981; **Fellow:** Pediatric Endocrinology, St Louis Chldns Hosp 1985

White, Neil H MD [PEn] - **Spec Exp:** Diabetes; Hypoglycemia; **Hospital:** St. Louis Chldns Hosp; **Address:** St Louis Chldns Hosp, One Children's Pl, CB 8116, St Louis, MO 63110-1010; **Phone:** 314-454-6051; **Board Cert:** Pediatrics 1981; Pediatric Endocrinology 1983; **Med School:** Albert Einstein Coll Med 1975; **Resid:** Pediatrics, St Louis Chldns Hosp 1977; **Fellow:** Endocrinology, Diabetes & Metabolism, Washington Univ 1979; **Fac Appt:** Prof Ped, Washington Univ, St Louis

Zimmerman, Donald MD [PEn] - **Spec Exp:** Growth Disorders in Childhood Cancer; Thyroid Cancer; Thyroid Disorders; Growth/Development Disorders; **Hospital:** Children's Mem Hosp - Chicago; **Address:** Children's Memorial Hosp, 2300 Children's Plaza, Div Endocrinology, Box 54, Chicago, IL 60614; **Phone:** 773-327-7740; **Board Cert:** Internal Medicine 1977; Endocrinology 1979; Pediatrics 1983; Pediatric Endocrinology 2001; **Med School:** Univ IL Coll Med 1974; **Resid:** Internal Medicine, Johns Hopkins Hosp 1977; Pediatrics, Mayo Clinic 1981; **Fellow:** Endocrinology, Diabetes & Metabolism, Mayo Clinic 1980; **Fac Appt:** Prof Ped, Northwestern Univ

Great Plains and Mountains

Foster, Carol M MD [PEn] - **Spec Exp:** Diabetes; Growth/Development Disorders; Pubertal Disorders; **Hospital:** Primary Children's Med Ctr, Univ Utah Hlth Care; **Address:** Utah Diabetes Ctr, 615 Arapeen Drive, Ste 100, Salt Lake City, UT 84108; **Phone:** 801-581-7761; **Board Cert:** Pediatrics 1983; Pediatric Endocrinology 1983; **Med School:** Washington Univ, St Louis 1978; **Resid:** Pediatrics, Univ Utah Hlth Scis Ctr 1981; **Fellow:** Pediatric Endocrinology, Natl Inst Hlth 1984; **Fac Appt:** Prof Med, Univ Utah

Kappy, Michael S MD/PhD [PEn] - **Spec Exp:** Growth/Development Disorders; Thyroid Disorders; Pubertal Disorders; **Hospital:** Chldn's Hosp - Aurora (CO); **Address:** Chldns Hosp-Dept Endocrinology, 13123 E 16th Ave, Box B265, Aurora, CO 80045; **Phone:** 720-777-6128; **Board Cert:** Pediatrics 1972; Pediatric Endocrinology 1980; **Med School:** Univ Wisc 1967; **Resid:** Pediatrics, Univ Colorado Med Ctr 1972; **Fellow:** Pediatric Endocrinology, Johns Hopkins Hosp 1980; **Fac Appt:** Prof Ped, Univ Colorado

Klingensmith, Georgeanna J MD [PEn] - **Spec Exp:** Diabetes; **Hospital:** Chldn's Hosp - Aurora (CO); **Address:** Barbara Davis Ctr, 1775 Aurora Court, MS A140, Aurora, CO 80045; **Phone:** 303-724-2323; **Board Cert:** Pediatrics 1976; Pediatric Endocrinology 2000; **Med School:** Duke Univ 1971; **Resid:** Pediatrics, Childrens Hosp 1974; **Fellow:** Pediatric Endocrinology, Johns Hopkins Hosp 1976; **Fac Appt:** Prof Ped, Univ Colorado

West Coast and Pacific

Geffner, Mitchell E MD [PEn] - **Spec Exp:** Growth Disorders; Pubertal Disorders; Thyroid Disorders; Pituitary Disorders; **Hospital:** Chldns Hosp - Los Angeles; **Address:** Chlds Hosp LA, Div Endocrinology, 4650 Sunset Blvd, MS 61, Los Angeles, CA 90027; **Phone:** 323-361-2185; **Board Cert:** Pediatrics 1980; Pediatric Endocrinology 2006; **Med School:** Albert Einstein Coll Med 1975; **Resid:** Pediatrics, LAC-USC Med Ctr 1979; **Fellow:** Pediatric Endocrinology, UCLA Med Ctr 1982; **Fac Appt:** Prof Ped, USC Sch Med

Pediatric Endocrinology

Gitelman, Stephen E MD [PEn] - **Spec Exp:** Diabetes; **Hospital:** UCSF Med Ctr; **Address:** UCSF Med Ctr, Pediatric Endocrinology, 513 Parnassus Ave, S-679, Box 0434, San Francisco, CA 94143; **Phone:** 415-353-2813; **Board Cert:** Pediatric Endocrinology 2006; **Med School:** Univ NC Sch Med 1984; **Resid:** Pediatrics, UCSF Med Ctr 1987; **Fellow:** Pediatric Endocrinology, UCSF Med Ctr 1990; **Fac Appt:** Clin Prof Ped, UCSF

Lustig, Robert H MD [PEn] - **Spec Exp:** Obesity; Metabolic Syndrome; Weight Management; Hyperinsulinism; **Hospital:** UCSF Med Ctr; **Address:** UCSF Medical Ctr, Div Pediatric Endocrinology, 513 Parnassus Ave, CB 0434, S-679, San Francisco, CA 94143; **Phone:** 415-353-2813; **Board Cert:** Pediatrics 1984; Pediatric Endocrinology 1986; **Med School:** Cornell Univ-Weill Med Coll 1980; **Resid:** Pediatrics, St Louis Children's Hosp 1983; **Fellow:** Pediatric Endocrinology, UCSF Medical Ctr 1984; **Fac Appt:** Prof Ped, UCSF

Rosenthal, Stephen M MD [PEn] - **Spec Exp:** Diabetes; **Hospital:** UCSF Med Ctr; **Address:** UCSF Medical Ctr, Dept Pediatric Endocrinology, 500 Parnassus Ave, Box 0434, San Fransisco, CA 94143; **Phone:** 415-476-2266; **Board Cert:** Pediatrics 1982; Pediatric Endocrinology 1983; **Med School:** Columbia P&S 1976; **Resid:** Pediatrics, NY Presby-Columbia Med Ctr 1979; **Fellow:** Pediatric Endocrinology, UCSF Med Ctr 1982; **Fac Appt:** Prof Ped, UCSF

Wilson, Darrell M MD [PEn] - **Spec Exp:** Diabetes; Growth Disorders; Weight Management; **Hospital:** Stanford Univ Hosp & Clinics, Lucile Packard Chldn's Hosp; **Address:** Stanford Univ Med Ctr - Pediatrics, 300 Pasteur Drive, Ste G-313, Stanford, CA 94305-5208; **Phone:** 650-723-5791; **Board Cert:** Pediatrics 1982; Pediatric Endocrinology 2010; **Med School:** UCSD 1977; **Resid:** Pediatrics, Stanford Univ Med Ctr 1980; **Fellow:** Endocrinology, Diabetes & Metabolism, Stanford Univ 1984; **Fac Appt:** Prof Ped, Stanford Univ

PEDIATRIC GASTROENTEROLOGY

New England

Jonas, Maureen M MD [PGe] - **Spec Exp:** Liver Disease; Transplant Medicine-Liver; Hepatitis; **Hospital:** Children's Hospital - Boston, Brigham and Women's Hosp (page 57); **Address:** Chldns Hosp, Dept Ped Gastroenterology, 300 Longwood Ave, Boston, MA 02115; **Phone:** 617-355-5837; **Board Cert:** Pediatrics 1982; Pediatric Gastroenterology 2005; Pediatric Transplant Hepatology 2006; **Med School:** Univ Miami Sch Med 1977; **Resid:** Pediatrics, Chldns Hosp 1980; **Fellow:** Pediatric Gastroenterology, Chldns Hosp 1982; **Fac Appt:** Assoc Prof Ped, Harvard Med Sch

Kleinman, Ronald E MD [PGe] - **Spec Exp:** Transplant Medicine-Liver; Nutrition; **Hospital:** Mass Genl Hosp, N Shore Children's Hosp; **Address:** Mass Genl Hosp, Div Ped GI/Nutrition, 55 Fruit St, VBK 107, Boston, MA 02114; **Phone:** 617-726-8705; **Board Cert:** Pediatrics 1992; Pediatric Gastroenterology 2005; **Med School:** NY Med Coll 1972; **Resid:** Pediatrics, Montefiore Med Ctr 1977; **Fellow:** Pediatric Gastroenterology, Mass Genl Hosp 1980; **Fac Appt:** Prof Ped, Harvard Med Sch

Leichtner, Alan M MD [PGe] - **Spec Exp:** Inflammatory Bowel Disease; Celiac Disease; Nutrition; **Hospital:** Children's Hospital - Boston; **Address:** Chldns Hosp, Div Gastroenterology, 300 Longwood Ave, Hunnewell-Ground, Boston, MA 02115; **Phone:** 617-355-2946; **Board Cert:** Pediatrics 1982; Pediatric Gastroenterology 2005; **Med School:** Harvard Med Sch 1977; **Resid:** Pediatrics, Chldn's Hosp 1980; **Fellow:** Pediatric Gastroenterology, Chldn's Hosp 1983; **Fac Appt:** Assoc Prof Ped, Harvard Med Sch

Mid Atlantic

Baker Jr, Robert D MD/PhD [PGe] - **Spec Exp:** Gastroesophageal Reflux Disease (GERD); Cystic Fibrosis; Nutrition; Malabsorption Syndrome; **Hospital:** Women's & Chldn's Hosp of Buffalo, The; **Address:** Childrens Hospital, Div Gastroenterology, 239 Bryant St Fl 2, Buffalo, NY 14222-2006; **Phone:** 716-878-7793; **Board Cert:** Pediatrics 1978; Pediatric Gastroenterology 2010; **Med School:** Temple Univ 1972; **Resid:** Pediatrics, Buffalo Chldns Hosp 1975; **Fellow:** Gastroenterology, Mass Genl Hosp/Chldns Hosp Med Ctr 1983; Nutritional Biochemistry, MIT 1984; **Fac Appt:** Prof Ped, SUNY Buffalo

Baker, Susan S MD/PhD [PGe] - **Spec Exp:** Nutrition; Obesity; Liver Disease; Gastroesophageal Reflux Disease (GERD); **Hospital:** Women's & Chldn's Hosp of Buffalo, The; **Address:** Childrens Hospital, Div Gastroenterology, 239 Bryant St Fl 2, Buffalo, NY 14201-2099; **Phone:** 716-878-7793; **Board Cert:** Pediatrics 1978; Pediatric Gastroenterology 2010; **Med School:** Temple Univ 1972; **Resid:** Pediatrics, Buffalo Chldns Hosp 1975; **Fellow:** Nutrition, MIT 1981; Gastroenterology, Mass Genl Hosp/Harvard 1984; **Fac Appt:** Prof Ped, SUNY Buffalo

Baldassano, Robert N MD [PGe] - **Spec Exp:** Inflammatory Bowel Disease; Ulcerative Colitis; Crohn's Disease; **Hospital:** Chldns Hosp of Philadelphia; **Address:** Chldns Hosp of Philadelphia, GI/Nutrition, 324 S 34th St, Philadelphia, PA 19104-4399; **Phone:** 215-590-3630; **Board Cert:** Pediatric Gastroenterology 2007; **Med School:** SUNY Downstate 1984; **Resid:** Pediatrics, Childrens Hosp 1988; **Fellow:** Pediatric Gastroenterology, Childrens Hosp 1991; **Fac Appt:** Prof Ped, Univ Pennsylvania

Baldridge, Alan D MD [PGe] - **Spec Exp:** Inflammatory Bowel Disease; Celiac Disease; **Hospital:** Cooper Univ Hosp; **Address:** 3 Cooper Plaza, Ste 200, Div Pediatric Gastroenterology, Camden, NJ 08034; **Phone:** 856-342-2001; **Board Cert:** Pediatrics 2008; Pediatric Gastroenterology 2005; **Med School:** Med Coll VA 1988; **Resid:** Pediatrics, Boston City Hosp 1991; **Fellow:** Pediatric Gastroenterology, Mass Genl Hosp 1994; **Fac Appt:** Asst Prof Med, Drexel Univ Coll Med

Benkov, Keith J MD [PGe] - **Spec Exp:** Inflammatory Bowel Disease/Crohn's; Liver Disease; Celiac Disease; **Hospital:** Mount Sinai Med Ctr (page 63), Englewood Hosp & Med Ctr; **Address:** Mt Sinai Div Ped Gastroenterology, 5 E 98th St Fl 10, Box 1656, New York, NY 10029; **Phone:** 212-241-5415; **Board Cert:** Pediatrics 1984; Pediatric Gastroenterology 2005; **Med School:** Mount Sinai Sch Med 1979; **Resid:** Pediatrics, Mt Sinai Hosp 1982; **Fellow:** Pediatric Gastroenterology, Mt Sinai Hosp 1984; **Fac Appt:** Assoc Prof Ped, Mount Sinai Sch Med

Fasano, Alessio MD [PGe] - **Spec Exp:** Celiac Disease; Diarrheal Diseases; Nutrition; **Hospital:** Univ of MD Med Ctr; **Address:** 20 Penn St, rm 351, Baltimore, MD 21201; **Phone:** 410-328-6749; **Med School:** Italy 1981; **Resid:** Pediatrics, Univ Naples 1985; **Fac Appt:** Prof Med, Univ MD Sch Med

Levy, Joseph MD [PGe] - **Spec Exp:** Celiac Disease; Irritable Bowel Syndrome; Gastroesophageal Reflux Disease (GERD); Nutrition in Autism; **Hospital:** NYU Langone Med Ctr (page 66); **Address:** 160 E 32nd St Fl 2, L-2 Medical, New York, NY 10016; **Phone:** 212-263-5407; **Board Cert:** Pediatrics 1981; Pediatric Gastroenterology 2005; **Med School:** Israel 1973; **Resid:** Pediatrics, Beth Israel Med Ctr 1977; **Fellow:** Research, Columbia-Presby Med Ctr 1975; Pediatric Gastroenterology, Columbia-Presby Med Ctr 1979; **Fac Appt:** Prof Ped, NYU Sch Med

Newman, Leonard MD [PGe] - **Spec Exp:** Inflammatory Bowel Disease; Celiac Disease; **Hospital:** Westchester Med Ctr, Children's & Women's Phys.of Westchester; **Address:** NY Med College, Dept Ped, Munger Pavillion - rm 123, Valhalla, NY 10595; **Phone:** 914-367-0000; **Board Cert:** Pediatrics 1975; Pediatric Gastroenterology 1990; **Med School:** NY Med Coll 1970; **Resid:** Pediatrics, UCSD Med Ctr 1972; Pediatrics, NY Med Coll 1973; **Fellow:** Gastroenterology, Bronx Lebanon Hosp/Einstein 1974; **Fac Appt:** Prof Ped, NY Med Coll

Pediatric Gastroenterology

Oliva-Hemker, Maria M MD [PGe] - **Spec Exp:** Inflammatory Bowel Disease/Crohn's; Ulcerative Colitis; Malabsorption Syndrome; **Hospital:** Johns Hopkins Hosp (page 61), Greater Baltimore Med Ctr; **Address:** Johns Hopkins Hosp, Ped GI & Nutrition, 600 N Wolfe St, Brady 320, Baltimore, MD 21287-2631; **Phone:** 410-955-8765; **Board Cert:** Pediatrics 2007; Pediatric Gastroenterology 2007; **Med School:** Johns Hopkins Univ 1986; **Resid:** Pediatrics, Johns Hopkins Hosp 1989; **Fellow:** Gastroenterology, Johns Hopkins Hosp 1992; **Fac Appt:** Assoc Prof Ped, Johns Hopkins Univ

Piccoli, David A MD [PGe] - **Spec Exp:** Liver Disease; **Hospital:** Chldns Hosp of Philadelphia; **Address:** Chlds Hosp of Philadelphia, Div Gastroenterology/Nutrition, 324 S 34th St, Philadelphia, PA 19104; **Phone:** 215-590-3630; **Board Cert:** Pediatrics 1984; Pediatric Gastroenterology 2005; **Med School:** Harvard Med Sch 1979; **Resid:** Pediatrics, Chldns Hosp Med Ctr 1983; **Fellow:** Gastroenterology, Chldns Hosp 1986; **Fac Appt:** Prof Ped, Univ Pennsylvania

Schwarz, Kathleen B MD [PGe] - **Spec Exp:** Hepatitis B & C; Transplant Medicine-Liver; Liver Disease; **Hospital:** Johns Hopkins Hosp (page 61); **Address:** Johns Hopkins Pediatric GI, 600 N Wolfe St, Brady 320, Baltimore, MD 21287-0005; **Phone:** 410-955-8769; **Board Cert:** Pediatrics 1977; Pediatric Gastroenterology 2005; Pediatric Transplant Hepatology 2006; **Med School:** Washington Univ, St Louis 1972; **Resid:** Pediatrics, St Louis Chldns Hosp 1974; **Fellow:** Pediatric Gastroenterology, St Louis Chldns Hosp 1976; **Fac Appt:** Prof Ped, Johns Hopkins Univ

Schwarz, Steven M MD [PGe] - **Spec Exp:** Gastroesophageal Reflux Disease (GERD); Nutrition; Endoscopy; Inflammatory Bowel Disease; **Hospital:** SUNY Downstate Med Ctr, Beth Israel Med Ctr - Petrie Division (page 55); **Address:** Children's Hosp at SUNY Downstate, 445 Lenox Rd, Box 49, Brooklyn, NY 11203; **Phone:** 718-270-4714; **Board Cert:** Pediatrics 1979; Pediatric Gastroenterology 2005; **Med School:** Columbia P&S 1974; **Resid:** Pediatrics, Columbia-Presby Med Ctr 1977; **Fellow:** Pediatric Gastroenterology, Stanford Univ Med Ctr 1978; Pediatric Gastroenterology, Columbia-Presby Med Ctr 1980; **Fac Appt:** Prof Ped, SUNY Downstate

Snyder, John David MD [PGe] - **Spec Exp:** Celiac Disease; Gastroesophageal Reflux Disease (GERD); **Hospital:** Chldns Natl Med Ctr; **Address:** Children's National Med Ctr, 11 Michigan Ave NW, Washington, DC 20010; **Phone:** 202-476-5000; **Board Cert:** Pediatrics 1982; Pediatric Gastroenterology 2005; **Med School:** UCLA 1975; **Resid:** Pediatrics, Duke Univ Med Ctr 1978; **Fellow:** Pediatric Gastroenterology, Mass Genl Hosp 1984

Spivak, William MD [PGe] - **Spec Exp:** Inflammatory Bowel Disease/Crohn's; Ulcerative Colitis; Gastroesophageal Reflux Disease (GERD); Feeding Disorders; **Hospital:** NY-Presby/Weill Cornell Med Ctr, NY (page 65), Lenox Hill Hosp; **Address:** 177 E 87th St, Ste 305, New York, NY 10128; **Phone:** 212-369-7700; **Board Cert:** Pediatrics 1981; Pediatric Gastroenterology 2005; **Med School:** Albert Einstein Coll Med 1976; **Resid:** Pediatrics, Jacobi Med Ctr 1979; **Fellow:** Gastroenterology, Childrens Hosp 1982; Research, Brigham & Womens Hosp 1982; **Fac Appt:** Clin Prof Ped, Cornell Univ-Weill Med Coll

Squires, Robert H MD [PGe] - **Spec Exp:** Liver Disease; Intestinal Disorders; **Hospital:** Chldns Hosp of Pittsburgh - UPMC; **Address:** Children's Hosp Pittsburgh, Pediatric Gastroenterology, 4401 Penn Ave, Pittsburgh, PA 15201; **Phone:** 412-692-5180; **Board Cert:** Pediatrics 1981; Pediatric Gastroenterology 2005; Pediatric Transplant Hepatology 2006; **Med School:** Univ Tex Med Br, Galveston 1977; **Resid:** Pediatrics, Children's Hosp 1979; **Fellow:** Pediatric Gastroenterology, Children's Hosp 1982; **Fac Appt:** Prof Ped, Univ Pittsburgh

Southeast

Black, Dennis D MD [PGe] - **Spec Exp:** Nutrition; Obesity; **Hospital:** Le Bonheur Chldns Med Ctr; **Address:** 777 Washington Ave, Ste P110, Memphis, TN 38105; **Phone:** 901-448-2000; **Board Cert:** Pediatrics 1983; Pediatric Gastroenterology 2005; **Med School:** Univ Tenn Coll Med 1978; **Resid:** Pediatrics, Le Bonheur Chldns Med Ctr 1981; **Fellow:** Pediatric Gastroenterology, Univ Tenn Hlth Sci Ctr 1984; **Fac Appt:** Prof Ped, Univ Tenn Coll Med

Hill, Ivor D MD [PGe] - **Spec Exp:** Celiac Disease; Inflammatory Bowel Disease; Malabsorption Syndrome; Diarrheal Diseases; **Hospital:** Wake Forest Univ Baptist Med Ctr; **Address:** Wake Forest Univ Sch Med, Div Pediatric Gastroenterology, Medical Center Blvd, Winston-Salem, NC 27157; **Phone:** 336-716-3009; **Board Cert:** Pediatrics 2007; Pediatric Gastroenterology 2003; **Med School:** South Africa 1972; **Resid:** Pediatrics, Addington Hosp 1976; Pediatrics, Red Cross Chldns Hosp 1977; **Fellow:** Pediatric Gastroenterology, Red Cross Chlds Hosp 1980; **Fac Appt:** Prof Ped, Wake Forest Univ

Novak, Donald A MD [PGe] - **Spec Exp:** Liver Disease; **Hospital:** Shands at Univ of FL; **Address:** UF Pediatrics, 1600 SW Archer Rd, rm RG120, Gainesville, FL 32610; **Phone:** 352-273-9350; **Board Cert:** Pediatrics 1988; Pediatric Gastroenterology 2010; **Med School:** Univ S Fla Coll Med 1981; **Resid:** Pediatrics, Univ South Fla 1984; **Fellow:** Pediatric Gastroenterology, Chldn's Hosp 1987; **Fac Appt:** Prof Ped, Univ Fla Coll Med

Ulshen, Martin H MD [PGe] - **Spec Exp:** Liver Disease; Inflammatory Bowel Disease; Irritable Bowel Syndrome; **Hospital:** Duke Univ Hosp; **Address:** Duke Univ Med Ctr, Box 102375, Durham, NC 27710; **Phone:** 919-684-5068; **Board Cert:** Pediatrics 1993; Pediatric Gastroenterology 2005; **Med School:** Univ Rochester 1969; **Resid:** Pediatrics, Univ Colorado Med Ctr 1974; **Fellow:** Pediatric Gastroenterology, Univ Colorado Med Ctr 1975; Pediatric Gastroenterology, Chldns Hosp 1977; **Fac Appt:** Prof Ped, Duke Univ

Midwest

Berman, James MD [PGe] - **Spec Exp:** Inflammatory Bowel Disease/Crohn's; Nutrition; Ulcerative Colitis; **Hospital:** Loyola Univ Med Ctr, Adv Luth Genl Hosp; **Address:** Loyola Univ Med Ctr, Dept Ped Gastro, 2160 S 1st Ave Bldg 105 Fl 3, Outpatient Ctr, Maywood, IL 60153-3304; **Phone:** 708-327-9073; **Board Cert:** Pediatrics 1986; Pediatric Gastroenterology 2005; **Med School:** Univ Pittsburgh 1981; **Resid:** Pediatrics, Chldns Hosp 1984; **Fellow:** Pediatric Gastroenterology, Mass Genl Hosp/Chldns Hosp 1987; **Fac Appt:** Asst Prof Ped, Loyola Univ-Stritch Sch Med

Bishop, Warren P MD [PGe] - **Spec Exp:** Liver Disease; Constipation; Diarrheal Diseases; Inflammatory Bowel Disease; **Hospital:** Univ Iowa Hosp & Clinics; **Address:** UIHC Dept of Pediatrics, GI, 200 Hawkins Drive 2869 JPP, Iowa City, IA 52242; **Phone:** 319-356-2229; **Board Cert:** Pediatrics 1984; Pediatric Gastroenterology 2005; **Med School:** Univ Wisc 1979; **Resid:** Pediatrics, Univ Michigan Hlth Sys 1982; **Fellow:** Pediatric Gastroenterology, Univ NC Affil Hosp 1989; **Fac Appt:** Prof Ped, Univ Iowa Coll Med

Cohen, Mitchell B MD [PGe] - **Spec Exp:** Inflammatory Bowel Disease; Diarrheal Diseases; Celiac Disease; **Hospital:** Cincinnati Chldns Hosp Med Ctr; **Address:** Chldns Hosp Med Ctr, Gastroenterology Div, 3333 Burnet Ave, MC 2010, Cincinnati, OH 45229; **Phone:** 513-636-4415; **Board Cert:** Pediatrics 1981; Pediatric Gastroenterology 2005; **Med School:** Mount Sinai Sch Med 1977; **Resid:** Pediatrics, Johns Hopkins Hosp 1980; **Fellow:** Pediatric Gastroenterology, Chldns Hosp Med Ctr 1986; **Fac Appt:** Prof Ped, Univ Cincinnati

Pediatric Gastroenterology

Di Lorenzo, Carlo MD [PGe] - **Spec Exp:** Gastrointestinal Motility Disorders; Gastrointestinal Functional Disorders; **Hospital:** Nationwide Chldn's Hosp; **Address:** Nationwide Children's Hospital, Div Gastroenterology & Nutrition, 700 Children's Drive, Columbus, OH 43205; **Phone:** 614-722-3450; **Board Cert:** Pediatric Gastroenterology 2005; **Med School:** Italy 1984; **Resid:** Pediatrics, Univ Naples Medical Ctr 1988; **Fellow:** Pediatric Gastroenterology, Harbor-UCLA Medical Ctr 1989; **Fac Appt:** Prof Ped, Ohio State Univ

El-Youssef, Mounif MD [PGe] - **Spec Exp:** Liver Disease; **Hospital:** Mayo Med Ctr & Clin - Rochester; **Address:** Mayo Clinic, Div Ped Gastroenterology, 200 First St SW, Rochester, MN 55905; **Phone:** 507-284-2141; **Board Cert:** Pediatric Gastroenterology 2005; Pediatric Transplant Hepatology 2008; **Med School:** Belgium 1982; **Resid:** Pediatrics, Cleveland Clin 1987; **Fellow:** Pediatric Gastroenterology, Harvard Med Sch 1990

Guandalini, Stefano MD [PGe] - **Spec Exp:** Celiac Disease; Digestive Disorders; Diarrheal Diseases; **Hospital:** Univ Chicago-Comer Chldn's Hosp; **Address:** Univ Chicago Med Ctr, 5841 S Maryland Ave, MC 4065, Chicago, IL 60637; **Phone:** 773-702-6418; **Med School:** Italy ; **Resid:** Pediatrics, Univ Messina Affil Hosp; **Fellow:** Pediatric Gastroenterology, Univ Naples Affil Hosp; **Fac Appt:** Prof Ped, Univ Chicago-Pritzker Sch Med

Gunasekaran, T S MD [PGe] - **Spec Exp:** Gastroesophageal Reflux Disease (GERD); Esophageal Disorders; Inflammatory Bowel Disease; Pain-Abdominal Recurrent; **Hospital:** Adv Luth Genl Hosp, Loyola Univ Med Ctr; **Address:** Lutheran Genl Chldns Hosp, Dept Ped GI, 1675 Dempster St, Park Ridge, IL 60068; **Phone:** 847-723-7700; **Board Cert:** Pediatric Gastroenterology 2007; **Med School:** India 1977; **Resid:** Pediatrics 1982; Pediatrics 1987; **Fellow:** Pediatric Gastroenterology, BC Childrens Hosp 1992; **Fac Appt:** Assoc Clin Prof Ped, Loyola Univ-Stritch Sch Med

Gupta, Sandeep K MD [PGe] - **Spec Exp:** Eosinophilic Esophagitis; Gastroesophageal Reflux Disease (GERD); Nutrition; Obesity; **Hospital:** Riley Hosp for Children; **Address:** Riley Hosp for Children, Div Pediatric Gastroenterology, 705 Riley Hospital Drive, ROC 4210, Indianapolis, IN 46202; **Phone:** 317-944-3774; **Board Cert:** Pediatric Gastroenterology 2005; **Med School:** Nigeria 1986; **Resid:** Pediatrics, Univ Conn Hlth Ctr; **Fellow:** Pediatric Gastroenterology, Indiana Univ; **Fac Appt:** Clin Prof Ped, Indiana Univ

Kirschner, Barbara S MD [PGe] - **Spec Exp:** Ulcerative Colitis; Pain-Abdominal Recurrent; Inflammatory Bowel Disease/Crohn's; **Hospital:** Univ Chicago-Comer Chldn's Hosp; **Address:** Univ Chicago Med Ctr, 5839 S Maryland Ave, MC 4065, Chicago, IL 60637; **Phone:** 773-702-6418; **Board Cert:** Pediatrics 1972; Pediatric Gastroenterology 2005; **Med School:** Med Coll PA 1967; **Resid:** Pediatrics, Univ Chicago Hosps 1970; **Fellow:** Pediatric Gastroenterology, Univ Chicago Hosps 1977; **Fac Appt:** Prof Ped, Univ Chicago-Pritzker Sch Med

Molleston, Jean P MD [PGe] - **Spec Exp:** Liver Disease; Hepatitis; Transplant Medicine-Liver; Graft vs Host Disease; **Hospital:** Riley Hosp for Children, IU Health North Hosp; **Address:** Indiana Univ-Riley Chldns Hosp, Div Ped Gastroenterology, 705 Riley Hospital Drive, ROC 4210, Indianapolis, IN 46202-5225; **Phone:** 317-944-3774; **Board Cert:** Pediatrics 2009; Pediatric Gastroenterology 2010; Pediatric Transplant Hepatology 2006; **Med School:** Washington Univ, St Louis 1986; **Resid:** Pediatrics, Chldns Hosp 1988; **Fellow:** Pediatric Gastroenterology, Washington Univ 1991; **Fac Appt:** Clin Prof Ped, Indiana Univ

Mousa, Hayat M MD [PGe] - **Spec Exp:** Gastroesophageal Reflux Disease (GERD); Gastrointestinal Motility Disorders; Gastrointestinal Functional Disorders; **Hospital:** Nationwide Chldn's Hosp; **Address:** Nationwide Children's Hospital, Div Gastroenterology & Nutrition, 700 Children's Drive, Columbus, OH 43205; **Phone:** 614-722-3450; **Board Cert:** Pediatric Gastroenterology 2007; **Med School:** Syria 1982; **Resid:** Pediatrics, Henry Ford Hosp 1993; **Fellow:** Pediatric Gastroenterology, Chldns Hosp 1998; **Fac Appt:** Assoc Clin Prof Ped, Ohio State Univ

Rothbaum, Robert J MD [PGe] - **Spec Exp:** Inflammatory Bowel Disease; **Hospital:** St. Louis Chldns Hosp, Barnes-Jewish Hosp; **Address:** 1 Children's Pl, NWT Bldg Fl 9, Box 8116, St Louis, MO 63110; **Phone:** 314-454-6173; **Board Cert:** Pediatrics 1981; Pediatric Gastroenterology 2005; **Med School:** Univ Chicago-Pritzker Sch Med 1976; **Resid:** Pediatrics, St Louis Chldns Hosp 1978; **Fellow:** Ambulatory Pediatrics, St Louis Chldns Hosp 1979; Pediatric Gastroenterology, Chldns Hosp Med Ctr 1982; **Fac Appt:** Prof Ped, Washington Univ, St Louis

Rudolph, Colin D MD [PGe] - **Spec Exp:** Feeding Disorders; Nutrition; Gastrointestinal Motility Disorders; Gastrointestinal Functional Disorders; **Hospital:** Chldns Hosp - Wisconsin; **Address:** 9000 W Wisconsin Ave, Milwaukee, WI 53201; **Phone:** 414-266-3690; **Board Cert:** Pediatrics 1987; Pediatric Gastroenterology 2005; **Med School:** Case West Res Univ 1982; **Resid:** Pediatrics, Chldn's Hosp 1984; **Fellow:** Pediatric Gastroenterology, UCSF Med Ctr 1986; **Fac Appt:** Assoc Prof Ped, Univ Wisc

Whitington, Peter F MD [PGe] - **Spec Exp:** Transplant Medicine-Liver; Liver Disease; **Hospital:** Children's Mem Hosp -Chicago; **Address:** Chldns Meml Hosp, Div Ped Gastro, 2300 Children's Plaza, Box 57, Chicago, IL 60614; **Phone:** 773-880-4643; **Board Cert:** Pediatrics 1977; Pediatric Gastroenterology 2005; Pediatric Transplant Hepatology 2006; **Med School:** Univ Tenn Coll Med 1971; **Resid:** Pediatrics, Univ Tenn Hosp 1975; **Fellow:** Gastroenterology, Johns Hopkins Hosp 1977; Gastroenterology, Univ Wisconsin Affil Hosp 1978; **Fac Appt:** Prof Ped, Northwestern Univ

Wyllie, Robert MD [PGe] - **Spec Exp:** Inflammatory Bowel Disease/Crohn's; Ulcerative Colitis; **Hospital:** Cleveland Clin (page 56); **Address:** Cleveland Clinic, 9500 Euclid Ave, Desk A111, Cleveland, OH 44195; **Phone:** 216-444-2237; **Board Cert:** Pediatrics 1982; Pediatric Gastroenterology 2005; **Med School:** Indiana Univ 1976; **Resid:** Pediatrics, Indiana Univ Med Ctr 1979; **Fellow:** Pediatric Gastroenterology, Indiana Univ Med Ctr 1980

Great Plains and Mountains

Hoffenberg, Edward J MD [PGe] - **Spec Exp:** Inflammatory Bowel Disease; Celiac Disease; Liver Disease; Pancreatic Disease; **Hospital:** Chldn's Hosp - Aurora (CO); **Address:** Chldns Hosp-Div Gastroenterology, 13123 E 16th Ave, Box B290, Aurora, CO 80045; **Phone:** 303-777-6669; **Board Cert:** Pediatric Gastroenterology 2007; **Med School:** Case West Res Univ 1986; **Resid:** Pediatrics, Rainbow Babies & Chldns Hosp 1989; **Fellow:** Pediatric Gastroenterology, Chldns Hosp 1992; **Fac Appt:** Assoc Prof Ped, Univ Colorado

Krebs, Nancy F MD [PGe] - **Spec Exp:** Obesity; Nutrition; Weight Management; **Hospital:** Chldn's Hosp - Aurora (CO); **Address:** 12700 E 19th Ave, Box C225, Aurora, CO 80045; **Phone:** 303-724-3260; **Board Cert:** Pediatrics 2009; Pediatric Gastroenterology 2010; **Med School:** Univ Colorado 1987; **Resid:** Pediatrics, Univ Colorado Affil Hosp 1990; **Fellow:** Pediatric Gastroenterology, Univ Colorado 1992; Nutrition, Univ Colorado 1993; **Fac Appt:** Prof Ped, Univ Colorado

Narkewicz, Michael R MD [PGe] - **Spec Exp:** Transplant Medicine-Liver; Liver Disease; **Hospital:** Chldn's Hosp - Aurora (CO); **Address:** Children's Hospital, Dept Liver Disease and Nutrition, 13123 E 16th Ave, Aurora, CO 80045; **Phone:** 720-777-6669; **Board Cert:** Pediatrics 1988; Pediatric Gastroenterology 2005; Pediatric Transplant Hepatology 2006; **Med School:** Univ VT Coll Med 1983; **Resid:** Pediatrics, Univ Colorado Med Ctr 1986; **Fellow:** Pediatric Gastroenterology, Univ Colorado Med Ctr 1989; **Fac Appt:** Prof Ped, Univ Colorado

Pediatric Gastroenterology

Sokol, Ronald Jay MD [PGe] - **Spec Exp:** Liver Disease; **Hospital:** Chldn's Hosp - Aurora (CO); **Address:** Chldn's Hosp-Gastro, Hepatol, Nutrition, 13123 E 16th Ave, Ste B290, Aurora, CO 80045; **Phone:** 720-777-6669; **Board Cert:** Pediatrics 1981; Pediatric Gastroenterology 2005; Pediatric Transplant Hepatology 2010; **Med School:** Univ Chicago-Pritzker Sch Med 1976; **Resid:** Pediatrics, Univ Colo Med Ctr 1980; **Fellow:** Pediatric Gastroenterology, Chldns Hosp 1983; **Fac Appt:** Prof Ped, Univ Colorado

Suchy, Frederick J MD [PGe] - **Spec Exp:** Hepatitis; Liver Disease; Neonatal Cholestasis; **Hospital:** Chldn's Hosp - Aurora (CO); **Address:** Children's Hosp Colorado, 13123 E 16th Ave, Box B290, Aurora, CO 80045; **Phone:** 720-777-6669; **Board Cert:** Pediatrics 1982; Pediatric Gastroenterology 2005; Pediatric Transplant Hepatology 2006; **Med School:** Univ Cincinnati 1974; **Resid:** Pediatrics, Chldns Hosp Med Ctr 1978; **Fellow:** Pediatric Gastroenterology, Chldns Hosp Med Ctr 1981; **Fac Appt:** Prof Ped, Mount Sinai Sch Med

Vanderhoof, Jon A MD [PGe] - **Spec Exp:** Nutrition; Short Bowel Syndrome; **Hospital:** Boys Town Natl Rsch Hosp, Children's Hosp - Omaha; **Address:** Boystown Hosp & Clin, 14040 Hosp Rd, Boystown, NE 68010; **Phone:** 402-778-6820; **Board Cert:** Pediatrics 1993; Pediatric Gastroenterology 2005; **Med School:** Univ Nebr Coll Med 1972; **Resid:** Pediatrics, Univ Nebr Coll Med 1974; **Fellow:** Pediatric Gastroenterology, UCLA Med Ctr 1976; **Fac Appt:** Prof Ped, Univ Nebr Coll Med

Southwest

Rhoads, J Marc MD [PGe] - **Spec Exp:** Diarrheal Diseases; Inflammatory Bowel Disease; Intestinal Disorders; **Hospital:** Meml Hermann Hosp - Texas Med Ctr; **Address:** Univ Texas Hlth Sci Ctr, Dept Pediatrics-Gastroenterology, 6410 Fannin St, Ste 500, Houston, TX 77030; **Phone:** 832-325-6516; **Board Cert:** Pediatrics 1986; Pediatric Gastroenterology 2005; **Med School:** Johns Hopkins Univ 1980; **Resid:** Pediatrics, UCLA Med Ctr 1983; **Fellow:** Pediatric Gastroenterology, Hosp for Sick Chldn 1986; **Fac Appt:** Prof Ped, Univ Tex, Houston

West Coast and Pacific

Christie, Dennis L MD [PGe] - **Spec Exp:** Inflammatory Bowel Disease; **Hospital:** Seattle Chldns Hosp; **Address:** Chldns Hosp Med Ctr, Div Gastroenterology, 4800 Sand Point Way NE, MS 7830, Seattle, WA 98105-3901; **Phone:** 206-987-2521; **Board Cert:** Pediatrics 1992; Pediatric Gastroenterology 2005; **Med School:** Northwestern Univ 1968; **Resid:** Pediatrics, Univ Wash Med Ctr 1971; **Fellow:** Pediatric Gastroenterology, UCLA Ctr Hlth Sci 1976; **Fac Appt:** Prof Ped, Univ Wash

Dubinsky, Marla C MD [PGe] - **Spec Exp:** Inflammatory Bowel Disease; Crohn's Disease; Ulcerative Colitis; Clinical Trials; **Hospital:** Cedars-Sinai Med Ctr; **Address:** 8635 W 3rd St, Ste 1165W, Los Angeles, CA 90048; **Phone:** 310-423-7100; **Board Cert:** Pediatric Gastroenterology 2009; **Med School:** Canada 1993; **Fac Appt:** Asst Prof Ped, UCLA

Heyman, Melvin B MD [PGe] - **Spec Exp:** Inflammatory Bowel Disease/Crohn's; Short Bowel Syndrome; Gastroesophageal Reflux Disease (GERD); Gastrointestinal Functional Disorders; **Hospital:** UCSF Med Ctr; **Address:** UCSF, Dept Ped Gastroenterology, 500 Parnassus Ave, Ste MU 406E, Box 0136, San Francisco, CA 94143-0136; **Phone:** 415-476-5892; **Board Cert:** Pediatrics 1981; Pediatric Gastroenterology 2005; **Med School:** UCLA 1976; **Resid:** Pediatrics, LAC-USC Med Ctr 1979; **Fellow:** Gastroenterology, UCLA Med Ctr 1981; Nutrition, Human Nutrition Res Ctr 1990; **Fac Appt:** Prof Ped, UCSF

McDiarmid, Suzanne V MD [PGe] - **Spec Exp:** Transplant Medicine-Liver; Transplant Medicine-Bowel; Transplant Immunology; Liver Disease; **Hospital:** UCLA Ronald Reagan Med Ctr; **Address:** UCLA Pediatric Gastroenterology, 18033 Le Conte Ave, Room 12-383 MDCC, Los Angeles, CA 90095; **Phone:** 310-206-6136; **Board Cert:** Pediatrics 1984; Pediatric Gastroenterology 2007; **Med School:** New Zealand 1976; **Resid:** Pediatrics, Chldns Hosp Kings Daughters 1982; Pediatrics, Valley Med Ctr 1983; **Fellow:** Pediatric Gastroenterology, UCLA 1988; **Fac Appt:** Prof Ped, UCLA

Murray, Karen MD [PGe] - **Spec Exp:** Transplant Medicine-Liver; Liver Disease; Hepatitis B & C; **Hospital:** Seattle Chldns Hosp; **Address:** Gastroenterology, MS 7830, 4800 Sand Point Way NE, Seattle, WA 98105; **Phone:** 206-987-2521; **Board Cert:** Pediatrics 2008; Pediatric Gastroenterology 2005; Transplant Hepatology 2006; **Med School:** Johns Hopkins Univ 1990; **Resid:** Pediatrics, Chldn's Hosp & Med Ctr 1993; **Fellow:** Gastroenterology, Chldn's Hosp 1996; **Fac Appt:** Prof Med, Univ Wash

PEDIATRIC HEMATOLOGY-ONCOLOGY

New England

Altman, Arnold MD [PHO] - **Spec Exp:** Leukemia; **Hospital:** CT Chldns Med Ctr; **Address:** CT Childrens Med Ctr, Hematology/Oncology, 282 Washington St, Ste 2J, Hartford, CT 06106; **Phone:** 860-545-9630; **Board Cert:** Pediatrics 1971; Pediatric Hematology-Oncology 1974; **Med School:** Johns Hopkins Univ 1965; **Resid:** Pediatrics, Chldns Hosp Med Ctr 1970; **Fellow:** Pediatric Hematology-Oncology, Chldns Hosp Med Ctr 1972; **Fac Appt:** Prof Ped, Univ Conn

Billett, Amy L MD [PHO] - **Spec Exp:** Hodgkin's Disease; Lymphoma, Non-Hodgkin's; **Hospital:** Children's Hospital - Boston; **Address:** 450 Brookline Ave, Boston, MA 02215; **Phone:** 617-632-5640; **Board Cert:** Pediatric Hematology-Oncology 2009; **Med School:** Harvard Med Sch 1984; **Resid:** Pediatrics, Univ Wash Affil Hosps 1987; **Fellow:** Pediatric Hematology-Oncology, Children's Hosp 1990; **Fac Appt:** Assoc Prof Ped, Harvard Med Sch

Diller, Lisa R MD [PHO] - **Spec Exp:** Neuroblastoma; Cancer Survivors-Late Effects of Therapy; **Hospital:** Children's Hospital - Boston, Dana-Farber Cancer Inst (page 57); **Address:** Dana-Farber Cancer Inst, 450 Brookline Ave, MS SW 312, Boston, MA 02115; **Phone:** 617-632-5642; **Board Cert:** Pediatric Hematology-Oncology 2007; **Med School:** UCSD 1985; **Resid:** Pediatrics, Chldns Hosp 1988; **Fellow:** Pediatric Hematology-Oncology, Chldns Hosp-Dana Farber Cancer Inst 1991; **Fac Appt:** Assoc Prof Ped, Harvard Med Sch

Guinan, Eva C MD [PHO] - **Spec Exp:** Bone Marrow Transplant; **Hospital:** Dana-Farber Cancer Inst (page 57), Children's Hospital - Boston; **Address:** Dana Faber Cancer Inst, 44 Binney St, Boston, MA 02115; **Phone:** 617-632-4932; **Board Cert:** Pediatrics 1986; Pediatric Hematology-Oncology 1998; **Med School:** Harvard Med Sch 1980; **Resid:** Internal Medicine, Children's Hosp 1982; **Fellow:** Pediatric Hematology-Oncology, Dana Farber Cancer Inst 1985; **Fac Appt:** Assoc Prof Med, Harvard Med Sch

Homans, Alan C MD [PHO] - **Spec Exp:** Leukemia; **Hospital:** Fletcher Allen Health Care-Med Ctr Campus; **Address:** Fletcher Allen Healthcare, 111 Colchester Ave Smith Bldg - Ste 559A, Burlington, VT 05401; **Phone:** 802-847-2850; **Board Cert:** Pediatrics 1985; Pediatric Hematology-Oncology 1987; **Med School:** Ohio State Univ 1979; **Resid:** Pediatrics, Med Ctr Hosp 1981; Pediatrics, Univ Mass Med Ctr 1982; **Fellow:** Pediatric Hematology-Oncology, Rhode Island Hosp 1985; **Fac Appt:** Prof Ped, Univ VT Coll Med

Pediatric Hematology-Oncology

Kieran, Mark W MD/PhD [PHO] - **Spec Exp:** Brain Tumors; Neuro-Oncology; **Hospital:** Dana-Farber Cancer Inst (page 57), Children's Hospital - Boston; **Address:** Dana Farber Cancer Inst, 44 Binney St, Shields Warren Ste 331, Boston, MA 02115; **Phone:** 617-632-4386; **Board Cert:** Pediatric Hematology-Oncology 2004; **Med School:** Univ Calgary 1986; **Resid:** Pediatrics, Montreal Chldns Hosp 1992; **Fellow:** Pediatric Hematology-Oncology, Chldns Hosp 1995; **Fac Appt:** Asst Prof Ped, Harvard Med Sch

Sallan, Stephen E MD [PHO] - **Spec Exp:** Pediatric Cancers; Leukemia; **Hospital:** Children's Hospital - Boston, Dana-Farber Cancer Inst (page 57); **Address:** Dana Farber Cancer Inst, 450 Brookline Ave, MS Dana 1642, Boston, MA 02215; **Phone:** 617-632-5508; **Board Cert:** Pediatrics 1972; **Med School:** Wayne State Univ 1967; **Resid:** Pediatrics, Chldns Hosp 1969; Pediatrics, Hosp Sick Chldn 1970; **Fellow:** Pediatric Oncology, Chldns Hosp Med Ctr 1975; **Fac Appt:** Prof Ped, Harvard Med Sch

Schwartz, Cindy Lee MD [PHO] - **Spec Exp:** Hodgkin's Disease; Bone Cancer; Cancer Survivors-Late Effects of Therapy; **Hospital:** Rhode Island Hosp; **Address:** RI Hospital, Div Ped Hem/Onc, 593 Eddy St, MPS rm 117, Providence, RI 02903-4923; **Phone:** 401-444-5171; **Board Cert:** Pediatrics 1985; Pediatric Hematology-Oncology 2009; **Med School:** Brown Univ 1979; **Resid:** Pediatrics, Johns Hopkins Hosp 1982; **Fellow:** Pediatric Hematology-Oncology, Johns Hopkins Hosp 1985; **Fac Appt:** Prof Med, Brown Univ

van Hoff, Jack MD [PHO] - **Spec Exp:** Brain Tumors; Clinical Trials; **Hospital:** Dartmouth - Hitchcock Med Ctr; **Address:** DHMC, Dept Pediatric Hem/Onc, One Medical Center Drive, Lebanon, NH 03756; **Phone:** 603-650-5541; **Board Cert:** Pediatrics 1985; Pediatric Hematology-Oncology 1987; **Med School:** UMDNJ-NJ Med Sch, Newark 1981; **Resid:** Pediatrics, Yale New Haven Hosp 1984; **Fellow:** Pediatric Hematology-Oncology, Yale New Haven Hosp 1986

Weinstein, Howard J MD [PHO] - **Spec Exp:** Bone Marrow Transplant; Leukemia; Lymphoma; **Hospital:** Mass Genl Hosp, Dana-Farber Cancer Inst (page 57); **Address:** 55 Fruit St, Yawkey 8B-8893, Boston, MA 02114-2622; **Phone:** 617-724-3315; **Board Cert:** Pediatrics 1977; **Med School:** Univ MD Sch Med 1972; **Resid:** Pediatrics, Mass Genl Hosp 1974; **Fellow:** Pediatric Hematology-Oncology, Dana Farber Cancer Inst/Chldns Hosp 1977; **Fac Appt:** Prof Ped, Harvard Med Sch

Mid Atlantic

Adamson, Peter C MD [PHO] - **Spec Exp:** Drug Development; Clinical Trials; Rhabdomyosarcoma; Pediatric Cancers; **Hospital:** Chldns Hosp of Philadelphia; **Address:** Chldns Hosp of Philadelphia, Div Onc, 34th St & Civic Ctr Blvd Abramson Bldg, Philadelphia, PA 19104; **Phone:** 215-590-3025; **Board Cert:** Pediatric Hematology-Oncology 2005; **Med School:** Cornell Univ-Weill Med Coll 1984; **Resid:** Pediatrics, Chldns Hosp 1987; **Fellow:** Pediatric Hematology-Oncology, Natl Cancer Inst 1990; **Fac Appt:** Clin Prof Ped, Univ Pennsylvania

Aledo, Alexander MD [PHO] - **Spec Exp:** Leukemia; Lymphoma; Bone Tumors; **Hospital:** NY-Presby/Weill Cornell Med Ctr, NY (page 65), NY Hosp Queens; **Address:** 525 E 68th St, rm P695, New York, NY 10021-4870; **Phone:** 212-746-3447; **Board Cert:** Pediatric Hematology-Oncology 2004; **Med School:** NYU Sch Med 1984; **Resid:** Pediatrics, NY Hosp 1987; **Fellow:** Pediatric Hematology-Oncology, Meml Sloan Kettering Cancer Ctr 1990; **Fac Appt:** Assoc Clin Prof Ped, Cornell Univ-Weill Med Coll

Angiolillo, Anne L MD [PHO] - **Spec Exp:** Leukemia; Lymphoma; **Hospital:** Chldns Natl Med Ctr; **Address:** Chldns Natl Med Ctr-Hem/Onc, 111 Michigan Ave NW, Washington, DC 20010; **Phone:** 202-884-2800; **Board Cert:** Pediatrics 2001; Pediatric Hematology-Oncology 2004; **Med School:** NY Med Coll 1989; **Resid:** Pediatrics, Chldns Natl Med Ctr 1992; **Fellow:** Pediatric Hematology-Oncology, Chldns Natl Med Ctr 1995

Arceci, Robert J MD/PhD [PHO] - **Spec Exp:** Leukemia; Histiocytoma; Bone Marrow Transplant; **Hospital:** Johns Hopkins Hosp (page 61); **Address:** Kimmel Cancer Ctr, Bunting-Blaustein Bldg, 1650 Orleans St, I-207, Baltimore, MD 21231; **Phone:** 410-502-7519; **Board Cert:** Pediatrics 1987; Pediatric Hematology-Oncology 2005; **Med School:** Univ Rochester 1981; **Resid:** Pediatrics, Chldns Hosp 1983; **Fellow:** Pediatric Hematology-Oncology, Chldns Hosp/Dana Farber Cancer Ctr 1986; **Fac Appt:** Prof Ped, Johns Hopkins Univ

Brecher, Martin L MD [PHO] - **Spec Exp:** Brain Tumors; Lymphoma; Hodgkin's Disease; Leukemia; **Hospital:** Roswell Park Cancer Inst, Women's & Chldn's Hosp of Buffalo, The; **Address:** Roswell Park Cancer Inst, Dept Pediatrics, Elm & Carlton Sts, Buffalo, NY 14263; **Phone:** 716-845-2333; **Board Cert:** Pediatrics 1977; Pediatric Hematology-Oncology 1978; **Med School:** SUNY Buffalo 1972; **Resid:** Pediatrics, Buffalo Chldns Hosp 1975; **Fellow:** Hematology & Oncology, Buffalo Chldns Hosp/Roswell Park Cancer Inst 1977; **Fac Appt:** Assoc Prof Ped, SUNY Buffalo

Bussel, James MD [PHO] - **Spec Exp:** Autoimmune Disease; Bleeding/Coagulation Disorders; Platelet Disorders; Wiskott-Aldrich Syndrome; **Hospital:** NY-Presby/Weill Cornell Med Ctr, NY (page 65), Lenox Hill Hosp; **Address:** 525 E 68th St, rm P-695, New York, NY 10065; **Phone:** 212-746-3474; **Board Cert:** Pediatrics 1979; Pediatric Hematology-Oncology 1980; **Med School:** Columbia P&S 1975; **Resid:** Pediatrics, Chldns Hosp 1978; **Fellow:** Pediatric Hematology-Oncology, NY Presby Hosp/Cornell 1981; **Fac Appt:** Prof Ped, Cornell Univ-Weill Med Coll

Cairo, Mitchell S MD [PHO] - **Spec Exp:** Bone Marrow Transplant; Stem Cell Transplant; Leukemia; Lymphoma; **Hospital:** Westchester Med Ctr; **Address:** New York Medical College, Munger Pavilion, rm 110, Valhalla, NY 10595; **Phone:** 914-594-3650; **Board Cert:** Pediatrics 1980; Pediatric Hematology-Oncology 1982; **Med School:** UCSF 1976; **Resid:** Pediatrics, UCLA Med Ctr 1979; **Fellow:** Pediatric Hematology-Oncology, Indiana Univ Med Ctr 1981; **Fac Appt:** Prof Ped, NY Med Coll

Carroll, William L MD [PHO] - **Spec Exp:** Leukemia; **Hospital:** NYU Langone Med Ctr (page 66); **Address:** NYU Med Ctr, Div Ped Hem/Onc, 160 E 32nd St, Fl 2, New York, NY 10016; **Phone:** 212-263-8400; **Board Cert:** Pediatrics 1984; Pediatric Hematology-Oncology 1987; **Med School:** UC Irvine 1978; **Resid:** Pediatrics, Chldns Hosp Med Ctr 1981; **Fellow:** Pediatric Hematology-Oncology, Stanford Univ 1987; **Fac Appt:** Prof Ped, NYU Sch Med

Chen, Allen R MD/PhD [PHO] - **Spec Exp:** Bone Marrow Transplant; Hodgkin's Disease; Immunotherapy; Graft vs Host Disease; **Hospital:** Johns Hopkins Hosp (page 61); **Address:** Johns Hopkins Hosp, Div Peds Oncology, 1650 Orleans St CRB Bldg Fl 2M - rm 53, Baltimore, MD 21231; **Phone:** 410-955-7385; **Board Cert:** Pediatric Hematology-Oncology 2006; **Med School:** Duke Univ 1986; **Resid:** Pediatrics, Chldns Hosp Med Ctr 1989; **Fellow:** Pediatric Hematology-Oncology, Fred Hutchinson Canc Ctr 1993; Bone Marrow Transplant, Fred Hutchinson Canc Ctr 1994; **Fac Appt:** Assoc Prof Ped, Johns Hopkins Univ

Cheung, Nai-Kong V MD/PhD [PHO] - **Spec Exp:** Neuroblastoma; **Hospital:** Meml Sloan-Kettering Cancer Ctr; **Address:** 1275 York Ave, Box 170, New York, NY 10065; **Phone:** 212-639-8401; **Board Cert:** Pediatrics 1987; Pediatric Hematology-Oncology 1998; **Med School:** Harvard Med Sch 1978; **Resid:** Pediatrics, Stanford Univ Hosp 1980; **Fellow:** Pediatric Hematology-Oncology, Stanford Univ Hosp 1982; **Fac Appt:** Assoc Prof Ped, Cornell Univ-Weill Med Coll

Pediatric Hematology-Oncology

Civin, Curt I MD [PHO] - **Spec Exp:** Pediatric Cancers; Leukemia; Bone Marrow Transplant; **Hospital:** Univ of MD Med Ctr; **Address:** Univ Maryland Office of Assoc Dean, 655 W Baltimore St, rm 14-023, Baltimore, MD 21201; **Phone:** 410-706-1181; **Board Cert:** Pediatrics 1979; Pediatric Hematology-Oncology 1980; **Med School:** Harvard Med Sch 1974; **Resid:** Pediatrics, Chldns Hosp 1976; **Fellow:** Pediatric Hematology-Oncology, Natl Cancer Inst 1979; **Fac Appt:** Prof Ped, Univ MD Sch Med

Cohen, Kenneth J MD [PHO] - **Spec Exp:** Brain Tumors; Spinal Tumors; **Hospital:** Johns Hopkins Hosp (page 61); **Address:** Johns Hopkins Hosp, 600 N Wolfe St, rm CMSC-800, Baltimore, MD 21287; **Phone:** 410-614-5055; **Board Cert:** Pediatrics 1990; Pediatric Hematology-Oncology 2002; **Med School:** SUNY Upstate Med Univ 1987; **Resid:** Pediatrics, Univ Colo Hlth Sci Ctr 1990; **Fellow:** Pediatric Hematology-Oncology, Johns Hopkins Hospital 1994; **Fac Appt:** Assoc Prof Ped, Johns Hopkins Univ

Drachtman, Richard A MD [PHO] - **Spec Exp:** Pediatric Cancers; Sickle Cell Disease; **Hospital:** Robert Wood Johnson Univ Hosp - New Brunswick, Jersey Shore Univ Med Ctr; **Address:** Cancer Inst of New Jersey, 195 Little Albany St, rm 3507, New Brunswick, NJ 08903; **Phone:** 732-235-5437; **Board Cert:** Pediatric Hematology-Oncology 2007; **Med School:** Ros Franklin Univ/Chicago Med Sch 1984; **Resid:** Pediatrics, N Shore Univ Hosp 1988; **Fellow:** Pediatric Hematology-Oncology, Mount Sinai Hosp 1991; **Fac Appt:** Prof Ped, UMDNJ-RW Johnson Med Sch

Dunkel, Ira J MD [PHO] - **Spec Exp:** Retinoblastoma; Brain & Spinal Cord Tumors; Brain Tumors; Pediatric Cancers; **Hospital:** Meml Sloan-Kettering Cancer Ctr; **Address:** 1275 York Ave, Box 185, New York, NY 10065; **Phone:** 212-639-2153; **Board Cert:** Pediatric Hematology-Oncology 2007; **Med School:** Duke Univ 1985; **Resid:** Pediatrics, Duke Univ Med Ctr 1988; **Fellow:** Pediatric Hematology-Oncology, Memorial-Sloan Kettering 1992; **Fac Appt:** Assoc Prof Ped, Cornell Univ-Weill Med Coll

Felix, Carolyn A MD [PHO] - **Spec Exp:** Leukemia; Leukemia in Infants; **Hospital:** Chldns Hosp of Philadelphia; **Address:** Colket Translational Research Bldg, 3501 Civic Ctr Blvd, Philadelphia, PA 19104; **Phone:** 215-590-2831; **Board Cert:** Pediatrics 1987; Pediatric Hematology-Oncology 1987; **Med School:** Boston Univ 1981; **Resid:** Pediatrics, Chldns Hosp 1984; **Fellow:** Pediatric Hematology-Oncology, Natl Cancer Inst-Pediatric Br 1987; **Fac Appt:** Prof Ped, Univ Pennsylvania

Frantz, Christopher N MD [PHO] - **Spec Exp:** Solid Tumors; Neuroblastoma; Leukemia; **Hospital:** Alfred I duPont Hosp for Children, Wilmington Hosp; **Address:** Alfred I duPont Hosp for Chldn, 1600 Rockland Rd, Box 269, Wilmington, DE 19899; **Phone:** 302-651-5500; **Board Cert:** Pediatrics 1977; Pediatric Hematology-Oncology 2005; **Med School:** Albert Einstein Coll Med 1971; **Resid:** Pediatrics, Chldns Hosp 1976; **Fellow:** Pediatric Hematology-Oncology, Chldns Hosp/Dana Farber Cancer Inst 1979

Friedman, Alan D MD [PHO] - **Spec Exp:** Leukemia; **Hospital:** Johns Hopkins Hosp (page 61); **Address:** 1650 Orleans St CRB1 Bldg - rm 253, Baltimore, MD 21231; **Phone:** 410-955-8817; **Board Cert:** Pediatrics 1987; Pediatric Hematology-Oncology 2005; **Med School:** Harvard Med Sch 1983; **Resid:** Pediatrics, Childrens Hosp 1986; **Fellow:** Pediatric Hematology-Oncology, Johns Hopkins Hosp 1987; **Fac Appt:** Prof Ped, Johns Hopkins Univ

Garvin, James H MD/PhD [PHO] - **Spec Exp:** Brain Tumors; Pediatric Cancers; Bone Marrow Transplant; **Hospital:** Morgan Stanley Children's Hosp of NY-Presby, NY (page 65); **Address:** 161 Fort Washington Ave Fl 7 - rm 708, New York, NY 10032-3729; **Phone:** 212-305-8685; **Board Cert:** Pediatrics 1982; Pediatric Hematology-Oncology 1984; **Med School:** Jefferson Med Coll 1976; **Resid:** Pediatrics, Chldns Hosp 1978; Pediatrics, Middlesex Hosp 1979; **Fellow:** Pediatric Hematology-Oncology, Dana Farber Cancer Inst/Childrens Hosp 1982; **Fac Appt:** Clin Prof Ped, Columbia P&S

Giardina, Patricia J V MD [PHO] - **Spec Exp:** Thalassemia; **Hospital:** NY-Presby/Weill Cornell Med Ctr, NY (page 65); **Address:** 525 E 68th St, Payson Pavilion 695, New York, NY 10065; **Phone:** 212-746-3400; **Board Cert:** Pediatrics 1973; Pediatric Hematology-Oncology 1974; **Med School:** NY Med Coll 1968; **Resid:** Pediatrics, New York Hosp 1971; **Fellow:** Pediatric Hematology-Oncology, New York Hosp-Cornell 1974; **Fac Appt:** Clin Prof Ped, Cornell Univ-Weill Med Coll

Greenberg, Jay N MD [PHO] - **Hospital:** Chldns Natl Med Ctr, Inova Fairfax Hosp; **Address:** Pediatric Hematology/Oncology, 111 Michigan Ave NW Fl 4 W Wing, Washington, DC 20010; **Phone:** 202-476-2140; **Board Cert:** Pediatrics 1981; Pediatric Hematology-Oncology 1982; **Med School:** Univ Pennsylvania 1976; **Resid:** Pediatrics, Univ MI Hosp 1978; Pediatrics, Chldns Hosp 1979; **Fellow:** Pediatric Hematology-Oncology, Chldns Hosp 1982

Grupp, Stephan A MD/PhD [PHO] - **Spec Exp:** Stem Cell Transplant; Neuroblastoma; Bone Marrow Transplant; **Hospital:** Chldns Hosp of Philadelphia; **Address:** Childrens Hosp - Oncology, 34th St & Civic Ctr Blvd Abramson Bldg, Philadelphia, PA 19104; **Phone:** 215-590-2821; **Board Cert:** Pediatric Hematology-Oncology 2009; **Med School:** Univ Cincinnati 1987; **Resid:** Pediatrics, Chldns Hosp 1990; **Fellow:** Pediatric Hematology-Oncology, Dana Farber Cancer Inst/Chldns Hosp 1992; **Fac Appt:** Asst Prof Ped, Univ Pennsylvania

Guarini, Ludovico MD [PHO] - **Spec Exp:** Leukemia; Solid Tumors; Sickle Cell Disease; **Hospital:** Maimonides Med Ctr (page 62); **Address:** 4802 10th Ave, Dept of Pediatrics, Brooklyn, NY 11219; **Phone:** 718-765-2671; **Board Cert:** Pediatrics 1984; Pediatric Hematology-Oncology 2007; **Med School:** Italy 1974; **Resid:** Pediatrics, Beth Israel Hosp 1981; **Fellow:** Pediatric Hematology-Oncology, Columbia-Presby Med Ctr 1984; **Fac Appt:** Assoc Prof Ped, Mount Sinai Sch Med

Halligan, Gregory E MD [PHO] - **Spec Exp:** Clinical Trials; Solid Tumors; **Hospital:** St. Christopher's Hosp for Chldn; **Address:** St Christophers Hosp for Children, Dept Oncology, 3601 A St, Philadelphia, PA 19134; **Phone:** 215-427-4447; **Board Cert:** Pediatrics 1982; Pediatric Hematology-Oncology 1984; **Med School:** Belgium 1977; **Resid:** Pediatrics, St Christophers Hosp for Chldn 1981; **Fellow:** Pediatric Hematology-Oncology, St Christophers Hosp for Chldn 1984; **Fac Appt:** Assoc Prof Ped, Drexel Univ Coll Med

Halpern, Steven MD [PHO] - **Spec Exp:** Leukemia & Lymphoma; Brain Tumors; Hodgkin's Disease; Hemophilia; **Hospital:** Morristown Med Ctr, Overlook Med Ctr; **Address:** 100 Madison Ave, Morristown, NJ 07960; **Phone:** 973-971-6720; **Board Cert:** Pediatrics 1981; Pediatric Hematology-Oncology 1982; **Med School:** Ros Franklin Univ/Chicago Med Sch 1976; **Resid:** Pediatrics, St Christophers Hosp for Children 1979; **Fellow:** Pediatric Hematology-Oncology, Childrens Hosp 1982; **Fac Appt:** Asst Prof Ped, UMDNJ-NJ Med Sch, Newark

Harris, Michael B MD [PHO] - **Spec Exp:** Leukemia & Lymphoma; Bone Tumors; Cancer Survivors-Late Effects of Therapy; **Hospital:** Hackensack Univ Med Ctr; **Address:** Tomorrows Chldns Inst, JM Sanzari Chldns Hosp, 30 Prospect Ave, Imus 1-TCI, rm PC116, Hackensack, NJ 07601; **Phone:** 201-996-5437; **Board Cert:** Pediatrics 1974; Pediatric Hematology-Oncology 1974; **Med School:** Albert Einstein Coll Med 1969; **Resid:** Pediatrics, Chldns Hosp 1971; **Fellow:** Pediatric Hematology-Oncology, Chldns Hosp 1974; **Fac Appt:** Prof Ped, UMDNJ-NJ Med Sch, Newark

Helman, Lee Jay MD [PHO] - **Spec Exp:** Solid Tumors; **Hospital:** Natl Inst of Hlth - Clin Ctr; **Address:** National Cancer Inst, NIH, 31 Center Drive, rm 3A11, Bethesda, MD 20892; **Phone:** 301-496-4257; **Board Cert:** Internal Medicine 1983; Medical Oncology 1985; **Med School:** Univ MD Sch Med 1980; **Resid:** Internal Medicine, Barnes Hosp 1983; **Fellow:** Oncology, Natl Inst Hlth 1986

Pediatric Hematology-Oncology

Hoots, William K MD [PHO] - **Spec Exp:** Hemophilia; **Hospital:** Natl Inst of Hlth - Clin Ctr; **Address:** Nat Inst Hlth-Clin Ctr, 6701 Rockledge Drive, Ste 9030 - rm 9136, Bethesda, MD 20892; **Phone:** 301-435-0080; **Board Cert:** Pediatrics 1980; Pediatric Hematology-Oncology 1980; **Med School:** Univ NC Sch Med 1975; **Resid:** Pediatrics, Chldns Med Ctr 1978; **Fellow:** Pediatric Hematology-Oncology, Univ NC Med Ctr 1980; **Fac Appt:** Prof Ped, Univ Tex, Houston

Jakacki, Regina I MD [PHO] - **Spec Exp:** Neuro-Oncology; Clinical Trials; Palliative Care; **Hospital:** Chldns Hosp of Pittsburgh - UPMC; **Address:** Children's Hospital Pittsburgh, 45th & Penn Drive, Pittsburgh, PA 15201; **Phone:** 412-692-8864; **Board Cert:** Pediatric Hematology-Oncology 2007; **Med School:** Univ Pennsylvania 1985; **Resid:** Pediatrics, Childrens Hosp 1988; **Fellow:** Pediatric Hematology-Oncology, Childrens Hosp 1991; **Fac Appt:** Assoc Prof Ped, Univ Pittsburgh

Kamen, Barton A MD/PhD [PHO] - **Spec Exp:** Drug Development; Leukemia; **Hospital:** Robert Wood Johnson Univ Hosp - New Brunswick; **Address:** Cancer Inst of New Jersey, 195 Little Albany St, rm 3549, New Brunswick, NJ 08903; **Phone:** 732-235-8864; **Board Cert:** Pediatrics 1981; Pediatric Hematology-Oncology 1987; **Med School:** Case West Res Univ 1976; **Resid:** Pediatrics, Yale-New Haven Hosp 1978; **Fellow:** Pediatric Hematology-Oncology, Yale-New Haven Hosp 1980; **Fac Appt:** Prof Ped, UMDNJ-RW Johnson Med Sch

Korones, David N MD [PHO] - **Spec Exp:** Brain Tumors; Palliative Care; Pediatric Cancers; **Hospital:** Univ of Rochester Strong Meml Hosp; **Address:** Golisano Childrens Hosp at Strong, 601 Elmwood Ave, Box 777, Rochester, NY 14642-8777; **Phone:** 585-275-2981; **Board Cert:** Pediatrics 1987; Pediatric Hematology-Oncology 2006; Hospice & Palliative Medicine 2002; **Med School:** Vanderbilt Univ 1983; **Resid:** Pediatrics, Strong Meml Hosp 1986; **Fellow:** Pediatrics, Yale Univ 1988; Pediatric Hematology-Oncology, Strong Meml Hosp 1991; **Fac Appt:** Prof Ped, Univ Rochester

Kushner, Brian H MD [PHO] - **Spec Exp:** Neuroblastoma; Bone Marrow Transplant; Immunotherapy; **Hospital:** Meml Sloan-Kettering Cancer Ctr; **Address:** 1275 York Avenue, New York, NY 10065; **Phone:** 800-525-2225; **Board Cert:** Pediatrics 1983; Pediatric Hematology-Oncology 1987; **Med School:** Johns Hopkins Univ 1976; **Resid:** Pediatrics, Columbia-Presby Med Ctr 1978; Pediatrics, NY Hosp 1979; **Fellow:** Pediatric Hematology-Oncology, Boston Chldns Hosp 1980; Pediatric Hematology-Oncology, Meml Sloan Kettering Cancer Ctr 1986; **Fac Appt:** Prof Ped, Cornell Univ-Weill Med Coll

Kuttesch, John F MD [PHO] - **Spec Exp:** Brain Tumors; Brain Tumors-Recurrent; Solid Tumors; **Hospital:** Penn State Chldns Hosp; **Address:** Penn State College of Medicine, Div Ped Hem/Onc & Stem Cell Transplant, 500 University Drive, MC HO85, Hershey, PA 17033-0850; **Phone:** 717-531-6012; **Board Cert:** Pediatrics 2008; Pediatric Hematology-Oncology 2007; **Med School:** Univ Tex, Houston 1985; **Resid:** Pediatrics, Vanderbilt Univ Med Ctr 1988; **Fellow:** Pediatric Hematology-Oncology, St Judes Chldns Hosp 1992; **Fac Appt:** Prof Ped

Lange, Beverly J MD [PHO] - **Spec Exp:** Leukemia; Brain & Spinal Cord Tumors; Cognitive Rehabilitation; **Hospital:** Chldns Hosp of Philadelphia; **Address:** Chldns Hosp Phila, Medical Oncology, 34th St & Civic Ctr Blvd, Wood Center Fl 4, Philadelphia, PA 19104; **Phone:** 215-590-3025; **Board Cert:** Pediatrics 1976; Pediatric Hematology-Oncology 1997; **Med School:** Temple Univ 1971; **Resid:** Pediatrics, Philadelphia Genl Hosp 1973; **Fellow:** Pediatric Oncology, Chldns Hosp; **Fac Appt:** Prof Ped, Univ Pennsylvania

Lipton, Jeffrey M MD/PhD [PHO] - **Spec Exp:** Bone Marrow Failure Disorders; Stem Cell Transplant; Bone Marrow Transplant; **Hospital:** Steven & Alexandra Cohen Chldn's Med Ctr of NY; **Address:** Steven & Alexandra Cohen Chldn's Med Ctr, Division, Hematology/Oncology, 269-01 76th Ave Ave, rm 255, New Hyde Park, NY 11040-1433; **Phone:** 718-470-3460; **Board Cert:** Pediatrics 1981; **Med School:** St Louis Univ 1975; **Resid:** Pediatrics, Boston Chldns Hosp 1977; **Fellow:** Pediatric Hematology-Oncology, Boston Chldns Hosp/Dana Farber Cancer Inst 1979; **Fac Appt:** Prof Ped, Albert Einstein Coll Med

Loeb, David M MD/PhD [PHO] - **Spec Exp:** Bone Marrow Transplant; Bone Cancer; **Hospital:** Johns Hopkins Hosp (page 61); **Address:** 601 N Caroline St, Baltimore, MD 21287; **Phone:** 410-955-8751; **Board Cert:** Pediatrics 2005; Pediatric Hematology-Oncology 2000; **Med School:** Columbia P&S 1994; **Resid:** Pediatrics, John Hopkins Hosp 1997; **Fellow:** Pediatric Oncology, John Hopkins Hosp 1997; **Fac Appt:** Asst Prof Ped, Johns Hopkins Univ

Luchtman-Jones, Lori MD [PHO] - **Spec Exp:** Leukemia; Bleeding/Coagulation Disorders; **Hospital:** Chldns Natl Med Ctr; **Address:** Chldn's Natl Med Ctr, 111 Michigan Ave NW Fl 4 - Ste 4043, Washington, DC 20010; **Phone:** 202-476-2140; **Board Cert:** Pediatric Hematology-Oncology 2004; **Med School:** UCSD 1987; **Resid:** Pediatrics, UCSD School Med 1990; **Fellow:** Pediatric Hematology-Oncology, Washington Univ 1995; **Fac Appt:** Asst Prof Ped, Washington Univ, St Louis

Marcus, Judith R MD [PHO] - **Spec Exp:** Leukemia; Lymphoma; Bleeding/Coagulation Disorders; Solid Tumors-Pediatric; **Hospital:** Morgan Stanley Children's Hosp of NY-Presby, NY (page 65), White Plains Hosp Ctr; **Address:** 161 Ft Wasthington Ave, Ste 7I, New York, NY 10032; **Phone:** 914-684-0220; **Board Cert:** Pediatrics 1997; Pediatric Hematology-Oncology 1997; **Med School:** NYU Sch Med 1971; **Resid:** Pediatrics, Bronx Muni Hosp-Albert Einstein 1974; **Fellow:** Pediatric Hematology-Oncology, Meml Sloan Kettering Cancer Ctr 1979; **Fac Appt:** Clin Prof Ped, Columbia P&S

Maris, John M MD [PHO] - **Spec Exp:** Neuroblastoma; Clinical Trials; **Hospital:** Chldns Hosp of Philadelphia; **Address:** Chldns Hosp Philadelphia - Oncology, 3501 Civic Ctr Blvd CTRB Bldg - rm 3060, Philadelphia, PA 19104-4318; **Phone:** 215-590-5244; **Board Cert:** Pediatric Hematology-Oncology 2004; **Med School:** Univ Pennsylvania 1989; **Resid:** Pediatrics, Chldns Hosp 1992; **Fellow:** Pediatric Hematology-Oncology, Chldns Hosp 1996

Meyers, Paul A MD [PHO] - **Spec Exp:** Pediatric Cancers; Bone Tumors; Sarcoma; **Hospital:** Meml Sloan-Kettering Cancer Ctr, NY-Presby/Weill Cornell Med Ctr, NY (page 65); **Address:** 1275 York Ave, New York, NY 10065; **Phone:** 800-525-2225; **Board Cert:** Pediatrics 1978; Pediatric Hematology-Oncology 1978; **Med School:** Mount Sinai Sch Med 1973; **Resid:** Pediatrics, Mt Sinai Hosp 1976; **Fellow:** Pediatric Hematology-Oncology, NY Hosp-Cornell Med Ctr 1979; **Fac Appt:** Prof Ped, Cornell Univ-Weill Med Coll

O'Reilly, Richard MD [PHO] - **Spec Exp:** Bone Marrow Transplant; **Hospital:** Meml Sloan-Kettering Cancer Ctr, NY-Presby/Weill Cornell Med Ctr, NY (page 65); **Address:** 1275 York Avenue, New York, NY 10065; **Phone:** 800-525-2225; **Board Cert:** Pediatrics 1974; **Med School:** Univ Rochester 1968; **Resid:** Pediatrics, Chldrns Hosp 1972; **Fellow:** Infectious Disease, Chldrns Hosp 1973; **Fac Appt:** Prof Ped, Cornell Univ-Weill Med Coll

Parker, Robert MD [PHO] - **Spec Exp:** Pediatric Cancers; Bleeding/Coagulation Disorders; Platelet Disorders; Lymphoma; **Hospital:** Stony Brook Univ Med Ctr; **Address:** Stony Brook Univ Hosp, Dept Peds, HSC T-11, Rm 029, Stony Brook, NY 11794-8111; **Phone:** 631-444-7720; **Board Cert:** Pediatrics 1983; Pediatric Hematology-Oncology 1984; **Med School:** Brown Univ 1976; **Resid:** Internal Medicine, Roger Williams Med Ctr 1977; Pediatrics, Rhode Island Hosp 1979; **Fellow:** Pediatric Hematology-Oncology, Natl Cancer Inst 1981; Hematology, Natl Cancer Inst 1984; **Fac Appt:** Prof Ped, SUNY Stony Brook

Pediatric Hematology-Oncology

Rausen, Aaron R MD [PHO] - **Spec Exp:** Leukemia & Lymphoma; Bone Tumors; Retinoblastoma; **Hospital:** NYU Langone Med Ctr (page 66), Lenox Hill Hosp; **Address:** NYU Medical Ctr, 160 E 32nd St Fl 2, New York, NY 10016; **Phone:** 212-263-7144; **Board Cert:** Pediatrics 1960; Pediatric Hematology-Oncology 1974; **Med School:** SUNY Downstate 1954; **Resid:** Pediatrics, Bellevue Hosp 1956; Pediatrics, Mount Sinai 1959; **Fellow:** Hematology, Chldns Hosp 1961; **Fac Appt:** Prof Ped, NYU Sch Med

Reaman, Gregory H MD [PHO] - **Spec Exp:** Leukemia; Lymphoma; Cancer Survivors-Late Effects of Therapy; **Hospital:** Chldns Natl Med Ctr; **Address:** 111 Michigan Ave NW, West Bldg Fl 4 - Ste 600, Washington, DC 20010-2916; **Phone:** 202-476-2800; **Board Cert:** Pediatrics 1978; Pediatric Hematology-Oncology 1978; **Med School:** Loyola Univ-Stritch Sch Med 1973; **Resid:** Hematology, Montreal Chldns Hosp 1975; Pediatrics, Montreal Chldns Hosp 1976; **Fellow:** Pediatric Oncology, Natl Cancer Inst 1979; **Fac Appt:** Prof Ped, Geo Wash Univ

Rheingold, Susan R MD [PHO] - **Spec Exp:** Leukemia; Clinical Trials; **Hospital:** Chldns Hosp of Philadelphia; **Address:** Chldns Hosp Phila - Div Oncology, 3501 Civic Ctr Blvd CTRB Bldg Fl 10, Philadelphia, PA 19104; **Phone:** 215-590-5244; **Board Cert:** Pediatrics 2010; Pediatric Hematology-Oncology 2008; **Med School:** Univ Pennsylvania 1992; **Resid:** Pediatrics, Johns Hopkins Hosp 1995; **Fellow:** Pediatric Hematology-Oncology, Chldns Hosp 1999; **Fac Appt:** Assoc Clin Prof Ped, Univ Pennsylvania

Ritchey, A Kim MD [PHO] - **Spec Exp:** Leukemia; Bleeding/Coagulation Disorders; Hematologic Malignancies; **Hospital:** Chldns Hosp of Pittsburgh - UPMC; **Address:** Chldns Hosp, Div Hematology/Oncology, One Children's Hosp Drive, 4401 Penn Ave, Faculty Pavilion Fl 8, Pittsburgh, PA 15224; **Phone:** 412-692-5055; **Board Cert:** Pediatrics 1977; Pediatric Hematology-Oncology 2007; **Med School:** Univ Cincinnati 1972; **Resid:** Pediatrics, Johns Hopkins Hosp 1975; **Fellow:** Pediatric Hematology-Oncology, Yale-New Haven Hosp 1980; **Fac Appt:** Prof Ped, Univ Pittsburgh

Rood, Brian R MD [PHO] - **Spec Exp:** Brain Tumors; **Hospital:** Chldns Natl Med Ctr; **Address:** CNMC Div Ped Onc, 111 Michigan Ave NW, Washington, DC 20010; **Phone:** 202-476-2140; **Board Cert:** Pediatrics 2006; Pediatric Hematology-Oncology 2010; **Med School:** Jefferson Med Coll 1995; **Resid:** Pediatrics, Univ VT Hosp 1998; **Fellow:** Pediatric Hematology-Oncology, Chldns Natl Med Ctr 1998; Research, Chldns Natl Med Ctr 2001

Small, Donald MD [PHO] - **Spec Exp:** Leukemia; Lymphoma; **Hospital:** Johns Hopkins Hosp (page 61); **Address:** Johns Hopkins Univ, 1650 Orleans St CRB-1 Bldg - rm 251, Baltimore, MD 21231; **Phone:** 410-614-0994; **Board Cert:** Pediatric Hematology-Oncology 2002; **Med School:** Johns Hopkins Univ 1985; **Resid:** Pediatrics, Johns Hopkins Hosp 1987; **Fellow:** Pediatric Hematology-Oncology, Johns Hopkins Hosp 1990; **Fac Appt:** Prof Ped, Johns Hopkins Univ

Steinherz, Peter G MD [PHO] - **Spec Exp:** Leukemia & Lymphoma; Pediatric Cancers; Wilms' Tumor; **Hospital:** Meml Sloan-Kettering Cancer Ctr, NY-Presby/Weill Cornell Med Ctr, NY (page 65); **Address:** 1275 York Avenue, New York, NY 10065; **Phone:** 212-639-7951; **Board Cert:** Pediatrics 1973; Pediatric Hematology-Oncology 1978; **Med School:** Albert Einstein Coll Med 1968; **Resid:** Pediatrics, NY Hosp-Cornell 1971; **Fellow:** Pediatric Hematology-Oncology, NY Hosp-Cornell 1975; **Fac Appt:** Prof Ped, Cornell Univ-Weill Med Coll

Weinblatt, Mark E MD [PHO] - **Spec Exp:** Leukemia & Lymphoma; Sickle Cell Disease; Bleeding/Coagulation Disorders; Thalassemia; **Hospital:** Winthrop Univ Hosp; **Address:** Winthrop Univ Hosp, 120 Mineola Blvd, Ste 460, Mineola, NY 11501; **Phone:** 516-663-9400; **Board Cert:** Pediatrics 1980; Pediatric Hematology-Oncology 1982; **Med School:** Albert Einstein Coll Med 1976; **Resid:** Pediatrics, Jacobi Med Ctr 1979; **Fellow:** Pediatric Hematology-Oncology, Children's Hosp 1981; **Fac Appt:** Prof Ped, SUNY Stony Brook

Weiner, Michael MD [PHO] - **Spec Exp:** Hodgkin's Disease; Lymphoma; Leukemia; **Hospital:** NY-Presby/Columbia Univ Med Ctr, NY (page 65); **Address:** 161 Fort Washington Ave, Irving Pavilion-FL 7, New York, NY 10032-3710; **Phone:** 212-305-9770; **Board Cert:** Pediatrics 1980; Pediatric Hematology-Oncology 1980; **Med School:** SUNY Hlth Sci Ctr 1972; **Resid:** Pediatrics, Montefiore Med Ctr 1974; **Fellow:** Pediatric Hematology-Oncology, NYU Med Ctr 1976; Pediatric Hematology-Oncology, Johns Hopkins Hosp 1977; **Fac Appt:** Prof Ped, Columbia P&S

Wexler, Leonard MD [PHO] - **Spec Exp:** Rhabdomyosarcoma; Bone Cancer; Gastrointestinal Stromal Tumors; Sarcoma-Soft Tissue; **Hospital:** Meml Sloan-Kettering Cancer Ctr; **Address:** 1275 York Avenue, New York, NY 10065; **Phone:** 800-525-2225; **Board Cert:** Pediatrics 2007; Pediatric Hematology-Oncology 2007; **Med School:** Boston Univ 1985; **Resid:** Pediatrics, Montefiore Med Ctr 1988; **Fellow:** Pediatric Hematology-Oncology, National Cancer Inst 1991; **Fac Appt:** Assoc Prof Ped, Columbia P&S

Wiley, Joseph M MD [PHO] - **Hospital:** Sinai Hosp - Baltimore; **Address:** Sinai Hospital, Div Pediattic Hematology/Oncology, 2401 W Belvedrer Ave, Baltimore, MD 21215; **Phone:** 410-601-5864; **Board Cert:** Pediatrics 1986; Pediatric Hematology-Oncology 2005; **Med School:** Univ MD Sch Med 1982; **Resid:** Pediatrics, Johns Hopkins Hosp 1995; **Fellow:** Pediatric Hematology-Oncology, Johns Hopkins Hosp 1998; **Fac Appt:** Assoc Prof Ped, Johns Hopkins Univ

Wolfe, Lawrence C MD [PHO] - **Spec Exp:** Palliative Care; Adrenal Cancer; Congenital Hemolytic Anemia; Hemochromatosis; **Hospital:** Steven & Alexandra Cohen Chldn's Med Ctr of NY; **Address:** Steven & Alexandra Cohen Chldn's Med Ctr, Div Pediatric Hematology/Oncology, 269-01 76th Ave, New Hyde Park, NY 11040; **Phone:** 718-470-3460; **Board Cert:** Pediatrics 1981; Pediatric Hematology-Oncology 1987; Hospice & Palliative Medicine 2011; **Med School:** Harvard Med Sch 1976; **Resid:** Pediatrics, Chldns Hosp 1978; **Fellow:** Pediatric Hematology-Oncology, Chldns Hosp 1991; **Fac Appt:** Prof Ped

York, Teresa A MD [PHO] - **Spec Exp:** Leukemia; **Hospital:** Univ of MD Med Ctr; **Address:** Greenebaum Cancer Center, 22 S Greene St, rm N5E16, Baltimore, MD 21201; **Phone:** 410-328-2808; **Board Cert:** Pediatric Hematology-Oncology 2004; **Med School:** W VA Univ 1997; **Resid:** Pediatrics, W Va Univ Chldns Hosp 2000; **Fellow:** Pediatric Hematology-Oncology, Med Univ SC Hosp 2000; **Fac Appt:** Asst Prof Ped, Univ MD Sch Med

Southeast

Barredo, Julio C MD [PHO] - **Spec Exp:** Leukemia; Bone Marrow Transplant; Cancer Survivors-Late Effects of Therapy; Stem Cell Transplant; **Hospital:** Univ of Miami Hosp & Clins/Sylvester Comp Canc Ctr (page 73); **Address:** Univ Miami Dept Pediatrics (R-131), PO Box 016960, Miami, FL 33101; **Phone:** 305-585-5635; **Board Cert:** Pediatric Hematology-Oncology 2007; **Med School:** Peru 1982; **Resid:** Pediatrics, Kings Co Hosp 1987; **Fellow:** Pediatric Hematology-Oncology, Chldns Hosp/USC 1988; **Fac Appt:** Prof Ped, Univ Miami Sch Med

Bertolone, Salvatore MD [PHO] - **Spec Exp:** Bone Marrow Transplant; Kasabach-Merritt Syndrome (KMS); Sickle Cell Disease; **Hospital:** Kosair Chldn's Hosp, Norton Hosp; **Address:** Pediatric Hematology/Oncology, 601 S Floyd St, Ste 403, Louisville, KY 40202; **Phone:** 502-629-7750; **Board Cert:** Pediatrics 1975; Pediatric Hematology-Oncology 1976; **Med School:** Univ Louisville Sch Med 1970; **Resid:** Pediatrics, Univ Louisville 1972; **Fellow:** Pediatric Hematology-Oncology, Univ Colorado 1974; **Fac Appt:** Prof Ped, Univ Louisville Sch Med

Pediatric Hematology-Oncology

Blatt, Julie MD [PHO] - **Spec Exp:** Neuroblastoma; Cancer Survivors-Late Effects of Therapy; **Hospital:** NC Memorial Hosp - UNC; **Address:** UNC, Dept Ped Hematology Oncology, 170 Manning Drive, Campus Box 7236, Chapel Hill, NC 27599-7236; **Phone:** 919-966-1178; **Board Cert:** Pediatrics 1981; Pediatric Hematology-Oncology 1982; **Med School:** Johns Hopkins Univ 1976; **Resid:** Pediatrics, Columbia-Presby Hosp 1978; **Fellow:** Pediatric Oncology, Natl Cancer Inst 1982; **Fac Appt:** Prof Ped, Univ NC Sch Med

Castellino, Sharon M MD [PHO] - **Spec Exp:** Cancer Survivors-Late Effects of Therapy; Leukemia; Lymphoma; **Hospital:** Brenner Chldrn's Hosp; **Address:** Wake Forest Univ Baptist Med Ctr, Div Pediatric Hematology/Oncology, Medical Center Blvd, Winston-Salem, NC 27157; **Phone:** 336-716-4324; **Board Cert:** Pediatrics 2003; Pediatric Hematology-Oncology 2006; **Med School:** Duke Univ 1992; **Resid:** Pediatrics, Childrens Hosp 1994; Pediatrics, Duke Univ Med Ctr 1995; **Fellow:** Pediatric Hematology-Oncology, Duke Univ 1997; **Fac Appt:** Asst Prof Ped, Wake Forest Univ

Frangoul, Haydar A MD [PHO] - **Spec Exp:** Stem Cell Transplant; **Hospital:** Vanderbilt Monroe Carrell Jr. Chldn's Hosp (page 76); **Address:** 1215 21st Ave S, 397 Preston Rsch Bldg, Nashville, TN 37232-6310; **Phone:** 615-936-1762; **Board Cert:** Pediatric Hematology-Oncology 2008; **Med School:** Amer Univ Beirut 1990; **Resid:** Pediatrics, Duke Univ Med Ctr 1993; **Fellow:** Pediatric Hematology-Oncology, Duke Univ Med Ctr 1994; Pediatric Hematology-Oncology, Seattle Chldns/Fred Hutchinson Cancer Ctr 1996; **Fac Appt:** Assoc Prof Ped, Vanderbilt Univ

Friedman, Debra L MD [PHO] - **Spec Exp:** Cancer Survivors-Late Effects of Therapy; Hodgkin's Disease; Retinoblastoma; **Hospital:** Vanderbilt Monroe Carrell Jr. Chldn's Hosp (page 76), Vanderbilt Univ Med Ctr (page 76); **Address:** 1215 21st Ave S, 397 Preston Research Bldg, Nashville, TN 37232-6310; **Phone:** 615-936-1762; **Board Cert:** Pediatric Hematology-Oncology 2006; **Med School:** UMDNJ-RW Johnson Med Sch 1991; **Resid:** Pediatrics, Chldns Hosp 1994; **Fellow:** Pediatric Hematology-Oncology, Chldns Hosp 1997; Cancer Epidemiology, Univ Penn; **Fac Appt:** Asst Prof Ped, Vanderbilt Univ

Furman, Wayne L MD [PHO] - **Spec Exp:** Neuroblastoma; Liver Cancer; Drug Development; **Hospital:** St. Jude Children's Research Hosp; **Address:** St Jude Children's Research Hospital, 262 Danny Thomas Pl, Memphis, TN 38105; **Phone:** 901-595-2800; **Board Cert:** Pediatrics 1985; Pediatric Hematology-Oncology 1987; **Med School:** Ohio State Univ 1979; **Resid:** Pediatrics, Children's Hosp 1983; **Fellow:** Pediatric Hematology-Oncology, St Jude Chldn's Rsch Hosp 1985; **Fac Appt:** Prof Ped, Univ Tenn Coll Med

Gajjar, Amar J MD [PHO] - **Spec Exp:** Brain Tumors; Medulloblastoma; Neuro-Oncology; Drug Development; **Hospital:** St. Jude Children's Research Hosp; **Address:** St Judes Children's Hosp, Dept Oncology, 262 Danny Thomas Pl, rm C6024, MS 260, Memphis, TN 38105-2794; **Phone:** 901-595-4599; **Board Cert:** Pediatric Hematology-Oncology 2007; **Med School:** India 1984; **Resid:** Pediatrics, All Chldns Hosp 1989; **Fellow:** Hematology & Oncology, St Jude Chldns Hosp 1990; **Fac Appt:** Prof Ped, Univ Tenn Coll Med

Godder, Kamar MD/PhD [PHO] - **Spec Exp:** Stem Cell Transplant; Leukemia; Palliative Care; **Hospital:** Med Coll of VA Hosp; **Address:** 401-09 N 11th St, Richmond, VA 23298; **Phone:** 804-828-9300; **Board Cert:** Pediatric Hematology-Oncology 2005; **Med School:** Israel 1980; **Resid:** Pediatrics, Hadassah-Mt Scopus 1984; **Fellow:** Pediatric Hematology-Oncology, Meml Sloan Kettering Cancer Ctr 1988; **Fac Appt:** Prof Ped, Va Commonwealth Univ Sch Med

Gold, Stuart H MD [PHO] - **Spec Exp:** Leukemia; Brain Tumors; Cancer Survivors-Late Effects of Therapy; **Hospital:** NC Memorial Hosp - UNC; **Address:** UNC, Dept Ped Hem-Onc, 1185A Physicians Office Bldg, 170 Manning Drive, Campus Box 7236, Chapel Hill, NC 27599-7236; **Phone:** 919-966-1178; **Board Cert:** Pediatrics 1986; Pediatric Hematology-Oncology 1987; **Med School:** Vanderbilt Univ 1981; **Resid:** Pediatrics, Univ Colorado Hlth Sci Ctr 1984; **Fellow:** Pediatric Hematology-Oncology, Univ Colorado Hlth Sci Ctr 1989; **Fac Appt:** Prof Ped, Univ NC Sch Med

Green, Daniel M MD [PHO] - **Spec Exp:** Wilms' Tumor; Fertility in Cancer Survivors; Cancer Survivors-Late Effects of Therapy; **Hospital:** St. Jude Children's Research Hosp; **Address:** Dept Epidemiology & Cancer Control, St Jude Children's Research Hosp, 262 Danny Thomas Pl, MS 735, Memphis, TN 38105-2794; **Phone:** 901-595-5915; **Board Cert:** Pediatrics 1986; Pediatric Hematology-Oncology 1997; **Med School:** St Louis Univ 1973; **Resid:** Pediatrics, Boston City Hosp 1975; **Fellow:** Pediatric Hematology-Oncology, Chldns Hosp Med Ctr 1978

Gururangan, Sridharan MD [PHO] - **Spec Exp:** Brain Tumors; Spinal Cord Tumors; Neuro-Oncology; **Hospital:** Duke Univ Hosp; **Address:** Robert Tisch Brain Tumor Ctr at Duke, DUMC Box 3624, Durham, NC 27710; **Phone:** 919-684-3506; **Med School:** India 1958; **Resid:** Pediatrics, Le Bonheur Children's Med Ctr 1992; **Fellow:** Pediatric Hematology-Oncology, St Jude Children's Hosp 1993; Pediatric Hematology-Oncology, Meml Sloan Kettering Cancer Ctr 1996; **Fac Appt:** Prof Ped, Duke Univ

Hudson, Melissa M MD [PHO] - **Spec Exp:** Cancer Survivors-Late Effects of Therapy; Hodgkin's Disease; **Hospital:** St. Jude Children's Research Hosp; **Address:** St Jude Children's Research Hosp, 262 Danny Thomas Pl, MS 735, Memphis, TN 38105; **Phone:** 901-595-3384; **Board Cert:** Pediatrics 1988; Pediatric Hematology-Oncology 2006; **Med School:** Univ Tex SW, Dallas 1983; **Resid:** Pediatrics, Univ Texas Affil Hosps 1986; **Fellow:** Pediatric Hematology-Oncology, MD Anderson Cancer Ctr 1989

Johnston, J Martin MD [PHO] - **Spec Exp:** Leukemia; Lymphoma; Hemophilia; **Hospital:** Meml Hlth Univ Med Ctr - Savannah; **Address:** Backus Children's Hosp Outpatient Ctr, 4700 Waters Ave, PO Box 23089, Savannah, GA 31403-3089; **Phone:** 912-350-8194; **Board Cert:** Pediatric Hematology-Oncology 2009; **Med School:** Duke Univ 1984; **Resid:** Pediatrics, Univ Utah Med Ctr 1988; **Fellow:** Pediatric Hematology-Oncology, Barnes Jewish Hosp 1991; **Fac Appt:** Assoc Prof Ped, Mercer Univ Sch Med

Kane, Javier R MD [PHO] - **Spec Exp:** Palliative Care; **Hospital:** St. Jude Children's Research Hosp; **Address:** St Jude Chldns Rsch Hosp, Dept Oncology, 262 Danny Thomas Pl, MS 260, Memphis, TN 38105-2794; **Phone:** 901-595-4152; **Board Cert:** Pediatrics 2007; Pediatric Hematology-Oncology 2004; Hospice & Palliative Medicine 2008; **Med School:** Mexico 1986; **Resid:** Pediatrics, Austin Med Ed Prog 1992; **Fellow:** Pediatric Hematology-Oncology, Univ Tennessee

Keller Jr, Frank G MD [PHO] - **Spec Exp:** Leukemia; Hodgkin's Disease; **Hospital:** Chldns Hlthcare Atlanta @ Egleston; **Address:** Aflac Cancer Ctr at Egleston, 1405 Clifton Rd NE, Tower 1, 4th Fl, Atlanta, GA 30322; **Phone:** 404-785-1200; **Board Cert:** Pediatric Hematology-Oncology 2009; **Med School:** Univ NC Sch Med 1986; **Resid:** Pediatrics, Vanderbilt Univ Med Ctr 1990; **Fellow:** Pediatric Hematology-Oncology, Duke Univ Med Ctr 1993; **Fac Appt:** Assoc Prof Ped, Emory Univ

Kreissman, Susan G MD [PHO] - **Spec Exp:** Neuroblastoma; Clinical Trials; **Hospital:** Duke Univ Hosp; **Address:** Duke Univ Med Ctr, Box 102382, Durham, NC 27710; **Phone:** 919-684-3401; **Board Cert:** Pediatric Hematology-Oncology 2004; **Med School:** Mount Sinai Sch Med 1985; **Resid:** Pediatrics, Chldns Hosp 1988; **Fellow:** Pediatric Hematology-Oncology, Chldns Hosp/Dana Farber Cancer Inst 1991; **Fac Appt:** Assoc Prof Ped, Duke Univ

Kurtzberg, Joanne MD [PHO] - **Spec Exp:** Stem Cell Transplant; Bone Marrow Transplant; **Hospital:** Duke Univ Hosp; **Address:** Duke Univ Med Ctr, 1400 Morreene Rd, Durham, NC 27705; **Phone:** 919-668-1100; **Board Cert:** Pediatrics 1982; Pediatric Hematology-Oncology 1982; **Med School:** NY Med Coll 1976; **Resid:** Pediatrics, Dartmouth Med Ctr 1977; Pediatrics, Upstate Med Ctr 1979; **Fellow:** Pediatric Hematology-Oncology, Upstate Med Ctr 1980; Pediatric Hematology-Oncology, Duke Med Ctr 1983; **Fac Appt:** Prof Ped, Duke Univ

Pediatric Hematology-Oncology

Laver, Joseph H MD [PHO] - **Spec Exp:** Stem Cell Transplant; Lymphoma, Non-Hodgkin's; **Hospital:** St. Jude Children's Research Hosp; **Address:** St Jude's Chldns Rsch Hosp, rm C-7045E, 262 Danny Thomas Pl, Memphis, TN 38105-3678; **Phone:** 901-595-3532; **Board Cert:** Pediatrics 1985; Pediatric Hematology-Oncology 1987; **Med School:** Israel 1979; **Resid:** Pediatrics, Assaf Harofeh Med Ctr 1982; **Fellow:** Pediatric Hematology-Oncology, Meml Slaon Kettering 1985

Leung, Wing H MD/PhD [PHO] - **Spec Exp:** Bone Marrow & Stem Cell Transplant; **Hospital:** St. Jude Children's Research Hosp; **Address:** 262 Danny Thomas Pl, Bone Marrow Transplant& Cellular Therapy, Memphis, TN 38105-3678; **Phone:** 901-495-3300; **Board Cert:** Pediatrics 2008; Pediatric Hematology-Oncology 2006; **Med School:** Hong Kong 1988; **Resid:** Pediatrics, Kings Co Hosp 1994; **Fellow:** Hematology & Oncology, Johns Hopkins Hosp 1997; **Fac Appt:** Prof Ped, Johns Hopkins Univ

McLean, Thomas W MD [PHO] - **Hospital:** Wake Forest Univ Baptist Med Ctr; **Address:** Wake Forest Univ Scho Medicine, Dept Ped/Onc, Medical Center Blvd, Winston Salem, NC 27157; **Phone:** 336-716-4085; **Board Cert:** Pediatrics 2009; Pediatric Hematology-Oncology 2006; **Med School:** Med Univ SC 1990; **Resid:** Pediatrics, Chldns Hosp 1993; **Fellow:** Pediatric Hematology-Oncology, Great Ormons St Hosp for Sick Chldn 1994; Pediatric Hematology-Oncology, Dana Farber Chldns Hosp 1997; **Fac Appt:** Assoc Prof Ped, Wake Forest Univ

Moscow, Jeffrey A MD [PHO] - **Spec Exp:** Pediatric Cancers; **Hospital:** Univ of Kentucky Albert B. Chandler Hosp; **Address:** Univ Kentucky - Kentucky Clinic, 740 S Limestone, rm J457, Lexington, KY 40536-0284; **Phone:** 859-323-0239; **Board Cert:** Pediatrics 1988; Pediatric Hematology-Oncology 2007; **Med School:** Dartmouth Med Sch 1982; **Resid:** Pediatrics, Univ Texas SW Med Ctr 1985; **Fellow:** Pediatric Hematology-Oncology, Natl Cancer Inst 1989; **Fac Appt:** Prof Ped, Univ KY Coll Med

Neuberg, Ronnie W MD [PHO] - **Spec Exp:** Pediatric Cancers; Gene Therapy; Clinical Trials; Brain Tumors; **Hospital:** Palmetto Health Richland Mem Hosp, MUSC Chldns Hosp; **Address:** Palmetto Health Richland, 7 Richland Medical Park Drive, Ste 7215, Columbia, SC 29203; **Phone:** 803-434-3533; **Board Cert:** Pediatrics 1982; Pediatric Hematology-Oncology 1982; **Med School:** SUNY Buffalo 1977; **Resid:** Pediatrics, Chldns Hosp 1980; **Fellow:** Pediatric Hematology-Oncology, SUNY Upstate Med Ctr 1982; **Fac Appt:** Assoc Prof Ped, Univ SC Sch Med

Nieder, Michael L MD [PHO] - **Spec Exp:** Bone Marrow Transplant; Inborn Errors of Metabolism; **Hospital:** All Children's Hosp; **Address:** 601 5th St S, Dept 7865, St Petersburg, FL 33701-4816; **Phone:** 727-767-6856; **Board Cert:** Pediatrics 1986; Pediatric Hematology-Oncology 2009; **Med School:** Univ IL Coll Med 1982; **Resid:** Pediatrics, Chldns Meml Hosp 1985; **Fellow:** Pediatric Hematology-Oncology, Chldns Meml Hosp 1988; **Fac Appt:** Prof Ped, Univ S Fla Coll Med

Olson, Thomas A MD [PHO] - **Spec Exp:** Platelet Disorders; Germ Cell Tumors; Retinoblastoma; Sarcoma; **Hospital:** Chldns Hlthcare Atlanta @ Egleston; **Address:** Childrens at Egleston Aflac Cancer Ctr, 1405 Clifton Rd NE, Tower 1, 4th Fl, Atlanta, GA 30322; **Phone:** 404-785-1200; **Board Cert:** Pediatrics 1982; Pediatric Hematology-Oncology 1984; **Med School:** Loyola Univ-Stritch Sch Med 1978; **Resid:** Pediatrics, Walter Reed AMC 1981; **Fellow:** Pediatric Hematology-Oncology, Walter Reed AMC 1983; **Fac Appt:** Assoc Prof Ped, Emory Univ

Pui, Ching-Hon MD [PHO] - **Spec Exp:** Leukemia; Lymphoma; **Hospital:** St. Jude Children's Research Hosp; **Address:** St Jude Chldns Rsch Hosp, 262 Danny Thomas Pl, Memphis, TN 38105; **Phone:** 901-595-3606; **Board Cert:** Pediatrics 1980; Pediatric Hematology-Oncology 1982; **Med School:** Taiwan 1976; **Resid:** Pediatrics, St Jude Chldns Rsch Hosp 1979; **Fellow:** Hematology & Oncology, St Jude Chldns Rsch Hosp 1981; **Fac Appt:** Prof Ped, Univ Tenn Coll Med

Ribeiro, Raul MD [PHO] - **Spec Exp:** Leukemia & Lymphoma; **Hospital:** St. Jude Children's Research Hosp; **Address:** St Jude's Chldns Rsch Hosp, 262 Danny Thomas Pl, rm S-2012, MS 721, Memphis, TN 38105-3678; **Phone:** 901-595-3694; **Board Cert:** Pediatric Hematology-Oncology 2009; **Med School:** Brazil 1975; **Resid:** Pediatrics, Univ Parana Sch Med 1978; **Fellow:** Hematology & Oncology, St Jude's Chldns Rsch Hosp 1987; **Fac Appt:** Prof Ped, Univ Tenn Coll Med

Rosoff, Philip M MD [PHO] - **Spec Exp:** Cancer Survivors-Late Effects of Therapy; Down Syndrome; Leukemia; **Hospital:** Duke Univ Hosp; **Address:** Duke Univ Med Ctr, Box 10238, Durham, NC 27710-0001; **Phone:** 919-684-3401; **Board Cert:** Pediatrics 1984; Pediatric Hematology-Oncology 2009; **Med School:** Case West Res Univ 1978; **Resid:** Pediatrics, Chldns Hosp 1980; **Fellow:** Pediatric Hematology-Oncology, Chldns Hosp/Dana Farber Cancer Inst 1984; **Fac Appt:** Assoc Prof Ped, Duke Univ

Russo, Carolyn MD [PHO] - **Spec Exp:** Brain Tumors; Cancer Survivors-Late Effects of Therapy; Palliative Care; **Hospital:** Huntsville Hosp, The; **Address:** 910 Adams St, Ste 310, huntsville, AL 35801; **Phone:** 256-265-5834; **Board Cert:** Pediatric Hematology-Oncology 2005; **Med School:** UCLA 1984; **Resid:** Pediatrics, Harbor-UCLA Med Ctr 1987; **Fellow:** Pediatric Hematology-Oncology, Stanford Med Ctr 1990

Sandler, Eric MD [PHO] - **Spec Exp:** Bone Marrow Transplant; Leukemia; Bone Tumors; Sickle Cell Disease; **Hospital:** Wolfson Chldns Hosp; **Address:** 807 Childrens Way, Jacksonville, FL 32207; **Phone:** 904-697-3793; **Board Cert:** Pediatrics 2008; Pediatric Hematology-Oncology 2007; **Med School:** Univ VT Coll Med 1985; **Resid:** Pediatrics, UCSF Med Ctr 1988; **Fellow:** Pediatric Hematology-Oncology, Univ Fla Med Sch 1991; **Fac Appt:** Assoc Prof Ped, Mayo Med Sch

Sandlund Jr, John T MD [PHO] - **Spec Exp:** Lymphoma, Non-Hodgkin's; Leukemia & Lymphoma; Ataxia Telangiectasia; **Hospital:** St. Jude Children's Research Hosp, Le Bonheur Chldns Med Ctr; **Address:** St Jude Children's Research Hosp, 262 Danny Thomas Pl, MS 260, Memphis, TN 38105; **Phone:** 901-595-2153; **Board Cert:** Pediatrics 1986; Pediatric Hematology-Oncology 1987; **Med School:** Ohio State Univ 1980; **Resid:** Pediatrics, Columbus Chldns Hosp 1983; **Fellow:** Hematology, Natl Cancer Inst 1986; Research, Natl Cancer Inst 1987; **Fac Appt:** Prof Ped, Univ Tenn Coll Med

Santana, Victor M MD [PHO] - **Spec Exp:** Solid Tumors; **Hospital:** St. Jude Children's Research Hosp; **Address:** St Jude Chldn's Rsch Hosp, Dept Oncology, 262 Danny Thomas Pl, rm C6041, MS 274, Memphis, TN 38105-2794; **Phone:** 901-595-2801; **Board Cert:** Pediatrics 1982; Pediatric Hematology-Oncology 1984; **Med School:** Puerto Rico 1978; **Resid:** Pediatrics, Johns Hopkins Hosp 1981; **Fellow:** Pediatric Hematology-Oncology, Johns Hopkins Hosp 1984; **Fac Appt:** Prof Ped, Univ Tenn Coll Med

Shearer, Patricia C MD [PHO] - **Spec Exp:** Cancer Survivors-Late Effects of Therapy; **Hospital:** Shands at Univ of FL; **Address:** Univ Florida/Shands Cancer Ctr, Cancer Survivorship Program, PO Box 103633, Gainesville, FL 32610; **Phone:** 352-273-8021; **Board Cert:** Pediatric Hematology-Oncology 2007; **Med School:** Louisiana State U, New Orleans 1986; **Resid:** Pediatrics, Johns Hopkins Hosp 1989; **Fellow:** Pediatric Hematology-Oncology, St Jude Chldns Rsch Hosp 1992; **Fac Appt:** Assoc Clin Prof Ped, Univ Fla Coll Med

Tebbi, Cameron MD [PHO] - **Spec Exp:** Hemophilia; Hodgkin's Disease; Leukemia; Sickle Cell Disease; **Hospital:** St. Josephs Chldns Hosp, Tampa Genl Hosp; **Address:** 4019 Carrollwood Village Drive, Tampa, FL 33607; **Phone:** 813-601-4400; **Board Cert:** Pediatrics 1974; Pediatric Hematology-Oncology 1980; **Med School:** Iran 1968; **Resid:** Pediatrics, Cincinnati Chldns Hosp 1972; Pediatric Hematology-Oncology, MD Anderson Cancer Inst 1972; **Fellow:** Pediatric Hematology-Oncology, St Louis Chldns Hosp 1973; Medical Oncology, Ontario Cancer Inst 1974

Pediatric Hematology-Oncology

Wang, Winfred C MD [PHO] - **Spec Exp:** Sickle Cell Disease; Bone Marrow Failure Disorders; Anemia-Aplastic; **Hospital:** St. Jude Children's Research Hosp, Le Bonheur Chldns Med Ctr; **Address:** St Jude Chldn Rsch Hosp, 262 Danny Thomas Pl, MS 800, Memphis, TN 38105-2729; **Phone:** 901-595-2051; **Board Cert:** Pediatrics 1972; Pediatric Hematology-Oncology 1974; **Med School:** Univ Chicago-Pritzker Sch Med 1967; **Resid:** Pediatrics, Montefiore Med Ctr 1969; Pediatrics, Kauikeolani Chldns Hosp 1970; **Fellow:** Pediatric Hematology-Oncology, UCSF Med Ctr 1975; **Fac Appt:** Prof Ped, Univ Tenn Coll Med

Wechsler, Daniel S MD/PhD [PHO] - **Spec Exp:** Leukemia & Lymphoma; Neuroblastoma; **Hospital:** Duke Univ Hosp; **Address:** Duke Univ Med Ctr-Ped Hem/Onc, Box 102382, Durham, NC 27710; **Phone:** 919-684-3401; **Board Cert:** Pediatric Hematology-Oncology 2009; **Med School:** Canada 1987; **Resid:** Pediatrics, Johns Hopkins Hosp 1990; **Fellow:** Pediatric Hematology-Oncology, Johns Hopkins Hosp 1994; **Fac Appt:** Assoc Prof Ped, Duke Univ

Midwest

Arndt, Carola A MD [PHO] - **Spec Exp:** Sarcoma; Brain Tumors; Stem Cell Transplant; **Hospital:** Mayo Med Ctr & Clin - Rochester; **Address:** Mayo Clinic, Dept Pediatrics, 200 1st St SW, Rochester, MN 55905; **Phone:** 507-284-2652; **Board Cert:** Pediatrics 1982; Pediatric Hematology-Oncology 1987; **Med School:** Boston Univ 1978; **Resid:** Pediatrics, Naval Reg Med Ctr 1981; **Fellow:** Pediatric Hematology-Oncology, Natl Inst Hlth 1984

Beyer, Eric C MD/PhD [PHO] - **Spec Exp:** Pediatric Cancers; Bleeding/Coagulation Disorders; Anemia; **Hospital:** Univ of Chicago Med Ctr; **Address:** University of Chicago Hospitals, 5841 S Maryland Ave, 900 E 57th St, Chicago, IL 60637; **Phone:** 773-702-6808; **Board Cert:** Pediatrics 1987; **Med School:** UCSD 1982; **Resid:** Pediatrics, Chldns Hosp 1984; **Fellow:** Hematology & Oncology, Dana Farber Cancer Inst 1987; **Fac Appt:** Prof Ped, Univ Chicago-Pritzker Sch Med

Blum, Kristie MD [PHO] - **Spec Exp:** Lymphoma; Lymphoma, Non-Hodgkin's; Lymphomas-Rare; **Hospital:** Ohio St Univ Med Ctr; **Address:** B315 Starling-Loving Hall, 320 W 10th Ave, Columbus, OH 43210; **Phone:** 614-293-8508; **Board Cert:** Internal Medicine 2000; Hematology 2004; Medical Oncology 2004; **Med School:** Univ Miami Sch Med 1997; **Resid:** Internal Medicine, Univ VA Hlth Sci Ctr 2000; **Fellow:** Hematology & Oncology, Vanderbilt Univ Med Ctr 2001; Hematology & Oncology, Wash Univ Affil Hosp 2003; **Fac Appt:** Asst Prof Med, Ohio State Univ

Boxer, Laurence MD [PHO] - **Spec Exp:** Congenital Neutropenia-Severe; Anemias & Red Cell Disorders; Bone Marrow Failure Disorders; Anemia-Aplastic; **Hospital:** Univ of Michigan Hosp; **Address:** Univ Michigan, L-2110 Womens Hosp, 1500 E Medical Ctr Dr, Box 0238, Ann Arbor, MI 48109-0238; **Phone:** 734-764-7126; **Board Cert:** Pediatrics 1971; Pediatric Hematology-Oncology 2010; **Med School:** Stanford Univ 1966; **Resid:** Pediatrics, Yale-New Haven Hosp 1968; Pediatrics, Stanford Univ Hosp 1969; **Fellow:** Hematology & Oncology, Chldns Hosp-Harvard 1974; **Fac Appt:** Prof Ped, Univ Mich Med Sch

Camitta, Bruce M MD [PHO] - **Spec Exp:** Leukemia; Anemia-Aplastic; Bone Marrow Transplant; **Hospital:** Chldns Hosp - Wisconsin; **Address:** MACC Fund Ctr for Cancer/Blood Disorders, 8701 Watertown Plank Rd, Ste 3018, Milwaukee, WI 53226; **Phone:** 414-456-4170; **Board Cert:** Pediatrics 1971; Pediatric Hematology-Oncology 1976; **Med School:** Johns Hopkins Univ 1966; **Resid:** Pediatrics, Chldns Hosp 1968; Pediatrics, Johns Hopkins Hosp 1969; **Fellow:** Pediatric Hematology-Oncology, Chldns Hosp 1973; **Fac Appt:** Prof Ped, Med Coll Wisc

Castle, Valerie P MD [PHO] - **Spec Exp:** Neuroblastoma; Bleeding/Coagulation Disorders; Cancer Survivors-Late Effects of Therapy; **Hospital:** Univ of Michigan Hosp; **Address:** Univ Mich Comp Cancer Ctr, 1500 E Medical Center Drive, Level B1-258, Reception B, Ann Arbor, MI 48109-0911; **Phone:** 734-936-9814; **Board Cert:** Pediatric Hematology-Oncology 2006; **Med School:** McMaster Univ 1983; **Resid:** Pediatrics, McMaster Univ Med Ctr 1986; **Fellow:** Pediatric Hematology-Oncology, Univ Mich Hosps 1989; **Fac Appt:** Prof Ped, Univ Mich Med Sch

Cohn, Susan L MD [PHO] - **Spec Exp:** Neuroblastoma; **Hospital:** Univ of Chicago Med Ctr; **Address:** Univ Chicago Medical Ctr, 900 E 57th St, rm 5100, Chicago, IL 60637; **Phone:** 773-702-2571; **Board Cert:** Pediatrics 1985; Pediatric Hematology-Oncology 1987; **Med School:** Univ IL Coll Med 1980; **Resid:** Pediatrics, Michael Reese Hosp 1984; **Fellow:** Hematology & Oncology, Chldns Meml Hosp 1985; **Fac Appt:** Prof Ped, Univ Chicago-Pritzker Sch Med

Corey, Seth J MD [PHO] - **Spec Exp:** Bone Marrow Failure Disorders; Leukemia; Myelodysplastic Syndromes; Ataxia Telangiectasia; **Hospital:** Children's Mem Hosp -Chicago; **Address:** Robert Lurie Comp Cancer Ctr, 303 E Superior St, Chicago, IL 60611; **Phone:** 312-503-6694; **Board Cert:** Pediatrics 1986; Pediatric Hematology-Oncology 2004; **Med School:** Tulane Univ 1982; **Resid:** Pediatrics, St Louis Chldns Hosp 1985; **Fellow:** Hematology & Oncology, Tufts Univ 1992; Renal Pathology, Boston Chldns-Dana Farber Ctr 1989; **Fac Appt:** Prof Ped, Northwestern Univ-Feinberg Sch Med

Croop, James M MD/PhD [PHO] - **Spec Exp:** Solid Tumors; Clinical Trials; **Hospital:** Riley Hosp for Children; **Address:** Riley Hosp for Children, Hem/Onc, 702 Riley Hospital Drive, Ste 4340, Indianapolis, IN 46202; **Phone:** 317-944-2143; **Board Cert:** Pediatrics 1985; Pediatric Hematology-Oncology 2010; **Med School:** Univ Pennsylvania 1980; **Resid:** Pediatrics, Childrens Hosp 1983; **Fellow:** Pediatric Hematology-Oncology, Childrens Hosp 1985; **Fac Appt:** Prof Ped, Indiana Univ

Cunningham, John M MD [PHO] - **Spec Exp:** Stem Cell Transplant; Sickle Cell Disease; Thalassemia; Clinical Trials; **Hospital:** Univ of Chicago Med Ctr; **Address:** 5841 S Maryland Ave, MC 4060, Chicago, IL 60637; **Phone:** 773-702-2616; **Med School:** Ireland 1982; **Resid:** Pediatrics, St Laurence's Hosp 1985; Pediatrics, Mater Misericordiae Hosp 1987; **Fellow:** Pediatric Hematology-Oncology, Royal Free Hosp 1991; Transplant Surgery, Natl Heart, Lung, & Blood Inst/NIH 1993; **Fac Appt:** Prof Ped, Univ Chicago-Pritzker Sch Med

Davies, Stella M MD/PhD [PHO] - **Spec Exp:** Leukemia; Bone Marrow Transplant; Stem Cell Transplant; **Hospital:** Cincinnati Chldns Hosp Med Ctr; **Address:** Cincinnati Chldns Hosp Med Ctr, 3333 Burnet Ave, MLC 7015, Cincinnati, OH 45229-3039; **Phone:** 513-636-2469; **Med School:** England, UK 1981; **Resid:** Pediatrics, Univ Newcastle Med Ctr 1985; **Fellow:** Pediatric Hematology-Oncology, Univ Minn Med Ctr 1993; **Fac Appt:** Prof Ped, Univ Cincinnati

Fallon, Robert J MD/PhD [PHO] - **Spec Exp:** Lymphoma; Hodgkin's Disease; Stem Cell Transplant; **Hospital:** Riley Hosp for Children; **Address:** Riley Childrens Hospital, 705 Riley Hospital Drive, rm 4340, Indianapolis, IN 46202; **Phone:** 317-944-2143; **Board Cert:** Internal Medicine 1983; Medical Oncology 1985; **Med School:** NYU Sch Med 1980; **Resid:** Internal Medicine, Brigham & Womens Hosp 1983; **Fellow:** Hematology & Oncology, Brigham & Womens Hosp/Dana Farber Cancer Inst 1985; **Fac Appt:** Prof Ped, Indiana Univ

Ferrara, James MD [PHO] - **Spec Exp:** Bone Marrow Transplant; Graft vs Host Disease; Inflammatory Cytokines; **Hospital:** Univ of Michigan Hosp; **Address:** Univ Michigan Comprehensive Cancer Ctr, 1500 E Medical Center Drive, Ste 6308, Ann Arbor, MI 48109-5942; **Phone:** 734-615-1340; **Board Cert:** Pediatrics 2005; Pediatric Hematology-Oncology 2006; **Med School:** Georgetown Univ 1980; **Resid:** Pediatrics, Children's Hosp 1982; **Fellow:** Pediatric Hematology-Oncology, Children's Hosp 1985; **Fac Appt:** Prof Ped, Univ Mich Med Sch

Pediatric Hematology-Oncology

Friebert, Sarah E MD [PHO] - **Spec Exp:** Palliative Care; Cancer Survivors-Late Effects of Therapy; **Hospital:** Akron Children's Hosp; **Address:** Children's Hosp Med Ctr of Akron, One Perkins Sq Fl 5, Akron, OH 44308; **Phone:** 330-543-3343; **Board Cert:** Pediatrics 2004; Pediatric Hematology-Oncology 2008; Hospice & Palliative Medicine 2008; **Med School:** Case West Res Univ 1993; **Resid:** Pediatrics, Chldns Hosp 1996; **Fellow:** Pediatric Hematology-Oncology, Rainbow Babies-Chldns Hosp 1999; **Fac Appt:** Asst Prof Ped, NE Ohio Univ

Goldman, Stewart MD [PHO] - **Spec Exp:** Neuro-Oncology; Brain Tumors; Clinical Trials; **Hospital:** Children's Mem Hosp -Chicago; **Address:** Childrens Meml Hosp, Div Hem/Onc, 2300 Childrens Plaza, Box 30, Chicago, IL 60614; **Phone:** 773-880-3004; **Board Cert:** Pediatric Hematology-Oncology 2011; **Med School:** Loyola Univ-Stritch Sch Med 1985; **Resid:** Pediatrics, Univ Chicago Hosps 1988; **Fellow:** Pediatric Hematology-Oncology, Univ Chicago Hosps 1991

Haut, Paul R MD [PHO] - **Spec Exp:** Stem Cell Transplant; Bone Marrow Transplant; Leukemia; **Hospital:** Riley Hosp for Children, IU Health North Hosp; **Address:** Riley Hospital for Children, 705 Riley Hospital Drive, rm 4340, Indianapolis, IN 46202; **Phone:** 317-944-2143; **Board Cert:** Pediatric Hematology-Oncology 2008; **Med School:** Univ Ark 1990; **Resid:** Pediatrics, Arkansas Childrens Hosp 1994; **Fellow:** Pediatric Hematology-Oncology, Children's Meml Hosp 1997; **Fac Appt:** Prof Ped, Indiana Univ

Hayani, Ammar MD [PHO] - **Spec Exp:** Leukemia; Solid Tumors; Lymphoma; **Hospital:** Adv Christ Med Ctr, Adv Good Samaritan Hosp; **Address:** Hope Childrens Hosp, 4440 W 95th St, Oak Lawn, IL 60453-2600; **Phone:** 708-684-4094; **Board Cert:** Pediatric Hematology-Oncology 2005; **Med School:** Syria 1982; **Resid:** Pediatrics, LSU Hosp 1987; **Fellow:** Pediatric Hematology-Oncology, Baylor Affil Hosp 1991

Hayashi, Robert J MD [PHO] - **Spec Exp:** Bone Marrow Transplant; Cancer Survivors-Late Effects of Therapy; Leukemia; **Hospital:** St. Louis Chldns Hosp; **Address:** St Louis Chldns Hosp, Div Ped Hem Onc, One Children's Pl, Ste 9 South, Box 8116, St Louis, MO 63110; **Phone:** 314-454-6018; **Board Cert:** Pediatrics 2007; Pediatric Hematology-Oncology 2007; **Med School:** Washington Univ, St Louis 1986; **Resid:** Pediatrics, St Louis Childrens Hosp 1989; **Fellow:** Pediatric Hematology-Oncology, Johns Hopkins Hosp 1992; **Fac Appt:** Assoc Prof Ped, Washington Univ, St Louis

Hetherington, Maxine MD [PHO] - **Spec Exp:** Brain Tumors; **Hospital:** Chldns Mercy Hosps & Clinics; **Address:** Childrens Mercy Hosptial, 2401 Gillham Rd, Kansas City, MO 64108; **Phone:** 816-234-3265; **Board Cert:** Pediatrics 1983; Pediatric Hematology-Oncology 1987; **Med School:** Univ Tenn Coll Med 1978; **Resid:** Pediatrics, Childrens Med Ctr 1981; **Fellow:** Pediatric Hematology-Oncology, Univ Texas Hlth Sci Ctr 1987; **Fac Appt:** Assoc Prof Ped, Univ MO-Kansas City

Hord, Jeffrey D MD [PHO] - **Spec Exp:** Hematologic Malignancies; Bone Marrow Failure Disorders; Sickle Cell Disease; Pediatric Cancers; **Hospital:** Akron Children's Hosp; **Address:** Akron Childrens Hosp, Hematology/Oncology, One Perkins Square, Akron, OH 44308; **Phone:** 330-543-8580; **Board Cert:** Pediatric Hematology-Oncology 2004; **Med School:** Univ KY Coll Med 1989; **Resid:** Pediatrics, Childrens Hosp 1992; **Fellow:** Pediatric Hematology-Oncology, Vanderbilt Univ Med Ctr 1995; **Fac Appt:** Prof Ped, NE Ohio Univ

Hutchinson, Raymond MD [PHO] - **Spec Exp:** Leukemia; Hodgkin's Disease; **Hospital:** Univ of Michigan Hosp; **Address:** Univ Michigan Hosp, 1500 E Med Ctr Drive, rm L2110, Level B1, 258 Reception B, Ann Arbor, MI 48109-5238; **Phone:** 734-936-9814; **Board Cert:** Pediatrics 1979; Pediatric Hematology-Oncology 1980; **Med School:** Harvard Med Sch 1973; **Resid:** Pediatrics, New England Med Ctr 1975; **Fellow:** Pediatric Hematology-Oncology, Childrens Hosp 1978; **Fac Appt:** Prof Ped, Univ Mich Med Sch

Lusher, Jeanne M MD [PHO] - **Hospital:** Chldns Hosp of Michigan; **Address:** Children's Hospital Michigan, Div Hem/Onc, 3901 Beaubien Blvd, Detroit, MI 48201; **Phone:** 313-745-5515; **Board Cert:** Pediatrics 1986; Pediatric Hematology-Oncology 1986; **Med School:** Univ Cincinnati 1960; **Resid:** Pediatrics, Charity Hosp/Tulane Univ 1963; **Fellow:** Hematology & Oncology, Charity Hosp/Tulane Univ 1965; Hematology & Oncology, Saint Louis Children's Hosp 1966; **Fac Appt:** Prof Ped, Wayne State Univ

Manera, Ricarchito B MD [PHO] - **Spec Exp:** Leukemia & Lymphoma; Brain Tumors; **Hospital:** Loyola Univ Med Ctr; **Address:** Loyola University Med Ctr, Div Pediatric Hematology/Oncology, 2160 S First Ave, Maywood, IL 60611; **Phone:** 708-327-9136; **Board Cert:** Pediatrics 2010; Pediatric Hematology-Oncology 2011; **Med School:** Philippines 1984; **Resid:** Pediatrics, Bronx-Lebanon Hosp Ctr 1995; **Fellow:** Pediatric Hematology-Oncology, MD Anderson Cancer Ctr 1994; Pediatric Hematology-Oncology, Columbia-Presby Med Ctr 1996; **Fac Appt:** Assoc Prof Ped, Loyola Univ-Stritch Sch Med

Morgan, Elaine MD [PHO] - **Spec Exp:** Leukemia; Palliative Care; Ethics; Hemophagocytic Syndrome; **Hospital:** Children's Mem Hosp -Chicago; **Address:** Children's Meml Hosp, Div Hem/Onc, 2300 Children's Plaza, Box 30, Chicago, IL 60614; **Phone:** 773-880-4562; **Board Cert:** Pediatrics 1976; Pediatric Hematology-Oncology 2009; Hospice & Palliative Medicine 2008; **Med School:** Univ Pennsylvania 1971; **Resid:** Pediatrics, Chldns Hosp 1974; **Fellow:** Pediatric Hematology-Oncology, Chldns Hosp Med Ctr 1975; Pediatric Hematology-Oncology, Chldns Meml Med Ctr 1976; **Fac Appt:** Prof Ped, Northwestern Univ-Feinberg Sch Med

Neglia, Joseph MD [PHO] - **Spec Exp:** Cancer Survivors-Late Effects of Therapy; **Address:** Univ Minnesota-Div Ped Hem/Oncology, 420 Delaware St SE, MMC 391, PWB 13-118, Minneapolis, MN 55455; **Phone:** 612-624-3113; **Board Cert:** Pediatrics 1986; Pediatric Hematology-Oncology 1987; **Med School:** Loma Linda Univ 1981; **Resid:** Pediatrics, Baylor Coll Med 1984; **Fellow:** Pediatric Hematology-Oncology, Univ Minn Hosp 1987; **Fac Appt:** Prof Ped, Univ Minn

O'Dorisio, M Sue MD/PhD [PHO] - **Spec Exp:** Neuroblastoma; Medulloblastoma; Neuroendocrine Tumors; **Hospital:** Univ Iowa Hosp & Clinics; **Address:** UIHC Dept Pediatrics, Div Hematology/Oncology, 200 Hawkins Drive, 2520 JCP, Iowa City, IA 52242; **Phone:** 319-356-7873; **Board Cert:** Pediatrics 2007; Pediatric Hematology-Oncology 2009; **Med School:** Ohio State Univ 1985; **Resid:** Pediatrics, Chldns Hosp 1988; **Fellow:** Pediatric Hematology-Oncology, Chldns Hosp 1992; **Fac Appt:** Prof Ped, Univ Iowa Coll Med

Olshefski, Randal S MD [PHO] - **Spec Exp:** Brain Tumors; **Hospital:** Nationwide Chldn's Hosp; **Address:** Nationwide Chldn's Hosp: Hemology/Onc, 700 Children's Drive, Columbus, OH 43205; **Phone:** 614-722-3552; **Board Cert:** Pediatric Hematology-Oncology 2004; **Med School:** Univ Pittsburgh 1988; **Resid:** Pediatrics, Nationwide Chldn's Hosp 1991; **Fellow:** Hematology & Oncology, Children's Natl Med Ctr 1995; **Fac Appt:** Clin Prof Ped, Ohio State Univ

Plautz, Gregory E MD [PHO] - **Spec Exp:** Brain Tumors; Leukemia & Lymphoma; Wilms' Tumor; Cancer Survivors-Late Effects of Therapy; **Hospital:** Cleveland Clin (page 56); **Address:** Cleveland Clinic Fdn - Div Ped Hem Onc, 9500 Euclid Ave, Cleveland, OH 44195; **Phone:** 216-445-4044; **Board Cert:** Pediatric Hematology-Oncology 2005; **Med School:** Indiana Univ 1984; **Resid:** Pediatrics, Johns Hopkins Hosp 1987; **Fellow:** Pediatric Hematology-Oncology, Univ Michigan Affil Hosp 1990; **Fac Appt:** Assoc Prof Ped, Case West Res Univ

Puccetti, Diane M MD [PHO] - **Spec Exp:** Brain Tumors; Neuro-Oncology; Cancer Survivors-Late Effects of Therapy; **Hospital:** Univ WI Hosp & Clins; **Address:** Univ Wisconsin Childrens Hosp, 1111 Highland Ave, 4105 WIMR, Madison, WI 53792; **Phone:** 608-263-6420; **Board Cert:** Pediatric Hematology-Oncology 2007; **Med School:** Med Coll OH 1985; **Resid:** Pediatrics, UC-Irvine Med Ctr 1986; Pediatrics, Med Coll Ohio 1988; **Fellow:** Pediatric Hematology-Oncology, Riley Hosp Chldn 1991; **Fac Appt:** Assoc Clin Prof Ped, Univ Wisc

Pediatric Hematology-Oncology

Razzouk, Bassem I MD [PHO] - **Spec Exp:** Leukemia; Clinical Trials; Lymphoma; Langerhans Cell Histiocytosis (LCH); **Hospital:** Peyton Manning Children's Hosp at St. Vincent; **Address:** Peyton Manning Chldns Hosp, Center for Cancer & Blood Diseases, 2001 W 86th St, Indianapolis, IN 46260; **Phone:** 317-338-4673; **Board Cert:** Pediatrics 2008; Pediatric Hematology-Oncology 2011; **Med School:** Lebanon 1987; **Resid:** Pediatrics, American Univ Med Ctr 1990; Pediatrics, SUNY Hlth Sci Ctr 1992; **Fellow:** Hematology & Oncology, St. Jude Chldns Rsch Hosp 1995

Rubin, Charles M MD [PHO] - **Spec Exp:** Brain Tumors; Retinoblastoma; Bone Marrow Transplant; **Hospital:** Univ Chicago-Comer Chldn's Hosp; **Address:** Univ Chicago Med Ctr, 5841 S Maryland Ave, MC 4060, Chicago, IL 60637; **Phone:** 773-702-6808; **Board Cert:** Pediatrics 1984; Clinical Cytogenetics 1987; Pediatric Hematology-Oncology 1984; **Med School:** Tufts Univ 1979; **Resid:** Pediatrics, Chldn's Hosp 1982; Pediatric Hematology-Oncology, Univ Minnesota Hosp 1985; **Fellow:** Cytogenetics, Univ Chicago-Pritzker School of Med 1987; **Fac Appt:** Assoc Prof Ped, Univ Chicago-Pritzker Sch Med

Salvi, Sharad MD [PHO] - **Spec Exp:** Leukemia & Lymphoma; Bleeding/Coagulation Disorders; Anemia; Solid Tumors; **Hospital:** Adv Christ Med Ctr, Central DuPage Hosp; **Address:** Hope Chldns Hosp, 4440 W 95th St, Oak Lawn, IL 60453; **Phone:** 708-684-4094; **Board Cert:** Pediatrics 1982; Pediatric Hematology-Oncology 1982; **Med School:** India 1974; **Resid:** Pediatrics, Lincoln Meml Hosp 1979; **Fellow:** Pediatric Hematology-Oncology, Chldns Hosp/Roswell Park Meml Cancer Inst 1981

Sencer, Susan F MD [PHO] - **Spec Exp:** Pediatric Cancers; Complementary Medicine; **Hospital:** Chldns Hosp and Clinics - Minneapolis; **Address:** Chldns Specialty Clinic, Hem/Onc Clin, 2525 Chicago Ave S, Ste CSC-175, Minneapolis, MN 55404; **Phone:** 612-813-5940; **Board Cert:** Pediatric Hematology-Oncology 2007; **Med School:** Univ Minn 1984; **Resid:** Pediatrics, Univ Minnesota Affil Hosp 1988; **Fellow:** Pediatric Hematology-Oncology, Univ Minnesota Affil Hosp 1991

Shapiro, Amy D MD [PHO] - **Spec Exp:** Hemophilia; Bleeding/Coagulation Disorders; **Hospital:** Peyton Manning Children's Hosp at St. Vincent; **Address:** Indiana Hemophilia & Thrombosis Ctr, 8402 Harcourt Rd, Ste 500, Indianapolis, IN 46260; **Phone:** 317-871-0011; **Board Cert:** Pediatrics 1986; Pediatric Hematology-Oncology 1987; **Med School:** NYU Sch Med 1980; **Resid:** Pediatrics, Univ Colo Affil Hosp 1982; **Fellow:** Pediatric Hematology-Oncology, Univ Colo Hlth Sci Ctr 1983

Sondel, Paul M MD/PhD [PHO] - **Spec Exp:** Immunotherapy; Stem Cell Transplant; Pediatric Cancers; **Hospital:** Univ WI Hosp & Clins; **Address:** 4159 WIMR, 1111 Highland Ave, Madison, WI 53705; **Phone:** 608-263-6200; **Board Cert:** Pediatrics 1981; **Med School:** Harvard Med Sch 1977; **Resid:** Pediatrics, Univ MN Hosp 1978; Pediatrics, Univ Wisconsin Hosp 1980; **Fellow:** Research, Sidney Farber Cancer Inst/Harvard 1977; **Fac Appt:** Prof Ped, Univ Wisc

Tannous, Raymond MD [PHO] - **Spec Exp:** Wilms' Tumor; Leukemia & Lymphoma; Pain-Cancer; **Hospital:** Univ Iowa Hosp & Clinics; **Address:** Univ Iowa Hosps & Clinics, Dept Peds, 200 Hawkins Drive, rm 2528 JCP, Iowa City, IA 52242; **Phone:** 319-356-2229; **Board Cert:** Pediatrics 1976; Pediatric Hematology-Oncology 1978; **Med School:** France 1972; **Resid:** Pediatrics, St Jude Chldns Rsch Hosp 1976; **Fellow:** Pediatric Hematology-Oncology, St Jude Chldns Rsch Hosp 1977; **Fac Appt:** Assoc Prof Ped, Univ Iowa Coll Med

Valentino, Leonard Anthony MD [PHO] - **Spec Exp:** Bleeding/Coagulation Disorders; Thrombotic Disorders; Hemophilia; Hereditary Hemorrhagic Telangiectasia; **Hospital:** Rush Univ Med Ctr, Rush Copley Med Ctr; **Address:** 1653 W Congress Pkwy, Chicago, IL 60612-3828; **Phone:** 312-942-5983; **Board Cert:** Pediatrics 2007; Pediatric Hematology-Oncology 2005; **Med School:** Creighton Univ 1984; **Resid:** Pediatrics, Univ Illinios Med Ctr 1987; **Fellow:** Pediatric Hematology-Oncology, UCLA Med Ctr 1990; **Fac Appt:** Prof Ped, Rush Med Coll

Vik, Terry A MD [PHO] - **Spec Exp:** Neuroblastoma; Cancer Survivors-Late Effects of Therapy; Leukemia; Drug Development; **Hospital:** Riley Hosp for Children; **Address:** Riley Hosp Children, 705 Riley Hospital Drive, rm 4340, Indianapolis, IN 46202; **Phone:** 317-944-2143; **Board Cert:** Pediatrics 1987; Pediatric Hematology-Oncology 2011; **Med School:** Johns Hopkins Univ 1983; **Resid:** Pediatrics, UCLA Med Ctr 1986; **Fellow:** Pediatric Hematology-Oncology, Chldns Hosp/Dana Farber 1989; **Fac Appt:** Assoc Prof Ped, Indiana Univ

Yaddanapudi, Ravindranath MD [PHO] - **Spec Exp:** Leukemia; **Hospital:** Chldns Hosp of Michigan; **Address:** Children's Hospital Michigan, Div Hem/Onc, 3901 Beaubien Blvd, Detroit, MI 48201; **Phone:** 313-745-5515; **Board Cert:** Pediatrics 1970; Pediatric Hematology-Oncology 1974; **Med School:** India 1964; **Resid:** Pathology, Western Penn Hosp 1967; Pediatrics, Children's Hosp 1969; **Fellow:** Pediatric Hematology-Oncology, Children's Hosp Michigan 1971; **Fac Appt:** Prof Ped, Wayne State Univ

Great Plains and Mountains

Abromowitch, Minnie MD [PHO] - **Hospital:** Children's Hosp - Omaha; **Address:** Children's Hosp & Med Ctr, Dept Pediatric Hem Onc, 8200 Dodge St, Omaha, NE 68114; **Phone:** 402-955-3950; **Board Cert:** Pediatrics 1980; Pediatric Hematology-Oncology 1982; **Med School:** Univ Manitoba 1973; **Resid:** Pediatrics, Hospital for Sick Children 1976; Pediatric Hematology-Oncology, Univ Manitoba 1978; **Fellow:** Pediatric Hematology-Oncology, St Jude Chldns Research Hosp 1980; **Fac Appt:** Assoc Prof Ped, Univ Nebr Coll Med

Bruggers, Carol S MD [PHO] - **Spec Exp:** Brain Tumors; Clinical Trials; **Hospital:** Primary Children's Med Ctr, Univ Utah Hlth Care; **Address:** Primary Children's Medical Ctr, 100 Mario Capecchi Drive, Salt Lake City, UT 84113; **Phone:** 801-662-4700; **Board Cert:** Pediatrics 2008; Pediatric Hematology-Oncology 2008; **Med School:** Mich State Univ 1984; **Resid:** Pediatrics, Univ Colorado Health Sci Ctr 1987; **Fellow:** Pediatric Hematology-Oncology, Duke Univ Med Ctr 1991; **Fac Appt:** Prof Ped, Univ Utah

Coccia, Peter F MD [PHO] - **Spec Exp:** Bone Marrow Transplant; Leukemia & Lymphoma; Solid Tumors; **Hospital:** Nebraska Med Ctr, Children's Hosp - Omaha; **Address:** Univ Nebr Med Ctr, Dept Pediatrics, 982168 Nebraska Med Ctr, Omaha, NE 68198-2168; **Phone:** 402-559-7257; **Board Cert:** Clinical Pathology 1972; Hematology 1975; Pediatrics 1976; Pediatric Hematology-Oncology 1976; **Med School:** SUNY Upstate Med Univ 1968; **Resid:** Pathology, Upstate Med Ctr 1970; Pediatrics, Univ Minn 1973; **Fellow:** Pediatric Hematology-Oncology, Univ Minn 1974; **Fac Appt:** Prof Ped, Univ Nebr Coll Med

Hilden, Joanne M MD [PHO] - **Spec Exp:** Leukemia in Infants; Brain Tumors; Leukemia & Lymphoma; Leukemia in Down Syndrome; **Hospital:** Children's Hosp - Denver; **Address:** Childrens Hosp Colorado, 13123 E 16th St, Ste B115, Aurora, CO 80045; **Phone:** 720-777-8857; **Board Cert:** Pediatrics 2006; Pediatric Hematology-Oncology 2009; Hospice & Palliative Medicine 2008; **Med School:** Univ Minn 1988; **Resid:** Pediatrics, Univ Minn Med Ctr 1991; **Fellow:** Pediatric Hematology-Oncology, Univ Minnesota 1994; **Fac Appt:** Assoc Prof Ped, Univ Colorado

Kobrinsky, Nathan L MD [PHO] - **Spec Exp:** Pediatric Cancers; Immunotherapy; Hemophilia; Bleeding/Coagulation Disorders; **Hospital:** Sanford Med Ctr Fargo; **Address:** Sanford Roger Maris Cancer Ctr, 820 4th St N, Fargo, ND 58122; **Phone:** 701-234-7544; **Board Cert:** Pediatrics 1981; Pediatric Hematology-Oncology 1982; **Med School:** Univ Manitoba 1976; **Resid:** Pediatrics, Chldns Hlth Sci Ctr 1978; **Fellow:** Pediatric Hematology-Oncology, Chldns Hlth Sci Ctr 1979; Pediatric Hematology-Oncology, Univ Minn 1981; **Fac Appt:** Prof Ped, Univ ND Sch Med

Pediatric Hematology-Oncology

Manco-Johnson, Marilyn MD [PHO] - **Spec Exp:** Hemophilia; Thrombotic Disorders; **Hospital:** Chldn's Hosp - Aurora (CO), Univ of CO Hosp - Anschutz Inpatient Pav; **Address:** Univ Colorado Hemophilia Ctr, 13199 E Montview Blvd, Ste 100, MS F416, Aurora, CO 80045; **Phone:** 303-724-0365; **Board Cert:** Pediatrics 1979; Pediatric Hematology-Oncology 1980; **Med School:** Jefferson Med Coll 1974; **Resid:** Pediatrics, Univ Colorado Affil Hosps 1977; **Fellow:** Pediatric Hematology-Oncology, Chldns Hosp 1981; **Fac Appt:** Prof Ped, Univ Colorado

Southwest

Albritton, Karen H MD [PHO] - **Spec Exp:** Sarcoma; **Hospital:** Cook Chldns Med Ctr, Harris Methodist Hosp - Fort Worth; **Address:** Cook Childrens Med Ctr, Hematology/Oncology Clinic, 901 7th Ave, Ste 220, Fort Worth, TX 76104; **Phone:** 682-885-4007; **Board Cert:** Pediatric Hematology-Oncology 2002; Medical Oncology 2001; **Med School:** Univ Tex, San Antonio 1992; **Resid:** Internal Medicine & Pediatrics, Univ NC Hosps 1996; **Fellow:** Hematology & Oncology, Univ NC Hosps 2000; Pediatric Hematology-Oncology, Univ NC Hosps 2000; **Fac Appt:** Assoc Prof Ped, Univ N Tex Hlth Sci Ctr, Coll Osteo Med

Berg, Stacey MD [PHO] - **Spec Exp:** Drug Discovery & Development; Brain Tumors; Solid Tumors; **Hospital:** Texas Chldns Hosp; **Address:** Texas Chldns Cancer Ctr, Dept Ped Hem-Onc, 6701 Fannin St, Ste CC 1400, Houston, TX 77030; **Phone:** 832-822-4242; **Board Cert:** Pediatrics 2007; Pediatric Hematology-Oncology 2007; **Med School:** Univ Pittsburgh 1985; **Resid:** Pediatrics, Chldns Hosp 1988; **Fellow:** Pediatric Hematology-Oncology, Natl Inst Hlth 1991; **Fac Appt:** Prof Ped, Baylor Coll Med

Blaney, Susan MD [PHO] - **Spec Exp:** Brain Tumors; Neuro-Oncology; Drug Development; Clinical Trials; **Hospital:** Texas Chldns Hosp; **Address:** 6701 Fannin St, Ste 1410.00, Houston, TX 77030; **Phone:** 832-822-1482; **Board Cert:** Pediatric Hematology-Oncology 2005; **Med School:** Med Coll OH 1984; **Resid:** Pediatrics, Letterman AMC 1987; **Fellow:** Pediatric Oncology, Walter Reed AMC 1990; **Fac Appt:** Prof Ped, Baylor Coll Med

Buchanan, George R MD [PHO] - **Spec Exp:** Sickle Cell Disease; Thrombotic Disorders; Hemophilia; Leukemia; **Hospital:** Chldns Med Ctr of Dallas; **Address:** Univ Texas SW Med Ctr, Peds Hem Onc, 5323 Harry Hines Blvd, MC 9063, Dallas, TX 75390-9063; **Phone:** 214-456-2978; **Board Cert:** Pediatrics 1975; Pediatric Hematology-Oncology 2000; **Med School:** Univ Chicago-Pritzker Sch Med 1970; **Resid:** Pediatrics, Chldns Meml Hosp 1973; **Fellow:** Hematology & Oncology, Chldns Meml Hosp 1975; **Fac Appt:** Prof Ped, Univ Tex SW, Dallas

Dreyer, ZoAnn E MD [PHO] - **Spec Exp:** Cancer Survivors-Late Effects of Therapy; Leukemia in Infants; **Hospital:** Texas Chldns Hosp; **Address:** Texas Childrens Hosp, Clinical Care Ctr, 6701 Fannin St Fl 14, MC CC1400, Houston, TX 77030; **Phone:** 832-822-4242; **Board Cert:** Pediatrics 1988; Pediatric Hematology-Oncology 2005; **Med School:** UC Davis 1982; **Resid:** Pediatrics, Baylor Affil Hosps 1985; **Fellow:** Pediatric Hematology-Oncology, Baylor Coll Med 1988; **Fac Appt:** Assoc Prof Ped, Baylor Coll Med

Goldman, Stanton C MD [PHO] - **Spec Exp:** Leukemia; Lymphoma; Stem Cell Transplant; **Hospital:** Med City Dallas Hosp; **Address:** 7777 Forest Ln, Ste D400, Dallas, TX 75230; **Phone:** 972-566-6647; **Board Cert:** Pediatric Hematology-Oncology 2004; Pediatrics 2008; **Med School:** Boston Univ 1990; **Resid:** Pediatrics, Chldns Natl Med Ctr 1996; **Fellow:** Pediatric Hematology-Oncology, Johns Hopkins Hosp

Graham, Michael L MD [PHO] - **Spec Exp:** Bone Marrow Transplant; Leukemia; Stem Cell Transplant; **Hospital:** Banner Desert Med Ctr; **Address:** Cardon Chldns Med Ctr, Div Pediatric Hematology/Oncology, 1432 S Dobson Rd, Ste 107, Mesa, AZ 85202; **Phone:** 480-412-4100; **Board Cert:** Pediatrics 1980; Pediatric Hematology-Oncology 1984; **Med School:** Brown Univ 1975; **Resid:** Pediatrics, Johns Hopkins Hosp 1978; Pediatric Hematology-Oncology, Johns Hopkins Hosp 1980; **Fellow:** Medical Oncology, Yale-New Haven Hosp 1982; **Fac Appt:** Assoc Prof Ped, Univ Ariz Coll Med

Meyer, William H MD [PHO] - **Spec Exp:** Sarcoma; Pediatric Cancers; **Hospital:** Chldns Hosp OU Med Ctr; **Address:** OU Childrens Physicians, 1200 N Phillips Ave, Ste 10000, Oklahoma City, OK 73104; **Phone:** 405-271-4412; **Board Cert:** Pediatrics 1980; Pediatric Hematology-Oncology 1980; **Med School:** Jefferson Med Coll 1974; **Resid:** Pediatrics, Wilmington Med Ctr 1977; **Fellow:** Pediatric Hematology-Oncology, Johns Hopkins Hosp 1980; **Fac Appt:** Prof Ped, Univ Okla Coll Med

Tomlinson, Gail E MD [PHO] - **Spec Exp:** Cancer Survivors-Late Effects of Therapy; Cancer Genetics; Liver Cancer; Kidney Cancer; **Hospital:** Christus Santa Rosa Children's Hosp, Univ Hlth Syst-San Antonio; **Address:** UT HSC at San Antonio, 7703 Floyd Curl Drive, MC 7810, San Antonio, TX 78229; **Phone:** 210-704-3405; **Board Cert:** Pediatrics 2008; Pediatric Hematology-Oncology 2009; **Med School:** Geo Wash Univ 1984; **Resid:** Pediatrics, Chldns Hosp Natl Med Ctr 1987; **Fellow:** Pediatric Hematology-Oncology, MD Anderson Cancer Ctr 1989; Pediatric Hematology-On-cology, Univ Texas SW Med Ctr 1992; **Fac Appt:** Prof Ped, Univ Tex, San Antonio

Williams, James A MD [PHO] - **Spec Exp:** Sarcoma; Leukemia; **Hospital:** Banner Desert Med Ctr, St. Joseph's Hosp & Med Ctr - Phoenix; **Address:** 1919 E Thomas Rd, Phoenix, AZ 85016; **Phone:** 602-546-0920; **Board Cert:** Pediatric Hematology-Oncology 2008; **Med School:** Wayne State Univ 1993; **Resid:** Pediatrics, Wayne St Univ Med Ctr 1996; **Fellow:** Pediatric Hematology-On-cology, Wayne St Univ Med Ctr 1999

Winick, Naomi J MD [PHO] - **Spec Exp:** Leukemia; **Hospital:** Chldns Med Ctr of Dallas; **Address:** Ctr for Cancer & Blood Disorders, 1935 Med District Drive Brides Bldg Fl 3, Dallas, TX 75235-7794; **Phone:** 214-456-2382; **Board Cert:** Pediatrics 1984; Pediatric Hematology-Oncology 1987; **Med School:** Northwestern Univ 1978; **Resid:** Pediatrics, Babies Hosp-Columbia Presbyterian Med Ctr 1981; **Fellow:** Pediatric Hematology-Oncology, Sloan-Kettering Cancer Ctr 1983; **Fac Appt:** Prof Ped, Univ Tex SW, Dallas

West Coast and Pacific

Andrews, Robert G MD [PHO] - **Spec Exp:** Bone Marrow Transplant; Leukemia; Lymphoma; **Hospital:** Seattle Chldns Hosp; **Address:** 1100 Fairview Ave N, D2-373, PO Box 19024, Seattle, WA 98109; **Phone:** 206-667-5000; **Board Cert:** Pediatrics 1984; Pediatric Hematology-Oncology 1984; **Med School:** Univ Minn 1976; **Resid:** Pediatrics, New England Med Ctr 1979; **Fellow:** Pe-diatric Hematology-Oncology, Children's Hosp Med Ctr 1983; **Fac Appt:** Assoc Prof Ped, Univ Wash

Banerjee, Anuradha MD [PHO] - **Spec Exp:** Brain Tumors; **Hospital:** UCSF Med Ctr; **Address:** UC San Francisco, Div Ped Oncology/Neuro Oncology, 400 Parnassus Ave, rm A808, Box 0372, San Francisco, CA 94107; **Phone:** 415-353-2986; **Board Cert:** Pediatrics 2004; Pediatric Hematology-Oncology 2004; **Med School:** Tulane Univ 1992; **Resid:** Pediatrics, UCSF Med Ctr 1996; **Fellow:** Pediatric Hematology-Oncology, UCSF Med Ctr 1997; **Fac Appt:** Assoc Clin Prof Ped, UCSF

Pediatric Hematology-Oncology

Ducore, Jonathan M MD [PHO] - **Spec Exp:** Brain Tumors; Bone & Soft Tissue Tumors; Bleeding/Coagulation Disorders; **Hospital:** UC Davis Med Ctr; **Address:** UC Davis Med Ctr, Dept Pediatrics, Div Pediatric Hematology/Oncology, 2521 Stockton Blvd, Sacramento, CA 95817; **Phone:** 916-734-8336; **Board Cert:** Pediatrics 1978; Pediatric Hematology-Oncology 1978; **Med School:** Duke Univ 1973; **Resid:** Pediatrics, Chldns Med Ctr 1975; **Fellow:** Pediatric Hematology-Oncology, Univ Colorado Med Ctr 1977; Cancer Research, Natl Cancer Inst 1980; **Fac Appt:** Assoc Prof Ped, UC Davis

Finklestein, Jerry Z MD [PHO] - **Spec Exp:** Cancer Survivors-Late Effects of Therapy; Anemias & Red Cell Disorders; **Hospital:** Long Beach Meml Med Ctr, LAC - Harbor - UCLA Med Ctr; **Address:** 2653 Elm Ave, Ste 200, Long Beach, CA 90806-1652; **Phone:** 562-728-5000; **Board Cert:** Pediatrics 1980; Pediatric Hematology-Oncology 1974; **Med School:** McGill Univ 1963; **Resid:** Pediatrics, Montreal Chldns Hosp 1966; **Fellow:** Pediatric Hematology-Oncology, LA Chldns Hosp 1968; **Fac Appt:** Clin Prof Ped, UCLA

Finlay, Jonathan MD [PHO] - **Spec Exp:** Brain Tumors; **Hospital:** Chldns Hosp - Los Angeles, Chldns Hosp - Oakland; **Address:** 4650 Sunset Blvd, MS 54, Los Angeles, CA 90027-6016; **Phone:** 323-361-8147; **Board Cert:** Pediatrics 1984; Pediatric Hematology-Oncology 1987; **Med School:** England, UK 1973; **Resid:** Pediatrics, Univ Birmingham 1975; Pediatrics, Christie Hosp 1976; **Fellow:** Pediatric Allergy & Immunology, Univ Wisconsin Hosp 1978; Pediatric Hematology-Oncology, Univ Wisconsin Hosp 1980; **Fac Appt:** Prof Ped, USC-Keck School of Medicine

Geyer, J Russell MD [PHO] - **Spec Exp:** Pediatric Cancers; Neuro-Oncology; Brain Tumors; **Hospital:** Seattle Chldns Hosp, Univ Wash Med Ctr; **Address:** Seattle Chldns Hosp - Div Hem/Onc, 4800 Sand Point Way NE, MS B-6553, Seattle, WA 98105; **Phone:** 206-987-2106; **Board Cert:** Pediatrics 1983; Pediatric Hematology-Oncology 1987; **Med School:** Wayne State Univ 1977; **Resid:** Pediatrics, Chldns Hosp Michigan 1980; **Fellow:** Pediatric Hematology-Oncology, Univ Michigan Med Ctr 1981; **Fac Appt:** Prof Ped, Univ Wash

Glader, Bertil MD/PhD [PHO] - **Spec Exp:** Genetic Disorders-Blood; Hemophilia; **Hospital:** Lucile Packard Chldn's Hosp; **Address:** Pediatric Hematology/Oncology, 1000 Welch Rd, Ste 300, Box 5798, Palo Alto, CA 94304; **Phone:** 650-497-8953; **Board Cert:** Pediatrics 1982; Pediatric Hematology-Oncology 2005; Hematology 1983; **Med School:** Northwestern Univ 1968; **Resid:** Pediatrics, Chldns Hosp Med Ctr 1973; **Fellow:** Hematology, Chldns Hosp Med Ctr 1975; **Fac Appt:** Prof Ped, Stanford Univ

Hawkins, Douglas MD [PHO] - **Spec Exp:** Bone Tumors; Ewing's Sarcoma; Leukemia; Rhabdomyosarcoma; **Hospital:** Seattle Chldns Hosp; **Address:** Children's Hosp & Regl Med Ctr, 4800 Sand Point Way NE, MS B6553, Seattle, WA 98105; **Phone:** 206-987-2106; **Board Cert:** Pediatric Hematology-Oncology 2004; **Med School:** Harvard Med Sch 1990; **Resid:** Pediatrics, Univ Washington Med Ctr 1993; **Fellow:** Pediatric Hematology-Oncology, Fred Hutchinson Cancer Research Ctr 1996; **Fac Appt:** Assoc Prof Ped, Univ Wash

Horn, Biljana N MD [PHO] - **Spec Exp:** Bone Marrow Transplant; Brain Tumors; Stem Cell Transplant; Immunotherapy; **Hospital:** UCSF Med Ctr; **Address:** UCSF Med Ctr, Pediatric BMT Prgm, 505 Parnassus Ave, rm M-659, San Francisco, CA 94143; **Phone:** 415-476-2188; **Board Cert:** Pediatrics 2006; Pediatric Hematology-Oncology 2004; **Med School:** Croatia 1983; **Resid:** Pediatrics, Rainbow Babies & Chldns Hosp 1991; **Fellow:** Pediatric Hematology-Oncology, Natl Cancer Inst 1994; Pediatric Neuro-Oncology, UCSF Med Ctr 1998; **Fac Appt:** Assoc Prof Ped, UCSF

Kapoor, Neena MD [PHO] - **Spec Exp:** Bone Marrow Transplant; Immune Deficiency; **Hospital:** Chldns Hosp - Los Angeles; **Address:** Chlds Hosp LA-Rsch Immunology/BMT, 4650 Sunset Blvd, MS 62, Los Angeles, CA 90027; **Phone:** 323-361-2546; **Board Cert:** Pediatrics 1978; **Med School:** India 1972; **Resid:** Pediatrics, Rhode Island Hosp 1976; **Fellow:** Pediatric Hematology-Oncology, Meml Sloan-Kettering Cancer Ctr 1978; **Fac Appt:** Prof Ped, USC Sch Med

Kung, Faith H MD [PHO] - **Spec Exp:** Leukemia & Lymphoma; Bleeding/Coagulation Disorders; Sickle Cell Disease; Hemophilia; **Hospital:** Rady Children's Hosp - San Diego; **Address:** UCSD Med Ctr, Div Ped Hem/Oncology, 200 W Arbor Drive, San Diego, CA 92103-8447; **Phone:** 619-543-6844; **Board Cert:** Pediatrics 1967; Pediatric Hematology-Oncology 1974; **Med School:** Univ VA Sch Med 1957; **Resid:** Pediatrics, NC Meml Hosp 1960; **Fellow:** Pediatric Hematology-Oncology, Chldns Hosp/Babies Hosp 1962; **Fac Appt:** Prof Ped, UCSD

Link, Michael P MD [PHO] - **Spec Exp:** Stem Cell Transplant; **Hospital:** Lucile Packard Chldn's Hosp, Stanford Univ Hosp & Clinics; **Address:** 1000 Welch Rd, Ste 300, Palo Alto, CA 94304; **Phone:** 650-723-5535; **Board Cert:** Pediatrics 1979; Pediatric Hematology-Oncology 1980; **Med School:** Stanford Univ 1974; **Resid:** Pediatrics, Chldns Hosp Med Ctr 1976; **Fellow:** Hematology & Oncology, Dana Farber Cancer Inst 1979; **Fac Appt:** Prof Ped, Stanford Univ

Marina, Neyssa MD [PHO] - **Spec Exp:** Sarcoma; Cancer Survivors-Late Effects of Therapy; Germ Cell Tumors; **Hospital:** Lucile Packard Chldn's Hosp; **Address:** Pediatric Hematology & Oncology, 725 Walsh Rd, Palo Alto, CA 94304; **Phone:** 650-497-8953; **Board Cert:** Pediatrics 1987; Pediatric Hematology-Oncology 2005; **Med School:** Puerto Rico 1983; **Resid:** Pediatrics, Univ Pediatric Hosp 1986; **Fellow:** Pediatric Hematology-Oncology, St Jude Children's Hosp 1989; **Fac Appt:** Prof Ped, Stanford Univ

Matthay, Katherine K MD [PHO] - **Spec Exp:** Neuroblastoma; Bone Marrow & Stem Cell Transplant; **Hospital:** UCSF Med Ctr; **Address:** UCSF, Dept Ped Onc, 505 Parnassus Ave, Box 0106, San Francisco, CA 94143; **Phone:** 415-476-0603; **Board Cert:** Pediatrics 1979; Pediatric Hematology-Oncology 1980; **Med School:** Univ Pennsylvania 1973; **Resid:** Pediatrics, Univ Colorado 1976; **Fellow:** Pediatric Hematology-Oncology, UCSF 1979; **Fac Appt:** Prof Ped, UCSF

Nicholson, H Stacy MD [PHO] - **Spec Exp:** Brain Tumors; Cancer Survivors-Late Effects of Therapy; Histiocytoma; **Hospital:** Doernbecher Chldns Hosp/OHSU, OR Hlth & Sci Univ; **Address:** OR Hlth Scis Univ, 707 SW Gaines Rd, CDRCP, Portland, OR 97239; **Phone:** 503-494-4265; **Board Cert:** Pediatrics 2008; Pediatric Hematology-Oncology 2007; **Med School:** Med Coll GA 1985; **Resid:** Pediatrics, Chldns National Med Ctr 1988; **Fellow:** Pediatric Hematology-Oncology, Chldns National Med Ctr 1991; **Fac Appt:** Prof Ped, Oregon Hlth & Sci Univ

Olson, Janice MD [PHO] - **Spec Exp:** Hodgkin's Disease; Neuro-Oncology; Bone Marrow Transplant; **Hospital:** Legacy Emanuel Chldn's Hosp; **Address:** Chldn's Cancer & Blood Disorders Program, Chldn's Hosp at Legacy Emanuel, 501 N Graham St, Ste 355, Portland, OR 97227; **Phone:** 503-413-2560; **Board Cert:** Pediatrics 2005; Pediatric Hematology-Oncology 2009; **Med School:** Univ Utah 1985; **Resid:** Pediatrics, Baylor/TX Chldn's Hosp 1988; **Fellow:** Hematology & Oncology, Duke Univ Med Ctr 1992

Park, Julie MD [PHO] - **Spec Exp:** Pediatric Cancers; Neuroblastoma; Lymphoma, Non-Hodgkin's; **Hospital:** Seattle Chldns Hosp; **Address:** Seattle Chldn's-Hem/Onc Dept, 4800 Sandpoint Way NE, Box B6553, Seattle, WA 98105; **Phone:** 206-987-2106; **Board Cert:** Pediatric Hematology-Oncology 2004; **Med School:** Univ VT Coll Med 1988; **Resid:** Pediatrics, Univ Wash Affil Hosp 1991; **Fellow:** Pediatric Hematology-Oncology, Univ Wash/Fred Hutchinson Cancer Rsch Ctr 1994; Pediatric Hematology-Oncology, Leukemia Soc/Fred Hutchinson Cancer Rsch Ctr 1996; **Fac Appt:** Assoc Prof Ped, Univ Wash

Pendergrass, Thomas W MD [PHO] - **Spec Exp:** Pediatric Cancers; Hematologic Disorders; Retinoblastoma; **Hospital:** Seattle Chldns Hosp, Univ Wash Med Ctr; **Address:** Seattle Chldn's Hosp, 4800 Sandpoint Way NE, Box 5371, MS B6553, Seattle, WA 98105; **Phone:** 206-987-2106; **Board Cert:** Pediatrics 1978; **Med School:** Univ Tenn Coll Med 1971; **Resid:** Pediatrics, Children's Memorial Hosp 1973; **Fellow:** Pediatric Hematology-Oncology, Children's Hosp Med Ctr 1977; **Fac Appt:** Prof Ped, Univ Wash

Pediatric Hematology-Oncology

Recht, Michael MD/PhD [PHO] - **Spec Exp:** Hemophilia; Bleeding/Coagulation Disorders; Hematologic Disorders; **Hospital:** Doernbecher Chldns Hosp/OHSU; **Address:** Peds Hem/Onc 10C, 3181 SW Sam Jackson Park Rd, MC CDRC, Portland, OR 97239; **Phone:** 503-494-8716; **Board Cert:** Pediatrics 2003; Pediatric Hematology-Oncology 2006; **Med School:** Univ Wisc 1992; **Resid:** Pediatrics, Yale/New Haven Hosp 1995; **Fellow:** Pediatric Hematology-Oncology, Yale/New Haven Hosp 1998

Rosenthal, Joseph MD [PHO] - **Spec Exp:** Bone Marrow Transplant; Clinical Trials; **Hospital:** Chldns Hosp Central CA; **Address:** Valley Children's Hospital, 9300 Valley Children's Pl, Madera, CA 93636; **Phone:** 559-353-5490 x68442; **Board Cert:** Pediatrics 2003; Pediatric Hematology-Oncology 2004; **Med School:** Israel 1984; **Resid:** Pediatrics, Soroka Med Ctr 1988; Pediatrics, Chldn Hosp 1995; **Fellow:** Pediatric Hematology-Oncology, Univ Colorado Affil Hosp 1991; Pediatric Hematology-Oncology, Chldn Hosp 1994; **Fac Appt:** Assoc Prof Ped, USC-Keck School of Medicine

Sakamoto, Kathleen M MD [PHO] - **Spec Exp:** Leukemia; Pediatric Cancers; Bone Marrow Transplant; **Hospital:** Mattel Chldns Hosp at UCLA; **Address:** Mattel Chldns Hosp UCLA, Div Hem-Onc, David Geffen Sch Med, 10833 Le Conte Ave, Los Angeles, CA 90095-1752; **Phone:** 310-825-6708; **Board Cert:** Pediatrics 2007; Pediatric Hematology-Oncology 2007; **Med School:** Univ Cincinnati 1985; **Resid:** Pediatrics, Chldn's Hosp 1988; **Fellow:** Pediatric Hematology-Oncology, Chldn's Hosp 1991; **Fac Appt:** Prof Ped, UCLA

Siegel, Stuart E MD [PHO] - **Spec Exp:** Leukemia & Lymphoma; Infections in Cancer Patients; Psychosocial Support in Childhood Cancer; Solid Tumors; **Hospital:** Chldns Hosp - Los Angeles, Ventura Cnty Med Ctr; **Address:** Chldns Hosp, 4650 Sunset Blvd, MS 54, Los Angeles, CA 90027-6062; **Phone:** 323-361-2205; **Board Cert:** Pediatrics 1973; Pediatric Hematology-Oncology 1976; **Med School:** Boston Univ 1967; **Resid:** Pediatrics, Univ Minnesota Hosps 1969; **Fellow:** Pediatric Hematology-Oncology, Natl Cancer Inst 1972; **Fac Appt:** Prof Ped, USC-Keck School of Medicine

Thomas, Gregory A MD [PHO] - **Spec Exp:** Palliative Care; Anemias & Red Cell Disorders; Bleeding/Coagulation Disorders; **Hospital:** Doernbecher Chldns Hosp/OHSU; **Address:** 707 SW Gaines Rd, MC 1104-CDRCP, Portland, OR 97239; **Phone:** 503-346-0644; **Board Cert:** Pediatrics 1986; Pediatric Hematology-Oncology 2005; **Med School:** Oregon Hlth & Sci Univ 1981; **Resid:** Pediatrics, Univ Utah Med Ctr 1984; **Fellow:** Pediatric Hematology-Oncology, Univ Utah Med Ctr 1987; **Fac Appt:** Assoc Prof Ped, Oregon Hlth & Sci Univ

PEDIATRIC INFECTIOUS DISEASE

New England

Andiman, Warren A MD [PInf] - **Spec Exp:** AIDS/HIV; Viral Infections; Lyme Disease; Infectious Mononucleosis; **Hospital:** Yale-New Haven Hosp, Yale Med Group; **Address:** 333 Cedar St, Box 208064, Yale Univ Sch Med, New Haven, CT 06520-8064; **Phone:** 203-785-4730; **Board Cert:** Pediatrics 1975; **Med School:** Albert Einstein Coll Med 1969; **Resid:** Pediatrics, Babies Hosp-Columbia Presby 1971; **Fellow:** Pediatric Infectious Disease, Yale Univ Sch Med 1973; **Fac Appt:** Prof Ped, Yale Univ

Baltimore, Robert MD [PInf] - **Spec Exp:** Neonatal Infections; Hospital Acquired Infections; Tuberculosis; **Hospital:** Yale-New Haven Hosp, Yale Med Group; **Address:** Yale Univ Sch Med, Dept Pediatrics, 333 Cedar St, Box 208064, New Haven, CT 06520-8064; **Phone:** 203-785-4750; **Board Cert:** Pediatrics 1975; Pediatric Infectious Disease 2009; **Med School:** SUNY Buffalo 1968; **Resid:** Pediatrics, Univ Chicago Hosps 1971; **Fellow:** Infectious Disease, Boston City Hosp-Harvard 1976; **Fac Appt:** Prof Ped, Yale Univ

Durbin Jr, William Applebee MD [PInf] - **Hospital:** UMass Meml Med Ctr - Univ Campus; **Address:** 55 Lake Ave N, Worcester, MA 01655; **Phone:** 508-856-2650; **Board Cert:** Pediatrics 1978; Pediatric Infectious Disease 2009; **Med School:** Columbia P&S 1972; **Resid:** Pediatrics, Boston Chldns Hosp 1977; **Fellow:** Infectious Disease, Boston Chldns Hosp/Beth Israel 1979; **Fac Appt:** Prof Ped, Univ Mass Sch Med

Raszka Jr, William V MD [PInf] - **Hospital:** Fletcher Allen Health Care- Med Ctr Campus; **Address:** Chldns Specialty Clin, Dept Ped Infect Disease, 111 Colchester Avenue, Burlington, VT 05401; **Phone:** 802-847-8200; **Board Cert:** Pediatrics 2008; Pediatric Infectious Disease 2009; **Med School:** Boston Univ 1985; **Resid:** Pediatrics, Tripler Army Med Ctr 1988; **Fellow:** Pediatric Infectious Disease, Uniformed Servs Hlth Ctr 1993; **Fac Appt:** Prof Ped, Univ VT Coll Med

Shapiro, Eugene D MD [PInf] - **Spec Exp:** Lyme Disease; Vaccines; **Hospital:** Yale-New Haven Hosp, Yale Med Group; **Address:** Yale Univ, Dept Pediatrics, 333 Cedar St, Box 208064, New Haven, CT 06520-8064; **Phone:** 203-688-4518; **Board Cert:** Pediatrics 1980; Pediatric Infectious Disease 2009; **Med School:** UCSF 1976; **Resid:** Pediatrics, Chldns Hosp 1979; **Fellow:** Pediatric Infectious Disease, Chldns Hosp 1981; Research, Yale Univ 1983; **Fac Appt:** Prof Ped, Yale Univ

Mid Atlantic

Borkowsky, William MD [PInf] - **Spec Exp:** AIDS/HIV; **Hospital:** NYU Langone Med Ctr (page 66), Bellevue Hosp Ctr; **Address:** 550 1st Ave, Dept Pediatrics, New York, NY 10016; **Phone:** 212-263-6513; **Board Cert:** Pediatrics 1979; Pediatric Infectious Disease 2009; **Med School:** NYU Sch Med 1972; **Resid:** Pediatrics, Bellevue Hosp Ctr 1975; **Fellow:** Infectious Disease, Bellevue Hosp Ctr-NYU 1978; **Fac Appt:** Prof Ped, NYU Sch Med

Green, Michael D MD [PInf] - **Spec Exp:** Infections-Transplant; **Hospital:** Chldns Hosp of Pittsburgh - UPMC; **Address:** University of Pittsburgh Physicians, 4401 Penn Ave, Pittsburgh, PA 15224; **Phone:** 412-692-7885; **Board Cert:** Pediatrics 1987; Pediatric Infectious Disease 2009; **Med School:** Univ IL Coll Med 1983; **Resid:** Pediatrics, Children's Hosp 1986; **Fellow:** Pediatric Infectious Disease, Children's Hosp 1989; **Fac Appt:** Assoc Prof Ped, Univ Pittsburgh

Kotloff, Karen MD [PInf] - **Spec Exp:** Diarrheal Diseases; Infectious Disease; Sexually Transmitted Diseases; **Hospital:** Univ of MD Med Ctr; **Address:** Ctr for Vaccine Development, 685 W Baltimore St HSF Bldg - Ste 480, Baltimore, MD 21201; **Phone:** 410-706-5328; **Board Cert:** Pediatrics 1985; Pediatric Infectious Disease 2002; **Med School:** Temple Univ 1979; **Resid:** Pediatrics, Chldn's Hosp 1983; **Fellow:** Pediatric Infectious Disease, Univ Maryland Med Ctr 1986; **Fac Appt:** Prof Ped, Univ MD Sch Med

Krilov, Leonard MD [PInf] - **Spec Exp:** Infections-Respiratory; Infections in Int'l Adopted Children; Chronic Fatigue Syndrome; Lyme Disease; **Hospital:** Winthrop Univ Hosp; **Address:** 120 Mineola Blvd, Ste 210, Mineola, NY 11501; **Phone:** 516-663-4600; **Board Cert:** Pediatrics 1983; Pediatric Infectious Disease 2009; **Med School:** Columbia P&S 1978; **Resid:** Pediatrics, Johns Hopkins Hosp 1981; **Fellow:** Pediatric Infectious Disease, Children's Hosp 1984; **Fac Appt:** Prof Ped, SUNY Stony Brook

Long, Sarah S MD [PInf] - **Spec Exp:** Whooping Cough; Vaccines; Antibiotic Resistance; **Hospital:** St. Christopher's Hosp for Chldn; **Address:** St Christopher's Hosp for Children, 3601 A St, Ste 1112, Philadelphia, PA 19134; **Phone:** 215-427-5201; **Board Cert:** Pediatrics 2002; Pediatric Infectious Disease 2009; **Med School:** Jefferson Med Coll 1970; **Resid:** Pediatrics, St Christophers Hosp Chldn 1973; **Fellow:** Pediatric Infectious Disease, Temple Univ Sch Med 1975; **Fac Appt:** Prof Ped, Drexel Univ Coll Med

Pediatric Infectious Disease

Michaels, Marian G MD [PInf] - **Spec Exp:** AIDS/HIV; Infections in Immunocompromised Patients; **Hospital:** Chldns Hosp of Pittsburgh - UPMC, Magee-Womens Hosp - UPMC; **Address:** Children's Hosp Pittsburgh, 4401 Penn Ave Fl 3, Pittsburgh, PA 15224; **Phone:** 412-692-7438; **Board Cert:** Pediatrics 2005; Pediatric Infectious Disease 2009; **Med School:** Univ Pennsylvania 1985; **Resid:** Pediatrics, Children's Hosp 1988; Pediatrics, Hosp for Sick Children 1989; **Fellow:** Pediatric Infectious Disease, Univ Pittsburgh 1992; **Fac Appt:** Prof Ped, Univ Pittsburgh

Munoz, Jose Luis MD [PInf] - **Spec Exp:** Lyme Disease; Immune Deficiency; Tick-borne Diseases; **Hospital:** Westchester Med Ctr, Children's & Women's Phys.of Westchester; **Address:** Pediatric Infectious Disease, 19 Bradhurst Ave, Ste 1400, Hawthorne, NY 10532; **Phone:** 914-493-8333; **Board Cert:** Pediatric Infectious Disease 2009; **Med School:** Yale Univ 1978; **Resid:** Pediatrics, Yale New Haven Hosp 1981; **Fellow:** Pediatric Infectious Disease, Univ Rochester 1984; **Fac Appt:** Assoc Prof Ped, NY Med Coll

Offit, Paul A MD [PInf] - **Spec Exp:** Vaccines; **Hospital:** Chldns Hosp of Philadelphia; **Address:** Children's Hospital of Philadelphia, Abramson Bldg, 34th St & Civic Center Blvd, Ste 1202D, Philadelphia, PA 19104; **Phone:** 215-590-2017; **Board Cert:** Pediatrics 1982; **Med School:** Univ MD Sch Med 1977; **Resid:** Pediatrics, Children's Hosp 1980; **Fac Appt:** Prof Ped, Univ Pennsylvania

Saiman, Lisa MD [PInf] - **Spec Exp:** Cystic Fibrosis Infection; Fungal Infections; Tick-borne Diseases; Tuberculosis; **Hospital:** Morgan Stanley Children's Hosp of NY-Presby, NY (page 65); **Address:** Columbia University, 622 W 168th St Fl 4 PH4 W - rm 470, New York, NY 10032; **Phone:** 212-305-4558; **Board Cert:** Pediatrics 1987; Pediatric Infectious Disease 2009; **Med School:** Albert Einstein Coll Med 1983; **Resid:** Pediatrics, Babies Hosp/NY Presby 1986; **Fellow:** Infectious Disease, Babies Hosp/NY Presby 1989; **Fac Appt:** Assoc Clin Prof Ped, Columbia P&S

Singh, Nalini MD [PInf] - **Hospital:** Chldns Natl Med Ctr; **Address:** Div Infectious Disease, 111 Michigan Ave NW, Ste 3450, Washington, DC 20010; **Phone:** 202-476-5051; **Board Cert:** Pediatrics 1982; Pediatric Infectious Disease 2005; **Med School:** India 1973; **Resid:** Pediatrics, Univ Mass Med Ctr 1979; **Fellow:** Infectious Disease, Natl Inst Hlth 1981; **Fac Appt:** Assoc Prof Ped, Geo Wash Univ

Southeast

Edwards, Kathryn M MD [PInf] - **Spec Exp:** Vaccines; Clinical Trials; **Hospital:** Vanderbilt Univ Med Ctr (page 76); **Address:** Vanderbilt Div Infectious Diseases, 1161 21st Ave S, CCC-5311, Med Ctr North, Nashville, TN 37232; **Phone:** 615-322-2250; **Board Cert:** Pediatrics 1978; Pediatric Infectious Disease 2005; **Med School:** Univ Iowa Coll Med 1973; **Resid:** Pediatrics, Chldns Meml Hosp 1976; **Fellow:** Pediatric Infectious Disease, Chldns Meml Hosp 1980; **Fac Appt:** Prof Ped, Vanderbilt Univ

Emmanuel, Patricia MD [PInf] - **Spec Exp:** Infections in Immunocompromised Patients; AIDS/HIV; Congenital Infections; **Hospital:** Tampa Genl Hosp, All Children's Hosp; **Address:** 17 Davis Blvd, Ste 200, Tampa, FL 33604; **Phone:** 813-259-8800; **Board Cert:** Pediatrics 2005; Pediatric Infectious Disease 2009; **Med School:** Univ Fla Coll Med 1986; **Resid:** Pediatrics, Univ S Florida Affil Hosp 1989; **Fellow:** Infectious Disease, Univ S Florida Affil Hosp 1993; **Fac Appt:** Assoc Prof Ped, Univ S Fla Coll Med

Flynn, Patricia M MD [PInf] - **Spec Exp:** AIDS/HIV; Infections in Immunocompromised Patients; Clinical Trials; **Hospital:** St. Jude Children's Research Hosp; **Address:** St Jude Chldns Rsch Hosp, 262 Danny Thomas Pl, rm Q1114, MS 600, Memphis, TN 38105; **Phone:** 901-595-2338; **Board Cert:** Pediatrics 1986; Pediatric Infectious Disease 2009; **Med School:** Louisiana State U, New Orleans 1981; **Resid:** Pediatrics, LeBonheur Chldns Med Ctr 1984; **Fellow:** Pediatric Infectious Disease, St Judes Chldns Rsch Hosp 1987; **Fac Appt:** Prof PrM, Univ Tenn Coll Med

Givner, Laurence B MD [PInf] - **Spec Exp:** Streptococcal Infections; Rocky Mountain Spotted Fever; **Hospital:** Wake Forest Univ Baptist Med Ctr, Brenner Chldrn's Hosp; **Address:** Wake Forest Univ Sch Med, Dept Ped, Medical Center Blvd, Winston-Salem, NC 27157-0001; **Phone:** 336-716-6568; **Board Cert:** Pediatrics 1984; Pediatric Infectious Disease 2009; **Med School:** Univ MD Sch Med 1978; **Resid:** Pediatrics, Univ Maryland 1982; **Fellow:** Infectious Disease, Baylor Coll Med 1984; **Fac Appt:** Prof Ped, Wake Forest Univ

Ingram, David MD [PInf] - **Hospital:** WakeMed-Raleigh Campus; **Address:** WakeMed Faculty Physicians, Pediatrics, 3024 New Bern Ave, Ste 307, Raleigh, NC 27610; **Phone:** 919-350-8009; **Board Cert:** Pediatrics 1980; Pediatric Infectious Disease 2009; **Med School:** Yale Univ 1967; **Resid:** Pediatrics, Yale-New Haven Hosp 1971; **Fellow:** Pediatric Infectious Disease, Chldns Hosp Med Ctr 1973; **Fac Appt:** Prof Ped, Univ NC Sch Med

McKinney Jr, Ross E MD [PInf] - **Spec Exp:** Infections in Immunocompromised Patients; Fevers of Unknown Origin; AIDS/HIV; **Hospital:** Duke Univ Hosp; **Address:** Duke Univ Med Ctr, Box 399, Durham, NC 27710; **Phone:** 919-668-9000; **Board Cert:** Pediatrics 1983; Pediatric Infectious Disease 2009; **Med School:** Univ Rochester 1979; **Resid:** Pediatrics, Duke Univ Med Ctr 1982; **Fellow:** Pediatric Infectious Disease, Duke Univ Med Ctr 1985; **Fac Appt:** Prof Ped, Duke Univ

Mitchell, Charles D MD [PInf] - **Spec Exp:** AIDS/HIV; Viral Infections; **Hospital:** Jackson Meml Hosp (page 70); **Address:** Univ Miami Div Ped Inf Disease, PO Box 016960 (D4-4), Miami, FL 33101; **Phone:** 305-243-2700; **Board Cert:** Pediatrics 1986; Pediatric Infectious Disease 2009; **Med School:** Univ Tex Med Br, Galveston 1977; **Resid:** Pediatrics, Univ Minn Hosp 1981; **Fellow:** Pediatric Infectious Disease, Univ Minn Hosp 1984; **Fac Appt:** Clin Prof Ped, Univ Miami Sch Med

Scott, Gwendolyn B MD [PInf] - **Spec Exp:** AIDS/HIV; **Hospital:** Jackson Meml Hosp (page 70), Univ of Miami Hosp & Clins/Sylvester Comp Canc Ctr (page 73); **Address:** Univ Miami Div Ped Inf Disease, 1580 NW 10th Ave, rm BCRI 286 (D4-4), Miami, FL 33136; **Phone:** 305-243-6522; **Board Cert:** Pediatrics 1978; Pediatric Infectious Disease 2009; **Med School:** UCSF 1972; **Resid:** Pediatrics, San Francisco Genl Hosp 1973; Pediatrics, Univ Maryland Hosp 1975; **Fellow:** Pediatric Infectious Disease, Univ Miami Hosp 1978; **Fac Appt:** Prof Ped, Univ Miami Sch Med

Midwest

Alexander, Kenneth MD/PhD [PInf] - **Spec Exp:** HPV-Human Papilloma Virus; Infections in Immunocompromised Patients; Fevers of Unknown Origin; Antibiotic Resistance; **Hospital:** Univ of Chicago Med Ctr; **Address:** 5841 S Maryland Ave, MC 6054, Chicago, IL 60637; **Phone:** 773-702-6176; **Board Cert:** Pediatric Infectious Disease 2005; **Med School:** Univ Wash 1989; **Resid:** Pediatrics, Chldn's Hosp 1992; **Fellow:** Pediatric Infectious Disease, Duke Univ Hosp 1995; **Fac Appt:** Assoc Prof Ped, Univ Chicago-Pritzker Sch Med

Bernstein, David I MD [PInf] - **Spec Exp:** Vaccines; Viral Infections; **Hospital:** Cincinnati Chldns Hosp Med Ctr; **Address:** Cincinnatti Children's Hosp, Dept Infectious Diseases, 3333 Burnet Ave, Cincinnati, OH 45229-3039; **Phone:** 513-636-7625; **Board Cert:** Pediatrics 1982; **Med School:** SUNY Buffalo 1977; **Resid:** Pediatrics, Tufts-New Englan Med Ctr 1981; **Fellow:** Infectious Disease, UCLA Med Ctr 1981; **Fac Appt:** Prof Ped, Univ Cincinnati

Christenson, John C MD [PInf] - **Spec Exp:** Travel Medicine; Lyme Disease; Viral Infections; Histoplasmosis; **Hospital:** Riley Hosp for Children; **Address:** Riley Childrens Hosp, Div Infectious Disease, 705 Riley Hospital Drive, ROC 4380, Indianapolis, IN 46202; **Phone:** 317-944-7260; **Board Cert:** Pediatrics 1986; Pediatric Infectious Disease 2009; **Med School:** Univ Puerto Rico 1981; **Resid:** Pediatrics, Univ Pediatric Hosp 1984; **Fellow:** Pediatric Infectious Disease, Okla Chldns Meml Hosp 1987; **Fac Appt:** Clin Prof Ped, Indiana Univ

Pediatric Infectious Disease

Kleiman, Martin B MD [PInf] - **Spec Exp:** Histoplasmosis; Blastomycosis; Meningitis; AIDS/HIV; **Hospital:** Riley Hosp for Children; **Address:** Riley Hosp for Children, 705 Riley Hospital Drive, ROC 4380, Indianapolis, IN 46202; **Phone:** 317-944-7260; **Board Cert:** Pediatrics 1973; Pediatric Infectious Disease 2009; **Med School:** SUNY Upstate Med Univ 1968; **Resid:** Pediatrics, Upstate Med Ctr 1971; **Fellow:** Infectious Disease, Johns Hopkins Hosp 1976; **Fac Appt:** Prof Emeritus Ped, Indiana Univ

Leonard, Ethan G MD [PInf] - **Hospital:** UH Rainbow Babies & Chldns Hosp (page 74); **Address:** UH Rainbow Babies & Children's Hospital, Pediatric Infectious Disease, 11100 Euclid Ave, Cleveland, OH 44106; **Phone:** 216-844-3645; **Board Cert:** Pediatrics 2007; Pediatric Infectious Disease 2003; **Med School:** Case West Res Univ 1996; **Resid:** Pediatrics, Univ Hosps 2000; **Fellow:** Pediatric Infectious Disease, Univ Hosps 2003; **Fac Appt:** Assoc Prof Ped, Case West Res Univ

McComsey, Grace A MD [PInf] - **Spec Exp:** AIDS/HIV; **Hospital:** UH Rainbow Babies & Chldns Hosp (page 74); **Address:** UH Rainbow Babies & Children's Hospital, Pediatric Infectious Disease, 11100 Euclid Ave, Cleveland, OH 44106; **Phone:** 216-844-3645; **Board Cert:** Internal Medicine 2005; Pediatric Infectious Disease 2005; Infectious Disease 2007; **Med School:** Lebanon 1989; **Resid:** Pediatrics, Metrohealth Med Ctr 1994; **Fellow:** Infectious Disease, Univ Hosps 1997; **Fac Appt:** Prof Med, Case West Res Univ

Shulman, Stanford MD [PInf] - **Spec Exp:** Kawasaki Disease; Streptococcal Infections; **Hospital:** Children's Mem Hosp -Chicago, Northwestern Meml Hosp; **Address:** 2300 Children's Plaza, Box 20, Chicago, IL 60614-3318; **Phone:** 773-880-4187; **Board Cert:** Pediatrics 1972; **Med School:** Univ Chicago-Pritzker Sch Med 1967; **Resid:** Pediatrics, Univ Chicago Hosps 1970; **Fellow:** Infectious Disease, Shands Hosp 1973; **Fac Appt:** Prof Ped, Northwestern Univ

Wald, Ellen MD [PInf] - **Spec Exp:** Urinary Tract Infections; Infections-Respiratory; Meningitis; Ear Infections; **Hospital:** Univ WI Hosp & Clins; **Address:** American Family Childrens Hosp, Dept Pediatrics, Box 4108, 600 Highland Ave, Madison, WI 57392; **Phone:** 608-263-8558; **Board Cert:** Pediatrics 1973; Pediatric Infectious Disease 2009; **Med School:** SUNY Downstate 1968; **Resid:** Pediatrics, Kings Co Hosp 1971; **Fellow:** Infectious Disease, Univ Maryland Hosp 1973; **Fac Appt:** Prof Ped, Univ Wisc

Southwest

Baker, Carol J MD [PInf] - **Spec Exp:** Streptococcal Infections; Neonatal Infections; Vaccines; **Hospital:** Texas Chldns Hosp, Ben Taub Genl Hosp; **Address:** 1102 Bates St, Ste 1150, Houston, TX 77030; **Phone:** 832-824-4330; **Board Cert:** Pediatrics 1973; Pediatric Infectious Disease 2009; **Med School:** Baylor Coll Med 1968; **Resid:** Pediatrics, Baylor Coll Med 1971; **Fellow:** Pediatric Infectious Disease, Baylor Coll Med 1973; Infectious Disease, Boston City Hosp/Harvard Med Sch 1974; **Fac Appt:** Prof Ped, Baylor Coll Med

Jacobs, Richard F MD [PInf] - **Spec Exp:** Viral Infections; Drug Discovery & Development; Neonatal Infections; **Hospital:** Arkansas Chldns Hosp, UAMS Med Ctr; **Address:** 800 Marshall St, Slot 512-11, Little Rock, AR 72202-3591; **Phone:** 501-364-1416; **Board Cert:** Pediatrics 1982; Pediatric Infectious Disease 2009; **Med School:** Univ Ark 1977; **Resid:** Pediatrics, Ark Chldns Hosp 1980; **Fellow:** Infectious Disease, Univ Washington 1982; **Fac Appt:** Prof Ped, Univ Ark

Kaplan, Sheldon MD [PInf] - **Spec Exp:** Pneumococcal Infections; Meningitis; **Hospital:** Texas Chldns Hosp; **Address:** Div Infectious Disease, 1102 Bates St, Houston, TX 77030; **Phone:** 832-824-4330; **Board Cert:** Pediatrics 1978; Pediatric Infectious Disease 2009; **Med School:** Univ MO-Columbia Sch Med 1973; **Resid:** Pediatrics, St Louis Chldns Hosp 1975; **Fellow:** Pediatric Infectious Disease, St Louis Chldns Hosp 1977; **Fac Appt:** Prof Ped, Baylor Coll Med

Kline, Mark MD [PInf] - **Spec Exp:** AIDS/HIV; **Hospital:** Texas Chldns Hosp; **Address:** Texas Children's Hosp, 6621 Fannin St, MC CCC1210, Houston, TX 77030; **Phone:** 832-822-1038; **Board Cert:** Pediatrics 1987; Pediatric Infectious Disease 2009; **Med School:** Baylor Coll Med 1981; **Resid:** Pediatrics, Baylor Coll Med 1985; **Fellow:** Pediatric Infectious Disease, Baylor Coll Med 1987; **Fac Appt:** Prof Ped, Baylor Coll Med

McCracken Jr, George H MD [PInf] - **Spec Exp:** Meningitis; Antibiotic Resistance; **Hospital:** UT Southwestern Med Ctr at Dallas; **Address:** Dept Pediatric Infectious Disease, 1935 Med District Drive, Dallas, TX 75235; **Phone:** 214-456-6500; **Board Cert:** Pediatrics 1966; Pediatric Infectious Disease 2002; **Med School:** Cornell Univ-Weill Med Coll 1962; **Resid:** Pediatrics, NY-Cornell Med Ctr 1965; Pediatrics, Univ Texas SW Med Ctr 1966

West Coast and Pacific

Bradley, John S MD [PInf] - **Spec Exp:** Meningitis; Brain Infections; **Hospital:** Rady Children's Hosp - San Diego, UCSD Med Ctr; **Address:** 3020 Chldns Way, MC 5041, San Diego, CA 92123; **Phone:** 858-966-7785; **Board Cert:** Pediatrics 1981; Pediatric Infectious Disease 2009; **Med School:** UC Davis 1976; **Resid:** Pediatrics, UC Davis Med Ctr 1980; **Fellow:** Pediatric Infectious Disease, Stanford Univ Hosp 1981; **Fac Appt:** Assoc Clin Prof Ped, UCSD

Bryson, Yvonne J MD [PInf] - **Spec Exp:** AIDS/HIV; Herpes Simplex; Clinical Trials; Toxoplasmosis; **Hospital:** UCLA Ronald Reagan Med Ctr; **Address:** UCLA Pediatric Infectious Disease, 10833 Le Conte Ave, rm 22-442 MDCC, Los Angeles, CA 90095-1752; **Phone:** 310-825-5235; **Board Cert:** Pediatrics 1976; **Med School:** Univ Tex SW, Dallas 1970; **Resid:** Pediatrics, UCSD Med Ctr 1974; **Fellow:** Pediatric Infectious Disease, UCSD Med Ctr 1976; **Fac Appt:** Prof Ped, UCLA

Mason, Wilbert H MD [PInf] - **Spec Exp:** Kawasaki Disease; **Hospital:** Chldns Hosp - Los Angeles, Keck Med Ctr of USC (page 75); **Address:** Chldns Hosp, Div Inf Dis, 4650 West Sunset Blvd, MS 51, Los Angeles, CA 90027-6062; **Phone:** 323-361-2509; **Board Cert:** Pediatrics 1975; Pediatric Infectious Disease 2009; **Med School:** UC Irvine 1970; **Resid:** Pediatrics, Chldns Hosp 1973; **Fellow:** Infectious Disease, Chldns Hosp 1974; **Fac Appt:** Assoc Clin Prof Ped, USC Sch Med

Petru, Ann MD [PInf] - **Spec Exp:** AIDS/HIV; **Hospital:** Chldns Hosp - Oakland; **Address:** Chldns Hosp, Div Infectious Disease, 744 52nd St, Oakland, CA 94609; **Phone:** 510-428-3336; **Board Cert:** Pediatrics 1983; Pediatric Infectious Disease 2002; **Med School:** UCSF 1978; **Resid:** Pediatrics, Chldns Hosp Med Ctr 1982; **Fellow:** Pediatric Infectious Disease, Chldns Hosp Med Ctr 1983; **Fac Appt:** Asst Clin Prof Med, UCSF

PEDIATRIC NEPHROLOGY

New England

Harmon, William E MD [PNep] - **Spec Exp:** Nephrotic Syndrome; **Hospital:** Children's Hospital - Boston; **Address:** Chldns Hosp, Div Nephrology, 300 Longwood Ave, Hunnewell 319, Boston, MA 02115; **Phone:** 617-355-6129; **Board Cert:** Pediatrics 1976; **Med School:** Case West Res Univ 1971; **Resid:** Pediatrics, Chldns Hosp Med Ctr 1976; **Fellow:** Pediatric Nephrology, Chldns Hosp Med Ctr 1979; **Fac Appt:** Prof Ped, Harvard Med Sch

Pediatric Nephrology

Mid Atlantic

Conley, Susan B MD [PNep] - Spec Exp: Transplant Medicine-Kidney; **Hospital:** St. Christopher's Hosp for Chldn; **Address:** St Christophers Hosp for Children, Nephrology Section Fl 1, 3601 A St, Philadelphia, PA 19134; **Phone:** 215-427-5190; **Board Cert:** Pediatrics 1978; Pediatric Nephrology 1979; **Med School:** Univ Mich Med Sch 1973; **Resid:** Pediatrics, Children's Hosp 1975; **Fellow:** Pediatric Nephrology, Children's Hosp 1977; **Fac Appt:** Prof Ped, Drexel Univ Coll Med

Dabbagh, Shermine MD [PNep] - Spec Exp: Kidney Disease; Kidney Failure-Chronic; Transplant Medicine-Kidney; **Hospital:** Alfred I duPont Hosp for Children; **Address:** Dupont Hosp for Children, Div Nephrology, 1600 Rockland Rd, PO Box 269, Wilmington, DE 19803; **Phone:** 302-651-4426; **Board Cert:** Pediatrics 1985; Pediatric Nephrology 1985; **Med School:** Lebanon 1979; **Resid:** Pediatrics, Univ Virginia Hosp 1981; **Fellow:** Pediatric Nephrology, Univ Wisconsin 1984

Ellis, Demetrius MD [PNep] - Spec Exp: Transplant Medicine-Kidney; Hypertension; **Hospital:** Chldns Hosp of Pittsburgh - UPMC; **Address:** Children's Hospital, Dept Nephrology, 4401 Penn Ave, Pittsburgh, PA 15224; **Phone:** 412-692-5182; **Board Cert:** Pediatrics 1978; Pediatric Nephrology 1979; **Med School:** SUNY Buffalo 1973; **Resid:** Pediatrics, Chldns Hosp 1975; **Fellow:** Pediatric Nephrology, Chldns Hosp-Natl Med Ctr 1977; **Fac Appt:** Prof Ped, Univ Pittsburgh

Fivush, Barbara A MD [PNep] - Spec Exp: Transplant Medicine-Kidney; **Hospital:** Johns Hopkins Hosp (page 61); **Address:** Johns Hopkins Hosp-Div Nephrology, 200 N Wolfe St, rm 3055, Baltimore, MD 21287; **Phone:** 410-955-2467; **Board Cert:** Pediatrics 1984; Pediatric Nephrology 2010; **Med School:** Boston Univ 1978; **Resid:** Pediatrics, Johns Hopkins Hosp 1981; **Fellow:** Pediatric Nephrology, Johns Hopkins Hosp 1983; Pediatric Nephrology, Chldns Hosp Natl Med Ctr 1984; **Fac Appt:** Assoc Prof Ped, Johns Hopkins Univ

Kaplan, Bernard S MD [PNep] - Spec Exp: Hemolytic Uremic Syndrome; Polycystic Kidney Disease; **Hospital:** Chldns Hosp of Philadelphia; **Address:** Chldns Hosp of Philadelphia, Div Nephrology, 34 St & Civic Ctr Blvd, rm 2143, Philadelphia, PA 19104; **Phone:** 215-590-2449; **Board Cert:** Pediatrics 1972; Pediatric Nephrology 1974; **Med School:** South Africa 1964; **Resid:** Pediatrics, Baragwanath Hosp, Transvaal Meml Hosp 1970; Nephrology, Royal Victoria Hosp 1973; **Fellow:** Nephrology, Montreal Chldns Hosp 1972; **Fac Appt:** Prof Ped, Univ Pennsylvania

Mendley, Susan MD [PNep] - Spec Exp: Transplant Medicine-Kidney; Hypertension; Dialysis Care; Glomerulonephritis; **Hospital:** Univ of MD Med Ctr; **Address:** Univ Maryland Med Ctr, 22 S Greene St, Pediatric Nephrol N5W67, Baltimore, MD 21201; **Phone:** 410-328-5303; **Board Cert:** Internal Medicine 1988; Nephrology 2000; **Med School:** Boston Univ 1984; **Resid:** Internal Medicine, Univ Chicago Hosps 1987; **Fellow:** Nephrology, Univ Chicago 1990; Pediatric Nephrology, Chldns Meml Hosp/Northwestern Univ 1991; **Fac Appt:** Assoc Prof Ped, Univ MD Sch Med

Roskes, Saul David MD [PNep] - Hospital: Johns Hopkins Hosp (page 61); **Address:** 10807 Falls Rd, Ste 200, Lutherville, MD 21093; **Phone:** 410-321-9393; **Board Cert:** Pediatrics 1970; Pediatric Nephrology 1976; **Med School:** Johns Hopkins Univ 1963; **Resid:** Pediatrics, Bronx Muni Hosp Ctr 1965; Pediatrics, Johns Hopkins Hosp 1968; **Fac Appt:** Assoc Prof Ped, Johns Hopkins Univ

Southeast

Ault, Bettina H MD [PNep] - **Spec Exp:** Hemolytic Uremic Syndrome; Kidney Failure; Anemia; **Hospital:** Le Bonheur Chldns Med Ctr; **Address:** 777 Washington Ave, Ste P110, Memphis, TN 38105; **Phone:** 901-866-8822; **Board Cert:** Pediatrics 2006; Pediatric Nephrology 2006; **Med School:** Univ Tenn Coll Med 1984; **Resid:** Pediatrics, Johns Hopkins Hosp 1987; **Fellow:** Pediatric Nephrology, Univ Tn Med Ctr 1990; **Fac Appt:** Assoc Prof

Benfield, Mark R MD [PNep] - **Spec Exp:** Hypertension; Glomerulonephritis; Nephrotic Syndrome; Transplant Medicine-Kidney; **Hospital:** Children's Hospital - Birmingham; **Address:** Pediatric Nephrology of Alabama, 1425 Richard Arrington Jr Blvd S, Ste 206, Birmingham, AL 35205; **Phone:** 205-558-3200; **Board Cert:** Pediatric Nephrology 2006; **Med School:** Tulane Univ 1984; **Resid:** Pediatrics, Chldn's Hosp 1987; **Fellow:** Pediatric Nephrology, Univ Minnesota 1990; **Fac Appt:** Prof Ped, Univ Alabama

Chandar, Jayanthi J MD [PNep] - **Spec Exp:** Kidney Disease; Transplant Medicine-Kidney; Renal Replacement Therapy; **Hospital:** Jackson Meml Hosp (page 70); **Address:** Univ Miami Div Ped Nephrology, PO Box 016960 (M-714), Miami, FL 33101; **Phone:** 305-585-6726; **Board Cert:** Pediatrics 2005; Pediatric Nephrology 2003; **Med School:** India 1983; **Resid:** Pediatrics, Jackson Memorial Hosp 1987; **Fellow:** Pediatric Nephrology, Jackson Memorial Hosp 1993; **Fac Appt:** Assoc Prof Ped, Univ Miami Sch Med

Jabs, Kathy L MD [PNep] - **Spec Exp:** Transplant Medicine-Kidney; Kidney Failure-Chronic; Dialysis Care; Hypertension; **Hospital:** Vanderbilt Monroe Carrell Jr. Chldn's Hosp (page 76); **Address:** Vanderbilt Chldns Hosp, Div Ped Nephrology, 6102 Doctor's Office Towers, Nashville, TN 37232-9306; **Phone:** 615-322-7416; **Board Cert:** Pediatrics 1987; Pediatric Nephrology 2010; **Med School:** Columbia P&S 1982; **Resid:** Pediatrics, Columbia-Presby Hosp 1985; **Fellow:** Pediatric Nephrology, Chldns Hosp 1988; **Fac Appt:** Assoc Prof Ped, Vanderbilt Univ

Neiberger, Richard E MD/PhD [PNep] - **Spec Exp:** Kidney Disease-Genetic; Hypertension; Kidney Failure; **Hospital:** Shands at Univ of FL; **Address:** Univ Florida College of Medicine, Div Pediatric Nephrology, 1600 SW Archer Rd, Box 100296, Gainesville, FL 32610; **Phone:** 352-273-9180; **Board Cert:** Pediatrics 2006; Nephrology 2006; **Med School:** Univ Louisville Sch Med 1982; **Resid:** Pediatrics, Montefiore Med Ctr 1985; **Fellow:** Pediatric Nephrology, Montefiore Med Ctr 1988; **Fac Appt:** Assoc Prof Ped, Univ Fla Coll Med

Wyatt, Robert J MD [PNep] - **Spec Exp:** Kidney Disease-Autoimmune; Berger's Disease (IgA Nephropathy); **Hospital:** Le Bonheur Chldns Med Ctr; **Address:** Univ Tennessee, Dept Peds, 777 Washington Ave, Ste P110, Memphis, TN 38105; **Phone:** 901-866-8822; **Board Cert:** Pediatrics 1978; Pediatric Nephrology 1979; **Med School:** Med Coll GA 1973; **Resid:** Pediatrics, Kentucky Med Ctr 1975; Pediatric Nephrology, Kentucky Med Ctr 1976; **Fellow:** Pediatric Nephrology, Cincinnati Chldns Hosp 1979; **Fac Appt:** Prof Ped, Univ Tenn Coll Med

Zilleruelo, Gaston E MD [PNep] - **Spec Exp:** Transplant Medicine-Kidney; Nephrotic Syndrome; Congenital Anomalies-Genitourinary; **Hospital:** Jackson Meml Hosp (page 70), Broward General Med Ctr; **Address:** Univ Miami, Dept Peds-Div Nephrology, PO Box 016960 (M-714), Miami, FL 33136; **Phone:** 305-585-6726; **Board Cert:** Pediatrics 1979; Pediatric Nephrology 1991; **Med School:** Chile 1969; **Resid:** Pediatrics, L Calvo-Mackenna Chldns Hosp 1972; Pediatrics, Jackson Meml Hosp 1977; **Fellow:** Pediatric Nephrology, Jackson Meml Hosp 1978; **Fac Appt:** Prof Ped, Univ Miami Sch Med

Pediatric Nephrology

Midwest

Andreoli, Sharon P MD [PNep] - **Spec Exp:** Kidney Failure; Kidney Failure-Chronic; Osteodystrophy; Glomerulonephritis; **Hospital:** Riley Hosp for Children, IU Health Methodist Hosp; **Address:** Riley Childrens Hosp-Ped Nephrology, 699 Riley Hosp Drive, rm RR230, Indianapolis, IN 46202; **Phone:** 317-274-2563; **Board Cert:** Pediatrics 1983; Pediatric Nephrology 1985; **Med School:** Indiana Univ 1978; **Resid:** Pediatrics, Riley Hosp Chldn 1981; **Fellow:** Pediatric Nephrology, Univ Minnesota 1981; Pediatric Nephrology, Indiana Univ 1984; **Fac Appt:** Prof Ped, Indiana Univ

Brophy, Patrick D MD [PNep] - **Spec Exp:** Polycystic Kidney Disease; Transplant Medicine-Kidney; Dialysis Care; **Hospital:** Univ Iowa Hosp & Clinics; **Address:** U of Iowa Children's Hospital, 200 Hawkins Drive, Iowa City, IA 52242; **Phone:** 319-384-3090; **Board Cert:** Pediatrics 2005; Pediatric Nephrology 2009; **Med School:** Canada 1994; **Resid:** Pediatrics, Univ Manitoba Affil Hosp 1998; **Fellow:** Pediatric Nephrology, Univ Michigan Hosps 2001; **Fac Appt:** Assoc Prof Ped, Univ Iowa Coll Med

Cohn, Richard MD [PNep] - **Spec Exp:** Transplant Medicine-Kidney; Nephrotic Syndrome; Kidney Disease-Chronic; **Hospital:** Children's Mem Hosp -Chicago; **Address:** Childrens Meml Hosp, 2300 Children's Plaza, Box 37, Chicago, IL 60614-3394; **Phone:** 773-327-3930; **Board Cert:** Pediatrics 1978; Pediatric Nephrology 1979; **Med School:** Albert Einstein Coll Med 1972; **Resid:** Pediatrics, Johns Hopkins Hosp 1975; **Fellow:** Pediatric Nephrology, Univ Minnesota Hosp 1978; **Fac Appt:** Prof Ped, Northwestern Univ

Friedman, Aaron L MD [PNep] - **Spec Exp:** Hypertension; Transplant Medicine-Kidney; Growth Disorders; Fanconi Syndrome; **Address:** 2450 Riverside Ave, Riverside East Bldg, Minneapolis, MN 55455; **Phone:** 612-365-6777; **Board Cert:** Pediatrics 1979; Pediatric Nephrology 2003; **Med School:** SUNY Upstate Med Univ 1974; **Resid:** Pediatrics, Univ Wisconsin Med Ctr 1976; **Fellow:** Pediatric Nephrology, Univ Wisconsin 1980; **Fac Appt:** Prof Ped, Univ Minn

Kashtan, Clifford E MD [PNep] - **Spec Exp:** Transplant Medicine-Kidney; Kidney Disease-Genetic; **Address:** Univ Minn Amplatz Chldns Hosp, Pediatric Spec Clinic, 2512 S 7th St Fl 3, Minneapolis, MN 55454; **Phone:** 612-626-2922; **Board Cert:** Pediatrics 1983; Pediatric Nephrology 2003; **Med School:** Wayne State Univ 1978; **Resid:** Pediatrics, Boston City Hosp 1981; **Fellow:** Pediatric Nephrology, Mass Genl Hosp 1984; Pediatric Nephrology, Univ Minnesota Hosp 1987; **Fac Appt:** Prof Ped, Univ Minn

Langman, Craig MD [PNep] - **Spec Exp:** Kidney Stones; Osteoporosis-Juvenile; Oxalosis; **Hospital:** Children's Mem Hosp -Chicago, Evanston/North Shore Univ Hlth Sys; **Address:** Children's Meml Hosp, 2300 N Children's Plaza, Box 37, Chicago, IL 60614-3394; **Phone:** 773-327-3930; **Board Cert:** Pediatrics 1982; Pediatric Nephrology 1992; **Med School:** Hahnemann Univ 1977; **Resid:** Pediatrics, Chldns Hosp 1979; **Fellow:** Pediatric Nephrology, Chldns Hosp 1981; **Fac Appt:** Prof Ped, Northwestern Univ

Mentser, Mark I MD [PNep] - **Hospital:** Nationwide Chldn's Hosp; **Address:** Nationwide Chldn's Hosp, Education Bldg, 700 Children's Drive Fl 6th, Columbus, OH 43205; **Phone:** 614-722-4360; **Board Cert:** Pediatrics 1978; Pediatric Nephrology 1979; **Med School:** Ohio State Univ 1973; **Resid:** Pediatrics, Children's Hosp LA 1975; **Fellow:** Pediatric Nephrology, Children's Hosp LA 1978; **Fac Appt:** Assoc Clin Prof Ped, Ohio State Univ

Nevins, Thomas E MD [PNep] - **Spec Exp:** Kidney Failure-Chronic; Transplant Medicine-Kidney; Hypertension; Dialysis Care; **Address:** Pediatric Spec Clinic, 3rd Fl, 2512 Bldg, 2512 S 7th St, Minneapolis, MN 55454; **Phone:** 612-626-2922; **Board Cert:** Pediatrics 1975; Pediatric Nephrology 1992; **Med School:** Washington Univ, St Louis 1969; **Resid:** Pediatrics, Univ Minnesota Hosps 1972; **Fellow:** Nephrology, Univ Minnesota Hosps 1978; **Fac Appt:** Prof Ped, Univ Minn

Warady, Bradley MD [PNep] - **Spec Exp:** Dialysis Care; Transplant Medicine-Kidney; Kidney Disease-Chronic; Birth Defects; **Hospital:** Chldns Mercy Hosps & Clinics; **Address:** Chldns Mercy Hosps & Clins, Dept Ped Nephrology, 2401 Gillham Rd, Kansas City, MO 64108; **Phone:** 816-234-3010; **Board Cert:** Pediatrics 1984; Pediatric Nephrology 1985; **Med School:** Univ IL Coll Med 1979; **Resid:** Pediatrics, Chldns Mercy Hosp 1982; **Fellow:** Pediatric Nephrology, Colorado Univ Med Ctr 1984; **Fac Appt:** Prof Ped, Univ MO-Kansas City

West Coast and Pacific

Alexander, Steven R MD [PNep] - **Spec Exp:** Kidney Failure; Transplant Medicine-Kidney; Nephrotic Syndrome; Dialysis Care; **Hospital:** Lucile Packard Chldn's Hosp; **Address:** Stanford Univ Med Ctr, Dept Peds, 300 Pasteur Drive, rm G306, Stanford, CA 94305-5208; **Phone:** 650-723-7903; **Board Cert:** Pediatrics 1986; Pediatric Nephrology 1986; **Med School:** Baylor Coll Med 1971; **Resid:** Pediatrics, Baylor Affil Hosps 1976; **Fellow:** Pediatric Nephrology, Baylor Affil Hosps 1978; **Fac Appt:** Prof Ped, Stanford Univ

Eddy, Allison MD [PNep] - **Spec Exp:** Kidney Disease; Glomerulonephritis; **Hospital:** Seattle Chldns Hosp; **Address:** 4800 Sand Point Way NE, MS A-7931, Seattle, WA 98105; **Phone:** 206-987-2524; **Board Cert:** Pediatrics 1981; Pediatric Nephrology 2002; **Med School:** Canada 1975; **Resid:** Pediatrics, Mc Gill Univ Affil Hosp 1980; **Fellow:** Pediatric Nephrology, Univ Minnesota Hosp 1985; **Fac Appt:** Prof Ped, Univ Wash

Ettenger, Robert B MD [PNep] - **Spec Exp:** Transplant Medicine-Kidney; Hypertension in Children; Urinary Tract Infections; Kidney Disease; **Hospital:** UCLA Ronald Reagan Med Ctr, Mattel Chldns Hosp at UCLA; **Address:** UCLA Pediatric Nephrology, 10833 Le Conte Ave, Box 951752, A2-383 MDCC, Los Angeles, CA 90095; **Phone:** 310-206-6987; **Board Cert:** Pediatrics 1986; Pediatric Nephrology 1986; **Med School:** Univ Pennsylvania 1968; **Resid:** Pediatrics, St Christophers Hosp Chldn 1971; **Fellow:** Pediatric Nephrology, Chldns Hosp 1975; **Fac Appt:** Prof Ped, UCLA

Flynn, Joseph T MD [PNep] - **Spec Exp:** Hypertension; Dialysis Care; Kidney Disease; Obesity; **Hospital:** Seattle Chldns Hosp; **Address:** Children's Hospital, Ped Nephrology, 4800 Sand Point Way NE, MS A-7931, Seattle, WA 98105; **Phone:** 206-987-2524; **Board Cert:** Pediatric Nephrology 2008; **Med School:** SUNY Upstate Med Univ 1987; **Resid:** Pediatrics, St Christophers Hosp 1990; **Fellow:** Pediatric Nephrology, St Christophers Hosp 1993; **Fac Appt:** Prof Ped, Univ Wash

Fouser, Laurie S MD [PNep] - **Spec Exp:** Congenital Kidney Disease; Glomerulonephritis; Hypertension in Children; Kidney Failure; **Hospital:** Swedish Med Ctr-First Hill-Seattle; **Address:** Swedish Ped Spec Care, 1101 Madison Ln, Ste 800, Seattle, WA 98104; **Phone:** 206-215-2700; **Board Cert:** Pediatrics 1985; Pediatric Nephrology 2003; **Med School:** Univ Nebr Coll Med 1979; **Resid:** Pediatrics, Chldns Ortho Hosp-Univ WA 1982; **Fellow:** Pediatric Nephrology, Univ Minnesota Hosp 1987; Research, Univ Washington Med Ctr 1989; **Fac Appt:** Asst Prof Ped, Univ Wash

Jordan, Stanley C MD [PNep] - **Spec Exp:** Transplant Medicine-Kidney; **Hospital:** Cedars-Sinai Med Ctr; **Address:** Cedars Sinai Med Ctr, Div Ped Nephrology, 8635 W 3rd St, Ste 590W, Los Angeles, CA 90048; **Phone:** 310-423-2641; **Board Cert:** Pediatrics 1978; Pediatric Nephrology 1979; Clinical & Laboratory Immunology 1988; **Med School:** Univ NC Sch Med 1973; **Resid:** Pediatrics, UCLA Med Ctr 1976; Pediatric Nephrology, UCLA Med Ctr 1977; **Fellow:** Renal Immunology, Scripps Clinic 1978; Dialysis & Tranplantation, Chldns Hosp 1980; **Fac Appt:** Prof Ped, UCLA

Pediatric Nephrology

McDonald, Ruth A MD [PNep] - **Spec Exp:** Transplant Medicine-Kidney; Kidney Disease; **Hospital:** Seattle Chldns Hosp; **Address:** 4800 Sand Point Way NE, MS A-7931, Seattle, WA 98105; **Phone:** 206-987-2524; **Board Cert:** Pediatric Nephrology 2005; **Med School:** Univ Minn 1987; **Resid:** Pediatrics, Chldns Hosp & Med Ctr 1990; **Fellow:** Pediatric Nephrology, Chldns Hosp & Med Ctr 1993; **Fac Appt:** Assoc Prof Ped, Univ Wash

PEDIATRIC OTOLARYNGOLOGY

New England

Cunningham, Michael J MD [PO] - **Spec Exp:** Head & Neck Tumors; Sinus Disorders; Hemangiomas; Vascular Malformations; **Hospital:** Mass Eye & Ear Infirmary, Mass Genl Hosp; **Address:** Chldns Hosp Boston, Dept otolaryngology, 300 Longwood Ave, Ste Lo-367, Boston, MA 02114; **Phone:** 617-355-6460; **Board Cert:** Otolaryngology 1988; **Med School:** Univ Rochester 1981; **Resid:** Pediatrics, Mass Genl Hosp 1983; Otolaryngology, Univ Pittsburgh Eye & Ear Hosp 1988; **Fellow:** Pediatric Otolaryngology, Mass Eye & Ear Infirm 1989; **Fac Appt:** Prof Oto, Harvard Med Sch

McGill, Trevor J MD [PO] - **Spec Exp:** Head & Neck Tumors; Cholesteatoma; Lymphatic Malformations-Head & Neck; Hemangiomas; **Hospital:** Children's Hospital - Boston; **Address:** Childrens Hosp, Dept Otolaryngology, 300 Longwood Ave, LO-367, Boston, MA 02115; **Phone:** 617-355-6460; **Board Cert:** Otolaryngology 1988; **Med School:** Ireland 1967; **Resid:** Otolaryngology, Royal Natl Throat Nose & Ear Hosp 1974; **Fellow:** Otolaryngology, Mass Eye & Ear Infirm 1976; **Fac Appt:** Prof Oto, Harvard Med Sch

Poe, Dennis MD [PO] - **Spec Exp:** Cochlear Implants; Neuro-Otology; Ear Disorders/Surgery; **Hospital:** Children's Hospital - Boston; **Address:** Chldns Hosp, Dept Otolaryngology, 300 Longwood Ave, Box 00367, Boston, MA 02115-5724; **Phone:** 617-355-3794; **Board Cert:** Otolaryngology 1987; Neurotology 2004; **Med School:** SUNY Upstate Med Univ 1982; **Resid:** Surgery, Univ Mass Med Ctr 1983; Otolaryngology, Univ Chicago Hosps 1987; **Fellow:** Otology & Neurotology, Otology Group 1988; **Fac Appt:** Assoc Prof Oto, Harvard Med Sch

Mid Atlantic

April, Max M MD [PO] - **Spec Exp:** Sinus Disorders; Neck Masses; Laryngeal Disorders; Sleep Apnea; **Hospital:** NY-Presby/Weill Cornell Med Ctr, NY (page 65), Long Island Jewish Med Ctr; **Address:** 428 E 72nd St, Ste 100, New York, NY 10021; **Phone:** 646-962-2224; **Board Cert:** Otolaryngology 1990; **Med School:** Boston Univ 1985; **Resid:** Otolaryngology, Boston Univ Med Ctr 1990; **Fellow:** Pediatric Otolaryngology, Johns Hopkins Hosp 1991; **Fac Appt:** Clin Prof Oto, Cornell Univ-Weill Med Coll

Casselbrant, Margaretha L MD/PhD [PO] - **Spec Exp:** Ear Infections; **Hospital:** Chldns Hosp of Pittsburgh - UPMC; **Address:** Children's Hospital, Dept Otolaryngology, 4401 Penn Ave, Children's Hospital Drive, Pittsburgh, PA 15224; **Phone:** 412-692-5460; **Board Cert:** Otolaryngology 1992; **Med School:** Sweden 1973; **Resid:** Otolaryngology, Malmo Genl Hosp-Univ Lund 1978; **Fellow:** Otolaryngology, Univ Pittsburgh Med Ctr 1982; **Fac Appt:** Prof Oto, Univ Pittsburgh

Dolitsky, Jay MD [PO] - **Spec Exp:** Ear Infections; Neck Masses; Tonsil/Adenoid Disorders; Sleep Disorders; **Hospital:** New York Eye & Ear Infirm (page 64); **Address:** 404 Park Ave S Fl 12, New York, NY 10016; **Phone:** 212-679-3499; **Board Cert:** Otolaryngology 1990; **Med School:** SUNY Downstate 1981; **Resid:** Otolaryngology, Manhattan EET Hosp 1990; **Fellow:** Pediatric Otolaryngology, Children's Hosp 1992; **Fac Appt:** Assoc Prof Oto, NY Med Coll

Goldsmith, Ari J MD [PO] - **Spec Exp:** Voice Disorders; Airway Disorders; Hearing Loss; Sleep Apnea; **Hospital:** Univ Hosp of Bklyn at Long Island Coll Hosp; **Address:** LICH-Dept Otolaryngology, 134 Atlantic Ave, Brooklyn, NY 11201-5502; **Phone:** 718-780-1498; **Board Cert:** Otolaryngology 1994; **Med School:** Albert Einstein Coll Med 1988; **Resid:** Otolaryngology, LI Jewish Hosp 1993; **Fellow:** Pediatric Otolaryngology, Chldns Hosp 1994; **Fac Appt:** Assoc Prof Oto, SUNY Hlth Sci Ctr

Haddad Jr, Joseph MD [PO] - **Spec Exp:** Ear Infections; Sinus Disorders; Cleft Palate/Lip; **Hospital:** Morgan Stanley Children's Hosp of NY-Presby, NY (page 65); **Address:** Morgan Stanley Chldns Hosp of NY-Presby, 3959 Broadway, Ste 501N, New York, NY 10032-1559; **Phone:** 212-305-8933; **Board Cert:** Otolaryngology 1988; **Med School:** NYU Sch Med 1983; **Resid:** Surgery, Columbia-Presby Hosp 1985; Otolaryngology, Columbia-Presby Hosp 1988; **Fellow:** Pediatric Otolaryngology, Chldns Hosp 1990; **Fac Appt:** Clin Prof Oto, Columbia P&S

Harley, Earl H MD [PO] - **Spec Exp:** Infectious Disease; **Hospital:** Georgetown Univ Hosp; **Address:** Georgetown Univ Hosp, 3800 Reservoir Rd NW, Gorman Bldg Fl 1, Washington, DC 20007; **Phone:** 202-444-8186; **Board Cert:** Otolaryngology 1984; **Med School:** Howard Univ 1971; **Resid:** Pediatrics, San Diego Naval Hosp 1973; Otolaryngology, Oakland Naval Hosp 1984; **Fellow:** Pediatric Otolaryngology, Chldn's Hosp Natl Med Ctr 1988; Pediatric Otolaryngology, Mass EE Infirm/Harvard Med Sch 1989; **Fac Appt:** Asst Prof Oto, Georgetown Univ

Jones, Jacqueline MD [PO] - **Spec Exp:** Sinus Disorders/Surgery; Ear Infections; **Hospital:** NY-Presby/Weill Cornell Med Ctr, NY (page 65), Lenox Hill Hosp; **Address:** 1175 Park Ave, Ste 1A, New York, NY 10128; **Phone:** 212-996-2559; **Board Cert:** Otolaryngology 1989; **Med School:** Cornell Univ-Weill Med Coll 1984; **Resid:** Otolaryngology, Hosp Univ Penn 1989; **Fellow:** Pediatric Otolaryngology, Chldns Hosp 1990; **Fac Appt:** Assoc Prof Oto, Cornell Univ-Weill Med Coll

Kazahaya, Ken MD [PO] - **Spec Exp:** Cochlear Implants; Skull Base Surgery; Otology; Thyroid Surgery; **Hospital:** Chldns Hosp of Philadelphia, Hosp Univ Penn - UPHS (page 68); **Address:** Children's Hosp of Philadelphia, Div Pediatric Otolaryngology, 34th St & Civic Ctr Blvd Wood Bldg Fl 1, Philadelphia, PA 19104; **Phone:** 215-590-3440; **Board Cert:** Otolaryngology 1999; **Med School:** Univ Pennsylvania 1993; **Resid:** Otolaryngology, Hosp U Penn 1998; **Fellow:** Pediatric Otolaryngology, Children's Hosp 2000; **Fac Appt:** Assoc Clin Prof Oto, Univ Pennsylvania

Rosenfeld, Richard M MD [PO] - **Spec Exp:** Sinus Disorders/Surgery; Head & Neck Surgery; Ear Disorders/Surgery; **Hospital:** SUNY Downstate Med Ctr, Univ Hosp of Bklyn at Long Island Coll Hosp; **Address:** Univ Otolaryngologists, 134 Atlantic Ave, Brooklyn, NY 11201; **Phone:** 718-780-1498; **Board Cert:** Otolaryngology 1989; **Med School:** SUNY Buffalo 1984; **Resid:** Otolaryngology, Mount Sinai Med Ctr 1989; **Fellow:** Pediatric Otolaryngology, Chldn's Hosp 1991; **Fac Appt:** Prof Oto, SUNY Downstate

Tunkel, David E MD [PO] - **Spec Exp:** Laryngeal Disorders; Otology; Head & Neck Surgery; **Hospital:** Johns Hopkins Hosp (page 61), Greater Baltimore Med Ctr; **Address:** 601 N Caroline St, rm 6161, Baltimore, MD 21287; **Phone:** 410-955-1559; **Board Cert:** Otolaryngology 1990; **Med School:** Johns Hopkins Univ 1984; **Resid:** Surgery, Johns Hopkins Hosp 1986; Otolaryngology, Johns Hopkins Hosp 1990; **Fellow:** Pediatric Otolaryngology, Chldns Natl Med Ctr 1991; **Fac Appt:** Assoc Prof Oto, Johns Hopkins Univ

Ward, Robert MD [PO] - **Spec Exp:** Airway Disorders; Sinus Disorders/Surgery; Choanal Atresia; **Hospital:** NY-Presby/Weill Cornell Med Ctr, NY (page 65), Lenox Hill Hosp (Manh Eye, Ear & Throat Hosp); **Address:** Weill Cornell Med Ctr, Otolaryngology, 428 E 72nd St, Ste 100, New York, NY 10021; **Phone:** 646-962-2224; **Board Cert:** Otolaryngology 1986; **Med School:** Cornell Univ-Weill Med Coll 1981; **Resid:** Surgery, NY Hosp 1983; Otolaryngology, NY Hosp 1986; **Fellow:** Pediatric Otolaryngology, Chldns Hosp 1986; **Fac Appt:** Assoc Clin Prof Oto, Cornell Univ-Weill Med Coll

Pediatric Otolaryngology

Southeast

Darrow, David H MD/DDS [PO] - **Spec Exp:** Airway Disorders; Sinus Disorders; Otology; Neck Masses; **Hospital:** Chldns Hosp of King's Daughters; **Address:** Chldns Hosp of Kings Daughters, Div Otolaryngology, 601 Childrens Lane, Norfolk, VA 23507; **Phone:** 757-668-9327; **Board Cert:** Otolaryngology 1994; **Med School:** Duke Univ 1987; **Resid:** Otolaryngology, UCSD Med Ctr 1993; **Fellow:** Pediatric Otolaryngology, Chldns Meml Hosp 1994; **Fac Appt:** Assoc Prof Oto, Eastern VA Med Sch

Drake, Amelia F MD [PO] - **Spec Exp:** Head & Neck Surgery; **Hospital:** NC Memorial Hosp - UNC; **Address:** 101 Manning Drive, Physicians Bldg, CB 7070, Chapel Hill, NC 27599; **Phone:** 919-966-6483; **Board Cert:** Otolaryngology 1987; **Med School:** Univ NC Sch Med 1981; **Resid:** Otolaryngology, Univ Michigan Hosps 1986; **Fac Appt:** Prof Oto, Univ NC Sch Med

Eavey, Roland D MD [PO] - **Spec Exp:** Ear Reconstruction/Microtia; Ear Disorders/Surgery; Otology; Hearing Loss; **Hospital:** Vanderbilt Monroe Carrell Jr. Chldn's Hosp (page 76); **Address:** Vanderbilt Pediatric Otolaryngology, 2200 Childrens Way, 7th Fl, Doctors Office Tower, Nashville, TN 37232; **Phone:** 615-936-8176; **Board Cert:** Pediatrics 1982; Otolaryngology 1981; **Med School:** Univ Pennsylvania 1975; **Resid:** Pediatrics, Chldns Hosp 1977; Surgery, Kaiser Fdn Hosp 1978; **Fellow:** Otolaryngology, Mass EE Infirm 1981; **Fac Appt:** Prof Oto, Vanderbilt Univ

Midwest

Arjmand, Ellis M MD/PhD [PO] - **Spec Exp:** Hearing Loss; Cochlear Implants; Sinus Disorders; **Hospital:** Cincinnati Chldns Hosp Med Ctr; **Address:** Cinncinatti Chldns Hosp-Otolaryngology, 3333 Burnet Ave, Fl C3, MS 2018, Cincinnati, OH 45229; **Phone:** 513-636-4355; **Board Cert:** Otolaryngology 1994; **Med School:** Northwestern Univ 1986; **Resid:** Otolaryngology, Barnes Jewish Hosp 1993; **Fellow:** Pediatric Otolaryngology, St Louis Chldns Hosp 1994; **Fac Appt:** Prof Oto, Univ Cincinnati

Arnold, James E MD [PO] - **Spec Exp:** Airway Disorders; Otology; Ear Tumors; **Hospital:** UH Rainbow Babies & Chldns Hosp (page 74), Univ Hosps Case Med Ctr (page 74); **Address:** 11100 Euclid Ave, Lakeside Bldg Fl 4, Cleveland, OH 44106-5045; **Phone:** 216-844-5031; **Board Cert:** Otolaryngology 1982; **Med School:** Univ Tex, San Antonio 1977; **Resid:** Otolaryngology, Fitzsimons Army Med Ctr 1982; **Fellow:** Pediatric Otolaryngology, Childrens Hosp 1987; **Fac Appt:** Prof Oto, Case West Res Univ

Belenky, Walter MD [PO] - **Spec Exp:** Cochlear Implants; Airway Disorders; **Hospital:** Chldns Hosp of Michigan; **Address:** Chldns Hosp, Dept Ped Oto, 3901 Beaubien Fl 3, Detroit, MI 48201; **Phone:** 313-745-9048; **Board Cert:** Otolaryngology 1970; **Med School:** Univ Mich Med Sch 1963; **Resid:** Surgery, William Beaumont Hosps 1965; Otolaryngology, Wayne Affil Hosp 1968

Cotton, Robin MD [PO] - **Spec Exp:** Tracheal Surgery; Head & Neck Surgery; Airway Reconstruction; **Hospital:** Cincinnati Chldns Hosp Med Ctr; **Address:** Cincinnati Chldns Hosp-Otolaryngology, 3333 Burnet Ave, Fl C3, MS 2018, Cincinnati, OH 45229; **Phone:** 513-636-4355; **Board Cert:** Otolaryngology 1972; **Med School:** England, UK 1965; **Resid:** Otolaryngology, Univ Birmingham 1968; Otolaryngology, Univ Toronto Med Ctr 1972; **Fellow:** Head and Neck Surgery, Univ Cincinnati Med Ctr 1973; **Fac Appt:** Prof Oto, Univ Cincinnati

Holinger, Lauren D MD [PO] - **Spec Exp:** Airway Disorders; Swallowing Disorders; Cough-Chronic; Voice Disorders; **Hospital:** Children's Mem Hosp -Chicago; **Address:** Chldns Meml Hosp, Dept Otolaryngology, 2300 Childrens Plaza, Box 25, Chicago, IL 60614-3394; **Phone:** 773-880-4457; **Board Cert:** Otolaryngology 1975; **Med School:** Ros Franklin Univ/Chicago Med Sch 1971; **Resid:** Surgery, Univ Colorado Affil Hosp 1972; Otolaryngology, Univ Colorado Affil Hosp 1975; **Fellow:** Pediatric Otolaryngology, Chldns Meml Hosp 1976; **Fac Appt:** Prof Oto, Northwestern Univ

Katz, Robert L MD [PO] - **Spec Exp:** Ear Infections; Sinus Disorders/Surgery; Hearing Loss; **Hospital:** Cleveland Clin (page 56); **Address:** Twinsburg Family Health & Surg Ctr, 8701 Darrow Rd, Twinsburg, OH 44087; **Phone:** 330-888-4000; **Board Cert:** Otolaryngology 1968; **Med School:** Case West Res Univ 1963; **Resid:** Surgery, Mount Sinai Hosp 1965; Otolaryngology, Mass EE Infirm/Chldns Hosp 1968; **Fac Appt:** Clin Prof Oto, Case West Res Univ

Miller, Robert P MD [PO] - **Spec Exp:** Ear Disorders/Surgery; Airway Disorders; Sinus Disorders; Tonsil/Adenoid Disorders; **Hospital:** Adv Luth Genl Hosp, Children's Mem Hosp -Chicago; **Address:** 8780 W Golf Rd, Ste 200, Niles, IL 60714; **Phone:** 847-674-5585; **Board Cert:** Otolaryngology 1978; **Med School:** Loyola Univ-Stritch Sch Med 1974; **Resid:** Otolaryngology, Univ Illinois Hosps 1978; **Fellow:** Pediatric Otolaryngology, Chldns Hosp Med Ctr 1987; **Fac Appt:** Asst Clin Prof Oto, Univ IL Coll Med

Myer III, Charles M MD [PO] - **Spec Exp:** Airway Disorders; Head & Neck Tumors; Neck Masses; **Hospital:** Cincinnati Chldns Hosp Med Ctr, Univ Hosp - Cincinnati; **Address:** Cincinnati Chldns Hosp-Otolaryngology, 3333 Burnet Ave, Fl C3, MS 2018, Cincinnati, OH 45229; **Phone:** 513-636-4355; **Board Cert:** Otolaryngology 1984; **Med School:** Univ Alabama 1978; **Resid:** Otolaryngology, Univ Cincinnati Med Ctr 1984; **Fellow:** Pediatric Otolaryngology, Chldns Hosp 1985; **Fac Appt:** Prof Oto, Univ Cincinnati

Great Plains and Mountains

Chan, Kenny H MD [PO] - **Spec Exp:** Ear Infections; Sinusitis; Hearing Disorders; **Hospital:** Chldn's Hosp - Aurora (CO), Parker Adventist Hosp; **Address:** Chldns Hosp, Dept Otolaryngology, 13123 E 16th Ave, Box B455, Aurora, CO 80045; **Phone:** 720-777-8501; **Board Cert:** Otolaryngology 1984; **Med School:** Loma Linda Univ 1977; **Resid:** Otolaryngology, Loma Linda Univ Hosp 1983; **Fellow:** Pediatric Otolaryngology, Chldns Hosp 1987; **Fac Appt:** Prof Oto, Univ Colorado

Lusk, Rodney P MD [PO] - **Spec Exp:** Cochlear Implants; Sinus Disorders/Surgery; Sleep Disorders/Apnea; **Hospital:** Boys Town Natl Rsch Hosp, Children's Hosp - Omaha; **Address:** Boystown National Research Hosp, 555 N 30th St, Omaha, NE 68131; **Phone:** 402-498-6502; **Board Cert:** Otolaryngology 1982; **Med School:** Univ MO-Columbia Sch Med 1977; **Resid:** Head and Neck Surgery, Univ Iowa Hosp & Clinics 1982; **Fellow:** Pediatric Otolaryngology, Chldns Hosp 1983

Southwest

Bower, Charles MD [PO] - **Spec Exp:** Airway Disorders; Sleep Disorders/Apnea; Sinus Disorders/Surgery; **Hospital:** Arkansas Chldns Hosp; **Address:** Arkansas Chldns Hosp, Dept Ped Oto, 1 Children's Way, Slot 836, Little Rock, AR 72202-3510; **Phone:** 501-364-1047; **Board Cert:** Otolaryngology 1990; **Med School:** Univ Ark 1985; **Resid:** Otolaryngology, Univ Ark Med Ctr 1991; **Fellow:** Pediatric Otolaryngology, Chldns Hosp 1992; **Fac Appt:** Assoc Prof Oto, Univ Ark

Pediatric Otolaryngology

Duncan III, Newton O MD [PO] - **Spec Exp:** Sinus Disorders; Airway Disorders; Head & Neck Surgery; **Hospital:** Texas Chldns Hosp, Methodist Hosp - Houston; **Address:** Childrens Ear Nose & Throat, 6550 Fannin St, Ste 2001, Houston, TX 77030-2709; **Phone:** 713-796-2001; **Board Cert:** Otolaryngology 1986; **Med School:** Baylor Coll Med 1978; **Resid:** Surgery, Baylor Coll Med 1983; Otolaryngology, Baylor Coll Med 1986; **Fellow:** Pediatric Otolaryngology, Univ Wash 1991; Pediatric Otolaryngology, Royal Alexandra Hosp Chld 1992; **Fac Appt:** Asst Clin Prof Oto, Baylor Coll Med

Friedman, Ellen M MD [PO] - **Spec Exp:** Airway Disorders; Lymphatic Malformations-Head & Neck; **Hospital:** Texas Chldns Hosp; **Address:** 67010 Fannin, Ste 540, MC CC6102, Houston, TX 77030; **Phone:** 832-822-3250; **Board Cert:** Otolaryngology 1981; **Med School:** Albert Einstein Coll Med 1975; **Resid:** Surgery, Montefiore Hosp 1976; Otolaryngology, Washington Hosp Ctr 1979; **Fellow:** Pediatric Otolaryngology, Boston Chldns Hosp; **Fac Appt:** Prof Oto, Baylor Coll Med

West Coast and Pacific

Crockett, Dennis M MD [PO] - **Spec Exp:** Head & Neck Cancer; Airway Disorders; **Hospital:** Keck Med Ctr of USC (page 75); **Address:** 26726 Crown Valley Pkwy, Ste 200, Mission Viejo, CA 92691; **Phone:** 949-364-4361; **Board Cert:** Otolaryngology 1985; **Med School:** USC Sch Med 1979; **Resid:** Otolaryngology, LAC-USC Med Ctr 1984; **Fellow:** Pediatrics, Boston Chldns Hosp 1985; **Fac Appt:** Assoc Prof Oto, USC Sch Med

Geller, Kenneth Allen MD [PO] - **Spec Exp:** Airway Disorders; Sinus Disorders/Surgery; Head & Neck Cancer; **Hospital:** Chldns Hosp - Los Angeles, Huntington Memorial Hosp; **Address:** Chldns Hosp, Div Otolaryngology, 4650 Sunset Blvd, MS 58, Los Angeles, CA 90027; **Phone:** 323-361-2145; **Board Cert:** Otolaryngology 1978; **Med School:** USC Sch Med 1972; **Resid:** Surgery, Wadsworth VA Hosp 1975; Otolaryngology, UCLA Hlth Scis Ctr 1978; **Fellow:** Pediatric Otolaryngology, Chldns Hosp 1979; **Fac Appt:** Assoc Clin Prof Oto, USC Sch Med

Inglis, Andrew MD [PO] - **Spec Exp:** Airway Disorders; Voice Disorders; **Hospital:** Seattle Chldns Hosp; **Address:** Children's Hospital & Medical Ctr, 4800 Sand Point Way NE, MS W6640, Seattle, WA 98105-0371; **Phone:** 206-987-2105; **Board Cert:** Otolaryngology 1987; **Med School:** Med Coll PA Hahnemann 1981; **Resid:** Surgery, Virginia Mason Hosp 1983; Otolaryngology, Univ Washington Hosps 1987; **Fellow:** Pediatric Otolaryngology, Royal Alexandria Hosp Chldn 1987; **Fac Appt:** Assoc Prof Oto, Univ Wash

Parikh, Sanjay R MD [PO] - **Spec Exp:** Airway Reconstruction; Cochlear Implants; Endoscopic Sinus Surgery; **Hospital:** Seattle Chldns Hosp; **Address:** Seattle Children's Hosp, Div Pediatric Otolaryngology, 4800 Sand Point Way, NE, W-7729, Seattle, WA 98105; **Phone:** 206-987-2105; **Board Cert:** Otolaryngology 2000; **Med School:** Rush Med Coll 1994; **Resid:** Surgery, Harbor UCLA Med Ctr 1996; Otolaryngology, Univ Toronto 1999; **Fellow:** Pediatric Otolaryngology, Chldns Hosp 2001; **Fac Appt:** Assoc Prof Oto, Univ Wash

Richardson, Mark A MD [PO] - **Spec Exp:** Sinus Disorders; Airway Disorders; Lymphatic Malformations-Head & Neck; **Hospital:** Doernbecher Chldns Hosp/OHSU; **Address:** 3181 SW Sam Jackson Park Rd, MC PV01, Portland, OR 97239; **Phone:** 503-494-5350; **Board Cert:** Otolaryngology 1979; **Med School:** Med Univ SC 1975; **Resid:** Otolaryngology, Med Univ Hosp 1979; **Fellow:** Pediatric Otolaryngology, Chldns Hosp Med Ctr 1980; **Fac Appt:** Prof Oto, Oregon Hlth & Sci Univ

Rosbe, Kristina W MD [PO] - **Spec Exp:** Airway Disorders; Sinus Disorders/Surgery; Cochlear Implants; Neck Masses; **Hospital:** UCSF Med Ctr; **Address:** UCSF Med Ctr, Dept Otolaryngology, 2380 Sutter St, San Francisco, CA 94115; **Phone:** 415-353-2757; **Board Cert:** Otolaryngology 1999; **Med School:** Dartmouth Med Sch 1993; **Resid:** Surgery, Univ N Carolina Hosps 1994; Otolaryngology, Univ N Carolina Hosps 1998; **Fellow:** Pediatric Otolaryngology, Chldns Hosp 2000; **Fac Appt:** Assoc Prof Ped, UCSF

PEDIATRIC PULMONOLOGY

New England

Dorkin, Henry L MD [PPul] - **Spec Exp:** Cystic Fibrosis; **Hospital:** Children's Hospital - Boston; **Address:** Chldn's Hosp Boston, Div Respiratory Diseases, 300 Longwood Ave, Box 343, Boston, MA 02111-1854; **Phone:** 617-355-1900; **Board Cert:** Pediatrics 1993; Pediatric Pulmonology 2003; **Med School:** Johns Hopkins Univ 1974; **Resid:** Pediatrics, Johns Hopkins Hosp 1977; **Fellow:** Pulmonary Disease, Chldn's Hosp Med Ctr 1980; **Fac Appt:** Assoc Prof Ped, Harvard Med Sch

Lapey, Allen MD [PPul] - **Spec Exp:** Cystic Fibrosis; Asthma; Food Allergy; **Hospital:** Mass Genl Hosp; **Address:** 275 Cambridge St, Ste 530, Professional Office Bldg, Boston, MA 02114; **Phone:** 617-726-8707; **Board Cert:** Pediatrics 1972; Allergy & Immunology 1979; Pediatric Pulmonology 2003; **Med School:** Univ Rochester 1966; **Resid:** Pediatrics, Chldns Hosp 1968; **Fellow:** Pediatric Pulmonology, Mass Genl Hosp 1972; Allergy & Immunology, Mass Genl Hosp 1972; **Fac Appt:** Asst Clin Prof Ped, Harvard Med Sch

Mid Atlantic

Borowitz, Drucy S MD [PPul] - **Spec Exp:** Cystic Fibrosis; Clinical Trials; Nutrition; **Hospital:** Women's & Chldn's Hosp of Buffalo, The; **Address:** Women & Childrens Hospital, The Lung Center, 219 Bryant St, Buffalo, NY 14222; **Phone:** 716-878-7561; **Board Cert:** Pediatrics 1984; Pediatric Gastroenterology 2007; **Med School:** Cornell Univ-Weill Med Coll 1979; **Resid:** Pediatrics, UCSF Med Ctr 1982; **Fellow:** Nutrition, UCSF 1983; **Fac Appt:** Clin Prof Ped, SUNY Buffalo

Dovey, Mark E MD [PPul] - **Spec Exp:** Cystic Fibrosis; **Hospital:** St. Christopher's Hosp for Chldn; **Address:** St Christopher's Hosp for Children, Div Pediatric Pulmonology, 3601 A St, Ste 2215, Philadelphia, PA 19134; **Phone:** 215-427-5183; **Board Cert:** Pediatric Pulmonology 2006; **Med School:** Duke Univ 1989; **Resid:** Pediatrics, Johns Hopkins Hosp 1992; **Fellow:** Pediatric Pulmonology, Childrens Hosp 1995; **Fac Appt:** Assoc Prof Ped, Temple Univ

Dozor, Allen J MD [PPul] - **Spec Exp:** Asthma; Cystic Fibrosis; **Hospital:** Westchester Med Ctr, Children's & Women's Phys.of Westchester; **Address:** NY Med College, Munger Pavilion, Pediatric Pulmonology, Ste 106, Valhalla, NY 10595-1600; **Phone:** 914-493-7585; **Board Cert:** Pediatrics 1981; Pediatric Pulmonology 2003; **Med School:** Penn State Coll Med 1977; **Resid:** Pediatrics, St Vincent's Hosp & Med Ctr 1980; **Fellow:** Pediatric Pulmonology, Chldns Hosp 1982; **Fac Appt:** Prof Ped, NY Med Coll

Kattan, Meyer MD [PPul] - **Spec Exp:** Asthma; Cystic Fibrosis; Chronic Lung Disease; **Hospital:** NY-Presby/Columbia Univ Med Ctr, NY (page 65), Englewood Hosp & Med Ctr; **Address:** 3959 Broadway, CHC 7-701, New York, NY 10032; **Phone:** 212-305-5122; **Board Cert:** Pediatrics 1980; Pediatric Pulmonology 2010; **Med School:** McGill Univ 1973; **Resid:** Pediatrics, Chldns Hosp 1975; Pediatrics, Hosp for Sick Chldn 1976; **Fellow:** Pulmonary Disease, Hosp for Sick Chldn 1978; **Fac Appt:** Prof Ped, Columbia P&S

Pediatric Pulmonology

Kurland, Geoffrey MD [PPul] - **Spec Exp:** Transplant Medicine-Lung; **Hospital:** Chldns Hosp of Pittsburgh - UPMC; **Address:** UPMC, Ped Pulmonology Dept, 4401 Penn Ave AOB Bldg - Ste 3300, Pittsburgh, PA 15224; **Phone:** 412-692-5630; **Board Cert:** Pediatrics 1978; Allergy & Immunology 1979; Pediatric Pulmonology 2010; **Med School:** Stanford Univ 1973; **Resid:** Pediatrics, Stanford Affil Hosps 1976; **Fellow:** Allergy & Immunology, Stanford Affil Hosps 1978; **Fac Appt:** Prof Ped, Univ Pittsburgh

Loughlin, Gerald M MD [PPul] - **Spec Exp:** Sleep Disorders/Apnea; Swallowing Disorders; Asthma & Chronic Lung Disease; Breathing Disorders; **Hospital:** NY-Presby/Weill Cornell Med Ctr, NY (page 65); **Address:** Cornell Med Coll, Dept Peds, 525 E 68th St, rm M-622, New York, NY 10021-4870; **Phone:** 212-746-4111; **Board Cert:** Pediatrics 1993; Pediatric Pulmonology 2010; **Med School:** Univ Rochester 1973; **Resid:** Pediatrics, Univ Ariz Med Ctr 1973; **Fellow:** Pediatric Pulmonology, Univ Ariz Med Ctr 1977; **Fac Appt:** Prof Ped, Cornell Univ-Weill Med Coll

Marcus, Carole L MD [PPul] - **Spec Exp:** Sleep Disorders/Apnea; **Hospital:** Chldns Hosp of Philadelphia; **Address:** Div of Pulmonology, 34th & Civic Ctr Blvd Wood Bldg Fl 5, Philadelphia, PA 19104; **Phone:** 215-590-3749; **Board Cert:** Pediatric Pulmonology 2007; Sleep Medicine 2007; **Med School:** South Africa 1982; **Resid:** Pediatrics, LIJ/SUNY Brooklyn Med Ctr 1986; **Fellow:** Pediatric Pulmonology, Chldns Hosp 1991; **Fac Appt:** Prof Ped, Univ Pennsylvania

Mcgrath-Morrow, Sharon A MD [PPul] - **Spec Exp:** Lung Injury-Neonatal; Bronchopulmonary Dysplasia; Ataxia Telangiectasia; Swallowing Disorders; **Hospital:** Johns Hopkins Hosp (page 61); **Address:** Johns Hopkins Ped Pulmonology, Rubenstein Chldns Hlth Bldg, 200 N Wolfe St, Ste 3029, Baltimore, MD 21287; **Phone:** 410-955-2035; **Board Cert:** Pediatrics 2007; Pediatric Pulmonology 2007; **Med School:** Univ VA Sch Med 1985; **Resid:** Pediatrics, Johns Hopkins Hosp 1988; **Fellow:** Pulmonary Critical Care Medicine, Johns Hopkins 1992; **Fac Appt:** Assoc Prof Ped, Johns Hopkins Univ

Orenstein, David M MD [PPul] - **Spec Exp:** Cystic Fibrosis; **Hospital:** Chldns Hosp of Pittsburgh - UPMC; **Address:** Children's Hospital Drive, Dept Pediatric Pulmonology, 4401 Penn Ave, Pittsburgh, PA 15224; **Phone:** 412-692-5630; **Board Cert:** Pediatrics 1979; Pediatric Pulmonology 2004; **Med School:** Case West Res Univ 1973; **Resid:** Pediatrics, Rainbow Babies & Chldn's Hosp 1975; **Fellow:** Pediatric Pulmonology, Rainbow Babies & Chldn's Hosp 1977; **Fac Appt:** Prof Ped, Univ Pittsburgh

Panitch, Howard B MD [PPul] - **Spec Exp:** Chronic Obstructive Lung Disease (COPD); Cystic Fibrosis; **Hospital:** Chldns Hosp of Philadelphia; **Address:** Div Pulmonology, 34th & Civic Ctr Blvd Wood Bldg Fl 5, Philadelphia, PA 19104; **Phone:** 215-590-3749; **Board Cert:** Pediatrics 1987; Pediatric Pulmonology 2011; **Med School:** Univ Pittsburgh 1982; **Resid:** Pediatrics, Children's Hosp 1985; **Fellow:** Pediatric Pulmonology, St Christopher's Hosp 1988; **Fac Appt:** Prof Ped, Univ Pennsylvania

Quittell, Lynne MD [PPul] - **Spec Exp:** Cystic Fibrosis; Asthma; **Hospital:** Northern Westchester Hosp; **Address:** 480 Bedford Rd, Chappaqua, NY 10514; **Phone:** 914-458-8800; **Board Cert:** Pediatrics 1986; Pediatric Pulmonology 2011; **Med School:** Israel 1981; **Resid:** Pediatrics, Schneider Chldns Hosp 1984; **Fellow:** Pediatric Pulmonology, St Christopher's Hosp 1988; **Fac Appt:** Assoc Prof Ped, Columbia P&S

Schidlow, Daniel V MD [PPul] - **Spec Exp:** Cystic Fibrosis; Lung Disease; **Hospital:** St. Christopher's Hosp for Chldn; **Address:** St Christopher's Hosp for Chldn, 3601 A St, Ste 2215, Philadelphia, PA 19134; **Phone:** 215-427-5183; **Board Cert:** Pediatrics 1979; Pediatric Pulmonology 2004; **Med School:** Chile 1972; **Resid:** Pediatrics, EG Cortes Hosp for Chldn 1974; Pediatrics, Bronx-Lebanon Hosp 1976; **Fellow:** Pediatric Pulmonology, St Christopher's Hosp for Chldn 1978; **Fac Appt:** Prof Ped, Drexel Univ Coll Med

Tauber, Danna MD [PPul] - **Spec Exp:** Sleep Disorders; Cystic Fibrosis; **Hospital:** St. Christopher's Hosp for Chldn; **Address:** St. Christopher's Hosp for Chldn, 3601 A St, Phildelphia, PA 19134; **Phone:** 215-427-5000; **Board Cert:** Pediatric Pulmonology 2004; Sleep Medicine 2009; **Med School:** Tulane Univ 1997; **Resid:** Pediatrics, Montefiore Med Ctr 2000; **Fellow:** Pediatric Pulmonology, Chldn's Hosp Phildelphia 2003; **Fac Appt:** Asst Prof Ped, Drexel Univ Coll Med

Zeitlin, Pamela L MD [PPul] - **Spec Exp:** Cystic Fibrosis; **Hospital:** Johns Hopkins Hosp (page 61), Mt Washington Ped Hosp; **Address:** Johns Hopkins Ped Pulmonology, 200 N Wolfe St, Baltimore, MD 21287; **Phone:** 410-955-2035; **Board Cert:** Pediatrics 1988; Pediatric Pulmonology 2007; **Med School:** Yale Univ 1983; **Resid:** Pediatrics, Johns Hopkins Hosp 1986; **Fellow:** Pediatric Pulmonology, Johns Hopkins Hosp 1989; **Fac Appt:** Prof Ped, Johns Hopkins Univ

Southeast

Murphy, Thomas M MD [PPul] - **Spec Exp:** Cystic Fibrosis; Asthma; Chronic Lung Disease of Infancy; Pneumonia-Recurrent; **Hospital:** Duke Univ Hosp; **Address:** Duke Univ Med Ctr, Box 102360, Durham, NC 27710; **Phone:** 919-684-3364; **Board Cert:** Internal Medicine 1976; Pediatrics 2003; Pediatric Pulmonology 2004; **Med School:** Univ Rochester 1973; **Resid:** Internal Medicine, Georgetown Univ Hosp 1976; **Fellow:** Pediatric Pulmonology, Georgetown Univ Hosp 1978; **Fac Appt:** Assoc Prof Ped, Duke Univ

Rubin, Bruce MD [PPul] - **Spec Exp:** Asthma; Cystic Fibrosis; Mucus Clearance Disorders; Cough-Chronic; **Hospital:** VCU Med Ctr; **Address:** VCU Med Ctr, PO Box 980646, Richmond, VA 23298; **Phone:** 804-828-2980; **Board Cert:** Pediatrics 1984; Pediatric Pulmonology 2005; **Med School:** Tulane Univ 1979; **Resid:** Pediatrics, Tulane Univ 1981; **Fellow:** Pediatric Pulmonary & Critical Care, Hosp for Sick Children 1983; **Fac Appt:** Prof Ped, Wake Forest Univ

Sallent, Jorge A MD [PPul] - **Spec Exp:** Chronic Lung Disease of Infancy; Asthma & Chronic Lung Disease; Lung Injuries-RSV related; **Hospital:** St. Mary's Med Ctr - W Palm Bch, Palms - West Hosp; **Address:** Pediatric Respiratory Ctr, 500 Federal Highway (US 1), Lake Park, FL 33403-3598; **Phone:** 561-863-0105; **Board Cert:** Pediatrics 1984; Pediatric Pulmonology 2010; **Med School:** Dominican Republic 1978; **Resid:** Pediatrics, Orlando Regional Med Ctr 1983; **Fellow:** Pediatric Pulmonology, Univ Florida 1986; **Fac Appt:** Asst Clin Prof Ped, Univ Fla Coll Med

Sherman, James MD [PPul] - **Spec Exp:** Asthma; Airway Disorders; Cough-Chronic; **Hospital:** Carilion Roanoke Meml Hosp; **Address:** 102 Highland Ave, Ste 203, Roanoke, VA 24013; **Phone:** 540-985-9835; **Board Cert:** Pediatrics 1981; Pediatric Pulmonology 2003; **Med School:** Univ S Fla Coll Med 1975; **Resid:** Pediatrics, SUNY Upstate Med Ctr 1977; Pediatrics, Tampa Genl Hosp- Univ So Florida 1978; **Fellow:** Pediatric Pulmonology, Rainbow Babies & Children's Hosp 1981; **Fac Appt:** Prof Ped, Univ Fla Coll Med

Midwest

Givan, Deborah C MD [PPul] - **Spec Exp:** Sleep Disorders/Apnea; Apnea in Infants; Asthma; Pulmonary Complications-Neurodisability; **Hospital:** Riley Hosp for Children; **Address:** Riley Hospital for Children, Pulmonary Medicine, 705 Riley Hospital Drive, #4270, Indianapolis, IN 46202; **Phone:** 317-274-7208; **Board Cert:** Pediatrics 1982; Pediatric Pulmonology 2010; Sleep Medicine 1997; **Med School:** Indiana Univ 1977; **Resid:** Pediatrics, Meethodist Hosp 1980; **Fellow:** Pediatric Pulmonology, Riley Chldns Hosp 1981; Pediatric Pulmonology, Texas Chldns Hosp 1982; **Fac Appt:** Clin Prof Ped, Indiana Univ

Pediatric Pulmonology

Green, Thomas P MD [PPul] - **Spec Exp:** Respiratory Failure; Breathing Disorders; **Hospital:** Children's Mem Hosp -Chicago, Northwestern Meml Hosp; **Address:** Dept Pulm-Crit Care Med, 2300 Chldns Pl, Box 86, Chicago, IL 60614; **Phone:** 773-880-8150; **Board Cert:** Pediatrics 1992; Pediatric Pulmonology 2009; Pediatric Critical Care Medicine 2010; **Med School:** Stanford Univ 1974; **Resid:** Pediatrics, Univ Minn Med Ctr 1977; **Fellow:** Pharmacology, Univ Minn Med Ctr 1979; Pediatric Pulmonology, Univ Minn Med Ctr 1994; **Fac Appt:** Prof Ped, Northwestern Univ

Kemp, James S MD [PPul] - **Spec Exp:** Sudden Infant Death Syndrome (SIDS); Breathing Disorders; Sleep Disorders; **Hospital:** St. Louis Chldns Hosp; **Address:** 660 S Euclid Ave, Box 8116, St Louis, MO 63141; **Phone:** 314-454-2694; **Board Cert:** Pediatrics 1981; Sleep Medicine 2007; **Med School:** Creighton Univ 1976; **Resid:** Pediatrics, Cardinal Glennon Chldns Hosp 1978; Pediatrics, Baylor Univ 1979; **Fellow:** Pediatric Pulmonology, Texas Chldns Hosp 1988; **Fac Appt:** Assoc Prof Ped, Washington Univ, St Louis

Kim, Young-Jee MD [PPul] - **Spec Exp:** Interstitial Lung Disease; Rare Lung Disease-Pediatric; Pulmonary Complications-Sickle Cell Dis; Pulmonary Complications-Cancer Therapy; **Hospital:** Riley Hosp for Children; **Address:** Riley Chldns Hosp - Dept Ped Pulm, 705 Riley Hospital Drive, ROC 4270, Indianapolis, IN 46202-5128; **Phone:** 317-274-7208; **Board Cert:** Pediatric Pulmonology 2006; **Med School:** South Korea 1982; **Resid:** Pediatrics, Duke Univ Med Ctr 1995; **Fellow:** Pediatric Pulmonology, Yale Univ Med Sch 1991; Pediatric Pulmonology, Riley Hosp Chldn 1998; **Fac Appt:** Assoc Clin Prof Ped, Indiana Univ

Konstan, Michael W MD [PPul] - **Spec Exp:** Cystic Fibrosis; Asthma; **Hospital:** UH Rainbow Babies & Chldns Hosp (page 74); **Address:** Div Ped Pulmonology, 11100 Euclid Ave, MS RBC6040, Cleveland, OH 44106; **Phone:** 216-844-1997; **Board Cert:** Pediatrics 1986; Pediatric Pulmonology 2011; **Med School:** Case West Res Univ 1982; **Resid:** Pediatrics, Chldn's Hosp 1985; **Fellow:** Pediatric Pulmonology, Rainbow Babies & Chldns Hosp 1988; **Fac Appt:** Prof Ped, Case West Res Univ

Kurachek, Stephen MD [PPul] - **Spec Exp:** Critical Care; Asthma; **Hospital:** Chldns Hosp and Clinics - Minneapolis; **Address:** 2530 Chicago Ave S, Ste 400, Minneapolis, MN 55404; **Phone:** 612-813-3300; **Board Cert:** Pediatrics 1985; Pediatric Critical Care Medicine 2003; Pediatric Pulmonology 2004; **Med School:** Univ Miami Sch Med 1978; **Resid:** Pediatrics, Univ Hosp 1981; **Fellow:** Pulmonary Disease, Boston Chldns Hosp 1984; **Fac Appt:** Asst Clin Prof Ped, Univ Minn

McCoy, Karen S MD [PPul] - **Spec Exp:** Cystic Fibrosis; Asthma; **Hospital:** Nationwide Chldn's Hosp; **Address:** Nationwide Children's Hosp, Section of Pulmonary Medicine, 555 S 18th St, Columbus, OH 43205; **Phone:** 614-722-4766; **Board Cert:** Pediatrics 1991; Pediatric Pulmonology 2010; **Med School:** Univ NC Sch Med 1975; **Resid:** Pediatrics, NC Meml Hosp 1979; **Fellow:** Pulmonary Disease, Arizona Hlth Scis Ctr 1982; **Fac Appt:** Assoc Prof Ped, Ohio State Univ

Great Plains and Mountains

Accurso, Frank J MD [PPul] - **Spec Exp:** Cystic Fibrosis; **Hospital:** Chldn's Hosp - Aurora (CO); **Address:** Chldn's Hosp Pulmonary Medicine, 13123 E 16th Ave, Box B395, Aurora, CO 80045; **Phone:** 720-777-2522; **Board Cert:** Pediatrics 1980; Pediatric Pulmonology 2010; **Med School:** Albert Einstein Coll Med 1974; **Resid:** Pediatrics, Univ Colo Affil Hosp 1977; **Fellow:** Pulmonary Disease, Univ Colo 1980; **Fac Appt:** Prof Ped, Univ Colorado

Fan, Leland Lane MD [PPul] - **Spec Exp:** Interstitial Lung Disease; **Hospital:** Chldn's Hosp - Aurora (CO); **Address:** The Chldn's Hosp Pulmonary Med, 13123 E 16th Ave, Ste B395, Aurora, CO 80045; **Phone:** 720-777-6181; **Board Cert:** Pediatrics 1978; Pediatric Pulmonology 2010; Pediatric Critical Care Medicine 2010; **Med School:** Baylor Coll Med 1973; **Resid:** Pediatrics, UCSF Med Ctr 1975; Pediatrics, Univ Colo Hlth Sci Ctr 1976; **Fellow:** Pediatric Pulmonary & Critical Care, Univ Colo Hlth Sci Ctr 1978; **Fac Appt:** Prof Ped, Baylor Coll Med

Southwest

Morgan, Wayne J MD [PPul] - **Spec Exp:** Cystic Fibrosis; Asthma; **Hospital:** Univ Med Ctr - Tucson, Tucson Med Ctr; **Address:** Univ Arizona Hlth Sci Ctr, Div Pediatric Pulmonology, 1501 N Campbell Ave, Box 245073, Tucson, AZ 85724; **Phone:** 520-626-7780; **Board Cert:** Pediatrics 1982; Pediatric Pulmonology 2010; **Med School:** McGill Univ 1976; **Resid:** Pediatrics, Montreal Chldns Hosp 1980; **Fellow:** Pediatric Pulmonology, Univ Ariz Hlth Sci 1982; **Fac Appt:** Prof Ped, Univ Ariz Coll Med

Warren, Robert H MD [PPul] - **Spec Exp:** Pulmonary Complications-Neurodisability; Pulmonary Rehabilitation; Ventilation Management-Long Term; **Hospital:** Arkansas Chldns Hosp; **Address:** Arkansas Chldns Hosp, Pulmonary Med, 1 Children's Way, Ste 512-17, Little Rock, AR 72202; **Phone:** 501-364-1006; **Board Cert:** Pediatrics 1973; Pediatric Pulmonology 2010; **Med School:** Univ Ark 1967; **Resid:** Pediatrics, LSU Med Ctr 1971; **Fellow:** Pediatric Pulmonology, Tulane Univ Sch Med 1974; Pediatric Pulmonary & Critical Care, Children's Meml Hosp 1974; **Fac Appt:** Assoc Prof Ped, Univ Ark

West Coast and Pacific

Cooper, Dan M MD [PPul] - **Hospital:** Chldns Hosp Orange Co; **Address:** Chldns Hosp Orange Co, Dept Ped Pulmology, 455 S Main St, Orange, CA 92868; **Phone:** 714-532-7983; **Board Cert:** Pediatrics 1980; Pediatric Pulmonology 2009; **Med School:** UCSF 1974; **Resid:** Internal Medicine, Hadassah Hosp; Pediatrics, Chldns Hosp Med Ctr 1980; **Fellow:** Pediatric Pulmonology, Babies Hosp-Columbia Univ 1994; **Fac Appt:** Prof Ped, UC Irvine

Keens, Thomas G MD [PPul] - **Spec Exp:** Sudden Infant Death Syndrome (SIDS); Breathing Disorders; **Hospital:** Chldns Hosp - Los Angeles; **Address:** Chldns Hosp, Div Pulmonology, 4650 W Sunset Blvd, MS 127, Los Angeles, CA 90027-6062; **Phone:** 323-361-2101; **Board Cert:** Pediatrics 1978; Neonatal-Perinatal Medicine 1983; Pediatric Pulmonology 2010; **Med School:** UCSD 1972; **Resid:** Pediatrics, Chldns Hosp 1975; **Fellow:** Pediatric Pulmonology, Hosp Sick Chldn 1977; **Fac Appt:** Prof Ped, USC Sch Med

Nielson, Dennis W MD/PhD [PPul] - **Spec Exp:** Cystic Fibrosis; **Hospital:** UCSF Med Ctr; **Address:** UCSF Dept Padiatric Pulmonology, 521 Parnassus Ave, rm C344, San Francisco, CA 94143; **Phone:** 415-476-2072; **Board Cert:** Pediatrics 1986; Pediatric Pulmonology 2003; **Med School:** Univ Utah 1976; **Resid:** Pediatrics, UCSF Med Ctr 1978; **Fellow:** Pediatric Pulmonology, UCSF Med Ctr 1981; **Fac Appt:** Clin Prof Ped, UCSF

Platzker, Arnold CG MD [PPul] - **Spec Exp:** Asthma; Chronic Lung Disease; Cystic Fibrosis; HIV and Lung Disease; **Hospital:** Chldns Hosp - Los Angeles, Mattel Chldns Hosp at UCLA; **Address:** Chldns Hosp, Div Ped Pulmonology, 4650 Sunset Blvd, Box 83, Los Angeles, CA 90027-6062; **Phone:** 323-361-2101; **Board Cert:** Pediatrics 1967; Neonatal-Perinatal Medicine 1975; Pediatric Pulmonology 2010; **Med School:** Tufts Univ 1962; **Resid:** Pediatrics, City Hosp 1964; Pediatrics, Stanford Univ Med Ctr 1966; **Fellow:** Pediatric Pulmonology, UCSF Med Ctr 1971; Neonatal-Perinatal Medicine, UCSF Med Ctr 1971; **Fac Appt:** Prof Ped, USC Sch Med

Pediatric Pulmonology

Ramsey, Bonnie W MD [PPul] - **Spec Exp:** Cystic Fibrosis; **Hospital:** Seattle Chldns Hosp; **Address:** 4800 Sand Point Way NE, MS A-5937, Seattle, WA 98105; **Phone:** 206-987-2024; **Board Cert:** Pediatrics 1981; Pediatric Pulmonology 2007; **Med School:** Harvard Med Sch 1976; **Resid:** Pediatrics, Chldns Hosp 1978; Pediatrics, Chldns Hosp 1979; **Fellow:** Pediatric Critical Care Medicine, Chldns Hosp 1981; **Fac Appt:** Prof Ped, Univ Wash

Redding, Gregory MD [PPul] - **Spec Exp:** Asthma; Chest Wall Deformities; Interstitial Lung Disease; **Hospital:** Seattle Chldns Hosp; **Address:** Pulmonary Division, 4800 Sand Point Way NE, rm A-5937, Seattle, WA 98105; **Phone:** 206-987-2174; **Board Cert:** Pediatrics 1992; Pediatric Pulmonology 2003; **Med School:** Stanford Univ 1974; **Resid:** Pediatrics, Harbor-UCLA Affil Hosps 1977; **Fellow:** Pediatric Pulmonology, Univ Colo Affil Hosps 1979; **Fac Appt:** Prof Ped, Univ Wash

Wall, Michael A MD [PPul] - **Spec Exp:** Cystic Fibrosis; Asthma; Pneumonia; **Hospital:** Doernbecher Chldns Hosp/OHSU, OR Hlth & Sci Univ; **Address:** OHSU, MC CDRC-P, 707 SW Gaines St, Portland, OR 97239; **Phone:** 503-494-8023; **Board Cert:** Pediatrics 1992; Pediatric Pulmonology 2010; **Med School:** Univ NC Sch Med 1973; **Resid:** Pediatrics, Mass Genl Hosp 1976; **Fellow:** Pulmonary Disease, Chldns Hosp 1978; **Fac Appt:** Prof Ped, Oregon Hlth & Sci Univ

PEDIATRIC RHEUMATOLOGY

New England

McCarthy, Paul L MD [PRhu] - **Spec Exp:** Lupus/SLE; Juvenile Arthritis; Dermatomyositis; Vasculitis; **Hospital:** Yale-New Haven Hosp, Yale Med Group; **Address:** Yale Schl Med, 333 Cedar St, Box 208064, New Haven, CT 06520-3206; **Phone:** 203-688-2475; **Board Cert:** Pediatrics 1974; Pediatric Rheumatology 2007; **Med School:** Georgetown Univ 1969; **Resid:** Pediatrics, Chldns Hosp 1972; **Fellow:** Pediatrics, Chldns Hosp 1974; **Fac Appt:** Prof Ped, Yale Univ

Mid Atlantic

Finkel, Terri H MD [PRhu] - **Spec Exp:** Juvenile Arthritis; Lupus/SLE; Vasculitis; **Hospital:** Chldns Hosp of Philadelphia; **Address:** Chldns Hosp of Philadelphia, Div Rheum, 3405 Civic Ctr Blvd, Philadelphia, PA 19104; **Phone:** 215-590-2547; **Board Cert:** Pediatrics 1988; Pediatric Rheumatology 2009; **Med School:** Stanford Univ 1982; **Resid:** Pediatrics, Univ Colorado Med Ctr 1985; **Fellow:** Pediatric Rheumatology, Natl Jewish Med Ctr 1990; **Fac Appt:** Prof Ped, Univ Pennsylvania

Goldsmith, Donald P MD [PRhu] - **Spec Exp:** Arthritis; Juvenile Arthritis; Vasculitis; **Hospital:** St. Christopher's Hosp for Chldn; **Address:** St Christophers Hosp for Children, Rheumatology Section, 3601 A St, Philadelphia, PA 19134; **Phone:** 215-427-5051; **Board Cert:** Pediatrics 1974; Allergy & Immunology 1975; Pediatric Rheumatology 2007; **Med School:** Univ VT Coll Med 1967; **Resid:** Pediatrics, St Christophers Hosp for Chldn 1973; **Fellow:** Allergy Immunology & Rheumatology, St Christophers Hosp for Chldn 1975; **Fac Appt:** Prof Ped, Drexel Univ Coll Med

Haines, Kathleen A MD [PRhu] - **Spec Exp:** Juvenile Arthritis; Lupus/SLE; Immune Deficiency; Scleroderma; **Hospital:** Hackensack Univ Med Ctr, NYU Langone Med Ctr (page 66); **Address:** Hackensack Univ Med Ctr, Don Imus Pediatric Ctr, 30 Prospect Ave Fl 3, Hackensack, NJ 07601; **Phone:** 201-996-5306; **Board Cert:** Pediatrics 1980; Allergy & Immunology 1981; Pediatric Rheumatology 2007; **Med School:** Albert Einstein Coll Med 1975; **Resid:** Pediatrics, New York Hosp 1977; **Fellow:** Allergy & Immunology, New York Hosp 1980; Rheumatology, NYU Med Sch 1982; **Fac Appt:** Assoc Prof Ped, UMDNJ-NJ Med Sch, Newark

Ilowite, Norman T MD [PRhu] - **Spec Exp:** Juvenile Arthritis; Lyme Disease; Lupus/SLE; Dermatomyositis; **Hospital:** Montefiore Med Ctr - Div. Moses, Jacobi Med Ctr; **Address:** Chldns Hosp-Montefiore, Rheumatology, 3415 Bainbridge Ave, Bronx, NY 10467; **Phone:** 718-741-2456; **Board Cert:** Pediatrics 1985; Clinical & Laboratory Immunology 1990; Pediatric Rheumatology 2007; **Med School:** SUNY Downstate 1979; **Resid:** Pediatrics, Chldns Hosp Natl Med Ctr 1982; **Fellow:** Pediatric Rheumatology, Univ WA Med Ctr 1984; **Fac Appt:** Prof Ped, Albert Einstein Coll Med

Lehman, Thomas MD [PRhu] - **Spec Exp:** Arthritis; Scleroderma; Lupus/SLE; Rheumatoid Arthritis; **Hospital:** Hosp For Special Surgery (page 60), NY-Presby/Weill Cornell Med Ctr, NY (page 65); **Address:** 535 E 70th St, New York, NY 10021-4872; **Phone:** 212-606-1151; **Board Cert:** Pediatrics 1979; Pediatric Rheumatology 2007; **Med School:** Jefferson Med Coll 1974; **Resid:** Pediatrics, Chldns Hosp 1976; Pediatrics, UCSF Med Ctr 1977; **Fellow:** Pediatric Rheumatology, Chldns Hosp 1979; Rheumatology, Natl Inst Hlth 1983; **Fac Appt:** Prof Ped, Cornell Univ-Weill Med Coll

Sherry, David D MD [PRhu] - **Spec Exp:** Pain-Musculoskeletal; Reflex Sympathetic Dystrophy (RSD); Juvenile Arthritis; Lupus/SLE; **Hospital:** Chldns Hosp of Philadelphia; **Address:** Chldns Hosp of Phildelphia, Div Rheum, 3405 Civic Ctr Blvd, Philadelphia, PA 19104; **Phone:** 215-590-2547; **Board Cert:** Pediatrics 1981; Pediatric Rheumatology 2007; **Med School:** Texas Tech Univ 1977; **Resid:** Pediatrics, Duke Univ Med Ctr 1980; **Fellow:** Pediatric Rheumatology, Univ British Columbia 1982; **Fac Appt:** Prof Ped, Univ Pennsylvania

Sills, Edward M MD [PRhu] - **Spec Exp:** Juvenile Arthritis; Lupus/SLE; Dermatomyositis; Vasculitis; **Hospital:** Johns Hopkins Hosp (page 61); **Address:** Johns Hopkins Hosp, 200 N Wolfe St, Ste 2-127, Baltimore, MD 21205; **Phone:** 410-955-6145; **Board Cert:** Pediatrics 1968; **Med School:** NYU Sch Med 1963; **Resid:** Pediatrics, Bronx Muni Hosp 1967; **Fac Appt:** Assoc Prof Ped, Johns Hopkins Univ

Southeast

Passo, Murray H MD [PRhu] - **Hospital:** MUSC Med Ctr; **Address:** MUSC, Dept Pediatrics, Div Pediatric Rheumatology, 135 Rutledge Ave, MSC 561, Charleston, SC 29425-5610; **Phone:** 843-792-5696; **Board Cert:** Pediatrics 1979; Pediatric Rheumatology 2007; **Med School:** Indiana Univ 1974; **Resid:** Pediatrics, Riley Chldns Hosp 1977; **Fellow:** Rheumatology, Indiana Univ Hosps 1979

Schanberg, Laura E MD [PRhu] - **Spec Exp:** Lupus/SLE; Juvenile Arthritis; Dermatomyositis; Spondyloarthropathies; **Hospital:** Duke Univ Hosp; **Address:** Duke Univ Med Ctr, Ste T-0909, Box 3212, Durham, NC 27710; **Phone:** 919-684-6627; **Board Cert:** Pediatric Rheumatology 2007; **Med School:** Duke Univ 1984; **Resid:** Pediatrics, Duke Univ Med Ctr 1987; **Fellow:** Pediatric Rheumatology, Duke Univ Med Ctr 1991; **Fac Appt:** Asst Prof Ped, Duke Univ

Warren, Robert W MD/PhD [PRhu] - **Spec Exp:** Juvenile Arthritis; Lupus/SLE; **Hospital:** MUSC Med Ctr; **Address:** 261 Calhoun St, rm 316 MSC186, Charleston, SC 29425; **Phone:** 843-876-1985; **Board Cert:** Pediatrics 1983; Allergy & Immunology 1983; Pediatric Rheumatology 2007; **Med School:** Washington Univ, St Louis 1978; **Resid:** Pediatrics, Duke Univ Med Ctr 1980; **Fellow:** Rheumatology, Duke Univ Med Ctr 1983; **Fac Appt:** Assoc Prof Ped, Baylor Coll Med

Pediatric Rheumatology

Midwest

Klein-Gitelman, Marisa MD [PRhu] - **Spec Exp:** Lupus/SLE; Juvenile Arthritis; **Hospital:** Children's Mem Hosp -Chicago; **Address:** Chldns Meml Hosp, 2300 Children's Plaza, Box 50, Chicago, IL 60614; **Phone:** 773-880-4360; **Board Cert:** Pediatrics 2006; Pediatric Rheumatology 2009; **Med School:** Washington Univ, St Louis 1985; **Resid:** Pediatrics, Columbia-Presby Med Ctr 1989; **Fellow:** Pediatric Rheumatology, New England Med Ctr 1993; **Fac Appt:** Assoc Prof Ped, Northwestern Univ

Wagner-Weiner, Linda MD [PRhu] - **Spec Exp:** Lupus/SLE; Juvenile Arthritis; Vasculitis; Dermatomyositis; **Hospital:** Univ Chicago-Comer Chldn's Hosp, La Rabida Chlds Hosp; **Address:** 5841 S Maryland, rm C101, MC 5044, Chicago, IL 60637; **Phone:** 773-702-2406; **Board Cert:** Pediatrics 1984; Pediatric Rheumatology 2007; **Med School:** Rush Med Coll 1979; **Resid:** Pediatrics, Univ Chicago Hosps 1982; **Fellow:** Pediatric Rheumatology, Univ Chicago/La Rabida Chldns Hosp 1984; **Fac Appt:** Assoc Prof Ped, Univ Chicago-Pritzker Sch Med

Southwest

Myones, Barry Lee MD [PRhu] - **Spec Exp:** Vasculitis; Kawasaki Disease; Dermatomyositis; Scleroderma; **Hospital:** Texas Chldns Hosp; **Address:** Ped Rheumatology Ctr, 6701 Fannin St Fl 11, Houston, TX 77030; **Phone:** 832-824-3830; **Board Cert:** Pediatrics 1983; Pediatric Rheumatology 2007; **Med School:** Albany Med Coll 1977; **Resid:** Pediatrics, Duke Univ Med Ctr 1980; **Fellow:** Pediatric Rheumatology, Chldns Hosp-Stanford 1983; Rheumatology, Univ N Carolina 1988; **Fac Appt:** Assoc Clin Prof Ped, Baylor Coll Med

Wilking, Andrew MD [PRhu] - **Spec Exp:** Arthritis; Lupus/SLE; Dermatomyositis; **Hospital:** Texas Chldns Hosp, Driscoll Chldn's Hosp; **Address:** Ped Rheumatology Ctr, 6701 Fannin St Fl 11, Houston, TX 77030; **Phone:** 832-824-3830; **Board Cert:** Pediatrics 1985; **Med School:** Columbia P&S 1978; **Resid:** Pediatrics, Babies Hosp 1981; **Fellow:** Pediatric Rheumatology, Tex Chldns Hosp 1983; **Fac Appt:** Prof Ped, Baylor Coll Med

West Coast and Pacific

Emery, Helen M MD [PRhu] - **Spec Exp:** Rheumatic Diseases of Childhood; Kidney Disease-Autoimmune; **Hospital:** Seattle Chldns Hosp, Univ Wash Med Ctr; **Address:** Chldns Hosp & Regl Med Ctr, Ped Rheum, 4800 Sand Point Way NE, MS R-5420, PO Box 5371, Seattle, WA 98105; **Phone:** 206-987-2057; **Board Cert:** Pediatrics 1992; Pediatric Rheumatology 2007; **Med School:** Australia 1971; **Resid:** Pediatrics, Chldns Orth Hosp-Univ Wash 1975; **Fellow:** Pediatric Rheumatology, Chldns Orth Hosp-Univ Wash 1977; **Fac Appt:** Prof Ped, Univ Wash

PEDIATRIC SURGERY

New England

Chwals, Walter J MD [PS] - **Spec Exp:** Nutrition/Critical Care; Necrotizing Enterocolitis; Cancer Surgery; Endocrine Surgery; **Hospital:** Tufts Med Ctr; **Address:** Tufts Med Ctr, Floating Hosp, 800 Washington St, Ste 207, Box 344, Boston, MA 02111; **Phone:** 617-636-5025; **Board Cert:** Pediatric Surgery 2007; **Med School:** Poland 1980; **Resid:** Surgery, Univ Mass Med Ctr 1985; **Fellow:** Nutrition, New England Deaconess Hosp 1986; Pediatric Surgery, Chldns Hosp 1988; **Fac Appt:** Prof S, Case West Res Univ

Doody, Daniel P MD [PS] - **Spec Exp:** Neonatal Surgery; Inflammatory Bowel Disease; Hirschsprung's Disease; Minimally Invasive Surgery; **Hospital:** Mass Genl Hosp, Newton - Wellesley Hosp; **Address:** MGH, Dept Pediatric Surgery, 55 Fruit St, Warren Bldg Fl 11, Boston, MA 02114-2621; **Phone:** 617-726-2913; **Board Cert:** Surgery 2006; Pediatric Surgery 2007; **Med School:** Univ IL Coll Med 1977; **Resid:** Surgery, Univ Illinois Hosps 1984; Pediatric Surgery, Chldn's Hosp 1987; **Fellow:** Transplant Research, Mass Genl Hosp 1985; **Fac Appt:** Assoc Prof S, Harvard Med Sch

Jennings, Russell W MD [PS] - **Spec Exp:** Fetal Surgery; Pediatric Cardiac Surgery; Robotic Surgery; **Hospital:** Children's Hospital - Boston, Brigham and Women's Hosp (page 57); **Address:** Children's Hospital, Fegan 3, 300 Longwood Ave, Boston, MA 02115; **Phone:** 617-355-3038; **Board Cert:** Surgery 2005; Pediatric Surgery 2007; **Med School:** UCSF 1986; **Resid:** Surgery, UCSF Med Ctr 1991; **Fellow:** Fetal Surgery, Fetal Trmt Ctr/UCSF Med Ctr 1994; Pediatric Surgery, Chldns Hosp 1996; **Fac Appt:** Asst Prof S, Harvard Med Sch

Latchaw, Laurie MD [PS] - **Spec Exp:** Pediatric Thoracic Surgery; Cancer Surgery; Neonatal Surgery; Lung Disease in Newborns; **Hospital:** Dartmouth - Hitchcock Med Ctr; **Address:** DHMC, Clinic 6M, One Medical Center Drive, Lebanon, NH 03756; **Phone:** 603-653-9883; **Board Cert:** Surgery 2001; Pediatric Surgery 2003; **Med School:** Rush Med Coll 1976; **Resid:** Surgery, Univ Texas 1981; **Fellow:** Pediatric Surgery, Montreal Chldns Hosp 1983; **Fac Appt:** Assoc Prof S, Dartmouth Med Sch

Lillehei, Craig W MD [PS] - **Spec Exp:** Transplant-Kidney; Transplant-Liver; Transplant-Lung; **Hospital:** Children's Hospital - Boston; **Address:** Chldns Hosp, Dept Surgery-Fagen Bldg, 300 Longwood Ave Fl 3, Boston, MA 02115; **Phone:** 617-355-3039; **Board Cert:** Surgery 2006; Pediatric Surgery 2007; Surgical Critical Care 2001; **Med School:** Harvard Med Sch 1976; **Resid:** Surgery, Mass Genl Hosp 1984; **Fellow:** Pediatric Surgery, Mass Genl Hosp 1986

Shamberger, Robert C MD [PS] - **Spec Exp:** Wilms' Tumor; Neuroblastoma; Inflammatory Bowel Disease; **Hospital:** Children's Hospital - Boston; **Address:** Children's Hosp-Dept Surgery, 300 Longwood Ave, Fegan - 3, Boston, MA 02115; **Phone:** 617-355-8326; **Board Cert:** Surgery 2002; Pediatric Surgery 2003; Surgical Critical Care 1999; **Med School:** Harvard Med Sch 1975; **Resid:** Surgery, Massachusetts Genl Hosp 1978; Pediatric Surgery, Children's Hosp 1985; **Fellow:** Surgical Oncology, NCI-Surgical Branch 1980; **Fac Appt:** Prof S, Harvard Med Sch

Tracy Jr, Thomas F MD [PS] - **Spec Exp:** Hepatobiliary Surgery; Endoscopic Surgery; Fetal Surgery; Hirschsprung's Disease; **Hospital:** Rhode Island Hosp, Women & Infants Hosp of RI; **Address:** 2 Dudley St, Ste 190, Providence, RI 02905; **Phone:** 401-421-1939; **Board Cert:** Surgery 2006; Pediatric Surgery 2006; **Med School:** Israel 1981; **Resid:** Surgery, Med Coll Virginia 1986; **Fellow:** Pediatric Surgery, Columbia Presby Med Ctr 1988; **Fac Appt:** Prof S, Brown Univ

Mid Atlantic

Adzick, N Scott MD [PS] - **Spec Exp:** Fetal Surgery; Congenital Hyperinsulinism; Neonatal Surgery; Twin to Twin Transfusion Syndrome (TTTS); **Hospital:** Chldns Hosp of Philadelphia; **Address:** 34th St & Civic Center Blvd, Wood Bldg Fl 5 - Ste 5113, Philadelphia, PA 19104-4399; **Phone:** 215-590-2727; **Board Cert:** Surgery 2006; Pediatric Surgery 2007; **Med School:** Harvard Med Sch 1979; **Resid:** Surgery, Mass Genl Hosp 1986; Pediatric Surgery, Chldns Hosp 1988; **Fellow:** Research, UCSF Med Ctr 1985; **Fac Appt:** Prof S, Univ Pennsylvania

Pediatric Surgery

Alexander, Frederick MD [PS] - **Spec Exp:** Inflammatory Bowel Disease; Solid Tumors; Congenital Anomalies-Gastrointestinal; **Hospital:** Hackensack Univ Med Ctr; **Address:** Joseph M Sanzari Chldns Hosp-HUMC, 30 Prospect Ave, Ste PC311, Hackensack, NJ 07601; **Phone:** 201-996-2921; **Board Cert:** Pediatric Surgery 1999; **Med School:** Columbia P&S 1977; **Resid:** Surgery, Brigham-Womens Hosp 1984; **Fellow:** Pediatric Surgery, Chldns Hosp 1986; **Fac Appt:** Clin Prof S

Colombani, Paul M MD [PS] - **Spec Exp:** Pediatric Thoracic Surgery; Transplant-Kidney; Transplant-Liver; Cancer Surgery; **Hospital:** Johns Hopkins Hosp (page 61); **Address:** 600 N Wolfe St, Harvey 319, Baltimore, MD 21287; **Phone:** 410-955-5210; **Board Cert:** Surgery 2003; Pediatric Surgery 2003; **Med School:** Univ KY Coll Med 1976; **Resid:** Surgery, Geo Wash Univ Hosp 1981; **Fellow:** Pediatric Surgery, Johns Hopkins Hosp 1983; **Fac Appt:** Prof S, Johns Hopkins Univ

Dolgin, Stephen MD [PS] - **Spec Exp:** Neonatal Surgery; Ulcerative Colitis; Inflammatory Bowel Disease/Crohn's; Ovarian Masses in Children/Adolescents; **Hospital:** Steven & Alexandra Cohen Chldn's Med Ctr of NY, N Shore Univ Hosp; **Address:** Cohen Chldn's Med Ctr, Pediatric Surgery, 269-01 76th Ave, Ste 158, New Hyde Park, NY 11040; **Phone:** 718-470-3636; **Board Cert:** Surgery 2000; Pediatric Surgery 2003; Surgical Critical Care 2000; **Med School:** NYU Sch Med 1977; **Resid:** Surgery, Peter Bent Brigham Hosp 1982; **Fellow:** Pediatric Surgery, Chldns Meml Hosp 1984; **Fac Appt:** Prof S, Albert Einstein Coll Med

Eichelberger, Martin R MD [PS] - **Spec Exp:** Trauma; **Hospital:** Chldns Natl Med Ctr; **Address:** Childrens National Med Ctr, 111 Michigan Ave NW, Washington, DC 20010; **Phone:** 202-476-2778; **Board Cert:** Pediatric Surgery 2003; **Med School:** Hahnemann Univ 1971; **Resid:** Surgery, Case-Western Res Hosp 1978; **Fellow:** Pediatric Surgery, Chldns Hosp 1980; **Fac Appt:** Prof S, Geo Wash Univ

Flake, Alan W MD [PS] - **Spec Exp:** Fetal Surgery; Stem Cell Transplant-Fetal; Neonatal Surgery; **Hospital:** Chldns Hosp of Philadelphia; **Address:** Dept Pediatric Surgery, 34th St & Civic Center Blvd, Wood Bldg - Ste 5113, Philadelphia, PA 19104; **Phone:** 215-590-2727; **Board Cert:** Surgery 2010; Pediatric Surgery 1999; **Med School:** Univ Ark 1981; **Resid:** Surgery, UCSF Med Ctr 1988; **Fellow:** Pediatric Surgery, Chldns Hosp Med Ctr 1990; **Fac Appt:** Prof S, Univ Pennsylvania

Gaines, Barbara A MD [PS] - **Spec Exp:** Trauma; Critical Care; Minimally Invasive Surgery; **Hospital:** Chldns Hosp of Pittsburgh - UPMC; **Address:** Children's Hosp of Pittsburgh, One Children's Hosp Drive, 4401 Penn, Faculty Pavilion Fl 7, Pittsburgh, PA 15224; **Phone:** 412-692-8288; **Board Cert:** Surgery 2007; Surgical Critical Care 2007; Pediatric Surgery 2009; **Med School:** Univ VA Sch Med 1990; **Resid:** Surgery, Vanderbilt Univ Hosp 1995; **Fellow:** Pediatric Surgery, Children's Hosp 1998; **Fac Appt:** Asst Prof S, Univ Pittsburgh

Ginsburg, Howard B MD [PS] - **Spec Exp:** Neonatal Surgery; Tumor Surgery; Pediatric Urology; Gastrointestinal Surgery; **Hospital:** NYU Langone Med Ctr (page 66), Bellevue Hosp Ctr; **Address:** 530 First Ave, Ste 10W, New York, NY 10016-6402; **Phone:** 212-263-7391; **Board Cert:** Pediatric Surgery 2001; **Med School:** Univ Cincinnati 1972; **Resid:** Surgery, NYU-Bellvue Hosp 1977; Pediatric Surgery, Columbia-Presby Med Ctr 1979; **Fellow:** Pediatric Surgery, Mass Genl Hosp 1980; **Fac Appt:** Assoc Prof PS, NYU Sch Med

Gittes, George K MD [PS] - **Spec Exp:** Gastrointestinal Surgery; **Hospital:** Chldns Hosp of Pittsburgh - UPMC; **Address:** Childrens Hosp Pittsburgh, Dept Surgery, 4401 Penn Ave, Pittsburgh, PA 15224; **Phone:** 412-692-7291; **Board Cert:** Surgery 2003; Pediatric Surgery 2007; **Med School:** Harvard Med Sch 1987; **Resid:** Surgery, UCSF Med Ctr 1994; **Fellow:** Pediatric Surgery, Childrens Mercy Hosp 1995; **Fac Appt:** Prof S, Univ Pittsburgh

Glick, Philip L MD [PS] - **Spec Exp:** Robotic Surgery; Neonatal Surgery; Fetal Surgery; Chest Wall Deformities; **Hospital:** Women's & Chldn's Hosp of Buffalo, The, Roswell Park Cancer Inst; **Address:** Womens & Childrens Hosp, Dept Pediatric Surgery, 219 Bryant St, Buffalo, NY 14222-2006; **Phone:** 716-878-7449; **Board Cert:** Surgery 2006; Pediatric Surgery 2009; Surgical Critical Care 1999; **Med School:** UCSF 1979; **Resid:** Surgery, UCSF Med Ctr 1985; **Fellow:** Fetal Surgery, UCSF Med Ctr 1984; Pediatric Surgery, Chldns Hosp Med Ctr 1988; **Fac Appt:** Prof S, SUNY Buffalo

Kane, Timothy D MD [PS] - **Spec Exp:** Minimally Invasive Surgery; Neonatal Surgery; **Hospital:** Chldns Natl Med Ctr; **Address:** Children's National Medical Ctr, Dept Surgery, 111 Michigan Ave NW, Ste W4-200, Washington, DC 20010; **Phone:** 202-476-2151; **Board Cert:** Surgery 2001; Pediatric Surgery 2004; **Med School:** SUNY Upstate Med Univ 1992; **Resid:** Surgery, Univ Cincinnati Hosp 1999; **Fellow:** Pediatric Surgery, UAB Chldns Hosp 2001; **Fac Appt:** Assoc Prof S, Univ Wash

La Quaglia, Michael MD [PS] - **Spec Exp:** Cancer Surgery; Neuroblastoma; Liver Cancer; Colon & Rectal Cancer; **Hospital:** Meml Sloan-Kettering Cancer Ctr, NY-Presby/Weill Cornell Med Ctr, NY (page 65); **Address:** 1275 York Ave, Ste H1315, New York, NY 10065; **Phone:** 212-639-7002; **Board Cert:** Surgery 2003; Pediatric Surgery 2007; **Med School:** UMDNJ-NJ Med Sch, Newark 1976; **Resid:** Surgery, Mass Genl Hosp 1983; **Fellow:** Cardiothoracic Surgery, Broadgreen Ctr 1984; Pediatric Surgery, Chldns Hosp 1985; **Fac Appt:** Prof S, Cornell Univ-Weill Med Coll

Nance, Michael L MD [PS] - **Spec Exp:** Trauma; Neonatal Surgery; Brain Injury; Congenital Anomalies; **Hospital:** Chldns Hosp of Philadelphia; **Address:** Chldns Hosp of Philadelphia, Dept Surgery, 34th & Civic Ctr Blvd, Philadelphia, PA 19104; **Phone:** 215-590-5932; **Board Cert:** Surgery 2005; Surgical Critical Care 2008; Pediatric Surgery 2007; **Med School:** Louisiana State U, New Orleans 1988; **Resid:** Surgery, Hosp Univ Penn 1995; **Fellow:** Surgical Critical Care, Hosp Univ Penn 1996; Pediatric Surgery, Chldns Hosp 1997; **Fac Appt:** Prof S, Univ Pennsylvania

Quaegebeur, Jan M MD [PS] - **Spec Exp:** Arterial Switch; Heart Valve Surgery; Pediatric Cardiac Surgery; **Hospital:** Morgan Stanley Children's Hosp of NY-Presby, NY (page 65); **Address:** Morgan Stanley Chlds Hosp of NY-Presby, 3959 Broadway, Ste BN276, New York, NY 10032; **Phone:** 212-305-5975; **Med School:** Belgium 1969; **Resid:** Surgery, St Michel Clinic 1973; **Fellow:** Thoracic Surgery, Baylor Coll Med 1974; Thoracic Surgery, Univ Hosp 1978; **Fac Appt:** Prof S, Columbia P&S

Schwartz, Marshall Z MD [PS] - **Spec Exp:** Gastrointestinal Surgery; Neonatal Surgery; Transplant-Kidney; Inflammatory Bowel Disease; **Hospital:** St. Christopher's Hosp for Chldn, St. Luke's Hosp - Bethlehem; **Address:** St Christopher's Hosp for Chldn, Dept of Surgery, 3601 A St, Ste 2204, Philadelphia, PA 19134; **Phone:** 215-427-5292; **Board Cert:** Surgery 2009; Pediatric Surgery 1999; **Med School:** Univ Minn 1970; **Resid:** Surgery, Univ Minnesota Hosp 1972; Pediatric Surgery, Chldns Hosp Med Ctr - Harvard Med Sch 1974; **Fellow:** Surgery, Univ Minnesota Hosp 1975; **Fac Appt:** Prof S, Jefferson Med Coll

Spigland, Nitsana A MD [PS] - **Spec Exp:** Congenital Anomalies; Pediatric Thoracic Surgery; Cancer Surgery; Minimally Invasive Surgery; **Hospital:** NY-Presby/Weill Cornell Med Ctr, NY (page 65); **Address:** NY Hosp-Cornell Med Ctr, 525 E 68th St, Box 209, New York, NY 10021; **Phone:** 212-746-5648; **Board Cert:** Pediatric Surgery 2003; **Med School:** NY Med Coll 1982; **Resid:** Surgery, Lenox Hill Hosp 1987; **Fellow:** Pediatric Surgery, St Justine Chldn's Hosp 1989; **Fac Appt:** Assoc Prof S, Cornell Univ-Weill Med Coll

Pediatric Surgery

Stolar, Charles J H MD [PS] - **Spec Exp:** Neonatal Surgery; Hernia; Pediatric Cancers; **Hospital:** Morgan Stanley Children's Hosp of NY-Presby, NY (page 65); **Address:** Morgan Stanley Chldns Hosp NY-Presby, 3959 Broadway, Fl 2 - rm 215 North, New York, NY 10032; **Phone:** 212-342-8586; **Board Cert:** Surgery 2001; Pediatric Surgery 2007; **Med School:** Georgetown Univ 1974; **Resid:** Surgery, Univ Illinois Hosp 1980; **Fellow:** Pediatric Surgery, Chldns Hosp Natl Med Ctr 1982; **Fac Appt:** Prof S, Columbia P&S

Strauch, Eric D MD [PS] - **Spec Exp:** Pediatric Cancers; Neonatal Surgery; Conjoined Twins; **Hospital:** Univ of MD Med Ctr; **Address:** UMMC, Dept Pediatric Surgery, 22 S Greene St, N4E37, Baltimore, MD 21201; **Phone:** 410-328-5730; **Board Cert:** Surgery 2003; Pediatric Surgery 2005; **Med School:** Univ MD Sch Med 1988; **Resid:** Surgery, Univ Maryland Med Ctr; **Fellow:** Pediatric Surgery, ¡OHNS hOPKINS hOSP 1996; **Fac Appt:** Assoc Prof S, Univ MD Sch Med

Stylianos, Steven MD [PS] - **Spec Exp:** Trauma; Neonatal Surgery; Chest Wall Deformities; Congenital Anomalies; **Hospital:** Steven & Alexandra Cohen Chldn's Med Ctr of NY; **Address:** 269-01 76th Ave, New Hyde Park, NY 11040; **Phone:** 718-470-3636; **Board Cert:** Surgery 2002; Pediatric Surgery 2003; **Med School:** NYU Sch Med 1983; **Resid:** Surgery, Columbia-Presby Med Ctr 1988; Pediatric Surgery, Chldns Hosp 1992; **Fellow:** Pediatric Trauma, New England Med Ctr 1990; **Fac Appt:** Prof S, FIU Coll Med

Velcek, Francisca T MD [PS] - **Spec Exp:** Anorectal Malformations; Pediatric Gynecology; Neonatal Surgery; Hernia; **Hospital:** Lenox Hill Hosp, Univ Hosp of Bklyn at Long Island Coll Hosp; **Address:** 965 5th Ave, New York, NY 10075; **Phone:** 212-744-9396; **Board Cert:** Surgery 1974; Pediatric Surgery 2007; **Med School:** Philippines 1966; **Resid:** Surgery, St Clares Hosp 1971; Pediatric Surgery, SUNY Downstate Med Ctr 1975; **Fellow:** Pediatric Surgery, SUNY Downstate Med Ctr 1973; **Fac Appt:** Prof S, SUNY Hlth Sci Ctr

Voigt, Roger W MD [PS] - **Spec Exp:** Minimally Invasive Surgery; Neonatal Surgery; Pediatric Urology; **Hospital:** Univ of MD Med Ctr; **Address:** UMMC, Dept Pediatric Surgery, 22 S Greene St, N4E37, Baltimore, MD 21201; **Phone:** 410-328-5730; **Med School:** New Zealand 1980; **Resid:** Surgery, Univ Aukland 1984; **Fellow:** Pediatric Surgery, Royal Children's Hosp; Pediatric Urology, Univ Maryland Med Ctr; **Fac Appt:** Asst Prof S, Univ MD Sch Med

Southeast

Bond, Sheldon J MD [PS] - **Spec Exp:** Pediatric Cancers; Fetal Surgery; Trauma; **Hospital:** Kosair Chldn's Hosp; **Address:** University Pediatric Surgery Assocs, 234 E Gray St, Ste 766, Louisville, KY 40202; **Phone:** 502-583-7337; **Board Cert:** Surgery 2008; Pediatric Surgery 2009; Surgical Critical Care 2001; **Med School:** Med Coll Wisc 1983; **Resid:** Surgery, Univ Louisville Med Ctr 1989; **Fellow:** Fetal Surgery, UCSF Med Ctr; Pediatric Surgery, Chldns Natl Med Ctr 1991; **Fac Appt:** Prof S, Univ Louisville Sch Med

Chen, Mike K MD [PS] - **Spec Exp:** Gastrointestinal Surgery; Transplant Surgery-Pediatric; **Hospital:** Children's Hospital - Birmingham; **Address:** UAB Pediatric Surgery, 1600 7th Ave S, ACC 300, Birmingham, AL 35233; **Phone:** 205-939-9688; **Board Cert:** Surgery 2003; Pediatric Surgery 2007; **Med School:** Univ Tex, Houston 1987; **Resid:** Surgery, Univ Fla/Shands Med Ctr 1993; **Fellow:** Transplant Surgery, Univ Fla/Shands Med Ctr 1994; Pediatric Surgery, Univ Tennessee Med Ctr 1996

Davidoff, Andrew M MD [PS] - **Spec Exp:** Neuroblastoma; Cancer Surgery; **Hospital:** St. Jude Children's Research Hosp, Le Bonheur Chldns Med Ctr; **Address:** St Jude Chldns Rsch Hosp, Dept Surg, 262 Danny Thomas Pl, MS 133, Memphis, TN 38105; **Phone:** 901-595-4060; **Board Cert:** Surgery 2005; Pediatric Surgery 2007; **Med School:** Univ Pennsylvania 1987; **Resid:** Surgery, Duke Med Ctr 1994; **Fellow:** Pediatric Surgery, Chldns Hosp 1996; **Fac Appt:** Assoc Prof S, Univ Tenn Coll Med

Fallat, Mary E MD [PS] - **Spec Exp:** Trauma; Burn Care; **Hospital:** Kosair Chldn's Hosp, Univ of Louisville Hosp; **Address:** University Pediatric Surgery Assocs, 234 E Gray St, Ste 766, Louisville, KY 40202; **Phone:** 502-583-7337; **Board Cert:** Surgery 2005; **Med School:** SUNY Upstate Med Univ 1979; **Resid:** Surgery, Univ Louisville Med Ctr 1985; **Fellow:** Research, Mass Genl Hosp 1983; Pediatric Surgery, Chldns Natl Med Ctr 1987; **Fac Appt:** Prof S, Univ Louisville Sch Med

Morgan III, Walter M MD [PS] - **Spec Exp:** Germ Cell Tumors; Neuroblastoma; Bone Cancer; Congenital Anomalies; **Hospital:** Vanderbilt Monroe Carrell Jr. Chldn's Hosp (page 76), Vanderbilt Univ Med Ctr (page 76); **Address:** Vanderbilt Dept Pediatric Surgery, 2200 Children's Way, 7100 Doctors Office Tower, Nashville, TN 37232-9780; **Phone:** 615-936-1050; **Board Cert:** Pediatric Surgery 2001; **Med School:** Vanderbilt Univ 1982; **Resid:** Surgery, Johns Hopkins Hosp 1988; **Fellow:** Pediatric Surgery, Johns Hopkins Hosp 1990; **Fac Appt:** Asst Prof S, Vanderbilt Univ

Nakayama, Don K MD [PS] - **Spec Exp:** Neonatal Surgery; Minimally Invasive Surgery; **Hospital:** Med Ctr of Central GA; **Address:** 777 Hemlock St, MSC 140, Macon, GA 31201; **Phone:** 478-633-1367; **Board Cert:** Surgery 2003; Pediatric Surgery 2005; **Med School:** UCSF 1978; **Resid:** Surgery, UCSF Hosps 1984; **Fellow:** Pediatric Surgery, Childrens Hosp 1986; **Fac Appt:** Prof S, Mercer Univ Sch Med

Paidas, Charles N MD [PS] - **Spec Exp:** Pediatric Cancers; Chest Wall Deformities; Transplant Surgery-Pediatric; Hernia; **Hospital:** Tampa Genl Hosp; **Address:** USF Dept Surgery, 12901 Bruce B Downs Blvd, Box MDC33, Tampa, FL 33612; **Phone:** 813-259-0929; **Board Cert:** Surgery 1999; Pediatric Surgery 2001; Surgical Critical Care 2002; **Med School:** NY Med Coll 1981; **Resid:** Surgery, NY Med Coll Affil Hosps 1987; **Fellow:** Pediatric Surgery, Johns Hopkins Hosp 1991; **Fac Appt:** Prof S, Univ S Fla Coll Med

Rice, Henry MD [PS] - **Spec Exp:** Neonatal Surgery; Cancer Surgery; **Hospital:** Duke Univ Hosp; **Address:** Duke Univ Med Ctr, Dept Ped Surg, DUMC, Box 3815, Durham, NC 27710; **Phone:** 919-681-5077; **Board Cert:** Surgery 2006; Pediatric Surgery 2009; **Med School:** Yale Univ 1988; **Resid:** Surgery, Univ Wash Affil Hosps 1996; **Fellow:** Pediatric Surgery, Chldns Hosp of Buffalo 1998; **Fac Appt:** Assoc Prof S, Duke Univ

Ricketts, Richard R MD [PS] - **Spec Exp:** Neonatal Surgery; Cancer Surgery; Gastrointestinal Surgery; Hirschsprung's Disease; **Hospital:** Chldns Hlthcare Atlanta @ Egleston, Chldns Hlthcare Atlanta @ Scottish Rite; **Address:** Atlanta Pediatric Surgery, 1975 Century Blvd, Ste 6, Atlanta, GA 30345; **Phone:** 404-982-9938; **Board Cert:** Surgery 2004; Pediatric Surgery 2001; **Med School:** Northwestern Univ 1973; **Resid:** Surgery, LAC-USC Med Ctr 1978; **Fellow:** Pediatric Surgery, Chldns Meml Hosp 1980; **Fac Appt:** Prof S, Emory Univ

Rodgers, Bradley M MD [PS] - **Spec Exp:** Pediatric Thoracic Surgery; Neonatal Surgery; Minimally Invasive Surgery; **Hospital:** Univ of Virginia Health Sys; **Address:** U VA Chldns Hosp, Dept Surgery, PO Box 800709, Charlottesville, VA 22908; **Phone:** 434-924-2673; **Board Cert:** Surgery 1997; Pediatric Surgery 2005; Thoracic Surgery 1975; **Med School:** Johns Hopkins Univ 1966; **Resid:** Surgery, Duke Univ Med Ctr 1968; Cardiothoracic Surgery, Duke Univ Med Ctr 1973; **Fellow:** Pediatric Surgery, Chldns Hosp 1974; **Fac Appt:** Prof S, Univ VA Sch Med

Pediatric Surgery

Shochat, Stephen J MD [PS] - **Spec Exp:** Cancer Surgery; Chest Wall Deformities; Pediatric Cancers; **Hospital:** St. Jude Children's Research Hosp; **Address:** St Jude Childrens Research Hosp, Dept Surgery, 262 Danny Thomas Pl, Memphis, TN 38105; **Phone:** 901-595-4060; **Board Cert:** Surgery 1969; Thoracic Surgery 1975; Pediatric Surgery 2005; **Med School:** Med Coll VA 1963; **Resid:** Surgery, Barnes Hosp 1968; Pediatric Surgery, Boston Chldns Hosp 1970; **Fellow:** Thoracic Surgery, George Washington Univ Med Ctr 1974; **Fac Appt:** Prof S, Univ Tenn Coll Med

Midwest

Aiken, John J MD [PS] - **Spec Exp:** Tumor Surgery; Chest Wall Deformities; Hernia; Solid Tumors; **Hospital:** Chldns Hosp - Wisconsin; **Address:** 999 N 92nd St, Ste C-320, Milwaukee, WI 53226; **Phone:** 414-266-6550; **Board Cert:** Surgery 2004; Pediatric Surgery 2000; **Med School:** Univ Cincinnati 1984; **Resid:** Surgery, Mass Genl Hosp 1991; **Fellow:** Pediatric Surgery, Chldns Hosp 1993; **Fac Appt:** Assoc Prof S, Med Coll Wisc

Andrews, Walter S MD [PS] - **Spec Exp:** Transplant-Liver; Transplant-Kidney; **Hospital:** Chldns Mercy Hosps & Clinics; **Address:** Chldn's Mercy Hosp, 2401 Gillham Rd, Kansaas City, MO 64108; **Phone:** 816-234-3199; **Board Cert:** Surgery 2002; Pediatric Surgery 2003; **Med School:** Boston Univ 1975; **Resid:** Surgery, Univ CO Hlth Science Ctr 1981; Pediatric Surgery, Univ Pittsburgh Med Ctr 1983; **Fellow:** Transplant Surgery, Univ Pittsburgh Med Ctr 1984; **Fac Appt:** Prof S, Univ MO-Kansas City

Arensman, Robert MD [PS] - **Spec Exp:** Congenital Anomalies; **Hospital:** Alexian Brothers Med Ctr; **Address:** 1555 Barrington Rd DOB 1 Bldg - Ste 415, Hoffman Estates, IL 60169; **Phone:** 847-490-4222; **Board Cert:** Pediatric Surgery 2010; **Med School:** Univ IL Coll Med 1969; **Resid:** Surgery, Univ Illinois Med Ctr 1972; Surgery, Univ Illinois Med Ctr 1976; **Fellow:** Pediatric Surgery, Chldns Natl Med Ctr 1978; Surgical Research, Boston Chldn's Hosp

Barksdale Jr, Edward M MD [PS] - **Spec Exp:** Gastrointestinal Surgery; Nutrition in Bowel Disorders; Neuroblastoma; Minimally Invasive Surgery; **Hospital:** UH Rainbow Babies & Chldns Hosp (page 74); **Address:** Rainbow Babies & Children's Hosp, 11100 Euclid Ave, rm 122, Cleveland, OH 44106; **Phone:** 216-844-8623; **Board Cert:** Surgery 2002; Pediatric Surgery 2003; **Med School:** Harvard Med Sch 1984; **Resid:** Surgery, Mass Genl Hosp 1992; Pediatric Surgery, Chldns Hosp 1994; **Fellow:** Surgical Research, Mass Genl Hosp 1989; **Fac Appt:** Prof S, Ohio State Univ

Bove, Edward L MD [PS] - **Spec Exp:** Pediatric Cardiothoracic Surgery; Hypoplastic Left Heart Syndrome; Congenital Heart Surgery; **Hospital:** Univ of Michigan Hosp; **Address:** 1500 E Med Ctr Drive, 5144 CVC, Ann Arbor, MI 48109-5864; **Phone:** 734-936-4980; **Board Cert:** Thoracic Surgery 2009; **Med School:** Albany Med Coll 1972; **Resid:** Surgery, Univ Mich Med Ctr 1976; Thoracic Surgery, Univ Mich Med Ctr 1979; **Fellow:** Pediatric Cardiac Surgery, Hosp Sick Chldn 1980; **Fac Appt:** Prof S, Univ Mich Med Sch

Crombleholme, Timothy M MD [PS] - **Spec Exp:** Fetal Surgery; Twin to Twin Transfusion Syndrome (TTTS); **Hospital:** Cincinnati Chldns Hosp Med Ctr, Univ Hosp - Cincinnati; **Address:** Fetal Care Center of Cincinnati, 3333 Burnet Ave, MC 11020, Cincinnati, OH 45229; **Phone:** 513-636-9608; **Board Cert:** Surgery 2003; Pediatric Surgery 2007; **Med School:** Tufts Univ 1984; **Resid:** Surgery, UCSF Med Ctr 1991; **Fellow:** Pediatric Surgery, Tufts-New England Med Ctr 1993; **Fac Appt:** Prof S, Univ Cincinnati

Dillon, Patrick A MD [PS] - **Spec Exp:** Pediatric Cancers; Trauma; Gastrointestinal Disorders; Congenital Anomalies; **Hospital:** St. Louis Chldns Hosp, Barnes-Jewish Hosp; **Address:** St Louis Chldn's Hosp, One Children's Place, Suite 5 South 40, St Louis, MO 63110; **Phone:** 314-454-6022; **Board Cert:** Surgery 2004; Pediatric Surgery 2007; **Med School:** Georgetown Univ 1988; **Resid:** Surgery, Barnes Hosp 1995; **Fellow:** Pediatric Surgery, John Hopkins Hosp 1997; **Fac Appt:** Assoc Prof S, Washington Univ, St Louis

Ehrlich, Peter F MD [PS] - **Spec Exp:** Pediatric Cancers; Wilms' Tumor; Thyroid Cancer; **Hospital:** Mott Chldns Hosp, Hurley Med Ctr-Mich St Univ; **Address:** Mott Children's Hospital, 1500 E Medical Ctr Drive, rm MOTT F3970, Ann Arbor, MI 48109; **Phone:** 734-764-4151; **Board Cert:** Surgery 2007; Pediatric Surgery 2009; **Med School:** Canada 1989; **Resid:** Surgery, Univ Toronto Med Ctr 1996; **Fellow:** Pediatric Surgery, Children's Natl Med Ctr 1998; **Fac Appt:** Assoc Clin Prof S, Univ Mich Med Sch

Holterman, Mark J MD [PS] - **Spec Exp:** Minimally Invasive Surgery; Neonatal Surgery; Head & Neck Surgery; Congenital Anomalies; **Hospital:** OSF Saint Francis Med Ctr; **Address:** Children's Hospital of Illinois, 420 NE Glen Oak Ave, Peoria, IL 61637; **Phone:** 309-655-2343; **Board Cert:** Surgery 2001; Pediatric Surgery 2007; **Med School:** Univ VA Sch Med 1988; **Resid:** Surgery, Univ Virginia Hosp 1993; **Fellow:** Pediatric Surgery, Chldns Hosp & Med Ctr 1993

Liu, Donald C MD [PS] - **Spec Exp:** Minimally Invasive Surgery; Cancer Surgery; Gastrointestinal Surgery; Inflammatory Bowel Disease/Crohn's; **Hospital:** Univ Chicago-Comer Chldn's Hosp; **Address:** 5839 S Maryland Ave, MC 4062, Chicago, IL 60637; **Phone:** 773-702-6175; **Board Cert:** Surgery 2005; Pediatric Surgery 2007; **Med School:** Thomas Jefferson Univ 1990; **Resid:** Surgery, Hosp Univ Penn 1995; **Fellow:** Pediatric Surgery, Univ Michigan Affil Hosp 1997; **Fac Appt:** Prof S, Univ Chicago-Pritzker Sch Med

Moss, R Lawrence MD [PS] - **Spec Exp:** Congenital Anomalies; Cancer Surgery; Minimally Invasive Surgery; **Hospital:** Nationwide Chldn's Hosp; **Address:** Nationwide Children's Hosp, Dept Surgery, Surgeon-in-Chief, 700 Children's Drive, Columbus, OH 43205; **Phone:** 614-722-3900; **Board Cert:** Surgery 1999; Pediatric Surgery 2003; Surgical Critical Care 2000; **Med School:** UCSD 1986; **Resid:** Surgery, Virginia Mason Med Ctr 1991; Surgical Critical Care, Chldns Meml Hosp 1992; **Fellow:** Pediatric Surgery, Chldns Meml Hosp 1994; **Fac Appt:** Prof S, Yale Univ

Oldham, Keith T MD [PS] - **Spec Exp:** Neonatal Surgery; Pediatric Thoracic Surgery; Gastrointestinal Surgery; **Hospital:** Chldns Hosp - Wisconsin; **Address:** 9000 W Wisconsin Ave, Milwaukee, WI 53201; **Phone:** 414-607-5280; **Board Cert:** Surgery 2000; Pediatric Surgery 2009; **Med School:** Med Coll VA 1976; **Resid:** Surgery, Univ Wash Med Ctr 1981; **Fellow:** Pediatric Surgery, Univ Cincinnati Chldns Hosp 1983; **Fac Appt:** Prof S, Med Coll Wisc

Pena, Alberto MD [PS] - **Spec Exp:** Imperforate Anus; Anorectal Malformations; Colon & Rectal Surgery; **Hospital:** Cincinnati Chldns Hosp Med Ctr; **Address:** Cincinnati Chlds Hosp Med Ctr, 3333 Burnet Ave, MLC 2023, Cincinnati, OH 45229; **Phone:** 513-636-3240; **Med School:** Mexico 1962; **Resid:** Surgery, Military Hosp 1966; **Fellow:** Pediatric Surgery, Childrens Hosp 1971; Cardiovascular Surgery, Childrens Hosp 1969

Rescorla, Frederick J MD [PS] - **Spec Exp:** Neonatal Surgery; Cancer Surgery; Head & Neck Surgery; Gastrointestinal Surgery; **Hospital:** Riley Hosp for Children; **Address:** Riley Hospital for Children, 705 Riley Hospital Drive, rm 2500, Indianapolis, IN 46202; **Phone:** 317-274-4681; **Board Cert:** Surgery 2004; Surgical Critical Care 2009; Pediatric Surgery 2007; **Med School:** Univ Wisc 1981; **Resid:** Surgery, Indiana Univ Med Ctr 1986; Pediatric Surgery, Indiana Univ Med Ctr 1988; **Fac Appt:** Prof S, Indiana Univ

Pediatric Surgery

Reynolds, Marleta MD [PS] - **Spec Exp:** Critical Care; Trauma; Congenital Anomalies; Pediatric Cancers; **Hospital:** Children's Mem Hosp -Chicago; **Address:** Chldns Meml Hosp, Dept Ped Surg, 2300 Children's Plaza, Box 63, Chicago, IL 60614; **Phone:** 773-880-4292; **Board Cert:** Surgery 2001; Thoracic Surgery 2006; Pediatric Surgery 2003; **Med School:** Tulane Univ 1976; **Resid:** Surgery, Tulane Univ Affil Hosp 1981; Pediatric Surgery, Chldns Meml Hosp 1983; **Fellow:** Cardiothoracic Surgery, Northwestern Univ 1985; **Fac Appt:** Prof S, Northwestern Univ

Sato, Thomas T MD [PS] - **Spec Exp:** Neonatal Surgery; Congenital Anomalies; **Hospital:** Chldns Hosp - Wisconsin; **Address:** 9000 W Wisconsin Ave, Milwaukee, WI 53201; **Phone:** 414-607-5280; **Board Cert:** Surgery 2006; Pediatric Surgery 2007; **Med School:** USC Sch Med 1988; **Resid:** Surgery, Univ Wash Med Ctr 1995; **Fellow:** Surgery, Harborview Med Ctr 1993; Pediatric Surgery, Chldns Natl Med Ctr 1997; **Fac Appt:** Prof S, Med Coll Wisc

Warner, Brad MD [PS] - **Spec Exp:** Gastrointestinal Surgery; Neonatal Surgery; Pediatric Cancers; Short Bowel Syndrome; **Hospital:** St. Louis Chldns Hosp; **Address:** 1 Children's Pl, Ste 5S40, St Louis, MO 63110; **Phone:** 314-454-6022; **Board Cert:** Surgery 2009; Pediatric Surgery 2001; **Med School:** Univ MO-Kansas City 1982; **Resid:** Surgery, Univ Cincinnati Med Ctr 1989; **Fellow:** Pediatric Surgery, Chldns Hosp Med Ctr 1991; **Fac Appt:** Prof S, Univ Cincinnati

Weber, Thomas R MD [PS] - **Spec Exp:** Neonatal Surgery; Short Bowel Syndrome; Chest Wall Deformities; **Hospital:** Adv Christ Med Ctr, St. Alexius Med Ctr; **Address:** 4440 W 95th St, Chicago, IL 60612; **Phone:** 708-684-2016; **Board Cert:** Surgery 2001; Surgical Critical Care 2002; **Med School:** Ohio State Univ 1971; **Resid:** Surgery, Univ MI Hosp & Hlth Ctr 1977; **Fellow:** Pediatric Surgery, Chldns Natl Med Ctr 1979; **Fac Appt:** Prof S, Univ IL Coll Med

Great Plains and Mountains

Bensard, Denis D MD [PS] - **Spec Exp:** Neonatal Surgery; Trauma; Minimally Invasive Surgery; Critical Care; **Hospital:** Denver Health Med Ctr; **Address:** Denver Health Medical Ctr, 777 Bannock St, MC 0206, Denver, CO 80204; **Phone:** 303-436-3034; **Board Cert:** Surgery 2002; Pediatric Surgery 2005; Surgical Critical Care 2003; **Med School:** Univ Colorado 1986; **Resid:** Surgery, Univ Colorado Med Ctr 1992; **Fellow:** Pediatric Surgery, Ohio State Univ 1995; **Fac Appt:** Prof S, Univ Colorado

Karrer, Frederick M MD [PS] - **Spec Exp:** Liver Surgery; Transplant-Liver; Critical Care; Neonatal Surgery; **Hospital:** Chldn's Hosp - Aurora (CO), Denver Health Med Ctr; **Address:** Chldn's Hosp, Dept Surgery, 13123 E 16th Ave, Box B323, Aurora, CO 80045; **Phone:** 720-777-6571; **Board Cert:** Surgery 2007; Pediatric Surgery 2009; Surgical Critical Care 1998; **Med School:** Univ Nebr Coll Med 1979; **Resid:** Surgery, Univ Ariz Med Ctr 1984; Pediatric Surgery, Chldns Meml Hosp 1986; **Fellow:** Transplant Surgery, Univ Pittsburgh Affil Hosp 1988; **Fac Appt:** Prof S, Univ Colorado

Meyers, Rebecca L MD [PS] - **Spec Exp:** Transplant-Liver; Tumor Surgery; Biliary Surgery; Pancreatic Surgery; **Hospital:** Primary Children's Med Ctr, Univ Utah Hlth Care; **Address:** Primary Chlds Med Ctr, Dept Ped Surg, 100 N Mario Capecchi Drive, Ste 2600, Salt Lake City, UT 84113-1103; **Phone:** 801-662-2950; **Board Cert:** Surgery 2003; Pediatric Surgery 2005; **Med School:** Oregon Hlth & Sci Univ 1985; **Resid:** Surgery, UCSF Med Ctr 1990; **Fellow:** Research, Cardio Rsch Inst-UCSF 1992; Pediatric Surgery, St Christophers Hosp for Chldn 1994; **Fac Appt:** Assoc Prof S, Univ Utah

Southwest

Black, C Thomas MD [PS] - **Spec Exp:** Neonatal Surgery; Minimally Invasive Surgery; Chest Wall Deformities; **Hospital:** Cook Chldns Med Ctr; **Address:** Ped Surg Assocs Ft Worth, 901 7th Ave, Ste 210, Fort Worth, TX 76104; **Phone:** 817-336-7881; **Board Cert:** Pediatric Surgery 2007; Surgery 2005; **Med School:** Baylor Coll Med 1979; **Resid:** Surgery, Baylor College Affil Hosp 1984; **Fellow:** Pediatric Surgery, Riley Childrens Hospital 1985; Pediatric Surgery-ECMO, Chldn's Meml Hosp 1987

Foglia, Robert P MD [PS] - **Spec Exp:** Congenital Anomalies; Burn Care; Gastroesophageal Reflux Disease (GERD); **Hospital:** Chldns Med Ctr of Dallas; **Address:** 1935 Medical District Drive, Ste B3250, Dallas, TX 75235; **Phone:** 214-456-6040; **Board Cert:** Surgery 2002; Pediatric Surgery 2005; Surgical Critical Care 1993; **Med School:** Georgetown Univ 1974; **Resid:** Surgery, UCLA Med Ctr 1981; **Fellow:** Pediatric Surgery, Chldns Hosp Natl Med Ctr 1983; **Fac Appt:** Prof S, Univ Tex SW, Dallas

Jackson, Richard J MD [PS] - **Spec Exp:** Pediatric Cancers; Neonatal Surgery; Robotic Surgery; **Hospital:** Arkansas Chldns Hosp; **Address:** Arkansas Children's Hospital, 1 Children's Way, Slot 837, Little Rock, AR 72202-3591; **Phone:** 501-364-1446; **Board Cert:** Surgery 2008; Pediatric Surgery 2001; Surgical Critical Care 1998; **Med School:** W VA Univ 1983; **Resid:** Surgery, W Va Univ Hosps 1988; Pediatric Surgery, Chldns Hosp 1989; **Fellow:** Surgical Critical Care, Chldns Hosp-Univ Pittsburgh 1990; Pediatric Surgery, Chldns Hosp-Univ Pittsburgh 1992

Notrica, David MD [PS] - **Spec Exp:** Biliary Surgery; Inflammatory Bowel Disease; Laparoscopic Surgery-Complex; Hirschsprung's Disease; **Hospital:** Phoenix Children's Hosp; **Address:** 1920 E Cambridge Ave, Ste 201, Phoenix, AZ 85006; **Phone:** 602-254-5561; **Board Cert:** Surgery 2005; Pediatric Surgery 2000; **Med School:** Emory Univ 1992; **Resid:** Surgery, Emory Univ 1997; **Fellow:** Pediatric Surgery, Texas Chldns Hosp 1997; **Fac Appt:** Asst Clin Prof S, Univ Ariz Coll Med

Nuchtern, Jed MD [PS] - **Spec Exp:** Pediatric Thoracic Surgery; Cancer Surgery; Laparoscopic Surgery; **Hospital:** Texas Chldns Hosp, Ben Taub Genl Hosp; **Address:** Texas Children's Hosp, 6621 Fannin St, MC CC650, Houston, TX 77030; **Phone:** 832-822-3135; **Board Cert:** Surgery 2003; Surgical Critical Care 2002; Pediatric Surgery 2007; **Med School:** Harvard Med Sch 1985; **Resid:** Surgery, Univ Washington 1992; Pediatric Surgery, Baylor Coll Med 1995; **Fellow:** Cellular Molecular Biology, Natl Inst Hlth 1990; **Fac Appt:** Prof S, Baylor Coll Med

Skinner, Michael A MD [PS] - **Spec Exp:** Endocrine Cancers; Thyroid Cancer; **Hospital:** UT Southwestern Med Ctr at Dallas; **Address:** UT Southwestern Med Ctr at Dallas, 1935 Med District Drive, Ste B3250, Dallas, TX 75235; **Phone:** 214-456-6040; **Board Cert:** Surgery 2000; Pediatric Surgery 2003; **Med School:** Rush Med Coll 1984; **Resid:** Surgery, Duke Univ Med Ctr 1991; **Fellow:** Pediatric Surgery, Indiana Univ 1993; **Fac Appt:** Assoc Prof S, Univ Tex SW, Dallas

Tuggle, David W MD [PS] - **Spec Exp:** Trauma; Critical Care; Reconstructive Surgery; **Hospital:** Chldns Hosp OU Med Ctr; **Address:** OU Div Pediatric Surgery, 1200 N Phillips Ave, Ste 2700, Oklahoma City, OK 73104; **Phone:** 405-271-4357; **Board Cert:** Surgery 2004; Pediatric Surgery 2005; Surgical Critical Care 2007; **Med School:** Univ Tex SW, Dallas 1979; **Resid:** Surgery, Parkland Meml Hosp 1985; Pediatric Surgery, Chldns Meml Hosp 1987; **Fac Appt:** Prof S, Univ Okla Coll Med

Pediatric Surgery

West Coast and Pacific

Albanese, Craig T MD [PS] - **Spec Exp:** Fetal Surgery; Laparoscopic Surgery; Twin to Twin Transfusion Syndrome (TTTS); **Hospital:** Lucile Packard Chldn's Hosp; **Address:** 780 Welch Rd, Ste 206, MC 5733, Palo Alto, CA 94304; **Phone:** 650-723-6439; **Board Cert:** Surgery 2000; Pediatric Surgery 2003; **Med School:** SUNY Hlth Sci Ctr 1986; **Resid:** Surgery, Mt Sinai Med Ctr 1991; **Fellow:** Pediatric Surgery, Chldns Hosp 1994; **Fac Appt:** Prof S, Stanford Univ

Farmer, Diana MD [PS] - **Spec Exp:** Pediatric Cancers; Fetal Surgery; Spina Bifida; Twin to Twin Transfusion Syndrome (TTTS); **Hospital:** UCSF Med Ctr; **Address:** 513 Parnassus Ave, Ste HNW1601, Box 0570, San Francisco, CA 94143-0570; **Phone:** 415-476-2538; **Board Cert:** Surgery 2001; Pediatric Surgery 2005; **Med School:** Univ Wash 1983; **Resid:** Surgery, UCSF Med Ctr 1993; **Fellow:** Pediatric Surgery, Childrens Hosp 1995; **Fac Appt:** Assoc Prof S, UCSF

Ford, Henri R MD [PS] - **Spec Exp:** Minimally Invasive Surgery; Trauma; **Hospital:** Chldns Hosp - Los Angeles, Long Beach Meml Med Ctr; **Address:** 4650 Sunset Blvd, MS 72, Los Angeles, CA 90027; **Phone:** 323-361-2104; **Board Cert:** Surgery 2002; Pediatric Surgery 2005; **Med School:** Harvard Med Sch 1984; **Resid:** Surgery, NY Hosp 1991; **Fellow:** Pediatric Surgery, Chldns Hosp Pittsburgh 1995

Healey, Patrick J MD [PS] - **Spec Exp:** Transplant Surgery-Pediatric; Transplant-Kidney; Transplant-Liver; Congenital Anomalies; **Hospital:** Seattle Chldns Hosp; **Address:** 4800 Sand Point Way, Dept Surgery, Box 359300, MS W7800, Seattle, WA 98105; **Phone:** 206-987-1800; **Board Cert:** Surgery 2002; Pediatric Surgery 2009; **Med School:** Boston Univ 1987; **Resid:** Surgery, Hartford Hosp 1992; **Fellow:** Transplant Surgery, Univ WA Med Ctr 1995; Pediatric Surgery, Chldns Hosp 1997; **Fac Appt:** Asst Prof S, Univ Wash

Hilfiker, Mary L MD/PhD [PS] - **Hospital:** Rady Children's Hosp - San Diego; **Address:** 8010 Frost St, Ste 414, San Diego, CA 92123; **Phone:** 858-966-7711; **Board Cert:** Surgery 2004; Pediatric Surgery 2007; **Med School:** Wright State Univ 1988; **Resid:** Surgery, Univ New Mexico Med Ctr 1993; **Fellow:** Pediatric Surgery, SUNY-Children's Hosp 1995; **Fac Appt:** Assoc Clin Prof S, UCSD

Krummel, Thomas M MD [PS] - **Spec Exp:** Minimally Invasive Surgery; Robotic Surgery; Fetal Surgery; **Hospital:** Lucile Packard Chldn's Hosp, Stanford Univ Hosp & Clinics; **Address:** 300 Pasteur Drive, MC 5115, Stanford, CA 94305-2200; **Phone:** 650-723-6439; **Board Cert:** Surgery 2004; Pediatric Surgery 2007; **Med School:** Univ Wisc 1977; **Resid:** Surgery, Med Coll Va Hosp 1983; Pediatric Surgery, Chldns Hosp 1985; **Fellow:** Fetal Surgery, UCSF Med Ctr 1985; **Fac Appt:** Prof S, Stanford Univ

Lobe, Thom E MD [PS] - **Spec Exp:** Minimally Invasive Surgery; Robotic Surgery; Pediatric Urology; **Address:** 50 N La Cienega, Ste 215, Beverly Hills, CA 90211; **Phone:** 310-289-2800; **Board Cert:** Surgery 2000; Pediatric Surgery 2001; **Med School:** Univ MD Sch Med 1975; **Resid:** Surgery, Ohio State Univ Med Ctr 1979; Pediatric Surgery, Childrens Hosp 1981

Proctor, Monja L MD [PS] - **Spec Exp:** Fetal Surgery; Neonatal Surgery; Hirschsprung's Disease; **Hospital:** Swedish Med Ctr-First Hill-Seattle; **Address:** Swedish Med Ctr-Ped Spec Care, 1101 Madison St, Ste 800, Seattle, WA 98104; **Phone:** 206-215-2700; **Board Cert:** Pediatrics 2003; Pediatric Surgery 2004; **Med School:** Univ Tex SW, Dallas 1993; **Resid:** Pediatrics, Univ TX SW Meml Med Ctr 2000; **Fellow:** Pediatric Surgery, Hosp For Sick Chldn 2002

Sawin, Robert S MD [PS] - **Spec Exp:** Pediatric Cancers; Pediatric Thoracic Surgery; Neonatal Surgery-Gastrointestinal; Transplant-Liver; **Hospital:** Seattle Chldns Hosp; **Address:** Seattle Chldn's Hosp, 4800 Sand Point Way NE, MS W7729, Seattle, WA 98145-5005; **Phone:** 206-987-2039; **Board Cert:** Surgical Critical Care 2001; Pediatric Surgery 2009; **Med School:** Univ Pittsburgh 1982; **Resid:** Surgery, Brigham Women's Hosp 1987; **Fellow:** Pediatric Surgery, Chldns Hosp 1989; **Fac Appt:** Prof S, Univ Wash

Stein, James E MD [PS] - **Hospital:** Chldns Hosp - Los Angeles; **Address:** Chdns Hosp-LA, Dept Pedisatric Surgery, 4650 Sunset Blvd, MS 106, Los Angeles, CA 90027; **Phone:** 323-361-2322; **Board Cert:** Surgery 2004; Pediatric Surgery 2005; **Med School:** Tufts Univ 1986; **Resid:** Surgery, Tufts New England Med Ctr 1993; **Fellow:** Pediatric Surgery, Royal Chldns Hosp 1994; Pediatric Surgery, Babies Hosp/Columbia Presby 1996; **Fac Appt:** Assoc Prof S, USC Sch Med

Waldhausen, John HT MD [PS] - **Spec Exp:** Minimally Invasive Surgery; Laparoscopic Surgery; Neonatal Surgery; Congenital Anomalies; **Hospital:** Seattle Chldns Hosp; **Address:** 4800 Sand Point Way, Dept Surgery, MS W-7729, Seattle, WA 98105; **Phone:** 206-526-2039; **Board Cert:** Surgery 2002; Pediatric Surgery 2005; **Med School:** Penn State Coll Med 1986; **Resid:** Surgery, Univ Virginia Med Ctr 1992; **Fellow:** Pediatric Surgery, Chldns Hosp Med Ctr - Washington Univ 1994; **Fac Appt:** Prof S, Univ Wash

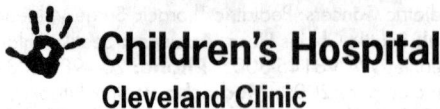

Children's Hospital
Cleveland Clinic

Cleveland Clinic
Children's Hospital
9500 Euclid Avenue
Cleveland, OH 44195

clevelandclinic.org/
childrenstopdocs

Pediatrics

Cleveland Clinic Children's Hospital is ranked among the best pediatric hospitals in the nation by *U.S.News & World Report*, and more than 80 pediatricians and pediatric specialists are recognized as "Best Doctors in America." Our specialists are nationally recognized for sophisticated diagnosis and innovative care for complex or chronic medical conditions, and nationally funded research initiatives that are leading to advanced treatments for young patients.

Our Center for Pediatric and Congenital Heart Diseases, the largest and most experienced in Northern Ohio, is known for groundbreaking catheter and surgical treatments. Our Department of Pediatric Gastroenterology offers breakthrough technology to diagnose and treat gastrointestinal problems. Our pediatric epilepsy specialists offer specialized diagnosis and surgery for different seizure disorders.

Children's Hospital oncologists are national leaders in the treatment of childhood cancers. Our Fetal Care Center is staffed by pediatric specialists and maternal-fetal medicine specialists who diagnose fetal problems and can treat them immediately after birth or in the womb. Our new Special Delivery Unit and adjoining Pediatric Cardiac Catheterization Laboratory are key components of the Fetal Care Center.

Cleveland Clinic Children's Hospital has the only comprehensive pediatric transplant center in Northern Ohio, offering heart, lung, liver, kidney, pancreas, bone marrow and intestinal transplantation and follow-up.

Our Pediatric ICU offers outstanding outcomes, saving many more young lives than the national standard, largely due to the 24-hour presence of seasoned critical care specialists.

Our expertise in specialty pediatrics extends into the realm of long-term care for developmental, behavioral and rehabilitation needs.

Offering Same-Day Appointments
Call 800.274.2009.

Treatment Guides

Cleveland Clinic has developed comprehensive treatment guides for many diseases and conditions. To download our free treatment guides, visit clevelandclinic.org/treatmentguides.

Online Medical Second Opinion

Cleveland Clinic's My**Consult** Online Medical Second Opinion program securely connects patients to our physician specialists for more than 1,000 life-changing or life-threatening diagnoses all by the click of a mouse. To learn more, log onto eclevelandclinic.org/myconsult or call 800.223.2273, ext. 43223.

Special Assistance for Out-of-State Patients

Cleveland Clinic Global Patient Services offers a complimentary Medical Concierge service for patients who travel from outside of Ohio. Call 800.223.2273, ext. 55580 or email medicalconcierge@ccf.org.

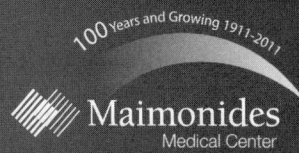

100 Years and Growing 1911-2011

Maimonides
Medical Center

The Maimonides Infants & Children's Hospital is a NACHRI-certified children's hospital-within-a-hospital. Offering over 30 sub-specialty divisions as well as primary care, the Pediatrics program is unrivaled in the region and serves one of the largest pediatric populations in the nation.

Danielle Laraque, MD, Vice President of the Infants & Children's Hospital, leads a family-centered pediatrics program in a state-of-the-art medical environment, where babies, children and adolescents receive the best and most appropriate care. For most children, this involves preventing illness and promoting healthy growth. For those whose problems are more complicated, Maimonides specialists can treat every manner of childhood disorder, no matter how rare or complex. The level and quality of critical care provided is evidenced by the demand for the Maimonides Pediatric Transport Program, through which critically ill children from other hospitals are transferred to Maimonides.

In recognition of its excellence in obstetrics and pediatrics, Maimonides was designated a Regional Perinatal Center by the New York State Department of Health.

Pediatric specialties include:

Allergy
Behavioral & Developmental
Pediatrics
Cardiology
Critical Care Medicine
Dentistry & Dental Surgery
Emergency Medicine
Endocrinology
Gastroenterology
Genetics
Hematology/Oncology
Immunology

Infectious Disease
Neonatology
Nephrology
Neurology
Ophthalmology
Orthopedic Surgery
Otolaryngology
Psychiatry/Psychology
Pulmonology
Rheumatology
Surgery
Urology

Relying heavily on evidence-based medicine, Maimonides Medical Center has been commended for outstanding services by a number of independent rating organizations. Earlier this year, Maimonides was named a Distinguished Hospital for Clinical Excellence by Healthgrades – one of only three hospitals in the metropolitan area; the American Stroke Association bestowed its Gold Plus Achievement Award on the hospital; and the American Hospital Association once again named it a Most Wired Hospital.

Maimonides Medical Center
Passionate about medicine.
Compassionate about people.

www.maimonidesmed.org/pediatrics

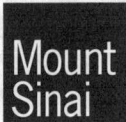 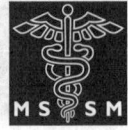

MOUNT SINAI
SCHOOL OF
MEDICINE

THE MOUNT SINAI MEDICAL CENTER
PEDIATRIC DIABETES AND ENDOCRINOLOGY
One Gustave L. Levy Place
Fifth Avenue and 100th Street
New York, NY 10029-6574
Physician Referral: 1-800-MD-SINAI (637-4624)
www.kravischildrenshospital.org

PEDIATRIC DIABETES AND ENDOCRINOLOGY
INNOVATIVE MEDICINE, FAMILY-CENTERED CARE

The Hall Family Center for Pediatric Endocrinology and Diabetes at the Kravis Children's Hospital at Mount Sinai is dedicated to excellence in clinical care, education and research – a fact that has led to our being **named among the top 50 pediatric diabetes and endocrinology services in America,** according to *The U.S. News & World Report's* 2011-2012 ranking of "Best Children's Hospitals."

Under the direction of Robert Rapaport, M.D., Division Chief, we use a team approach, which is patient and family centered, to manage:

- Diabetes (type 1 and type 2, medication-related, monogenic and pre-diabetes)

- Short stature

- Growth disorders, including growth hormone deficiency, growth in children born small for gestational age, and early and late puberty

- Genetic disorders, including Turner Syndrome and Noonan Syndrome

- Congenital and acquired hypothyroidism and hyperthyroidism

- Hyperparathyroidism

- Congenital adrenal hyperplasia/hypoplasia

- Obesity and other nutritional disorders, including Vitamin D deficiency.

Diabetes – We offer the complete spectrum of high level diagnostic and treatment services, including simulation testing, for children and adolescents and bring families into their circle of care. Since education and support are vital to managing diabetes, we offer a variety of programs for patients and their families, including "Toddlers and Grandparents," "College Prep," for teens entering college, and a free one-week day camp in Central Park in conjunction with the Barton Center for Diabetes Education.

We are currently collaborating with four other medical centers on the **R.O.A.D. (Reduce Obesity and Diabetes) Project**, to study and educate middle school children in Harlem. By identifying the metabolic factors that lead from obesity to diabetes, we will develop a protocol for detecting which children will most likely develop diabetes, allowing us to streamline interventions and identify where best to allocate resources.

Endocrine Disorders and Growth - With our faculty leading investigations into both international and multi-center trials, we enjoy a stellar reputation for identifying and treating a host of common and complex endocrine disorders, including growth hormone deficiency, growth in children born small for gestational age, and other disorders caused by Turner or Noonan Syndrome, and congenital hypothyroidism. In addition to offering expert consultations, we employ early screening methods and breakthrough growth hormone therapy that enables children to grow and develop normally.

We also excel at diagnosing and treating children with **precocious or delayed puberty** and have developed methods to identify and manage these conditions before they appear clinically obvious.

ANNUAL SYMPOSIUM

Our physician-scientists conduct investigations into the causes and treatments of childhood endocrine conditions, and we are committed to translating research into better methods of clinical care. To that end, we hold an annual symposium to update pediatricians practicing within the community on the latest advances in pediatric endocrinology and diabetes.

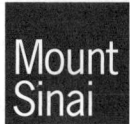
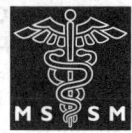

THE MOUNT SINAI MEDICAL CENTER
PEDIATRIC GASTROENTEROLOGY
One Gustave L. Levy Place
Fifth Avenue and 100th Street
New York, NY 10029-6574
Physician Referral: 1-800-MD-SINAI (637-4624)
www.kravischildrenshospital.org

PEDIATRIC GASTROENTEROLOGY
Innovative Medicine, Family-Centered Care

In recognition of our tradition of excellence in patient care, research and education, **Mount Sinai's Kravis Children's Hospital was named among the country's best in Pediatric Gastroenterology**, according to *U.S. News and World Report's* 2011-2012 edition of "America's Best Children's Hospitals."

Under the direction of Keith Benkov, M.D., Chief of Pediatric Gastroenterology, we deliver expert consultation and compassionate, evidence-based care to pediatric patients with common and complex digestive disorders, including inflammatory bowel disease, celiac disease, gastroesophageal reflux disease and irritable bowel syndrome.

With a reputation for providing the highest level of innovative and comprehensive care to patients with Crohn's disease and ulcerative colitis, our nationally recognized **Children's IBD Center** receives referrals from across the country. We are currently following over 500 children and have seen over 1700 patients with IBD in the last 10 years. The combination of this extensive experience, our focus on basic science and clinical research, and our collaboration with Mount Sinai's internationally renowned adult IBD program, enables us to deliver a unique approach to IBD care in children.

To optimize outcomes, our entire team of healthcare professionals participates in every patient's circle of care. We address each patient's specific needs, including management, nutrition, growth, body image and coping methods for a chronic illness. The center fosters family participation and encourages patients to gather to share ideas. Lectures, discussions and support groups are open to all families.

In addition, we continually strive to advance our knowledge of IBD and its treatments through research. In conjunction with Department of Pediatric Allergy and Immunology, we are currently investigating the benefits of an herbal medicine developed as a complementary therapy for children with Crohn's disease.

IBD runs the spectrum from mild to severe disease. No matter how seriously a child is affected, our ultimate goal is to help children with IBD lead normal, productive lives and achieve all their personal aspirations.

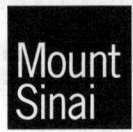
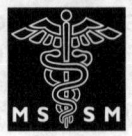

THE MOUNT SINAI MEDICAL CENTER
PEDIATRIC NEPHROLOGY AND HYPERTENSION
One Gustave L. Levy Place
Fifth Avenue and 100th Street
New York, NY 10029-6574
Physician Referral: 1-800-MD-SINAI (637-4624)
www.kravischildrenshospital.org

MOUNT SINAI
SCHOOL OF
MEDICINE

Pediatric Nephrology and Hypertension
Innovative Medicine, Family-Centered Care

Mount Sinai's Kravis Children's Hospital's Division of Pediatric Nephrology and Hypertension is recognized as one of America's best by *U.S .News & World Report's* **2011-2012 ranking of "Best Children's Hospitals."**

As one of our country's largest and most respected centers for pediatric kidney care and a pioneer in research and education, we deliver specialized, evidence-based care to children with kidney disease, high blood pressure, urinary tract infections and a wide variety of related conditions, both common and complex.

At our **Children's Center for Complete Kidney Care**, patients receive A to Z services, benefitting from a multidisciplinary team of pediatric nephrologists, urologists, transplantation specialists, psychiatrists, registered nurses, social workers, nutritionists and child life specialists working together to deliver the most effective treatment. Understanding that children require a special level of support and service, we bring families into their circle of care, and, as our patients become young adults, we help transition them into our excellent adult kidney program, which has also been recognized as one of our nation's best by *U.S. News & World Report .*

Our teaching and research programs in pediatric kidney disease serve to drive and maintain our expertise at the highest level. Working closely with our colleagues in diagnostic radiology, pediatric urology, and transplant surgery, we offer advanced diagnostic services and confident and experienced care for all kidney-related conditions, including every type of treatment for kidney failure:

- Dialysis (hemodialysis or peritoneal dialysis)

- Hemofiltration

- Kidney transplant, multiple organ transplant

We are a major referral center for children with high blood pressure, offering state-of-the art diagnostics such as ambulatory blood pressure monitoring (ABPM), a home-based measure that allows us to be sure hypertension is present, and we provide comprehensive treatment plans that include a focus on diet, physical activity, and stress factors.

As a **Center of Excellence in Transplantation**, we are one of the most sought after pediatric kidney transplant centers in the country. During the past five years, we provided kidney transplants to twice as many children as any other hospital in the tri-state region, and, even more significant, the outcomes of those transplants were superior, as verified by the U.S. Department of Health and Human Services (data publically available at srtr.org and optn.transplant.hrsa.gov).

We offer fast appointments and a streamlined consultation process for patients and their physicians.

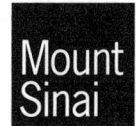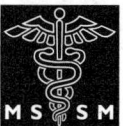

**MOUNT SINAI
SCHOOL OF
MEDICINE**

**THE MOUNT SINAI MEDICAL CENTER
PEDIATRIC PULMONOLOGY**
One Gustave L. Levy Place
Fifth Avenue and 100th Street
New York, NY 10029-6574
Physician Referral: 1-800-MD-SINAI (637-4624)
www.kravischildrenshospital.org

PEDIATRIC PULMONOLOGY
Innovative Medicine, Family-Centered Care

At Mount Sinai's **Kravis Children's Hospital's Division of Pediatric Pulmonology,** we are dedicated to treating the full spectrum of children's respiratory illnesses, both common and complex, with a high level of skill and compassion. This dedication has led to our being **named among the top 50 pediatric pulmonary services in America**, according to *U.S. News & World* Report's 2011-2012 ranking of "Best Children's Hospitals."

Under the direction of Andrew Ting, M.D., Acting Division Chief, our team of award winning pediatric pulmonologists, nurse practitioners, nurse educators, nutritionists, social workers and respiratory therapists deliver evidence-based care to children with asthma, cystic fibrosis, chronic respiratory failure, bronchopulmonary dysplasia and other respiratory conditions.

Offering medical support and guidance, our **Children's Asthma Center** provides advanced pulmonary function testing, allergy testing, environmental assessment, nutritional evaluation, education, and family services. We teach patients and their parents or guardians to identify asthma triggers and offer a personalized asthma action plan for each patient—a process that has our patients experiencing fewer emergency department visits and hospitalizations, missing less school and enjoying more active lives. In addition, through outreach efforts and care delivered to children from East Harlem—an area with one of the highest asthma rates in the country—we have succeeded in empowering these patients to manage their disease and face the future with confidence.

As an accredited **Cystic Fibrosis Foundation Care Center**, we offer the latest therapies and participate in multi-center trials. With our team specially trained in caring for cystic fibrosis patients, we treat all aspects of the disease, ranging from the latest antimicrobial strategies to nutritional optimization. We offer services that include pediatric spirometry, plethysmography, and comprehensive psychosocial support and evaluation.

Our **Chronic Ventilator Program** provides the most advanced and compassionate management of children with chronic respiratory failure as well as those with muscular dystrophies and other conditions that require mechanical ventilation. Our **Bronchopulmonary Dysplasia Program** offers the highest level of care for premature infants while they are in the hospital and, as outpatients, once they are discharged.

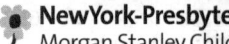

NewYork-Presbyterian
The University Hospital of Columbia and Cornell

Affiliated with Columbia University College of Physicians and Surgeons and Weill Cornell Medical College

NewYork-Presbyterian
Morgan Stanley Children's Hospital
Columbia University Medical Center
3959 Broadway
New York, NY 10032

NewYork-Presbyterian
Phyllis and David Komansky
Center for Children's Health
Weill Cornell Medical Center
525 East 68th Street
New York, NY 10065

1-800-245-KIDS (1-800-245-5437) www.childrensnyp.org

Accreditation: The Joint Commission

Overview

The pediatric services of NewYork-Presbyterian Hospital are comprised of NewYork-Presbyterian Morgan Stanley Children's Hospital, which is affiliated with Columbia University College of Physicians and Surgeons, and the NewYork-Presbyterian Phyllis and David Komansky Center for Children's Health, which is affiliated with Weill Cornell Medical College. Together, they serve as one of the nation's premier centers for comprehensive pediatric care. Skilled and experienced physicians, surgeons, nurses and other pediatric healthcare professionals manage some of the most complex medical conditions of children at every stage of development. Their expertise includes general pediatric care and the full range of medical and surgical subspecialties:

- Adolescent Medicine
- Allergy and Immunology
- Anesthesiology
- Blood Disorders
- Blood and Marrow Transplantation
- Cancer
- Cardiology and Cardiac Surgery
- Craniofacial and Plastic Surgery
- Critical Care
- Dermatology
- Digestive Disease
- Ear, Nose and Throat
- Emergency Department, including specialized units for burns and trauma injuries
- Endocrinology, Diabetes and Metabolism
- Epilepsy
- Genetics
- Infectious Diseases

- Kidney Disease
- Liver Disease
- Lung Disease
- Neonatal Medicine
- Neurology and Neurological Surgery
- Nutrition
- Obesity and Bariatric Surgery
- Ophthalmology
- Oral and Maxillofacial Surgery and Pediatric Dentistry
- Organ Transplantation
- Orthopaedic Surgery
- Pain Medicine
- Pediatric Surgery
- Pregnancy and Newborn Services
- Primary Care/General Pediatrics
- Psychiatry
- Radiology
- Rheumatology
- Urology

Highlights at a Glance:

- A national leader in pediatric open-heart surgery with one the largest pediatric heart transplant programs in the nation.
- A pediatric kidney transplant program, which includes a Living Donor Program and leading edge therapies to help reduce the side effects of anti-rejection drugs.
- Pediatric cardiac surgeons at the forefront of ventricular assist devices for infants and small children as a bridge to recovery or transplantation.
- One of three Level 1-designated Regional Pediatric Trauma Centers in New York State and the only one in New York City.
- A New York State Department of Health-designated Regional Perinatal Center of Expertise for the care of women with high-risk pregnancies.
- One of the largest Type 1 diabetes programs in New York State.
- Outstanding neonatal intensive care programs setting standards of care nationwide for extremely ill newborns.
- The only program in the New York tri-state area that has active programs in both liver and small bowel transplantation.

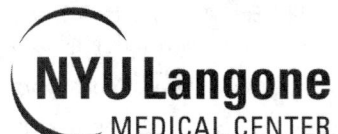

HASSENFELD PEDIATRIC CENTER

The new Hassenfeld Pediatric Center (HPC) is a full-service specialty children's hospital that works as a cohesive team across all children's health services provided at NYU Langone Medical Center. At HPC, newborns, children, adolescents and young adults receive the most comprehensive and advanced care possible from a team of pediatricians and pediatric specialists across more than 30 medical and surgical disciplines. With more than 150 full-time pediatric specialists, as well as pediatric nurses, child life specialists and social workers, the Hassenfeld Pediatric Center is uniquely equipped to provide innovative pediatric subspecialty care in a highly personalized manner.

About Children's Services at NYU Langone

NYU Langone Medical Center is nationally recognized in many pediatric specialty fields, including craniofacial anomalies, cardiac surgery, orthopaedic surgery, rehabilitation medicine, brain tumors, leukemia, sarcoma, and epilepsy. Our specialists work collaboratively to optimize care for each child, from the operating room and pediatric intensive care unit to the Emergency Department and pediatric inpatient unit.

A Family-Centered Approach

Integral to the care we provide is a myriad of support services for children and their families. We recognize that the best outcomes are achieved when the child's family is actively involved in every step of care. For that reason, our trained specialists address the needs of not just the patient, but of parents and siblings through ongoing education and communication.

The Future Shape of Pediatric Care at HPC

In 2017, a 160,000 square foot pediatric hospital, on the Medical Center's main campus, will become the inpatient centerpiece of the Hassenfeld Pediatric Center. This state-of-the-art facility will enhance the Center's ability to deliver world-class care through all private rooms, a feature that increases patient safety by decreasing exposure to infections, while providing a private, supportive environment for the patients and their families. HPC will be the only pediatric inpatient facility in Manhattan with this amenity, which will also include a "family zone" offering a sleep-in couch, storage, and Web access for each room.

The new pediatric hospital will also include a child-friendly pre-operative unit along with recovery bays where parents can be by the child's bedside during post-operation. Rounding out the new hospital will be a Family Center for orientation activities geared to patients, space for child-life activities and performances, as well as support, education and respite services for families.

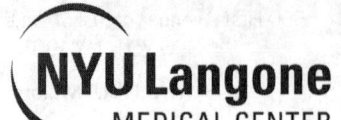
PEDIATRIC CARDIOLOGY

Pediatric Cardiology is part of the Hassenfeld Pediatric Center, a full service specialty Children's Hospital, which supports the array of children's health services across the Medical Center where newborns, children, adolescents and young adults receive the most comprehensive and advanced care by a team of pediatricians and pediatric specialists.

Pediatric Cardiology is at the forefront of innovation in clinical care, research and teaching. Special emphasize on early and accurate diagnosis during fetal life allows for better preparation and quicker response for treatment of newborns with congenital heart disease. Surgical and Congenital Cardiovascular Care Unit capabilities result in better outcomes for a wide range of patients with congenital heart disease, from the fetus to the adult.

Cardiothoracic Surgery
The Division offers corrective and palliative procedures for all types of congenital and acquired heart disease for a wide range of ages, from fetal life to adult.

Pediatric Cardiac Critical Care
We provide cardiac intensive care for children with heart disease. Our staff of pediatric cardiologists, pediatric cardiac intensivists, neonatologists, cardiac anesthesiologists, respiratory therapists and pediatric intensive care nurses are highly skilled and compassionate.

Pediatric Cardiac Electrophysiology
Specialists in the Division provide a wide array of diagnostic and therapeutic services, including arrhythmia detection, cardiac ablation and pacemaker placement.

Pediatric Cardiopulmonary Exercise Laboratory
Our lab assesses the cardio-respiratory response of exercise in children as young as three and four. It features some of the most sophisticated equipment in the region for measuring oxygen consumption, cardiac output and lung capacity.

Pediatric Interventional Cardiac Catheterization
We offer diagnosis and treatment of complex heart conditions in both nonsurgical and surgical settings. A full range of interventional procedures, including stent implantation and transcatheter device closure, are available.

Pediatric Non-Invasive Cardiac Imaging
The Division offers Cardiac Echocardiography, Magnetic Resonance Imaging (MRI) and Computer Tomography (CT) to diagnose and monitor a wide range of cardiac abnormalities.

Fetal Cardiac Program
An active program of fetal cardiac imaging works in close partnership with NYU Langone Neonatologists, Geneticists and the OB/GYN department.

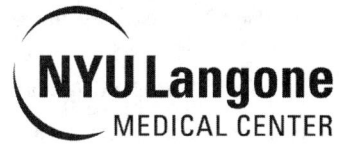
PEDIATRIC CRITICAL CARE

Pediatric Critical Care is part of the Hassenfeld Pediatric Center, a full service specialty Children's Hospital, which supports the array of children's health services across the Medical Center where newborns, children, adolescents and young adults receive the most comprehensive and advanced care by a team of pediatricians and pediatric specialists.

About the Pediatric Critical Care Team
Pediatric critical care specialists at NYU Langone Medical Center are highly trained and experienced in the treatment of seriously ill children, providing a supportive environment for patients and their families. In addition to these dedicated pediatric intensivists, the Medical Center's 12-bed Laurence D. and Lori Weider Fink Pediatric Intensive Care Unit (PICU) is staffed by a team of specially trained pediatric nurses who care for children from babies through young adults. In addition to managing children who require days or weeks of intense therapy, the Pediatric Critical Care team's responsibilities include caring for children recovering from postsurgical anesthesia, as well as overnight monitoring of patients after surgery or other procedures in the PICU. The Pediatric Critical Care team collaborates with all of the pediatric surgical specialties at NYU Langone, as well as with medical specialties and pediatric anesthesia. Social workers dedicated to the PICU are also an integral part of the team. We specialize in the following areas:

Ventilator Support
Children who require ventilator support benefit from the knowledge and experience of physicians who assess and carefully negotiate the proper timing of extubation. They are also skilled in the management of pain for each young patient.

Parent Education
Educating parents of critical ill children is a very important part of our services. The Pediatric Critical Care team is committed to fostering a supportive environment by continually engaging parents in dialogue. This includes "demystifying" the PICU, which can be an intimidating environment for children given its elaborate equipment and unfamiliar sounds. Parents are also encouraged to participate in daily rounds, and to listen and contribute to medical updates regarding their child's condition. Particularly comforting to the parents of critically ill children is the availability of round-the-clock, unlimited visitation.

Children with Complex Conditions
Because of their expertise with various congenital and acquired conditions, pediatric critical care specialists at NYU Langone are highly experienced in caring for children with complex conditions, including severely handicapped youngsters with special needs. Primary care pediatricians are encouraged to visit their patients at the PICU, and our team of caregivers communicates frequently with these physicians in-person and by telephone.

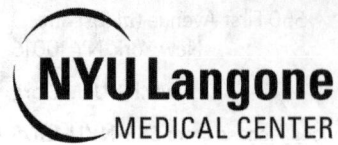

550 First Avenue *(at 31st Street)*
New York, NY 10016
www.NYULMC.org
Children's Services Access Line: **855-NYU-KIDS**

PEDIATRIC EMERGENCY MEDICINE

Pediatric Emergency Medicine is part of the Hassenfeld Pediatric Center, a full service specialty Children's Hospital, which supports the array of children's health services across the Medical Center where newborns, children, adolescents and young adults receive the most comprehensive and advanced care by a team of pediatricians and pediatric specialists.

About the Division of Pediatric Emergency Medicine, Department of Pediatrics

The Division of Pediatric Emergency Medicine at NYU Langone Medical Center offers patients compassionate, state-of-the-art emergency medical care. Our physicians are specially trained in pediatric emergency medicine and are expert in managing emergencies specific to infants, children, adolescents and young adults. They are recognized as national leaders for the training of Pediatric Emergency Medicine physicians, as well as for their research and advocacy. We specialize in the following areas:

Pediatric Emergency Medicine

The Tisch Hospital Pediatric Emergency Medicine Program at NYU Langone Medical Center provides the highest level of care to all pediatric patients. Ill and injured children receive treatment in an atmosphere that is child-friendly and family-focused. Pediatric sub-specialty physicians and pediatric surgeons are available for consultation in the Emergency Department 24 hours a day, 365 days a year.

Pediatric Emergency Services

Pediatric Emergency Services (PES) at Bellevue Hospital Center, an affiliate of NYU Langone Medical Center, is dedicated to the care of acutely ill and injured children. Each year approximately 25,000 children and young adults are evaluated by PES, which is staffed around the clock by board-certified pediatric emergency medicine physicians and nurses who specialize in the emergency care of children. PES manages patients with a wide range of medical, surgical and psychiatric problems, including asthma, appendicitis, child abuse, orthopaedic injuries, major trauma, poisoning and suicide.

Pediatric Transport

The Pediatric Transport Program at NYU Langone Medical Center transfers critically ill pediatric patients from outlying facilities to the Medical Center. In-house teams are available 24 hours a day, 7 days a week to allow a rapid response to medical transports from more than 50 hospitals. The transport team includes a physician as well as a respiratory therapist and pediatric critical care nurse. Patients are provided with the most advanced care possible from the beginning of the transport at the referring facility to their final destination.

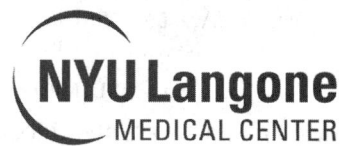
PEDIATRIC GASTROENTEROLOGY

Pediatric Gastroenterology is part of the Hassenfeld Pediatric Center, a full service specialty Children's Hospital, which supports the array of children's health services across the Medical Center where newborns, children, adolescents and young adults receive the most comprehensive and advanced care by a team of pediatricians and pediatric specialists.

About the Division of Pediatric Gastroenterology, Department of Pediatrics

Pediatric gastroenterologists at NYU Langone Medical Center are committed to the highest quality medical care and state-of-the-art techniques in the evaluation and management of gastrointestinal, liver and nutritional disorders from infancy to young adulthood. With access to the latest in endoscopic procedures performed at one of the country's leading academic medical centers, patients receive comprehensive and multidisciplinary treatments for a wide range of conditions. Our pediatric gastroenterologists are particularly adept at providing family-centered, integrated care with a focus on the physical and psychological well-being of the child. We specialize in the following areas:

Clinical Care

Most children will occasionally experience one or more gastrointestinal symptoms during their childhood years. Some children, however, develop recurrent symptoms, which interrupt their normal lives and are the presenting features of serious but treatable diseases. The gastrointestinal and nutritional concerns impacting on the health and quality of life of children on the autism spectrum is an area of particular interest at NYU Langone. We are in the forefront of the evaluation and management of celiac disease and food allergies, including allergic involvement of the esophagus (eosinophilic esophagitis), and our experts use the latest techniques to pinpoint problems and determine the most effective therapy. We offer a vast range of therapeutic services, as well as access to clinical nutrition services, pediatric rehabilitation and some of the country's best surgeons.

Specialty Care

Pediatric gastroenterologists at NYU Langone Medical Center evaluate and treat a variety of disorders including abdominal pain, celiac spruce, congenital bowel dysfunction, congenital liver disorders and chronic liver disease, chronic constipation, feeding problems in infants, failure to thrive, food allergies, lactose intolerance, gastrointestinal bleeding, gastroesophageal reflux, hepatitis, malabsorption syndromes, pancreatitis, peptic ulcer disease, ulcerative colitis and Crohn's disease.

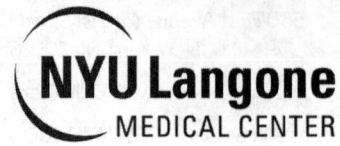
PEDIATRIC HEMATOLOGY/ONCOLOGY

Pediatric Hemaology/Oncology is part of the Hassenfeld Pediatric Center, a full service specialty Children's Hospital, which supports the array of children's health services across the Medical Center where newborns, children, adolescents and young adults receive the most comprehensive and advanced care by a team of pediatricians and pediatric specialists.

We are committed to providing modern, family-centered and highly personalized care to children with cancer and blood disorders. Teams of specialists deliver personalized care in a healing environment promoting physical, emotional and spiritual well-being of children and their families.

Hematologic Malignancies
We offer new treatments for childhood acute lymphoblastic leukemia (ALL) and are a national leader in clinical trials for children with newly diagnosed leukemia and recurrent diseases.

Hematology
We provide treatment for children and adolescents with all types of blood disorders including Sickle Cell Disease, other hemoglobinopathies, bleeding disorders and aplastic anemia.

Pediatric Neuro-Oncology
We provide multidisciplinary comprehensive care for children from infants to young adults with primary central nervous system, slow-growing and malignant tumors assuring the safest and most effective treatments for newly diagnosed or recurrent tumors.

Pediatric Special Hematology Laboratory
NYU Langone offers comprehensive homeostasis and red cell testing incorporating the latest developments in the field.

Psychosocial Services
Our holistic approach to care includes art therapy, relaxation training, play therapy, psychiatric evaluation, neuropsychological assessment, individual/group counseling and patient education.

Sarcoma and Solid Tumor Program
We offer cutting-edge medical, surgical and radiotherapy treatments for bone and soft tissue sarcomas, and all pediatric solid tumors including Wilms' Tumor and neuroblastoma and are developing national trials for the treatment of sarcomas and offer a number of clinical trials.

Stephen D. Hassenfeld Children's Center for Cancer and Blood Disorders
As a member of the NCI-designated NYU Cancer Institute, we are constantly developing new ways to treat childhood cancer. Our unique interdisciplinary and family-centered approach combines the most advanced medical treatments with psychosocial and emotional support.

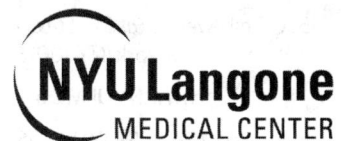

550 First Avenue *(at 31st Street)*
New York, NY 10016
www.NYULMC.org
Children's Services Access Line: **855-NYU-KIDS**

PEDIATRIC PULMONOLOGY

Pediatric Pulmonology is part of the Hassenfeld Pediatric Center, a full service specialty Children's Hospital, which supports the array of children's health services across the Medical Center where newborns, children, adolescents and young adults receive the most comprehensive and advanced care by a team of pediatricians and pediatric specialists.

About Pediatric Pulmonology, Department of Pediatrics

The Division of Pediatric Pulmonology provides comprehensive care to children -- from infancy to adolescence to young adulthood -- with a variety of conditions affecting the respiratory system. Physicians in the Division are committed to providing both family-centered and multidisciplinary care, collaborating with specialists in other divisions throughout NYU Langone Medical Center. For example, physicians in the Division work closely with the Infant Apnea/SIDS Program to follow children discharged from the Neonatal Intensive Care Unit; with the Division of Pediatric Gastroenterology and the Swallowing Center to follow children with feeding difficulties and swallowing dysfunction; with the Division of Pediatric Surgery to follow children with congenital lung lesions through minimally invasive surgery; and with the Division of Orthopaedics to optimize the care of children with neuromuscular disease undergoing spine surgery. We specialize in the following areas:

Pulmonologists in the Division care for children with a wide range of problems, including asthma, bronchopulmonary dysplasia (chronic lung disease of prematurity), cystic fibrosis, chronic respiratory failure and pulmonary complications of neuromuscular disease, congenital lung malformations, chest wall deformities, interstitial lung disease, and obstructive sleep apnea. Consultation for chronic cough, noisy breathing, and exercise intolerance is also provided.

Flexible bronchoscopy

Using specialized pediatric equipment, the airways of even the tiniest infants can be examined in the state-of-the-art endoscopy suite at NYU Langone Medical Center, with multiple specialists often involved in the procedure. Because the equipment is mobile, procedures can also be performed at bedside in the Pediatric Intensive Care Unit.

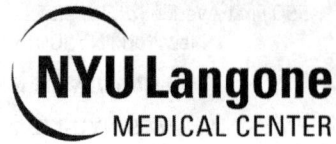

550 First Avenue *(at 31st Street)*
New York, NY 10016
www.NYULMC.org
Children's Services Access Line: **855-NYU-KIDS**

PEDIATRIC RHEUMATOLOGY

Pediatric Rheumatology is part of the Hassenfeld Pediatric Center, a full service specialty Children's Hospital, which supports the array of children's health services across the Medical Center where newborns, children, adolescents and young adults receive the most comprehensive and advanced care by a team of pediatricians and pediatric specialists.

About the Division of Pediatric Rheumatology, Department of Pediatrics

Pediatric rheumatology specialists at the NYU Langone Medical Center are dedicated to the complete care of children with rheumatic disease. In conjunction with our multidisciplinary team of specialists, we treat children with a variety of rheumatologic conditions, including Juvenile Idiopathic Arthritis (JIA), systemic lupus erythematosus, juvenile dermatomyositis, Kawasaki's disease, and others. Through early diagnosis and appropriately intensive treatment we aim to achieve disease quiescence as quickly and safely as possible, with the ultimate goal of returning children to full physical functionality.

In addition to our clinical services, we are committed to the continued formal education of residents, rheumatology fellows and medical students, as well as the general public through our community outreach programs and in collaboration with the adult Rheumatology Division, we have initiated an annual pediatric rheumatology CME course which is well-attended by general physicians and rheumatologists. Our emphasis on providing high-level clinical services and teaching is complemented by the Division's collaboration with national pediatric rheumatology research organizations in several clinical research projects pertaining to drug exposure in children with rheumatic disease. We specialize in the following areas:

Juvenile Idiopathic Arthritis

An umbrella term for several different patterns of arthritis in children, juvenile idiopathic arthritis (JIA) refers to arthritic disorders caused by an autoimmune reaction. Our Pediatric rheumatologists diagnose and treat different types of JIA. The use of methotrexate in combination with newly discovered biologic agents, such as Etanercept and Infliximab, gives even greater reason for optimism. Juvenile arthritis, once a crippler of children, is fast becoming a highly manageable disease.

Pediatric Arthritis

A bacterial joint infection in children, known as septic arthritis, is a painful condition requiring urgent care to prevent the spread of infection and the possibility of permanent damage to the joint. At the first sign of septic arthritis, NYU Langone's Pediatric staff takes quick action to fight the infection at its source.

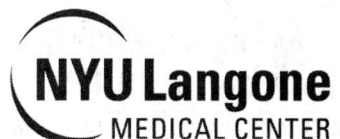
PEDIATRIC SURGERY

Pediatric Surgery is part of the Hassenfeld Pediatric Center, a full service specialty Children's Hospital, which supports the array of children's health services across the Medical Center where newborns, children, adolescents and young adults receive the most comprehensive and advanced care by a team of pediatricians and pediatric specialists.

The Division of Pediatric Surgery at NYU Langone Medical Center provides comprehensive pediatric surgical care for the smallest preterm infant to the adolescent. Our surgeons are experts at minimally invasive procedures (resulting in shorter hospitals stays and faster recoveries), as well as in conventional surgical techniques. In addition to highly-skilled surgeons and surgical nurses, we offer a wide array of Child Life Services to help children and their families become familiar with the hospital environment and lessen fears.

Surgical Expertise
NYU Langone Medical Center is renowned for its achievements in the full spectrum of pediatric surgical specialties, including abdominal and thoracic surgery, neonatal surgery, surgery for all congenital anomalies, cancer surgery, urology, cardiac surgery, neurosurgery, orthopaedics, plastic and reconstructive surgery, repair of cleft lips and palates, ophthalmology, and ENT, among others.

Pediatric Anesthesia
We are proud of our expert team of fellowship-trained pediatric anesthesiologists who serve the pediatric population. These anesthesiologists are involved in preoperative and postoperative care as well as in administering anesthesia, and they have close working relationships with our pediatric surgeons.

Child Life Services
The pediatric unit is home to The Child Life Program which is focused on creating a supportive environment for children undergoing surgery and their families through a total care approach. Child Life personnel meet with parents and their child prior to surgery and provide a continuum of care to the entire family throughout the hospital experience.

Pre-Admission Orientation and Information
Informational packets about what to expect are given to families during the pre-admission testing process. Parents and their children are also encouraged to attend an orientation session.

Facilities
Day surgery facilities include an expansive playroom with computers, games and Child Life personnel to care for the family. A separate recovery room area provides a calming environment for children during their emergence from anesthesia.

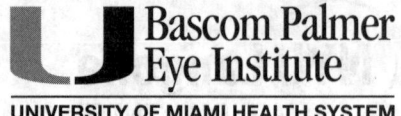

UNIVERSITY OF MIAMI HEALTH SYSTEM

INTERNATIONALLY ACCLAIMED

Bascom Palmer Eye Institute is committed to the protection and preservation of the treasured gift of sight and is recognized as one of the world's finest and most progressive centers for ophthalmic care, vision research and education. Each of our 65 clinical faculty members specializes in a specific area of ophthalmology and is board-certified by the American Board of Ophthalmology. In addition to providing care to more than 250,000 patients annually, all clinical faculty members have research and teaching responsibilities at the University of Miami Miller School of Medicine.

BASCOM PALMER EYE INSTITUTE EARNS TOP RATINGS

Bascom Palmer Eye Institute continues to be ranked as one of the nation's best ophthalmic hospitals by board-certified ophthalmologists from across the United States. In 2011, Bascom Palmer was named the #1 eye hospital in the United States by *U.S.News & World Report* for the eighth year in a row. Bascom Palmer is also recognized as having the Best Overall Program, Best Clinical (Patient) Care and Best Residency Education Program by *Ophthalmology Times*, which annually ranks the top ophthalmology programs in the United States.

PEDIATRIC OPHTHALMOLOGISTS DIAGNOSE AND TREAT CHILDHOOD EYE DISEASE AND DISORDERS

Bascom Palmer Eye Institute is one of only a few centers giving special attention to the diverse ophthalmic needs of children from infancy through adolescence- a critical time when clear vision plays an important role in mental, physical and social development. As a major referral center serving the southeastern United States, Caribbean and South America, we treat approximately 7,000 children annually in our children's clinic designed specifically for pediatric care. Our outpatient clinic is specifically designed to meet the unique ophthalmic and social needs of children with visual deficiencies as well as adults with strabismus. The clinic's diagnostic and treatment services encompass common eye disorders of childhood, such as amblyopia and strabismus, as well as rare disorders affecting infants and children. With the support of the extensive resources of the entire Bascom Palmer Eye Institute, we specialize in the blinding and visually-impairing diseases of childhood including congenital cataracts, congenital glaucoma, retinopathy of prematurity, detached retinas, ocular infections, hereditary disorders and tumors.

To schedule an appointment please call (800) 329-7000 or visit www.bascompalmer.org

Miami	Palm Beach Gardens	Naples	Plantation
900 NW 17th Street	7101 Fairway Drive,	311 9th Street North	1000 South Pine Island Road
Miami, FL 33136	Palm Beach Gardens, FL 33418	Naples, FL 34102	Plantation, FL 33324
(305) 326-6000	(561) 515-1500	(239) 659-3937	(954) 465-2700

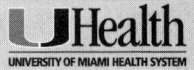

UNIVERSITY OF MIAMI
MILLER SCHOOL
of MEDICINE

www.uhealthsystem.com

UHealth: Top-ranked doctors and hospitals providing the finest health care at more than 30 convenient South Florida locations, including our hospitals: University of Miami Hospital, Bascom Palmer Eye Institute, and Sylvester Comprehensive Cancer Center. UHealth is powered by the research and education of the University of Miami Miller School of Medicine.

Monroe Carell Jr. Children's Hospital at Vanderbilt

Vanderbilt University Medical Center
2200 Children's Way
Nashville, TN 37232
(800) 288-5000

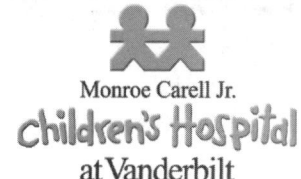

Overview

Monroe Carell Jr. Children's Hospital at Vanderbilt is a nationally recognized leader in pediatric health care. Children's Hospital offers an extremely high level of care within an elite teaching and research facility. A recent 33-bed expansion to our 243-bed facility will help meet the growing demands for pediatric care in our region.

While Children's Hospital primarily serves children in Middle Tennessee, southern Kentucky and northern Alabama, patients from across the country seek treatment here. Every child who needs our services is given care, regardless of ability to pay.

Among the Nation's Best

Children's Hospital is ranked as one of the top children's hospitals in the nation by *U.S. News & World Report* in 10 out of 10 possible specialties:

Cancer

Cardiology and heart surgery

Diabetes and endocrinology

Gastroenterology

Neurology and neurosurgery

Neonatology

Orthopaedics

Pulmonology

Urology

Junior League Fetal Center at Vanderbilt

The Junior League Fetal Center at Vanderbilt gives babies and their families the best care possible. Patients from across the country turn to us for care of complications during pregnancy. Our internationally recognized experts offer superior care that leads to very high patient satisfaction.

Fetal Repair of Spina Bifida

A landmark study co-led by experts at Vanderbilt has proven that babies who have surgery to repair spina bifida while still in the womb have better outcomes than babies who have surgery after birth. Members of the fetal surgery team at Vanderbilt pioneered the surgery to repair myelomeningocele, the most serious form of spina bifida. Noel Tulipan, M.D., internationally renowned neurosurgeon and director of pediatric neurosurgery, has performed more than 200 prenatal surgeries to repair the spina bifida defect. Learn more.

Family-centered Care

At Children's Hospital, your family is our family. Children heal faster with their loved ones nearby, and staying at a place that doesn't feel like a hospital helps families focus on rest and recuperation. We offer a robust Family Resource Center, serenity gardens, quiet rooms for families, a beautiful chapel and other features to promote healing and reduce stress. Learn more.

ChildrensHospital.Vanderbilt.org

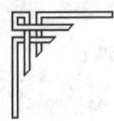

The Best in American Medicine
www.CastleConnolly.com

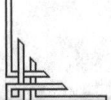
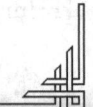

Physical Medicine
& Rehabilitation

Physical medicine and rehabilitation, also referred to as rehabilitation medicine, is the medical specialty concerned with diagnosing, evaluating and treating patients with physical disabilities. These disabilities may arise from conditions affecting the musculoskeletal system such as neck and back pain, sports injuries, or other painful conditions affecting the limbs, for example carpal tunnel syndrome. Alternatively, the disabilities may result from neurological trauma or disease such as spinal cord injury, head injury or stroke.

A physician certified in physical medicine and rehabilitation is often called a physiatrist. The primary goal of the physiatrist is to achieve maximal restoration of physical, psychological, social and vocational function through comprehensive rehabilitation. Pain management is often an important part of the role of the physiatrist. For diagnosis and evaluation, a physiatrist may include the techniques of electromyography to supplement the standard history, physical, X-ray and laboratory examinations. The physiatrist has expertise in the appropriate use of therapeutic exercise, prosthetics (artificial limbs), orthotics and mechanical and electrical devices.

Training Required: Four years *plus* one year clinical practice.

Certification in the following subspecialty requires additional training and examination.

Spinal Cord Injury Medicine: A physician who addresses the prevention, diagnosis, treatment and management of traumatic spinal cord injury and non-traumatic etiologies of spinal cord dysfunction by working in an interdisciplinary manner. Care is provided to patients of all ages on a lifelong basis and covers related medical, physical, psychological and vocational disabilities and complications.

PHYSICAL MEDICINE & REHABILITATION

New England

Bloch, Rina M MD [PMR] - **Spec Exp:** Spinal Cord Injury; Brain Injury Rehabilitation; Geriatric Rehabilitation; Musculoskeletal Disorders; **Hospital:** Tufts Med Ctr; **Address:** Tufts Medical Ctr, Rehab Medicine, 750 Washington St, Box 400, Boston, MA 02111; **Phone:** 617-636-3003; **Board Cert:** Physical Medicine & Rehabilitation 1989; Spinal Cord Injury Medicine 2008; Electrodiagnostic Medicine 1997; **Med School:** Univ Louisville Sch Med 1983; **Resid:** Physical Medicine & Rehabilitation, Rehab Inst of Chicago 1987

Borg-Stein, Joanne MD [PMR] - **Spec Exp:** Pain Management; Sports Medicine; Acupuncture; Spinal Rehabilitation; **Hospital:** Spaulding Rehab Hosp, Newton - Wellesley Hosp; **Address:** Spaulding-Wellesley Outpatient Center, 65 Walnut St, Wellesley, MA 02481; **Phone:** 781-431-9144; **Board Cert:** Physical Medicine & Rehabilitation 1990; Pain Medicine 2000; Sports Medicine 2008; **Med School:** Albert Einstein Coll Med 1984; **Resid:** Physical Medicine & Rehabilitation, Columbia-Presby Med Ctr 1988; **Fac Appt:** Asst Prof PMR, Harvard Med Sch

Glenn, Mel B MD [PMR] - **Spec Exp:** Brain Injury Rehabilitation; Spasticity Management; **Hospital:** Spaulding Rehab Hosp, Mass Genl Hosp; **Address:** Spaulding Rehab Hosp, 125 Nashua St, Boston, MA 02114; **Phone:** 617-573-2200; **Board Cert:** Physical Medicine & Rehabilitation 1982; **Med School:** NYU Sch Med 1978; **Resid:** Physical Medicine & Rehabilitation, NYU Med Ctr 1981; **Fellow:** Spinal Cord Injury Medicine, NYU Med Ctr 1982; **Fac Appt:** Assoc Prof PMR, Harvard Med Sch

Richter, Edwin MD [PMR] - **Spec Exp:** Neuro-Rehabilitation; Musculoskeletal Injuries; Amputee Rehabilitation; Lymphedema; **Hospital:** Stamford Hosp; **Address:** 166 W Broad St, Ste 305, Stamford, CT 06902; **Phone:** 203-316-0610; **Board Cert:** Physical Medicine & Rehabilitation 1992; **Med School:** NYU Sch Med 1987; **Resid:** Physical Medicine & Rehabilitation, NYU Med Ctr 1991; **Fac Appt:** Asst Clin Prof PMR, NYU Sch Med

Silver, Julie K MD [PMR] - **Spec Exp:** Post Polio Syndrome/Rehabilitation; **Hospital:** UMass Memorial Med Ctr; **Address:** 154 E Main St, West Borough, MA 01581; **Phone:** 508-871-2389; **Board Cert:** Physical Medicine & Rehabilitation 2006; **Med School:** Georgetown Univ 1991; **Resid:** Physical Medicine & Rehabilitation, Natl Rehab Hosp 1995; **Fac Appt:** Asst Prof PMR, Harvard Med Sch

Webster, Harry C MD [PMR] - **Spec Exp:** Pediatric Rehabilitation; Cerebral Palsy; Muscular Dystrophy; Spasticity Management; **Hospital:** Tufts Med Ctr; **Address:** Tufts Med Ctr, 800 Washington St, Box 387, Boston, MA 02111; **Phone:** 617-636-5626; **Board Cert:** Pediatrics 1983; Physical Medicine & Rehabilitation 1988; **Med School:** UCSF 1977; **Resid:** Pediatrics, Chldns Hosp 1980; Physical Medicine & Rehabilitation, Tufts Med Ctr 1987; **Fac Appt:** Asst Prof PMR, Tufts Univ

Zafonte, Ross D DO [PMR] - **Spec Exp:** Brain Injury Rehabilitation; Spinal Cord Injury; **Hospital:** Spaulding Rehab Hosp; **Address:** Spaulding Rehab Hosp, 125 Nashua St, rm 707, Boston, MA 02114; **Phone:** 617-573-2754; **Board Cert:** Physical Medicine & Rehabilitation 1990; **Med School:** Nova SE Univ, Coll Osteo Med 1985; **Resid:** Physical Medicine & Rehabilitation, Mt Sinai Med Ctr 1989; **Fac Appt:** Clin Prof PMR, Boston Univ

Mid Atlantic

Ahn, Jung Hwan MD [PMR] - **Spec Exp:** Spinal Cord Injury; Stroke Rehabilitation; Neuro-logic Rehabilitation; **Hospital:** NYU Langone Med Ctr (page 66); **Address:** 400 E 34th St, rm 421, New York, NY 10016-4901; **Phone:** 212-263-6122; **Board Cert:** Physical Medicine & Rehabilita-tion 1980; Spinal Cord Injury Medicine 2008; **Med School:** South Korea 1970; **Resid:** Obstetrics & Gynecology, Elmhurst City Hosp - Mt Sinai 1976; Physical Medicine & Rehabilitation, NYU Med Ctr 1979; **Fellow:** Spinal Cord Injury Medicine, NYU Med Ctr 1980; **Fac Appt:** Clin Prof PMR, NYU Sch Med

Aseff, John N MD [PMR] - **Spec Exp:** Electrodiagnosis; Pain-Soft Tissue; **Hospital:** Natl Rehab Hosp, Washington Hosp Ctr; **Address:** National Rehabilitation Hosp, 102 Irving St NW, Washington, DC 20010; **Phone:** 202-877-1916; **Board Cert:** Physical Medicine & Rehabilitation 1978; **Med School:** Ohio State Univ 1973; **Resid:** Surgery, Univ Hosps Cleveland 1975; Physical Medicine & Rehabilitation, Ohio State Univ Hosps 1977; **Fac Appt:** Assoc Clin Prof PMR, Georgetown Univ

Bach, John MD [PMR] - **Spec Exp:** Neuromuscular Disorders; Amyotrophic Lateral Sclerosis (ALS); Post Polio Syndrome/Rehabilitation; **Hospital:** Univ Hosp-UMDNJ—Newark; **Address:** 150 Bergen St, Ste B403, Newark, NJ 07103; **Phone:** 973-972-7195; **Board Cert:** Physical Medicine & Rehabilitation 1986; **Med School:** UMDNJ-NJ Med Sch, Newark 1976; **Resid:** Physical Medicine & Rehabilitation, NYU Med Ctr 1980; **Fellow:** Neuromuscular Disease, Univ Hosp 1983; **Fac Appt:** Prof PMR, UMDNJ-NJ Med Sch, Newark

Ballard, Pamela H MD [PMR] - **Spec Exp:** Spinal Cord Injury; Spasticity Management; Neu-romuscular Disorders; **Hospital:** Natl Rehab Hosp; **Address:** 102 Irving St NW, Washington, DC 20010; **Phone:** 202-877-1621; **Board Cert:** Physical Medicine & Rehabilitation 1991; Spinal Cord Injury Medicine 2009; **Med School:** Howard Univ 1986; **Resid:** Physical Medicine & Rehabilitation, Sinai Hosp 1990

Braddom, Randall L MD [PMR] - **Spec Exp:** Electromyography; Pain-Neck; Pain-Low Back; Musculoskeletal Disorders; **Hospital:** Riverview Med Ctr; **Address:** Orthopaedic, Sports Medicine & Rehab Ctr, 25 Kilmer Drive, Ste 105, Morganville, NJ 07751; **Phone:** 732-617-9111; **Board Cert:** Physical Medicine & Rehabilitation 1974; **Med School:** Ohio State Univ 1968; **Resid:** Physical Med-icine & Rehabilitation, Ohio State Univ Hosp 1973; **Fac Appt:** Clin Prof PMR, UMDNJ-NJ Med Sch, Newark

De Lateur, Barbara J MD [PMR] - **Spec Exp:** Frailty Syndrome; **Hospital:** Johns Hopkins Bayview Med Ctr (page 61), Good Samaritan Hosp; **Address:** Johns Hopkins Bayview Med Ctr, Rehab, 4940 Eastern Ave, Baltimore, MD 21224; **Phone:** 410-550-5299; **Board Cert:** Physical Medicine & Rehabilitation 1970; **Med School:** Univ Wash 1963; **Resid:** Physical Medicine & Reha-bilitation, Univ Wash Hosp 1968; **Fac Appt:** Prof PMR, Johns Hopkins Univ

Dillard, James N MD [PMR] - **Spec Exp:** Pain Management; Acupuncture; Complementary Medicine; Nutrition; **Hospital:** Southampton Hosp; **Address:** 110 E 59th St, Ste 10A, New York, NY 10022; **Phone:** 212-265-4038; **Board Cert:** Physical Medicine & Rehabilitation 2005; **Med School:** Rush Med Coll 1990; **Resid:** Physical Medicine & Rehabilitation, Columbia-Presby Med Ctr 1994; **Fac Appt:** Asst Clin Prof PMR, Columbia P&S

Esquenazi, Alberto M MD [PMR] - **Spec Exp:** Amputee Rehabilitation; Mobility Evaluation & Treatment; Post Polio Syndrome/Rehabilitation; Spasticity Management; **Hospital:** Moss Rehab Hosp; **Address:** Moss Rehab Hosp, 60 Township Line Rd, Elkins Park, PA 19027; **Phone:** 215-663-6676; **Board Cert:** Physical Medicine & Rehabilitation 1986; **Med School:** Mexico 1981; **Resid:** Physical Medicine & Rehabilitation, Temple Univ Hosp 1985; **Fellow:** Gait and Prosthetics, Moss Rehab Hosp 1986; **Fac Appt:** Prof PMR, Jefferson Med Coll

Physical Medicine & Rehabilitation

Evans, Sarah H MD [PMR] - **Spec Exp:** Pediatric Rehabilitation; White Matter Disorders; Encephalitis; **Hospital:** Chldns Natl Med Ctr, Natl Rehab Hosp; **Address:** Children's National Medical Ctr, Pediatric Rehabilitation, 111 Michigan Ave NW, Ste 1090, Washington, DC 20010; **Phone:** 202-476-3080; **Board Cert:** Physical Medicine & Rehabilitation 1992; Pediatrics 2002; Pediatric Rehabilitation Medicine 2003; **Med School:** Univ MD Sch Med 1984; **Resid:** Pediatrics, Univ Colorado Hlth Sci Ctr 1987; **Fellow:** Physical Medicine & Rehabilitation, Univ Colorado Hlth Sci Ctr 1988; Pediatric Rehabilitation Medicine, Chldns Hosp 1989; **Fac Appt:** Assoc Prof PMR, Univ Colorado

Feinberg, Joseph H MD [PMR] - **Spec Exp:** Peripheral Neuropathy; Spinal Rehabilitation; Electrodiagnosis; Sports Medicine; **Hospital:** Hosp For Special Surgery (page 60), Kessler Inst for Rehab - W Orange; **Address:** 535 E 70th St, New York, NY 10021-4872; **Phone:** 212-606-1568; **Board Cert:** Physical Medicine & Rehabilitation 1991; Sports Medicine 2009; **Med School:** Albany Med Coll 1983; **Resid:** Surgery, Mt Sinai Hosp 1985; Physical Medicine & Rehabilitation, Rusk Inst Rehab 1990; **Fellow:** Orthopaedic Pathology, Hosp Spec Surg 1986; Orthopaedic Biomechanics, Univ Iowa Hosp & Clins 1987; **Fac Appt:** Assoc Prof PMR, Cornell Univ-Weill Med Coll

Flanagan, Steven R MD [PMR] - **Spec Exp:** Brain Injury Rehabilitation; Stroke Rehabilitation; **Hospital:** NYU Langone Med Ctr (page 66), NYU Hosp For Joint Diseases; **Address:** Rusk Institute, 400 E 34th St, Ste 600, New York, NY 10016; **Phone:** 212-267-6037; **Board Cert:** Physical Medicine & Rehabilitation 2003; **Med School:** UMDNJ-NJ Med Sch, Newark 1988; **Resid:** Physical Medicine & Rehabilitation, Mt Sinai Hosp 1992; **Fac Appt:** Prof PMR, NYU Sch Med

Francis, Kathleen D MD [PMR] - **Spec Exp:** Lymphedema; **Address:** Lymphedema Physician Services, 200 S Orange Ave, Ste 111, Livingston, NJ 07039; **Phone:** 973-322-7366; **Board Cert:** Physical Medicine & Rehabilitation 2004; **Med School:** UMDNJ-NJ Med Sch, Newark 1989; **Resid:** Physical Medicine & Rehabilitation, UMDNJ-Kessler Inst Rehab 1993; **Fac Appt:** Asst Clin Prof PMR, UMDNJ-NJ Med Sch, Newark

Fried, Guy W MD [PMR] - **Spec Exp:** Brain Injury Rehabilitation; Spinal Cord Injury; Neurogenic Bladder; **Hospital:** Magee Rehab Hosp; **Address:** 1513 Race St, Philadelphia, PA 19102-1177; **Phone:** 215-587-3394; **Board Cert:** Physical Medicine & Rehabilitation 1990; Spinal Cord Injury Medicine 2009; Pain Medicine 2011; **Med School:** Yale Univ 1985; **Resid:** Physical Medicine & Rehabilitation, Thomas Jefferson Univ Hosp 1988; Preventive Medicine, Thomas Jefferson Univ Hosp 1989; **Fac Appt:** Asst Prof PMR, Thomas Jefferson Univ

Kirshblum, Steven C MD [PMR] - **Spec Exp:** Spinal Cord Injury; Spasticity Management; **Hospital:** Kessler Inst for Rehab - W Orange, Saint Barnabas Med Ctr; **Address:** Kessler Institute, 1199 Pleasant Valley Way, West Orange, NJ 07052-1424; **Phone:** 973-731-3600 x2258; **Board Cert:** Physical Medicine & Rehabilitation 1991; Spinal Cord Injury Medicine 2008; **Med School:** Univ Hlth Scis, Chicago Med Sch 1986; **Resid:** Physical Medicine & Rehabilitation, Mount Sinai Med Ctr 1990; **Fac Appt:** Prof PMR, UMDNJ-NJ Med Sch, Newark

Lutz, Gregory MD [PMR] - **Spec Exp:** Spinal Rehabilitation; Sports Medicine; Pain-Low Back; **Hospital:** Hosp For Special Surgery (page 60), Univ Med Ctr - Princeton; **Address:** 535 E 70th St, New York, NY 10021; **Phone:** 212-606-1648; **Board Cert:** Physical Medicine & Rehabilitation 2003; **Med School:** Georgetown Univ 1988; **Resid:** Physical Medicine & Rehabilitation, Mayo Clinic 1992; **Fellow:** Sports Medicine, Hosp For Spec Surg 1993; **Fac Appt:** Assoc Prof PMR, Cornell Univ-Weill Med Coll

Ma, Dong M MD [PMR] - **Spec Exp:** Electromyography; Musculoskeletal Disorders; **Hospital:** NYU Rusk Inst (page 67), NYU Langone Med Ctr (page 66); **Address:** Rusk Institute, 400 E 34th St, rm 211, New York, NY 10016; **Phone:** 212-263-6338; **Board Cert:** Physical Medicine & Rehabilitation 1979; **Med School:** South Korea 1968; **Resid:** Physical Medicine & Rehabilitation, NYU Med Ctr 1975; **Fellow:** Physical Medicine & Rehabilitation, NYU Med Ctr 1977; **Fac Appt:** Clin Prof PMR, NYU Sch Med

Marino, Ralph J MD [PMR] - **Spec Exp:** Spinal Cord Injury; Spasticity Management; **Hospital:** Thomas Jefferson Univ Hosp; **Address:** 132 S 10th St, 375 Main Bldg, Philadelphia, PA 19107; **Phone:** 215-955-1200; **Board Cert:** Physical Medicine & Rehabilitation 1988; Spinal Cord Injury Medicine 2010; **Med School:** Jefferson Med Coll 1982; **Resid:** Physical Medicine & Rehabilitation, Thos Jefferson Univ Hosp 1987; **Fac Appt:** Assoc Prof PMR, Jefferson Med Coll

Mayer, Nathaniel H MD [PMR] - **Spec Exp:** Motor Control Analysis; Spasticity Management; Brain Injury Rehabilitation; **Hospital:** Moss Rehab Hosp; **Address:** Drucker Brain Injury Ctr, 60 Township Line Rd, Elkins Park, PA 19027; **Phone:** 215-663-6681; **Board Cert:** Physical Medicine & Rehabilitation 1976; **Med School:** Albert Einstein Coll Med 1968; **Resid:** Physical Medicine & Rehabilitation, Temple Univ Hosp 1973; **Fac Appt:** Prof PMR, Temple Univ

Miknevich, Mary Ann MD [PMR] - **Spec Exp:** Prosthesis Control; Electrodiagnosis; **Hospital:** UPMC Mercy, Pittsburgh, UPMC McKeesport; **Address:** Mercy Rehabilitation, 1350 Locust St, Ste 409, Pittsburgh, PA 15219; **Phone:** 412-232-7608; **Board Cert:** Physical Medicine & Rehabilitation 1985; **Med School:** Univ Pittsburgh 1980; **Resid:** Physical Medicine & Rehabilitation, UPMC Mercy Hosp 1983; **Fac Appt:** Asst Clin Prof PMR, Univ Pittsburgh

Munin, Michael C MD [PMR] - **Spec Exp:** Spasticity Management; Amputee Rehabilitation; Hip Surgery Rehabilitation; Electrodiagnosis; **Hospital:** UPMC Presby, Pittsburgh, UPMC Inst Rehab & Rsch; **Address:** UPMC Shadyside, 3471 Fifth Ave, Kaufman Bldg Ste 1103, Pittsburgh, PA 15213; **Phone:** 412-692-4400; **Board Cert:** Physical Medicine & Rehabilitation 2003; **Med School:** Jefferson Med Coll 1988; **Resid:** Physical Medicine & Rehabilitation, Thomas Jefferson Univ Hosp 1992; **Fac Appt:** Assoc Prof PMR, Univ Pittsburgh

Palmer, Jeffrey B MD [PMR] - **Hospital:** Johns Hopkins Hosp (page 61); **Address:** Johns Hopkins Hosp-Physical Med & Rehab, 600 N Wolfe St, Phipps 160, Baltimore, MD 21287; **Phone:** 410-502-2446; **Board Cert:** Physical Medicine & Rehabilitation 1984; **Med School:** NYU Sch Med 1980; **Resid:** Physical Medicine & Rehabilitation, Univ Wash Med Ctr 1983; **Fac Appt:** Prof PMR, Johns Hopkins Univ

Ragnarsson, Kristjan T MD [PMR] - **Spec Exp:** Spinal Cord Injury; Brain Injury Rehabilitation; Pain-Back & Neck; **Hospital:** Mount Sinai Med Ctr (page 63); **Address:** 5 E 98th St Fl 6, New York, NY 10029-6501; **Phone:** 212-659-9370; **Board Cert:** Physical Medicine & Rehabilitation 1976; **Med School:** Iceland 1969; **Resid:** Physical Medicine & Rehabilitation, NYU Med Ctr 1974; **Fellow:** Spinal Cord & Brain Injury Rehab, NYU Med Ctr 1975; **Fac Appt:** Prof PMR, Mount Sinai Sch Med

Schwartz, L Matthew MD [PMR] - **Spec Exp:** Pain-Musculoskeletal; Cancer Rehabilitation; Lymphedema; Head & Neck Cancer; **Hospital:** Chestnut Hill Hosp; **Address:** Montgomery Rehab Assocs, 8601 Stenton Ave, Wyndmoor, PA 19038; **Phone:** 215-233-6226; **Board Cert:** Physical Medicine & Rehabilitation 1992; Pain Medicine 2003; **Med School:** UMDNJ-NJ Med Sch, Newark 1987; **Resid:** Physical Medicine & Rehabilitation, Hosp Univ Penn 1989; Physical Medicine & Rehabilitation, Thos Jefferson Univ Hosp 1991; **Fac Appt:** Asst Clin Prof PMR, Univ Pennsylvania

Physical Medicine & Rehabilitation

Stubblefield, Michael Dean MD [PMR] - **Spec Exp:** Cancer Rehabilitation; Pain-Cancer; Pain-Neuropathic; Pain-Musculoskeletal; **Hospital:** Meml Sloan-Kettering Cancer Ctr; **Address:** 515 Madison Ave, Fl 5th Floor, Meml Sloan-Kettering Cancer Ctr, Outpatient Rehabilitation Ctr, New York, NY 10022; **Phone:** 646-888-1936; **Board Cert:** Internal Medicine 2001; Physical Medicine & Rehabilitation 2002; Electrodiagnostic Medicine 2003; **Med School:** Columbia P&S 1996; **Resid:** Internal Medicine, Columbia Presby Med Ctr 2001; Physical Medicine & Rehabilitation, Columbia Presby Med Ctr 2001; **Fac Appt:** Asst Prof PMR, Cornell Univ-Weill Med Coll

Southeast

Alexander, Joshua MD [PMR] - **Spec Exp:** Pediatric Rehabilitation; Cerebral Palsy; Spina Bifida; **Hospital:** NC Memorial Hosp - UNC; **Address:** UNC- Physical Med & Rehab, 101 Manning Drive, Campus Box 7200, Chapel Hill, NC 27599-7200; **Phone:** 919-966-5165; **Board Cert:** Pediatrics 2010; Physical Medicine & Rehabilitation 2006; Pediatric Rehabilitation Medicine 2005; **Med School:** Temple Univ 1990; **Resid:** Pediatrics, Baylor Coll of Med 1995; Physical Medicine & Rehabilitation, Baylor Coll of Med 1995; **Fac Appt:** Assoc Prof PMR, Univ NC Sch Med

Cardenas, Diana D MD [PMR] - **Spec Exp:** Spinal Cord Injury; Spina Bifida; Neurogenic Bladder; Urinary Tract Infections; **Hospital:** Univ of Miami Hosp & Clins/Sylvester Comp Canc Ctr (page 73), Jackson Meml Hosp (page 70); **Address:** The Miami Project to Cure Paralysis, U Health, PO Box 016960 (C-206), Miami, FL 33136; **Phone:** 305-243-9516; **Board Cert:** Physical Medicine & Rehabilitation 1977; Electrodiagnostic Medicine 1989; **Med School:** Univ Tex SW, Dallas 1973; **Resid:** Physical Medicine & Rehabilitation, Univ Wash Affil Hosps 1976; **Fac Appt:** Prof PMR, Univ Miami Sch Med

Creamer, Michael DO [PMR] - **Spec Exp:** Spinal Cord Injury; Pain Management; Electrodiagnosis; **Hospital:** Florida Hosp - Orlando, Orlando Regl Med Ctr; **Address:** 100 W Gore St, Ste 500, Orlando, FL 32826; **Phone:** 407-649-8707; **Board Cert:** Physical Medicine & Rehabilitation 1992; Spinal Cord Injury Medicine 2008; Pain Medicine 2011; **Med School:** Chicago Coll Osteo Med 1987; **Resid:** Physical Medicine & Rehabilitation, Rehab Inst Chicago 1991; **Fac Appt:** Asst Prof Med, Univ Fla Coll Med

Diamond, Paul T MD [PMR] - **Spec Exp:** Neuro-Rehabilitation; Geriatric Rehabilitation; **Hospital:** Univ of Virginia Health Sys; **Address:** Univ of Virginia Hlth Sci Ctr, Dept Rehabilitation, Box 801004, Charlottesville, VA 22908-1004; **Phone:** 434-243-5622; **Board Cert:** Internal Medicine 1989; Physical Medicine & Rehabilitation 2003; **Med School:** Univ VA Sch Med 1986; **Resid:** Internal Medicine, Johns Hospkins Bayview Hosp 1989; Physical Medicine & Rehabilitation, Sinai/Johns Hopkins Hosp 1992; **Fac Appt:** Assoc Prof PMR, Univ VA Sch Med

Gater Jr, David R MD/PhD [PMR] - **Spec Exp:** Spinal Cord Injury; Exercise Physiology; Electrodiagnosis; **Hospital:** Hunter Holmes McGuire VA Med Ctr - Richmond, VCU Med Ctr; **Address:** 1201 Broadrock Blvd, Richmond, VA 23249; **Phone:** 804-675-5000 x6583; **Board Cert:** Physical Medicine & Rehabilitation 2007; Spinal Cord Injury Medicine 2009; Electrodiagnostic Medicine 1998; **Med School:** Univ Ariz Coll Med 1992; **Resid:** Physical Medicine & Rehabilitation, UC Davis Med Ctr 1994; **Fac Appt:** Prof PMR, Va Commonwealth Univ Sch Med

Jackson, Amie B MD [PMR] - **Spec Exp:** Spinal Cord Injury; **Hospital:** UAB Spain Rehab Ctr, Univ of Ala Hosp at Birmingham; **Address:** UAB Spain Rehab Ctr, 619 19th St S, SRC 190, Birmingham, AL 35249-7330; **Phone:** 205-934-3330; **Board Cert:** Physical Medicine & Rehabilitation 1990; **Med School:** Univ Alabama 1984; **Resid:** Physical Medicine & Rehabilitation, Univ Alabama Med Ctr 1987; **Fac Appt:** Prof PMR, Univ Alabama

Kezar, Laura B MD [PMR] - **Spec Exp:** Pain-Back; Pain-Spine; **Hospital:** UAB Spain Rehab Ctr; **Address:** Spain Rehabilitation Ctr, 1717 6th Ave S, Birmingham, AL 35249; **Phone:** 205-934-4179; **Board Cert:** Physical Medicine & Rehabilitation 2006; **Med School:** Emory Univ 1985; **Resid:** Physical Medicine & Rehabilitation, Univ Alabama Hosp 1994; **Fac Appt:** Assoc Prof PMR, Univ Alabama

King Jr, Richard W MD [PMR] - **Spec Exp:** Cancer Rehabilitation; Lymphedema; Soft Tissue Radiation Necrosis; Soft Tissue Radiation Necrosis-Breast; **Hospital:** WellStar Windy Hill Hosp, Well-Star Cobb Hosp; **Address:** HyOx Medical Treatment Ctr, 2550 Windy Hill Rd, Ste 110, Marietta, GA 30067; **Phone:** 678-303-3200; **Board Cert:** Physical Medicine & Rehabilitation 1988; Undersea & Hyperbaric Medicine 2002; **Med School:** Emory Univ 1979; **Resid:** Physical Medicine & Rehabilitation, Emory Univ Hosp 1987; **Fac Appt:** Asst Clin Prof PMR, Emory Univ

Leslie, Donald P MD [PMR] - **Spec Exp:** Brain/Spinal Cord Injury; **Hospital:** Shepherd Ctr - Atlanta; **Address:** Shepherd Center, 2020 Peachtree Rd NW, Atlanta, GA 30309; **Phone:** 404-352-2020; **Board Cert:** Physical Medicine & Rehabilitation 1989; **Med School:** Univ Tenn Coll Med 1972; **Resid:** Internal Medicine, Mayo Clinic 1975; Physical Medicine & Rehabilitation, Emory Univ Hosp 1986

Lipkin, David L MD [PMR] - **Spec Exp:** Geriatric Rehabilitation; Pain-Back; Rheumatology; **Hospital:** Mount Sinai Med Ctr - Miami, Aventura Hosp & Med Ctr; **Address:** 4701 N Meridian Ave, Miami Beach, FL 33140; **Phone:** 305-672-1256; **Board Cert:** Physical Medicine & Rehabilitation 1971; **Med School:** Belgium 1964; **Resid:** Pediatrics, Jersey City Med Ctr 1966; Physical Medicine & Rehabilitation, Bronx Muni Hosp 1969; **Fellow:** Research, Natl Inst Hlth-Einstein Coll Med 1969; **Fac Appt:** Assoc Clin Prof PMR, Univ Miami Sch Med

McKinley, William MD [PMR] - **Spec Exp:** Spinal Cord Injury; **Hospital:** Hunter Holmes McGuire VA Med Ctr - Richmond; **Address:** Ambulatory Care Ctr, 417 N 11th St, Richmond, VA 23298; **Phone:** 804-828-4097; **Board Cert:** Physical Medicine & Rehabilitation 1990; Spinal Cord Injury Medicine 2008; **Med School:** Albany Med Coll 1985; **Resid:** Physical Medicine & Rehabilitation, Med Coll Va 1989; **Fac Appt:** Prof PMR, Va Commonwealth Univ Sch Med

Stewart, Paula JB MD [PMR] - **Spec Exp:** Lymphedema; Brain Tumors; Spinal Cord Tumors; Cancer Rehabilitation; **Hospital:** Healthsouth Lakeshore Rehab Hosp; **Address:** Healthsouth Lakeshore Rehab Hosp, 3800 Ridgeway Drive, Birmingham, AL 35209; **Phone:** 205-868-2347; **Board Cert:** Physical Medicine & Rehabilitation 2006; Spinal Cord Injury Medicine 2000; **Med School:** Univ Minn 1987; **Resid:** Physical Medicine & Rehabilitation, Mayo Clinic 1991

Midwest

Chen, David MD [PMR] - **Spec Exp:** Spinal Cord Injury; **Hospital:** Rehab Inst of Chicago; **Address:** 345 E Superior St, Ste 1146, Chicago, IL 60611; **Phone:** 312-238-1000; **Board Cert:** Physical Medicine & Rehabilitation 1992; Spinal Cord Injury Medicine 2008; **Med School:** Univ IL Coll Med 1987; **Resid:** Physical Medicine & Rehabilitation, Northwestern Med Sch 1991; **Fac Appt:** Asst Prof PMR, Northwestern Univ

Cheville, Andrea L MD [PMR] - **Spec Exp:** Lymphedema; Cancer Rehabilitation; Pain-Cancer; **Hospital:** Mayo Med Ctr & Clin - Rochester; **Address:** Mayo Clinic, Dept Physical Med & Rehab, 200 1st St SW, Rochester, MN 55905; **Phone:** 507-284-2747; **Board Cert:** Physical Medicine & Rehabilitation 2008; Pain Medicine 2004; Hospice & Palliative Medicine 2008; **Med School:** Harvard Med Sch 1993; **Resid:** Physical Medicine & Rehabilitation, UMDNJ Med Ctr 1997; **Fellow:** Pain & Palliative Care, Meml Sloan Kettering Cancer Ctr 1999; **Fac Appt:** Asst Prof PMR, Mayo Med Sch

Physical Medicine & Rehabilitation

Clairmont, Albert C MD [PMR] - **Spec Exp:** Spasticity Management; Electrodiagnosis; **Hospital:** Ohio St Univ Med Ctr; **Address:** 480 Medical Center Drive, Columbus, OH 43210; **Phone:** 614-293-7604; **Board Cert:** Physical Medicine & Rehabilitation 1985; Pediatrics 1985; **Med School:** Jamaica 1974; **Resid:** Pediatrics, Columbus Chldns Hosp 1981; Physical Medicine & Rehabilitation, Ohio St Univ Hosps 1983; **Fac Appt:** Assoc Clin Prof PMR, Ohio State Univ

Colachis III, Samuel C MD [PMR] - **Spec Exp:** Spinal Cord Injury; Electrodiagnosis; **Hospital:** Ohio St Univ Med Ctr; **Address:** 480 Medical Center Drive, Columbus, OH 43210; **Phone:** 614-293-7604; **Board Cert:** Physical Medicine & Rehabilitation 1988; Spinal Cord Injury Medicine 2003; **Med School:** USC Sch Med 1984; **Resid:** Physical Medicine & Rehabilitation, Ohio State Univ Hosps 1987; **Fellow:** Electrodiagnosis, Ohio State Univ Hosps 1988; **Fac Appt:** Assoc Prof PMR, Ohio State Univ

DePompolo, Robert W MD [PMR] - **Spec Exp:** Cancer Rehabilitation; Lymphedema; **Hospital:** St. Mary's Hosp - Rochester MN (Mayo), Mayo Med Ctr & Clin - Rochester; **Address:** Mayo Clinic, Dept Phys Med & Rehab, 200 1st St SW, Rochester, MN 55905; **Phone:** 507-255-3116; **Board Cert:** Physical Medicine & Rehabilitation 1981; **Med School:** Wayne State Univ 1977; **Resid:** Physical Medicine & Rehabilitation, Univ Minnesota Affil Hosp 1980

Dillingham, Timothy R MD [PMR] - **Spec Exp:** Electrodiagnosis; Electromyography; Amputee Rehabilitation; **Hospital:** Froedtert and Med Ctr of WI; **Address:** Dept Physical Med & Rehab, 9200 W Wisconsin Ave, rm 2103, Milwaukee, WI 53226; **Phone:** 414-805-7343; **Board Cert:** Physical Medicine & Rehabilitation 1991; **Med School:** Univ Wash 1986; **Resid:** Physical Medicine & Rehabilitation, Univ Wash Affil Hosps 1990; **Fac Appt:** Prof PMR, Med Coll Wisc

Feldman, Joseph L MD [PMR] - **Spec Exp:** Lymphedema; **Hospital:** Evanston/North Shore Univ Hlth Sys; **Address:** 1000 Central St, Ste 800, Evanston, IL 60201; **Phone:** 847-570-2066; **Board Cert:** Physical Medicine & Rehabilitation 1971; **Med School:** Univ IL Coll Med 1965; **Resid:** Physical Medicine & Rehabilitation, Univ Ilinois Med Ctr 1969; **Fac Appt:** Asst Prof PMR, Northwestern Univ

Frost, Frederick S MD [PMR] - **Spec Exp:** Spinal Cord Injury; Stroke Rehabilitation; Geriatric Rehabilitation; **Hospital:** Cleveland Clin (page 56); **Address:** Cleveland Clinic Fdn, 9500 Euclid Ave, MC S-31, Cleveland, OH 44195; **Phone:** 216-445-2006; **Board Cert:** Physical Medicine & Rehabilitation 1988; Spinal Cord Injury Medicine 2008; **Med School:** Northwestern Univ 1983; **Resid:** Physical Medicine & Rehabilitation, Northwestern Meml Hosp 1987; **Fellow:** Spinal Cord Injury Medicine, Rehab Inst Chicago; **Fac Appt:** Asst Prof PMR, Cleveland Cl Coll Med/Case West Res

Gamble, Gail L MD [PMR] - **Spec Exp:** Lymphedema; Cancer Rehabilitation; **Hospital:** Rehab Inst of Chicago; **Address:** Rehab Inst of Chicago, 345 E Superior St, Ste 1136, Chicago, IL 60611; **Phone:** 312-238-7670; **Board Cert:** Physical Medicine & Rehabilitation 1985; **Med School:** Mayo Med Sch 1979; **Resid:** Physical Medicine & Rehabilitation, Mayo Clinic 1983

Gittler, Michelle S MD [PMR] - **Spec Exp:** Spinal Cord Injury; Amputee Rehabilitation; **Hospital:** Schwab Rehab Hosp, Univ of Chicago Med Ctr; **Address:** 1401 S California Blvd, Chicago, IL 60608; **Phone:** 773-522-5853; **Board Cert:** Physical Medicine & Rehabilitation 2003; Spinal Cord Injury Medicine 2008; **Med School:** Univ IL Coll Med 1988; **Resid:** Physical Medicine & Rehabilitation, Rehab Inst Chicago 1992; **Fac Appt:** Assoc Clin Prof S, Univ Chicago-Pritzker Sch Med

Haig, Andrew MD [PMR] - **Spec Exp:** International Health; Pain-Back & Neck; Electrodiagnosis; **Hospital:** Univ of Michigan Hosp, VA Ann Arbor Healthcare Sys; **Address:** Univ Michigan Spine Program, 325 E Eisenhower, Burlington Bldg - Ste 100, Ann Arbor, MI 48108-3346; **Phone:** 734-763-4200; **Board Cert:** Physical Medicine & Rehabilitation 1987; Pain Medicine 2002; **Med School:** Med Coll Wisc 1983; **Resid:** Physical Medicine & Rehabilitation, Northwestern Univ 1986; **Fac Appt:** Prof PMR, Univ Mich Med Sch

Keen, Mary MD [PMR] - **Spec Exp:** Pediatric Rehabilitation; Spasticity Management; Neurode-velopmental Disability; Autism; **Hospital:** Marianjoy Rehab Hosp, Central DuPage Hosp; **Address:** Marianjoy Rehab Medical Clinic, 26 W 171 Roosevelt Rd, Wheaton, IL 60187; **Phone:** 630-909-7000 x2; **Board Cert:** Physical Medicine & Rehabilitation 1984; Pediatrics 2005; Neurodevelopmental Disabilities 2001; Pediatric Rehabilitation Medicine 2003; **Med School:** Northwestern Univ 1979; **Resid:** Physical Medicine & Rehabilitation, Univ Wash Med Ctr 1983; Pediatrics, Loyola Univ Med Ctr 1990; **Fac Appt:** Assoc Clin Prof Ped, Loyola Univ-Stritch Sch Med

Kirschner, Kristi MD [PMR] - **Spec Exp:** Spina Bifida-Adult; Neuromuscular Disorders; Women's Health/Disabilities; **Hospital:** Schwab Rehab Hosp, Northwestern Meml Hosp; **Address:** Schwab Rehab Hosp, 1401 S California Ave, Chicago, IL 60608; **Phone:** 773-522-5853; **Board Cert:** Physical Medicine & Rehabilitation 1991; **Med School:** Northwestern Univ-Feinberg Sch Med 1986; **Resid:** Physical Medicine & Rehabilitation, Rehab Inst of Chicago/Northwestern Univ 1990; **Fellow:** Clinical Ethics, Maclean Ctr/Univ Chicago 1995; **Fac Appt:** Prof PMR, Northwestern Univ-Feinberg Sch Med

Kuiken, Todd A MD/PhD [PMR] - **Spec Exp:** Amputee Rehabilitation; Prosthesis Control; Gait Disorders; **Hospital:** Rehab Inst of Chicago; **Address:** Rehab Inst of Chicago, 345 E Superior St, rm 1309, Chicago, IL 60611; **Phone:** 312-238-8072; **Board Cert:** Physical Medicine & Rehabilitation 2006; **Med School:** Northwestern Univ 1990; **Resid:** Physical Medicine & Rehabilitation, Rehab Inst Chicago 1995; **Fac Appt:** Assoc Prof PMR, Northwestern Univ

La Ban, Myron M MD [PMR] - **Spec Exp:** Pain-Back; Electromyography; Neuromuscular Disorders; **Hospital:** Beaumont Hosp-Royal Oak; **Address:** 3535 W Thirteen Mile Rd, Ste 437, Royal Oak, MI 48073; **Phone:** 248-288-2237; **Board Cert:** Physical Medicine & Rehabilitation 1967; **Med School:** Univ Mich Med Sch 1961; **Resid:** Physical Medicine & Rehabilitation, Univ Ohio Hosps 1965; **Fac Appt:** Clin Prof PMR, Ohio State Univ

Leonard Jr, James A MD [PMR] - **Spec Exp:** Amputee Rehabilitation; Electrodiagnosis; **Hospital:** Univ of Michigan Hosp; **Address:** Univ Michigan, Dept Physical Med & Rehab, 325 E Eisenhower Pkwy, Ste 100, Ann Arbor, MI 48108; **Phone:** 734-936-7175; **Board Cert:** Physical Medicine & Rehabilitation 1977; **Med School:** Univ Mich Med Sch 1972; **Resid:** Physical Medicine & Rehabilitation, Univ Mich Med Ctr 1975; **Fac Appt:** Clin Prof PMR, Univ Mich Med Sch

Mysiw, W Jerry MD [PMR] - **Spec Exp:** Brain Injury Rehabilitation; **Hospital:** Ohio St Univ Med Ctr; **Address:** 480 Medical Center Drive, Columbus, OH 43210-1245; **Phone:** 614-293-7604; **Board Cert:** Physical Medicine & Rehabilitation 1985; **Med School:** Ohio State Univ 1981; **Resid:** Physical Medicine & Rehabilitation, Ohio State Univ Med Ctr 1984; **Fac Appt:** Assoc Prof PMR, Ohio State Univ

Nieshoff, Edward MD [PMR] - **Spec Exp:** Spinal Cord Injury; Spinal Rehabilitation; **Hospital:** Rehab Inst of Mich; **Address:** Rehab Inst Mich, 261 Mack Ave, Detroit, MI 48201; **Phone:** 313-745-4600; **Board Cert:** Physical Medicine & Rehabilitation 2006; Spinal Cord Injury Medicine 2009; **Med School:** Med Coll OH 1991; **Resid:** Physical Medicine & Rehabilitation, Detroit Med Ctr/Wayne State Univ 1995; **Fac Appt:** Asst Prof PMR, Wayne State Univ

Nobunaga, Austin MD [PMR] - **Spec Exp:** Spinal Cord Injury; Electrodiagnosis; **Hospital:** Univ Hosp - Cincinnati; **Address:** Drake Center, 151 W Galbraith Rd, South Pavillion, Cincinnati, OH 45216; **Phone:** 513-418-2707; **Board Cert:** Physical Medicine & Rehabilitation 1990; Spinal Cord Injury Medicine 2009; **Med School:** Univ Mich Med Sch 1985; **Resid:** Physical Medicine & Rehabilitation, Rehab Inst Chicago 1989

Physical Medicine & Rehabilitation

Press, Joel MD [PMR] - **Spec Exp:** Sports Medicine; Pain-Back; Musculoskeletal Injuries; **Hospital:** Rehab Inst of Chicago; **Address:** Ctr for Spine, Sports & Occup Rehab, 1030 N Clark St, Ste 500, Chicago, IL 60610; **Phone:** 312-238-7767; **Board Cert:** Physical Medicine & Rehabilitation 1989; Sports Medicine 2009; **Med School:** Univ IL Coll Med 1984; **Resid:** Physical Medicine & Rehabilitation, Northwestern Meml Hosp 1988; **Fac Appt:** Assoc Clin Prof PMR, Northwestern Univ

Roth, Elliot MD [PMR] - **Spec Exp:** Stroke Rehabilitation; Neurologic Rehabilitation; Geriatric Rehabilitation; **Hospital:** Rehab Inst of Chicago, Northwestern Meml Hosp; **Address:** Rehab Inst Chicago, 345 E Superior St, Chicago, IL 60611-2654; **Phone:** 312-238-1000; **Board Cert:** Physical Medicine & Rehabilitation 1987; **Med School:** Northwestern Univ 1982; **Resid:** Physical Medicine & Rehabilitation, Northwestern Univ 1985; **Fellow:** Physical Medicine & Rehabilitation, Rehab Inst Chicago 1986; **Fac Appt:** Prof PMR, Northwestern Univ

Sisung, Charles MD [PMR] - **Spec Exp:** Rheumatic Diseases of Childhood; Trauma Rehabilitation; Burn Care; **Hospital:** Rehab Inst of Chicago; **Address:** 345 E Superior St, rm 1158, Chicago, IL 60611; **Phone:** 312-238-1246; **Board Cert:** Pediatrics 2011; Physical Medicine & Rehabilitation 1991; Pediatric Rehabilitation Medicine 2003; **Med School:** Univ Mich Med Sch 1981; **Resid:** Pediatrics, Mott Chldns Hosp/Univ Mich 1984; Physical Medicine & Rehabilitation, Schwab Rehab Hosp 1989; **Fellow:** Pediatric Rheumatology, Univ Chicago Hosps 1991; **Fac Appt:** Asst Prof PMR, Northwestern Univ

Sliwa, James A DO [PMR] - **Spec Exp:** Post Polio Syndrome/Rehabilitation; Multiple Sclerosis; Pain-Back; **Hospital:** Rehab Inst of Chicago; **Address:** Rehab Inst Chicago, 345 E Superior St, rm 1108, Chicago, IL 60611-3015; **Phone:** 312-238-4093; **Board Cert:** Physical Medicine & Rehabilitation 2005; **Med School:** Chicago Coll Osteo Med 1980; **Resid:** Physical Medicine & Rehabilitation, Rehab Institute Chicago 1984; **Fac Appt:** Prof PMR, Northwestern Univ

Smith, Joanne MD [PMR] - **Spec Exp:** Pain-Pelvic; Pain-Back; **Hospital:** Rehab Inst of Chicago, Northwestern Meml Hosp; **Address:** Rehab Inst of Chicago, 345 E Superior St, Ste 1507, Chicago, IL 60611; **Phone:** 312-238-0815; **Board Cert:** Physical Medicine & Rehabilitation 2003; **Med School:** Mich State Univ 1988; **Resid:** Physical Medicine & Rehabilitation, Northwestern Univ 1992; **Fac Appt:** Asst Prof PMR, Northwestern Univ

Volshteyn, Oksana MD [PMR] - **Spec Exp:** Spinal Cord Injury; Amputee Rehabilitation; **Hospital:** Rehab Inst St. Louis, Barnes-Jewish Hosp; **Address:** 4444 Forest Park, Box 8518, St Louis, MO 63108; **Phone:** 314-362-4503; **Board Cert:** Physical Medicine & Rehabilitation 1986; Spinal Cord Injury Medicine 2009; **Med School:** Russia 1976; **Resid:** Physical Medicine & Rehabilitation, Barnes Jewish Hosp 1985; **Fac Appt:** Assoc Prof N, Washington Univ, St Louis

Great Plains and Mountains

Mason, Kristin D MD [PMR] - **Spec Exp:** Neurologic Rehabilitation; Electrodiagnosis; Musculoskeletal Injuries; **Hospital:** Swedish Med Ctr - Englewood; **Address:** Rehab Assocs Colorado, 9025 Grant St, Ste 103, Thornton, CO 80229; **Phone:** 303-286-2888; **Board Cert:** Physical Medicine & Rehabilitation 2003; **Med School:** Baylor Coll Med 1988; **Resid:** Physical Medicine & Rehabilitation, Rehab Inst Chicago 1992

Matthews, Dennis J MD [PMR] - **Spec Exp:** Pediatric Rehabilitation; Brain Injury Rehabilitation; Neuromuscular Disorders; Cerebral Palsy; **Hospital:** Chldn's Hosp - Aurora (CO); **Address:** Chldns Hosp, Dept Rehabilitation, 13123 E 16th Ave, Box 285, Aurora, CO 80045; **Phone:** 720-777-3907; **Board Cert:** Physical Medicine & Rehabilitation 1979; Pediatric Rehabilitation Medicine 2003; Neuromuscular Medicine 2008; **Med School:** Univ Colorado 1975; **Resid:** Physical Medicine & Rehabilitation, Univ Minnesota Hosps 1978; **Fellow:** Research, Univ Minnesota Hosps 1978; **Fac Appt:** Prof PMR, Univ Colorado

Southwest

Currie, Donald M MD [PMR] - **Spec Exp:** Pediatric Rehabilitation; Neuro-Rehabilitation; **Hospital:** Christus Santa Rosa Children's Hosp, Univ Hlth Syst-San Antonio; **Address:** Univ Hospital, 4502 Medical Drive, MS 64-1, San Antonio, TX 78229; **Phone:** 210-358-0500; **Board Cert:** Physical Medicine & Rehabilitation 1978; **Med School:** Univ Tex SW, Dallas 1972; **Resid:** Physical Medicine & Rehabilitation, Baylor Univ Med Ctr 1975; Physical Medicine & Rehabilitation, Univ Washington Affil Hosp 1977; **Fac Appt:** Prof PMR, Univ Tex, San Antonio

Dumitru, Daniel MD/PhD [PMR] - **Spec Exp:** Electrodiagnosis; **Hospital:** Univ Hlth Syst-San Antonio; **Address:** 4502 Med Drive, MS 33-1, San Antonio, TX 78229-3900; **Phone:** 210-358-0770; **Board Cert:** Physical Medicine & Rehabilitation 1984; **Med School:** Univ Cincinnati 1980; **Resid:** Physical Medicine & Rehabilitation, VA Hosp 1983; **Fac Appt:** Prof PMR, Univ Tex, San Antonio

Francisco, Gerard E MD [PMR] - **Spec Exp:** Spasticity Management; Brain Injury Rehabilitation; Stroke Rehabilitation; **Hospital:** TIRR-Inst for Rehab and Research, Meml Hermann Hosp - Texas Med Ctr; **Address:** The Inst of Rehab & Research, 1333 Moursund St, Houston, TX 77030; **Phone:** 713-797-5246; **Board Cert:** Physical Medicine & Rehabilitation 2005; **Med School:** Philippines 1989; **Resid:** Physical Medicine & Rehabilitation, UMDNJ-Univ Hosp 1994; **Fellow:** Physical Medicine & Rehabilitation, Baylor Coll Med 1995; **Fac Appt:** Clin Prof PMR, Univ Tex, Houston

Harris, David K MD [PMR] - **Spec Exp:** Spinal Rehabilitation; Spinal Cord Injury; Pain-Back; Pain-Spine; **Address:** Ctr for Healing & Regenerative Med, 7307 Creekbluff Drive, Austin, TX 78750; **Phone:** 512-614-3300; **Board Cert:** Physical Medicine & Rehabilitation 2004; Pain Medicine 2004; **Med School:** Univ Tex SW, Dallas 1988; **Resid:** Physical Medicine & Rehabilitation, Univ Colorado Hlth Sci Ctr 1992

Ivanhoe, Cindy MD [PMR] - **Spec Exp:** Brain Injury Rehabilitation; Spasticity Management; Movement Disorders; **Hospital:** TIRR-Inst for Rehab and Research, Meml Hermann Hosp - Texas Med Ctr; **Address:** 2211 Norfolk, Ste 220, Houston, TX 77098; **Phone:** 713-942-7300; **Board Cert:** Physical Medicine & Rehabilitation 2003; **Med School:** Mexico 1984; **Resid:** Physical Medicine & Rehabilitation, Univ Illinois Affil Hosp 1992; **Fellow:** Brain Injury, Baylor Coll Med 1993; **Fac Appt:** Assoc Prof PMR, Baylor Coll Med

Kevorkian, Charles G MD [PMR] - **Spec Exp:** Stroke Rehabilitation; Neuromuscular Disorders; Electrodiagnosis; **Hospital:** St. Luke's Episcopal Hosp-Houston; **Address:** Dept Physical Med & Rehab, 6624 Fannin St, Ste 2330, Houston, TX 77030-2335; **Phone:** 713-798-4061; **Board Cert:** Physical Medicine & Rehabilitation 1980; **Med School:** Australia 1972; **Resid:** Physical Medicine & Rehabilitation, Prince Henry Hosp 1976; Physical Medicine & Rehabilitation, Mayo Clinic 1979; **Fac Appt:** Assoc Prof PMR, Baylor Coll Med

King, John C MD [PMR] - **Spec Exp:** Stroke Rehabilitation; Pain-Chronic; Spinal Cord Injury; Electrodiagnosis; **Hospital:** Univ Hlth Syst-San Antonio; **Address:** Dept Rehab Med, 7703 Floyd Curl Drive, MC 7798, San Antonio, TX 78229-3900; **Phone:** 210-358-4253; **Board Cert:** Physical Medicine & Rehabilitation 1987; Spinal Cord Injury Medicine 2000; Pain Medicine 2002; **Med School:** Oral Roberts Sch Med 1983; **Resid:** Physical Medicine & Rehabilitation, Baylor Coll Med 1986; **Fac Appt:** Prof PMR, Univ Tex, San Antonio

Nelson, Maureen R MD [PMR] - **Spec Exp:** Pediatric Rehabilitation; Brachial Plexus Palsy; Electrodiagnosis; **Hospital:** Dell Children's Med Ctr of Central Texas; **Address:** 6811 Austin Center Blvd, Ste 420, Austin, TX 78731; **Phone:** 512-324-2715; **Board Cert:** Physical Medicine & Rehabilitation 1990; Pediatric Rehabilitation Medicine 2003; **Med School:** Univ IL Coll Med 1985; **Resid:** Physical Medicine & Rehabilitation, Univ Tex Hlth Scis Ctr 1989; **Fellow:** Pediatric Rehabilitation Medicine, Alfred I Dupont Inst 1990

Physical Medicine & Rehabilitation

Wilson, Amy J MD [PMR] - **Spec Exp:** Amputee Rehabilitation; Stroke Rehabilitation; **Hospital:** Baylor Inst for Rehabilitation; **Address:** Baylor Institute for Rehabilitation, 909 N Washington Ave, Dallas, TX 75246; **Phone:** 214-820-9300; **Board Cert:** Physical Medicine & Rehabilitation 2007; **Med School:** Univ Tex, Houston 1992; **Resid:** Physical Medicine & Rehabilitation, Baylor Univ Med Ctr 1996

West Coast and Pacific

Herring, Stanley A MD [PMR] - **Spec Exp:** Sports Medicine; Pain-Back; Spinal Rehabilitation; **Hospital:** Harborview Med Ctr; **Address:** 908 Jefferson St Fl 5, Seattle, WA 98104; **Phone:** 206-744-0401; **Board Cert:** Physical Medicine & Rehabilitation 1983; **Med School:** Univ Tex SW, Dallas 1979; **Resid:** Physical Medicine & Rehabilitation, Univ Washington Med Ctr 1982; **Fac Appt:** Clin Prof PMR, Univ Wash

Kraft, George H MD [PMR] - **Spec Exp:** Multiple Sclerosis; Spinal Cord Injury; Electrodiagnosis; **Hospital:** Univ Wash Med Ctr; **Address:** 1959 NE Pacific St, Box 356157, Seattle, WA 98195; **Phone:** 206-598-3344; **Board Cert:** Physical Medicine & Rehabilitation 1969; **Med School:** Ohio State Univ 1963; **Resid:** Physical Medicine & Rehabilitation, UCSF-Moffitt Hosp 1965; Physical Medicine & Rehabilitation, Ohio State Univ Med Ctr 1967; **Fac Appt:** Prof PMR, Univ Wash

Massagli, Teresa L MD [PMR] - **Spec Exp:** Spinal Cord Injury-Pediatric; Brain Injury Rehabilitation-Pediatric; Neuromuscular Disorders; Pediatric Rehabilitation; **Hospital:** Seattle Chldns Hosp, Harborview Med Ctr; **Address:** Seattle Children's Hosp, 4800 Sand Point Way NE, PO Box 50010, MS W6847, Seattle, WA 98145; **Phone:** 206-987-2180; **Board Cert:** Pediatrics 1987; Physical Medicine & Rehabilitation 2009; Spinal Cord Injury Medicine 2008; Pediatric Rehabilitation Medicine 2009; **Med School:** Yale Univ 1982; **Resid:** Pediatrics, Yale-New Haven Hosp 1985; **Fellow:** Physical Medicine & Rehabilitation, Univ Washington Med Ctr 1988; **Fac Appt:** Prof PMR, Univ Wash

Robinson, Lawrence R MD [PMR] - **Spec Exp:** Electrodiagnosis; Electromyography; Botox Therapy; **Hospital:** Harborview Med Ctr, Univ Wash Med Ctr; **Address:** Harborview Medical Ctr, Phys Med & Rehab, 325 Ninth Ave, Maleng Bldg, Box 359859, Seattle, WA 98104; **Phone:** 206-744-5862; **Board Cert:** Physical Medicine & Rehabilitation 1987; **Med School:** Baylor Coll Med 1982; **Resid:** Physical Medicine & Rehabilitation, Northwestern Meml Hosp 1985; **Fac Appt:** Prof PMR, Univ Wash

Saal, Jeffrey A MD [PMR] - **Spec Exp:** Pain-Lower Back (IDET procedure); Spinal Rehabilitation; Sports Medicine; **Address:** 500 Arguello St, Ste 100, Redwood City, CA 94063; **Phone:** 650-851-4900; **Board Cert:** Internal Medicine 1978; Physical Medicine & Rehabilitation 1982; **Med School:** Tulane Univ 1975; **Resid:** Internal Medicine, VA Med Ctr 1978; Physical Medicine & Rehabilitation, Stanford Univ Affil Hosps 1981; **Fac Appt:** Assoc Clin Prof PMR, UC Irvine

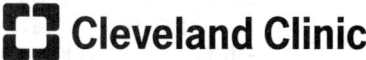

Cleveland Clinic

Every life deserves world class care.

Physical Medicine & Rehabilitation

Comprehensive rehabilitation programs can help patients regain lost skills, improve function, relearn tasks and maximize independence. The Cleveland Clinic Department of Physical Medicine & Rehabilitation, part of the Cleveland Clinic Neurological Institute, engages innovative treatments through disease-specific physician evaluations combined with physical, occupational and speech therapy programs.

Our physician faculty members serve as medical directors to nearly 100 acute inpatient rehabilitation beds throughout Greater Cleveland. Consulting services are provided to inpatient, outpatient and sub-acute settings. Patients benefit from rapid access to Cleveland Clinic medical and surgical specialists.

Our senior therapists have achieved certifications and qualifications in more than a dozen subspecialties. Advanced staff training and certification in Neuro-Developmental Treatment (NDT) offers special benefits for our patients with disorders such as stroke. Cleveland Clinic has more NDT-trained therapists than any other center in the region.

Primary conditions we see:
- Stroke, brain tumors and aneurysms
- Brain injury
- Orthopedic conditions
- Back and neck pain
- Spinal cord injury
- Cancer
- Parkinson's disease
- Organ transplant
- Cardiac disorders
- MS and transverse myelitis
- Vestibular Rehabilitation
- Osteoporosis Rehabilitation
- Falls and Injury Prevention

clevelandclinic.org/
rehabtopdocs

Offering Same-Day Appointments
Call 800.274.2009.

Treatment Guides
Cleveland Clinic has developed comprehensive treatment guides for many diseases and conditions. To download our free treatment guides, visit clevelandclinic.org/treatmentguides.

Online Medical Second Opinion
Cleveland Clinic's My**Consult** Online Medical Second Opinion program securely connects patients to our physician specialists for more than 1,000 life-changing or life-threatening diagnoses all by the click of a mouse. To learn more, log onto eclevelandclinic.org/myconsult or call 800.223.2273, ext. 43223.

Special Assistance for Out-of-State Patients
Cleveland Clinic Global Patient Services offers a complimentary Medical Concierge service for patients who travel from outside of Ohio. Call 800.223.2273, ext. 55580 or email medicalconcierge@ccf.org.

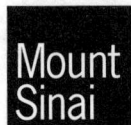
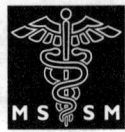

Mount Sinai

MSSM

MOUNT SINAI
SCHOOL OF
MEDICINE

THE MOUNT SINAI MEDICAL CENTER
REHABILITATION MEDICINE

One Gustave L. Levy Place
Fifth Avenue and 100th Street
New York, NY 10029-6574
Physician Referral: 1-800-MD-SINAI (637-4624)
www.mountsinai.org/rehab

THE DEPARTMENT OF REHABILITATION MEDICINE at Mount Sinai is a Center of Excellence in the delivery of complete care for people with disabilities. A wide range of comprehensive patient care services is available for individuals with spinal cord injuries, brain injuries, and a variety of neuromuscular, musculoskeletal, and chronic conditions. We are accredited by the Commission on Accreditation of Rehabilitation Facilities (CARF) for our inpatient spinal cord and brain injury programs—the only such accredited programs at non-VA hospitals in New York City—as well as for our comprehensive rehabilitation medicine program.

Pivotal to successful rehabilitation, the multidisciplinary team approach at Mount Sinai takes advantage of all areas of expertise to provide the highest quality of coordinated care. Our experienced professionals evaluate each patient and meet regularly to develop and implement individualized treatment plans in partnership with patients and their families. Our goal is to make each individual with a disability maximally self-sufficient and mobile, and able to return to community life.

The Mount Sinai Rehabilitation Center team is led by Kristjan T. Ragnarsson, MD, whose leadership and innovative approach to patient care has had a major impact in the field of rehabilitation medicine. The Center includes physicians, primary rehabilitation nurses, nurse practitioners, and professional staff in physical therapy, occupational therapy, speech therapy, nutrition, social work, psychology, therapeutic recreation, and vocational counseling. Special rehabilitation medicine programs include the following:

- **The Spinal Cord Injury Rehabilitation Program** provides comprehensive care to individuals with spinal cord injuries. This includes a full range of innovative medical and rehabilitation services. For example, our "Do It" program is a unique outpatient program that facilitates community integration.

- **The Brain Injury Rehabilitation Program** provides comprehensive care to individuals with brain injuries. It is well recognized that the treatment of individuals with cognitive and behavioral challenges is critical to community integration. Our program contains specialists uniquely qualified to meet these challenges.

- **The Sports Therapy Center** is a comprehensive outpatient physical and occupational therapy facility offering individualized treatments for people with a variety of musculoskeletal conditions. It is conveniently located in midtown Manhattan.

MODEL SYSTEMS OF CARE

The Department of Rehabilitation Medicine provides comprehensive services that serve as national models of care.

- Consistently ranked among the top rehabilitation centers by *U.S. News & World Report.*

- One of 14 programs designated by the National Institute of Disability and Rehabilitation Research (NIDRR) as a Model System of Care for Spinal Cord Injury, the only such designated program in New York State.

- One of 14 programs designated by NIDRR as a Model System of Care for Traumatic Brain Injury, the only such designated program in New York State.

- The only NIDRR-designated Research and Training Center for Traumatic Brain Injury Intervention.

- The first CDC Injury Control Research Center focusing on traumatic brain injury research.

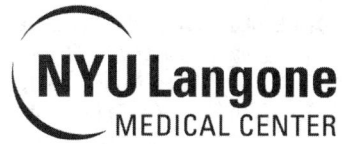

RUSK INSTITUTE OF REHABILITATION MEDICINE
400 East 34th Street *(between 1st Avenue and FDR Drive)*
New York, NY 10016
HJD: 301 East 17th Street *(at 2nd Avenue)*
New York, NY 10003
www.RUSKINSTITUTE.org
Children's Services Access Line: **855-NYU-KIDS**

PEDIATRIC REHABILITATION MEDICINE

Pediatric Rehabilitation is part of the Hassenfeld Pediatric Center, a full service special-ty Children's Hospital, which supports the array of children's health services across the Medical Center where newborns, children, adolescents and young adults receive the most comprehensive and advanced care by a team of pediatricians and pediatric specialists.

About the Pediatric Rehabilitation Program

The Pediatric Rehabilitation Medicine Division is a key component of the Rusk Institute of Rehabilitation Medicine at NYU Langone (Rusk), providing world-class inpatient and outpatient rehabilitation services for children, from birth through early adulthood. Rusk has been ranked the best rehabilitation hospital in New York and among the top ten in the country by U.S. News & World Report for 22 consecutive years. At Rusk, the focus is on early intervention and a family-centered approach that includes sibling and family support groups and counseling.

Areas of Expertise

The pediatric rehabilitation team is particularly skilled in treating the multiple challenges of children with developmental disorders such as cerebral palsy, spina bifida, muscu-lar dystrophy, reflex sympathetic dystrophy, limb deficiencies, arthrogryposis, and spinal cord injuries. Children with traumatic brain injuries, brain tumors, and oncologic diagno-ses (such as bone tumors or musculoskeletal disease) also benefit from our specialized services, as do youngsters affected by stroke or cerebrovascular accidents, viral infec-tions or inflammatory diseases, and rheumatic disease. In addition to inpatient services, we offer extensive outpatient programs for young patients, including physical therapy, occupational therapy, speech therapy, feeding and swallowing, vocational services, psy-chological services, and other specialized therapies.

Spanning the Continuum of Care

Rusk's pediatric outpatient services are delivered at NYU Langone Medical Center's Hos-pital for Joint Diseases. Moreover, specialized rehabilitation care for premature infants is provided by the Medical Center's neonatal intensive care unit.

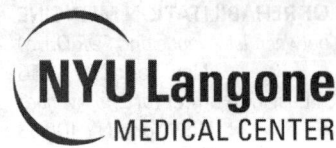

RUSK INSTITUTE OF REHABILITATION MEDICINE
400 East 34th Street *(between 1st Avenue and FDR Drive)*
New York, NY 10016
HJD: 301 East 17th Street *(at 2nd Avenue)*
New York, NY 10003
www.RUSKINSTITUTE.org • 212-263-8830

RUSK INSTITUTE OF REHABILITATION MEDICINE

The Rusk Institute of Rehabilitation Medicine at NYU Langone Medical Center (Rusk) is ranked among the nation's top 10 "Best Hospitals" for the 22nd consecutive year in U.S. News & World Report, as well as #1 rehabilitation program in New York. Rusk is internationally renowned for the treatment of adults and children with disabilities, providing the full continuum of inpatient and outpatient rehabilitation care across all specialties: physical, occupational, speech/swallowing and vocational therapy, psychology, music and recreational therapy, nutrition, nursing, and social work.

Rusk's CARF-Accredited Brain Injury Rehabilitation Program is tailored for patients who have medical, physical, cognitive, and behavioral changes as a result of a brain injury or neurological illness.

The Amputee Program provides specialized limb deficiency rehabilitation to patients who have undergone amputations.

The Joan and Joel Smilow Cardiac and Pulmonary Rehabilitation & Prevention Center offers a model of transitional care for patients with cardiac and lung conditions.

Orthopaedic/Musculoskeletal Rehabilitation is offered for patients with back, neck, hip, elbow and shoulder disorders, arthritis-related joint pain, conditions affecting the bones, tendon, ligaments and muscles, and for pre- and post-surgical patients.

The Spinal Cord Injury program offers a comprehensive, patient-centered array of specialized and innovative clinical and educational programs to optimize quality of life.

Sports Injury Rehabilitation addresses the needs of patients with sports-related conditions, including post-operative rehabilitation for patients who require orthopaedic surgery.

Rusk's CARF-Accredited Stroke Program offers an interdisciplinary team with specialized training in the medical, nursing or therapeutic care and treatment of stroke patients.

Vestibular Rehabilitation addresses the evaluation and treatment of patients suffering from dizziness and imbalance.

The Women's Health Program addresses issues that uniquely affect women, including pelvic floor muscle dysfunction/pain, urinary incontinence, cancer rehabilitation and lymphedema, and prenatal and postpartum musculoskeletal conditions.

Chest Physical Therapy cares for individuals with lung congestion, secretion retention or areas of lung collapse.

The Outpatient Rehabilitation Psychology Service provides care to patients with neurological and medical conditions on an outpatient basis.

Speech-Language Pathology & Swallowing is dedicated to patients with communication disorders due to neurological problems as well as diagnosis and management of swallowing and feeding disorders.

Vocational Services provides disabled individuals with the competencies needed to return to school or work and to lead a productive life.

Plastic Surgery

A plastic surgeon deals with the repair, reconstruction or replacement of physical defects of form or function involving the skin, musculoskeletal system, craniomaxillofacial structures, hand, extremities, breast and trunk and external genitalia. He/she uses aesthetic surgical principles not only to improve undesirable qualities of normal structures (commonly called "cosmetic surgery") but in all reconstructive procedures as well.

A plastic surgeon possesses special knowledge and skill in the design and surgery of grafts, flaps, free tissue transfer and replantation. Competence in the management of complex wounds, the use of implantable materials, and in tumor surgery is required.

Training Required: Five to seven years

Certification in one of the following subspecialties requires additional training and examination.

Plastic Surgery within the Head and Neck: A plastic surgeon with additional training in plastic and reconstructive procedures within the head, face, neck and associated structures, including cutaneous head and neck oncology and reconstruction, management of maxillofacial trauma, soft tissue repair and neural surgery.

The field is diverse and involves a wide age range of patients, from the newborn to the aged. While both cosmetic and reconstructive surgery are practiced, there are many additional procedures which interface with them.

Surgery of the Hand (see Hand Surgery)

PLASTIC SURGERY

New England

Collins, Dale MD [PlS] - **Spec Exp:** Breast Cancer; Breast Reconstruction; **Hospital:** Dartmouth - Hitchcock Med Ctr; **Address:** Div Plastic Surgery, 1 Medical Center Drive, Lebanon, NH 03756; **Phone:** 603-653-3500; **Board Cert:** Plastic Surgery 2007; **Med School:** Emory Univ 1989; **Resid:** Plastic Surgery, Washington Univ Med Ctr 1994; **Fellow:** Microsurgery, Washington Univ Med Ctr 1995; **Fac Appt:** Prof S, Dartmouth Med Sch

Constantian, Mark B MD [PlS] - **Spec Exp:** Rhinoplasty; Rhinoplasty Revision; Cosmetic Surgery-Face; Breast Surgery; **Hospital:** St. Joseph Hosp & Trauma Ctr, Southern NH Med Ctr; **Address:** 19 Tyler St, Ste 302, Nashua, NH 03060-2951; **Phone:** 603-880-7700; **Board Cert:** Plastic Surgery 1979; **Med School:** Univ VA Sch Med 1972; **Resid:** Surgery, Boston Univ Med Ctr 1976; **Fellow:** Plastic/Reconstructive Surgery, Medical Coll VA 1978

Eriksson, Elof K MD [PlS] - **Spec Exp:** Abdominoplasty; Cosmetic Surgery-Breast; Facial Plastic & Reconstructive Surgery; **Hospital:** Brigham and Women's Hosp (page 57), Children's Hospital - Boston; **Address:** Brigham & Women's Hosp, Div Plas Surg, 75 Francis St, Boston, MA 02115; **Phone:** 617-732-5093; **Board Cert:** Plastic Surgery 1980; **Med School:** Sweden 1969; **Resid:** Surgery, Chicago Affil Hosps 1977; **Fellow:** Plastic Surgery, Med Coll Va 1979; **Fac Appt:** Prof PlS, Harvard Med Sch

Feldman, Joel J MD [PlS] - **Spec Exp:** Cosmetic Surgery-Face & Neck; Burns-Reconstructive Plastic Surgery; Reconstructive Surgery; **Hospital:** Mount Auburn Hosp, Mass Genl Hosp; **Address:** Doctors Office Bldg, 300 Mt Auburn St, Ste 304, Cambridge, MA 02138; **Phone:** 617-661-5998; **Board Cert:** Surgery 1975; Plastic Surgery 1977; **Med School:** Harvard Med Sch 1969; **Resid:** Surgery, Mass Genl Hosp 1974; Plastic Surgery, Johns Hopkins Hosp 1976; **Fac Appt:** Assoc Clin Prof PlS, Harvard Med Sch

Gallico III, G Gregory MD [PlS] - **Spec Exp:** Liposuction & Body Contouring; Rhinoplasty; Abdominoplasty; Breast Surgery; **Hospital:** Mass Genl Hosp, Mass Eye & Ear Infirmary; **Address:** Boston Ctr for Ambulatory Surgery, 170 Commonwealth Ave, Boston, MA 02116; **Phone:** 617-267-5553; **Board Cert:** Plastic Surgery 1982; **Med School:** Harvard Med Sch 1973; **Resid:** Surgery, Mass Genl Hosp 1980; Plastic Surgery, Mass Genl Hosp 1981; **Fellow:** Immunology, Oxford Univ Med Sch 1977; **Fac Appt:** Assoc Clin Prof S, Harvard Med Sch

Meara, John MD/DMD [PlS] - **Spec Exp:** Cleft Palate/Lip; Craniofacial Surgery-Pediatric; **Hospital:** Children's Hospital - Boston; **Address:** Dept Plastic Surgery, 300 Longwood Ave, Enders 1, Boston, MA 02115; **Phone:** 617-355-4401; **Board Cert:** Plastic Surgery 2001; Otolaryngology 1998; **Med School:** Univ Mich Med Sch 1990; **Resid:** Plastic Surgery, Brigham & Womens & The Chldns Hosps 1999; Otolaryngology, Mass Eye & Ear Infirmary 1997; **Fellow:** Craniofacial Surgery, Royal Chldns Hosp 2000; **Fac Appt:** Assoc Prof PlS, Harvard Med Sch

Mulliken, John B MD [PlS] - **Spec Exp:** Pediatric Plastic Surgery; Cleft Palate/Lip; Vascular Malformations; **Hospital:** Children's Hospital - Boston; **Address:** Chldns Hosp, Div Plastic Surgery, 300 Longwood Ave, Hunnewell-1, Boston, MA 02115-5724; **Phone:** 617-355-7686; **Board Cert:** Surgery 1972; Plastic Surgery 1975; **Med School:** Columbia P&S 1964; **Resid:** Surgery, Mass Genl Hosp 1970; Plastic Surgery, Johns Hopkins Hosp 1974; **Fac Appt:** Prof S, Harvard Med Sch

Orgill, Dennis MD [PlS] - **Spec Exp:** Wound Healing/Care; Burns-Reconstructive Plastic Surgery; **Hospital:** Brigham and Women's Hosp (page 57); **Address:** Brigham & Women's Hosp, Dept Plas Surg, 75 Francis St, Boston, MA 02115; **Phone:** 617-732-5456; **Board Cert:** Surgery 2000; Plastic Surgery 1994; **Med School:** Harvard Med Sch 1985; **Resid:** Surgery, Brigham & Women's Hosp 1990; **Fellow:** Plastic Surgery, Brigham & Women's Hosp 1992; **Fac Appt:** Prof S, Harvard Med Sch

Persing, John A MD [PlS] - **Spec Exp:** Craniofacial Surgery; Vascular Malformations; Cosmetic Surgery; **Hospital:** Yale-New Haven Hosp, Yale Med Group; **Address:** Yale Plastic Surgery, 330 Cedar St Boardroom Bldg Fl 3, New Haven, CT 06519-3218; **Phone:** 203-785-2570; **Board Cert:** Plastic Surgery 1985; Neurological Surgery 1986; **Med School:** Univ VT Coll Med 1974; **Resid:** Surgery, Univ Arizona Med Ctr 1976; Neurological Surgery, Univ Virginia Med Ctr 1982; **Fellow:** Plastic Surgery, Univ Virginia Med Ctr 1984; **Fac Appt:** Prof PlS, Yale Univ

Slavin, Sumner MD [PlS] - **Spec Exp:** Breast Reconstruction; Cosmetic Surgery-Face; Liposuction & Body Contouring; **Hospital:** Beth Israel Deaconess Med Ctr - Boston; **Address:** 1101 Beacon St, Ste 7E, Brookline, MA 02446; **Phone:** 617-277-7010; **Board Cert:** Plastic Surgery 1983; **Med School:** Univ VT Coll Med 1973; **Resid:** Surgery, Beth Israel Hosp 1978; Plastic Surgery, NYU Med Ctr 1980; **Fellow:** Hand & Microvascular Surgery, Bellevue Hosp-NYU Med Ctr 1981; **Fac Appt:** Assoc Clin Prof S, Harvard Med Sch

Stadelmann, Wayne K MD [PlS] - **Spec Exp:** Melanoma-Head & Neck; Breast Reconstruction; Breast Augmentation; **Hospital:** Concord Hospital, New London Hosp; **Address:** 246 Pleasant St, Ste 210, MS 03301, Concord, NH 03301; **Phone:** 603-224-5200; **Board Cert:** Plastic Surgery 2009; **Med School:** Univ Chicago-Pritzker Sch Med 1990; **Resid:** Surgery, Univ Chicago Hosps 1994; Plastic Surgery, Univ S Florida/H Lee Moffit Cancer Ctr 1997

Stahl, Richard S MD [PlS] - **Spec Exp:** Abdominal Wall Reconstruction; Chest Wall Reconstruction; Breast Reconstruction; Chest Wall Deformities; **Hospital:** Yale-New Haven Hosp, Hosp of St Raphael; **Address:** 5 Durham Rd, Guilford, CT 06437; **Phone:** 203-458-4440; **Board Cert:** Surgery 2001; Plastic Surgery 1984; **Med School:** Vanderbilt Univ 1976; **Resid:** Surgery, Yale New Haven Hosp 1981; **Fellow:** Plastic Surgery, Emory Univ Med Ctr 1983; **Fac Appt:** Clin Prof S, Yale Univ

Stotland, Mitchell A MD [PlS] - **Spec Exp:** Cleft Palate/Lip; Craniofacial Surgery-Pediatric; Pediatric Plastic Surgery; **Hospital:** Dartmouth - Hitchcock Med Ctr; **Address:** DHMC, Dept Plastic Surgery, 1 Med Ctr Drive, Lebanon, NH 03756-1000; **Phone:** 603-650-8068; **Board Cert:** Plastic Surgery 2000; **Med School:** McGill Univ 1989; **Resid:** Surgery, McGill Univ Med Ctr 1994; Plastic Surgery, UCLA Med Ctr 1997; **Fac Appt:** Assoc Prof S, Dartmouth Med Sch

Sullivan, Patrick K MD [PlS] - **Spec Exp:** Cosmetic Surgery-Face; Cosmetic Surgery-Breast; Rhinoplasty; Eyelid Surgery; **Hospital:** Rhode Island Hosp; **Address:** 235 Plain St, Ste 502, Providence, RI 02905; **Phone:** 401-831-8300; **Board Cert:** Otolaryngology 1985; Plastic Surgery 1989; **Med School:** Mayo Med Sch 1979; **Resid:** Otolaryngology, Univ Colo Hlth Scis Ctr 1984; Plastic Surgery, Rhode Island Hosp 1986; **Fellow:** Craniofacial Surgery, Dr Paul Tessier & Dr Hugo Obwegeser 1987; **Fac Appt:** Assoc Prof PlS, Brown Univ

Plastic Surgery

Mid Atlantic

Ascherman, Jeffrey MD [PlS] - **Spec Exp:** Breast Cosmetic & Reconstructive Surgery; Craniofacial Surgery; Cleft Palate/Lip; Cosmetic Surgery; **Hospital:** NY-Presby/Columbia Univ Med Ctr, NY (page 65), New York Eye & Ear Infirm (page 64); **Address:** 161 Ft Washington Ave, Ste 509, New York, NY 10032-3713; **Phone:** 212-305-9612; **Board Cert:** Plastic Surgery 2007; **Med School:** Columbia P&S 1988; **Resid:** Surgery, Columbia-Presby Med Ctr 1991; Plastic Surgery, Columbia-Presby Med Ctr 1994; **Fellow:** Craniofacial Surgery, Hosp Necke-Enfants Malades 1995; **Fac Appt:** Prof S, Columbia P&S

Aston, Sherrell MD [PlS] - **Spec Exp:** Cosmetic Surgery-Face & Body; Rhinoplasty; Cosmetic Surgery-Breast; Liposuction & Body Contouring; **Hospital:** Lenox Hill Hosp, NYU Langone Med Ctr (page 66); **Address:** 728 Park Ave, New York, NY 10021; **Phone:** 212-249-6000; **Board Cert:** Surgery 1974; Plastic Surgery 1978; **Med School:** Univ VA Sch Med 1968; **Resid:** Surgery, UCLA Med Ctr 1973; Plastic Surgery, NY Univ 1975; **Fellow:** Surgery, Johns Hopkins Hosp 1970; **Fac Appt:** Prof PlS, NYU Sch Med

Attinger, Christopher E MD [PlS] - **Spec Exp:** Limb Surgery/Reconstruction; Diabetic Leg/Foot; Wound Healing/Care; Lower Limb Reconstruction; **Hospital:** Georgetown Univ Hosp; **Address:** Georgetown Univ Hosp-Wound Healing Ctr, 3800 Reservoir Rd NW 1 Bles Bldg, Washington, DC 20007; **Phone:** 202-444-6161; **Board Cert:** Plastic Surgery 1992; **Med School:** Yale Univ 1981; **Resid:** Surgery, Brigham & Women's Hosp 1986; Plastic Surgery, NYU Med Ctr 1989; **Fellow:** Vascular Surgery, Brigham & Women's Hosp 1987; Hand Surgery, NYU Med Ctr 1990; **Fac Appt:** Prof PlS, Georgetown Univ

Baker, Daniel MD [PlS] - **Spec Exp:** Cosmetic Surgery-Face; Reconstructive Surgery-Face; Rhinoplasty; **Hospital:** Lenox Hill Hosp (Manh Eye, Ear & Throat Hosp); **Address:** 65 E 66th St, New York, NY 10065; **Phone:** 212-734-9695; **Board Cert:** Plastic Surgery 1978; **Med School:** Columbia P&S 1968; **Resid:** Surgery, UCSF Med Ctr 1975; Plastic Surgery, NYU Med Ctr 1977; **Fellow:** Head and Neck Surgery, NYU Med Ctr/St Vincents Hosp 1978; **Fac Appt:** Assoc Prof PlS, NYU Sch Med

Baker, Stephen B MD/DDS [PlS] - **Spec Exp:** Craniofacial Surgery/Reconstruction; Facial Trauma/Fractures; Cosmetic Surgery-Face; Cleft Palate/Lip; **Hospital:** Georgetown Univ Hosp, Inova Fairfax Hosp; **Address:** Georgetown Univ-Div Plastic Surgery, 3800 Reservoir Rd NW, PHC-1, Washington, DC 20007; **Phone:** 202-444-9302; **Board Cert:** Plastic Surgery 2002; **Med School:** Univ Pennsylvania 1993; **Resid:** Oral & Maxillofacial Surgery, Hosp Univ Penn 1996; Plastic Surgery, Hosp Univ Penn 2000; **Fellow:** Craniofacial Surgery, Childrens Hosp 2001; **Fac Appt:** Assoc Prof PlS, Georgetown Univ

Bartlett, Scott P MD [PlS] - **Spec Exp:** Craniofacial Surgery/Reconstruction; Cosmetic Surgery-Face; Reconstructive Surgery-Face; Pediatric Plastic Surgery; **Hospital:** Hosp Univ Penn - UPHS (page 68), Chldns Hosp of Philadelphia; **Address:** 3400 Spruce St, 10 Penn Tower, Philadelphia, PA 19104-4227; **Phone:** 215-662-2096; **Board Cert:** Plastic Surgery 1987; **Med School:** Washington Univ, St Louis 1975; **Resid:** Surgery, Mass Genl Hosp 1983; Plastic Surgery, Mass Genl Hosp 1985; **Fellow:** Craniofacial Surgery, Hosp Univ Penn 1986; **Fac Appt:** Prof S, Univ Pennsylvania

Boyajian, Michael J MD [PlS] - **Spec Exp:** Pediatric Plastic Surgery; Craniofacial Surgery; Cleft Palate/Lip; Vascular Malformations; **Hospital:** Chldns Natl Med Ctr; **Address:** 111 Michigan Ave NW, Ste 4W-100, Washington, DC 20010-2978; **Phone:** 202-476-2157; **Board Cert:** Plastic Surgery 1984; **Med School:** NYU Sch Med 1976; **Resid:** Surgery, Univ Colo Med Ctr 1979; Surgery, Univ Cincinnati Hosp 1981; **Fellow:** Plastic Surgery, Brigham & Women's Hosp 1983; Craniofacial Surgery, Chldns Hosp 1983; **Fac Appt:** Asst Prof S, Geo Wash Univ

Bucky, Louis P MD [PlS] - **Spec Exp:** Cosmetic Surgery-Face; Cosmetic Surgery-Breast; Liposuction & Body Contouring; Breast Reconstruction; **Hospital:** Pennsylvania Hosp-UPHS (page 68), Hosp Univ Penn - UPHS (page 68); **Address:** 230 W Washington Square, Ste 101, Philadelphia, PA 19106; **Phone:** 215-829-6320; **Board Cert:** Plastic Surgery 2006; **Med School:** Harvard Med Sch 1986; **Resid:** Surgery, Mass Genl Hosp 1992; Plastic Surgery, Mass Genl Hosp 1994; **Fellow:** Microsurgery, Meml Sloan Kettering Cancer Ctr 1995; Craniofacial Surgery, Miami Chldns Hosp 1996; **Fac Appt:** Clin Prof S, Univ Pennsylvania

Chang, Benjamin MD [PlS] - **Spec Exp:** Hand Surgery; Melanoma; Microsurgery; **Hospital:** Hosp Univ Penn - UPHS (page 68), Chldns Hosp of Philadelphia; **Address:** Univ Penn Med Ctr, Div Plastic Surgery, 10 Penn Tower, 3400 Spruce St, Philadelphia, PA 19104-4306; **Phone:** 215-662-4283; **Board Cert:** Plastic Surgery 2006; Hand Surgery 2006; **Med School:** Harvard Med Sch 1986; **Resid:** Surgery, NYU Med Ctr 1992; Plastic Surgery, NYU Med Ctr 1994; **Fellow:** Hand Surgery, NYU Med Ctr 1995; **Fac Appt:** Assoc Clin Prof S, Univ Pennsylvania

Chiu, David T W MD [PlS] - **Spec Exp:** Hand & Microvascular Surgery; Cosmetic Surgery-Face; Peripheral Nerve Surgery; **Hospital:** NYU Langone Med Ctr (page 66), Lenox Hill Hosp; **Address:** 900 Park Ave, New York, NY 10075; **Phone:** 212-879-8880; **Board Cert:** Plastic Surgery 1982; Hand Surgery 2010; **Med School:** Columbia P&S 1973; **Resid:** Surgery, Barnes Jewish Hosp 1977; Plastic Surgery, Columbia-Presby Med Ctr 1979; **Fellow:** Hand Surgery, NYU Med Ctr 1980; **Fac Appt:** Prof S, NYU Sch Med

Chun, Jin K MD [PlS] - **Spec Exp:** Breast Cosmetic & Reconstructive Surgery; Facial Deformities/Reconstruction; Microsurgery; Body Contouring; **Hospital:** Mount Sinai Med Ctr (page 63); **Address:** Mount Sinai School of Medicine, 5 E 98 St Fl 14, Box 1259, New York, NY 10029-6501; **Phone:** 212-241-9161; **Board Cert:** Plastic Surgery 1993; **Med School:** Univ VA Sch Med 1983; **Resid:** Surgery, Eastern VA Med Coll Affil Hosp 1986; Plastic Surgery, Albany Meml Hosp 1990; **Fellow:** Microsurgery, Micro Surgery Rsrch Ctr 1987; Burn Surgery, Westchester Med Ctr 1988; **Fac Appt:** Assoc Prof PlS, Mount Sinai Sch Med

Cordeiro, Peter G MD [PlS] - **Spec Exp:** Reconstructive Surgery; Breast Reconstruction; Facial Plastic & Reconstructive Surgery; **Hospital:** Meml Sloan-Kettering Cancer Ctr, Lenox Hill Hosp (Manh Eye, Ear & Throat Hosp); **Address:** 1275 York Avenue, New York, NY 10065; **Phone:** 800-525-2225; **Board Cert:** Surgery 2008; Plastic Surgery 1994; **Med School:** Harvard Med Sch 1983; **Resid:** Surgery, New Eng Deaconess Hosp-Harvard 1989; Plastic Surgery, NYU Med Ctr 1991; **Fellow:** Microsurgery, Meml Sloan-Kettering Cancer Ctr. 1992; Craniofacial Surgery, Univ Miami 1992; **Fac Appt:** Prof S, Cornell Univ-Weill Med Coll

Cutting, Court MD [PlS] - **Spec Exp:** Cleft Palate/Lip; Reconstructive Plastic Surgery; Rhinoplasty; Craniofacial Surgery/Reconstruction; **Hospital:** NYU Langone Med Ctr (page 66); **Address:** 333 E 34th St, Ste 1K, New York, NY 10016-6481; **Phone:** 212-447-6229; **Board Cert:** Otolaryngology 1980; Plastic Surgery 1986; **Med School:** Univ Chicago-Pritzker Sch Med 1975; **Resid:** Otolaryngology, Univ Iowa Hosps 1980; Plastic Surgery, NYU Langone Med Ctr 1983; **Fellow:** Craniofacial Surgery, NYU Langone Med Ctr 1984; **Fac Appt:** Prof PlS, NYU Sch Med

Dagum, Alexander B MD [PlS] - **Spec Exp:** Reconstructive Plastic Surgery; Cleft Palate/Lip; Hand Surgery; Microsurgery; **Hospital:** Stony Brook Univ Med Ctr; **Address:** SUNY Health Science Ctr, T19-060, Box 8191, Stony Brook, NY 11794-8191; **Phone:** 631-444-8210; **Board Cert:** Plastic Surgery 2003; Hand Surgery 2004; **Med School:** Canada 1987; **Resid:** Surgery, Univ Ottawa Civic Hosp 1988; Plastic Surgery, Univ Toronto Med Ctr 1993; **Fellow:** Microsurgery, Univ Toronto Med Ctr 1984; Hand Surgery, Stony Brook Univ Hosp 1995; **Fac Appt:** Prof S, SUNY Stony Brook

Dick, Gregory O MD [PlS] - **Spec Exp:** Cosmetic Surgery-Face; Facial Rejuvenation; Cosmetic Surgery-Breast; Liposuction & Body Contouring; **Hospital:** Shady Grove Adven Hosp; **Address:** 9711 Medical Ctr Drive, Ste 100, Rockville, MD 20850; **Phone:** 301-251-2600; **Board Cert:** Plastic Surgery 1989; **Med School:** NY Med Coll 1980; **Resid:** Surgery, New Britain Genl Hosp 1985; Plastic Surgery, Univ Pittsbugh Med Ctr 1987; **Fac Appt:** Clin Prof S, Uniformed Srvs Univ, Bethesda

Disa, Joseph MD [PlS] - **Spec Exp:** Cancer Reconstruction; Breast Reconstruction; Head & Neck Reconstruction; Microsurgery; **Hospital:** Meml Sloan-Kettering Cancer Ctr; **Address:** 1275 York Ave, New York, NY 10065; **Phone:** 212-639-5022; **Board Cert:** Surgery 2005; Plastic Surgery 2009; **Med School:** Univ Mass Sch Med 1988; **Resid:** Surgery, Univ Md Med Ctr 1994; Plastic Surgery, Johns Hopkins Univ 1996; **Fellow:** Reconstructive Microsurgery, Meml Sloan-Kettering Cancer Ctr.; **Fac Appt:** Prof PlS, Cornell Univ-Weill Med Coll

Ducic, Ivica MD/PhD [PlS] - **Spec Exp:** Reconstructive Surgery; Peripheral Nerve Surgery; **Hospital:** Georgetown Univ Hosp; **Address:** Dept of Plastic Surgery, 3800 Reservoir Rd NW Fl 1, 1PHC, Washington, DC 20007; **Phone:** 202-444-8929; **Board Cert:** Plastic Surgery 2004; **Med School:** Croatia 1991; **Resid:** Plastic Surgery, Georgetown Univ Hosp 2002; **Fellow:** Peripheral Nerve Surgery, Inst Peripheral Nerve Surg 2003; **Fac Appt:** Prof PlS, Georgetown Univ

Dufresne, Craig R MD [PlS] - **Spec Exp:** Craniofacial Surgery; Reconstructive Surgery; Cosmetic Surgery-Face; Liposuction & Body Contouring; **Hospital:** Inova Fairfax Hosp, Sibley Mem Hosp; **Address:** 5530 Wisconsin Ave, Ste 1208, Chevy Chase, MD 20815; **Phone:** 301-654-9151; **Board Cert:** Plastic Surgery 1986; **Med School:** Columbia P&S 1977; **Resid:** Surgery, Johns Hopkins Hosp 1982; Plastic Surgery, NYU Med Ctr 1984; **Fellow:** Craniofacial Surgery, NYU Med Ctr 1985; **Fac Appt:** Clin Prof PlS, Georgetown Univ

Fox IV, James W MD [PlS] - **Spec Exp:** Breast Cancer & Surgery; Breast Cosmetic & Reconstructive Surgery; Cosmetic Surgery-Face; Facial Rejuvenation; **Hospital:** Thomas Jefferson Univ Hosp; **Address:** 840 Walnut St Fl 15, Philadelphia, PA 19107; **Phone:** 215-625-6630; **Board Cert:** Plastic Surgery 1978; **Med School:** Jefferson Med Coll 1970; **Resid:** Surgery, Jefferson Hosp 1974; **Fellow:** Plastic Surgery, Univ Virginia Med Ctr 1976; **Fac Appt:** Prof S, Jefferson Med Coll

Glat, Paul M MD [PlS] - **Spec Exp:** Pediatric & Adult Plastic Surgery; Burns-Reconstructive Plastic Surgery; Craniofacial Surgery; Cleft Palate/Lip; **Hospital:** St. Christopher's Hosp for Chldn, Bryn Mawr Hosp; **Address:** 191 Presidential Blvd, Ste 101, Bala Cynwyd, PA 19004; **Phone:** 866-472-6009; **Board Cert:** Plastic Surgery 2009; **Med School:** NYU Sch Med 1988; **Resid:** Surgery, NYU Med Ctr 1994; Plastic Surgery, NYU Med Ctr 1996; **Fellow:** Craniofacial Surgery, Univ Penn 1997; **Fac Appt:** Assoc Prof PlS, Drexel Univ Coll Med

Hidalgo, David MD [PlS] - **Spec Exp:** Cosmetic Surgery-Face; Cosmetic Surgery-Breast; Rhinoplasty; Reconstructive Surgery; **Hospital:** NY-Presby/Weill Cornell Med Ctr, NY (page 65), Lenox Hill Hosp; **Address:** 655 Park Ave, New York, NY 10065; **Phone:** 212-517-9777; **Board Cert:** Plastic Surgery 1987; **Med School:** Georgetown Univ 1978; **Resid:** Surgery, NYU Med Ctr 1983; Plastic Surgery, NYU Med Ctr 1985; **Fellow:** Microsurgery, NYU Med Ctr 1986; **Fac Appt:** Clin Prof S, Cornell Univ-Weill Med Coll

Hoffman, Lloyd A MD [PlS] - **Spec Exp:** Cosmetic Surgery-Face; Liposuction & Body Contouring; Breast Reconstruction; Facial Rejuvenation; **Hospital:** NY-Presby/Columbia Univ Med Ctr, NY (page 65), Lenox Hill Hosp; **Address:** 12A E 68th St, New York, NY 10021; **Phone:** 212-861-1640; **Board Cert:** Plastic Surgery 1989; **Med School:** Northwestern Univ 1978; **Resid:** Surgery, New York Hosp 1983; Plastic Surgery, NYU Med Ctr 1986; **Fellow:** Hand Surgery, NYU Med Ctr 1987; **Fac Appt:** Assoc Prof PlS, Cornell Univ-Weill Med Coll

Hurwitz, Dennis J MD [PlS] - **Spec Exp:** Body Contouring; Cosmetic Surgery-Face; Rhinoplasty; Breast Cosmetic & Reconstructive Surgery; **Hospital:** Magee-Womens Hosp - UPMC; **Address:** 3109 Forbes Ave, Ste 500, Pittsburgh, PA 15213; **Phone:** 412-802-6100; **Board Cert:** Plastic Surgery 2005; **Med School:** Univ MD Sch Med 1970; **Resid:** Surgery, Dartmouth Med Ctr 1975; Plastic Surgery, Univ Pittsburgh Med Ctr 1977; **Fac Appt:** Prof S, Univ Pittsburgh

Imber, Gerald MD [PlS] - **Spec Exp:** Cosmetic Surgery-Face; Eyelid Surgery; **Hospital:** NY-Presby/Weill Cornell Med Ctr, NY (page 65); **Address:** 121A E 83rd St, New York, NY 10028; **Phone:** 212-472-1800; **Board Cert:** Plastic Surgery 1976; **Med School:** SUNY Downstate 1966; **Resid:** Surgery, LI Jewish Med Ctr 1972; Plastic Surgery, NY Hosp 1974; **Fac Appt:** Asst Clin Prof S, Cornell Univ-Weill Med Coll

Leipziger, Lyle S MD [PlS] - **Spec Exp:** Cosmetic Surgery-Face & Eyes; Cosmetic Surgery-Breast; Breast Reconstruction; Liposuction & Body Contouring; **Hospital:** N Shore Univ Hosp, Long Island Jewish Med Ctr; **Address:** 825 Northern Blvd Fl 3, Great Neck, NY 11021; **Phone:** 516-465-8787; **Board Cert:** Plastic Surgery 1994; **Med School:** Cornell Univ-Weill Med Coll 1985; **Resid:** Plastic Surgery, New York Hosp 1990; **Fellow:** Craniofacial Surgery, Johns Hopkins Hosp 1991; **Fac Appt:** Asst Prof S, Albert Einstein Coll Med

Levin, Lawrence Scott MD [PlS] - **Spec Exp:** Toe-to-Hand Transfer; Reconstructive Microvascular Surgery; Microsurgery; **Hospital:** Penn Presby Med Ctr - UPHS (page 68), Pennsylvania Hosp-UPHS (page 68); **Address:** Univ Penn Hlth System-Orth Surgery Dept, 2 Silverstein, 3400 Spruce St, Philadelphia, PA 19104; **Phone:** 215-349-5803; **Board Cert:** Plastic Surgery 1993; Orthopaedic Surgery 2004; Hand Surgery 2004; **Med School:** Temple Univ 1982; **Resid:** Orthopaedic Surgery, Duke Univ Med Ctr 1988; Plastic Surgery, Duke Univ Med Ctr 1989; **Fac Appt:** Prof S, Univ Pennsylvania

Levine, Joshua L MD [PlS] - **Spec Exp:** Breast Reconstruction; Microsurgery; **Hospital:** New York Eye & Ear Infirm (page 64), Montefiore Med Ctr - Div. Weiler; **Address:** 1776 Broadway at 57th St, Ste 1200, New York, NY 10019; **Phone:** 212-245-8140; **Board Cert:** Plastic Surgery 2005; **Med School:** Med Coll GA 1994; **Resid:** Plastic Surgery, Montefiore Med Ctr 2000; Plastic Surgery, Montefiore Med Ctr 2001; **Fellow:** Cosmetic Plastic Surgery, NY Eye & Ear Infirm 2003; Reconstructive Microsurgery, Louisiana State Univ 2004

Little, John W MD [PlS] - **Spec Exp:** Cosmetic Surgery-Face; **Hospital:** Georgetown Univ Hosp, G Washington Univ Hosp; **Address:** 1145 19th St NW, Ste 802, Washington, DC 20036; **Phone:** 202-467-6700; **Board Cert:** Surgery 1975; Plastic Surgery 1977; **Med School:** Harvard Med Sch 1969; **Resid:** Surgery, Case Western Reserve Affil Hosps 1974; Plastic Surgery, Case Western Reserve Affil Hosps 1975; **Fellow:** Plastic Surgery, Jackson Meml Hosp 1977; **Fac Appt:** Clin Prof PlS, Georgetown Univ

Loree, Thom R MD [PlS] - **Spec Exp:** Head & Neck Cancer; Thyroid Cancer; Reconstructive Surgery; Breast Reconstruction; **Hospital:** Erie County Med Ctr; **Address:** Erie County Med Ctr, Dept Plastic/Head & Neck Surgery, 462 Grider St, Buffalo, NY 14215; **Phone:** 716-898-3698; **Board Cert:** Surgery 2010; Plastic Surgery 2004; **Med School:** Geo Wash Univ 1982; **Resid:** Surgery, St Lukes-Roosevelt Hosp 1987; Plastic Surgery, St Lukes-Roosevelt Hosp 1989; **Fellow:** Head & Neck Surgical Oncology, Meml Sloan-Kettering Cancer Ctr 1990; **Fac Appt:** Assoc Prof S, SUNY Buffalo

Losee, Joseph E MD [PlS] - **Spec Exp:** Pediatric Plastic Surgery; Cleft Palate/Lip; Craniofacial Surgery/Reconstruction; **Hospital:** Chldns Hosp of Pittsburgh - UPMC; **Address:** Dept of Pediatric Surgery, 1 Chldn's Hosp Plaza, 4401 Penn Ave Fl 3, Pittsburgh, PA 15224; **Phone:** 412-692-7949; **Board Cert:** Plastic Surgery 2011; **Med School:** Univ Rochester 1994; **Resid:** Plastic Surgery, Strong Meml Hosp 1999; **Fellow:** Pediatric Plastic Surgery, Childrens Hosp 2000; Craniofacial Surgery, Hosp Univ Penn 2000; **Fac Appt:** Assoc Prof S, Univ Pittsburgh

Plastic Surgery

Low, David W MD [PlS] - **Spec Exp:** Microsurgery; Cosmetic & Reconstructive Surgery; Vascular Malformations; Cleft Palate/Lip; **Hospital:** Hosp Univ Penn - UPHS (page 68), Chldns Hosp of Philadelphia; **Address:** Perelman Ctr for Advanced Medicine, 3400 Civic Ctr Blvd, 10 Penn Tower, Philadelphia, PA 19104; **Phone:** 215-662-2040; **Board Cert:** Plastic Surgery 1991; **Med School:** Harvard Med Sch 1980; **Resid:** Surgery, Hosp Univ Penn 1986; **Fellow:** Plastic/Reconstructive Surgery, Hosp Univ Penn 1989; **Fac Appt:** Prof S, Univ Pennsylvania

Mackay, Donald R MD/DDS [PlS] - **Spec Exp:** Pediatric Plastic Surgery; Craniofacial Surgery; Cleft Palate/Lip; Cosmetic Surgery-Face; **Hospital:** Penn State Milton S Hershey Med Ctr; **Address:** MS Hershey Med Ctr Plastic Surgery, 500 University Drive, MC H071, PO Box 850, Hershey, PA 17033; **Phone:** 717-531-8952; **Board Cert:** Plastic Surgery 2006; **Med School:** South Africa 1980; **Resid:** Plastic Surgery, Univ Teaching Hosps 1984; Plastic Surgery, MS Hershey Med Ctr 1995; **Fac Appt:** Prof PlS

Manders, Ernest K MD [PlS] - **Spec Exp:** Facial Nerve Disorders; **Hospital:** UPMC Presby, Pittsburgh, Magee-Womens Hosp - UPMC; **Address:** UPMC Presbyterian, 3601 Fifth Ave, Ste 6B, Pittsburgh, PA 15213; **Phone:** 412-648-9670; **Board Cert:** Surgery 2009; Plastic Surgery 1982; **Med School:** Harvard Med Sch 1972; **Resid:** Surgery, Univ Michigan Med Ctr 1979; Plastic Surgery, Univ Michigan Med Ctr 1981; **Fellow:** Viral Oncology, Natl Insts of Allergy-Infectious Disease 1975; **Fac Appt:** Prof S, Univ Pittsburgh

Manson, Paul MD [PlS] - **Spec Exp:** Facial Trauma/Fractures; Skin Cancer; Reconstructive Surgery; Cosmetic Surgery-Face; **Hospital:** Johns Hopkins Hosp (page 61), Univ of MD Med Ctr; **Address:** 601 N Caroline St, McElderry-8152F, Baltimore, MD 21287; **Phone:** 410-955-9470; **Board Cert:** Plastic Surgery 1979; **Med School:** Northwestern Univ 1968; **Resid:** Surgery, New Eng Deaconess Hosp 1971; Plastic Surgery, Johns Hopkins Hosp 1978; **Fellow:** Surgery, Lahey Clinic 1974; **Fac Appt:** Prof PlS, Johns Hopkins Univ

Matarasso, Alan MD [PlS] - **Spec Exp:** Cosmetic Surgery-Face & Eyes; Rhinoplasty; Liposuction; Abdominoplasty; **Hospital:** Lenox Hill Hosp (Manh Eye, Ear & Throat Hosp); **Address:** 1009 Park Ave, New York, NY 10028-0936; **Phone:** 212-249-7500; **Board Cert:** Plastic Surgery 1986; **Med School:** Univ Miami Sch Med 1979; **Resid:** Surgery, Montefiore Med Ctr 1983; Plastic Surgery, Montefiore Med Ctr 1985; **Fellow:** Plastic Surgery, Manhattan EET Hosp/NYU 1985; **Fac Appt:** Clin Prof PlS, Albert Einstein Coll Med

McCarthy, Joseph G MD [PlS] - **Spec Exp:** Craniofacial Surgery-Pediatric; Reconstructive Surgery-Face; Cosmetic Surgery-Face; **Hospital:** NYU Langone Med Ctr (page 66), Lenox Hill Hosp (Manh Eye, Ear & Throat Hosp); **Address:** 722 Park Ave, New York, NY 10021-4954; **Phone:** 212-628-4420; **Board Cert:** Surgery 1972; Plastic Surgery 1978; **Med School:** Columbia P&S 1964; **Resid:** Surgery, Columbia-Presby Med Ctr 1971; Plastic Surgery, NYU Med Ctr 1973; **Fac Appt:** Prof PlS, NYU Sch Med

Mehrara, Babak J MD [PlS] - **Spec Exp:** Breast Reconstruction; Cancer Reconstruction; Microsurgery; Reconstructive Surgery-Face; **Hospital:** Meml Sloan-Kettering Cancer Ctr; **Address:** 1275 York Ave, New York, NY 10065; **Phone:** 212-639-8639; **Board Cert:** Plastic Surgery 2003; **Med School:** Columbia P&S 1993; **Resid:** Surgery, NYU Med Ctr 1996; Plastic Surgery, NYU Med Ctr 2001; **Fellow:** Microsurgery, UCLA Med Ctr 2002; **Fac Appt:** Assoc Prof S, Cornell Univ-Weill Med Coll

Nahabedian, Maurice Yervant MD [PlS] - **Spec Exp:** Breast Reconstruction & Augmentation; Cosmetic Surgery-Face; Abdominoplasty; **Hospital:** Georgetown Univ Hosp; **Address:** Georgetown Univ Hosp, Dept Plastic Surgery, 3800 Reservoir Rd NW Fl 1PHC, Washington, DC 20007; **Phone:** 202-444-6576; **Board Cert:** Plastic Surgery 2005; **Med School:** UC Irvine 1987; **Resid:** Surgery, UC Irvine Med Ctr 1992; Plastic Surgery, Johns Hopkins Univ Hosp 1995; **Fac Appt:** Assoc Prof PlS, Geo Wash Univ

Napoli, Joseph A MD/DDS [PlS] - **Spec Exp:** Cleft Palate/Lip; Maxillofacial Surgery; Cranio-facial Surgery-Pediatric; Beckwith-Wiedemann Syndrome; **Hospital:** Alfred I duPont Hosp for Children, Wilmington Hosp; **Address:** AI duPont Hosp for Children, Div Plastic Surgery, 1600 Rockland Rd, Wilmington, DE 19803; **Phone:** 302-651-6301; **Board Cert:** Plastic Surgery 2004; **Med School:** Columbia P&S 1987; **Resid:** Oral & Maxillofacial Surgery, Columbia-Presby Med Ctr 1985; Plastic/Reconstructive Surgery, Dartmouth-Hitchcock Med Ctr 2001; **Fellow:** Craniofacial Surgery, Royal Chldns Hosp 2002; Pediatric Plastic Surgery, Royal Chldns Hosp 2002; **Fac Appt:** Asst Prof S, Jefferson Med Coll

Noone, R Barrett MD [PlS] - **Spec Exp:** Breast Reconstruction; Cosmetic Surgery; Skin Cancer; **Hospital:** Bryn Mawr Hosp, Lankenau Hosp; **Address:** 888 Glenbrook Ave, Bryn Mawr, PA 19010-2506; **Phone:** 610-527-4833; **Board Cert:** Surgery 1972; Plastic Surgery 1974; **Med School:** Univ Pennsylvania 1965; **Resid:** Surgery, Hosp Univ Penn 1971; Plastic Surgery, Hosp Univ Penn 1973; **Fac Appt:** Clin Prof S, Univ Pennsylvania

Olding, Michael Joseph MD [PlS] - **Spec Exp:** Breast Reconstruction; Liposuction & Body Contouring; Cosmetic Surgery-Face & Breast; **Hospital:** G Washington Univ Hosp; **Address:** GWU Med Faculty Assocs, 2150 Pennsylvania Ave NW Fl 9, Washington, DC 20037; **Phone:** 202-741-3241; **Board Cert:** Plastic Surgery 1986; **Med School:** Univ KY Coll Med 1980; **Resid:** Surgery, NY Presy Hosp/Weill Cornell 1982; Plastic Surgery, Mcgill Univ Hosps 1985; **Fac Appt:** Prof PlS, Geo Wash Univ

Pitman, Gerald H MD [PlS] - **Spec Exp:** Cosmetic Surgery-Face; Liposuction; Abdominoplasty; **Hospital:** Lenox Hill Hosp (Manh Eye, Ear & Throat Hosp), NYU Langone Med Ctr (page 66); **Address:** 170 E 73rd St, New York, NY 10021; **Phone:** 212-517-2600; **Board Cert:** Plastic Surgery 1978; **Med School:** Univ Pennsylvania 1968; **Resid:** Surgery, Columbia-Presby Hosp 1975; Plastic Surgery, NYU Med Ctr 1977; **Fellow:** Microsurgery, NYU Med Ctr 1981; **Fac Appt:** Clin Prof PlS, NYU Sch Med

Posnick, Jeffrey C MD/DMD [PlS] - **Spec Exp:** Cosmetic Surgery-Face; Craniofacial Surgery/Reconstruction; Maxillofacial Surgery; **Hospital:** Georgetown Univ Hosp; **Address:** 5530 Wisconsin Ave, Ste 1250, Chevy Chase, MD 20815; **Phone:** 301-986-9475; **Board Cert:** Plastic Surgery 1988; **Med School:** Vanderbilt Univ 1979; **Resid:** Surgery, Mass Genl Hosp 1983; Plastic Surgery, Eastern Va Affil HOsp 1986; **Fellow:** Craniofacial Surgery, Hosp Univ Penn/Chldns Hosp 1983; **Fac Appt:** Clin Prof PlS, Georgetown Univ

Price, G Wesley MD [PlS] - **Spec Exp:** Cosmetic Surgery-Face & Breast; Liposuction & Body Contouring; **Hospital:** Sibley Mem Hosp; **Address:** Center for Plastic Surgery, 5550 Friendshop Blvd, Ste 130, Chevy Chase, MD 20815; **Phone:** 301-652-7700; **Board Cert:** Plastic Surgery 1987; **Med School:** Bowman Gray 1977; **Resid:** Surgery, Geo Wash Univ Hosp 1982; Plastic Surgery, NYU Med Ctr 1984; **Fellow:** Facial Plastic & Reconstr Surgery, Univ Miami 1985

Serletti, Joseph M MD [PlS] - **Spec Exp:** Breast Reconstruction; Reconstructive Surgery; Cosmetic Surgery; **Hospital:** Hosp Univ Penn - UPHS (page 68); **Address:** Hosp Univ Penn, Dept Plastic Surgery, 10 Penn Tower, 3400 Spruce St, Philadelphia, PA 19104; **Phone:** 215-662-3743; **Board Cert:** Plastic Surgery 2003; **Med School:** Univ Rochester 1982; **Resid:** Surgery, Strong Meml Hosp 1986; Plastic Surgery, Strong Meml Hosp 1988; **Fellow:** Reconstructive Surgery, Johns Hopkins Hosp 1990; **Fac Appt:** Prof PlS, Univ Pennsylvania

Seyfer, Alan MD [PlS] - **Spec Exp:** Chest Wall Reconstruction; Cleft Palate/Lip; Reconstructive Surgery; Abdominal Wall Reconstruction; **Hospital:** Walter Reed Natl Military Med Ctr; **Address:** USUHS-School of Medicine, 4301 Jones Bridge Rd, Bethesda, MD 20814; **Phone:** 301-295-0441; **Board Cert:** Hand Surgery 1999; Plastic Surgery 1982; **Med School:** Louisiana State U, New Orleans 1973; **Resid:** Surgery, Fitzsimons AMC 1978; Plastic Surgery, Walter Reed AMC 1981; **Fellow:** Hand Surgery, Duke Univ Med Ctr 1980; **Fac Appt:** Prof S, Uniformed Srvs Univ, Bethesda

Silver, Lester MD [PlS] - **Spec Exp:** Cleft Palate/Lip; Pediatric Plastic Surgery; Reconstructive Surgery; **Hospital:** Mount Sinai Med Ctr (page 63); **Address:** 5 E 98th St, Box 1259, New York, NY 10029-6574; **Phone:** 212-241-1968; **Board Cert:** Plastic Surgery 1978; **Med School:** Ros Franklin Univ/Chicago Med Sch 1960; **Resid:** Surgery, Montefiore Med Ctr 1966; Plastic Surgery, Mt Sinai Med Ctr 1969; **Fac Appt:** Prof PlS, Mount Sinai Sch Med

Singh, Navin MD [PlS] - **Spec Exp:** Cosmetic Surgery-Face & Breast; Liposuction & Body Contouring; Abdominoplasty; Facial Rejuvenation; **Hospital:** Sibley Mem Hosp; **Address:** Washington Plastic Surgery, 5454 Wisconsin Ave, Ste 1710, Chevy Chase, MD 20815; **Phone:** 301-244-0277; **Board Cert:** Plastic Surgery 2011; **Med School:** Brown Univ 1993; **Resid:** Surgery, Johns Hopkins Hosp 1997; Plastic/Reconstructive Surgery, Johns Hopkins Hosp 1999; **Fellow:** Craniofacial Surgery, Johns Hopkins Hosp 2000; **Fac Appt:** Asst Prof PlS, Johns Hopkins Univ

Slezak, Sheri MD [PlS] - **Spec Exp:** Breast Reconstruction; Cosmetic Surgery-Breast; **Hospital:** Univ of MD Med Ctr; **Address:** Univ Maryland, Dept Plastic Surgery, 22 S Greene St, rm S8D18, Baltimore, MD 21201; **Phone:** 410-328-2360; **Board Cert:** Plastic Surgery 1991; **Med School:** Harvard Med Sch 1980; **Resid:** Surgery, Columbia-Presby Med Ctr 1985; Plastic Surgery, Johns Hopkins Hosp 1989; **Fac Appt:** Assoc Prof PlS, Univ MD Sch Med

Spence, Robert J MD [PlS] - **Spec Exp:** Burns-Reconstructive Plastic Surgery; Burn Care; Tissue Banking; **Hospital:** Good Samaritan Hosp; **Address:** 5601 Loch Raven Blvd, Baltimore, MD 21239; **Phone:** 443-444-2876; **Board Cert:** Plastic Surgery 1981; **Med School:** Johns Hopkins Univ 1972; **Resid:** Surgery, Johns Hopkins Hops 1974; Surgery, Hershey Med Ctr 1978; **Fellow:** Plastic Surgery, Johns Hopkins Hosp 1980; **Fac Appt:** Assoc Prof S, Johns Hopkins Univ

Spinelli, Henry M MD [PlS] - **Spec Exp:** Cosmetic Surgery-Face; Craniofacial Surgery/Reconstruction; Oculoplastic & Orbital Surgery; Eyelid Surgery/Blepharoplasty; **Hospital:** NY-Presby/Weill Cornell Med Ctr, NY (page 65), Lenox Hill Hosp (Manh Eye, Ear & Throat Hosp); **Address:** 875 Fifth Ave, New York, NY 10021-4952; **Phone:** 212-570-6235; **Board Cert:** Ophthalmology 1987; Plastic Surgery 1993; **Med School:** NYU Sch Med 1981; **Resid:** Ophthalmology, Manhattan EET Hosp 1985; Plastic/Reconstructive Surgery, NYU-Bellevue Hosp 1990; **Fellow:** Craniofacial Surgery, NYU Med Ctr 1991; **Fac Appt:** Clin Prof S, Cornell Univ-Weill Med Coll

Staffenberg, David A MD [PlS] - **Spec Exp:** Craniofacial Surgery/Reconstruction; Pediatric Plastic Surgery; Ear Reconstruction/Microtia; Cosmetic Surgery-Face; **Hospital:** NYU Langone Med Ctr (page 66); **Address:** NYU Med Ctr, 530 First Ave, Ste 8Y, New York, NY 10016; **Phone:** 212-263-8065; **Board Cert:** Plastic Surgery 2009; **Med School:** NY Med Coll 1989; **Resid:** Surgery, Maimonides Med Ctr 1995; Plastic Surgery, Emory Univ Med Ctr 1997; **Fellow:** Craniofacial Surgery, UCLA Med Ctr 1998; **Fac Appt:** Assoc Prof PlS, Albert Einstein Coll Med

Sultan, Mark R MD [PlS] - **Spec Exp:** Breast Reconstruction; Cosmetic Surgery-Breast; Cosmetic Surgery-Face; Liposuction & Body Contouring; **Hospital:** St. Luke's - Roosevelt Hosp Ctr - Roosevelt Div (page 55); **Address:** 1100 Park Ave, New York, NY 10128; **Phone:** 212-360-0700; **Board Cert:** Plastic Surgery 1992; **Med School:** Columbia P&S 1982; **Resid:** Surgery, Columbia-Presby Hosp 1987; Plastic Surgery, Columbia-Presby Hosp 1990; **Fellow:** Head and Neck Surgery, Emory Univ Hosp 1989; **Fac Appt:** Assoc Prof S, Columbia P&S

Tabbal, Nicolas MD [PlS] - **Spec Exp:** Rhinoplasty; Cosmetic Surgery-Face; Eyelid Surgery; **Hospital:** Lenox Hill Hosp (Manh Eye, Ear & Throat Hosp), NYU Langone Med Ctr (page 66); **Address:** 521 Park Ave, rm 1, New York, NY 10021-8140; **Phone:** 212-644-5800; **Board Cert:** Plastic Surgery 1980; **Med School:** Lebanon 1972; **Resid:** Surgery, Am Univ Med Ctr 1976; Plastic Surgery, Akron City Hosp 1979; **Fellow:** Surgery, Upstate Med Ctr 1977; Reconstructive Microsurgery, NYU Med Ctr 1980

Taub, Peter J MD [PlS] - **Spec Exp:** Pediatric Plastic Surgery; Craniofacial Surgery; Cosmetic Surgery; Maxillofacial Surgery; **Hospital:** Mount Sinai Med Ctr (page 63), Westchester Med Ctr; **Address:** Mount Sinai Medical Ctr, 5 E 98th St Fl 14, Box 1259, New York, NY 10029-6574; **Phone:** 212-241-4178; **Board Cert:** Surgery 2009; Plastic Surgery 2003; **Med School:** Albert Einstein Coll Med 1993; **Resid:** Surgery, Mt Sinai Med Ctr 1999; Plastic Surgery, UCLA Med Ctr 2001; **Fellow:** Craniofacial Surgery, UCLA Med Ctr 2002; **Fac Appt:** Assoc Prof PlS, Mount Sinai Sch Med

Thorne, Charles H MD [PlS] - **Spec Exp:** Cosmetic Surgery-Face; Ear Reconstruction/Microtia; Craniofacial Surgery; Rhinoplasty; **Hospital:** NYU Langone Med Ctr (page 66), Lenox Hill Hosp (Manh Eye, Ear & Throat Hosp); **Address:** 812 Park Ave, New York, NY 10021-2759; **Phone:** 212-794-0044; **Board Cert:** Plastic Surgery 1991; **Med School:** UCLA 1981; **Resid:** Surgery, Mass Genl Hosp 1986; Plastic Surgery, NYU Med Ctr 1988; **Fellow:** Craniofacial Surgery, NYU Med Ctr 1989; **Fac Appt:** Assoc Prof PlS, NYU Sch Med

Ting, Jess MD [PlS] - **Spec Exp:** Breast Reconstruction; Cosmetic Surgery; **Hospital:** Mount Sinai Med Ctr (page 63), Mount Sinai Hosp of Queens (page 63); **Address:** 5 E 98th St, Fl 14, Ste B, Box 1259, New York, NY 10029; **Phone:** 212-241-4410; **Board Cert:** Plastic Surgery 2002; Hand Surgery 2003; **Med School:** Columbia P&S 1995; **Resid:** Surgery, Columbia Presby Med Ctr 1998; Plastic Surgery, Univ Pittsburgh Med Ctr 2000; **Fellow:** Hand Surgery, Hosp Special Surgery 2001; **Fac Appt:** Asst Prof S, Mount Sinai Sch Med

Topham, Neal MD [PlS] - **Spec Exp:** Breast Reconstruction; Head & Neck Reconstruction; Reconstructive Surgery; Microsurgery; **Hospital:** Fox Chase Cancer Ctr (page 58); **Address:** Fox Chase Cancer Center, Dept Surgical Oncology, 333 Cottman Ave, C308, Philadelphia, PA 19111; **Phone:** 215-728-2662; **Board Cert:** Plastic Surgery 2005; **Med School:** Case West Res Univ 1994; **Resid:** Surgery, Akron Med Ctr 1998; Plastic Surgery, Case Western Reserve Univ 2000; **Fellow:** Microvascular Surgery, MD Anderson Cancer Ctr 2003; **Fac Appt:** Asst Clin Prof S, Univ Pennsylvania

Tufaro, Anthony P MD/DDS [PlS] - **Spec Exp:** Head & Neck Cancer; Skin Cancer-Head & Neck; Merkel Cell Carcinoma; Craniofacial Surgery/Reconstruction; **Hospital:** Johns Hopkins Hosp (page 61); **Address:** Johns Hopkins Plastic Surgery, 601 N Caroline St Fl 8, Baltimore, MD 21287; **Phone:** 410-955-9846; **Board Cert:** Plastic Surgery 2000; **Med School:** Hahnemann Univ 1993; **Resid:** Surgery, Johns Hopkins Hosp 1995; **Fellow:** Plastic Surgery, Johns Hopkins Hosp 1997; Head and Neck Surgery, Meml Sloan Kettering Cancer Ctr 1999; **Fac Appt:** Assoc Prof S, Johns Hopkins Univ

Vander Kolk, Craig A MD [PlS] - **Spec Exp:** Cosmetic Surgery-Face; Cleft Palate/Lip; Craniofacial Surgery/Reconstruction; Cosmetic Surgery-Breast; **Hospital:** Mercy Med Ctr - Baltimore; **Address:** Cosmetic Medicine at Mercy, 227 St Paul Place Fl 6, Baltimore, MD 21202; **Phone:** 410-332-9700; **Board Cert:** Plastic Surgery 1989; **Med School:** Univ Mich Med Sch 1980; **Resid:** Surgery, Univ Mich Med Ctr 1983; Plastic Surgery, Univ Mich Med Ctr 1986; **Fellow:** Hand Surgery, St Vincents Hosp 1985; Craniofacial Surgery, Chldns Hosp 1987; **Fac Appt:** Prof PlS, Johns Hopkins Univ

Whitaker, Linton A MD [PlS] - **Spec Exp:** Cosmetic Surgery-Face; Craniofacial Surgery-Pediatric; Eyelid Surgery; **Hospital:** Hosp Univ Penn - UPHS (page 68), Chldns Hosp of Philadelphia; **Address:** Hosp Univ Penn-10 Penn Tower, 3400 Spruce St, Philadelphia, PA 19104; **Phone:** 215-662-2048; **Board Cert:** Surgery 1970; Plastic Surgery 1978; **Med School:** Tulane Univ 1962; **Resid:** Surgery, Dartmouth Affl Hosp 1969; Plastic Surgery, Hosp Univ Penn 1971; **Fac Appt:** Prof Emeritus PlS, Univ Pennsylvania

Plastic Surgery

Zide, Barry M MD/DMD [PlS] - **Spec Exp:** Facial Surgery-Chin & Lip; Birthmarks/Heman-giomas; Reconstructive Plastic Surgery; Melanoma; **Hospital:** NYU Langone Med Ctr (page 66), Lenox Hill Hosp; **Address:** 420 E 55th St, Ste 1D, New York, NY 10022-5140; **Phone:** 212-421-2424; **Board Cert:** Plastic Surgery 1981; **Med School:** Tufts Univ 1973; **Resid:** Surgery, Stanford Med Ctr 1976; Plastic Surgery, Univ NC Hosp 1978; **Fellow:** Head & Neck Oncology, Roswell Park Cancer Inst 1979; Craniofacial Surgery, NYU Med Ctr 1980; **Fac Appt:** Prof PlS, NYU Sch Med

Southeast

Allen, Robert J MD [PlS] - **Spec Exp:** Breast Reconstruction; Microsurgery; **Hospital:** Roper Hosp; **Address:** 125 Doughty St, Ste 590, Charleston, SC 29403; **Phone:** 888-890-3437; **Board Cert:** Plastic Surgery 1985; **Med School:** Med Univ SC 1976; **Resid:** Surgery, LSU Med Ctr 1982; Plastic Surgery, LSU Med Ctr 1981; **Fellow:** Microsurgery, NYU Med Ctr 1983; **Fac Appt:** Assoc Clin Prof PlS, Louisiana State U, New Orleans

Argenta, Louis C MD [PlS] - **Spec Exp:** Pediatric Plastic Surgery; Craniofacial Surgery; Wound Healing/Care; **Hospital:** Wake Forest Univ Baptist Med Ctr; **Address:** WFU Bapt Med Ctr, Dept Plastic Surg, Medical Center Blvd, Winston-Salem, NC 27157-1075; **Phone:** 336-716-4171; **Board Cert:** Plastic Surgery 1982; **Med School:** Univ Mich Med Sch 1969; **Resid:** Surgery, Univ Mich Hosp 1977; Plastic Surgery, Univ Mich Hosp 1979; **Fellow:** Craniofacial Surgery, Hosp Foch 1982; **Fac Appt:** Prof PlS, Wake Forest Univ

Beasley, Michael E MD [PlS] - **Spec Exp:** Breast Reconstruction & Augmentation; Liposuction; Body Contouring; Facial Rejuvenation; **Hospital:** Presby Hosp - Charlotte; **Address:** Charlotte Plastic Surgery, 2215 Randolph Rd, Charlotte, NC 28207-1523; **Phone:** 704-372-6846; **Board Cert:** Plastic Surgery 1989; **Med School:** Univ NC Sch Med 1980; **Resid:** Surgery, NC Meml Hosp 1985; Plastic Surgery, Emory Univ Hosp 1987; **Fellow:** Plastic Surgery, St Joseph's Hosp 1987; **Fac Appt:** Clin Prof PlS, Univ NC Sch Med

Burstein, Fernando D MD [PlS] - **Spec Exp:** Craniofacial Surgery-Pediatric; Cosmetic Surgery-Face; Maxillofacial Surgery; Rhinoplasty; **Hospital:** Chldns Hlthcare Atlanta @ Scottish Rite, Northside Hosp; **Address:** Atlanta Plastic Surgery, 975 Johnson Ferry Rd NE, Ste 100, Atlanta, GA 30342; **Phone:** 404-256-1311; **Board Cert:** Otolaryngology 1986; Plastic Surgery 1991; **Med School:** Univ Kansas 1980; **Resid:** Otolaryngology, UCLA Med Ctr 1986; Plastic Surgery, Yale Univ 1988; **Fellow:** Craniofacial Surgery, UCLA Med Ctr 1989; **Fac Appt:** Clin Prof PlS, Emory Univ

Carraway, James Howard MD [PlS] - **Spec Exp:** Oculoplastic Surgery; Cosmetic Surgery-Face; Eyelid Surgery; Breast Surgery; **Hospital:** Sentara Leigh Hosp; **Address:** 5589 Greenwich Rd, Ste 100, Virginia Beach, VA 23462; **Phone:** 757-557-0300; **Board Cert:** Surgery 1972; Plastic Surgery 1974; **Med School:** Univ VA Sch Med 1962; **Resid:** Surgery, Norfolk Med Ctr 1970; Plastic Surgery, Eastern VA Med Ctr 1973; **Fellow:** Plastic Surgery, Glasgow Royal Infirmary 1970; **Fac Appt:** Prof PlS, Eastern VA Med Sch

Cruse, C Wayne MD [PlS] - **Spec Exp:** Burns-Reconstructive Plastic Surgery; Cancer Reconstruction; **Hospital:** Tampa Genl Hosp, H Lee Moffitt Cancer Ctr & Research Inst (page 59); **Address:** 12902 Magnolia Dr, Ste 4035, Tampa, FL 33612; **Phone:** 813-844-8546; **Board Cert:** Plastic Surgery 1981; **Med School:** Univ Louisville Sch Med 1972; **Resid:** Surgery, Univ S Fla Hosp 1977; Plastic Surgery, Univ KY Hosp-Chandler Med Ctr 1979; **Fac Appt:** Prof S, Univ S Fla Coll Med

Davis, Glenn M MD [PlS] - **Spec Exp:** Cosmetic Surgery-Face; Cosmetic Surgery-Breast; Liposuction & Body Contouring; Facial Rejuvenation; **Hospital:** Rex HlthCare, WakeMed-Raleigh Campus; **Address:** 2304 Wesvill Court, Ste 360, Raleigh, NC 27607-2981; **Phone:** 919-785-1220; **Board Cert:** Plastic Surgery 1986; **Med School:** Med Univ SC 1974; **Resid:** Surgery, National Naval Med Ctr 1982; Plastic Surgery, Eastern Va Affil Hosp 1985; **Fac Appt:** Assoc Clin Prof PlS, Univ NC Sch Med

Erdmann, Detlev MD/PhD [PlS] - **Spec Exp:** Body Contouring after Weight Loss; Abdominoplasty; Cosmetic Surgery-Breast; Hand Surgery; **Hospital:** Duke Univ Hosp; **Address:** Duke Univ Medical Ctr, Box 3181, Durham, NC 27710; **Phone:** 919-684-3320; **Board Cert:** Plastic Surgery 2000; Hand Surgery 2003; **Med School:** Germany 1990; **Resid:** Surgery, Univ Heidelberg Affil Hosp 1998; **Fellow:** Plastic Surgery, Univ Heidelberg 2000; Hand Surgery, Univ Heidelberg 2003; **Fac Appt:** Assoc Prof S, Duke Univ

Fix, R Jobe MD [PlS] - **Spec Exp:** Breast Reconstruction; Hand Surgery; Microsurgery; **Hospital:** Univ of Ala Hosp at Birmingham, Children's Hospital - Birmingham; **Address:** Univ of Alabama Hosp, Div Plastic Surg, 1530 3rd Ave S, Ste FOT-1102, Birmingham, AL 35294; **Phone:** 205-801-8500; **Board Cert:** Surgery 2009; Plastic Surgery 1991; Hand Surgery 2001; **Med School:** Univ Nebr Coll Med 1982; **Resid:** Surgery, Valley Med Ctr 1987; Plastic Surgery, Univ Ala Hosp 1989; **Fac Appt:** Prof PlS, Univ Alabama

Georgiade, Gregory S MD [PlS] - **Spec Exp:** Breast Reconstruction; Cleft Palate/Lip; **Hospital:** Duke Univ Hosp; **Address:** Duke Univ Med Ctr, Box 3960, Durham, NC 27710; **Phone:** 919-684-3039; **Board Cert:** Surgery 2001; Plastic Surgery 1981; **Med School:** Duke Univ 1973; **Resid:** Surgery, Duke Univ Med Ctr 1978; Plastic Surgery, Duke Univ Med Ctr 1980; **Fac Appt:** Prof S, Duke Univ

Gregory, Richard O MD [PlS] - **Spec Exp:** Skin Laser Surgery; Cosmetic Surgery-Face; Facial Rejuvenation; Liposuction & Body Contouring; **Hospital:** Florida Hosp Celebration Hlth, Florida Hosp - Orlando; **Address:** 400 Celebration Pl, Ste A320, Kissimmee, FL 34747; **Phone:** 407-303-4250; **Board Cert:** Plastic Surgery 1981; **Med School:** Indiana Univ 1971; **Resid:** Surgery, Duke Univ Med Ctr 1977; Plastic Surgery, Duke Univ Med Ctr 1979; **Fellow:** Hand Surgery, Univ Louisville 1979; **Fac Appt:** Assoc Clin Prof PlS, Univ S Fla Coll Med

Grotting, James S MD [PlS] - **Spec Exp:** Cosmetic Surgery-Face & Body; Cosmetic Surgery-Breast; Breast Reconstruction; Liposuction & Body Contouring; **Hospital:** UAB Highlands Hosp, St. Vincent's Hosp - Birmingham; **Address:** One Inverness Center Pkwy, Ste 100, Birmingham, AL 35242-4865; **Phone:** 205-930-1600; **Board Cert:** Plastic Surgery 1986; **Med School:** Univ Minn 1978; **Resid:** Surgery, Univ Wash Affil Hosp 1983; Plastic Surgery, UCSF Med Ctr 1985; **Fac Appt:** Clin Prof PlS, Univ Alabama

Hagan, Kevin F MD [PlS] - **Spec Exp:** Reconstructive Surgery; Cosmetic Surgery-Breast; Cosmetic Surgery; **Hospital:** Vanderbilt Univ Med Ctr (page 76); **Address:** Vanderbilt Univ Med Ctr, Dept Plastic Surg, D-4207 Medical Center N, Nashville, TN 37232-2345; **Phone:** 615-936-3574; **Board Cert:** Plastic Surgery 1983; **Med School:** Johns Hopkins Univ 1974; **Resid:** Surgery, Med Coll VA Hosps 1979; Plastic Surgery, UCSF Med Ctr 1982; **Fellow:** Microsurgery, Dr Harry Buncke Med Clinic 1980; **Fac Appt:** Assoc Prof PlS, Vanderbilt Univ

Hester Jr, T Roderick MD [PlS] - **Spec Exp:** Cosmetic Surgery-Face; **Hospital:** Emory Univ Hosp, Northside Hosp; **Address:** Paces Plastic Surgery, 3200 Downwood Cir, Ste 640, Atlanta, GA 30327-1610; **Phone:** 404-351-0051; **Board Cert:** Surgery 1973; Plastic Surgery 1980; **Med School:** Emory Univ 1967; **Resid:** Surgery, Emory Affil Hosps 1972; Plastic/Reconstructive Surgery, Emory Affil Hosps 1978; **Fac Appt:** Assoc Prof S, Emory Univ

Plastic Surgery

Hultman, C Scott MD [PlS] - **Spec Exp:** Breast Reconstruction; Burns-Reconstructive Plastic Surgery; Reconstructive Plastic Surgery; Cosmetic Surgery; **Hospital:** NC Memorial Hosp - UNC; **Address:** UNC Div Plastic & Reconstructive Surgery, CB 7195, Chapel Hill, NC 27599-7195; **Phone:** 919-966-2300; **Board Cert:** Surgery 1999; Plastic Surgery 2001; Surgical Critical Care 2002; **Med School:** Univ Pittsburgh 1990; **Resid:** Surgery, Univ NC Hosps 1996; Plastic Surgery, Emory Univ Med Ctr 2000; **Fellow:** Surgical Critical Care, Univ N Carolina 1998; **Fac Appt:** Assoc Prof S, Univ NC Sch Med

Hunstad, Joseph P MD [PlS] - **Spec Exp:** Facial Plastic & Reconstructive Surgery; Body Contouring after Weight Loss; Abdominoplasty; **Hospital:** Carolinas Med Ctr-Univ, Presby Hosp - Charlotte; **Address:** 11208 Statesville Rd, Ste 300, Huntersville, NC 28078; **Phone:** 704-659-9000; **Board Cert:** Plastic Surgery 1989; **Med School:** Mich State Univ 1981; **Resid:** Surgery, Butterworth Hosp 1984; Plastic Surgery, Grand Rapids Area Med Ed Ct 1986; **Fellow:** Reconstructive Microsurgery, MECOM MicSurg Inst 1987

Kelly, Kevin J MD/DDS [PlS] - **Spec Exp:** Craniofacial Surgery; Pediatric Plastic Surgery; Cleft Palate/Lip; Ear Reshaping (Otoplasty); **Hospital:** Vanderbilt Univ Med Ctr (page 76), Vanderbilt Monroe Carrell Jr. Chldn's Hosp (page 76); **Address:** Vanderbilt Univ Med Ctr, Dept Plastic Surgery, D-4207 Med Ctr North, Nashville, TN 37232-2345; **Phone:** 615-322-2350; **Board Cert:** Plastic Surgery 1991; **Med School:** SUNY Downstate 1982; **Resid:** Surgery, Albany Med Ctr 1986; Plastic Surgery, Albany Med Ctr 1988; **Fellow:** Craniofacial Surgery, Johns Hopkins Med Ctr 1989; **Fac Appt:** Assoc Prof PlS, Vanderbilt Univ

Mast, Bruce A MD [PlS] - **Spec Exp:** Breast Cosmetic & Reconstructive Surgery; Body Contouring; Cosmetic Surgery-Face; Hidradenitis-Chronic; **Hospital:** Shands at Univ of FL, North Florida Regl Med Ctr; **Address:** 4340 W Newberry Rd, Ste 203, Gainesville, FL 32607; **Phone:** 352-271-5367; **Board Cert:** Plastic Surgery 2008; **Med School:** UMDNJ-RW Johnson Med Sch 1987; **Resid:** Surgery, Med Coll Virginia Hosp 1993; **Fellow:** Plastic Surgery, Univ Pittsburgh Med Ctr 1995; **Fac Appt:** Assoc Prof PlS, Univ Fla Coll Med

Matthews, David C MD [PlS] - **Spec Exp:** Craniofacial Surgery/Reconstruction; Facial Trauma/Fractures; Cosmetic Surgery-Face; Cleft Palate/Lip; **Hospital:** Carolinas Med Ctr; **Address:** 1719 South Blvd, Ste B, Charlotte, NC 28203-2747; **Phone:** 704-375-2955; **Board Cert:** Plastic Surgery 1983; **Med School:** Univ Cincinnati 1974; **Resid:** Surgery, Hosp Univ Penn 1980; Plastic Surgery, Hosp Univ Penn 1982; **Fellow:** Craniofacial Surgery, Royal Melbourne Hosp 1982; **Fac Appt:** Clin Prof PlS, Univ NC Sch Med

Maxwell, G Patrick MD [PlS] - **Spec Exp:** Cosmetic Surgery-Breast; Cosmetic Surgery-Face; Breast Reconstruction; Liposuction & Body Contouring; **Hospital:** Baptist Hosp - Nashville, Centennial Med Ctr; **Address:** 2020 21st Ave S, Nashville, TN 37212; **Phone:** 615-932-7700; **Board Cert:** Plastic Surgery 1981; **Med School:** Vanderbilt Univ 1972; **Resid:** Surgery, Johns Hopkins Hosp 1976; Plastic Surgery, Johns Hopkins Hosp 1979; **Fellow:** Microsurgery, Davies Med Ctr 1975; **Fac Appt:** Asst Clin Prof PlS, Vanderbilt Univ

McCraw, John MD [PlS] - **Spec Exp:** Breast Reconstruction; **Hospital:** Univ Mississippi Med Ctr; **Address:** Univ Mississippi Med Ctr, Div Plastic Surg, 2500 N State St, Jackson, MS 39216; **Phone:** 601-815-1343; **Board Cert:** Surgery 1972; Plastic Surgery 1974; **Med School:** Univ MO-Columbia Sch Med 1966; **Resid:** Orthopaedic Surgery, Duke U Med Ctr 1969; Surgery, Univ Florida Med Ctr 1971; **Fellow:** Plastic Surgery, Univ Florida Med Ctr 1973; **Fac Appt:** Prof PlS, Univ Miss

Molnar, Joseph MD/PhD [PlS] - **Spec Exp:** Burns-Reconstructive Plastic Surgery; Reconstructive Microvascular Surgery; Hand Surgery; Wound Healing/Care; **Hospital:** Wake Forest Univ Baptist Med Ctr, Moses H Cone Mem Hosp; **Address:** Wake Forest Univ Sch Med, Dept Plastic Surgery, Medical Center Blvd, Winston-Salem, NC 27157-1075; **Phone:** 336-716-4171; **Board Cert:** Plastic Surgery 2005; Hand Surgery 2000; **Med School:** Ohio State Univ 1977; **Resid:** Surgery, Univ Wash Med Ctr 1989; Plastic Surgery, Med Coll VA 1992; **Fellow:** Microsurgery, Med Coll Wisc 1199; Hand Surgery, Med Coll Wisc 1994; **Fac Appt:** Assoc Prof PlS, Wake Forest Univ

Morgan, Raymond F MD [PlS] - **Spec Exp:** Cosmetic Surgery; Laser Surgery; Hand Surgery; **Hospital:** Univ of Virginia Health Sys; **Address:** Univ VA Hlth Sys, Dept Plas Surg, PO Box 800376, Charlottesville, VA 22908; **Phone:** 434-924-2413; **Board Cert:** Plastic Surgery 1983; Hand Surgery 2005; **Med School:** W VA Univ 1976; **Resid:** Surgery, Johns Hopkins Hosp 1980; Plastic Surgery, Johns Hopkins Hosp 1982; **Fellow:** Hand Surgery, Union Meml Hosp; **Fac Appt:** Prof PlS, Univ VA Sch Med

Smith Jr, David J MD [PlS] - **Spec Exp:** Breast Reconstruction; Burns-Reconstructive Plastic Surgery; Reconstructive Surgery; Body Contouring after Weight Loss; **Hospital:** Tampa Genl Hosp; **Address:** USF Dept Plastic Surgery, 2 Tampa General Circle Fl 7, Tampa, FL 33606; **Phone:** 813-259-0842; **Board Cert:** Plastic Surgery 1981; **Med School:** Indiana Univ 1973; **Resid:** Surgery, Grady Hosp 1988; Plastic Surgery, Indiana Univ Med Ctr 1980; **Fellow:** Hand Surgery, Univ Louisville 1979; **Fac Appt:** Prof S, Univ S Fla Coll Med

Smith, Paul D MD [PlS] - **Spec Exp:** Facial Plastic Surgery; Reconstructive Surgery-Face; Breast Reconstruction; **Hospital:** H Lee Moffitt Cancer Ctr & Research Inst (page 59); **Address:** 2 Tampa Genl Cir Fl 7, Tampa, FL 33606-3589; **Phone:** 813-259-0964; **Board Cert:** Plastic Surgery 2002; **Med School:** Univ IL Coll Med 1994; **Resid:** Surgery, Univ IL Med Ctr 1999; **Fellow:** Plastic Surgery, Univ Texas SW Med Ctr 2001; **Fac Appt:** Prof PlS, Univ S Fla Coll Med

Stuzin, James M MD [PlS] - **Spec Exp:** Facial Rejuvenation; Skin Laser Surgery-Resurfacing; Cosmetic Surgery-Face & Neck; Rhinoplasty; **Hospital:** Mercy Hosp; **Address:** 3225 Aviation Ave, Ste 100, Coconut Grove, FL 33133; **Phone:** 305-854-8828; **Board Cert:** Plastic Surgery 1989; **Med School:** Univ Fla Coll Med 1978; **Resid:** Surgery, Univ Wash Affil Hosp 1983; Plastic Surgery, NYU Med Ctr 1986; **Fellow:** Craniofacial Surgery, UCLA Med Ctr 1987

Thaller, Seth R MD/DMD [PlS] - **Spec Exp:** Cosmetic Surgery-Face; Rhinoplasty; Pediatric Plastic Surgery; Reconstructive Plastic Surgery; **Hospital:** Jackson Meml Hosp (page 70), Univ of Miami Hosp (page 72); **Address:** Univ Miami Dept Plastic Surgery, 1120 NW 14th St Fl 4, Miami, FL 33136; **Phone:** 305-243-4500; **Board Cert:** Otolaryngology 1985; Plastic Surgery 1987; **Med School:** Univ Louisville Sch Med 1975; **Resid:** Otolaryngology, Mass Eye & Ear Infirmary 1983; Plastic Surgery, Montefiore Med Ctr 1985; **Fellow:** Craniofacial Surgery, UCLA Med Ctr 1986; **Fac Appt:** Prof PlS, Univ Miami Sch Med

Tobin, Gordon R MD [PlS] - **Spec Exp:** Reconstructive Plastic Surgery; Transplant-Hand; Cosmetic Surgery; Pelvic Reconstruction After Cancer; **Hospital:** Univ of Louisville Hosp, Jewish Hosp; **Address:** 401 E Chestnut St, Ste 710, Louisville, KY 40202; **Phone:** 502-583-8303; **Board Cert:** Plastic Surgery 1978; **Med School:** UCSF 1969; **Resid:** Surgery, Univ Ariz Affil Hosps 1975; Plastic Surgery, Univ Ariz Affil Hosps 1976; **Fellow:** Pediatric Plastic Surgery, Univ Miami 1973; Cosmetic Plastic Surgery, Univ Miami 1973; **Fac Appt:** Prof PlS, Univ Louisville Sch Med

Vasconez, Henry C MD [PlS] - **Spec Exp:** Craniofacial Surgery/Reconstruction; Pediatric Plastic Surgery; Breast Reconstruction; Cosmetic Surgery; **Hospital:** Univ of Kentucky Albert B. Chandler Hosp; **Address:** 740 S Limestone St, Ste E101, Lexington, KY 40536; **Phone:** 859-257-7171; **Board Cert:** Plastic Surgery 1989; **Med School:** Ecuador 1978; **Resid:** Surgery, Cook Co Hosp 1984; Plastic Surgery, Emory Univ Med Ctr 1986; **Fellow:** Craniofacial Surgery, Baylor Med Ctr/International Craniofacial Inst 1987; **Fac Appt:** Prof S, Univ KY Coll Med

Plastic Surgery

Wilhelmi, Bradon J MD [PlS] - **Spec Exp:** Cosmetic Surgery; Hand Surgery; Reconstructive Plastic Surgery; **Hospital:** Norton Hosp, Univ of Louisville Hosp; **Address:** University Surgical Assocs, 401 E Chestnut St, Ste 710, Louisville, KY 40202; **Phone:** 502-583-8303; **Board Cert:** Plastic Surgery 2011; Hand Surgery 2002; **Med School:** Rush Med Coll 1992; **Resid:** Surgery, Northwestern Univ 1996; Plastic Surgery, Univ Texas Med Ctr 1998; **Fellow:** Hand & Microvascular Surgery, Mass General Hosp 1999; **Fac Appt:** Prof PlS, Univ Louisville Sch Med

Wolfe, S Anthony MD [PlS] - **Spec Exp:** Craniofacial Surgery/Reconstruction; Maxillofacial Surgery; Cosmetic Surgery; **Hospital:** South Miami Hosp, Miami Children's Hosp; **Address:** 3100 SW 62nd Ave, Ste 2230, Miami, FL 33155; **Phone:** 305-662-4111; **Board Cert:** Surgery 1973; Plastic Surgery 2003; **Med School:** Harvard Med Sch 1965; **Resid:** Surgery, Peter Bent Brigham Hosp 1972; Plastic Surgery, Jackson Meml Hosp 1974; **Fac Appt:** Assoc Clin Prof PlS, Univ Miami Sch Med

Yu, Jack C MD/DMD [PlS] - **Spec Exp:** Facial Plastic & Reconstructive Surgery; Facial Tumors; Craniofacial Surgery; Cleft Palate/Lip; **Hospital:** Med Coll of GA Hosp and Clin (MCG Health Inc); **Address:** Med College of Georgia Health, Dept Plastic Surgery, HB 5040, 1467 Harper St, Augusta, GA 30912; **Phone:** 706-721-4147; **Board Cert:** Surgery 2003; Plastic Surgery 2004; **Med School:** Univ Pennsylvania 1985; **Resid:** Surgery, Hosp Univ Penn 1991; Plastic Surgery, Hosp Univ Penn 1993; **Fellow:** Craniofacial Surgery, Chldn's Hosp 1994; **Fac Appt:** Prof PlS, Med Coll GA

Midwest

Bauer, Bruce S MD [PlS] - **Spec Exp:** Cleft Palate/Lip; Vascular Birthmarks; Ear Reconstruction/Microtia; Pigmented Lesions; **Hospital:** Highland Park/North Shore Univ Hlth Syst, Children's Mem Hosp -Chicago; **Address:** 501 Skokie Blvd, Northbrook, IL 60062; **Phone:** 847-504-2300; **Board Cert:** Plastic Surgery 1980; **Med School:** Northwestern Univ 1974; **Resid:** Surgery, Northwestern Meml Hosp 1977; Plastic Surgery, Northwestern Meml Hosp 1979; **Fac Appt:** Clin Prof S, Northwestern Univ

Bentz, Michael L MD [PlS] - **Spec Exp:** Pediatric Plastic Surgery; Facial Deformities/Reconstruction; Pediatric Hand Surgery; Reconstructive Surgery; **Hospital:** Univ WI Hosp & Clins, Meriter Hosp; **Address:** Univ Wisconsin Hosp, 600 Highland Ave, CSC, rm G5-361, Madison, WI 53792-3236; **Phone:** 608-263-1367; **Board Cert:** Surgery 2009; Plastic Surgery 1994; **Med School:** Temple Univ 1984; **Resid:** Surgery, Temple Univ Hosp 1989; Plastic Surgery, Univ Pittsburgh Med Ctr 1992; **Fellow:** Research, Univ Pittsburgh 1990; **Fac Appt:** Prof S, Univ Wisc

Billmire, David A MD [PlS] - **Spec Exp:** Cleft Palate/Lip; Reconstructive Plastic Surgery; **Hospital:** Cincinnati Chldns Hosp Med Ctr, Univ Hosp - Cincinnati; **Address:** 3333 Burnet Ave, MC 2020, Cincinnati, OH 45229; **Phone:** 513-636-7181; **Board Cert:** Plastic Surgery 1985; **Med School:** Ohio State Univ 1975; **Resid:** Surgery, Univ Hosp 1982; Plastic Surgery, Univ Hosp 1984; **Fellow:** Craniofacial Surgery, Texas Craniofacial Fdn 1985; **Fac Appt:** Assoc Clin Prof S, Univ Cincinnati

Brandt, Keith E MD [PlS] - **Spec Exp:** Breast Reconstruction; Cancer Reconstruction; Microsurgery; Reconstructive Surgery-Complex; **Hospital:** Barnes-Jewish Hosp, Barnes-Jewish West County Hosp; **Address:** 4921 Parkview Pl, Ste 6G, St Louis, MO 63110-1010; **Phone:** 314-362-7388; **Board Cert:** Surgery 1999; Plastic Surgery 2003; Hand Surgery 2005; **Med School:** Univ Tex, Houston 1983; **Resid:** Surgery, Univ Nebraska Med Ctr 1989; Plastic Surgery, Univ Tennessee 1991; **Fellow:** Hand Surgery, Wash Univ 1992; Microsurgery, Wash Univ 1993; **Fac Appt:** Prof S, Washington Univ, St Louis

Buchman, Steven R MD [PIS] - **Spec Exp:** Pediatric Plastic Surgery; Craniofacial Surgery-Pediatric; Craniofacial Surgery; **Hospital:** Mott Chldns Hosp, Univ of Michigan Hosp; **Address:** Mott Chldns Hosp, 1500 E Med Ctr Drive, rm 7859, Ann Arbor, MI 48109-5219; **Phone:** 734-763-8063; **Board Cert:** Plastic Surgery 2005; **Med School:** Univ VA Sch Med 1985; **Resid:** Surgery, Hosp Univ Penn 1990; Plastic Surgery, Hosp Univ Penn 1992; **Fellow:** Craniofacial Surgery, UCLA Med Ctr 1993; **Fac Appt:** Prof PIS, Univ Mich Med Sch

Cederna, Paul S MD [PIS] - **Spec Exp:** Burns-Reconstructive Plastic Surgery; Cosmetic Surgery-Face; Facial Rejuvenation; Body Contouring; **Hospital:** Univ of Michigan Hosp; **Address:** 2130 Taubman Center, 1500 E Medical Center Drive, Ann Arbor, MI 48109-0340; **Phone:** 734-998-6022; **Board Cert:** Plastic Surgery 2009; **Med School:** Univ Mich Med Sch 1989; **Resid:** Surgery, Univ Iowa Hosp & Clin 1994; **Fellow:** Microsurgery, Univ Iowa Hosp & Clin 1995; Plastic Surgery, Univ Michigan Hosps 1997; **Fac Appt:** Prof PIS, Univ Mich Med Sch

Coleman III, John J MD [PIS] - **Spec Exp:** Cancer Reconstruction; Breast Reconstruction; Head & Neck Surgery; Pediatric Plastic Surgery; **Hospital:** IU Health University Hosp, Riley Hosp for Children; **Address:** 545 Barnhill Dr, Emerson Hall, Ste 232, Indianapolis, IN 46202-5120; **Phone:** 317-274-8106; **Board Cert:** Surgery 1998; Plastic Surgery 1981; **Med School:** Harvard Med Sch 1973; **Resid:** Surgery, Emory Univ Affil Hosp 1978; Plastic Surgery, Emory Univ Affil Hosp 1979; **Fellow:** Surgical Oncology, Univ Maryland Med Ctr 1981; **Fac Appt:** Prof S, Indiana Univ

Gottlieb, Lawrence Jay MD [PIS] - **Spec Exp:** Burn Care; Reconstructive Plastic Surgery; **Hospital:** Univ of Chicago Med Ctr; **Address:** Univ Chicago Hosps, 5841 S Maryland Ave, MC 6035, Chicago, IL 60637-1447; **Phone:** 773-702-6302; **Board Cert:** Plastic Surgery 1986; **Med School:** Penn State Coll Med 1977; **Resid:** Surgery, Yale-New Haven Hosp 1982; Plastic Surgery, LAC-USC Med Ctr 1984; **Fac Appt:** Prof S, Univ Chicago-Pritzker Sch Med

Hammond, Dennis C MD [PIS] - **Spec Exp:** Cosmetic Surgery-Breast; Breast Reconstruction; Body Contouring after Weight Loss; **Hospital:** Spectrum Hlth Blodgett Campus; **Address:** 4070 Lake Drive SE, Ste 202, Grand Rapids, MI 49546; **Phone:** 616-464-4420; **Board Cert:** Plastic Surgery 1994; **Med School:** Univ Mich Med Sch 1985; **Resid:** Surgery, Blodgett Meml Med Ctr 1988; Plastic/Reconstructive Surgery, Grand Rapids Area Med Educ Ctr 1990; **Fellow:** Plastic Surgery, Baptist Hosp 1991; Hand & Microvascular Surgery, Med Coll Wisconsin 1992; **Fac Appt:** Prof PIS, Univ Mich Med Sch

Kirschner, Richard Eugene MD [PIS] - **Spec Exp:** Cleft Palate/Lip; Craniofacial Surgery; **Hospital:** Nationwide Chldn's Hosp; **Address:** Nationwide Chldn's Hosp: Education Bldg, 700 Children's Drive Fl 2nd - Ste 260, Columbus, OH 43205; **Phone:** 614-722-6692; **Board Cert:** Plastic Surgery 2009; Surgery 2006; **Med School:** Univ Miami Sch Med 1989; **Resid:** Surgery, NY-Presby Hosp/Cornell 1995; Plastic Surgery, Univ Penn 1997; **Fellow:** Plastic Surgery, Chldn's Hosp Philadelphia 1997

Kuzon Jr, William M MD/PhD [PIS] - **Spec Exp:** Facial Paralysis Reconstruction; Abdominal Wall Reconstruction; Gender Reassignment Surgery; **Hospital:** Univ of Michigan Hosp, John D. Dingell VA Med Ctr, Detroit; **Address:** 1500 E Med Ctr Drive, 2130 Taubman Ctr, Ann Arbor, MI 48109-0340; **Phone:** 734-998-6022; **Board Cert:** Plastic Surgery 2006; **Med School:** Univ Rochester 1981; **Resid:** Plastic Surgery, Univ Toronto Med Ctr 1990; **Fellow:** Microvascular Surgery, Univ Toronto Med Ctr 1991; Hand & Microvascular Surgery, Univ Pittsburgh Med Ctr 1992; **Fac Appt:** Prof PIS, Univ Mich Med Sch

Plastic Surgery

Lee, Raphael MD [PlS] - **Spec Exp:** Reconstructive Surgery; Trauma-Reconstructive Plastic Surgery; Burns-Reconstructive Plastic Surgery; Nerve Injuries/Surgery; **Hospital:** Univ of Chicago Med Ctr; **Address:** 5841 S Maryland Ave, MC 6035, Chicago, IL 60637; **Phone:** 773-702-6302; **Board Cert:** Plastic Surgery 1989; **Med School:** Temple Univ 1975; **Resid:** Surgery, Univ Chicago Hosp 1981; Plastic Surgery, Mass Genl Hosp 1983; **Fellow:** Research, Harvard Med School 1979; **Fac Appt:** Prof PlS, Univ Chicago-Pritzker Sch Med

MacKinnon, Susan E MD [PlS] - **Spec Exp:** Nerve Surgery & Transplantation; Hand Surgery; Reconstructive Surgery; Peripheral Nerve Surgery; **Hospital:** Barnes-Jewish Hosp; **Address:** Washington Univ Sch Med, 660 S Euclid Ave, Box 8238, St Louis, MO 63110; **Phone:** 314-362-4586; **Med School:** Canada 1975; **Resid:** Surgery, Queens Univ-Kingston 1978; Plastic Surgery, Univ Toronto Med Ctr 1980; **Fellow:** Neurological Surgery, Univ Toronto Med Ctr 1981; Hand Surgery, Union Meml Hosp 1982; **Fac Appt:** Prof S, Washington Univ, St Louis

Marsh, Jeffrey L MD [PlS] - **Spec Exp:** Cleft Palate/Lip; Craniofacial Surgery/Reconstruction; Pediatric Plastic Surgery; **Hospital:** St. John's Mercy Med Ctr - St Louis; **Address:** 621 S New Ballas Rd, Ste 260A, St Louis, MO 63141; **Phone:** 314-251-4772; **Board Cert:** Plastic Surgery 1979; **Med School:** Johns Hopkins Univ 1970; **Resid:** Surgery, UCLA Med Ctr 1975; Plastic Surgery, Univ Va Hosp 1977; **Fellow:** Craniofacial Surgery, Cannisburn Hosp; Craniofacial Surgery, Clinic Belvedere Hosp; **Fac Appt:** Clin Prof PlS, St Louis Univ

Medalie, Daniel A MD [PlS] - **Spec Exp:** Cosmetic Surgery-Breast; Liposuction & Body Contouring; Genital Enhancement; Gender Reassignment Surgery; **Hospital:** MetroHealth Med Ctr; **Address:** MetroHealth Medical Ctr, 2500 MetroHealth Drive, Ste H953, Cleveland, OH 44109; **Phone:** 216-778-4450; **Board Cert:** Plastic Surgery 2010; **Med School:** Cornell Univ 1991; **Resid:** Surgery, Univ Pittsburgh Med Ctr 1995; Plastic Surgery, Univ Pittsburgh Med Ctr 1997; **Fellow:** Research, Mass Genl Hosp 1999; **Fac Appt:** Asst Prof PlS, Case West Res Univ

Miller, Michael J MD [PlS] - **Spec Exp:** Cancer Reconstruction; Breast Reconstruction; Head & Neck Reconstruction; **Hospital:** Ohio St Univ Med Ctr; **Address:** OSU Div of Plastic Surgery, 915 Olentangy River Rd, Ste 2100, Columbus, OH 43212; **Phone:** 614-293-8566; **Board Cert:** Plastic Surgery 1993; **Med School:** Univ Mass Sch Med 1983; **Resid:** Surgery, Berkshire Med Ctr 1987; **Fellow:** Plastic Surgery, Ohio State Univ Med Ctr 1989; **Fac Appt:** Prof S, Ohio State Univ

Mustoe, Thomas A MD [PlS] - **Spec Exp:** Cosmetic Surgery-Face; Cosmetic Surgery-Breast; Rhinoplasty; Body Contouring; **Hospital:** Northwestern Meml Hosp; **Address:** NW Med Faculty Fdn-Plastic Surgery, 675 N St Clair St Fl 19 - Ste 250, Chicago, IL 60611-5975; **Phone:** 312-695-6022; **Board Cert:** Otolaryngology 1983; Plastic Surgery 1987; **Med School:** Harvard Med Sch 1978; **Resid:** Surgery, Brigham & Womens Hosp 1980; Otolaryngology, Mass Eye & Ear Infirm 1983; **Fellow:** Plastic Surgery, Brigham & Womens Hosp 1985; **Fac Appt:** Prof S, Northwestern Univ

Ness, John A MD [PlS] - **Spec Exp:** Cosmetic Surgery-Breast; Facial Plastic Surgery; Abdominoplasty; Cosmetic Surgery-Face; **Hospital:** Maple Grove Hosp; **Address:** 2805 Campus Drive, Ste 485, Plymouth, MN 55441; **Phone:** 763-559-4500; **Board Cert:** Otolaryngology 1992; Plastic Surgery 2009; Facial Plastic & Reconstr Surgery 1996; **Med School:** Univ Minn 1986; **Resid:** Otolaryngology, Loyola Univ Med Ctr 1991; Plastic Surgery, UC Davis Med Ctr 1998; **Fellow:** Facial Plastic & Reconstr Surgery, UC Davis 1993; Craniofacial Surgery, Australian Craniofacial Inst 1996; **Fac Appt:** Asst Clin Prof PlS, Univ Minn

Neumeister, Michael W MD [PlS] - **Spec Exp:** Hand Surgery; Microsurgery; Breast Reconstruction & Augmentation; Cleft Palate/Lip; **Hospital:** Memorial Med Ctr-Springfield; **Address:** SIU Div Plastic Surgery, PO Box 19653, Springfield, IL 62794-9653; **Phone:** 217-545-6314; **Board Cert:** Plastic Surgery 2005; Hand Surgery 2006; **Med School:** Univ Toronto 1988; **Resid:** Surgery, Dalhousie Univ Affil Hosp 1991; Plastic Surgery, Univ Manitoba Affil Hosp 1994; **Fellow:** Microsurgery, Brigham & Womens Hosp; Hand & Microvascular Surgery, Southern Illinois Univ; **Fac Appt:** Prof S, Southern IL Univ

Papay, Francis A MD [PlS] - **Spec Exp:** Craniofacial Surgery/Reconstruction; Maxillofacial Surgery; Cosmetic Surgery-Face; Pediatric Plastic Surgery; **Hospital:** Cleveland Clin (page 56); **Address:** Cleveland Clinic, 9500 Euclid Ave, MC A51, Cleveland, OH 44195; **Phone:** 216-444-6900; **Board Cert:** Plastic Surgery 1994; Otolaryngology 1989; **Med School:** NE Ohio Univ 1983; **Resid:** Otolaryngology, Cleveland Clinic 1989; Plastic/Reconstructive Surgery, Cleveland Clinic 1991; **Fellow:** Craniofacial & Maxillofacial Surgery, Primary Chldns Med Ctr 1992; **Fac Appt:** Assoc Prof S, Cleveland Cl Coll Med/Case West Res

Patel, Pravin K MD [PlS] - **Spec Exp:** Pediatric Plastic Surgery; Craniofacial Surgery; Cleft Palate/Lip; Reconstructive Surgery-Complex; **Hospital:** Children's Mem Hosp -Chicago, Shriners Hosp for Children-Chicago; **Address:** Childrens Memorial Hosp, Div Plastic Surgery, 2300 Childrens Plaza, Box 93, Chicago, IL 60614; **Phone:** 773-327-2440; **Board Cert:** Plastic Surgery 2009; **Med School:** Hahnemann Univ 1985; **Resid:** Surgery, Mayo Clinic 1989; Plastic Surgery, Northwestern Univ 1993; **Fellow:** Craniofacial Surgery, UCLA Med Ctr 1994; **Fac Appt:** Assoc Prof S, Northwestern Univ-Feinberg Sch Med

Polley, John W MD [PlS] - **Spec Exp:** Craniofacial Surgery; Pediatric Plastic Surgery; Maxillofacial Surgery; **Hospital:** Rush Univ Med Ctr; **Address:** Rush Univ Med Ctr, Plastic Surgery, 1725 W Harrison St, Ste 425, Professional Bldg 1, Chicago, IL 60612; **Phone:** 312-563-3000; **Board Cert:** Plastic Surgery 1992; **Med School:** Northwestern Univ 1983; **Resid:** Surgery, Mich State Univ Med Ctr 1986; Plastic Surgery, Mich State Univ Med Ctr 1988; **Fellow:** Craniofacial & Maxillofacial Surgery, Chang Gung Meml Hosp 1989; Pediatric Craniofacial Surgery, Hosp for Sick Chldn 1990; **Fac Appt:** Prof PlS, Rush Med Coll

Puckett, Charles L MD [PlS] - **Spec Exp:** Cosmetic & Reconstructive Surgery; Breast Surgery; **Hospital:** Univ of Missouri Hosp, Columbia Regional Hosp; **Address:** 1 Hospital Drive, Ste M349, Columbia, MO 65212-5276; **Phone:** 573-882-2275; **Board Cert:** Surgery 1972; Plastic Surgery 1977; **Med School:** Wake Forest Univ 1966; **Resid:** Surgery, Duke Univ Med Ctr 1971; Plastic Surgery, Duke Univ Med Ctr 1976; **Fellow:** Hand Surgery, Kleinert Hand Fellowship; **Fac Appt:** Prof S, Univ MO-Columbia Sch Med

Rees, Riley S MD [PlS] - **Spec Exp:** Wound Healing/Care; Melanoma; **Hospital:** Univ of Michigan Hosp, VA Ann Arbor Healthcare Sys; **Address:** 2130 Taubman, 1500 E Med Ctr Drive, Ann Arbor, MI 48109-0340; **Phone:** 734-998-6022; **Board Cert:** Plastic Surgery 1981; **Med School:** Univ Utah 1973; **Resid:** Surgery, LSU Med Ctr 1978; Plastic Surgery, Vanderbilt Univ Med Ctr 1980; **Fac Appt:** Prof S, Univ Mich Med Sch

Sanger, James R MD [PlS] - **Spec Exp:** Reconstructive Surgery; Hand Surgery; Microsurgery; **Hospital:** Froedtert and Med Ctr of WI, Chldns Hosp - Wisconsin; **Address:** 8700 Watertown Plank Rd, Dept Plastic Surg, Milwaukee, WI 53226-3595; **Phone:** 414-805-5451; **Board Cert:** Plastic Surgery 1982; Hand Surgery 2009; **Med School:** Univ Wisc 1974; **Resid:** Surgery, LAC-Harbor UCLA Med Ctr 1979; Plastic Surgery, Med Coll Wisc Affil Hosps 1981; **Fellow:** Hand Surgery, Med Coll Wisc Affil Hosps 1982; **Fac Appt:** Prof PlS, Med Coll Wisc

Plastic Surgery

Siebert, John W MD [PIS] - **Spec Exp:** Facial Plastic & Reconstructive Surgery; Microsurgery; Cosmetic Surgery-Face; **Hospital:** Univ WI Hosp & Clins, New York Eye & Ear Infirm (page 64); **Address:** UW Hospital and Clinics, Div of Plastic & Reconstructive Surgery, 600 Highland Ave, Madison, WI 53792; **Phone:** 212-737-8300; **Board Cert:** Plastic Surgery 1991; **Med School:** Univ Wisc 1981; **Resid:** Surgery, Mass Genl Hosp 1986; Plastic Surgery, NYU Med Ctr 1988; **Fellow:** Microsurgery, NYU Med Ctr 1989; **Fac Appt:** Assoc Prof S, Univ Wisc

Siemionow, Maria MD/PhD [PIS] - **Spec Exp:** Microsurgery; Peripheral Nerve Surgery; Reconstructive Plastic Surgery; Transplant-Face; **Hospital:** Cleveland Clin (page 56); **Address:** Cleveland Clin Fdn, 9500 Euclid Ave, Desk A60, Cleveland, OH 44195; **Phone:** 216-445-2405; **Med School:** Poland 1974; **Resid:** Surgery, Inst Orth & Rehab Med; **Fellow:** Plastic Surgery, Univ Hosp; Microsurgery, Univ Louisville Hosp

Sood, Rajiv MD [PIS] - **Spec Exp:** Burns-Reconstructive Plastic Surgery; Pediatric Hand Surgery; Breast Cosmetic & Reconstructive Surgery; Body Contouring after Weight Loss; **Hospital:** IU Health University Hosp, Riley Hosp for Children; **Address:** Richard Fairbanks Burn Center, 1001 W 10th St, Dunlap Bldg Fl 4, Indianapolis, IN 46202; **Phone:** 317-278-1022; **Board Cert:** Plastic Surgery 1994; Hand Surgery 2006; **Med School:** Albany Med Coll 1984; **Resid:** Surgery, Temple Univ Hosp 1989; **Fellow:** Plastic Surgery, Cleveland Clinic Fdn 1991; Hand Surgery, Union Meml Hosp 1992; **Fac Appt:** Prof S, Indiana Univ

Vogt, Peter MD [PIS] - **Spec Exp:** Cosmetic Surgery; **Hospital:** Mercy Hosp - Coon Rapids, Unity Hosp - Fridley; **Address:** 319 Barry Ave S, Ste 300, Wayzata, MN 55391; **Phone:** 952-473-1111; **Board Cert:** Plastic Surgery 1974; **Med School:** Univ Manitoba 1965; **Resid:** Surgery, Montreal Genl Hosp 1970; Plastic Surgery, Winnipeg Hlth Scis Ctr 1973

Walton Jr, Robert L MD [PIS] - **Spec Exp:** Nasal Reconstruction; Breast Reconstruction; Ear Reconstruction/Microtia; Cosmetic Surgery-Face; **Hospital:** Resurrection Hlth Care St Joseph Hosp, Children's Mem Hosp -Chicago; **Address:** 60 E Delaware Place, Ste 1430, Chicago, IL 60611-1495; **Phone:** 312-337-7795; **Board Cert:** Plastic Surgery 1980; **Med School:** Univ Kansas 1972; **Resid:** Surgery, Johns Hopkins Hosp 1974; Plastic Surgery, Yale-New Haven Hosp 1978; **Fellow:** Hand Surgery, Hartford Hosp 1978; **Fac Appt:** Prof PlS, Northwestern Univ-Feinberg Sch Med

Wilkins, Edwin G MD [PIS] - **Spec Exp:** Breast Reconstruction; Lower Limb Reconstruction; Microsurgery; **Hospital:** Univ of Michigan Hosp; **Address:** Univ Mich, Div Plastic Surg, 1500 E Med Ctr Drive, rm 2130 Taubman Ctr, Ann Arbor, MI 48109-5340; **Phone:** 734-998-6022; **Board Cert:** Plastic Surgery 1991; **Med School:** Wake Forest Univ 1981; **Resid:** Surgery, Charlotte Meml Hosp 1986; Plastic Surgery, Vanderbilt Univ Med Ctr 1988; **Fellow:** Reconstructive Microsurgery, Univ Louisville Sch Med 1989; **Fac Appt:** Assoc Prof PlS, Univ Mich Med Sch

Yetman, Randall MD [PIS] - **Spec Exp:** Breast Reconstruction; Melanoma; Microsurgery; **Hospital:** Cleveland Clin (page 56); **Address:** 9500 Euclid Ave, Desk A60, Cleveland, OH 44195; **Phone:** 216-444-6908; **Board Cert:** Plastic Surgery 1984; **Med School:** Univ Miami Sch Med 1975; **Resid:** Surgery, Montefiore Med Ctr 1979; Plastic Surgery, NY Cornell Med Ctr 1981; **Fellow:** Plastic Surgery, Cleveland Clin Fdn 1982

Young, V Leroy MD [PIS] - **Spec Exp:** Breast Augmentation; Skin Laser Surgery-Resurfacing; Body Contouring after Weight Loss; **Hospital:** Barnes-Jewish West County Hosp; **Address:** 969 N Mason Rd, Ste 170, St Louis, MO 63141; **Phone:** 314-628-8200; **Board Cert:** Plastic Surgery 1981; **Med School:** Univ KY Coll Med 1970; **Resid:** Surgery, Univ KY Med Ctr 1977; Plastic Surgery, Barnes Hosp-Wash Univ 1979; **Fac Appt:** Prof S, Washington Univ, St Louis

Zins, James E MD [PIS] - **Spec Exp:** Cosmetic Surgery-Face; Rhinoplasty; Facial Rejuvenation; Maxillofacial Surgery; **Hospital:** Cleveland Clin (page 56); **Address:** Department of Plastic Surgery, 9500 Euclid Ave, Desk A-60, Cleveland, OH 44195; **Phone:** 216-444-6901; **Board Cert:** Plastic Surgery 1985; **Med School:** Univ Pennsylvania 1974; **Resid:** Surgery, Hosp Univ Penn 1980; Plastic Surgery, Hosp Univ Penn 1982; **Fellow:** Craniofacial Surgery, Hosp Univ Penn 1978; Maxillofacial Surgery, Hosp Sick Chldn 1983

Great Plains and Mountains

Deleyiannis, Frederic W B MD [PIS] - **Spec Exp:** Head & Neck Reconstruction; Maxillofacial Surgery; Craniofacial Surgery; Pediatric Plastic Surgery; **Hospital:** Univ of CO Hosp - Anschutz Inpatient Pav, Chldn's Hosp - Aurora (CO); **Address:** 13123 E 16th Ave, Box B467, Aurora, CO 80045; **Phone:** 720-777-3880; **Board Cert:** Otolaryngology 2000; Plastic Surgery 2003; **Med School:** Yale Univ 1992; **Resid:** Otolaryngology, Univ Washington Med Ctr 1999; Plastic Surgery, Univ Pittsburgh Med Ctr 2002; **Fellow:** Head and Neck Surgery, Univ Oviedo Med Ctr 2000; **Fac Appt:** Assoc Prof PlS, Univ Colorado

Grossman, John A MD [PIS] - **Spec Exp:** Cosmetic Surgery; **Hospital:** Rose Med Ctr, Cedars-Sinai Med Ctr; **Address:** 4600 Hale Pkwy, Ste 100, Denver, CO 80220; **Phone:** 303-320-5566; **Board Cert:** Surgery 1974; Plastic Surgery 1976; **Med School:** Cornell Univ-Weill Med Coll 1967; **Resid:** Surgery, Boston City Hosp 1973; Plastic Surgery, Univ Colo Hlth Scis Ctr 1975; **Fellow:** Surgery, Harvard Med Sch 1973

Rockwell, William MD [PIS] - **Spec Exp:** Microsurgery; Sarcoma; Breast Reconstruction; Hand Surgery; **Hospital:** Univ Utah Hlth Care; **Address:** 30 N 1900 E, rm 3B400, Salt Lake City, UT 84132; **Phone:** 801-585-3253; **Board Cert:** Plastic Surgery 1994; Hand Surgery 2006; **Med School:** Washington Univ, St Louis 1984; **Resid:** Surgery, Univ Washington/Barnes Hosp 1987; Plastic Surgery, Univ Rochester Affil Hosp 1991; **Fellow:** Hand Surgery, Univ Rochester Affil Hosp 1992; **Fac Appt:** Assoc Prof PlS, Univ Utah

Southwest

Barone, Constance M MD [PIS] - **Spec Exp:** Cosmetic Surgery; Breast Augmentation; Rhinoplasty; Craniofacial Surgery; **Hospital:** Christus Santa Rosa Med Ctr Hosp, Univ Hlth Syst-San Antonio; **Address:** 2829 Babcock Rd, Ste 615, San Antonio, TX 78229; **Phone:** 210-614-0400; **Board Cert:** Plastic Surgery 1991; **Med School:** Mount Sinai Sch Med 1982; **Resid:** Surgery, Temple Univ Hosp 1987; Plastic Surgery, NYU Med Ctr 1989; **Fellow:** Craniofacial Surgery, Montefiore-Weiler Einstein Div 1992; **Fac Appt:** Prof NS, Univ Tex, San Antonio

Barton Jr, Fritz E MD [PIS] - **Spec Exp:** Cosmetic Surgery-Face; Liposuction & Body Contouring; Cosmetic Surgery-Breast; Facial Rejuvenation; **Hospital:** Baylor Univ Medical Ctr-Dallas; **Address:** Dallas Plastic Surgery Inst, 9101 N Central Expresswy, Ste 600, Dallas, TX 75231; **Phone:** 214-821-9355; **Board Cert:** Surgery 1975; Plastic Surgery 1977; **Med School:** Univ Tex SW, Dallas 1967; **Resid:** Surgery, Parkland Meml Hosp 1974; Plastic/Reconstructive Surgery, NYU Med Ctr 1976; **Fac Appt:** Clin Prof PlS, Univ Tex SW, Dallas

Beals, Stephen P MD [PIS] - **Spec Exp:** Craniofacial Surgery; Pediatric Plastic Surgery; Cosmetic Surgery-Face & Breast; Liposuction & Body Contouring; **Hospital:** St. Joseph's Hosp & Med Ctr - Phoenix, Phoenix Children's Hosp; **Address:** 500 W Thomas Rd, Ste 960, Phoenix, AZ 85013-4223; **Phone:** 602-266-9066; **Board Cert:** Plastic Surgery 1986; **Med School:** Wayne State Univ 1978; **Resid:** Surgery, William Beaumont Hosp 1983; Plastic Surgery, Phoenix Plastic Surgery Inst 1985; **Fellow:** Craniofacial Surgery, Hospital for Sick Chldn 1985; **Fac Appt:** Assoc Prof PlS, Mayo Med Sch

Plastic Surgery

Burns, A Jay MD [PlS] - **Spec Exp:** Cosmetic Surgery-Face; Cosmetic Surgery-Breast; Facial Rejuvenation; Vascular Birthmarks; **Hospital:** Baylor Univ Medical Ctr-Dallas, Chldns Med Ctr of Dallas; **Address:** 9101 N Central Expresswy St, Ste 600, Dallas, TX 75231; **Phone:** 214-823-1978; **Board Cert:** Plastic Surgery 1990; **Med School:** Univ Tex SW, Dallas 1981; **Resid:** Surgery, Univ Utah Hosp 1986; Plastic Surgery, Univ Tex SW Med Ctr 1988; **Fellow:** Vascular Anomalies, Chldns Hosp 1988; **Fac Appt:** Asst Prof PlS, Univ Tex SW, Dallas

Butler, Charles E MD [PlS] - **Spec Exp:** Breast Reconstruction; **Hospital:** UT MD Anderson Cancer Ctr; **Address:** Univ Texas- M.D. Anderson Cancer Ctr, 1515 Holcombe Blvd, Ste 1488, P.O. Box 301402, Houston, TX 77030; **Phone:** 713-794-1247; **Board Cert:** Plastic Surgery 2010; Surgery 2008; **Med School:** Univ Pennsylvania 1990; **Resid:** Surgery, Mass Genl Hosp 1993; Plastic Surgery, Brigham & Women's Hosp 1995; **Fellow:** Research, Brigham & Women's Hosp 1998; **Fac Appt:** Prof PlS, Case West Res Univ

Byrd, H Stephenson MD [PlS] - **Spec Exp:** Rhinoplasty; Cosmetic Surgery-Face; Cosmetic Surgery-Breast; Liposuction & Body Contouring; **Hospital:** Baylor Univ Medical Ctr-Dallas; **Address:** 9101 N Central Expressway, Ste 600, Dallas, TX 75231; **Phone:** 214-821-9662; **Board Cert:** Plastic Surgery 1980; **Med School:** Univ Tex Med Br, Galveston 1972; **Resid:** Surgery, Univ Utah Med Ctr 1977; Plastic Surgery, Dallas Co Hosp-Parkland Meml 1979; **Fac Appt:** Clin Prof PlS, Univ Tex SW, Dallas

Gunter, Jack MD [PlS] - **Spec Exp:** Rhinoplasty; Rhinoplasty Revision; **Hospital:** TX Hlth Presby Hosp Dallas; **Address:** 8144 Walnut Hill Lane, Ste 170, Dallas, TX 75231-4218; **Phone:** 214-369-8123; **Board Cert:** Otolaryngology 1969; Plastic Surgery 1981; **Med School:** Univ Okla Coll Med 1963; **Resid:** Surgery, Univ Ark Med Ctr 1965; Otolaryngology, Tulane Univ Hosp 1968; **Fellow:** Mercy Hosp 1969; Plastic Surgery, Univ Mich Hosp 1980; **Fac Appt:** Clin Prof PlS, Univ Tex SW, Dallas

Hamra, Sameer T MD [PlS] - **Spec Exp:** Cosmetic Surgery-Face; Rhinoplasty; **Hospital:** Mary Shiels Hosp; **Address:** 9301 N Central Expressway, Ste 551, Tower 2, Dallas, TX 75231; **Phone:** 214-754-9001; **Board Cert:** Surgery 1970; Plastic Surgery 1977; **Med School:** Univ Okla Coll Med 1963; **Resid:** Surgery, Univ Okla 1968; Plastic Surgery, NYU Med Ctr 1973; **Fellow:** Surgery, Univ Lausanne 1966; **Fac Appt:** Clin Prof S, Univ Tex SW, Dallas

Kane, Alex A MD [PlS] - **Spec Exp:** Pediatric Plastic Surgery; Craniofacial Surgery; Cleft Palate/Lip; Hemangiomas/Birthmarks; **Hospital:** Chldns Med Ctr of Dallas; **Address:** 2350 N Demmons Freeway, Ambulatory Care Pavilion Fl 4, Dallas, TX 75207; **Phone:** 214-456-2240; **Board Cert:** Plastic Surgery 2001; **Med School:** Dartmouth Med Sch 1991; **Resid:** Surgery, Barnes Jewish Hosp 1994; Plastic Surgery, Barnes Jewish Hosp 1998; **Fellow:** Craniofacial Surgery, Chang-Gung Meml Hosp 1999; Craniofacial Imaging, Nat'l Lab for Diagnostic Rsch 1999; **Fac Appt:** Prof S, Univ Tex SW, Dallas

Kenkel, Jeffrey M MD [PlS] - **Spec Exp:** Cosmetic Surgery-Face; Laser Surgery; Cosmetic Surgery-Breast; Body Contouring after Weight Loss; **Hospital:** UT Southwestern Med Ctr at Dallas; **Address:** UTSW Plastic Surgery, 1801 Inwood Rd Fl 5, Dallas, TX 75390; **Phone:** 214-645-2353; **Board Cert:** Plastic Surgery 2008; **Med School:** Georgetown Univ 1990; **Resid:** Surgery, Georgetown Univ Med Ctr 1994; Plastic Surgery, UT Southwestern Med Ctr 1996; **Fac Appt:** Prof PlS, Univ Tex SW, Dallas

Meltzer, Toby R MD [PlS] - **Spec Exp:** Gender Reassignment Surgery; Penile Inversion Technique; Breast Augmentation; Cosmetic Surgery-Face & Breast; **Hospital:** Scottsdale Hlthcare - Osborn; **Address:** 7025 N Scottsdale Rd, Ste 302, Scottsdale, AZ 85253; **Phone:** 480-657-7006; **Board Cert:** Plastic Surgery 1992; **Med School:** Louisiana State U, New Orleans 1983; **Resid:** Surgery, Charity Hosp Louisiana 1988; Plastic Surgery, Univ Michigan Med Ctr 1990; **Fellow:** Burn Surgery, Wayne State Univ 1987; **Fac Appt:** Asst Clin Prof S, Univ Ariz Coll Med

Menick, Frederick J MD [PlS] - **Spec Exp:** Reconstructive Surgery-Face; Nasal Reconstruction; Cancer Reconstruction; Rhinoplasty; **Hospital:** St. Joseph's Hosp - Tucson; **Address:** 1102 N Eldorado Pl, Tucson, AZ 85715; **Phone:** 520-881-4525; **Board Cert:** Plastic Surgery 1983; **Med School:** Yale Univ 1970; **Resid:** Surgery, Stanford Med Ctr 1974; Surgery, Univ Ariz Med Ctr 1979; **Fellow:** Plastic Surgery, UC Irvine 1981; Plastic Surgery, Univ Miami 1982; **Fac Appt:** Assoc Clin Prof S, Univ Ariz Coll Med

Metzinger, Stephen E MD [PlS] - **Spec Exp:** Rhinoplasty; Eyelid Surgery/Blepharoplasty; Cosmetic Surgery-Face; Cosmetic Surgery-Breast; **Hospital:** E Jefferson Genl Hosp; **Address:** Aesthetic Surgery Assocs, 3223 8th St, Ste 200, Metairie, LA 70002; **Phone:** 504-309-7061; **Board Cert:** Otolaryngology 1994; Plastic Surgery 2008; Facial Plastic & Reconstr Surgery 1998; **Med School:** Louisiana State U, New Orleans 1987; **Resid:** Otolaryngology, LSU Med Ctr 1993; Plastic Surgery, Johns Hopkins Affil Hosp 1996; **Fellow:** Facial Plastic & Reconstr Surgery, McCollough Aesthetic Med Ctr 1994; Craniofacial Surgery, Univ Maryland Trauma Ctr 1996; **Fac Appt:** Assoc Prof PlS, Louisiana State U, New Orleans

Moses, Michael H MD [PlS] - **Spec Exp:** Cosmetic Surgery-Face; Cosmetic Surgery-Breast; Liposuction & Body Contouring; Rhinoplasty; **Hospital:** Touro Infirmary, Children's Hospital - New Orleans; **Address:** 1603 2nd St, New Orleans, LA 70130; **Phone:** 504-895-7200; **Board Cert:** Plastic Surgery 1985; **Med School:** Tulane Univ 1977; **Resid:** Surgery, Yale-New Haven Hosp 1982; Plastic Surgery, Mass Genl Hosp 1984; **Fellow:** Craniofacial Surgery, Childrens Hosp 1985; **Fac Appt:** Assoc Clin Prof S, Tulane Univ

Rappaport, Norman H MD/DDS [PlS] - **Spec Exp:** Cosmetic Surgery-Face; Breast Cosmetic & Reconstructive Surgery; Body Contouring after Weight Loss; Facial Rejuvenation; **Hospital:** Methodist Hosp - Houston, St. Luke's Episcopal Hosp-Houston; **Address:** Houston Center for Plastic Surgey, 6560 Fannin St, Ste 1812 Scurlock Tower, Houston, TX 77030-2775; **Phone:** 713-790-4500; **Board Cert:** Plastic Surgery 1981; **Med School:** Hahnemann Univ 1975; **Resid:** Surgery, Abingdon Meml Hosp 1978; Plastic Surgery, Baylor Coll Med 1980; **Fellow:** Plastic Surgery, Hosp Univ Penn 1978; **Fac Appt:** Assoc Clin Prof S, Baylor Coll Med

Robb, Geoffrey L MD [PlS] - **Spec Exp:** Breast Reconstruction; Head & Neck Cancer Reconstruction; Facial Plastic & Reconstructive Surgery; **Hospital:** UT MD Anderson Cancer Ctr, St. Luke's Episcopal Hosp-Houston; **Address:** 1515 Holcombe Blvd, Unit 1488, Houston, TX 77030; **Phone:** 713-794-1247; **Board Cert:** Otolaryngology 1979; Plastic Surgery 1986; **Med School:** Univ Miami Sch Med 1974; **Resid:** Otolaryngology, Naval Reg Med Ctr 1979; Plastic Surgery, Univ Pittsburgh 1985; **Fellow:** Microvascular Surgery, Univ Pittsburgh 1986; **Fac Appt:** Prof PlS, Univ Tex, Houston

Rohrich, Rod J MD [PlS] - **Spec Exp:** Rhinoplasty; Cosmetic Surgery-Face; Facial Rejuvenation; Liposuction & Body Contouring; **Hospital:** UT Southwestern Med Ctr at Dallas, Baylor Univ Medical Ctr-Dallas; **Address:** Univ Tex SW Med Ctr, Plastic Surgery, 1801 Inwood Rd, MS 9132, Dallas, TX 75390-9132; **Phone:** 214-645-3119; **Board Cert:** Plastic Surgery 1987; Hand Surgery 1990; **Med School:** Baylor Coll Med 1979; **Resid:** Plastic Surgery, Univ Mich Hosp 1985; Plastic Surgery, Radcliffe Infirm/Oxford 1983; **Fellow:** Hand Surgery, Mass Genl Hosp 1987; **Fac Appt:** Prof PlS, Univ Tex SW, Dallas

Schusterman, Mark A MD [PlS] - **Spec Exp:** Breast Reconstruction; Cancer Reconstruction; Cosmetic Surgery-Face & Breast; Body Contouring; **Hospital:** Methodist Hosp - Houston, St. Luke's Episcopal Hosp-Houston; **Address:** 1200 Binz St, Ste 1200, Houston, TX 77004; **Phone:** 713-794-0368; **Board Cert:** Plastic Surgery 1989; **Med School:** Univ Louisville Sch Med 1980; **Resid:** Surgery, Univ Hosp 1985; Plastic Surgery, Univ Pittsburgh Med Ctr 1987; **Fellow:** Microsurgery, Univ Pittsburgh 1988; **Fac Appt:** Clin Prof PlS, Baylor Coll Med

Plastic Surgery

Stal, Samuel MD [PlS] - **Spec Exp:** Pediatric Plastic Surgery; Craniofacial Surgery; Cleft Palate/Lip; Maxillofacial Surgery; **Hospital:** Texas Chldns Hosp; **Address:** Texas Children's Hosp, Clinical Care Ctr, 6701 Fannin St, Ste 610, Houston, TX 77030; **Phone:** 832-822-3180; **Board Cert:** Otolaryngology 1981; Plastic Surgery 1982; **Med School:** Loyola Univ-Stritch Sch Med 1974; **Resid:** Otolaryngology, Univ Chicago Hosps 1979; Plastic Surgery, Baylor College Med 1981; **Fellow:** Craniofacial Surgery, Enfant Malade Hosp 1982; **Fac Appt:** Prof Oto, Baylor Coll Med

Tebbetts, John B MD [PlS] - **Spec Exp:** Cosmetic Surgery-Breast; Rhinoplasty; Liposuction; **Hospital:** Mary Shiels Hosp, Baylor Univ Medical Ctr-Dallas; **Address:** 2801 Lemmon Ave W, Ste 300, Dallas, TX 75204; **Phone:** 214-220-2712; **Board Cert:** Plastic Surgery 1980; **Med School:** Univ Tex Med Br, Galveston 1972; **Resid:** Surgery, Univ Utah Med Ctr 1977; Plastic Surgery, Dallas Co Hosp-Parkland Meml Hosp 1979; **Fac Appt:** Asst Clin Prof PlS, Univ Tex SW, Dallas

Wilcox, Robert D MD [PlS] - **Spec Exp:** Cosmetic Surgery-Face; Cosmetic Surgery-Breast; Liposuction & Body Contouring; **Hospital:** Columbia Med Ctr - Plano; **Address:** Plastic & Cosmetic Surgery Ctr of Texas, 5316 W Plano Pkwy, Plano, TX 75093; **Phone:** 972-620-1700; **Board Cert:** Plastic Surgery 1994; Hand Surgery 2003; **Med School:** Univ Tex SW, Dallas 1984; **Resid:** Surgery, Univ Florida Hlth Sci Ctr 1989; Plastic/Reconstructive Surgery, Univ Texas-SW Med Sch 1991; **Fellow:** Hand Surgery, Univ Texas-SW Med Sch 1992

Yuen, James C MD [PlS] - **Spec Exp:** Hand Reconstruction; Breast Reconstruction; Head & Neck Cancer Reconstruction; Chest Wall Reconstruction; **Hospital:** UAMS Med Ctr; **Address:** 4301 W Markham, Ste 720, Little Rock, AR 72205; **Phone:** 501-686-8711; **Board Cert:** Surgery 2001; Plastic Surgery 2004; **Med School:** Med Coll VA 1985; **Resid:** Surgery, West Va Med Ctr 1990; Plastic/Reconstructive Surgery, Duke Univ Med Ctr 1993; **Fellow:** Hand & Microvascular Surgery, Kleinert Inst of Hand & Microsurgery 1991; **Fac Appt:** Assoc Prof S, Univ Ark

West Coast and Pacific

Alter, Gary J MD [PlS] - **Spec Exp:** Genitourinary Reconstruction; Gender Reassignment Surgery; Genital Enhancement; **Hospital:** Cedars-Sinai Med Ctr, UCLA Ronald Reagan Med Ctr; **Address:** 416 N Bedford Drive, Ste 400, Beverly Hills, CA 90210-4318; **Phone:** 310-275-5566; **Board Cert:** Urology 1981; Plastic Surgery 2007; **Med School:** UCLA 1973; **Resid:** Urology, Baylor Med Ctr 1979; Plastic Surgery, Mayo Clin 1992; **Fellow:** Genitourinary Surgery, Eastern Va Med Sch 1992; **Fac Appt:** Clin Prof PlS, UCLA

Andersen, James S MD [PlS] - **Spec Exp:** Breast Reconstruction; Head & Neck Reconstruction; Microsurgery; **Hospital:** City of Hope Natl Med Ctr, Huntington Memorial Hosp; **Address:** City Hope Natl Cancer Ctr, Div Plastic Surgery, 1500 E Duarte Rd, Duarte, CA 91010; **Phone:** 626-471-7100; **Board Cert:** Plastic Surgery 1994; **Med School:** Jefferson Med Coll 1983; **Resid:** Surgery, Hosp Univ Penn 1989; Plastic Surgery, Hosp Univ Penn 1991; **Fellow:** Microsurgery, USC Med Ctr 1992; **Fac Appt:** Assoc Clin Prof S, USC Sch Med

Brent, Burton D MD [PlS] - **Spec Exp:** Ear Reconstruction/Microtia; **Hospital:** El Camino Hosp; **Address:** 2995 Woodside Rd, Ste 300, Woodside, CA 94062-2401; **Phone:** 650-851-5300; **Board Cert:** Plastic Surgery 1974; **Med School:** Ros Franklin Univ/Chicago Med Sch 1963; **Resid:** Surgery, University Hosp 1970; Plastic Surgery, Loyola Univ Med Ctr 1973; **Fellow:** Plastic Surgery, Canniesburn Hosp; **Fac Appt:** Assoc Clin Prof PlS, Stanford Univ

Chang, James MD [PlS] - **Spec Exp:** Hand & Upper Extremity Surgery; Reconstructive Surgery; Pediatric Hand Surgery; Peripheral Nerve Surgery; **Hospital:** Stanford Univ Hosp & Clinics; **Address:** SUMC Hand & Upper Extremity Surgery, 450 Broadway St, Pavilion A, Fl 2, Redwood City, CA 94063-6120; **Phone:** 650-723-5256; **Board Cert:** Plastic Surgery 2009; Hand Surgery 2002; **Med School:** Yale Univ 1993; **Resid:** Plastic Surgery, Stanford Univ Med Ctr 1998; **Fellow:** Hand Surgery, UCLA Med Ctr 2000; **Fac Appt:** Prof PlS, Stanford Univ

Cohen, Steven R MD [PlS] - **Spec Exp:** Craniofacial Surgery-Pediatric; Craniofacial Surgery/Reconstruction; Cosmetic Surgery-Face; Rhinoplasty; **Hospital:** Rady Children's Hosp - San Diego, UCSD Med Ctr; **Address:** 4510 Executive Drive, Ste 200, San Diego, CA 92121; **Phone:** 858-453-7224; **Board Cert:** Plastic Surgery 1992; **Med School:** Geo Wash Univ 1980; **Resid:** Surgery, Dartmouth-Hitchcock Med Ctr 1987; Plastic Surgery, Hosp Univ Penn/Chldns Hosp 1989; **Fellow:** Craniofacial Surgery, UCLA Med Ctr 1990; **Fac Appt:** Clin Prof PlS, UCSD

Daniel, Rollin K MD [PlS] - **Spec Exp:** Rhinoplasty; **Hospital:** Hoag Meml Hosp Presby; **Address:** 1441 Avocado Ave, Ste 308, Newport Beach, CA 92660; **Phone:** 949-721-0494; **Board Cert:** Plastic Surgery 1977; **Med School:** Columbia P&S 1972; **Resid:** Plastic Surgery, McGill Univ Affil Hosps 1975; Hand Surgery, Univ Louisville Hosp 1976; **Fellow:** Craniofacial Surgery, Univ Toronto 1984

Edwards, Michael C MD [PlS] - **Spec Exp:** Breast Cosmetic & Reconstructive Surgery; Liposuction & Body Contouring; Body Contouring after Weight Loss; **Hospital:** Summerlin Hosp Med Ctr; **Address:** 653 N Town Center Drive, Ste 214, Las Vegas, NV 89144; **Phone:** 702-248-8989; **Board Cert:** Surgery 2006; Plastic Surgery 2008; **Med School:** Uniformed Srvs Univ, Bethesda 1988; **Resid:** Surgery, David Grant Med Ctr 1993; **Fellow:** Plastic Surgery, Wilford Hall Med Ctr 1996

Evans, Gregory R MD [PlS] - **Spec Exp:** Cosmetic Surgery-Face; Cosmetic Surgery-Breast; Body Contouring; Cancer Reconstruction; **Hospital:** UC Irvine Med Ctr; **Address:** Aesthetic & Plastic Surgery Inst, 200 S Manchester Ave, Ste 650, Orange, CA 92868; **Phone:** 714-456-3077; **Board Cert:** Surgery 2001; Plastic Surgery 2008; **Med School:** USC Sch Med 1985; **Resid:** Surgery, LAC/USC Med Ctr 1990; Plastic Surgery, Johns Hopkins Hosp 1993; **Fac Appt:** Prof S, UC Irvine

Fisher, Garth MD [PlS] - **Spec Exp:** Cosmetic Surgery-Face; Cosmetic Surgery-Breast; Rhinoplasty; Body Contouring; **Hospital:** St. John's Hlth Ctr, Santa Monica; **Address:** 120 S Spalding Drive, Ste 222, Beverly Hills, CA 90212; **Phone:** 310-273-5995; **Board Cert:** Plastic Surgery 1993; **Med School:** Univ Miss 1984; **Resid:** Surgery, UC Irvine Med Ctr 1989; Plastic Surgery, UC Irvine Med Ctr 1991; **Fellow:** Plastic Surgery, Bruce Connelly 1992

Fodor, Peter B MD [PlS] - **Spec Exp:** Facial Rejuvenation; Liposuction & Body Contouring; Cosmetic Surgery-Breast; **Hospital:** Olympia Med Ctr; **Address:** 2080 Century Park East, Ste 710, Los Angeles, CA 90067; **Phone:** 310-203-9818; **Board Cert:** Plastic Surgery 1977; **Med School:** Univ Wisc 1966; **Resid:** Surgery, Columbia-Presby Med Ctr 1968; Plastic Surgery, St Luke's Hosp 1976; **Fac Appt:** Assoc Clin Prof S, UCLA

Garner, Warren L MD [PlS] - **Spec Exp:** Burns-Reconstructive Plastic Surgery; Wound Healing/Care; Skin Healing; **Hospital:** LAC & USC Med Ctr, Keck Med Ctr of USC (page 75); **Address:** 1510 San Pablo St, Ste 415, Los Angeles, CA 90033; **Phone:** 323-442-7920; **Board Cert:** Plastic Surgery 1991; Surgical Critical Care 2001; **Med School:** Univ Kansas 1978; **Resid:** Surgery, Ohio State Univ Hosp 1985; Plastic Surgery, Wash Univ Hosp 1989; **Fellow:** Critical Care Medicine, Ohio State Univ Hosp 1986; **Fac Appt:** Assoc Prof PlS, USC Sch Med

Plastic Surgery

Gruss, Joseph MD [PlS] - **Spec Exp:** Maxillofacial & Craniofacial Surgery; Facial Trauma/Fractures; Cleft Palate/Lip; Pediatric Plastic Surgery; **Hospital:** Seattle Chldns Hosp; **Address:** Seattle Children's, 4800 Sand Point Way NE, MS 7729, Seattle, WA 98105; **Phone:** 206-987-2039; **Board Cert:** Plastic Surgery 1977; **Med School:** South Africa 1969; **Resid:** Plastic Surgery, Toronto Western Hosp 1976; Plastic Surgery, Hosp for Sick Children 1976; **Fellow:** Surgical Oncology, Princess Margaret Hosp 1977; Head and Neck Surgery, Princess Margaret Hosp 1977; **Fac Appt:** Prof PlS, Univ Wash

Hansen, Juliana MD [PlS] - **Spec Exp:** Breast Reconstruction; Cancer Reconstruction; **Hospital:** OR Hlth & Sci Univ; **Address:** 3303 SW Bond Ave, MC CH5P, Portland, OR 97239; **Phone:** 503-494-6687; **Board Cert:** Plastic Surgery 2008; **Med School:** Univ Wash 1988; **Resid:** Surgery, UCSF Med Ctr 1994; Plastic Surgery, UCSF Med Ctr 1996

Hardesty, Robert MD [PlS] - **Spec Exp:** Cosmetic Surgery-Face & Body; Reconstructive Surgery; Body Contouring; Cosmetic Surgery-Breast; **Hospital:** Riverside Comm Hosp, Loma Linda Univ Med Ctr; **Address:** 4646 Brockton Ave, Ste 302, Riverside, CA 92506; **Phone:** 951-686-7600; **Board Cert:** Plastic Surgery 1989; **Med School:** Loma Linda Univ 1978; **Resid:** Surgery, Loma Linda Univ Med Ctr 1983; Plastic Surgery, Univ Pittsburgh Med Ctr 1986; **Fellow:** Pediatric Plastic Surgery, Washington Univ 1987; **Fac Appt:** Clin Prof PlS, Loma Linda Univ

Hoffman, William Y MD [PlS] - **Spec Exp:** Pediatric Plastic Surgery; Cleft Palate/Lip; Craniofacial Surgery; Reconstructive Surgery; **Hospital:** UCSF Med Ctr, CA Pacific Med Ctr-Pacific Campus; **Address:** UCSF Plastic Surgery, 350 Parnassus Ave, Ste 509, Box 0932, San Francisco, CA 94117; **Phone:** 415-353-4287; **Board Cert:** Plastic Surgery 1987; **Med School:** Univ Rochester 1977; **Resid:** Surgery, UCSF Med Ctr 1983; Plastic Surgery, UCSF Med Ctr 1985; **Fellow:** Craniofacial Surgery, NYU Med Ctr 1986; **Fac Appt:** Prof PlS, UCSF

Horowitz, Jed H MD [PlS] - **Spec Exp:** Cosmetic Surgery-Breast; Cosmetic Surgery-Face; Transumbilical Breast Augmentation(TUBA); **Hospital:** Hoag Meml Hosp Presby, Orange Coast Memorial Med Ctr; **Address:** 7677 Center Ave, Ste 401, Huntington Beach, CA 92647-3098; **Phone:** 714-902-1100; **Board Cert:** Plastic Surgery 1986; **Med School:** SUNY Buffalo 1977; **Resid:** Surgery, Grady Meml Hosp 1983; **Fellow:** Plastic Surgery, Univ Virginia 1985; **Fac Appt:** Asst Clin Prof PlS, USC Sch Med

Isik, Ferda Frank MD [PlS] - **Spec Exp:** Cosmetic Surgery-Face; Breast Reconstruction; Cosmetic Surgery-Breast; Liposuction & Body Contouring; **Hospital:** Swedish Med Ctr-First Hill-Seattle; **Address:** The Polyclinic, 1145 Broadway, Seattle, WA 98122; **Phone:** 206-860-4566; **Board Cert:** Surgery 2001; Plastic Surgery 2007; **Med School:** Mount Sinai Sch Med 1985; **Resid:** Surgery, Boston Univ Hosps 1990; Plastic Surgery, Univ Wash Affil Hosp 1995; **Fellow:** Research, NIH / Univ Washington 1992

Jewell, Mark L MD [PlS] - **Spec Exp:** Liposuction & Body Contouring; Cosmetic Surgery-Face; Breast Reconstruction; Cosmetic Surgery-Breast; **Hospital:** Sacred Heart Med Ctr; **Address:** 10 Coburg Rd, Ste 300, Eugene, OR 97401; **Phone:** 541-683-3234; **Board Cert:** Plastic Surgery 1981; **Med School:** Univ Kansas 1973; **Resid:** Surgery, LAC-Harbor Med Ctr 1976; Plastic Surgery, Erlanger Hosp 1979; **Fellow:** Burn Surgery, LAC-USC Med Ctr 1977; **Fac Appt:** Asst Clin Prof PlS, Oregon Hlth & Sci Univ

Jones, Neil F MD [PlS] - **Spec Exp:** Hand Reconstruction-Pediatric; Nerve Disorders/Surgery; Tendon Surgery; Hand Surgery; **Hospital:** UC Irvine Med Ctr, Chldns Hosp Orange Co; **Address:** 101 The City Drive S, Route 94, Orthopaedic Spine Ctr, Orange, CA 92868; **Phone:** 714-456-7012; **Board Cert:** Plastic Surgery 1985; **Med School:** England, UK 1974; **Resid:** Surgery, Radcliffe Infirmary 1979; Plastic Surgery, Univ Mich Med Ctr 1981; **Fellow:** Plastic Surgery, St Bartholomew's Hosp 1982; Hand & Microvascular Surgery, Mass Gen Hosp 1983; **Fac Appt:** Prof S, UC Irvine

Kawamoto Jr, Henry K MD/DDS [PlS] - **Spec Exp:** Cosmetic Surgery-Face & Neck; Craniofacial Surgery; Maxillofacial Surgery; **Hospital:** UCLA Ronald Reagan Med Ctr, St. John's Hlth Ctr, Santa Monica; **Address:** 1301 20th St, Ste 460, Santa Monica, CA 90404; **Phone:** 310-829-0391; **Board Cert:** Surgery 1972; Plastic Surgery 1976; **Med School:** USC Sch Med 1964; **Resid:** Surgery, Columbia-Presby Med Ctr 1971; Plastic Surgery, NYU Med Ctr 1973; **Fellow:** Craniofacial Surgery, Dr Paul Tessier 1974; **Fac Appt:** Clin Prof S, UCLA

Koplin, Lawrence M MD [PlS] - **Spec Exp:** Cosmetic Surgery-Face; Breast Cosmetic & Reconstructive Surgery; Facial Rejuvenation; Liposuction & Body Contouring; **Hospital:** Cedars-Sinai Med Ctr; **Address:** 465 N Roxbury Drive, Ste 800, Beverly Hills, CA 90210; **Phone:** 310-277-3223; **Board Cert:** Plastic Surgery 1985; **Med School:** Baylor Coll Med 1976; **Resid:** Surgery, Kaiser Fdn Hosp 1981; Plastic Surgery, St Joseph Hosp 1983

Leaf, Norman MD [PlS] - **Spec Exp:** Cosmetic Surgery-Face & Neck; Cosmetic Surgery-Breast; Eyelid Surgery/Blepharoplasty; **Hospital:** Cedars-Sinai Med Ctr, UCLA Ronald Reagan Med Ctr; **Address:** 436 N Bedford Drive, Ste 104, Beverly Hills, CA 90210-4310; **Phone:** 310-274-8001; **Board Cert:** Surgery 1973; Plastic Surgery 1974; **Med School:** Univ Chicago-Pritzker Sch Med 1966; **Resid:** Surgery, Univ Chicago Hosps 1972; Plastic Surgery, Univ Chicago Hosps 1973; **Fellow:** Research, Univ Chicago Hosps 1969; **Fac Appt:** Asst Clin Prof PlS, UCLA

Lesavoy, Malcolm A MD [PlS] - **Spec Exp:** Cosmetic Surgery-Face & Neck; Cosmetic Surgery-Breast; Abdominoplasty; Reconstructive Surgery; **Hospital:** UCLA Ronald Reagan Med Ctr; **Address:** 16311 Ventura Blvd, Ste 555, Encino, CA 91436-4314; **Phone:** 818-986-8270; **Board Cert:** Plastic Surgery 1977; **Med School:** Ros Franklin Univ/Chicago Med Sch 1969; **Resid:** Surgery, Univ Chicago Hosps 1974; Plastic Surgery, Univ Miami Hosp/Clinics 1976; **Fac Appt:** Clin Prof PlS, UCLA

Markowitz, Bernard L MD [PlS] - **Spec Exp:** Cosmetic Surgery-Face & Body; Abdominoplasty; Facial Rejuvenation; Craniofacial Surgery/Reconstruction; **Hospital:** UCLA Ronald Reagan Med Ctr, Cedars-Sinai Med Ctr; **Address:** 9675 Brighton Way, Ste 350, Beverly Hills, CA 90210; **Phone:** 310-205-5557; **Board Cert:** Plastic Surgery 1989; **Med School:** NYU Sch Med 1979; **Resid:** Surgery, NYU Med Ctr 1984; Plastic Surgery, NYU Med Ctr 1986; **Fellow:** Maxillofacial Surgery, Johns Hopkins Hosp 1987; Microvascular Surgery, Johns Hopkins Hosp 1987; **Fac Appt:** Clin Prof PlS, UCLA

Marten, Timothy J MD [PlS] - **Spec Exp:** Cosmetic Surgery-Face & Neck; Facial Rejuvenation; **Hospital:** CA Pacific Med Ctr-Pacific Campus, St. Mary's Med Ctr - San Fran; **Address:** 450 Sutter St, Ste 2222, San Francisco, CA 94108-4207; **Phone:** 415-677-9937; **Board Cert:** Plastic Surgery 1993; **Med School:** UC Davis 1982; **Resid:** Surgery, Kaiser Fdn Hosp 1987; Plastic Surgery, Univ Illinois Chicago Hosp 1989; **Fellow:** Cosmetic Plastic Surgery, Connell Aesthetic Network 1990; Cosmetic Plastic Surgery, Baker, Gordon, & Stuzin 1990

Miller, Timothy A MD [PlS] - **Spec Exp:** Cosmetic Surgery-Face; Eyelid Cancer & Reconstruction; Skin Cancer; Nasal Reconstruction; **Hospital:** UCLA Ronald Reagan Med Ctr; **Address:** 200 UCLA Medical Plaza, Ste 465, Los Angeles, CA 90095-8344; **Phone:** 310-825-5644; **Board Cert:** Surgery 1971; Plastic Surgery 1973; **Med School:** UCLA 1963; **Resid:** Surgery, Johns Hopkins Hosp 1967; Thoracic Surgery, UCLA Med Ctr 1969; **Fellow:** Plastic Surgery, Univ Pittsburgh 1971; **Fac Appt:** Prof S, UCLA

Nichter, Larry S MD [PlS] - **Spec Exp:** Cosmetic Surgery-Face & Body; Cosmetic Surgery-Breast; Liposuction & Body Contouring; Congenital Breast Anomalies; **Hospital:** Hoag Meml Hosp Presby, Orange Coast Memorial Med Ctr; **Address:** 7677 Center Ave, Ste 401, Huntington Beach, CA 92647-3098; **Phone:** 714-902-1100; **Board Cert:** Plastic Surgery 1986; **Med School:** Boston Univ 1978; **Resid:** Surgery, UCLA Medical Ctr 1982; Plastic Surgery, Univ Virginia Med Ctr 1985; **Fellow:** Hand & Microvascular Surgery, Univ Virginia 1983; Craniofacial Surgery, Univ Virginia 1985; **Fac Appt:** Clin Prof PlS, USC-Keck School of Medicine

Plastic Surgery

Ousterhout, Douglas K MD/DDS [PlS] - **Spec Exp:** Cosmetic Surgery-Face; Gender Reassignment Surgery; Craniofacial Surgery; Facial Feminization Surgery (FFS); **Hospital:** CA Pacific Med Ctr - Davies Campus; **Address:** 45 Castro St, Ste 150, San Francisco, CA 94114; **Phone:** 415-626-2888; **Board Cert:** Plastic Surgery 1974; **Med School:** Univ Mich Med Sch 1965; **Resid:** Surgery, Univ Mich Hosps 1969; Plastic Surgery, Stanford Univ 1972; **Fellow:** Craniofacial Surgery, Clinic Belvedere 1973; **Fac Appt:** Clin Prof PlS, UCSF

Paul, Malcolm D MD [PlS] - **Spec Exp:** Cosmetic Surgery-Face & Neck; Cosmetic Surgery-Breast; Liposuction & Body Contouring; **Hospital:** Hoag Meml Hosp Presby; **Address:** 1401 Avocado Ave, Ste 810, Newport Beach, CA 92660-8708; **Phone:** 949-760-5047; **Board Cert:** Plastic Surgery 1976; **Med School:** Univ MD Sch Med 1969; **Resid:** Surgery, Geo Wash Med Ctr 1973; Plastic Surgery, Geo Wash Med Ctr 1975; **Fac Appt:** Clin Prof S, UC Irvine

Rand, Richard P MD [PlS] - **Spec Exp:** Cosmetic Surgery-Face; Cosmetic Surgery-Breast; Liposuction & Body Contouring; Facial Rejuvenation; **Hospital:** Overlake Hosp Med Ctr; **Address:** 1135 116th Ave NE, Ste 630, Bellevue, WA 98005; **Phone:** 425-688-8828; **Board Cert:** Plastic Surgery 1991; **Med School:** Univ Mich Med Sch 1981; **Resid:** Surgery, Tufts-New England Med Ctr 1986; Plastic Surgery, Emory Univ Hosp 1989; **Fellow:** Craniofacial Surgery, Univ Miami 1989; **Fac Appt:** Assoc Prof S, Univ Wash

Reinisch, John F MD [PlS] - **Spec Exp:** Birthmarks/Hemangiomas; Ear Reconstruction/Microtia; Pediatric Plastic Surgery; **Hospital:** Cedars-Sinai Med Ctr; **Address:** 250 N Robertson Blvd, Ste 506, Beverly Hills, CA 90211; **Phone:** 310-385-6090; **Board Cert:** Plastic Surgery 1980; **Med School:** Harvard Med Sch 1970; **Resid:** Surgery, Univ Mich Med Ctr 1975; Plastic Surgery, Univ Virginia Hosp 1978; **Fac Appt:** Prof S, USC Sch Med

Ristow, Brunno MD [PlS] - **Spec Exp:** Cosmetic Surgery-Face; Facial Plastic & Reconstructive Surgery; Rhinoplasty; Nasal Reconstruction; **Hospital:** CA Pacific Med Ctr-Pacific Campus; **Address:** 2100 Webster St, Ste 501, San Francisco, CA 94115-2381; **Phone:** 415-202-1507; **Board Cert:** Plastic Surgery 1975; **Med School:** Brazil 1966; **Resid:** Surgery, New York Hosp 1971; Plastic Surgery, NYU Med Ctr 1973; **Fellow:** Plastic Surgery, NYU Med Ctr 1968

Romano, James John MD [PlS] - **Spec Exp:** Body Contouring; Cosmetic Surgery-Breast; Tuberous Breasts; Facial Rejuvenation; **Hospital:** CA Pacific Med Ctr - CA Campus, Seton Med Ctr; **Address:** 1650 Jackson St, Ste 101, San Francisco, CA 94109; **Phone:** 415-981-3911; **Board Cert:** Plastic Surgery 1990; **Med School:** Eastern VA Med Sch 1980; **Resid:** Surgery, Georgetown Univ Hosp 1985; Plastic Surgery, Johns Hopkins Hosp 1988; **Fac Appt:** Asst Prof PlS, USC Sch Med

Rosenberg, Howard L MD [PlS] - **Spec Exp:** Cosmetic Surgery-Face; Cosmetic Surgery-Breast; Liposuction & Body Contouring; Facial Rejuvenation; **Hospital:** El Camino Hosp; **Address:** 2204 Grant Rd, Ste 201, Mountain View, CA 94040; **Phone:** 650-961-2652; **Board Cert:** Surgery 1975; Plastic Surgery 1977; **Med School:** Johns Hopkins Univ 1969; **Resid:** Surgery, UCLA Med Ctr 1974; Plastic Surgery, Stanford Univ Med Ctr 1976; **Fac Appt:** Asst Clin Prof PlS, Stanford Univ

Sherman, Randolph MD [PlS] - **Spec Exp:** Facial Paralysis; Breast Reconstruction; Limb Surgery/Reconstruction; **Hospital:** Cedars-Sinai Med Ctr; **Address:** 8635 W 3rd St, Ste 650-W, Los Angeles, CA 90048; **Phone:** 310-423-2129; **Board Cert:** Surgery 2004; Plastic Surgery 1986; Hand Surgery 2000; **Med School:** Univ MO-Columbia Sch Med 1977; **Resid:** Surgery, UCSF Hosps 1981; Surgery, State Univ of New York 1983; **Fellow:** Plastic Surgery, USC Med Ctr 1985; **Fac Appt:** Prof S, USC Sch Med

Singer, Robert MD [PlS] - **Spec Exp:** Cosmetic Surgery-Face; Cosmetic Surgery-Breast; Liposuction & Body Contouring; **Hospital:** Scripps Meml Hosp - La Jolla; **Address:** 9834 Genesee Ave, Ste 100, La Jolla, CA 92037-1214; **Phone:** 858-455-0290; **Board Cert:** Plastic Surgery 1977; **Med School:** SUNY Buffalo 1967; **Resid:** Surgery, Stanford Univ Med Ctr 1969; Plastic Surgery, Vanderbilt Univ Hosp 1976; **Fellow:** Neurological Surgery, Rigs Hosp-Kommunes Hosp 1976

Stevens, W Grant MD [PlS] - **Spec Exp:** Cosmetic Surgery-Breast; Liposuction & Body Contouring; Cosmetic Surgery-Face; **Hospital:** St. John's Hlth Ctr, Santa Monica, Marina Del Rey Hosp; **Address:** 4644 Lincoln Blvd, Ste 552, Marina Del Rey, CA 90292-6391; **Phone:** 310-827-2653; **Board Cert:** Plastic Surgery 1989; **Med School:** Washington Univ, St Louis 1980; **Resid:** Surgery, Harbor/UCLA Med Ctr 1983; **Fellow:** Hand Surgery, Washington Univ Sch Med 1984; Plastic Surgery, Washington Univ Sch Med 1986; **Fac Appt:** Assoc Clin Prof PlS, USC Sch Med

Urata, Mark M MD/DDS [PlS] - **Spec Exp:** Craniofacial Surgery-Pediatric; Maxillofacial Surgery; Head & Neck Surgery; **Hospital:** Chldns Hosp - Los Angeles, Keck Med Ctr of USC (page 75); **Address:** Chldns Hosp LA, Dept Plastic Surgery, 4650 W Sunset Blvd, MS 96, Los Angeles, CA 90027; **Phone:** 323-361-2154; **Board Cert:** Plastic Surgery 2005; **Med School:** USC Sch Med 1996; **Resid:** Oral & Maxillofacial Surgery, USC Med Ctr 1993; Plastic Surgery, USC Med Ctr 2002; **Fellow:** Craniofacial Surgery, UCLA Med Ctr 2003; **Fac Appt:** Prof PlS, USC-Keck School of Medicine

Wells, James H MD [PlS] - **Spec Exp:** Cleft Palate/Lip; Breast Surgery; **Hospital:** Long Beach Meml Med Ctr; **Address:** 2880 Atlantic Ave, Ste 290, Long Beach, CA 90806; **Phone:** 562-595-6543; **Board Cert:** Plastic Surgery 1978; **Med School:** Univ Tex Med Br, Galveston 1966; **Resid:** Surgery, Ochsner Fdn Hosp 1971; Plastic Surgery, Univ Virginia Hosp 1975

▪ Cleveland Clinic

Every life deserves world class care.

Plastic Surgery

Cleveland Clinic's Department of Plastic Surgery, part of the Cleveland Clinic Dermatology & Plastic Surgery Institute, offers a full array of subspecialized care for adult and pediatric patients. Among the department's major advancements is the successful completion in 2008 of the first near-total face transplant in the United States. This achievement has progressed into our new Reconstructive Transplant Center which provides an alternative for patients seeking new avenues in reconstruction of difficult facial, abdominal, laryngeal and hand deformities and dysfunction. The department also includes a team of surgeons extremely adept at handling all types of traumatic, congenital and work-related hand, peripheral nerve and upper extremity problems. Pediatric surgery and craniofacial surgery are strong specialties in the department.

Cleveland Clinic plastic surgeons offer numerous methods of breast reconstruction that can be performed either at the time of mastectomy or as a secondary procedure. These techniques include breast implants and expanders; pedicled transverse rectus abdominis myocutaneous flaps (using abdominal skin and muscle); and free-tissue transfers such as deep inferior epigastric perforator flap.

The Department of Plastic Surgery focuses on minimally invasive techniques in facial cosmetic surgery. This includes alternatives to face lift and neck lift surgery, short-scar face lifts and minimally invasive face lift techniques. In addition to standard body contouring procedures including abdominoplasty and a wide variety of liposuction techniques, the department is particularly interested in plastic surgery after significant weight loss.

Cleveland Clinic
Dermatology & Plastic
Surgery Institute
9500 Euclid Avenue
Cleveland, OH 44195

clevelandclinic.org/
plasticstopdocs

Offering Same-Day Appointments
Call 800.274.2009.

Treatment Guides

Cleveland Clinic has developed comprehensive treatment guides for many diseases and conditions. To download our free treatment guides, visit clevelandclinic.org/treatmentguides.

Online Medical Second Opinion

Cleveland Clinic's My**Consult** Online Medical Second Opinion program securely connects patients to our physician specialists for more than 1,000 life-changing or life-threatening diagnoses all by the click of a mouse. To learn more, log onto eclevelandclinic.org/myconsult or call 800.223.2273, ext. 43223.

Special Assistance for Out-of-State Patients

Cleveland Clinic Global Patient Services offers a complimentary Medical Concierge service for patients who travel from outside of Ohio. Call 800.223.2273, ext. 55580 or email medicalconcierge@ccf.org.

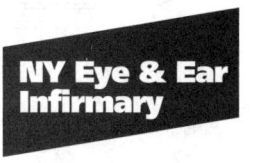

NY Eye & Ear Infirmary

Continuum Health Partners, Inc.

THE NEW YORK EYE AND EAR INFIRMARY

310 East 14th Street
New York, New York 10003
Tel. 212.979.4000   Fax. 212.228.0664
http://www.nyee.edu

PROVIDING EXCEPTIONAL CARE

The Department of Plastic & Reconstructive Surgery is one of the region's most comprehensive centers for surgery which restores the body and spirit. More than 1,500 procedures a year are performed here, and 50 of the most noted board-certified plastic surgeons located throughout New York City and tri-state area comprise the attending medical staff.

IN A HIGHLY SPECIALIZED SETTING

As a specialty hospital, the Infirmary is uniquely qualified to handle the most complicated cases. It serves as a nationwide referral center with a commitment to teaching, research, and high-technology based patient care. Highly experienced staff using state-of-the-art instrumentation have made the Infirmary's 17 operating rooms a national benchmark in efficiency. In addition, private premium patient accommodations are available to assure that the hospital experience is as comfortable and convenient as possible.

FOR PATIENTS OF ALL AGES

The Department treats more than 1,500 patients a year who seek reconstructive surgery of the body as well as facial area as a result of accident, birth defect or cancer, and those who elect cosmetic surgery. It is one of the few hospitals in the region to perform breast reconstruction after mastectomy with microvascular surgery to harvest tissue from patients' lower body to create living, natural, and normal looking breasts, often preferred to artificial implants. State-of-the-art lymph node transfer to cure post-mastectomy lymphedema is also available.

Childhood problems, such as cleft lip and palate and ear deformities also fall under the care of our surgeons.

Innovative cosmetic surgery procedures such as endoscopic and other minimally invasive operations are offered. The Center for Nasal Plastic specializes in closed (no scar) nasal plastic techniques as well as repair of previous nasal surgeries, the secondary nasal plasty. Liposuction using the latest instrumentation and fat grafting by the latest technology is also available as are the latest variants of the abdominoplasty (tummy tuck) operation.

The latest version of a skin tightening Fraxel Re:pair laser enables many patients to avoid a surgical face and eyelid plastic operation.

The hospital has a Post Graduate Cosmetic Surgery Program which offers a year of intensive cosmetic surgery training to surgeons who have completed a formal plastic surgery residency. The program is the largest and most sought-after in the US and also provides a source for affordable cosmetic surgery for the community.

Plastic Surgery Clinical Services

Facial plasty

Eyelid plastic operations

Nasal plastic operations

Breast augmentation
Breast reduction procedures and suspension

Breast reconstruction using patient's own tissue
(DIEP, S-GAP, I-GAP and SIEA flap procedures)

Liposuction

Abdominoplasty

Facial resurfacing and dermabrasion

Fraxel laser

Botox

About The New York Eye and Ear Infirmary

Founded in 1820, it is the nation's oldest, continuously operating specialty hospital Throughout its history, the Infirmary has led clinical advances and research in vision, hearing, speech and restoration of the physical appearance.

Physician Referral
1.800.449.HOPE (4673)

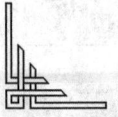
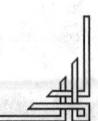

The Best in American Medicine
www.CastleConnolly.com

Preventive & Occupational Medicine

A preventive medicine specialist focuses on the health of individuals and defined populations in order to protect, promote and maintain health and well-being, and to prevent disease, disability and premature death. A preventive medicine physician may be a specialist in general preventive medicine, public health, occupational medicine, or aerospace medicine. This specialist works with large population groups as well as with individual patients to promote health and understand the risks of disease, injury, disability, and death, seeking to modify and eliminate these risks.

Training Required: Three years

OCCUPATIONAL MEDICINE

Mid Atlantic

Gochfeld, Michael MD/PhD [OM] - **Spec Exp:** Environmental Medicine; Occupational Medicine; Mercury Toxic Exposure; Toxic Exposure; **Hospital:** Robert Wood Johnson Univ Hosp - New Brunswick; **Address:** Enviro & Occupational Health - EOHSI, 170 Frelinghuysen Rd, Ste 200, Piscataway, NJ 08854; **Phone:** 732-445-0123 x627; **Board Cert:** Occupational Medicine 1983; **Med School:** Albert Einstein Coll Med 1965; **Resid:** Behavioral Medicine, Rockefeller Univ 1977; **Fac Appt:** Prof OM, UMDNJ-RW Johnson Med Sch

Kipen, Howard M MD [OM] - **Spec Exp:** Environmental Medicine; Occupational Medicine; Occupational Lung Disease; **Hospital:** Robert Wood Johnson Univ Hosp - New Brunswick; **Address:** UMDNJ-RWJ Med Sch, EOHSI, 170 Frelinghuysen Rd, Ste 200, Piscataway, NJ 08854; **Phone:** 732-445-0123 x601; **Board Cert:** Internal Medicine 1982; Occupational Medicine 1986; **Med School:** UCSF 1979; **Resid:** Internal Medicine, Columbia Presby Med Ctr 1982; Occupational Medicine, Mt Sinai Hosp 1984; **Fac Appt:** Prof Med, UMDNJ-RW Johnson Med Sch

Landrigan, Philip MD [OM] - **Spec Exp:** Environmental Health in Children; **Hospital:** Mount Sinai Med Ctr (page 63); **Address:** Dept Preventive Med, One Gustave L Levy Pl, Box 1057, New York, NY 10029-6500; **Phone:** 212-824-7018; **Board Cert:** Pediatrics 1973; Public Health & Genl Preventive Med 1979; Occupational Medicine 1983; **Med School:** Harvard Med Sch 1967; **Resid:** Internal Medicine, Metro Genl Hosp 1968; Pediatrics, Chldns Hosp 1970; **Fellow:** Epidemiology, Ctrs for Disease Control 1973; Occupational Medicine, Univ London 1977; **Fac Appt:** Prof Ped, Mount Sinai Sch Med

West Coast and Pacific

Harber, Philip I MD [OM] - **Spec Exp:** Occupational Lung Disease; Occupational Asthma; Beryllium-induced Lung Disease; Asbestos-related Lung Disease; **Address:** 7230 Medical Center Drive, Ste 300, West Hills, CA 91307; **Phone:** 310-433-5342; **Board Cert:** Internal Medicine 1979; Pulmonary Disease 1980; Occupational Medicine 1982; **Med School:** Univ Pennsylvania 1972; **Resid:** Internal Medicine, Georgetown Univ Med Ctr 1978; Occupational Medicine, Johns Hopkins Hosp 1980; **Fellow:** Pulmonary Disease, Johns Hopkins Hosp 1980; **Fac Appt:** Prof Public Hlth, Univ Ariz Coll Med

PREVENTIVE MEDICINE

Mid Atlantic

Cahill, John MD [PrM] - **Spec Exp:** Tropical Diseases; Travel Medicine; Parasitic Infections; International Health; **Hospital:** St. Luke's - Roosevelt Hosp Ctr - Roosevelt Div (page 55); **Address:** 425 W 59th St, Ste 8A, New York, NY 10019; **Phone:** 212-492-5500; **Board Cert:** Emergency Medicine 2001; **Med School:** Mount Sinai Sch Med 1996; **Resid:** Emergency Medicine, Rhode Island Hosp 1997; Emergency Medicine, Rhode Island Hosp 2000; **Fellow:** Tropical Medicine, Royal Coll Surgeons 1998; **Fac Appt:** Asst Clin Prof Med, Columbia P&S

Cahill, Kevin M MD [PrM] - **Spec Exp:** Tropical Diseases; International Health; Parasitic Infections; Tropical Diseases; **Hospital:** Lenox Hill Hosp; **Address:** 850 5th Ave, New York, NY 10065; **Phone:** 212-434-2477; **Board Cert:** Public Health & Genl Preventive Med 1970; **Med School:** Cornell Univ-Weill Med Coll 1961; **Resid:** Internal Medicine, US Navy Med Res Unit 1965; Public Health & Genl Preventive Med, US Navy Med Res Unit 1965; **Fac Appt:** Clin Prof Med, NYU Sch Med

Hoffman, Robert S MD [PrM] - **Spec Exp:** Poison Control; Disaster Preparedness; **Hospital:** NYU Langone Med Ctr (page 66), Bellevue Hosp Ctr; **Address:** NY Poison Control Ctr, 455 1st Ave, rm 123, New York, NY 10016; **Phone:** 212-340-4494; **Board Cert:** Internal Medicine 1987; Emergency Medicine 2005; Medical Toxicology 2008; **Med School:** NYU Sch Med 1984; **Resid:** Internal Medicine, NYU Med Ctr 1987; **Fellow:** Medical Toxicology, NYU Med Ctr 1989; **Fac Appt:** Assoc Prof Med, NYU Sch Med

Pearson, Thomas A MD/PhD [PrM] - **Spec Exp:** Preventive Cardiology; Cholesterol/Lipid Disorders; **Hospital:** Univ of Rochester Strong Meml Hosp; **Address:** Dept Community & Preventive Medicine, PO Box 278990, Rochester, NY 14627; **Phone:** 585-341-7759; **Board Cert:** Internal Medicine 1983; Preventive Medicine 1986; **Med School:** Johns Hopkins Univ 1976; **Resid:** Preventive Medicine, Johns Hopkins Hosp 1979; Internal Medicine, Johns Hopkins Hosp 1980; **Fellow:** Cardiovascular Disease, Johns Hopkins Hosp 1983; **Fac Appt:** Prof PrM, Univ Rochester

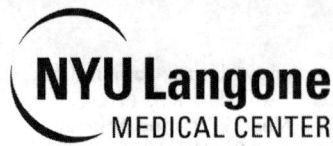

Joan H. Tisch Center for Women's Health
207 East 84th Street *(at 3rd Avenue)*
New York, NY
www.NYULMC.org
646-754-3300
Physician Referral: **888-7-NYU-MED** *(888-769-8633)*

THE JOAN H. TISCH CENTER FOR WOMEN'S HEALTH

About the Joan H. Tisch Center for Women's Health

Because many diseases and conditions impact women differently than men, NYU Langone Medical Center has created the Joan H. Tisch Center for Women's Health. Offering a comprehensive array of primary and specialty care, the Joan H. Tisch Center for Women's Health is New York City's premier destination for healthcare services tailored to the special needs of women. Conveniently located in the heart of Manhattan's Upper East Side, the Center combines NYU Langone's tradition of excellence with a multidisciplinary approach to providing individuals with the best possible medical care. At the Joan H. Tisch Center for Women's Health, the goal is maintaining excellent health and the vehicle is a caring, nurturing environment which understands that women are more than a collection of symptoms and medical conditions.

Expert Staff

Primary and specialty care physicians at the Joan H. Tisch Center for Women's Health have been carefully chosen for their ability to render quality, compassionate care to women. These healthcare professionals are focused on the holistic needs of patients in a state-of-the-art setting that relies heavily on teamwork. As part of a major academic medical institution, the Center is able to draw on additional healthcare resources and innovative research, when the need arises.

Comprehensive Range of Services

The Joan H. Tisch Center for Women's Health offers a wide range of primary and specialty medical care geared to women at a single location. Specialty services include breast health, cardiology, dermatology, endocrinology, ear/nose/throat, gastroenterology, gynecology, internal medicine, mental health, neurology, orthopaedics, plastic surgery, podiatry, pulmonary medicine, rehabilitation medicine, rheumatology, urology, vascular and women's imaging.

Technology Edge

The Joan H. Tisch Center for Women's Health has incorporated sophisticated technology into all levels of the patient experience. This ranges from the Center's informative website to its use of Epic, the Medical Center's up-to-the-minute electronic medical records system. In addition, patients can confidentially view their medical records and test results, as well as make appointment, request prescriptions and communicate with their physicians, through myNYULMC, a secure online service.

Psychiatry

A psychiatrist specializes in the prevention, diagnosis and treatment of mental, addictive and emotional disorders such as schizophrenia and other psychotic disorders, mood disorders, anxiety disorders, substance-related disorders, sexual and gender identity disorders and adjustment disorders. The psychiatrist is able to understand the biologic, psychologic and social components of illness, and therefore is uniquely prepared to treat the whole person. A psychiatrist is qualified to order diagnostic laboratory tests and to prescribe medications, evaluate and treat psychologic and interpersonal problems and to intervene with families who are coping with stress, crises and other problems in living.

Training Required: Four years

Certification in one of the following subspecialties requires additional training and examination.

Addiction Psychiatry: A psychiatrist who focuses on the evaluation and treatment of individuals with alcohol, drug, or other substance-related disorders and of individuals with the dual diagnosis of substance-related and other psychiatric disorders.

Child and Adolescent Psychiatry: A psychiatrist with additional training in the diagnosis and treatment of developmental, behavioral, emotional and mental disorders of childhood and adolescence.

Geriatric Psychiatry: A psychiatrist with expertise in the prevention, evaluation, diagnosis and treatment of mental and emotional disorders in the elderly. The geriatric psychiatrist seeks to improve the psychiatric care of the elderly both in health and in disease.

PSYCHIATRY

New England

Adler, David A MD [Psyc] - **Spec Exp:** Depression; Personality Disorders; Schizophrenia; **Hospital:** Tufts Med Ctr; **Address:** Tufts Med Ctr, Dept Psyc, 800 Washington St, Ste 1007, Boston, MA 02111; **Phone:** 617-636-8755; **Board Cert:** Psychiatry 1977; **Med School:** Yale Univ 1973; **Resid:** Psychiatry, Mass Mental Hlth Ctr 1976; **Fac Appt:** Prof Psyc, Tufts Univ

Benes, Francine M MD/PhD [Psyc] - **Spec Exp:** Schizophrenia; Bipolar/Mood Disorders; Neuro-Pathology; **Hospital:** McLean Hosp; **Address:** McLean Hosp, Harvard Brain Tissue Resource Ctr, 115 Mill St, Mailman Rsch Bldg, Belmont, MA 02478-1064; **Phone:** 617-855-2401; **Board Cert:** Psychiatry 1987; **Med School:** Yale Univ 1978; **Resid:** Psychiatry, McLean Hosp 1982; **Fac Appt:** Prof Psyc, Harvard Med Sch

Block, Susan D MD [Psyc] - **Spec Exp:** Psychiatry in Cancer; Palliative Care; **Hospital:** Dana-Farber Cancer Inst (page 57), Brigham and Women's Hosp (page 57); **Address:** Dana Farber Cancer Inst, 450 Brookline Ave, Shields Warren, Boston, MA 02115; **Phone:** 617-632-5788; **Board Cert:** Internal Medicine 1981; Psychiatry 1984; Hospice & Palliative Medicine 2003; **Med School:** Case West Res Univ 1977; **Resid:** Internal Medicine, Beth Israel Hosp 1980; Psychiatry, Beth Israel Hosp 1982; **Fac Appt:** Prof Psyc, Harvard Med Sch

Ellison, James M MD [Psyc] - **Spec Exp:** Geriatric Psychiatry; **Hospital:** McLean Hosp; **Address:** McLean Hospital, 115 Mill St, Belmont, MA 02478; **Phone:** 617-855-2532; **Board Cert:** Psychiatry 1984; Geriatric Psychiatry 2007; **Med School:** UCSF 1978; **Resid:** Psychiatry, Mass Genl Hosp 1982; **Fac Appt:** Assoc Prof Psyc, Harvard Med Sch

Friedman, Matthew J MD/PhD [Psyc] - **Spec Exp:** Post Traumatic Stress Disorder; Psychopharmacology; Anxiety & Mood Disorders; **Hospital:** White River Junction VA Med Ctr, Dartmouth - Hitchcock Med Ctr; **Address:** National Ctr for PTSD, VA Med Ctr, 215 N Main St, White River Junction, VT 05009; **Phone:** 802-296-5132; **Board Cert:** Psychiatry 1976; **Med School:** Univ KY Coll Med 1976; **Resid:** Psychiatry, Mass Genl Hosp 1972; Psychiatry, Dartmouth Hitchcock Med Ctr 1973; **Fac Appt:** Prof Psyc, Dartmouth Med Sch

Goff, Donald C MD [Psyc] - **Spec Exp:** Schizophrenia; Psychopharmacology; **Hospital:** Mass Genl Hosp; **Address:** Freedom Trail Clin, 25 Stainiford St, Boston, MA 02114; **Phone:** 617-912-7899; **Board Cert:** Psychiatry 1986; **Med School:** UCLA 1980; **Resid:** Psychiatry, Mass Genl Hosp 1984; **Fellow:** Psychopharmacology, Tufts-New England Med Ctr 1985; **Fac Appt:** Assoc Prof Psyc, Tufts Univ

Greenberg, Benjamin D MD/PhD [Psyc] - **Spec Exp:** Obsessive-Compulsive Disorder; **Hospital:** Butler Hosp; **Address:** 345 Blackstone Blvd, Providence, RI 02906; **Phone:** 401-455-6602; **Board Cert:** Psychiatry 1994; **Med School:** Univ Miami Sch Med 1987; **Resid:** Neurology, Columbian Univ/Presbyterian Hosp 1989; Psychiatry, Johns Hopkins Hosp 1992; **Fac Appt:** Psyc, Johns Hopkins Univ

Greenberg, Donna B MD [Psyc] - **Spec Exp:** Psychiatry in Cancer; **Hospital:** Mass Genl Hosp; **Address:** Mass General Hosp, 55 Fruit St, Yawkey 9A- Psych, Fatigue Dept, Boston, MA 02114-2696; **Phone:** 617-724-4800; **Board Cert:** Internal Medicine 1978; Psychiatry 1990; **Med School:** Univ Rochester 1975; **Resid:** Internal Medicine, Boston City Hosp 1978; Psychiatry, Mass Genl Hosp 1989; **Fellow:** Psychiatry, Mass Genl Hosp 1979; **Fac Appt:** Assoc Prof Psyc, Harvard Med Sch

Greenberg, William E MD [Psyc] - **Hospital:** Beth Israel Deaconess Med Ctr - Boston; **Address:** Beth Israel Deaconess Med Ctr, Dept Psychiatry, 330 Brookline Ave, Ste 205, Boston, MA 02215-5400; **Phone:** 617-667-2740; **Board Cert:** Psychiatry 1981; **Med School:** Univ Pennsylvania 1976; **Resid:** Psychiatry, Beth Israel Deaconess Med Ctr 1981; **Fac Appt:** Clin Prof Psyc, Harvard Med Sch

Gunderson, John G MD [Psyc] - **Spec Exp:** Personality Disorders; Personality Disorders-Borderline; Psychotherapy; **Hospital:** McLean Hosp; **Address:** McLean Hospital, 115 Mill St, Belmont, MA 02478; **Phone:** 617-855-2293; **Board Cert:** Psychiatry 1974; **Med School:** Harvard Med Sch 1967; **Resid:** Psychiatry, Mass Mental Hlth Ctr 1971; **Fac Appt:** Prof Psyc, Harvard Med Sch

Jenike, Michael A MD [Psyc] - **Spec Exp:** Obsessive-Compulsive Disorder; Geriatric Psychiatry; **Hospital:** Mass Genl Hosp; **Address:** Obsessive Compulsive Disorders Unit, 185 Cambridge St, Ste 2200, Boston, MA 02114; **Phone:** 617-726-6766; **Board Cert:** Psychiatry 1984; **Med School:** Univ Okla Coll Med 1978; **Resid:** Psychiatry, Mass Genl Hosp 1982; **Fellow:** Psychiatry, Harvard Med Sch; Psychiatry, Mass Genl Hosp; **Fac Appt:** Prof Psyc, Harvard Med Sch

Jimerson, David C MD [Psyc] - **Spec Exp:** Eating Disorders; **Hospital:** Beth Israel Deaconess Med Ctr - Boston; **Address:** Beth Israel Deaconess Med Ctr, Dept Psyc, 330 Brookline Ave, Boston, MA 02215-5400; **Phone:** 617-667-4667; **Board Cert:** Psychiatry 1977; **Med School:** Cornell Univ-Weill Med Coll 1972; **Resid:** Psychiatry, UC-San Diego 1974; Psychiatry, NIMH 1975; **Fac Appt:** Prof Psyc, Harvard Med Sch

McGlashan, Thomas H MD [Psyc] - **Spec Exp:** Schizophrenia-Early Detection/Treatment; Personality Disorders; Schizophrenia-Clinical Trials; Personality Disorders-Clinical Trials; **Hospital:** Connecticut Mental Hlth Ctr, Yale-New Haven Hosp; **Address:** Yale Univ Sch Med, Dept Psychiatry, 301 Cedar St, New Haven, CT 06519; **Phone:** 203-737-2077; **Board Cert:** Psychiatry 1973; **Med School:** Univ Pennsylvania 1967; **Resid:** Psychiatry, Mass Mental Hlth Ctr 1971; **Fac Appt:** Prof Psyc, Yale Univ

Phillips, Katharine A MD [Psyc] - **Spec Exp:** Body Dysmorphic Disorder (BDD); Obsessive-Compulsive Disorder; **Hospital:** Rhode Island Hosp; **Address:** Rhode Island Hospital, Coro Center West, 1 Hoppin St, Ste 2.030, Providence, RI 02903; **Phone:** 401-444-1646; **Board Cert:** Psychiatry 1992; **Med School:** Dartmouth Med Sch 1987; **Resid:** Psychiatry, McLean Hosp 1991; **Fellow:** Research, McLean Hosp 1994; **Fac Appt:** Prof Psyc, Brown Univ

Price, Lawrence H MD [Psyc] - **Spec Exp:** Anxiety & Mood Disorders; Depression; Bipolar/Mood Disorders; Obsessive-Compulsive Disorder; **Hospital:** Butler Hosp, Kent Hosp; **Address:** Butler Hospital, Dept Psychiatry, 345 Blackstone Blvd, Providence, RI 02906; **Phone:** 401-455-6533; **Board Cert:** Psychiatry 1983; **Med School:** Univ Mich Med Sch 1978; **Resid:** Psychiatry, Yale-New Haven Hosp 1982; **Fellow:** Psychiatry, Yale-New Haven Hosp 1983; **Fac Appt:** Prof Psyc, Brown Univ

Rasmussen, Steven A MD [Psyc] - **Spec Exp:** Obsessive-Compulsive Disorder; **Hospital:** Butler Hosp; **Address:** Butler Hosp, 345 Blackstone Blvd, Providence, RI 02906; **Phone:** 401-455-6209; **Board Cert:** Psychiatry 1983; **Med School:** Brown Univ 1977; **Resid:** Psychiatry, Yale Univ 1981; **Fac Appt:** Assoc Prof Psyc, Brown Univ

Rauch, Paula K MD [Psyc] - **Spec Exp:** Psychiatry in Childhood Cancer; Children/Families with Severe Illness; Parent Guidance in Parental Cancer; Psychiatry in Physical Illness; **Hospital:** Mass Genl Hosp; **Address:** Mass General Hosp, Dept Child Psychiatry, 55 Fruit St, Yawkey 6A, Boston, MA 02114; **Phone:** 617-724-5600; **Board Cert:** Psychiatry 1990; Child & Adolescent Psychiatry 1991; **Med School:** Univ Cincinnati 1981; **Resid:** Psychiatry, Mass Genl Hosp 1984; **Fac Appt:** Asst Prof Psyc, Harvard Med Sch

Psychiatry

Salzman, Carl MD [Psyc] - **Spec Exp:** Psychopharmacology; Geriatric Psychiatry; Psychotherapy; **Hospital:** MA Mental Hlth Ctr, Beth Israel Deaconess Med Ctr - Boston; **Address:** Havard Med Sch, Dept Psychiatry, 25 Shattuck St, Boston, MA 02115; **Phone:** 617-998-5006; **Board Cert:** Psychiatry 1970; **Med School:** SUNY Upstate Med Univ 1963; **Resid:** Psychiatry, Mass Mental Hlth Ctr 1967; Psychiatry, Natl Inst Mental Hlth 1969; **Fac Appt:** Prof Psyc, Harvard Med Sch

Shapiro, Edward R MD [Psyc] - **Spec Exp:** Psychoanalysis; **Hospital:** Austen Riggs Ctr; **Address:** Austen Riggs Ctr, 25 Main St, PO Box 962, Stockbridge, MA 01262; **Phone:** 413-298-5511; **Board Cert:** Psychiatry 1974; **Med School:** Harvard Med Sch 1968; **Resid:** Psychiatry, Mass Mental Hlth Ctr 1972; **Fellow:** Psychiatry, Natl Inst Mental Hlth 1974; **Fac Appt:** Assoc Clin Prof Psyc, Harvard Med Sch

Summergrad, Paul MD [Psyc] - **Hospital:** Tufts Med Ctr; **Address:** Tufts Med Ctr, 800 Washington St, Ste 1007, Boston, MA 02111; **Phone:** 617-636-5773; **Board Cert:** Internal Medicine 1981; Psychiatry 1986; Geriatric Psychiatry 2007; Psychosomatic Medicine 2005; **Med School:** SUNY Buffalo 1978; **Resid:** Internal Medicine, Boston City Hosp 1981; **Fellow:** Psychiatry, Mass Genl Hosp 1985; **Fac Appt:** Prof Psyc, Tufts Univ

Mid Atlantic

Akhtar, Salman MD [Psyc] - **Spec Exp:** Psychoanalysis; **Hospital:** Thomas Jefferson Univ Hosp; **Address:** Jefferson Med College, Dept Psychiatry, 833 Chestnut St, Ste 210, Philadelphia, PA 19107; **Phone:** 215-955-2547; **Board Cert:** Psychiatry 1977; **Med School:** India 1968; **Resid:** Psychiatry, UMDNJ Med Ctr 1974; Psychiatry, Univ Virginia Med Ctr 1976; **Fellow:** Psychoanalysis, Philadelphia Psych Inst 1986; **Fac Appt:** Prof Psyc, Thomas Jefferson Univ

Appelbaum, Paul S MD [Psyc] - **Spec Exp:** Forensic Psychiatry; Depression; Anxiety & Mood Disorders; **Hospital:** NY-Presby/Columbia Univ Med Ctr, NY (page 65); **Address:** NY State Psychiatric Inst, 1051 Riverside Drive, rm 6714, Box 122, New York, NY 10032; **Phone:** 212-543-4184; **Board Cert:** Psychiatry 1981; Forensic Psychiatry 2004; **Med School:** Harvard Med Sch 1976; **Resid:** Psychiatry, Mass Mental Health Ctr 1980; **Fac Appt:** Prof Psyc, Columbia P&S

Arnold, Steven E MD [Psyc] - **Spec Exp:** Alzheimer's Disease; **Hospital:** Hosp Univ Penn - UPHS (page 68); **Address:** Ralston House, 3615 Chestnut St, Philadelphia, PA 19104; **Phone:** 215-662-7810; **Board Cert:** Psychiatry 1988; Neurology 1991; **Med School:** Boston Univ 1983; **Resid:** Psychiatry, NYS Psych Inst/Columbia Presby Med Ctr 1987; Neurology, Univ IA Hosps & Clins 1990; **Fellow:** Behavioral Neurology, Univ IA Hosps & Clins 1990; **Fac Appt:** Prof Psyc, Univ Pennsylvania

Basch, Samuel MD [Psyc] - **Spec Exp:** Psychopharmacology; Psychiatry in Physical Illness; Psychiatry in Cancer; Psychoanalysis; **Hospital:** Mount Sinai Med Ctr (page 63); **Address:** 10 E 85th St, Ste 1B, New York, NY 10028-0412; **Phone:** 212-427-0344; **Board Cert:** Psychiatry 1970; **Med School:** Hahnemann Univ 1961; **Resid:** Psychiatry, Mount Sinai Hosp 1965; **Fellow:** Psychoanalysis, Columbia Presby Hosp 1976; **Fac Appt:** Clin Prof Psyc, Mount Sinai Sch Med

Boronow, John Joseph MD [Psyc] - **Spec Exp:** Psychotic Disorders; Schizophrenia; **Hospital:** Sheppard Pratt Hlth Sys; **Address:** 6501 N Charles St, rm TJ-113, Towson, MD 21284; **Phone:** 410-938-4306; **Board Cert:** Psychiatry 1983; **Med School:** Yale Univ 1977; **Resid:** Psychiatry, New York Hosp 1981; **Fellow:** Psychopharmacology, Natl Inst Mntl Hlth 1983; **Fac Appt:** Assoc Clin Prof Psyc, Univ MD Sch Med

Brandt, Harry A MD [Psyc] - **Spec Exp:** Eating Disorders; **Hospital:** St. Joseph Med Ctr, Sheppard Pratt Hlth Sys; **Address:** Ctr for Eating Disorders, 6535 N Charles St, Ste 300, Towson, MD 21204; **Phone:** 410-938-5252; **Board Cert:** Psychiatry 1989; **Med School:** Univ MD Sch Med 1983; **Resid:** Psychiatry, Univ Maryland Hosp 1986; **Fellow:** Biological Psychiatry, Natl Inst Mental Hlth 1988; **Fac Appt:** Assoc Clin Prof Psyc, Univ MD Sch Med

Breitbart, William MD [Psyc] - **Spec Exp:** Psychiatry in Cancer; AIDS Related Cancers; Pain-Cancer; Palliative Care; **Hospital:** Meml Sloan-Kettering Cancer Ctr; **Address:** 1275 York Avenue, New York, NY 10065; **Phone:** 646-888-0100; **Board Cert:** Internal Medicine 1982; Psychiatry 1986; Psychosomatic Medicine 2005; **Med School:** Albert Einstein Coll Med 1978; **Resid:** Internal Medicine, Bronx Muni Hosp Ctr 1982; Psychiatry, Bronx Muni Hosp Ctr 1984; **Fellow:** Psychiatric Oncology, Meml Sloan Kettering Cancer Ctr 1986; **Fac Appt:** Prof Psyc, Cornell Univ-Weill Med Coll

Brodkin, Edward S MD [Psyc] - **Spec Exp:** Autism; Asperger's Syndrome; **Hospital:** Hosp Univ Penn - UPHS (page 68), Pennsylvania Hosp-UPHS (page 68); **Address:** Univ Penn Sch Med, Translational Rsch Lab, 125 S 31st St, rm 2220, Philadelphia, PA 19104-3403; **Phone:** 215-746-0118; **Board Cert:** Psychiatry 2006; **Med School:** Harvard Med Sch 1992; **Resid:** Psychiatry, Yale-New Haven Hosp 1996; **Fellow:** Neurological Science, Yale Univ Sch Med 1998; Genetics, Princeton Univ 2002; **Fac Appt:** Asst Prof Psyc, Univ Pennsylvania

Bronheim, Harold MD [Psyc] - **Spec Exp:** Psychiatry in Body Image Awareness; Relationship Problems; Psychiatry in Physical Illness; Anxiety & Depression; **Hospital:** Mount Sinai Med Ctr (page 63); **Address:** 1155 Park Ave, New York, NY 10028; **Phone:** 212-996-5777; **Board Cert:** Psychiatry 1985; Internal Medicine 1986; Psychosomatic Medicine 2005; Geriatric Psychiatry 2001; **Med School:** SUNY Downstate 1980; **Resid:** Psychiatry, Mount Sinai Hosp 1984; **Fellow:** Internal Medicine, Beth Israel Hosp 1985; **Fac Appt:** Clin Prof Psyc, Mount Sinai Sch Med

Buysse, Daniel J MD [Psyc] - **Spec Exp:** Sleep Disorders; **Hospital:** UPMC Presby, Pittsburgh; **Address:** 3811 O'Hara St, rm E-1127, Pittsburgh, PA 15213; **Phone:** 412-246-6413; **Board Cert:** Psychiatry 1988; Sleep Medicine 2007; **Med School:** Univ Mich Med Sch 1983; **Resid:** Psychiatry, Western Psych Inst 1987; **Fellow:** Sleep Medicine, Univ of Pittsburgh; **Fac Appt:** Asst Prof Psyc, Univ Pittsburgh

Cohen, Mitchell Joseph MD [Psyc] - **Spec Exp:** Pain-Chronic; Psychiatry in Physical Illness; Anxiety Disorders; **Hospital:** Thomas Jefferson Univ Hosp; **Address:** 833 Chestnut St E, Ste 210B, Philadelphia, PA 19107; **Phone:** 215-955-6592; **Board Cert:** Psychiatry 1989; Pain Medicine 2002; **Med School:** Med Coll PA 1984; **Resid:** Psychiatry, Johns Hopkins Hosp 1988; **Fac Appt:** Prof Psyc, Thomas Jefferson Univ

DePaulo Jr, J Raymond MD [Psyc] - **Spec Exp:** Bipolar/Mood Disorders; Depression; **Hospital:** Johns Hopkins Hosp (page 61); **Address:** Johns Hopkins Hosp, Dept Psychiatry, 600 N Wolfe St, Meyer 4-113, Baltimore, MD 21287-7413; **Phone:** 410-955-3130; **Board Cert:** Psychiatry 1977; **Med School:** Johns Hopkins Univ 1972; **Resid:** Psychiatry, Johns Hopkins Hosp 1977; **Fac Appt:** Prof Psyc, Johns Hopkins Univ

Doghramji, Karl MD [Psyc] - **Spec Exp:** Sleep Disorders/Apnea; Narcolepsy; Restless Legs Syndrome; **Hospital:** Thomas Jefferson Univ Hosp; **Address:** 211 S Ninth St, Ste 500, Philadelphia, PA 19107; **Phone:** 215-955-6175; **Board Cert:** Psychiatry 1986; Sleep Medicine 1985; **Med School:** Thomas Jefferson Univ 1980; **Resid:** Psychiatry, Thomas Jefferson Univ Hosp 1984; **Fellow:** Sleep Medicine, Montefiore Med Ctr; **Fac Appt:** Prof Psyc, Thomas Jefferson Univ

Psychiatry

Eaton Jr, James S MD [Psyc] - **Spec Exp:** Anxiety Disorders; Sexual Identity Issues; Depression; Diagnostic Second Opinions; **Hospital:** Georgetown Univ Hosp, G Washington Univ Hosp; **Address:** 4214 50th St NW, Washington, DC 20016; **Phone:** 202-333-5796; **Board Cert:** Psychiatry 1976; **Med School:** Tulane Univ 1962; **Resid:** Internal Medicine, Tulane Univ Med Ctr 1966; Psychiatry, Tulane Univ Med Ctr 1968; **Fellow:** Psychoanalysis, Tulane Univ Med Ctr 1973; **Fac Appt:** Clin Prof Psyc, Georgetown Univ

Fallon, Brian A MD [Psyc] - **Spec Exp:** Lyme Disease-Neuro Complications; Psychosomatic Disorders; Obsessive-Compulsive Disorder; Psychiatry in Physical Illness; **Hospital:** NY-Presby/Columbia Univ Med Ctr, NY (page 65); **Address:** NYS Psychiatric Institute, 1051 Riverside Drive, Room 3724, Unit Box 69, New York, NY 10032; **Phone:** 212-543-5487; **Board Cert:** Psychiatry 1991; **Med School:** Columbia P&S 1985; **Resid:** Psychiatry, NYS Psychiatric Inst 1989; **Fellow:** Psychiatric Research, NYS Psychiatric Inst 1992; Psychodynamic Psychotherapy, Columbia Univ Psychoanalytic Inst 1990; **Fac Appt:** Asst Clin Prof Psyc, Columbia P&S

First, Michael B MD [Psyc] - **Spec Exp:** Psychotherapy; Psychopharmacology; Forensic Psychiatry; Sexual Addiction; **Hospital:** NY-Presby/Columbia Univ Med Ctr, NY (page 65); **Address:** NY State Psychiatric Inst, Unit 60, 1051 Riverside Drive, New York, NY 10032; **Phone:** 212-543-5531; **Board Cert:** Psychiatry 1989; **Med School:** Univ Pittsburgh 1983; **Resid:** Psychiatry, NY State Psych Inst 1987; **Fellow:** Psychiatric Research, NY State Psych Inst 1988; **Fac Appt:** Clin Prof Psyc, Columbia P&S

Fyer, Abby J MD [Psyc] - **Spec Exp:** Anxiety Disorders; Panic Disorder; **Hospital:** NY State Psychiatric Inst; **Address:** 1051 Riverside Dr, Box 82, New York, NY 10032; **Phone:** 212-543-5372; **Board Cert:** Psychiatry 1980; **Med School:** NYU Sch Med 1973; **Resid:** Psychiatry, Montefiore Med Ctr 1978; **Fac Appt:** Prof Psyc, Columbia P&S

Guarda, Angela S MD [Psyc] - **Spec Exp:** Eating Disorders; **Hospital:** Johns Hopkins Hosp (page 61); **Address:** Johns Hopkins Hosp, Eating Disorder Prgm, 600 N Wolfe St Myer Bldg - rm 101, Baltimore, MD 21287; **Phone:** 410-614-4624; **Board Cert:** Psychiatry 2006; **Med School:** Univ MD Sch Med 1991; **Resid:** Psychiatry, Johns Hopkins Hosp 1995; **Fac Appt:** Assoc Prof Psyc, Johns Hopkins Univ

Halmi, Katherine MD [Psyc] - **Spec Exp:** Eating Disorders; **Hospital:** NY-Presby/Westchester Div, NY (page 65); **Address:** NY Presby Hosp - Westchester Div, 21 Bloomingdale Rd, White Plains, NY 10605; **Phone:** 914-997-5875; **Board Cert:** Pediatrics 1970; Psychiatry 1977; **Med School:** Univ Iowa Coll Med 1965; **Resid:** Pediatrics, Univ Iowa Hosp 1968; Psychiatry, Univ Iowa Hosp 1972; **Fellow:** Child Development, Univ Iowa Hosp 1969; **Fac Appt:** Prof Psyc, Cornell Univ-Weill Med Coll

Hollander, Eric MD [Psyc] - **Spec Exp:** Obsessive-Compulsive Disorder; Anxiety Disorders; Autism; Body Dysmorphic Disorder (BDD); **Hospital:** Montefiore Med Ctr - Div. Moses; **Address:** 901 Fifth Ave, New York, NY 10021; **Phone:** 212-873-4051; **Board Cert:** Psychiatry 1987; **Med School:** SUNY Hlth Sci Ctr 1982; **Resid:** Internal Medicine, Mount Sinai Hosp 1983; Psychiatry, Mount Sinai Hosp 1986; **Fellow:** Psychiatry, Columbia-Presby Med Ctr 1988; **Fac Appt:** Prof Psyc, Albert Einstein Coll Med

Karasu, T Byram MD [Psyc] - **Spec Exp:** Depression; Personality Disorders; Psychotherapy; **Hospital:** Montefiore Med Ctr - Div. Moses; **Address:** 2 E 88th St, New York, NY 10128-0555; **Phone:** 212-426-5208; **Board Cert:** Psychiatry 1972; **Med School:** Turkey 1959; **Resid:** Psychiatry, Yale-New Haven Hosp 1968; **Fellow:** Psychiatry, Yale-New Haven Hosp 1969; **Fac Appt:** Prof Psyc, Albert Einstein Coll Med

Kavey, Neil B MD [Psyc] - **Spec Exp:** Sleep Medicine; Narcolepsy; Sleep Disorders/Apnea; **Hospital:** NY-Presby/Columbia Univ Med Ctr, NY (page 65), Rockefeller Univ; **Address:** Columbia Presby Med Ctr, Sleep Disorders Ctr, 161 Ft Washington Ave Fl 3 - rm 342, New York, NY 10032; **Phone:** 212-305-1860; **Board Cert:** Psychiatry 1976; Sleep Medicine 2003; **Med School:** Columbia P&S 1969; **Resid:** Psychiatry, Columbia Presby Med Ctr 1973; **Fac Appt:** Clin Prof Psyc, Columbia P&S

Klagsbrun, Samuel C MD [Psyc] - **Spec Exp:** Psychiatry in Cancer; Psychiatry in Terminal Illness; **Hospital:** Four Winds Hosp; **Address:** Four Winds Hospital, 800 Cross River Rd, Katonah, NY 10536; **Phone:** 914-763-8151 x2222; **Board Cert:** Psychiatry 1977; **Med School:** Ros Franklin Univ/Chicago Med Sch 1962; **Resid:** Psychiatry, Yale-New Haven Hosp 1966; **Fac Appt:** Clin Prof Psyc, Albert Einstein Coll Med

Krueger, Richard B MD [Psyc] - **Spec Exp:** Sexual Behavior-Compulsive; **Hospital:** NY-Presby/Columbia Univ Med Ctr, NY (page 65); **Address:** 210 E 68th St, Ste 1H, New York, NY 10021-6047; **Phone:** 212-517-6624; **Board Cert:** Psychiatry 1984; Internal Medicine 1980; Addiction Psychiatry 2007; Forensic Psychiatry 2006; **Med School:** Harvard Med Sch 1977; **Resid:** Internal Medicine, Boston VA Hosp 1980; **Fellow:** Psychiatry, Boston Univ Hosp 1983; **Fac Appt:** Assoc Prof Psyc, Columbia P&S

Kunkel, Elisabeth J MD [Psyc] - **Spec Exp:** Psychiatry in Cancer; Psychiatry in Physical Illness; **Hospital:** Thomas Jefferson Univ Hosp, Methodist Hosp; **Address:** Thomas Jefferson Univ, 1020 Samson St, Thompson Bldg, Ste 1652, Philadelphia, PA 19107; **Phone:** 215-955-9545; **Board Cert:** Psychiatry 1989; Psychosomatic Medicine 2005; **Med School:** McGill Univ 1983; **Resid:** Psychiatry, NYU Med Ctr 1987; **Fellow:** Liaison Psychiatry, Meml Sloan Kettering Cancer Ctr 1989; Consultation Psychiatry, Meml Sloan Kettering Cancer Ctr 1989; **Fac Appt:** Prof Psyc, Jefferson Med Coll

Kupfer, David J MD [Psyc] - **Spec Exp:** Bipolar/Mood Disorders; **Hospital:** Western Psych Inst & Clin-UPMC; **Address:** Western Psychiatric Inst & Clinic, 3811 O'Hara St, Pittsburgh, PA 15213-2593; **Phone:** 412-246-6777; **Board Cert:** Psychiatry 1978; **Med School:** Yale Univ 1965; **Resid:** Psychiatry, Yale-New Haven Hosp 1970; Psychiatry, Natl Inst Mental Hlth 1969; **Fellow:** Psychiatry, Yale-New Haven Hosp 1967; **Fac Appt:** Prof Psyc, Univ Pittsburgh

Lawson, William B MD [Psyc] - **Spec Exp:** Bipolar/Mood Disorders; Addiction/Substance Abuse; Dual Diagnosis; **Hospital:** Howard Univ Hosp; **Address:** Howard Univ Hosp, Dept Psychiatry, 2041 Georgia Ave NW, Ste 5B01, Washington, DC 20060; **Phone:** 202-865-6611; **Board Cert:** Psychiatry 1984; Addiction Psychiatry 2006; **Med School:** Univ Chicago-Pritzker Sch Med 1978; **Resid:** Psychiatry, Stanford Univ Med Ctr 1981; Psychiatry, Natl Inst Mental Hlth 1982; **Fellow:** Neuropsychiatry, Natl Inst Mental Hlth 1984; **Fac Appt:** Prof Psyc, Howard Univ

Loewenstein, Richard J. MD [Psyc] - **Spec Exp:** Trauma Psychiatry; Dissociative Disorders; Post Traumatic Stress Disorder; Psychopharmacology; **Hospital:** Sheppard Pratt Hlth Sys; **Address:** 6501 N Charles St, Ste PJ106, Baltimore, MD 21204; **Phone:** 410-938-5075; **Board Cert:** Psychiatry 1980; **Med School:** Yale Univ 1975; **Resid:** Psychiatry, Yale Affil Hosps 1979; **Fellow:** Psychiatry, NIH,NIMH-Biol Psych Br 1982; **Fac Appt:** Assoc Clin Prof Psyc, Univ MD Sch Med

Manevitz, Alan MD [Psyc] - **Spec Exp:** Marital/Family/Sex Therapy; Depression-TMS Therapy; ADD/PTSD; Frbromyalgia Syndrome (FMS); **Hospital:** NY-Presby/Weill Cornell Med Ctr, NY (page 65), Lenox Hill Hosp; **Address:** 60 Sutton Place South, Ste 1CN, New York, NY 10022; **Phone:** 212-751-5072; **Board Cert:** Psychiatry 1987; **Med School:** Columbia P&S 1980; **Resid:** Psychiatry, NY Hosp 1984; **Fellow:** Psychopharmacology, NY Hosp 1985; **Fac Appt:** Assoc Clin Prof Psyc, Cornell Univ-Weill Med Coll

Psychiatry

Mann, J John MD/PhD [Psyc] - **Spec Exp:** Mood Disorders; Clinical Trials; Suicide; **Hospital:** NY-Presby/Columbia Univ Med Ctr, NY (page 65); **Address:** NYS Psychiatric Institute, 1051 Riverside Drive, Box 42, New York, NY 10032 **Phone:** 212-543-5571; **Board Cert:** Psychiatry 1980; **Med School:** Australia 1978; **Resid:** Psychiatry, Royal Melbourne Hosp 1976; **Fac Appt:** Prof Psyc, Columbia P&S

Marin, Deborah B MD [Psyc] - **Spec Exp:** Memory Disorders; Depression; Depression in the Elderly; Geriatric Psychiatry; **Hospital:** Mount Sinai Med Ctr (page 63); **Address:** Mount Sinai Hospital, One Gustave L Levy Pl, Box 1230, New York, NY 10029; **Phone:** 212-659-8092; **Board Cert:** Psychiatry 1990; **Med School:** Mount Sinai Sch Med 1984; **Resid:** Psychiatry, Mount Sinai Hosp 1988; **Fellow:** Psychiatry, NY Hosp-Cornell Med Ctr 1991; **Fac Appt:** Prof Psyc, Mount Sinai Sch Med

McCann, Merle C MD [Psyc] - **Hospital:** Sheppard Pratt Hlth Sys; **Address:** Sheppard & Enoch Pratt Hosp, 6501 N Charles St,, rm PJ-111, Baltimore, MD 21204; **Phone:** 410-938-3000; **Board Cert:** Psychiatry 1986; **Med School:** Med Coll VA 1981; **Resid:** Psychiatry, Geo Wash Univ Hosp 1985; **Fac Appt:** Asst Clin Prof Psyc, Univ MD Sch Med

Roose, Steven MD [Psyc] - **Spec Exp:** Depression in the Elderly; **Hospital:** NY-Presby/Columbia Univ Med Ctr, NY (page 65); **Address:** NY State Psychiatric Institute, 1051 Riverside Drive, New York, NY 10032; **Phone:** 212-831-8644; **Board Cert:** Psychiatry 1979; **Med School:** Mount Sinai Sch Med 1974; **Resid:** Psychiatry, NY Psychiatric Inst 1978; **Fellow:** Research, Columbia-Presby Med Ctr 1981; **Fac Appt:** Clin Prof Psyc, Columbia P&S

Rosenthal, Norman E MD [Psyc] - ; **Address:** 11110 Stephalee Ln, Rockville, MD 20852; **Phone:** 301-770-3843; **Board Cert:** Psychiatry 1980; **Med School:** South Africa 1973; **Resid:** Psychiatry, NY State Psych Inst 1979; **Fellow:** Psychiatry, Natl Inst Mental Health 1981; **Fac Appt:** Clin Prof Psyc, Georgetown Univ

Rosenthal, Richard N MD [Psyc] - **Spec Exp:** Anxiety & Mood Disorders; Addiction/Substance Abuse; **Hospital:** St. Luke's - Roosevelt Hosp Ctr - Roosevelt Div (page 55), Beth Israel Med Ctr - Petrie Division (page 55); **Address:** 1090 Amerstdam Ave Fl 16 - Ste G, New York, NY 10025; **Phone:** 212-523-5366; **Board Cert:** Psychiatry 1985; Addiction Psychiatry 2002; **Med School:** SUNY Hlth Sci Ctr 1980; **Resid:** Psychiatry, Mount Sinai Hosp 1984; **Fac Appt:** Prof Psyc, Columbia P&S

Rosse, Richard B MD [Psyc] - **Hospital:** VA Med Ctr - Washington; **Address:** Mental Health Dept (116A), 50 Irving St NW, Washington, DC 20422-0001; **Phone:** 202-745-8156; **Board Cert:** Psychiatry 1986; **Med School:** Univ MD Sch Med 1980; **Resid:** Psychiatry, Georgetown Univ Med Ctr 1984; **Fac Appt:** Prof Psyc, Howard Univ

Roth, Andrew J MD [Psyc] - **Spec Exp:** Psychiatry of Prostate Cancer; Geriatic Psychiatry; **Hospital:** Meml Sloan-Kettering Cancer Ctr; **Address:** 641 Lexington Ave Fl 7, New York, NY 10022; **Phone:** 646-888-0024; **Board Cert:** Psychiatry 1993; Geriatric Psychiatry 2007; Psychosomatic Medicine 2005; **Med School:** NY Med Coll 1988; **Resid:** Psychiatry, Mt Sinai Med Ctr 1992; **Fellow:** Liaison Psychiatry, Meml Sloan-Kettering Canc Ctr 1994; **Fac Appt:** Clin Prof Psyc, Cornell Univ-Weill Med Coll

Sadock, Virginia MD [Psyc] - **Spec Exp:** Psychotherapy; Sexual Dysfunction; Anxiety & Depression; Marital/Family/Sex Therapy; **Hospital:** NYU Langone Med Ctr (page 66); **Address:** 4 E 89th St, Ste 1E, New York, NY 10128; **Phone:** 212-427-0885; **Board Cert:** Psychiatry 1975; **Med School:** NY Med Coll 1970; **Resid:** Psychiatry, Metropolitan Hosp 1973; **Fac Appt:** Clin Prof Psyc, NYU Sch Med

Samberg, Eslee MD [Psyc] - **Spec Exp:** Psychoanalysis; **Hospital:** NY-Presby/Weill Cornell Med Ctr, NY (page 65); **Address:** 165 W End Ave, Ste 1M, New York, NY 10024; **Phone:** 212-874-7725; **Board Cert:** Psychiatry 1983; **Med School:** Cornell Univ-Weill Med Coll 1978; **Resid:** Psychiatry, NY Hosp-Cornell Med Ctr 1982; **Fac Appt:** Assoc Clin Prof Psyc, Cornell Univ-Weill Med Coll

Scott, C Paul MD [Psyc] - **Spec Exp:** Anxiety & Mood Disorders; Psychoanalysis; **Hospital:** UPMC Presby, Pittsburgh; **Address:** 401 Shady Ave, Ste C202, Pittsburgh, PA 15206; **Phone:** 412-661-2354; **Board Cert:** Psychiatry 1976; **Med School:** Case West Res Univ 1968; **Resid:** Internal Medicine, Univ Cleveland Hosps 1970; Psychiatry, Western Psych Inst 1974; **Fellow:** Psychoanalysis, Western Psych Inst 1982; **Fac Appt:** Clin Prof Psyc, Univ Pittsburgh

Stone, Michael H MD [Psyc] - **Spec Exp:** Personality Disorders; Psychoanalysis; Forensic Psychiatry; Addiction/Substance Abuse; **Hospital:** NY-Presby/Columbia Univ Med Ctr, NY (page 65); **Address:** 225 Central Park West, Ste 114, New York, NY 10024-6027; **Phone:** 212-758-2000; **Board Cert:** Psychiatry 1971; **Med School:** Cornell Univ-Weill Med Coll 1958; **Resid:** Internal Medicine, Bellevue Hosp 1961; Psychiatry, NYS Psych Inst 1966; **Fellow:** Hematology, Meml Sloan Kettering Cancer Ctr 1962; Medical Oncology, Meml Sloan Kettering Cancer Ctr 1963; **Fac Appt:** Clin Prof Psyc, Columbia P&S

Sussman, Norman MD [Psyc] - **Spec Exp:** Psychopharmacology; Anxiety & Mood Disorders; Bipolar/Mood Disorders; **Hospital:** NYU Langone Med Ctr (page 66); **Address:** 150 E 58th St, Fl 27, New York, NY 10155; **Phone:** 212-588-9722; **Board Cert:** Psychiatry 1980; **Med School:** NY Med Coll 1975; **Resid:** Psychiatry, Metropolitan Hosp Ctr 1977; Psychiatry, Westchester Co Med Ctr 1978; **Fac Appt:** Prof Psyc, NYU Sch Med

Thase, Michael E MD [Psyc] - **Spec Exp:** Anxiety & Mood Disorders; Psychopharmacology; Depression; **Hospital:** Hosp Univ Penn - UPHS (page 68); **Address:** Univ Penn, Dept Psychiatry, 3535 Market St, Ste 670, Philadelphia, PA 19104; **Phone:** 215-746-6680; **Board Cert:** Psychiatry 1984; **Med School:** Ohio State Univ 1979; **Resid:** Psychiatry, Western Psych Inst 1983; **Fellow:** Research, Univ Pittsburgh Sch Med 1984; **Fac Appt:** Prof Psyc, Univ Pennsylvania

Wait, Susan B MD [Psyc] - **Spec Exp:** Post Traumatic Stress Disorder; Dissociative Disorders; Anxiety & Mood Disorders; Dialectical Behavioral Therapy; **Hospital:** Sheppard Pratt Hlth Sys; **Address:** Sheppard Pratt Hlth Sys, 6501 N Charles St, Baltimore, MD 21285; **Phone:** 410-938-5076; **Board Cert:** Psychiatry 1993; **Med School:** Med Coll PA Hahnemann 1987; **Resid:** Psychiatry, Sheppard Pratt Hosp 1991; **Fac Appt:** Assoc Clin Prof Psyc, Univ MD Sch Med

Walsh, B Timothy MD [Psyc] - **Spec Exp:** Eating Disorders; **Hospital:** NY State Psychiatric Inst, NY-Presby/Columbia Univ Med Ctr, NY (page 65); **Address:** NY State Psychiatric Inst-Unit 98, 1051 Riverside Dr, New York, NY 10032-2695; **Phone:** 212-543-5739; **Board Cert:** Psychiatry 1978; **Med School:** Harvard Med Sch 1972; **Resid:** Internal Medicine, Dartmouth Affil Hosps 1973; Psychiatry, Bronx Muni Hosp Ctr 1977; **Fac Appt:** Prof Psyc, Columbia P&S

Southeast

Blazer II, Dan G MD/PhD [Psyc] - **Spec Exp:** Geriatric Psychiatry; Mood Disorders; **Hospital:** Duke Univ Hosp; **Address:** Duke Univ Med Ctr, Dept Psychiatary, 3521 Hospital South, Box 3003, Durham, NC 27710-3003; **Phone:** 919-684-4128; **Board Cert:** Psychiatry 1977; Geriatric Psychiatry 2000; **Med School:** Univ Tenn Coll Med 1969; **Resid:** Psychiatry, Duke Univ Med Ctr 1975; **Fellow:** Liaison Psychiatry, Montefiore Hosp 1976; **Fac Appt:** Prof Psyc, Duke Univ

Psychiatry

Canterbury II, Randolph J MD [Psyc] - **Spec Exp:** Panic Disorder; Depression; Substance Abuse; **Hospital:** Univ of Virginia Health Sys; **Address:** Univ Virginia Dept Psychiatry, Div Outpatient Psychiatry, Box 800623, Charlottesville, VA 22908-0623; **Phone:** 434-924-2241; **Board Cert:** Internal Medicine 1983; Psychiatry 1985; Psychosomatic Medicine 2005; **Med School:** W VA Univ 1979; **Resid:** Internal Medicine, Univ Va Hosp 1983; Psychiatry, Univ Va Hosp 1985; **Fac Appt:** Prof Psyc, Univ VA Sch Med

Eth, Spencer MD [Psyc] - **Spec Exp:** Forensic Psychiatry; Post Traumatic Stress Disorder; **Hospital:** Univ of Miami Hosp (page 72); **Address:** UM-Jackson Memorial Hosp, 1695 NW 9th Ave Fl 3, Miami, FL 33136; **Phone:** 305-575-3301; **Board Cert:** Child & Adolescent Psychiatry 1982; Geriatric Psychiatry 2010; Forensic Psychiatry 2005; Addiction Psychiatry 2009; **Med School:** UCLA 1976; **Resid:** Psychiatry, NY Cornell Med Ctr 1979; **Fellow:** Child & Adolescent Psychiatry, Cedars-Sinai Med Ctr 1981; **Fac Appt:** Prof Psyc, Univ Miami Sch Med

Giustra Jr, Lawrence J MD [Psyc] - **Spec Exp:** Psychotherapy; Marital/Family/Sex Therapy; Depression; **Hospital:** Emory Univ Hosp; **Address:** 1945 Cliff Valley Way NE, Ste 202, Atlanta, GA 30329; **Phone:** 404-325-2139; **Board Cert:** Psychiatry 1982; **Med School:** Johns Hopkins Univ 1976; **Resid:** Psychiatry, Mass Genl Hosp 1980; **Fac Appt:** Asst Prof Psyc, Emory Univ

Klapheke, Martin M MD [Psyc] - **Spec Exp:** Transplantation Psychiatry; Psychoanalysis; **Address:** College of Medicine Rm427, 6850 Lake Nona Blvd, Orlando, FL 32827; **Phone:** 407-266-1100; **Board Cert:** Psychiatry 1985; **Med School:** Univ KY Coll Med 1979; **Resid:** Psychiatry, Mayo Grad Sch Med 1982; **Fellow:** Child & Adolescent Psychiatry, Mayo Grad Sch Med 1984; Psychoanalysis, Topeka Inst Psychoanalysis 1994; **Fac Appt:** Prof Psyc, Univ C Fla Coll Med

Levy, Steven T MD [Psyc] - **Spec Exp:** Depression; Anxiety & Mood Disorders; Bipolar/Mood Disorders; **Hospital:** Emory Univ Hosp, Grady Hlth Sys; **Address:** Emory Univ Psychoanalytic Inst, 2004 Ridgewood Drive, Ste 300, Atlanta, GA 30322; **Phone:** 404-727-5886; **Board Cert:** Psychiatry 1976; **Med School:** Duke Univ 1969; **Resid:** Psychiatry, Yale-New Haven Hosp 1973; **Fac Appt:** Prof Psyc, Emory Univ

McCall, William V MD [Psyc] - **Spec Exp:** Sleep Disorders; Electroconvulsive Therapy (ECT); Depression; **Hospital:** Wake Forest Univ Baptist Med Ctr; **Address:** Wake Forest Univ Dept Psychiatry, Medical Center Blvd, Winston-Salem, NC 27157; **Phone:** 336-716-2911; **Board Cert:** Psychiatry 1990; Geriatric Psychiatry 2005; Sleep Medicine 2007; **Med School:** Duke Univ 1984; **Resid:** Psychiatry, Duke Univ Med Ctr 1987; **Fac Appt:** Prof Psyc, Wake Forest Univ

Powers, Pauline MD [Psyc] - **Spec Exp:** Eating Disorders; **Hospital:** Tampa Genl Hosp; **Address:** 2304 W Cleveland St, Tampa, FL 33609; **Phone:** 813-253-3094; **Board Cert:** Psychiatry 1977; **Med School:** Univ Iowa Coll Med 1971; **Resid:** Psychiatry, Univ Iowa Med Ctr 1974; Psychiatry, UC Davis Med Ctr 1975; **Fac Appt:** Prof Psyc, Univ S Fla Coll Med

Salloum, Ihsan M MD [Psyc] - **Spec Exp:** Bipolar/Mood Disorders; Addiction/Substance Abuse; **Hospital:** Univ of Miami Hosp (page 72); **Address:** 1120 NW 14th St, Ste 1450, Miami, FL 33136; **Phone:** 305-243-7931; **Board Cert:** Psychiatry 1994; Addiction Psychiatry 2007; **Med School:** Italy 1980; **Resid:** Psychiatry, Univ Hlth Sci Ctr 1988; **Fellow:** Research, Univ Pittsburgh Med Ctr 1989; **Fac Appt:** Prof Psyc, Univ Miami Sch Med

Weiner, Richard D MD/PhD [Psyc] - **Spec Exp:** Bipolar/Mood Disorders; Electroconvulsive Therapy (ECT); Depression; Schizophrenia; **Hospital:** Duke Univ Hosp, Durham VA Med Ctr; **Address:** Duke Univ Medical Ctr, Box 3309, Durham, NC 27710; **Phone:** 919-681-8742; **Board Cert:** Psychiatry 1979; Clinical Neurophysiology 2003; **Med School:** Duke Univ 1973; **Resid:** Psychiatry, Duke Univ Med Ctr 1976; **Fellow:** Electroencephalography, Duke Univ Med Ctr 1977; **Fac Appt:** Prof Psyc, Duke Univ

Weisler, Richard H MD [Psyc] - **Spec Exp:** Depression; Bipolar/Mood Disorders; Clinical Trials; **Hospital:** NC Memorial Hosp - UNC; **Address:** 700 Spring Forest Rd, Ste 125, Raleigh, NC 27609; **Phone:** 919-872-5900; **Board Cert:** Psychiatry 1982; **Med School:** Univ NC Sch Med 1977; **Resid:** Psychiatry, Duke Univ Med Ctr 1982; **Fac Appt:** Assoc Prof Psyc, Duke Univ

Midwest

Black, Donald W MD [Psyc] - **Spec Exp:** Obsessive-Compulsive Disorder; Personality Disorders; Bipolar/Mood Disorders; Psychotic Disorders; **Hospital:** Univ Iowa Hosp & Clinics; **Address:** University of Iowa Hospital & Clinics, MEB Bldg - rm 2-126B, 500 Newton Rd, Iowa City, IA 52242; **Phone:** 319-353-4431; **Board Cert:** Psychiatry 1988; **Med School:** Univ Utah 1982; **Resid:** Psychiatry, Univ Iowa Hosp & Clincs 1988; **Fellow:** Epidemiology, Univ Iowa Hosp & Clincs 1989; **Fac Appt:** Prof Psyc, Univ Iowa Coll Med

Black, Kevin J MD [Psyc] - **Spec Exp:** Neuro-Psychiatry; **Hospital:** Barnes-Jewish Hosp; **Address:** 517 S Euclid Ave, CB 8111, St Louis, MO 63110; **Phone:** 314-362-6908; **Board Cert:** Psychiatry 2005; **Med School:** Duke Univ 1990; **Resid:** Psychiatry, Barnes Hosp-Washington Univ 1994; **Fellow:** Movement Disorders, Barnes Hosp-Washington Univ 1996; **Fac Appt:** Assoc Prof Psyc, Washington Univ, St Louis

Calabrese, Joseph R MD [Psyc] - **Spec Exp:** Bipolar/Mood Disorders; **Hospital:** Univ Hosps Case Med Ctr (page 74); **Address:** Case Western Reserve Univ, 10524 Euclid Ave, Ste 12-135, Cleveland, OH 44106; **Phone:** 216-844-2865; **Board Cert:** Psychiatry 1989; **Med School:** Ohio State Univ 1980; **Resid:** Psychiatry, Cleveland Clinic 1984; **Fellow:** Biological Psychiatry, Natl Inst Mental Hlth 1986; **Fac Appt:** Prof Psyc, Case West Res Univ

Cloninger, C Robert MD [Psyc] - **Spec Exp:** Personality Disorders; **Hospital:** Barnes-Jewish Hosp; **Address:** Wash Univ Sch Med, Dept Psyc, 660 S Euclid Ave, Box 8134, St Louis, MO 63110; **Phone:** 314-362-7005; **Board Cert:** Psychiatry 1975; **Med School:** Washington Univ, St Louis 1970; **Resid:** Psychiatry, Barnes Hosp 1973; Psychiatry, Renard Hosp-Wash Univ 1973; **Fac Appt:** Prof Psyc, Washington Univ, St Louis

Crow, Scott J MD [Psyc] - **Spec Exp:** Eating Disorders; Obesity; **Address:** The Emily Program, 2265 Como Ave, St Paul, MN 55108; **Phone:** 651-645-5323; **Board Cert:** Psychiatry 1994; **Med School:** Univ Minn 1988; **Resid:** Psychiatry, Univ Minn Hosp 1992; **Fellow:** Psychiatry, Univ Minn Hosp 1992; **Fac Appt:** Prof Psyc, Univ Minn

Greden, John F MD [Psyc] - **Spec Exp:** Depression; **Hospital:** Univ of Michigan Hosp; **Address:** Univ Michigan Comp Depression Ctr, Rachel Upjohn Bldg, 4250 Plymouth Rd, Ann Arbor, MI 48109-2700; **Phone:** 734-763-9629; **Board Cert:** Psychiatry 1975; **Med School:** Univ Minn 1967; **Resid:** Psychiatry, Univ Minn Med Ctr 1969; Psychiatry, Walter Reed AMC 1972; **Fac Appt:** Prof Psyc, Univ Mich Med Sch

Janicak, Philip G MD [Psyc] - **Spec Exp:** Psychopharmacology; Mood Disorders; Psychotic Disorders; **Hospital:** Rush Univ Med Ctr; **Address:** Rush Univ Med Ctr, Dept Psych, 2150 W Harrison St, rm 253, Chicago, IL 60612; **Phone:** 312-942-7287; **Board Cert:** Psychiatry 1978; **Med School:** Loyola Univ-Stritch Sch Med 1973; **Resid:** Psychiatry, McGaw Hosp/Loyola Med Ctr 1976; **Fac Appt:** Prof Psyc, Rush Med Coll

Levine, Stephen B MD [Psyc] - **Spec Exp:** Sexual Dysfunction; Relationship Problems; Sexual Identity Issues; **Hospital:** Univ Hosps Case Med Ctr (page 74); **Address:** 23230 Chagrin Blvd, Ste 350, Beachwood, OH 44122-5446; **Phone:** 216-831-2900; **Board Cert:** Psychiatry 1976; **Med School:** Case West Res Univ 1967; **Resid:** Psychiatry, Univ Hosps Cleveland 1973; **Fac Appt:** Clin Prof Psyc, Case West Res Univ

Psychiatry

Locala, Joseph MD [Psyc] - **Spec Exp:** Psychiatry in Transplant Patients; Psychiatry in Physical Illness; Anxiety & Mood Disorders; Neuro-Psychiatry; **Hospital:** Univ Hosps Case Med Ctr (page 74); **Address:** WO Walker Ctr, 10524 Euclid Ave Fl 13, Cleveland, OH 44106; **Phone:** 216-844-2400; **Board Cert:** Psychiatry 2006; Psychosomatic Medicine 2006; **Med School:** Temple Univ 1990; **Resid:** Psychiatry, Medical Ctr Hosp 1994; **Fellow:** Psychosomatic Medicine, Cleveland Clinic 1995; **Fac Appt:** Assoc Prof Psyc, Case West Res Univ

McCallum, Kimberli E MD [Psyc] - **Spec Exp:** Eating Disorders; **Hospital:** St. Louis Univ Hosp; **Address:** McCallum Place, 231 W Lockwood Ave, Ste 201, Webster Groves, MO 63119; **Phone:** 314-968-1900; **Board Cert:** Psychiatry 1993; Child & Adolescent Psychiatry 1994; **Med School:** Yale Univ 1986; **Resid:** Psychiatry, UCLA Neuropsyc Inst 1991; **Fellow:** Child Psychiatry, Washington Univ 1993; **Fac Appt:** Assoc Clin Prof Psyc, Washington Univ, St Louis

Nurnberger Jr, John I MD/PhD [Psyc] - **Spec Exp:** Bipolar/Mood Disorders; Depression; Psychiatric Genetics; **Hospital:** IU Health University Hosp, Wishard Hlth Srvs; **Address:** Institute Psychiatric Research-IUMC, 791 Union Dr, Indianapolis, IN 46202-4887; **Phone:** 317-944-7422; **Board Cert:** Psychiatry 1981; **Med School:** Indiana Univ 1975; **Resid:** Psychiatry, Columbia-Presby Med Ctr 1978; **Fellow:** Psychiatry & Genetics, NIMH Clinical Ctr 1983; **Fac Appt:** Prof Psyc, Indiana Univ

Riba, Michelle B MD [Psyc] - **Spec Exp:** Psychiatry in Cancer; **Hospital:** Univ of Michigan Hosp; **Address:** Comprehensive Depression Ctr, 4250 Plymouth Rd, 1533 Rachel Upjohn Bldg, MC 5763, Ann Arbor, MI 48109-0295; **Phone:** 734-764-6879; **Board Cert:** Psychiatry 1991; Psychosomatic Medicine 2005; **Med School:** Univ Conn 1985; **Resid:** Psychiatry, Univ Connecticut 1988; **Fac Appt:** Clin Prof Psyc, Univ Mich Med Sch

Strakowski, Stephen M MD [Psyc] - **Spec Exp:** Bipolar/Mood Disorders; Psychotic Disorders; Dual Diagnosis; Addiction/Substance Abuse; **Hospital:** Univ Hosp - Cincinnati, Cincinnati Chldns Hosp Med Ctr; **Address:** Univ Cincinnati, Dept Psych, PO Box 670559, 231 Albert Sabin Way, Cincinnati, OH 45267-0559; **Phone:** 513-558-4274; **Board Cert:** Psychiatry 1993; **Med School:** Vanderbilt Univ 1988; **Resid:** Psychiatry, McLean Hosp-Harvard Med Sch 1992; **Fac Appt:** Prof Psyc, Univ Cincinnati

Wooten, Virgil D MD [Psyc] - **Spec Exp:** Sleep Disorders only; **Hospital:** Univ Hosp - Cincinnati, University Pointe Surgical Hosp; **Address:** 231 Albert Sabin Way, Box ML 0564, Pulmonary, Crit Care & Sleep Medicine, Cincinnati, OH 45267; **Phone:** 513-558-4831; **Board Cert:** Sleep Medicine 2007; Psychiatry 1985; **Med School:** Univ Ark 1980; **Resid:** Psychiatry, Univ Hosp-VA Hosp 1984; **Fellow:** Sleep Medicine, Univ Hosp 1985; **Fac Appt:** Prof Psyc, Univ Cincinnati

Great Plains and Mountains

Freedman, Robert MD [Psyc] - **Spec Exp:** Schizophrenia; **Hospital:** Univ of CO Hosp - Anschutz Inpatient Pav; **Address:** Univ Colorado, Dept Psychiatry, 13001 E 17th Place, Campus Box F546, Aurora, CO 80045; **Phone:** 303-724-4940; **Board Cert:** Psychiatry 1980; **Med School:** Harvard Med Sch 1972; **Resid:** Psychiatry, Univ Chicago Hosps 1978; **Fellow:** Neuropharmacology, NIMH/St Elizabeth's Hosp 1975; **Fac Appt:** Prof Psyc, Univ Colorado

Greiner, Carl B MD [Psyc] - **Spec Exp:** Psychiatry in Cancer; Psychiatry in Physical Illness; Palliative Care; Post Traumatic Stress Disorder; **Hospital:** Nebraska Med Ctr; **Address:** UNMC, dept Psychiatry, 985575 Nebraska Medical Ctr, Omaha, NE 68198-5575; **Phone:** 402-552-6002; **Board Cert:** Psychiatry 1984; Forensic Psychiatry 2008; **Med School:** Univ Cincinnati 1978; **Resid:** Psychiatry, Univ Cincinnati Med Ctr 1982; **Fac Appt:** Prof Psyc, Univ Nebr Coll Med

Hoffman, Daniel A MD [Psyc] - **Spec Exp:** ADD/ADHD; Mood Disorders; **Hospital:** Rose Med Ctr; **Address:** Neuro-Therapy Clinic, 7800 E Orchard Rd, Ste 340, Greenwood Village, CO 80111; **Phone:** 303-741-4800; **Board Cert:** Psychiatry 1981; **Med School:** Wayne State Univ 1974; **Resid:** Psychiatry, Univ Colo Affil Hosp 1977

McIntosh, J Michael MD [Psyc] - **Spec Exp:** Depression; Schizophrenia; Anxiety Disorders; Bipolar/Mood Disorders; **Hospital:** Univ Utah Hlth Care; **Address:** 30 N 1900 East, rm 5R110, Salt Lake City, UT 84108; **Phone:** 801-581-7951; **Board Cert:** Psychiatry 1994; **Med School:** UCLA 1987; **Resid:** Psychiatry, Univ Colo Hlth Sci Ctr 1991; Psychiatry, Univ Utah Hosps 1992; **Fac Appt:** Clin Prof Psyc, Univ Utah

Mitchell, James E MD [Psyc] - **Spec Exp:** Eating Disorders; **Hospital:** Sanford Med Ctr Fargo; **Address:** NeuroPsychiatric Research Inst, 120 S 8th St, Fargo, ND 58103; **Phone:** 701-293-1335; **Board Cert:** Psychiatry 1979; **Med School:** Northwestern Univ 1972; **Resid:** Psychiatry, Fairview-Univ Med Ctr 1976; **Fac Appt:** Prof Psyc, Univ ND Sch Med

Moench, Louis A MD [Psyc] - **Hospital:** LDS Hosp; **Address:** 324 Kent Ave, Ste 178, Salt Lake City, UT 84103; **Phone:** 801-408-8500; **Board Cert:** Psychiatry 1978; Forensic Psychiatry 2004; **Med School:** Univ Utah 1970; **Resid:** Psychiatry, Hosp U Penn 1976; **Fellow:** Forensic Psychiatry, Hosp U Penn 1976; **Fac Appt:** Clin Prof Psyc, Univ Utah

Weiner, Kenneth L MD [Psyc] - **Spec Exp:** Eating Disorders; **Hospital:** Univ of CO Hosp - Anschutz Inpatient Pav; **Address:** Eating Recovery Center, 1830 Franklin St, Ste 500, Denver, CO 80218; **Phone:** 303-825-8584; **Board Cert:** Psychiatry 1983; **Med School:** Tufts Univ 1977; **Resid:** Psychiatry, Univ Colorado Hlth Sci Ctr 1981; **Fac Appt:** Asst Clin Prof Psyc, Univ Colorado

Wilson, Daniel R MD/PhD [Psyc] - **Spec Exp:** Psychopharmacology; Forensic Psychiatry; Neuro-Psychiatry; **Hospital:** Creighton Univ Med Ctr, Alegent Hlth - Immanuel Med Ctr; **Address:** Creighton Psychiatry, 3528 Dodge St, Omaha, NE 68131; **Phone:** 402-345-8828; **Board Cert:** Psychiatry 1989; Forensic Psychiatry 2009; **Med School:** Univ Iowa Coll Med 1983; **Resid:** Psychiatry, McLean Hosp 1986; **Fellow:** Geriatric Psychiatry, McLean Hosp 1987; Genetics, Cambridge Univ 1993; **Fac Appt:** Prof Psyc, Creighton Univ

Southwest

Avery, Eric N MD [Psyc] - **Spec Exp:** Depression; Dementia; Arts in the Healing Process; AIDS/HIV Liaison Psychiatry; **Hospital:** UT Med Br at Galveston; **Address:** Dept Psychiatry, 301 University Blvd, Galveston, TX 77555-0193; **Phone:** 409-747-9789; **Board Cert:** Psychiatry 2003; **Med School:** Univ Tex Med Br, Galveston 1974; **Resid:** Psychiatry, NY State Psych Inst 1978; **Fellow:** Liaison Psychiatry for AIDS/HIV, NY State Psych Inst 1994; **Fac Appt:** Asst Prof Psyc, Univ Tex Med Br, Galveston

Baile, Walter F MD [Psyc] - **Spec Exp:** Psychiatry in Cancer; **Hospital:** UT MD Anderson Cancer Ctr; **Address:** PO Box 301402, Unit 1426, Texas, TX 77230; **Phone:** 713-563-1484; **Board Cert:** Psychiatry 1980; **Med School:** Italy 1973; **Resid:** Psychiatry, Johns Hopkins Hosp 1976; **Fellow:** Behavioral Medicine, Natl Inst Aging 1978; **Fac Appt:** Prof Psyc, Univ Tex, Houston

Bowden, Charles L MD [Psyc] - **Spec Exp:** Bipolar/Mood Disorders; **Hospital:** Univ Hlth Syst-San Antonio; **Address:** Univ Tex Hlth Sci Ctr, Dept Psychiatry, 7526 Louis Pasteur, San Antonio, TX 78229-3900; **Phone:** 210-567-5555; **Board Cert:** Psychiatry 1970; **Med School:** Baylor Coll Med 1964; **Resid:** Psychiatry, NY State Psyc Inst/Columbia-Presby Med Ctr 1968; **Fac Appt:** Prof Psyc, Univ Tex, San Antonio

Psychiatry

Davidson, Joyce E MD [Psyc] - **Spec Exp:** Obsessive-Compulsive Disorder; Bipolar/Mood Disorders; Schizophrenia; **Hospital:** Menninger Clinic; **Address:** The Menninger Clinic, 2801 Gessner Drive, Houston, TX 77080; **Phone:** 713-275-5000; **Board Cert:** Psychiatry 1988; **Med School:** Univ MO-Kansas City 1979; **Resid:** Psychiatry, Karl Menninger Sch Psyc 1982; **Fellow:** Child & Adolescent Psychiatry, Karl Menninger Sch Psyc 1984; **Fac Appt:** Asst Prof Psyc, Baylor Coll Med

Gabbard, Glen O MD [Psyc] - **Spec Exp:** Personality Disorders-Borderline; Cognitive Psychotherapy; Psychoanalysis; **Hospital:** Baylor Univ Medical Ctr-Dallas; **Address:** 1799 Butler Blvd, Ste 400, Houston, TX 77030; **Phone:** 713-798-6397; **Board Cert:** Psychiatry 1979; **Med School:** Rush Med Coll 1975; **Resid:** Psychiatry, Menninger Sch Psyc 1978; **Fellow:** Psychoanalysis, Topeka Inst Psychoanalysis 1984; **Fac Appt:** Clin Prof Psyc, Univ Kansas

Haque, Waheedul MD [Psyc] - **Spec Exp:** Depression; Panic Disorder; **Hospital:** UT Med Br at Galveston; **Address:** Dept Psychiatry, 301 University Blvd, Route 0190, Galveston, TX 77555; **Phone:** 409-747-9722; **Board Cert:** Psychiatry 1970; **Med School:** India 1962; **Resid:** Psychiatry, Barnes Jewish Med Ctr 1969; **Fac Appt:** Prof Psyc, Univ Tex Med Br, Galveston

Hirschfeld, Robert M A MD [Psyc] - **Spec Exp:** Bipolar/Mood Disorders; Schizophrenia; Depression; Suicide; **Hospital:** UT Med Br at Galveston; **Address:** Dept Psychiatry, 301 University Blvd, Route 0188, Galveston, TX 77555-0188; **Phone:** 409-747-9791; **Board Cert:** Psychiatry 1975; **Med School:** Univ Mich Med Sch 1968; **Resid:** Psychiatry, Stanford Univ Med Ctr 1972; **Fac Appt:** Prof Psyc, Univ Tex Med Br, Galveston

Mohl, Paul C MD [Psyc] - **Spec Exp:** Psychopharmacology; Psychotherapy; **Hospital:** UT Southwestern Med Ctr at Dallas; **Address:** 5323 Harry Hines Blvd, Dallas, TX 75390-9070; **Phone:** 214-648-7312; **Board Cert:** Psychiatry 1977; **Med School:** Duke Univ 1971; **Resid:** Psychiatry, Duke Univ Hosp 1974; **Fac Appt:** Prof Psyc, Univ Tex SW, Dallas

Valentine, Alan D MD [Psyc] - **Spec Exp:** Psychiatry in Cancer; Palliative Care; **Hospital:** UT MD Anderson Cancer Ctr; **Address:** MD Anderson Cancer Center, Dept Psychiatry Unit 1454, PO Box 301402, Houston, TX 77230-1402; **Phone:** 713-745-3344; **Board Cert:** Psychiatry 1992; Geriatric Psychiatry 2006; Psychosomatic Medicine 2005; **Med School:** Univ Tex, Houston 1986; **Resid:** Psychiatry, Univ Texas Affil Hosps; **Fac Appt:** Assoc Prof Psyc, Univ Tex, Houston

Weiner, Myron MD [Psyc] - **Spec Exp:** Geriatric Psychiatry; Alzheimer's Disease; Dementia; Memory Disorders; **Hospital:** UT Southwestern Med Ctr at Dallas; **Address:** Univ Texas SW Med Ctr, 5323 Harry Hines Blvd, Dallas, TX 75390-9129; **Phone:** 214-648-9353; **Board Cert:** Psychiatry 1966; Geriatric Psychiatry 2001; **Med School:** Tulane Univ 1957; **Resid:** Psychiatry, Parkland Hosp 1963; **Fellow:** Geriatric Psychiatry, Mt Sinai Med Ctr 1985; **Fac Appt:** Prof Psyc, Univ Tex SW, Dallas

West Coast and Pacific

Blumenfield, Michael MD [Psyc] - **Spec Exp:** Psychotherapy; Psychopharmacology; Psychosomatic Disorders; Disaster Psychiatry; **Address:** 5901 Nita Ave, Woodland Hills, CA 91367; **Phone:** 818-564-4207; **Board Cert:** Psychiatry 1970; Psychosomatic Medicine 2005; **Med School:** SUNY Downstate 1964; **Resid:** Psychiatry, Kings County Hosp 1968; **Fellow:** Psychosomatic Medicine, Kings County Hosp 1971; **Fac Appt:** Prof Emeritus Psyc, NY Med Coll

Burt, Vivien K MD/PhD [Psyc] - **Spec Exp:** Women's Health-Mental Health; Impulse-Control Disorders; Psychiatry in Pregnancy; Postpartum Depression; **Hospital:** Resnick Neuropsychiatric Hosp at UCLA; **Address:** 300 UCLA Medical Plaza, Ste 2337, Los Angeles, CA 90095; **Phone:** 310-562-4942; **Board Cert:** Psychiatry 1990; **Med School:** McGill Univ 1984; **Resid:** Psychiatry, UCLA-Neurpsyc Inst 1988; **Fac Appt:** Assoc Prof Psyc, UCLA

Bystritsky, Alexander MD/PhD [Psyc] - **Spec Exp:** Obsessive-Compulsive Disorder; Anxiety Disorders; Psychopharmacology; Body Dysmorphic Disorder (BDD); **Hospital:** Resnick Neuropsychiatric Hosp at UCLA; **Address:** 300 UCLA Med Plaza, Ste 2200, Box 956968, Los Angeles, CA 90095-6968; **Phone:** 310-206-5133; **Board Cert:** Psychiatry 1988; **Med School:** Russia 1977; **Resid:** Psychiatry, NYU Med Ctr 1985; **Fellow:** Psychiatry, UCLA 1987; **Fac Appt:** Prof Psyc, UCLA

Eisendrath, Stuart J MD [Psyc] - **Spec Exp:** Depression; Munchausen Syndrome; Cognitive Psychotherapy; **Hospital:** UCSF Med Ctr; **Address:** UCSF Med Ctr, 401 Parnassus Ave, Ste 278, MS 0984, San Francisco, CA 94143-0984; **Phone:** 415-476-7868; **Board Cert:** Psychiatry 1980; Psychosomatic Medicine 2008; **Med School:** Med Coll Wisc 1974; **Resid:** Psychiatry, Langley Porter Neuropsych Inst 1978; **Fellow:** Liaison Psychiatry, Langley Porter Neuropsych Inst 1979; **Fac Appt:** Prof Psyc, UCSF

Fann, Jesse R MD [Psyc] - **Spec Exp:** Psychiatry in Physical Illness; Psychiatry in Cancer; Neuro-Psychiatry; **Hospital:** Univ Wash Med Ctr, Harborview Med Ctr; **Address:** 1959 NE Pacific St, Box 356560, Seattle, WA 98195-6560; **Phone:** 206-685-4280; **Board Cert:** Psychiatry 2005; **Med School:** Northwestern Univ 1989; **Resid:** Psychiatry, Univ Washington Med Ctr 1993; **Fellow:** Liaison Psychiatry, Univ Washington Med Ctr 1995; Epidemiology, Univ Washington Med Ctr 1996; **Fac Appt:** Assoc Prof Psyc, Univ Wash

Friedman, Barry MD [Psyc] - **Spec Exp:** Psychopharmacology; Psychoanalysis; **Address:** 9171 Wilshire Blvd, Ste 310, Beverly Hills, CA 90210; **Phone:** 310-274-4372; **Board Cert:** Psychiatry 1974; **Med School:** UCSF 1965; **Resid:** Psychiatry, UCLA Med Ctr 1971; **Fellow:** Psychoanalysis, Los Angeles Psychoanalytic Inst 1992; **Fac Appt:** Assoc Clin Prof Psyc, UCLA

Gitlin, Michael Jay MD [Psyc] - **Spec Exp:** Mood Disorders; **Hospital:** Resnick Neuropsychiatric Hosp at UCLA; **Address:** UCLA NPI-Mood Disorders Clin, 300 Med Plaza, Ste 2200, Los Angeles, CA 90095-6968; **Phone:** 310-206-3654; **Board Cert:** Psychiatry 1981; **Med School:** Univ Pennsylvania 1975; **Resid:** Psychiatry, UCLA Med Ctr 1979; **Fac Appt:** Prof Psyc, UCLA

Keepers, George MD [Psyc] - **Spec Exp:** Neuro-Psychiatry; ADD/ADHD; **Hospital:** OR Hlth & Sci Univ; **Address:** Dept of Psychiatry, 3181 SW Sam Jackson Park Rd, MC UHN80, Portland, OR 97239; **Phone:** 503-494-8144; **Board Cert:** Psychiatry 1984; **Med School:** Baylor Coll Med 1977; **Resid:** Psychiatry, Oregon Hlth Sci Univ 1981; **Fac Appt:** Prof Psyc, Oregon Hlth & Sci Univ

Kerrihard, Thomas N MD [Psyc] - **Spec Exp:** Psychiatry in Physical Illness; Psychiatry in Cancer; **Hospital:** Cedars-Sinai Med Ctr; **Address:** Cedars Sinai Medical Ctr, Dept Psychiatry, 8700 Beverly Blvd, Ste AC1004, Los Angeles, CA 90048; **Phone:** 310-423-8030; **Board Cert:** Psychiatry 2009; Pain Medicine 2005; Hospice & Palliative Medicine 2008; **Med School:** Harvard Med Sch 1994; **Resid:** Psychiatry, Mass Genl Hosp 1998; **Fellow:** Liaison Psychiatry, Meml Sloan Kettering Cancer Ctr 1999

Leuchter, Andrew F MD [Psyc] - **Spec Exp:** Depression; **Hospital:** Resnick Neuropsychiatric Hosp at UCLA; **Address:** 760 Westwood Pl, rm 37-452, Los Angeles, CA 90024; **Phone:** 310-825-0207; **Board Cert:** Psychiatry 1986; Geriatric Psychiatry 2001; **Med School:** Baylor Coll Med 1980; **Resid:** Psychiatry, UCLA-Neuro Psyc Inst & Hosp 1984; **Fellow:** Geriatric Psychiatry, UCLA Med Ctr 1986; **Fac Appt:** Prof Psyc, UCLA

Psychiatry

Liberman, Robert Paul MD [Psyc] - **Spec Exp:** Schizophrenia; Psychotic Disorders; Psychiatric Rehabilitation; Family Therapy; **Hospital:** Resnick Neuropsychiatric Hosp at UCLA; **Address:** UCLA Neuropsychiatric Inst, 760 Westwood Plaza, Ste C9-400, Los Angeles, CA 90024; **Phone:** 310-206-1616; **Board Cert:** Psychiatry 1969; **Med School:** Johns Hopkins Univ 1963; **Resid:** Psychiatry, Mass Mntl Hlth Ctr 1968; **Fellow:** Pharmacology, UCSF Med Ctr 1961; Research, Harvard Med Sch 1968; **Fac Appt:** Prof Psyc, UCLA

Marder, Stephen R MD [Psyc] - **Spec Exp:** Schizophrenia; Psychopharmacology; **Hospital:** VA Greater Los Angeles Hthecare Sys, UCLA Ronald Reagan Med Ctr; **Address:** West Los Angeles VA - Gr LA Hlth Svcs, 11301 Wilshire Blvd, Bldg MIRECC 210A, Los Angeles, CA 90073; **Phone:** 310-268-3647; **Board Cert:** Psychiatry 1977; **Med School:** SUNY Buffalo 1971; **Resid:** Psychiatry, LAC-USC Med Ctr 1975; **Fac Appt:** Prof Psyc, UCLA

Nelson, J Craig MD [Psyc] - **Spec Exp:** Geriatric Psychiatry; Dementia; Depression; Psychopharmacology; **Hospital:** UCSF Med Ctr; **Address:** UCSF-Langley Porter Psychiatric Inst, 401 Parnassus Ave, Box 0984, San Francisco, CA 94143-0984; **Phone:** 415-476-7405; **Board Cert:** Psychiatry 1974; Geriatric Psychiatry 2002; **Med School:** Univ Wisc 1968; **Resid:** Psychiatry, Yale-New Haven Hosp 1970; Psychiatry, Yale-New Haven Hosp 1974; **Fac Appt:** Prof Psyc, UCSF

Neppe, Vernon M MD/PhD [Psyc] - **Spec Exp:** Behavioral Neurology; Neuro-Psychiatry; Psychopharmacology; Forensic Psychiatry; **Hospital:** Overlake Hosp Med Ctr, Northwest Hosp - Seattle; **Address:** 6300 Ninth Ave NE, Ste 353, Seattle, WA 98115; **Phone:** 206-527-6289; **Board Cert:** Psychiatry 1988; Geriatric Psychiatry 2001; Behavioral Neurology & Neuropsychiatry 2006; **Med School:** South Africa 1973; **Resid:** Neurology, Univ Witwatersrand 1979; Psychiatry, Univ Witwatersrand 1980; **Fellow:** Psychopharmacology, Cornell Med Ctr 1983; Neuropsychiatry, Cornell Med Ctr 1983

Norman, Kim P MD [Psyc] - **Spec Exp:** Eating Disorders/Obesity; Personality Disorders; Dual Diagnosis; **Hospital:** UCSF Med Ctr; **Address:** UCSF-Langley Porter Psychiatric Inst, 401 Parnassus Ave, Box CAF-0984, San Francisco, CA 94143-0984; **Phone:** 415-476-7365; **Board Cert:** Psychiatry 1983; **Med School:** Albert Einstein Coll Med 1977; **Resid:** Psychiatry, Langley Porter Psych Inst 1981; **Fac Appt:** Clin Prof Psyc, UCSF

Pi, Edmond H MD [Psyc] - **Spec Exp:** Psychopharmacology; Cross Cultural Psychiatry; Anxiety Disorders; Mood Disorders; **Hospital:** LAC & USC Med Ctr; **Address:** LAC USC Healthcare Network, 2010 Zonal Ave OPD Bldg - Ste 1P-1, Los Angeles, CA 90033; **Phone:** 310-668-2000; **Board Cert:** Psychiatry 1980; Psychosomatic Medicine 2008; **Med School:** South Korea 1972; **Resid:** Psychiatry, SUNY-Stony Brook Affil Hosp 1977; Psychiatry, Univ Kentucky Hosp-Chandler Med Ctr 1978; **Fac Appt:** Clin Prof Psyc, USC Sch Med

Pynoos, Robert S MD [Psyc] - **Spec Exp:** Post Traumatic Stress Clinical Trials; **Hospital:** Resnick Neuropsychiatric Hosp at UCLA; **Address:** Natl Ctr for Chld Traumatic Stress-UCLA, 11150 W Olympic Blvd, Ste 650, Los Angeles, CA 90064; **Phone:** 310-235-2633; **Board Cert:** Psychiatry 1980; **Med School:** Columbia P&S 1972; **Resid:** Pediatrics, Mt Sinai Hosp; Psychiatry, NY Presby-Cornell Med Ctr; **Fac Appt:** Prof Psyc, UCLA

Raskind, Murray MD [Psyc] - **Spec Exp:** Geriatric Psychiatry; Alzheimer's Disease; Post Traumatic Stress Disorder; **Hospital:** VA Puget Sound Hlth Care Sys, Univ Wash Med Ctr; **Address:** VA Puget Sound Health Care System, Mental Hlth Svc 1166-E, 1660 S Columbian Way, Seattle, WA 98108; **Phone:** 206-764-2702; **Board Cert:** Psychiatry 1976; Geriatric Psychiatry 2001; **Med School:** Columbia P&S 1968; **Resid:** Internal Medicine, Harlem Hosp Ctr 1970; Psychiatry, Univ Wash Affil Hosps 1973; **Fac Appt:** Prof Psyc, Univ Wash

Reus, Victor I MD [Psyc] - **Spec Exp:** Psychopharmacology; Bipolar/Mood Disorders; Behavioral Disorders; Depression; **Hospital:** UCSF Med Ctr; **Address:** UCSF, Dept Psychiatry, Langley Porter Psych Inst, 401 Parnussus Ave, Box 0984, San Francisco, CA 94143-0984; **Phone:** 415-476-7478; **Board Cert:** Psychiatry 1977; Geriatric Psychiatry 2010; **Med School:** Univ MD Sch Med 1973; **Resid:** Psychiatry, Univ Wisc Med Ctr 1976; **Fellow:** Biological Psychiatry, Natl Inst Mntl Hlth 1978; **Fac Appt:** Prof Psyc, UCSF

Roy-Byrne, Peter P MD [Psyc] - **Spec Exp:** Anxiety & Mood Disorders; Panic Disorder; Bipolar/Mood Disorders; Post Traumatic Stress Disorder; **Hospital:** Harborview Med Ctr, Univ Wash Med Ctr; **Address:** Psychiatric Medicine Assoc, 1501-05 West Lake Ave N, Seattle, WA 98199; **Phone:** 206-386-3103; **Board Cert:** Psychiatry 1983; **Med School:** Tufts Univ 1978; **Resid:** Psychiatry, UCLA Neuropsych Inst 1982; **Fellow:** Biological Psychiatry, Natl Inst Hlth - NIMH 1984; **Fac Appt:** Prof Psyc, Univ Wash

Saxena, Sanjaya MD [Psyc] - **Spec Exp:** Obsessive-Compulsive Disorder; **Hospital:** UCSD Med Ctr; **Address:** La Jolla Professional Building, 5060 Shoreham Pl, Ste 200, San Diego, CA 92122; **Phone:** 858-334-4640; **Board Cert:** Psychiatry 2006; **Med School:** Univ Minn 1990; **Resid:** Psychiatry, UCLA Neuropsychiatric Hosp 1994; **Fellow:** Neuroimaging, Charles A. Dana Fdn 1996; **Fac Appt:** Asst Prof Psyc, UCSD

Schatzberg, Alan F MD [Psyc] - **Spec Exp:** Psychopharmacology; Anxiety & Mood Disorders; Depression; **Hospital:** Stanford Univ Hosp & Clinics; **Address:** Stanford Univ Dept Psychiatry, 401 Quarry Rd, Stanford, CA 94305-5797; **Phone:** 650-723-6811; **Board Cert:** Psychiatry 1975; **Med School:** NYU Sch Med 1968; **Resid:** Psychiatry, Mass Mental Hlth Ctr 1972; **Fellow:** Psychiatry, Mass Mental Hlth Ctr/Harvard 1972; **Fac Appt:** Prof Psyc, Stanford Univ

Spiegel, David MD [Psyc] - **Spec Exp:** Hypnosis; Psychiatry in Cancer; Post Traumatic Stress Disorder; **Hospital:** Stanford Univ Hosp & Clinics; **Address:** Stanford Univ School of Medicine, Dept Psychiatry & Behavioral Sciences, 401 Quarry Rd PBS Bldg - rm 2325, Stanford, CA 94305-5718; **Phone:** 650-723-6421; **Board Cert:** Psychiatry 1976; **Med School:** Harvard Med Sch 1971; **Resid:** Psychiatry, Harvard Univ/Mass Mental Hlth Ctr 1974; Psychiatry, Cambridge Hosp-Harvard Med Sch 1974; **Fellow:** Community Psychiatry, Harvard Univ Med School 1974; **Fac Appt:** Prof Psyc, Stanford Univ

Stein, Murray B MD [Psyc] - **Spec Exp:** Anxiety Disorders; Panic Disorder; Post Traumatic Stress Disorder; **Hospital:** UCSD Med Ctr, VA San Diego Hlthcre Sys; **Address:** UCSD Dept Psychiatry, 8939 Villa La Jolla Drive, Ste 200, MS 0855, La Jolla, CA 92037; **Phone:** 858-534-6400; **Board Cert:** Psychiatry 1989; **Med School:** Univ Manitoba 1983; **Resid:** Psychiatry, Univ Toronto Hosp 1986; Psychiatry, Natl Inst Mental Hlth-NIH 1987; **Fellow:** Anxiety Disorder, Natl Inst Mental Hlth-NIH 1990; **Fac Appt:** Prof Psyc, UCSD

Strouse, Thomas B MD [Psyc] - **Spec Exp:** Psychiatry in Cancer; Pain-Cancer; Psychiatry in Physical Illness; Palliative Care; **Hospital:** UCLA Ronald Reagan Med Ctr, Cedars-Sinai Med Ctr; **Address:** UCLA Resnick Neuropsychiatric Hosp, 757 Westwood Plaza, Ste 4230B, Los Angeles, CA 90095; **Phone:** 310-267-9159; **Board Cert:** Psychiatry 1993; Pain Medicine 2000; Hospice & Palliative Medicine 2008; Psychosomatic Medicine 2009; **Med School:** Case West Res Univ 1987; **Resid:** Psychiatry, UCLA Med Ctr 1991; **Fac Appt:** Clin Prof Psyc, UCLA

Weinstock, Robert MD [Psyc] - **Spec Exp:** Adolescent Psychiatry; Addiction/Substance Abuse; **Hospital:** Cedars-Sinai Med Ctr; **Address:** 1823 Sawtelle Blvd, Los Angeles, CA 90025; **Phone:** 310-477-9933; **Board Cert:** Psychiatry 1975; Forensic Psychiatry 2004; **Med School:** NYU Sch Med 1966; **Resid:** Psychiatry, McLean Hosp 1970; McLean Hosp 1972; **Fellow:** Psychiatric Research, Boston Univ 1974; **Fac Appt:** Clin Prof Psyc, UCLA

Psychiatry

Zerbe, Kathryn J MD [Psyc] - **Spec Exp:** Eating Disorders; Women's Health-Mental Health; Psychoanalysis; **Address:** 4800 SW Macadam Ave, Ste 340, Portland, OR 97239; **Phone:** 503-295-9909; **Board Cert:** Psychiatry 1984; **Med School:** Temple Univ 1978; **Resid:** Psychiatry, Menninger Clin 1982; Psychoanalysis, Topeka Inst for Psychoanalysis 1992; **Fac Appt:** Prof Psyc, Oregon Hlth & Sci Univ

ADDICTION PSYCHIATRY

New England

Ciraulo, Domenic A MD [AdP] - **Spec Exp:** Alcohol Abuse; Psychopharmacology; Anxiety & Depression; **Hospital:** Boston Med Ctr; **Address:** Boston Univ, Div Psychiatry, 720 Harrison Ave, Ste 914, Boston, MA 02118; **Phone:** 617-414-1995; **Board Cert:** Psychiatry 1980; Addiction Psychiatry 2003; **Med School:** Georgetown Univ 1975; **Resid:** Psychiatry, Inst Living 1977; **Fellow:** Psychopharmacology, Mass Mental Hlth Ctr 1978; **Fac Appt:** Prof Psyc, Boston Univ

Greenfield, Shelly F MD [AdP] - **Spec Exp:** Addiction/Substance Abuse; Alcohol Abuse; Women & Addiction; **Hospital:** McLean Hosp; **Address:** McLean Hospital, 115 Mill St, Belmont, MA 02478; **Phone:** 617-855-2241; **Board Cert:** Psychiatry 1992; Addiction Psychiatry 2006; **Med School:** Harvard Med Sch 1986; **Resid:** Psychiatry, McLean Hosp 1990; **Fellow:** Epidemiology, Univ North Carolina 1992; Research, NIH-Natl Inst Drug Abuse 1993; **Fac Appt:** Assoc Prof Psyc, Harvard Med Sch

Nitenson, Nancy C MD [AdP] - **Spec Exp:** Alcohol Abuse; Addiction/Substance Abuse; **Address:** 10 Post Office Square Fl 8, Boston, MA 02109; **Phone:** 617-850-9005; **Board Cert:** Psychiatry 1998; Addiction Psychiatry 2006; **Med School:** Univ Mass Sch Med 1986; **Resid:** Psychiatry, U Mass Med Ctr 1990; **Fellow:** Psychopharmacology, McLean Hosp 1991

Schottenfeld, Richard MD [AdP] - **Spec Exp:** Drug Abuse-Consultation; Alcohol Abuse-Consultation; **Hospital:** Yale-New Haven Hosp, Connecticut Mental Hlth Ctr; **Address:** Connecticut Mental Health Ctr, 34 Park St, rm S-204, New Haven, CT 06519; **Phone:** 203-974-7349; **Board Cert:** Psychiatry 1984; **Med School:** Yale Univ 1976; **Resid:** Psychiatry, Yale Psych Inst 1982; **Fellow:** Epidemiology, Yale Univ 1984; **Fac Appt:** Prof Psyc, Yale Univ

Weiss, Roger D MD [AdP] - **Spec Exp:** Alcohol Abuse-Consultation; Drug Abuse-Consultation; Dual Diagnosis-Consultation; **Hospital:** McLean Hosp; **Address:** McLean Hospital, 115 Mill St, Belmont, MA 02478; **Phone:** 617-855-2242; **Board Cert:** Psychiatry 1980; Addiction Psychiatry 2002; **Med School:** Tufts Univ 1976; **Resid:** Psychiatry, McLean Hosp 1979; **Fac Appt:** Prof Psyc, Harvard Med Sch

Ziedonis, Douglas M MD [AdP] - **Spec Exp:** Tobacco Abuse; **Hospital:** UMass Memorial Med Ctr; **Address:** Univ Mass Med Sch, Dept Psychiatry, 55 Lake Ave N, Worcester, MA 01655; **Phone:** 508-856-3066; **Board Cert:** Psychiatry 1994; Addiction Psychiatry 2006; **Med School:** Penn State Coll Med 1985; **Resid:** Psychiatry, UCLA Med Ctr 1989; **Fellow:** Addiction Psychiatry, UCLA Med Ctr 1990; **Fac Appt:** Prof Psyc, Univ Mass Sch Med

Mid Atlantic

Frances, Richard J MD [AdP] - **Spec Exp:** Addiction/Substance Abuse; Anxiety & Mood Disorders; Forensic Psychiatry; **Hospital:** Silver Hill Hosp, NYU Langone Med Ctr (page 66); **Address:** 510 E 86th St, Ste 1D, New York, NY 10028; **Phone:** 212-861-0570; **Board Cert:** Psychiatry 1976; Addiction Psychiatry 2002; **Med School:** NYU Sch Med 1971; **Resid:** Psychiatry, Bronx Meml Hosp 1974; **Fellow:** Psychoanalysis, NY Psychoanalitic Inst 1984; **Fac Appt:** Clin Prof Psyc, NYU Sch Med

Galanter, Marc MD [AdP] - **Spec Exp:** Alcohol Abuse; Drug Abuse; **Hospital:** NYU Langone Med Ctr (page 66), Bellevue Hosp Ctr; **Address:** 285 Central Park West, New York, NY 10024-3006; **Phone:** 212-877-4093; **Board Cert:** Psychiatry 1974; Addiction Psychiatry 2002; **Med School:** Albert Einstein Coll Med 1967; **Resid:** Psychiatry, Bronx Muni Hosp-Einstein 1971; **Fac Appt:** Prof Psyc, NYU Sch Med

Kampman, Kyle M MD [AdP] - **Spec Exp:** Addiction/Substance Abuse; Cocaine Addiction; Opiate Addiction; Alcohol Abuse; **Hospital:** Hosp Univ Penn - UPHS (page 68); **Address:** UPHS Treatment Ctr, 3900 Chesnut St Fl Ground, Philadelphia, PA 19104; **Phone:** 215-222-3200; **Board Cert:** Psychiatry 2004; Addiction Psychiatry 2006; **Med School:** Tulane Univ 1985; **Resid:** Psychiatry, Hosp Univ Penn 1993; **Fellow:** Substance Abuse, Hosp Univ Penn 1994; **Fac Appt:** Assoc Prof Psyc, Univ Pennsylvania

Kleber, Herbert MD [AdP] - **Spec Exp:** Opiate Addiction; Cocaine Addiction; Drug Abuse; **Hospital:** NY-Presby/Columbia Univ Med Ctr, NY (page 65), NY State Psychiatric Inst; **Address:** NY State Psychiatric Inst, 1051 Riverside Drive, Room 3713, Unit 66, New York, NY 10032-1007; **Phone:** 212-543-5570; **Med School:** Jefferson Med Coll 1960; **Resid:** Psychiatry, Yale-New Haven Hosp 1964; **Fac Appt:** Prof Psyc, Columbia P&S

Serota, Ronald D MD [AdP] - **Spec Exp:** Addiction/Substance Abuse; **Hospital:** Thomas Jefferson Univ Hosp; **Address:** 833 Chestnut St, Ste 210, Philadelphia, PA 19107; **Phone:** 215-955-8780; **Board Cert:** Internal Medicine 1974; Psychiatry 1990; **Med School:** Thomas Jefferson Univ 1968; **Resid:** Internal Medicine, Mt Zion Hosp 1972; Psychiatry, Thomas Jefferson Univ Hosp 1981; **Fac Appt:** Asst Prof Psyc, Thomas Jefferson Univ

Strain, Eric C MD [AdP] - **Spec Exp:** Addiction/Substance Abuse; Dual Diagnosis; Opiate Addiction; **Hospital:** Johns Hopkins Bayview Med Ctr (page 61); **Address:** 5510 Mathen Shock Drive Fl 3 - Ste 3046, Baltimore, MD 21224; **Phone:** 410-550-1191; **Board Cert:** Psychiatry 1989; Addiction Psychiatry 2002; **Med School:** Ohio State Univ 1984; **Resid:** Psychiatry, Johns Hopkins Hosp 1988; **Fellow:** Addiction Psychiatry, Johns Hopkins Hosp 1990; **Fac Appt:** Prof Psyc, Johns Hopkins Univ

Southeast

Anton, Raymond F MD [AdP] - **Spec Exp:** Alcohol Abuse; Clinical Trials; **Hospital:** MUSC Med Ctr; **Address:** MUSC Dept Psychiatry, 67 President St, Box 250861, Charleston, SC 29425; **Phone:** 843-792-1226; **Board Cert:** Psychiatry 1982; **Med School:** UMDNJ-Rutgers Med Sch 1976; **Resid:** Psychiatry, Yale-New Haven Hosp/CT Mental Health Ctr 1980; **Fac Appt:** Prof Psyc, Med Univ SC

Addiction Psychiatry

Midwest

Stine, Susan M MD/PhD [AdP] - **Spec Exp:** Addiction/Substance Abuse; Opiate Addiction; **Hospital:** John D. Dingell VA Med Ctr, Detroit; **Address:** Wayne State Univ Sch Med, Dept Psychiatry, 2761 E Jefferson Ave, Detroit, MI 48207; **Phone:** 313-993-9879; **Board Cert:** Psychiatry 1993; Addiction Psychiatry 2002; **Med School:** Univ Miami Sch Med 1983; **Resid:** Psychiatry, Yale-New Haven Hosp 1987; **Fac Appt:** Assoc Prof Psyc, Wayne State Univ

Great Plains and Mountains

Howell, Elizabeth F MD [AdP] - **Spec Exp:** Opiate Addiction; Alcohol Abuse; Addiction/Substance Abuse; Pain Management; **Hospital:** Univ Utah Hlth Care; **Address:** Univ Utah Neuropsychiatric Inst, 501 Chipeta Way, Salt Lake City, UT 84108; **Phone:** 801-585-1575; **Board Cert:** Psychiatry 1985; Addiction Psychiatry 2003; Addiction Medicine 1998; **Med School:** Med Univ SC 1980; **Resid:** Pediatrics, Univ S Carolina Med Ctr 1981; Psychiatry, Univ S Carolina Med Ctr 1984; **Fellow:** Psychiatric Research, Univ S Carolina 1985; **Fac Appt:** Assoc Clin Prof Psyc, Univ Utah

Southwest

Kosten, Thomas MD [AdP] - **Spec Exp:** Cocaine Addiction; Alcohol Abuse; Psychopharmacology; Opiate Addiction; **Hospital:** DeBakey VA Med Ctr-Houston, UT MD Anderson Cancer Ctr; **Address:** Michael DeBakey VA Medical Ctr, 2002 Holcombe Blvd, Research - Building 110, Houston, TX 77030; **Phone:** 713-794-7032; **Board Cert:** Psychiatry 1984; Addiction Psychiatry 2002; **Med School:** Cornell Univ-Weill Med Coll 1977; **Resid:** Psychiatry, Yale-New Haven Hosp 1981; **Fellow:** Epidemiology, Yale-New Haven Hosp 1983; **Fac Appt:** Prof Psyc, Baylor Coll Med

West Coast and Pacific

Schuckit, Marc A MD [AdP] - **Spec Exp:** Alcohol Abuse; Substance Abuse; Psychopharmacology; **Hospital:** UCSD Med Ctr; **Address:** UCSD Dept Psychiatry, 8950 Villa La Jolla Drive, Ste B-218, San Diego, CA 92037; **Phone:** 858-822-0880; **Board Cert:** Psychiatry 1974; **Med School:** Washington Univ, St Louis 1968; **Resid:** Psychiatry, Wash Univ Affil Hosp 1971; Psychiatry, UCSD Med Ctr 1972; **Fac Appt:** Prof Psyc, UCSD

Walker, R Dale MD [AdP] - **Spec Exp:** Alcohol Abuse-Consultation; Drug Abuse-Consultation; Substance Abuse-Consultation; **Hospital:** OR Hlth & Sci Univ; **Address:** OHSU/One Sky Ctr, 3181 SW Sam Jackson Pk Rd, GH 151, Portland, OR 97239; **Phone:** 503-494-3703; **Board Cert:** Psychiatry 1982; **Med School:** Univ Okla Coll Med 1972; **Resid:** Psychiatry, Univ Oklahoma Med Ctr 1973; Psychiatry, UCSD Med Ctr 1977; **Fellow:** Public Health & Genl Preventive Med, Andriga Stampur; **Fac Appt:** Prof Psyc, Oregon Hlth & Sci Univ

CHILD & ADOLESCENT PSYCHIATRY

New England

Biederman, Joseph MD [ChAP] - **Spec Exp:** ADD/ADHD; Anxiety & Mood Disorders; Psychopharmacology; **Hospital:** Mass Genl Hosp; **Address:** 55 Fruit St Yawkey Bldg - rm 6900, Boston, MA 02114; **Phone:** 617-726-1743; **Board Cert:** Psychiatry 1983; Child & Adolescent Psychiatry 1984; **Med School:** Argentina 1971; **Resid:** Psychiatry, Hadassah Univ Hosp 1977; Psychiatry, Mass Genl Hosp 1981; **Fellow:** Child Psychiatry, Childrens Hosp 1979; **Fac Appt:** Prof Psyc, Harvard Med Sch

Herzog, David B MD [ChAP] - **Spec Exp:** Eating Disorders; Psychiatry in Physical Illness; **Hospital:** Mass Genl Hosp; **Address:** 2 Longfellow Place, Ste 200, Boston, MA 02114; **Phone:** 617-726-8470; **Board Cert:** Pediatrics 1980; Psychiatry 1982; Child & Adolescent Psychiatry 1986; **Med School:** Mexico 1973; **Resid:** Pediatrics, Univ Wisc 1975; Pediatrics, Boston City Hosp 1976; **Fellow:** Child & Adolescent Psychiatry, Chldns Hosp 1978; Psychiatry, Mass Genl Hosp 1980; **Fac Appt:** Prof Psyc, Harvard Med Sch

Hudziak, James MD [ChAP] - **Spec Exp:** ADD/ADHD; Obsessive-Compulsive Disorder; Psychopharmacology; **Hospital:** Fletcher Allen Health Care- Med Ctr Campus; **Address:** Univ Hlth Ctr, Dept Psychiatry, St Joseph's, rm 3213, Box 364SJ3, 1 S Prospect Drive, Burlington, VT 05401; **Phone:** 802-656-1084; **Board Cert:** Psychiatry 2005; Child & Adolescent Psychiatry 2005; **Med School:** Univ Minn 1988; **Resid:** Psychiatry, St Louis Chldns Hosp 1991; **Fac Appt:** Assoc Prof Psyc, Univ VT Coll Med

King, Robert A MD [ChAP] - **Spec Exp:** Tourette's Syndrome; Obsessive-Compulsive Disorder; Psychoanalysis; **Hospital:** Yale-New Haven Hosp, Yale Med Group; **Address:** Yale Child Study Ctr, 230 S Frontage Rd, Box 207900, New Haven, CT 06520; **Phone:** 203-785-5880; **Board Cert:** Psychiatry 1974; Child & Adolescent Psychiatry 1981; **Med School:** Harvard Med Sch 1968; **Resid:** Pediatrics, Chldns Hosp 1969; Psychiatry, Mass Mental Hlth Ctr 1971; **Fellow:** Child Psychiatry, Chldns Hosp 1972; Child Psychiatry, Chldns Hosp Natl Med Ctr 1974; **Fac Appt:** Prof ChAP, Yale Univ

Leckman, James F MD [ChAP] - **Spec Exp:** Tourette's Syndrome; Obsessive-Compulsive Disorder; Autism; **Hospital:** Yale-New Haven Hosp, Yale Med Group; **Address:** Yale Child Study Ctr, 230 S Frontage Rd, Box 207900, New Haven, CT 06520-7900; **Phone:** 203-785-7971; **Board Cert:** Psychiatry 1980; Child & Adolescent Psychiatry 1982; **Med School:** Univ New Mexico 1973; **Resid:** Psychiatry, Yale Univ 1979; Child Psychiatry, Yale Chld Stdy Ctr 1980; **Fellow:** Psychiatry, Natl Inst Mental Hlth 1976; **Fac Appt:** Prof Psyc, Yale Univ

McDougle, Christopher J MD [ChAP] - **Spec Exp:** Autism & Developmental Disorders; Obsessive-Compulsive Disorder; Mental Retardation; **Hospital:** Mass Genl Hosp; **Address:** Lurie Center for Autism, 1 Maguire Rd, Lexington, MA 02421; **Phone:** 781-860-1700; **Board Cert:** Psychiatry 1992; Child & Adolescent Psychiatry 2006; **Med School:** Indiana Univ 1986; **Resid:** Psychiatry, Yale Univ Affil Hosp 1990; **Fellow:** Child & Adolescent Psychiatry, Yale Child Study Ctr 1995; **Fac Appt:** Prof Psyc, Harvard Med Sch

Sargent III, Albert John MD [ChAP] - **Spec Exp:** Eating Disorders; Suicide; Family Therapy; Trauma Psychiatry; **Hospital:** Tufts Med Ctr; **Address:** Tufts Medical Center, 800 Washington St, Box 1007, Boston, MA 02111; **Phone:** 617-636-8768; **Board Cert:** Pediatrics 1979; Psychiatry 1988; Child & Adolescent Psychiatry 1989; **Med School:** Univ Rochester 1973; **Resid:** Pediatrics, Univ Wisc Hosp 1977; Child Psychiatry, Phila Child Guidance Ctr 1980; **Fellow:** Ambulatory Pediatrics, Univ Wisconsin Hosp 1976; **Fac Appt:** Prof Psyc, Tufts Univ

Child & Adolescent Psychiatry

Spencer, Thomas MD [ChAP] - **Spec Exp:** ADD/ADHD; **Hospital:** Mass Genl Hosp; **Address:** Mass Gen Hosp, 55 Fruit St, Ste YAW 6A, Boston, MA 02114; **Phone:** 617-724-5600; **Board Cert:** Psychiatry 1984; Child & Adolescent Psychiatry 1992; **Med School:** Univ Wisc 1978; **Resid:** Psychiatry, New England Med Ctr 1984; **Fellow:** Child & Adolescent Psychiatry, Mass Genl Hosp 1992; **Fac Appt:** Assoc Prof Psyc, Harvard Med Sch

Volkmar, Fred R MD [ChAP] - **Spec Exp:** Autism; Asperger's Syndrome; Developmental Disorders; Childhood Disintegrative Disorder; **Hospital:** Yale-New Haven Hosp, Greenwich Hosp; **Address:** Yale Child Study Ctr, 230 S Frontage Rd, Box 207900, New Haven, CT 06520-7900; **Phone:** 203-785-5759; **Board Cert:** Psychiatry 1981; Child & Adolescent Psychiatry 1988; **Med School:** Stanford Univ 1976; **Resid:** Psychiatry, Stanford Univ 1980; Child Psychiatry, Yale Child Study Ctr 1982; **Fac Appt:** Prof Psyc, Yale Univ

Wilens, Timothy MD [ChAP] - **Spec Exp:** ADD/ADHD; Bipolar/Mood Disorders; Addiction/Substance Abuse; **Hospital:** Mass Genl Hosp; **Address:** Mass Genl Hosp, Dept Psyc, 55 Fruit St Yawkey Bldg - Ste 6A, Boston, MA 02114; **Phone:** 617-724-5600; **Board Cert:** Psychiatry 1990; Child & Adolescent Psychiatry 1991; Addiction Psychiatry 2004; **Med School:** Univ Mich Med Sch 1985; **Resid:** Internal Medicine, Henry Ford Hosp 1986; Psychiatry, Mass Genl Hosp 1988; **Fellow:** Child & Adolescent Psychiatry, Mass Genl Hosp 1990; **Fac Appt:** Assoc Prof Psyc, Harvard Med Sch

Mid Atlantic

Abright, A Reese MD [ChAP] - **Spec Exp:** Mood Disorders; ADD/ADHD; Anxiety Disorders; **Hospital:** Elmhurst Hosp Ctr; **Address:** 140 E 40th St, Ste 1B, New York, NY 10016; **Phone:** 212-867-3131; **Board Cert:** Psychiatry 1978; Child & Adolescent Psychiatry 1981; **Med School:** Univ Tex SW, Dallas 1973; **Resid:** Psychiatry, St Vincent's Hosp 1974; Psychiatry, NY Hosp-Cornell Med Ctr 1977; **Fellow:** Child & Adolescent Psychiatry, NY Hosp-Cornell Med Ctr 1979; **Fac Appt:** Clin Prof Psyc, NY Med Coll

Bird, Hector MD [ChAP] - **Spec Exp:** ADD/ADHD; Anxiety & Depression; Personality Disorders; **Hospital:** NY-Presby/Columbia Univ Med Ctr, NY (page 65); **Address:** 300 W 72nd St, Ste 1F, New York, NY 10023-2004; **Phone:** 212-874-5311; **Board Cert:** Psychiatry 1975; Child & Adolescent Psychiatry 1977; **Med School:** Yale Univ 1965; **Resid:** Psychiatry, NY State Psych Inst 1971; NY State Psych Inst 1972; **Fellow:** Psychoanalysis, WA White Institute 1977; **Fac Appt:** Prof Emeritus Psyc, Columbia P&S

Birmaher, Boris MD [ChAP] - **Spec Exp:** Bipolar/Mood Disorders; Anxiety Disorders; **Hospital:** Western Psych Inst & Clin-UPMC; **Address:** Western Psych Inst & Clinic-UPMC, 3811 O'Hara St, Pittsburgh, PA 15213; **Phone:** 412-246-5788; **Board Cert:** Psychiatry 1989; Child & Adolescent Psychiatry 1990; **Med School:** Colombia 1975; **Resid:** Psychiatry, Haddassah Med Coll-Hebrew U 1983; Psychiatry, Montefiore Med Ctr 1984; **Fellow:** Child Psychiatry, NY Presby-Columbia Med Ctr 1986; Child Psychiatry, NY Psych Inst-Columbia U 1987; **Fac Appt:** Prof Psyc, Univ Pittsburgh

Bogrov, Michael MD [ChAP] - **Spec Exp:** ADD/ADHD; Mood Disorders; **Hospital:** Sheppard Pratt Hlth Sys, Johns Hopkins Hosp (page 61); **Address:** 6501 N Charles St, P.O. Box 6815, Towson, MD 21204-6815; **Phone:** 410-938-4913; **Board Cert:** Psychiatry 1993; Child & Adolescent Psychiatry 1994; **Med School:** Emory Univ 1987; **Resid:** Psychiatry, Univ Maryland 1990; Critical Care Obstetrics, Johns Hopkins Hosp 1992; **Fac Appt:** Asst Prof Psyc, Johns Hopkins Univ

Brent, David A MD [ChAP] - **Spec Exp:** Suicide; **Hospital:** Western Psych Inst & Clin-UPMC; **Address:** Western Psych Inst & Clin, 3811 O'Hara St, Ste 315 BFT, Pittsburgh, PA 15213-2593; **Phone:** 412-246-5596; **Board Cert:** Pediatrics 1981; Psychiatry 1982; Child & Adolescent Psychiatry 1983; **Med School:** Jefferson Med Coll 1974; **Resid:** Psychiatry, Western Psych Inst 1982; **Fellow:** Psychiatry, Univ Colorado Med Ctr 1976; **Fac Appt:** Prof Psyc, Univ Pittsburgh

Coffey, Barbara J MD [ChAP] - **Spec Exp:** Tourette's Syndrome; ADD/ADHD; Obsessive-Compulsive Disorder; Psychopharmacology; **Hospital:** NYU Langone Med Ctr (page 66); **Address:** NYU Child Study Ctr, 577 1st Ave, New York, NY 10016; **Phone:** 212-263-3926; **Board Cert:** Psychiatry 1981; Child & Adolescent Psychiatry 1986; **Med School:** Tufts Univ 1975; **Resid:** Psychiatry, Boston Univ Med Ctr 1978; **Fellow:** Child & Adolescent Psychiatry, Tufts Univ 1980; **Fac Appt:** Assoc Prof Psyc, NYU Sch Med

Foley, Carmel A MD [ChAP] - **Spec Exp:** Mood Disorders; **Hospital:** Steven & Alexandra Cohen Chldn's Med Ctr of NY; **Address:** 420 Lakeville Rd, 1st Floor, New Hyde Park, NY 11040; **Phone:** 718-470-3550; **Board Cert:** Psychiatry 1979; Child & Adolescent Psychiatry 1981; Forensic Psychiatry 1999; Psychosomatic Medicine 2009; **Med School:** Ireland 1972; **Resid:** Psychiatry, St Patrick's Hosp 1976; Psychiatry, Lafayette Clinic 1977; **Fellow:** Child & Adolescent Psychiatry, Lafayette Clinic 1979; **Fac Appt:** Assoc Prof Psyc, Albert Einstein Coll Med

Fornari, Victor MD [ChAP] - **Spec Exp:** Eating Disorders; Trauma Psychiatry; Post Traumatic Stress Disorder; **Hospital:** Zucker Hillside Hosp; **Address:** Zucker Hillside Hospital, Ambulatory Care Pavilion Lower Level, 75-59 263rd St, Glen Oaks, NY 11004; **Phone:** 718-470-3510; **Board Cert:** Psychiatry 1984; Child & Adolescent Psychiatry 1985; **Med School:** SUNY Downstate 1979; **Resid:** Psychiatry, Hosp Univ Penn 1982; **Fellow:** Child & Adolescent Psychiatry, LIJ Med Ctr 1984; **Fac Appt:** Prof Psyc, NYU Sch Med

Hertzig, Margaret MD [ChAP] - **Spec Exp:** Developmental Disorders; ADD/ADHD; **Hospital:** NY-Presby/Weill Cornell Med Ctr, NY (page 65); **Address:** 525 E 68th St, Box 140, New York, NY 10021-4870; **Phone:** 212-746-5712; **Board Cert:** Psychiatry 1968; Child & Adolescent Psychiatry 1975; **Med School:** NYU Sch Med 1960; **Resid:** Pediatrics, Jewish Hosp 1962; Psychiatry, Bellevue Psych Hosp 1964; **Fellow:** Psychiatric Research, NYU Sch Med 1966; **Fac Appt:** Prof Psyc, Cornell Univ-Weill Med Coll

Hirsch, Glenn S MD [ChAP] - **Spec Exp:** Anxiety & Mood Disorders; Tourette's Syndrome; Bipolar/Mood Disorders; ADD/ADHD; **Hospital:** NYU Langone Med Ctr (page 66), Bellevue Hosp Ctr; **Address:** NYU Child Study Center, 577 First Ave, New York, NY 10016; **Phone:** 212-263-8704; **Board Cert:** Psychiatry 1984; Child & Adolescent Psychiatry 1985; **Med School:** Albert Einstein Coll Med 1979; **Resid:** Psychiatry, New York Hosp-Cornell 1982; **Fellow:** Child & Adolescent Psychiatry, Columbia-Presby Med Ctr 1984; **Fac Appt:** Asst Prof ChAP, NYU Sch Med

Koplewicz, Harold S MD [ChAP] - **Spec Exp:** Anxiety & Mood Disorders; Psychopharmacology; ADD/ADHD; **Address:** Child Mind Inst, 445 Park Ave at 56th St, New York, NY 10022; **Phone:** 212-308-3118; **Board Cert:** Psychiatry 1983; Child & Adolescent Psychiatry 1984; **Med School:** Albert Einstein Coll Med 1978; **Resid:** Psychiatry, New York Hosp-Westchester Div 1981; Psychiatry, NY State Psych Inst 1983; **Fellow:** Psychiatric Research, NY State Psych Inst 1985

Leventhal, Bennett MD [ChAP] - **Spec Exp:** Autism; ADD/ADHD; Psychopharmacology; **Hospital:** NYU Langone Med Ctr (page 66); **Address:** 577 First Ave, New York, NY 10016; **Phone:** 212-263-8696; **Board Cert:** Psychiatry 1979; Child & Adolescent Psychiatry 1980; **Med School:** Louisiana State U, New Orleans 1974; **Resid:** Psychiatry, Duke Univ Med Ctr 1978; **Fellow:** Child & Adolescent Psychiatry, Duke Univ Med Ctr 1977; **Fac Appt:** Prof Psyc, NYU Sch Med

Pomeroy, John C MD [ChAP] - **Spec Exp:** Autism; Mental Retardation; Developmental Disorders; **Hospital:** Stony Brook Univ Med Ctr; **Address:** The Cody Center for Autism, 5 Medical Drive, Port Jefferson Stn, NY 11776; **Phone:** 631-632-3070; **Board Cert:** Psychiatry 1984; Child & Adolescent Psychiatry 1988; **Med School:** England, UK 1973; **Resid:** Psychiatry, St Mary's Hosp 1979; **Fellow:** Child & Adolescent Psychiatry, Univ Iowa Hosps 1981; **Fac Appt:** Assoc Prof Psyc, SUNY Stony Brook

Child & Adolescent Psychiatry

Rapoport, Judith MD [ChAP] - **Spec Exp:** Schizophrenia; Obsessive-Compulsive Disorder; **Hospital:** Natl Inst of Hlth - Clin Ctr; **Address:** 3010 44th Place NW, Washington, DC 20016; **Phone:** 202-966-7355; **Board Cert:** Psychiatry 1969; Child & Adolescent Psychiatry 1969; **Med School:** Harvard Med Sch 1959; **Resid:** Psychiatry, Mass Mental Hlth Ctr 1961; Psychiatry, St Elizabeth Hosp 1962; **Fellow:** Psychiatry, Karolinska Inst 1964; Child & Adolescent Psychiatry, Childns Hosp 1966

Riddle, Mark A MD [ChAP] - **Spec Exp:** Psychopharmacology; Anxiety Disorders; Mood Disorders; **Hospital:** Johns Hopkins Hosp (page 61); **Address:** 600 N Wolfe St, CMSC-346, Baltimore, MD 21287-3325; **Phone:** 410-955-2320; **Board Cert:** Psychiatry 1982; Child & Adolescent Psychiatry 1986; **Med School:** Indiana Univ 1977; **Resid:** Psychiatry, Yale-New Haven Hosp 1981; **Fellow:** Child & Adolescent Psychiatry, Yale Child Study Ctr 1983; **Fac Appt:** Prof Psyc, Johns Hopkins Univ

Rostain, Anthony L MD [ChAP] - **Spec Exp:** ADD/ADHD; Autism; Tourette's Syndrome; Asperger's Syndrome; **Hospital:** Chldns Hosp of Philadelphia, Penn Presby Med Ctr - UPHS (page 68); **Address:** Hosp Univ Penn, Dept Psychiatry, 3535 Market St Fl 2, Philadelphia, PA 19104; **Phone:** 215-746-7210; **Board Cert:** Pediatrics 1985; Psychiatry 1988; Child & Adolescent Psychiatry 1989; **Med School:** NYU Sch Med 1980; **Resid:** Pediatrics, Chldn's Hosp 1983; Psychiatry, Hosp Univ Penn 1987; **Fellow:** Child Psychiatry, Philadelphia Child Guidance Clin 1985; **Fac Appt:** Prof Psyc, Univ Pennsylvania

Turecki, Stanley K MD [ChAP] - **Spec Exp:** Temperamentally Difficult Child; ADD/ADHD; Parenting Issues; **Hospital:** Lenox Hill Hosp, Beth Israel Med Ctr - Petrie Division (page 55); **Address:** 136 E 64th St, Ste 1B, New York, NY 10065; **Phone:** 212-355-2535; **Board Cert:** Psychiatry 1978; Child & Adolescent Psychiatry 1981; **Med School:** South Africa 1961; **Resid:** Psychiatry, Tara Hospital 1969; Psychiatry, Mt Sinai Hosp 1971

Walkup, John MD [ChAP] - **Spec Exp:** Anxiety Disorders; **Hospital:** NY-Presby/Weill Cornell Med Ctr, NY (page 65); **Address:** NY Presby Hosp-Weill Cornell, Dept Psych, 525 E 68th St, Box 140, New York, NY 10065; **Phone:** 212-746-1891; **Board Cert:** Psychiatry 1987; Child & Adolescent Psychiatry 1992; **Med School:** Univ Minn 1982; **Resid:** Psychiatry, Yale Univ Med Sch 1985; Child Psychiatry, Yale Chld Study Ctr 1988; **Fac Appt:** Asst Prof Psyc, Johns Hopkins Univ

Southeast

Deas, Deborah V MD [ChAP] - **Spec Exp:** Addiction/Substance Abuse; Dual Diagnosis; Substance Abuse in ADHD Patients; **Hospital:** MUSC Med Ctr; **Address:** MUSC, Ctr for Drug & Alcohol Programs, 67 President St, Charleston, SC 29425; **Phone:** 843-792-5214; **Board Cert:** Psychiatry 2005; Child & Adolescent Psychiatry 2007; **Med School:** Med Univ SC 1989; **Resid:** Psychiatry, MUSC Med Ctr 1992; **Fellow:** Child & Adolescent Psychiatry, MUSC Med Ctr 1994; Addiction Psychiatry, MUSC/Natl Inst Alcohol Abuse & Alcoholism 1994; **Fac Appt:** Prof Psyc, Med Univ SC

Heston, Jerry D MD [ChAP] - **Spec Exp:** ADD/ADHD; Depression; Asperger's Syndrome; **Hospital:** Le Bonheur Chldns Med Ctr, St. Jude Children's Research Hosp; **Address:** Child & Adolescent Psychiatric Assocs, 1135 Cully Rd, Ste 100, Cordova, TN 38016; **Phone:** 901-752-1980; **Board Cert:** Psychiatry 1988; Pediatrics 2004; Child & Adolescent Psychiatry 1989; **Med School:** Univ S Fla Coll Med 1981; **Resid:** Pediatrics, LeBonheur Chldns Hosp 1984; Psychiatry, Univ Tennessee Affil Hosp 1986; **Fellow:** Child & Adolescent Psychiatry, Univ Tennessee Affil Hosp 1988; **Fac Appt:** Clin Prof Psyc, Univ Tenn Coll Med

Sexson, Sandra G B MD [ChAP] - **Spec Exp:** Psychiatry in Transplant Patients; Death & Dying; **Hospital:** Med Coll of GA Hosp and Clin (MCG Health Inc); **Address:** Medical College Georgia, Dept Psych & Health Behavior, 997 St Sebastian Way, Augusta, GA 30912; **Phone:** 706-721-6699; **Board Cert:** Psychiatry 1980; Child & Adolescent Psychiatry 2004; **Med School:** Univ Miss 1971; **Resid:** Psychiatry, Tex Hlth Sci Ctr 1974; Child Psychiatry, Washington Univ Affil Hosp 1978; **Fac Appt:** Prof Psyc, Med Coll GA

Midwest

Alessi, Norman E MD [ChAP] - **Spec Exp:** Mood Disorders; Autism; Cognitive Psychotherapy; ADD/ADHD; **Hospital:** Univ of Michigan Hosp; **Address:** 325 E Eisenhower Pkwy, Ste 6, Ann Arbor, MI 48108; **Phone:** 734-222-6222; **Board Cert:** Psychiatry 1982; Child & Adolescent Psychiatry 1985; **Med School:** Emory Univ 1976; **Resid:** Psychiatry, Univ Mich Med Ctr 1980; Child Psychiatry, Univ Mich Med Ctr 1981; **Fellow:** Child & Adolescent Psychiatry, Univ Mich Med Ctr 1983; **Fac Appt:** Prof Emeritus Psyc, Univ Mich Med Sch

Boxer, Gary H MD [ChAP] - **Spec Exp:** ADD/ADHD; Parenting Issues; Mood Disorders; Behavioral Disorders; **Hospital:** St. Louis Chldns Hosp, Barnes-Jewish Hosp; **Address:** St Louis Chldns Hosp, Dept Psychiatry, 24 S Kingshighway Blvd, St Louis, MO 63108; **Phone:** 314-286-1700; **Board Cert:** Psychiatry 1986; Child & Adolescent Psychiatry 1988; **Med School:** Univ Colorado 1980; **Resid:** Psychiatry, Univ Michigan Med Ctr 1983; **Fellow:** Child Psychiatry, Univ Colorado 1985; **Fac Appt:** Assoc Prof Psyc, Washington Univ, St Louis

Campo, John V MD [ChAP] - **Spec Exp:** Psychosomatic Disorders; Psychiatry in Physical Illness; **Hospital:** Nationwide Chldn's Hosp, Ohio St Univ Med Ctr; **Address:** Columbus Chldn's Hosp, 700 Childrens Drive, Dept Psychiatry, Columbus, OH 43205; **Phone:** 614-722-2291; **Board Cert:** Pediatrics 1986; Psychiatry 1989; Child & Adolescent Psychiatry 1993; **Med School:** Univ Pennsylvania 1982; **Resid:** Pediatrics, Childrens Hosp 1985; Psychiatry, West Psych Inst Clin 1989; **Fac Appt:** Prof Psyc, Ohio State Univ

Dulcan, Mina K MD [ChAP] - **Spec Exp:** ADD/ADHD; **Hospital:** Children's Mem Hosp - Chicago, Northwestern Meml Hosp; **Address:** Chldns Meml Hosp, Dept Psyc, 2300 Children's Plaza, Box 10, Chicago, IL 60614; **Phone:** 773-880-4811; **Board Cert:** Psychiatry 1978; Child & Adolescent Psychiatry 1979; **Med School:** Penn State Coll Med 1974; **Resid:** Psychiatry, Western Psych Inst/Clinic 1977; **Fellow:** Child Psychiatry, Western Psych Inst 1978; **Fac Appt:** Prof Psyc, Northwestern Univ

Luby, Joan L MD [ChAP] - **Spec Exp:** Mood Disorders; **Hospital:** Barnes-Jewish Hosp; **Address:** Wash Univ Sch Med, Dept Psychiatry, 660 S Euclid Ave, Box 8134, St Louis, MO 63110; **Phone:** 314-286-2730; **Board Cert:** Psychiatry 1993; Child & Adolescent Psychiatry 1993; **Med School:** Wayne State Univ 1985; **Resid:** Psychiatry, Stanford Univ Sch Med 1988; **Fellow:** Child & Adolescent Psychiatry, Stanford Univ Sch Med 1990; **Fac Appt:** Assoc Prof Psyc, Washington Univ, St Louis

Slomowitz, Marcia MD [ChAP] - **Spec Exp:** ADD/ADHD; Bipolar/Mood Disorders; Anxiety & Depression; **Hospital:** Northwestern Meml Hosp; **Address:** 333 N Michigan Ave, Ste 1125, Chicago, IL 60601; **Phone:** 312-726-1083; **Board Cert:** Psychiatry 1982; Child & Adolescent Psychiatry 1983; **Med School:** Univ Wisc 1977; **Resid:** Psychiatry, Univ Cincinnati Affil Hosp 1980; **Fellow:** Child & Adolescent Psychiatry, Univ Cincinnati Affil Hosp 1982; **Fac Appt:** Asst Prof Psyc, Northwestern Univ

Child & Adolescent Psychiatry

Great Plains and Mountains

Hagman, Jennifer O MD [ChAP] - **Spec Exp:** Eating Disorders; Depression; Anxiety Disorders; **Hospital:** Chldn's Hosp - Aurora (CO); **Address:** Chldns Hosp, Dept Psychiatry, 13123 E 16th Ave, B130, Aurora, CO 80045; **Phone:** 720-777-2539; **Board Cert:** Psychiatry 1992; Child & Adolescent Psychiatry 1992; **Med School:** Univ Kansas 1986; **Resid:** Psychiatry, UC Irvine Med Ctr 1990; **Fellow:** Child & Adolescent Psychiatry, UC Irvine Med Ctr 1991; **Fac Appt:** Assoc Prof Psyc, Univ Colorado

Martini, D Richard MD [ChAP] - **Spec Exp:** Psychiatry in Physical Illness; Post Traumatic Stress Disorder; ADD/ADHD; Brain Injury; **Hospital:** Primary Children's Med Ctr; **Address:** Primary Chldns Med Ctr, 100 N Mario Capecchi Drive, Salt Lake City, UT 84113; **Phone:** 801-662-6755; **Board Cert:** Psychiatry 1987; Child & Adolescent Psychiatry 1990; **Med School:** Univ Nebr Coll Med 1982; **Resid:** Psychiatry, Univ Pittsburgh Med Ctr 1985; Child Psychiatry, Univ Pittsburgh Med Ctr 1987; **Fac Appt:** Prof Psyc, Univ Utah

Wamboldt, Marianne Z MD [ChAP] - **Hospital:** Chldn's Hosp - Aurora (CO); **Address:** Children's Hosp, Dept Psychiatry, 13123 E 16th Ave, B130, Aurora, CO 80045; **Phone:** 720-777-6096; **Board Cert:** Psychiatry 1986; Child & Adolescent Psychiatry 1991; **Med School:** Univ Wisc 1982; **Resid:** Psychiatry, Univ Wisconsin 1986

Southwest

Bleiberg, Efrain MD [ChAP] - **Spec Exp:** Trauma Psychiatry; Personality Disorders; **Hospital:** Menninger Clinic; **Address:** Menninger Hosp & Clinic, 2801 Gessner Drive, Box 809045, Houston, TX 77280-9045; **Phone:** 713-275-5213; **Board Cert:** Psychiatry 1985; Child & Adolescent Psychiatry 1986; **Med School:** Mexico 1976; **Resid:** Psychiatry, Menninger Fdn 1980; **Fellow:** Child & Adolescent Psychiatry, Menninger Fdn 1981

Emslie, Graham J MD [ChAP] - **Spec Exp:** Depression; **Hospital:** Chldns Med Ctr of Dallas; **Address:** UT SW Med Ctr at Dallas, 6300 Harry Hines Blvd, Dallas, TX 75235; **Phone:** 214-456-5900; **Board Cert:** Psychiatry 1981; **Med School:** Scotland, UK 1974; **Resid:** Psychiatry, Univ Rochester 1978; Child Psychiatry, Stanford Med Ctr 1981; **Fac Appt:** Prof Psyc, Univ Tex SW, Dallas

Zeanah Jr, Charles H MD [ChAP] - **Spec Exp:** Attachment Disorders; Abuse/Neglect; Post Traumatic Stress Disorder; Infant-Toddler Psychiatry; **Hospital:** Tulane Med Ctr; **Address:** Tulane Dept Child Psychiatry, 1430 Tulane Ave, #8055, 144, New Orleans, LA 70112; **Phone:** 504-988-5402; **Board Cert:** Psychiatry 1983; Child & Adolescent Psychiatry 1983; **Med School:** Tulane Univ 1977; **Resid:** Psychiatry, Duke Univ Med Ctr 1980; Child Psychiatry, Stanford Univ Med Ctr 1982; **Fellow:** Research, Stanford Univ 1984; **Fac Appt:** Prof Psyc, Tulane Univ

West Coast and Pacific

King, Bryan H MD [ChAP] - **Spec Exp:** Autism; Developmental Disorders; Behavioral Disorders; **Hospital:** Seattle Chldns Hosp; **Address:** Chldns Hosp & Regl Med Ctr, Dept Psych, PO Box 5371, MS W3636, Seattle, WA 98105; **Phone:** 206-987-4080; **Board Cert:** Psychiatry 1991; Child & Adolescent Psychiatry 2004; **Med School:** Med Coll Wisc 1983; **Resid:** Psychiatry, UCLA Neuropsych Inst 1987; **Fellow:** Child & Adolescent Psychiatry, UCLA Neuropsych Inst 1990; **Fac Appt:** Prof Psyc, Univ Wash

Kwon, Hower MD [ChAP] - **Spec Exp:** Anxiety & Mood Disorders; ADD/ADHD; Developmental Disorders; **Hospital:** Univ Wash Med Ctr; **Address:** Bellevue Child Behavior Ctr, 365 118th Ave SE, Ste 118, Bellevue, WA 98005; **Phone:** 425-454-2911; **Board Cert:** Psychiatry 2009; Child & Adolescent Psychiatry 2009; **Med School:** NYU Sch Med 1993; **Resid:** Psychiatry, UCLA Neuropsychiatric Ins 1996; **Fellow:** Child & Adolescent Psychiatry, UCLA Neuropsychiatric Inst 1999; **Fac Appt:** Asst Clin Prof Psyc, Univ Wash

McCracken, James T MD [ChAP] - **Spec Exp:** Obsessive-Compulsive Disorder; Tourette's Syndrome; **Hospital:** Resnick Neuropsychiatric Hosp at UCLA; **Address:** UCLA Neuropsychiatric Inst, 760 Westwood Plaza, Ste 48-270, Los Angeles, CA 90024; **Phone:** 310-825-0470; **Board Cert:** Psychiatry 1986; Child & Adolescent Psychiatry 1988; **Med School:** Baylor Coll Med 1980; **Resid:** Psychiatry, Duke Univ Med Ctr 1984; **Fellow:** Child & Adolescent Psychiatry, UCLA Neuropsych Inst 1985; **Fac Appt:** Prof Psyc, UCLA

McKelvey, Robert S MD [ChAP] - **Spec Exp:** Suicide; Depression; Cross Cultural Psychiatry; **Hospital:** Doernbecher Chldns Hosp/OHSU; **Address:** 5520 SW Macadam Ave, Ste 265, Portland, OR 97239; **Phone:** 971-219-8363; **Board Cert:** Psychiatry 1980; Child & Adolescent Psychiatry 1982; **Med School:** Dartmouth Med Sch 1974; **Resid:** Psychiatry, Cambridge Hosp 1977; **Fellow:** Child Psychiatry, McLean Hosp 1979; **Fac Appt:** Prof Psyc, Oregon Hlth & Sci Univ

Ponton, Lynn Elisabeth MD [ChAP] - **Spec Exp:** Behavioral Disorders; Eating Disorders; **Hospital:** UCSF Med Ctr; **Address:** 201 Edgewood Ave, San Francisco, CA 94117; **Phone:** 415-664-3039; **Board Cert:** Psychiatry 1985; Child & Adolescent Psychiatry 1985; **Med School:** Univ Wisc 1978; **Resid:** Psychiatry, Hosp Univ Penn 1980; Psychiatry, UCSF Med Ctr 1981; **Fellow:** Child & Adolescent Psychiatry, UCSF Med Ctr 1983; **Fac Appt:** Prof Psyc, UCSF

Russell, Andrew T MD [ChAP] - **Spec Exp:** ADD/ADHD; Schizophrenia; Developmental Disorders; **Hospital:** Resnick Neuropsychiatric Hosp at UCLA; **Address:** UCLA-NPI Semel Institute, 760 Westwood Plaza, Los Angeles, CA 90024; **Phone:** 310-825-0389; **Board Cert:** Psychiatry 1980; Child & Adolescent Psychiatry 2004; **Med School:** Univ Colorado 1970; **Resid:** Psychiatry, UCLA Med Ctr 1973; **Fellow:** Child & Adolescent Psychiatry, UCLA Med Ctr 1977; **Fac Appt:** Clin Prof Psyc, UCLA

Steiner, Hans MD [ChAP] - **Spec Exp:** Aggression Disorders; Eating Disorders; Trauma Psychiatry; Psychosomatic Disorders; **Hospital:** Stanford Univ Hosp & Clinics, Lucile Packard Chldn's Hosp; **Address:** Child & Adolescent Psychiatry, 401 Quarry Rd, MC 5719, Stanford, CA 94305-5719; **Phone:** 650-723-5511; **Board Cert:** Psychiatry 1979; Child & Adolescent Psychiatry 1981; **Med School:** Austria 1972; **Resid:** Psychiatry, SUNY Syracuse Med Ctr 1976; **Fellow:** Child & Adolescent Psychiatry, Univ Mich Hosps 1978; **Fac Appt:** Prof Emeritus Psyc, Stanford Univ

Terr, Lenore MD [ChAP] - **Spec Exp:** Trauma Psychiatry; **Hospital:** UCSF Med Ctr; **Address:** 450 Sutter St, Ste 1336, San Francisco, CA 94108-4204; **Phone:** 415-433-7800; **Board Cert:** Psychiatry 1968; Child & Adolescent Psychiatry 1969; **Med School:** Univ Mich Med Sch 1961; **Resid:** Psychiatry, Univ Mich Med Ctr 1964; **Fellow:** Child & Adolescent Psychiatry, Univ Mich 1966; **Fac Appt:** Clin Prof Psyc, UCSF

GERIATRIC PSYCHIATRY

Mid Atlantic

Greenwald, Blaine MD [GerPsy] - **Spec Exp:** Depression; Dementia; **Hospital:** Zucker Hillside Hosp, N Shore Univ Hosp; **Address:** Zudker Hillside Hospital, Ambulatory Care Pavilion, 75-59 263rd St, rm 2102, Glen Oaks, NY 11004; **Phone:** 718-470-8159; **Board Cert:** Psychiatry 1983; Geriatric Psychiatry 2000; **Med School:** NY Med Coll 1978; **Resid:** Psychiatry, Mt Sinai Hosp 1982; **Fellow:** Geriatric Psychiatry, Mt Sinai Hosp/Bronx VA Hosp 1983; **Fac Appt:** Assoc Prof Psyc, Albert Einstein Coll Med

Kennedy, Gary MD [GerPsy] - **Spec Exp:** Alzheimer's Disease; Dementia; Depression; **Hospital:** Montefiore Med Ctr - Div. Moses; **Address:** Dept Psyc & Behav Science, Montefiore Medical Center, 111 E 210th St, Bronx, NY 10467; **Phone:** 718-920-6270; **Board Cert:** Psychiatry 1980; Geriatric Psychiatry 2010; Psychosomatic Medicine 2005; **Med School:** Univ Tex, San Antonio 1975; **Resid:** Psychiatry, VA Hosp-Univ Texas 1979; **Fellow:** Geriatric Psychiatry, Montefiore Med Ctr 1981; Psychosomatic Medicine, Montefiore Med Ctr 1983; **Fac Appt:** Prof Psyc, Albert Einstein Coll Med

Lyketsos, Constantine G MD [GerPsy] - **Spec Exp:** Alzheimer's Disease; Neuro-Psychiatry; Depression; Dementia; **Hospital:** Johns Hopkins Bayview Med Ctr (page 61), Johns Hopkins Hosp (page 61); **Address:** Johns Hopkins Bayview Med Ctr, 5300 Alpha Commons Drive Fl 4th, Baltimore, MD 21224; **Phone:** 410-550-0062; **Board Cert:** Psychiatry 1994; Psychosomatic Medicine 2005; **Med School:** Washington Univ, St Louis 1988; **Resid:** Psychiatry, Johns Hopkins Hosp 1992; **Fellow:** Neuropsychiatry, Johns Hopkins Hosp 1994; **Fac Appt:** Prof Psyc, Johns Hopkins Univ

Reisberg, Barry MD [GerPsy] - **Spec Exp:** Alzheimer's Disease; Dementia; Cognitive Loss in Aging; Depression; **Hospital:** NYU Langone Med Ctr (page 66); **Address:** Aging & Dementia Rsch Ctr - NYU, 145 E 32nd St, rm 508, New York, NY 10016-6055; **Phone:** 212-263-8550; **Board Cert:** Psychiatry 1976; Geriatric Psychiatry 2000; **Med School:** NY Med Coll 1972; **Resid:** Psychiatry, Metropolitan Hosp 1975; **Fellow:** Psychiatric Research, Univ London 1975; **Fac Appt:** Prof Psyc, NYU Sch Med

Rosen, Jules MD [GerPsy] - **Spec Exp:** Alzheimer's Disease; Dementia; **Hospital:** Western Psych Inst & Clin-UPMC, UPMC Presby, Pittsburgh; **Address:** Western Psych Inst & Clin, 3811 O'Hara St, Pittsburgh, PA 15213; **Phone:** 412-246-5900; **Board Cert:** Psychiatry 1984; Geriatric Psychiatry 2003; **Med School:** Univ Cincinnati 1978; **Resid:** Psychiatry, Univ Mich Med Ctr 1982; **Fac Appt:** Prof Psyc, Univ Pittsburgh

Rovner, Barry W MD [GerPsy] - **Spec Exp:** Alzheimer's Disease; Behavioral Problems & Dementia; **Hospital:** Thomas Jefferson Univ Hosp; **Address:** Jefferson Hosp Neuroscience, 900 Walnut St, Ste 200, Philadelphia, PA 19107; **Phone:** 215-503-1254; **Board Cert:** Psychiatry 1985; **Med School:** Jefferson Med Coll 1980; **Resid:** Psychiatry, Johns Hopkins Hosp 1984; **Fac Appt:** Assoc Prof Psyc, Jefferson Med Coll

Streim, Joel E MD [GerPsy] - **Spec Exp:** Psychiatry in Physical Illness; Psychiatric Barriers to Physical Rehab; Alzheimer's Disease; **Hospital:** Hosp Univ Penn - UPHS (page 68), VA Med Ctr - Philadelphia; **Address:** Univ Penn, Dept Geriatric Psychiatry, 3535 Market St, rm 3053, Philadelphia, PA 19104; **Phone:** 215-615-3086; **Board Cert:** Psychiatry 1988; Geriatric Psychiatry 2009; **Med School:** Univ Rochester 1978; **Resid:** Psychiatry, Univ Wisconsin 1985; **Fellow:** Liaison Psychiatry, Univ Rochester/Strong Mem 1981; Geriatric Psychiatry, VA Med Ctr 1988; **Fac Appt:** Prof Psyc, Univ Pennsylvania

Southeast

Holroyd, Suzanne MD [GerPsy] - **Spec Exp:** Dementia; Psychoses-Late Onset; Mood Disorders; **Hospital:** Univ of Virginia Health Sys; **Address:** Univ of Virginia Health Sys, Dept Psych, Box 800623, Charlottesville, VA 22908; **Phone:** 434-924-2241; **Board Cert:** Psychiatry 1992; Geriatric Psychiatry 2004; **Med School:** Univ VA Sch Med 1986; **Resid:** Psychiatry, Johns Hopkins Hosp 1990; **Fellow:** Geriatric Psychiatry, Johns Hopkins Hosp 1991; **Fac Appt:** Prof Psyc, Univ VA Sch Med

Tune, Larry E MD [GerPsy] - **Spec Exp:** Alzheimer's Disease; Dementia; Psychopharmacology; Psychoses-Late Onset; **Hospital:** Wesley Woods Ger Hosp, Emory Univ Hosp; **Address:** Wesley Woods Ctr, Dept Psychiatry, 1841 Clifton Rd NE, Atlanta, GA 30329; **Phone:** 404-728-6690; **Board Cert:** Psychiatry 1991; Geriatric Psychiatry 2004; **Med School:** Univ VA Sch Med 1975; **Resid:** Psychiatry, Johns Hopkins Hosp 1979; Neurology, Johns Hopkins Hosp 1983; **Fellow:** Psychopharmacology, Johns Hopkins Univ 1981; **Fac Appt:** Prof Psyc, Emory Univ

Midwest

Grossberg, George MD [GerPsy] - **Spec Exp:** Alzheimer's Disease; Depression; Behavioral Problems & Dementia; **Hospital:** St. Louis Univ Hosp; **Address:** St Louis Univ Sch Med, Dept Neurology & Psychiatry, 1438 S Grand Blvd, St Louis, MO 63104; **Phone:** 314-977-4850; **Board Cert:** Psychiatry 1982; Geriatric Psychiatry 2001; **Med School:** St Louis Univ 1975; **Resid:** Psychiatry, St Louis Univ Med Ctr 1979; **Fac Appt:** Prof N, St Louis Univ

Manepalli, Jothika M MD [GerPsy] - **Spec Exp:** Mood Disorders; Dementia; Depression; Palliative Care; **Hospital:** St. Louis Univ Hosp; **Address:** St Louis Univ Hosp, Dept Psychiatry, 14838 S Grand Blvd, St Louis, MO 63104; **Phone:** 314-977-4815; **Board Cert:** Psychiatry 1994; Geriatric Psychiatry 1995; **Med School:** India 1977; **Resid:** Psychiatry, Duke Univ Med Ctr 1987; Psychiatry, Barnes Hosp 1989; **Fellow:** Geriatric Psychiatry, St Louis Univ Hosp 1990; **Fac Appt:** Prof Psyc, St Louis Univ

Mellow, Alan M MD/PhD [GerPsy] - **Spec Exp:** Dementia; Depression; **Hospital:** VA Ann Arbor Healthcare Sys, Univ of Michigan Hosp; **Address:** Dept VA Affairs, (10N11), VISN Office, PO Box 134002, Ann Arbor, MI 48113-4002; **Phone:** 734-222-4350; **Board Cert:** Psychiatry 1988; Geriatric Psychiatry 2002; **Med School:** Northwestern Univ 1981; **Resid:** Internal Medicine, Univ Chicago Hosp 1982; Psychiatry, McLean Hosp-Harvard 1985; **Fellow:** Psychiatry, Natl Inst Mental Hlth 1988; **Fac Appt:** Prof Psyc, Univ Mich Med Sch

Great Plains and Mountains

Burke, William J MD [GerPsy] - **Spec Exp:** Depression; Dementia; Alzheimer's Disease; Panic Disorder; **Hospital:** Nebraska Med Ctr; **Address:** Nebraska Medical Ctr, Dept Psychiatry, 985580 Nebraska Medical Ctr, Omaha, NE 68198-5580; **Phone:** 402-552-6062; **Board Cert:** Psychiatry 1986; Geriatric Psychiatry 2001; **Med School:** Univ Nebr Coll Med 1980; **Resid:** Internal Medicine, Univ Nebraska Med Ctr 1981; Psychiatry, Wash Univ Barnes Hosp 1984; **Fac Appt:** Prof Psyc, Univ Nebr Coll Med

Geriatric Psychiatry

West Coast and Pacific

Borson, Soo MD [GerPsy] - **Spec Exp:** Alzheimer's Disease; Psychiatry in Physical Illness; Dementia; Memory Disorders; **Hospital:** Univ Wash Med Ctr; **Address:** Univ Washington Med Ctr, 4225 Roosevelt Way NE, Ste 306, Seattle, WA 98105-6099; **Phone:** 206-598-7792; **Board Cert:** Psychiatry 1985; **Med School:** Stanford Univ 1969; **Resid:** Psychiatry, Univ Washington Med Ctr 1979; **Fellow:** Geriatric Psychiatry, Univ Washington Med Ctr 1981; **Fac Appt:** Prof Psyc, Univ Wash

Kramer, Barry A MD [GerPsy] - **Spec Exp:** Electroconvulsive Therapy (ECT); Depression; **Hospital:** Cedars-Sinai Med Ctr, Kaiser Permanente LA Med Ctr; **Address:** PO Box 5792, Beverly Hills, CA 90209; **Phone:** 310-423-4014; **Board Cert:** Psychiatry 1978; Geriatric Psychiatry 2001; **Med School:** Hahnemann Univ 1974; **Resid:** Psychiatry, Montefiore Hosp Med Ctr 1977; **Fellow:** Geriatric Psychiatry, UCLA-USC Long Term Gero Ctr 1986

Small, Gary W MD [GerPsy] - **Spec Exp:** Dementia; Alzheimer's Disease; Memory Disorders; **Hospital:** UCLA Ronald Reagan Med Ctr; **Address:** 760 Westwood Plaza, 38-251 Semel Inst, Los Angeles, CA 90095-1759; **Phone:** 310-825-0291; **Board Cert:** Psychiatry 1983; Geriatric Psychiatry 2001; **Med School:** USC Sch Med 1977; **Resid:** Psychiatry, Mass Genl Hosp 1981; **Fellow:** Psychiatry, UCLA Med Ctr 1983; **Fac Appt:** Prof Psyc, UCLA

Stein, Elliott M MD [GerPsy] - **Spec Exp:** Anxiety & Depression; Memory Disorders; Dementia; Stress Management; **Address:** Jewish Home of San Francisco, 302 Silver Ave, San Francisco, CA 94112; **Phone:** 415-406-1516; **Board Cert:** Psychiatry 1979; Geriatric Psychiatry 2001; **Med School:** Univ Miami Sch Med 1973; **Resid:** Psychiatry, Herrick Meml Hosp 1976; **Fac Appt:** Assoc Clin Prof Psyc, Univ Miami Sch Med

Veith, Richard C MD [GerPsy] - **Spec Exp:** Depression in Cardiovascular Disease; **Hospital:** Univ Wash Med Ctr; **Address:** Univ Washington Med Ctr, BB 1644, Box 356560, 1959 NE Pacific St, Seattle, WA 98195; **Phone:** 206-543-3752; **Board Cert:** Psychiatry 1979; Geriatric Psychiatry 2000; **Med School:** Univ Wash 1973; **Resid:** Psychiatry, Univ Wash Med Ctr 1977; **Fac Appt:** Prof Psyc, Univ Wash

Cleveland Clinic

Every life deserves world class care.

Psychiatry and Psychology

Cleveland Clinic Center for Behavioral Health offers the full range of mental health and behavioral services for children, adolescents and adults. Our staff, who offer expert clinical evaluation and treatment, includes psychiatrists, psychologists, clinical nurse specialists, social workers, counselors and therapists. In addition to evaluating and treating patients, our proven staff educates trainees, professionals and the public on the latest developments in psychiatry and the behavioral sciences.

The Center for Behavioral Health includes:

- Adult psychiatry
- Child and adolescent psychiatry
- Chemical dependency
- General psychology
- Habit management
- Neuropsychology
- Psychosomatic medicine
- Psychiatric occupational therapy

The center is part of Cleveland Clinic Neurological Institute, a fully integrated entity with a disease-specific focus, combining medical, surgical and research specialists who treat children and adults with neurological and neurobehavioral disorders. Our staff of more than 300 specialists works with one of the largest and most diverse patient populations in the country. Our clinical expertise, academic achievement and innovative research has earned Cleveland Clinic Neurological Institute an international reputation for excellence and advanced patient care.

Our staff also serves as consultants for patients admitted to Cleveland Clinic medical and surgical units, and as key team members in the treatment of many conditions including epilepsy, movement disorders, organ transplantation, morbid obesity, chronic pain, headaches and cancer.

Cleveland Clinic
Center for Behavioral Health
9500 Euclid Avenue
Cleveland, OH 44195

clevelandclinic.org/
psychtopdocs

Offering Same-Day Appointments
Call 800.274.2009.

Treatment Guides

Cleveland Clinic has developed comprehensive treatment guides for many diseases and conditions. To download our free treatment guides, visit clevelandclinic.org/treatmentguides.

Online Medical Second Opinion

Cleveland Clinic's My**Consult** Online Medical Second Opinion program securely connects patients to our physician specialists for more than 1,000 life-changing or life-threatening diagnoses all by the click of a mouse. To learn more, log onto eclevelandclinic.org/myconsult or call 800.223.2273, ext. 43223.

Special Assistance for Out-of-State Patients

Cleveland Clinic Global Patient Services offers a complimentary Medical Concierge service for patients who travel from outside of Ohio. Call 800.223.2273, ext. 55580 or email medicalconcierge@ccf.org.

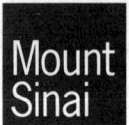 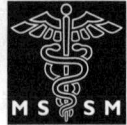

MOUNT SINAI
SCHOOL OF
MEDICINE

THE MOUNT SINAI MEDICAL CENTER
PSYCHIATRY

One Gustave L. Levy Place
Fifth Avenue and 100th Street
New York, NY 10029-6574
Physician Referral: 1-800-MD-SINAI (637-4624)
www.mountsinai.org/psychiatry

THE DEPARTMENT OF PSYCHIATRY at Mount Sinai strives to bring tomorrow's breakthrough treatments from clinical neuroscience research to clinical care today. We provide services for infants, children, adolescents, adults, and seniors, offering mental health evaluation and treatment for autism, attention-deficit hyperactivity disorder (ADHD), behavioral disorders, schizophrenia, Alzheimer's disease, mood and anxiety disorders, obsessive-compulsive disorder (OCD), substance abuse, post-traumatic stress disorder (PTSD), eating disorders, and personality disorders.

Clinical Services – The Department of Psychiatry is organized around key Centers of Excellence that link academic thought leaders to clinicians throughout the department. We offer a full range of diagnostic and treatment services, including psychotherapy, psychopharmacology, emergency services, electroconvulsive therapy, neuropsychological testing, and management of difficult clinical cases. We also provide mental health services in the Mount Sinai's World Trade Center Medical Monitoring and Treatment Program.

Specialty Programs – The Seaver Autism Center of Excellence offers a comprehensive assessment and treatment program that provides the finest patient care informed by the latest research. Our expert clinical staff is experienced in autism spectrum disorders, specializing in personalized and evidence-based treatment for very young children and high-functioning adults, as well as those individuals considered most difficult to assess and treat. The Attention-Deficit Hyperactivity Disorder (ADHD) Center serves children and adults providing state-of-the-art psychiatric evaluation, psychological testing, behavioral and cognitive-behavioral treatments, and medication management. Our Center for Eating and Weight Disorders serves adults and children, offering innovative, and evidence based treatment for anorexia nervosa, bulimia nervosa, binge eating disorder, and obesity.

The Mood and Anxiety Disorders Program (MAP) is devoted to understanding the causes of mood and anxiety disorders and aims to advance the latest integrative treatment strategies for patients who suffer from major depression, bipolar disorder, PTSD, panic attacks, generalized anxiety disorder, and social phobia. MAP at Mount Sinai uses state-of-the-art brain imaging, and genetic, and clinical trials methods to enhance our understanding of brain processes associated with these disorders.

TRANSLATING KNOWLEDGE INTO NEW SOLUTIONS
Mount Sinai is at the forefront of unlocking the interactions between biological processes and the myriad states of the human mind. Among our major research programs in psychiatry are the Alzheimer's Disease Research Center, which conducts both basic science and clinical research, and The Seaver Autism Center for Research and Treatment, which is dedicated to unraveling the biological causes of this disorder and to developing innovative treatment strategies. In shedding important new light on mental illness, psychiatrists at Mount Sinai are frequently able to offer the treatments of tomorrow—therapies that will not be widely available for years.

The Obsessive Compulsive Disorders (OCD) Center of Excellence provides state-of-the-art diagnostic evaluation and specializes in treating severe or treatment-resistant OCD. The Center offers comprehensive evaluations, expert consultations, novel and evidence-based treatments, and research studies. We offer outpatient services for children, adolescents, and adults. We specialize in biological interventions for patients who have not responded to conventional therapies.

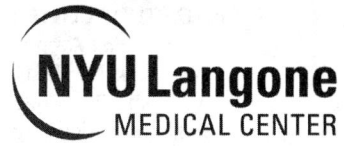

550 First Avenue *(at 31st Street)*
New York, NY 10016

www.NYULMC.org

Physician Referral: **888-7-NYU-MED** *(888-769-8633)*

BEHAVIORAL HEALTH

About the Behavioral Health Program

The Behavioral Health Program at NYU Langone Medical Center offers the most up-to-date treatments available for a wide range of disorders, including stress/anxiety, schizophrenia, depression (including medicine resistant depression), shyness, insomnia, low self-esteem, women's issues, sexual difficulties, panic attacks and phobias, manic-depression, obsession and compulsions and attention-deficit/hyperactivity disorder. The program serves its patients through a variety of approaches, including career counseling, assertiveness training, marital/couples counseling, and individual, group or family therapy. We specialize in the following areas:

Inpatient Services

An inpatient unit serves an adult population and includes a special Young Adult Program. The service combines comprehensive diagnostic assessment and treatment, including psychopharmacology, neuropsychology, psychotherapies and electroconvulsive therapy (a treatment in which seizures are electronically induced in anesthetized patients for therapeutic effect). A multidisciplinary team approach provides a continuum of behavioral and therapeutic modalities.

Outpatient Psychiatry

The Outpatient Psychiatry Program at Tisch Hospital provides expert treatment to individuals suffering from a broad range of mental disorders and emotional problems, including anxiety, depression (including medicine resistant depression), insomnia, manic-depression, reproductive psychiatry, attention-deficit hyperactivity disorder and schizophrenia. Our multidisciplinary team of licensed psychiatrists, psychologists and social workers offers the most up-to-date and scientifically validated treatments, such as psychotherapy, medication, or a combination of the two. Direct treatment with a member of faculty is also available as an option.

Scientific Innovation

At NYU Langone Medical Center, scientific innovation goes hand-in-hand with patient care. Our physician-scientists continue to lead the way in psychopharmacology and test new treatments for depression and bipolar disorder, with potentially life-altering results for the millions who suffer from these debilitating illnesses.

Sleep Disorders

The Sleep Disorders Consultation and Treatment Service provides thorough evaluation for a full range of sleep problems, including insomnia, nightmares, narcolepsy, sleepwalking and restless leg syndrome. Both behavioral and medication treatments are available to treat sleep disorders.

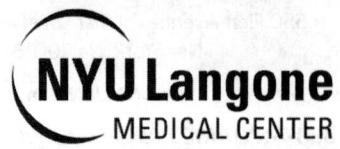
CHILD STUDY CENTER

The Child Study Center is the world's leading institution for transformative science and innovation in the diagnosis and treatment of children with mental illness and learning disabilities. Since 1997, The Child Study Center has treated thousands of children from around the world at its Faculty Group Practices in Manhattan and satellite clinical campuses in New Jersey and Long Island. Through its website, www.AboutOurKids.org, and through professional education programs, parents and practitioners are provided with the tools and knowledge needed to promote children's mental health. The Child Study Center, part of NYU Langone's Department of Child and Adolescent Psychiatry, provides the following services:

Anxiety and Mood Disorders
The Anita Saltz Institute for Anxiety and Mood Disorders offers the most advanced treatment and evaluation of children, adolescents and young adults. Our psychopharmacologists are experts in understanding the issues of treating children with bipolar disorder and our researchers explore treatments for children with severe temper outbursts and adolescent depression.

Attention Deficit Hyperactivity and Behavior Disorders
The Institute for Attention Deficit Hyperactivity and Behavior Disorders focuses on the treatment of ADHD. Our Parent-Child Interaction Therapy Program (PCIT) offers state-of-the-art treatment for behavioral problems in young children and is the largest program of its kind in the Northeast.

Autism, Asperger's Syndrome and Communication Disorders
The Autism Spectrum programs at the Child Study Center provide extensive evaluations for toddlers and preschoolers with social and communication difficulties. Our Early Social Interaction treatment is a home-based intervention for children identified with symptoms of autism. Center specialists are also experienced at supporting the needs of teens and young adults who have been diagnosed with Asperger's.

Learning Disorders
The Institute for Learning and Academic Achievement evaluates children with suspected learning weaknesses or poor academic achievement using a multidisciplinary team-based approach.

Tics and Tourette Disorder
The Center's Tics and Tourette Clinical and Research programs are dedicated to the evaluation and treatment of individuals with tics, Tourette disorder and related problems. Treatment includes Habit Reversal Therapy (HRT).

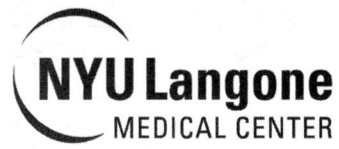

PSYCHIATRY

About the Department of Psychiatry

The Department of Psychiatry is dedicated to improving the health and well-being of patients by delivering peerless psychiatric services and care. The Department is home to some of the nation's most respected clinical psychiatrists and psychologists, with specialties in psychoanalysis, psychopharmacology, behavioral therapy, child psychiatry, geriatric psychiatry and neuropsychiatry. We specialize in the following areas:

Inpatient Services

The Inpatient Services Unit combines comprehensive diagnostic assessment and treatment, including psychopharmacology, neuropsychology, psychotherapies and electroconvulsive therapy.

Outpatient Psychiatry

The Outpatient Psychiatry Program provides expert treatment to individuals suffering from a broad range of mental disorders and emotional problems, including anxiety, depression (including medicine resistant depression), insomnia, manic-depression, reproductive psychiatry, attention-deficit hyperactivity disorder and schizophrenia. Multidisciplinary teams of licensed psychiatrists, psychologists and social workers offer the most up-to-date, scientifically validated treatments, such as psychotherapy, medication, or a combination of both.

Post-Traumatic Stress Disorder

The Department of Psychiatry offers assessment and treatment of PTSD for victims of sexual and physical assault, natural disasters, terrorism and combat trauma. Treatment includes end-based cognitive behavioral therapy and evaluation of strategies for the prevention of insomnia, stress, anxiety and depression.

Memory Impairment

The Pearl Barlow Center for Memory Evaluation and Treatment specializes in treating patients with memory impairments caused by neurological, psychological and physical ailments, as well as memory issues resulting from medication side effects, anxiety, depression and the effects of normal aging from illnesses like Alzheimer's disease. The Center's multidisciplinary medical approach, integrated with advanced research, represents a first-of-its-kind in New York City for the treatment of memory disorders.

Human Sexuality

The Human Sexuality Treatment Program provides comprehensive evaluation of a full range of sexual dysfunction, including erectile disorder, premature ejaculation, male orgasmic disorder, female orgasmic and arousal disorders, vaginismus, dyspareunia, lack of desire, and unconsummated marriage and sexual incompatibility between partners.

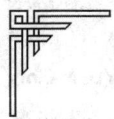

The Best in American Medicine
www.CastleConnolly.com

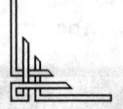
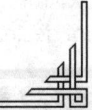

Pulmonary Disease

a subspecialty of Internal Medicine

An internist who treats diseases of the lungs and airways. The pulmonologist diagnoses and treats cancer, pneumonia, pleurisy, asthma, occupational diseases, bronchitis, sleep disorders, emphysema and other complex disorders of the lungs.

Training Required: Three years in internal medicine *plus* additional training and examination for certification in pulmonary disease.

PULMONARY DISEASE

New England

Berk, John L MD [Pul] - **Spec Exp:** Interstitial Lung Disease; Amyloidosis; Pulmonary Fibrosis; **Hospital:** Boston Med Ctr; **Address:** The Pulmonary Ctr, 72 E Concord St, Ste R-304, Boston, MA 02118-2371; **Phone:** 671-638-4860; **Board Cert:** Critical Care Medicine 2002; Internal Medicine 1986; Pulmonary Disease 2000; **Med School:** Case West Res Univ 1983; **Resid:** Internal Medicine, Univ Hosp/VAMC 1986; **Fellow:** Pulmonary Critical Care Medicine, Boston Univ Med Ctr 1991; **Fac Appt:** Assoc Prof Med, Boston Univ

Celli, Bartolome MD [Pul] - **Spec Exp:** Chronic Obstructive Lung Disease (COPD); Mechanical Ventilation; Respiratory Failure; **Hospital:** Brigham and Women's Hosp (page 57); **Address:** Brigham & Women's Hosp, Pulmonary Div, 75 Francis St, PBB Clin 3, Boston, MA 02115; **Phone:** 617-132-6770; **Board Cert:** Internal Medicine 1975; Pulmonary Disease 1978; **Med School:** Venezuela 1971; **Resid:** Internal Medicine, St Vincent Hosp 1973; Internal Medicine, Boston City Hosp 1976; **Fellow:** Pulmonary Disease, Boston Univ Med Ctr 1977; **Fac Appt:** Prof Med, Tufts Univ

Christiani, David MD [Pul] - **Spec Exp:** Occupational Lung Disease; **Hospital:** Mass Genl Hosp; **Address:** Mass Genl Hosp, Pulmonary Assocs, 55 Fruit St Cox 201B, Boston, MA 02114; **Phone:** 617-726-1721; **Board Cert:** Internal Medicine 1979; Occupational Medicine 1984; Pulmonary Disease 1988; **Med School:** Tufts Univ 1976; **Resid:** Internal Medicine, Boston City Hosp 1979; Occupational Medicine, Harvard Sch Public Hlth 1981; **Fellow:** Pulmonary Disease, Mass Genl Hosp 1987; **Fac Appt:** Prof Med, Harvard Med Sch

Enelow, Richard Ian MD [Pul] - **Spec Exp:** Interstitial Lung Disease; Lung Disease; **Hospital:** Dartmouth - Hitchcock Med Ctr; **Address:** Section Chief, Pulmonary & Critical Care, Dartmouth-Hitchcock Medical Ctr, 1 Med Ctr Drive, Lebanon, NH 03756; **Phone:** 603-650-5533; **Board Cert:** Internal Medicine 1986; Pulmonary Disease 2002; **Med School:** Boston Univ 1983; **Resid:** Internal Medicine, New England Deaconess Med Ctr 1986; **Fellow:** Pulmonary Disease, Univ VA Hlth Scis Ctr 1992; **Fac Appt:** Prof Med, Dartmouth Med Sch

Ernst, Armin MD [Pul] - **Spec Exp:** Interventional Pulmonology; Tracheal Stenosis; Airway Disorders; Lung Cancer; **Hospital:** Caritas St Elizabeth's Med Ctr-Boston; **Address:** 736 Cambridge St, Seton 6 East, Brighton, MA 02135; **Phone:** 617-789-2936; **Board Cert:** Internal Medicine 2003; Pulmonary Disease 2006; Critical Care Medicine 2007; **Med School:** Germany 1988; **Resid:** Internal Medicine, Thoraxklinik-Univ Heidelberg; Internal Medicine, Univ Tex Hlth Sci Ctr 1993; **Fellow:** Pulmonary Critical Care Medicine, Deaconess Med Ctr/Brigham & Women's 1996; Interventional Pulmonology, Thoraxklinik-Univ Heidelberg; **Fac Appt:** Assoc Prof Med, Harvard Med Sch

Fanta, Christopher MD [Pul] - **Spec Exp:** Asthma; Chronic Obstructive Lung Disease (COPD); Bronchiectasis; **Hospital:** Brigham and Women's Hosp (page 57), Faulkner Hosp; **Address:** 75 Francis St, Boston, MA 02115; **Phone:** 617-732-6770; **Board Cert:** Internal Medicine 1978; Pulmonary Disease 1980; **Med School:** Harvard Med Sch 1975; **Resid:** Internal Medicine, Peter Bent Brigham Hosp 1978; **Fellow:** Pulmonary Disease, Peter Bent Brigham Hosp 1980; **Fac Appt:** Assoc Prof Med, Harvard Med Sch

Friedman, Lloyd Neal MD [Pul] - **Spec Exp:** Tuberculosis; **Hospital:** Milford Hosp, Yale-New Haven Hosp; **Address:** Milford Hospital, 300 Seaside Ave, Milford, CT 06460; **Phone:** 203-876-4288; **Board Cert:** Internal Medicine 1983; Pulmonary Disease 1988; Critical Care Medicine 2009; **Med School:** Yale Univ 1979; **Resid:** Internal Medicine, Beth Israel Med Ctr 1980; Internal Medicine, Oregon Hlth Scis Univ 1983; **Fellow:** Pulmonary Intensive Care, Yale-New Haven Hosp 1988; **Fac Appt:** Clin Prof Med, Yale Univ

Hill, Nicholas S MD [Pul] - **Spec Exp:** Pulmonary Hypertension; **Hospital:** Tufts Med Ctr; **Address:** Tufts Med Ctr, 800 Washington St, Ste 257, Boston, MA 02111; **Phone:** 617-636-4288; **Board Cert:** Internal Medicine 1978; Pulmonary Disease 1982; Critical Care Medicine 2009; **Med School:** Dartmouth Med Sch 1975; **Resid:** Internal Medicine, New England Med Ctr 1977; Cardiovascular Disease, Boston VA Med Ctr 1978; **Fellow:** Pulmonary Disease, Univ Mass Med Ctr 1979; Critical Care Medicine, Boston Univ Med Ctr 1982; **Fac Appt:** Prof Med, Tufts Univ

Irwin, Richard S MD [Pul] - **Spec Exp:** Cough; Asthma; Chronic Obstructive Lung Disease (COPD); Critical Care; **Hospital:** UMass Meml Med Ctr - Univ Campus; **Address:** 55 Lake Ave N, Worcester, MA 01655-0002; **Phone:** 508-856-1919; **Board Cert:** Internal Medicine 1972; Pulmonary Disease 1974; Critical Care Medicine 2007; **Med School:** Tufts Univ 1968; **Resid:** Internal Medicine, Tufts-New England Med Ctr 1970; **Fellow:** Pulmonary Disease, Columbia-Presby Hosp 1972; **Fac Appt:** Prof Med, Univ Mass Sch Med

Mahler, Donald A MD [Pul] - **Spec Exp:** Chronic Obstructive Lung Disease (COPD); Asthma; Breathing Disorders; **Hospital:** Dartmouth - Hitchcock Med Ctr; **Address:** Dartmouth-Hitchcock Med Ctr, Div Pulmonary Med, 1 Med Ctr Drive, Lebanon, NH 03756-0001; **Phone:** 603-650-5533; **Board Cert:** Internal Medicine 1978; Pulmonary Disease 1980; **Med School:** Loyola Univ-Stritch Sch Med 1972; **Resid:** Internal Medicine, Dartmouth-Hitchcock Med Ctr 1977; **Fellow:** Pulmonary Disease, Yale-New Haven Hosp 1980; **Fac Appt:** Prof Med, Dartmouth Med Sch

Metersky, Mark L MD [Pul] - **Spec Exp:** Pulmonary Infections; Asthma; Bronchiectasis; **Hospital:** Univ of Conn Hlth Ctr, John Dempsey Hosp; **Address:** Univ Conn Hlth Ctr, 263 Farmington Ave, Farmington, CT 06030-2204; **Phone:** 860-679-8300; **Board Cert:** Internal Medicine 1988; Pulmonary Disease 2003; Critical Care Medicine 2003; Sleep Medicine 2009; **Med School:** NYU Sch Med 1985; **Resid:** Internal Medicine, Boston City Hosp 1988; **Fellow:** Pulmonary Critical Care Medicine, UCSD Med Ctr 1992; **Fac Appt:** Prof Med, Univ Conn

Millman, Richard P MD [Pul] - **Spec Exp:** Sleep Disorders/Apnea; **Hospital:** Rhode Island Hosp, Miriam Hosp; **Address:** 1 James P Murphy Hwy, West Warwick, RI 02893; **Phone:** 401-615-5878; **Board Cert:** Internal Medicine 1979; Pulmonary Disease 1982; Critical Care Medicine 1999; Sleep Medicine 2009; **Med School:** Univ Pennsylvania 1976; **Resid:** Internal Medicine, Univ Mich Hosp 1979; **Fellow:** Pulmonary Disease, Univ Penn 1981; **Fac Appt:** Prof Med, Brown Univ

Nardell, Edward MD [Pul] - **Spec Exp:** Tuberculosis; Mycobacterial Infections; **Hospital:** Brigham and Women's Hosp (page 57); **Address:** Brigham & Women's Hosp, 15 Francis St, Boston, MA 02115; **Phone:** 617-732-6770; **Board Cert:** Internal Medicine 1975; Pulmonary Disease 1982; **Med School:** Hahnemann Univ 1972; **Resid:** Internal Medicine, Hahnemann Univ Hosp 1975; **Fellow:** Pulmonary Disease, Mass Genl Hosp 1977; **Fac Appt:** Assoc Prof Med, Harvard Med Sch

Parsons, Polly E MD [Pul] - **Spec Exp:** Critical Care; Lung Injury-Acute; **Hospital:** Fletcher Allen Health Care- Med Ctr Campus; **Address:** Fletcher Allen Health Care, 111 Colchester Ave, Fletcher 311, Burlington, VT 05401; **Phone:** 802-847-6177; **Board Cert:** Internal Medicine 1981; Pulmonary Disease 1986; Critical Care Medicine 2005; **Med School:** Univ Ariz Coll Med 1978; **Resid:** Internal Medicine, Univ Colorado Hosp 1981; **Fellow:** Pulmonary Disease, Univ Colorado Hosp 1985; **Fac Appt:** Prof Med, Univ VT Coll Med

Redlich, Carrie MD [Pul] - **Spec Exp:** Occupational Lung Disease; **Hospital:** Yale-New Haven Hosp, Yale Med Group; **Address:** Yale Occupational & Environmental Med, 135 College St Fl 3 - Ste 392, New Haven, CT 06510; **Phone:** 203-785-4197; **Board Cert:** Internal Medicine 1986; Occupational Medicine 1990; Pulmonary Disease 2002; **Med School:** Yale Univ 1982; **Resid:** Internal Medicine, Yale-New Haven Hosp 1986; Occupational Medicine, Yale-New Haven Hosp 1987; **Fellow:** Pulmonary Disease, Univ Washington 1989; **Fac Appt:** Assoc Prof Med, Yale Univ

Pulmonary Disease

Rochester, Carolyn L MD [Pul] - **Spec Exp:** Chronic Obstructive Lung Disease (COPD); **Hospital:** VA Conn Hlthcre Sys-W Haven Campus, Yale-New Haven Hosp; **Address:** Yale Univ Sch Med, Pulm & Crit Care Sect, 300 Cedar St, Box 208057, New Haven, CT 06520-8057; **Phone:** 203-785-3207; **Board Cert:** Internal Medicine 1986; Pulmonary Disease 2002; Critical Care Medicine 2006; **Med School:** Columbia P&S 1983; **Resid:** Internal Medicine, Columbia Presby Med Ctr 1986; **Fellow:** Pulmonary Disease, Columbia Presby Med Ctr 1988; **Fac Appt:** Asst Prof Med, Yale Univ

Villanueva, Andrew G MD [Pul] - **Spec Exp:** Asthma; Chronic Obstructive Lung Disease (COPD); Interstitial Lung Disease; **Hospital:** Lahey Clin; **Address:** Lahey Clinic, 41 Mall Rd, Burlington, MA 01805; **Phone:** 781-744-8480; **Board Cert:** Internal Medicine 1983; Pulmonary Disease 1986; Critical Care Medicine 2007; **Med School:** UCSD 1980; **Resid:** Internal Medicine, Boston Univ Med Ctr 1984; **Fellow:** Pulmonary Disease, Boston Univ Med Ctr 1986; **Fac Appt:** Asst Clin Prof Med, Tufts Univ

White, David P MD [Pul] - **Spec Exp:** Sleep Disorders/Apnea; **Hospital:** Brigham and Women's Hosp (page 57); **Address:** Brigham & Women's Hosp, Division of Sleep Med, 75 Francis St, Boston, MA 02115; **Phone:** 617-732-5778; **Board Cert:** Internal Medicine 1978; Pulmonary Disease 1982; Sleep Medicine 2007; **Med School:** Emory Univ 1975; **Resid:** Internal Medicine, Univ Colo Med Ctr 1978; **Fellow:** Pulmonary Disease, Univ Colo Med Ctr 1982; **Fac Appt:** Prof Med, Harvard Med Sch

Mid Atlantic

Ahya, Vivek N MD [Pul] - **Spec Exp:** Transplant Medicine-Lung; Lymphangioleiomyomatosis (LAM); **Hospital:** Hosp Univ Penn - UPHS (page 68); **Address:** 832 W Gates Bldg, 3400 Spruce St, St, Philadelphia, PA 19104; **Phone:** 215-662-4202; **Board Cert:** Pulmonary Disease 2000; Critical Care Medicine 2001; **Med School:** Boston Univ 1994; **Resid:** Internal Medicine, Barnes Jewish Hosp 1997; **Fellow:** Pulmonary Critical Care Medicine, Hosp U Penn 1998 **Fac Appt:** Assoc Prof Med, Univ Pennsylvania

Arcasoy, Selim M MD [Pul] - **Spec Exp:** Transplant Medicine-Lung; Chronic Obstructive Lung Disease (COPD); Interstitial Lung Disease; Pulmonary Embolism; **Hospital:** NY-Presby/Columbia Univ Med Ctr, NY (page 65); **Address:** Ctr for Advanced Lung Dis/Transp, 622 W 168th St PH Bldg Fl 14E - rm 104, New York, NY 10032-3720; **Phone:** 212-305-6589; **Board Cert:** Internal Medicine 2003; Pulmonary Disease 2006; Critical Care Medicine 2007; **Med School:** Turkey 1990; **Resid:** Internal Medicine, SUNY Downstate Med Ctr 1994; **Fellow:** Pulmonary Critical Care Medicine, Univ Pittsburgh Med Ctr 1998; **Fac Appt:** Prof Med, Columbia P&S

Bascom, Rebecca MD [Pul] - **Spec Exp:** Environmental Medicine; Chemical Exposure; Occupational Medicine; Pulmonary Fibrosis; **Hospital:** Penn State Milton S Hershey Med Ctr; **Address:** Hershey Med Ctr, Dept Pulmonary Disease, 500 University Drive, MC HO41, Hershey, PA 17033-0850; **Phone:** 717-531-6525; **Board Cert:** Internal Medicine 1982; Occupational Medicine 1987; Pulmonary Disease 1988; **Med School:** Oregon Hlth & Sci Univ 1979; **Resid:** Internal Medicine, Johns Hopkins Hosp 1982; **Fellow:** Pulmonary Disease, Johns Hopkins 1986; Occupational Medicine, Johns Hopkins 1985; **Fac Appt:** Prof Med

Burschtin, Omar E MD [Pul] - **Spec Exp:** Sleep Disorders/Apnea; Airway Disorders; Asthma; **Hospital:** NYU Langone Med Ctr (page 66); **Address:** Sleep Medicine Assocs NYC, 11 E 26th St Fl 13, New York, NY 10010; **Phone:** 212-481-1818; **Board Cert:** Pulmonary Disease 2008; Sleep Medicine 2009; **Med School:** Uruguay 1988; **Resid:** Internal Medicine, NYU Downtown Hosp 1994; **Fellow:** Pulmonary Critical Care Medicine, NYU 1998; **Fac Appt:** Asst Prof Med, NYU Sch Med

Christie, Jason D MD [Pul] - **Spec Exp:** Transplant Medicine-Lung; **Hospital:** Penn Presby Med Ctr - UPHS (page 68); **Address:** Penn Lung Ctr, Pearlman Ctr, West Pavilion Fl 1, 3400 Civic Ctr Blvd, Philadelphia, PA 19104; **Phone:** 215-573-3209; **Board Cert:** Internal Medicine 2006; Pulmonary Disease 2009; Critical Care Medicine 2010; **Med School:** Columbia P&S 1993; **Resid:** Internal Medicine, Hosp U Penn 1996; **Fellow:** Pulmonary Disease, Hosp U Penn 1998; **Fac Appt:** Assoc Prof Med, Univ Pennsylvania

Criner, Gerard J MD [Pul] - **Spec Exp:** Chronic Obstructive Lung Disease (COPD); Pulmonary Fibrosis; Pulmonary Hypertension; Critical Care; **Hospital:** Temple Univ Hosp; **Address:** Temple Univ Hosp, Pulmonary Med, 3401 N Broad St Fl 5, Philadelphia, PA 19140; **Phone:** 215-707-5555; **Board Cert:** Internal Medicine 1982; Pulmonary Disease 1986; Critical Care Medicine 2007; **Med School:** Temple Univ 1979; **Resid:** Internal Medicine, Temple Univ Hosp 1983; **Fellow:** Pulmonary Disease, Boston Univ 1986; **Fac Appt:** Prof Med, Temple Univ

Deitz, Joel L MD [Pul] - **Spec Exp:** Respiratory Failure; Chronic Obstructive Lung Disease (COPD); Cough; **Hospital:** Penn Presby Med Ctr - UPHS (page 68), Hosp Univ Penn - UPHS (page 68); **Address:** Penn-Presby Med Ctr, Pulmonology, 51 N 39th St, Philadelphia Heart Inst Fl 1 Rear, Philadelphia, PA 19104; **Phone:** 215-662-8585; **Board Cert:** Internal Medicine 1980; Pulmonary Disease 1984; Critical Care Medicine 2007; **Med School:** Tufts Univ 1977; **Resid:** Internal Medicine, Med Coll Va Med Ctr 1980; **Fellow:** Pulmonary Disease, Duke Univ Med Ctr 1984; **Fac Appt:** Assoc Clin Prof Med, Univ Pennsylvania

Donahoe, Michael MD [Pul] - **Spec Exp:** Critical Care; Respiratory Distress Syndrome (ARDS); Chronic Obstructive Lung Disease (COPD); **Hospital:** UPMC Montefiore; **Address:** UPMC Montefiore Hosp, NW628, 3459 Fifth Ave, Pittsburgh, PA 15213; **Phone:** 412-648-6161; **Board Cert:** Internal Medicine 1986; Pulmonary Disease 1988; Critical Care Medicine 2000; **Med School:** Hahnemann Univ 1983; **Resid:** Internal Medicine, UPMC Presbyterian 1086; **Fellow:** Pulmonary Critical Care Medicine, UPMC Presbyterian 1989; **Fac Appt:** Assoc Prof Med, Univ Pittsburgh

Greenberg, Harly MD [Pul] - **Spec Exp:** Sleep Disorders/Apnea; Lung Disease; Critical Care; **Hospital:** Long Island Jewish Med Ctr, N Shore Univ Hosp; **Address:** North Shore LIJ Sleep Disorders Ctr, 410 Lakeville Rd, Ste 107, New Hyde Park, NY 11040; **Phone:** 516-465-3899; **Board Cert:** Internal Medicine 1985; Pulmonary Disease 1988; **Med School:** NYU Sch Med 1982; **Resid:** Internal Medicine, North Shore Univ Hosp 1985; **Fellow:** Pulmonary Disease, NYU-Bellevue Hosp Ctr 1987; **Fac Appt:** Assoc Prof Med, Albert Einstein Coll Med

Hansen-Flaschen, John MD [Pul] - **Spec Exp:** Diagnostic Problems; Interstitial Lung Disease; Chronic Obstructive Lung Disease (COPD); **Hospital:** Hosp Univ Penn - UPHS (page 68); **Address:** Perelman Center for Advanced Medicine, 34th & Civic Center Blvd, Philadelphia, PA 19104; **Phone:** 215-662-6003; **Board Cert:** Internal Medicine 1979; Pulmonary Disease 1982; **Med School:** NYU Sch Med 1976; **Resid:** Internal Medicine, Hosp Univ Penn 1981; **Fellow:** Pulmonary Disease, Hosp Univ Penn 1981; Critical Care Medicine, Hosp Univ Penn 1982; **Fac Appt:** Prof Med, Univ Pennsylvania

Kamelhar, David L MD [Pul] - **Spec Exp:** Chronic Obstructive Lung Disease (COPD); Bronchiectasis; Mycobacterial Infections; **Hospital:** NYU Langone Med Ctr (page 66); **Address:** 404 Park Ave S, Ste 701, New York, NY 10016; **Phone:** 212-685-6611; **Board Cert:** Internal Medicine 1977; Pulmonary Disease 1980; **Med School:** NYU Sch Med 1974; **Resid:** Internal Medicine, VA Hosp 1978; **Fellow:** Pulmonary Disease, Bellevue/NYU Med Ctr 1980; **Fac Appt:** Assoc Prof Med, NYU Sch Med

Pulmonary Disease

King, Earl D MD [Pul] - **Spec Exp:** Lung Cancer; Critical Care; **Hospital:** Fox Chase Cancer Ctr (page 58); **Address:** Fox Chase Cancer Center, 333 Cottman Ave, Philadelphia, PA 19111; **Phone:** 215-728-5703; **Board Cert:** Internal Medicine 1989; Pulmonary Disease 2002; Critical Care Medicine 2003; Sleep Medicine 1995; **Med School:** Penn State Coll Med 1986; **Resid:** Internal Medicine, Temple Univ Med Ctr 1989; **Fellow:** Pulmonary Critical Care Medicine, Johns Hopkins Hosp 1993; Sleep Medicine, Johns Hopkins Hosp 1993

Kotloff, Robert M MD [Pul] - **Spec Exp:** Transplant Medicine-Lung; Lung Disease-Complex; Interstitial Lung Disease; **Hospital:** Hosp Univ Penn - UPHS (page 68); **Address:** Perelman Center for Advanced Medicine, West Pavilion, Fl 1, 3400 Civic Center Blvd, Philadelphia, PA 19104; **Phone:** 215-662-3202; **Board Cert:** Internal Medicine 1986; Pulmonary Disease 2005; Critical Care Medicine 2005; **Med School:** Yale Univ 1983; **Resid:** Internal Medicine, Temple Univ Hosp 1986; **Fellow:** Pulmonary Disease, Hosp Univ Penn 1990; **Fac Appt:** Prof Med, Univ Pennsylvania

Libby, Daniel M MD [Pul] - **Spec Exp:** Asthma; Lung Cancer; Interstitial Lung Disease; Chronic Obstructive Lung Disease (COPD); **Hospital:** NY-Presby/Weill Cornell Med Ctr, NY (page 65); **Address:** 635 Madison Ave, Ste 1101, New York, NY 10022; **Phone:** 212-628-6611; **Board Cert:** Internal Medicine 1977; Pulmonary Disease 1980; **Med School:** Baylor Coll Med 1974; **Resid:** Internal Medicine, NY Hosp 1977; **Fellow:** Pulmonary Disease, NY Hosp 1979; **Fac Appt:** Clin Prof Med, Cornell Univ-Weill Med Coll

Maxfield, Roger MD [Pul] - **Spec Exp:** Emphysema & Asthma; Occupational Lung Disease; Lung Cancer; Bronchoscopy; **Hospital:** NY-Presby/Columbia Univ Med Ctr, NY (page 65); **Address:** Columbia Presbyterian Eastside, 16 E 60th St, Ste 320, New York, NY 10022-1002; **Phone:** 212-326-8415; **Board Cert:** Internal Medicine 1980; Pulmonary Disease 1986; **Med School:** Brown Univ 1977; **Resid:** Internal Medicine, Georgetown Univ Hosp 1980; **Fellow:** Pulmonary Disease, Bellevue-NYU Med Ctr 1985; **Fac Appt:** Clin Prof Med, Columbia P&S

Nash, Thomas MD [Pul] - **Spec Exp:** Asthma; Cough; Pneumonia; **Hospital:** NY-Presby/Weill Cornell Med Ctr, NY (page 65), Hosp For Special Surgery (page 60); **Address:** 310 E 72nd St, New York, NY 10021-4726; **Phone:** 212-734-6612; **Board Cert:** Internal Medicine 1981; Infectious Disease 1984; Pulmonary Disease 1988; **Med School:** NYU Sch Med 1978; **Resid:** Internal Medicine, New York Hosp-Cornell 1981; **Fellow:** Infectious Disease, New York Hosp-Cornell 1983; Pulmonary Disease, Meml Sloan Kettering Cancer Ctr 1985; **Fac Appt:** Assoc Clin Prof Med, NYU Sch Med

Nelson, Judith E MD [Pul] - **Spec Exp:** Palliative Care; Critical Care; **Hospital:** Mount Sinai Med Ctr (page 63); **Address:** Mt Sinai Medical Ctr, One Gustave Levy Pl, Box 1232, New York, NY 10029; **Phone:** 212-241-2587; **Board Cert:** Internal Medicine 1989; Pulmonary Disease 2002; Critical Care Medicine 2003; Hospice & Palliative Medicine 2005; **Med School:** NYU Sch Med 1986; **Resid:** Internal Medicine, Mt Sinai Med Ctr 1989; **Fellow:** Pulmonary Critical Care Medicine, Mt Sinai Med Ctr 1992; **Fac Appt:** Assoc Prof Med, Mount Sinai Sch Med

Niederman, Michael S MD [Pul] - **Spec Exp:** Infections-Respiratory; Emphysema; Respiratory Failure; Pneumonia; **Hospital:** Winthrop Univ Hosp; **Address:** 222 Station Plaza N, Ste 400, Mineola, NY 11501-3893; **Phone:** 516-663-2834; **Board Cert:** Internal Medicine 1980; Pulmonary Disease 1982; Critical Care Medicine 2007; **Med School:** Boston Univ 1977; **Resid:** Internal Medicine, Northwestern Univ Med Ctr 1980; **Fellow:** Pulmonary Disease, Yale-New Haven Hosp 1983; **Fac Appt:** Prof Med, SUNY Stony Brook

Pack, Allan MD/PhD [Pul] - **Spec Exp:** Sleep Disorders/Apnea; **Hospital:** Hosp Univ Penn - UPHS (page 68); **Address:** Penn Sleep Ctr, 3624 Market St, Ste 201, Philadelphia, PA 19104; **Phone:** 215-662-7772; **Med School:** Scotland, UK 1967; **Resid:** Internal Medicine, Univ Glasgow Med Ctr 1972; **Fellow:** Pulmonary Disease, Univ Glasgow Med Ctr 1975; **Fac Appt:** Prof Med, Univ Pennsylvania

Padilla, Maria L MD [Pul] - **Spec Exp:** Pulmonary Fibrosis; Transplant Medicine-Lung; Sarcoidosis; Pulmonary Hypertension; **Hospital:** Mount Sinai Med Ctr (page 63); **Address:** Mt Sinai Med Ctr, Div Pulmonology, One Gustave L Levy Pl, Box 1232, New York, NY 10029-6574; **Phone:** 212-241-5656; **Board Cert:** Internal Medicine 1978; Pulmonary Disease 1980; **Med School:** Mount Sinai Sch Med 1975; **Resid:** Internal Medicine, Mt Sinai Hosp 1978; **Fellow:** Pulmonary Disease, Mt Sinai Hosp 1980; Critical Care Medicine, Mt Sinai Hosp 1991; **Fac Appt:** Prof Med, Mount Sinai Sch Med

Palevsky, Harold I MD [Pul] - **Spec Exp:** Pulmonary Hypertension; Pulmonary Vascular Disease; Thromboembolic Disorders; Pulmonary Embolism; **Hospital:** Penn Presby Med Ctr - UPHS (page 68), Hosp Univ Penn - UPHS (page 68); **Address:** Penn Lung Center at Presbyterian, Philadelphia Heart Inst Bldg Fl 1 Rear, 51 N 39th St, Philadelphia, PA 19104; **Phone:** 215-662-8585; **Board Cert:** Internal Medicine 2007; Pulmonary Disease 2007; Critical Care Medicine 2007; **Med School:** Med Coll VA 1978; **Resid:** Internal Medicine, Hosp Univ Penn 1981; **Fellow:** Pulmonary Critical Care Medicine, Hosp Univ Penn 1984; **Fac Appt:** Prof Med, Univ Pennsylvania

Reilly Jr, John Joseph MD [Pul] - **Spec Exp:** Transplant Medicine-Lung; Emphysema; Chronic Obstructive Lung Disease (COPD); **Hospital:** UPMC Presby, Pittsburgh; **Address:** 1220 Scaife Hall, 3550 Terrace St, Pittsburgh, PA 15261; **Phone:** 412-648-9091; **Board Cert:** Internal Medicine 1984; Pulmonary Disease 1986; **Med School:** Harvard Med Sch 1981; **Resid:** Internal Medicine, Brigham & Women's Hosp 1984; **Fellow:** Pulmonary Disease, Brigham & Women's Hosp 1987; **Fac Appt:** Assoc Prof Med, Harvard Med Sch

Rossman, Milton D MD [Pul] - **Spec Exp:** Beryllium-induced Lung Disease; Sarcoidosis; Interstitial Lung Disease; **Hospital:** Hosp Univ Penn - UPHS (page 68); **Address:** Perelman Center for Advanced Medicine, West Pavilion, Fl 1, 3400 Civic Center Blvd, Philadelphia, PA 19104-4283; **Phone:** 215-662-3202; **Board Cert:** Internal Medicine 1975; Pulmonary Disease 1978; **Med School:** Jefferson Med Coll 1970; **Resid:** Internal Medicine, Univ Hosps 1975; **Fellow:** Pulmonary Disease, Hosp Univ Penn 1977; **Fac Appt:** Prof Med, Univ Pennsylvania

Schluger, Neil MD [Pul] - **Spec Exp:** Tuberculosis; **Hospital:** NY-Presby/Columbia Univ Med Ctr, NY (page 65); **Address:** Div Pulm, Allergy & Crit Care Med, 630 W 168th St, PH-8 East, Rm 101, New York, NY 10032; **Phone:** 212-305-1544; **Board Cert:** Internal Medicine 1988; Pulmonary Disease 2003; **Med School:** Univ Pennsylvania 1985; **Resid:** Internal Medicine, St Lukes Hosp 1989; **Fellow:** Pulmonary Critical Care Medicine, NY Hosp-Cornell 1992; **Fac Appt:** Prof Med, Columbia P&S

Schwab, Richard MD [Pul] - **Spec Exp:** Sleep Disorders/Apnea; **Hospital:** Hosp Univ Penn - UPHS (page 68); **Address:** Penn Sleep Ctr, 3624 Market St Fl 2 - Ste 201, Philadelphia, PA 19104; **Phone:** 215-662-7772; **Board Cert:** Internal Medicine 1986; Pulmonary Disease 2000; Critical Care Medicine 2000; Sleep Medicine 2009; **Med School:** Univ Pennsylvania 1983; **Resid:** Internal Medicine, Hosp Univ Penn 1986; **Fellow:** Pulmonary Critical Care Medicine, Hosp Univ Penn 1991; **Fac Appt:** Prof Med, Univ Pennsylvania

Steiger, David MD [Pul] - **Spec Exp:** Rheumatologic Diseases of the Lung; Thromboembolic Disorders; Pulmonary Hypertension; Critical Care; **Hospital:** NYU Hosp For Joint Diseases, NYU Langone Med Ctr (page 66); **Address:** 305 2nd Ave, Ste 16, New York, NY 10003; **Phone:** 212-598-6091; **Board Cert:** Internal Medicine 1987; Pulmonary Disease 2002; Critical Care Medicine 2005; **Med School:** England, UK 1981; **Resid:** Internal Medicine, St Thomas's Hosp 1984; Internal Medicine, St Lukes Hosp 1989; **Fellow:** Pulmonary Disease, UCSF Med Ctr 1994; **Fac Appt:** Asst Prof Med, NYU Sch Med

Pulmonary Disease

Steinberg, Harry MD [Pul] - **Spec Exp:** Asthma; Emphysema; Lung Cancer; **Hospital:** Long Island Jewish Med Ctr, N Shore Univ Hosp; **Address:** LI Jewish Med Ctr, Dept Med, 270-05 76th Ave, New Hyde Park, NY 11040-1433; **Phone:** 516-465-5400; **Med School:** Temple Univ 1966; **Resid:** Internal Medicine, LI Jewish Med Ctr 1969; Pulmonary Critical Care Medicine, LI Jewish Med Ctr 1970; **Fellow:** Pulmonary Disease, Hosp Univ Penn 1974; **Fac Appt:** Clin Prof Med, Albert Einstein Coll Med

Sterman, Daniel H MD [Pul] - **Spec Exp:** Interventional Pulmonology; Lung Cancer; Mesothelioma; Gene Therapy; **Hospital:** Hosp Univ Penn - UPHS (page 68); **Address:** Perelman Center for Advanced Medicine, West Pavilion, Fl 1, 3400 Civic Ctr Blvd, Philadelphia, PA 19104-4283; **Phone:** 215-662-3202; **Board Cert:** Internal Medicine 2007; Pulmonary Disease 2007; Critical Care Medicine 2007; **Med School:** Cornell Univ-Weill Med Coll 1989; **Resid:** Internal Medicine, Hosp Univ Penn 1992; **Fellow:** Pulmonary Critical Care Medicine, Hosp Univ Penn 1997; **Fac Appt:** Assoc Prof Med, Univ Pennsylvania

Stover-Pepe, Diane E MD [Pul] - **Spec Exp:** Interstitial Lung Disease; Pulmonary Infections; Pulmonary Disease/Immunocompromised; **Hospital:** Meml Sloan-Kettering Cancer Ctr; **Address:** 1275 York Avenue, New York, NY 10065; **Phone:** 212-639-8380; **Board Cert:** Internal Medicine 1975; Pulmonary Disease 1978; **Med School:** Albert Einstein Coll Med 1970; **Resid:** Internal Medicine, Harlem Hosp Ctr 1972; Internal Medicine, NY Hosp-Cornell Med Ctr 1975; **Fellow:** Pulmonary Disease, Montefiore Med Ctr 1977; **Fac Appt:** Prof Med, Cornell Univ-Weill Med Coll

Strollo, Patrick J MD [Pul] - **Spec Exp:** Sleep Disorders/Apnea; Respiratory Failure; **Hospital:** UPMC Montefiore, UPMC Presby, Pittsburgh; **Address:** Montefiore Univ Hosp, 3459 5th Ave, Ste S639.11, Pittsburgh, PA 15213; **Phone:** 412-692-2880; **Board Cert:** Internal Medicine 1984; Pulmonary Disease 1988; Sleep Medicine 2007; **Med School:** Uniformed Srvs Univ, Bethesda 1981; **Resid:** Internal Medicine, Wilford Hall Med Ctr 1984; **Fellow:** Pulmonary Disease, Wilford Hall Med Ctr 1987; **Fac Appt:** Assoc Prof Med, Univ Pittsburgh

Teirstein, Alvin S MD [Pul] - **Spec Exp:** Sarcoidosis; Interstitial Lung Disease; Occupational Lung Disease; Lung Cancer; **Hospital:** Mount Sinai Med Ctr (page 63), James J. Peters VA Med Ctr-Bronx; **Address:** Mount Sinai Med Ctr, 1 Gustave Levy Pl, Box 1232, New York, NY 10029; **Phone:** 212-241-5656; **Board Cert:** Internal Medicine 1961; Pulmonary Disease 1969; **Med School:** SUNY Downstate 1953; **Resid:** Internal Medicine, Mt Sinai Med Ctr 1957; **Fellow:** Pulmonary Disease, Mt Sinai Med Ctr 1954; Pulmonary Disease, VA Med Ctr 1956; **Fac Appt:** Prof Med, Mount Sinai Sch Med

Thomashow, Byron MD [Pul] - **Spec Exp:** Emphysema; Asthma; Respiratory Failure; Chronic Obstructive Lung Disease (COPD); **Hospital:** NY-Presby/Columbia Univ Med Ctr, NY (page 65); **Address:** 161 Fort Washington Ave, rm 311, New York, NY 10032; **Phone:** 212-305-5261; **Board Cert:** Internal Medicine 1977; Pulmonary Disease 1980; **Med School:** Columbia P&S 1974; **Resid:** Internal Medicine, Roosevelt Hosp 1977; Pulmonary Disease, Roosevelt Hosp 1978; **Fellow:** Pulmonary Disease, Harlem Hosp Ctr 1979; **Fac Appt:** Clin Prof Med, Columbia P&S

Tino, Gregory MD [Pul] - **Spec Exp:** Emphysema-Lung Volume Reduction; Interstitial Lung Disease; Bronchiectasis; Chronic Obstructive Lung Disease (COPD); **Hospital:** Hosp Univ Penn - UPHS (page 68); **Address:** Perelman Center for Advanced Medicine, West Pavilion, Fl 1, 3400 Civic Ctr Blvd, Philadelphia, PA 19104; **Phone:** 215-662-3202; **Board Cert:** Internal Medicine 1989; Pulmonary Disease 2009; Critical Care Medicine 2009; **Med School:** Mount Sinai Sch Med 1986; **Resid:** Internal Medicine, Hosp Univ Penn 1989; **Fellow:** Pulmonary Disease, Hosp Univ Penn 1992; **Fac Appt:** Assoc Prof Med, Univ Pennsylvania

Unger, Michael MD [Pul] - **Spec Exp:** Lung Cancer; Bronchoscopy; Cancer Prevention; Interventional Pulmonology; **Hospital:** Fox Chase Cancer Ctr (page 58); **Address:** Fox Chase Cancer Center, 333 Cottman Ave, Philadelphia, PA 19111; **Phone:** 215-728-6900; **Board Cert:** Internal Medicine 1977; Pulmonary Disease 1978; **Med School:** France 1971; **Resid:** Internal Medicine, Mt Sinai Hosp 1974; **Fellow:** Pulmonary Disease, NY Hosp-Cornell 1976; **Fac Appt:** Clin Prof Med, Thomas Jefferson Univ

Wenzel, Sally E MD [Pul] - **Spec Exp:** Asthma; Bronchiolitis Obliterans; Allergy; Inflammatory Pulmonary Diseases; **Hospital:** UPMC Montefiore; **Address:** UPMC Montefiore, 3601 Fifth Ave, Falk Medical Bldg Fl 4, Pittsburgh, PA 15213; **Phone:** 412-692-2139; **Board Cert:** Internal Medicine 1984; Pulmonary Disease 1986; **Med School:** Univ Fla Coll Med 1981; **Resid:** Internal Medicine, NC Baptist Hosp 1984; **Fellow:** Pulmonary Disease, Med Coll VA Hosp 1986; **Fac Appt:** Prof Med, Univ Colorado

Young Jr, K Randall MD [Pul] - **Spec Exp:** Transplant Medicine-Lung; Cystic Fibrosis; **Hospital:** Albert Einstein Med Ctr; **Address:** Albert Einstein Med Ctr, 5401 Old York Rd, Ste 363, Philadelphia, PA 19141; **Phone:** 215-456-6950; **Board Cert:** Internal Medicine 1982; Pulmonary Disease 2009; Allergy & Immunology 1987; **Med School:** Jefferson Med Coll 1978; **Resid:** Internal Medicine, Yale-New Haven Hosp 1982; Pulmonary Critical Care Medicine, Yale-New Haven Hosp 1985; **Fellow:** Allergy & Immunology, Nat Inst Hlth 1988

Southeast

Alberts, W Michael MD [Pul] - **Spec Exp:** Lung Cancer; **Hospital:** H Lee Moffitt Cancer Ctr & Research Inst (page 59); **Address:** H Lee Moffitt Cancer Ctr, Thoracic Onc, 12902 Magnolia Drive, MCC VP Suite, Tampa, FL 33612; **Phone:** 813-979-3067; **Board Cert:** Internal Medicine 1980; Pulmonary Disease 1982; **Med School:** Univ IL Coll Med 1977; **Resid:** Internal Medicine, Ohio State Univ Hosp 1980; **Fellow:** Pulmonary Critical Care Medicine, UCSD Med Ctr 1983; **Fac Appt:** Prof Med, Univ S Fla Coll Med

Brooks, Stuart M MD [Pul] - **Spec Exp:** Occupational Lung Disease; Asthma; Lung Injuries-Inhalation Induced; **Hospital:** Tampa Genl Hosp, H Lee Moffitt Cancer Ctr & Research Inst (page 59); **Address:** 4572 Bardsdale Drive, Palm Harbor, FL 34685; **Phone:** 813-389-6000; **Board Cert:** Internal Medicine 1977; Pulmonary Disease 1969; Occupational Medicine 1987; **Med School:** Univ Cincinnati 1962; **Resid:** Internal Medicine, Boston City Hosp 1967; **Fellow:** Pulmonary Disease, Boston City Hosp 1969; **Fac Appt:** Prof Med, Univ S Fla Coll Med

Campbell Jr, G Douglas MD [Pul] - **Spec Exp:** Infectious Disease-Lung; **Hospital:** Univ Mississippi Med Ctr, G.V. (Sonny) Montgomery VA Med Ctr - Jackson; **Address:** G.V. (Sonny) Montgomery VA Med Ctr, 1500 E Woodrow Wilson Drive, Jackson, MS 39216; **Phone:** 601-362-4471; **Board Cert:** Internal Medicine 1979; Pulmonary Disease 1986; **Med School:** Univ Miss 1976; **Resid:** Internal Medicine, Univ Miss Hosp 1979; **Fellow:** Pulmonary Disease, Univ Tex Hlth Sci Ctr 1983; Infectious Disease, Univ Calgary HSC 1985; **Fac Appt:** Prof Med, Univ Miss

Christman, Brian W MD [Pul] - **Spec Exp:** Chronic Obstructive Lung Disease (COPD); Sepsis; Critical Care; Respiratory Distress Syndrome (ARDS); **Hospital:** TN Valley Healthcare Sys-Nashville; **Address:** VA Tennessee Valley Hlth Care Sys, 1310 24th Ave So (111), Nashville, TN 37212; **Phone:** 615-327-4751 x5349; **Board Cert:** Internal Medicine 1984; Pulmonary Disease 1986; Critical Care Medicine 2010; **Med School:** Univ Okla Coll Med 1981; **Resid:** Internal Medicine, Vanderbilt Univ Med Ctr 1984; **Fellow:** Pulmonary Disease, Vanderbilt Univ Med Ctr 1987; **Fac Appt:** Prof Med, Vanderbilt Univ

Pulmonary Disease

Cooper, J Allen D MD [Pul] - **Spec Exp:** Drug Induced Lung Disease; Chronic Obstructive Lung Disease (COPD); **Hospital:** Univ of Ala Hosp at Birmingham, Birmingham, Alabama VA Med Ctr; **Address:** UAB Pulmonary Medicine, 1530 3rd Ave S, TNT 422, Birmingham, AL 35294; **Phone:** 205-934-5400; **Board Cert:** Internal Medicine 1981; Pulmonary Disease 1984; **Med School:** Duke Univ 1978; **Resid:** Internal Medicine, Univ Virginia Hosp 1981; **Fellow:** Pulmonary Disease, Yale Univ 1985; **Fac Appt:** Prof Med, Univ Alabama

Cooper, William R MD [Pul] - **Spec Exp:** Lung Cancer; Asthma; Chronic Obstructive Lung Disease (COPD); **Hospital:** Sentara VA Beach Genl Hosp; **Address:** 1008 First Colonial Rd, Virginia Beach, VA 23454-3071; **Phone:** 757-481-2515; **Board Cert:** Internal Medicine 1972; Pulmonary Disease 1974; Critical Care Medicine 2009; **Med School:** Univ VA Sch Med 1969; **Resid:** Internal Medicine, Cleveland Metro Genl Hosp 1971; Pulmonary Disease, Univ Va Hosp 1973; **Fellow:** Pulmonary Disease, Mt Sinai Med Ctr 1974

Doherty, Dennis E MD [Pul] - **Spec Exp:** Asthma; Chronic Obstructive Lung Disease (COPD); Interstitial Lung Disease; **Hospital:** Univ of Kentucky Albert B. Chandler Hosp, Lexington VA Med Ctr-Leestown Div; **Address:** Univ Kentucky Med Ctr, Div Pulm & Crit Care, 740 S Limestone, rm L-543, Lexington, KY 40536; **Phone:** 859-323-5045; **Board Cert:** Internal Medicine 1985; Pulmonary Disease 1988; **Med School:** Ohio State Univ 1980; **Resid:** Internal Medicine, Ohio State Univ Hosp 1983; **Fellow:** Pulmonary Disease, Univ Colorado Hlth Sci Ctr 1986; **Fac Appt:** Prof Med, Univ KY Coll Med

Donohue, James Francis MD [Pul] - **Spec Exp:** Asthma; Chronic Obstructive Lung Disease (COPD); Sarcoidosis; **Hospital:** NC Memorial Hosp - UNC; **Address:** Univ NC, Div Pulmonary Disease, 102 Mason Farm Rd, CB 7020, Chapel Hill, NC 27599-7020; **Phone:** 919-966-6838; **Board Cert:** Internal Medicine 1975; Pulmonary Disease 1976; **Med School:** UMDNJ-NJ Med Sch, Newark 1969; **Resid:** Internal Medicine, UMDNJ-Newark 1971; Internal Medicine, NC Meml Hosp 1974; **Fellow:** Pulmonary Disease, Univ North Carolina 1976; **Fac Appt:** Prof Med, Univ NC Sch Med

Fulkerson Jr, William J MD [Pul] - **Spec Exp:** Respiratory Failure; Lung Injury/ARDS; **Hospital:** Duke Univ Hosp; **Address:** Duke Univ Med Ctr, Box 3708, Durham, NC 27710; **Phone:** 919-684-1860; **Board Cert:** Internal Medicine 1981; Pulmonary Disease 1984; **Med School:** Univ NC Sch Med 1977; **Resid:** Internal Medicine, Vanderbilt Univ Hosp 1980; **Fellow:** Pulmonary Disease, Vanderbilt Univ Hosp 1983; **Fac Appt:** Prof Med, Duke Univ

Garver Jr, Robert MD [Pul] - **Spec Exp:** Lung Cancer; Lung Disease; **Hospital:** Mobile Infirmary Med Ctr; **Address:** 109 Med Park Drive, Ste C, Andalusia, AL 36420; **Phone:** 888-681-5864; **Board Cert:** Internal Medicine 1984; Pulmonary Disease 1986; **Med School:** Johns Hopkins Univ 1981; **Resid:** Internal Medicine, Johns Hopkins Hosp 1984; **Fellow:** Pulmonary Disease, NHLBI 1985; **Fac Appt:** Prof Med, Univ Alabama

Goldman, Allan L MD [Pul] - **Spec Exp:** Occupational Lung Disease; Airway Disorders; Lung Cancer; **Hospital:** Tampa Genl Hosp, James A Haley VA Hosp; **Address:** USF Coll Med, Dept Internal Medicine, 12901 Bruce B Downs Blvd, Box MDC19, Tampa, FL 33612-4742; **Phone:** 813-974-2271; **Board Cert:** Internal Medicine 1972; Pulmonary Disease 1972; **Med School:** Univ Minn 1968; **Resid:** Internal Medicine, Brooke Army Hosp 1970; **Fellow:** Pulmonary Disease, Walter Reed Army Hosp 1972; **Fac Appt:** Prof Med, Univ S Fla Coll Med

Harman, Eloise M MD [Pul] - **Spec Exp:** Critical Care; Diagnostic Problems; Mechanical Ventilation; **Hospital:** Shands at Univ of FL; **Address:** Shands at Univ of Florida, 1600 SW Archer Rd, Box 100225, Gainesville, FL 32610-0225; **Phone:** 352-273-8740; **Board Cert:** Internal Medicine 1973; Pulmonary Disease 1976; Critical Care Medicine 2007; **Med School:** Johns Hopkins Univ 1970; **Resid:** Internal Medicine, Johns Hopkins Hosp 1972; **Fellow:** Pulmonary Disease, NY Hosp-Cornell Med Ctr 1974; **Fac Appt:** Prof Med, Univ Fla Coll Med

Haynes Jr, Johnson MD [Pul] - **Spec Exp:** Sickle Cell Disease-Lung; Chronic Obstructive Lung Disease (COPD); **Hospital:** Univ of S AL Med Ctr; **Address:** USA Comprehensive Sickle Cell Ctr, 2451 Fillingim St, MCSB 1530, Mobile, AL 36617; **Phone:** 251-470-5893; **Board Cert:** Internal Medicine 1983; Pulmonary Disease 1986; **Med School:** Univ S Ala Coll Med 1980; **Resid:** Internal Medicine, Univ S Alabama Med Ctr 1983; **Fellow:** Pulmonary Disease, Univ S Alabama 1986; Univ Colorado 1988; **Fac Appt:** Prof Med, Univ S Ala Coll Med

Henke, David C MD [Pul] - **Spec Exp:** Asthma; Chronic Obstructive Lung Disease (COPD); Vasculitis; **Hospital:** NC Memorial Hosp - UNC; **Address:** Univ NC Med Sch, Div Pulm Dis & Crit Care Med, 130 Mason Farm Rd, Box 7020, Chapel Hill, NC 27599-7020; **Phone:** 919-966-7933; **Board Cert:** Internal Medicine 1980; Dermatology 1983; Pulmonary Disease 1988; **Med School:** Univ NC Sch Med 1977; **Resid:** Internal Medicine, NC Memorial Hosp 1980; Dermatology, NC Meml NIEHS 1984; **Fellow:** Pulmonary Disease, NC Memorial Hosp 1987; **Fac Appt:** Assoc Prof Med, Univ NC Sch Med

Johnson, Bruce Ellsworth MD [Pul] - **Spec Exp:** Sleep Disorders/Apnea; **Hospital:** Sentara VA Beach Genl Hosp; **Address:** 1008 First Colonial Rd, Virginia Beach, VA 23454-3002; **Phone:** 757-481-2515; **Board Cert:** Internal Medicine 1981; Pulmonary Disease 1986; Critical Care Medicine 2001; Sleep Medicine 2009; **Med School:** Med Coll GA 1978; **Resid:** Internal Medicine, Univ VA Med Ctr 1981; **Fellow:** Pulmonary Disease, Univ VA Med Ctr 1983

Light, Richard W MD [Pul] - **Spec Exp:** Pleural Disease; **Hospital:** Vanderbilt Univ Med Ctr (page 76); **Address:** Vanderbilt Univ Med Ctr-Pulmonary Medicine, 1161 21st Ave S, T1218 MCN, Nashville, TN 37232-2650; **Phone:** 615-322-3412; **Board Cert:** Internal Medicine 1972; Pulmonary Disease 1974; **Med School:** Johns Hopkins Univ 1968; **Resid:** Internal Medicine, Johns Hopkins Hosp 1970; **Fellow:** Pulmonary Disease, Johns Hopkins Hosp 1972; **Fac Appt:** Prof Med, Vanderbilt Univ

LoRusso, Thomas J MD [Pul] - **Spec Exp:** Critical Care; Sleep Disorders/Apnea; **Hospital:** Inova Fairfax Hosp; **Address:** 1800 Town Ctr Drive, Ste 419, Reston, VA 20190; **Phone:** 703-620-3926; **Board Cert:** Internal Medicine 2001; Pulmonary Disease 2002; Critical Care Medicine 2003; Sleep Medicine 2009; **Med School:** SUNY Upstate Med Univ 1987; **Resid:** Internal Medicine, Univ Hosp-SUNY 1990; **Fellow:** Pulmonary Disease, Cedars Sinai Med Ctr 1993

Loyd, James E MD [Pul] - **Spec Exp:** Pulmonary Fibrosis; Interstitial Lung Disease; Transplant Medicine-Lung; Pulmonary Hypertension; **Hospital:** Vanderbilt Univ Med Ctr (page 76); **Address:** Vanderbilt Univ Div Pulmonary Medicine, 1161 21st Ave S, T-1218 Medical Center N, Nashville, TN 37232-2650; **Phone:** 615-322-3412; **Board Cert:** Internal Medicine 1978; Pulmonary Disease 1984; **Med School:** W VA Univ 1973; **Resid:** Internal Medicine, Vanderbilt Univ Hosp 1976; **Fellow:** Pulmonary Disease, Vanderbilt Univ Hosp 1978; **Fac Appt:** Prof Med, Vanderbilt Univ

Sahn, Steven A MD [Pul] - **Spec Exp:** Pleural Disease; Interstitial Lung Disease; Chronic Obstructive Lung Disease (COPD); Pulmonary Fibrosis; **Hospital:** MUSC Med Ctr, R H Johnson VA Med Ctr - charleston; **Address:** MUSC, Div Pulm & Crit Care Med, 96 Jonathan Lucas St, Box 250630, Charleston, SC 29425-8900; **Phone:** 843-792-3167; **Board Cert:** Internal Medicine 1974; Pulmonary Disease 1974; **Med School:** Univ Louisville Sch Med 1968; **Resid:** Internal Medicine, Univ Iowa Hosp 1971; **Fellow:** Pulmonary Disease, Univ CO Hlth Sci Ctr 1973; **Fac Appt:** Prof Med, Med Univ SC

Staton Jr, Gerald W MD [Pul] - **Spec Exp:** Interstitial Lung Disease; Chronic Obstructive Lung Disease (COPD); Pulmonary Fibrosis; Sarcoidosis; **Hospital:** Emory Univ Hosp Midtown, Wesley Woods Ger Hosp; **Address:** 550 Peachtree St NE Fl 6, Atlanta, GA 30308; **Phone:** 404-686-2505; **Board Cert:** Internal Medicine 1979; Pulmonary Disease 1982; Critical Care Medicine 2007; **Med School:** Med Coll GA 1976; **Resid:** Internal Medicine, Stanford Univ Med Ctr 1979; **Fellow:** Pulmonary Disease, Mass Genl Hosp 1981; **Fac Appt:** Prof Med, Emory Univ

Pulmonary Disease

Tapson, Victor MD [Pul] - **Spec Exp:** Pulmonary Hypertension; Thromboembolic Disorders; Chronic Obstructive Lung Disease (COPD); Emphysema; **Hospital:** Duke Univ Hosp; **Address:** Duke Univ Med Ctr, Box 102351, Durham, NC 27710; **Phone:** 919-684-6237; **Board Cert:** Internal Medicine 1986; Pulmonary Disease 2000; **Med School:** Hahnemann Univ 1982; **Resid:** Internal Medicine, Duke Univ Med Ctr 1986; **Fellow:** Pulmonary Disease, Boston Univ 1989; **Fac Appt:** Prof Med, Duke Univ

Vaughey, Ellen MD [Pul] - **Spec Exp:** Critical Care; Sleep Disorders/Apnea; Asthma; **Hospital:** Inova Fairfax Hosp, Virginia Hosp Ctr - Arlington; **Address:** 3289 Woodburn Rd, Ste 350, Annandale, VA 22003; **Phone:** 703-641-8616; **Board Cert:** Internal Medicine 2001; Pulmonary Disease 2002; Critical Care Medicine 2003; **Med School:** Georgetown Univ 1987; **Resid:** Internal Medicine, Thomas Jefferson Univ Hosp 1990; **Fellow:** Pulmonary Disease, Roger Williams Hosp-Brown Univ 1993

Voelkel, Norbert F MD [Pul] - **Spec Exp:** Pulmonary Hypertension; Asthma; Emphysema; **Hospital:** Med Coll of VA Hosp; **Address:** Heart-Lung Transplant Dept, West Hosp, 1200 E Broad St, West 10 East, Richmond, VA 23298; **Phone:** 804-628-9614; **Med School:** Germany 1972; **Resid:** Internal Medicine, Univ Hamburg 1977; **Fellow:** Research, Univ Colorado 1978; Pulmonary Disease, Univ Colorado 1981; **Fac Appt:** Prof Med, Univ Colorado

Wanner, Adam MD [Pul] - **Spec Exp:** Asthma; **Hospital:** Jackson Meml Hosp (page 70), Univ of Miami Hosp (page 72); **Address:** Univ Miami Sch Med, Div Pulm & Crit Care, 1600 NW 10th Ave, rm 7056, Miami, FL 33136; **Phone:** 305-243-3045; **Board Cert:** Internal Medicine 1973; Pulmonary Disease 1974; **Med School:** Switzerland 1966; **Resid:** Internal Medicine, Kantonsspital Aarau 1970; **Fellow:** Pulmonary Disease, Mt Sinai Med Ctr 1972; **Fac Appt:** Prof Med, Univ Miami Sch Med

Wheeler, Arthur P MD [Pul] - **Spec Exp:** Critical Care; Sepsis; Respiratory Distress Syndrome (ARDS); **Hospital:** Vanderbilt Univ Med Ctr (page 76); **Address:** Vanderbilt Univ Medical Ctr, 1161 21st Ave S, rm T-1218 MCN, Nashville, TN 37232-2650; **Phone:** 615-322-3412; **Board Cert:** Internal Medicine 1985; Pulmonary Disease 1988; **Med School:** Univ MD Sch Med 1982; **Resid:** Internal Medicine, Vanderbilt Univ Med Ctr 1985; **Fellow:** Pulmonary Disease, Vanderbilt Univ Med Ctr 1986; **Fac Appt:** Assoc Prof Med, Vanderbilt Univ

Midwest

Balk, Robert A MD [Pul] - **Spec Exp:** Asthma; Cystic Fibrosis; Respiratory Failure; Lung Injury/ARDS; **Hospital:** Rush Univ Med Ctr; **Address:** 1725 W Harrison St, Ste 054, Chicago, IL 60612; **Phone:** 312-942-6744; **Board Cert:** Internal Medicine 1981; Pulmonary Disease 1986; Critical Care Medicine 2008; **Med School:** Univ MO-Kansas City 1978; **Resid:** Internal Medicine, Univ MO-Kansas City Affil Hosps 1981; **Fellow:** Pulmonary Critical Care Medicine, Univ Ark Hosp 1983; **Fac Appt:** Prof Med, Rush Med Coll

Bijwadia, Jagdeep S MD [Pul] - **Spec Exp:** Sleep Medicine; **Address:** HealthPartners Spec Ctr, 401 Phalen Blvd, St Paul, MN 55130; **Phone:** 651-254-7670 x3; **Board Cert:** Internal Medicine 2001; Pulmonary Disease 2004; Sleep Medicine 2007; **Med School:** India 1986; **Resid:** Internal Medicine, Nassau Co MC 1992; **Fellow:** Pulmonary Critical Care Medicine, USC Univ Hosp 1992; **Fac Appt:** Asst Prof Med, Univ Minn

Fahey, Patrick J MD [Pul] - **Hospital:** Loyola Univ Med Ctr, Edward Hines, Jr. VA Hosp; **Address:** Loyola Univ Med Ctr-Pulmonary Disease, 2160 S 1st Ave Bldg 54 - rm 124, Maywood, IL 60153-3304; **Phone:** 708-216-8563; **Board Cert:** Internal Medicine 1976; Pulmonary Disease 1978; **Med School:** Univ Wisc 1973; **Resid:** Internal Medicine, St Elizabeth's Hosp 1976; **Fellow:** Pulmonary Disease, Strong Meml Hosp 1980; **Fac Appt:** Prof Med, Loyola Univ-Stritch Sch Med

Fletcher, Eugene MD [Pul] - **Spec Exp:** Chronic Obstructive Lung Disease (COPD); Sleep Disorders/Apnea; **Hospital:** Floyd Meml Hosp & Hlth Svcs; **Address:** 428 Vincennes St, New Albany, IN 47150; **Phone:** 812-948-5841; **Board Cert:** Internal Medicine 1974; Pulmonary Disease 1980; Critical Care Medicine 2010; **Med School:** Temple Univ 1971; **Resid:** Internal Medicine, Univ Colo Affil Hosp 1973; Internal Medicine, Fitzsimons Army Med Ctr 1974; **Fellow:** Pulmonary Disease, Univ Okla Hlth Scis Ctr 1974

Garrity Jr, Edward MD [Pul] - **Spec Exp:** Transplant Medicine-Lung; Pulmonary Vascular Disease; Asthma; Cystic Fibrosis; **Hospital:** Univ of Chicago Med Ctr; **Address:** Lung Transplant Prgrm, 5841 S Maryland Ave, MC 0999, Chicago, IL 60637; **Phone:** 773-834-1119; **Board Cert:** Internal Medicine 2003; Pulmonary Disease 1984; **Med School:** Loyola Univ-Stritch Sch Med 1976; **Resid:** Internal Medicine, Loyola Univ Med Ctr 1979; **Fellow:** Pulmonary Disease, Univ Chicago Hosps 1983; **Fac Appt:** Prof Med, Univ Chicago-Pritzker Sch Med

Grum, Cyril M MD [Pul] - **Spec Exp:** Asthma; Cystic Fibrosis; **Hospital:** Univ of Michigan Hosp; **Address:** Univ Mich, Div Pulm & Crit Care Med, 1500 E Med Ctr Drive, 3916 TC, Ann Arbor, MI 48109; **Phone:** 734-647-9342; **Board Cert:** Internal Medicine 1980; Pulmonary Disease 1982; **Med School:** Med Coll Wisc 1977; **Resid:** Internal Medicine, Cleveland Clin; **Fellow:** Pulmonary Disease, Univ Mich Hosps; **Fac Appt:** Asst Prof Med, Univ Mich Med Sch

Hall, Jesse MD [Pul] - **Spec Exp:** Respiratory Failure; Critical Care; **Hospital:** Univ of Chicago Med Ctr; **Address:** 5841 S Maryland Ave, rm W656, MC 6076, Chicago, IL 60637; **Phone:** 773-702-1454; **Board Cert:** Internal Medicine 1980; **Med School:** Univ Chicago-Pritzker Sch Med 1977; **Resid:** Internal Medicine, Univ Chicago Hosps 1982; **Fac Appt:** Prof Med, Univ Chicago-Pritzker Sch Med

Hertz, Marshall I MD [Pul] - **Spec Exp:** Transplant Medicine-Lung; Transplant Medicine-Heart & Lung; Pulmonary Hypertension; **Address:** Pulmonary, Allergy & Critical Care Med, 420 Delaware St SE, MMC 276, Minneapolis, MN 55455; **Phone:** 612-624-0999; **Board Cert:** Internal Medicine 1981; Pulmonary Disease 1984; **Med School:** Univ Mich Med Sch 1978; **Resid:** Internal Medicine, Univ Minn Med Ctr 1982; **Fellow:** Pulmonary Critical Care Medicine, Univ Minn Med Ctr 1984; **Fac Appt:** Prof Med, Univ Minn

Hyers, Thomas M MD [Pul] - **Spec Exp:** Thromboembolic Disorders; Chronic Obstructive Lung Disease (COPD); Occupational Medicine; **Hospital:** SSM St. Clare Hlth Ctr, St. John's Mercy Med Ctr - St Louis; **Address:** CARE Clin Research, 522 N New Ballas Rd, Ste 350, St Louis, MO 63141; **Phone:** 314-699-9383; **Board Cert:** Internal Medicine 1974; Pulmonary Disease 1980; **Med School:** Duke Univ 1968; **Resid:** Internal Medicine, Univ Wash Med Ctr 1975; Pulmonary Disease, Univ Colorado Hosp 1977; **Fellow:** Pulmonary Disease, Natl Inst Hlth 1972; **Fac Appt:** Clin Prof Med, St Louis Univ

Ingbar, David H MD [Pul] - **Spec Exp:** Critical Care; Pulmonary Infections; Respiratory Failure; **Hospital:** Univ Minn Med Ctr, Fairview - Riverside Campus, Fairview Southdale Hosp; **Address:** University of Minnesota; MMC 276 Pulmonary and Critical Care, 420 Delaware St SE, Minneapolis, MN 55455; **Phone:** 612-626-6100; **Board Cert:** Internal Medicine 1981; Critical Care Medicine 2007; Pulmonary Disease 1984; **Med School:** Harvard Med Sch 1978; **Resid:** Internal Medicine, Univ Wash Med Ctr 1981; **Fellow:** Pulmonary Disease, Yale Univ-New Haven Hosp 1985; **Fac Appt:** Prof Med, Univ Minn

Kaye, Mitchell MD [Pul] - **Spec Exp:** Chronic Obstructive Lung Disease (COPD); Asthma; **Hospital:** Abbott - Northwestern Hosp; **Address:** Minnesota Lung and Sleep Ctr, 920 E 28th St, Ste 700, Minneapolis, MN 55407; **Phone:** 952-567-7400; **Board Cert:** Internal Medicine 1987; Pulmonary Disease 2000; Critical Care Medicine 2001; **Med School:** Univ Minn 1984; **Resid:** Internal Medicine, Univ Ill Hosps & Clins 1987; **Fellow:** Pulmonary Disease, Northwestern Univ Med Sch 1989

Kovitz, Kevin L MD [Pul] - **Spec Exp:** Interventional Pulmonology; **Hospital:** Central DuPage Hosp, Alexian Brothers Med Ctr; **Address:** Chicago Chest Ctr/Suburban Lung Assocs, 800 Biesterfield Rd, Ste 510, Elk Grove Village, IL 60007; **Phone:** 847-498-5864; **Board Cert:** Internal Medicine 1988; Pulmonary Disease 2002; Critical Care Medicine 2005; **Med School:** Israel 1985; **Resid:** Internal Medicine, Univ Maryland Hosps 1988; **Fellow:** Pulmonary Intensive Care, Johns Hopkins Hosp 1992; Interventional Pulmonology, Sainte Marguerite Hosp 1993

Krowka, Michael J MD [Pul] - **Spec Exp:** Hepatopulmonary Syndrome; Pulmonary Hypertension; Chronic Obstructive Lung Disease (COPD); **Hospital:** Mayo Med Ctr & Clin - Rochester; **Address:** Mayo Clinic, Pulm & Crit Care Med, 200 First St SW, Rochester, MN 55905; **Phone:** 507-538-3270; **Board Cert:** Internal Medicine 1983; Pulmonary Disease 1986; **Med School:** Univ Nevada 1980; **Resid:** Internal Medicine, Evanston Hosp 1983; **Fellow:** Pulmonary Disease, Mayo Clinic 1986; **Fac Appt:** Prof Med, Mayo Med Sch

Lem, Vincent M MD [Pul] - **Spec Exp:** Asthma; **Hospital:** St. Luke's Hosp of Kansas City; **Address:** 4321 Washington St, Ste 6000, Kansas City, MO 64111; **Phone:** 816-756-2255; **Board Cert:** Internal Medicine 1982; Pulmonary Disease 1984; Critical Care Medicine 2004; **Med School:** Univ Kansas 1978; **Resid:** Internal Medicine, St Luke's Hosp 1982; **Fellow:** Pulmonary Disease, Univ Texas Hlth Sci Ctr 1984; **Fac Appt:** Assoc Clin Prof Med, Univ MO-Kansas City

Marini, John Joseph MD [Pul] - **Spec Exp:** Critical Care; Mechanical Ventilation; Chronic Obstructive Lung Disease (COPD); **Hospital:** Regions Hosp - St Paul; **Address:** 401 Phelon Blvd, St Paul, MN 55130; **Phone:** 952-967-7616; **Board Cert:** Internal Medicine 2003; Pulmonary Disease 2003; Critical Care Medicine 2002; **Med School:** Johns Hopkins Univ 1973; **Resid:** Internal Medicine, Univ Washington Med Ctr 1976; **Fellow:** Pulmonary Disease, Univ Washington Med Ctr 1978; **Fac Appt:** Prof Med, Univ Minn

Martinez, Fernando J MD [Pul] - **Spec Exp:** Lung Disease; Critical Care; **Hospital:** Univ of Michigan Hosp; **Address:** 1500 E Med Ctr Dr, 3916 TC, Ann Arbor, MI 48109; **Phone:** 734-647-9342; **Board Cert:** Internal Medicine 1986; Pulmonary Disease 1988; Critical Care Medicine 2000; **Med School:** Univ Fla Coll Med 1983; **Resid:** Internal Medicine, Beth Israel Hosp 1986; **Fellow:** Pulmonary Disease, Boston Univ 1989; **Fac Appt:** Prof Med, Univ Mich Med Sch

Matuschak, George M MD [Pul] - **Spec Exp:** Chronic Obstructive Lung Disease (COPD); Asthma; **Address:** 621 S New Ballas Rd, Ste 228A, St. Louis, MO 63141; **Phone:** 314-251-4966; **Board Cert:** Internal Medicine 1980; Critical Care Medicine 2008; Pulmonary Disease 2008; **Med School:** Temple Univ 1977; **Resid:** Internal Medicine, Strong Meml Hosp 1980; **Fellow:** Critical Care Medicine, Univ Htlh Ctr 1981; Pulmonary Disease, Univ Hlth Ctr 1984; **Fac Appt:** Prof Med, St Louis Univ

Popovich Jr, John MD [Pul] - **Spec Exp:** Lung Disease; Pulmonary Embolism; Interstitial Lung Disease; Critical Care; **Hospital:** Henry Ford Hosp; **Address:** Henry Ford Hosp, Dept Int Med, 2799 W Grand Blvd, Detroit, MI 48202; **Phone:** 313-916-8058; **Board Cert:** Internal Medicine 1978; Pulmonary Disease 1980; **Med School:** Univ Mich Med Sch 1975; **Resid:** Internal Medicine, Henry Ford Hosp 1978; **Fellow:** Pulmonary Disease, Henry Ford Hosp 1980; **Fac Appt:** Prof Med, Wayne State Univ

Prakash, Udaya MD [Pul] - **Spec Exp:** Bronchoscopy; **Hospital:** Mayo Med Ctr & Clin - Rochester; **Address:** Mayo Clin, Div Pulm & Crit Care Med, 200 First St SW, Rochester, MN 55905; **Phone:** 507-284-2158; **Board Cert:** Internal Medicine 1987; Pulmonary Disease 1976; **Med School:** India 1970; **Resid:** Internal Medicine, Mayo Clin 1973; **Fellow:** Pulmonary Disease, Mayo Clin 1976; **Fac Appt:** Prof Med, Mayo Med Sch

Rosenbluth, Daniel B MD [Pul] - **Spec Exp:** Cystic Fibrosis; **Hospital:** Barnes-Jewish Hosp; **Address:** Washington Univ Sch Med, 660 S Euclid, Box 8052, St Louis, MO 63110; **Phone:** 314-454-8762; **Board Cert:** Internal Medicine 2002; Pulmonary Disease 2004; Critical Care Medicine 2005; **Med School:** Mount Sinai Sch Med 1989; **Resid:** Internal Medicine, Northwestern Meml Hosp 1992; **Fellow:** Pulmonary Critical Care Medicine, Barnes Hosp 1995; **Fac Appt:** Prof Med, Washington Univ, St Louis

Shore, Bernard L MD [Pul] - **Spec Exp:** Lung Disease; Palliative Care; Pain Management; **Hospital:** Barnes-Jewish Hosp; **Address:** 1110 Highland Plaza Drive E, Ste 375, St Louis, MO 63110; **Phone:** 314-367-3113; **Board Cert:** Internal Medicine 1980; Pulmonary Disease 1982; **Med School:** Washington Univ, St Louis 1977; **Resid:** Internal Medicine, Barnes Hosp 1980; **Fellow:** Pulmonary Disease, Wash Univ Med Ctr 1982; **Fac Appt:** Assoc Clin Prof Med, Washington Univ, St Louis

Silver, Michael R MD [Pul] - **Spec Exp:** Chronic Obstructive Lung Disease (COPD); Lung Cancer; Asthma; **Hospital:** Rush Univ Med Ctr, Rush Oak Park Hosp; **Address:** Rush Univ Med Ctr, Professional Office Bldg 3, 1725 W Harrison St, Ste 054, Chicago, IL 60612; **Phone:** 312-942-6744; **Board Cert:** Internal Medicine 1984; Pulmonary Disease 1988; Critical Care Medicine 2009; **Med School:** Albany Med Coll 1981; **Resid:** Internal Medicine, Rush-Presby-St Lukes Med Ctr 1985; **Fellow:** Pulmonary Critical Care Medicine, Rush-Presby-St Lukes Med Ctr 1987; **Fac Appt:** Assoc Prof Med, Rush Med Coll

Simon, Richard H MD [Pul] - **Spec Exp:** Cystic Fibrosis; **Hospital:** Univ of Michigan Hosp; **Address:** Univ Michigan Div Pulmonary Medicine, 1500 E Med Ctr Drive, 3916 TC, Ann Arbor, MI 48109; **Phone:** 734-647-9342; **Board Cert:** Internal Medicine 1976; Pulmonary Disease 1980; **Med School:** Duke Univ 1972; **Resid:** Internal Medicine, UCSF Med Ctr 1975; Internal Medicine, Univ Colorado Affil Hosps 1976; **Fellow:** Pulmonary Disease, Univ Colorado 1981; **Fac Appt:** Prof Med, Univ Mich Med Sch

Stoller, James MD [Pul] - **Spec Exp:** Emphysema/Alpha-1 Antitrypsin Deficiency; **Hospital:** Cleveland Clin (page 56); **Address:** Cleveland Clinic, Dept Education, 9500 Euclid Ave, Desk NA22, Cleveland, OH 44195; **Phone:** 216-444-1960; **Board Cert:** Internal Medicine 1982; Pulmonary Disease 1984; Critical Care Medicine 2007; **Med School:** Yale Univ 1979; **Resid:** Internal Medicine, Peter Bent Brigham Hosp 1982; **Fellow:** Pulmonary Disease, Brigham & Women's Hosp 1983; Critical Care Medicine, Mass Genl Hosp 1985; **Fac Appt:** Prof Med, Cleveland Cl Coll Med/Case West Res

Tobin, Martin MD [Pul] - **Spec Exp:** Mechanical Ventilation; Chronic Obstructive Lung Disease (COPD); **Hospital:** Edward Hines, Jr. VA Hosp, Loyola Univ Med Ctr; **Address:** Hines VA Hosp (111N), Fifth Ave and Roosevelt Rd, Bldg 1 - rm E438, Hines, IL 60141; **Phone:** 708-202-2705; **Board Cert:** Internal Medicine 1983; Pulmonary Disease 1984; **Med School:** Ireland 1975; **Resid:** Internal Medicine, Trinity Coll Hosps 1979; Pulmonary Disease, Kings Coll Hosp 1980; **Fellow:** Pulmonary Critical Care Medicine, Mt Sinai Hosp 1983; Pulmonary Critical Care Medicine, Univ Pittsburgh 1983; **Fac Appt:** Prof Med, Loyola Univ-Stritch Sch Med

Trulock, Elbert MD [Pul] - **Spec Exp:** Transplant Medicine-Lung; Emphysema-Lung Volume Reduction; Pulmonary Hypertension; Cystic Fibrosis; **Hospital:** Barnes-Jewish Hosp; **Address:** 216 S Kings Hwy, MS 90-32-680, St Louis, MO 63110; **Phone:** 314-362-5378; **Board Cert:** Internal Medicine 1981; Pulmonary Disease 1984; **Med School:** Emory Univ 1978; **Resid:** Internal Medicine, Barnes Hosp 1981; **Fellow:** Pulmonary Disease, Wash Univ Med Ctr 1983; **Fac Appt:** Prof Med, Washington Univ, St Louis

Pulmonary Disease

Wiedemann, Herbert P MD [Pul] - **Spec Exp:** Respiratory Distress Syndrome (ARDS); Asthma; Emphysema; **Hospital:** Cleveland Clin (page 56); **Address:** Cleveland Clinic-Pulmonary & Allergy, 9500 Euclid Ave, Desk A90, Cleveland, OH 44195; **Phone:** 216-444-8335; **Board Cert:** Internal Medicine 1980; Pulmonary Disease 1984; **Med School:** Cornell Univ 1977; **Resid:** Internal Medicine, Univ Wash Hosps 1980; Internal Medicine, Harborview Hosp 1981; **Fellow:** Pulmonary Disease, Yale Univ 1984

Great Plains and Mountains

Brown, Kevin K MD [Pul] - **Spec Exp:** Pulmonary Fibrosis; Interstitial Lung Disease; Autoimmune Lung Disease; Clinical Trials; **Hospital:** Natl Jewish Med & Rsch Ctr, Univ of CO Hosp - Anschutz Inpatient Pav; **Address:** Natl Jewish Health, 1400 Jackson St, Denver, CO 80206-2762; **Phone:** 303-398-1621; **Board Cert:** Internal Medicine 1989; Pulmonary Disease 2005; **Med School:** Univ Minn 1984; **Resid:** Internal Medicine, Providence Med Ctr 1989; **Fellow:** Pulmonary Disease, Maine Med Ctr 1992; Pulmonary Disease, Univ Colo Hlth Scis Ctr 1994; **Fac Appt:** Assoc Prof Med, Univ Colorado

Elliott, C Gregory MD [Pul] - **Spec Exp:** Pulmonary Hypertension; Thromboembolic Disorders; **Hospital:** Intermountain Med Ctr, LDS Hosp; **Address:** Intermountain Med Ctr, Dept Medicine, 5121 S Cottonwood St, Ste 307, Murray, UT 84157; **Phone:** 801-507-3373; **Board Cert:** Internal Medicine 1976; Pulmonary Disease 1978; **Med School:** Univ MD Sch Med 1973; **Resid:** Internal Medicine, Univ Maryland Hosp 1976; **Fellow:** Pulmonary Disease, Univ Utah 1978; **Fac Appt:** Prof Med, Univ Utah

Iseman, Michael MD [Pul] - **Spec Exp:** Tuberculosis; Mycobacterial Infections; **Hospital:** Natl Jewish Med & Rsch Ctr; **Address:** Natl Jewish Med & Rsch Ctr, 1400 Jackson St, rm J223, Denver, CO 80206; **Phone:** 303-398-1667; **Board Cert:** Internal Medicine 1972; Pulmonary Disease 1976; **Med School:** Columbia P&S 1965; **Resid:** Internal Medicine, Bellevue Hosp 1967; Internal Medicine, Harlem Hosp 1970; **Fellow:** Pulmonary Disease, Harlem Hosp 1972; **Fac Appt:** Prof Med, Univ Colorado

Kaplan, James MD [Pul] - **Spec Exp:** Critical Care; Sleep Disorders/Apnea; **Hospital:** Overland Pk Regl Med Ctr; **Address:** 10550 Quivira, Ste 335, Overland Park, KS 66215-2304; **Phone:** 913-599-3800; **Board Cert:** Internal Medicine 1987; Pulmonary Disease 2010; Critical Care Medicine 2003; **Med School:** Univ MO-Kansas City 1984; **Resid:** Internal Medicine, Barnes Hosp 1987; **Fellow:** Pulmonary Disease, Barnes Hosp-Wash Univ 1987

Kern, Jeffrey A MD [Pul] - **Spec Exp:** Lung Cancer; **Hospital:** Natl Jewish Med & Rsch Ctr; **Address:** National Jewish Health, 1400 Jackson St, Denver, CO 80206; **Phone:** 877-225-5654; **Board Cert:** Internal Medicine 1982; Pulmonary Disease 1986; **Med School:** Univ Wisc 1979; **Resid:** Internal Medicine, Parkland Meml Hosp 1982; **Fellow:** Pulmonary Critical Care Medicine, Hosp Univ of Penn 1984

Martin, Richard J MD [Pul] - **Spec Exp:** Asthma; Vocal Cord Disorders; Chronic Obstructive Lung Disease (COPD); **Hospital:** Natl Jewish Med & Rsch Ctr, Univ of CO Hosp - Anschutz Inpatient Pav; **Address:** 1400 Jackson St, Denver, CO 80206-2762; **Phone:** 303-398-1847; **Board Cert:** Internal Medicine 1976; Pulmonary Disease 1978; **Med School:** Univ Mich Med Sch 1971; **Resid:** Internal Medicine, Tulane Univ Affil Hosp 1976; **Fellow:** Pulmonary Disease, Univ Oklahoma 1978; **Fac Appt:** Prof Med, Univ Colorado

Rennard, Stephen I MD [Pul] - **Spec Exp:** Chronic Obstructive Lung Disease (COPD); Emphysema; **Hospital:** Nebraska Med Ctr; **Address:** 985910 Nebraska Med Ctr, Omaha, NE 68198-5910; **Phone:** 402-559-7313; **Board Cert:** Internal Medicine 1978; Pulmonary Disease 1982; **Med School:** Baylor Coll Med 1975; **Resid:** Internal Medicine, Barnes Hosp-Washington Univ 1977; **Fac Appt:** Prof Med, Univ Nebr Coll Med

Rose, Cecile MD [Pul] - **Spec Exp:** Occupational Lung Disease; Sarcoidosis; Pneumoconiosis; Asbestos-related Lung Disease; **Hospital:** Natl Jewish Med & Rsch Ctr, Univ of CO Hosp - Anschutz Inpatient Pav; **Address:** 1400 Jackson St, rm G-211, Denver, CO 80206-2761; **Phone:** 303-398-1867; **Board Cert:** Internal Medicine 1983; Pulmonary Disease 1986; Occupational Medicine 1987; **Med School:** Univ IL Coll Med 1980; **Resid:** Internal Medicine, Med Coll Virginia Hosp 1983; **Fellow:** Pulmonary Disease, Med Coll Virginia Hosp 1985; **Fac Appt:** Assoc Prof Med, Univ Colorado

Schwartz, David A MD [Pul] - **Spec Exp:** Occupational Lung Disease; Pulmonary Fibrosis; Asthma; **Hospital:** Denver Health Med Ctr, Univ of CO Hosp - Anschutz Inpatient Pav; **Address:** 12631 E 17th Ave, MS B178, Aurora, CO 80045; **Phone:** 303-724-1783; **Board Cert:** Internal Medicine 1984; Occupational Medicine 1987; Pulmonary Disease 1988; **Med School:** UCSD 1979; **Resid:** Internal Medicine, Boston City Hosp 1984; Preventive Medicine, Harvard Sch Public Health 1986; **Fellow:** Pulmonary Disease, Univ Seattle Medical Ctr 1988; **Fac Appt:** Prof Med

Schwarz, Marvin I MD [Pul] - **Spec Exp:** Interstitial Lung Disease; Pulmonary Vascular Disease; Pulmonary Fibrosis; **Hospital:** Univ of CO Hosp - Anschutz Inpatient Pav, Natl Jewish Med & Rsch Ctr; **Address:** Div Pulmonary Science & Critical Care, 12700 E 19th Ave, MS C-272, Aurora, CO 80045; **Phone:** 303-724-4075; **Board Cert:** Internal Medicine 1970; Pulmonary Disease 1971; **Med School:** Tulane Univ 1964; **Resid:** Internal Medicine, Charity Hosp 1967; **Fellow:** Pulmonary Disease, Charity Hosp/Tulane Univ 1969; **Fac Appt:** Prof Med, Univ Colorado

Sutherland, Everett Rand MD [Pul] - **Spec Exp:** Allergy; Occupational Asthma; Chronic Obstructive Lung Disease (COPD); **Hospital:** Natl Jewish Med & Rsch Ctr; **Address:** 1400 Jackson St, Denver, CO 80206; **Phone:** 303-398-1355; **Board Cert:** Internal Medicine 2007; Pulmonary Disease 2010; Critical Care Medicine 2001; **Med School:** Univ Chicago-Pritzker Sch Med 1994; **Resid:** Internal Medicine, UCSF 1997; **Fellow:** Pulmonary Critical Care Medicine, Univ Colorado Denver 2001; **Fac Appt:** Assoc Prof Med, Univ Colorado

Southwest

Arroliga, Alejandro C MD [Pul] - **Spec Exp:** Pulmonary Hypertension; Respiratory Distress Syndrome (ARDS); Critical Care; **Hospital:** Scott & White Mem Hosp; **Address:** 2401 S 31st St, Temple, TX 76508; **Phone:** 254-724-4069; **Board Cert:** Internal Medicine 2010; Pulmonary Disease 2000; Critical Care Medicine 2003; **Med School:** Mexico 1984; **Resid:** Internal Medicine, Coney Island Hosp 1990; **Fellow:** Pulmonary Critical Care Medicine, Yale-New Haven Hosp 1993; **Fac Appt:** Prof Med, Cleveland Cl Coll Med/Case West Res

Guidry, George G MD [Pul] - **Spec Exp:** Chronic Obstructive Lung Disease (COPD); Asthma; Pneumonia; Lung Cancer; **Hospital:** Lafayette Genl Med Ctr; **Address:** 155 Hospital Drive, Ste 206, Lafayette, LA 70503-2852; **Phone:** 337-234-3204; **Board Cert:** Internal Medicine 1988; Pulmonary Disease 2010; **Med School:** Louisiana State U, New Orleans 1985; **Resid:** Internal Medicine, LSU Med Ctr 1988; **Fellow:** Pulmonary Disease, LSU Med Ctr 1991; **Fac Appt:** Assoc Clin Prof Med, Louisiana State U, New Orleans

Pulmonary Disease

Levin, David C MD [Pul] - **Spec Exp:** Asthma; Chronic Obstructive Lung Disease (COPD); **Hospital:** OU Med Ctr, VA Med Ctr - Oklahoma City; **Address:** OU Physicians Building, 825 NE 10th St, Ste 2500, Oklahoma City, OK 73104; **Phone:** 405-271-7001; **Board Cert:** Internal Medicine 1973; Pulmonary Disease 1976; **Med School:** Case West Res Univ 1970; **Resid:** Internal Medicine, Univ Colorado Affil Hosp 1974; **Fellow:** Pulmonary Disease, Univ Colorado 1975; **Fac Appt:** Prof Med, Univ Okla Coll Med

Perret, Philip S MD [Pul] - **Spec Exp:** Chronic Obstructive Lung Disease (COPD); **Hospital:** Our Lady of Lourdes Reg Med Ctr - Lafayette, Lafayette Genl Med Ctr; **Address:** 614 W St Mary Blvd, Lafayette, LA 70506; **Phone:** 337-232-6435; **Board Cert:** Internal Medicine 1978; Pulmonary Disease 1980; **Med School:** Emory Univ 1974; **Resid:** Internal Medicine, Emory Univ Hosp 1977; **Fellow:** Pulmonary Disease, Emory Univ 1979

Shellito, Judd E MD [Pul] - **Spec Exp:** Pulmonary Infections; Occupational Lung Disease; **Hospital:** Ochsner Med Ctr-New Orleans; **Address:** LSU Pulmonary Medicine, 1901 Perdido St, Ste 3205, New Orleans, LA 70112; **Phone:** 504-568-4634; **Board Cert:** Internal Medicine 1977; Pulmonary Disease 1980; **Med School:** Tulane Univ 1974; **Resid:** Internal Medicine, Evanston Hosp 1978; **Fellow:** Pulmonary Critical Care Medicine, Univ New Mexico Hosp 1980; **Fac Appt:** Prof Med, Louisiana State U, New Orleans

Weissler, Jonathan C MD [Pul] - **Spec Exp:** Interstitial Lung Disease; Asthma; **Hospital:** UT Southwestern Med Ctr at Dallas, Parkland Hlth & Hosp Sys; **Address:** 5323 Harry Hines Blvd, Dallas, TX 75390-9034; **Phone:** 214-645-1825; **Board Cert:** Internal Medicine 1982; Pulmonary Disease 1984; Critical Care Medicine 2007; **Med School:** NYU Sch Med 1979; **Resid:** Internal Medicine, Univ Texas Hlth Sci Ctr 1982; **Fellow:** Pulmonary Disease, Univ Texas Hlth Sci Ctr 1985; **Fac Appt:** Prof Med, Univ Tex SW, Dallas

West Coast and Pacific

Albertson, Timothy MD/PhD [Pul] - **Spec Exp:** Critical Care; Toxicology; **Hospital:** UC Davis Med Ctr; **Address:** UC Davis, Div Pulm Crit Care, 4150 V St, Ste 3400, Patient Support Svcs Bldg, Sacramento, CA 95817-9002; **Phone:** 916-734-3564; **Board Cert:** Pulmonary Disease 1984; Critical Care Medicine 2007; Emergency Medicine 2007; Medical Toxicology 2005; **Med School:** UC Davis 1977; **Resid:** Internal Medicine, Univ Arizona 1980; Internal Medicine, UC Davis Med Ctr 1981; **Fellow:** Pulmonary Critical Care Medicine, UC Davis Med Ctr 1983; **Fac Appt:** Prof Med, UC Davis

Auger, William R MD [Pul] - **Spec Exp:** Thromboembolic Disorders; Pulmonary Hypertension; **Hospital:** UCSD Med Ctr; **Address:** Thorton Hosp, UCSD, 9330 Campus Pt Drive, MC 7381, La Jolla, CA 92037; **Phone:** 858-657-7140; **Board Cert:** Internal Medicine 1986; Pulmonary Disease 1988; **Med School:** Univ Rochester 1982; **Resid:** Internal Medicine, Strong Meml Hosp 1985; **Fellow:** Critical Care Medicine, Ellis Hosp 1986; Pulmonary Disease, UCSD Med Ctr 1989; **Fac Appt:** Clin Prof Med, UCSD

Balmes, John Randolph MD [Pul] - **Spec Exp:** Beryllium-induced Lung Disease; **Hospital:** San Francisco Genl Hosp, UCSF Med Ctr; **Address:** UCSF, Div Occup & Envr Med, Campus Box 0843, 1001 Potrero Ave, rm 5K1, San Francisco, CA 94110; **Phone:** 415-206-8314; **Board Cert:** Internal Medicine 1979; Pulmonary Disease 1984; **Med School:** Mount Sinai Sch Med 1976; **Resid:** Internal Medicine, Mount Sinai Hosp 1979; **Fellow:** Pulmonary Disease, Yale-New Haven Hosp 1981; **Fac Appt:** Prof Med, UCSF

Bellamy, Paul E MD [Pul] - **Spec Exp:** Critical Care; **Hospital:** Kaiser Permanente Woodland Hills Med Ctr; **Address:** Kaiser Woodland Hills Med Ctr, Pulm Div, 5601 De Soto Ave, Med Office Twr, Fl 4, Woodland Hills, CA 91367; **Phone:** 818-719-3530; **Board Cert:** Internal Medicine 1978; Pulmonary Disease 1980; Critical Care Medicine 2007; **Med School:** SUNY Buffalo 1975; **Resid:** Internal Medicine, Univ Hosps-Case West Res 1978; **Fellow:** Pulmonary Disease, UCLA Med Ctr 1980; **Fac Appt:** Clin Prof Med, UCLA

Boushey Jr, Homer A MD [Pul] - **Spec Exp:** Asthma; Lung Injuries-Inhalation Induced; **Hospital:** UCSF Med Ctr; **Address:** UCSF Med Ctr, Pulmonary Medicine, 505 Parnassus Ave, Box 0130, Room M1292, San Francisco, CA 94143; **Phone:** 415-476-8019; **Board Cert:** Internal Medicine 1972; Pulmonary Disease 1974; **Med School:** UCSF 1968; **Resid:** Internal Medicine, UCSF Med Ctr 1970; Internal Medicine, Beth Israel Hosp 1971; **Fellow:** Pulmonary Disease, Oxford Univ 1972; Pulmonary Disease, UCSF Hosp 1974; **Fac Appt:** Prof Med, UCSF

Catanzaro, Antonino MD [Pul] - **Spec Exp:** Tuberculosis; Coccidioidomycosis; Mycobacterial Infections; **Hospital:** UCSD Med Ctr; **Address:** 200 W Arbor Drive, MC 8374, San Diego, CA 92103; **Phone:** 619-543-5550; **Board Cert:** Internal Medicine 1972; Pulmonary Disease 1976; **Med School:** SUNY Buffalo 1965; **Resid:** Internal Medicine, Georgetown Univ Hosp 1970; **Fellow:** Pulmonary Critical Care Medicine, UCSD Med Ctr 1972; Research, Scripps Clin Rsch Fdn 1972; **Fac Appt:** Prof Med, UCSD

Gerboth, Gregory D MD [Pul] - **Spec Exp:** Asthma; Critical Care; **Hospital:** Providence Alaska Med Ctr; **Address:** Internal Medicine Assocs, 2841 De Barre Rd, Ste 50, Anchorage, AK 99508; **Phone:** 907-276-2811; **Board Cert:** Internal Medicine 2000; Pulmonary Disease 2000; Critical Care Medicine 2000; **Med School:** Med Coll Wisc 1987; **Resid:** Internal Medicine, Med Coll Wisc Med Ctr 1990; **Fellow:** Pulmonary Critical Care Medicine, Med Coll Wisc Med Ctr 1991

Gibson, Ronald MD/PhD [Pul] - **Spec Exp:** Pulmonary Infections; Cystic Fibrosis; Asthma; **Hospital:** Seattle Chldns Hosp; **Address:** Seattle Children's, A-5937 - Pulmonary, 4800 Sand Point Way NE, Seattle, WA 98105; **Phone:** 206-987-2174; **Board Cert:** Pediatrics 1988; Pediatric Pulmonology 2007; **Med School:** Washington Univ, St Louis 1982; **Resid:** Pediatrics, Univ Washington Med Ctr 1985; **Fellow:** Pediatric Pulmonology, Univ Washington Med Ctr 1988; **Fac Appt:** Prof Ped, Univ Wash

Heffner, John E MD [Pul] - **Spec Exp:** Critical Care; Respiratory Failure; **Hospital:** Providence Portland Med Ctr; **Address:** 5050 NE Hoyt St, Ste 540, Portland, OR 97213; **Phone:** 503-215-6258; **Board Cert:** Internal Medicine 1977; Pulmonary Disease 1982; Critical Care Medicine 2005; **Med School:** UCLA 1974; **Resid:** Internal Medicine, Univ Colo Med Ctr 1978; **Fac Appt:** Prof Med, Med Univ SC

Hopewell, Philip C MD [Pul] - **Spec Exp:** AIDS/HIV; Tuberculosis; Infectious Disease-Lung; **Hospital:** San Francisco Genl Hosp; **Address:** San Francisco Genl Hosp, 1001 Potrero Ave, 5K1, San Francisco, CA 94110; **Phone:** 415-206-8314; **Board Cert:** Internal Medicine 1973; Pulmonary Disease 1974; **Med School:** W VA Univ 1965; **Resid:** Internal Medicine, UCSF Med Ctr 1971; **Fellow:** Pulmonary Disease, UCSF Med Ctr 1973; **Fac Appt:** Prof Med, UCSF

Huang, Laurence MD [Pul] - **Spec Exp:** AIDS/HIV; Pneumocystis Carinii Pneumonia (PCP); **Hospital:** San Francisco Genl Hosp; **Address:** UCSF Positive Health Program-SFGH, 995 Potrero Ave, Bldg 80-Ward 84, San Francisco, CA 94110; **Phone:** 415-206-2400; **Board Cert:** Internal Medicine 2003; Pulmonary Disease 2006; Critical Care Medicine 2007; **Med School:** Columbia P&S 1989; **Resid:** Internal Medicine, Columbia-Presby Hosp 1992; Pulmonary Critical Care Medicine, UCSF Med Ctr 1995; **Fac Appt:** Assoc Clin Prof Med, UCSF

Pulmonary Disease

Jacoby, David MD [Pul] - **Spec Exp:** Viral Infections; Infections-Respiratory; Asthma; **Hospital:** OR Hlth & Sci Univ; **Address:** 3181 SW Sam Jackson Park Rd, MC UHN67, Dept Pulmonary/Crit Care, Portland, OR 97239; **Phone:** 503-494-6158; **Board Cert:** Internal Medicine 1983; Pulmonary Disease 1986; **Med School:** NY Med Coll 1980; **Resid:** Internal Medicine, Temple Univ Hosp 1984; **Fellow:** Pulmonary Critical Care Medicine, UCSF Hosp 1987; **Fac Appt:** Prof Med, Oregon Hlth & Sci Univ

King Jr, Talmadge E MD [Pul] - **Spec Exp:** Interstitial Lung Disease; Sarcoidosis; Asthma; Pulmonary Fibrosis; **Hospital:** UCSF Med Ctr; **Address:** UCSF Dept Medicine, 505 Parnassus Ave, M994, Box 0120, San Francisco, CA 94143-0120; **Phone:** 415-476-0909; **Board Cert:** Internal Medicine 1977; Pulmonary Disease 2009; **Med School:** Harvard Med Sch 1974; **Resid:** Internal Medicine, Emory Univ Affil Hosps 1977; **Fellow:** Pulmonary Critical Care Medicine, Univ Colorado 1979; **Fac Appt:** Prof Med, UCSF

Lynch, Joseph P MD [Pul] - **Spec Exp:** Transplant Medicine-Lung; Interstitial Lung Disease; Pulmonary Fibrosis; Lymphangioleiomyomatosis(LAM); **Hospital:** UCLA Ronald Reagan Med Ctr; **Address:** UCLA - Div Pulmonary Medicine, 10833 Le Conte Ave, CHS Bldg - rm 37-131, Los Angeles, CA 90095-1690; **Phone:** 310-825-8599; **Board Cert:** Internal Medicine 1976; Pulmonary Disease 1980; **Med School:** Harvard Med Sch 1973; **Resid:** Internal Medicine, Univ Mich Med Ctr 1976; **Fellow:** Pulmonary Disease, Univ Mich 1978; **Fac Appt:** Prof Med, UCLA

Mosenifar, Zab MD [Pul] - **Spec Exp:** Chronic Obstructive Lung Disease (COPD); Interstitial Lung Disease; Asthma; Pulmonary Hypertension; **Hospital:** Cedars-Sinai Med Ctr; **Address:** Cedars-Sinai Med Ctr, Div Pulmonary Med, 8700 Beverly Blvd, rm 6732 South Twr, Los Angeles, CA 90048-1804; **Phone:** 310-423-4685; **Board Cert:** Internal Medicine 1978; Pulmonary Disease 1980; **Med School:** Iran 1973; **Resid:** Internal Medicine, Thomas Jefferson Univ Hosp; Internal Medicine, UCLA Med Ctr; **Fellow:** Pulmonary Disease, UCLA Med Ctr; **Fac Appt:** Prof Med, UCLA

Patterson, James R MD [Pul] - **Spec Exp:** Sleep Disorders/Apnea; **Hospital:** Providence Portland Med Ctr; **Address:** 1111 NE 99th Ave, Ste 200, Portland, OR 97220; **Phone:** 503-963-3030; **Board Cert:** Internal Medicine 1972; Pulmonary Disease 2001; **Med School:** Columbia P&S 1968; **Resid:** Internal Medicine, Columbia-Presby Med Ctr 1970; **Fellow:** Pulmonary Disease, Fitzsimons Army Med Ctr 1973; **Fac Appt:** Clin Prof Med, Oregon Hlth & Sci Univ

Raghu, Ganesh MD [Pul] - **Spec Exp:** Interstitial Lung Disease; Pulmonary Fibrosis; Sarcoidosis; Transplant-Lung; **Hospital:** Univ Wash Med Ctr; **Address:** 1959 NE Pacific St, Box 356166, Seattle, WA 98195-6166; **Phone:** 206-598-4615; **Board Cert:** Internal Medicine 1982; **Med School:** India 1974; **Resid:** Internal Medicine, Univ Rochester-Strong Meml Hosp 1978; Internal Medicine, SUNY Buffalo Med Ctr 1981; **Fellow:** Pulmonary Critical Care Medicine, Univ Washington Med Ctr 1984; **Fac Appt:** Prof Med, Univ Wash

Rizk, Norman W MD [Pul] - **Spec Exp:** Critical Care; Asthma; Pulmonary Infections; **Hospital:** Stanford Univ Hosp & Clinics; **Address:** 300 Pasteur Drive, rm H3142, Stanford, CA 94305-5236; **Phone:** 650-725-7061; **Board Cert:** Internal Medicine 1979; Pulmonary Disease 1984; Critical Care Medicine 2007; **Med School:** Yale Univ 1976; **Resid:** Internal Medicine, San Fran Genl Hosp 1980; **Fellow:** Pulmonary Disease, Moffitt Hosp-UCSF 1983; **Fac Appt:** Prof Med, Stanford Univ

Rubin, Lewis J MD [Pul] - **Spec Exp:** Pulmonary Hypertension; Pulmonary Vascular Disease; **Hospital:** UCSD Med Ctr; **Address:** UCSD Med Ctr, Pulmonary & Crit Care, 9300 Campus Point Drive, MC 7381, La Jolla, CA 92037-7381; **Phone:** 858-657-8700; **Board Cert:** Internal Medicine 1978; Pulmonary Disease 1980; **Med School:** Albert Einstein Coll Med 1975; **Resid:** Internal Medicine, Duke Univ Med Ctr 1978; **Fellow:** Pulmonary Disease, Duke Univ Med Ctr 1979; **Fac Appt:** Prof Med, UCSD

America's Top Doctors® 11th Edition

Sharma, Om Prakash MD [Pul] - **Spec Exp:** Sarcoidosis; Interstitial Lung Disease; Hypersensitivity Pneumonitis; **Hospital:** LAC & USC Med Ctr, Keck Med Ctr of USC (page 75); **Address:** IRD/178, 2020 Zonal Ave, Los Angeles, CA 90033; **Phone:** 323-226-7923; **Board Cert:** Internal Medicine 1987; **Med School:** India 1959; **Resid:** Internal Medicine, Norwalk Hosp 1963; Internal Medicine, Montefiore Med Ctr 1965; **Fellow:** Pulmonary Disease, Montefiore Med Ctr 1966; Research, Royal Coll Physicians 1969; **Fac Appt:** Prof Med, USC Sch Med

Tharratt, Robert S MD [Pul] - **Spec Exp:** Disaster Preparedness; Critical Care; Toxicology; **Hospital:** UC Davis Med Ctr; **Address:** UC Davis Div Pulmonary/Critical Care, 4150 V St, PSSB 3400, Sacramento, CA 95817-2214; **Phone:** 916-734-3564; **Board Cert:** Pulmonary Disease 1988; Critical Care Medicine 2009; Medical Toxicology 2004; Emergency Medicine 2007; **Med School:** UCLA 1983; **Resid:** Internal Medicine, UC Davis Med Ctr 1986; **Fellow:** Pulmonary Critical Care Medicine, UC Davis Med Ctr 1989; **Fac Appt:** Prof Med, UC Davis

Wallace, Jeanne M MD [Pul] - **Spec Exp:** Pulmonary Infections; Sleep Disorders/Apnea; Asthma; **Hospital:** Olive View-UCLA Med Ctr; **Address:** Olive View UCLA Med Ctr, 14445 Olive View Dr, Dept Medicine 2B 182, Sylmar, CA 91342-1437; **Phone:** 818-364-3205; **Board Cert:** Internal Medicine 1977; Pulmonary Disease 1980; Sleep Medicine 2007; **Med School:** UCLA 1974; **Resid:** Internal Medicine, UCSF Med Ctr 1977; **Fellow:** Pulmonary Disease, UCSD Med Ctr 1980; **Fac Appt:** Assoc Prof Med, UCLA

◼️ Cleveland Clinic

Every life deserves world class care.

Pulmonary Disease

Individuals with all types of acute or chronic lung diseases, as well as sleep disordered breathing (sleep apnea) can access specialty care at Cleveland Clinic. In 2010, physicians in the Department of Pulmonary, Allergy and Critical Care Medicine provided more than 95,000 outpatient visits.

Lung Transplantation

Cleveland Clinic's Lung Transplant Program is the largest in Ohio and among the largest in the United States. In 2010 our program performed 122 lung transplants. The average wait time for a lung transplantation at Cleveland Clinic is significantly lower than the national average.

Sarcoidosis Center of Excellence

Cleveland Clinic established a Sarcoidosis Center of Excellence in 2003. The only such center in Northeastern Ohio, the center aims to raise awareness of pulmonary sarcoidosis, improve the quality of sarcoidosis care and minimize the degree to which it can affect quality of life.

Areas of Expertise

Cleveland Clinic specializes in diagnosing and curing acute respiratory distress syndrome, allergic rhinitis and allergies (drug and food; latex) We have doctors and specialists in the field of aspirin desensitization, asthma and Beryllium-induced lung disease.

In collaboration with Cleveland Clinic thoracic surgeons, patients are evaluated for:

- Lung transplantation
- Lung volume reduction surgery (LVRS) for emphysema
- Pulmonary thromboendarterectomy (for chronic pulmonary hypertension secondary to thromboemboli)

Cleveland Clinic
Pulmonology, Allergy and
Critical Care Medicine
9500 Euclid Avenue
Cleveland, OH 44195

clevelandclinic.org/
pulmonarytopdocs

Offering Same-Day Appointments
Call 800.274.2009.

Treatment Guides

Cleveland Clinic has developed comprehensive treatment guides for many diseases and conditions. To download our free treatment guides, visit clevelandclinic.org/treatmentguides.

Online Medical Second Opinion

Cleveland Clinic's My**Consult** Online Medical Second Opinion program securely connects patients to our physician specialists for more than 1,000 life-changing or life-threatening diagnoses all by the click of a mouse. To learn more, log onto eclevelandclinic.org/myconsult or call 800.223.2273, ext. 43223.

Special Assistance for Out-of-State Patients

Cleveland Clinic Global Patient Services offers a complimentary Medical Concierge service for patients who travel from outside of Ohio. Call 800.223.2273, ext. 55580 or email medicalconcierge@ccf.org.

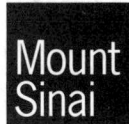 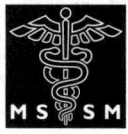

MOUNT SINAI
SCHOOL OF
MEDICINE

THE MOUNT SINAI MEDICAL CENTER
PULMONARY MEDICINE
One Gustave L. Levy Place
Fifth Avenue and 100th Street
New York, NY 10029-6574
Physician Referral: 1-800-MD-SINAI (637-4624)
www.mountsinai.org/pulmonary

The mission of Mount Sinai's **DIVISION OF PULMONARY, CRITICAL CARE, AND SLEEP MEDICINE** is to offer state-of-the-art clinical care to patients with all forms of lung disease and critical illness, cutting-edge research that will translate into improved patient care and outcomes, and hands-on training of future leaders in the field.

To achieve this goal, every faculty member is charged with the success of a specific program. Mount Sinai's Pulmonary Division has a long history of providing specialized care and key research in several disease areas that include Sarcoidosis and Occupational Lung Diseases. Mount Sinai's Sarcoidosis Service, the largest of its kind in the world, is a Center of Excellence for sarcoidosis research. It is the only site in the United States that performs the diagnostic Kveim- Siltzbach skin test for sarcoidosis, which eliminates the need for more invasive, uncomfortable, and expensive procedures. Through its Pulmonary Physiology Laboratory, Mount Sinai has been instrumental in establishing normal values for various pulmonary function tests and is currently conducting clinical studies of new tests for obesity, sarcoidosis, asthma, and lung cancer.

Pulmonary specialists at Mount Sinai are investigating asthma and emphysema, lung cancer, collagen vascular diseases, pulmonary infections, and occupational lung diseases. Mount Sinai has the largest screening program for workers and anyone in the general population exposed to polluted air at the World Trade Center catastrophe site. Our critical care physicians are experts in treating liver disease and acute and chronic respiratory failure, using the most modern forms of delivery of intensive care and providing compassionate end-of-life care.

The Asthma Program uses a multidisciplinary team approach, focusing on patient education and skill-building to foster self-management.

The Chronic Obstructive Pulmonary Disease Program offers a screening and a coordinated approach of exercise, treatment, and education that improves symptoms and quality of life, for one of the nation's most underdiagnosed conditions.

The Critical Care Medicine Program features state-of-the-art medical intensive care and respiratory care units.

The Interventional Pulmonary Service performs cutting-edge diagnostic and therapeutic procedures for patients with advanced pulmonary diseases.

The Lung Cancer/Thoracic Oncology Service provides specialized care for lung cancer diagnosis and staging and for coordinating multidisciplinary medical care for lung cancer.

The Occupational Lung Disorders Program specializes in the diagnosis and management of occupational lung disorders, such as occupational asthma and bronchitis, asbestosis, silicosis, and heavy metal lung injury.

The Pulmonary Fibrosis/Interstitial Lung Disease Program treats patients with chronic inflammatory and scarring disorders of the lungs, including idiopathic pulmonary fibrosis and collagen vascular-associated pulmonary diseases.

The Pulmonary Physiology Laboratory, performs the full range of physiological lung function and cardiopulmonary exercise testing for lung disease.

The Pulmonary Rehabilitation Program provides occupational, physical, and cardiopulmonary rehabilitation programs for patients with disabling lung disorders, as well as pre- and post-operative consultation and therapy.

The Thoracic Oncology Service provides multidisciplinary medical care for lung cancer, as a joint effort with the Department of Cardiothoracic Surgery.

The Sarcoidosis Service, which has passed its 20,000 enrollee count, offers standard care as well as the opportunity to participate in new clinical trials to 60 new enrollees per week.

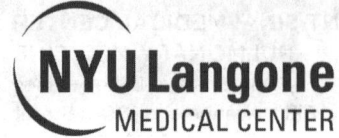

550 First Avenue *(at 31st Street)*
New York, NY 10016
www.NYULMC.org
Physician Referral: **888-7-NYU-MED** *(888-769-8633)*

PULMONOLOGY

About the Division of Pulmonary, Critical Care and Sleep Medicine

NYU Langone's Pulmonary, Critical Care and Sleep Medicine Division offers a full range of services for the diagnosis and treatment of inpatient and ambulatory patients. Services include pulmonary function laboratories; specialized medical critical care units at Tisch Hospital and the Hospital for Joint Diseases; and a multidisciplinary interventional bronchoscopy program integrated with thoracic radiology at Tisch Hospital. Research grant support includes the National Institutes of Health and the Centers for Disease Control and Prevention. We specialize in the following areas:

Asthma

The Division of Pulmonary Medicine is experienced in treating all aspects of asthma and airway disorders. The Bellevue Asthma Clinic at Bellevue Hospital Center, an affiliate of NYU Langone Medical Center, offers an active research program dealing exclusively with particulate matter pollution and asthma.

Pulmonary Services

The Division of Pulmonary Medicine provides clinical chest services at Tisch Hospital which care for patients with tuberculosis, lung cancer, asthma and interstitial fibrosis. Hospital consultation services are available for interstitial lung diseases, sarcoidosis, pulmonary hypertension, COPD, lung cancer, occupational lung diseases, bronchiectasis, and myobacterial other than TB.

Interventional Bronchoscopy

The Interventional Bronchoscopy Program at Tisch Hospital employs leading-edge techniques to diagnose and treat tumors and inflammatory conditions of the lung.

Lung Cancer Screening Program

Individuals at high risk for lung cancer may schedule a CT-scan as part of our lung cancer screening program. Eligible patients are also choose to contribute to our research efforts by participating in our lung cancer biomarker screening study.

Sleep Disorders

The Sleep Disorders Center at NYU Langone Medical Center offers clinical and research services for physicians and patients in the diagnosis and treatment of severe or prolonged sleeping difficulties. The Center is also equipped for limited home or in-hospital patient monitoring.

Radiation Oncology

a subspecialty of Radiology

A radiation oncologist deals with the therapeutic applications of radiant energy and its modifiers and the study and management of disease, especially malignant tumors.

Training Required: Four years in radiology *plus* additional training and examination.

RADIATION ONCOLOGY

New England

Choi, Noah C MD [RadRO] - **Spec Exp:** Lung Cancer; Esophageal Cancer; Mesothelioma; **Hospital:** Mass Genl Hosp; **Address:** Mass Genl Hosp, Dept Rad Oncology, 100 Blossom St, Cox 3, Boston, MA 02114; **Phone:** 617-726-6050; **Board Cert:** Therapeutic Radiology 1970; **Med School:** South Korea 1963; **Resid:** Radiation Oncology, Princess Margaret Hosp 1970; **Fac Appt:** Prof RadRO, Harvard Med Sch

D'Amico, Anthony V MD/PhD [RadRO] - **Spec Exp:** Prostate Cancer; Brachytherapy; Urologic Cancer; **Hospital:** Dana-Farber Cancer Inst (page 57), Brigham and Women's Hosp (page 57); **Address:** Brigham & Women's Hosp, Radiation Oncology, L2, 75 Francis St, Boston, MA 02115; **Phone:** 617-632-6328; **Board Cert:** Radiation Oncology 2010; **Med School:** Univ Pennsylvania 1990; **Resid:** Radiation Oncology, Hosp Univ Penn 1994; **Fac Appt:** Prof RadRO, Harvard Med Sch

DeLaney, Thomas F MD [RadRO] - **Spec Exp:** Sarcoma; Proton Beam Therapy; **Hospital:** Mass Genl Hosp; **Address:** Francis H. Burr Proton Therapy Ctr, MGH Radiation Oncology, 30 Fruit St, Boston, MA 02114; **Phone:** 617-726-6876; **Board Cert:** Therapeutic Radiology 1986; Radiation Oncology 1999; **Med School:** Harvard Med Sch 1982; **Resid:** Therapeutic Radiology, Mass Genl Hosp 1986; **Fac Appt:** Assoc Prof RadRO, Harvard Med Sch

Harris, Jay R MD [RadRO] - **Spec Exp:** Breast Cancer; **Hospital:** Brigham and Women's Hosp (page 57), Dana-Farber Cancer Inst (page 57); **Address:** Dana Farber Cancer Inst, 44 Binney St, Dana 1622, Boston, MA 02115; **Phone:** 617-632-2291; **Board Cert:** Therapeutic Radiology 1976; **Med School:** Stanford Univ 1970; **Resid:** Radiation Therapy, Joint Ctr Rad Ther 1976; **Fellow:** Radiation Therapy, Harvard Med Sch 1977; **Fac Appt:** Prof RadRO, Harvard Med Sch

Hartford, Alan C MD/PhD [RadRO] - **Spec Exp:** Prostate Cancer; Brain & Spinal Tumors; **Hospital:** Dartmouth - Hitchcock Med Ctr; **Address:** Darthmouth-Hitchcock Med Ctr, 1 Med Ctr Drive, Lebanon, NH 03756; **Phone:** 603-650-6602; **Board Cert:** Radiation Oncology 2010; **Med School:** Harvard Med Sch 1992; **Resid:** Radiation Oncology, Mass Genl Hosp 1998; **Fellow:** Radiation Oncology, Mass Genl Hosp 1999; **Fac Appt:** Assoc Prof RadRO, Dartmouth Med Sch

Heimann, Ruth MD [RadRO] - **Spec Exp:** Breast Cancer; Gastrointestinal Cancer; Lung Cancer; **Hospital:** Fletcher Allen Health Care- Med Ctr Campus; **Address:** Fletcher Allen Radiation Medicine, 111 Colchester Ave, Burlington, VT 05401; **Phone:** 802-847-3506; **Board Cert:** Radiation Oncology 1995; **Med School:** UMDNJ-NJ Med Sch, Newark 1989; **Resid:** Radiation Oncology, Meml Sloan-Kettering Cancer Ctr 1993; **Fac Appt:** Prof Med, Univ VT Coll Med

Kachnic, Lisa A MD [RadRO] - **Spec Exp:** Breast Cancer; Gastrointestinal Cancer; Thoracic Cancers; **Hospital:** Boston Med Ctr; **Address:** Boston Medical Ctr, Dept Rad/Onc, 830 Harrison Ave, lower level, Boston, MA 02118; **Phone:** 617-638-7070; **Board Cert:** Radiation Oncology 2006; **Med School:** Tufts Univ 1991; **Resid:** Radiation Oncology, Mass Genl Hosp 1996; **Fac Appt:** Assoc Prof RadRO, Boston Univ

Kaplan, Irving D MD [RadRO] - **Spec Exp:** Prostate Cancer; Brachytherapy; **Hospital:** Beth Israel Deaconess Med Ctr - Boston; **Address:** Beth Israel Deaconess Med Ctr, Dept Radiation Oncology, 330 Brookline Ave, Boston, MA 02215; **Phone:** 617-667-2345; **Board Cert:** Radiation Oncology 1989; **Med School:** Stanford Univ 1985; **Resid:** Radiation Oncology, Stanford Univ Med Ctr 1989; **Fac Appt:** Asst Prof RadRO, Harvard Med Sch

Loeffler, Jay S MD [RadRO] - **Spec Exp:** Stereotactic Radiosurgery; Brain Tumors-Benign; Meningioma; Acoustic Neuroma; **Hospital:** Mass Genl Hosp; **Address:** Mass Genl Hosp, Radiation Oncology, 100 Blossom St, Boston, MA 02114; **Phone:** 617-724-1548; **Board Cert:** Therapeutic Radiology 1986; **Med School:** Brown Univ 1982; **Resid:** Radiation Oncology, Harvard Joint Ctr for Rad Ther 1986; **Fellow:** Cancer Biology, Harvard Sch Pub Hlth 1985; **Fac Appt:** Prof RadRO, Harvard Med Sch

Mauch, Peter M MD [RadRO] - **Spec Exp:** Lymphoma; Hodgkin's Disease; **Hospital:** Dana-Farber Cancer Inst (page 57); **Address:** Brigham & Womens Hosp, 75 Francis St, Radiation Oncology ASB1/L2, Boston, MA 02115; **Phone:** 617-732-6310; **Board Cert:** Therapeutic Radiology 1978; **Med School:** St Louis Univ 1974; **Resid:** Radiation Therapy, Harvard Joint Ctr 1978; **Fac Appt:** Prof RadRO, Harvard Med Sch

Peschel, Richard E MD [RadRO] - **Spec Exp:** Prostate Cancer; Testicular Cancer; **Hospital:** Yale-New Haven Hosp, Yale Med Group; **Address:** Yale-New Haven Hosp, Dept Therapeutic Radiology, 15 York St, rm HRT 142, New Haven, CT 06510; **Phone:** 203-785-2957; **Board Cert:** Therapeutic Radiology 1982; **Med School:** Yale Univ 1977; **Resid:** Radiation Oncology, Yale-New Haven Hosp 1981; **Fac Appt:** Prof RadRO, Yale Univ

Recht, Abram MD [RadRO] - **Spec Exp:** Breast Cancer; Gastrointestinal Cancer; Gynecologic Cancer; **Hospital:** Beth Israel Deaconess Med Ctr - Boston; **Address:** 330 Brookline Ave Finard Bldg - rm B25, Beth Israel Deaconess Med Ctr, Boston, MA 02215; **Phone:** 617-667-2345; **Board Cert:** Therapeutic Radiology 1984; **Med School:** Johns Hopkins Univ 1980; **Resid:** Radiation Oncology, Joint Ctr Radiation Therapy 1984; **Fac Appt:** Prof RadRO, Harvard Med Sch

Roberts, Kenneth MD [RadRO] - **Spec Exp:** Pediatric Cancers; Lymphoma; Hodgkin's Disease; **Hospital:** Yale-New Haven Hosp, Yale Med Group; **Address:** Yale Univ Sch Med, Dept Radiation Therapy, 15 York St, New Haven, CT 06520-8040; **Phone:** 203-785-2957; **Board Cert:** Internal Medicine 1987; Medical Oncology 1989; Radiation Oncology 1995; **Med School:** Duke Univ 1984; **Resid:** Internal Medicine, Ohio State Univ Hosps 1987; Radiation Oncology, Duke Univ Med Ctr 1992; **Fellow:** Hematology & Oncology, Duke Univ Med Ctr 1989; **Fac Appt:** Assoc Prof Rad, Yale Univ

Russell, Anthony Henryk MD [RadRO] - **Spec Exp:** Gynecologic Cancer; Intensity Modulated Radiotherapy (IMRT); Proton Beam Therapy; **Hospital:** Mass Genl Hosp; **Address:** Clark Ctr for Radiology, 100 Blossom St, COX 3, Boston, MA 02114; **Phone:** 617-726-5184; **Board Cert:** Therapeutic Radiology 1978; **Med School:** Harvard Med Sch 1974; **Resid:** Radiation Oncology, Mass Genl Hosp 1978

Taghian, Alphonse G MD/PhD [RadRO] - **Spec Exp:** Breast Cancer; **Hospital:** Mass Genl Hosp; **Address:** MGH Dept Radiation Oncology, 100 Blossom St, COX 3, Boston, MA 02114; **Phone:** 617-726-6050; **Board Cert:** Radiation Oncology 2006; **Med School:** Egypt 1980; **Resid:** Radiation Oncology, Vautrin Cancer Ctr 1987; Radiation Oncology, Inst Gustave Roussy 1989; **Fellow:** Radiation Oncology, Mass Genl Hosp 1993; **Fac Appt:** Assoc Prof RadRO, Harvard Med Sch

Tarbell, Nancy MD [RadRO] - **Spec Exp:** Brain Tumors-Pediatric; Proton Beam Therapy; **Hospital:** Mass Genl Hosp; **Address:** Massachusetts Genl Hosp, Proton Ctr, 55 Fruit St, Boston, MA 02114; **Phone:** 617-724-1836; **Board Cert:** Therapeutic Radiology 1983; **Med School:** SUNY Upstate Med Univ 1979; **Resid:** Radiation Therapy, Harvard Med School 1983; **Fac Appt:** Prof RadRO, Harvard Med Sch

Radiation Oncology

Wazer, David E MD [RadRO] - **Spec Exp:** Breast Cancer; Melanoma; **Hospital:** Rhode Island Hosp, Tufts Med Ctr; **Address:** 593 Eddy St, Providence, RI 02903; **Phone:** 401-444-8311; **Board Cert:** Radiation Oncology 1988; **Med School:** NYU Sch Med 1982; **Resid:** Radiation Oncology, Tufts New Eng Med Ctr 1988; **Fellow:** Neurological Chemistry, NYU Med Ctr 1984; **Fac Appt:** Prof RadRO, Tufts Univ

Wilson, Lynn D MD [RadRO] - **Spec Exp:** Lymphoma, Cutaneous T Cell (CTCL); Lymphoma, Cutaneous B Cell (CBCL); Lung Cancer; Head & Neck Cancer; **Hospital:** Yale-New Haven Hosp, Yale Med Group; **Address:** Yale Univ Sch Med, Dept Therapeutic Rad, PO Box 208040, New Haven, CT 06520-8040; **Phone:** 203-688-4344; **Board Cert:** Radiation Oncology 2004; **Med School:** Geo Wash Univ 1990; **Resid:** Therapeutic Radiology, Yale-New Haven Hosp 1994; **Fac Appt:** Prof RadRO, Yale Univ

Zietman, Anthony L MD [RadRO] - **Spec Exp:** Prostate Cancer; Urologic Cancer; Proton Beam Therapy; **Hospital:** Mass Genl Hosp; **Address:** Mass General Hosp, Yawkey Ste 7E, 55 Fruit St, Boston, MA 02114; **Phone:** 617-724-1158; **Board Cert:** Radiation Oncology 1994; **Med School:** England, UK 1983; **Resid:** Internal Medicine, St Stephens & Westminster Hosp 1986; Radiation Oncology, Mass Genl Hosp 1989; **Fellow:** Radiation Oncology, Middlesex Hosp 1991; Radiation Oncology, Mass Genl Hosp; **Fac Appt:** Prof RadRO, Harvard Med Sch

Mid Atlantic

Berg, Christine D MD [RadRO] - **Spec Exp:** Breast Cancer-Early Detection; Breast Cancer-High Risk Women; **Hospital:** Natl Inst of Hlth - Clin Ctr; **Address:** 6130 Executive Blvd, Bethesda, MD 20892; **Phone:** 301-496-8544; **Board Cert:** Internal Medicine 1980; Medical Oncology 1983; Therapeutic Radiology 1986; Radiation Oncology 1999; **Med School:** Northwestern Univ 1977; **Resid:** Internal Medicine, Northwestern Meml Hosp 1981; Radiation Oncology, Georgetown Univ Hosp 1986; **Fellow:** Medical Oncology, Natl Cancer Inst-NIH 1984

Bogart, Jeffrey A MD [RadRO] - **Spec Exp:** Lung Cancer; Thoracic Cancers; Prostate Cancer; Clinical Trials; **Hospital:** SUNY Upstate Med Univ Shos; **Address:** SUNY Upstate Medical Ctr, Dept Radiation Oncology, 750 E Adams St, Syracuse, NY 13210; **Phone:** 315-464-5276; **Board Cert:** Radiation Oncology 1994; **Med School:** SUNY Upstate Med Univ 1989; **Resid:** Radiation Oncology, SUNY Hlth Sci Ctr 1993; **Fac Appt:** Prof RadRO, SUNY Upstate Med Univ

Chao, KS Clifford MD [RadRO] - **Spec Exp:** Intensity Modulated Radiotherapy (IMRT); **Hospital:** NY-Presby/Weill Cornell Med Ctr, NY (page 65); **Address:** 622 W 168th St, New York, NY 10032; **Phone:** 212-305-9987; **Board Cert:** Radiation Oncology 2010; **Med School:** Taiwan 1982; **Resid:** Radiation Oncology, Mallinckrodt Inst Rad-Wash Med Ctr 1993; **Fellow:** Radiation Oncology, Mallinckrodt Inst Rad-Wash Med Ctr 1994; **Fac Appt:** Prof RadRO, Cornell Univ-Weill Med Coll

Constine, Louis Sanders MD [RadRO] - **Spec Exp:** Pediatric Cancers; Lymphoma; Cancer Survivors-Late Effects of Therapy; Sarcoma; **Hospital:** Univ of Rochester Strong Meml Hosp; **Address:** 601 Elmwood Ave, Box 647, Rochester, NY 14642; **Phone:** 585-275-5622; **Board Cert:** Pediatrics 1978; Therapeutic Radiology 1981; Pediatric Hematology-Oncology 1978; **Med School:** Johns Hopkins Univ 1973; **Resid:** Pediatrics, Moffitt Hosp-UCSF Med Ctr 1975; Pediatrics, Stanford Hosp Med Ctr 1976; **Fellow:** Therapeutic Radiology, Stanford Hosp Med Ctr 1981; Pediatric Hematology-Oncology, Univ Wash/Chldns Ortho Hosp 1978; **Fac Appt:** Prof RadRO, Univ Rochester

Cooper, Jay MD [RadRO] - **Spec Exp:** Head & Neck Cancer; Skin Cancer; Chemo-Radiation Combined Therapy; **Hospital:** Maimonides Med Ctr (page 62); **Address:** 6300 8th Ave, Brooklyn, NY 11220; **Phone:** 718-765-2700; **Board Cert:** Therapeutic Radiology 1977; **Med School:** NYU Sch Med 1973; **Resid:** Radiation Oncology, NYU Med Ctr 1977; **Fac Appt:** Prof RadRO, Albert Einstein Coll Med

DeWeese, Theodore L MD [RadRO] - **Spec Exp:** Urologic Cancer; Prostate Cancer; Testicular Cancer; **Hospital:** Johns Hopkins Hosp (page 61); **Address:** Johns Hopkins Hosp, Weinberg Bldg, 401 N Broadway, rm 1363, Baltimore, MD 21231; **Phone:** 410-955-8964; **Board Cert:** Radiation Oncology 2005; **Med School:** Univ Colorado 1990; **Resid:** Radiation Oncology, Johns Hopkins Hosp 1994; **Fellow:** Urologic Oncology, Johns Hopkins Hosp 1995; **Fac Appt:** Prof RadRO, Johns Hopkins Univ

Dicker, Adam P MD/PhD [RadRO] - **Spec Exp:** Prostate Cancer; **Hospital:** Thomas Jefferson Univ Hosp; **Address:** Bodine Cancer Treatment Ctr, 111 South 11th St, Philadelphia, PA 19107-5097; **Phone:** 215-955-6527; **Board Cert:** Radiation Oncology 2000; **Med School:** Cornell Univ-Weill Med Coll 1992; **Resid:** Surgery, Lenox Hill Hosp 1994; Radiation Oncology, Meml Sloan Kettering Cancer Ctr 1997; **Fac Appt:** Prof RadRO, Thomas Jefferson Univ

Donahue, Bernadine R MD [RadRO] - **Spec Exp:** Brain Tumors; Gastrointestinal Cancer; Pediatric Cancers; Solid Tumors; **Hospital:** Maimonides Med Ctr (page 62); **Address:** Maimonides Med Ctr, Dept Radiation Oncology, 6300 8th Ave, Lower Level, Brooklyn, NY 11220; **Phone:** 718-765-2700; **Board Cert:** Internal Medicine 1987; Radiation Oncology 1991; **Med School:** Boston Univ 1984; **Resid:** Internal Medicine, Boston Univ Med Ctr 1987; **Fellow:** Radiation Oncology, NYU Med Ctr 1990

Dritschilo, Anatoly MD [RadRO] - **Spec Exp:** Prostate Cancer; **Hospital:** Georgetown Univ Hosp; **Address:** Georgetown Univ Hosp, Dept Radiation Medicine, LL-Bles, 3800 Reservoir Rd NW, Washington, DC 20007; **Phone:** 202-687-2144; **Board Cert:** Therapeutic Radiology 1977; **Med School:** UMDNJ-NJ Med Sch, Newark 1973; **Resid:** Radiation Therapy, Harvard Joint Rad Ther Ctr 1977; **Fac Appt:** Prof Med, Georgetown Univ

Ennis, Ronald D MD [RadRO] - **Spec Exp:** Prostate Cancer; Brachytherapy; Breast Cancer; **Hospital:** St. Luke's - Roosevelt Hosp Ctr - Roosevelt Div (page 55), Beth Israel Med Ctr - Petrie Division (page 55); **Address:** 1000 10th Ave, Lower Level, New York, NY 10019; **Phone:** 212-523-7165; **Board Cert:** Radiation Oncology 2005; **Med School:** Yale Univ 1990; **Resid:** Therapeutic Radiology, Yale-New Haven Hosp 1994

Flickinger, John C MD [RadRO] - **Spec Exp:** Neuro-Oncology; Brain & Spinal Tumors; **Hospital:** UPMC Presby, Pittsburgh; **Address:** UPMC Cancer Ctr, Radiation Oncology, 5230 Centre Ave, Pittsburgh, PA 15213; **Phone:** 412-647-3600; **Board Cert:** Therapeutic Radiology 1985; **Med School:** Univ Chicago-Pritzker Sch Med 1981; **Resid:** Radiation Therapy, Mass Genl Hosp 1985; **Fac Appt:** Prof RadRO, Univ Pittsburgh

Formenti, Silvia C MD [RadRO] - **Spec Exp:** Breast Cancer; Chemo-Radiation Combined Therapy; **Hospital:** NYU Langone Med Ctr (page 66); **Address:** NYU Med Ctr, Dept Radiation Oncology, 160 E 34th St, New York, NY 10016; **Phone:** 212-263-2601; **Board Cert:** Radiation Oncology 1991; **Med School:** Italy 1980; **Resid:** Internal Medicine, San Carlo Borromeo Hosp 1983; Medical Oncology, Univ of Pavia Med Ctr 1985; **Fellow:** Radiation Oncology, USC Med Ctr 1990; **Fac Appt:** Prof RadRO, NYU Sch Med

Freedman, Gary M MD [RadRO] - **Spec Exp:** Breast Cancer; **Hospital:** Hosp Univ Penn - UPHS (page 68); **Address:** Hosp Univ Penn, Dept Radiation Oncology, 3400 Spruce St, Philadelphia, PA 19104; **Phone:** 215-615-6767; **Board Cert:** Radiation Oncology 2000; **Med School:** Temple Univ 1993; **Resid:** Radiation Oncology, Fox Chase Cancer Ctr 1997; **Fac Appt:** Assoc Prof RadRO, Univ Pennsylvania

Gejerman, Glen MD [RadRO] - **Spec Exp:** Prostate Cancer; Intensity Modulated Radiotherapy (IMRT); Breast Cancer; Brachytherapy; **Hospital:** Hackensack Univ Med Ctr; **Address:** Hackensack Univ Med Ctr, Radiation Onc, 30 Prospect Ave, Hackensack, NJ 07601; **Phone:** 201-996-2464; **Board Cert:** Radiation Oncology 2006; **Med School:** UMDNJ-NJ Med Sch, Newark 1990; **Resid:** Radiation Oncology, Montefiore Med Ctr 1995; **Fac Appt:** Asst Clin Prof RadRO, Albert Einstein Coll Med

Goodman, Robert L MD [RadRO] - **Spec Exp:** Breast Cancer; Lymphoma; Prostate Cancer; Brain Tumors; **Hospital:** Saint Barnabas Med Ctr; **Address:** St Barnabas Med Ctr, Dept Rad Oncology, 94 Old Short Hills Rd, Livingston, NJ 07039; **Phone:** 973-322-5133; **Board Cert:** Internal Medicine 1971; Therapeutic Radiology 1974; Medical Oncology 1975; **Med School:** Columbia P&S 1966; **Resid:** Internal Medicine, Beth Israel Hosp 1970; Radiation Therapy, Harvard Joint Ctr Rad Therapy 1974; **Fellow:** Hematology, NY-Presby Hosp 1969

Greenberger, Joel S MD [RadRO] - **Spec Exp:** Lung Cancer; Esophageal Cancer; **Hospital:** UPMC Presby, Pittsburgh; **Address:** UPMC Cancer Ctr, Cancer Pavilion, 5230 Centre Ave, Pittsburgh, PA 15232; **Phone:** 412-647-3600; **Board Cert:** Therapeutic Radiology 1977; **Med School:** Harvard Med Sch 1971; **Resid:** Radiation Therapy, Mass General Hosp 1977; **Fac Appt:** Prof RadRO, Univ Pittsburgh

Haffty, Bruce MD [RadRO] - **Spec Exp:** Breast Cancer; Head & Neck Cancer; Lung Cancer; **Hospital:** Robert Wood Johnson Univ Hosp - New Brunswick, Robert Wood Johnson Univ Hosp Hamilton; **Address:** The Cancer Institute of New Jersey, 195 Little Albany St, rm 2038, New Brunswick, NJ 08903; **Phone:** 732-253-3939; **Board Cert:** Radiation Oncology 1988; **Med School:** Yale Univ 1984; **Resid:** Radiation Oncology, Yale-New Haven Hosp 1988; **Fac Appt:** Prof RadRO

Hahn, Stephen M MD [RadRO] - **Spec Exp:** Lung Cancer; Prostate Cancer; Sarcoma; Photodynamic Therapy; **Hospital:** Hosp Univ Penn - UPHS (page 68), Penn Presby Med Ctr - UPHS (page 68); **Address:** Hosp of the Univ of Penn, 3400 Spruce St Donner Bldg Fl 2, Philadelphia, PA 19104; **Phone:** 215-662-7296; **Board Cert:** Internal Medicine 1987; Medical Oncology 2001; Radiation Oncology 2004; **Med School:** Temple Univ 1984; **Resid:** Internal Medicine, UCSF Med Ctr 1988; Medical Oncology, Natl Inst Hlth 1991; **Fellow:** Radiation Oncology, Natl Inst Hlth 1994; **Fac Appt:** Prof RadRO, Univ Pennsylvania

Harrison, Louis B MD [RadRO] - **Spec Exp:** Brachytherapy; Head & Neck Cancer; Radiation Therapy-Intraoperative; **Hospital:** Beth Israel Med Ctr - Petrie Division (page 55), St. Luke's - Roosevelt Hosp Ctr - Roosevelt Div (page 55); **Address:** Beth Israel Med Ctr, Dept Rad Onc, 10 Union Square East, Ste 4G, New York, NY 10003-3314; **Phone:** 212-844-8087; **Board Cert:** Therapeutic Radiology 1986; **Med School:** SUNY Downstate 1982; **Resid:** Therapeutic Radiology, Yale-New Haven Hosp 1986; **Fac Appt:** Prof RadRO, Albert Einstein Coll Med

Horwitz, Eric MD [RadRO] - **Spec Exp:** Prostate Cancer; Intensity Modulated Radiotherapy (IMRT); Brachytherapy; **Hospital:** Fox Chase Cancer Ctr (page 58); **Address:** Fox Chase Cancer Ctr, Dept Radiation Oncology, 333 Cottman Ave, Philadelphia, PA 19111; **Phone:** 215-728-2995; **Board Cert:** Radiation Oncology 2010; **Med School:** Albany Med Coll 1992; **Resid:** Radiation Oncology, William Beaumont Hosp 1997

Isaacson, Steven R MD [RadRO] - **Spec Exp:** Brain Tumors; Neuro-Oncology; Stereotactic Radiosurgery; Arteriovenous Malformations; **Hospital:** NY-Presby/Columbia Univ Med Ctr, NY (page 65); **Address:** NY Presbyterian-Columbia Med Ctr, Dept Radiation Oncology, 622 W 168th St BHN Bldg - rm B-11, New York, NY 10032-3720; **Phone:** 212-305-2611; **Board Cert:** Radiation Oncology 1988; Otolaryngology 1978; **Med School:** Jefferson Med Coll 1973; **Resid:** Otolaryngology, Hosp Univ Penn 1978; Radiation Oncology, SUNY Hlth Sci Ctr 1988; **Fac Appt:** Clin Prof RadRO, Columbia P&S

Kleinberg, Lawrence MD [RadRO] - **Spec Exp:** Brain & Spinal Cord Tumors; Brain Tumors-Metastatic; Stereotactic Radiosurgery; Esophageal Cancer; **Hospital:** Johns Hopkins Hosp (page 61); **Address:** Johns Hopkins Oncology Ctr Weinberg Bldg, 401 N Broadway, Ste 1440, Baltimore, MD 21231; **Phone:** 410-614-2597; **Board Cert:** Radiation Oncology 1994; **Med School:** Yale Univ 1989; **Resid:** Radiation Oncology, Meml Sloan-Kettering Canc Ctr 1993; **Fac Appt:** Assoc Prof RadRO, Johns Hopkins Univ

Kuettel, Michael R MD/PhD [RadRO] - **Spec Exp:** Prostate Cancer; **Hospital:** Roswell Park Cancer Inst; **Address:** Roswell Park Cancer Inst, Radiation Med, Elm and Carlton St, Buffalo, NY 14263; **Phone:** 716-845-1562; **Board Cert:** Radiation Oncology 1992; **Med School:** Northwestern Univ 1985; **Resid:** Internal Medicine, Northwestern Hosp 1986; Radiation Oncology, Johns Hopkins Hosp 1990; **Fac Appt:** Prof RadRO, SUNY Buffalo

Lepanto, Philip B MD [RadRO] - **Hospital:** St. Mary's Med Ctr - Huntington, Cabell Huntington Hosp; **Address:** St Mary's Med Ctr, Dept Radiation Oncology, 2900 First Ave, Huntington, WV 25702; **Phone:** 304-526-1143; **Board Cert:** Therapeutic Radiology 1975; **Med School:** Univ Louisville Sch Med 1970; **Resid:** Diagnostic Radiology, Graduate Hosp 1972; Radiation Therapy, Hosp Univ Penn 1975; **Fac Appt:** Clin Prof Rad, Marshall Univ

McCormick, Beryl MD [RadRO] - **Spec Exp:** Breast Cancer; Eye Tumors/Cancer; **Hospital:** Meml Sloan-Kettering Cancer Ctr, NY-Presby/Weill Cornell Med Ctr, NY (page 65); **Address:** 1275 York Avenue, New York, NY 10065; **Phone:** 800-525-2225; **Board Cert:** Therapeutic Radiology 1977; **Med School:** UMDNJ-NJ Med Sch, Newark 1973; **Resid:** Therapeutic Radiology, Meml Sloan Kettering Cancer Ctr 1977; **Fac Appt:** Prof RadRO, Cornell Univ-Weill Med Coll

Nicolaou, Nicos MD [RadRO] - **Spec Exp:** Lymphoma; Hodgkin's Disease; Urologic Cancer; Breast Cancer; **Address:** Phila Cancer Treatment, 1 Presidential Blvd, Ste 100, Bala Cynwyd, PA 19004; **Phone:** 610-632-4100; **Board Cert:** Radiation Oncology 2010; **Med School:** South Africa 1984; **Resid:** Radiation Oncology, Univ British Columbia Cancer Ctr 1994; **Fellow:** Radiation Oncology, Fox Chase Cancer Ctr 1995

Nori, Dattatreyudu MD [RadRO] - **Spec Exp:** Prostate Cancer; Brachytherapy; Lung Cancer; Breast Cancer; **Hospital:** NY-Presby/Weill Cornell Med Ctr, NY (page 65), NY Hosp Queens; **Address:** 525 E 68th St, Box 575, New York, NY 10065; **Phone:** 212-746-3679; **Board Cert:** Therapeutic Radiology 1979; **Med School:** India 1970; **Resid:** Radiation Oncology, Meml Sloan Kettering Cancer Ctr 1975; **Fellow:** Radiation Oncology, Meml Sloan Kettering Cancer Ctr 1978; **Fac Appt:** Prof RadRO, Cornell Univ-Weill Med Coll

Porrazzo, Michael S MD [RadRO] - **Spec Exp:** Prostate Cancer; Central Nervous System Cancer; Breast Cancer; Stereotactic Radiosurgery; **Hospital:** Washington Hosp Ctr; **Address:** Wash Hosp Ctr-Dept. Radiation Onc, 110 Irving St NW, Rm CG-107, Washington, DC 20010; **Phone:** 202-877-3925; **Board Cert:** Radiation Oncology 1990; **Med School:** Meharry Med Coll 1985; **Resid:** Radiation Oncology, SUNY Hlth Sci Ctr 1989

Radiation Oncology

Randolph-Jackson, Pamela D MD [RadRO] - **Spec Exp:** Breast Cancer; Lung Cancer; Gastrointestinal Cancer; **Hospital:** Washington Hosp Ctr; **Address:** 110 Irving St NW, CG 116, Washington, DC 20010; **Phone:** 202-877-3925; **Board Cert:** Radiation Oncology 2004; **Med School:** E Tenn State Univ 1988; **Resid:** Radiology, Howard Univ Hosp 1992; **Fellow:** Radiation Oncology, Jefferson Med Coll 1993

Regine, William F MD [RadRO] - **Spec Exp:** Stereotactic Radiosurgery; Brain & Spinal Tumors; Gastrointestinal Cancer; **Hospital:** Univ of MD Med Ctr; **Address:** Univ MD Med System-Greenbaum Cancer Ctr, 22 S Green St Guldelsky Bldg, Baltimore, MD 21201; **Phone:** 410-328-6080; **Board Cert:** Radiation Oncology 1992; **Med School:** SUNY Upstate Med Univ 1987; **Resid:** Radiation Oncology, Thomas Jefferson Univ Hosp 1991; **Fellow:** Radiation Oncology, Thomas Jefferson Univ Hosp 1992; **Fac Appt:** Prof RadRO, Univ MD Sch Med

Rotman, Marvin MD [RadRO] - **Spec Exp:** Bladder Cancer; Gynecologic Cancer; Eye Tumors/Cancer; Prostate Cancer; **Hospital:** SUNY Downstate Med Ctr, Univ Hosp of Bklyn at Long Island Coll Hosp; **Address:** 450 Clarkson Ave, Box 1211, Brooklyn, NY 11203-2056; **Phone:** 718-270-2181; **Board Cert:** Diagnostic Radiology 1966; Radiation Oncology 1999; **Med School:** Jefferson Med Coll 1958; **Resid:** Internal Medicine, Albert Einstein Med Ctr 1960; Radiation Oncology, Montefiore Hosp Med Ctr 1965; **Fac Appt:** Prof RadRO, SUNY Downstate

Schiff, Peter B MD/PhD [RadRO] - **Spec Exp:** Prostate Cancer; Gynecologic Cancer; Breast Cancer; **Hospital:** NYU Langone Med Ctr (page 66); **Address:** NYU Clinical Cancer Ctr, 160 E 34th St Fl 1, New York, NY 10016; **Phone:** 212-731-5003; **Board Cert:** Radiation Oncology 1990; **Med School:** Albert Einstein Coll Med 1984; **Resid:** Radiation Oncology, Meml Sloan Kettering Cancer Ctr 1988; **Fac Appt:** Prof RadRO, NYU Sch Med

Solin, Lawrence J MD [RadRO] - **Spec Exp:** Breast Cancer; **Hospital:** Albert Einstein Med Ctr; **Address:** Albert Einstein Medical Center, Dept Radiation Oncology, 5501 Old York Rd, Philadelphia, PA 19141; **Phone:** 215-456-6280; **Board Cert:** Therapeutic Radiology 1984; **Med School:** Brown Univ 1978; **Resid:** Surgery, Thos Jefferson Univ Hosp 1981; Radiation Oncology, Thos Jefferson Univ Hosp 1982; **Fellow:** Radiation Oncology, Hosp Univ Penn 1984; **Fac Appt:** Prof Emeritus RadRO, Univ Pennsylvania

Stock, Richard MD [RadRO] - **Spec Exp:** Prostate Cancer; **Hospital:** Mount Sinai Med Ctr (page 63); **Address:** Dept Radiation Oncology, 1184 5th Ave, Box 1236, New York, NY 10029; **Phone:** 212-241-7502; **Board Cert:** Radiation Oncology 1993; **Med School:** Mount Sinai Sch Med 1988; **Resid:** Radiation Oncology, Meml Sloan Kettering Cancer Ctr 1992; **Fac Appt:** Prof RadRO, Mount Sinai Sch Med

Streeter Jr, Oscar E MD [RadRO] - **Spec Exp:** Lung Cancer; Head & Neck Cancer; **Hospital:** Howard Univ Hosp; **Address:** Howard Univ Hosp, Dept Radiation Onc, 2041 Georgia Ave NW, Washington, DC 20060; **Phone:** 202-865-6100; **Board Cert:** Radiation Oncology 1989; **Med School:** Howard Univ 1982; **Resid:** Radiation Oncology, Howard Univ 1986; Radiation Oncology, USC Sch Med 1994; **Fac Appt:** Assoc Prof RadRO, USC Sch Med

Suntharalingam, Mohan MD [RadRO] - **Spec Exp:** Head & Neck Cancer; Lung Cancer; Esophageal Cancer; **Hospital:** Univ of MD Med Ctr; **Address:** 22 S Greene St, Baltimore, MD 21201; **Phone:** 410-328-2331; **Board Cert:** Radiation Oncology 2005; **Med School:** Thomas Jefferson Univ 1990; **Resid:** Radiation Oncology, Univ Maryland Med Ctr 1993; **Fellow:** Radiation Oncology, Univ Maryland Med Ctr 1994; **Fac Appt:** Prof RadRO, Univ MD Sch Med

Weiss, Marisa C MD [RadRO] - **Spec Exp:** Breast Cancer; **Hospital:** Lankenau Hosp; **Address:** Lankenau Hospital, Dept Rad Oncology, 100 E Lancaster Ave, Wynnewood, PA 19096; **Phone:** 484-476-2433; **Board Cert:** Radiation Oncology 1988; **Med School:** Univ Pennsylvania 1984; **Resid:** Radiation Oncology, Hosp Univ Penn 1988; **Fellow:** Radiological Biology, Hosp Univ Penn 1990

Werner-Wasik, Maria MD [RadRO] - **Spec Exp:** Brain Tumors; Lung Cancer; Melanoma; Breast Cancer; **Hospital:** Thomas Jefferson Univ Hosp; **Address:** Thomas Jefferson Univ Hosp, Dept Radiation Oncology, 111 S 11 St, Philadelphia, PA 19107; **Phone:** 215-955-6702; **Board Cert:** Radiation Oncology 1994; **Med School:** Poland 1979; **Resid:** Internal Medicine, Framingham Union Hosp 1990; Radiation Oncology, Tufts/New England Med Ctr 1993; **Fellow:** Radiation Oncology, Hosp Univ Penn 1994; **Fac Appt:** Assoc Prof RadRO, Thomas Jefferson Univ

Wharam Jr, Moody D MD [RadRO] - **Spec Exp:** Pediatric Cancers; Brain Tumors; Sarcoma-Soft Tissue; **Hospital:** Johns Hopkins Hosp (page 61); **Address:** Kimmel Cancer Ctr, Dept Rad Oncology, 401 N Broadway St, Ste 1440, Baltimore, MD 21231-2410; **Phone:** 410-955-8964; **Board Cert:** Therapeutic Radiology 1974; **Med School:** Univ VA Sch Med 1969; **Resid:** Radiation Oncology, UCSF Med Ctr 1973; **Fac Appt:** Prof RadRO, Johns Hopkins Univ

Yahalom, Joachim MD [RadRO] - **Spec Exp:** Lymphoma; Hodgkin's Disease; Multiple Myeloma; **Hospital:** Meml Sloan-Kettering Cancer Ctr; **Address:** 1275 York Ave, SM03, Dept Radiation Onc, New York, NY 10065; **Phone:** 212-639-5999; **Board Cert:** Radiation Oncology 1988; **Med School:** Israel 1976; **Resid:** Internal Medicine, Hadassah Hosp 1979; Radiation Oncology, Hadassah Hosp 1984; **Fellow:** Radiation Oncology, Meml Sloan Kettering Canc Ctr 1986; **Fac Appt:** Prof RadRO, Cornell Univ-Weill Med Coll

Zelefsky, Michael J MD [RadRO] - **Spec Exp:** Prostate Cancer; Brachytherapy; Head & Neck Cancer; **Hospital:** Meml Sloan-Kettering Cancer Ctr; **Address:** 1275 York Avenue, New York, NY 10065; **Phone:** 800-525-2225; **Board Cert:** Radiation Oncology 1991; **Med School:** Albert Einstein Coll Med 1986; **Resid:** Radiation Oncology, Meml Sloan Kettering Cancer Ctr 1990; **Fac Appt:** Prof RadRO, Cornell Univ-Weill Med Coll

Southeast

Anscher, Mitchell S MD [RadRO] - **Spec Exp:** Prostate Cancer; Brachytherapy; Penile Cancer; Testicular Cancer; **Hospital:** Med Coll of VA Hosp, Hunter Holmes McGuire VA Med Ctr - Richmond; **Address:** 401 College St, Box 980058, Department of Radiation Oncology, Richmond, VA 23298-0058; **Phone:** 804-828-7238; **Board Cert:** Internal Medicine 1984; Radiation Oncology 1987; **Med School:** Med Coll VA 1981; **Resid:** Internal Medicine, St Marys Hosp 1984; Radiation Oncology, Duke Univ Med Ctr 1987; **Fac Appt:** Prof RadRO, Va Commonwealth Univ Sch Med

Beitler, Jonathan J MD [RadRO] - **Spec Exp:** Head & Neck Cancer; Breast Cancer; Lung Cancer; Brachytherapy; **Hospital:** Emory Univ Hosp; **Address:** Winship Cancer Institute, Dept Radiation Oncology, 1365C Clifton Rd NE, Atlanta, GA 30322; **Phone:** 404-778-3473; **Board Cert:** Radiation Oncology 2000; **Med School:** Med Coll PA Hahnemann 1982; **Resid:** Surgery, Downstate Med Ctr 1985; Radiation Oncology, Meml Sloan Kettering Cancer Ctr 1988; **Fac Appt:** Prof RadRO, Emory Univ

Blackstock, A William MD [RadRO] - **Spec Exp:** Lung Cancer; Gastrointestinal Cancer; Clinical Trials; **Hospital:** Wake Forest Univ Baptist Med Ctr; **Address:** Wake Forest, Comprehensive Cancer Ctr, Dept Radiation Oncology, Medical Center Blvd, Winston-Salem, NC 27157; **Phone:** 336-713-3600; **Board Cert:** Radiation Oncology 2006; **Med School:** E Carolina Univ 1989; **Resid:** Radiation Oncology, Univ NC Hosps 1994; **Fac Appt:** Prof RadRO, Wake Forest Univ

Radiation Oncology

Bonner, James Alan MD [RadRO] - **Spec Exp:** Head & Neck Cancer; Lung Cancer; **Hospital:** Univ of Ala Hosp at Birmingham; **Address:** UAB- Birmingham, Dept Rad Onc, 1700 6th Ave S, rm 2262, Birmingham, AL 35294; **Phone:** 205-934-2761; **Board Cert:** Radiation Oncology 1990; **Med School:** Wayne State Univ 1985; **Resid:** Radiation Oncology, Univ Michigan Med Ctr 1989; **Fac Appt:** Prof RadRO, Univ Alabama

Brizel, David M MD [RadRO] - **Spec Exp:** Head & Neck Cancer; Sarcoma; **Hospital:** Duke Univ Hosp; **Address:** Duke Univ Med Ctr, Dept Rad Onc, Box 3085, Durham, NC 27710-0001; **Phone:** 919-668-5637; **Board Cert:** Radiation Oncology 1987; **Med School:** Northwestern Univ 1983; **Resid:** Radiation Oncology, Harvard Joint Ctr Radiation Ther 1987; **Fac Appt:** Prof RadRO, Duke Univ

Chakravarthy, Anuradha M MD [RadRO] - **Spec Exp:** Breast Cancer; Gastrointestinal Cancer; **Hospital:** Vanderbilt Univ Med Ctr (page 76); **Address:** Vanderbilt Radiation Oncology, 22nd St at Pierce Ave, B-1003 TVC Bldg, Nashville, TN 37232; **Phone:** 615-322-2555; **Board Cert:** Radiation Oncology 1994; Internal Medicine 1986; Medical Oncology 1989; **Med School:** Geo Wash Univ 1983; **Resid:** Internal Medicine, Mayo Clinic 1986; Medical Oncology, Univ MD Cancer Ctr 1990; **Fellow:** Radiation Oncology, Johns Hopkins Hosp 1993; **Fac Appt:** Assoc Prof RadRO, Vanderbilt Univ

Cmelak, Anthony J MD [RadRO] - **Spec Exp:** Brain Cancer; Stereotactic Radiosurgery; **Hospital:** Vanderbilt Univ Med Ctr (page 76); **Address:** Vanderbilt Dept of Radiation Oncology, B-1003 TVC, 22nd Pierce Ave, Nashville, TN 37232-5671; **Phone:** 615-322-2555; **Board Cert:** Radiation Oncology 2008; **Med School:** Northwestern Univ 1992; **Resid:** Radiation Oncology, Stanford Univ Med Ctr 1996; **Fac Appt:** Assoc Prof RadRO, Vanderbilt Univ

Crocker, Ian R MD [RadRO] - **Spec Exp:** Brain Tumors; Eye Tumors/Cancer; Melanoma-Choroidal (eye); **Hospital:** Emory Univ Hosp, Emory Univ Hosp Midtown; **Address:** The Emory Clinic, Dept Radiation Onc, 1365C Clifton Rd NE, CT-104, Atlanta, GA 30322; **Phone:** 404-778-3473; **Board Cert:** Therapeutic Radiology 1983; Internal Medicine 1980; **Med School:** Univ Saskatchewan 1976; **Resid:** Internal Medicine, Univ Hosp-Univ West Ontario 1980; **Fellow:** Radiation Oncology, Princess Margaret Hosp-Univ Toronto 1983; **Fac Appt:** Prof RadRO, Emory Univ

Fiveash, John MD [RadRO] - **Spec Exp:** Brain Tumors; Pediatric Cancers; **Hospital:** Univ of Ala Hosp at Birmingham; **Address:** Hazelrig-Salter Radiation-Oncology Ctr, 1700 6th Ave, Birmingham, AL 35249; **Phone:** 205-934-9999; **Board Cert:** Radiation Oncology 2009; **Med School:** Med Coll GA 1993; **Resid:** Radiation Oncology, GA Hlth Sci Univ 1997

Halle, Jan MD [RadRO] - **Spec Exp:** Breast Cancer; Lung Cancer; **Hospital:** NC Memorial Hosp - UNC, Rex HlthCare; **Address:** Univ North Carolina Sch Med, Dept Rad Onc, 101 Manning Drive, CB 7512, Chapel Hill, NC 27514; **Phone:** 919-445-5218; **Board Cert:** Therapeutic Radiology 1982; **Med School:** Tufts Univ 1975; **Resid:** Radiation Oncology, North Carolina Meml Hosp 1981; **Fac Appt:** Assoc Prof RadRO, Univ NC Sch Med

Henderson, Randal H MD [RadRO] - **Spec Exp:** Gynecologic Cancer; Prostate Cancer; Brachytherapy; Proton Beam Therapy; **Hospital:** Shands at Univ of FL; **Address:** Univ Florida Proton Therapy Inst, 2015 N Jefferson St, Jacksonville, FL 32206; **Phone:** 904-588-1800; **Board Cert:** Therapeutic Radiology 1984; **Med School:** Texas Tech Univ 1979; **Resid:** Radiation Oncology, Univ Florida/Shands Hosp 1983; **Fac Appt:** Prof RadRO, Univ Fla Coll Med

Jose, Baby Oliapuram MD [RadRO] - **Spec Exp:** Head & Neck Cancer; Lung Cancer; Gynecologic Cancer; Prostate Cancer; **Hospital:** Univ of Louisville Hosp, Floyd Meml Hosp & Hlth Svcs; **Address:** James G Brown Cancer Center, 529 S Jackson St Fl 4, Louisville, KY 40202; **Phone:** 502-562-4759; **Board Cert:** Therapeutic Radiology 1978; **Med School:** India 1971; **Resid:** Surgery, CMC Hosp 1974; Radiation Oncology, CMC Hosp 1976; **Fellow:** Radiation Oncology, Brown Univ-RI Hosp 1979; **Fac Appt:** Prof RadRO, Univ Louisville Sch Med

Kudrimoti, Mahesh R MD [RadRO] - **Spec Exp:** Lung Cancer; Head & Neck Cancer; Brachytherapy; **Hospital:** Univ of Kentucky Albert B. Chandler Hosp; **Address:** UKMC, Dept Radiation Oncology, 800 Rose St, C-113, Lexington, KY 40536; **Phone:** 859-323-6486; **Board Cert:** Radiation Oncology 2003; **Med School:** India 1992; **Resid:** Radiation Oncology, Univ KY Chandler Med Ctr 2001; **Fac Appt:** Assoc Prof RadRO, Univ KY Coll Med

Kun, Larry E MD [RadRO] - **Spec Exp:** Brain Tumors; Pediatric Cancers; **Hospital:** St. Jude Children's Research Hosp, Le Bonheur Chldns Med Ctr; **Address:** St Jude Chldns Research Hosp, 262 Danny Thomas Pl, MS 220, Memphis, TN 38105; **Phone:** 901-595-3565; **Board Cert:** Therapeutic Radiology 1973; **Med School:** Jefferson Med Coll 1968; **Resid:** Therapeutic Radiology, Penrose Cancer Hosp 1972; **Fellow:** Radiation Oncology, Natl Cancer Inst 1974; Radiation Oncology, Rotterdam Radiotherapy Inst 1975; **Fac Appt:** Prof, Univ Tenn Coll Med

Landry, Jerome C MD [RadRO] - **Spec Exp:** Gastrointestinal Cancer; Sarcoma-Soft Tissue; **Hospital:** Emory Univ Hosp, Grady Hlth Sys; **Address:** Emory Dept Radiation Oncology, 1365C Clifton Rd NE, Atlanta, GA 30322; **Phone:** 404-778-3473; **Board Cert:** Radiation Oncology 1988; **Med School:** Harvard Med Sch 1983; **Resid:** Radiation Oncology, Mass Genl Hosp 1987; **Fac Appt:** Prof RadRO, Emory Univ

Larner, James M MD [RadRO] - **Spec Exp:** Neuro-Oncology; Brain Tumors; **Hospital:** Univ of Virginia Health Sys; **Address:** Univ Virginia Medical Ctr, Dept Radiation Oncology, 1240 Lee St, PO Box 800383, Charlottesville, VA 22908; **Phone:** 434-924-5191; **Board Cert:** Internal Medicine 1983; Medical Oncology 1987; Hematology 1988; Radiation Oncology 1989; **Med School:** Univ VA Sch Med 1980; **Resid:** Internal Medicine, Thos Jefferson Univ Hosp 1983; Radiation Oncology, Montefiore-Einstein Med Ctr 1989; **Fellow:** Hematology & Oncology, Thos Jefferson Univ Hosp 1986; **Fac Appt:** Assoc Prof Med, Univ VA Sch Med

Lee, W Robert MD [RadRO] - **Spec Exp:** Prostate Cancer; Brachytherapy; Intensity Modulated Radiotherapy (IMRT); **Hospital:** Duke Univ Hosp; **Address:** Duke Univ Med Ctr, Div Radiation Oncology, Box 3085, Durham, NC 27710; **Phone:** 919-668-5640; **Board Cert:** Radiation Oncology 1994; **Med School:** Univ VA Sch Med 1989; **Resid:** Radiation Oncology, Univ Florida 1993; **Fac Appt:** Prof RadRO, Duke Univ

Lewin, Alan A MD [RadRO] - **Spec Exp:** Breast Cancer; Lung Cancer; Brain & Spinal Cord Tumors; **Hospital:** Baptist Hosp of Miami; **Address:** Baptist Hosp Miami, Dept Radiation Oncology, 8900 N Kendall Drive, Miami, FL 33176-2118; **Phone:** 786-596-6566; **Board Cert:** Therapeutic Radiology 1982; Internal Medicine 1976; Hematology 1978; Medical Oncology 1981; **Med School:** Geo Wash Univ 1973; **Resid:** Internal Medicine, Mt Sinai Hosp 1976; **Fellow:** Hematology & Oncology, Beth Israel Med Ctr 1978; Radiation Oncology, Joint Ctr Radiation Therapy 1980; **Fac Appt:** Clin Prof RadRO, Univ Miami Sch Med

Malcolm, Arnold MD [RadRO] - **Spec Exp:** Prostate Cancer; Gynecologic Cancer; Brachytherapy; **Hospital:** Vanderbilt Univ Med Ctr (page 76); **Address:** Vanderbilt Radiation Oncology, 22nd St At Pierce Ave, B-1003 TVC Bldg, Nashville, TN 37232; **Phone:** 615-322-2555; **Board Cert:** Radiation Oncology 1977; **Med School:** Meharry Med Coll 1973; **Resid:** Radiation Oncology, Joint Ctr Radiation Therapy 1977; **Fac Appt:** Assoc Prof RadRO, Vanderbilt Univ

Radiation Oncology

Marcus Jr, Robert B MD [RadRO] - **Spec Exp:** Pediatric Cancers; Proton Beam Therapy; Bone Cancer; Brain & Spinal Cord Tumors; **Hospital:** Shands Jacksonville; **Address:** 2015 N Jefferson St, Jacksonville, FL 32206; **Phone:** 904-588-1800; **Board Cert:** Therapeutic Radiology 1980; **Med School:** Univ Fla Coll Med 1975; **Resid:** Radiation Oncology, Shands Hosp 1979; **Fac Appt:** Prof RadRO, Univ Fla Coll Med

Markoe, Arnold M MD [RadRO] - **Spec Exp:** Eye Tumors/Cancer; Orbital Tumors/Cancer; Central Nervous System Cancer; Lymphoma; **Hospital:** Univ of Miami Hosp & Clins/Sylvester Comp Canc Ctr (page 73), Jackson Meml Hosp (page 70); **Address:** Univ of Miami Sylvester Comp Cancer Ctr, 1475 NW 12th Ave Ave NW, MC D-31, Miami, FL 33136; **Phone:** 305-243-4319; **Board Cert:** Therapeutic Radiology 1983; **Med School:** Hahnemann Univ 1977; **Resid:** Radiation Oncology, Hahnemann Hosp 1981; **Fac Appt:** Prof RadRO, Univ Miami Sch Med

Marks, Lawrence MD [RadRO] - **Spec Exp:** Breast Cancer; Lung Cancer; **Hospital:** NC Memorial Hosp - UNC; **Address:** UNC Cancer Hosp, Dept Rad Onc, 101 Manning Drive, rm CB 295, Level B, Campus Box 7512, Chapel Hill, NC 27514; **Phone:** 919-966-0400; **Board Cert:** Radiation Oncology 1989; **Med School:** Univ Rochester 1985; **Resid:** Radiation Oncology, Mass Genl Hosp 1989; **Fac Appt:** Prof RadRO, Univ NC Sch Med

McGarry, Ronald C MD/PhD [RadRO] - **Spec Exp:** Lung Cancer; Lymphoma; Clinical Trials; Stereotactic Radiosurgery; **Hospital:** Univ of Kentucky Albert B. Chandler Hosp; **Address:** Chandler Medical Ctr, Radiation Medicine, 800 Rose St, rm C114C, Lexington, KY 40536; **Phone:** 859-323-6486; **Board Cert:** Radiation Oncology 1999; **Med School:** Canada 1992; **Resid:** Radiation Oncology, Univ W Ontario Regl Cancer Ctr 1997; **Fac Appt:** Prof RadRO, Univ KY Coll Med

Mendenhall, Nancy P MD [RadRO] - **Spec Exp:** Breast Cancer; Lymphoma; Hodgkin's Disease; Prostate Cancer; **Hospital:** Shands at Univ of FL; **Address:** Univ Florida, Proton Therapy Inst, 2015 N Jefferson St, Jacksonville, FL 32206; **Phone:** 904-588-1800; **Board Cert:** Therapeutic Radiology 1985; **Med School:** Univ Fla Coll Med 1980; **Resid:** Diagnostic Radiology, Shands-Univ of Florida 1984; **Fac Appt:** Prof RadRO, Univ Fla Coll Med

Mendenhall, William M MD [RadRO] - **Spec Exp:** Head & Neck Cancer; Stereotactic Radiosurgery; Gastrointestinal Cancer; Gynecologic Cancer; **Hospital:** Shands at Univ of FL; **Address:** Univ Florida, Dept Radiation Oncology, Box 100385, Gainesville, FL 32610-0385; **Phone:** 352-265-0287; **Board Cert:** Therapeutic Radiology 1983; **Med School:** Univ S Fla Coll Med 1978; **Resid:** Radiation Oncology, Univ Fla Affil Hosp 1983; **Fac Appt:** Prof RadRO, Univ Fla Coll Med

Merchant, Thomas E DO [RadRO] - **Spec Exp:** Brain Tumors-Pediatric; **Hospital:** St. Jude Children's Research Hosp; **Address:** St Jude Chldns Rsch Hosp, 262 Danny Thomas Pl, MS 220, Memphis, TN 38105; **Phone:** 901-595-3565; **Board Cert:** Radiation Oncology 2004; **Med School:** Chicago Coll Osteo Med 1989; **Resid:** Radiation Oncology, Meml Sloan Kettering Cancer Ctr 1994

Meredith, Ruby F MD [RadRO] - **Spec Exp:** Multiple Myeloma; Breast Cancer; Radionuclide Therapy; Bone Tumors-Metastatic; **Hospital:** Univ of Ala Hosp at Birmingham; **Address:** Univ Alabama Hosps-Radiation Oncology, 619 19th St S, 1700 6th Ave S, Birmingham, AL 35249; **Phone:** 205-934-2763; **Board Cert:** Radiation Oncology 1987; **Med School:** Ohio State Univ 1983; **Resid:** Radiation Oncology, Med College Va Hosps 1987; **Fac Appt:** Prof RadRO, Univ Alabama

Morris, Monica M MD [RadRO] - **Spec Exp:** Breast Cancer; Lung Cancer; **Hospital:** Univ of Virginia Health Sys; **Address:** Univ VA Hlth Sciences-Radiation Onc, PO Box 800383, Charlottesville, VA 22908; **Phone:** 434-924-5192; **Board Cert:** Radiation Oncology 2008; **Med School:** Baylor Coll Med 1993; **Resid:** Radiation Oncology, Mass Genl Hosp 1998; **Fac Appt:** Assoc Prof RadRO, Univ VA Sch Med

Pollack, Alan MD/PhD [RadRO] - **Spec Exp:** Prostate Cancer; Genitourinary Cancer; Sarcoma; **Hospital:** Univ of Miami Hosp & Clins/Sylvester Comp Canc Ctr (page 73); **Address:** 1475 NW 12th Ave, Ste 1501, Miami, FL 33136; **Phone:** 305-243-4916; **Board Cert:** Radiation Oncology 1993; **Med School:** Univ Miami Sch Med 1987; **Resid:** Radiation Oncology, MD Anderson Cancer Ctr 1992; **Fac Appt:** Prof RadRO, Univ Miami Sch Med

Prosnitz, Leonard MD [RadRO] - **Spec Exp:** Lymphoma; Breast Cancer; Hyperthermia Treatment of Cancer; Sarcoma; **Hospital:** Duke Univ Hosp; **Address:** Duke Univ Med Ctr, Dept Rad Onc, Box 3085, Durham, NC 27710; **Phone:** 919-668-5637; **Board Cert:** Therapeutic Radiology 1970; **Med School:** SUNY Downstate 1961; **Resid:** Internal Medicine, Dartmouth Affil Hosps 1963; Radiation Oncology, Yale-New Haven Hosp 1969; **Fellow:** Hematology & Oncology, Yale-New Haven Hosp 1967; **Fac Appt:** Prof RadRO, Duke Univ

Randall, Marcus E MD [RadRO] - **Spec Exp:** Gynecologic Cancer; Stereotactic Radiosurgery; **Hospital:** Univ of Kentucky Albert B. Chandler Hosp; **Address:** Univ Kentucky Medical Ctr, 800 Rose St, rm C11-14D, Office of Radiation Medicine, Lexington, KY 40536-0001; **Phone:** 859-323-6487; **Board Cert:** Therapeutic Radiology 1986; **Med School:** Univ NC Sch Med 1982; **Resid:** Radiation Oncology, Univ Va Med Ctr 1986; **Fellow:** Radiation Oncology, Univ Va Med Ctr 1986; **Fac Appt:** Prof RadRO, Univ KY Coll Med

Rich, Tyvin A MD [RadRO] - **Spec Exp:** Colon & Rectal Cancer; Chemo-Radiation Combined Therapy; Gastrointestinal Cancer; Gallbladder & Biliary Cancer; **Hospital:** Univ of Virginia Health Sys; **Address:** Univ Va Hlth Sys, Dept Rad Onc, 1240 Lee St, PO Box 800383, Charlottesville, VA 22908-0383; **Phone:** 434-924-5191; **Board Cert:** Radiation Oncology 1978; **Med School:** Univ VA Sch Med 1973; **Resid:** Radiation Oncology, Mass Genl Hosp 1978; **Fellow:** Radiation Oncology, Mt Vernon Hosp/Gray Lab 1978; **Fac Appt:** Prof RadRO, Univ VA Sch Med

Rosenman, Julian MD/PhD [RadRO] - **Spec Exp:** Lung Cancer; Breast Cancer; Prostate Cancer; **Hospital:** NC Memorial Hosp - UNC; **Address:** UNC Cancer Hosp, Dept Rad Onc, 101 Manning Drive, rm CB 295, Level B, Campus Box 7512, Chapel Hill, NC 27514; **Phone:** 919-966-0400; **Board Cert:** Therapeutic Radiology 1981; **Med School:** Univ Tex SW, Dallas 1977; **Resid:** Therapeutic Radiology, Mass Genl Hosp 1981; **Fac Appt:** Prof RadRO, Univ NC Sch Med

Sailer, Scott MD [RadRO] - **Spec Exp:** Breast Cancer; Genitourinary Cancer; Head & Neck Cancer; **Hospital:** WakeMed Cary, WakeMed-Raleigh Campus; **Address:** 300 Ashville Ave, Ste 110, Cary, NC 27518; **Phone:** 919-854-4588; **Board Cert:** Radiation Oncology 1988; **Med School:** Harvard Med Sch 1984; **Resid:** Radiation Therapy, Mass Genl Hosp 1988

Shaw, Edward G MD [RadRO] - **Spec Exp:** Stereotactic Radiosurgery; Brain Tumors; **Hospital:** Wake Forest Univ Baptist Med Ctr; **Address:** Wake Forest Baptist Health, Research Base Fl 4, Piedmont Plaza Two, Winston-Salem, NC 27104; **Phone:** 336-713-6506; **Board Cert:** Radiation Oncology 1987; **Med School:** Rush Med Coll 1983; **Resid:** Radiation Oncology, Mayo Grad Sch Med 1987; **Fac Appt:** Prof RadRO, Wake Forest Univ

Song, Shiyu MD/PhD [RadRO] - **Spec Exp:** Head & Neck Cancer; **Hospital:** VCU Med Ctr; **Address:** 401 College St, Box 980058, Richmond, VA 23298-0037; **Phone:** 804-828-7232; **Board Cert:** Radiation Oncology 2006; **Med School:** China 1983; **Resid:** Radiation Oncology, Univ Wisc Hosp & Clins; **Fellow:** Radiation Oncology, Johns Hopkins Hosp; **Fac Appt:** Asst Prof RadRO, Va Commonwealth Univ Sch Med

St Clair, William H MD/PhD [RadRO] - **Hospital:** Univ of Kentucky Albert B. Chandler Hosp; **Address:** 800 Rose St, Lexington, KY 40536; **Phone:** 859-323-6486; **Board Cert:** Radiation Oncology 2000; **Med School:** Univ KY Coll Med 1995; **Resid:** Radiation Oncology, Mass Genl Hosp 2000; **Fellow:** Radiation Oncology, Mass Genl Hosp 2000

Radiation Oncology

Tepper, Joel E MD [RadRO] - **Spec Exp:** Gastrointestinal Cancer; Sarcoma; Rectal Cancer; **Hospital:** NC Memorial Hosp - UNC; **Address:** UNC Cancer Hosp, Dept Rad Onc, 101 Manning Drive, rm CB 295, Level B, Campus Box 7512, Chapel Hill, NC 27514; **Phone:** 919-966-0400; **Board Cert:** Therapeutic Radiology 1976; **Med School:** Washington Univ, St Louis 1972; **Resid:** Therapeutic Radiology, Mass Genl Hosp 1976; **Fellow:** Therapeutic Radiology, Mass Genl Hosp 1977; **Fac Appt:** Prof RadRO, Univ NC Sch Med

Toonkel, Leonard M MD [RadRO] - **Spec Exp:** Prostate Cancer; Breast Cancer; Brachytherapy; **Hospital:** Mount Sinai Med Ctr - Miami; **Address:** Dept Radiation Oncology, 4300 Alton Rd, Miami Beach, FL 33140; **Phone:** 305-535-3400; **Board Cert:** Therapeutic Radiology 1979; **Med School:** Univ Miami Sch Med 1975; **Resid:** Radiation Therapy, Jackson Meml Hosp 1977; Diagnostic Radiology, MD Anderson Hosp 1978; **Fellow:** Radiation Oncology, MD Anderson Hosp 1979; **Fac Appt:** Assoc Clin Prof Rad, Univ Miami Sch Med

Vijayakumar, Srinivasan MD [RadRO] - **Spec Exp:** Brachytherapy; Prostate Cancer; **Hospital:** Univ Mississippi Med Ctr; **Address:** 350 Woodrow Wilson Drive, Jackson, MS 39213; **Phone:** 601-984-2550; **Board Cert:** Therapeutic Radiology 1986; **Med School:** India 1978; **Resid:** Radiation Oncology, Madras Univ Med Ctr 1981; Radiation Oncology, Michael Reese Hosp 1984; **Fellow:** Brachytherapy, Univ Chicago Hosps 1985; **Fac Appt:** Prof RadRO, Univ Miss

Willett, Christopher MD [RadRO] - **Spec Exp:** Gastrointestinal Cancer; Clinical Trials; **Hospital:** Duke Univ Hosp; **Address:** Duke Univ Med Ctr, PO Box 3085, Durham, NC 27710; **Phone:** 919-668-5640; **Board Cert:** Therapeutic Radiology 1985; **Med School:** Tufts Univ 1981; **Resid:** Radiation Oncology, Mass Genl Hosp 1986; **Fac Appt:** Prof RadRO, Duke Univ

Wolfson, Aaron H MD [RadRO] - **Spec Exp:** Gynecologic Cancer; Sarcoma; Gastrointestinal Cancer; **Hospital:** Univ of Miami Hosp & Clins/Sylvester Comp Canc Ctr (page 73); **Address:** UMHC Sylvester Comp Cancer Ctr, 1475 NW 12th Ave, Box D31, Miami, FL 33136; **Phone:** 305-243-4210; **Board Cert:** Radiation Oncology 1999; **Med School:** Univ Fla Coll Med 1982; **Resid:** Radiation Oncology, Med Coll of Virginia 1989; **Fac Appt:** Prof RadRO, Univ Miami Sch Med

Woo, Shiao Y MD [RadRO] - **Spec Exp:** Brain Tumors-Adult & Pediatric; Proton Beam Therapy; Stereotactic Radiosurgery; Pediatric Cancers; **Hospital:** Univ of Louisville Hosp; **Address:** Univ Louisville-Radiation Onc, 5295 S Jackson St, Louisville, KY 40202; **Phone:** 502-562-4759; **Board Cert:** Radiation Oncology 1988; Pediatrics 1980; **Med School:** Malaysia 1972; **Resid:** Pediatrics, Georgetown Univ Hosp 1978; **Fellow:** Pediatric Hematology-Oncology, Georgetown Univ Hosp 1980; Radiation Oncology, Georgetown Univ Hosp 1988; **Fac Appt:** Prof RadRO, Univ Louisville Sch Med

Midwest

Abrams, Ross A MD [RadRO] - **Spec Exp:** Gastrointestinal Cancer; Lymphoma; **Hospital:** Rush Univ Med Ctr; **Address:** Women's Board Ctr for Radiation Therapy, 500 S Paulina, Ground Floor Atrium, Chicago, IL 60612; **Phone:** 312-942-5751; **Board Cert:** Internal Medicine 1976; Medical Oncology 1979; Hematology 1982; Radiation Oncology 1987; **Med School:** Univ Pennsylvania 1973; **Resid:** Internal Medicine, Pennsylvania Hosp 1975; Hematology & Oncology, Hosp Univ Penn 1976; **Fellow:** Hematology & Oncology, Natl Cancer Inst 1978; Radiation Oncology, Med Coll Wisconsin 1987; **Fac Appt:** Prof RadRO, Rush Med Coll

Awan, Azhar M MD [RadRO] - **Spec Exp:** Brain Tumors; Prostate Cancer; Breast Cancer; **Hospital:** Sherman Hosp, Univ of Chicago Med Ctr; **Address:** Sherman Hosp Cancer Care Ctr, 1425 N Randall Rd, Elgin, IL 60123; **Phone:** 224-783-8746; **Board Cert:** Therapeutic Radiology 1985; **Med School:** Loyola Univ-Stritch Sch Med 1981; **Resid:** Therapeutic Radiology, Rush Med Ctr 1985; **Fac Appt:** Assoc Prof RadRO, Univ Chicago-Pritzker Sch Med

Ben-Josef, Edgar MD [RadRO] - **Spec Exp:** Bone Cancer; Gastrointestinal Cancer; Pancreatic Cancer; Intensity Modulated Radiotherapy (IMRT); **Hospital:** Univ of Michigan Hosp; **Address:** Univ of Mich Hosp, 1500 E Medical Ctr Drive, rm UH B2C490, Ann Arbor, MI 48109-0010; **Phone:** 734-936-8207; **Board Cert:** Radiation Oncology 1994; **Med School:** Israel 1986; **Resid:** Radiation Oncology, Wayne State Univ Hosp 1994; **Fellow:** Cancer Biology, Wayne State Univ Hosp 1995; **Fac Appt:** Assoc Prof RadRO, Univ Mich Med Sch

Bradley, Jeffrey D MD [RadRO] - **Spec Exp:** Lung Cancer; Esophageal Cancer; Thoracic Cancers; Clinical Trials; **Hospital:** Barnes-Jewish Hosp; **Address:** Ctr for Advanced Medicine, Rad Oncology, 4921 Parkview Pl Fl LL, St Louis, MO 63110; **Phone:** 314-747-7236; **Board Cert:** Radiation Oncology 2008; **Med School:** Univ Ark 1993; **Resid:** Radiation Oncology, Univ Chicago 1998; **Fac Appt:** Assoc Prof RadRO, Washington Univ, St Louis

Buatti, John M MD [RadRO] - **Spec Exp:** Central Nervous System Cancer; **Hospital:** Univ Iowa Hosp & Clinics; **Address:** 200 Hawkins Drive, rm 01626 PFP, Iowa City, IA 52242; **Phone:** 319-356-2699; **Board Cert:** Radiation Oncology 1994; **Med School:** Georgetown Univ 1986; **Resid:** Internal Medicine, Georgetown Univ 1989; **Fellow:** Radiation Oncology, Univ Arizona 1993; **Fac Appt:** Prof RadRO, Univ Iowa Coll Med

Ciezki, Jay P MD [RadRO] - **Spec Exp:** Brachytherapy; Prostate Cancer; Genitourinary Cancer; **Hospital:** Cleveland Clin (page 56); **Address:** Cleveland Clinic Fdn, 9500 Euclid Ave, MC T28, Cleveland, OH 44195; **Phone:** 216-445-9465; **Board Cert:** Radiation Oncology 2005; **Med School:** Med Coll Wisc 1991; **Resid:** Radiation Oncology, Cleveland Clinic 1995; **Fellow:** Brachytherapy, Cleveland Clinic 1996

Eisbruch, Avraham MD [RadRO] - **Spec Exp:** Head & Neck Cancer; **Hospital:** Univ of Michigan Hosp; **Address:** Univ MI Hlth Sys, 1500 E Med Ctr Drive, Fl B2 - rm C490, Ann Arbor, MI 48109; **Phone:** 734-936-4319; **Board Cert:** Radiation Oncology 1992; **Med School:** Israel 1979; **Resid:** Radiology, Washington Univ 1992; **Fellow:** Medical Oncology, Univ TX MD Anderson Cancer Ctr 1996; **Fac Appt:** Assoc Clin Prof RadRO, Univ Mich Med Sch

Emami, Bahman MD [RadRO] - **Spec Exp:** Head & Neck Cancer; Lung Cancer; **Hospital:** Loyola Univ Med Ctr, Edward Hines, Jr. VA Hosp; **Address:** Loyola Univ Med Ctr, Dept Rad Onc, 2160 S First Ave Bldg 150 - rm 0300, Maywood, IL 60153-3328; **Phone:** 708-216-2729; **Board Cert:** Therapeutic Radiology 1976; **Med School:** Iran 1968; **Resid:** Radiation Therapy, St Vincents Hosp 1973; Radiation Therapy, New England Med Ctr 1977; **Fac Appt:** Prof RadRO, Loyola Univ-Stritch Sch Med

Forman, Jeffrey D MD [RadRO] - **Spec Exp:** Neutron Therapy for Advanced Cancer; Genitourinary Cancer; Prostate Cancer; **Address:** 70 Fulton St, Pontiac, MI 48341; **Phone:** 248-338-0300; **Board Cert:** Radiation Oncology 1986; **Med School:** NYU Sch Med 1982; **Resid:** Radiation Oncology, Johns Hopkins Hosp 1986; **Fellow:** Therapeutic Radiology, Johns Hopkins Hosp 1987; **Fac Appt:** Prof RadRO, Wayne State Univ

Grigsby, Perry W MD [RadRO] - **Spec Exp:** Gynecologic Cancer; Thyroid Cancer; **Hospital:** Barnes-Jewish Hosp, St. Louis Chldns Hosp; **Address:** Ctr for Advanced Medicine, Rad Oncology, 4921 Parkview Pl Fl LL, St Louis, MO 63110; **Phone:** 314-747-7236; **Board Cert:** Radiation Oncology 1987; **Med School:** Univ KY Coll Med 1982; **Resid:** Radiation Oncology, Barnes Jewish Hosp 1985; **Fac Appt:** Prof RadRO, Washington Univ, St Louis

Halpern, Howard J MD/PhD [RadRO] - **Spec Exp:** Breast Cancer; Esophageal Cancer; Gynecologic Cancer; **Hospital:** Univ of Chicago Med Ctr, Univ of IL Med Ctr at Chicago; **Address:** Univ Chicago Dept Radiation Oncology, 5758 S Maryland Ave, MC 9006, Chicago, IL 60637; **Phone:** 773-702-6870; **Board Cert:** Therapeutic Radiology 1984; **Med School:** Univ Miami Sch Med 1980; **Resid:** Therapeutic Radiology, Harvard Jnt Ctr Rad Ther 1984; **Fellow:** Therapeutic Radiology, Harvard Jnt Ctr Rad Ther 1985; **Fac Appt:** Prof RadRO, Univ Chicago-Pritzker Sch Med

Haraf, Daniel J MD [RadRO] - **Spec Exp:** Head & Neck Cancer; Lung Cancer; Prostate Cancer; **Hospital:** Univ of Chicago Med Ctr; **Address:** Univ Chicago Medical Center, 5841 S Maryland Ave, Chicago, IL 60637; **Phone:** 773-702-6870; **Board Cert:** Internal Medicine 1985; Radiation Oncology 1990; **Med School:** Ros Franklin Univ/Chicago Med Sch 1982; **Resid:** Internal Medicine, Michael Reese Hosp 1985; **Fellow:** Radiation Oncology, Michael Reese Hosp 1988; **Fac Appt:** Prof RadRO, Univ Chicago-Pritzker Sch Med

Harari, Paul M MD [RadRO] - **Spec Exp:** Head & Neck Cancer; **Hospital:** Univ WI Hosp & Clins; **Address:** Dept of Human Oncology, 600 Highland Ave, Ste K4/336, Madison, WI 53792; **Phone:** 608-263-5009; **Board Cert:** Radiation Oncology 1990; **Med School:** Univ VA Sch Med 1984; **Resid:** Radiation Oncology, Univ Arizona Med Ctr 1990; **Fac Appt:** Prof RadRO, Univ Wisc

Hayman, James A MD [RadRO] - **Spec Exp:** Breast Cancer; Stomach Cancer; Lung Cancer; Brain Tumors; **Hospital:** Univ of Michigan Hosp; **Address:** Univ Michigan Hosp, 1500 E Medical Ctr Drive, rm UH B2C490, Ann Arbor, MI 48109-0010; **Phone:** 734-647-9956; **Board Cert:** Radiation Oncology 2004; **Med School:** Univ Chicago-Pritzker Sch Med 1991; **Resid:** Radiation Therapy, Joint Ctr for Radiation Therapy 1996; **Fac Appt:** Assoc Prof RadRO, Univ Mich Med Sch

Johnstone, Peter A S MD [RadRO] - **Spec Exp:** Prostate Cancer; Proton Beam Therapy; Head & Neck Cancer; **Hospital:** IU Health University Hosp; **Address:** IU Dept Radiation Oncology, 535 Barnhill Drive, RT 041, Indianapolis, IN 46202; **Phone:** 317-944-2524; **Board Cert:** Radiation Oncology 2010; **Med School:** Uniformed Srvs Univ, Bethesda 1989; **Resid:** Radiation Oncology, Natl Cancer Inst 1993; **Fac Appt:** Prof RadRO, Indiana Univ

Kim, Jae Ho MD [RadRO] - **Spec Exp:** Brain Tumors; Spinal Cord Tumors; Breast Cancer; Lymphoma; **Hospital:** Henry Ford Hosp; **Address:** Radiation Oncology, 2799 W Grand Blvd, Detroit, MI 48202; **Phone:** 313-916-1029; **Board Cert:** Therapeutic Radiology 1973; **Med School:** Korea 1959; **Resid:** Therapeutic Radiology, Meml-Sloan-Kettering 1972; **Fellow:** Medical Biophysics, Meml-Sloan-Kettering 1968; **Fac Appt:** Prof RadRO, Wayne State Univ

Konski, Andre MD [RadRO] - **Spec Exp:** Esophageal Cancer; Rectal Cancer; Pancreatic Cancer; Gastrointestinal Cancer; **Hospital:** Barbara Ann Karmanos Cancer Inst; **Address:** Dept Radiation Oncology, 4100 John R, Detroit, MI 48201; **Phone:** 313-745-2560; **Board Cert:** Radiation Oncology 2000; **Med School:** NY Med Coll 1984; **Resid:** Radiation Oncology, Stong Meml/Genesee Hosp 1988; **Fac Appt:** Prof RadRO, Wayne State Univ

Lawrence, Theodore S MD/PhD [RadRO] - **Spec Exp:** Gastrointestinal Cancer; Liver Cancer; Pancreatic Cancer; **Hospital:** Univ of Michigan Hosp; **Address:** Univ of Mich Hosp, Dept Rad Onc, 1500 E Med Ctr Dr, SPC5010, Box 5010, UH-B2-C502, Ann Arbor, MI 48109-5010; **Phone:** 734-936-4300; **Board Cert:** Internal Medicine 1983; Medical Oncology 1985; Radiation Oncology 1987; **Med School:** Cornell Univ-Weill Med Coll 1980; **Resid:** Internal Medicine, Stanford Univ Hosp 1983; Radiation Oncology, Natl Cancer Inst 1987; **Fellow:** Medical Oncology, Natl Cancer Inst 1986; **Fac Appt:** Prof RadRO, Univ Mich Med Sch

Lee, Chung K MD [RadRO] - **Spec Exp:** Head & Neck Cancer; Breast Cancer; Lymphoma; Gastrointestinal Cancer; **Address:** Univ Minn, Dept Radiation Oncology, 420 Delaware St SE, MMC 400, Minneapolis, MN 55455; **Phone:** 612-273-6700; **Board Cert:** Therapeutic Radiology 1976; **Med School:** Korea 1965; **Resid:** Radiation Oncology, Yonsei Univ Hosp 1971; Therapeutic Radiology, Univ of Minn Hosp 1976; **Fellow:** Yonsei Univ Hosp; **Fac Appt:** Prof RadRO, Univ Minn

Machtay, Mitchell MD [RadRO] - **Spec Exp:** Head & Neck Cancer; Skin Cancer; Skull Base Tumors; **Hospital:** Univ Hosps Case Med Ctr (page 74); **Address:** UH Case Med Ctr, Dept Rad Oncology, 11100 Euclid Ave, Lerner Tower B-181, Cleveland, OH 44106; **Phone:** 216-844-2530; **Board Cert:** Radiation Oncology 1994; **Med School:** NYU Sch Med 1989; **Resid:** Radiation Oncology, Hosp Univ Penn 1993; **Fac Appt:** Assoc Prof RadRO, Jefferson Med Coll

Macklis, Roger M MD [RadRO] - **Spec Exp:** Radioimmunotherapy of Cancer; Breast Cancer; Lymphoma; **Hospital:** Cleveland Clin (page 56); **Address:** Cleveland Cin Fdn, Dept Rad Onc, 9500 Euclid Ave, Desk T28, Cleveland, OH 44195; **Phone:** 216-444-5576; **Board Cert:** Radiation Oncology 1989; **Med School:** Harvard Med Sch 1983; **Resid:** Radiation Oncology, Joint Ctr Radiotherapy Inst 1987; **Fellow:** Research, Dana Farber Cancer Inst 1987; **Fac Appt:** Prof RadRO, Case West Res Univ

Mansur, David B MD [RadRO] - **Spec Exp:** Pediatric Cancers; Breast Cancer; Genitourinary Cancer; **Hospital:** St. Louis Chldns Hosp, Barnes-Jewish Hosp; **Address:** Washington University School of Medicine, Dept Radiation Oncology, 4921 Parkview Pl, St Louis, MO 63110; **Phone:** 314-362-4633; **Board Cert:** Radiation Oncology 2009; **Med School:** Univ Kansas 1992; **Resid:** Radiation Oncology, Unic Chicago Hosps 1997; **Fac Appt:** Assoc Prof RadRO, Washington Univ, St Louis

Martenson Jr, James A MD [RadRO] - **Spec Exp:** Mucositis; Esophageal Cancer; **Hospital:** Mayo Med Ctr & Clin - Rochester; **Address:** Mayo Clinic, Dept Rad/Onc, 200 First St SW, Rochester, MN 55905; **Phone:** 507-284-4561; **Board Cert:** Therapeutic Radiology 1985; **Med School:** Univ Wash 1981; **Resid:** Radiation Oncology, Mayo Clinic 1985; **Fac Appt:** Assoc Prof, Mayo Med Sch

Michalski, Jeff M MD [RadRO] - **Spec Exp:** Prostate Cancer; Sarcoma; Pediatric Cancers; **Hospital:** Barnes-Jewish Hosp, St. Louis Chldns Hosp; **Address:** Ctr for Advanced Medicine, Rad Oncology, 4921 Parkview Pl Fl LL, St Louis, MO 63110; **Phone:** 314-747-7236; **Board Cert:** Radiation Oncology 1991; **Med School:** Med Coll Wisc 1986; **Resid:** Radiation Oncology, Columbia Presby Med Ctr 1988; Radiation Oncology, Mallinckrodt Inst of Radiology 1990; **Fellow:** Radiation Oncology, Mallinckrodt Inst of Radiology 1991; **Fac Appt:** Prof RadRO, Washington Univ, St Louis

Minsky, Bruce MD [RadRO] - **Spec Exp:** Gastrointestinal Cancer; Esophageal Cancer; Colon & Rectal Cancer; Pancreatic Cancer; **Hospital:** Univ of Chicago Med Ctr; **Address:** Univ Chicago Hosp, 5841 S Maryland Ave, Chicago, IL 60637; **Phone:** 773-834-1180; **Board Cert:** Radiation Oncology 1987; **Med School:** Univ Mass Sch Med 1982; **Resid:** Radiation Oncology, Harvard Jt Ctr Rad Ther 1986; **Fac Appt:** Prof RadRO, Univ Chicago-Pritzker Sch Med

Mittal, Bharat B MD [RadRO] - **Spec Exp:** Head & Neck Cancer; Lymphoma; Skin Cancer; **Hospital:** Northwestern Meml Hosp; **Address:** 251 E Huron St, Galter LC-178, Chicago, IL 60611; **Phone:** 312-926-2520; **Board Cert:** Therapeutic Radiology 1981; **Med School:** India 1975; **Resid:** Internal Medicine, Christian Med Coll 1976; Radiation Oncology, Northwestern Meml Hosp 1980; **Fellow:** Radiation Oncology, Mallinckrodt Inst 1981; **Fac Appt:** Prof RadRO, Northwestern Univ

Radiation Oncology

Movsas, Benjamin MD [RadRO] - **Spec Exp:** Lung Cancer; Brain Tumors; Prostate Cancer; Stereotactic Radiosurgery; **Hospital:** Henry Ford Hosp; **Address:** Henry Ford Health Sys, Dept Rad Oncology, 2799 W Grand Blvd, Detroit, MI 48202-2608; **Phone:** 313-916-1029; **Board Cert:** Radiation Oncology 2010; **Med School:** Washington Univ, St Louis 1990; **Resid:** Radiation Oncology, National Cancer Inst 1995

Myerson, Robert J MD [RadRO] - **Spec Exp:** Gastrointestinal Cancer; Breast Cancer; Hyperthermia Treatment of Cancer; **Hospital:** Barnes-Jewish Hosp; **Address:** Ctr for Advanced Med, Rad Oncology, 4921 Parkview Pl Fl LL, St Louis, MO 63110; **Phone:** 314-747-7236; **Board Cert:** Therapeutic Radiology 1985; **Med School:** Univ Miami Sch Med 1980; **Resid:** Radiation Therapy, Hosp Univ Penn 1984; **Fac Appt:** Prof RadRO, Washington Univ, St Louis

Pierce, Lori J MD [RadRO] - **Spec Exp:** Breast Cancer; **Hospital:** Univ of Michigan Hosp; **Address:** Univ Hosp, Dept Radiation Oncology, 1500 E Med Ctr, rm B2C440, Box 5010, Ann Arbor, MI 48109-5099; **Phone:** 734-936-4300; **Board Cert:** Radiation Oncology 1989; **Med School:** Duke Univ 1985; **Resid:** Radiation Oncology, Hosp Univ Penn 1989; **Fac Appt:** Prof RadRO, Univ Mich Med Sch

Schomberg, Paula J MD [RadRO] - **Spec Exp:** Brain Tumors; Pediatric Cancers; **Hospital:** Mayo Med Ctr & Clin - Rochester; **Address:** Mayo Clinic - Charlton Bldg, Desk R, 200 1st St SW, Rochester, MN 55905; **Phone:** 507-284-4561; **Board Cert:** Therapeutic Radiology 1984; **Med School:** Med Coll Wisc 1979; **Resid:** Radiation Therapy, Mayo Clinic 1983; **Fac Appt:** Prof RadRO, Mayo Med Sch

Small Jr, William MD [RadRO] - **Spec Exp:** Gynecologic Cancer; Gastrointestinal Cancer; Breast Cancer; Pancreatic Cancer; **Hospital:** Northwestern Meml Hosp; **Address:** Northwestern Meml Hosp, Rad Oncology, Prentice Pavilion, rm 00-2101, 250 E Superior St, Chicago, IL 60611; **Phone:** 312-472-3650; **Board Cert:** Radiation Oncology 2004; **Med School:** Northwestern Univ 1990; **Resid:** Radiation Oncology, Northwestern Univ 1994; **Fac Appt:** Prof RadRO, Northwestern Univ

Suh, John H MD [RadRO] - **Spec Exp:** Brain Tumors-Adult & Pediatric; Stereotactic Radiosurgery; Stereotactic Body Radiation Therapy; **Hospital:** Cleveland Clin (page 56); **Address:** Cleveland Clinic, Dept Rad/Onc, 9500 Euclid Ave, Desk T28, Cleveland, OH 44195-0001; **Phone:** 216-444-5574; **Board Cert:** Radiation Oncology 2000; **Med School:** Univ Miami Sch Med 1990; **Resid:** Radiation Oncology, Cleveland Clinic 1994; **Fellow:** Radiation Oncology, Cleveland Clinic 1995

Taylor, Marie E MD [RadRO] - **Spec Exp:** Breast Cancer; **Hospital:** Barnes-Jewish Hosp, Barnes-Jewish West County Hosp; **Address:** Center for Advanced Med, Rad Oncology, 4921 Parkview Pl Fl LL, St Louis, MO 63110; **Phone:** 314-747-7236; **Board Cert:** Radiation Oncology 1987; **Med School:** Univ Wash 1982; **Resid:** Radiation Oncology, Univ Wash Med Ctr 1986

Vicini, Frank A MD [RadRO] - **Spec Exp:** Breast Cancer; Prostate Cancer; Brachytherapy; **Hospital:** Beaumont Hosp-Royal Oak; **Address:** William Beaumont Hospital, 3601 W 13 Mile Rd, Royal Oak, MI 48073; **Phone:** 248-551-1219; **Board Cert:** Radiation Oncology 1999; **Med School:** Wayne State Univ 1985; **Resid:** Radiation Oncology, William Beaumont Hosp 1989; **Fellow:** Radiation Oncology, Harvard Med Sch/Joint Ctr for Rad Ther 1990; **Fac Appt:** Clin Prof RadRO, Oakland Univ-William Beaumont Med Sch

Videtic, Gregory M MD [RadRO] - **Spec Exp:** Lung Cancer; Mesothelioma; Esophageal Cancer; Thymoma; **Hospital:** Cleveland Clin (page 56); **Address:** Cleveland Clinic, Radiation Oncology, 9500 Euclid Ave, Cleveland, OH 44195; **Phone:** 216-444-9797; **Board Cert:** Radiation Oncology 2008; **Med School:** McGill Univ 1986; **Resid:** Radiation Oncology, Dalhousie Univ 1988; Radiation Oncology, London Regl Cancer Ctr 1997; **Fellow:** Radiation Oncology, Wayne State Univ 1998; **Fac Appt:** Assoc Prof Rad, Cleveland Cl Coll Med/Case West Res

Weichselbaum, Ralph R MD [RadRO] - **Spec Exp:** Gene Targeted Radiotherapy; Pancreatic Cancer; Rectal Cancer; **Hospital:** Univ of Chicago Med Ctr; **Address:** Univ Chicago Medical Center, 5841 S Maryland Ave, MC 9006, Chicago, IL 60637; **Phone:** 773-702-6870; **Board Cert:** Therapeutic Radiology 1975; **Med School:** Univ IL Coll Med 1971; **Resid:** Therapeutic Radiology, Harvard Jt Ctr Rad Therapy 1975; **Fellow:** Harvard Univ 1976; **Fac Appt:** Prof RadRO, Univ Chicago-Pritzker Sch Med

Wilson, J Frank MD [RadRO] - **Spec Exp:** Breast Cancer; Skin Cancer; **Hospital:** Froedtert and Med Ctr of WI; **Address:** Dept Radiation Oncology, 9200 W Wisconsin Ave, Milwaukee, WI 53226; **Phone:** 414-805-4400; **Board Cert:** Therapeutic Radiology 1971; **Med School:** Univ MO-Columbia Sch Med 1965; **Resid:** Radiation Therapy, Penrose Cancer Hosp 1969; **Fellow:** Radiation Therapy, Natl Cancer Inst/NIH 1971; **Fac Appt:** Prof RadRO, Med Coll Wisc

Great Plains and Mountains

Gaffney, David K MD/PhD [RadRO] - **Spec Exp:** Breast Cancer; Gynecologic Cancer; **Hospital:** Univ Utah Hlth Care; **Address:** Huntsman Cancer Hosp, Dept Rad Oncology, 1950 Circle of Hope, rm 1440, Salt Lake City, UT 84112-5560; **Phone:** 801-581-2396; **Board Cert:** Radiation Oncology 2007; **Med School:** Med Coll Wisc 1992; **Resid:** Radiation Oncology, Univ Utah Hosps 1996; **Fac Appt:** Assoc Prof, Univ Utah

Rabinovitch, Rachel A MD [RadRO] - **Spec Exp:** Breast Cancer; Lymphoma; **Hospital:** Univ of CO Hosp - Anschutz Inpatient Pav; **Address:** Anschutz Cancer Pavilion, Dept Rad Oncology, 1665 Aurora Court, Ste 1032, MS F-706, Aurora, CO 80045; **Phone:** 720-848-0156; **Board Cert:** Radiation Oncology 1994; **Med School:** Albert Einstein Coll Med 1989; **Resid:** Radiation Oncology, Meml Sloan Kettering Cancer Ctr 1993; **Fac Appt:** Assoc Prof RadRO, Univ Colorado

Shrieve, Dennis C MD [RadRO] - **Spec Exp:** Brain Tumors-Adult & Pediatric; Genitourinary Cancer; Gastrointestinal Cancer; **Hospital:** Univ Utah Hlth Care, Primary Children's Med Ctr; **Address:** Huntsman Cancer Inst, Dept Rad Oncology, 1950 Circle of Hope, rm 1440, Salt Lake City, UT 84112; **Phone:** 801-581-2396; **Board Cert:** Radiation Oncology 1993; **Med School:** Univ Miami Sch Med 1989; **Resid:** Radiation Oncology, UCSF Med Ctr; **Fac Appt:** Prof RadRO, Univ Utah

Smalley, Stephen R MD [RadRO] - **Spec Exp:** Colon Cancer; Gastrointestinal Cancer; **Hospital:** Olathe Med Ctr; **Address:** Olathe Medical Center, 20375 W 151st St, Doctors Bldg - Ste 180, Olathe, KS 66061-4575; **Phone:** 913-768-7200; **Board Cert:** Internal Medicine 1982; Radiation Oncology 1987; Medical Oncology 1985; **Med School:** Univ MO-Kansas City 1979; **Resid:** Internal Medicine, Mayo Clinic 1982; Radiation Oncology, Mayo Clinic 1986; **Fellow:** Medical Oncology, Mayo Clinic 1984; **Fac Appt:** Prof RadRO, Univ Kansas

Southwest

Ang, Kie-Kian MD/PhD [RadRO] - **Spec Exp:** Head & Neck Cancer; **Hospital:** UT MD Anderson Cancer Ctr; **Address:** UT MD Anderson Cancer Ctr, 1515 Holcombe Blvd, Unit 97, Houston, TX 77030; **Phone:** 713-563-8400; **Board Cert:** Radiation Oncology 1987; **Med School:** Belgium 1975; **Resid:** Radiation Oncology, Univ Hosp Louvian 1980; **Fac Appt:** Prof, Univ Tex, Houston

Radiation Oncology

Buchholz, Thomas A MD [RadRO] - **Spec Exp:** Breast Cancer; **Hospital:** UT MD Anderson Cancer Ctr; **Address:** Univ Texas MD Anderson Cancer Ctr, 1515 Holcombe Blvd, Unit 97, Houston, TX 77030; **Phone:** 713-794-4892; **Board Cert:** Radiation Oncology 1993; **Med School:** Tufts Univ 1988; **Resid:** Radiation Oncology, Univ Washington Med Ctr 1993; **Fellow:** Research, Univ Washington Med Ctr 1994; **Fac Appt:** Prof RadRO, Univ Tex, Houston

Choy, Hak MD [RadRO] - **Spec Exp:** Lung Cancer; **Hospital:** UT Southwestern Med Ctr at Dallas; **Address:** UT SW Med Ctr - Dallas, Dept Rad-Onc, 5801 Forest Park Rd, Dallas, TX 75390-9183; **Phone:** 214-645-7600; **Board Cert:** Radiation Oncology 1993; **Med School:** Univ Tex Med Br, Galveston 1987; **Resid:** Radiation Oncology, Ohio State Univ Hosp 1989; Radiation Oncology, Univ Texas Hlth Sci Ctr 1991; **Fac Appt:** Prof RadRO, Univ Tex SW, Dallas

Cox, James D MD [RadRO] - **Spec Exp:** Lung Cancer; Esophageal Cancer; Thymoma; Thoracic Cancers; **Hospital:** UT MD Anderson Cancer Ctr; **Address:** Univ Tex MD Anderson Cancer Ctr, 1515 Holcombe Blvd, Unit 97, Houston, TX 77030; **Phone:** 713-563-2316; **Board Cert:** Therapeutic Radiology 1971; **Med School:** Univ Rochester 1965; **Resid:** Diagnostic Radiology, Penrose Cancer Hosp 1969; **Fellow:** Therapeutic Radiology, Inst Gustave-Roussy 1970; **Fac Appt:** Prof RadRO, Univ Tex, Houston

Eifel, Patricia J MD [RadRO] - **Spec Exp:** Cervical Cancer; Uterine Cancer; Vulvar Disease/Cancer; Vaginal Cancer; **Hospital:** UT MD Anderson Cancer Ctr; **Address:** MD Anderson Cancer Ctr, Dept Rad Onc, 1515 Holcombe Blvd, Unit 1202, Houston, TX 77030-4009; **Phone:** 713-563-6900; **Board Cert:** Therapeutic Radiology 1983; **Med School:** Stanford Univ 1977; **Resid:** Radiation Oncology, Stanford Univ Med Ctr 1981; **Fellow:** Therapeutic Radiology, Stanford Univ Med Ctr 1982

Grado, Gordon L MD [RadRO] - **Spec Exp:** Prostate Cancer; Brachytherapy; **Hospital:** Scottsdale Hlthcare - Shea; **Address:** 2926 N Civic Center Plaza, Scottsdale, AZ 85251; **Phone:** 480-614-6300; **Board Cert:** Therapeutic Radiology 1981; Radiation Oncology 1999; **Med School:** Southern IL Univ 1977; **Resid:** Therapeutic Radiology, Mayo Clinic 1981; **Fac Appt:** Assoc Prof RadRO, Univ Minn

Halyard, Michele MD [RadRO] - **Spec Exp:** Breast Cancer; Head & Neck Cancer; **Hospital:** Mayo Clinic - Scottsdale; **Address:** Mayo Clinic, Dept Radiation Oncology, 13400 E Shea Blvd, Scottsdale, AZ 85259-5404; **Phone:** 480-301-8120; **Board Cert:** Radiation Oncology 1989; **Med School:** Howard Univ 1984; **Resid:** Radiation Therapy, Howard Univ Hosp 1987; **Fellow:** Radiation Oncology, Mayo Clinic 1989

Herman, Terence S MD [RadRO] - **Spec Exp:** Breast Cancer; Sarcoma; Brain Tumors; **Hospital:** OU Med Ctr; **Address:** Oklahoma Univ Health Sci Ctr, 825 NE 10th St, Ste 1430, Oklahoma City, OK 73104-5417; **Phone:** 405-271-5641; **Board Cert:** Internal Medicine 1975; Medical Oncology 1977; Therapeutic Radiology 1985; **Med School:** Univ Conn 1972; **Resid:** Internal Medicine, Univ Arizona Med Ctr 1975; Radiation Oncology, Stanford Univ Med Ctr 1985; **Fellow:** Medical Oncology, Univ Arizona 1977; **Fac Appt:** Prof RadRO, Univ Okla Coll Med

Jhingran, Anuja MD [RadRO] - **Spec Exp:** Gynecologic Cancer; Brachytherapy; **Hospital:** UT MD Anderson Cancer Ctr; **Address:** MD Anderson Cancer Ctr, 1515 Holcombe Blvd, Box 1202, Houston, TX 77030; **Phone:** 713-563-6900; **Board Cert:** Radiation Oncology 1993; **Med School:** Texas Tech Univ 1988; **Resid:** Radiation Oncology, Baylor College Med 1993; **Fac Appt:** Assoc Prof RadRO, Univ Tex, Houston

Komaki, Ritsuko U MD [RadRO] - **Spec Exp:** Lung Cancer; Thymoma; Esophageal Cancer; **Hospital:** UT MD Anderson Cancer Ctr; **Address:** UT-MD Anderson Cancer Ctr, Dept Rad Onc, 1515 Holcombe Blvd, Unit 97, Houston, TX 77030; **Phone:** 713-563-2300; **Board Cert:** Therapeutic Radiology 1977; Radiation Oncology 2001; **Med School:** Japan 1969; **Resid:** Radiation Oncology, Med Coll Wisc 1978; **Fac Appt:** Prof RadRO, Univ Tex, Houston

Kuske, Robert R MD [RadRO] - **Spec Exp:** Breast Cancer; **Hospital:** Scottsdale Hlthcare - Shea; **Address:** 9055 E Del Camino Drive, Ste 200, Scottsdale, AZ 85258; **Phone:** 480-922-4600; **Board Cert:** Therapeutic Radiology 1985; **Med School:** Univ Cincinnati 1980; **Resid:** Radiation Oncology, Univ Cincinnati Med Ctr 1984

Lee, Andrew K MD [RadRO] - **Spec Exp:** Prostate Cancer; Proton Beam Therapy; Genitourinary Cancer; **Hospital:** UT MD Anderson Cancer Ctr; **Address:** MD Anderson Cancer Ctr, 1515 Holcombe Blvd, Unit 1150, Houston, TX 77030; **Phone:** 713-563-2348; **Board Cert:** Radiation Oncology 2001; **Med School:** Univ Minn 1996; **Resid:** Radiation Oncology, Joint Ctr for Radiation Therapy/Harvard 2001; **Fac Appt:** Assoc Prof RadRO, Univ Tex, Houston

Medbery, Clinton A MD [RadRO] - **Spec Exp:** Breast Cancer; Prostate Cancer; Brachytherapy; Stereotactic Radiosurgery; **Hospital:** St. Anthony Hosp -Oklahoma City; **Address:** Southwest Radiation Oncology, 1011 N Dewey Ave, Ste 101, Oklahoma City, OK 73101; **Phone:** 405-272-7311; **Board Cert:** Internal Medicine 1980; Medical Oncology 1983; Radiation Oncology 1987; **Med School:** Med Univ SC 1976; **Resid:** Internal Medicine, Naval Hosp 1980; Radiation Oncology, Natl Cancer Inst 1987; **Fellow:** Medical Oncology, Naval Hosp 1982

Morrison, William H MD [RadRO] - **Spec Exp:** Head & Neck Cancer; **Hospital:** UT MD Anderson Cancer Ctr; **Address:** 1515 Holcombe Blvd, Unit 97, Houston, TX 77030-4000; **Phone:** 713-794-1974; **Board Cert:** Internal Medicine 1981; Therapeutic Radiology 1985; **Med School:** Johns Hopkins Univ 1978; **Resid:** Internal Medicine, Rush Presby/St Lukes Med Ctr 1981; **Fellow:** Therapeutic Radiology, Stanford Univ Hosp 1985; **Fac Appt:** Prof RadRO, Univ Tex, Houston

Schild, Steven E MD [RadRO] - **Spec Exp:** Lung Cancer; Prostate Cancer; Clinical Trials; **Hospital:** Mayo Clinic - Scottsdale; **Address:** Mayo Clinic, Dept Radiation Oncology, 13400 E Shea Blvd, Scottsdale, AZ 85259; **Phone:** 480-342-1262; **Board Cert:** Radiation Oncology 1989; **Med School:** Creighton Univ 1985; **Resid:** Radiation Oncology, Mayo Clin 1989; **Fac Appt:** Prof RadRO, Mayo Med Sch

Senzer, Neil N MD [RadRO] - **Spec Exp:** Clinical Trials; Gene Therapy; **Hospital:** Med City Dallas Hosp, Baylor Univ Medical Ctr-Dallas; **Address:** Mary Crowley Cancer Research Ctr, 7777 Forest Ln C Bldg - Ste 707, Dallas, TX 75230; **Phone:** 972-566-3000; **Board Cert:** Pediatrics 1976; Pediatric Hematology-Oncology 1978; Therapeutic Radiology 1985; **Med School:** SUNY Buffalo 1971; **Resid:** Pediatrics, Johns Hopkins Hosp 1974; Radiation Oncology, St Barnabas Med Ctr 1985; **Fellow:** Pediatric Hematology-Oncology, St Jude Chldns Rsch Hosp 1978

Shina, Donald C MD [RadRO] - **Spec Exp:** Breast Cancer; **Hospital:** Christus St Vincent Reg Med Ctr-Santa Fe; **Address:** Santa Fe Cancer Ctr at St Vincent Hosp, 455 Saint Michael's Drive, Santa Fe, NM 87505; **Phone:** 505-820-5233; **Board Cert:** Internal Medicine 1977; Medical Oncology 1979; Therapeutic Radiology 1981; **Med School:** Case West Res Univ 1974; **Resid:** Internal Medicine, Univ Hosps 1977; **Fellow:** Radiation Oncology, Univ Hosps 1980; Medical Oncology, Univ Hosps 1980

Stea, Baldassarre MD/PhD [RadRO] - **Spec Exp:** Brain Tumors; Stereotactic Radiosurgery; Pediatric Cancers; Lymphoma; **Hospital:** Univ Med Ctr - Tucson, St. Joseph's Hosp - Tucson; **Address:** Univ Hlth Scis Ctr, Dept Rad Onc, 1501 N Campbell Ave, Tucson, AZ 85724-0001; **Phone:** 520-626-6724; **Board Cert:** Radiation Oncology 1987; **Med School:** Geo Wash Univ 1983; **Resid:** Radiation Oncology, Natl Cancer Inst 1987; **Fac Appt:** Prof RadRO, Univ Ariz Coll Med

Radiation Oncology

West Coast and Pacific

Donaldson, Sarah S MD [RadRO] - **Spec Exp:** Pediatric Cancers; Hodgkin's Disease; Sarcoma; Breast Cancer; **Hospital:** Stanford Univ Hosp & Clinics; **Address:** 875 Blake Wilbur Drive, CC Bldg Fl G - rm 226, MC 5847, Stanford, CA 94305-5847; **Phone:** 650-723-6195; **Board Cert:** Therapeutic Radiology 1974; **Med School:** Harvard Med Sch 1968; **Resid:** Radiation Oncology, Stanford Univ Med Ctr 1972; **Fellow:** Pediatric Hematology-Oncology, Inst Gustave-Roussy 1973; Pediatric Hematology-Oncology, MD Anderson Cancer Ctr 1971; **Fac Appt:** Prof RadRO, Stanford Univ

Fowble, Barbara MD [RadRO] - **Spec Exp:** Breast Cancer; **Hospital:** UCSF Med Ctr; **Address:** 1600 Divisadero St, Ste H1031, San Francisco, CA 94115; **Phone:** 415-353-9819; **Board Cert:** Therapeutic Radiology 1976; **Med School:** Jefferson Med Coll 1972; **Resid:** Therapeutic Radiology, Bellevue Hosp Ctr-NYU 1975; Therapeutic Radiology, Hahnemann 1976; **Fellow:** Radiation Therapy, Jefferson Hosp 1977; **Fac Appt:** Prof RadRO, UCSF

Fuss, Martin MD/PhD [RadRO] - **Spec Exp:** Intensity Modulated Radiotherapy (IMRT); Stereotactic Body Radiation Therapy; Stereotactic Radiosurgery; Bladder Cancer; **Hospital:** OR Hlth & Sci Univ; **Address:** Dept of Radiation Medicine, 3181 SW Sam Jackson Park Rd, MC KPV4, Portland, OR 97239; **Phone:** 503-494-8756; **Med School:** Germany 1994; **Resid:** Radiation Oncology, Univ of Heidelberg; **Fellow:** Radiation Therapy, Loma Linda Univ; **Fac Appt:** Prof RadRO, Oregon Hlth & Sci Univ

Halberg, Francine MD [RadRO] - **Spec Exp:** Breast Cancer; **Hospital:** Marin Genl Hosp, UCSF Med Ctr; **Address:** Marin Cancer Inst-Dept of Rad.Oncology, 1350 S Eliseo Drive, Ste 100, Greenbrae, CA 94904; **Phone:** 415-925-7326; **Board Cert:** Internal Medicine 1981; Therapeutic Radiology 1984; **Med School:** Cornell Univ-Weill Med Coll 1978; **Resid:** Internal Medicine, USPHS Hosp 1981; **Fellow:** Radiation Oncology, Stanford Univ Med Ctr 1984; **Fac Appt:** Assoc Prof RadRO, UCSF

Hancock, Steven MD [RadRO] - **Spec Exp:** Prostate Cancer; Breast Cancer; Cancer Survivors-Late Effects of Therapy; **Hospital:** Stanford Univ Hosp & Clinics; **Address:** Stanford Cancer Center-Dept Rad Onc, 875 Blake Wilbur Drive, MC 5847, Stanford, CA 94305; **Phone:** 650-723-6440; **Board Cert:** Internal Medicine 1980; Therapeutic Radiology 1982; **Med School:** Stanford Univ 1976; **Resid:** Radiation Therapy, Stanford Univ Med Ctr 1981; Internal Medicine, Stanford Univ Med Ctr 1979; **Fac Appt:** Prof RadRO, Stanford Univ

Hoppe, Richard T MD [RadRO] - **Spec Exp:** Lymphoma; Hodgkin's Disease; Cutaneous Lymphoma; **Hospital:** Stanford Univ Hosp & Clinics; **Address:** 875 Blake Wilbur Drive, rm CC-G224, Stanford, CA 94305-5847; **Phone:** 650-723-5510; **Board Cert:** Therapeutic Radiology 1976; **Med School:** Cornell Univ-Weill Med Coll 1971; **Resid:** Radiation Therapy, Stanford Univ Med Ctr 1976; **Fac Appt:** Prof, Stanford Univ

Koh, Wui-Jin MD [RadRO] - **Spec Exp:** Gynecologic Cancer; Brachytherapy; Clinical Trials; **Hospital:** Univ Wash Med Ctr; **Address:** Seattle Cancer Care Alliance, 825 Eastlake Ave E, Box 19023, MS G1-101, Seattle, WA 98109; **Phone:** 206-288-7318; **Board Cert:** Radiation Oncology 1988; **Med School:** Loma Linda Univ 1984; **Resid:** Radiation Oncology, Univ Washington Med Ctr 1988; **Fellow:** Tumor Imaging, Univ Washington Med Ctr 1988; **Fac Appt:** Prof RadRO, Univ Wash

Kupelian, Patrick A MD [RadRO] - **Spec Exp:** Genitourinary Cancer; Clinical Trials; Stereotactic Body Radiation Therapy; Stereotactic Radiosurgery; **Hospital:** UCLA Ronald Reagan Med Ctr; **Address:** UCLA Jonsson Comprehensive Cancer Center, 200 UCLA Medical Plaza, Ste B265, Los Angeles, CA 90095-6951; **Phone:** 310-825-9775; **Board Cert:** Radiation Oncology 2004; **Med School:** Lebanon 1989; **Resid:** Radiation Oncology, MD Anderson Cancer Ctr 1994; **Fellow:** Radiation Oncology, Cleveland Clin 1995; **Fac Appt:** Prof RadRO, UCLA

Laramore, George E MD/PhD [RadRO] - **Spec Exp:** Neutron Therapy for Advanced Cancer; Salivary Gland Tumors; Head & Neck Cancer; Skin Cancer; **Hospital:** Univ Wash Med Ctr, Harborview Med Ctr; **Address:** Univ Washington Med Ctr, Dept Rad Onc Box 356043, Seattle, WA 98195; **Phone:** 206-598-4121; **Board Cert:** Therapeutic Radiology 1980; Radiation Oncology 2000; **Med School:** Univ Miami Sch Med 1976; **Resid:** Radiation Oncology, Univ Washington Med Ctr 1980; **Fac Appt:** Prof RadRO, Univ Wash

Larson, David A MD/PhD [RadRO] - **Spec Exp:** Neuro-Oncology; Brain Tumors; Stereotactic Radiosurgery; **Hospital:** UCSF Med Ctr; **Address:** UCSF Med Ctr, Dept Rad Onc, 505 Parnassus Ave, rm L-08, San Francisco, CA 94143-0226; **Phone:** 415-353-8900; **Board Cert:** Therapeutic Radiology 1986; **Med School:** Univ Miami Sch Med 1981; **Resid:** Radiation Therapy, Joint Ctr RadTherapy 1985; **Fac Appt:** Prof RadRO, UCSF

Le, Quynh-Thu Xuan MD [RadRO] - **Spec Exp:** Head & Neck Cancer; Lung Cancer; Thoracic Cancers; Clinical Trials; **Hospital:** Stanford Univ Hosp & Clinics; **Address:** Stanford Univ, Dept Rad Oncology, 875 Blake Wilbur Drive, MC 5847, Ground Flr, Stanford, CA 94305; **Phone:** 650-498-5032; **Board Cert:** Radiation Oncology 2008; **Med School:** UCSF 1993; **Resid:** Radiation Oncology, UCSF Med Ctr 1997; **Fac Appt:** Prof RadRO, Stanford Univ

Mundt, Arno J MD [RadRO] - **Spec Exp:** Gynecologic Cancer; Intensity Modulated Radiotherapy (IMRT); **Hospital:** UCSD Med Ctr; **Address:** Moores UCSD Cancer Ctr, Radiation Oncology Dept, 3855 Health Sciences Drive, MC 0843, La Jolla, CA 92093-0843; **Phone:** 858-822-6046; **Board Cert:** Radiation Oncology 1994; **Med School:** Univ Mich Med Sch 1987; **Resid:** Physical Medicine & Rehabilitation, George Washington Univ Hosp 1990; Radiation Oncology, Univ Chicago Hosps 1993; **Fellow:** Physical Medicine & Rehabilitation, Univ Chicago Hosps 1994; **Fac Appt:** Assoc Prof RadRO, Univ Chicago-Pritzker Sch Med

Park, Catherine C MD [RadRO] - **Spec Exp:** Breast Cancer; Lymphoma; **Hospital:** UCSF Med Ctr; **Address:** UCSF Radiation Oncology, 1600 Divisadero St, Ste H1031, San Francisco, CA 94115; **Phone:** 415-353-7175; **Board Cert:** Radiation Oncology 2000; **Med School:** UCLA 1995; **Resid:** Radiation Oncology, Mass Genl Hosp 2000; **Fac Appt:** Assoc Prof RadRO, UCSF

Pezner, Richard D MD [RadRO] - **Spec Exp:** Sarcoma-Soft Tissue; Breast Cancer; Stereotactic Radiosurgery; **Hospital:** City of Hope Natl Med Ctr; **Address:** City of Hope Med Ctr-Div Radiation Onc, 1500 E Duarte Rd, Duarte, CA 91010-3000; **Phone:** 626-301-8247; **Board Cert:** Therapeutic Radiology 1979; **Med School:** Northwestern Univ 1975; **Resid:** Radiation Oncology, Oregon Health Sci Ctr 1979; **Fac Appt:** Clin Prof RadRO, UC Irvine

Quivey, Jeanne M MD [RadRO] - **Spec Exp:** Head & Neck Cancer; Breast Cancer; Eye Tumors/Cancer; Intensity Modulated Radiotherapy (IMRT); **Hospital:** UCSF Med Ctr; **Address:** UCSF Med Ctr @ Mt Zion, Radiation Onc Dept, 1600 Divisadero St, Ste H1031, Box 1708, San Francisco, CA 94115-3010; **Phone:** 415-353-7175; **Board Cert:** Therapeutic Radiology 1974; **Med School:** UCSF 1970; **Resid:** Radiation Therapy, UCSF Med Ctr 1974; **Fac Appt:** Prof RadRO, UCSF

Roach III, Mack MD [RadRO] - **Spec Exp:** Prostate Cancer; Genitourinary Cancer; Lung Cancer; **Hospital:** UCSF - Mt Zion Med Ctr, UCSF Med Ctr; **Address:** UCSF Radiation Oncology, 1600 Divisadero St, Ste H1031, San Francisco, CA 94143-1708; **Phone:** 415-353-7181; **Board Cert:** Internal Medicine 1984; Medical Oncology 1985; Radiation Oncology 1987; **Med School:** Stanford Univ 1979; **Resid:** Internal Medicine, ML King Genl Hosp 1981; Radiation Oncology, Stanford Univ Med Ctr 1987; **Fellow:** Medical Oncology, UCSF Med Ctr 1983; **Fac Appt:** Prof RadRO, UCSF

Radiation Oncology

Rose, Christopher M MD [RadRO] - **Spec Exp:** Prostate Cancer; Breast Cancer; Intensity Modulated Radiotherapy (IMRT); **Hospital:** Providence St Joseph Med Ctr, Providence Tarzana Med Ctr; **Address:** Valley Radiotherapy Assocs, The Ctr for Radiation Therapy, 9229 Wilshire Blvd, Beverly Hills, CA 90210; **Phone:** 310-205-5777; **Board Cert:** Radiation Oncology 1999; **Med School:** Harvard Med Sch 1974; **Resid:** Internal Medicine, Beth Israel Deaconess 1976; Radiation Oncology, Joint Ctr Rad Therapy 1979; **Fellow:** Cancer Research, British Inst Cancer Rsch 1979; **Fac Appt:** Clin Prof RadRO, USC Sch Med

Rossi, Carl John MD [RadRO] - **Spec Exp:** Prostate Cancer; Proton Beam Therapy; **Hospital:** Loma Linda Univ Med Ctr; **Address:** Loma Linda Univ Med Ctr, 11234 Anderson St, rm B124, Loma Linda, CA 92354; **Phone:** 909-558-4280; **Board Cert:** Radiation Oncology 1994; **Med School:** Loyola Univ-Stritch Sch Med 1988; **Resid:** Radiation Oncology, Loma Linda Univ Med Ctr 1992; **Fac Appt:** Asst Prof RadRO, Loma Linda Univ

Russell, Kenneth J MD [RadRO] - **Spec Exp:** Genitourinary Cancer; Prostate Cancer; Lymphoma; **Hospital:** Univ Wash Med Ctr; **Address:** Seattle Cancer Care Alliance, 825 Eastlake Ave E, Box 19023, MS G1-101, Seattle, WA 98109; **Phone:** 206-288-7318; **Board Cert:** Therapeutic Radiology 1984; **Med School:** Harvard Med Sch 1979; **Resid:** Radiation Therapy, Stanford Univ Med Ctr 1983; **Fellow:** Radiological Biology, Stanford Univ Med Ctr 1985; **Fac Appt:** Prof Rad, Univ Wash

Sandler, Howard M MD [RadRO] - **Spec Exp:** Prostate Cancer; Genitourinary Cancer; Brain Tumors; **Hospital:** Cedars-Sinai Med Ctr; **Address:** S Oschin Comprehensive Cancer Inst, Cedars-Sinai Med Ctr, 8700 Beverly Blvd, Los Angeles, CA 90048; **Phone:** 310-423-4234; **Board Cert:** Radiation Oncology 1989; **Med School:** Univ Conn 1985; **Resid:** Radiation Oncology, Hosp Univ Penn 1989

Seung, Steven K MD/PhD [RadRO] - **Spec Exp:** Stereotactic Radiosurgery; Brain Tumors; Esophageal Cancer; Lung Cancer; **Hospital:** Providence Portland Med Ctr; **Address:** 4805 NE Glisan St, Garden Level, Portland, OR 97213; **Phone:** 503-215-6029; **Board Cert:** Radiation Oncology 2010; **Med School:** Univ Chicago-Pritzker Sch Med 1994; **Resid:** Radiation Oncology, UCSF Med Ctr 1998

Thomas Jr, Charles R MD [RadRO] - **Spec Exp:** Gastrointestinal Cancer; Esophageal Cancer; Colon & Rectal Cancer; **Hospital:** OR Hlth & Sci Univ; **Address:** 3181 SW Sam Jackson Park Rd, MC KPV4, Portland, OR 97239; **Phone:** 503-494-8756; **Board Cert:** Internal Medicine 2010; Radiation Oncology 1999; **Med School:** Univ IL Coll Med 1985; **Resid:** Internal Medicine, Baylor Coll Med 1988; Radiation Oncology, Univ Wash Med Ctr 1997; **Fellow:** Medical Oncology, Rush Univ Med Ctr 1999; **Fac Appt:** Prof RadRO, Oregon Hlth & Sci Univ

Tripuraneni, Prabhakar MD [RadRO] - **Spec Exp:** Prostate Cancer; Head & Neck Cancer; Lymphoma; **Hospital:** Scripps Green Hosp, Scripps Meml Hosp - La Jolla; **Address:** Scripps Clinic, Div Radiation Oncology, 10666 N Torrey Pines Rd, MSB 1, La Jolla, CA 92037; **Phone:** 858-554-2000; **Board Cert:** Therapeutic Radiology 1983; **Med School:** India 1976; **Resid:** Radiation Oncology, Univ Alberta 1981; Radiation Oncology, UCSF Med Ctr 1983; **Fac Appt:** Clin Prof RadRO, UCSD

Wara, William M MD [RadRO] - **Spec Exp:** Brain & Spinal Tumors; Sarcoma; Pediatric Cancers; **Hospital:** Kaiser Permanente S San Francisco Med Ctr; **Address:** Cancer Treatment Ctr, 220 Oyster Pt Blvd, South San Francisco, CA 94080; **Phone:** 650-827-6500; **Board Cert:** Therapeutic Radiology 1974; **Med School:** UC Irvine 1969; **Resid:** Therapeutic Radiology, UCSF Medical Ctr 1973; **Fac Appt:** Prof RadRO, UCSF

Wong, Jeffrey Y C MD [RadRO] - **Spec Exp:** Radioimmunotherapy of Cancer; Prostate Cancer; Intensity Modulated Radiotherapy (IMRT); Multiple Myeloma; **Hospital:** City of Hope Natl Med Ctr; **Address:** City of Hope Med Ctr-Dept Radiation Onc, 1500 E Duarte Rd, Duarte, CA 91768-3012; **Phone:** 626-359-8111 x62969; **Board Cert:** Therapeutic Radiology 1985; **Med School:** Johns Hopkins Univ 1981; **Resid:** Radiation Oncology, UCSF Med Ctr 1985; **Fac Appt:** Prof RadRO, UC Irvine

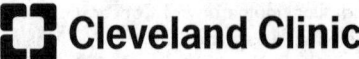
Cleveland Clinic

Every life deserves world class care.

Radiation Oncology

At Cleveland Clinic Taussig Cancer Institute, more than 250 top cancer specialists, researchers, nurses and technicians are dedicated to delivering the most effective medical treatments and offering access to the latest clinical trials for more than 13,000 new cancer patients every year. Our doctors are known nationally and internationally for their contributions to cancer breakthroughs and their ability to deliver superior outcomes for our patients. *U.S.News & World Report* has ranked Cleveland Clinic one of the top cancer centers in the nation.

The Taussig Cancer Institute offers a full range of advanced technology equipment, including 15 linear accelerators, fully integrated CT simulators and various image-guided treatment technologies. Using multiple imaging modalities including PET/CT, SPECT/CT and MRI, we offer patients accurately targeted treatment, and our state-of-the-art computer technologies provide precise external beam radiation. The department is equipped with a combined X-ray and optical imaging tracking system; kilovoltage and mega-voltage cone-beam computerized tomography; electromagnetic emission detectors and ultrasound imaging to provide optimal cancer treatment.

Our program was one of the first to implement intensity-modulated radiation therapy, image-guided radiation therapy and radioimmunotherapy. In addition to intra-cavitary and intraluminal treatments, we have developed many novel approaches to brachytherapy, especially with prostate cancer.

Cleveland Clinic is active in a number of in-house pharmaceutical and cooperative group trials. We are one of the leading enrollers in national studies and in combining novel agents such as radiation sensitizers with radiation therapy. In addition, the Department of Radiation Oncology houses one of the largest prostate cancer databases in the nation.

clevelandclinic.org/radonctopdocs

Offering Same-Day Appointments
Call 800.274.2009.

Treatment Guides

Cleveland Clinic has developed comprehensive treatment guides for many diseases and conditions. To download our free treatment guides, visit clevelandclinic.org/treatmentguides.

Online Medical Second Opinion

Cleveland Clinic's My**Consult** Online Medical Second Opinion program securely connects patients to our physician specialists for more than 1,000 life-changing or life-threatening diagnoses all by the click of a mouse. To learn more, log onto eclevelandclinic.org/myconsult or call 800.223.2273, ext. 43223.

Special Assistance for Out-of-State Patients

Cleveland Clinic Global Patient Services offers a complimentary Medical Concierge service for patients who travel from outside of Ohio. Call 800.223.2273, ext. 55580 or email medicalconcierge@ccf.org.

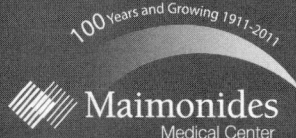
Maimonides Cancer Center offers a fully integrated, multi-modal approach to cancer care that includes prevention, education, screening, diagnostics, treatment, palliative care and clinical research. The Lena Cymbrowitz Pavilion contains the following specialty divisions:

Radiation Oncology: equipped with state-of-the art imaging and treatment delivery technologies; offers patients the most precise treatments available, yet does so in an airy, life-affirming environment.

Medical Oncology: provides comprehensive diagnosis, oral drug therapies, intravenous chemotherapy infusions, and biological and hormonal therapies.

Pediatric Oncology: treats children with cancer and diseases of the blood in a child-friendly environment, and features special areas set aside for parent conferences.

Surgical Oncology: provides a convenient location for minor surgical procedures, as well as innovative surgical techniques such as sentinel node mapping and biopsy, skin/tissue-sparing mastectomy, and nerve-sparing prostatectomy.

Research Center: conducts basic science and genetic research, as well as clinical trials that offer appropriately screened patients, who wish to volunteer, new therapies and medications.

Resource Center: offers access to integrative (complementary) oncology services, dietary advice, as well as psychological and social services.

Located around the block from the Maimonides Cancer Center, the newly opened Rivera Pavilion houses the **Maimonides Breast Cancer Center**. With a spa-like decor and life-affirming environment, the Center provides digital mammography, sonography, computerized interpretation, digital stereotactic biopsies, breast-specific gamma imaging, and treatment plans tailored to each patient. A genetics counselor is also on-site.

Clinicians at the Maimonides Cancer Center – Brooklyn's only dedicated cancer center – are talented specialists, recruited specifically for their expertise. Our doctors emphasize multimodal care, which means that multiple methods of treatment are available to patients, sometimes simultaneously. Every week, physicians from radiology, surgery, pathology, radiation oncology, and medical oncology meet to discuss patient treatment at our case management meetings. The patient's needs, as well as the disease, are considered from many angles.

Maimonides Medical Center
Passionate about medicine.
Compassionate about people.

www.maimonidesmed.org/cancer

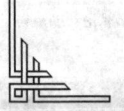
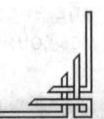

The Best in American Medicine
www.CastleConnolly.com

Radiology

A radiologist utilizes radiologic methodologies to diagnose and treat disease. Physicians practicing in the field of radiology most often specialize in radiology, diagnostic radiology, radiation oncology or radiological physics.

Diagnostic Radiology: A radiologist who utilizes X-ray, radionuclides, ultrasound and electromagnetic radiation to diagnose and treat disease.

Training Required: Four years

Radiation Oncology: A radiologist who deals with the therapeutic applications of radiant energy and its modifiers and the study and management of disease, especially malignant tumors.

Certification in one of the following subspecialties requires additional training and examination.

Neuroradiology: A radiologist who diagnoses and treats diseases utilizing imaging procedures as they relate to the brain, spine and spinal cord, head, neck and organs of special sense in adults and children.

Pediatric Radiology: A radiologist who is proficient in all forms of diagnostic imaging as it pertains to the treatment of diseases in the newborn, infant, child and adolescent. This specialist has knowledge of both imaging and interventional procedures related to the care and management of diseases of children. A pediatric radiologist must be highly knowledgeable of all organ systems as they relate to growth and development, congenital malformations, diseases peculiar to infants and children and diseases that begin in childhood but cause substantial residual impairment in adulthood.

Vascular and Interventional Radiology: A radiologist who diagnoses and treats diseases by various radiologic imaging modalities. These include fluoroscopy, digital radiography, computed tomography, sonography and magnetic resonance imaging.

DIAGNOSTIC RADIOLOGY

New England

Benson, Carol MD [DR] - **Spec Exp:** Obstetric Ultrasound; Thyroid Ultrasound; Fetal Surgical Imaging; Gynecologic Imaging; **Hospital:** Brigham and Women's Hosp (page 57); **Address:** Brigham & Women's Hosp, Dept Radiology, 75 Francis St, Boston, MA 02115; **Phone:** 617-732-6280; **Board Cert:** Diagnostic Radiology 1984; **Med School:** Univ Pennsylvania 1980; **Resid:** Diagnostic Radiology, New York Hosp-Cornell 1984; **Fellow:** Ultrasound, Brigham & Womens Hosp 1985; **Fac Appt:** Prof Rad, Harvard Med Sch

Black, William C MD [DR] - **Spec Exp:** Chest Radiology; Lung Cancer; CT Chest Scan; **Hospital:** Dartmouth - Hitchcock Med Ctr; **Address:** Dartmouth Hitchcock Med Ctr, Dept Radiology, 1 Med Ctr Drive, Lebanon, NH 03756; **Phone:** 603-650-7443; **Board Cert:** Diagnostic Radiology 1983; **Med School:** Med Coll VA 1979; **Resid:** Diagnostic Radiology, Univ Virginia Hosp 1983; **Fellow:** Ultrasound/CT, Univ Virginia Hosp 1984; **Fac Appt:** Prof Rad, Dartmouth Med Sch

Doubilet, Peter MD [DR] - **Spec Exp:** Ultrasound; Obstetric Ultrasound; **Hospital:** Brigham and Women's Hosp (page 57); **Address:** Brigham & Women's Hosp, Dept Radiology, 75 Francis St, Boston, MA 02115; **Phone:** 617-732-6757; **Board Cert:** Diagnostic Radiology 1981; **Med School:** Columbia P&S 1977; **Resid:** Diagnostic Radiology, Brigham Women's Hosp 1981; **Fac Appt:** Prof Rad, Harvard Med Sch

Kopans, Daniel B MD [DR] - **Spec Exp:** Breast Imaging; Breast Cancer; **Hospital:** Mass Genl Hosp; **Address:** Mass Genl Hosp, Avon Comprehensive Breast Ctr, 15 Parkman St, WAC 240, Boston, MA 02114; **Phone:** 617-726-3093; **Board Cert:** Diagnostic Radiology 1977; **Med School:** Harvard Med Sch 1973; **Resid:** Diagnostic Radiology, Mass Genl Hosp 1977; **Fac Appt:** Prof Rad, Harvard Med Sch

McCarthy, Shirley M MD/PhD [DR] - **Spec Exp:** Gynecologic Cancer; Pelvic Imaging; **Hospital:** Yale-New Haven Hosp, Yale Med Group; **Address:** Yale-New Haven Hosp, 333 Cedar St, Ste TE2, PO Box 208042, New Haven, CT 06520-3206; **Phone:** 203-785-2384; **Board Cert:** Diagnostic Radiology 1983; **Med School:** Yale Univ 1979; **Resid:** Diagnostic Radiology, Yale-New Haven Hosp 1983; **Fellow:** Cross Sectional Imaging, UCSF Med Ctr 1984; **Fac Appt:** Prof Rad, Yale Univ

Palmer, William E MD [DR] - **Spec Exp:** Musculoskeletal Imaging; Sports Medicine Radiology; Pain Management; Musculoskeletal Imaging; **Hospital:** Mass Genl Hosp; **Address:** 55 Fruit St, YAW 6030, Boston, MA 02114; **Phone:** 617-726-7717; **Board Cert:** Internal Medicine 1987; Diagnostic Radiology 1991; **Med School:** Yale Univ 1984; **Resid:** Internal Medicine, Hosp Univ Penn 1987; Diagnostic Radiology, Mass Genl Hosp 1991

Weinreb, Jeffrey C MD [DR] - **Spec Exp:** MRI; Breast Cancer; Abdominal Imaging; CT Body Scan; **Hospital:** Yale-New Haven Hosp, Yale Med Group; **Address:** Yale Univ Sch Medicine, Dept Radiology, 333 Cedar St, rm MRC147, Box 208042, New Haven, CT 06520-8042; **Phone:** 203-785-5913; **Board Cert:** Diagnostic Radiology 1983; **Med School:** Mount Sinai Sch Med 1978; **Resid:** Diagnostic Radiology, LI Jewish Med Ctr 1982; **Fellow:** Ultrasound/CT, Hosp Univ Penn 1983; **Fac Appt:** Prof Rad, Yale Univ

Mid Atlantic

Adler, Ronald S MD/PhD [DR] - **Spec Exp:** Musculoskeletal Imaging; Ultrasound; Power Doppler Imaging; **Hospital:** Hosp For Special Surgery (page 60), NY-Presby/Weill Cornell Med Ctr, NY (page 65); **Address:** Hosp for Special Surgery, 535 E 70th St, New York, NY 10021; **Phone:** 212-606-1635; **Board Cert:** Diagnostic Radiology 1988; **Med School:** Wayne State Univ 1984; **Resid:** Diagnostic Radiology, Univ Mich Med Ctr 1988; **Fellow:** Ultrasound/CT/MRI, Univ Mich Med Ctr 1989; **Fac Appt:** Prof Rad, Cornell Univ-Weill Med Coll

Austin, John H M MD [DR] - **Spec Exp:** Lung Cancer; Thoracic Radiology; **Hospital:** NY-Presby/Columbia Univ Med Ctr, NY (page 65); **Address:** Columbia Presby Hosp, Dept Radiology, 622 W 168th St, HP 3-305, New York, NY 10032-3784; **Phone:** 212-305-2986; **Board Cert:** Diagnostic Radiology 1970; **Med School:** Yale Univ 1965; **Resid:** Diagnostic Radiology, UCSF Med Ctr 1968; **Fellow:** Diagnostic Radiology, UCSF Med Ctr 1970; **Fac Appt:** Prof Emeritus Rad, Columbia P&S

Bluemke, David A MD/PhD [DR] - **Spec Exp:** Cardiac Imaging; MRI; **Hospital:** Natl Inst of Hlth - Clin Ctr; **Address:** 9000 Rockville Pike, Bldg 10 - Ste 1C351, Betheseda, MD 20892; **Phone:** 301-402-1854; **Board Cert:** Diagnostic Radiology 1993; **Med School:** Univ Chicago-Pritzker Sch Med 1989; **Resid:** Diagnostic Radiology, Johns Hopkins Hosp 1993; **Fellow:** Diagnostic Imaging, Johns Hopkins Hosp 1994; **Fac Appt:** Prof Rad, Johns Hopkins Univ

Brem, Rachel F MD [DR] - **Spec Exp:** Breast Imaging; Breast Cancer; **Hospital:** G Washington Univ Hosp; **Address:** GWU Med Faculty Assocs, Mammography Clin, 2150 Pennsylvania Ave NW, DC Level, Washington, DC 20037; **Phone:** 202-741-3036; **Board Cert:** Diagnostic Radiology 1990; **Med School:** Columbia P&S 1984; **Resid:** Diagnostic Radiology, Johns Hopkins Hosp 1989; **Fellow:** Mammography, Johns Hopkins Hosp 1990; **Fac Appt:** Prof Rad, Geo Wash Univ

Cohen, Burton A MD [DR] - **Spec Exp:** CT Scan; MRI; PET Imaging; **Hospital:** Mount Sinai Med Ctr (page 63); **Address:** 165 E 84th St, New York, NY 10028; **Phone:** 212-535-9770; **Board Cert:** Diagnostic Radiology 1979; **Med School:** NY Med Coll 1975; **Resid:** Diagnostic Radiology, Mt Sinai Hosp 1979; **Fac Appt:** Assoc Clin Prof Rad, Mount Sinai Sch Med

Coleman, Beverly G MD [DR] - **Spec Exp:** Ultrasound; **Hospital:** Hosp Univ Penn - UPHS (page 68); **Address:** Univ Penn Radiology, Ground Dulles, 3400 Spruce St, Philadelphia, PA 19104; **Phone:** 215-662-3046; **Board Cert:** Diagnostic Radiology 1978; **Med School:** Harvard Med Sch 1974; **Resid:** Diagnostic Radiology, Univ Penn Hosp 1975; Diagnostic Radiology, Univ Mich Hosp 1977; **Fellow:** Ultrasound, Univ Penn Hosp 1979; **Fac Appt:** Prof Rad, Univ Pennsylvania

Conant, Emily F MD [DR] - **Spec Exp:** Breast Cancer; Breast Imaging; **Hospital:** Hosp Univ Penn - UPHS (page 68); **Address:** Dept Radiology (Breast Imaging), 3400 Spruce St, 1 Silverstein, Philadelphia, PA 19104; **Phone:** 215-662-4032; **Board Cert:** Diagnostic Radiology 1989; **Med School:** Univ Pennsylvania 1984; **Resid:** Diagnostic Radiology, Hosp Univ Penn 1986; **Fellow:** Breast Imaging, Hosp Univ Penn 1989; **Fac Appt:** Prof Rad, Univ Pennsylvania

Dalinka, Murray MD [DR] - **Spec Exp:** Bone Disorders-Metabolic; Musculoskeletal Imaging; MRI; **Hospital:** Hosp Univ Penn - UPHS (page 68); **Address:** Hosp Univ Penn, Dept Radiology, 3400 Spruce St, Philadelphia, PA 19104; **Phone:** 215-662-3019; **Board Cert:** Diagnostic Radiology 1969; **Med School:** Univ Mich Med Sch 1964; **Resid:** Diagnostic Radiology, Montefiore Med Ctr 1968; **Fac Appt:** Prof Emeritus Rad, Univ Pennsylvania

Dershaw, D David MD [DR] - **Spec Exp:** Breast Imaging; Breast Cancer; Mammography; **Hospital:** Meml Sloan-Kettering Cancer Ctr; **Address:** 300 E 66th St, New York, NY 10065; **Phone:** 800-525-2225; **Board Cert:** Diagnostic Radiology 1978; **Med School:** Jefferson Med Coll 1974; **Resid:** Diagnostic Radiology, New York Hosp 1978; **Fellow:** Ultrasound, Thos Jefferson Univ Hosp 1979; **Fac Appt:** Prof Rad, Cornell Univ-Weill Med Coll

Edelstein, Barbara A MD [DR] - **Spec Exp:** Breast Cancer; Women's Imaging; **Address:** 1045 Park Ave, New York, NY 10028; **Phone:** 212-860-7700; **Board Cert:** Diagnostic Radiology 1983; **Med School:** NY Med Coll 1977; **Resid:** Diagnostic Radiology, Montefiore Hosp 1982

Evers, Kathryn A MD [DR] - **Spec Exp:** Breast Cancer; Mammography; MRI-Breast; **Hospital:** Fox Chase Cancer Ctr (page 58); **Address:** Fox Chase Cancer Ctr, Diagnostic Imaging, 333 Cottman Ave, Philadelphia, PA 19111; **Phone:** 215-728-2646; **Board Cert:** Diagnostic Radiology 1980; **Med School:** NYU Sch Med 1975; **Resid:** Diagnostic Radiology, Hosp Univ Penn 1980; **Fellow:** Diagnostic Radiology, Hosp Univ Penn 1981; **Fac Appt:** Asst Clin Prof Rad, Temple Univ

Fishman, Elliot MD [DR] - **Spec Exp:** CT Body Scan; Abdominal Imaging; Cardiac Imaging; Cancer Imaging; **Hospital:** Johns Hopkins Hosp (page 61); **Address:** Johns Hopkins Hosp, Dept Radiology, 601 N Caroline St, JHOC 3254, Baltimore, MD 21287-0006; **Phone:** 410-955-5173; **Board Cert:** Diagnostic Radiology 1981; **Med School:** Univ MD Sch Med 1977; **Resid:** Diagnostic Radiology, Sinai Hosp 1980; **Fellow:** Computerized Tomography, Johns Hopkins Hosp 1981; **Fac Appt:** Prof Rad, Johns Hopkins Univ

Fuhrman, Carl R MD [DR] - **Spec Exp:** Thoracic Imaging; **Hospital:** UPMC Presby, Pittsburgh; **Address:** UPMC-Dept Radiology, 200 Lothrop St, rm E177-PUH, Pittsburgh, PA 15213; **Phone:** 412-647-7288; **Board Cert:** Diagnostic Radiology 1983; **Med School:** Univ Pittsburgh 1979; **Resid:** Diagnostic Radiology, Presby Univ Hosp 1983; **Fac Appt:** Prof Rad, Univ Pittsburgh

Gefter, Warren B MD [DR] - **Spec Exp:** Thoracic Imaging; **Hospital:** Hosp Univ Penn - UPHS (page 68); **Address:** Hospital Univ Penn, 1 Silverstein, 3400 Spruce St, Philadelphia, PA 19104; **Phone:** 215-662-6724; **Board Cert:** Diagnostic Radiology 1978; **Med School:** Univ Pennsylvania 1974; **Resid:** Diagnostic Radiology, Hosp Univ Penn 1978; **Fac Appt:** Prof Rad, Univ Pennsylvania

Henschke, Claudia L MD/PhD [DR] - **Spec Exp:** Lung Cancer; Lung Disease; Thoracic Radiology; **Hospital:** Mount Sinai Med Ctr (page 63); **Address:** Mt Sinai Med Ctr, Radiology Dept, 1 Gustave Levy Pl, Box 1234, New York, NY 10029; **Phone:** 212-241-2420; **Board Cert:** Diagnostic Radiology 1981; **Med School:** Howard Univ 1977; **Resid:** Diagnostic Radiology, Brigham & Womens Hosp 1983; **Fac Appt:** Prof Rad, Cornell Univ-Weill Med Coll

Holliday, Roy MD [DR] - **Spec Exp:** Head & Neck Radiology; **Hospital:** New York Eye & Ear Infirm (page 64), Beth Israel Med Ctr - Petrie Division (page 55); **Address:** 310 E 14th St, New York, NY 10003; **Phone:** 212-979-4397; **Board Cert:** Diagnostic Radiology 1986; **Med School:** NYU Sch Med 1982; **Resid:** Diagnostic Radiology, NYU Med Ctr 1986; **Fellow:** Neurological Radiology, NYU Med Ctr 1987; **Fac Appt:** Clin Prof Rad, NYU Sch Med

Hricak, Hedvig MD/PhD [DR] - **Spec Exp:** Prostate Cancer-MR Spectroscopy (MRSI); Breast Imaging; Breast Cancer; **Hospital:** Meml Sloan-Kettering Cancer Ctr; **Address:** 1275 York Ave, Ste C278, New York, NY 10065; **Phone:** 800-525-2225; **Board Cert:** Diagnostic Radiology 1978; **Med School:** Yugoslavia 1970; **Resid:** Diagnostic Radiology, St Joseph Mercy Hosp 1977; **Fellow:** Ultrasound/CT, Henry Ford Hosp 1978; **Fac Appt:** Prof Rad, Cornell Univ-Weill Med Coll

Diagnostic Radiology

Jaramillo, Diego MD [DR] - **Spec Exp:** Pediatric Radiology; **Hospital:** Chldns Hosp of Philadelphia; **Address:** CHOP, Dept Radiology, 34th & Civic Center Blvd, rm 3NW-17, Philadelphia, PA 19104; **Phone:** 267-425-7110; **Board Cert:** Diagnostic Radiology 1987; Pediatric Radiology 2005; **Med School:** Colombia 1981; **Resid:** Diagnostic Radiology, Univ Texas 1987; **Fellow:** Pediatric Radiology, Children's Hosp 1989; **Fac Appt:** Prof Rad, Univ Pennsylvania

Kanal, Emanuel MD [DR] - **Spec Exp:** Neuroradiology; MRI; **Hospital:** UPMC Presby, Pittsburgh; **Address:** Univ Pittsburgh Med Ctr, Dept Radiology, 200 Lothrop St, rm D132, Pittsburgh, PA 15213-2582; **Phone:** 412-647-3540; **Board Cert:** Diagnostic Radiology 1985; **Med School:** Univ Pittsburgh 1981; **Resid:** Diagnostic Radiology, Univ Pittsburgh Med Ctr 1985; **Fellow:** Magnetic Resonance Imaging, Pittsburgh NMR Inst 1986; Neurological Radiology, Univ Pittsburgh Med Ctr 1993; **Fac Appt:** Prof Rad, Univ Pittsburgh

Kurtz, Alfred B MD [DR] - **Spec Exp:** Obstetric Ultrasound; **Hospital:** Thomas Jefferson Univ Hosp; **Address:** Thomas Jefferson Univ Hosp, Radiology, 111 S 11th St, Ste 3350A-B, Philadelphia, PA 19107; **Phone:** 215-955-6343; **Board Cert:** Diagnostic Radiology 1977; **Med School:** Stanford Univ 1972; **Resid:** Internal Medicine, Montefiore Med Ctr 1974; Diagnostic Radiology, Montefiore Med Ctr 1977; **Fellow:** Ultrasound, Thomas Jefferson Univ Hosp 1978; **Fac Appt:** Prof Rad, Jefferson Med Coll

Levy, Angela D MD [DR] - **Spec Exp:** Abdominal Imaging; **Hospital:** Georgetown Univ Hosp, Armed Forces Inst of Path; **Address:** Georgetown University Hospital, 3800 Reservoir Rd NW, Ground Floor, Washington, DC 20007; **Phone:** 202-444-3380; **Board Cert:** Diagnostic Radiology 1993; **Med School:** Uniformed Srvs Univ, Bethesda 1988; **Resid:** Diagnostic Radiology, Walter Reed Army Hosp 1992; **Fac Appt:** Assoc Prof Rad, Uniformed Srvs Univ, Bethesda

Megibow, Alec J MD [DR] - **Spec Exp:** Abdominal Imaging; Gastrointestinal Imaging; CT Body Scan; **Hospital:** NYU Langone Med Ctr (page 66), Bellevue Hosp Ctr; **Address:** 550 1st Ave, HHC 232, New York, NY 10016; **Phone:** 212-263-5222; **Board Cert:** Diagnostic Radiology 1978; **Med School:** SUNY Upstate Med Univ 1974; **Resid:** Diagnostic Radiology, Bellevue/NYU Med Ctr 1978; **Fellow:** Abdominal Imaging, NYU Med Ctr 1978; **Fac Appt:** Prof Rad, NYU Sch Med

Mirvis, Stuart E MD [DR] - **Spec Exp:** Trauma Radiology; **Hospital:** Univ of MD Med Ctr; **Address:** Univ Maryland Med Ctr, Dept Radiology, 22 S Greene St, Baltimore, MD 21201; **Phone:** 410-328-8845; **Board Cert:** Diagnostic Radiology 1984; **Med School:** Johns Hopkins Univ 1979; **Resid:** Diagnostic Radiology, Univ Maryland Med Ctr 1984; **Fellow:** Trauma Radiology, Univ Maryland Med Ctr 1985; **Fac Appt:** Prof Rad, Univ MD Sch Med

Mitnick, Julie MD [DR] - **Spec Exp:** Mammography; Breast Cancer; **Address:** 650 1st Ave, New York, NY 10016; **Phone:** 212-686-4440; **Board Cert:** Diagnostic Radiology 1977; **Med School:** NYU Sch Med 1973; **Resid:** Diagnostic Radiology, NYU Med Ctr 1977; **Fellow:** Pediatric Radiology, NYU Med Ctr 1978; **Fac Appt:** Assoc Clin Prof Rad, NYU Sch Med

Panicek, David M MD [DR] - **Spec Exp:** Bone Cancer; Soft Tissue Tumors; Musculoskeletal Tumor Imaging; **Hospital:** Meml Sloan-Kettering Cancer Ctr; **Address:** Department of Radiology, 1275 York Ave, New York, NY 10065; **Phone:** 800-525-2225; **Board Cert:** Diagnostic Radiology 1984; **Med School:** Cornell Univ-Weill Med Coll 1980; **Resid:** Diagnostic Radiology, NY Hosp-Cornell Med Ctr 1984; **Fac Appt:** Prof Rad, Cornell Univ-Weill Med Coll

Parsons, Rosaleen B MD [DR] - **Spec Exp:** CT Body Scan; Genitourinary Cancer; Genitourinary Radiology; **Hospital:** Fox Chase Cancer Ctr (page 58); **Address:** Fox Chase Cancer Ctr, Dept of Diagnostic Imaging, 333 Cottman Ave, Philadelphia, PA 19111; **Phone:** 215-728-3024; **Board Cert:** Diagnostic Radiology 1991; **Med School:** Med Coll PA Hahnemann 1986; **Resid:** Diagnostic Radiology, Med Coll Penn Affil Hosp 1991; **Fac Appt:** Assoc Clin Prof Rad, Temple Univ

Pavlov, Helene MD [DR] - **Spec Exp:** Sports Medicine Radiology; Musculoskeletal Imaging; Orthopaedic Imaging; **Hospital:** Hosp For Special Surgery (page 60), NY-Presby/Weill Cornell Med Ctr, NY (page 65); **Address:** Hosp for Special Surgery, 535 E 70th St, New York, NY 10021-4892; **Phone:** 212-606-1132; **Board Cert:** Diagnostic Radiology 1976; **Med School:** Temple Univ 1972; **Resid:** Diagnostic Radiology, Germantown Hosp 1976; **Fellow:** Musculoskeletal Imaging, Hosp For Special Surg 1977; **Fac Appt:** Prof Rad, Cornell Univ-Weill Med Coll

Potter, Hollis G MD [DR] - **Spec Exp:** Musculoskeletal Imaging; Cartilage Damage; Arthroplasty Imaging; **Hospital:** Hosp For Special Surgery (page 60); **Address:** Hosp for Special Surgery, MRI-basement, 535 E 70th St, New York, NY 10021-4892; **Phone:** 212-606-1882; **Board Cert:** Diagnostic Radiology 1990; **Med School:** NY Med Coll 1985; **Resid:** Diagnostic Radiology, North Shore Univ Hosp 1990; **Fellow:** Diagnostic Radiology, Hosp Special Surgery 1991; **Fac Appt:** Prof Rad, Cornell Univ-Weill Med Coll

Rao, Vijay M MD [DR] - **Spec Exp:** Head & Neck Tumors Imaging; TMJ Imaging; Ear Nose & Throat Imaging; **Hospital:** Thomas Jefferson Univ Hosp; **Address:** 132 S 10th St, 1087 Main Bldg, Philadelphia, PA 19107-4824; **Phone:** 215-955-4804; **Board Cert:** Diagnostic Radiology 1978; **Med School:** India 1973; **Resid:** Diagnostic Radiology, Thomas Jefferson Univ Hosp 1978; **Fac Appt:** Prof Rad, Thomas Jefferson Univ

Reinus, William R MD [DR] - **Spec Exp:** Musculoskeletal Imaging; MRI; **Hospital:** Temple Univ Hosp; **Address:** Temple Univ Hosp, Dept Radiology, 3401 N Broad St, Philadelphia, PA 19140; **Phone:** 215-707-9745; **Board Cert:** Diagnostic Radiology 1983; **Med School:** NYU Sch Med 1979; **Resid:** Radiology, Mallinkradt Inst Rad 1983; **Fellow:** Musculoskeletal Imaging, Mallinkradt Inst Rad 1984; **Fac Appt:** Assoc Prof Rad, Temple Univ

Roth, Susan G MD [DR] - **Spec Exp:** Breast Imaging; Breast Cancer; **Hospital:** Hosp Univ Penn - UPHS (page 68); **Address:** Hosp Univ Penn, Dept Radiology, 3400 Spruce St, Philadelphia, PA 19104; **Phone:** 215-614-0124; **Board Cert:** Diagnostic Radiology 1989; **Med School:** Univ Pennsylvania 1986; **Resid:** Diagnostic Radiology, Johns Hopkins Hosp 1989; **Fac Appt:** Prof Rad, Univ Pennsylvania

Teal, James S MD [DR] - **Spec Exp:** Interventional Radiology; **Hospital:** Howard Univ Hosp; **Address:** Howard Univ Hosp, Dept Radiology, 2041 Georgia Ave NW, Washington, DC 20060; **Phone:** 202-865-1571; **Board Cert:** Diagnostic Radiology 1970; **Med School:** Univ Tex Med Br, Galveston 1964; **Resid:** Diagnostic Radiology, Mt Zion Hosp 1969; **Fellow:** Neuroradiology, LAC-USC Med Ctr 1970; **Fac Appt:** Prof Rad, Howard Univ

White, Charles S MD [DR] - **Spec Exp:** Thoracic Imaging; **Hospital:** Univ of MD Med Ctr; **Address:** Univ Maryland Med Ctr, Dept Radiology, 22 S Greene St, Baltimore, MD 21201; **Phone:** 410-328-3477; **Board Cert:** Diagnostic Radiology 1991; Internal Medicine 1987; **Med School:** SUNY Buffalo 1984; **Resid:** Internal Medicine, Columbia-Presby Hosp 1987; Diagnostic Radiology, Columbia-Presby Hosp 1991; **Fellow:** Thoracic Radiology, Columbia-Presby Med Ctr; **Fac Appt:** Prof, Univ MD Sch Med

Yankelevitz, David MD [DR] - **Spec Exp:** Lung Cancer; Thoracic Radiology; **Hospital:** Mount Sinai Med Ctr (page 63); **Address:** Mt Sinai Med Ctr, Radiology Dept, 1 Gustave Levy Pl, Box 1234, New York, NY 10029; **Phone:** 212-241-2420; **Board Cert:** Diagnostic Radiology 1987; Nuclear Medicine 1987; **Med School:** SUNY Hlth Sci Ctr 1981; **Resid:** Diagnostic Radiology, Long Island Coll Hosp 1984; Nuclear Medicine, NY-Cornell Med Ctr 1987; **Fellow:** Diagnostic Radiology, NY-Cornell Med Ctr 1987; **Fac Appt:** Prof Rad, Cornell Univ-Weill Med Coll

Diagnostic Radiology

Yoon, Sydney S MD [DR] - Spec Exp: MRI; CT Scan; Neuroradiology; Interventional Radiology; **Hospital:** South Nassau Comm Hosp; **Address:** 1 Healthy Way, Dept of Radiology, Oceanside, NY 11572; **Phone:** 516-632-4660; **Board Cert:** Internal Medicine 1989; Diagnostic Radiology 1993; Vascular & Interventional Radiology 2011; Neuroradiology 2006; **Med School:** Univ Chicago-Pritzker Sch Med 1986; **Resid:** Internal Medicine, Johns Hopkins Hosp 1989; Diagnostic Radiology, UCLA Med Ctr 1993; **Fellow:** Neuroradiology, Columbia Presby Med Ctr 1995; Vascular & Interventional Radiology, UCLA Med Ctr 1997

Zeman, Robert K MD [DR] - Spec Exp: Cardiovascular Imaging; Cardiac CT Angiography; Nuclear Medicine; **Hospital:** G Washington Univ Hosp; **Address:** GM Medical Faculty Associates, Diagnostic Radiology, 900 23rd St NW, Washington, DC 20037; **Phone:** 202-715-5154; **Board Cert:** Diagnostic Radiology 1980; **Med School:** Northwestern Univ 1976; **Resid:** Diagnostic Radiology, Yale-New Haven Hosp 1980; **Fellow:** Nuclear Medicine, Yale-New Haven Hosp 1980; **Fac Appt:** Prof Rad, Geo Wash Univ

Southeast

Abbitt, Patricia L MD [DR] - Spec Exp: Ultrasound; Interventional Radiology; Breast Imaging; Breast Cancer; **Hospital:** Shands at Univ of FL; **Address:** Shands Healthcare, Dept Radiology, 1600 SW Archer Rd, PO Box 100374, Gainesville, FL 32610; **Phone:** 352-265-0291; **Board Cert:** Diagnostic Radiology 1986; **Med School:** Tufts Univ 1981; **Resid:** Diagnostic Radiology, Univ VA Med Ctr 1986; **Fellow:** Breast Imaging, Univ VA Med Ctr 1987; **Fac Appt:** Prof Rad, Univ Fla Coll Med

Berland, Lincoln L MD [DR] - Spec Exp: Abdominal Imaging; Gastrointestinal Imaging; **Hospital:** Univ of Ala Hosp at Birmingham; **Address:** UAB Diagnostic Radiology, N348 Jefferson Tower Bldg, 619 19th St S, Birmingham, AL 35249-6830; **Phone:** 205-934-7978; **Board Cert:** Diagnostic Radiology 1980; **Med School:** Washington Univ, St Louis 1975; **Resid:** Diagnostic Radiology, Med Coll Wisconsin Hosps 1979; **Fellow:** Ultrasound/CT, Med Coll Wisconsin Hosps 1980; **Fac Appt:** Prof Rad, Univ Alabama

Cardenosa, Gilda MD [DR] - Spec Exp: Breast Imaging; **Hospital:** Med Coll of VA Hosp; **Address:** VCU Med Ctr at Stony Point, Dept Radiology, 9000 Stony Point Pkwy, Richmond, VA 23235; **Phone:** 804-560-8906 x7862; **Board Cert:** Diagnostic Radiology 1989; **Med School:** Columbia P&S 1984; **Resid:** Diagnostic Radiology, Mass Genl Hosp 1989; **Fac Appt:** Prof Rad, Med Coll VA

Chiles, Caroline MD [DR] - Spec Exp: Thoracic Radiology; Lung Cancer; **Hospital:** Wake Forest Univ Baptist Med Ctr; **Address:** Medical Center Blvd, Winston-Salem, NC 27157; **Phone:** 336-716-4316; **Board Cert:** Diagnostic Radiology 1984; **Med School:** Duke Univ 1979; **Resid:** Diagnostic Radiology, Stanford Univ Hosp 1984; **Fellow:** Thoracic Radiology, Duke Univ Med Ctr 1985; **Fac Appt:** Assoc Prof Rad, Bowman Gray

Cohen, Harris L MD [DR] - Spec Exp: Pediatric Radiology; Fetal Ultrasound/Obstetrical Imaging; Ultrasound; **Hospital:** Le Bonheur Chldns Med Ctr; **Address:** Le Bonheur Children's Hosp, Dept Radiology Fl Ground, 50 N Dunlap St, Memphis, TN 38103-2807; **Phone:** 901-287-6938; **Board Cert:** Diagnostic Radiology 1980; Pediatric Radiology 2005; **Med School:** SUNY Downstate 1976; **Resid:** Diagnostic Radiology, Univ Hosp 1980; **Fellow:** Pediatric Radiology, Chldns Hosp 1981; **Fac Appt:** Prof Rad, Univ Tenn Coll Med

Elster, Allen D MD [DR] - **Spec Exp:** MRI; Neurologic Imaging; Brain Tumors; Spinal Tumors; **Hospital:** Wake Forest Univ Baptist Med Ctr; **Address:** Wake Forest Univ Baptist Med Ctr, 1 Medical Center Blvd, Dept Radiology, Winston Salem, NC 27157-1088; **Phone:** 336-716-7095; **Board Cert:** Diagnostic Radiology 1987; Neuroradiology 2005; **Med School:** Baylor Coll Med 1980; **Resid:** Surgery, Mass Genl Hosp 1983; Diagnostic Radiology, Univ Texas 1986; **Fellow:** Neuroradiology, Bowman Gray Sch Med 1987; **Fac Appt:** Prof Rad, Wake Forest Univ

Freimanis, Rita I MD [DR] - **Spec Exp:** Breast Cancer; Breast Imaging; **Hospital:** Wake Forest Univ Baptist Med Ctr; **Address:** Wake Forest Univ Bapt Med Ctr, One Medical Center Blvd, Winston-Salem, NC 27157; **Phone:** 336-713-4019; **Board Cert:** Diagnostic Radiology 1990; **Med School:** Bowman Gray 1985; **Resid:** Diagnostic Radiology, NC Bapt Hosp 1990; **Fac Appt:** Assoc Prof Rad, Wake Forest Univ

Mancuso, Anthony A MD [DR] - **Spec Exp:** Head & Neck Radiology; Neuroradiology; **Hospital:** Shands at Univ of FL; **Address:** Shands Hosp, Univ Florida, Dept Radiology, 1600 SW Archer Rd, Ste G393, Gainesville, FL 32610; **Phone:** 352-265-0296; **Board Cert:** Diagnostic Radiology 1978; **Med School:** Univ Miami Sch Med 1973; **Resid:** Diagnostic Radiology, UCLA Med Ctr 1977; **Fellow:** Neuroradiology, UCLA Med Ctr 1978; **Fac Appt:** Prof Rad, Univ Fla Coll Med

Partain, Clarence L MD/PhD [DR] - **Spec Exp:** MRI; Nuclear Radiology; Chest Radiology; **Hospital:** Vanderbilt Univ Med Ctr (page 76); **Address:** Vanderbilt Univ Med Ctr, Dept Radiology, 1161 21st Ave S, rm RR1223 MCN, Nashville, TN 37232-2675; **Phone:** 615-343-3588; **Board Cert:** Nuclear Medicine 1979; Diagnostic Radiology 1980; Nuclear Radiology 1981; **Med School:** Washington Univ, St Louis 1975; **Resid:** Diagnostic Radiology, Univ North Carolina 1979; Nuclear Medicine, Univ North Carolina 1979; **Fac Appt:** Prof, Vanderbilt Univ

Patz, Edward F MD [DR] - **Spec Exp:** Thoracic Radiology; PET Imaging; Lung Cancer; **Hospital:** Duke Univ Hosp; **Address:** Duke Univ Med Ctr, Dept Radiology, Box 3808, Durham, NC 27710; **Phone:** 919-684-7999; **Board Cert:** Diagnostic Radiology 1990; **Med School:** Univ MD Sch Med 1985; **Resid:** Diagnostic Radiology, Brigham & Womens Hosp 1990; **Fellow:** Thoracic Radiology, Brigham & Womens Hosp 1990; **Fac Appt:** Prof, Duke Univ

Rubin, Geoffrey D MD [DR] - **Spec Exp:** Cardiovascular Imaging; Cardiac Imaging; Thoracic Imaging; **Hospital:** Duke Univ Hosp; **Address:** Duke Univ Med Ctr, 2301 Erwin Rd, rm 1529, DUMC 3808, Durham, NC 27710-3808; **Phone:** 919-684-7289; **Board Cert:** Diagnostic Radiology 1992; **Med School:** UCSD 1987; **Resid:** Diagnostic Radiology, Stanford Univ Med Ctr 1992; **Fellow:** Body Imaging, Stanford Univ Med Ctr 1993; **Fac Appt:** Prof Rad, Duke Univ

Zagoria, Ronald J MD [DR] - **Spec Exp:** Abdominal Imaging; Genitourinary Radiology; Interventional Radiology; MRI; **Hospital:** Wake Forest Univ Baptist Med Ctr; **Address:** Wake Forest Univ Bapt Med Ctr, Medical Center Blvd, MRI Bldg Fl 3, Winston-Salem, NC 27157; **Phone:** 336-716-2471; **Board Cert:** Diagnostic Radiology 1987; Vascular & Interventional Radiology 2004; **Med School:** Univ MD Sch Med 1983; **Resid:** Radiology, Bowman Gray Med Ctr 1987; **Fellow:** Abdominal Imaging, Bowman Gray Med Ctr 1987; **Fac Appt:** Prof Rad, Wake Forest Univ

Midwest

Charboneau, J William MD [DR] - **Spec Exp:** Radiofrequency Tumor Ablation; Liver Cancer; Thyroid Cancer; Radiation Oncology; **Hospital:** Mayo Med Ctr & Clin - Rochester; **Address:** Mayo Clinic Dept of Radiology, 200 First St SW, Rochester, MN 55905-0002; **Phone:** 507-284-2097; **Board Cert:** Diagnostic Radiology 1980; **Med School:** Univ Wisc 1976; **Resid:** Diagnostic Radiology, Mayo Clin 1980; **Fac Appt:** Prof, Mayo Med Sch

Diagnostic Radiology

Edelman, Robert R MD [DR] - **Spec Exp:** MRI; Cardiac CT Angiography; **Hospital:** Evanston/North Shore Univ Hlth Sys; **Address:** Evanston Hosp, Dept Radiology, 2650 Ridge Ave, rm 5108, Evanston, IL 60201; **Phone:** 847-570-2475; **Board Cert:** Diagnostic Radiology 1984; **Med School:** Boston Univ 1980; **Resid:** Diagnostic Radiology, Beth Israel Deaconess Med Ctr 1984; **Fac Appt:** Prof Rad, Northwestern Univ

Fidler, Jeff L MD [DR] - **Spec Exp:** Gastrointestinal Imaging; CT Colonography; MRI; **Hospital:** Mayo Med Ctr & Clin - Rochester; **Address:** Mayo Clinic-Rochester, 200 First St SW, Rochester, MN 55905-0002; **Phone:** 507-284-2311; **Board Cert:** Diagnostic Radiology 1993; **Med School:** Univ Nebr Coll Med 1988; **Resid:** Radiology, Duke Univ Med Ctr; **Fellow:** Diagnostic Radiology, Duke Univ Med Ctr; **Fac Appt:** Assoc Prof Rad, Mayo Med Sch

Flamm, Scott D MD [DR] - **Spec Exp:** Cardiac MRI; Cardiovascular Imaging; Congenital Heart Disease; **Hospital:** Cleveland Clin (page 56); **Address:** Cleveland Clinic, 9500 Euclid Ave, MC J1-4, Cleveland, OH 44195; **Phone:** 216-444-2740; **Board Cert:** Diagnostic Radiology 1993; **Med School:** Geo Wash Univ 1988; **Resid:** Diagnostic Radiology, UCLA Med Ctr 1993; **Fellow:** Cardiovascular Disease, UCSF Med Ctr 1994; **Fac Appt:** Assoc Prof Rad, Case West Res Univ

Goodman, Lawrence R MD [DR] - **Spec Exp:** Thoracic Imaging; Pulmonary Embolism; Lung Disease; **Hospital:** Froedtert and Med Ctr of WI; **Address:** Dept Radiology, 9200 W Wisconsin Ave, Milwaukee, WI 53226; **Phone:** 414-805-2060; **Board Cert:** Diagnostic Radiology 1973; **Med School:** SUNY Downstate 1968; **Resid:** Diagnostic Radiology, Boston Univ/City Hosp 1972; **Fellow:** Thoracic Radiology, UCSF Med Ctr 1973; **Fac Appt:** Prof Rad, Med Coll Wisc

Helvie, Mark A MD [DR] - **Spec Exp:** Breast Imaging; Breast Cancer; Mammography; **Hospital:** Univ of Michigan Hosp; **Address:** Univ Of Michigan Hospital, Taubman Center, rm 2910N, 1500 E Medical Center Drive, Ann Arbor, MI 48109-0326; **Phone:** 734-936-4367; **Board Cert:** Internal Medicine 1983; Diagnostic Radiology 1986; **Med School:** Univ NC Sch Med 1980; **Resid:** Internal Medicine, Univ Michigan Hosps 1983; Diagnostic Radiology, Univ Michigan Hosps 1986; **Fellow:** Breast Imaging, Univ Michigan Hosps 1987; **Fac Appt:** Prof, Univ Mich Med Sch

Jackson, Valerie P MD [DR] - **Spec Exp:** Breast Imaging; **Hospital:** IU Health University Hosp, Wishard Hlth Srvs; **Address:** Indiana Univ Dept Radiology, 550 N University Blvd, rm 0663, Indianapolis, IN 46202; **Phone:** 317-944-1866; **Board Cert:** Diagnostic Radiology 1982; **Med School:** Indiana Univ 1978; **Resid:** Diagnostic Radiology, Indiana Univ Med Ctr 1982; **Fac Appt:** Prof Rad, Indiana Univ

Monsees, Barbara MD [DR] - **Spec Exp:** Mammography; Breast Cancer; **Hospital:** Barnes-Jewish Hosp; **Address:** 510 S Kingshighway Blvd, Campus Box 8131, St Louis, MO 63110; **Phone:** 314-454-7500; **Board Cert:** Diagnostic Radiology 1980; **Med School:** Washington Univ, St Louis 1975; **Resid:** Pediatrics, St Louis Chldns Hosp 1977; Diagnostic Radiology, Mallinckrodt Inst Radiology 1980; **Fac Appt:** Prof, Washington Univ, St Louis

Sagel, Stuart S MD [DR] - **Spec Exp:** Lung Cancer; Pulmonary Embolism; Occupational Lung Disease; **Hospital:** Barnes-Jewish Hosp, Barnes-Jewish West County Hosp; **Address:** Mallinckrodt Inst Rad-Barnes Hosp, 510 S Kingshighway Blvd, Box 8131, St Louis, MO 63110-1016; **Phone:** 314-362-2927; **Board Cert:** Diagnostic Radiology 1970; **Med School:** Temple Univ 1965; **Resid:** Diagnostic Radiology, Yale New Haven Hosp 1968; Diagnostic Radiology, UCSF Med Ctr 1970; **Fac Appt:** Prof Rad, Washington Univ, St Louis

Sivit, Carlos J MD [DR] - **Spec Exp:** Pediatric Radiology; Abdominal Imaging; Trauma Radiology; **Hospital:** UH Rainbow Babies & Chldns Hosp (page 74); **Address:** Dept Radiology, 11100 Euclid Ave, Cleveland, OH 44106-1736; **Phone:** 216-844-1172; **Board Cert:** Pediatrics 1987; Diagnostic Radiology 1987; **Med School:** Univ VA Sch Med 1981; **Resid:** Pediatrics, Vanderbilt Univ Hosp 1984; Diagnostic Radiology, George Washington Univ Hosp 1987; **Fellow:** Pediatric Radiology, Chldns Natl Med Ctr 1989; **Fac Appt:** Prof Rad, Case West Res Univ

Swensen, Stephen J MD [DR] - **Spec Exp:** Lung Cancer; Lung Disease; **Hospital:** Mayo Med Ctr & Clin - Rochester; **Address:** Mayo Clinic - Diagnostic Radiology, 200 1st St SW, Rochester, MN 55905; **Phone:** 507-284-8550; **Board Cert:** Diagnostic Radiology 1986; **Med School:** Univ Wisc 1981; **Resid:** Diagnostic Radiology, Mayo Clinic 1986; **Fellow:** Pulmonary Radiology, Brigham & Womens Hosp 1987; **Fac Appt:** Prof Rad, Mayo Med Sch

Thompson, Brad H MD [DR] - **Spec Exp:** Cardiovascular Imaging; **Hospital:** Univ Iowa Hosp & Clinics; **Address:** University of Iowa, 200 Hawkins Drive, 3960 JPP, Iowa City, IA 52242; **Phone:** 319-356-3444; **Board Cert:** Diagnostic Radiology 1990; **Med School:** Univ Iowa Coll Med 1986; **Resid:** Diagnostic Radiology, Univ Iowa Hosp & Clins 1990; **Fac Appt:** Assoc Prof Rad, Univ Iowa Coll Med

Wells, Robert G MD [DR] - **Spec Exp:** Pediatric Radiology; **Hospital:** Chldns Hosp - Wisconsin, Northwestern Lake Forest Hosp; **Address:** Pediatric Diagnostic Imaging, 150500 W Loomis Rd, Ste 120, Franklin, WI 53132; **Phone:** 414-529-3100; **Board Cert:** Diagnostic Radiology 1984; Pediatric Radiology 2004; Vascular & Interventional Radiology 2004; **Med School:** Med Coll Wisc 1980; **Resid:** Diagnostic Radiology, St Lukes Hosp 1984; **Fellow:** Pediatric Radiology, Milwaukee Chldns Hosp 1985; **Fac Appt:** Assoc Clin Prof Rad, Med Coll Wisc

White, Richard D MD [DR] - **Spec Exp:** Cardiovascular Imaging; Congenital Heart Disease-Adult & Child; **Hospital:** Ohio St Univ Med Ctr; **Address:** 358 W 12th Ave, Ste 452A, Columbus, OH 43210; **Phone:** 614-293-8382; **Board Cert:** Diagnostic Radiology 1986; **Med School:** Duke Univ 1981; **Resid:** Diagnostic Radiology, UCSF Med Ctr 1985; **Fellow:** Cardiovascular Radiology, UCSF Med Ctr 1987; **Fac Appt:** Prof, Univ Fla Coll Med

Great Plains and Mountains

Dodd III, Gerald Dewey MD [DR] - **Hospital:** Univ of CO Hosp - Anschutz Inpatient Pav; **Address:** 12401 E 17th Ave, MS L954, Aurora, CO 80045; **Phone:** 720-848-6608; **Board Cert:** Diagnostic Radiology 1987; **Med School:** Univ Tex, Houston 1983; **Resid:** Diagnostic Radiology, Univ Hosp 1987; **Fellow:** Abdominal Imaging & Angio-Interventional, Univ Hosp 1988; **Fac Appt:** Prof, Univ Tex, San Antonio

Hubbard, Anne M MD [DR] - **Spec Exp:** Pediatric Radiology; Fetal MRI; Fetal Imaging; **Hospital:** Nebraska Med Ctr; **Address:** 981045 Nebraska Medical Ctr, Omaha, NE 68198-1045; **Phone:** 402-559-1010; **Board Cert:** Diagnostic Radiology 1983; Pediatric Radiology 2005; **Med School:** Univ Nebr Coll Med 1977; **Resid:** Internal Medicine, Mayo Clinic 1980; Diagnostic Radiology, Med Coll Wisc Affil Hosp 1983; **Fellow:** Pediatric Radiology, Milwaukee Chldns Hosp 1984; **Fac Appt:** Prof Rad, Univ Nebr Coll Med

Diagnostic Radiology

Southwest

Erasmus, Jeremy J MD [DR] - **Spec Exp:** Lung Cancer; CT Body Scan; PET Imaging; **Hospital:** UT MD Anderson Cancer Ctr; **Address:** MD Anderson Cancer Ctr, Dept of Rad, 1515 Holcombe Blvd, Unit 1478, Houston, TX 77030; **Phone:** 713-792-5878; **Board Cert:** Diagnostic Radiology 1993; **Med School:** South Africa 1982; **Resid:** Diagnostic Radiology, Queens Univ 1993; **Fac Appt:** Prof Rad, Univ Tex, Houston

Huynh, Phan Tuong MD [DR] - **Spec Exp:** Mammography; Breast Cancer; **Hospital:** St. Luke's Episcopal Hosp-Houston; **Address:** 6624 Fannin St, St Luke's Tower, Womens Ctr Fl 10, Houston, TX 77030; **Phone:** 832-355-8130; **Board Cert:** Diagnostic Radiology 1994; **Med School:** Univ VA Sch Med 1989; **Resid:** Diagnostic Radiology, Univ Virginia Med Ctr 1994; **Fellow:** Mammography, Univ Virginia 1995; **Fac Appt:** Assoc Clin Prof Rad, Baylor Coll Med

Otto, Pamela MD [DR] - **Spec Exp:** Breast Imaging; Breast Cancer; **Hospital:** Univ Hlth Syst-San Antonio, Audie L Murphy Meml Vets Hosp - San Antonio; **Address:** 7703 Floyd Curl Drive, MC 7800, San Antonio, TX 78229; **Phone:** 210-567-3448; **Board Cert:** Diagnostic Radiology 1993; **Med School:** Univ MO-Columbia Sch Med 1988; **Resid:** Diagnostic Radiology, Univ Texas Hlth Sci Ctr 1993; **Fellow:** Breast Imaging, Univ Texas Hlth Sci Ctr 1993; **Fac Appt:** Assoc Prof Rad, Univ Tex, San Antonio

Stough, Rebecca G MD [DR] - **Spec Exp:** MRI-Breast; Breast Cancer; **Hospital:** Mercy Hlth Ctr - Oklahoma City; **Address:** Mercy Womens Center, Breast MRI of Oklahoma, 4300 McAuley Blvd, Oklahoma City, OK 73120; **Phone:** 405-749-7077; **Board Cert:** Diagnostic Radiology 1981; **Med School:** Univ Okla Coll Med 1975; **Resid:** Diagnostic Radiology, Univ Oklahoma Affil Hosp 1980

Ulissey, Michael J MD [DR] - **Spec Exp:** Breast Imaging; Breast Cancer; Mammography; **Hospital:** UT Southwestern Med Ctr at Dallas; **Address:** Univ SW Med Ctr, 5701 Maple Drive, Ste 300, Dallas, TX 75235; **Phone:** 214-266-3300; **Board Cert:** Diagnostic Radiology 1998; **Med School:** Texas A&M Univ 1991; **Resid:** Diagnostic Radiology, Univ Oklahoma Hlth Ctr 1998; **Fellow:** Radiology, Univ TX SW Clin Breast Radiology 1999; Magnetic Resonance Imaging, UT Southwestern Med Ctr 2004; **Fac Appt:** Assoc Prof Rad, Univ Tex SW, Dallas

West Coast and Pacific

Bahn, Duke K MD [DR] - **Spec Exp:** Prostate Cancer-Cryosurgery; Ultrasound; Immunotherapy; **Hospital:** Comm Meml Hosp - Ventura; **Address:** Prostate Inst of America, 168 N Brent St, Ste 402, Ventura, CA 93003; **Phone:** 805-585-3082; **Board Cert:** Diagnostic Radiology 1978; **Med School:** Korea 1970; **Resid:** Diagnostic Radiology, Wayne State Univ Med Ctr 1978; **Fac Appt:** Clin Prof Rad

Bassett, Lawrence W MD [DR] - **Spec Exp:** Breast Imaging; **Hospital:** UCLA Ronald Reagan Med Ctr; **Address:** 200 UCLA Med Plaza, rm 165-47, Los Angeles, CA 90095; **Phone:** 310-206-9608; **Board Cert:** Diagnostic Radiology 1975; **Med School:** UC Irvine 1968; **Resid:** Diagnostic Radiology, UCLA Med Ctr 1972; **Fac Appt:** Prof, UCLA

Coakley, Fergus V MD [DR] - **Spec Exp:** Abdominal Imaging; Anal Cancer; Liver Cancer; Esophageal Cancer; **Hospital:** UCSF Med Ctr; **Address:** UCSF Medical Ctr, 505 Parnassus Ave Fl 3 - rm M372, San Francisco, CA 94143; **Phone:** 415-353-1821; **Board Cert:** Diagnostic Radiology 2001; **Med School:** Ireland 1988; **Resid:** Internal Medicine, Mater & St. Vincents Hosp 1991; Radiology, Leicester Univ Hosp 1996; **Fellow:** Body Imaging, Meml Sloan-Kettering Cancer Ctr 1997; **Fac Appt:** Prof Rad, UCSF

Federle, Michael P MD [DR] - **Spec Exp:** Abdominal Imaging; Gastrointestinal Imaging; **Hospital:** Stanford Univ Hosp & Clinics; **Address:** Diagnostic Radiology, 300 Pasteur Drive, SO92, MC 5105, Stanford, CA 94305; **Phone:** 650-721-6411; **Board Cert:** Diagnostic Radiology 1978; **Med School:** Georgetown Univ 1974; **Resid:** Diagnostic Radiology, Univ Cincinnati Hosp 1978; **Fellow:** Body Imaging, UCSF Med Ctr 1979; **Fac Appt:** Prof Rad, Stanford Univ

Feig, Stephen Albert MD [DR] - **Spec Exp:** Breast Imaging; Breast Cancer; **Hospital:** UC Irvine Med Ctr; **Address:** UCI Medical Ctr, 101 City Drive South Route 140, Orange, CA 92868-3298; **Phone:** 714-456-6905; **Board Cert:** Diagnostic Radiology 1972; **Med School:** NYU Sch Med 1967; **Resid:** Radiology, Bronx Muni Hosp-Einstein 1971; **Fac Appt:** Prof Rad, UC Irvine

Filly, Roy A MD [DR] - **Spec Exp:** Obstetric Ultrasound; **Hospital:** UCSF Med Ctr; **Address:** UCSF Med Ctr, Dept Diagnostic Radiology, 505 Parnassus Ave, Box 0628, San Francisco, CA 94143-0628; **Phone:** 415-353-1628; **Board Cert:** Diagnostic Radiology 1974; **Med School:** Ohio State Univ 1970; **Resid:** Diagnostic Radiology, Stanford Univ Med Ctr 1974; **Fac Appt:** Prof Rad, UCSF

Gilsanz, Vicente MD [DR] - **Spec Exp:** Pediatric Radiology; Bone Disorders-Metabolic; **Hospital:** Chldns Hosp - Los Angeles; **Address:** Chdns Hosp LA, 4650 Sunset Blvd, MS 81, Los Angeles, CA 90027; **Phone:** 323-361-4571; **Board Cert:** Internal Medicine 1973; Diagnostic Radiology 1976; Pediatric Radiology 2004; **Med School:** Spain 1969; **Resid:** Internal Medicine, Mayo Clin 1973; Diagnostic Radiology, Mt Sinai Hosp 1976; **Fellow:** Pediatric Radiology, Chldns Hosp 1978; **Fac Appt:** Prof Rad, USC Sch Med

Lehman, Constance D MD/PhD [DR] - **Spec Exp:** Breast Imaging; Breast Cancer; MRI-Breast; Mammography; **Hospital:** Univ Wash Med Ctr, Swedish Med Ctr-First Hill-Seattle; **Address:** Seattle Cancer Care Alliance, 825 Eastlake Ave E, MS G2600, Seattle, WA 98109-1023; **Phone:** 206-288-2046; **Board Cert:** Diagnostic Radiology 1995; **Med School:** Yale Univ 1990; **Resid:** Diagnostic Radiology, Univ Washington Med Ctr 1995; **Fellow:** Breast Imaging, Univ Washington Med Ctr 1996; **Fac Appt:** Prof Rad, Univ Wash

Parikh, Jay Rajendra MD [DR] - **Spec Exp:** Breast Imaging; Breast Cancer; Mammography; **Hospital:** Swedish Med Ctr-First Hill-Seattle; **Address:** 1221 Madison St, Ste 520, Seattle, WA 98104; **Phone:** 206-215-3939; **Board Cert:** Diagnostic Radiology 1996; **Med School:** Univ Ottawa 1990; **Resid:** Diagnostic Radiology, Queens Univ Faculty Hlth Scics 1996; **Fac Appt:** Assoc Clin Prof Rad, Univ Wash

Pathria, Mini N MD [DR] - **Spec Exp:** Musculoskeletal Imaging; **Hospital:** UCSD Med Ctr; **Address:** UCSD Med Ctr, Dept Radiology, 200 W Arbor Drive, San Diego, CA 92103-8756; **Phone:** 619-543-6222; **Board Cert:** Diagnostic Radiology 1986; **Med School:** McMaster Univ 1982; **Resid:** Diagnostic Radiology, Mcmaster Univ 1983; **Fellow:** Skeletal Radiology, UCSD Med Ctr 1987; **Fac Appt:** Clin Prof Rad, UCSD

Shaw, Dennis MD [DR] - **Spec Exp:** Pediatric Neuroradiology; Interventional Radiology; **Hospital:** Seattle Chldns Hosp; **Address:** 4800 Sand Point Way NE, R-5417 Radiology, Seattle, WA 98105; **Phone:** 206-987-2133; **Board Cert:** Diagnostic Radiology 1990; Pediatric Radiology 2006; **Med School:** Univ Wash 1983; **Resid:** Neurological Surgery, Univ Washington Med Ctr 1985; Diagnostic Radiology, Univ Washington Med Ctr 1990; **Fellow:** Pediatric Radiology, Chldn's Hosp & Med Ctr 1991; **Fac Appt:** Prof Rad, Univ Wash

Thurmond, Amy S MD [DR] - **Spec Exp:** Women's Imaging; Gynecologic Imaging; **Hospital:** OR Hlth & Sci Univ; **Address:** Siker Medical Imaging, 1800 NE 2nd Ave, Portland, OR 97212; **Phone:** 503-595-3967; **Board Cert:** Diagnostic Radiology 1987; **Med School:** UCLA 1982; **Resid:** Cardiovascular Disease, St Vincent Hosp Med Ctr 1984; Diagnostic Radiology, Oreg Hlth Scis Univ 1987; **Fellow:** Interventional Radiology, Oreg Hlth Scis Univ 1988; **Fac Appt:** Assoc Prof Rad, Oregon Hlth & Sci Univ

Diagnostic Radiology

Wood, Beverly MD/PhD [DR] - **Spec Exp:** Pediatric Radiology; **Hospital:** LAC & USC Med Ctr, Loma Linda Chldns Hosp; **Address:** Loma Linda Univ Chldns Hosp, Div Pediatric Radiology, 11234 Anderson St, rm 2851, Loma Linda, CA 92354; **Phone:** 909-558-8205; **Board Cert:** Diagnostic Radiology 1972; Pediatric Radiology 2003; **Med School:** Univ Rochester 1965; **Resid:** Diagnostic Radiology, Strong Meml Hosp 1971; **Fellow:** Pediatric Radiology, Strong Meml Hosp 1972; **Fac Appt:** Prof Rad, USC Sch Med

NEURORADIOLOGY

New England

Curtin, Hugh D MD [NRad] - **Spec Exp:** Head & Neck Radiology; **Hospital:** Mass Eye & Ear Infirmary; **Address:** Mass Eye & Ear Infirmary, Dept Radiology, 243 Charles St, Lobby, Boston, MA 02114; **Phone:** 617-573-3563 x4; **Board Cert:** Diagnostic Radiology 1976; Neuroradiology 1999; **Med School:** SUNY Upstate Med Univ 1972; **Resid:** Diagnostic Radiology, Presby Univ Hosp 1976; **Fellow:** Neuroradiology, Foundation Rothschild; **Fac Appt:** Prof Rad, Harvard Med Sch

Hackney, David B MD [NRad] - **Hospital:** Beth Israel Deaconess Med Ctr - Boston; **Address:** BIDMC, Dept Radiology, 330 Brookline Ave, Boston, MA 02215; **Phone:** 617-754-2009; **Board Cert:** Diagnostic Radiology 1984; Neuroradiology 2005; **Med School:** Cornell Univ 1980; **Resid:** Diagnostic Radiology, UCSD Med Ctr 1983; **Fellow:** Neurological Radiology, Mass Genl Hosp 1985; **Fac Appt:** Prof Rad, Harvard Med Sch

Hirsch, Joshua A MD [NRad] - **Spec Exp:** Interventional Neuroradiology; Endovascular Surgery; Minimally Invasive Spinal Surgery; Osteoporosis Spine-Vertebroplasty; **Hospital:** Mass Genl Hosp; **Address:** Mass General Hosp, Interventional Neuroradiology GRB-241, 55 Fruit St, Boston, MA 02114; **Phone:** 617-726-1767; **Board Cert:** Diagnostic Radiology 1996; **Med School:** Univ Pennsylvania 1991; **Resid:** Diagnostic Radiology, Hosp Univ Penn 1996; **Fellow:** Neuroradiology, Hosp Univ Penn 1995; Interventional Neuroradiology, Lahey Clinic 1998; **Fac Appt:** Asst Prof Rad, Harvard Med Sch

Norbash, Alexander M MD [NRad] - **Spec Exp:** Interventional Neuroradiology; Aneurysm-Cerebral; Osteoporosis Spine-Kyphoplasty; Arteriovenous Malformations; **Hospital:** Boston Med Ctr; **Address:** BMC, Dept Radiology, 820 Harrison Ave, Boston, MA 02118; **Phone:** 617-638-6610; **Board Cert:** Diagnostic Radiology 1991; Neuroradiology 2004; **Med School:** Univ MO-Kansas City 1986; **Resid:** Diagnostic Radiology, St Francis Hosp 1990; Diagnostic Radiology, Presby Univ Hosp 1991; **Fellow:** Neurological Radiology, Stanford Univ Hosp 1993; Interventional Radiology, Stanford Univ Hosp 1994; **Fac Appt:** Prof Rad, Boston Univ

Orbach, Darren MD/PhD [NRad] - **Spec Exp:** Stroke in Children; Vascular Malformations; Interventional Neuroradiology; **Hospital:** Children's Hospital - Boston; **Address:** Chldn's Hosp-Boston, Interventional Radiology Dept, 300 Longwood Ave, Boston, MA 02115; **Phone:** 617-355-6579; **Board Cert:** Diagnostic Radiology 2004; Neurology 2004; Neuroradiology 2005; **Med School:** Cornell Univ 1998; **Resid:** Diagnostic Radiology, NYU Med Ctr 2002; Neurology, NYU Med Ctr 2004; **Fellow:** Neuroradiology, NYU Med Ctr 2005

Sze, Gordon K MD [NRad] - **Spec Exp:** Brain Tumors; Spinal Cord Tumors; Head & Neck Cancer; MRI; **Hospital:** Yale-New Haven Hosp, Yale Med Group; **Address:** Yale-New Haven Hospital, Yale Diagnostic Radiology, 20 York St, New Haven, CT 06510; **Phone:** 203-785-3667; **Board Cert:** Diagnostic Radiology 1985; Neuroradiology 2008; **Med School:** Harvard Med Sch 1981; **Resid:** Diagnostic Radiology, UCSF Med Ctr 1985; **Fellow:** Neuroradiology, UCSF Med Ctr 1986; **Fac Appt:** Prof Rad, Yale Univ

Mid Atlantic

Berenstein, Alejandro MD [NRad] - **Spec Exp:** Interventional Neuroradiology; Aneurysm-Cerebral; Endovascular Surgery; Vascular Malformations; **Hospital:** St. Luke's - Roosevelt Hosp Ctr - Roosevelt Div (page 55); **Address:** Center for Endovascular Surgery, 1000 10th Ave, 10th Fl, Ste 10G - INN, New York, NY 10019; **Phone:** 212-636-3400; **Board Cert:** Diagnostic Radiology 1976; **Med School:** Mexico 1970; **Resid:** Diagnostic Radiology, Mt Sinai Med Ctr 1976; **Fellow:** Neuroradiology, NYU Med Ctr 1978; **Fac Appt:** Prof Rad, Albert Einstein Coll Med

Drayer, Burton P MD [NRad] - **Spec Exp:** Stroke; Parkinson's Disease/Aging Brain; MRI & CT of Brain & Spine; **Hospital:** Mount Sinai Med Ctr (page 63); **Address:** 1 Gustave Levy Pl, Box 1234, New York, NY 10029; **Phone:** 212-241-6403; **Board Cert:** Neurology 1976; Diagnostic Radiology 1978; Neuroradiology 2006; **Med School:** Ros Franklin Univ/Chicago Med Sch 1971; **Resid:** Neurology, Univ Vt Med Ctr 1975; Diagnostic Radiology, Univ Pitt Hlth Ctr 1978; **Fellow:** Neuroradiology, Univ Pitt Hlth Ctr 1978; **Fac Appt:** Prof Rad, Mount Sinai Sch Med

Faro, Scott H MD [NRad] - **Spec Exp:** Brain Mapping; Brain Tumors; Epilepsy; Spinal Cord Injury; **Hospital:** Temple Univ Hosp; **Address:** 3401 N Broad St, Philadelphia, PA 19140; **Phone:** 215-707-5003; **Board Cert:** Diagnostic Radiology 1993; Neuroradiology 2006; **Med School:** UMDNJ-Rutgers Med Sch 1986; **Resid:** Diagnostic Radiology, Med Ctr Delaware 1991; **Fellow:** Neuroradiology, Jefferson Med Ctr 1992; Neuroradiology, Hosp U Penn 1993; **Fac Appt:** Prof Rad, Temple Univ

Flanders, Adam E MD [NRad] - **Spec Exp:** Spinal Trauma; Head Injury; **Hospital:** Thomas Jefferson Univ Hosp; **Address:** 132 10th St, Main Bldg - Ste 1080B, Philadelphia, PA 19107; **Phone:** 215-955-2430; **Board Cert:** Diagnostic Radiology 1987; Neuroradiology 2006; **Med School:** Rush Med Coll 1983; **Resid:** Diagnostic Radiology, Univ Illinois Hosps 1987; **Fellow:** Neuroradiology, Thos Jefferson Univ Hosp 1989; **Fac Appt:** Prof Rad, Thomas Jefferson Univ

Hurst, Robert W MD [NRad] - **Spec Exp:** Interventional Neuroradiology; Aneurysm; Carotid Artery Stent Placement; Intracranial Angioplasty & Stent; **Hospital:** Hosp Univ Penn - UPHS (page 68); **Address:** Dept Radiology/Neuroradiology, HUP, 3400 Spruce St, 1 Silverstein, Philadelphia, PA 19104; **Phone:** 215-662-3064; **Board Cert:** Neurology 1986; Diagnostic Radiology 1989; Neuroradiology 2005; Vascular Neurology 2009; **Med School:** Univ Tex, Houston 1981; **Resid:** Neurology, Univ Virginia Hosp 1985; Diagnostic Radiology, Univ Virginia Hosp 1989; **Fellow:** Neurological Radiology, Hosp Univ Penn 1990; Interventional Radiology, NYU Med Ctr 1991; **Fac Appt:** Prof Rad, Univ Pennsylvania

Khandji, Alexander G MD [NRad] - **Spec Exp:** Pituitary Disorders; Spine Imaging & Intervention; MRI; Brain Tumors; **Hospital:** NY-Presby/Columbia Univ Med Ctr, NY (page 65); **Address:** 177 Ft Washington Ave, Ste 4-156, New York, NY 10032-3173; **Phone:** 212-305-7669; **Board Cert:** Diagnostic Radiology 1985; Neuroradiology 2006; **Med School:** SUNY Downstate 1980; **Resid:** Surgery, MS Hershey Med Ctr 1982; Diagnostic Radiology, Columbia-Presby Med Ctr 1985; **Fellow:** Neuroradiology, Columbia-Presby Med Ctr 1987; **Fac Appt:** Clin Prof Rad, Columbia P&S

Loevner, Laurie A MD [NRad] - **Spec Exp:** Head & Neck Cancer; Thyroid Cancer; Brain Tumor Imaging; Spinal Tumor Imaging; **Hospital:** Hosp Univ Penn - UPHS (page 68), Pennsylvania Hosp-UPHS (page 68); **Address:** 3400 Spruce St Dulles Bldg Fl 2nd, Philadelphia, PA 19104; **Phone:** 215-662-3020; **Board Cert:** Diagnostic Radiology 1993; Neuroradiology 2006; **Med School:** Univ Pennsylvania 1988; **Resid:** Diagnostic Radiology, Univ Michigan Hosps 1993; **Fellow:** Neuroradiology, Hosp Univ Penn 1995; **Fac Appt:** Prof Rad, Univ Pennsylvania

Neuroradiology

Pile-Spellman, John MD [NRad] - **Spec Exp:** Interventional Neuroradiology; Cerebrovascular Disease; Aneurysm; Arteriovenous Malformations; **Hospital:** Winthrop Univ Hosp; **Address:** Neurological Surgery, PC, 1991 Marcus Ave, Ste 108, Lake Success, NY 11042; **Phone:** 516-442-2250; **Board Cert:** Diagnostic Radiology 1984; **Med School:** Tufts Univ 1978; **Resid:** Neurological Surgery, New England Med Ctr 1981; Neurological Radiology, Mass Genl Hosp 1984; **Fellow:** Interventional Neuroradiology, NYU Med Ctr 1986; **Fac Appt:** Prof Rad, Columbia P&S

Tenner, Michael MD [NRad] - **Spec Exp:** Stroke; Brain & Spinal Tumors; Carotid Artery Stent Placement; **Hospital:** Westchester Med Ctr; **Address:** NY Med Coll, Dept Radiology, 95 Grasslands Rd, Valhalla, NY 10595; **Phone:** 914-493-8158; **Board Cert:** Diagnostic Radiology 1967; Neuroradiology 2007; **Med School:** Univ MD Sch Med 1960; **Resid:** Diagnostic Radiology, Univ Maryland Hosp 1962; Diagnostic Radiology, Univ Maryland Hosp 1966; **Fellow:** Neuroradiology, Neurological Inst-Columbia Presby 1968; **Fac Appt:** Prof Rad, NY Med Coll

Vezina, L Gilbert MD [NRad] - **Spec Exp:** Pediatric Neuroradiology; Brain Tumors; Neurofibromatosis; **Hospital:** Chldns Natl Med Ctr; **Address:** Chldns Natl Med Ctr, Dept Radiology, 111 Michigan Ave NW, Washington, DC 20010-2970; **Phone:** 202-476-3651; **Board Cert:** Diagnostic Radiology 1987; Neuroradiology 2008; **Med School:** McGill Univ 1983; **Resid:** Diagnostic Radiology, Mass Genl Hosp 1987; **Fellow:** Neurological Radiology, Mass Genl Hosp 1989; Pediatric Neuroradiology, Chldns Natl Med Ctr 1991; **Fac Appt:** Prof, Geo Wash Univ

Yousem, David M MD [NRad] - **Hospital:** Johns Hopkins Hosp (page 61); **Address:** Johns Hopkins Hosp, Div Neuroradiology, 600 N Wolfe St Phipps Bldg - rm B-100, Baltimore, MD 21287; **Phone:** 410-955-2353; **Board Cert:** Diagnostic Radiology 1987; Neuroradiology 2005; **Med School:** Univ Mich Med Sch 1983; **Resid:** Diagnostic Radiology, Johns Hopkins Hosp 1987; **Fellow:** Neuroradiology, Hosp Univ Penn 1990; **Fac Appt:** Prof Rad, Johns Hopkins Univ

Zimmerman, Robert A MD [NRad] - **Spec Exp:** Pediatric Neuroradiology; **Hospital:** Chldns Hosp of Philadelphia; **Address:** Childrens Hosp Philadelphia, Radiology, 324 S 34th St Wood Bldg - rm 215, Philadelphia, PA 19104; **Phone:** 215-590-2569; **Board Cert:** Diagnostic Radiology 1970; Neuroradiology 2005; **Med School:** Georgetown Univ 1964; **Resid:** Diagnostic Radiology, Hosp Univ Penn 1969; **Fac Appt:** Prof Rad, Univ Pennsylvania

Zinreich, S James MD [NRad] - **Spec Exp:** Head & Neck Radiology; **Hospital:** Johns Hopkins Hosp (page 61); **Address:** Johns Hopkins Hosp, 600 N Wolfe St Phipps Bldg - rm B-100, Baltimore, MD 21287; **Phone:** 410-614-3020; **Board Cert:** Diagnostic Radiology 1982; Neuroradiology 2006; **Med School:** Belgium 1976; **Resid:** Diagnostic Radiology, Sinai Hosp; **Fac Appt:** Prof Oto, Johns Hopkins Univ

Southeast

Burdette, Jonathan Hill MD [NRad] - **Spec Exp:** Brain Injury; MRI; **Hospital:** Wake Forest Univ Baptist Med Ctr; **Address:** Medical Center Blvd, Winston-Salem, NC 27157; **Phone:** 336-716-1286; **Board Cert:** Diagnostic Radiology 1997; Neuroradiology 2000; **Med School:** Univ Tenn Coll Med 1993; **Resid:** Diagnostic Radiology, Univ Mich Affil Hosps 1997; **Fellow:** Neurological Radiology, Wake Forest Univ Med Ctr 1999

Dion, Jacques E MD [NRad] - **Spec Exp:** Interventional Neuroradiology; Aneurysm-Cerebral; Intracranial Angioplasty & Stent; **Hospital:** Emory Univ Hosp; **Address:** Emory Univ Hosp, Dept Radiology, 1364 Clifton Rd NE, rm AG21, Atlanta, GA 30322; **Phone:** 404-712-4991; **Board Cert:** Diagnostic Radiology 1982; Neuroradiology 2009; **Med School:** Univ Ottawa 1978; **Resid:** Diagnostic Radiology, Harbor-UCLA Med Ctr 1981; Diagnostic Radiology, Notre Dame Hosp 1983; **Fellow:** Neuroradiology, Univ Hospital 1985; **Fac Appt:** Prof Rad, Emory Univ

Jensen, Mary E MD [NRad] - **Spec Exp:** Interventional Neuroradiology; Osteoporosis Spine-Vertebroplasty; Aneurysm-Cerebral; **Hospital:** Univ of Virginia Health Sys; **Address:** Univ of Virginia Med Ctr, Dept Radiology, Box 800170, Charlottsville, VA 22908; **Phone:** 434-924-9719; **Board Cert:** Diagnostic Radiology 1987; **Med School:** Med Coll VA 1982; **Resid:** Diagnostic Radiology, Univ Virginia Med Ctr 1991; **Fellow:** Interventional Neuroradiology, UCLA Med Ctr 1992; **Fac Appt:** Prof Rad, Univ VA Sch Med

Johnson, Annette MD [NRad] - **Spec Exp:** Brain Tumors; MRI; **Hospital:** Wake Forest Univ Baptist Med Ctr; **Address:** Medical Center Blvd, Wake Forest Baptist Hlth, Dept Radiology, Winston-Salem, NC 27157; **Phone:** 336-716-2872; **Board Cert:** Diagnostic Radiology 1996; Neuroradiology 2008; **Med School:** Med Coll VA 1992; **Resid:** Diagnostic Radiology, Geisinger Med Ctr 1996; **Fellow:** Diagnostic Radiology, Mallinckrodt Inst Radiology/Washingtno Univ 1998; **Fac Appt:** Assoc Prof Rad, Wake Forest Univ

Joseph, Gregory J MD [NRad] - **Spec Exp:** Stroke; Aneurysm-Cerebral; Intracranial Angioplasty & Stent; **Hospital:** Presby Hosp - Charlotte; **Address:** Presbyterian Hosp, Dept Radiology, 200 Hawthrne Ln, Charlotte, NC 28204; **Phone:** 704-384-9654; **Board Cert:** Diagnostic Radiology 1989; Neuroradiology 2010; **Med School:** Georgetown Univ 1984; **Resid:** Diagnostic Radiology, Georgetown Univ Hosp 1989; Vascular & Interventional Radiology, Emory Univ Hosp 1990; **Fellow:** Neuroradiology, Emory Univ Hosp 1991

Maldjian, Joseph MD [NRad] - **Spec Exp:** Brain Tumors; Stroke; **Hospital:** Wake Forest Univ Baptist Med Ctr; **Address:** Wake Forest Univ Med Ctr, Dept Radiology, Medical Center Blvd MRI Bldg Fl 3, Winston-Salem, NC 27157; **Phone:** 336-716-7849; **Board Cert:** Diagnostic Radiology 1993; Neuroradiology 2005; **Med School:** UMDNJ-NJ Med Sch, Newark 1988; **Resid:** Diagnostic Radiology, Mount Sinai Med Ctr 1993; **Fellow:** Neuroradiology, Hosp U Penn 1995

Morris, P Pearse MD [NRad] - **Spec Exp:** Interventional Neuroradiology; Endovascular Neurosurgery; Aneurysm-Cerebral; Arteriovenous Malformations; **Hospital:** Wake Forest Univ Baptist Med Ctr; **Address:** Wake Forest Univ Bapt Med Ctr, Medical Center, MRI Bldg, Fl 3, Winston-Salem, NC 27157; **Phone:** 336-716-7849; **Board Cert:** Psychiatry 1989; Diagnostic Radiology 1994; Neuroradiology 2007; **Med School:** Ireland 1983; **Resid:** Psychiatry, Johns Hopkins Hosp 1987; Diagnostic Radiology, Mass Genl Hosp 1994; **Fellow:** Geriatric Psychiatry, Cornell Univ 1988; Neuroradiology, Mass Genl Hosp 1995; **Fac Appt:** Prof Rad, Wake Forest Univ

Murtagh, F Reed MD [NRad] - **Spec Exp:** Neuro-Oncology; Brain Tumor Imaging; Spinal Tumor Imaging; Memory Disorders; **Hospital:** H Lee Moffitt Cancer Ctr & Research Inst (page 59); **Address:** Univ Diagnostic Institute-USF, 3301 Alumni Drive, Tampa, FL 33612; **Phone:** 813-975-0725; **Board Cert:** Diagnostic Radiology 1978; Neuroradiology 2004; **Med School:** Temple Univ 1971; **Resid:** Diagnostic Radiology, Jackson Meml Hosp 1978; **Fellow:** Neurological Radiology, Univ Miami 1979; **Fac Appt:** Prof Rad, Univ S Fla Coll Med

Provenzale, James M MD [NRad] - **Spec Exp:** Brain Tumor Imaging; Multiple Sclerosis Imaging; Brain Imaging-Pediatric; **Hospital:** Duke Univ Hosp, Durham VA Med Ctr; **Address:** Duke University Medical Ctr, Dept Radiology, Box 3808, Durham, NC 27710; **Phone:** 919-684-7218; **Board Cert:** Neurology 1988; Diagnostic Radiology 1991; Neuroradiology 2001; **Med School:** Albany Med Coll 1983; **Resid:** Neurology, NC Memorial Hosp 1987; Diagnostic Radiology, Mass Genl Hosp 1991; **Fellow:** Neuroradiology, Mass Genl Hosp 1992; **Fac Appt:** Prof Rad, Duke Univ

Quencer, Robert MD [NRad] - **Spec Exp:** Spinal Cord Injury; **Hospital:** Univ of Miami Hosp & Clins/Sylvester Comp Canc Ctr (page 73); **Address:** Univ Miami, Dept Radiology, 1150 NW 14th St, Ste 511, MC M828, Miami, FL 33136-2116; **Phone:** 305-243-4701; **Board Cert:** Diagnostic Radiology 1972; Neuroradiology 2006; **Med School:** SUNY Upstate Med Univ 1967; **Resid:** Diagnostic Radiology, Columbia-Presbyterian Med Ctr 1971; **Fellow:** Neuroradiology, Neurological Inst 1972; **Fac Appt:** Prof, Univ Miami Sch Med

Neuroradiology

Midwest

Ball Jr, William S MD [NRad] - **Spec Exp:** Pediatric Neuroradiology; **Hospital:** Cincinnati Chldns Hosp Med Ctr; **Address:** Cincinnati Chldns Hosp, Dept Neuroradiology, 3333 Burnet Ave, ML 5031, Cincinnati, OH 45229-3039; **Phone:** 513-636-8574; **Board Cert:** Diagnostic Radiology 1982; Pediatrics 1982; Neuroradiology 1999; **Med School:** Tulane Univ 1974; **Resid:** Pediatrics, Oschner Fdn Hosp 1977; Diagnostic Radiology, Univ New Mexico 1978; **Fellow:** Pediatric Radiology, Chldns Hosp Med Ctr 1981; Neuroradiology, Univ New Mexico Med Ctr 1979; **Fac Appt:** Prof, Univ Cincinnati

Cross III, DeWitte T MD [NRad] - **Spec Exp:** Interventional Neuroradiology; Aneurysm-Cerebral; Stroke; **Hospital:** Barnes-Jewish Hosp, St. Louis Chldns Hosp; **Address:** Wash Univ, Dept Radiology, 510 S Kingshighway Blvd, Box 8131, St Louis, MO 63110-1016; **Phone:** 314-362-5949; **Board Cert:** Diagnostic Radiology 1985; Neuroradiology 2006; **Med School:** Univ Alabama 1980; **Resid:** Diagnostic Radiology, Naval Hosp 1985; **Fellow:** Neuroradiology, NY Med Coll 1988; Neuroradiology, Columbia Univ 1989; **Fac Appt:** Assoc Prof Rad, Washington Univ, St Louis

Grobelny, Thomas MD [NRad] - **Spec Exp:** Interventional Neuroradiology; Aneurysm-Cerebral; Stroke; Arteriovenous Malformations; **Hospital:** Evanston/North Shore Univ Hlth Sys, Adv Christ Med Ctr; **Address:** 9669 Kenton Ave, Ste 500, Skokie, IL 60076; **Phone:** 847-933-3700; **Board Cert:** Diagnostic Radiology 1996; Neuroradiology 2010; **Med School:** Poland 1986; **Resid:** Diagnostic Radiology, Harlem Hospital 1995; **Fellow:** Neurocritical Care, Thos Jefferson Univ Hosp 1998; Interventional Neuroradiology, UCLA Med Ctr 1989

Haughton III, Victor M MD [NRad] - **Spec Exp:** Spinal Imaging; **Hospital:** Univ WI Hosp & Clins; **Address:** Univ WI Hosps & Clins, Dept Radiology, 600 Highland Ave, MC 3252, Madison, WI 53792; **Phone:** 608-263-9179; **Board Cert:** Diagnostic Radiology 1974; **Med School:** Yale Univ 1967; **Resid:** Diagnostic Radiology, Peter Bent Brigham Hosp 1973; **Fellow:** Neurological Radiology, Peter Bent Brigham Hosp 1974; **Fac Appt:** Prof Rad, Univ Wisc

Kallmes, David F MD [NRad] - **Spec Exp:** Aneurysm-Cerebral; Stroke; Osteoporosis Spine-Vertebroplasty; **Hospital:** Mayo Med Ctr & Clin - Rochester; **Address:** Mayo Clinic, 200 First St SW, OL 1-115, Rochester, MN 55905; **Phone:** 507-266-3350; **Board Cert:** Diagnostic Radiology 1994; Neuroradiology 1998; **Med School:** Univ Mass Sch Med 1989; **Resid:** Diagnostic Radiology, Duke Univ Med Ctr 1993; **Fellow:** Neuroradiology, Univ Virginia Med Ctr 1995; **Fac Appt:** Assoc Prof Rad, Mayo Med Sch

Koeller, Kelly K MD [NRad] - **Spec Exp:** Brain Tumor Imaging; Head & Neck Tumors Imaging; Spinal Tumor Imaging; **Hospital:** Mayo Med Ctr & Clin - Rochester; **Address:** Mayo Clinic, 200 First St SW, Charlton Bldg, rm 2-290, Rochester, MN 55905; **Phone:** 507-266-3412; **Board Cert:** Diagnostic Radiology 1990; Neuroradiology 2004; **Med School:** Univ Tenn Coll Med 1982; **Resid:** Diagnostic Radiology, Naval Hosp 1990; **Fellow:** Neuroradiology, UCSF Med Ctr 1992

Masaryk, Thomas MD [NRad] - **Spec Exp:** Cerebrovascular Disease; Aneurysm-Cerebral; Vascular Lesions of the CNS; Carotid Artery Stent Placement; **Hospital:** Cleveland Clin (page 56); **Address:** Cleveland Clinic, Dept Radiology, 9500 Euclid Ave, MC P34, Cleveland, OH 44195; **Phone:** 216-444-6653; **Board Cert:** Diagnostic Radiology 1985; Neuroradiology 2005; **Med School:** Med Coll OH 1981; **Resid:** Diagnostic Radiology, Cleveland Clinic 1984; **Fellow:** Neurological Radiology, Cleveland Clinic 1985

Modic, Michael MD [NRad] - **Spec Exp:** MRI; Spinal Imaging; **Hospital:** Cleveland Clin (page 56); **Address:** 9500 Euclid Ave Desk T13, Cleveland, OH 44195; **Phone:** 216-444-9308; **Board Cert:** Diagnostic Radiology 1979; Neuroradiology 2003; **Med School:** Case West Res Univ 1975; **Resid:** Diagnostic Radiology, Cleveland Clin Fdn 1978; **Fellow:** Neuroradiology, Cleveland Clin Fdn 1979; **Fac Appt:** Prof Rad, Cleveland Cl Coll Med/Case West Res

Moran, Christopher J MD [NRad] - **Spec Exp:** Aneurysm-Cerebral; Cerebrovascular Disease/Stroke; Carotid Artery Stent Placement; Interventional Neuroradiology; **Hospital:** Barnes-Jewish Hosp; **Address:** Mallinckrodt Inst Radiology, Wash Univ Sch Med, Campus Box 8131, 510 S Kingshighway Blvd, St Louis, MO 63110; **Phone:** 314-362-5949; **Board Cert:** Diagnostic Radiology 1978; Neuroradiology 2004; **Med School:** St Louis Univ 1974; **Resid:** Diagnostic Radiology, Mallinckrodt Inst Rad/Wash U 1978; **Fellow:** Neuroradiology, Mallinckrodt Inst Rad/Wash U 1979; **Fac Appt:** Prof Rad, Washington Univ, St Louis

Mukherji, Suresh K MD [NRad] - **Spec Exp:** Head & Neck Radiology; Head & Neck Tumors Imaging; **Hospital:** Univ of Michigan Hosp; **Address:** Univ of Michigan-Dept Radiology, 1500 E Medical Ctr Drive, UH-B2A209B, Ann Arbor, MI 48109-0030; **Phone:** 734-936-8865; **Board Cert:** Diagnostic Radiology 1992; Neuroradiology 2006; **Med School:** Georgetown Univ 1987; **Resid:** Diagnostic Radiology, Brigham & Women's Hosp 1992; **Fellow:** Neuroradiology, Univ Florida 1994; **Fac Appt:** Prof Rad, Univ Mich Med Sch

Rowley, Howard A MD [NRad] - **Spec Exp:** Epilepsy; Cerebrovascular Disease/Stroke; **Hospital:** Univ WI Hosp & Clins; **Address:** Dept Neuroradiology, 600 Highland Ave, MC 3252, Madison, WI 53792; **Phone:** 608-263-9179; **Board Cert:** Neurology 1991; Diagnostic Radiology 1993; Neuroradiology 2008; **Med School:** Washington Univ, St Louis 1985; **Resid:** Neurology, UCSF Med Ctr 1989; Diagnostic Radiology, UCSF Med Ctr 1991; **Fellow:** Neurological Radiology, UCSF Med Ctr 1991; **Fac Appt:** Prof Rad, Univ Wisc

Thulborn, Keith R MD/PhD [NRad] - **Spec Exp:** MRI; **Hospital:** Univ of IL Med Ctr at Chicago; **Address:** Univ Illinois Chicago, 1801 W Taylor St, Ste 1A, Chicago, IL 60612; **Phone:** 312-355-3755; **Board Cert:** Diagnostic Radiology 1989; **Med School:** Washington Univ, St Louis 1984; **Resid:** Diagnostic Radiology, Mass Genl Hosp 1989; **Fellow:** Neuroradiology, Mass Genl Hosp 1991; **Fac Appt:** Prof Rad, Univ IL Coll Med

Great Plains and Mountains

Osborn, Anne G MD [NRad] - **Spec Exp:** Spinal Imaging; Brain Imaging; Head & Neck Radiology; **Hospital:** Univ Utah Hlth Care; **Address:** Dept Radiology, 30 N 1900 E, rm 1A71, Salt Lake City, UT 84132-2140; **Phone:** 801-581-7553; **Board Cert:** Diagnostic Radiology 1974; Neuroradiology 2004; **Med School:** Stanford Univ 1970; **Resid:** Diagnostic Radiology, Stanford Univ Hosp 1974; **Fellow:** Diagnostic Radiology, Univ Utah Hosp 1977; **Fac Appt:** Prof, Univ Utah

Southwest

Hunter, Jill V MD [NRad] - **Spec Exp:** Pediatric Neuroradiology; Brain Injury-Pediatric; Autism; **Hospital:** Texas Chldns Hosp, St. Luke's Episcopal Hosp-Houston; **Address:** 6621 Fannin, West Twr, Ste B120, MC 2-2521, Houston, TX 77030; **Phone:** 832-822-5324; **Board Cert:** Diagnostic Radiology 1997; Neuroradiology 2009; **Med School:** England, UK 1975; **Resid:** Diagnostic Radiology, Baylor Coll Med 1978; **Fellow:** Neuroradiology, Queen Square Hosp 1992; **Fac Appt:** Assoc Prof Rad, Baylor Coll Med

Mawad, Michel E MD [NRad] - **Spec Exp:** Interventional Neuroradiology; **Hospital:** St. Luke's Episcopal Hosp-Houston; **Address:** BCM Neurovascular, 6720 Bertner Ave, MC 4-267, Houston, TX 77030; **Phone:** 713-798-2200; **Board Cert:** Diagnostic Radiology 1980; Neuroradiology 2006; **Med School:** Lebanon 1976; **Resid:** Diagnostic Radiology, St Luke's-Roosevelt Hosp 1979; **Fellow:** Neurological Radiology, Columbia-Presby Med Ctr 1980; **Fac Appt:** Prof, Baylor Coll Med

Neuroradiology

West Coast and Pacific

Atlas, Scott W MD [NRad] - **Spec Exp:** MRI-Brain & Spine; Brain Tumors; **Hospital:** Stanford Univ Hosp & Clinics; **Address:** Stanford Univ Med Ctr, Dept Rad, 300 Pasteur Drive, rm S-047, Stanford, CA 94305-5105; **Phone:** 650-498-7152; **Board Cert:** Diagnostic Radiology 1985; Neuroradiology 2005; **Med School:** Univ Chicago-Pritzker Sch Med 1981; **Resid:** Diagnostic Radiology, Northwestern Univ Med Ctr 1985; **Fellow:** Neuroradiology, Hosp Univ Penn 1987; **Fac Appt:** Prof Rad, Stanford Univ

Barkovich, A James MD [NRad] - **Spec Exp:** Pediatric Neuroradiology; MRI; Brain Development Abnormalities; Stroke-Neonatal; **Hospital:** UCSF Med Ctr; **Address:** UCSF Med Ctr, Div Neuroradiology, 505 Parnassus Ave, rm L371, Box 0628, San Francisco, CA 94143-0628; **Phone:** 415-353-1668; **Board Cert:** Diagnostic Radiology 1984; Neuroradiology 2006; **Med School:** Geo Wash Univ 1980; **Resid:** Diagnostic Radiology, Letterman AMC 1984; **Fellow:** Neuroradiology, Walter Reed AMC 1986; **Fac Appt:** Prof Rad, UCSF

Barnes, Patrick D MD [NRad] - **Spec Exp:** Pediatric Neuroradiology; Brain Injury-Pediatric; Brain Development Abnormalities; Fetal Neuroradiology; **Hospital:** Lucile Packard Chldn's Hosp; **Address:** Lucile Packard Chldns Hosp, Pediatric Radiology, 725 Welch Rd, Palo Alto, CA 94304; **Phone:** 650-497-8376; **Board Cert:** Diagnostic Radiology 1977; Neuroradiology 2008; **Med School:** Univ Okla Coll Med 1973; **Resid:** Diagnostic Radiology, Univ Okla Coll Med 1976; **Fellow:** Pediatric Neuroradiology, Chldns Hosp/Harvard Med Sch 1977; **Fac Appt:** Assoc Prof, Stanford Univ

Cha, Soonmee MD [NRad] - **Spec Exp:** Brain Tumors; **Hospital:** UCSF Med Ctr; **Address:** 350 Parnassus Ave, Ste 307, Neuroradiology Section, San Francisco, CA 94117; **Phone:** 415-353-8913; **Board Cert:** Diagnostic Radiology 1996; Neuroradiology 2008; **Med School:** Georgetown Univ 1991; **Resid:** Diagnostic Radiology, North Shore Univ Hosp 1996; **Fellow:** Neuroradiology, NYU Med Ctr 1998; **Fac Appt:** Assoc Prof Rad, UCSF

Dillon, William P MD [NRad] - **Spec Exp:** Brain Tumors; **Hospital:** UCSF Med Ctr; **Address:** 505 Parnassus Ave, rm L 371, San Francisco, CA 94143-0628; **Phone:** 415-353-1668; **Board Cert:** Diagnostic Radiology 1982; Neuroradiology 2006; **Med School:** Loyola Univ-Stritch Sch Med 1978; **Resid:** Diagnostic Radiology, Univ Utah Hosp 1982; **Fellow:** Neuroradiology, UCSF Med Ctr 1983; **Fac Appt:** Prof, UCSF

Hesselink, John R MD [NRad] - **Spec Exp:** MRI & CT of Brain & Spine; Stroke; Brain Tumor Imaging; **Hospital:** UCSD Med Ctr; **Address:** UCSD Med Ctr, Div Neuroradiology, 200 W Arbor Drive, MC 8749, San Diego, CA 92013; **Phone:** 619-543-3856; **Board Cert:** Diagnostic Radiology 1975; Neuroradiology 2005; **Med School:** Univ Wisc 1971; **Resid:** Diagnostic Radiology, Univ Wisconsin-Madison 1975; **Fellow:** Neuroradiology, Mass Genl Hosp- Harvard Univ 1979; **Fac Appt:** Prof Rad, UCSD

Higashida, Randall T MD [NRad] - **Spec Exp:** Aneurysm-Cerebral; Stroke; Intracranial Angioplasty & Stent; **Hospital:** UCSF Med Ctr; **Address:** UCSF Med Ctr, Dept Interven Neurorad, 505 Parnassus Ave, rm L352, Neurovascular Medical Group, San Francisco, CA 94143-0628; **Phone:** 415-353-1863; **Board Cert:** Diagnostic Radiology 1984; **Med School:** Tulane Univ 1980; **Resid:** Diagnostic Radiology, UCLA Med Ctr 1984; **Fellow:** Neuroradiology, UCLA Med Ctr 1985; **Fac Appt:** Clin Prof, UCSF

Jarvik, Jeffrey G MD [NRad] - **Hospital:** Harborview Med Ctr; **Address:** Harborview Med Ctr, 325 Ninth Ave, Box 359728, Seattle, WA 98104; **Phone:** 206-744-3561; **Board Cert:** Diagnostic Radiology 1992; Neuroradiology 2005; **Med School:** UCSD 1987; **Resid:** Diagnostic Radiology, Hosp Univ Penn 1992; **Fellow:** Neuroradiology, Hosp Univ Penn 1993; **Fac Appt:** Prof Rad, Univ Wash

Larsen, Donald W MD [NRad] - **Spec Exp:** Interventional Neuroradiology; Stroke; Stroke Prevention; Aneurysm-Cerebral; **Hospital:** Keck Med Ctr of USC (page 75); **Address:** 1520 San Pablo St, Ste 3800, Los Angeles, CA 90033; **Phone:** 323-442-5720; **Board Cert:** Diagnostic Radiology 1990; **Med School:** Ros Franklin Univ/Chicago Med Sch 1985; **Resid:** Diagnostic Radiology, USC Med Ctr 1990; **Fellow:** Vascular & Interventional Radiology, USC Med Ctr 1991; Neuroradiology, USF Med Ctr 1995; **Fac Appt:** Assoc Prof Rad, USC-Keck School of Medicine

Teitelbaum, George P MD [NRad] - **Spec Exp:** Interventional Neuroradiology; Aneurysm-Cerebral; Carotid Artery Stent Placement; Vascular Lesions of the CNS; **Hospital:** Providence St Joseph Med Ctr; **Address:** 501 S Buena Vista St, Burbank, CA 91505; **Phone:** 818-847-4835; **Board Cert:** Diagnostic Radiology 1984; Neuroradiology 2008; **Med School:** UCSD 1980; **Resid:** Diagnostic Radiology, UC Irvine Med Ctr 1984; Interventional Radiology, George Washington 1985; **Fellow:** Magnetic Resonance Imaging, Huntington Med Research Inst 1988; Interventional Radiology, UCSF Med Ctr 1994; **Fac Appt:** Prof NS, USC-Keck School of Medicine

Vinuela, Fernando MD [NRad] - **Spec Exp:** Stroke; Intracranial Angioplasty & Stent; Aneurysm-Cerebral; **Hospital:** UCLA Ronald Reagan Med Ctr; **Address:** 757 Westwood Plaza, rm 2129, Los Angeles, CA 90095-7437; **Phone:** 310-267-8765; **Board Cert:** Diagnostic Radiology 1979; **Med School:** Uruguay 1970; **Resid:** Diagnostic Radiology, Westminster Hosp 1975; Diagnostic Radiology, Victoria Hosp 1977; **Fellow:** Neuroradiology, Univ Hosp 1979; **Fac Appt:** Prof Rad, UCLA

VASCULAR & INTERVENTIONAL RADIOLOGY

New England

Aruny, John E MD [VIR] - **Spec Exp:** Thrombolytic Therapy; Dialysis Access; Vascular Disease; Vein Disorders; **Hospital:** Yale-New Haven Hosp, Yale Med Group; **Address:** Yale Univ School of Medicine, 333 Cedar St, New Haven, CT 06520; **Phone:** 203-785-7026; **Board Cert:** Diag Rad with Spec Comp in Nuc Rad 1989; Vascular & Interventional Radiology 2009; **Med School:** Mexico 1983; **Resid:** Diagnostic Radiology, Westch Co Med Ctr 1989; **Fellow:** Interventional Radiology, Brigham & Women's Hosp 1992; **Fac Appt:** Assoc Prof Rad, Yale Univ

Hallisey, Michael J MD [VIR] - **Spec Exp:** Uterine Fibroid Embolization; Liver Cancer/Chemoembolization; **Hospital:** Hartford Hosp; **Address:** 399 Farmington Ave, Farmington, CT 06032; **Phone:** 860-676-0110; **Board Cert:** Diagnostic Radiology 1991; Vascular & Interventional Radiology 2008; **Med School:** Univ Conn 1986; **Resid:** Diagnostic Radiology, Hospital of St Raphael 1991

Murphy, Timothy P MD [VIR] - **Spec Exp:** Uterine Fibroid Embolization; Aneurysm-Aortic; Hypertension-Renovascular; **Hospital:** Rhode Island Hosp; **Address:** RI Hosp, Diagnostic Imaging, 593 Eddy St Fl 3, Providence, RI 02903-4970; **Phone:** 401-444-5194; **Board Cert:** Diagnostic Radiology 1992; Vascular & Interventional Radiology 2005; **Med School:** Boston Univ 1987; **Resid:** Diagnostic Radiology, Rhode Island Hosp 1992; **Fellow:** Vascular & Interventional Radiology, Rhode Island Hosp 1993; **Fac Appt:** Prof Rad, Brown Univ

White, Robert I MD [VIR] - **Spec Exp:** Uterine Fibroid Embolization; Pelvic Congestion Syndrome; Varicocele Embolization; Hereditary Hemorrhagic Telangiectasia; **Hospital:** Yale-New Haven Hosp, Yale Med Group; **Address:** Yale Univ Sch Med, Vasc & Interventional Rad, PO Box 208042, New Haven, CT 06520-8042; **Phone:** 203-737-5395; **Board Cert:** Diagnostic Radiology 1970; **Med School:** Baylor Coll Med 1963; **Resid:** Internal Medicine, Johns Hopkins Hosp 1967; Diagnostic Radiology, Johns Hopkins Hosp 1969; **Fellow:** Cardiovascular Disease, Johns Hopkins Hosp 1958; Cardiovascular Radiology, Univ Minn Med Ctr 1971; **Fac Appt:** Prof Rad, Yale Univ

Vascular & Interventional Radiology

Mid Atlantic

Brown, Daniel B MD [VIR] - **Spec Exp:** Liver Cancer/Chemoembolization; **Hospital:** Thomas Jefferson Univ Hosp; **Address:** Thos Jefferson Univ Hosp, Dept Radiology, 132 S 10th St 766F Main Bldg, Philadelphia, PA 19107; **Phone:** 215-955-6440; **Board Cert:** Diagnostic Radiology 1997; Vascular & Interventional Radiology 2001; **Med School:** Hahnemann Univ 1993; **Resid:** Diagnostic Radiology, Bryn Mawr Hosp 1997; **Fellow:** Vascular & Interventional Radiology, Penn State 1999; **Fac Appt:** Assoc Prof Rad, Thomas Jefferson Univ

Brown, Karen T MD [VIR] - **Spec Exp:** Liver Cancer; Radiofrequency Tumor Ablation; Interventional Radiology; **Hospital:** Meml Sloan-Kettering Cancer Ctr; **Address:** 1275 York Avenue, New York, NY 10065; **Phone:** 800-525-2225; **Board Cert:** Diagnostic Radiology 1984; Vascular & Interventional Radiology 2004; **Med School:** Boston Univ 1979; **Resid:** Diagnostic Radiology, Mass Genl Hosp 1984; **Fellow:** Vascular & Interventional Radiology, Mass Genl Hosp 1985; **Fac Appt:** Prof Rad, Cornell Univ-Weill Med Coll

Cohen, Gary S MD [VIR] - **Spec Exp:** Uterine Fibroid Embolization; Cancer Chemoembolization; Liver Cancer/Chemoembolization; Portal Hypertension; **Hospital:** Temple Univ Hosp, Jeanes Hosp; **Address:** 3401 N Broad St, MS 19140, Parkinson Bldg Fl 1 - Ste C, Philadelphia, PA 19140; **Phone:** 215-707-7002; **Board Cert:** Diagnostic Radiology 1992; Vascular & Interventional Radiology 2006; **Med School:** Mount Sinai Sch Med 1988; **Resid:** Diagnostic Radiology, Temple Univ Hosp 1992; **Fellow:** Vascular & Interventional Radiology, Temple Univ Hosp 1993; **Fac Appt:** Prof Rad, Temple Univ

Denny, Donald F MD [VIR] - **Spec Exp:** Dialysis Access; Uterine Fibroids; **Hospital:** Univ Med Ctr - Princeton; **Address:** Princeton Radiology Assocs, 3674 Route 27, Kendall Park, NJ 08824; **Phone:** 609-497-4310; **Board Cert:** Diagnostic Radiology 1982; Vascular & Interventional Radiology 2005; **Med School:** Hahnemann Univ 1978; **Resid:** Diagnostic Radiology, Yale-New Haven Hosp 1982; **Fellow:** Diagnostic Radiology, Brigham & Womens Hosp 1983; **Fac Appt:** Assoc Clin Prof Rad, Yale Univ

Geschwind, Jean-Francois H MD [VIR] - **Spec Exp:** Liver Cancer/Chemoembolization; Cancer Chemoembolization; Cancer Radiotherapy; **Hospital:** Johns Hopkins Hosp (page 61); **Address:** Interventional Radiology, 600 N Wolfe St Blalock Bldg - rm 545, Baltimore, MD 21287; **Phone:** 410-614-2227; **Board Cert:** Diagnostic Radiology 1998; **Med School:** Boston Univ 1991; **Resid:** Diagnostic Radiology, UCSF Med Ctr 1996; **Fellow:** Interventional Radiology, Johns Hopkins Hosp 1998; **Fac Appt:** Assoc Prof, Johns Hopkins Univ

Haskal, Ziv MD [VIR] - **Spec Exp:** Uterine Fibroid Embolization; Vascular Malformations; Liver Cancer/Chemoembolization; **Hospital:** Univ of MD Med Ctr; **Address:** 22 S Greene St, rm G2K14, Baltimore, MD 21201; **Phone:** 410-328-7467; **Board Cert:** Diagnostic Radiology 1991; Vascular & Interventional Radiology 2010; **Med School:** Boston Univ 1986; **Resid:** Diagnostic Radiology, UCSF Med Ctr 1991; **Fellow:** Vascular & Interventional Radiology, UCSF Med Ctr 1992; **Fac Appt:** Prof Rad, Univ MD Sch Med

McLean, Gordon K MD [VIR] - **Spec Exp:** Uterine Fibroid Embolization; Angioplasty & Stent Placement; **Hospital:** Western Penn Hosp; **Address:** Western Pennsylvania Hosp, Dept Radiology, 4800 Friendship Ave, Pittsburgh, PA 15224-1722; **Phone:** 412-578-7412; **Board Cert:** Diagnostic Radiology 1979; Vascular & Interventional Radiology 2005; **Med School:** Dartmouth Med Sch 1975; **Resid:** Diagnostic Radiology, Hosp Univ Penn 1979; **Fellow:** Angiography, Hosp Univ Penn 1980; **Fac Appt:** Prof Rad, Univ Pennsylvania

Shlansky-Goldberg, Richard MD [VIR] - **Spec Exp:** Uterine Fibroid Embolization; Varicocele Embolization; Pelvic Congestion Syndrome; **Hospital:** Hosp Univ Penn - UPHS (page 68); **Address:** Dept Radiology, 3400 Spruce St, 1 Silverstein Bldg, Philadelphia, PA 19104; **Phone:** 215-662-6839; **Board Cert:** Diagnostic Radiology 1989; Vascular & Interventional Radiology 2008; **Med School:** Univ Rochester 1984; **Resid:** Diagnostic Radiology, Thomas Jefferson Univ Hosp 1989; **Fellow:** Interventional Radiology, Hosp Univ Penn 1991; **Fac Appt:** Assoc Prof Rad, Univ Pennsylvania

Soulen, Michael C MD [VIR] - **Spec Exp:** Liver Cancer/Chemoembolization; Kidney Cancer; Radiofrequency Tumor Ablation; **Hospital:** Hosp Univ Penn - UPHS (page 68); **Address:** Hosp Univ Penn, Interventional Radiology, 3400 Spruce St Dulles Bldg Fl Ground, Philadelphia, PA 19104; **Phone:** 215-615-4135; **Board Cert:** Diagnostic Radiology 1989; Vascular & Interventional Radiology 2006; **Med School:** Univ Pennsylvania 1984; **Resid:** Diagnostic Radiology, Johns Hopkins Med Inst 1989; **Fellow:** Vascular & Interventional Radiology, Thomas Jefferson Univ Hosp 1991; **Fac Appt:** Prof Rad, Univ Pennsylvania

Trerotola, Scott O MD [VIR] - **Spec Exp:** Uterine Fibroid Embolization; Hereditary Hemorrhagic Telangiectasia; Varicocele Embolization; Hereditary Hemorrhagic Telangiectasia; **Hospital:** Hosp Univ Penn - UPHS (page 68), Penn Presby Med Ctr - UPHS (page 68); **Address:** Hosp Univ Penn, Div Interventional Rad, 3400 Spruce St, Dulles Bldg Fl Ground, Philadelphia, PA 19104; **Phone:** 215-615-3540; **Board Cert:** Diagnostic Radiology 1991; Vascular & Interventional Radiology 2005; **Med School:** Univ Pennsylvania 1986; **Resid:** Diagnostic Radiology, Johns Hopkins Hosp 1991; **Fellow:** Vascular & Interventional Radiology, Johns Hopkins Hosp 1992; **Fac Appt:** Prof Rad, Univ Pennsylvania

Weintraub, Joshua L MD [VIR] - **Spec Exp:** Gastrointestinal Cancer; Chemoembolization & Tumor Ablation; Uterine Fibroid Embolization; Vein Disorders; **Hospital:** Mount Sinai Med Ctr (page 63); **Address:** Mount Sinai Medical Ctr, Dept Radiology, One Gustave L Levy Pl, Box 1234, New York, NY 10029; **Phone:** 212-241-7409; **Board Cert:** Diagnostic Radiology 1996; Vascular & Interventional Radiology 1998; **Med School:** Wayne State Univ 1991; **Resid:** Diagnostic Radiology, Beth Israel Hosp 1996; **Fellow:** Vascular & Interventional Radiology, Hosp Univ Penn 1997; **Fac Appt:** Assoc Prof Rad, Mount Sinai Sch Med

Wood, Bradford J MD [VIR] - **Spec Exp:** Radiofrequency Tumor Ablation; Liver Cancer; Kidney Cancer; Gene Therapy Delivery Systems; **Hospital:** Natl Inst of Hlth - Clin Ctr; **Address:** National Inst Health, 9000 Rockville Pike, msc 1182, Bldg 10, rm 1C364, Bethesda, MD 20892; **Phone:** 301-594-4511; **Board Cert:** Diagnostic Radiology 1996; **Med School:** Univ VA Sch Med 1991; **Resid:** Diagnostic Radiology, Georgetown Univ Med Ctr 1996; **Fellow:** Abdominal/Interventional Radiology, Mass General Hosp 1997

Southeast

Benenati, James F MD [VIR] - **Spec Exp:** Uterine Fibroid Embolization; Aneurysm-Abdominal Aortic; Peripheral Vascular Disease; **Hospital:** Baptist Hosp of Miami; **Address:** 8900 N Kendall Drive Fl 3, Miami, FL 33176; **Phone:** 786-596-5990; **Board Cert:** Diagnostic Radiology 1988; Vascular & Interventional Radiology 2005; **Med School:** Univ S Fla Coll Med 1984; **Resid:** Diagnostic Radiology, Indiana Univ Hosp 1988; **Fellow:** Vascular & Interventional Radiology, Johns Hopkins Hosp 1989; **Fac Appt:** Prof Rad, Univ S Fla Coll Med

Vascular & Interventional Radiology

Bettmann, Michael A MD [VIR] - **Spec Exp:** Uterine Fibroid Embolization; Chemoemboliza-tion & Tumor Ablation; Carotid Artery Stent Placement; Arteriovenous Malformations; **Hospital:** Wake Forest Univ Baptist Med Ctr, Iredell Meml Hlthcare Sys; **Address:** Wake Forest Univ Baptist Med Ctr, Dept Radiology, Medical Center Blvd, Winston-Salem, NC 27157; **Phone:** 336-716-2463; **Board Cert:** Diagnostic Radiology 1975; Vascular & Interventional Radiology 2005; **Med School:** Albert Einstein Coll Med 1969; **Resid:** Diagnostic Radiology, Beth Israel Med Ctr-Harvard 1975; **Fellow:** Cardiovascular Radiology, Peter Bent Brigham Hosp-Harvard 1977; **Fac Appt:** Prof Rad, Wake Forest Univ

Katzen, Barry T MD [VIR] - **Spec Exp:** Peripheral Vascular Disease; Aneurysm-Aortic; Carotid Artery Disease; **Hospital:** Baptist Hosp of Miami; **Address:** Baptist Cardiac & Vascular Inst, 8900 N Kendall Drive, Miami, FL 33176-2118; **Phone:** 786-596-5990; **Board Cert:** Diagnostic Radiology 1974; Vascular & Interventional Radiology 2004; **Med School:** Univ Miami Sch Med 1970; **Resid:** Diagnostic Radiology, New York Hosp-Cornell Med Ctr 1974

Lewis, Curtis A MD [VIR] - **Spec Exp:** Interventional Radiology; Vein Disorders; **Hospital:** Grady Hlth Sys, Emory Univ Hosp; **Address:** Grady Meml Hosp, Dept Radiology, 80 Jesse Hill Jr Drive, 1B Admin Suite, Box 26298, Atlanta, GA 30303; **Phone:** 404-616-4261; **Board Cert:** Diag-nostic Radiology 1991; Vascular & Interventional Radiology 2007; **Med School:** Emory Univ 1986; **Resid:** Diagnostic Radiology, Emory Univ Affil Hosps 1991; **Fellow:** Interventional Radiology, Emory Univ Affil Hosps 1992; **Fac Appt:** Asst Prof Rad, Emory Univ

Mauro, Matthew A MD [VIR] - **Spec Exp:** Cancer Chemoembolization; Cancer Radiother-apy; Gastrointestinal Cancer; **Hospital:** NC Memorial Hosp - UNC; **Address:** University NC Hosps, Dept Radiology, CB 7510, 2006 Old Clinic Bldg, Chapel Hill, NC 27514-7590; **Phone:** 919-966-4238; **Board Cert:** Diagnostic Radiology 1981; Vascular & Interventional Radiology 2003; **Med School:** Cornell Univ-Weill Med Coll 1977; **Resid:** Diagnostic Radiology, Univ NC Hosps 1980; **Fel-low:** Interventional Radiology, Univ NC Hosp 1981; Abdominal/Interventional Radiology, Mallinck-rodt Inst 1982; **Fac Appt:** Prof Rad, Univ NC Sch Med

Midwest

Cho, Kyung J MD [VIR] - **Spec Exp:** Chemoembolization & Tumor Ablation; Vascular Malforma-tions; Peripheral Vascular Disease; **Hospital:** Univ of Michigan Hosp; **Address:** Univ Michigan Med Ctr, Dept Radiology, 1500 E Med Ctr Drive, CVC 5582, Ann Arbor, MI 48109-5868; **Phone:** 734-936-4466; **Board Cert:** Diagnostic Radiology 1974; Vascular & Interventional Radiology 2005; **Med School:** Korea 1966; **Resid:** Diagnostic Radiology, Wayne Med Ctr 1973; **Fellow:** Cardio-vascular Radiology, Univ Michigan 1975; **Fac Appt:** Prof Rad, Univ Mich Med Sch

Darcy, Michael MD [VIR] - **Spec Exp:** Portal Hypertension; Chemoembolization & Tumor Abla-tion; **Hospital:** Barnes-Jewish Hosp; **Address:** Washington Univ, Mallinckrodt Inst Radiology, 510 S Kingshighway Blvd, St Louis, MO 63110; **Phone:** 314-362-2900; **Board Cert:** Diagnostic Radiol-ogy 1985; Vascular & Interventional Radiology 2004; **Med School:** Ohio State Univ 1979; **Resid:** Surgery, Univ Minn Hosps 1982; Diagnostic Radiology, Univ Minn Hosps 1985; **Fellow:** Interven-tional Radiology, Univ Minn Hosps 1987; **Fac Appt:** Prof Rad, Washington Univ, St Louis

Johnson, Matthew S MD [VIR] - **Spec Exp:** Liver Tumors; Uterine Fibroid Embolization; Portal Hypertension; Varicocele Embolization; **Hospital:** IU Health University Hosp, IU Health Methodist Hosp; **Address:** Indiana Univ Hospital, Interventional Radiology, 550 N University Blvd, rm 0276, In-dianapolis, IN 46202-5253; **Phone:** 317-944-1837; **Board Cert:** Diagnostic Radiology 1992; Vas-cular & Interventional Radiology 2006; **Med School:** Univ Mich Med Sch 1986; **Resid:** Surgery, Loyola Univ Med Ctr 1988; Diagnostic Radiology, Loyola Univ Med Ctr 1992; **Fellow:** Interventional Radiology, Johns Hopkins Univ 1994; **Fac Appt:** Prof Rad, Indiana Univ

Ketcham, Douglas B MD [VIR] - **Spec Exp:** Uterine Fibroid Embolization; Varicocele Embolization; Osteoporosis Spine-Vertebroplasty; **Hospital:** United Hosp, Regions Hosp - St Paul; **Address:** 250 Thompson St, St Paul, MN 55102; **Phone:** 651-297-6504; **Board Cert:** Diagnostic Radiology 1972; Vascular & Interventional Radiology 2005; **Med School:** Univ Wisc 1965; **Resid:** Diagnostic Radiology, Univ Minn Hosp 1971; **Fellow:** Neuroradiology, Univ Minn Hosp 1972

Nemcek, Albert A MD [VIR] - **Spec Exp:** Radiofrequency Tumor Ablation; Vascular Disease; Liver Tumors; **Hospital:** Northwestern Meml Hosp; **Address:** Northwestern Meml Hosp, Dept Radiology, Feinberg Pavillion, 4-710T, 251 E Huron St, Chicago, IL 60611; **Phone:** 312-926-5302; **Board Cert:** Diagnostic Radiology 1986; Vascular & Interventional Radiology 2005; **Med School:** UCSD 1982; **Resid:** Diagnostic Radiology, UCSD Med Ctr 1986; **Fellow:** Interventional Radiology, Northwestern Meml Hosp 1987; **Fac Appt:** Assoc Prof Rad, Northwestern Univ

Rilling, William S MD [VIR] - **Spec Exp:** Liver Cancer/Chemoembolization; Arteriovenous Malformations; Uterine Fibroid Embolization; **Hospital:** Froedtert and Med Ctr of WI; **Address:** Froedtert Hosp, Dept Radiology, 9200 W Wisconsin Ave, Milwaukee, WI 53226; **Phone:** 414-805-3028; **Board Cert:** Diagnostic Radiology 1995; Vascular & Interventional Radiology 2007; **Med School:** Univ Wisc 1990; **Resid:** Diagnostic Radiology, Univ Wisc Affil Hosps 1995; **Fellow:** Vascular & Interventional Radiology, Northwestern Meml Hosp 1996; **Fac Appt:** Assoc Prof Rad, Univ Wisc

Salem, Riad MD [VIR] - **Spec Exp:** Cancer Radiotherapy; Cancer Chemoembolization; Liver Cancer/Chemoembolization; **Hospital:** Northwestern Meml Hosp; **Address:** Northwestern Univ Dept Radiology, 676 N St Clair St, Ste 800, Chicago, IL 60611; **Phone:** 312-695-5753; **Board Cert:** Diagnostic Radiology 1997; Vascular & Interventional Radiology 2010; **Med School:** McGill Univ 1993; **Resid:** Diagnostic Radiology, Geo Washington Univ Hosp 1997; **Fellow:** Interventional Radiology, Chldns Hosp 1998; Interventional Radiology, Hosp Univ Penn 1998; **Fac Appt:** Assoc Prof Rad, Northwestern Univ

Smith, Steven J MD [VIR] - **Spec Exp:** Angioplasty-Peripheral; Uterine Fibroid Embolization; Varicocele Embolization; Arteriovenous Malformations; **Hospital:** La Grange Meml Hosp, Adventist Hinsdale Hosp; **Address:** 911 N Elm St, Ste 327, Hinsdale, IL 60521; **Phone:** 630-856-7460; **Board Cert:** Diagnostic Radiology 1983; Vascular & Interventional Radiology 2006; **Med School:** Wayne State Univ 1979; **Resid:** Diagnostic Radiology, Henry Ford Hosp 1983; **Fellow:** Vascular & Interventional Radiology, Northwestern Meml Hosp 1984; **Fac Appt:** Assoc Clin Prof Rad, Northwestern Univ

Vogelzang, Robert MD [VIR] - **Spec Exp:** Uterine Fibroid Embolization; Varicocele Embolization; Vascular Malformations; **Hospital:** Northwestern Meml Hosp; **Address:** Northwestern Meml Hosp, Dept Radiology, 251 E Huron St, Chicago, IL 60611; **Phone:** 312-926-5113; **Board Cert:** Diagnostic Radiology 1981; Vascular & Interventional Radiology 2005; **Med School:** Ros Franklin Univ/Chicago Med Sch 1977; **Resid:** Diagnostic Radiology, Northwestern Meml Hosp 1982; **Fellow:** Interventional Radiology, Northwestern Meml Hosp; **Fac Appt:** Prof Rad, Northwestern Univ

Great Plains and Mountains

Durham, Janette D MD [VIR] - **Spec Exp:** Uterine Fibroid Embolization; Peripheral Vascular Disease; Liver Cancer; **Hospital:** Univ of CO Hosp - Anschutz Inpatient Pav; **Address:** Univ Colorado Dept Radiology, 12401 E 17th Ave, MS L954, Aurora, CO 80045; **Phone:** 303-724-3796; **Board Cert:** Diagnostic Radiology 1987; Vascular & Interventional Radiology 2006; **Med School:** Indiana Univ 1983; **Resid:** Diagnostic Radiology, Indiana Univ Hosp 1987; **Fellow:** Vascular & Interventional Radiology, Mass General Hosp 1988; **Fac Appt:** Prof Rad, Univ Colorado

Vascular & Interventional Radiology

Kumpe, David A MD [VIR] - **Spec Exp:** Aneurysm-Cerebral; Stroke; Arterial & Venous Stents; Interventional Neuroradiology; **Hospital:** Univ of CO Hosp - Anschutz Inpatient Pav, Chldn's Hosp - Aurora (CO); **Address:** Univ Hosp, Dept Radiology, 12605 E 16th Ave, Aurora, CO 80045; **Phone:** 720-848-7620; **Board Cert:** Diagnostic Radiology 1972; Vascular & Interventional Radiology 2005; **Med School:** Harvard Med Sch 1967; **Resid:** Diagnostic Radiology, Mass Genl Hosp 1971; **Fellow:** Neurological Radiology, Kantonsspital 1976; Angiography, Kantonsspital 1976; **Fac Appt:** Prof Rad, Univ Colorado

Yakes, Wayne F MD [VIR] - **Spec Exp:** Vascular Malformations; Interventional Neuroradiology; **Hospital:** Swedish Med Ctr - Englewood; **Address:** Vasacular Malformation Ctr, 501 E Hampden Ave, Ste 4600, Englewood, CO 80113; **Phone:** 303-788-4280; **Board Cert:** Diagnostic Radiology 1983; **Med School:** Creighton Univ 1979; **Resid:** Diagnostic Radiology, Fitzsimons Med Ctr 1983; **Fellow:** Angiography, Walter Reed Med Ctr 1984; Interventional Neuroradiology, Baptist Hosp 1992; **Fac Appt:** Clin Prof, Univ Colorado

Southwest

Kay, Dennis MD [VIR] - **Spec Exp:** Radiofrequency Tumor Ablation; **Hospital:** Ochsner Med Ctr-New Orleans; **Address:** Ochsner Clinic, Dept Radiology, 1514 Jefferson Hwy, New Orleans, LA 70121-2429; **Phone:** 504-842-3470; **Board Cert:** Diagnostic Radiology 1986; Vascular & Interventional Radiology 2004; **Med School:** Tulane Univ 1981; **Resid:** Diagnostic Radiology, Ochsner Fdn Hosp 1985; **Fellow:** Vascular & Interventional Radiology, Beth Israel Hosp 1986; **Fac Appt:** Assoc Clin Prof Rad, Tulane Univ

West Coast and Pacific

Dake, Michael D MD [VIR] - **Spec Exp:** Aortic Stent Grafts; Endovascular Stent Grafts; Vascular Disease; Aneurysm; **Hospital:** Stanford Univ Hosp & Clinics; **Address:** Stanford Dept Cardiothoracic Surgery, 300 Pasteur Drive, Falk Research Bldg, 2nd Fl, Stanford, CA 94305-5407; **Phone:** 650-724-0831; **Board Cert:** Internal Medicine 1981; Pulmonary Disease 1986; Diagnostic Radiology 1986; Vascular & Interventional Radiology 2006; **Med School:** Baylor Coll Med 1978; **Resid:** Internal Medicine, Baylor Affil Hosp 1982; Diagnostic Radiology, UCSF Med Ctr 1986; **Fellow:** Pulmonary Disease, UCSF 1983; Interventional Radiology, UCSF 1987; **Fac Appt:** Prof TS, Stanford Univ

Gomes, Antoinette S MD [VIR] - **Spec Exp:** Cardiovascular Interventional Radiology; Vascular Malformations; Chemoembolization & Tumor Ablation; **Hospital:** UCLA Ronald Reagan Med Ctr, Santa Clara Vly Med Ctr; **Address:** Dept Radiological Sciences, Ronald Reagan UCLA Med Ctr, 757 Westwood Plaza, Ste 2125, Los Angeles, CA 90095; **Phone:** 310-267-8769; **Board Cert:** Diagnostic Radiology 1975; Vascular & Interventional Radiology 2004; **Med School:** Med Coll PA Hahnemann 1969; **Resid:** Internal Medicine, LAC-USC Med Ctr 1972; Diagnostic Radiology, Stanford Univ Med Ctr 1975; **Fellow:** Cardiovascular Radiology, UCLA Med Ctr 1976; Cardiovascular Radiology, Univ Minn 1978; **Fac Appt:** Prof Rad, UCLA

Goodwin, Scott C MD [VIR] - **Spec Exp:** Uterine Fibroid Embolization; Liver Cancer/Chemoembolization; **Hospital:** UC Irvine Med Ctr; **Address:** 333 City Blvd W, Ste 1405, MC 5005, Orange, CA 92868; **Phone:** 714-456-7517; **Board Cert:** Diagnostic Radiology 1989; Vascular & Interventional Radiology 2007; **Med School:** Harvard Med Sch 1984; **Resid:** Diagnostic Radiology, UCLA Medical Ctr 1988; **Fellow:** Vascular & Interventional Radiology, UCLA Medical Ctr 1989; **Fac Appt:** Prof Rad, UCLA

Hovsepian, David M MD [VIR] - **Spec Exp:** Uterine Fibroid Embolization; Aneurysm-Aortic; Vascular Malformations; **Hospital:** Stanford Univ Hosp & Clinics; **Address:** Dept Interventional Radiology, 300 Pasteur Drive, rm H3649, Stanford, CA 94305-5642; **Phone:** 650-724-7362; **Board Cert:** Diagnostic Radiology 1991; Vascular & Interventional Radiology 2006; **Med School:** Columbia P&S 1986; **Resid:** Diagnostic Radiology, Columbia Presby Hosp 1991; **Fellow:** Interventional Radiology, Thomas Jefferson Univ Hosp 1993; **Fac Appt:** Prof Rad, Stanford Univ

Kaufman, John A MD [VIR] - **Spec Exp:** Uterine Fibroid Embolization; Angioplasty & Stent Placement; **Hospital:** OR Hlth & Sci Univ; **Address:** Dotter Interven Inst-OHSU Hosps & Clins, 3181 SW Sam Jackson Park Rd, MC L605, Portland, OR 97239; **Phone:** 503-494-7660; **Board Cert:** Diagnostic Radiology 1990; Vascular & Interventional Radiology 2005; **Med School:** Boston Univ 1982; **Resid:** Diagnostic Radiology, Boston Univ Med Ctr 1990; **Fellow:** Vascular & Interventional Radiology, Boston Univ Med Ctr 1991; **Fac Appt:** Prof Rad, Oregon Hlth & Sci Univ

Keller, Frederick S MD [VIR] - **Spec Exp:** Uterine Fibroid Embolization; Arterial & Venous Stents; Urinary Tract Interventions; **Hospital:** OR Hlth & Sci Univ; **Address:** Dotter Interventional Inst, L-605, 3181 SW Sam Jackson Park Rd, Portland, OR 97239; **Phone:** 503-494-7660; **Board Cert:** Diagnostic Radiology 1977; Vascular & Interventional Radiology 2003; **Med School:** Univ Pennsylvania 1968; **Resid:** Diagnostic Radiology, Univ Oreg Hlth Scis Ctr 1977; **Fac Appt:** Prof, Oregon Hlth & Sci Univ

McGahan, John P MD [VIR] - **Spec Exp:** Radiofrequency Tumor Ablation; Liver Cancer; Kidney Cancer; **Hospital:** UC Davis Med Ctr; **Address:** UC Davis Medical Ctr, Dept Radiology, 4860 Y St ACC3100, Sacramento, CA 95817; **Phone:** 916-734-3606; **Board Cert:** Diagnostic Radiology 1979; **Med School:** Oregon Hlth & Sci Univ 1974; **Resid:** Surgery, UC Davis Med Ctr 1976; Diagnostic Radiology, UC Davis Med Ctr 1979; **Fac Appt:** Prof Rad, UC Davis

Valji, Karim MD [VIR] - **Spec Exp:** Dialysis Access; **Hospital:** Univ Wash Med Ctr; **Address:** Univ of WA Med Ctr-Dept Rad, 1959 NE Pacific St, rm RR215, Box 357115, Seattle, WA 98195-7115; **Phone:** 206-543-3320; **Board Cert:** Diagnostic Radiology 1989; Vascular & Interventional Radiology 2008; **Med School:** Harvard Med Sch 1982; **Resid:** Internal Medicine, UCSF Med Ctr 1984; Diagnostic Radiology, UCSD Med Ctr 1988; **Fellow:** Angiography, UCSD Med Ctr 1989

◧ Cleveland Clinic

Every life deserves world class care.

Diagnostic Radiology, Neuroradiology

Cleveland Clinic Imaging Institute is one of the leading academic imaging centers in the world and one of the busiest clinical departments in the country. Each year, Cleveland Clinic imagers perform and interpret more than 1.8 million examinations, for which all images are acquired digitally.

Imaging Institute radiologists are leaders in their specialties. They are responsible for the publication of numerous peer-reviewed manuscripts each year, serve on committees of the most prestigious radiologic societies and are involved in cutting-edge research. This research encompasses treatment of acute stroke, magnetic resonance angiography, 3-D imaging, digital radiography, digital mammography, cardiac magnetic resonance, cartilage imaging, electronic image distribution and intravascular ultrasound.

Neuroradiology specializes in imaging and diagnosing neurological disorders such as epilepsy, brain tumors, multiple sclerosis and problems of the ear-nose-throat system. Patients are referred from around the United States and the world to seek the insights, treatments and opinions from our dedicated team of professionals.

Interventional Radiology supports some of the most cutting-edge therapies offered at Cleveland Clinic. Organ transplantation, thoracic surgery and hepato-biliary surgery have been developed in unison with image-guided techniques for the management of issues that arise during surgery. Interventional radiology performs more than 9,500 procedures annually.

Cardiovascular Imaging is equipped with state-of-the-art CT and MRI equipment. The staff is expert in the diagnosis and planning of treatment for conditions that include acquired cardiac disease in adults and congenital heart disease in children and adults. The advanced technology used includes two MRI scanners for cardiac analysis and two CT scanners.

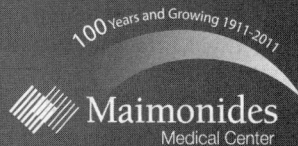
The Jaffe Stroke Center is ranked among the top 5% in the nation, and the top two in New York State. There are several other stroke centers in Brooklyn, but the services at Maimonides are far more advanced than at any other institution.

After the onset of stroke symptoms, there is a three-hour window of opportunity for the administration of a clot-busting drug. With highly specialized training, experts at certified stroke centers can administer that drug to appropriate patients. But there is a nine-hour window of opportunity for advanced treatment, and Maimonides is one of only a handful of hospitals in the New York metropolitan area with the capability of providing that treatment.

Dr. Jeffrey Farkas, Director of Interventional Neuroradiology, can insert a special instrument into a blood vessel, thread it up to the brain, and remove a stroke-causing blood clot. This procedure can greatly reduce stroke damage and, in some cases, has completely reversed all symptoms. Dr. Farkas is among an elite few in the nation with significant experience utilizing this advanced technology for stroke patients.

Dr. Steven Rudolph, the Director of the Jaffe Stroke Center, has been selected as investigator in two clinical trials for the newest medical stroke therapies. This distinction is bestowed only on the most respected clinicians in that specialty. These therapies, too, will be able to provide treatment up to nine hours after the onset of symptoms.

In addition, Maimonides has a multidisciplinary team of stroke experts that includes physicians and nurses from the Department of Emergency Medicine, providing the vital first line of defense in combating stroke. The ER at Maimonides is equipped with telemedicine, an interactive system which allows consultation with a stroke neurologist in real time, even when the doctor is at a remote location.

In our stroke unit and interventional neuroradiology suite, nurses are certified and experienced in these specialties, and they coordinate recovery plans that include numerous technicians and therapists.

The Jaffe Stroke Center at Maimonides Medical Center was awarded the Gold Plus Award for excellence in performance from the American Stroke Association's "Get With the Guidelines" Program. In addition, we have been named to the "Target: Stroke" Honor Roll – one of only 50 hospitals in the U.S. to achieve the recognition.

Maimonides Medical Center
Passionate about medicine.
Compassionate about people.

www.maimonidesmed.org/stroke

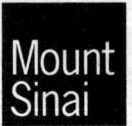 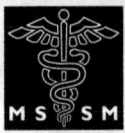

**MOUNT SINAI
SCHOOL OF
MEDICINE**

THE MOUNT SINAI MEDICAL CENTER
RADIOLOGY

One Gustave L. Levy Place
Fifth Avenue and 100th Street
New York, NY 10029-6574
Physician Referral: 1-800-MD-SINAI (637-4624)
www.mountsinai.org/imaging

THE DEPARTMENT OF RADIOLOGY at Mount Sinai offers patients one of the world's most comprehensive and sophisticated arrays of diagnostic and interventional radiology services. The department uses filmless digital technology that spans magnetic resonance imaging (MRI), multi-slice computed tomography (CT), positron emission tomography CT (PET-CT), single photon emission computed tomography CT (SPECT-CT), advanced ultrasound, conventional radiography, angiography, digital mammography, and state-of-the-art Picture Archiving Communication System (PACS) technology.

Comprehensive Diagnostic Services – Mount Sinai provides the entire range of diagnostic radiology services in a patient-friendly environment. Its nationally renowned radiologic physicians specialize in every area of disease diagnosis, as well as disease prevention and innovative therapeutic approaches. The combination of state-of-the-art imaging equipment with the finest imaging physicians makes Mount Sinai Radiology the place to go for all your imaging needs.

Early Detection Programs – We are committed to special screening approaches for early disease detection. We provide radiological screenings for colon, breast, and lung cancer and atherosclerosis. The early detection programs use a variety of imaging techniques, such as CT and MRI for atherosclerosis, CT for lung and colon cancer, PET for oncology, digital and 3D mammography, MRI, ultrasound, and computer-aided diagnosis for breast cancer.

Minimally Invasive Procedures – Radiology at Mount Sinai has moved beyond diagnosis to the most sophisticated therapeutic interventions. Interventional radiologists at Mount Sinai perform biopsies, vascular therapies, and uterine artery embolization for fibroids—an alternative to hysterectomy—as well as treatments for aneurysms, atherosclerosis, and many types of cancer. In addition, advanced CT and MR angiography techniques are widely utilized to diagnose vascular diseases in a minimally invasive yet highly accurate manner.

Oncology Imaging – Radiologists work closely with surgeons, oncologists, and other caregivers to optimize the diagnosis and treatment of patients with head and neck, liver, lung, breast, and gastrointestinal cancers. State of the art CT, MRI, ultrasound, SPECT and PET CT are utilized to make the most accurate, least invasive and lowest dose diagnosis.

DEVELOPING NEW DIAGNOSTIC TOOLS

Radiology at Mount Sinai is an active center of imaging research and development. Mount Sinai physicians and scientists developed a special form of MRI to diagnose heart disease and atherosclerosis noninvasively and thereby identify patients at greatest risk for stroke and heart attack. We actively collaborate with other disciplines to develop and refine imaging tools that will make prevention and diagnosis increasingly effective. That is the case, for example, in neuroscience, where the imaging innovations impact our understanding of neurodegenerative conditions, such as Parkinson's disease, multiple sclerosis, stroke, brain tumors, and various psychiatric disorders; cardiovascular disease, where studies are under way to predict the risk associated with atherosclerotic plaques and assess new therapies for aortic and cerebral artery aneurysms; and liver disease, where radiologists, transplant surgeons, and hepatologists collaborate closely to develop optimal therapeutic strategies.

NewYork-Presbyterian
The University Hospital of Columbia and Cornell

Affiliated with Columbia University College of Physicians and Surgeons and Weill Cornell Medical College

NewYork-Presbyterian Hospital
Columbia University Medical Center
622 West 168th Street
New York, NY 10032

NewYork-Presbyterian Hospital
Weill Cornell Medical Center
525 East 68th Street
New York, NY 10065

1-877-NYP-WELL (1-877-697-9355)   www.nyp.org/vascular

NewYork-Presbyterian Vascular Program

Vascular disease can affect people of all ages and requires a wide range of expertise for appropriate and effective therapies. NewYork-Presbyterian Hospital Vascular Services, encompassing Vascular Surgery, Interventional Cardiology, Interventional Radiology and Interventional Neuro Radiology at two premiere facilities offers a comprehensive program for the prevention, diagnosis and treatment of diverse problems relating to arteries and veins throughout the body, including the aorta, abdomen, kidneys, legs and neck.

The Vascular Program brings together medical and surgical experts of two internationally renowned academic medical centers— NewYork-Presbyterian Hospital/Columbia University Medical Center and NewYork-Presbyterian Hospital/Weill Cornell Medical Center— who have vast experience in the treatment of even the most unusual vascular conditions.

Patients benefit from the Vascular Programs' proven cutting-edge technologies, innovative programs and ground-breaking research.

- Innovative therapy for the management of complex lower extremity arterial, carotid and aortic disease;
- Cutting-edge technology enabling the management of complex arterial and venous disease including:
  - State-of-the-art robotic Siemens Artis zeego® medical imaging system;
  - Inventive applications of non-invasive diagnostic technologies, including CT scans, ultrasound, MRI and MRA;
- Innovative minimally invasive treatments of venous disease;
- Participation in ground-breaking trials for management of vascular disease;
- Increased awareness, management and treatment of blood clots (DVT);
- Rigorous screenings and integrated care for patients at risk for life-threatening vascular diseases such as strokes, aortic aneurysms and dissections;
- Advances in the latest drug therapies;
- Programs that emphasize prevention measures.

Comprehensive Services Include:

- Comprehensive Abdominal Aortic Aneurysm Program to detect and treat one of the leading causes of death.

- Treatment of Thoracic and Abdominal Aneurysms through surgical and minimally invasive repair.

- Amputation Prevention Program for treating vascular blockages leading to difficulty walking or the loss of a leg.

- Gene Therapy Center includes a program to treat blocked arteries in legs.

- Dedicated Wound Healing Program offering multiple therapy options for management of patients with chronic lower extremity wounds.

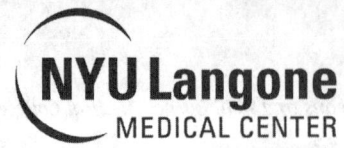

550 First Avenue *(at 31st Street)*
New York, NY 10016

www.NYULMC.org

Physician Referral: **888-7-NYU-MED** *(888-769-8633)*

RADIOLOGY

The Department of Radiology at NYU Langone Medical Center is committed to capturing the best images possible with the lowest dose of radiation. As an academic medical center, our radiologists are in a unique position to take the lead in helping to define and advance radiology in today's rapidly advancing technological environment.

Expertise
NYU Langone Medical Center's board certified radiologists and licensed technologists specialize in imaging and are involved in a variety of innovative collaborations and research initiatives. The Department consists of over 100 sub-specialized academic radiologists, many of them acknowledged leaders and innovators in their fields.

Advanced Technology
NYU Langone uses some of the most advanced imaging equipment in the world, including high and ultra high-field MRI imaging systems (known as 1.5T and 3T magnets). Its MRI scanners are shorter and wider than ever, making for a more patient-friendly experience. The Center for Biomedical Imaging, an advanced research facility, features a powerful 7T magnet.

Recognition for Safety and Quality
We continually follow a rigorous set of quality standards and maintain accreditation by the American College of Radiology (ACR). We are designated by the ACR as a "Breast Imaging Center of Excellence" and have achieved high practice standards in image quality, personal qualifications, facility equipment, quality control procedures and quality assurance programs.

Patient Focused Approach
We are conveniently located and participate in many insurance plans. We ensure timely delivery of reports and images and allow physicians to view patient exam status, reports and images online from their office. In addition to our convenient hours, weekend, evening and often same-day appointments are available. Language interpretation services are available as needed.

Our Areas of Specialization
We offer an extensive range of diagnostic services around MRI, CT, ultrasound, PET/CT, X-ray, interventional radiology and nuclear medicine. Sub-specialized radiologists provide diagnostic interpretation in abdominal, biomedical, breast, cardiac, chest, emergency, general, musculoskeletal, neuroradiology, neuro interventional, nuclear medicine, pediatric, vascular interventional and women's imaging. Specialty procedures include coronary artery disease and virtual colonoscopy screening, stereotactic biopsy capability, minimally invasive techniques including radiofrequency ablation, chemoembolization, radioimmunotherapy and bone densitometry.

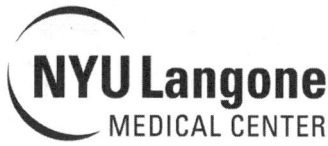

VASCULAR SURGERY

Staffed by one of the largest vascular surgery teams in the country, NYU Langone Medical Center emphasizes both expert patient care and minimally invasive therapies. Physicians have extensive experience performing the most advanced procedures, including stents and angioplasty for carotid artery disease, aortic aneurysms and blockages in arteries throughout the body. In addition to its expertise in arterial disease, NYU Langone is proud to offer one of the few academic Vein Centers in the United States. We specialize in the following areas:

Aortic Pathology
The Medical Center offers minimally invasive surgical solutions as well as treatments for complex aortic problems. Patients usually require no blood transfusions and are able to leave the hospital one or two days after surgery. We are also a training center for endovascular management of abdominal and thoracic aneurysms.

Carotid Artery Disease
NYU Langone remains a leader in both the screening for carotid disease and the prevention of stroke in patients being treated for carotid artery occlusive disease. Our physicians helped pioneer carotid endarterectomy as an open surgical procedure, and played a pivotal role in the development of the carotid stenting procedure.

Peripheral Arterial Disease
Vascular surgeons at the Medical Center draw on a wealth of experience in treating peripheral arterial disease (PAD). The team specializes in new and innovative technologies such as laser and "Silverhawk" atherectomy procedures, as well as cryoplasty. Additionally, we offer drug-eluting stents, which are coated with special medicines to prevent scar formation and re-occlusion of the stent.

Vascular Screenings
Our physicians are committed to improving public awareness and understanding of vascular disease through preventative screenings. The disease is among the leading causes of death in the U.S., yet is generally asymptomatic until a stroke or aneurysm occurs. Effective screening techniques at the Medical Center include ultrasound scans of the aorta, ultrasound scans of the carotid arteries, and blood pressure measurements.

Venous Disease
The Vein Center at NYU Langone is considered an authority in the minimally invasive treatment of venous disease. The Center treats patients with all forms of venous pathology, from venous insufficiency and varicose veins to occlusive disease and deep vein thrombosis.

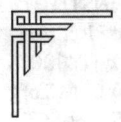

The Best in American Medicine
www.CastleConnolly.com

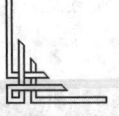
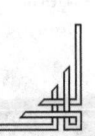

Reproductive Endocrinology
a subspecialty of Obstetrics & Gynecology

An obstetrician/gynecologist who is capable of managing complex problems relating to reproductive endocrinology and infertility.

Training Required: Four years *plus* two years in clinical practice before certification in obstetrics and gynecology is complete *plus* additional training and examination in reproductive endocrinology.

REPRODUCTIVE ENDOCRINOLOGY

New England

Buster, John E MD [RE] - **Spec Exp:** Infertility-IVF; Reproductive Surgery; **Hospital:** Tufts Med Ctr; **Address:** 800 Washington St, Boston, MA 02111; **Phone:** 617-636-0053; **Board Cert:** Obstetrics & Gynecology 2010; Reproductive Endocrinology 2010; **Med School:** UCLA 1966; **Resid:** Obstetrics & Gynecology, Harbor-UCLA Med Ctr 1971; **Fellow:** Reproductive Endocrinology, Harbor-UCLA Med Ctr 1973; **Fac Appt:** Prof ObG, Tufts Univ

Carson, Sandra A MD [RE] - **Spec Exp:** Infertility-IVF; Laparoscopic Surgery; Endometriosis; Sexual Dysfunction; **Hospital:** Women & Infants Hosp of RI; **Address:** Women & Infants Hosp of RI, 90 Plain St, Providence, RI 02903; **Phone:** 401-453-7500; **Board Cert:** Obstetrics & Gynecology 2005; Reproductive Endocrinology 2005; **Med School:** Northwestern Univ 1977; **Resid:** Obstetrics & Gynecology, Prentice Womens Hosp 1981; **Fellow:** Reproductive Endocrinology, Michael Reese Hosp 1983; **Fac Appt:** Prof ObG, Brown Univ

Crowley, William F MD [RE] - **Spec Exp:** Pituitary Disorders; Kallmann's Syndrome; Fertility Preservation in Cancer; **Hospital:** Mass Genl Hosp; **Address:** Mass Genl Hosp, Reproductive Sci Ctr, 55 Fruit St, Bartlett Hall-Ext 511, Boston, MA 02114; **Phone:** 617-726-5390; **Board Cert:** Internal Medicine 1974; Endocrinology 1977; **Med School:** Tufts Univ 1969; **Resid:** Internal Medicine, Mass Genl Hosp 1971; Internal Medicine, Mass Genl Hosp 1974; **Fellow:** Endocrinology, Mass Genl Hosp 1976; **Fac Appt:** Prof Med, Harvard Med Sch

Ginsburg, Elizabeth S MD [RE] - **Spec Exp:** Infertility-IVF; Fertility Preservation in Cancer; **Hospital:** Brigham and Women's Hosp (page 57), Dana-Farber Cancer Inst (page 57); **Address:** Brigham & Womens Hosp, Reproductive Med, 75 Francis St, ASB-1 3254, Boston, MA 02115; **Phone:** 617-732-4222; **Board Cert:** Obstetrics & Gynecology 2009; Reproductive Endocrinology 2009; **Med School:** Mount Sinai Sch Med 1985; **Resid:** Obstetrics & Gynecology, Brigham & Womens Hosp 1989; **Fellow:** Reproductive Endocrinology, Brigham & Womens Hosp 1991

Hill III, Joseph A MD [RE] - **Spec Exp:** Miscarriage-Recurrent; Infertility-Female; Gynecology; Infertility-IVF; **Hospital:** Portsmouth Regl Hosp, Winchester Hosp; **Address:** Fertility Ctr of New England, 875 Greenland Rd C Bldg, Unit 1, Portsmouth, NH 03801; **Phone:** 781-942-7000 x601; **Board Cert:** Obstetrics & Gynecology 2008; Reproductive Endocrinology 2008; **Med School:** Med Coll GA 1981; **Resid:** Obstetrics & Gynecology, Med Coll Ga 1985; **Fellow:** Reproductive Endocrinology, Brigham-Womens Hosp/Harvard 1987; Reproductive Immunology, Brigham-Womens Hosp/Harvard 1988; **Fac Appt:** Prof ObG, Harvard Med Sch

Hornstein, Mark D MD [RE] - **Spec Exp:** Infertility-IVF; Endometriosis; Laparoscopic Surgery; Hysteroscopic Surgery; **Hospital:** Brigham and Women's Hosp (page 57), Newton - Wellesley Hosp; **Address:** Brigham & Women's Hosp, 75 Francis St, Boston, MA 02115; **Phone:** 617-732-4648; **Board Cert:** Obstetrics & Gynecology 2010; Reproductive Endocrinology 2010; **Med School:** Univ Cincinnati 1982; **Resid:** Obstetrics & Gynecology, Brigham & Women's Hosp 1986; **Fellow:** Reproductive Endocrinology, Brigham & Women's Hosp 1988; **Fac Appt:** Assoc Prof ObG, Harvard Med Sch

Isaacson, Keith B MD [RE] - **Spec Exp:** Infertility; Endometriosis; Minimally Invasive Surgery; **Hospital:** Newton - Wellesley Hosp, Mass Genl Hosp; **Address:** 2014 Washington St Fl 2 West, Newton, MA 02462; **Phone:** 617-243-5205; **Board Cert:** Obstetrics & Gynecology 2009; Reproductive Endocrinology 2009; **Med School:** Med Coll GA 1983; **Resid:** Obstetrics & Gynecology, Ochsner Fdn Hosp 1987; **Fellow:** Reproductive Endocrinology, Hosp Univ Penn 1989; **Fac Appt:** Assoc Prof ObG, Harvard Med Sch

Johnson, Julia V MD [RE] - **Spec Exp:** Infertility-IVF; Endometriosis; Menopause Problems; **Hospital:** UMass Memorial Med Ctr; **Address:** U Mass Medical Ctr-Memorial Campus, 119 Belmont St, Worcester, MA 01605; **Phone:** 508-334-1345; **Board Cert:** Obstetrics & Gynecology 2010; Reproductive Endocrinology/Infertility 2010; **Med School:** Med Coll GA 1984; **Resid:** Obstetrics & Gynecology, Med Coll of Georgia 1988; **Fellow:** Reproductive Endocrinology, Univ Texas Hlth Sci Ctr 1990; **Fac Appt:** Prof ObG, Univ Mass Sch Med

Luciano, Anthony A MD [RE] - **Spec Exp:** Infertility; Endometriosis; Menopause Problems; Osteoporosis; **Hospital:** Hosp of Central CT at New Britain, Hartford Hosp; **Address:** Center for Fertility & Womens Health, 100 Grand St, Ste E3, New Britain, CT 06050; **Phone:** 860-224-5467; **Board Cert:** Obstetrics & Gynecology 1980; Reproductive Endocrinology 1981; **Med School:** Univ Conn 1973; **Resid:** Obstetrics & Gynecology, Univ Conn Hosp 1977; **Fellow:** Reproductive Endocrinology, Univ Conn Hosp 1979; **Fac Appt:** Prof ObG, Univ Conn

Manganiello, Paul D MD [RE] - **Spec Exp:** Infertility; Menopause Problems; **Hospital:** Dartmouth - Hitchcock Med Ctr; **Address:** Dartmouth-Hitchcock Med Ctr, Dept OB/Gyn, 1 Med Ctr Drive, Lebanon, NH 03756; **Phone:** 603-653-9240; **Board Cert:** Obstetrics & Gynecology 1980; Reproductive Endocrinology 1984; **Med School:** Jefferson Med Coll 1973; **Resid:** Obstetrics & Gynecology, Thomas Jefferson Univ Hosp 1977; **Fellow:** Reproductive Endocrinology, Med Coll Ga Hosp 1979; **Fac Appt:** Assoc Prof ObG, Dartmouth Med Sch

Oskowitz, Selwyn P MD [RE] - **Spec Exp:** Infertility-IVF; **Hospital:** Beth Israel Deaconess Med Ctr - Boston; **Address:** Boston IVF, 1 Brookline Pl, Ste 302, Brookline, MA 02445; **Phone:** 617-735-9000; **Board Cert:** Obstetrics & Gynecology 1981; **Med School:** South Africa 1970; **Resid:** Obstetrics & Gynecology, Univ Colorado Med Ctr 1977; **Fellow:** Reproductive Endocrinology, Beth Israel Deaconess Med Ctr 1984; **Fac Appt:** Asst Prof ObG, Harvard Med Sch

Patrizio, Pasquale MD [RE] - **Spec Exp:** Infertility-IVF; Fertility Preservation in Cancer; **Hospital:** Yale-New Haven Hosp, Yale Med Group; **Address:** Yale Fertility Ctr, Dept OB/GYN, 150 Sargent Drive, New Haven, CT 06511; **Phone:** 203-785-4708; **Board Cert:** Obstetrics & Gynecology 2007; Reproductive Endocrinology 2010; **Med School:** Italy 1983; **Resid:** Obstetrics & Gynecology, Univ Naples 1987; Reproductive Endocrinology, Univ Pisa 1990; **Fellow:** Infertility, UC Irvine 1995; **Fac Appt:** Prof ObG, Yale Univ

Petrozza, John C MD [RE] - **Spec Exp:** Pain-Chronic Pelvic; Endometriosis; Minimally Invasive Surgery; Infertility-IVF; **Hospital:** Mass Genl Hosp; **Address:** Mass Genl Hosp, Fetility Ctr, 55 Fruit St Yawkey Bldg - Ste 10-A, Boston, MA 02114; **Phone:** 617-726-8868; **Board Cert:** Obstetrics & Gynecology 2009; Reproductive Endocrinology/Infertility 2009; **Med School:** Univ Tex Med Br, Galveston 1990; **Resid:** Obstetrics & Gynecology, Univ Texas Affil Hosp 1994; **Fellow:** Reproductive Endocrinology, Tufts New England Med Ctr 1996; **Fac Appt:** Asst Prof ObG, Harvard Med Sch

Toth, Thomas L MD [RE] - **Spec Exp:** Infertility-IVF; **Hospital:** Mass Genl Hosp, Newton - Wellesley Hosp; **Address:** Mass Genl Hosp, Fertility Ctr, 55 Fruit St Yawkey Bldg - Ste 10A, Boston, MA 02114-2621; **Phone:** 617-726-8868; **Board Cert:** Obstetrics & Gynecology 2010; Reproductive Endocrinology/Infertility 2010; **Med School:** Univ MO-Kansas City 1986; **Resid:** Obstetrics & Gynecology, Mass Genl Hosp/Brigham & Womens Hosp 1990; **Fellow:** Reproductive Endocrinology, E Virginia Med Sch Hosps 1992; **Fac Appt:** Assoc Prof ObG, Harvard Med Sch

Zinaman, Michael J MD [RE] - **Spec Exp:** Endometriosis; Infertility; Uterine Fibroids; **Hospital:** Caritas St Elizabeth's Med Ctr-Boston; **Address:** Caritas St Elizabeth's Med Ctr SMC5, 736 Cambridge St, Boston, MA 02135; **Phone:** 617-562-7018; **Board Cert:** Obstetrics & Gynecology 2010; Reproductive Endocrinology 2010; **Med School:** SUNY Downstate 1981; **Resid:** Obstetrics & Gynecology, Univ Chicago Hosps 1985; **Fellow:** Reproductive Endocrinology, Georgetown Univ 1987

Reproductive Endocrinology

Mid Atlantic

Copperman, Alan B MD [RE] - **Spec Exp:** Infertility-IVF; Endometriosis; Laparoscopic Surgery; Hysteroscopic Surgery; **Hospital:** Mount Sinai Med Ctr (page 63); **Address:** 635 Madison Ave Fl 10, RMA of New York, New York, NY 10022; **Phone:** 212-756-5777; **Board Cert:** Obstetrics & Gynecology 2010; Reproductive Endocrinology 2010; **Med School:** NY Med Coll 1989; **Resid:** Obstetrics & Gynecology, Yale-New Haven Hosp 1993; **Fellow:** Reproductive Endocrinology, Mt Sinai Med Ctr 1995; **Fac Appt:** Clin Prof ObG, Mount Sinai Sch Med

Coutifaris, Christos MD/PhD [RE] - **Spec Exp:** Infertility-IVF; Fertility Preservation in Cancer; Polycystic Ovarian Syndrome; **Hospital:** Hosp Univ Penn - UPHS (page 68); **Address:** Penn Fertility Care, 3701 Market St Fl 8 - Ste 800, Philadelphia, PA 19104; **Phone:** 215-662-6100; **Board Cert:** Obstetrics & Gynecology 2009; Reproductive Endocrinology 2009; **Med School:** Univ Pennsylvania 1982; **Resid:** Obstetrics & Gynecology, Hosp Univ Penn 1986; **Fellow:** Reproductive Endocrinology, Hosp Univ Penn 1987; **Fac Appt:** Prof ObG, Univ Pennsylvania

Gracia, Clarisa R MD [RE] - **Spec Exp:** Gynecology in Cancer Patients; Infertility in Cancer Patients; Fertility Preservation in Cancer; **Hospital:** Hosp Univ Penn - UPHS (page 68); **Address:** Penn Fertility Care, 3701 Market St, Ste 800, Philadelphia, PA 19104; **Phone:** 215-662-6100; **Board Cert:** Obstetrics & Gynecology 2007; Reproductive Endocrinology 2007; **Med School:** SUNY Buffalo 1997; **Resid:** Obstetrics & Gynecology, Hosp U Penn 2000; **Fellow:** Reproductive Endocrinology, Hosp U Penn; **Fac Appt:** Asst Prof ObG, Univ Pennsylvania

Grazi, Richard MD [RE] - **Spec Exp:** Infertility-IVF; Preimplantation Genetic Diagnosis; Fertility Preservation in Cancer; **Hospital:** Maimonides Med Ctr (page 62), Richmond Univ Med Ctr; **Address:** 1355 84th St, Brooklyn, NY 11228-3030; **Phone:** 718-283-8600; **Board Cert:** Obstetrics & Gynecology 2006; Reproductive Endocrinology 2006; **Med School:** SUNY Buffalo 1981; **Resid:** Obstetrics & Gynecology, NYU Med Ctr 1985; **Fellow:** Reproductive Endocrinology, UMDNJ Med Ctr 1987; **Fac Appt:** Assoc Clin Prof ObG, Mount Sinai Sch Med

Grifo, James A MD/PhD [RE] - **Spec Exp:** Infertility-IVF; Prenatal Genetic Diagnosis; Hysteroscopic Surgery; Laparoscopic Surgery; **Hospital:** NYU Langone Med Ctr (page 66); **Address:** 660 1st Ave Fl 5, New York, NY 10016; **Phone:** 212-263-7978; **Board Cert:** Obstetrics & Gynecology 2010; Reproductive Endocrinology 2010; **Med School:** Case West Res Univ 1984; **Resid:** Obstetrics & Gynecology, NY Hosp-Cornell Med Ctr 1988; **Fellow:** Reproductive Endocrinology, Yale-New Haven Hosp 1990; **Fac Appt:** Prof ObG, NYU Sch Med

Grunfeld, Lawrence MD [RE] - **Spec Exp:** Infertility-IVF; Hysteroscopic Surgery; Laparoscopic Surgery; **Hospital:** Mount Sinai Med Ctr (page 63), Lenox Hill Hosp; **Address:** 635 Madison Ave Fl 10, RMA of New York, New York, NY 10022-1009; **Phone:** 212-756-5777; **Board Cert:** Obstetrics & Gynecology 2010; Reproductive Endocrinology 2010; **Med School:** Mount Sinai Sch Med 1979; **Resid:** Obstetrics & Gynecology, Montefiore Med Ctr 1984; **Fellow:** Reproductive Endocrinology, Montefiore Med Ctr 1987; **Fac Appt:** Assoc Clin Prof ObG, Mount Sinai Sch Med

Legro, Richard S MD [RE] - **Spec Exp:** Polycystic Ovarian Syndrome; Menstrual Disorders; Ovarian Failure; Infertility-IVF; **Hospital:** Penn State Milton S Hershey Med Ctr; **Address:** Hershey Med Ctr, 500 University Drive, PO Box 850, MC H103, Hershey, PA 17033; **Phone:** 717-531-8478; **Board Cert:** Obstetrics & Gynecology 2010; Reproductive Endocrinology 2010; **Med School:** Mount Sinai Sch Med 1987; **Resid:** Obstetrics & Gynecology, Magee Womens Hosp 1991; **Fellow:** Reproductive Endocrinology, USC Women's Hosp 1993; **Fac Appt:** Prof ObG

Licciardi, Frederick L MD [RE] - **Spec Exp:** Infertility-IVF; Infertility; Fertility Preservation in Cancer; **Hospital:** NYU Langone Med Ctr (page 66); **Address:** NYU Medical Ctr, 660 First Ave, 5th Fl, New York, NY 10016; **Phone:** 212-263-7754; **Board Cert:** Obstetrics & Gynecology 2007; Reproductive Endocrinology 2007; **Med School:** UMDNJ-Rutgers Med Sch 1986; **Resid:** Obstetrics & Gynecology, St Barnabas Med Ctr 1990; **Fellow:** Reproductive Endocrinology, NY Hosp-Cornell Med Ctr 1992; **Fac Appt:** Assoc Prof ObG, NYU Sch Med

McClamrock, Howard D MD [RE] - **Spec Exp:** Infertility-IVF; Prenatal Genetic Diagnosis; **Hospital:** Univ of MD Med Ctr, St. Joseph Med Ctr; **Address:** Univ Maryland Professional Bldg, 419 W Redwood St, Ste 500, Baltimore, MD 21201; **Phone:** 410-328-2304; **Board Cert:** Obstetrics & Gynecology 2009; Reproductive Endocrinology 2009; **Med School:** Univ NC Sch Med 1981; **Resid:** Obstetrics & Gynecology, Univ Maryland Affil Hosp 1986; **Fellow:** Reproductive Endocrinology, Univ Maryland 1988; **Fac Appt:** Assoc Prof ObG, Univ MD Sch Med

McGovern, Peter G MD [RE] - **Spec Exp:** Infertility-IVF; Fertility Preservation in Cancer; **Hospital:** Univ Hosp-UMDNJ—Newark, Hackensack Univ Med Ctr; **Address:** Univ Reproductive Assocs, 214 Terrace Ave, Hasbrouck Heights, NJ 07604; **Phone:** 201-288-6330; **Board Cert:** Obstetrics & Gynecology 2008; Reproductive Endocrinology/Infertility 2008; **Med School:** NYU Sch Med 1986; **Resid:** Obstetrics & Gynecology, NYU-Bellevue Hosp Ctr 1990; **Fellow:** Reproductive Endocrinology, UMDNJ-Newark 1992; **Fac Appt:** Assoc Prof ObG, UMDNJ-NJ Med Sch, Newark

Mukherjee, Tanmoy MD [RE] - **Spec Exp:** Infertility-IVF; Endometriosis; Uterine Fibroids; **Hospital:** Mount Sinai Med Ctr (page 63); **Address:** 635 Madison Ave Fl 10, RMA of New York, New York, NY 10022; **Phone:** 212-756-5777; **Board Cert:** Obstetrics & Gynecology 2010; Reproductive Endocrinology 2010; **Med School:** Albert Einstein Coll Med 1990; **Resid:** Obstetrics & Gynecology, Montefiore Med Ctr 1994; **Fellow:** Reproductive Endocrinology, Mt Sinai Hosp 1996

Noyes, Nicole MD [RE] - **Spec Exp:** Infertility-IVF; Fertility Preservation in Cancer; Reproductive Surgery; **Hospital:** NYU Langone Med Ctr (page 66); **Address:** NYU Med Ctr, 660 First Ave, 5th FL, New York, NY 10016; **Phone:** 212-263-7981; **Board Cert:** Obstetrics & Gynecology 2007; Reproductive Endocrinology 2007; **Med School:** Univ VT Coll Med 1986; **Resid:** Obstetrics & Gynecology, NY Hosp-Cornell Med Ctr 1990; **Fellow:** Reproductive Endocrinology, NY Hosp-Cornell Med Ctr 1992; **Fac Appt:** Assoc Prof ObG, NYU Sch Med

Rosenwaks, Zev MD [RE] - **Spec Exp:** Infertility-IVF; Genetic Disorders; Fertility Preservation in Cancer; **Hospital:** NY-Presby/Weill Cornell Med Ctr, NY (page 65); **Address:** Ctr For Reproductive Medicine & Infertility, 1305 York Ave Fl 6, New York, NY 10021-4872; **Phone:** 646-962-3743; **Board Cert:** Obstetrics & Gynecology 1978; Reproductive Endocrinology 1981; **Med School:** SUNY Downstate 1972; **Resid:** Obstetrics & Gynecology, LI Jewish Med Ctr 1976; **Fellow:** Reproductive Endocrinology, Johns Hopkins Hosp 1978; **Fac Appt:** Prof ObG, Cornell Univ-Weill Med Coll

Sanfilippo, Joseph S MD [RE] - **Spec Exp:** Adolescent Gynecology; Pediatric Gynecology; Minimally Invasive Surgery; Infertility; **Hospital:** Magee-Womens Hosp - UPMC, Chldns Hosp of Pittsburgh - UPMC; **Address:** Ctr for Fertility & Repro Endocrinology, Magee-Women's Hosp, 300 Halket St, rm 2309, Pittsburgh, PA 15213; **Phone:** 412-641-1204; **Board Cert:** Obstetrics & Gynecology 2007; Reproductive Endocrinology 2007; **Med School:** Univ Hlth Scis, Chicago Med Sch 1973; **Resid:** Obstetrics & Gynecology, SUNY Upstate Med Ctr 1977; **Fellow:** Reproductive Endocrinology, Univ Louisville 1979; **Fac Appt:** Prof ObG, Univ Pittsburgh

Sauer, Mark MD [RE] - **Spec Exp:** Infertility-IVF; **Hospital:** NY-Presby/Columbia Univ Med Ctr, NY (page 65); **Address:** 1790 Broadway Fl 2, New York, NY 10019; **Phone:** 646-756-8282; **Board Cert:** Obstetrics & Gynecology 2010; Reproductive Endocrinology 2010; **Med School:** Univ IL Coll Med 1980; **Resid:** Obstetrics & Gynecology, Univ Illinois Med Ctr 1984; **Fellow:** Reproductive Endocrinology, Harbor-UCLA Med Ctr 1986; **Fac Appt:** Prof ObG, Columbia P&S

Reproductive Endocrinology

Seifer, David B MD [RE] - **Spec Exp:** Infertility-IVF; Infertility-Advanced Maternal Age; Fertility Preservation in Cancer; **Hospital:** Maimonides Med Ctr (page 62), Richmond Univ Med Ctr; **Address:** 1355 84th St, Brooklyn, NY 11228; **Phone:** 718-283-8600; **Board Cert:** Obstetrics & Gynecology 2010; Reproductive Endocrinology/Infertility 2010; **Med School:** Univ IL Coll Med 1981; **Resid:** Obstetrics & Gynecology, Stanford Univ Hosp 1985; **Fellow:** Reproductive Endocrinology, Yale-New Haven Hosp 1991; **Fac Appt:** Prof ObG, Mount Sinai Sch Med

Sondheimer, Steven MD [RE] - **Spec Exp:** Infertility-Female; **Hospital:** Hosp Univ Penn - UPHS (page 68); **Address:** Penn Fertility Care, 3701 Market St Fl 8, Philadelphia, PA 19104; **Phone:** 215-662-6100; **Board Cert:** Obstetrics & Gynecology 2005; Reproductive Endocrinology 2005; **Med School:** Univ Pennsylvania 1974; **Resid:** Obstetrics & Gynecology, Hosp Univ Penn 1978; **Fellow:** Endocrinology, Hosp Univ Penn 1980; **Fac Appt:** Prof ObG, Univ Pennsylvania

Stangel, John MD [RE] - **Spec Exp:** Infertility-IVF; Endometriosis; Miscarriage-Recurrent; **Hospital:** Northern Westchester Hosp, Phelps Meml Hosp Ctr; **Address:** 70 Maple Ave, Rye, NY 10580-1568; **Phone:** 914-967-6800; **Board Cert:** Obstetrics & Gynecology 1976; Reproductive Endocrinology 1981; **Med School:** NY Med Coll 1969; **Resid:** Obstetrics & Gynecology, Mount Sinai Med Ctr 1974; **Fellow:** Reproductive Endocrinology, Metropolitan Hosp Ctr 1976

Wallach, Edward E MD [RE] - **Spec Exp:** Uterine Fibroids; Infertility-IVF; **Hospital:** Johns Hopkins Hosp (page 61), Johns Hopkins Bayview Med Ctr (page 61); **Address:** Johns Hopkins at Greenspring Station, 2330 W Joppa Rd, Ste 301, Lutherville, MD 21093; **Phone:** 410-583-2751; **Board Cert:** Obstetrics & Gynecology 1979; Reproductive Endocrinology 1975; **Med School:** Cornell Univ-Weill Med Coll 1958; **Resid:** Obstetrics & Gynecology, Kings Co Hosp 1963; **Fellow:** Reproductive Endocrinology, Worcester Fdn Exper Biol 1962; **Fac Appt:** Prof ObG, Johns Hopkins Univ

Weiss, Gerson MD [RE] - **Spec Exp:** Infertility; Menopause Problems; **Hospital:** Hackensack Univ Med Ctr, Univ Hosp-UMDNJ—Newark; **Address:** 214 Terrace Ave, Hasbrouck Heights, NJ 07604-1815; **Phone:** 201-288-6330; **Board Cert:** Obstetrics & Gynecology 1993; Reproductive Endocrinology 1974; **Med School:** NYU Sch Med 1964; **Resid:** Obstetrics & Gynecology, Bellevue Hosp Ctr 1969; **Fellow:** Reproductive Endocrinology, Univ Pittsburgh 1973; **Fac Appt:** Prof ObG, UMDNJ-NJ Med Sch, Newark

Widra, Eric A MD [RE] - **Spec Exp:** Infertility-IVF; **Hospital:** Georgetown Univ Hosp; **Address:** Shady Grove Fertility, 2021 K St NW, Ste 701, Washington, DC 20006; **Phone:** 202-296-2595; **Board Cert:** Obstetrics & Gynecology 2009; Reproductive Endocrinology/Infertility 2009; **Med School:** UMDNJ-RW Johnson Med Sch 1990; **Resid:** Obstetrics & Gynecology, Thomas Jefferson Univ Hosp 1994; **Fellow:** Reproductive Endocrinology, George Washington Univ Hosp 1996; **Fac Appt:** Assoc Prof ObG, Georgetown Univ

Zacur, Howard A MD/PhD [RE] - **Spec Exp:** Prolactin Disorders; Uterine Fibroids; Hormonal Disorders; Infertility-IVF; **Hospital:** Johns Hopkins Hosp (page 61); **Address:** Johns Hopkins at Green Spring Station, 10753 Falls Rd, Pavilion 2, Ste 335, Lutherville, MD 21093; **Phone:** 410-616-7140; **Board Cert:** Obstetrics & Gynecology 1994; Reproductive Endocrinology 1984; **Med School:** Univ Miami Sch Med 1973; **Resid:** Obstetrics & Gynecology, Johns Hopkins Hosp 1980; **Fellow:** Reproductive Endocrinology, Johns Hopkins Hosp 1982; **Fac Appt:** Prof ObG, Johns Hopkins Univ

Southeast

Azziz, Ricardo MD [RE] - **Spec Exp:** Infertility-Female; Reproductive Surgery; Polycystic Ovarian Syndrome; **Hospital:** Med Coll of GA Hosp and Clin (MCG Health Inc); **Address:** Med Coll GA, Kelly Admin Bldg, rm 311, 1120 15th St, Augusta, GA 30912; **Phone:** 706-721-2301; **Board Cert:** Obstetrics & Gynecology 2007; Reproductive Endocrinology 2007; **Med School:** Penn State Coll Med 1981; **Resid:** Obstetrics & Gynecology, Georgetown Univ Hosp 1985; **Fellow:** Reproductive Endocrinology, Johns Hopkins Hosp 1987; **Fac Appt:** Prof ObG, UCLA

Bateman, Bruce MD [RE] - **Spec Exp:** Infertility-IVF; **Hospital:** Univ of Virginia Health Sys; **Address:** 595 Martha Jefferson Drive, Ste 390, Charlottesville, VA 22911; **Phone:** 434-654-8520; **Board Cert:** Obstetrics & Gynecology 1977; Reproductive Endocrinology/Infertility 1985; **Med School:** Med Coll GA 1970; **Resid:** Obstetrics & Gynecology, Univ Va Med Ctr 1975; **Fellow:** Reproductive Endocrinology, Univ Va Med Ctr 1975

Blackwell, Richard E MD/PhD [RE] - **Spec Exp:** Infertility-Female; Women's Health; Menopause Problems; **Hospital:** Univ of Ala Hosp at Birmingham; **Address:** Women & Infants Ctr, 1700 6 Ave S, rm 10390, Birmingham, AL 35249; **Phone:** 205-801-8200; **Board Cert:** Obstetrics & Gynecology 1982; Reproductive Endocrinology 1987; **Med School:** Baylor Coll Med 1975; **Resid:** Obstetrics & Gynecology, Univ Alabama Hosp 1979; **Fellow:** Reproductive Endocrinology, Univ Alabama 1981; **Fac Appt:** Prof Emeritus ObG, Univ Alabama

DeVane, Gary W MD [RE] - **Spec Exp:** Infertility-IVF; Miscarriage-Recurrent; Endometriosis; Vaginal/Uterine Abnormalities; **Hospital:** Florida Hosp - Orlando, Winnie Palmer Hosp for Women & Babies; **Address:** 3435 Pinehurst Ave, Orlando, FL 32804-4049; **Phone:** 407-740-0909; **Board Cert:** Obstetrics & Gynecology 1977; Reproductive Endocrinology 1982; **Med School:** Baylor Coll Med 1971; **Resid:** Obstetrics & Gynecology, UCSD Hosp 1975; **Fellow:** Reproductive Endocrinology, Univ Texas SW Hosp 1980; **Fac Appt:** Assoc Clin Prof ObG, Univ Fla Coll Med

Durso, Nancy MD [RE] - **Spec Exp:** Infertility-IVF; Uterine Fibroids; Endometriosis; **Hospital:** Inova Fairfax Hosp; **Address:** 8501 Arlington Blvd, Ste 500, Fairfax, VA 22031; **Phone:** 703-876-6311; **Board Cert:** Obstetrics & Gynecology 2009; Reproductive Endocrinology/Infertility 2009; **Med School:** Univ VA Sch Med 1983; **Resid:** Obstetrics & Gynecology, St Louis/Washington Univ 1987; **Fellow:** Reproductive Endocrinology, Washington Univ Sch Med 1989

Fritz, Marc A MD [RE] - **Spec Exp:** Infertility-IVF; Menopause Problems; **Hospital:** NC Memorial Hosp - UNC; **Address:** Univ NC Sch Med, Dept Ob/Gyn, 4001 Old Clinic Bldg, CB 7570, Chapel Hill, NC 27599-7570; **Phone:** 919-966-5283; **Board Cert:** Obstetrics & Gynecology 1996; Reproductive Endocrinology 1996; **Med School:** Tulane Univ 1977; **Resid:** Obstetrics & Gynecology, Wright-Patterson USAF Med Ctr 1981; **Fellow:** Reproductive Endocrinology, Oregon Hlth Sci Univ 1983; **Fac Appt:** Prof ObG, Univ NC Sch Med

Kutteh, William H MD/PhD [RE] - **Spec Exp:** Miscarriage-Recurrent; Infertility; **Hospital:** Baptist Memorial Hospital-Memphis, Methodist LeBonheur Germantown Hosp; **Address:** 80 Humphrey's Ctr, Ste 307, Memphis, TN 38120-2363; **Phone:** 901-747-2229; **Board Cert:** Obstetrics & Gynecology 2008; Reproductive Endocrinology/Infertility 2008; **Med School:** Wake Forest Univ 1985; **Resid:** Obstetrics & Gynecology, UAB Med Ctr 1989; **Fellow:** Reproductive Endocrinology, Univ Tennessee Affil Hosp 1991; **Fac Appt:** Prof Med, Univ Tenn Coll Med

Murphy, Ana A MD [RE] - **Spec Exp:** Infertility; Endometriosis; Pelvic Surgery; **Hospital:** Med Coll of GA Hosp and Clin (MCG Health Inc); **Address:** Med Coll Ga-Dept Ob/Gyn, 1447 Harper St, Med Office Bldg Fl 5, Agusta, GA 30912; **Phone:** 706-722-4434; **Board Cert:** Obstetrics & Gynecology 2010; Reproductive Endocrinology 2009; **Med School:** Univ Mich Med Sch 1980; **Resid:** Obstetrics & Gynecology, Johns Hopkins Univ 1984; **Fellow:** Reproductive Endocrinology, Johns Hopkins Univ 1986; **Fac Appt:** Prof ObG, Med Coll GA

Reproductive Endocrinology

Ory, Steven J MD [RE] - **Spec Exp:** Infertility-IVF; Hormonal Disorders; Endometriosis; Uterine Fibroids; **Hospital:** Northwest Med Ctr, Meml Regl Hosp; **Address:** 2960 N State Road 7, Ste 300, Margate, FL 33063-5737; **Phone:** 954-247-6200; **Board Cert:** Obstetrics & Gynecology 2009; Reproductive Endocrinology 2008; **Med School:** Baylor Coll Med 1976; **Resid:** Obstetrics & Gynecology, Mayo Clinic 1980; **Fellow:** Reproductive Endocrinology, Duke Univ 1982; **Fac Appt:** Prof ObG, FIU Coll Med

Session, Donna R MD [RE] - **Spec Exp:** Infertility-IVF; Reproductive Surgery; Polycystic Ovarian Syndrome; Ultrasound; **Hospital:** Emory Univ Hosp, Emory Univ Hosp Midtown; **Address:** Emory Reproductive Center, 550 Peachtree St NE, 18th Fl MOT, Atlanta, GA 30308; **Phone:** 404-778-3401; **Board Cert:** Obstetrics & Gynecology 2004; Reproductive Endocrinology 2004; **Med School:** Eastern VA Med Sch 1986; **Resid:** Obstetrics & Gynecology, Winthrop Hosp 1990; **Fellow:** Reproductive Endocrinology, Columbia-Presby Med Ctr 1993; **Fac Appt:** Assoc Prof ObG, Emory Univ

Steinkampf, Michael P MD [RE] - **Spec Exp:** Infertility-IVF; **Hospital:** Brookwood Med Ctr, St. Vincent's Hosp - Birmingham; **Address:** Alabama Fertility Specialists, 2700 Highway 280 South, Ste 370 East, Birmingham, AL 35223; **Phone:** 205-874-0000; **Board Cert:** Obstetrics & Gynecology 2010; Reproductive Endocrinology 2010; **Med School:** Louisiana State U, New Orleans 1981; **Resid:** Obstetrics & Gynecology, Parkland Meml Hosp 1985; **Fellow:** Reproductive Endocrinology, Univ Texas SW Med Ctr 1987; **Fac Appt:** Prof ObG, Univ Alabama

Walmer, David K MD/PhD [RE] - **Spec Exp:** Infertility-IVF; Miscarriage-Recurrent; Polycystic Ovarian Syndrome; Asherman's Syndrome; **Hospital:** Duke Univ Hosp; **Address:** Duke Fertility Center, 5704 Fayetteville Rd, Durham, NC 27713; **Phone:** 919-572-4673; **Board Cert:** Obstetrics & Gynecology 2009; Reproductive Endocrinology 2009; **Med School:** Univ NC Sch Med 1983; **Resid:** Obstetrics & Gynecology, Univ Texas Affil Hosp 1987; **Fellow:** Reproductive Endocrinology, Duke Univ 1989; **Fac Appt:** Assoc Prof ObG, Duke Univ

Midwest

Barnes, Randall B MD [RE] - **Spec Exp:** Infertility-IVF; Polycystic Ovarian Syndrome; Miscarriage-Recurrent; **Hospital:** Northwestern Meml Hosp; **Address:** 675 N St Clair St Fl 14 - Ste 200, Chicago, IL 60611; **Phone:** 312-695-7269; **Board Cert:** Obstetrics & Gynecology 2009; Reproductive Endocrinology 2009; **Med School:** Johns Hopkins Univ 1979; **Resid:** Obstetrics & Gynecology, LAC-USC Med Ctr 1983; **Fellow:** Reproductive Endocrinology, LAC-USC Med Ctr 1985; **Fac Appt:** Assoc Prof ObG, Northwestern Univ

Christman, Gregory MD [RE] - **Spec Exp:** Infertility-IVF; Uterine Fibroids; Endometriosis; Microsurgery; **Hospital:** Univ of Michigan Hosp; **Address:** Ctr for Reproductive Med, 475 Market Pl, Ste B, Ann Arbor, MI 48108; **Phone:** 734-763-4323; **Board Cert:** Obstetrics & Gynecology 2002; Reproductive Endocrinology 2002; **Med School:** Univ Wisc 1983; **Resid:** Obstetrics & Gynecology, Univ Wisconsin Hosps 1987; **Fellow:** Reproductive Endocrinology, Univ North Carolina 1992; **Fac Appt:** Assoc Prof ObG, Univ Mich Med Sch

Coddington III, Charles C MD [RE] - **Spec Exp:** Reproductive Surgery; Endometriosis; Infertility-IVF; **Hospital:** Mayo Med Ctr & Clin - Rochester; **Address:** Mayo Clinic, Dept Reproductive Med, 200 First St SW, Rochester, MN 55905; **Phone:** 507-284-9792; **Board Cert:** Obstetrics & Gynecology 2006; Reproductive Endocrinology 2006; **Med School:** Med Univ SC 1977; **Resid:** Obstetrics & Gynecology, Natl Naval Med Ctr 1981; **Fellow:** Reproductive Endocrinology, Natl Inst Hlth 1985; **Fac Appt:** Prof ObG, Mayo Med Sch

Diamond, Michael P MD [RE] - **Spec Exp:** Infertility-IVF; Endometriosis; Polycystic Ovarian Syndrome; Hysteroscopic Surgery; **Hospital:** Hutzel Hosp - Detroit, Harper Univ Hosp; **Address:** Univ Physicians, 26400 W 12 Mile Rd, Southfield, MI 48034; **Phone:** 248-352-8200; **Board Cert:** Obstetrics & Gynecology 2009; Reproductive Endocrinology 2009; **Med School:** Vanderbilt Univ 1981; **Resid:** Obstetrics & Gynecology, Vanderbilt Univ Med Ctr 1985; **Fellow:** Reproductive Endocrinology, Yale-New Haven Hosp 1987; **Fac Appt:** Prof ObG, Wayne State Univ

Dodds, William G MD [RE] - **Spec Exp:** Infertility; Endometriosis; **Hospital:** Spectrum Hlth Butterworth Campus, Bronson Meth Hosp; **Address:** The Fertility Center, 3230 Eagle Park Drive NE, Grand Rapids, MI 49525; **Phone:** 616-988-2229; **Board Cert:** Obstetrics & Gynecology 2009; Reproductive Endocrinology 2009; **Med School:** Ohio State Univ 1982; **Resid:** Obstetrics & Gynecology, Ohio State Univ Med Ctr 1986; **Fellow:** Reproductive Endocrinology, Ohio State Univ 1988; **Fac Appt:** Assoc Prof ObG, Univ Mich Med Sch

Falcone, Tommaso MD [RE] - **Spec Exp:** Minimally Invasive Surgery; Infertility-IVF; Endometriosis; Hysteroscopic Surgery; **Hospital:** Cleveland Clin (page 56); **Address:** Cleveland Clinic, Dept Ob/Gyn, 9500 Euclid Ave, MC A81, Cleveland, OH 44195-0001; **Phone:** 216-444-1758; **Board Cert:** Obstetrics & Gynecology 2009; Reproductive Endocrinology 2009; **Med School:** McGill Univ 1981; **Resid:** Obstetrics & Gynecology, McGill Univ Hlth Ctr 1986; **Fellow:** Reproductive Endocrinology, McGill Univ 1989; **Fac Appt:** Prof ObG, Cleveland Cl Coll Med/Case West Res

Friedman, Chad MD [RE] - **Spec Exp:** Infertility-IVF; Polycystic Ovarian Syndrome; **Hospital:** Ohio St Univ Med Ctr; **Address:** 4830 Knightsbridge Blvd, Ste E, Columbus, OH 43214; **Phone:** 614-451-2280; **Board Cert:** Obstetrics & Gynecology 1982; Reproductive Endocrinology/Infertility 1983; **Med School:** Univ Chicago-Pritzker Sch Med 1975; **Resid:** Obstetrics & Gynecology, Ohio State Univ Hosp 1979; **Fellow:** Reproductive Endocrinology, Ohio State Univ Hosp 1981; **Fac Appt:** Assoc Prof ObG, Ohio State Univ

Goldberg, Jeffrey M MD [RE] - **Spec Exp:** Infertility-IVF; Endoscopic Surgery; Microsurgery; **Hospital:** Cleveland Clin (page 56); **Address:** Beachwood Family Health Ctr, 26900 Cedar Rd, MC BD20, Beechwood, OH 44122; **Phone:** 216-839-3150; **Board Cert:** Obstetrics & Gynecology 2009; Reproductive Endocrinology 2009; **Med School:** UMDNJ-NJ Med Sch, Newark 1983; **Resid:** Obstetrics & Gynecology, Emory Univ Med Ctr 1987; **Fellow:** Reproductive Endocrinology, Ohio State Univ 1989; **Fac Appt:** Prof ObG, Cleveland Cl Coll Med/Case West Res

Haney, Arthur F MD [RE] - **Spec Exp:** Infertility-Female; DES-Exposed Females; Minimally Invasive Gynecologic Surgery; **Hospital:** Univ of Chicago Med Ctr; **Address:** 5841 S Maryland Ave, MC 2050, Chicago, IL 60637; **Phone:** 773-702-6127; **Board Cert:** Obstetrics & Gynecology 2010; Reproductive Endocrinology 2010; **Med School:** Univ Ariz Coll Med 1972; **Resid:** Obstetrics & Gynecology, Duke Univ Med Ctr 1976; **Fellow:** Reproductive Endocrinology, Duke Univ Med Ctr 1978; **Fac Appt:** Prof ObG, Univ Chicago-Pritzker Sch Med

Jacobs, Laurence A MD [RE] - **Spec Exp:** Infertility-IVF; Polycystic Ovarian Syndrome; Endometriosis; **Hospital:** Adv Luth Genl Hosp, Northwest Comm Hosp; **Address:** 135 N Arlington Hts Rd, Ste 195, Buffalo Grove, IL 60089; **Phone:** 847-215-8899; **Board Cert:** Obstetrics & Gynecology 1981; **Med School:** Northwestern Univ 1975; **Resid:** Obstetrics & Gynecology, Northwestern Meml Hosp 1979; **Fellow:** Reproductive Endocrinology, Mayo Clinic 1988; **Fac Appt:** Assoc Prof ObG, Northwestern Univ

Kazer, Ralph R MD [RE] - **Spec Exp:** Polycystic Ovarian Syndrome; Infertility-IVF; **Hospital:** Northwestern Meml Hosp; **Address:** Northwestern Meml Hosp, 675 N St Clair St Fl 14 - Ste 200, Galter Pavillion, Chicago, IL 60611; **Phone:** 312-695-7269; **Board Cert:** Obstetrics & Gynecology 2010; Reproductive Endocrinology 2010; **Med School:** Tufts Univ 1979; **Resid:** Obstetrics & Gynecology, Tufts Univ Med Ctr 1983; **Fellow:** Reproductive Endocrinology, UC San Diego Med Ctr 1986; **Fac Appt:** Prof ObG, Northwestern Univ

Reproductive Endocrinology

Milad, Magdy P MD [RE] - **Spec Exp:** Reproductive Surgery; Infertility; Uterine Fibroids; **Hospital:** Northwestern Meml Hosp, Children's Mem Hosp -Chicago; **Address:** Northwestern Med Fac Fdn, 675 N St Clair St, Galter Pavilion Fl 14 - Ste 200, Chicago, IL 60611-5975; **Phone:** 312-695-7269; **Board Cert:** Obstetrics & Gynecology 2010; Reproductive Endocrinology 2010; **Med School:** Wayne State Univ 1987; **Resid:** Obstetrics & Gynecology, William Beaumont Hosp 1991; **Fellow:** Reproductive Endocrinology, Mayo Clinic 1993; **Fac Appt:** Prof ObG, Northwestern Univ

Miller, Charles E MD [RE] - **Spec Exp:** Infertility-IVF; Minimally Invasive Surgery; Endometriosis; Uterine Fibroids; **Hospital:** Edward Hosp, Adv Luth Genl Hosp; **Address:** 120 Osler Drive, Ste 100, Naperville, IL 60540; **Phone:** 630-428-2229; **Board Cert:** Obstetrics & Gynecology 1984; **Med School:** Northwestern Univ 1977; **Resid:** Obstetrics & Gynecology, Univ Texas SW Med Ctr 1980; **Fellow:** Reproductive Endocrinology, Hosp Univ Penn 1983; **Fac Appt:** Assoc Clin Prof ObG, Univ Chicago-Pritzker Sch Med

Molo, Mary W MD [RE] - **Spec Exp:** Infertility-IVF; Uterine Fibroids; Fertility Preservation in Cancer; **Hospital:** Rush Univ Med Ctr; **Address:** 1725 W Harrison St, Ste 408 East, Chicago, IL 60612; **Phone:** 312-997-2229; **Board Cert:** Obstetrics & Gynecology 2010; Reproductive Endocrinology 2010; **Med School:** Southern IL Univ 1982; **Resid:** Obstetrics & Gynecology, Southern Illinois Affil Hosps 1984; Obstetrics & Gynecology, Rush Presby St Lukes Hosp 1987; **Fellow:** Reproductive Endocrinology, Rush Presby St Lukes Hosp 1989; **Fac Appt:** Asst Prof ObG, Rush Med Coll

Nagel, Theodore C MD [RE] - **Spec Exp:** Infertility-IVF; Hysteroscopic Surgery; Vaginal/Uterine Abnormalities; Laparoscopic Surgery; **Hospital:** Univ Minn Med Ctr, Fairview - Riverside Campus; **Address:** Reproductive Med Ctr, Univ Minnesota, 606 24th Ave S, Ste 500, Minnneapolis, MN 55454; **Phone:** 612-372-7050; **Board Cert:** Internal Medicine 1970; Endocrinology 1975; Obstetrics & Gynecology 1981; Reproductive Endocrinology 1983; **Med School:** Cornell Univ-Weill Med Coll 1963; **Resid:** Internal Medicine, Bellevue Hosp Ctr 1968; Obstetrics & Gynecology, Univ Minn Hosps 1977; **Fellow:** Endocrinology, Diabetes & Metabolism, Northwestern Univ Med Sch 1972; Reproductive Endocrinology, Univ Minnesota 1980; **Fac Appt:** Assoc Clin Prof ObG, Univ Minn

Odem, Randall R MD [RE] - **Spec Exp:** Infertility; Reproductive Surgery; Miscarriage-Recurrent; Asherman's Syndrome; **Hospital:** Barnes-Jewish Hosp; **Address:** Reproductive Medicine Ctr, 4444 Forest Park Ave, Ste 3100, St Louis, MO 63108-2212; **Phone:** 314-286-2400; **Board Cert:** Obstetrics & Gynecology 2009; Reproductive Endocrinology 2009; **Med School:** Univ Iowa Coll Med 1981; **Resid:** Obstetrics & Gynecology, Univ Illinois Hosps 1985; **Fellow:** Reproductive Endocrinology, Wash Univ 1987; **Fac Appt:** Prof ObG, Washington Univ, St Louis

Ratts, Valerie S MD [RE] - **Spec Exp:** Infertility-IVF; Miscarriage-Recurrent; Uterine Fibroids; Polycystic Ovarian Syndrome; **Hospital:** Barnes-Jewish Hosp; **Address:** Reproductive Medicine Ctr, 4444 Forest Park Ave, Ste 3100, St Louis, MO 63108; **Phone:** 314-286-2400; **Board Cert:** Obstetrics & Gynecology 2009; Reproductive Endocrinology 2009; **Med School:** Johns Hopkins Univ 1987; **Resid:** Obstetrics & Gynecology, Johns Hopkins Hosp 1991; **Fellow:** Reproductive Endocrinology, Johns Hopkins Hosp 1993; **Fac Appt:** Assoc Prof ObG, Washington Univ, St Louis

Smith, Yolanda R MD [RE] - **Spec Exp:** Infertility-IVF; Pediatric & Adolescent Gynecology; Polycystic Ovarian Syndrome; Menopause Problems; **Hospital:** Univ of Michigan Hosp; **Address:** Ctr for Reproductive Medicine, 475 Market Pl, Ste B, Ann Arbor, MI 48108; **Phone:** 734-763-4323; **Board Cert:** Obstetrics & Gynecology 2009; Reproductive Endocrinology 2009; **Med School:** Wake Forest Univ 1989; **Resid:** Obstetrics & Gynecology, Univ Mich Hosp 1993; **Fellow:** Reproductive Endocrinology, Johns Hopkins Univ 1995; **Fac Appt:** Assoc Prof ObG, Univ Mich Med Sch

Stewart, Elizabeth A MD [RE] - **Spec Exp:** Uterine Fibroids; Hysteroscopic Surgery; Infertility-IVF; **Hospital:** Mayo Med Ctr & Clin - Rochester; **Address:** Mayo Clinic, Dept Reproductive Med, 200 First St SW, Rochester, MN 55905; **Phone:** 507-284-9792; **Board Cert:** Obstetrics & Gynecology 2009; Reproductive Endocrinology 2009; **Med School:** Harvard Med Sch 1985; **Resid:** Obstetrics & Gynecology, Brigham & Womens Hosp 1989; **Fellow:** Reproductive Endocrinology, Brigham & Womens Hosp 1992; **Fac Appt:** Prof ObG, Mayo Med Sch

Van Voorhis, Bradley MD [RE] - **Spec Exp:** Infertility; Endometriosis; Uterine Fibroids; **Hospital:** Univ Iowa Hosp & Clinics; **Address:** Univ Iowa Hosps & Clinics, 200 Hawkins Drive, Dept Reproductive Endocrinology, Iowa City, IA 52242; **Phone:** 319-356-1767; **Board Cert:** Obstetrics & Gynecology 2010; Reproductive Endocrinology 2010; **Med School:** Univ Iowa Coll Med 1984; **Resid:** Obstetrics & Gynecology, Med Coll Va 1988; **Fellow:** Reproductive Endocrinology, Brigham & Women's Hosp 1991; **Fac Appt:** Prof ObG, Univ Iowa Coll Med

Great Plains and Mountains

Richardson, Marilyn MD [RE] - **Spec Exp:** Menopause Problems; Infertility; Polycystic Ovarian Syndrome; **Hospital:** Univ of Kansas Hosp; **Address:** 12616 W 62nd Terr, Ste 112, Shawnee, KS 66216; **Phone:** 913-631-0277; **Board Cert:** Obstetrics & Gynecology 2010; **Med School:** Univ Kansas 1979; **Resid:** Obstetrics & Gynecology, Truman Med Ctr 1983; **Fellow:** Reproductive Endocrinology, Univ Texas Hlth Scis Ctr 1985; **Fac Appt:** Asst Clin Prof ObG, Univ Kansas

Schlaff, William D MD [RE] - **Spec Exp:** Infertility; Endometriosis; Vaginal/Uterine Abnormalities; **Hospital:** Univ of CO Hosp - Anschutz Inpatient Pav; **Address:** Dept of OB & Gyn, 1635 Aurora Ct, MS F701, Aurora, CO 80045; **Phone:** 719-314-3333; **Board Cert:** Obstetrics & Gynecology 2010; Reproductive Endocrinology 2010; **Med School:** Univ Mich Med Sch 1977; **Resid:** Obstetrics & Gynecology, Univ Mich Hosps 1981; **Fellow:** Reproductive Endocrinology, Johns Hopkins Med Ctr 1985; **Fac Appt:** Prof ObG, Univ Colorado

Surrey, Eric S MD [RE] - **Spec Exp:** Infertility-IVF; Endometriosis; **Hospital:** Sky Ridge Med Ctr, Swedish Med Ctr - Englewood; **Address:** 10290 RidgeGate Circle, Lone Tree, CO 80124; **Phone:** 303-788-8300; **Board Cert:** Obstetrics & Gynecology 2010; Reproductive Endocrinology 2010; **Med School:** Univ Pennsylvania 1981; **Resid:** Obstetrics & Gynecology, UCLA Med Ctr 1986; **Fellow:** Reproductive Endocrinology, UCLA Med Ctr 1988

Southwest

Carr, Bruce R MD [RE] - **Spec Exp:** Infertility-Female; **Hospital:** UT Southwestern Med Ctr at Dallas, Parkland Hlth & Hosp Sys; **Address:** 1801 Inwood Rd, rm WA6.616, Dallas, TX 75390; **Phone:** 214-645-3858; **Board Cert:** Obstetrics & Gynecology 2000; Reproductive Endocrinology 2000; **Med School:** Univ Mich Med Sch 1971; **Resid:** Obstetrics & Gynecology, Parkland Meml Hosp 1975; **Fellow:** Reproductive Endocrinology, Univ Texas SW Med Ctr 1980; **Fac Appt:** Prof ObG, Univ Tex SW, Dallas

Clisham, P Ronald MD [RE] - **Spec Exp:** Infertility-IVF; Endometriosis; Uterine Fibroids; Laparoscopic Surgery; **Hospital:** Tulane Med Ctr; **Address:** Audobon Fertility & Reproductive Med, 4321 Magnolia St, New Orleans, LA 70115; **Phone:** 504-891-1390; **Board Cert:** Obstetrics & Gynecology 2010; Reproductive Endocrinology 2010; **Med School:** Louisiana State U, New Orleans 1982; **Resid:** Obstetrics & Gynecology, Charity Hosp 1986; **Fellow:** Reproductive Endocrinology, UCLA Med Ctr 1988; **Fac Appt:** Prof ObG, Tulane Univ

Reproductive Endocrinology

Dickey, Richard P MD/PhD [RE] - **Spec Exp:** Infertility-IVF; **Hospital:** Tulane-Lakeside Hosp; **Address:** The Fertility Inst, 800 N Causeway Blvd, Ste 2C, Mandeville, LA 70448; **Phone:** 985-892-7621; **Board Cert:** Obstetrics & Gynecology 1967; Reproductive Endocrinology/Infertility 1976; **Med School:** Case West Res Univ 1960; **Resid:** Obstetrics & Gynecology, Ohio State Univ Hosp 1965; **Fellow:** Reproductive Endocrinology, Ohio State Univ Hosp 1966; **Fac Appt:** Clin Prof ObG, Louisiana State U, New Orleans

Huang, Jaou-Chen MD [RE] - **Spec Exp:** Infertility-IVF; Endometriosis; Hysteroscopic Surgery; Uterine Fibroids; **Hospital:** Meml Hermann Hosp - Texas Med Ctr; **Address:** UT Physicians Womens Center, 6410 Fannin St, Ste 250, Houston, TX 77030; **Phone:** 832-325-7131; **Board Cert:** Obstetrics & Gynecology 2010; Reproductive Endocrinology/Infertility 2010; **Med School:** Taiwan 1980; **Resid:** Obstetrics & Gynecology, Natl Taiwan Univ Hosp 1985; Obstetrics & Gynecology, Harlem Hosp 1992; **Fellow:** Reproductive Endocrinology, Brigham & Women's Hosp 1993

Moffitt, Drew MD [RE] - **Spec Exp:** Infertility-IVF; Reproductive Surgery; **Hospital:** Banner Good Samaritan Regl Med Ctr - Phoenix; **Address:** Arizona Reproductive Medicine, 1701 E Thomas Rd, Ste 101, Phoenix, AZ 85016; **Phone:** 602-343-2767; **Board Cert:** Obstetrics & Gynecology 2010; Reproductive Endocrinology/Infertility 2010; **Med School:** UCLA 1988; **Resid:** Obstetrics & Gynecology, UCLA Med Ctr 1992; **Fellow:** Reproductive Endocrinology, Jones Inst/Eastern Va Med Sch 1994; **Fac Appt:** Assoc Prof ObG, Univ Ariz Coll Med

Putman, John M MD [RE] - **Spec Exp:** Infertility-IVF; Uterine Fibroids; Endometriosis; Minimally Invasive Surgery; **Hospital:** Baylor Univ Medical Ctr-Dallas; **Address:** Fertility Center of Dallas, 3900 Junius St, Ste 610, Dallas, TX 75246; **Phone:** 214-823-2692; **Board Cert:** Obstetrics & Gynecology 1980; **Med School:** Med Coll GA 1979; **Resid:** Obstetrics & Gynecology, Baylor Univ Med Ctr 1977; **Fac Appt:** Assoc Clin Prof ObG, Univ Tex SW, Dallas

Schenken, Robert S MD [RE] - **Spec Exp:** Infertility-Female; Endometriosis; **Hospital:** Univ Hlth Syst-San Antonio, Baptist Hlth Sys; **Address:** Dept OB/GYN, 7703 Floyd Curl Dr, MSC 7836, San Antonio, TX 78229-3900; **Phone:** 210-567-4950; **Board Cert:** Obstetrics & Gynecology 1995; Reproductive Endocrinology 1995; **Med School:** Baylor Coll Med 1977; **Resid:** Obstetrics & Gynecology, Bexar Co Hosp 1981; **Fellow:** Reproductive Endocrinology, Natl Inst Hlth 1982; Reproductive Endocrinology, Univ Tex Hlth Sci Ctr 1983; **Fac Appt:** Prof ObG, Univ Tex, San Antonio

Wilson, Ellen E MD [RE] - **Spec Exp:** Infertility; Uterine Fibroids; Polycystic Ovarian Syndrome; Pediatric & Adolescent Gynecology; **Hospital:** UT Southwestern Med Ctr at Dallas; **Address:** UTSW Fertility & Reproductive Medicine, 5323 Harry Hines Blvd, Dallas, TX 75390-8539; **Phone:** 214-645-3858; **Board Cert:** Obstetrics & Gynecology 2009; Reproductive Endocrinology/Infertility 2009; **Med School:** Baylor Coll Med 1984; **Resid:** Obstetrics & Gynecology, George Washington Univ Hosp 1989; **Fellow:** Reproductive Endocrinology, UTSW Southwestern 1991; Laparoscopic Surgery, Womens Hosp 1992; **Fac Appt:** Assoc Prof ObG, Univ Tex SW, Dallas

West Coast and Pacific

Adamson, G David MD [RE] - **Spec Exp:** Infertility-Female; Endometriosis; Infertility-IVF; Laparoscopic Surgery; **Hospital:** Stanford Univ Hosp & Clinics, Good Samaritan Hosp - San Jose; **Address:** Fertility Phsyicians of N California, 540 University Ave, Ste 200, Palo Alto, CA 94301; **Phone:** 650-322-1900; **Board Cert:** Obstetrics & Gynecology 1980; Reproductive Endocrinology 1982; **Med School:** Univ Toronto 1973; **Resid:** Obstetrics & Gynecology, Toronto Genl Hosp 1977; **Fellow:** Obstetrics & Gynecology, Toronto Genl Hosp 1978; Reproductive Endocrinology, Stanford Univ 1980; **Fac Appt:** Clin Prof ObG, Stanford Univ

Agarwal, Sanjay K MD [RE] - **Spec Exp:** Infertility-IVF; Endometriosis; **Hospital:** UCSD Med Ctr; **Address:** 9500 Gilman Drive, MC 0633, La Jolla, CA 92093-0633; **Phone:** 858-552-9177; **Board Cert:** Obstetrics & Gynecology 2009; Reproductive Endocrinology/Infertility 2009; **Med School:** England, UK 1986; **Resid:** Obstetrics & Gynecology, Duke Univ Med Ctr 1993; **Fellow:** Reproductive Endocrinology, UCLA Med Ctr 1995; **Fac Appt:** Clin Prof ObG, UCSD

Cedars, Marcelle I MD [RE] - **Spec Exp:** Infertility-IVF; Polycystic Ovarian Syndrome; **Hospital:** UCSF Med Ctr; **Address:** UCSF Ctr for Reproductive Hlth, 2356 Sutter St Fl 7, San Francisco, CA 94115; **Phone:** 415-353-7475; **Board Cert:** Obstetrics & Gynecology 2010; Reproductive Endocrinology 2010; **Med School:** Univ Tex SW, Dallas 1981; **Resid:** Obstetrics & Gynecology, Parkland Meml Hosp 1985; **Fellow:** Reproductive Endocrinology, UCLA Med Ctr 1987; **Fac Appt:** Prof ObG, UCSF

Chang, R Jeffrey MD [RE] - **Spec Exp:** Polycystic Ovarian Syndrome; Hormonal Disorders; Menstrual Disorders; Pituitary Tumors; **Hospital:** UCSD Med Ctr; **Address:** UCSD Reproductive Medicine, 9500 Gilman Drive, MC 0633, La Jolla, CA 92093; **Phone:** 858-534-8930; **Board Cert:** Obstetrics & Gynecology 2002; Reproductive Endocrinology/Infertility 2002; **Med School:** Oregon Hlth & Sci Univ 1969; **Resid:** Obstetrics & Gynecology, Harbor Genl Hosp-UCLA 1974; **Fellow:** Reproductive Endocrinology, Harbor Genl Hosp-UCLA 1975; Reproductive Endocrinology, UCSF Med Ctr 1977; **Fac Appt:** Prof ObG, UCSD

Dumesic, Daniel A MD [RE] - **Spec Exp:** Infertility-Female; Hormonal Disorders; Polycystic Ovarian Syndrome; Hysteroscopic Surgery; **Hospital:** UCLA Ronald Reagan Med Ctr; **Address:** 200 UCLA Medical Plaza, Ste 220, Los Angeles, CA 90095; **Phone:** 310-794-7274; **Board Cert:** Obstetrics & Gynecology 2009; Reproductive Endocrinology 2009; **Med School:** Univ Wisc 1978; **Resid:** Obstetrics & Gynecology, UCSF Med Ctr 1982; **Fellow:** Reproductive Endocrinology, UCSF 1987

Giudice, Linda C MD/PhD [RE] - **Spec Exp:** Infertility-IVF; Endometriosis; **Hospital:** UCSF Med Ctr; **Address:** Center for Reproductive Health, 2356 Sutter St Fl 7, San Francisco, CA 94115; **Phone:** 415-353-7475; **Board Cert:** Obstetrics & Gynecology 2009; Reproductive Endocrinology 2009; **Med School:** Stanford Univ 1982; **Resid:** Obstetrics & Gynecology, Stanford Univ Med Ctr 1984; Obstetrics & Gynecology, Barnes Hosp-Wash Univ Med Ctr 1986; **Fellow:** Reproductive Endocrinology, Stanford Univ Med Ctr 1987; **Fac Appt:** Prof ObG, UCSF

Houmard, Brenda MD/PhD [RE] - **Spec Exp:** Infertility; Menstrual Disorders; **Hospital:** Univ Wash Med Ctr; **Address:** University Reproductive Care, 4245 Roosevelt Way NE, Box 354765, Seattle, WA 98105; **Phone:** 206-598-4225; **Board Cert:** Obstetrics & Gynecology 2006; **Med School:** Ohio State Univ 1994; **Resid:** Obstetrics & Gynecology, OSU Med Ctr 1998; **Fellow:** Reproductive Endocrinology, Univ Wash Med Ctr 2001; **Fac Appt:** Asst Prof ObG, Univ Wash

Marrs, Richard P MD [RE] - **Spec Exp:** Infertility-Female; Endometriosis; Uterine Fibroids; **Hospital:** Santa Monica - UCLA Med Ctr & Ortho Hosp; **Address:** 11818 Wilshire Blvd, Ste 300, Los Angeles, CA 90025; **Phone:** 310-828-4008; **Board Cert:** Obstetrics & Gynecology 1980; Reproductive Endocrinology 1983; **Med School:** Univ Tex Med Br, Galveston 1974; **Resid:** Obstetrics & Gynecology, Univ Tex Hosps 1977; **Fellow:** Reproductive Endocrinology, USC Med Ctr 1979

Paulson, Richard J MD [RE] - **Spec Exp:** Infertility-IVF; Infertility-Advanced Maternal Age; **Hospital:** LAC & USC Med Ctr, Good Samaritan Hosp - LA; **Address:** USC Fertility, 1127 Wilshire Blvd, Ste 1400, Los Angeles, CA 90017; **Phone:** 213-975-9990; **Board Cert:** Obstetrics & Gynecology 2010; Reproductive Endocrinology 2010; **Med School:** UCLA 1980; **Resid:** Obstetrics & Gynecology, Harbor-UCLA Med Ctr 1984; **Fellow:** Reproductive Endocrinology, LAC-USC Med Ctr 1986; **Fac Appt:** Prof ObG, USC Sch Med

Reproductive Endocrinology

Smikle, Collin B MD [RE] - **Spec Exp:** Infertility-IVF; Laparoscopic Surgery; Fertility Preservation in Cancer; **Hospital:** CA Pacific Med Ctr-Pacific Campus; **Address:** Laurel Fertility Care, 1700 California St, Ste 570, San Francisco, CA 94109; **Phone:** 415-673-9199; **Board Cert:** Obstetrics & Gynecology 2010; Reproductive Endocrinology/Infertility 2010; **Med School:** Yale Univ 1985; **Resid:** Obstetrics & Gynecology, Brigham & Women's Hosp 1989; **Fellow:** Reproductive Endocrinology, UCSF Med Ctr 1991

Soules, Michael R MD [RE] - **Spec Exp:** Infertility-IVF; Polycystic Ovarian Syndrome; Endometriosis; **Hospital:** Northwest Hosp - Seattle; **Address:** 1505 Westlake Ave N, Ste 400, Seattle, WA 98109; **Phone:** 206-301-5000; **Board Cert:** Obstetrics & Gynecology 2002; Reproductive Endocrinology 2002; **Med School:** UCLA 1972; **Resid:** Obstetrics & Gynecology, Univ Colorado Med Ctr 1976; **Fellow:** Reproductive Endocrinology, Duke Univ Hosp 1978; **Fac Appt:** Prof ObG, Univ Wash

Winer, Sharon A MD [RE] - **Spec Exp:** Hormonal Disorders; Infertility-Female; Vaginitis; Gynecology; **Hospital:** Cedars-Sinai Med Ctr, Keck Med Ctr of USC (page 75); **Address:** 9400 Brighton Way, Ste 206, Beverly Hills, CA 90210-4709; **Phone:** 310-274-9100; **Board Cert:** Obstetrics & Gynecology 2010; Reproductive Endocrinology 2010; **Med School:** USC Sch Med 1978; **Resid:** Obstetrics & Gynecology, LAC-USC Med Ctr 1982; **Fellow:** Microsurgery, Hammersmith Hosp 1983; Reproductive Endocrinology, LAC-USC Med Ctr 1985; **Fac Appt:** Clin Prof ObG, USC Sch Med

Yee, Billy MD [RE] - **Spec Exp:** Infertility-IVF; Microsurgery; Laparoscopic Surgery; Hysteroscopic Surgery; **Hospital:** Long Beach Meml Med Ctr, Torrance Memorial Med Ctr; **Address:** 13950 Milton Ave, Ste 100, Westminster, CA 92683; **Phone:** 714-702-3001; **Board Cert:** Obstetrics & Gynecology 2010; Reproductive Endocrinology 2010; **Med School:** UC Davis 1978; **Resid:** Obstetrics & Gynecology, LAC-USC Med Ctr 1982; **Fellow:** Reproductive Endocrinology, USC 1985; **Fac Appt:** Assoc Clin Prof ObG, UC Irvine

Cleveland Clinic

Every life deserves world class care.

Reproductive Endocrinology

Cleveland Clinic Ob/Gyn & Women's Health Institute. is designed to meet the unique and changing medical needs of women from adolescence to mature adulthood. Our team offers coordinated and supportive care. *U.S.News & World Report* has ranked our gynecology program No. 4 in the country. Our physicians are nationally and internationally known and many serve on leadership boards for professional physician societies.

Reproductive Endocrinology and Infertility Section physicians provide comprehensive evaluation for infertile couples. Treatments encompass all assisted reproductive technologies, including artificial insemination, ovulation induction, intracytoplasmic sperm injection, in vitro fertilization and reproductive surgery, including microsurgery (sterilization reversal) both robotic and conventional and advanced endoscopic techniques for problems such as stage IV endometriosis.

For maximum patient convenience, Cleveland Clinic's Fertility Center has several locations throughout the area. In vitro fertilization retrievals and transfers are performed at the Fertility Center at Beachwood, while initial fertility consultations and testing are available on the main campus, the Beachwood Fertility Center, the Fairview Fertility Center and the Solon, Strongsville and Twinsburg Family Health Centers.

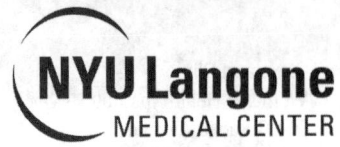
PROGRAM FOR IVF REPRODUCTIVE SURGERY AND INFERTILITY

About the Division of Reproductive Endocrinology and Infertility, Department of Obstetrics and Gynecology

The Division of Reproductive Endocrinology and Infertility offers the most advanced technology available to help infertile women and men realize their dreams of parenthood. The Division is highly experienced in all aspects of reproductive endocrinology, including the diagnosis and treatment of endometriosis, fibroids, problems with ovulation or sperm function, and recurring pregnancy loss. Its clinical staff includes seasoned technicians and physicians who have pioneered new innovations and been honored for their contributions to the field.

Patient-Centered Care

From the initial diagnosis through all stages of treatment, couples at NYU Langone Medical Center receive state-of-the-art, compassionate care tailored to their specific needs. After a comprehensive evaluation to determine the cause of infertility, couples are counseled on whether assisted reproduction is necessary.

In Vitro Fertilization (IVF)

When medical conditions prevent the sperm from reaching the egg, skilled physicians and laboratory staff at the Fertility Center assist patients with retrieving their eggs, insemination in the lab, and insertion back into the patient's uterus as embryos. Preimplantation Genetic Screening (PGS) at the Fertility Center offers tests for aneuploidy (an abnormal number of chromosomes). Some of the genetic disorders identified with PGS include cystic fibrosis, Down syndrome, hemophilia, Huntington's disease, Marfan's disease, muscular dystrophy and sickle cell anemia. State-of-the-art technology is also used to increase chances of delivery in some women with a history of recurrent miscarriage or previous IVF failures.

Complex Cases

The Center offers the most advanced care available for complex cases of infertility including those which may not have been successful in other centers and may even have been told there is no hope.

IVF for Male Factor Infertility

The Fertility Center provides male patients with experienced urologists who can provide expert fertility treatment. Men receive a complete evaluation, including a fertility history, physical exam, blood testing and semen analysis. Surgical treatment of male infertility is performed on-site at the Center's surgical suites on an outpatient basis and may include testicular biopsy, vasectomy reversal, epididymal tissue repair and varicose vein repair.

Rheumatology
a subspecialty of Internal Medicine

An internist who treats diseases of joints, muscle, bones and tendons. This specialist diagnoses and treats arthritis, back pain, muscle strains, common athletic injuries and "collagen" diseases.

Training Required: Three years in internal medicine *plus* additional training and examination for certification in rheumatology.

RHEUMATOLOGY

New England

Albert, Daniel A MD [Rhu] - **Spec Exp:** Juvenile Arthritis; Rheumatology-Adult & Pediatric; . **Hospital:** Dartmouth - Hitchcock Med Ctr; **Address:** Dartmouth-Hitchcock Med Ctr, Dept Rheumatology, One Medical Center Drive, Lebanon, NH 03756; **Phone:** 603-650-8622; **Board Cert:** Internal Medicine 1977; Rheumatology 1980; **Med School:** NYU Sch Med 1974; **Resid:** Internal Medicine, NC Meml Hosp 1977; **Fellow:** Rheumatology, UCSD Med Ctr 1981; **Fac Appt:** Prof Med, Univ Pennsylvania

Coblyn, Jonathan S MD [Rhu] - **Spec Exp:** Rheumatoid Arthritis; Lupus/SLE; Vasculitis; Musculoskeletal Disorders; **Hospital:** Brigham and Women's Hosp (page 57), New England Bapt Hosp; **Address:** Brigham & Women's Hosp, Div Rheumatology, 75 Francis St, PBB-B3, Boston, MA 02115; **Phone:** 617-732-5347; **Board Cert:** Internal Medicine 1977; Rheumatology 1980; **Med School:** Johns Hopkins Univ 1974; **Resid:** Internal Medicine, Peter Bent Brigham Hosp 1976; Internal Medicine, Stanford Univ Hosps 1977; **Fellow:** Rheumatology, Peter Bent Brigham Hosp 1979; **Fac Appt:** Assoc Prof Med, Harvard Med Sch

Kay, Jonathan MD [Rhu] - **Spec Exp:** Rheumatoid Arthritis; Psoriatic Arthritis; Ankylosing Spondylitis; Nephrogenic Systemic Fibrosis; **Hospital:** UMass Mem Med Ctr-Memorial Campus, UMass Meml Med Ctr - Univ Campus; **Address:** Rheumatology Ctr, Meml Campus, 119 Belmont St, Worcester, MA 01605; **Phone:** 508-334-6273; **Board Cert:** Internal Medicine 1986; Rheumatology 1988; **Med School:** UCSF 1983; **Resid:** Internal Medicine, Hosp Univ Penn 1986; **Fellow:** Rheumatology/Immunology, Brigham & Womens Hosp 1989; **Fac Appt:** Prof Med, Univ Mass Sch Med

Massarotti, Elena M MD [Rhu] - **Spec Exp:** Lupus/SLE; Rheumatoid Arthritis; Psoriatic Arthritis; Gout; **Hospital:** Brigham and Women's Hosp (page 57); **Address:** Brigham & Women's Hosp, Div Rheumatology, PBB-B3, 75 Francis St, Boston, MA 02115; **Phone:** 617-732-6523; **Board Cert:** Internal Medicine 1989; Rheumatology 2000; **Med School:** Tufts Univ 1984; **Resid:** Internal Medicine, Tufts-New England Med Ctr 1987; **Fellow:** Rheumatology, Tufts-New England Med Ctr 1989; **Fac Appt:** Assoc Prof Med, Tufts Univ

Polisson, Richard P MD [Rhu] - **Spec Exp:** Rheumatoid Arthritis; Lupus/SLE; **Hospital:** Mass Genl Hosp; **Address:** 55 Fruit St Yawkey Bldg - Ste 2C, Boston, MA 02114; **Phone:** 617-726-7938; **Board Cert:** Internal Medicine 1979; Rheumatology 1984; **Med School:** Duke Univ 1976; **Resid:** Internal Medicine, Duke Univ Med Ctr 1978; Internal Medicine, Natl Inst Hlth/NCI 1980; **Fellow:** Rheumatology, Mass Genl Hosp 1982; **Fac Appt:** Assoc Prof Med, Harvard Med Sch

Schoen, Robert T MD [Rhu] - **Spec Exp:** Rheumatoid Arthritis; Lyme Disease; Osteoporosis; **Hospital:** Yale-New Haven Hosp; **Address:** 60 Temple St, Ste 6A, New Haven, CT 06510-2716; **Phone:** 203-789-2255; **Board Cert:** Internal Medicine 1979; Rheumatology 1982; **Med School:** Columbia P&S 1976; **Resid:** Internal Medicine, Yale New Haven Hosp 1979; **Fellow:** Rheumatology, Brigham & Womens Hosp 1981; **Fac Appt:** Clin Prof Med, Yale Univ

Seton, Margaret P MD [Rhu] - **Spec Exp:** Paget's Disease of Bone; **Hospital:** Mass Genl Hosp; **Address:** Rheumatology Assocs, 55 Fruit St Yawkey Bldg - Ste 2C, Boston, MA 02114; **Phone:** 617-726-7938; **Board Cert:** Internal Medicine 1986; Rheumatology 2002; **Med School:** Med Coll VA 1980; **Resid:** Internal Medicine, Univ Hosp 1984; **Fellow:** Immunology, Mass Genl Hosp 1986; Rheumatology, Mass Genl Hosp 1991; **Fac Appt:** Asst Prof Med, Harvard Med Sch

Shadick, Nancy A MD [Rhu] - **Spec Exp:** Lyme Disease; Rheumatoid Arthritis; Osteoarthritis; **Hospital:** Brigham and Women's Hosp (page 57); **Address:** Brigham & Womens Hosp, Arthritis Ctr, Dept Rheumatology, 75 Francis St, Boston, MA 02115-6105; **Phone:** 617-732-5266; **Board Cert:** Internal Medicine 1989; Rheumatology 2002; **Med School:** NYU Sch Med 1986; **Resid:** Internal Medicine, Columbia-Presby Hosp 1989; **Fellow:** Rheumatology, Brigham & Womens Hosp 1992; **Fac Appt:** Asst Prof Med, Harvard Med Sch

Simms, Robert W MD [Rhu] - **Spec Exp:** Scleroderma; Rheumatoid Arthritis; Lyme Disease; **Hospital:** Boston Med Ctr; **Address:** Boston Univ Sch Med, Arthritis Ctr, 72 E Concord St, Evans-501, Boston, MA 02118; **Phone:** 617-638-4312; **Board Cert:** Internal Medicine 1985; Rheumatology 1988; **Med School:** Univ Rochester 1980; **Resid:** Internal Medicine, N Shore Hosp 1982; Internal Medicine, Brigham & Women's Hosp 1985; **Fellow:** Rheumatology, Boston Univ Med Ctr 1987; **Fac Appt:** Prof Med, Boston Univ

Tsokos, George MD [Rhu] - **Spec Exp:** Lupus/SLE; **Hospital:** Beth Israel Deaconess Med Ctr - Boston; **Address:** Beth Israel Deaconess Med Ctr, Dept Rheumatology, 110 Francis St, Ste 4B, Boston, MA 02215; **Phone:** 617-632-8658; **Board Cert:** Internal Medicine 1983; Diagnostic Lab Immunology 1986; Rheumatology 1984; **Med School:** Greece 1975; **Resid:** Internal Medicine, Natl Univ 1979; Immunology, NIH-NIADDK 1981; **Fellow:** Rheumatology, NIH-NIADDK 1983

Weinblatt, Michael E MD [Rhu] - **Spec Exp:** Rheumatoid Arthritis; **Hospital:** Brigham and Women's Hosp (page 57); **Address:** Brigham & Womens Hosp, Arthritis Ctr, 75 Francis St, Boston, MA 02115; **Phone:** 617-732-5331; **Board Cert:** Internal Medicine 1978; Rheumatology 1980; **Med School:** Univ MD Sch Med 1975; **Resid:** Internal Medicine, Univ Maryland Hosp 1978; **Fellow:** Rheumatology, Peter Bent Brigham Hosp 1980; **Fac Appt:** Prof Med, Harvard Med Sch

Mid Atlantic

Belmont, H Michael MD [Rhu] - **Spec Exp:** Lupus/SLE; Antiphospholipid Syndrome (APS); Wegener's Granulomatosis; Rheumatoid Arthritis; **Hospital:** NYU Hosp For Joint Diseases, NYU Langone Med Ctr (page 66); **Address:** 305 2nd Ave, Ste 16, New York, NY 10003-2739; **Phone:** 212-598-6516; **Board Cert:** Internal Medicine 1983; Rheumatology 1986; **Med School:** Univ Pittsburgh 1980; **Resid:** Internal Medicine, Mt Sinai Hosp 1983; **Fellow:** Rheumatology, NYU/Bellevue Hosp 1985; **Fac Appt:** Assoc Prof Med, NYU Sch Med

Blume, Ralph S MD [Rhu] - **Spec Exp:** Vasculitis; Lupus/SLE; Rheumatoid Arthritis; **Hospital:** NY-Presby/Columbia Univ Med Ctr, NY (page 65); **Address:** 161 Fort Washington Ave, Ste 537, New York, NY 10032-3713; **Phone:** 212-305-5512; **Board Cert:** Internal Medicine 1972; Rheumatology 1974; **Med School:** Columbia P&S 1964; **Resid:** Internal Medicine, Columbia-Presby Med Ctr 1968; **Fellow:** Rheumatology, Columbia-Presby Med Ctr 1970; **Fac Appt:** Clin Prof Med, Columbia P&S

Bunning, Robert D MD [Rhu] - **Spec Exp:** Exercise Physiology; Rheumatoid Arthritis; Musculoskeletal Disorders; **Hospital:** Natl Rehab Hosp; **Address:** National Rehab Hosp, 102 Irving St NW, Washington, DC 20010; **Phone:** 202-877-1660; **Board Cert:** Internal Medicine 1984; Rheumatology 1986; **Med School:** Univ Cincinnati 1979; **Resid:** Internal Medicine, Wash Hosp Ctr 1984; **Fellow:** Rheumatology, Wash Hosp Ctr 1983; **Fac Appt:** Asst Clin Prof Med, Geo Wash Univ

Buyon, Jill P MD [Rhu] - **Spec Exp:** Lupus/SLE in Pregnancy; Lupus/SLE in Menopause; **Hospital:** NYU Hosp For Joint Diseases, NYU Langone Med Ctr (page 66); **Address:** 246 E 20th St, New York, NY 10003; **Phone:** 646-356-9400; **Board Cert:** Internal Medicine 1981; Rheumatology 1984; **Med School:** Albert Einstein Coll Med 1978; **Resid:** Internal Medicine, Montefiore Med Ctr 1981; **Fellow:** Rheumatology, NYU Med Ctr 1983; **Fac Appt:** Prof Med, NYU Sch Med

Rheumatology

Cupps, Thomas R MD [Rhu] - **Spec Exp:** Vasculitis; Hepatitis B-Immune Response; **Hospital:** Georgetown Univ Hosp; **Address:** 3800 Resevoir Rd NW, George Univ Hosp, Dept of Med, Pasquerilla Bldg, Ste 3004, Washington, DC 20007; **Phone:** 202-444-6200; **Board Cert:** Internal Medicine 1978; Allergy & Immunology 1981; **Med School:** Stanford Univ 1975; **Resid:** Internal Medicine, Strong Meml Hosp 1978; **Fellow:** Allergy & Immunology, Natl Inst Allergy & Inf Dis 1980; **Fac Appt:** Assoc Prof Med, Georgetown Univ

Farber, Martin S MD/PhD [Rhu] - **Hospital:** Sunnyview Hosp & Rehab Ctr, Ellis Hosp; **Address:** Sunnyview Hospital, 124 Rosa Rd, Schenectady, NY 12308-2198; **Phone:** 518-386-3644; **Board Cert:** Internal Medicine 1982; Rheumatology 1984; **Med School:** Albert Einstein Coll Med 1979; **Resid:** Internal Medicine, Boston City Hosp 1982; **Fellow:** Rheumatology, Boston Univ Sch Med 1984; **Fac Appt:** Asst Clin Prof Med, Albany Med Coll

Fields, Theodore R MD [Rhu] - **Spec Exp:** Gout; Rheumatoid Arthritis; Osteoarthritis; **Hospital:** Hosp For Special Surgery (page 60), NY-Presby/Weill Cornell Med Ctr, NY (page 65); **Address:** Hosp Special Surg-Faculty Practice, 535 E 70th St Fl 8, New York, NY 10021-4872; **Phone:** 212-606-1286; **Board Cert:** Internal Medicine 1979; Rheumatology 1982; **Med School:** SUNY Downstate 1976; **Resid:** Internal Medicine, Nassau Co Med Ctr 1979; **Fellow:** Rheumatology, Univ Hosp 1982; **Fac Appt:** Clin Prof Med, Cornell Univ-Weill Med Coll

Gorevic, Peter D MD [Rhu] - **Spec Exp:** Autoimmune Disease; Amyloidosis/Joint Disease; Cryoglobulinemia; **Hospital:** Mount Sinai Med Ctr (page 63), Huntington Hosp; **Address:** Mount Sinai Medical Ctr, One Gustave L Levy Pl, Box 1244, New York, NY 10029; **Phone:** 212-241-1671; **Board Cert:** Allergy & Immunology 1977; Rheumatology 1976; Diagnostic Lab Immunology 1986; Internal Medicine 1973; **Med School:** NYU Sch Med 1970; **Resid:** Internal Medicine, NYU Med Ctr 1974; **Fellow:** Rheumatology, NYU Med Ctr 1976; Allergy & Immunology, NYU Med Ctr 1977; **Fac Appt:** Prof Med, Mount Sinai Sch Med

Gourley, Mark F MD [Rhu] - **Spec Exp:** Autoimmune Disease; Lupus/SLE; **Hospital:** Natl Inst of Hlth - Clin Ctr; **Address:** Natl Inst Hlth, 10 Center Drive Bldg 10 - rm 10/6N216F, Bethesda, MD 20892-1616; **Phone:** 301-451-6269; **Board Cert:** Internal Medicine 1988; Rheumatology 2002; **Med School:** Tulane Univ 1985; **Resid:** Internal Medicine, Univ Wisconsin Hosps 1988; **Fellow:** Rheumatology, Natl Inst Hlth 1996

Hochberg, Marc C MD [Rhu] - **Spec Exp:** Osteoporosis; Osteoarthritis; Rheumatoid Arthritis; **Hospital:** Univ of MD Med Ctr, Kernan Hosp; **Address:** Univ MD Sch Med, Div Rheum, 10 S Pine St, MSTF 8-34, Baltimore, MD 21201; **Phone:** 410-706-6474; **Board Cert:** Internal Medicine 1976; Rheumatology 1978; **Med School:** Johns Hopkins Univ 1973; **Resid:** Internal Medicine, Johns Hopkins Hosp 1975; **Fellow:** Rheumatology, Johns Hopkins Hosp 1977; **Fac Appt:** Prof Med, Univ MD Sch Med

Lahita, Robert G MD/PhD [Rhu] - **Spec Exp:** Lupus/SLE; Endocrinology & Joint Disorders; Immunodeficiency Disorders; Vasculitis; **Hospital:** Newark Beth Israel Med Ctr; **Address:** 201 Lyons Ave, Newark, NJ 07112; **Phone:** 973-926-7472; **Board Cert:** Internal Medicine 2004; Rheumatology 2007; **Med School:** Jefferson Med Coll 1973; **Resid:** Internal Medicine, New York Hosp-Cornell 1976; **Fellow:** Rheumatology, Rockefeller Hosp 1978; **Fac Appt:** Prof Med, Mount Sinai Sch Med

Lockshin, Michael D MD [Rhu] - **Spec Exp:** Lupus/SLE in Women; Antiphospholipid Syndrome (APS); Pregnancy & Rheumatic Disease; Lupus/SLE in Pregnancy; **Hospital:** Hosp For Special Surgery (page 60), NY-Presby/Weill Cornell Med Ctr, NY (page 65); **Address:** 535 E 70th St, rm 848, New York, NY 10021-4872; **Phone:** 212-606-1461; **Board Cert:** Internal Medicine 1969; Rheumatology 1972; **Med School:** Harvard Med Sch 1963; **Resid:** Internal Medicine, Bellevue Hosp 1968; **Fellow:** Rheumatology, Columbia-Presby Hosp 1970; **Fac Appt:** Prof Med, Cornell Univ-Weill Med Coll

Magid, Steven K MD [Rhu] - **Spec Exp:** Rheumatoid Arthritis; Osteoarthritis; Lyme Disease; Polymyalgia Rheumatica; **Hospital:** Hosp For Special Surgery (page 60), NY-Presby/Weill Cornell Med Ctr, NY (page 65); **Address:** 535 E 70th St Fl 8, New York, NY 10021; **Phone:** 212-606-1060; **Board Cert:** Internal Medicine 1979; Rheumatology 1984; **Med School:** Cornell Univ-Weill Med Coll 1976; **Resid:** Internal Medicine, New York Hosp 1979; **Fellow:** Rheumatology, Hosp For Special Surgery 1981; **Fac Appt:** Clin Prof Med, Cornell Univ-Weill Med Coll

Manzi, Susan MD [Rhu] - **Spec Exp:** Lupus/SLE; Lupus/SLE in Women; **Hospital:** Allegheny General Hosp, Western Penn Hosp; **Address:** Allegheny Genl Hosp, Dept Rheumatology, 320 E North Ave, Pittsburgh, PA 15212; **Phone:** 412-578-1152; **Board Cert:** Internal Medicine 1988; Rheumatology 2000; **Med School:** Univ Pittsburgh 1985; **Resid:** Internal Medicine, Duke Univ Med Ctr 1988; **Fellow:** Rheumatology, Univ Pittsburgh 1991; **Fac Appt:** Assoc Prof Med, Drexel Univ Coll Med

Medsger Jr, Thomas A MD [Rhu] - **Spec Exp:** Scleroderma; Raynaud's Disease; Polymyositis; Dermatomyositis; **Hospital:** UPMC Presby, Pittsburgh; **Address:** Arthritis & Autoimmunity Ctr, 3601 Fifth Ave, Suite 2B Falk Med Bldg, Pittsburgh, PA 15213; **Phone:** 412-647-6700; **Board Cert:** Internal Medicine 1972; Rheumatology 1972; **Med School:** Univ Pennsylvania 1962; **Resid:** Internal Medicine, Univ Pittsburgh 1968; **Fellow:** Rheumatology, Univ Pittsburgh 1966; Rheumatology, Univ Tenn Coll Med 1969; **Fac Appt:** Prof Med, Univ Pittsburgh

Mitnick, Hal J MD [Rhu] - **Spec Exp:** Rheumatoid Arthritis; Psoriatic Arthritis; Osteoporosis; Dermatomyositis; **Hospital:** NYU Langone Med Ctr (page 66); **Address:** 333 E 34th St, Ste 1C, New York, NY 10016-4977; **Phone:** 212-889-7217; **Board Cert:** Internal Medicine 1976; Rheumatology 1978; **Med School:** NYU Sch Med 1972; **Resid:** Internal Medicine, Bellevue Hosp 1976; **Fellow:** Rheumatology, NYU Med Ctr 1978; **Fac Appt:** Clin Prof Med, NYU Sch Med

Oddis, Chester V MD [Rhu] - **Spec Exp:** Polymyositis; Dermatomyositis; Connective Tissue Disorders; **Hospital:** UPMC Presby, Pittsburgh; **Address:** UPMC-Div Rheumatology, 3601 Fifth Ave Falk Med Bldg - Ste 2B, Pittsburgh, PA 15213; **Phone:** 412-647-6700; **Board Cert:** Internal Medicine 1983; Rheumatology 1986; **Med School:** Penn State Coll Med 1980; **Resid:** Internal Medicine, Hershey Med Ctr 1984; **Fellow:** Rheumatology, Univ Pittsburgh 1986; **Fac Appt:** Prof Med, Univ Pittsburgh

Paget, Stephen MD [Rhu] - **Spec Exp:** Rheumatoid Arthritis; Lupus/SLE; Vasculitis; Connective Tissue Disorders; **Hospital:** Hosp For Special Surgery (page 60), NY-Presby/Weill Cornell Med Ctr, NY (page 65); **Address:** 535 E 70th St, New York, NY 10021; **Phone:** 212-606-1845; **Board Cert:** Internal Medicine 1974; Rheumatology 2009; **Med School:** SUNY Downstate 1971; **Resid:** Internal Medicine, Johns Hopkins Hosp 1973; **Fellow:** Rheumatology, Hosp Special Surg 1975; **Fac Appt:** Prof Med, Cornell Univ-Weill Med Coll

Petri, Michelle A MD [Rhu] - **Spec Exp:** Lupus/SLE; Antiphospholipid Syndrome (APS); Autoimmune Disease; **Hospital:** Johns Hopkins Hosp (page 61); **Address:** Jonhs Hopkins Lupus Ctr, Div Rheumatology, 1830 E Monument St, Ste 7500, Baltimore, MD 21205-2100; **Phone:** 410-955-9114; **Board Cert:** Internal Medicine 1983; Allergy & Immunology 1985; Rheumatology 1986; **Med School:** Harvard Med Sch 1980; **Resid:** Internal Medicine, Mass Genl Hosp 1983; **Fellow:** Allergy & Immunology, UCSF Med Ctr 1985; Rheumatology, UCSF Med Ctr 1986; **Fac Appt:** Prof Med, Johns Hopkins Univ

Plotz, Paul MD [Rhu] - **Hospital:** Natl Inst of Hlth - Clin Ctr; **Address:** 50 S Drive, MC 8023, Louis B Stokes Lab, 1503 Bldg 50, Bethesda, MD 20892-1820; **Phone:** 301-496-9904; **Board Cert:** Internal Medicine 1970; **Med School:** Harvard Med Sch 1963; **Resid:** Internal Medicine, Beth Israel Hosp 1965; **Fellow:** Rheumatology, Clin Ctr- NIH 1968

Rheumatology

Rothenberg, Russell R MD [Rhu] - **Spec Exp:** Fibromyalgia; Lupus/SLE; Rheumatoid Arthritis; Preventive Medicine; **Hospital:** G Washington Univ Hosp; **Address:** 10215 Fernwood Rd, Ste 401, Bethesda, MD 20817; **Phone:** 301-571-2273; **Board Cert:** Internal Medicine 1980; Rheumatology 1982; **Med School:** Albany Med Coll 1977; **Resid:** Internal Medicine, LIJ Med Ctr 1980; **Fellow:** Rheumatology, Mt Sinai Med Ctr 1982; **Fac Appt:** Assoc Prof Med, Geo Wash Univ

Schubert, Richard D MD [Rhu] - **Spec Exp:** Arthritis; **Hospital:** Sibley Mem Hosp; **Address:** Foxhall Internists, 3301 New Mexico Ave NW, Ste 348, Washington, DC 20016; **Phone:** 202-362-4467; **Board Cert:** Rheumatology 1978; Internal Medicine 1975; **Med School:** SUNY Downstate 1972; **Resid:** Internal Medicine, Peter Bent Brigham Hosp 1975; **Fellow:** Rheumatology, Peter Bent Brigham Hosp 1978

Solitar, Bruce M MD [Rhu] - **Spec Exp:** Arthritis; Fibromyalgia; Reiter's Syndrome; Retroperitoneal Fibrosis; **Hospital:** NYU Langone Med Ctr (page 66), NYU Hosp For Joint Diseases; **Address:** 333 E 34th St, New York, NY 10016; **Phone:** 212-889-7217; **Board Cert:** Internal Medicine 2001; Rheumatology 2004; **Med School:** NYU Sch Med 1988; **Resid:** Internal Medicine, NYU/Bellevue Med Ctr 1992; **Fellow:** Rheumatology, NYU/Bellevue Med Ctr 1994; **Fac Appt:** Assoc Clin Prof Med, NYU Sch Med

Solomon, Gary MD [Rhu] - **Spec Exp:** Psoriatic Arthritis; Rheumatoid Arthritis; Autoimmune Disease; **Hospital:** NYU Hosp For Joint Diseases, NYU Langone Med Ctr (page 66); **Address:** Hosp Joint Diseases, Dept Rheumatology, 305 2nd Ave, Ste 16, New York, NY 10003-2747; **Phone:** 212-598-6516; **Board Cert:** Internal Medicine 1980; Rheumatology 1982; **Med School:** Mount Sinai Sch Med 1977; **Resid:** Internal Medicine, Mt Sinai Med Ctr 1980; **Fellow:** Rheumatology, Montefiore Med Ctr 1982; **Fac Appt:** Assoc Clin Prof Med, NYU Sch Med

Spiera, Harry MD [Rhu] - **Spec Exp:** Lupus/SLE; Scleroderma; Vasculitis; Behcet's Syndrome; **Hospital:** Mount Sinai Med Ctr (page 63), NY-Presby/Weill Cornell Med Ctr, NY (page 65); **Address:** 1088 Park Ave, New York, NY 10128-1132; **Phone:** 212-860-4000 x36; **Board Cert:** Internal Medicine 1965; Rheumatology 1972; **Med School:** NYU Sch Med 1958; **Resid:** Internal Medicine, VA Med Ctr 1960; Internal Medicine, Mt Sinai Hosp 1961; **Fellow:** Rheumatology, Columbia-Presby Med Ctr 1963; **Fac Appt:** Clin Prof Med, Mount Sinai Sch Med

Starz, Terence W MD [Rhu] - **Spec Exp:** Arthritis; **Hospital:** UPMC Shadyside, UPMC St Margaret; **Address:** Arthritis & Int Medicine Assocs-UPMC, 3500 Fifth Ave Hieber Bldg Fl 4, Pittsburgh, PA 15213; **Phone:** 412-682-2434; **Board Cert:** Internal Medicine 1975; Rheumatology 1978; **Med School:** Jefferson Med Coll 1971; **Resid:** Internal Medicine, Presby-Univ Hosp 1975; **Fellow:** Rheumatology, Presby-Univ Hosp 1977; **Fac Appt:** Clin Prof Med, Univ Pittsburgh

Steen, Virginia MD [Rhu] - **Spec Exp:** Scleroderma; Lupus/SLE; Polymyositis; **Hospital:** Georgetown Univ Hosp; **Address:** 3800 Reservoir Rd NW, Pasquerilla Bldg, Ste 3004, Washington, DC 20007; **Phone:** 202-444-6200; **Board Cert:** Internal Medicine 1978; Rheumatology 1980; **Med School:** Univ Pittsburgh 1975; **Resid:** Internal Medicine, Hosp Univ Penn 1978; **Fellow:** Rheumatology, Presby Hosp 1980; **Fac Appt:** Prof Med, Georgetown Univ

Vivino, Frederick B MD [Rhu] - **Spec Exp:** Sjogren's Syndrome; **Hospital:** Penn Presby Med Ctr - UPHS (page 68); **Address:** Presbyterian Med Ctr, 3910 Powelton Ave Fl 2, Philadelphia, PA 19104; **Phone:** 215-662-4333; **Board Cert:** Internal Medicine 1986; Rheumatology 1988; **Med School:** Temple Univ 1983; **Resid:** Internal Medicine, Hosp Univ Penn 1986; **Fellow:** Rheumatology, Hosp Univ Penn 1989; **Fac Appt:** Assoc Clin Prof Med, Univ Pennsylvania

Weinstein, Arthur MD [Rhu] - **Spec Exp:** Lyme Disease; Lupus/SLE; Vasculitis; Polymyositis; **Hospital:** Washington Hosp Ctr, Georgetown Univ Hosp; **Address:** Washington Hosp Ctr, Div Rheumatology, 110 Irving St NW, rm 2A-66, Washington, DC 20010; **Phone:** 202-877-0333; **Board Cert:** Rheumatology 1976; Diagnostic Lab Immunology 1986; **Med School:** Univ Toronto 1967; **Resid:** Internal Medicine, Toronto Wellesley Hosp 1972; Rheumatology, Hammersmith Hosp 1971; **Fellow:** Rheumatology, Toronto Wellesley Hosp 1973; **Fac Appt:** Prof Med, Georgetown Univ

Wigley, Frederick M MD [Rhu] - **Spec Exp:** Scleroderma; Raynaud's Disease; **Hospital:** Johns Hopkins Bayview Med Ctr (page 61), Johns Hopkins Hosp (page 61); **Address:** 5501 Hopkins Bayview Cir, Ste 1B32, Baltimore, MD 21224; **Phone:** 410-550-7715; **Board Cert:** Internal Medicine 1975; Rheumatology 1980; **Med School:** Univ Fla Coll Med 1972; **Resid:** Internal Medicine, Johns Hopkins Hosp 1975; **Fellow:** Rheumatology, Johns Hopkins Hosp 1979; **Fac Appt:** Prof Med, Johns Hopkins Univ

Southeast

Allen, Nancy B MD [Rhu] - **Spec Exp:** Vasculitis; Wegener's Granulomatosis; Lupus/SLE; Temporal Arteritis; **Hospital:** Duke Univ Hosp; **Address:** Duke Univ Med Ctr, Box 3440, Durham, NC 27710; **Phone:** 919-684-2965; **Board Cert:** Internal Medicine 1981; Rheumatology 1984; **Med School:** Tufts Univ 1978; **Resid:** Internal Medicine, Duke Univ Med Ctr 1981; **Fellow:** Rheumatology, Duke Univ Med Ctr 1983; **Fac Appt:** Prof Med, Duke Univ

Chatham, W Winn MD [Rhu] - **Spec Exp:** Lupus/SLE; Connective Tissue Disorders; Rheumatoid Arthritis; **Hospital:** Univ of Ala Hosp at Birmingham; **Address:** UAB Rheumatology, 1530 3rd Ave S, FOT 802D, Birmingham, AL 35294-3408; **Phone:** 205-934-4212; **Board Cert:** Internal Medicine 1983; Rheumatology 1988; **Med School:** Vanderbilt Univ 1980; **Resid:** Internal Medicine, North Carolina Meml Hosp 1983; **Fellow:** Rheumatology, Univ Alabama Birmingham 1988; **Fac Appt:** Prof Med, Univ Alabama

Crofford, Leslie J MD [Rhu] - **Spec Exp:** Fibromyalgia; Rheumatoid Arthritis; Lupus/SLE; **Hospital:** Univ of Kentucky Albert B. Chandler Hosp; **Address:** 740 S Limestone St, rm J509, Lexington, KY 40536-0284; **Phone:** 859-323-4939; **Board Cert:** Internal Medicine 1987; Rheumatology 2003; **Med School:** Univ Tenn Coll Med 1984; **Resid:** Internal Medicine, Barnes/Wash Univ 1987; **Fellow:** Rheumatology, Natl Inst Hlth Clin Ctr 1992; **Fac Appt:** Prof Med, Univ KY Coll Med

Hadler, Nortin MD [Rhu] - **Spec Exp:** Occupational Musculoskeletal Disorders; Musculoskeletal Disorders; Spondylitis; Pain-Back; **Hospital:** NC Memorial Hosp - UNC; **Address:** Univ North Carolina, Dept Medicine, 3300 Thurston Building, Box 7280, Chapel Hill, NC 27599-7280; **Phone:** 919-966-0566; **Board Cert:** Rheumatology 1974; Allergy & Immunology 1975; Internal Medicine 1987; **Med School:** Harvard Med Sch 1968; **Resid:** Internal Medicine, Mass Genl Hosp 1973; **Fellow:** Rheumatology, Natl Inst Hlth 1972; Allergy & Immunology, Clin Res Ctr 1974; **Fac Appt:** Prof Med, Univ NC Sch Med

Kimberly, Robert P MD [Rhu] - **Spec Exp:** Lupus/SLE; Rheumatoid Arthritis; Vasculitis; Autoimmune Disease; **Hospital:** Univ of Ala Hosp at Birmingham; **Address:** UAB Rheumatology, 1530 3rd Ave S, SHEL 172B, Birmingham, AL 35294; **Phone:** 205-934-0245; **Board Cert:** Internal Medicine 1976; Rheumatology 1978; **Med School:** Harvard Med Sch 1973; **Resid:** Internal Medicine, Hosp Univ Penn 1975; **Fellow:** Rheumatology, NIAMS, NIH 1977; Rheumatology, Hosp Special Surgery 1979; **Fac Appt:** Prof Med, Univ Alabama

Rheumatology

Moore, Walter J MD [Rhu] - **Spec Exp:** Rheumatoid Arthritis; Lupus/SLE; **Hospital:** Med Coll of GA Hosp and Clin (MCG Health Inc); **Address:** Medical College of Georgia, 1120 15th St, rm BI 5083, Augusta, GA 30912; **Phone:** 706-721-2981; **Board Cert:** Internal Medicine 1980; Rheumatology 1984; **Med School:** Georgetown Univ 1977; **Resid:** Internal Medicine, Walter Reed AMC 1980; **Fellow:** Rheumatology, Walter Reed AMC 1983; **Fac Appt:** Assoc Prof Med, Med Coll GA

Sergent, John S MD [Rhu] - **Spec Exp:** Vasculitis; **Hospital:** Vanderbilt Univ Med Ctr (page 76); **Address:** Vanderbilt Rheumatology, 1301 Medical Center Drive, Ste 2501, Nashville, TN 27232; **Phone:** 615-322-1900; **Board Cert:** Internal Medicine 1972; Rheumatology 1974; **Med School:** Vanderbilt Univ 1966; **Resid:** Internal Medicine, Johns Hopkins Hosp 1968; Internal Medicine, Vanderbilt Univ Hosp 1972; **Fellow:** Rheumatology, Hosp Special Surgery 1974; **Fac Appt:** Prof Med, Vanderbilt Univ

Silver, Richard M MD [Rhu] - **Spec Exp:** Scleroderma & Lung Disease; Pediatric Rheumatology; Connective Tissue Disorders; **Hospital:** MUSC Med Ctr; **Address:** MUSC Med Ctr, 96 Jonathan Lucas St, Ste 912, Charleston, SC 29425; **Phone:** 843-876-0500; **Board Cert:** Internal Medicine 1978; Rheumatology 1982; **Med School:** Vanderbilt Univ 1975; **Resid:** Internal Medicine, Univ NC Hosps 1978; **Fellow:** Rheumatology, UCSD Med Ctr 1981; **Fac Appt:** Prof Med, Med Univ SC

Wise, Christopher M MD [Rhu] - **Spec Exp:** Gout; Sjogren's Syndrome; Rheumatoid Arthritis; **Hospital:** Med Coll of VA Hosp; **Address:** Virginia Commonwealth Univ/MCV Campus, Box 980647, Richmond, VA 23298; **Phone:** 804-828-9341; **Board Cert:** Internal Medicine 1980; Rheumatology 1982; **Med School:** Univ NC Sch Med 1977; **Resid:** Internal Medicine, Med Coll Virginia Hosp 1980; **Fellow:** Rheumatology, Med Coll Virginia Hosp 1982; **Fac Appt:** Prof Med, Va Commonwealth Univ Sch Med

Midwest

Adams, Elaine MD [Rhu] - **Spec Exp:** Rheumatoid Arthritis; Lupus/SLE; Spondyloarthropathies; **Hospital:** Loyola Univ Med Ctr, Edward Hines, Jr. VA Hosp; **Address:** Loyola Univ Med Ctr, Dept Rheumatology, 2160 S 1st Ave, Bldg 54 - rm 121, Maywood, IL 60153-5590; **Phone:** 708-216-8563; **Board Cert:** Internal Medicine 1981; Rheumatology 1984; **Med School:** Loyola Univ-Stritch Sch Med 1978; **Resid:** Internal Medicine, Loyola Univ Med Ctr 1981; **Fellow:** Rheumatology, Univ Wisconsin Med Ctr 1983; **Fac Appt:** Prof Med, Loyola Univ-Stritch Sch Med

Brasington, Richard MD [Rhu] - **Hospital:** Barnes-Jewish Hosp; **Address:** 4921 Parkview Pl, Ste 5C, Box 8602, St Louis, MO 63110; **Phone:** 314-286-2635; **Board Cert:** Internal Medicine 1985; Rheumatology 1986; **Med School:** Duke Univ 1980; **Resid:** Internal Medicine, Univ Iowa Med Ctr 1982; Internal Medicine, Univ Iowa Med Ctr 1985; **Fellow:** Rheumatology, Univ Iowa 1986; **Fac Appt:** Assoc Prof Med, Washington Univ, St Louis

Chang, Rowland W MD [Rhu] - **Spec Exp:** Rheumatoid Arthritis; Arthritis; Ankylosing Spondylitis; **Hospital:** Rehab Inst of Chicago, Northwestern Meml Hosp; **Address:** Rehab Inst of Chicago Arthritis Ctr, 345 E Superior St Fl 9, Chicago, IL 60611-2654; **Phone:** 312-238-2784; **Board Cert:** Internal Medicine 1979; Rheumatology 1982; **Med School:** Tufts Univ 1976; **Resid:** Internal Medicine, Mt Auburn Hosp 1979; **Fellow:** Rheumatology, Hammersmith Hosp 1980; Rheumatology, Brigham & Womens Hosp 1982; **Fac Appt:** Prof Med, Northwestern Univ

Curran, James J MD [Rhu] - **Spec Exp:** Rheumatoid Arthritis; Polymyositis; Sjogren's Syndrome; Lupus/SLE; **Hospital:** Univ of Chicago Med Ctr; **Address:** 5841 S Maryland Ave, MC-0930, Chicago, IL 60637-1463; **Phone:** 773-702-1232; **Board Cert:** Internal Medicine 1980; Rheumatology 1982; **Med School:** Univ IL Coll Med 1976; **Resid:** Internal Medicine, Bethesda Naval Hosp 1980; **Fellow:** Rheumatology, Univ Chicago Hosps 1982; **Fac Appt:** Prof Med, Univ Chicago-Pritzker Sch Med

Fife, Rose S MD [Rhu] - **Spec Exp:** Women's Health; Arthritis; **Hospital:** IU Health University Hosp; **Address:** Gatch Clinical Bldg, rm 370, 541 N Clinical Drive, Indianapolis, IN 46202-7718; **Phone:** 317-944-7718; **Board Cert:** Internal Medicine 1978; Rheumatology 1982; **Med School:** Johns Hopkins Univ 1975; **Resid:** Internal Medicine, Johns Hopkins Hosp 1978; **Fellow:** Rheumatology, Univ Washington Med Ctr 1981; **Fac Appt:** Prof Med, Indiana Univ

Hugenberg, Steven T MD [Rhu] - **Spec Exp:** Rheumatoid Arthritis; Osteoarthritis; Psoriatic Arthritis; Ankylosing Spondylitis; **Hospital:** IU Health University Hosp; **Address:** IU Health Physicians Rheumatology, 550 N University Blvd, Ste 2180, Indianapolis, IN 46202; **Phone:** 317-944-8660; **Board Cert:** Internal Medicine 1985; Rheumatology 1988; **Med School:** Ohio State Univ 1982; **Resid:** Internal Medicine, Indiana Univ Med Ctr 1985; **Fellow:** Rheumatology, Indiana Univ Med Ctr 1987; **Fac Appt:** Assoc Prof Med, Indiana Univ

Katz, Robert S MD [Rhu] - **Spec Exp:** Rheumatoid Arthritis; Lupus/SLE; Fibromyalgia; Vasculitis; **Hospital:** Rush Univ Med Ctr, Northwestern Meml Hosp; **Address:** 1725 W Harrison St, Ste 365, Chicago, IL 60612-3841; **Phone:** 312-942-2159; **Board Cert:** Internal Medicine 1975; Rheumatology 1976; **Med School:** Univ MD Sch Med 1970; **Resid:** Internal Medicine, Washington Univ Med Ctr 1972; **Fellow:** Rheumatology, Johns Hopkins Hosp 1976; **Fac Appt:** Prof Med, Rush Med Coll

Langford, Carol MD [Rhu] - **Spec Exp:** Vasculitis; **Hospital:** Cleveland Clin (page 56); **Address:** Cleveland Clinic, 9500 Euclid Ave, Ste A50, Cleveland, OH 44195; **Phone:** 216-445-6056; **Board Cert:** Internal Medicine 2000; Rheumatology 2000; **Med School:** UCLA 1987; **Resid:** Internal Medicine, Univ Mich 1990; **Fellow:** Rheumatology, Duke Univ Med Ctr 1991

Luggen, Michael MD [Rhu] - **Hospital:** Univ Hosp - Cincinnati, Deaconess Hosp - Cincinnati; **Address:** 2123 Auburn Ave, Ste 630, Cincinnati, OH 45219; **Phone:** 513-585-1970; **Board Cert:** Internal Medicine 1978; Rheumatology 1982; **Med School:** Columbia P&S 1974; **Resid:** Internal Medicine, Cinn Genl Hosp 1977; **Fellow:** Rheumatology, Univ Cincinnati 1982; **Fac Appt:** Prof Med, Univ Cincinnati

Luthra, Harvinder Singh MD [Rhu] - **Spec Exp:** Rheumatoid Arthritis; Ankylosing Spondylitis; Relapsing Polychondritis; **Hospital:** St. Mary's Hosp - Rochester MN (Mayo), Rochester Methodist Hosp; **Address:** Mayo Clin, 200 First St SW, Rochester, MN 55905-0002; **Phone:** 507-266-4439; **Board Cert:** Internal Medicine 1973; Rheumatology 2002; **Med School:** India 1967; **Resid:** Ophthalmology, Christian Med Coll; Internal Medicine, Mount Sinai Hosp 1972; **Fellow:** Rheumatology, Mayo Grad Sch Affil Hosp 1974; **Fac Appt:** Prof Med, Mayo Med Sch

McCune, W Joseph MD [Rhu] - **Spec Exp:** Lupus/SLE; Rheumatoid Arthritis; **Hospital:** Univ of Michigan Hosp; **Address:** Univ Mich, Dept Rheum, 1500 E Med Ctr Drive, 3918 Taubman Ctr, Ann Arbor, MI 48109-0358; **Phone:** 734-647-5900; **Board Cert:** Internal Medicine 1978; Rheumatology 1982; **Med School:** Univ Cincinnati 1975; **Resid:** Internal Medicine, Univ Mich Hosps 1978; **Fellow:** Rheumatology, Brigham Womens Hosp 1981; **Fac Appt:** Prof Med, Univ Mich Med Sch

Moder, Kevin G MD [Rhu] - **Spec Exp:** Rheumatoid Arthritis; Lupus/SLE; **Hospital:** Mayo Med Ctr & Clin - Rochester; **Address:** Mayo Clin, Div Rheumatology, 200 First St SW, Rochester, MN 55905-0002; **Phone:** 507-284-4550; **Board Cert:** Internal Medicine 2000; Rheumatology 2000; **Med School:** Univ MO-Columbia Sch Med 1987; **Resid:** Internal Medicine, Mayo Clinic 1990; **Fellow:** Rheumatology, Mayo Clinic 1993; **Fac Appt:** Asst Prof Med, Mayo Med Sch

Rheumatology

Pope, Richard M MD [Rhu] - **Spec Exp:** Rheumatoid Arthritis; Sjogren's Syndrome; Psoriatic Arthritis; **Hospital:** Northwestern Meml Hosp; **Address:** 675 N St Clair, Ste 14-100, Chicago, IL 60611-5966; **Phone:** 312-695-8628; **Board Cert:** Internal Medicine 1973; Rheumatology 1976; Clinical & Laboratory Immunology 1986; **Med School:** Loyola Univ-Stritch Sch Med 1970; **Resid:** Internal Medicine, Michael Reese Hosp 1972; **Fellow:** Rheumatology, Univ Wash Med Ctr 1974; **Fac Appt:** Prof Med, Northwestern Univ

Warner, Ann E MD [Rhu] - **Hospital:** St. Luke's Hosp of Kansas City; **Address:** 4330 Wornall Rd, Ste 40, Kansas City, MO 64111-3210; **Phone:** 816-531-0930; **Board Cert:** Internal Medicine 1986; Rheumatology 1988; **Med School:** Univ Kansas 1983; **Resid:** Internal Medicine, St Luke's Hosp 1986; **Fellow:** Rheumatology, Univ Kansas Med Ctr 1989; **Fac Appt:** Asst Clin Prof Med, Univ MO-Kansas City

Great Plains and Mountains

O'Dell, James R MD [Rhu] - **Spec Exp:** Osteoarthritis; Rheumatoid Arthritis; **Hospital:** Nebraska Med Ctr; **Address:** 983025 Nebraska Med Ctr, Omaha, NE 68198-3025; **Phone:** 402-559-4015; **Board Cert:** Internal Medicine 1980; Rheumatology 1984; **Med School:** Univ Nebr Coll Med 1977; **Resid:** Internal Medicine, Univ Nebraska Med Ctr 1981; **Fellow:** Rheumatology, Univ Colorado 1984; **Fac Appt:** Prof Med, Univ Nebr Coll Med

West, Sterling G MD [Rhu] - **Spec Exp:** Lupus/SLE; Vasculitis; Osteoporosis; **Hospital:** Univ of CO Hosp - Anschutz Inpatient Pav; **Address:** Univ Colorado Rheumatology Practice, 1635 Aurora Court, MS F721, Box 6510, Aurora, CO 80045; **Phone:** 720-848-1940; **Board Cert:** Internal Medicine 1979; Rheumatology 2005; **Med School:** Emory Univ 1976; **Resid:** Internal Medicine, Fitzsimons Army Med Ctr 1979; **Fellow:** Rheumatology, Walter Reed Army Med Ctr 1981; **Fac Appt:** Prof Med, Univ Colorado

Southwest

Arnett Jr, Frank C MD [Rhu] - **Spec Exp:** Reiter's Syndrome; Spondylitis; Scleroderma; **Hospital:** Meml Hermann Hosp - Texas Med Ctr; **Address:** 6410 Fannin St UT Prof Bldg - Ste 600, Houston, TX 77030-5302; **Phone:** 832-325-7191; **Board Cert:** Internal Medicine 1972; Rheumatology 1976; Clinical & Laboratory Immunology 1990; **Med School:** Univ Cincinnati 1968; **Resid:** Internal Medicine, Johns Hopkins Hosp 1970; **Fellow:** Rheumatology, Johns Hopkins Hosp 1972; **Fac Appt:** Prof Med, Univ Tex, Houston

Chang-Miller, April MD [Rhu] - **Spec Exp:** Connective Tissue Disorders-Consult; Spondyloarthropathies-Consult; **Hospital:** Mayo Clinic - Scottsdale; **Address:** Mayo Clinic, Div Rheumatology, 13400 E Shea Blvd, Scottsdale, AZ 85259; **Phone:** 480-301-4342; **Board Cert:** Internal Medicine 1986; Rheumatology 2000; **Med School:** Yale Univ 1983; **Resid:** Internal Medicine, Mayo Clinic 1985; **Fellow:** Rheumatology, Mayo Clinic 1989; Biochemical and Molecular Biology, Mayo Clinic 1990; **Fac Appt:** Asst Prof Med, Mayo Med Sch

Davis, William E MD [Rhu] - **Spec Exp:** Lupus/SLE; Rheumatoid Arthritis; Gout; **Hospital:** Ochsner Med Ctr-New Orleans; **Address:** Ochsner Clinic, Rheumatology, 1514 Jefferson Hwy, New Orleans, LA 70121-2483; **Phone:** 504-842-3920; **Board Cert:** Internal Medicine 1987; Rheumatology 1988; **Med School:** Louisiana State U, New Orleans 1983; **Resid:** Internal Medicine, Ochsner Fdn Hosp 1986; **Fellow:** Rheumatology, Univ Michigan 1988

Lindsey, Stephen M MD [Rhu] - **Spec Exp:** Osteoporosis; Rheumatoid Arthritis; **Hospital:** Ochsner Med Ctr-Baton Rouge; **Address:** Ochsner Hlth Ctr, 9001 Summa Ave, Baton Rouge, LA 70809; **Phone:** 225-761-5481; **Board Cert:** Internal Medicine 1975; Rheumatology 1980; **Med School:** Louisiana State U, New Orleans 1972; **Resid:** Internal Medicine, Letterman AMC 1975; **Fellow:** Rheumatology, Walter Reed AMC 1979; **Fac Appt:** Clin Prof Med, Louisiana State U, New Orleans

Lipstate, James M MD [Rhu] - **Spec Exp:** Arthritis; Osteoporosis; **Hospital:** Our Lady of Lourdes Reg Med Ctr - Lafayette, Lafayette Genl Med Ctr; **Address:** 401 Audubon Blvd, Ste 102B, Lafayette, LA 70503; **Phone:** 337-237-7801; **Board Cert:** Internal Medicine 1983; Rheumatology 1986; **Med School:** Tulane Univ 1980; **Resid:** Internal Medicine, Univ Alabama Hosp 1983; **Fellow:** Rheumatology, Univ Alabama 1986; **Fac Appt:** Asst Clin Prof Med, Louisiana State U, New Orleans

Mayes, Maureen D MD [Rhu] - **Spec Exp:** Scleroderma; **Hospital:** Meml Hermann Hosp - Texas Med Ctr, LBJ General Hosp; **Address:** 6410 Fannin St UT Prof Bldg - Ste 600, Houston, TX 77030-1501; **Phone:** 832-325-7191; **Board Cert:** Internal Medicine 1980; Rheumatology 1982; **Med School:** Eastern VA Med Sch 1976; **Resid:** Internal Medicine, Cleveland Clinic Fnd 1979; **Fellow:** Rheumatology, Cleveland Clinic Fnd 1981; **Fac Appt:** Prof Med, Univ Tex, Houston

Sessoms, Sandra Lee MD [Rhu] - **Spec Exp:** Arthritis; Lupus/SLE; Autoimmune Disease; **Hospital:** Methodist Hosp - Houston, St. Luke's Episcopal Hosp-Houston; **Address:** 4100 S Shepherd Drive, Houston, TX 77030; **Phone:** 713-524-9800; **Board Cert:** Internal Medicine 1981; Rheumatology 1984; **Med School:** Baylor Coll Med 1978; **Resid:** Internal Medicine, Baylor Coll Med 1979; **Fellow:** Rheumatology, Baylor Coll Med 1983; **Fac Appt:** Assoc Prof Med, Baylor Coll Med

West Coast and Pacific

Bobrove, Arthur M MD [Rhu] - **Spec Exp:** Psoriatic Arthritis; Ankylosing Spondylitis; Sjogren's Syndrome; Lupus/SLE; **Hospital:** Stanford Univ Hosp & Clinics; **Address:** Palo Alto Medical Fdn, 795 El Camino Real, Palo Alto, CA 94301-2302; **Phone:** 650-853-2972; **Board Cert:** Internal Medicine 1972; Rheumatology 1976; **Med School:** Temple Univ 1967; **Resid:** Internal Medicine, Univ Mich Hosp 1969; Internal Medicine, Univ Mich Hosp 1972; **Fellow:** Immunology, Stanford Univ Hosp 1974; **Fac Appt:** Clin Prof Med, Stanford Univ

Clements, Philip J MD [Rhu] - **Spec Exp:** Scleroderma; Raynaud's Disease; **Hospital:** UCLA Ronald Reagan Med Ctr; **Address:** UCLA Sch Med, Rehab 32-59, 1000 Veteran Ave, Los Angeles, CA 90095-1670; **Phone:** 310-825-8414; **Board Cert:** Internal Medicine 1972; Rheumatology 1974; **Med School:** Indiana Univ 1965; **Resid:** Internal Medicine, Cedars-Sinai Med Ctr 1971; **Fellow:** Rheumatology, UCLA Med Ctr 1974; **Fac Appt:** Prof Med, UCLA

Ehresmann, Glenn R MD [Rhu] - **Spec Exp:** Rheumatoid Arthritis; Scleroderma; Rehabilitation for Rheumatic Diseases; Lupus/SLE; **Hospital:** Keck Med Ctr of USC (page 75); **Address:** 1520 San Pablo St, Ste 1000, Los Angeles, CA 90033; **Phone:** 323-442-5100; **Board Cert:** Internal Medicine 1977; Rheumatology 1978; **Med School:** UC Irvine 1973; **Resid:** Internal Medicine, LAC-USC Med Ctr 1976; **Fellow:** Rheumatology, LAC-USC Med Ctr 1978; **Fac Appt:** Assoc Prof Med, USC-Keck School of Medicine

Rheumatology

Gershwin, Merrill E MD [Rhu] - **Spec Exp:** Allergy; Rheumatoid Arthritis; **Hospital:** UC Davis Med Ctr; **Address:** UC Davis Sch Med, Div Rheum, 451 Health Sciences Drive, Ste 6510, Davis, CA 95616; **Phone:** 530-752-2884; **Board Cert:** Internal Medicine 1974; Rheumatology 1976; Allergy & Immunology 1979; **Med School:** Stanford Univ 1971; **Resid:** Internal Medicine, Tufts-New Eng Med Ctr 1972; Allergy & Immunology, Tufts-New Eng Med Ctr 1973; **Fellow:** Rheumatology, Natl Inst Hlth 1975; Allergy & Immunology, Natl Inst Hlth 1977; **Fac Appt:** Prof Med, UC Davis

Lawry, George V MD [Rhu] - **Hospital:** UC Irvine Med Ctr; **Address:** UC Irvine Med Ctr, 101 The City Drive S, South Orange, CA 92868; **Phone:** 714-456-7662; **Board Cert:** Internal Medicine 1978; Rheumatology 1982; **Med School:** Johns Hopkins Univ 1975; **Resid:** Internal Medicine, Mass Genl Hosp 1977; Internal Medicine, Stanford Hosp 1978; **Fellow:** Rheumatology, Wadsworth VA-UCLA Med Ctr 1981; **Fac Appt:** Clin Prof Med, Univ Iowa Coll Med

Mease, Philip J MD [Rhu] - **Spec Exp:** Arthritis; Autoimmune Disease; Fibromyalgia; Lupus/SLE; **Hospital:** Swedish Med Ctr-First Hill-Seattle, Swedish Med Ctr-Cherry Hill Campus; **Address:** 1101 Madison St, Ste 1000, Seattle, WA 98104; **Phone:** 206-386-2000; **Board Cert:** Internal Medicine 1980; Rheumatology 1982; **Med School:** Stanford Univ 1977; **Resid:** Internal Medicine, Univ Wash Med Ctr 1981; **Fellow:** Rheumatology, Univ Wash Med Ctr 1982; **Fac Appt:** Clin Prof Med, Univ Wash

Peng, Stanford L MD [Rhu] - **Spec Exp:** Lupus/SLE; Inflammatory Arthritis; Scleroderma; Vasculitis; **Hospital:** Virginia Mason Med Ctr; **Address:** Virginia Mason, 1100 9th Ave, Ste X6-RHE, Seattle, WA 98101; **Phone:** 206-223-6824; **Board Cert:** Rheumatology 2002; **Med School:** Yale Univ 1997; **Resid:** Internal Medicine, Univ Penn Hosp 1999; **Fellow:** Rheumatology, Brigham & Women's Hosp 2002

Wallace, Daniel J MD [Rhu] - **Spec Exp:** Lupus/SLE; Rheumatoid Arthritis; Scleroderma; **Hospital:** Cedars-Sinai Med Ctr, UCLA Ronald Reagan Med Ctr; **Address:** 8737 Beverly Blvd, Ste 302, Los Angeles, CA 90048-1828; **Phone:** 310-652-0920; **Board Cert:** Internal Medicine 1978; Rheumatology 1982; **Med School:** USC Sch Med 1974; **Resid:** Internal Medicine, Cedars-Sinai Med Ctr 1977; **Fellow:** Rheumatology, UCLA Med Ctr 1979; **Fac Appt:** Clin Prof Med, UCLA

Wener, Mark MD [Rhu] - **Spec Exp:** Lupus/SLE; Vasculitis; Scleroderma; Autoimmune Disease; **Hospital:** Univ Wash Med Ctr, Harborview Med Ctr; **Address:** Univ Washington Med Ctr, Medical Specialties, 1959 NE Pacific St, Box 356166, Seattle, WA 98195; **Phone:** 206-598-4615; **Board Cert:** Internal Medicine 1978; Rheumatology 1980; Clinical & Laboratory Immunology 1986; **Med School:** Washington Univ, St Louis 1974; **Resid:** Internal Medicine, Univ Iowa Hosps 1978; **Fellow:** Rheumatology, Univ Iowa Hosp 1980; Immunology, Univ Washington Med Ctr 1981; **Fac Appt:** Prof Med, Univ Wash

Wofsy, David MD [Rhu] - **Spec Exp:** Rheumatoid Arthritis; Lupus/SLE; Autoimmune Disease; Clinical Trials; **Hospital:** VA Med Ctr - San Francisco, UCSF Med Ctr; **Address:** 533 Parnassus Ave, Box 0633, San Francisco, CA 94143-0633; **Phone:** 415-750-2104; **Board Cert:** Internal Medicine 1977; Rheumatology 1980; **Med School:** UCSD 1974; **Resid:** Internal Medicine, UCSF Hosps 1977; **Fellow:** Rheumatology, UCSF 1979; **Fac Appt:** Prof Med, UCSF

Cleveland Clinic

Every life deserves world class care.

Rheumatology

Cleveland Clinic's Department of Rheumatic and Immunologic Diseases has a long-standing commitment to excellence and innovation in the research and care of patients with illnesses such as arthritis, osteoporosis and vasculitis. Since 1993, *U.S.News & World Report* has consistently ranked it among the nation's top 10 rheumatology programs.

Arthritis: Our department's Arthritis & Musculoskeletal Center is a multidisciplinary clinic combining the expertise of non-operative orthopaedists and rheumatologists in one location for patients with joint pain. Our doctors have a specific interest in joint pain problems, including rheumatoid arthritis and osteoarthritis, and work together to provide patients with the highest level of care so that they can return to their usual level of activity.

Osteoporosis: Our Center for Osteoporosis and Metabolic Bone Diseases is devoted to the evaluation and treatment of patients with osteoporosis and other diseases that affect bones. The Center's goal is to evaluate patients at an early stage to prevent the complications and additional disease manifestations of osteoporosis and other treatable diseases.

Vasculitis: Cleveland Clinic's Center for Vasculitis Care and Research aims to ensure the best possible care for patients with vasculitis, discover the causes of these diseases, identify improved therapies and alleviate discomfort. The department has established extensive collaborations with other Cleveland Clinic departments to bring complementary skills to both patient care and research.

Autoimmune Disease: Our Department of Rheumatic and Immunologic Diseases also provides expert care for autoimmune diseases, such as systemic lupus, scleroderma, myositis, polychondritis and vasculitis.

Cleveland Clinic
Rheumatic and Immunologic Diseases
9500 Euclid Avenue
Cleveland, OH 44195

clevelandclinic.org/rheumtopdocs

Offering Same-Day Appointments
Call 800.274.2009.

Treatment Guides
Cleveland Clinic has developed comprehensive treatment guides for many diseases and conditions. To download our free treatment guides, visit clevelandclinic.org/treatmentguides.

Online Medical Second Opinion
Cleveland Clinic's My**Consult** Online Medical Second Opinion program securely connects patients to our physician specialists for more than 1,000 life-changing or life-threatening diagnoses all by the click of a mouse. To learn more, log onto eclevelandclinic.org/myconsult or call 800.223.2273, ext. 43223.

Special Assistance for Out-of-State Patients
Cleveland Clinic Global Patient Services offers a complimentary Medical Concierge service for patients who travel from outside of Ohio. Call 800.223.2273, ext. 55580 or email medicalconcierge@ccf.org.

RHEUMATOLOGY

Rheumatologists at NYU Langone Medical Center are dedicated to the diagnosis and treatment of patients with rheumatic illnesses, particularly autoimmune diseases. U.S. News and World Report has repeatedly recognized the Division of Rheumatology as one of the best in the country, ranking #8 nationwide in the 2011-2012 "Best Hospitals" survey. The division provides care at NYU Langone's premier outpatient facility, the Center for Musculoskeletal Care, the Hospital for Joint Diseases, our internationally-renowned inpatient musculoskeletal facility, and at the medical center's Tisch Hospital.

Arthritis and Autoimmunity: We offer a comprehensive program for the prevention, diagnosis and treatment of all rheumatologic conditions. Patients also have access to complete rheumatologic evaluations, orthopaedic and neurological consultative services, and participation in clinical trials using the most advanced interventional therapies, highly sophisticated diagnostic testing, and complementary medicine.

Behçet's Syndrome: We have the largest North American Behçet's Center for research and the evaluation and treatment of patients with Behçet's Syndrome, a disease that involves inflammation of the blood vessels.

Biological Treatment: Biological treatments for inflammatory arthritis, rheumatoid arthritis, lupus, psoriatic arthritis, vasculitis, and osteoporosis are administered by the Medical Center's infusion centers.

Lupus: The Center for Lupus Care and Research is devoted to the treatment and research of patients with this autoimmune disease. Patients have access to world renowned specialists in lupus, lupus and pregnancy, and related sub-specialties.

Osteoporosis: We offer comprehensive care for the prevention, evaluation and treatment of osteoporosis, including state-of-the art bone densitometers, a range of advanced drug therapies, and programs in balance training and exercise.

Psoriatic Arthritis: Patients at the Psoriatic Arthritis Center, a collaborative effort with the Department of Dermatology, are seen by both a rheumatologist and dermatologist who specialize in psoriasis and psoriatic arthritis.

We are also leaders in rheumatology research, focusing on the study of drugs, drug delivery systems and protocols, and the roles genes play in the development and treatment of rheumatic diseases, positioning us at the forefront of basic science and translational research, personalized medicine and the genetics of rheumatic diseases. The Peter D. Seligman Center for Advanced Therapeutics, renowned for breakthrough research in arthritis and Systematic Lupus Erythematosus, conducts clinical studies using a wide variety of newly developed therapies.

Sports Medicine

a subspecialty of Internal Medicine, Family Practice, Pediatrics, Physical Medicine & Rehabilitation, or Orthopaedics

A specialist trained to be responsible for continuous care in the field of sports medicine, not only for the enhancement of health and fitness, but also for the prevention of injury and illness. A sports medicine physician must have knowledge and experience in the promotion of wellness and the prevention of injury. Knowledge about special areas of medicine such as exercise physiology, biomechanics, nutrition, psychology, physical rehabilitation, epidemiology, physical evaluation, injuries (treatment and prevention and referral practice) and the role of exercise in promoting a healthy life style are essential to the practice of sports medicine. The sports medicine physician requires special education to provide the knowledge to improve the healthcare of the individual engaged in physical exercise (sports) whether as an individual or in team participation.

Training Required: Three years in internal medicine, family practice, or pediatrics or seven years in orthopaedics *plus* additional training and examination for certification in sports medicine.

For more information about the main specialties of these physicians, see **Internal Medicine, Family Practice, Pediatrics, Physical Medicine & Rehabilitation, Orthopaedics** section(s).

Sports Medicine

New England

Asnis, Peter MD [SM] - **Spec Exp:** Arthroscopic Surgery-Hip; Shoulder Injuries; Rotator Cuff Surgery; Ligament Reconstruction; **Hospital:** Mass Genl Hosp; **Address:** Massachusetts General Hospital, 55 Fruit St, Yawkey 3200, Boston, MA 02114; **Phone:** 617-643-0803; **Board Cert:** Orthopaedic Surgery 2008; **Med School:** Cornell Univ-Weill Med Coll 1999; **Resid:** Orthopaedic Surgery, Hosp Special Surg 2005; **Fellow:** Orthopaedic Sports Medicine, Mass Genl Hosp 2006

Gill IV, Thomas J MD [SM] - **Spec Exp:** Knee Injuries; Shoulder Injuries; Arthroscopic Surgery; **Hospital:** Mass Genl Hosp; **Address:** MGH Sports Medicine Ctr, 175 Cambridge St Fl 4, CPZS 4, Boston, MA 02114-2723; **Phone:** 617-726-7797; **Board Cert:** Orthopaedic Surgery 2000; **Med School:** Harvard Med Sch 1990; **Resid:** Orthopaedic Surgery, Hosp Special Surgery 1992; Orthopaedic Surgery, Brigham & Women's Hosp 1996; **Fellow:** Sports Medicine, Steadman Hawkins Clinic 1998; **Fac Appt:** Assoc Prof OrS, Harvard Med Sch

Micheli, Lyle J MD [SM] - **Spec Exp:** Pediatric Sports Medicine; Dance/Ballet Injuries; Osteochondritis Dissecans (OCD); Knee Injuries/ACL; **Hospital:** Children's Hospital - Boston, Beth Israel Deaconess Med Ctr - Boston; **Address:** Chldns Hosp, Div Sports Medicine, 319 Longwood Ave, Boston, MA 02115; **Phone:** 617-355-3501; **Board Cert:** Orthopaedic Surgery 1973; **Med School:** Harvard Med Sch 1966; **Resid:** Surgery, Univ Hosps 1968; Orthopaedic Surgery, Mass Genl Hosp/Chldns Hosp 1972; **Fellow:** Pediatric Orthopaedic Surgery, Orth Rsch Soc-Traveling Fell 1973; **Fac Appt:** Assoc Clin Prof OrS, Harvard Med Sch

Scheller, Arnold D MD [SM] - **Spec Exp:** Sports Injuries; Ankle Surgery; Shoulder Surgery; Knee Surgery; **Hospital:** New England Bapt Hosp; **Address:** Pro Sports Orthopaedics, 235 Cypres St, Ste 300, Brookline, MA 02445; **Phone:** 617-738-8642; **Board Cert:** Orthopaedic Surgery 1983; **Med School:** Rush Med Coll 1973; **Resid:** Orthopaedic Surgery, New England Hosp 1983; **Fac Appt:** Asst Clin Prof OrS, Tufts Univ

Steiner, Mark E MD [SM] - **Spec Exp:** Shoulder Injuries; Knee Injuries; Arthroscopic Surgery; **Hospital:** New England Bapt Hosp; **Address:** 830 Boylston St, Ste 205, Chestnut Hill, MA 02467; **Phone:** 617-739-2003; **Board Cert:** Orthopaedic Surgery 2008; **Med School:** Columbia P&S 1978; **Resid:** Surgery, Mass General Hosp 1980; Orthopaedic Surgery, Mass General Hosp 1984; **Fellow:** Sports Medicine, U Oklahoma Med Ctr 1985

Mid Atlantic

Altchek, David MD [SM] - **Spec Exp:** Shoulder Surgery; Elbow Surgery; Knee Surgery; Arthroscopic Surgery; **Hospital:** Hosp For Special Surgery (page 60), NY-Presby/Weill Cornell Med Ctr, NY (page 65); **Address:** Hospital for Special Surgery, 535 E 70th St, New York, NY 10021; **Phone:** 212-606-1909; **Board Cert:** Orthopaedic Surgery 2011; **Med School:** Cornell Univ-Weill Med Coll 1982; **Resid:** Orthopaedic Surgery, Hosp for Special Surg 1987; **Fellow:** Sports Medicine, Hosp for Special Surg 1988; **Fac Appt:** Assoc Prof OrS, Cornell Univ-Weill Med Coll

Bradley, James P MD [SM] - **Spec Exp:** Reconstructive Surgery; Shoulder Surgery; Knee Surgery; **Hospital:** UPMC St Margaret, UPMC Shadyside; **Address:** 200 Delafield Rd, Ste 4010, Pittsburgh, PA 15215; **Phone:** 412-784-5783; **Board Cert:** Orthopaedic Surgery 2001; **Med School:** Georgetown Univ 1982; **Resid:** Surgery, Univ Tennessee Affil Hosp 1984; Orthopaedic Surgery, Univ Hlth Ctr 1987; **Fellow:** Sports Medicine, Kerlan-Jobe Ortho Clinic 1988; **Fac Appt:** Assoc Prof OrS, Univ Pittsburgh

Burke, Charles J MD [SM] - **Spec Exp:** Knee Injuries; Shoulder Injuries; **Hospital:** UPMC St Margaret, UPMC Shadyside; **Address:** 200 Delafield Rd, Ste 4010, Pittsburgh, PA 15215; **Phone:** 412-784-5783; **Board Cert:** Orthopaedic Surgery 2009; **Med School:** Univ Cincinnati 1981; **Resid:** Therapeutic Radiology, Univ Mass Med Ctr 1983; Orthopaedic Surgery, Univ Pittsburgh Med Ctr 1986; **Fac Appt:** Asst Prof OrS, Univ Pittsburgh

Ciccotti, Michael G MD [SM] - **Spec Exp:** Knee Reconstruction; Elbow Reconstruction; Shoulder Reconstruction; Arthroscopic Surgery; **Hospital:** Thomas Jefferson Univ Hosp, Bryn Mawr Hosp; **Address:** Rothman Institute, 925 Chestnut St Fl 5, Philadelphia, PA 19107; **Phone:** 800-321-9999; **Board Cert:** Orthopaedic Surgery 2005; **Med School:** Georgetown Univ 1986; **Resid:** Orthopaedic Surgery, Thos Jefferson Univ Med Ctr 1991; **Fellow:** Sports Medicine, Kerlan-Jobe Clinic/USC 1992; **Fac Appt:** Assoc Prof OrS, Jefferson Med Coll

Harner, Christopher D MD [SM] - **Spec Exp:** Knee Injuries; **Hospital:** UPMC South Side-Out Pt Ctr; **Address:** UPMC Ctr for Sports Med, 3200 S Water St, Pittsburgh, PA 15203; **Phone:** 412-432-3661; **Board Cert:** Orthopaedic Surgery 2010; Orthopaedic Sports Medicine 2007; **Med School:** Univ Mich Med Sch 1981; **Resid:** Orthopaedic Surgery, Univ Pittsburgh 1986; **Fellow:** Sports Medicine/Knee Surgery, Salt Lake City Knee & Sport 1987; **Fac Appt:** Prof OrS, Univ Pittsburgh

Hershman, Elliott MD [SM] - **Spec Exp:** Knee Injuries; Knee Surgery; Arthroscopic Surgery; Ligament Reconstruction; **Hospital:** Lenox Hill Hosp; **Address:** 130 E 77th St Fl 7, New York, NY 10075; **Phone:** 212-744-8114; **Board Cert:** Orthopaedic Surgery 2008; **Med School:** Univ Rochester 1979; **Resid:** Orthopaedic Surgery, Lenox Hill Hosp 1984; **Fellow:** Sports Medicine, Cleveland Clinic 1985; **Fac Appt:** Asst Clin Prof OrS, Mount Sinai Sch Med

Levine, William MD [SM] - **Spec Exp:** Arthroscopic Surgery; Shoulder & Elbow Surgery; Knee Injuries; **Hospital:** NY-Presby/Columbia Univ Med Ctr, NY (page 65); **Address:** 622 W 168th St, Ste PH-11, New York, NY 10032; **Phone:** 212-305-0762; **Board Cert:** Orthopaedic Surgery 2010; Orthopaedic Sports Medicine 2008; **Med School:** Case West Res Univ 1990; **Resid:** Surgery, Beth Israel Hosp 1991; Orthopaedic Surgery, New Eng Med Ctr Hosps 1995; **Fellow:** Shoulder Surgery, Columbia-Presby Med Ctr 1996; Sports Medicine, Univ MD Med Ctr 1998; **Fac Appt:** Clin Prof OrS, Columbia P&S

Metzl, Jordan D MD [SM] - **Spec Exp:** Adolescent Sports Medicine; Running Injuries; Dance/Ballet Injuries; **Hospital:** Hosp For Special Surgery (page 60); **Address:** 519 E 72nd St, Ste 206, New York, NY 10021; **Phone:** 212-606-1678; **Board Cert:** Sports Medicine 2001; **Med School:** Univ MO-Columbia Sch Med 1993; **Resid:** Pediatrics, New Eng Med Ctr 1996; **Fellow:** Sports Medicine, Vanderbilt Univ Med Ctr 1996; Sports Medicine, Hosp Special Surgery 1997; **Fac Appt:** Asst Prof Ped, Cornell Univ-Weill Med Coll

Nisonson, Barton MD [SM] - **Spec Exp:** Shoulder & Knee Surgery; Arthroscopic Surgery; Knee Replacement; **Hospital:** Lenox Hill Hosp; **Address:** 130 E 77th St, New York, NY 10021-1851; **Phone:** 212-570-9120; **Board Cert:** Orthopaedic Surgery 1974; **Med School:** Columbia P&S 1966; **Resid:** Surgery, Columbia-Presby Med Ctr 1968; Orthopaedic Surgery, Columbia-Presby Med Ctr 1973

Rodeo, Scott A MD [SM] - **Spec Exp:** Knee Injuries; Cartilage Damage; **Hospital:** Hosp For Special Surgery (page 60); **Address:** Hosp for Special Surgery, 535 E 70th St, New York, NY 10021; **Phone:** 212-606-1513; **Board Cert:** Orthopaedic Surgery 2009; Orthopaedic Sports Medicine 2007; **Med School:** Cornell Univ-Weill Med Coll 1989; **Resid:** Orthopaedic Surgery, Hosp Special Surgery 1994; **Fellow:** Sports Medicine, Hosp Special Surgery 1996; **Fac Appt:** Assoc Clin Prof OrS, Cornell Univ-Weill Med Coll

Sports Medicine

Sennett, Brian J MD [SM] - **Spec Exp:** Arthroscopic Surgery; Cartilage Damage; Sports Injuries; **Hospital:** Hosp Univ Penn - UPHS (page 68); **Address:** Penn Sports Medicine Center, Weightman Hall, Fl 1, 235 S 33rd St, Philadelphia, PA 19104; **Phone:** 800-789-7366; **Board Cert:** Orthopaedic Surgery 2009; Orthopaedic Sports Medicine 2008; **Med School:** Univ Pennsylvania 1988; **Resid:** Orthopaedic Surgery, Hosp Univ Penn 1993; **Fellow:** Sports Medicine, Univ Penn Sports Med Ctr 1994; Hand Surgery, Hosp Univ Penn 1994; **Fac Appt:** Assoc Prof OrS, Univ Pennsylvania

Southeast

Andrews, James R MD [SM] - **Spec Exp:** Shoulder Surgery; Elbow Surgery; Knee Surgery; **Hospital:** Baptist Hosp - Pensacola, St. Vincent's Hosp - Birmingham; **Address:** Inst Orthopaedics & Sports Medicine, 1040 Gulf Breeze Pkwy, Gulf Breeze, FL 32561; **Phone:** 850-916-8700; **Board Cert:** Orthopaedic Surgery 1974; **Med School:** Louisiana State U, New Orleans 1967; **Resid:** Orthopaedic Surgery, USPHS Hosp 1969; Orthopaedic Surgery, Touro Infirm-Tulane 1970; **Fellow:** Orthopaedic Sports Medicine, Univ Va Med Ctr 1972; **Fac Appt:** Clin Prof OrS, Univ Alabama

Byrd, J.W. Thomas MD [SM] - **Spec Exp:** Arthroscopic Surgery; **Hospital:** Baptist Hosp - Nashville; **Address:** Nashville Sports Med & Ortho Ctr, 2011 Church St, Ste 100, Nashville, TN 37203; **Phone:** 615-284-5800; **Board Cert:** Orthopaedic Surgery 2011; Orthopaedic Sports Medicine 2007; **Med School:** Vanderbilt Univ 1982; **Resid:** Orthopaedic Surgery, Univ Louisville Hosp 1987; **Fellow:** Sports Medicine, Amer Sprts Inst 1988; Joint Replacement Surgery, New England Baptist Hosp 1989

Estwanik, Joseph J MD [SM] - **Hospital:** Carolinas Specialty Hosp; **Address:** Metrolina Ortho & Sports Med Clinic, 335 Bellingsley Rd, Ste 201, Charlotte, NC 28211; **Phone:** 704-334-4663; **Board Cert:** Orthopaedic Surgery 1979; **Med School:** Wake Forest Univ 1973; **Resid:** Orthopaedic Surgery, Cleveland Clinic 1976; Orthopaedic Surgery, North Carolina Baptist Hosp 1978; **Fac Appt:** Asst Prof Oph, Wake Forest Univ

Garth Jr, William P MD [SM] - **Spec Exp:** Knee Ligament Reconstruction; Shoulder Reconstruction; **Hospital:** Univ of Ala Hosp at Birmingham, Children's Hospital - Birmingham; **Address:** UAB Sports Medicine, 1600 7th Ave S, Ste 402, Birmingham, AL 35233-1711; **Phone:** 205-934-1041; **Board Cert:** Orthopaedic Surgery 1980; Orthopaedic Sports Medicine 2007; **Med School:** Tulane Univ 1973; **Resid:** Surgery, Duke Univ Hosp 1975; Orthopaedic Surgery, Campbell Clinic 1979; **Fellow:** Sports Medicine, Sports Med Clinic 1984; **Fac Appt:** Prof OrS, Univ Alabama

Speer, Kevin P MD [SM] - **Spec Exp:** Shoulder Surgery; Arthroscopic Surgery; Shoulder Replacement; **Hospital:** Duke Health Raleigh; **Address:** Southeastern Ortho Sports Medicine, 3404 Wake Forest Rd, Ste 201, Raleigh, NC 27609; **Phone:** 919-256-1511; **Board Cert:** Orthopaedic Surgery 2005; **Med School:** Johns Hopkins Univ 1985; **Resid:** Orthopaedic Surgery, Duke Univ Med Ctr 1991; **Fellow:** Sports Medicine, Hosp Special Surgery 1992; **Fac Appt:** Assoc Prof OrS, Duke Univ

Xerogeanes, John W MD [SM] - **Spec Exp:** Knee Surgery; Shoulder Surgery; Knee Injuries/ACL; Arthroscopic Surgery; **Hospital:** Emory Univ Hosp; **Address:** Emory Sports Medicine Ctr, 59 Executive Park S, Ste 1000, Atlanta, GA 30029; **Phone:** 404-778-3350; **Board Cert:** Orthopaedic Surgery 2001; Orthopaedic Sports Medicine 2008; **Med School:** Emory Univ 1992; **Resid:** Orthopaedic Surgery, Univ Pittsburgh Med Ctr 1997; **Fellow:** Sports Medicine, Steadman-Hawkins Clinic 1998; **Fac Appt:** Assoc Prof OrS, Emory Univ

Midwest

Arendt, Elizabeth A MD [SM] - **Spec Exp:** Sports Medicine; Knee Ligament Reconstruction; Knee Injuries; **Hospital:** Univ Minn Med Ctr, Fairview - Riverside Campus; **Address:** 2512 S 7th St, rm 102, Minneapolis, MN 55454; **Phone:** 612-273-9400; **Board Cert:** Orthopaedic Surgery 2008; Orthopaedic Sports Medicine 2007; **Med School:** Univ Rochester 1979; **Resid:** Surgery, Univ Rochester Med Ctr 1981; Orthopaedic Surgery, Univ Rochester Med Ctr 1984; **Fellow:** Sports Medicine, Univ Minn Med Ctr 1985; **Fac Appt:** Prof OrS, Univ Miss

Bush-Joseph, Charles MD [SM] - **Spec Exp:** Knee Reconstruction; Cartilage Damage; Sports Medicine; Rotator Cuff Surgery; **Hospital:** Rush Univ Med Ctr, Rush Oak Park Hosp; **Address:** Midwest Orthopaedics at Rush, 1725 W Harrison St, Ste 1063, Chicago, IL 60612; **Phone:** 312-243-4244; **Board Cert:** Orthopaedic Surgery 2003; Orthopaedic Sports Medicine 2007; **Med School:** Univ Mich Med Sch 1983; **Resid:** Orthopaedic Surgery, Rush Med Ctr 1988; **Fellow:** Sports Medicine, Cincinnati Sports Med Ctr 1989; **Fac Appt:** Prof OrS, Rush Med Coll

Ho, Sherwin S W MD [SM] - **Spec Exp:** Shoulder & Knee Surgery; Arthroscopic Surgery; Cartilage Damage; **Hospital:** Univ of Chicago Med Ctr; **Address:** Univ Chicago Dept Surgery, 5841 S Maryland Ave, MC 3079, Chicago, IL 60637-3079; **Phone:** 773-702-5978; **Board Cert:** Orthopaedic Surgery 2005; Orthopaedic Sports Medicine 2008; **Med School:** Univ Hawaii JA Burns Sch Med 1985; **Resid:** Orthopaedic Surgery, Univ Hawaii Med Ctr 1991; **Fellow:** Sports Medicine, Univ Chicago 1992; **Fac Appt:** Assoc Prof S, Univ Chicago-Pritzker Sch Med

Miniaci, Anthony MD [SM] - **Spec Exp:** Shoulder Reconstruction; Shoulder Arthroscopic Surgery; Knee Reconstruction; Cartilage Damage; **Hospital:** Cleveland Clin (page 56); **Address:** Cleveland Clinic, Sports Hlth Ctr, 5555 Transportation Blvd, Garfield Heights, OH 44125; **Phone:** 216-518-3444; **Med School:** Univ Western Ontario 1982; **Resid:** Orthopaedic Surgery, Univ Western Ontario 1987; **Fellow:** Sports Medicine, Kerlan-Jobe Orthopaedic Clin 1989; Orthopaedic Research, Univ Calgary 1990; **Fac Appt:** Prof S, Case West Res Univ

Paletta, George A MD [SM] - **Spec Exp:** Ankle Surgery; Knee Surgery; Shoulder & Elbow Surgery; **Address:** The Orthopaedic Ctr of St Louis, 14825 N Outer Forty Rd, Ste 200, Chesterfield, MO 63017; **Phone:** 314-336-2555; **Board Cert:** Orthopaedic Surgery 2009; **Med School:** Johns Hopkins Univ 1988; **Resid:** Orthopaedic Surgery, Cornell Univ Med Ctr 1994; **Fellow:** Sports Medicine, Cleveland Clin Fnd 1995; Pediatric Sports Medicine, Chldns Hosp Michigan; **Fac Appt:** Assoc Prof OrS, Washington Univ, St Louis

Great Plains and Mountains

Saint-Phard, Deborah MD [SM] - **Spec Exp:** Sports Medicine-Women; Spinal Rehabilitation; **Hospital:** Univ of CO Hosp - Anschutz Inpatient Pav; **Address:** Univ Sports Med, 2000 S Colorado Blvd, Ste 4500, Denver, CO 80222; **Phone:** 720-848-8200; **Board Cert:** Physical Medicine & Rehabilitation 2007; Pain Medicine 2004; Sports Medicine 2008; **Med School:** Temple Univ 1992; **Resid:** Physical Medicine & Rehabilitation, Univ Colorado Med Ctr 1996; **Fellow:** Sports Medicine, Mayo Clin 1997; **Fac Appt:** Assoc Prof PMR, Univ Colorado

Sports Medicine

Southwest

Jones, Deryk G MD [SM] - **Spec Exp:** Arthroscopic Surgery; Cartilage Damage & Transplant; **Hospital:** Ochsner Med Ctr-Kenner; **Address:** Ochsner Sports Medicine, 1201 S Clearview Pkwy, Elmwood, LA 70123; **Phone:** 504-736-4800; **Board Cert:** Orthopaedic Surgery 2000; Orthopaedic Sports Medicine 2009; **Med School:** Stanford Univ 1991; **Resid:** Orthopaedic Surgery, Harvard Combined Prog 1997; **Fellow:** Sports Medicine, Univ Pittsburgh Med Ctr 1998; **Fac Appt:** Asst Clin Prof OrS, Tulane Univ

West Coast and Pacific

Fronek, Jan MD [SM] - **Spec Exp:** Knee Injuries; Shoulder Injuries; Arthroscopic Surgery; Rotator Cuff Surgery; **Hospital:** Scripps Green Hosp; **Address:** Scripps Clinic, 10666 N Torrey Pines Rd, MS B4, La Jolla, CA 92037; **Phone:** 858-554-9753; **Board Cert:** Orthopaedic Surgery 2009; **Med School:** Univ Rochester 1978; **Resid:** Orthopaedic Surgery, UCSD Med Ctr 1984; **Fellow:** Sports Medicine, Hosp Special Surgery 1985

Gambardella, Ralph A MD [SM] - **Spec Exp:** Cartilage Damage; Shoulder & Elbow Surgery; Knee Surgery; **Hospital:** Marina Del Rey Hosp, White Memorial Med Ctr; **Address:** Kerlan-Jobe Clinic, 6801 Park Terr, Ste 400, Los Angeles, CA 90045; **Phone:** 310-665-7200; **Board Cert:** Orthopaedic Surgery 1985; **Med School:** USC Sch Med 1977; **Resid:** Orthopaedic Surgery, USC Med Ctr 1982; **Fellow:** Sports Medicine, Southwestern Ortho Grp 1983; **Fac Appt:** Assoc Clin Prof S, USC Sch Med

Ma, C Benjamin MD [SM] - **Spec Exp:** Shoulder Surgery; Knee Surgery; Arthroscopic Surgery; **Hospital:** UCSF Med Ctr; **Address:** Sports Medicine Center, 1500 Owens St, San Francisco, CA 94158; **Phone:** 415-353-2808; **Board Cert:** Orthopaedic Surgery 2005; Orthopaedic Sports Medicine 2008; **Med School:** Johns Hopkins Univ 1996; **Resid:** Orthopaedic Surgery, Univ Pittsburgh Med Ctr 2002; **Fellow:** Shoulder Surgery, Hosp for Special Surg 2003; Macular Disease, Hosp for Special Surg 2003

Mirzayan, Raffy MD [SM] - **Spec Exp:** Arthroscopic Surgery; Shoulder & Elbow Surgery; Ligament Reconstruction; Knee Injuries; **Hospital:** Kaiser Permanente Baldwin Pk Med Ctr; **Address:** Kaiser Permanente Med Ctr, Orthopaedics, 1011 Baldwin Park Blvd, Baldwin Park, CA 91706; **Phone:** 626-851-5256; **Board Cert:** Orthopaedic Surgery 2003; Sports Medicine 2007; **Med School:** USC Sch Med 1995; **Resid:** Orthopaedic Surgery, LAC/USC Med Ctr 2000; **Fellow:** Sports Medicine, Kerlan Jobe Ortho Clin 2001; **Fac Appt:** Clin Prof OrS, USC-Keck School of Medicine

Schechter, David L MD [SM] - **Spec Exp:** Pain-Back; Sports Injuries; Muscle Pain-Stress Related; **Hospital:** Cedars-Sinai Med Ctr; **Address:** 8500 Wilshire Blvd, Ste 705, Beverly Hills, CA 90211; **Phone:** 310-657-1022; **Board Cert:** Family Medicine 2008; Sports Medicine 2003; **Med School:** NYU Sch Med 1984; **Resid:** Family Medicine, UCLA/Santa Monica Hosp 1987; **Fac Appt:** Assoc Clin Prof FMed, USC Sch Med

Teitz, Carol C MD [SM] - **Spec Exp:** Sports Injuries; Musculoskeletal Injuries in Dancers; **Hospital:** Univ Wash Med Ctr; **Address:** University of Washington, Box 354060, Bank of America Arena, 3950 Montlake Blvd NE, rm 148, Seattle, WA 98195; **Phone:** 206-543-1552; **Board Cert:** Orthopaedic Surgery 1981; Orthopaedic Sports Medicine 2007; **Med School:** Yale Univ 1974; **Resid:** Orthopaedic Surgery, Univ Wash Affil Hosps 1980; **Fellow:** Arthroscopic Surgery, J McGinty MD, Newton-Wellesley Hosp 1983; **Fac Appt:** Prof OrS, Univ Wash

Cleveland Clinic

Every life deserves world class care.

Cleveland Clinic
Sports Health
9500 Euclid Avenue
Cleveland, OH 44195

clevelandclinic.org/
sportstopdocs

Offering Same-Day Appointments
Call 800.274.2009.

Sports Health

Cleveland Clinic Sports Health brings together top orthopaedic surgeons, primary care sports medicine physicians, physical therapists, athletic trainers, nutritionists, radiologists and exercise physiologists to keep athletes in the game and get injured players back on the field sooner.

All athletes deserve the best sports-related care and treatment that is focused, one-on-one and state-of-the art.

At Cleveland Clinic Sports Health, our experts treat athletes in all sports and at all ages and skill levels.

Our comprehensive services include rehabilitation and injury prevention, athletic training, imaging, nutrition, evaluation and management for sports-related concussions, treating injuries and improving future performance. Our staff is involved in research every day to discover new treatments to improve the patient care of tomorrow.

Our world-renowned team of physicians is trained in diagnosing and treating the unique problems of amateur to high-performance athletes. We've provided the physicians for Cleveland's professional teams for more than 25 years.

Athletic Performance

Sports Rehabilitation and Injury Prevention Programs offer services such as motion analysis, injury prevention, sport-specific evaluations and rehabilitation programs — all tailored to particular sports.

Cleveland Clinic Sports Health is dedicated to building performance and strives to provide athletes with advanced understanding of body mechanics and capabilities, unique as each athlete. Performance Training Systems are strength- building and functional fitness training programs designed to meet the goals of each athlete.

Treatment Guides

Cleveland Clinic has developed comprehensive treatment guides for many diseases and conditions. To download our free treatment guides, visit clevelandclinic.org/treatmentguides.

Online Medical Second Opinion

Cleveland Clinic's My**Consult** Online Medical Second Opinion program securely connects patients to our physician specialists for more than 1,000 life-changing or life-threatening diagnoses all by the click of a mouse. To learn more, log onto eclevelandclinic.org/myconsult or call 800.223.2273, ext. 43223.

Special Assistance for Out-of-State Patients

Cleveland Clinic Global Patient Services offers a complimentary Medical Concierge service for patients who travel from outside of Ohio. Call 800.223.2273, ext. 55580 or email medicalconcierge@ccf.org.

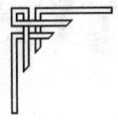

The Best in American Medicine
www.CastleConnolly.com

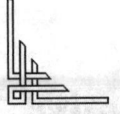
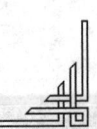

Surgery

A surgeon manages a broad spectrum of surgical conditions affecting almost any area of the body. The surgeon establishes the diagnosis and provides the preoperative, operative and postoperative care to surgical patients and is usually responsible for the comprehensive management of the trauma victim and the critically ill surgical patient.

The surgeon uses a variety of diagnostic techniques, including endoscopy, for observing internal structures and may use specialized instruments during operative procedures. A general surgeon is expected to be familiar with the salient features of other surgical specialties in order to recognize problems in those areas and to know when to refer a patient to another specialist.

Training Required: Five years

For a description of the subspecialty **Hand Surgery, Pediatric Surgery** and **Vascular Surgery** see the corresponding section(s).

SURGERY

New England

Ashley, Stanley W MD [S] - **Spec Exp:** Gastrointestinal Cancer & Surgery; **Hospital:** Brigham and Women's Hosp (page 57), Dana-Farber Cancer Inst (page 57); **Address:** Brigham & Womens Hosp, Dept Surgery, 75 Francis St, Boston, MA 02115; **Phone:** 617-732-6730; **Board Cert:** Surgery 2004; Surgical Critical Care 1999; **Med School:** Cornell Univ-Weill Med Coll 1981; **Resid:** Surgery, Barnes Jewish Med Ctr 1989; **Fac Appt:** Prof S, Harvard Med Sch

Ballantyne, Garth H MD [S] - **Spec Exp:** Laparoscopic Surgery; Gastroesophageal Reflux Disease (GERD); Colon Cancer; Obesity/Bariatric Surgery; **Hospital:** Lawrence & Meml Hosp; **Address:** 4 Shaw's Cove, Ste 201, New London, CT 06320; **Phone:** 860-444-7675; **Board Cert:** Surgery 2006; Colon & Rectal Surgery 1985; **Med School:** Columbia P&S 1977; **Resid:** Surgery, UCLA Med Ctr 1980; Surgery, Northwestern Meml Hosp 1982; **Fellow:** Colon & Rectal Surgery, Mayo Clinic 1984

Becker, James M MD [S] - **Spec Exp:** Inflammatory Bowel Disease; Gastrointestinal Cancer; Gastrointestinal Surgery; **Hospital:** Boston Med Ctr; **Address:** 88 E Newton St, rm C500, Boston, MA 02118-2393; **Phone:** 617-638-8600; **Board Cert:** Surgery 1999; **Med School:** Case West Res Univ 1975; **Resid:** Surgery, Univ Utah Med Ctr 1980; **Fellow:** Research, Mayo Clinic 1982; **Fac Appt:** Prof S, Boston Univ

Brooks, David C MD [S] - **Spec Exp:** Gastrointestinal Surgery; **Hospital:** Brigham and Women's Hosp (page 57); **Address:** Brigham & Women's Hospital, Dept Surgery, 75 Francis St, ASB II Fl 3, Boston, MA 02115; **Phone:** 617-732-6337; **Board Cert:** Surgery 2003; **Med School:** Brown Univ 1976; **Resid:** Surgery, Brigham & Women's Hosp 1983; **Fac Appt:** Assoc Prof S, Harvard Med Sch

Burke, Peter A MD [S] - **Spec Exp:** Trauma; Critical Care; **Hospital:** Boston Med Ctr; **Address:** Boston Med Ctr, 1 Boston Med Ctr Pl, Dowling Bldg 2 South, Boston, MA 02118; **Phone:** 617-414-8056; **Board Cert:** Surgery 1999; Surgical Critical Care 2001; **Med School:** Tufts Univ 1983; **Resid:** Surgery, New England Deaconess Med Ctr 1990; **Fac Appt:** Prof S, Boston Univ

Callery, Mark P MD [S] - **Spec Exp:** Pancreatic Cancer; Liver Cancer; Laparoscopic Surgery; **Hospital:** Beth Israel Deaconess Med Ctr - Boston; **Address:** Beth Israel Deaconess Med Ctr, Dept Surgery, 330 Brookline Ave, Ste 928, Boston, MA 02215; **Phone:** 617-667-3798; **Board Cert:** Surgery 2004; **Med School:** Albany Med Coll 1985; **Resid:** Surgery, Albany Med Coll Hosp 1987; Surgery, Barnes Jewish Med Ctr 1992; **Fellow:** Research, Wash Univ Sch Med 1990; **Fac Appt:** Assoc Prof S, Harvard Med Sch

Cioffi, William G MD [S] - **Spec Exp:** Trauma; Cancer Surgery; **Hospital:** Rhode Island Hosp; **Address:** Rhode Island Hosp, Dept Surg, 2 Dudley St, Ste 470, Providence, RI 02905; **Phone:** 401-553-8348; **Board Cert:** Surgery 2007; Surgical Critical Care 2008; **Med School:** Univ VT Coll Med 1981; **Resid:** Surgery, Med Ctr Hosp 1986; **Fac Appt:** Prof S, Brown Univ

Cusack Jr, James C MD [S] - **Spec Exp:** Gastrointestinal Cancer; Colon and Rectal Cancer; Melanoma; **Hospital:** Mass Genl Hosp; **Address:** Massachusetts General Hospital, Division of Surgical Oncology, 55 Fruit St, Yawkey Bldg - Fl 7, Boston, MA 02114-2621; **Phone:** 617-724-4093; **Board Cert:** Surgery 2001; **Med School:** Emory Univ 1986; **Resid:** Surgery, Tufts-New England Med Ctr 1991; **Fellow:** Surgical Oncology, Brigham & Women's Hosp 1992; Surgical Oncology, MD Anderson Cancer Ctr 1992; **Fac Appt:** Assoc Prof S, Harvard Med Sch

Cushing, Brad M MD [S] - **Spec Exp:** Trauma; Critical Care; **Hospital:** Maine Med Ctr; **Address:** Maine Medical Partners Surgical Assocs, 887 Congress St, Ste 210, Portland, ME 04102-3113; **Phone:** 207-774-2381; **Board Cert:** Surgery 2005; Surgical Critical Care 2003; **Med School:** Univ Rochester 1980; **Resid:** Surgery, St Francis Hosp 1985; **Fellow:** Trauma/Critical Care, Univ Maryland 1987; **Fac Appt:** Clin Prof S, Univ VT Coll Med

Eisenberg, Burton L MD [S] - **Spec Exp:** Breast Cancer; Melanoma; Sarcoma; **Hospital:** Dartmouth - Hitchcock Med Ctr; **Address:** DHMC, Dept General Surgery, One Medical Center Drive, Lebanon, NH 03756; **Phone:** 603-650-9479; **Board Cert:** Surgery 1999; **Med School:** Univ Tenn Coll Med 1974; **Resid:** Surgery, Wilford Hall USAF Med Ctr 1979; **Fellow:** Surgical Oncology, Meml Sloan-Kettering Cancer Ctr 1981; **Fac Appt:** Prof S, Dartmouth Med Sch

Emre, Sukru MD [S] - **Spec Exp:** Transplant-Liver-Adult & Pediatric; Hepatobiliary Surgery; Liver Cancer; Portal Hypertension; **Hospital:** Yale-New Haven Hosp, Yale Med Group; **Address:** PO BOX 208062, FMB 121, New Haven, CT 06520-8062; **Phone:** 203-785-2565; **Med School:** Turkey 1977; **Resid:** Surgery, Univ Istanbul 1982; **Fellow:** Hepatobiliary Surgery, Univ Istanbul 1988; Transplant Surgery, Mount Sinai Med Ctr 1994; **Fac Appt:** Prof S, Yale Univ

Gawande, Atul A MD [S] - **Spec Exp:** Endocrine Surgery; Cancer Surgery; Gastrointestinal Surgery; **Hospital:** Brigham and Women's Hosp (page 57), Dana-Farber Cancer Inst (page 57); **Address:** Brigham & Womens Hosp, Div Gnl Surgery, ASB2-3rd Fl, 75 Francis St, Boston, MA 02115; **Phone:** 617-732-6830; **Board Cert:** Surgery 2004; **Med School:** Harvard Med Sch 1995; **Resid:** Surgery, Brigham & Womens Hosp 2003; **Fac Appt:** Assoc Prof S, Harvard Med Sch

Goodman, Martin D MD [S] - **Spec Exp:** Gastrointestinal Cancer; Peritoneal Carcinomatosis; **Hospital:** Tufts Med Ctr; **Address:** Tufts Med Ctr, Surgical Oncology, 800 Washington St, Box 9248, Boston, MA 02111; **Phone:** 617-636-9248; **Board Cert:** Surgery 2001; **Med School:** UMDNJ-RW Johnson Med Sch 1994; **Resid:** Surgery, Cooper Hosp 2000; **Fellow:** Surgical Oncology, UPMC 2002

Gupta, Rajan MD [S] - **Spec Exp:** Trauma; Critical Care; **Hospital:** Dartmouth - Hitchcock Med Ctr; **Address:** Dartmouth Hitchcock Med Ctr, Dept Surgery, One Medical Center Drive, Lebanon, NH 03756; **Phone:** 603-650-8022; **Board Cert:** Surgery 2001; Surgical Critical Care 2003; **Med School:** Boston Univ 1991; **Resid:** Surgery, Dartmouth-Hitchcock Med Ctr 1997; **Fellow:** Trauma/Critical Care, Hosp U Penn 1999; **Fac Appt:** Asst Prof S, Dartmouth Med Sch

Hebert, James C MD [S] - **Spec Exp:** Biliary Surgery; Colon & Rectal Surgery; **Hospital:** Fletcher Allen Health Care- Med Ctr Campus; **Address:** Fletcher Allen Hlth Care, 111 Colchester Ave, Burlington, VT 05401; **Phone:** 802-847-3344; **Board Cert:** Surgery 2000; **Med School:** Univ VT Coll Med 1977; **Resid:** Surgery, Med Ctr Hosp 1982; **Fac Appt:** Prof S, Univ VT Coll Med

Hodin, Richard A MD [S] - **Spec Exp:** Thyroid Cancer; Parathyroid Cancer; Adrenal Tumors; Inflammatory Bowel Disease; **Hospital:** Mass Genl Hosp; **Address:** Mass Genl Hosp, Dept Surgery, Wang Bldg-#460, 15 Parkman Street, Boston, MA 02114; **Phone:** 617-724-2570; **Board Cert:** Surgery 2001; **Med School:** Tulane Univ 1984; **Resid:** Surgery, Beth Israel Med Ctr 1990; **Fellow:** Endocrine Surgery, Brigham & Women's Hosp 1989; **Fac Appt:** Prof S, Harvard Med Sch

Hughes, Kevin S MD [S] - **Spec Exp:** Breast Cancer; Ovarian Cancer; Breast Cancer-High Risk Women; Hereditary Cancer; **Hospital:** Mass Genl Hosp, Newton - Wellesley Hosp; **Address:** Mass Genl Hosp, Dept Surgery, 55 Fruit St, Yawkey Center Fl 7 - Ste B, Boston, MA 02114; **Phone:** 617-724-0048; **Board Cert:** Surgery 2006; **Med School:** Dartmouth Med Sch 1979; **Resid:** Surgery, Mercy Hosp 1984; **Fellow:** Surgical Oncology, National Cancer Inst 1986; **Fac Appt:** Assoc Prof S, Harvard Med Sch

Iglehart, J Dirk MD [S] - **Spec Exp:** Breast Cancer; **Hospital:** Brigham and Women's Hosp (page 57), Dana-Farber Cancer Inst (page 57); **Address:** Dana-Farber Cancer Inst, 450 Brookline Ave, Smith 1058, Boston, MA 02215; **Phone:** 617-632-5178 x1; **Board Cert:** Surgery 2005; **Med School:** Harvard Med Sch 1975; **Resid:** Surgery, Duke Univ Med Ctr 1981; Thoracic Surgery, Duke Univ Med Ctr 1984; **Fac Appt:** Prof S, Harvard Med Sch

Jenkins, Roger L MD [S] - **Spec Exp:** Transplant-Liver; Liver & Biliary Cancer; Pancreatic Cancer; **Hospital:** Lahey Clin, Children's Hospital - Boston; **Address:** 41 Mall Rd, Fl 4, Ste West, Burlington, MA 01805; **Phone:** 781-744-2500; **Board Cert:** Surgery 2005; **Med School:** Univ VT Coll Med 1977; **Resid:** Surgery, New Eng Deaconess Hosp 1982; **Fellow:** Cardiac Surgery, New Eng Deaconess Hosp 1983; Transplant Surgery, Univ Pittsburgh Hosp 1983; **Fac Appt:** Prof S, Tufts Univ

Kavanah, Maureen MD [S] - **Spec Exp:** Breast Cancer; Gynecologic Cancer; Melanoma; **Hospital:** Boston Med Ctr; **Address:** Boston Medical Ctr, 820 Harrison Ave, rm 5009, Bldg FGH, Boston, MA 02118; **Phone:** 617-638-8473; **Board Cert:** Surgery 2009; **Med School:** Tufts Univ 1975; **Resid:** Surgery, St Elizabeths Hosp 1979; **Fellow:** Surgical Oncology, Boston Univ Med Ctr 1981; **Fac Appt:** Assoc Prof S, Boston Univ

Krag, David N MD [S] - **Spec Exp:** Sentinel Node Surgery; Breast Cancer; Cancer Surgery; Melanoma; **Hospital:** Fletcher Allen Health Care- Med Ctr Campus; **Address:** Univ Vermont Coll Med, Dept Surgery, 89 Beaumont Ave, Given Bldg - E309C, Burlington, VT 05405; **Phone:** 802-656-5830; **Board Cert:** Surgery 2006; **Med School:** Loyola Univ-Stritch Sch Med 1980; **Resid:** Surgery, UC Davis Med Ctr 1983; **Fellow:** Surgical Oncology, UCLA Med Ctr 1984; **Fac Appt:** Assoc Prof S, Univ VT Coll Med

Lannin, Donald R MD [S] - **Spec Exp:** Breast Cancer; Breast Surgery; **Hospital:** Yale-New Haven Hosp, Yale Med Group; **Address:** Yale-New Haven Breast Ctr, 20 York St, New Haven, CT 06510; **Phone:** 203-785-2328; **Board Cert:** Surgery 2002; **Med School:** Univ Minn 1974; **Resid:** Surgery, Univ Minnesota Med Ctr 1982; **Fac Appt:** Prof S, Yale Univ

Lillemoe, Keith D MD [S] - **Spec Exp:** Pancreatic Cancer; Colon Cancer; Pancreatic & Biliary Surgery; Gastrointestinal Cancer; **Hospital:** Mass Genl Hosp; **Address:** Mass General Hosp, Dept Surgery, 55 Fruit St, White 506, Boston, MA 02114; **Phone:** 617-643-1010; **Board Cert:** Surgery 2007; **Med School:** Johns Hopkins Univ 1978; **Resid:** Surgery, Johns Hopkins Hosp 1985; **Fac Appt:** Prof S, Harvard Med Sch

Lipkowitz, George S MD [S] - **Spec Exp:** Transplant-Kidney; Dialysis Access; **Hospital:** Baystate Med Ctr, Mercy Med Ctr - Baltimore; **Address:** 208 Ashley Ave, West Springfield, MA 01089; **Phone:** 413-747-4170 x151; **Board Cert:** Surgery 2006; **Med School:** SUNY Downstate 1980; **Resid:** Surgery, SUNY Kings Co Hosp 1985; **Fellow:** Transplant Surgery, SUNY Hlth Scis Ctr 1986; **Fac Appt:** Assoc Prof S, Tufts Univ

Markmann, James F MD/PhD [S] - **Spec Exp:** Transplant-Liver; Transplant-Kidney; Transplant-Pancreas; Pancreatic Islet Cell Transplant; **Hospital:** Mass Genl Hosp; **Address:** MGH Transplantation Ctr, WHT 517, 55 Fruit St, Boston, MA 02114; **Phone:** 617-643-4533; **Board Cert:** Surgery 1997; **Med School:** Univ Pennsylvania 1986; **Resid:** Surgery, Hosp UPenn 1992; **Fellow:** Transplant Surgery, UCLA Med Ctr 1994; **Fac Appt:** Assoc Prof S, Harvard Med Sch

McAneny, David B MD [S] - **Spec Exp:** Gastrointestinal Cancer & Surgery; Endocrine Tumors; Pancreatic Cancer; Biliary Surgery; **Hospital:** Boston Med Ctr; **Address:** Boston Med Ctr, FGH Bldg - Ste 5008, 820 Harrison Ave, Boston, MA 02118; **Phone:** 617-638-8446; **Board Cert:** Surgery 2008; **Med School:** Georgetown Univ 1983; **Resid:** Surgery, Boston Med Ctr 1988; **Fellow:** Gastrointestinal Surgery, Lahey Clinic 1989; **Fac Appt:** Assoc Prof S, Boston Univ

McFadden, David W MD [S] - **Spec Exp:** Pancreatic Cancer; **Hospital:** Fletcher Allen Health Care- Med Ctr Campus; **Address:** Fletcher Allen Hlthcare, Fletcher House 301, 111 Colchester Ave, Burlington, VT 05401; **Phone:** 802-847-5354; **Board Cert:** Surgery 2007; Surgical Critical Care 2003; **Med School:** Univ VA Sch Med 1980; **Resid:** Surgery, Johns Hopkins Hosp 1986; **Fellow:** Surgery, Johns Hopkins Hosp 1988; **Fac Appt:** Prof S, Univ VT Coll Med

Moore Jr, Francis D MD [S] - **Spec Exp:** Endocrine Surgery; Thyroid Cancer; **Hospital:** Brigham and Women's Hosp (page 57); **Address:** Brigham & Womens Hosp, 75 Francis St, ASB11-3rd Fl, Boston, MA 02115; **Phone:** 617-732-6830; **Board Cert:** Surgery 2004; **Med School:** Harvard Med Sch 1976; **Resid:** Surgery, Brigham & Womens Hosp 1984; **Fellow:** Immunology, Harvard Med Sch 1981; **Fac Appt:** Prof S, Harvard Med Sch

Ponn, Teresa MD [S] - **Spec Exp:** Breast Cancer; **Hospital:** Elliot Hosp; **Address:** Elliot Breast Health Center, 275 Mammoth Rd, Manchester, NH 03109; **Phone:** 603-668-3067; **Board Cert:** Surgery 2000; **Med School:** Univ Fla Coll Med 1976; **Resid:** Surgery, Stanford Univ Med Ctr 1982

Rattner, David W MD [S] - **Spec Exp:** Gastrointestinal Cancer & Surgery; Minimally Invasive Surgery; Gastroesophageal Reflux Disease (GERD); Natural Orifice Surgery (NOTES); **Hospital:** Mass Genl Hosp; **Address:** Mass General Hosp, Dept Surgery, 15 Parkman St, WACC 460, Boston, MA 02114-3117; **Phone:** 617-726-1893; **Board Cert:** Surgery 2004; **Med School:** Johns Hopkins Univ 1978; **Resid:** Surgery, Mass General Hosp 1985; **Fac Appt:** Prof S, Harvard Med Sch

Ryan, Colleen M MD [S] - **Spec Exp:** Burn Care; Toxic Epidermal Neurolysis; Wound Healing/Care; **Hospital:** Mass Genl Hosp, Shriners Hosp for Chldn-Boston; **Address:** MGH Burn Assocs, 55 Fruit St GRB Bldg - Ste 1303, Boston, MA 02114-2621; **Phone:** 617-726-3712; **Board Cert:** Surgery 1999; Surgical Critical Care 2003; **Med School:** Georgetown Univ 1982; **Resid:** Surgery, NE Deaconess Hosp 1988; **Fellow:** Hepatology, Hammersmith Hosp 1986; Burn Surgery, Mass Genl Hosp 1989; **Fac Appt:** Assoc Prof S, Harvard Med Sch

Salem, Ronald R MD [S] - **Spec Exp:** Cancer Surgery; Liver & Biliary Surgery; Gastrointestinal Cancer; Liver Cancer; **Hospital:** Yale-New Haven Hosp, Yale Med Group; **Address:** Dept Surgery, 333 Cedar St, TMP 203, New Haven, CT 06520-8062; **Phone:** 203-785-3577; **Board Cert:** Surgery 2000; **Med School:** Zimbabwe 1978; **Resid:** Surgery, Hammersmith Hosp 1985; Surgery, New England Deaconess Hosp 1989; **Fac Appt:** Prof S, Yale Univ

Shikora, Scott A MD [S] - **Spec Exp:** Obesity/Bariatric Surgery; Laparoscopic Abdominal Surgery; **Hospital:** Tufts Med Ctr; **Address:** Tufts Med Ctr, 800 Washington St, Box 900, Boston, MA 02111; **Phone:** 617-636-6093; **Board Cert:** Surgery 2001; **Med School:** Columbia P&S 1985; **Resid:** Surgery, New England Deaconess Hosp 1991; **Fellow:** Nutrition & Metabolism, New England Deaconess Hos 1989; **Fac Appt:** Prof S, Tufts Univ

Smith, Barbara L MD/PhD [S] - **Spec Exp:** Breast Cancer; Breast Cancer-High Risk Women; **Hospital:** Mass Genl Hosp; **Address:** MGH Cancer Center, Yawkey 9A, 55 Fruit St, Boston, MA 02114; **Phone:** 617-724-4800; **Board Cert:** Surgery 2009; **Med School:** Harvard Med Sch 1983; **Resid:** Surgery, Brigham & Women's Hosp 1989; **Fac Appt:** Asst Prof S, Harvard Med Sch

Sosa, Julie A MD [S] - **Spec Exp:** Thyroid Cancer; Parathyroid Cancer; Endocrine Cancers; **Hospital:** Yale-New Haven Hosp; **Address:** Yale Univ Sch Med, Dept Surgery, 333 Cedar St, Box 208062, New Haven, CT 06520; **Phone:** 203-785-2314; **Board Cert:** Surgery 2004; **Med School:** Johns Hopkins Univ 1994; **Resid:** Surgery, Johns Hopkins Hosp 2001; **Fellow:** Surgical Oncology, Johns Hoplins Hosp 2002; **Fac Appt:** Assoc Prof S, Yale Univ

Surgery

Sutton, John E MD [S] - **Spec Exp:** Esophageal Cancer; Liver & Biliary Surgery; Pancreatic Cancer; **Hospital:** Dartmouth - Hitchcock Med Ctr; **Address:** One Medical Center Drive, Lebanon, NH 03756; **Phone:** 603-650-8022; **Board Cert:** Surgery 2001; Surgical Critical Care 2007; **Med School:** Georgetown Univ 1974; **Resid:** Surgery, Dartmouth-Hitchcock Med Ctr 1981; **Fellow:** Surgical Critical Care, Dartmouth-Hitchcock Med Ctr 1983; **Fac Appt:** Prof S, Dartmouth Med Sch

Tanabe, Kenneth K MD [S] - **Spec Exp:** Liver Cancer; Colon & Rectal Cancer; Melanoma; **Hospital:** Mass Genl Hosp; **Address:** Mass General Hosp, Div Surgical Oncology, 55 Fruit St, Yawkey 7B, Boston, MA 02114; **Phone:** 617-724-3868; **Board Cert:** Surgery 2010; **Med School:** UCSD 1985; **Resid:** Surgery, New York Hosp-Cornell 1990; **Fellow:** Surgical Oncology, MD Anderson Cancer Ctr 1993; **Fac Appt:** Prof S, Harvard Med Sch

Thayer, Sarah P MD/PhD [S] - **Spec Exp:** Pancreatic Cancer; Gastrointestinal Cancer & Surgery; Hepatobiliary Surgery; Breast Cancer & Surgery; **Hospital:** Mass Genl Hosp; **Address:** Mass Genl Hosp, 15 Parkman St, WAC 460, Boston, MA 02114; **Phone:** 617-726-0624; **Board Cert:** Surgery 2001; **Med School:** Univ VA Sch Med 1991; **Resid:** Surgery, Mass Genl Hosp 1994; Surgery, Mass Genl Hosp 2001; **Fellow:** Research, Meml Sloan Kettering Cancer Ctr 1998; **Fac Appt:** Assoc Prof Surg & Onc, Harvard Med Sch

Udelsman, Robert MD [S] - **Spec Exp:** Parathyroid Cancer; Adrenal Tumors; Thyroid Cancer; Parathyroid Disorders; **Hospital:** Yale-New Haven Hosp, Yale Med Group; **Address:** Yale School Medicine, Dept Surgery, PO Box 208062, New Haven, CT 06520-8062; **Phone:** 203-785-2697; **Board Cert:** Surgery 2009; **Med School:** Geo Wash Univ 1981; **Resid:** Surgery, Natl Inst Hlth 1986; Surgery, Johns Hopkins Hosp 1989; **Fellow:** Gastrointestinal Surgery, Johns Hopkins Hosp 1990; Surgical Oncology, Natl Cancer Inst 1985; **Fac Appt:** Prof S, Yale Univ

Ward, Barbara MD [S] - **Spec Exp:** Breast Cancer; Breast Surgery; Breast Disease; **Hospital:** Greenwich Hosp; **Address:** 77 Lafayette Pl, Ste 302, Greenwich, CT 06830-5426; **Phone:** 203-863-4250; **Board Cert:** Surgery 2002; **Med School:** Temple Univ 1983; **Resid:** Surgery, Yale-New Haven Hosp 1990; **Fellow:** Surgical Oncology, Natl Cancer Inst 1987; **Fac Appt:** Assoc Clin Prof S, Yale Univ

Winchell, Robert J MD [S] - **Spec Exp:** Critical Care; Trauma; Burn Care; **Hospital:** Maine Med Ctr; **Address:** Maine Medical Partners Surgical Assocs, 887 Congress St, Ste 210, Portland, ME 04102-3113; **Phone:** 207-774-2381; **Board Cert:** Surgery 2010; Surgical Critical Care 2001; **Med School:** Yale Univ 1984; **Resid:** Surgery, UCSD Med Ctr 1990; **Fellow:** Trauma/Critical Care, UCSD Med Ctr 1991; **Fac Appt:** Assoc Clin Prof S, Univ VT Coll Med

Zinner, Michael MD [S] - **Spec Exp:** Colon & Rectal Cancer & Surgery; Pancreatic Cancer; Stomach Cancer; Gastrointestinal Stromal Tumors; **Hospital:** Brigham and Women's Hosp (page 57), Dana-Farber Cancer Inst (page 57); **Address:** Brigham & Women's Hosp, Dept Surg, 75 Francis St, Twr 1, Ste 220, Boston, MA 02115; **Phone:** 617-732-8181; **Board Cert:** Surgery 2000; **Med School:** Univ Fla Coll Med 1971; **Resid:** Surgery, Johns Hopkins Hosp 1974; Surgery, Johns Hopkins Hosp 1980; **Fac Appt:** Prof S, Harvard Med Sch

Mid Atlantic

Alexander Jr, H Richard MD [S] - **Spec Exp:** Gastrointestinal Cancer & Surgery; Liver Cancer-Metastatic; Pancreatic Cancer; **Hospital:** Univ of MD Med Ctr; **Address:** UMMC, Dept Surgery, 22 S Greene St, rm S4B05, Baltimore, MD 21201; **Phone:** 410-328-2999; **Board Cert:** Surgery 2004; **Med School:** Georgetown Univ 1979; **Resid:** Surgery, Bethesda Naval Hosp 1985; **Fellow:** Surgical Oncology, Meml Sloan Kettering Cancer Ctr 1989; **Fac Appt:** Prof S, Univ MD Sch Med

Alfonso, Antonio E MD [S] - **Spec Exp:** Breast Cancer; Head & Neck Surgery; Thyroid Cancer; **Hospital:** Univ Hosp of Bklyn at Long Island Coll Hosp, SUNY Downstate Med Ctr; **Address:** Long Island Coll Hosp, 339 Hicks St, Brooklyn, NY 11201; **Phone:** 718-875-3244; **Board Cert:** Surgery 1973; **Med School:** Philippines 1968; **Resid:** Surgery, Temple Univ Hosp 1972; **Fellow:** Surgical Oncology, Meml Sloan Kettering Cancer Ctr 1974; **Fac Appt:** Prof S, SUNY Downstate

August, David MD [S] - **Spec Exp:** Pancreatic Cancer; Esophageal Cancer; Stomach Cancer; Sarcoma-Soft Tissue; **Hospital:** Robert Wood Johnson Univ Hosp - New Brunswick; **Address:** Cancer Institute of NJ, 195 Little Albany St, New Brunswick, NJ 08903; **Phone:** 732-235-7701; **Board Cert:** Surgery 2005; **Med School:** Yale Univ 1980; **Resid:** Surgery, Yale-New Haven Hosp 1986; **Fellow:** Surgical Oncology, Natl Cancer Inst 1984; **Fac Appt:** Prof S, UMDNJ-RW Johnson Med Sch

Axelrod, Deborah MD [S] - **Spec Exp:** Breast Cancer; Breast Disease; **Hospital:** NYU Langone Med Ctr (page 66); **Address:** NYU Clinical Cancer Ctr, 160 E 34th St, New York, NY 10016; **Phone:** 212-731-5366; **Board Cert:** Surgery 2008; **Med School:** Israel 1982; **Resid:** Surgery, Beth Israel Med Ctr 1988; **Fellow:** Surgical Oncology, Meml Sloan Kettering Cancer Ctr 1986; **Fac Appt:** Assoc Prof S, NYU Sch Med

Barie, Philip MD [S] - **Spec Exp:** Trauma; Critical Care; Hernia; Sepsis; **Hospital:** NY-Presby/Weill Cornell Med Ctr, NY (page 65), Hosp For Special Surgery (page 60); **Address:** Weill Med College-Cornell Univ, 525 E 68th St, Box 206, New York, NY 10021-4873; **Phone:** 212-746-5401; **Board Cert:** Surgery 2004; Surgical Critical Care 2005; **Med School:** Boston Univ 1977; **Resid:** Surgery, NY Hosp-Cornell Med Ctr 1984; **Fellow:** Trauma, Albany Med Coll 1981; **Fac Appt:** Prof S, Cornell Univ-Weill Med Coll

Bartlett, David L MD [S] - **Spec Exp:** Peritoneal Carcinomatosis; Pancreatic Cancer; Liver Cancer; Appendix Cancer; **Hospital:** UPMC Shadyside; **Address:** UPMC Cancer Pavilion, 5150 Centre Ave Fl 4 - rm 415, Pittsburgh, PA 15232; **Phone:** 412-692-2852; **Board Cert:** Surgery 2004; **Med School:** Univ Tex, Houston 1987; **Resid:** Surgery, Hosp Univ Penn 1993; **Fellow:** Surgical Oncology, Meml Sloan-Kettering Cancer Ctr 1995; **Fac Appt:** Assoc Prof S, Univ Pittsburgh

Bartlett, Stephen T MD [S] - **Spec Exp:** Transplant-Pancreas; Transplant-Kidney; **Hospital:** Univ of MD Med Ctr; **Address:** UMMC Transplant Ctr, 22 S Greene St, rm N4E40, Baltimore, MD 21201; **Phone:** 410-328-8407; **Board Cert:** Surgery 2004; Vascular Surgery 2007; **Med School:** Univ Chicago-Pritzker Sch Med 1979; **Resid:** Surgery, Hosp Univ Penn 1985; **Fellow:** Vascular Surgery, Northwestern Univ Affil Hosp 1986; **Fac Appt:** Prof S, Univ MD Sch Med

Bessey, Palmer Q MD [S] - **Spec Exp:** Burn Care; Wound Healing/Care; Nutrition; **Hospital:** NY-Presby/Weill Cornell Med Ctr, NY (page 65); **Address:** 525 E 68th St, Box 137, New York, NY 10065; **Phone:** 212-746-0242; **Board Cert:** Surgery 2000; Surgical Critical Care 2005; **Med School:** Univ VT Coll Med 1975; **Resid:** Surgery, Univ Alabama Hosp 1981; **Fellow:** Metabolism, Brigham & Women's Hosp 1983; **Fac Appt:** Prof S, Cornell Univ-Weill Med Coll

Bessler, Marc MD [S] - **Spec Exp:** Obesity/Bariatric Surgery; Laparoscopic Surgery; Gastrointestinal Metabolic Surgery; Natural Orifice Surgery (NOTES); **Hospital:** NY-Presby/Columbia Univ Med Ctr, NY (page 65); **Address:** NY Presby Med Ctr, Dept of Surgery, 161 Fort Washington Ave Fl 5 - rm 524, New York, NY 10032; **Phone:** 212-305-9506; **Board Cert:** Surgery 2007; **Med School:** NYU Sch Med 1989; **Resid:** Surgery, Columbia Presby Med Ctr 1995; **Fac Appt:** Clin Prof S, Columbia P&S

Boraas, Marcia MD [S] - **Spec Exp:** Breast Disease; Breast Cancer; **Hospital:** Fox Chase Cancer Ctr (page 58); **Address:** Fox Chase Cancer Ctr, Dept Surgery, 333 Cotman Ave, rm P2131, Philadelphia, PA 19111; **Phone:** 215-728-2982; **Board Cert:** Surgery 2005; **Med School:** Univ Pennsylvania 1977; **Resid:** Surgery, Hosp U Penn 1983

Surgery

Borgen, Patrick I MD [S] - **Spec Exp:** Breast Cancer; Breast Cancer & Surgery; **Hospital:** Maimonides Med Ctr (page 62); **Address:** Maimonides Breast Ctr, 6300 8th Ave, Brooklyn, NY 11220; **Phone:** 718-765-2570; **Board Cert:** Surgery 2002; **Med School:** Louisiana State U, New Orleans 1984; **Resid:** Surgery, Ochsner Fdn Hosp 1989; **Fellow:** Surgical Oncology, Meml Sloan Kettering Canc Ctr 1990; **Fac Appt:** Prof S, Cornell Univ-Weill Med Coll

Brennan, Murray F MD [S] - **Spec Exp:** Sarcoma; Pancreatic Cancer; Stomach Cancer; Endocrine Cancers; **Hospital:** Meml Sloan-Kettering Cancer Ctr; **Address:** 1275 York Ave, New York, NY 10065; **Phone:** 212-639-6586; **Board Cert:** Surgery 1975; **Med School:** New Zealand 1964; **Resid:** Surgery, Univ Otago Hosp 1969; **Fellow:** Surgery, Harvard Med Sch 1972; Surgery, Peter Bent Brigham Hosp 1975; **Fac Appt:** Prof S, Cornell Univ-Weill Med Coll

Brody, Fred J MD [S] - **Spec Exp:** Gastrointestinal Surgery; Laparoscopic Surgery; Hernia; **Hospital:** G Washington Univ Hosp; **Address:** George Washington Univ Dept Surgery, 2150 Pennsylvania Ave NW, Ste 6B, Washington, DC 20037; **Phone:** 202-741-2587; **Board Cert:** Surgery 2008; **Med School:** Univ NC Sch Med 1991; **Resid:** Surgery, George Washington Univ Med Ctr 1997; **Fellow:** Laparoscopic Surgery, Duke Univ Med Ctr 1998; **Fac Appt:** Assoc Prof S, Geo Wash Univ

Bromberg, Jonathan S MD/PhD [S] - **Spec Exp:** Transplant-Kidney; Transplant-Pancreas; **Hospital:** Univ of MD Med Ctr; **Address:** Univ Maryland Med Ctr, 29 S Greene St, Ste 200, Baltimore, MD 21201; **Phone:** 410-328-5408; **Board Cert:** Surgery 2009; **Med School:** Harvard Med Sch 1983; **Resid:** Surgery, Univ Washington Med Ctr 1988; **Fellow:** Transplant Surgery, Hosp U Penn 1990; **Fac Appt:** Prof S, Univ MD Sch Med

Brooks, Ari D MD [S] - **Spec Exp:** Breast Cancer; **Hospital:** Hahnemann Univ Hosp; **Address:** Drexel Surgical Assocs, 219 N Broad St Fl 8, Philadelphia, PA 19107; **Phone:** 215-762-2295; **Board Cert:** Surgery 2000; **Med School:** Hahnemann Univ 1992; **Resid:** Surgery, NYU Med Ctr 1999; **Fellow:** Surgical Oncology, Meml Sloan-Kettering Cancer Ctr 2001; **Fac Appt:** Assoc Prof S, Drexel Univ Coll Med

Cameron, John L MD [S] - **Spec Exp:** Pancreatic Cancer; Pancreatic Surgery; Biliary Cancer; Liver Cancer; **Hospital:** Johns Hopkins Hosp (page 61); **Address:** 600 N Wolfe St Blalock Bldg - Ste 679, Baltimore, MD 21287; **Phone:** 410-955-5166; **Board Cert:** Surgery 1970; Thoracic Surgery 1971; **Med School:** Johns Hopkins Univ 1962; **Resid:** Surgery, Johns Hopkins Hosp 1970; **Fellow:** Thoracic Surgery, Johns Hopkins Hosp 1971; **Fac Appt:** Prof S, Johns Hopkins Univ

Cance, William G MD [S] - **Spec Exp:** Pancreatic Cancer; Endocrine Cancers; Colon & Rectal Cancer; **Hospital:** Roswell Park Cancer Inst; **Address:** RPCI, Dept Surgical Oncology, Elm and Carlton Streets, Buffalo, NY 14263; **Phone:** 716-845-8204; **Board Cert:** Surgery 2009; **Med School:** Duke Univ 1982; **Resid:** Surgery, Barnes Jewish Hosp 1988; **Fellow:** Surgical Oncology, Meml Sloan Kettering Canc Ctr 1990; **Fac Appt:** Prof S, SUNY Buffalo

Carty, Sally E MD [S] - **Spec Exp:** Endocrine Surgery; Endocrine Tumors; Parathyroid Surgery; **Hospital:** UPMC Presby, Pittsburgh, UPMC Shadyside; **Address:** 3471 Fifth Ave, Ste 101, Pittsburgh, PA 15213; **Phone:** 412-647-0467; **Board Cert:** Surgery 1999; **Med School:** Penn State Coll Med 1984; **Resid:** Surgery, Penn State Hershey Med Ctr 1989; **Fellow:** Surgical Oncology, Natl Cancer Inst 1991; **Fac Appt:** Prof S, Univ Pittsburgh

Chabot, John A MD [S] - **Spec Exp:** Liver & Biliary Surgery; Pancreatic Cancer; Pancreatic Surgery; Thyroid & Parathyroid Surgery; **Hospital:** NY-Presby/Columbia Univ Med Ctr, NY (page 65); **Address:** NY Presby-Columbia Medical Ctr, 161 Ft Washington Ave Fl 8 - Ste 819, New York, NY 10032; **Phone:** 212-305-9468; **Board Cert:** Surgery 2000; **Med School:** Dartmouth Med Sch 1983; **Resid:** Surgery, Columbia-Presby Med Ctr 1990; **Fac Appt:** Prof S, Columbia P&S

Cherqui, Daniel MD [S] - **Spec Exp:** Transplant-Liver; Hepatobiliary Surgery; Liver Cancer; Minimally Invasive Surgery; **Hospital:** NY-Presby/Weill Cornell Med Ctr, NY (page 65); **Address:** 525 E 68th St, Box 287, New York, NY 10065; **Phone:** 212-746-2127; **Med School:** France 1980; **Resid:** Surgery, Hospitaux de Paris 1986; **Fellow:** Hepatobiliary Surgery, Paul Brousse Hosp 1987; Transplant Surgery, Univ Chicago Med Ctr; **Fac Appt:** Prof S, Cornell Univ-Weill Med Coll

Choti, Michael A MD [S] - **Spec Exp:** Pancreatic Cancer; Liver Cancer-Metastatic; Carcinoid Tumors; **Hospital:** Johns Hopkins Hosp (page 61); **Address:** Johns Hopkins Hosp, 600 N Wolfe St Blalock Bldg - rm 665, Baltimore, MD 21287; **Phone:** 410-955-7113; **Board Cert:** Surgery 2002; **Med School:** Yale Univ 1983; **Resid:** Surgery, Hosp Univ Penn 1990; **Fellow:** Surgical Oncology, Meml Sloan-Kettering Canc Ctr 1992; **Fac Appt:** Prof S, Johns Hopkins Univ

Cohen, Murray J MD [S] - **Spec Exp:** Trauma; **Hospital:** Thomas Jefferson Univ Hosp; **Address:** 1100 Walnut St, Ste 500, Philadelphia, PA 19107; **Phone:** 215-955-2600; **Board Cert:** Surgery 2006; Surgical Critical Care 2008; **Med School:** Temple Univ 1981; **Resid:** Surgery, Albert Einstein Med Ctr 1986; **Fellow:** Trauma, Hartford Hosp 1987; **Fac Appt:** Assoc Clin Prof S, Thomas Jefferson Univ

Coit, Daniel G MD [S] - **Spec Exp:** Melanoma; Pancreatic Cancer; Stomach Cancer; **Hospital:** Meml Sloan-Kettering Cancer Ctr; **Address:** 1275 York Avenue, New York, NY 10065; **Phone:** 800-525-2225; **Board Cert:** Surgery 2004; **Med School:** Univ Cincinnati 1976; **Resid:** Internal Medicine, New Eng Deaconess Hosp 1978; Surgery, New Eng Deaconess Hosp 1983; **Fellow:** Surgical Oncology, Meml Sloan Kettering Canc Ctr 1985; **Fac Appt:** Prof S, Cornell Univ-Weill Med Coll

Conti, David J MD [S] - **Spec Exp:** Transplant-Kidney; **Hospital:** Albany Med Ctr; **Address:** Albany Medical Center, 47 New Scotland Ave, MC 61GE, Albany, NY 12208; **Phone:** 518-262-5614; **Board Cert:** Surgery 2008; **Med School:** Northwestern Univ 1981; **Resid:** Surgery, Northwestern Meml Hosp 1987; **Fellow:** Transplant Surgery, Mass Genl Hosp 1989; **Fac Appt:** Prof S, Albany Med Coll

Cornwell III, Edward E MD [S] - **Spec Exp:** Trauma; **Hospital:** Howard Univ Hosp; **Address:** Howard Univ Hospital, 2041 Georgia Ave NW, Ste 4B02, Washington, DC 20060; **Phone:** 202-865-1441; **Board Cert:** Surgery 2006; Surgical Critical Care 1998; **Med School:** Howard Univ 1982; **Resid:** Surgery, LAC-USC Med Ctr 1987; **Fellow:** Trauma, Emer/Med Svcs System 1989; **Fac Appt:** Assoc Prof S, Johns Hopkins Univ

Courcoulas, Anita P MD [S] - **Spec Exp:** Obesity/Bariatric Surgery; Minimally Invasive Surgery; **Hospital:** Magee-Womens Hosp - UPMC, UPMC Shadyside; **Address:** Magee-Women's Hospital, 3380 Boulevard of the Allies, Ste 390, Pittsburgh, PA 15213; **Phone:** 412-641-3632; **Board Cert:** Surgery 2005; **Med School:** Boston Univ 1988; **Resid:** Surgery, Univ Pittsburgh Med Ctr 1996; **Fac Appt:** Assoc Prof S, Univ Pittsburgh

Curcillo, Paul G MD [S] - **Spec Exp:** Minimally Invasive Surgery; Gastrointestinal Cancer & Surgery; Natural Orifice Surgery (NOTES); **Hospital:** Fox Chase Cancer Ctr (page 58); **Address:** Fox Chase Cancer Ctr, Dept Surgery, 333 Cottman Ave, Philadelphia, PA 19111; **Phone:** 215-728-5363; **Board Cert:** Surgery 2007; **Med School:** Univ Pennsylvania 1989; **Resid:** Surgery, Thomas Jefferson Univ Hosp 1995; **Fac Appt:** Assoc Prof S, Drexel Univ Coll Med

Dayton, Merril T MD [S] - **Spec Exp:** Gastrointestinal Surgery; Inflammatory Bowel Disease; Pancreatic & Biliary Surgery; **Hospital:** Buffalo General Hosp; **Address:** Buffalo Genl Hosp, Dept Surgery, 100 High St, Buffalo, NY 14203; **Phone:** 716-859-3911; **Board Cert:** Surgery 2004; **Med School:** Univ Utah 1976; **Resid:** Surgery, UCLA Med Ctr 1982; **Fellow:** Gastrointestinal Surgery, Wadsworth VA Hosp 1980; **Fac Appt:** Prof S, SUNY Buffalo

Surgery

Deitch, Edwin A MD [S] - **Spec Exp:** Burn Care; Critical Care; Trauma; **Hospital:** Univ Hosp-UMDNJ—Newark; **Address:** 185 S Orange Ave, MSB, rm G530, Newark, NJ 07103; **Phone:** 973-972-6639; **Board Cert:** Surgery 1997; Surgical Critical Care 2006; **Med School:** Univ MD Sch Med 1973; **Resid:** Surgery, US Public Hlth Svc Hosp 1976; Surgery, US Public Hlth Svc Hosp 1978; **Fac Appt:** Prof S, UMDNJ-NJ Med Sch, Newark

Dempsey, Daniel T MD [S] - **Spec Exp:** Gastrointestinal Surgery; Laparoscopic Surgery; Gastroesophageal Reflux Disease (GERD); Esophageal Surgery; **Hospital:** Hosp Univ Penn - UPHS (page 68); **Address:** Hosp Univ Penn, Dept Gastro, 3400 Spruce St, 4 Silverstein Pavilion, Philadelphia, PA 19104; **Phone:** 215-662-2083; **Board Cert:** Surgery 2006; **Med School:** Univ Rochester 1979; **Resid:** Surgery, Hosp Univ Penn 1986; **Fac Appt:** Prof S, Univ Pennsylvania

Drebin, Jeffrey A MD/PhD [S] - **Spec Exp:** Pancreatic Cancer; Liver Cancer; Biliary Cancer; Gastrointestinal Cancer; **Hospital:** Hosp Univ Penn - UPHS (page 68); **Address:** Hosp Univ Penn, Dept Surgery, 3400 Spruce St, 4 Silverstein Pavilion, Philadelphia, PA 19104; **Phone:** 215-662-2165; **Board Cert:** Surgery 2004; **Med School:** Harvard Med Sch 1987; **Resid:** Surgery, Johns Hopkins Hosp 1994; **Fellow:** Medical Oncology, Johns Hopkins Hosp 1991; Surgical Oncology, Johns Hopkins Hosp 1995; **Fac Appt:** Prof S, Univ Pennsylvania

Duncan, Mark D MD [S] - **Spec Exp:** Gastrointestinal Cancer & Surgery; Minimally Invasive Surgery; **Hospital:** Johns Hopkins Bayview Med Ctr (page 61); **Address:** Johns Hopkins Bayview Med Ctr, 4940 Eastern Ave, Baltimore, MD 21224; **Phone:** 410-550-1226; **Board Cert:** Surgery 1997; **Med School:** Mayo Med Sch 1987; **Resid:** Surgery, Georgetown Univ Hosp 1994; **Fellow:** Surgery, VA Medical Ctr 1991

Edge, Stephen B MD [S] - **Spec Exp:** Breast Cancer; Cancer Surgery; **Hospital:** Roswell Park Cancer Inst; **Address:** Roswell Park Cancer Inst, Dept Surg Onc, Elm & Carlton Streets, Buffalo, NY 14263; **Phone:** 716-845-2918; **Board Cert:** Surgery 2006; **Med School:** Case West Res Univ 1979; **Resid:** Surgery, Univ Hosp 1986; **Fellow:** Surgical Oncology, Natl Cancer Inst 1984; **Fac Appt:** Prof S, SUNY Buffalo

Edington, Howard D MD [S] - **Spec Exp:** Melanoma; Breast Reconstruction; Reconstructive Surgery; **Hospital:** Magee-Womens Hosp - UPMC; **Address:** Magee-Women's Hospital, Dept Surgery, 300 Halket St, rm 2502, Pittsburgh, PA 15213; **Phone:** 412-641-1342; **Board Cert:** Surgery 2008; Plastic Surgery 1993; **Med School:** Temple Univ 1983; **Resid:** Surgery, Univ Pittsburgh Med Ctr 1989; Plastic Surgery, Univ Pittsburgh Med Ctr 1990; **Fellow:** Hand Surgery, Univ Pittsburgh Med Ctr 1991; Surgical Oncology, National Cancer Inst 1993; **Fac Appt:** Assoc Prof S, Univ Pittsburgh

Edye, Michael MD [S] - **Spec Exp:** Laparoscopic Abdominal Surgery; Colon Cancer; Diverticulitis; Obesity/Bariatric Surgery; **Hospital:** Mount Sinai Med Ctr (page 63); **Address:** 5 E 98th St, Box 1259, New York, NY 10029; **Phone:** 212-241-0872; **Med School:** Australia 1977; **Resid:** Surgery, St Vincents Hosp 1980; Surgery, Royal N Shore Hosp 1984; **Fellow:** Laparoscopic Surgery, Univ Bordeaux 1992; **Fac Appt:** Assoc Clin Prof S, Mount Sinai Sch Med

Emond, Jean C MD [S] - **Spec Exp:** Transplant-Liver; Liver Cancer; Liver & Biliary Cancer; Hepatobiliary Surgery; **Hospital:** NY-Presby/Columbia Univ Med Ctr, NY (page 65), Holy Name Med Ctr; **Address:** 622 W 168th St, PH - Fl 14, New York, NY 10032; **Phone:** 212-305-9691; **Board Cert:** Surgery 2006; **Med School:** Univ Chicago-Pritzker Sch Med 1979; **Resid:** Surgery, Cook Cty Hosp 1984; **Fellow:** Surgery, Hopital P Brousse/Univ de Paris Sud 1985; Transplant Surgery, Univ Chicago Hosps 1987; **Fac Appt:** Prof S, Columbia P&S

Estabrook, Alison MD [S] - **Spec Exp:** Breast Cancer; Breast Disease; Breast Cancer-High Risk Women; **Hospital:** St. Luke's - Roosevelt Hosp Ctr - Roosevelt Div (page 55); **Address:** 425 W 59th St, Ste 7A, New York, NY 10019-1104; **Phone:** 212-523-7500; **Board Cert:** Surgery 2004; **Med School:** NYU Sch Med 1978; **Resid:** Surgery, Columbia Presby Med Ctr 1984; **Fellow:** Surgical Oncology, Columbia Presby Med Ctr 1982; **Fac Appt:** Prof S, Columbia P&S

Fahey III, Thomas J MD [S] - **Spec Exp:** Endocrine Surgery; Pheochromocytoma; Pancreatic Cancer; Minimally Invasive Surgery; **Hospital:** NY-Presby/Weill Cornell Med Ctr, NY (page 65); **Address:** NY Presby Cornell Med Ctr, Dept Surgery, 525 E 68 St, rm F2024, Box 249, New York, NY 10065; **Phone:** 212-746-5130; **Board Cert:** Surgery 2002; **Med School:** Cornell Univ-Weill Med Coll 1986; **Resid:** Surgery, New York Hosp 1992; **Fellow:** Endocrine Surgery, Royal North Shore Hosp 1993; **Fac Appt:** Prof S, Cornell Univ-Weill Med Coll

Fong, Yuman MD [S] - **Spec Exp:** Pancreatic Cancer; Liver & Biliary Cancer; Stomach Cancer; **Hospital:** Meml Sloan-Kettering Cancer Ctr, NY-Presby/Weill Cornell Med Ctr, NY (page 65); **Address:** 1275 York Ave, rm C887, New York, NY 10065; **Phone:** 800-525-2225; **Board Cert:** Surgery 2002; **Med School:** Cornell Univ-Weill Med Coll 1984; **Resid:** Surgery, NY Hosp-Cornell Med Ctr 1992; **Fellow:** Surgical Oncology, Meml Sloan-Kettering Cancer Ctr 1994; **Fac Appt:** Prof S, Cornell Univ-Weill Med Coll

Fraker, Douglas L MD [S] - **Spec Exp:** Melanoma; Endocrine Tumors; Liver Cancer; Sarcoma; **Hospital:** Hosp Univ Penn - UPHS (page 68); **Address:** Hosp Univ Penn, Dept Surgery, 3400 Spruce St, 4 Silverstein Pavilion, Philadelphia, PA 19104; **Phone:** 215-662-7866; **Board Cert:** Surgery 2002; **Med School:** Harvard Med Sch 1983; **Resid:** Surgery, UCSF Med Ctr 1986; Surgery, UCSF Med Ctr 1991; **Fellow:** Surgical Oncology, National Cancer Inst 1989; **Fac Appt:** Prof S, Univ Pennsylvania

Frazier, Thomas G MD [S] - **Spec Exp:** Breast Cancer; Breast Disease; **Hospital:** Bryn Mawr Hosp; **Address:** 101 S Bryn Mawr Ave, Ste 201, Bryn Mawr, PA 19010; **Phone:** 610-520-0700; **Board Cert:** Surgery 2004; **Med School:** Univ Pennsylvania 1968; **Resid:** Surgery, Hosp Univ Penn 1975; **Fellow:** Surgical Oncology, MD Anderson Cancer Ctr 1976; **Fac Appt:** Clin Prof S, Drexel Univ Coll Med

Geller, David A MD [S] - **Spec Exp:** Liver Cancer; Laparoscopic Surgery; Liver & Biliary Cancer; **Hospital:** UPMC Presby, Pittsburgh, UPMC Passavant-McCandless; **Address:** UPMC Liver Cancer Center, 3459 5th Ave, Pittsburgh, PA 15213-2582; **Phone:** 412-692-2001; **Board Cert:** Surgery 2005; **Med School:** Northwestern Univ-Feinberg Sch Med 1988; **Resid:** Surgery, UPMC-Presbyterian 1993; **Fellow:** Hepatobiliary Surgery, UPMC-Presbyterian 1998; Transplant Surgery, UPMC-Presbyterian 1998; **Fac Appt:** Prof S, Univ Pittsburgh

Gibbs, John F MD [S] - **Spec Exp:** Gastrointestinal Cancer; Stomach Cancer; Pancreatic Cancer; Liver Cancer; **Hospital:** Buffalo General Hosp; **Address:** University Surgeons, 100 High St, C319, Buffalo, NY 14203; **Phone:** 716-859-2268; **Board Cert:** Surgery 2009; **Med School:** UCSD 1985; **Resid:** Surgery, Rush Presby-St Lukes Med Ctr 1990; **Fellow:** Transplant Surgery, Baylor Univ Med Ctr 1992; Surgical Oncology, Roswell Park Cancer Inst 1996; **Fac Appt:** Prof S, SUNY Buffalo

Hanna, Nader N MD [S] - **Spec Exp:** Pancreatic Cancer; Adrenal Tumors; Peritoneal Carcinomatosis; Sarcoma-Soft Tissue; **Hospital:** Univ of MD Med Ctr; **Address:** 22 S Greene St, Ste S4B-07, Baltimore, MD 21201; **Phone:** 410-328-7320; **Board Cert:** Surgery 2005; **Med School:** Egypt 1985; **Resid:** Surgery, St. Elizabeth's Med Ctr-Tuft's Univ 1994; **Fellow:** Surgical Oncology, Univ Chicago 1997; Research, Univ Chicago; **Fac Appt:** Assoc Prof S, Univ MD Sch Med

Surgery

Hiotis, Spiros P MD/PhD [S] - **Spec Exp:** Liver Cancer; Gallbladder & Biliary Cancer; Pancreatic Cancer; Stomach Cancer; **Hospital:** Mount Sinai Med Ctr (page 63); **Address:** Surgical Oncology Assocs, 5 E 98th St Fl 12, Box 1259, New York, NY 100 129; **Phone:** 212-241-2891; **Board Cert:** Surgery 2000; **Med School:** Univ MD Sch Med 1992; **Resid:** Surgery, USF Med Ctr 1998; **Fellow:** Surgical Oncology, Meml Sloan Kettering Cancer Ctr 2000; **Fac Appt:** Asst Prof S, Mount Sinai Sch Med

Hoffman, John P MD [S] - **Spec Exp:** Pancreatic Cancer; Gastrointestinal Cancer; Hepatobiliary Surgery; Liver Cancer; **Hospital:** Fox Chase Cancer Ctr (page 58); **Address:** Fox Chase Cancer Ctr, 333 Cottman Ave, Philadelphia, PA 19111-2497; **Phone:** 215-728-3518; **Board Cert:** Surgery 1998; **Med School:** Case West Res Univ 1970; **Resid:** Surgery, Virginia Mason Hosp 1977; **Fellow:** Surgical Oncology, Meml Sloan Kettering Cancer Ctr 1980; **Fac Appt:** Prof S, Temple Univ

Jarnagin, William MD [S] - **Spec Exp:** Hepatobiliary Surgery; Liver Cancer; Pancreatic Cancer; Gallbladder & Biliary Cancer; **Hospital:** Meml Sloan-Kettering Cancer Ctr; **Address:** 1275 York Ave, New York, NY 10065; **Phone:** 212-639-7601; **Board Cert:** Surgery 2006; **Med School:** Rush Med Coll 1988; **Resid:** Surgery, Univ Calif San Francisco 1996; **Fellow:** Hepatopancreatobiliary Surgery, Meml Sloan-Kettering Cancer Ctr 1997; **Fac Appt:** Prof S, Cornell Univ

Johnson, Ronald R MD [S] - **Spec Exp:** Breast Cancer; **Hospital:** Magee-Womens Hosp - UPMC; **Address:** Magee-Womens Hosp - UPMC, 300 Halket St, Ste 2601, Pittsburgh, PA 15213; **Phone:** 412-641-1225; **Board Cert:** Surgery 1999; **Med School:** Univ Pittsburgh 1983; **Resid:** Surgery, Univ Pittsburgh Med Ctr 1989; **Fac Appt:** Asst Prof S, Univ Pittsburgh

Julian, Thomas B MD [S] - **Spec Exp:** Breast Cancer & Surgery; Clinical Trials; **Hospital:** Allegheny General Hosp; **Address:** Allegheny Cancer Ctr, 320 E North Ave, Cancer Center Fl 5, Pittsburgh, PA 15212; **Phone:** 412-359-8229; **Board Cert:** Surgery 2001; **Med School:** Univ Pittsburgh 1976; **Resid:** Surgery, Univ Pittsburgh Med Ctr 1982; **Fac Appt:** Assoc Prof S, Drexel Univ Coll Med

Kapur, Sandip MD [S] - **Spec Exp:** Transplant-Kidney; Pancreatic Islet Cell Transplant; Hepatobiliary Surgery; Transplant-Pancreas; **Hospital:** NY-Presby/Weill Cornell Med Ctr, NY (page 65), NY-Presby/Columbia Univ Med Ctr, NY (page 65); **Address:** 525 E 68th St, Box 98, New York, NY 10065; **Phone:** 212-746-5330; **Board Cert:** Surgery 2007; **Med School:** Cornell Univ-Weill Med Coll 1990; **Resid:** Surgery, Cornell Univ Med Ctr 1996; **Fellow:** Research, The Rogosin Inst 1994; Transplant Surgery, Thomas E Starzl Transplant Inst 1998; **Fac Appt:** Assoc Prof S, Cornell Univ-Weill Med Coll

Karpeh Jr, Martin S MD [S] - **Spec Exp:** Gastrointestinal Cancer; Esophageal Cancer; Pancreatic Cancer; Liver Cancer; **Hospital:** Beth Israel Med Ctr - Petrie Division (page 55); **Address:** Beth Israel Med Ctr, Philips Ambulatory Ctr, 10 Union Square E, Ste 4D, New York, NY 10003; **Phone:** 212-420-4041; **Board Cert:** Surgery 1998; **Med School:** Penn State Coll Med 1983; **Resid:** Surgery, Hosp Univ Penn 1989; **Fellow:** Surgical Oncology, Meml Sloan Kettering Cancer Ctr 1991; **Fac Appt:** Prof S, Mount Sinai Sch Med

Kato, Tomoaki MD [S] - **Spec Exp:** Transplant-Liver; Transplant Surgery-Pediatric; Transplant-Multi Organ; Transplant-Auto Transplantation; **Hospital:** NY-Presby/Columbia Univ Med Ctr, NY (page 65); **Address:** Columbia Univ Med Ctr, PH 14 Bldg - rm 105, 622 W 168 St, New York, NY 10032; **Phone:** 212-305-5101; **Med School:** Japan 1991; **Resid:** Surgery, Itami City Hospital 1995; **Fellow:** Transplant Surgery, Jackson Meml Hosp 1997; **Fac Appt:** Prof S, Columbia P&S

Kinkhabwala, Milan M MD [S] - **Spec Exp:** Transplant-Liver; Hepatobiliary Surgery; Liver & Biliary Surgery; **Hospital:** Montefiore Med Ctr - Div. Moses, Montefiore Med Ctr - Div. Weiler; **Address:** 111 E 210th St, Bronx, NY 10467; **Phone:** 718-920-6659; **Board Cert:** Surgery 2004; **Med School:** Cornell Univ-Weill Med Coll 1989; **Resid:** Surgery, NY Presby/Weil Cornell 1994; **Fellow:** Hepatobiliary Surgery, UCLA Med Ctr; **Fac Appt:** Prof S, Albert Einstein Coll Med

Leach, Steven D MD [S] - **Spec Exp:** Pancreatic Cancer; **Hospital:** Johns Hopkins Hosp (page 61); **Address:** Johns Hopkins Med Outpatient Ctr, 601 N Caroline St, Baltimore, MD 21287; **Phone:** 410-933-1233; **Board Cert:** Surgery 2004; **Med School:** Emory Univ 1986; **Resid:** Surgery, Yale-New Haven Hosp 1993; **Fellow:** Surgical Oncology, MD Anderson Cancer Ctr 1995; **Fac Appt:** Prof S, Johns Hopkins Univ

Lee, Kenneth K W MD [S] - **Spec Exp:** Pancreatic Cancer; Gastrointestinal Cancer & Surgery; **Hospital:** UPMC Presby, Pittsburgh, UPMC Shadyside; **Address:** UPMC Presbyterian, 200 Lothrop St, Ste 497, Scaife Hall, Pittsburgh, PA 15261; **Phone:** 412-647-0457; **Board Cert:** Surgery 2008; **Med School:** Univ Chicago-Pritzker Sch Med 1981; **Resid:** Surgery, Univ Chicago Hosps 1988; **Fac Appt:** Assoc Prof S, Univ Pittsburgh

Libutti, Steven K MD [S] - **Spec Exp:** Liver Cancer; Neuroendocrine Tumors; Gastrointestinal Cancer; **Hospital:** Montefiore Med Ctr - Div. Weiler, Montefiore Med Ctr - Div. Moses; **Address:** 3400 Bainbridge Ave Fl 4th, Bronx, NY 10467; **Phone:** 718-920-4231; **Board Cert:** Surgery 2004; **Med School:** Columbia P&S 1990; **Resid:** Surgery, Columbia Presby Med Ctr 1995; **Fellow:** Surgical Oncology, Natl Cancer Inst 1996; **Fac Appt:** Prof S, Albert Einstein Coll Med

Lieberman, Michael D MD [S] - **Spec Exp:** Gastrointestinal Cancer; Colon & Rectal Cancer & Surgery; Hepatobiliary Surgery; Pancreatic Cancer; **Hospital:** NY-Presby/Weill Cornell Med Ctr, NY (page 65); **Address:** 1315 York Ave, Box 216, New York, NY 10021; **Phone:** 212-746-5434; **Board Cert:** Surgery 2003; **Med School:** UMDNJ-NJ Med Sch, Newark 1985; **Resid:** Surgery, Hosp Univ Penn 1992; **Fellow:** Surgical Oncology, Hosp Univ Penn 1990; Surgical Oncology, Meml Sloan-Kettering Cancer Ctr 1994; **Fac Appt:** Assoc Prof S, Cornell Univ-Weill Med Coll

Marsh Jr, James W MD [S] - **Spec Exp:** Transplant-Liver; Liver Cancer; Pancreatic Cancer; **Hospital:** UPMC Presby, Pittsburgh, Monongahela Valley Hosp; **Address:** UPMC, Starzl Transplantation Inst, 3459 Fifth Ave 7 South, Pittsburgh, PA 15213-2582; **Phone:** 412-647-5800; **Board Cert:** Surgery 2003; **Med School:** Univ Ark 1979; **Resid:** Surgery, St Paul Hosp 1984; **Fellow:** Transplant Surgery, Mayo Clinic 1985; Transplant Surgery, Univ Pittsburgh Hosps 1986; **Fac Appt:** Prof S, Univ Pittsburgh

Meyers, William C MD [S] - **Spec Exp:** Hernia; Liver & Biliary Surgery; **Address:** 4623 S Broad St, Philadelphia, PA 19112; **Phone:** 215-334-1274; **Board Cert:** Surgery 2004; **Med School:** Columbia P&S 1975; **Resid:** Surgery, Duke Univ Med Ctr 1982; Surgery, Duke Univ Med Ctr 1983; **Fellow:** Gastroenterology, Duke Univ Med Ctr 1983; **Fac Appt:** Prof S, Drexel Univ Coll Med

Michelassi, Fabrizio MD [S] - **Spec Exp:** Gastrointestinal Cancer; Crohn's Disease; Ulcerative Colitis; Colon Cancer; **Hospital:** NY-Presby/Weill Cornell Med Ctr, NY (page 65); **Address:** Weill Cornell Med College, Surg Dept, 525 E 68th St, rm F-739, New York, NY 10021; **Phone:** 212-746-6006; **Board Cert:** Surgery 2002; **Med School:** Italy 1975; **Resid:** Surgery, NYU Med Ctr 1981; **Fellow:** Research, Mass Genl Hosp 1983; **Fac Appt:** Prof S, Cornell Univ-Weill Med Coll

Montgomery, Robert A MD/PhD [S] - **Spec Exp:** Transplant-Kidney; **Hospital:** Johns Hopkins Hosp (page 61); **Address:** Johns Hopkins Hosp, Transplant Surgery, 720 Rutland Ave Ross Bldg - Ste 765, Baltimore, MD 21205; **Phone:** 410-614-8297; **Board Cert:** Surgery 2006; **Med School:** Univ Rochester 1987; **Resid:** Surgery, Johns Hopkins Hosp 1995; **Fellow:** Transplant Surgery, Johns Hopkins Hosp 1997; **Fac Appt:** Prof S, Johns Hopkins Univ

Surgery

Morrow, Monica MD [S] - **Spec Exp:** Breast Cancer; **Hospital:** Meml Sloan-Kettering Cancer Ctr; **Address:** 300 E 66th St, New York, NY 10065; **Phone:** 646-888-5350; **Board Cert:** Surgery 2001; **Med School:** Jefferson Med Coll 1976; **Resid:** Surgery, Med Ctr Hosp Vermont 1981; **Fellow:** Surgical Oncology, Meml Sloan Kettering Cancer Ctr 1983; **Fac Appt:** Prof S, Cornell Univ-Weill Med Coll

Nava-Villarreal, Hector MD [S] - **Spec Exp:** Esophageal Cancer; Stomach Cancer; Barrett's Esophagus; **Hospital:** Roswell Park Cancer Inst; **Address:** Roswell Park Cancer Inst, Elm & Carlton Sts, Buffalo, NY 14263; **Phone:** 716-845-5915; **Board Cert:** Surgery 2001; **Med School:** Mexico 1967; **Resid:** Surgery, Buffalo Genl Hosp 1974; **Fellow:** Surgical Oncology, Roswell Park Cancer Inst 1976; **Fac Appt:** Assoc Prof S, SUNY Buffalo

Newman, Elliot MD [S] - **Spec Exp:** Gastrointestinal Cancer; Pancreatic Cancer; Liver Cancer; Colon & Rectal Cancer; **Hospital:** NYU Langone Med Ctr (page 66); **Address:** NYU Medical Ctr, 530 1st Ave, Ste 6C, New York, NY 10016-6402; **Phone:** 212-263-7302; **Board Cert:** Surgery 2004; **Med School:** NYU Sch Med 1986; **Resid:** Surgery, NYU Med Ctr 1989; Surgery, NYU Med Ctr 1993; **Fellow:** Research, Meml Sloan Kettering Cancer Ctr 1991; Surgical Oncology, Meml Sloan Kettering Cancer Ctr 1995; **Fac Appt:** Assoc Prof S, NYU Sch Med

Nowak, Eugene J MD [S] - **Spec Exp:** Breast Cancer; Hernia; Gastrointestinal Surgery; Sentinel Node Surgery; **Hospital:** NY-Presby/Weill Cornell Med Ctr, NY (page 65); **Address:** 325 E 79th St, Ground Fl, New York, NY 10075-0954; **Phone:** 212-517-6693; **Board Cert:** Surgery 2002; **Med School:** UMDNJ-NJ Med Sch, Newark 1975; **Resid:** Surgery, New York Hosp 1980; **Fac Appt:** Asst Clin Prof S, Cornell Univ-Weill Med Coll

O'Hea, Brian J MD [S] - **Spec Exp:** Breast Cancer; Sentinel Node Surgery; **Hospital:** Stony Brook Univ Med Ctr; **Address:** SUNY Stony Brook, Dept Surgery, 3 Edmund D Pelligrino Rd, Stony Brook, NY 11794-8191; **Phone:** 631-444-1795; **Board Cert:** Surgery 2002; **Med School:** Georgetown Univ 1986; **Resid:** Surgery, St Vincent's Hosp 1991; **Fellow:** Breast Disease, Meml Sloan-Kettering Cancer Ctr 1996; **Fac Appt:** Asst Prof S, SUNY Stony Brook

Olthoff, Kim M MD [S] - **Spec Exp:** Transplant-Liver-Adult & Pediatric; Liver & Biliary Surgery; Liver Cancer; **Hospital:** Hosp Univ Penn - UPHS (page 68), Chldns Hosp of Philadelphia; **Address:** Hosp Univ Penn - Dept Surgery, 3400 Spruce St Dulles Bldg Fl 2, Philadelphia, PA 19104; **Phone:** 215-662-6136; **Board Cert:** Surgery 2003; **Med School:** Univ Chicago-Pritzker Sch Med 1986; **Resid:** Surgery, UCLA Med Ctr 1990; **Fellow:** Transplant Surgery, UCLA Med Ctr; **Fac Appt:** Prof S, Univ Pennsylvania

Osborne, Michael P MD [S] - **Spec Exp:** Breast Cancer & Surgery; Breast Disease; Breast Reconstruction; **Hospital:** Beth Israel Med Ctr - Petrie Division (page 55); **Address:** Beth Israel Comprehensive Cancer Center, 10 Union Square Ave E, Ste 4E, MS 10003, New York, NY 10011; **Phone:** 212-367-0133; **Med School:** England, UK 1970; **Resid:** Surgery, Charing Cross Hosp 1977; Surgery, Royal Marsden Hosp 1980; **Fellow:** Surgical Oncology, Meml Sloan-Kettering Canc Ctr 1981; **Fac Appt:** Prof S, Cornell Univ-Weill Med Coll

Pachter, H Leon MD [S] - **Spec Exp:** Adrenal Surgery; Gastrointestinal Surgery; Pancreatic Cancer; Hernia; **Hospital:** NYU Langone Med Ctr (page 66), Bellevue Hosp Ctr; **Address:** 530 1st Ave, Ste 6C, New York, NY 10016; **Phone:** 212-263-7302; **Board Cert:** Surgery 2010; **Med School:** NYU Sch Med 1971; **Resid:** Surgery, NYU Med Ctr 1976; **Fac Appt:** Prof S, NYU Sch Med

Paty, Philip B MD [S] - **Spec Exp:** Colon & Rectal Cancer; Pelvic Tumors; Appendix Cancer; **Hospital:** Meml Sloan-Kettering Cancer Ctr; **Address:** 1275 York Avenue, New York, NY 10065; **Phone:** 800-525-2225; **Board Cert:** Surgery 2001; **Med School:** Stanford Univ 1983; **Resid:** Surgery, UCSF Med Ctr 1990; **Fellow:** Surgical Oncology, Meml Sloan Kettering Cancer Ctr 1992; **Fac Appt:** Prof S, Cornell Univ-Weill Med Coll

Pawlik, Timothy M MD [S] - **Spec Exp:** Liver Cancer; Pancreatic Cancer; Gastrointestinal Cancer; Gallbladder & Biliary Cancer; **Hospital:** Johns Hopkins Hosp (page 61); **Address:** Johns Hopkins Hospital, 600 N Wolfe St, Harvey Bldg - rm 611, Baltimore, MD 21287; **Phone:** 410-502-2387; **Board Cert:** Surgery 2004; **Med School:** Tufts Univ 1995; **Resid:** Surgery, Univ Michigan Hosp 2002; **Fellow:** Research, Mass Genl Hosp 2004; Surgical Oncology, UT MD Anderson Cancert Ctr 2006; **Fac Appt:** Assoc Prof S, Johns Hopkins Univ

Peitzman, Andrew B MD [S] - **Spec Exp:** Trauma; **Hospital:** UPMC Presby, Pittsburgh, UPMC Shadyside; **Address:** UPMC, Dept Surg-F1281, 200 Lothrop St, Pittsburgh, PA 15213; **Phone:** 412-647-0635; **Board Cert:** Surgery 2003; **Med School:** Univ Pittsburgh 1976; **Resid:** Surgery, Univ Pittsburgh Med Ctr 1979; Surgery, Univ Pittsburgh Med Ctr 1984; **Fellow:** Surgery, NY Hosp-Cornell Med Ctr 1981; **Fac Appt:** Prof S, Univ Pittsburgh

Peters, Jeffrey H MD [S] - **Spec Exp:** Esophageal Surgery; Gastroesophageal Reflux Disease (GERD); **Hospital:** Univ of Rochester Strong Meml Hosp; **Address:** 601 Elmwood Ave, Box SURG, Rochester, NY 14642-8410; **Phone:** 585-275-2725; **Board Cert:** Surgery 2007; **Med School:** Ohio State Univ 1981; **Resid:** Surgery, Johns Hopkins Hosp 1988; **Fellow:** Allergy & Immunology, Johns Hopkins Hosp 1985; Esophageal Surgery, Creighton Univ; **Fac Appt:** Prof S, Univ Rochester

Philosophe, Benjamin MD [S] - **Spec Exp:** Transplant-Liver; Transplant-Pancreas; Hepatobiliary Surgery; Liver Cancer; **Hospital:** Univ of MD Med Ctr; **Address:** UMMC Transplant Ctr, 29 S Greene St, rm 200, Baltimore, MD 21201; **Phone:** 410-328-1145; **Board Cert:** Surgery 2001; **Med School:** Boston Univ 1990; **Resid:** Surgery, Barnes Jewish Hosp 1995; **Fellow:** Hepatopancreatobiliary Surgery, Toronto Hosp 1996; Transplant Surgery, Toronto Hosp 1997; **Fac Appt:** Assoc Prof S, Univ MD Sch Med

Pomp, Alfons MD [S] - **Spec Exp:** Obesity/Bariatric Surgery; Laparoscopic Abdominal Surgery; Hernia; **Hospital:** NY-Presby/Weill Cornell Med Ctr, NY (page 65); **Address:** Weill Cornell College of Medicine, 525 E 68th St, Box 294, New York, NY 10065; **Phone:** 212-746-5294; **Board Cert:** Surgery 2010; **Med School:** Univ Sherbrooke 1980; **Resid:** Surgery, Univ Montreal Med Ctr 1985; **Fellow:** Nutrition, Rhode Island Hosp 1988; **Fac Appt:** Prof S, Cornell Univ-Weill Med Coll

Ramanathan, Ramesh Chandran MD [S] - **Spec Exp:** Obesity/Bariatric Surgery; Minimally Invasive Surgery; Colon Cancer; Clinical Trials; **Hospital:** Magee-Womens Hosp - UPMC; **Address:** Magee-Women's Hospital, 3380 Boulevard of the Allies, Ste 390, Pittsburgh, PA 15213; **Phone:** 412-641-3632; **Board Cert:** Surgery 2004; **Med School:** India 1988; **Resid:** Surgery, Univ Pitt Med Ctr 2003; **Fellow:** Surgical Oncology, Univ Pitt Med Ctr 1999; Minimally Invasive Surgery, Univ Pitt Med Ctr 2000; **Fac Appt:** Asst Prof S, Univ Pittsburgh

Reich, David J MD [S] - **Spec Exp:** Transplant-Liver; Hepatobiliary Surgery; Liver Cancer; **Hospital:** Hahnemann Univ Hosp; **Address:** 216 N Broad St Fl 5, Philadelphia, PA 19102; **Phone:** 215-762-8153; **Board Cert:** Surgery 2003; **Med School:** McGill Univ 1989; **Resid:** Surgery, Beth Israel Med Ctr 1994; **Fellow:** Hepatobiliary Surgery, Mt Sinai Med Ctr 1996

Reiner, Mark MD [S] - **Spec Exp:** Laparoscopic Surgery; Hernia; Esophageal Surgery; Pancreatic Surgery; **Hospital:** Mount Sinai Med Ctr (page 63); **Address:** 1010 5th Ave, New York, NY 10028-0130; **Phone:** 212-879-6677; **Board Cert:** Surgery 2001; **Med School:** SUNY Downstate 1974; **Resid:** Surgery, Mt Sinai Hosp 1979; **Fac Appt:** Clin Prof S, Mount Sinai Sch Med

Ridge, John Andrew MD/PhD [S] - **Spec Exp:** Head & Neck Cancer & Surgery; Thyroid Cancer & Surgery; Laryngeal Cancer; **Hospital:** Fox Chase Cancer Ctr (page 58); **Address:** 333 Cottman Ave, Philadelphia, PA 19111; **Phone:** 215-728-3517; **Board Cert:** Surgery 2007; **Med School:** Stanford Univ 1982; **Resid:** Surgery, Univ Colorado Med Ctr 1987; **Fellow:** Surgical Oncology, Meml Sloan-Kettering Cancer Ctr 1989; **Fac Appt:** Prof S, Temple Univ

Rosenberg, Steven A MD [S] - **Spec Exp:** Melanoma; Kidney Cancer; **Hospital:** Natl Inst of Hlth - Clin Ctr; **Address:** National Cancer Inst, 9000 Rockville Pike CRC Bldg, rm 3W-3940, Bethesda, MD 20892; **Phone:** 301-496-4164; **Board Cert:** Surgery 1975; **Med School:** Johns Hopkins Univ 1964; **Resid:** Surgery, Peter Bent Brigham Hosp 1974

Roses, Daniel F MD [S] - **Spec Exp:** Breast Cancer; Melanoma; Thyroid & Parathyroid Surgery; **Hospital:** NYU Langone Med Ctr (page 66); **Address:** 530 First Ave, Ste 6B, New York, NY 10016-6402; **Phone:** 212-263-7329; **Board Cert:** Surgery 1975; **Med School:** NYU Sch Med 1969; **Resid:** Surgery, NYU-Bellevue Hosp 1974; **Fellow:** Surgical Oncology, NYU-Bellevue Hosp 1978; **Fac Appt:** Prof Surg & Onc, NYU Sch Med

Rubino, Francesco MD [S] - **Spec Exp:** Gastrointestinal Metabolic Surgery; Diabetes Surgery-Rubino's Procedure; Obesity/Bariatric Surgery; **Hospital:** NY-Presby/Weill Cornell Med Ctr, NY (page 65); **Address:** NY Presbyterian Hosp/Weill Cornell, 525 E 68th St, rm P714, New York, NY 10065; **Phone:** 212-746-5925; **Med School:** Italy 1994; **Resid:** Surgery, Catholic Univ/Policlinico Gemelli; **Fellow:** Laparoscopic Surgery, European Inst of Telesurgery; Research, Catholic Univ; **Fac Appt:** Asst Prof S, Cornell Univ-Weill Med Coll

Salky, Barry A MD [S] - **Spec Exp:** Laparoscopic Abdominal Surgery; Gastroesophageal Reflux Disease (GERD); Colon Cancer; Ulcerative Colitis; **Hospital:** Mount Sinai Med Ctr (page 63); **Address:** Mt Sinai Medical Center, Div of Laparoscopic Surgery, 5 E 98th St, Box 1259, New York, NY 10029; **Phone:** 212-241-6156; **Board Cert:** Surgery 2010; **Med School:** Univ Tenn Coll Med 1970; **Resid:** Surgery, Mount Sinai Hosp 1973; Surgery, Mount Sinai Hosp 1978; **Fac Appt:** Prof S, Mount Sinai Sch Med

Sataloff, Dahlia M MD [S] - **Spec Exp:** Breast Cancer; Breast Disease; **Hospital:** Pennsylvania Hosp-UPHS (page 68); **Address:** 700 Spruce St, Ste B03, Philadelphia, PA 19106; **Phone:** 215-829-8461; **Board Cert:** Surgery 2005; **Med School:** Univ Mich Med Sch 1978; **Resid:** Surgery, St Joseph Mercy Hosp 1980; Surgery, Pennsylvania Hosp 1985; **Fac Appt:** Clin Prof S, Univ Pennsylvania

Saunders Jr, John R MD [S] - **Spec Exp:** Head & Neck Cancer; Thyroid Cancer; **Hospital:** Greater Baltimore Med Ctr; **Address:** Johns Hopkins Head & Neck Ctr at GBMC, 6569 N Charles St, Ste 401, Physicians Pavilion West, Baltimore, MD 21204; **Phone:** 443-849-8940; **Board Cert:** Surgery 2008; **Med School:** Georgetown Univ 1971; **Resid:** Surgery, Walter Reed Army Hosp 1976; **Fellow:** Head and Neck Surgery, Walter Reed Army Hosp 1980; **Fac Appt:** Assoc Prof S, Johns Hopkins Univ

Scantlebury, Velma P MD [S] - **Spec Exp:** Transplant-Kidney; Kidney Disease; **Hospital:** Wilmington Hosp; **Address:** 4735 Ogletown-Stanton Rd, Med Arts Pavilion II, Ste 2224, Newark, DE 19713; **Phone:** 302-623-3866; **Board Cert:** Surgery 2001; **Med School:** Columbia P&S 1981; **Resid:** Surgery, Harlem Hosp 1986; **Fellow:** Transplant Surgery, Univ Pittsburgh Med Ctr 1988

Schnabel, Freya MD [S] - **Spec Exp:** Breast Cancer; Breast Cancer-High Risk Women; **Hospital:** NYU Langone Med Ctr (page 66); **Address:** 160 E 34th St Fl 3, New York, NY 10016; **Phone:** 212-731-5367; **Board Cert:** Surgery 2008; **Med School:** NYU Sch Med 1982; **Resid:** Surgery, NYU Med Ctr 1987; **Fellow:** Research, SUNY Hlth Sci Ctr 1988; **Fac Appt:** Prof S, NYU Sch Med

Schraut, Wolfgang H MD [S] - **Spec Exp:** Inflammatory Bowel Disease; Gastrointestinal Surgery; Colon & Rectal Cancer & Surgery; Laparoscopic Surgery; **Hospital:** UPMC Presby, Pittsburgh, Magee-Womens Hosp - UPMC; **Address:** Univ Pittsburgh Med Ctr, Dept Surgery, 200 Lothrop St, Ste 497, Scaife Hall, Pittsburgh, PA 15261; **Phone:** 412-647-0457; **Board Cert:** Surgery 2009; **Med School:** Germany 1970; **Resid:** Surgery, Univ Chicago Hosps 1978; **Fac Appt:** Prof S, Univ Pittsburgh

Schulick, Richard D MD [S] - **Spec Exp:** Liver Cancer; Biliary Cancer; Pancreatic Cancer; Adrenal Tumors; **Hospital:** Johns Hopkins Hosp (page 61); **Address:** Johns Hopkins Hosp-Dept Surgery, 600 N Wolfe St, Blalock 685, Baltimore, MD 21287; **Phone:** 410-614-9879; **Board Cert:** Surgery 2007; **Med School:** Johns Hopkins Univ 1989; **Resid:** Surgery, Johns Hopkins Hosp 1994; **Fellow:** Clinical Pharmacology, NIH 1995; Thyroid Oncology, Maml Sloan Kettering Cancer Ctr 1996; **Fac Appt:** Prof Surg & Onc, Johns Hopkins Univ

Shah, Jatin P MD/PhD [S] - **Spec Exp:** Head & Neck Cancer & Surgery; Thyroid Cancer; Skull Base Tumors; Salivary Gland Tumors & Surgery; **Hospital:** Meml Sloan-Kettering Cancer Ctr; **Address:** 1275 York Ave, New York, NY 10065; **Phone:** 212-639-7604; **Board Cert:** Surgery 1975; **Med School:** India 1964; **Resid:** Surgery, SSG Hosp 1967; Surgery, NY Eye & Ear Infirm 1974; **Fellow:** Head & Neck Surgical Oncology, Meml Sloan-Kettering Hosp 1972; **Fac Appt:** Prof S, Cornell Univ-Weill Med Coll

Shaked, Abraham MD/PhD [S] - **Spec Exp:** Transplant Surgery; Transplant-Liver; Hepatobiliary Surgery; **Hospital:** Hosp Univ Penn - UPHS (page 68); **Address:** Hosp Univ Pennsylvania, Transplant Unit, Dulles Bldg Fl 2, 3400 Spruce St, Philadelphia, PA 19104; **Phone:** 215-662-6723; **Board Cert:** Surgery 2010; **Med School:** Israel 1982; **Resid:** Surgery, Mt Sinai Hosp 1989; **Fellow:** Transplant Surgery, UCLA Med Ctr 1990; **Fac Appt:** Prof S, Univ Pennsylvania

Shapiro, Richard L MD [S] - **Spec Exp:** Breast Cancer; Melanoma; Thyroid & Parathyroid Surgery; Cancer Surgery; **Hospital:** NYU Langone Med Ctr (page 66); **Address:** NYU Medical Clinical Cancer Center, 160 E 34th St Fl 4, New York, NY 10016; **Phone:** 212-731-5347; **Board Cert:** Surgery 2004; **Med School:** NYU Sch Med 1988; **Resid:** Surgery, NYU Langone Med Ctr 1993; **Fellow:** Surgical Oncology, NYU Langone Med Ctr 1995; **Fac Appt:** Assoc Prof S, NYU Sch Med

Shapiro, Ron MD [S] - **Spec Exp:** Transplant-Kidney; Transplant-Pancreas; Pancreatic Islet Cell Transplant; **Hospital:** UPMC Presby, Pittsburgh, Chldns Hosp of Pittsburgh - UPMC; **Address:** Starzl Transplantation Inst, UPMC Montefiore - 7 South, 3459 Fifth Ave, Pittsburgh, PA 15213-2582; **Phone:** 412-647-5800; **Board Cert:** Surgery 2005; **Med School:** Stanford Univ 1980; **Resid:** Surgery, Mt Sinai Hosp 1986; **Fellow:** Transplant Surgery, Univ Pittsburgh 1988; **Fac Appt:** Prof S, Univ Pittsburgh

Sigurdson, Elin R MD [S] - **Spec Exp:** Breast Cancer; Colon & Rectal Cancer; Melanoma; Gastrointestinal Cancer; **Hospital:** Fox Chase Cancer Ctr (page 58); **Address:** 333 Cottman Ave, Philadelphia, PA 19111-2412; **Phone:** 215-728-3519; **Board Cert:** Surgery 2006; **Med School:** Univ Toronto 1980; **Resid:** Surgery, Univ Toronto Med Ctr 1984; **Fellow:** Surgical Oncology, Meml Sloan-Kettering Cancer Ctr 1987; **Fac Appt:** Assoc Prof S

Simmons, Rache M MD [S] - **Spec Exp:** Breast Cancer & Surgery; Minimally Invasive Surgery; **Hospital:** NY-Presby/Weill Cornell Med Ctr, NY (page 65); **Address:** Weill Cornell Breast Ctr, 425 E 61st St Fl 10, New York, NY 10065; **Phone:** 212-821-0853; **Board Cert:** Surgery 2005; **Med School:** Duke Univ 1988; **Resid:** Surgery, Univ NC Hosp 1993; **Fellow:** Surgical Oncology, NY Hosp-Cornell Hosp 1994; **Fac Appt:** Assoc Prof S, Cornell Univ-Weill Med Coll

Singer, Samuel MD [S] - **Spec Exp:** Sarcoma-Soft Tissue; **Hospital:** Meml Sloan-Kettering Cancer Ctr; **Address:** 1275 York Avenue, New York, NY 10065; **Phone:** 646-497-9072; **Board Cert:** Surgery 2010; **Med School:** Harvard Med Sch 1982; **Resid:** Surgery, Brigham & Women's Hosp 1988; **Fellow:** Surgical Oncology, Dana Farber Cancer Inst 1990; **Fac Appt:** Assoc Prof S, Cornell Univ-Weill Med Coll

Skinner, Kristin A MD [S] - **Spec Exp:** Breast Cancer; **Hospital:** Univ of Rochester Strong Meml Hosp; **Address:** Univ Rochester Med Ctr, 601 Elmwood Ave, Box SURG, Rochester, NY 14642; **Phone:** 585-276-3332; **Board Cert:** Surgery 2005; **Med School:** Johns Hopkins Univ 1988; **Resid:** Surgery, UCLA Med Ctr 1995; **Fellow:** Surgical Oncology, UCLA Med Ctr 1994; **Fac Appt:** Assoc Prof S, Univ Rochester

Sugarbaker, Paul H MD [S] - **Spec Exp:** Appendix Cancer; Peritoneal Carcinomatosis; Cystadenocarcinoma; Ovarian Cancer; **Hospital:** Washington Hosp Ctr; **Address:** Washington Hosp Ctr, 106 Irving St NW, Ste 3900N, Washington, DC 20010; **Phone:** 202-877-3908; **Board Cert:** Surgery 1973; **Med School:** Cornell Univ-Weill Med Coll 1967; **Resid:** Surgery, Peter Bent Brigham Hosp 1973; **Fellow:** Surgical Oncology, Mass Genl Hosp 1976; **Fac Appt:** Prof S, Univ Wash

Sundaram, Magesh MD [S] - **Spec Exp:** Gastrointestinal Cancer & Surgery; Pancreatic Cancer; Stomach Cancer; Liver & Biliary Cancer; **Hospital:** Ruby Memorial - WVU Hosp; **Address:** WV Univ Hosp-Dept Surgery, PO Box 9238, Morgantown, WV 26506; **Phone:** 304-293-7095; **Board Cert:** Surgery 2006; **Med School:** Univ MD Sch Med 1990; **Resid:** Surgery, Delaware Med Ctr 1995; **Fellow:** Surgical Oncology, Jackson Meml Hosp 1997; **Fac Appt:** Assoc Prof Surg & Onc, W VA Univ

Swistel, Alexander J MD [S] - **Spec Exp:** Breast Cancer; Breast Disease; Sentinel Node Surgery; Nipple Sparing Mastectomy; **Hospital:** NY-Presby/Weill Cornell Med Ctr, NY (page 65), St. Luke's - Roosevelt Hosp Ctr - Roosevelt Div (page 55); **Address:** 425 E 61st St, Fl 10, New York, NY 10065; **Phone:** 212-821-0602; **Board Cert:** Surgery 2005; **Med School:** Brown Univ 1975; **Resid:** Surgery, St Luke's Roosevelt Hosp Ctr 1981; **Fellow:** Surgical Oncology, Meml Sloan Kettering Canc Ctr 1983; **Fac Appt:** Assoc Clin Prof S, Cornell Univ-Weill Med Coll

Tafra, Lorraine MD [S] - **Spec Exp:** Breast Cancer; **Hospital:** Anne Arundel Med Ctr; **Address:** 2000 Medical Parkway, Ste 200, Annapolis, MD 21401; **Phone:** 443-481-5300; **Board Cert:** Surgery 2005; **Med School:** Case West Res Univ 1986; **Resid:** Surgery, Rhode Island Hosp 1988; Surgery, Hosp Univ Penn 1992; **Fellow:** Surgical Oncology, John Wayne Cancer Inst 1994

Tartter, Paul MD [S] - **Spec Exp:** Breast Cancer; Breast Cancer in Elderly; Sentinel Node Surgery; **Hospital:** St. Luke's - Roosevelt Hosp Ctr - Roosevelt Div (page 55), Mount Sinai Med Ctr (page 63); **Address:** 425 W 59th St, Ste 7A, New York, NY 10019-1104; **Phone:** 212-523-7500; **Board Cert:** Surgery 2003; **Med School:** Brown Univ 1977; **Resid:** Surgery, Mt Sinai Hosp 1982; **Fac Appt:** Assoc Prof S, Columbia P&S

Tchou, Julia Chok-Moua MD/PhD [S] - **Spec Exp:** Breast Cancer; Breast Disease; Breast Cancer Risk Assessment; **Hospital:** Hosp Univ Penn - UPHS (page 68); **Address:** Abramson Cancer Ctr, Rena Rowan Breast Ctr Fl 3 West, 3400 Civic Ctr Blvd, Philadelphia, PA 19104; **Phone:** 215-615-7575; **Board Cert:** Surgery 2002; **Med School:** SUNY Stony Brook 1995; **Resid:** Surgery, Johns Hopkins Hosp 2001; **Fellow:** Gastrointestinal Surgery, Johns Hopkins Hosp 2002; Breast Surgery, Northwestern Meml Hosp 2003; **Fac Appt:** Asst Prof S, Univ Pennsylvania

Teperman, Lewis W MD [S] - **Spec Exp:** Transplant-Liver; Transplant-Kidney; Liver Cancer; **Hospital:** NYU Langone Med Ctr (page 66); **Address:** 403 E 34th St Fl 3, Transplant Assocs, New York, NY 10016; **Phone:** 212-263-8134; **Board Cert:** Surgery 2007; **Med School:** Mount Sinai Sch Med 1981; **Resid:** Surgery, Columbia Presby Med Ctr 1984; Surgery, LI Jewish Med Ctr 1986; **Fellow:** Transplant Surgery, Univ Pittsburgh 1988; **Fac Appt:** Assoc Prof S, NYU Sch Med

Tsangaris, Theodore N MD [S] - **Spec Exp:** Breast Cancer; **Hospital:** Johns Hopkins Hosp (page 61); **Address:** Johns Hopkins Hospital, 600 N Wolfe St, Carnegie 686, Baltimore, MD 21287; **Phone:** 410-955-2615; **Board Cert:** Surgery 2005; **Med School:** Geo Wash Univ 1983; **Resid:** Surgery, Geo Washington Univ Med Ctr 1989; **Fellow:** Surgical Oncology, Baylor Univ Med Ctr 1990; **Fac Appt:** Assoc Prof S, Johns Hopkins Univ

Van Zee, Kimberly J MD [S] - **Spec Exp:** Breast Cancer; **Hospital:** Meml Sloan-Kettering Cancer Ctr; **Address:** Meml Sloan Kettering Cancer Ctr, Evelyn H Lauder Breast Center, 300 E 66th St, New York, NY 10065; **Phone:** 800-525-2225; **Board Cert:** Surgery 2003; **Med School:** Harvard Med Sch 1987; **Resid:** Surgery, New York Hosp-Cornell 1990; Surgery, New York Hosp-Cornell 1994; **Fellow:** Research, New York Hosp-Cornell 1993; **Fac Appt:** Prof S, Cornell Univ-Weill Med Coll

Willey, Shawna C MD [S] - **Spec Exp:** Breast Cancer; Clinical Trials; **Hospital:** Georgetown Univ Hosp; **Address:** 3800 Reservoir Rd NW, PHC Bldg Fl 4, Washington, DC 20007; **Phone:** 202-444-0241; **Board Cert:** Surgery 2009; **Med School:** Univ Iowa Coll Med 1982; **Resid:** Surgery, George Washington Univ Med Ctr 1988; **Fac Appt:** Asst Prof S, Georgetown Univ

Yang, James C MD [S] - **Spec Exp:** Kidney Cancer; Kidney Cancer Clinical Trials; Clinical Trials; Immunotherapy; **Hospital:** Natl Inst of Hlth - Clin Ctr; **Address:** National Cancer Inst, 9000 Rockville Pike CRC Bldg - rm 3-5952, Bethesda, MD 20892; **Phone:** 301-496-1574; **Board Cert:** Surgery 2005; **Med School:** UCSD 1978; **Resid:** Surgery, UCSD Med Ctr 1984; **Fellow:** Surgical Oncology, Natl Cancer Inst 1986

Yeo, Charles J MD [S] - **Spec Exp:** Pancreatic Cancer; Biliary Cancer; Gastrointestinal Surgery; Pancreatic Endocrine Tumors; **Hospital:** Thomas Jefferson Univ Hosp; **Address:** 1015 Walnut St, Ste 620, Philadelphia, PA 19107; **Phone:** 215-955-9402; **Board Cert:** Surgery 2005; **Med School:** Johns Hopkins Univ 1979; **Resid:** Surgery, Johns Hopkins Hosp 1985; **Fellow:** Research, SUNY Downstate 1982; **Fac Appt:** Prof S, Thomas Jefferson Univ

Yurt, Roger W MD [S] - **Spec Exp:** Burn Care; Wound Healing/Care; Hyperbaric Medicine; Critical Care; **Hospital:** NY-Presby/Weill Cornell Med Ctr, NY (page 65); **Address:** 525 E 68th St, rm L706, New York, NY 10021-4885; **Phone:** 212-746-5410; **Board Cert:** Surgery 2008; **Med School:** Univ Miami Sch Med 1972; **Resid:** Surgery, Parkland Meml Hosp 1974; Surgery, New York Hosp-Cornell Med Ctr 1980; **Fellow:** Internal Medicine, Brigham & Womens Hosp 1978; **Fac Appt:** Prof S, Cornell Univ-Weill Med Coll

Southeast

Adams, Reid B MD [S] - **Spec Exp:** Hepatobiliary Surgery; Liver Cancer; Pancreatic & Biliary Surgery; **Hospital:** Univ of Virginia Health Sys; **Address:** UVA Health System, Dept Surgery, PO Box 800709, Charlottesville, VA 22908; **Phone:** 434-924-2839; **Board Cert:** Surgery 2003; **Med School:** Univ VA Sch Med 1987; **Resid:** Surgery, Univ Va Hlth Sci Ctr 1994; **Fellow:** Hepatopancreatobiliary Surgery, Univ Toronto Med Ctr 1995; **Fac Appt:** Assoc Prof S, Univ VA Sch Med

Baker, Christopher C MD [S] - **Spec Exp:** Trauma/Critical Care; Colon & Rectal Surgery; Hernia; Incontinence-Fecal; **Hospital:** Carilion Roanoke Meml Hosp; **Address:** Carillion Clinic, General Surgery, 3 Riverside Cir, Roanoke, VA 24016; **Phone:** 540-224-5170; **Board Cert:** Surgery 2002; Surgical Critical Care 2007; **Med School:** Harvard Med Sch 1974; **Resid:** Surgery, UCSF Med Ctr 1981; **Fellow:** Trauma, San Francisco Genl Hosp 1979; **Fac Appt:** Prof S, Louisiana State U, New Orleans

Bear, Harry D MD/PhD [S] - **Spec Exp:** Breast Cancer; Melanoma; Gastrointestinal Cancer; **Hospital:** Med Coll of VA Hosp; **Address:** Med Coll Virginia - VCU, PO Box 980011, Richmond, VA 23298; **Phone:** 804-828-9325; **Board Cert:** Surgery 2003; **Med School:** Med Coll VA 1975; **Resid:** Surgery, Brigham & Women's Hosp 1983; **Fellow:** Surgical Oncology, Med Coll Virgina 1984; **Fac Appt:** Prof Surg & Onc, Med Coll VA

Surgery

Beauchamp, Robert D MD [S] - **Spec Exp:** Esophageal Cancer; Colon & Rectal Cancer; Gastrointestinal Cancer; Breast Cancer; **Hospital:** Vanderbilt Univ Med Ctr (page 76), TN Valley Healthcare Sys-Nashville; **Address:** Vanderbilt Dept Surgery, Medical Center North D-4316, 1161 21st Ave S, Nashville, TN 37232-2730; **Phone:** 615-322-2363; **Board Cert:** Surgery 2007; **Med School:** Univ Tex Med Br, Galveston 1982; **Resid:** Surgery, Univ Tex Med Br 1987; **Fellow:** Cellular Molecular Biology, Vanderbilt Univ 1989; **Fac Appt:** Prof S, Vanderbilt Univ

Behrns, Kevin E MD [S] - **Spec Exp:** Pancreatic Cancer; Gastrointestinal Cancer & Surgery; **Hospital:** Shands at Univ of FL; **Address:** Shands Healthcare at Univ Florida, PO Box 100109, Gainesville, FL 32610-0109; **Phone:** 352-265-0604; **Board Cert:** Surgery 2005; **Med School:** Mayo Med Sch 1988; **Resid:** Surgery, Mayo Clinic 1995; **Fac Appt:** Prof S, Univ Fla Coll Med

Bland, Kirby MD [S] - **Spec Exp:** Breast Cancer; Colon Cancer; Thyroid & Parathyroid Cancer & Surgery; **Hospital:** Univ of Ala Hosp at Birmingham; **Address:** UAB, Dept Surgery, 1530 3rd Ave S, BDB 502, Birmingham, AL 35294-0002; **Phone:** 205-975-2193; **Board Cert:** Surgery 2000; **Med School:** Univ Alabama 1968; **Resid:** Surgery, Univ Fla Hosp 1970; Surgery, Univ Fla Hosp 1976; **Fellow:** Surgical Oncology, MD Anderson Cancer Ctr 1977; **Fac Appt:** Prof S, Univ Alabama

Britt, L D MD [S] - **Spec Exp:** Trauma; Head Injury; Thyroid Surgery; **Hospital:** Sentara Norfolk Genl Hosp; **Address:** Eastern Virginia Med Sch, Dept Surgery, 825 Fairfax Ave, Ste 610, Norfolk, VA 23507; **Phone:** 757-446-8950; **Board Cert:** Surgery 2003; Surgical Critical Care 2006; **Med School:** Harvard Med Sch 1977; **Resid:** Surgery, Barnes Hosp-Wash Univ 1979; Surgery, Univ Illinois Chicago Med Ctr 1984; **Fellow:** Trauma, Md Inst Emer Med Serv Sys 1986; **Fac Appt:** Prof S, Eastern VA Med Sch

Buchman, Timothy G MD/PhD [S] - **Spec Exp:** Critical Care; Pilonidal Disease; Wound Healing/Care; Sepsis; **Hospital:** Emory Univ Hosp, Emory Univ Hosp Midtown; **Address:** Emory Ctr for Crtical Care, 1364 Clifton Rd NE, Ste F524, Atlanta, GA 30322; **Phone:** 404-712-2609; **Board Cert:** Surgery 2004; Surgical Critical Care 2005; **Med School:** Univ Chicago-Pritzker Sch Med 1980; **Resid:** Surgery, Johns Hopkins Hosp 1985; **Fellow:** Trauma, Maryland Inst for Emergency Med 1987; **Fac Appt:** Prof S, Emory Univ

Cairns, Bruce A MD [S] - **Spec Exp:** Burn Care; Wound Healing/Care; Electrical Injury; **Hospital:** NC Memorial Hosp - UNC; **Address:** Univ N Carolina Dept Surgery, N Carolina Jaycee Burn Ctr, Box 7600, Chapel Hill, NC 27599-7212; **Phone:** 919-966-3693; **Board Cert:** Surgery 2005; Surgical Critical Care 2000; **Med School:** Univ Pennsylvania 1989; **Resid:** Surgery, Univ NC Hosps 1994; **Fellow:** Surgical Critical Care, Univ NC Hosps 1996; **Fac Appt:** Assoc Prof S, Univ NC Sch Med

Calvo, Benjamin MD [S] - **Spec Exp:** Colon Cancer; Endocrine Cancers; Breast Cancer; **Hospital:** NC Memorial Hosp - UNC; **Address:** UNC, Dept of Surgery, 170 Manning Drive, 1150 POB, CB #7213, Chapel Hill, NC 27599; **Phone:** 919-966-5221; **Board Cert:** Surgery 1999; **Med School:** Univ MD Sch Med 1981; **Resid:** Surgery, George Washington Univ Hosp 1988; Surgery, Natl Inst Hlth 1991; **Fellow:** Surgery, Meml Sloan Kettering Cancer Ctr 1993; **Fac Appt:** Assoc Prof S, Univ NC Sch Med

Chari, Ravi S MD [S] - **Spec Exp:** Liver Cancer; Biliary Cancer; Transplant-Liver; **Hospital:** Centennial Med Ctr; **Address:** Centennial Med Ctr, 2300 Patterson St, Nashville, TN 37203; **Phone:** 615-342-1050; **Board Cert:** Surgery 2005; **Med School:** Canada 1989; **Resid:** Surgery, Duke Univ Med Ctr 1996; **Fellow:** Transplant Surgery, Univ Toronto-Toronto Hosp 1998; **Fac Appt:** Prof S, Vanderbilt Univ

Cole, David J MD [S] - **Spec Exp:** Breast Cancer; Gastrointestinal Cancer; Vaccine Therapy; Gene Therapy; **Hospital:** MUSC Med Ctr; **Address:** 96 Jonathan Lucas St, MSC 613 /CSB 420, Charleston, SC 29425; **Phone:** 843-792-4638; **Board Cert:** Surgery 2000; **Med School:** Cornell Univ-Weill Med Coll 1986; **Resid:** Surgery, Emory Univ Affil Hosp 1991; **Fellow:** Surgical Oncology, Natl Cancer Institute 1994; **Fac Appt:** Prof S, Med Univ SC

Daneker, George W MD/PhD [S] - **Spec Exp:** Gastrointestinal Surgery; Cancer Surgery; Melanoma; Laparoscopic Surgery; **Hospital:** St. Joseph's Hosp - Atlanta, Northside Hosp; **Address:** 5673 Peachtree Dunwoody Rd, Ste 300, Atlanta, GA 30342; **Phone:** 404-252-6118; **Board Cert:** Surgery 2002; **Med School:** Univ MD Sch Med 1983; **Resid:** Surgery, Univ Cincinnati Med Ctr 1990; **Fellow:** Cancer Research, New Engl Deaconess Med Ctr 1988; Surgical Oncology, UT MD Anderson Cancer Ctr 1992

Eason, James D MD [S] - **Spec Exp:** Transplant-Kidney; Transplant-Pancreas & Liver; Liver Cancer; **Hospital:** Methodist Univ Hosp - Memphis; **Address:** Transplant Inst, 1265 Union Ave, rm S1011, Memphis, TN 38104; **Phone:** 901-516-7469; **Board Cert:** Surgery 2002; **Med School:** Univ Tenn Coll Med 1987; **Resid:** Surgery, Wilford Hall USAF Med Ctr 1992; **Fellow:** Transplant Surgery, Mass Genl Hosp 1994; **Fac Appt:** Prof S, Univ Tenn Coll Med

Eckhoff, Devin E MD [S] - **Spec Exp:** Transplant-Liver; Hepatobiliary Surgery; Transplant-Kidney; Pancreatic Islet Cell Transplant; **Hospital:** Univ of Ala Hosp at Birmingham; **Address:** UAB Transplant Surgery, 1530 3rd Ave S, LHRB 710, Birmingham, AL 35294-0007; **Phone:** 205-975-7622; **Board Cert:** Surgery 2010; Surgical Critical Care 2001; **Med School:** Univ Minn 1986; **Resid:** Surgery, Univ Wisconsin Med Ctr 1992; **Fellow:** Transplant Surgery, Univ Wisconsin 1994; **Fac Appt:** Prof S, Univ Alabama

Feliciano, David V MD [S] - **Spec Exp:** Vascular Surgery; Trauma; **Hospital:** Grady Hlth Sys, Emory Univ Hosp; **Address:** Emory Univ Dept Surgery, 69 Jesse Hill Jr Dr SE, rm 104, Atlanta, GA 30303; **Phone:** 404-251-8914; **Board Cert:** Surgery 2008; **Med School:** Georgetown Univ 1970; **Resid:** Surgery, Mayo Clinic 1977; **Fellow:** Cardiovascular Surgery, Texas Med Ctr/Baylor 1978; **Fac Appt:** Prof S, Emory Univ

Flynn, Michael B MD [S] - **Spec Exp:** Head & Neck Cancer; Head & Neck Surgery; Thyroid & Parathyroid Surgery; **Hospital:** Univ of Louisville Hosp, Norton Hosp; **Address:** 401 E Chestnut St, Ste 710, Louisville, KY 40202; **Phone:** 502-583-8303; **Board Cert:** Surgery 1972; **Med School:** Ireland 1962; **Resid:** Surgery, Univ Maryland Hosp 1969; **Fellow:** Surgical Oncology, MD Anderson Hosp 1970; Head and Neck Surgery, MD Anderson Hosp 1971; **Fac Appt:** Prof S, Univ Louisville Sch Med

Gabram, Sheryl G A MD [S] - **Spec Exp:** Breast Cancer; Breast Cancer-High Risk Women; Breast Disease; **Hospital:** Emory Univ Hosp, Grady Hlth Sys; **Address:** Winship Cancer Institute, 1365 Clifton Rd NE C Bldg Fl 2, Atlanta, GA 30322; **Phone:** 404-778-1230; **Board Cert:** Surgery 2006; **Med School:** Georgetown Univ 1982; **Resid:** Surgery, Washington Hosp Ctr 1987; **Fellow:** Trauma, Hartford Hosp 1988; **Fac Appt:** Prof S, Emory Univ

Galloway, John R MD [S] - **Spec Exp:** Gastrointestinal Surgery; Pancreatic Surgery; Pancreatic Islet Cell Transplant; Hepatobiliary Surgery; **Hospital:** Emory Univ Hosp; **Address:** Emory Univ Hosp, Dept Surgery, 1365A Clifton Rd NE, Atlanta, GA 30322; **Phone:** 404-778-3712; **Board Cert:** Surgery 2008; **Med School:** Emory Univ 1981; **Resid:** Surgery, Emory Affil Hosps 1986; **Fellow:** Emory Univ Hosp 1987; **Fac Appt:** Prof S, Emory Univ

Greene, Frederick L MD [S] - **Spec Exp:** Gastrointestinal Surgery; Gastrointestinal Cancer; Hernia; **Hospital:** Carolinas Med Ctr; **Address:** Carolinas Medical Ctr, 1025 Morehead Medical Drive, Ste 300, Charlotte, NC 28204; **Phone:** 704-355-1813; **Board Cert:** Surgery 2009; **Med School:** Univ VA Sch Med 1970; **Resid:** Surgery, Yale-New Haven Hosp 1976; **Fellow:** Surgical Oncology, Yale-New Haven Hosp 1973; **Fac Appt:** Prof S, Univ NC Sch Med

Hanks, John B MD [S] - **Spec Exp:** Endocrine Cancers; Breast Cancer; Thyroid Cancer & Surgery; Endocrine Surgery; **Hospital:** Univ of Virginia Health Sys; **Address:** Univ VA Hlth Sys, Dept Surgery, PO Box 800709, Charlottesville, VA 22908-0709; **Phone:** 434-924-0376; **Board Cert:** Surgery 2001; **Med School:** Univ Rochester 1973; **Resid:** Surgery, Duke Univ Med Ctr 1982; **Fac Appt:** Prof S, Univ VA Sch Med

Herrmann, Virginia M MD [S] - **Spec Exp:** Breast Cancer; Nutrition & Cancer Prevention/Control; **Hospital:** Hilton Head Reg Med Ctr, MUSC Med Ctr; **Address:** Hilton Head Reg Med Ctr, 25 Hospital Center Blvd, Ste 300, Hilton Head Isl, SC 29926; **Phone:** 843-682-7377; **Board Cert:** Surgery 2009; **Med School:** St Louis Univ 1974; **Resid:** Surgery, St Louis Univ Hosps 1979; **Fellow:** Surgery, Brigham & Women's Hosp 1980; **Fac Appt:** Prof S, Med Univ SC

Heslin, Martin J MD [S] - **Spec Exp:** Gastrointestinal Cancer; Pancreatic Cancer; Biliary Cancer; Sarcoma-Soft Tissue; **Hospital:** Univ of Ala Hosp at Birmingham; **Address:** Univ Alabama, 1922 7th Ave S, Ste 321, Birmingham, AL 35294-0016; **Phone:** 205-934-3064; **Board Cert:** Surgery 2006; **Med School:** SUNY Upstate Med Univ 1987; **Resid:** Surgery, NYU Med Ctr 1994; Surgery, Meml Sloan-Kettering Canc Ctr 1991; **Fellow:** Surgical Oncology, Meml Sloan-Kettering Cancer Ctr 1996; **Fac Appt:** Prof S, Univ Alabama

Howerton, Russell M MD [S] - **Spec Exp:** Hepatobiliary Surgery; Pancreatic Surgery; Colon & Rectal Surgery; Laparoscopic Surgery; **Hospital:** Wake Forest Univ Baptist Med Ctr; **Address:** Wake Forest Univ Sch Med, Dept Surgery, Medical Center Blvd, Winston-Salem, NC 27157; **Phone:** 336-716-0664; **Board Cert:** Surgery 2008; **Med School:** Vanderbilt Univ 1983; **Resid:** Surgery, Tufts/New England Med Ctr 1989; **Fellow:** Hepatobiliary Surgery, Hammersmith Hosp 1992; **Fac Appt:** Assoc Prof S, Wake Forest Univ

Kelley, Mark C MD [S] - **Spec Exp:** Breast Cancer; Melanoma; **Hospital:** Vanderbilt Univ Med Ctr (page 76), TN Valley Healthcare Sys-Nashville; **Address:** Vanderbilt Div Surgical Oncology, 2220 Pierce Ave, 597 Preston Rsch Bldg, Nashville, TN 37232-6860; **Phone:** 615-322-2391; **Board Cert:** Surgery 2005; **Med School:** Univ Fla Coll Med 1989; **Resid:** Surgery, Shands Hosp 1995; **Fellow:** Surgical Oncology, John Wayne Cancer Inst 1997; **Fac Appt:** Assoc Prof S, Vanderbilt Univ

Knechtle, Stuart J MD [S] - **Spec Exp:** Transplant-Liver; Transplant-Kidney; Transplant Immunology; Hepatobiliary Surgery; **Hospital:** Emory Univ Hosp; **Address:** Emory Transplant Surgery Program, 1365 Clifton Rd NE, Ste 6400, Atlanta, GA 30322; **Phone:** 404-712-5676; **Board Cert:** Surgery 2009; **Med School:** Cornell Univ 1982; **Resid:** Surgery, Duke Univ Med Ctr 1989; **Fellow:** Transplant Surgery, Univ Wisconsin Hosp 1991; **Fac Appt:** Prof S, Emory Univ

Koruda, Mark J MD [S] - **Spec Exp:** Gastrointestinal Surgery; Minimally Invasive Surgery; Inflammatory Bowel Disease; **Hospital:** NC Memorial Hosp - UNC; **Address:** Div Gastorintestinal Surgery, 4035 Burnett-Womack Bldg, Campus Box 7081, Chapel Hill, NC 27599-7081; **Phone:** 919-966-8436; **Board Cert:** Surgery 1999; **Med School:** Yale Univ 1981; **Resid:** Surgery, Hosp Univ Penn 1988; **Fac Appt:** Prof S, Univ NC Sch Med

Krontiras, Helen MD [S] - **Spec Exp:** Breast Cancer; **Hospital:** Univ of Ala Hosp at Birmingham; **Address:** The Kirklin Clinic, 2000 6th Ave S, Birmingham, AL 35233; **Phone:** 205-801-8266; **Board Cert:** Surgery 2010; **Med School:** Univ Alabama 1991; **Resid:** Surgery, Univ AL Hosp 2000; **Fellow:** Surgical Oncology, Northwestern Univ Med Ctr 2001; **Fac Appt:** Assoc Prof S, Univ Alabama

Larsen, Christian P MD/PhD [S] - **Spec Exp:** Pancreatic Islet Cell Transplant; Transplant-Pancreas; Transplant-Kidney; Transplant Immunology; **Hospital:** Emory Univ Hosp; **Address:** Emory Kidney Transplant Prgm, 1364 Clifton Rd NE B Bldg - Ste 6400, Atlanta, GA 30322; **Phone:** 404-727-0717; **Board Cert:** Surgery 2001; **Med School:** Emory Univ 1984; **Resid:** Surgery, Emory Univ Hosp 1988; **Fellow:** Surgical Research, Oxford Univ 1990; Transplant Surgery, Emory Univ Hosp 1993; **Fac Appt:** Prof S, Emory Univ

Levi, Joe U MD [S] - **Spec Exp:** Pancreatic Cancer; Liver Disease; Liver Cancer; Biliary Surgery; **Hospital:** Jackson Meml Hosp (page 70), Univ of Miami Hosp & Clins/Sylvester Comp Canc Ctr (page 73); **Address:** 1120 NW 14th St, M875, Clinical Research Bldg, Miami, FL 33136; **Phone:** 305-243-4211; **Board Cert:** Surgery 1975; **Med School:** Univ Fla Coll Med 1967; **Resid:** Surgery, Johns Hopkins Hosp 1969; Surgery, Jackson Meml Hosp 1974; **Fac Appt:** Prof S, Univ Miami Sch Med

Levine, Edward A MD [S] - **Spec Exp:** Breast Cancer; Esophageal Cancer; Peritoneal Carcinomatosis; Sarcoma; **Hospital:** Wake Forest Univ Baptist Med Ctr; **Address:** Wake Forest Univ Baptist Med Ctr, Dept Surgery, Med Ctr Blvd Fl 5, Winston-Salem, NC 27157; **Phone:** 336-716-4276; **Board Cert:** Surgery 1999; **Med School:** Ros Franklin Univ/Chicago Med Sch 1985; **Resid:** Surgery, Michael Reese Hosp 1990; **Fellow:** Surgical Oncology, Univ Illinois 1992; **Fac Appt:** Prof S, Wake Forest Univ

Lind, David S MD [S] - **Spec Exp:** Breast Cancer; Melanoma; Sarcoma; **Hospital:** Med Coll of GA Hosp and Clin (MCG Health Inc); **Address:** MCG Health, Div Surgical Oncology, 1120 15th St, Augusta, GA 30912; **Phone:** 706-721-6744; **Board Cert:** Surgery 2000; **Med School:** Eastern VA Med Sch 1984; **Resid:** Surgery, Univ Texas Affil Hosp 1989; **Fellow:** Medical Oncology, Med Coll Virginia 1992; **Fac Appt:** Prof S, Med Coll GA

Livingstone, Alan S MD [S] - **Spec Exp:** Liver & Biliary Cancer; Stomach Cancer; Esophageal Cancer; Pancreatic Cancer; **Hospital:** Jackson Meml Hosp (page 70), Univ of Miami Hosp & Clins/Sylvester Comp Canc Ctr (page 73); **Address:** 1150 NW 14th St Fl 4, Miami, FL 33136; **Phone:** 305-243-4902; **Board Cert:** Surgery 2007; **Med School:** McGill Univ 1971; **Resid:** Surgery, Montreal Genl Hosp 1976; Surgery, Jackson Meml Hosp 1975; **Fac Appt:** Prof S, Univ Miami Sch Med

Luterman, Arnold MD [S] - **Spec Exp:** Burn Care; Wound Healing/Care; Critical Care; **Hospital:** Univ of S AL Med Ctr; **Address:** Univ of S Alabama Med Ctr, Mastin Bldg, 2451 Fillingim St, Ste 101, Mobile, AL 36617; **Phone:** 251-445-8282; **Board Cert:** Surgery 2006; **Med School:** McGill Univ 1970; **Resid:** Surgery, Jewish Gen Hosp 1976; Surgery, Sinai Hospital 1973; **Fellow:** Burn Surgery, Univ Washington 1976; **Fac Appt:** Prof S, Univ S Ala Coll Med

MacDonald Jr, Kenneth G MD [S] - **Spec Exp:** Gastrointestinal Surgery; Obesity/Bariatric Surgery; Pancreatic Surgery; **Hospital:** Univ Hlth Sys-Pitt Co Meml Hosp, Nash Genl Hosp; **Address:** Physicians East, P.A., 1850 W Arlington Blvd, East Entrance, Greenville, NC 27834; **Phone:** 252-413-6735; **Board Cert:** Surgery 1998; **Med School:** W VA Univ 1981; **Resid:** Surgery, NC Baptist Hosp 1984; Surgery, Univ Med Ctr E Carolina 1987; **Fac Appt:** Prof S, E Carolina Univ

MacFadyen Jr, Bruce V MD [S] - **Spec Exp:** Laparoscopic Surgery; Gastrointestinal Surgery; Endoscopy; **Hospital:** Med Coll of GA Hosp and Clin (MCG Health Inc); **Address:** Medical College GA, Dept Surgery, 1120 15th St, Ste 4076, Augusta, GA 30912; **Phone:** 706-721-4651; **Board Cert:** Surgery 1975; **Med School:** Hahnemann Univ 1968; **Resid:** Surgery, Hosp Univ Penn 1972; Surgery, Hermann Hosp 1974; **Fellow:** MD Anderson Cancer Ctr 1978; **Fac Appt:** Prof S, Med Coll GA

McGrath, Patrick C MD [S] - **Spec Exp:** Breast Cancer; Cancer Surgery; **Hospital:** Univ of Kentucky Albert B. Chandler Hosp; **Address:** Univ Kentucky Hospital, Dept General Surgery, 800 Rose St, rm C224, Lexington, KY 40536-0293; **Phone:** 859-323-6346 x240; **Board Cert:** Surgery 2008; **Med School:** Univ IL Coll Med 1980; **Resid:** Surgery, Med Coll Virginia Hosp 1986; **Fellow:** Surgical Oncology, Med Coll Virginia Hosp 1988; **Fac Appt:** Prof S, Univ KY Coll Med

McMasters, Kelly M MD [S] - **Spec Exp:** Melanoma; Breast Cancer; Liver Cancer; **Hospital:** Univ of Louisville Hosp; **Address:** 401 S Chestnut St, Ste 710, Louisville, KY 40202; **Phone:** 502-583-8303; **Board Cert:** Surgery 2005; **Med School:** UMDNJ-RW Johnson Med Sch 1989; **Resid:** Surgery, Univ Louisville Sch Med 1994; **Fellow:** Surgical Oncology, Texas-MD Anderson Cancer Ctr 1995; **Fac Appt:** Prof S, Univ Louisville Sch Med

Meyer, Anthony A MD [S] - **Spec Exp:** Trauma/Critical Care; Burn Care; **Hospital:** NC Memorial Hosp - UNC; **Address:** Univ NC-Sch Med, Dept Surgery, 4041 Burnett-Womack Bldg, CB7050, Chapel Hill, NC 27599-7050; **Phone:** 919-966-4321; **Board Cert:** Surgery 2001; Surgical Critical Care 2005; **Med School:** Univ Chicago-Pritzker Sch Med 1977; **Resid:** Surgery, UCSF Med Ctr 1982; **Fac Appt:** Prof S, Univ NC Sch Med

Neifeld, James P MD [S] - **Spec Exp:** Melanoma; Head & Neck Cancer; Gastrointestinal Cancer; Cancers-Rare & Unusual; **Hospital:** Med Coll of VA Hosp; **Address:** Medical College Virginia Hosp, PO Box 980645, Richmond, VA 23298-0645; **Phone:** 804-828-9324; **Board Cert:** Surgery 2008; **Med School:** Med Coll VA 1972; **Resid:** Surgery, Med Coll Va Hosps 1978; **Fac Appt:** Prof S, Va Commonwealth Univ Sch Med

Newell, Kenneth A MD/PhD [S] - **Spec Exp:** Transplant-Kidney; Transplant-Pancreas; **Hospital:** Emory Univ Hosp; **Address:** Emory Kidney Transplant Prgm, 1364 Clifton Rd NE B Bldg - Ste 6400, Atlanta, GA 30322; **Phone:** 404-727-0717; **Board Cert:** Surgery 2008; **Med School:** Univ Mich Med Sch 1984; **Resid:** Surgery, Loyola Univ Med Ctr 1989; **Fellow:** Transplant Surgery, Univ Chicago 1994; **Fac Appt:** Prof S, Emory Univ

Norman Jr, James G MD [S] - **Spec Exp:** Parathyroid Surgery; **Hospital:** Tampa Genl Hosp; **Address:** 2400 Cypress Glen Drive, Wesley Chapel, FL 33544; **Phone:** 813-972-0000; **Board Cert:** Surgery 2002; **Med School:** Oral Roberts Sch Med 1986; **Resid:** Surgery, Univ S Fla 1991; **Fellow:** Univ S Fla 1992

Olson, John A MD [S] - **Spec Exp:** Endocrine Cancers; Breast Cancer; Melanoma; Clinical Trials; **Hospital:** Duke Univ Hosp; **Address:** Duke Univ Med Ctr, Box 2945, Durham, NC 27710; **Phone:** 919-684-6849; **Board Cert:** Surgery 2009; **Med School:** Univ Fla Coll Med 1992; **Resid:** Surgery, Barnes Hospital/Wash Univ 1998; **Fellow:** Endocrine Surgery, Royal Infirmary 1997; Surgical Oncology, Meml Sloan-Kettering Cancer Ctr 2000; **Fac Appt:** Assoc Prof S, Duke Univ

Pappas, Theodore N MD [S] - **Spec Exp:** Pancreatic Surgery; Laparoscopic Surgery; **Hospital:** Duke Univ Hosp; **Address:** Duke Univ Med Ctr, Dept Surgery, DUMC Box 3479, Durham, NC 27710; **Phone:** 919-681-3442; **Board Cert:** Surgery 1997; **Med School:** Ohio State Univ 1981; **Resid:** Surgery, Brigham & Womens Hosp 1988; **Fellow:** Research, Wadworth VA Med Ctr 1985; **Fac Appt:** Prof S, Duke Univ

Pinson, C Wright MD [S] - **Spec Exp:** Transplant-Liver; Liver & Biliary Cancer; Pancreatic Cancer; Liver & Biliary Surgery; **Hospital:** Vanderbilt Univ Med Ctr (page 76); **Address:** Vanderbilt Univ Med Ctr, TVC 3810A, 1301 Med Center Drive, Nashville, TN 37232-5545; **Phone:** 615-343-9324; **Board Cert:** Surgery 2007; Surgical Critical Care 2007; **Med School:** Vanderbilt Univ 1980; **Resid:** Surgery, Oregon Health Sci Ctr 1986; **Fellow:** Gastrointestinal Surgery, Lahey Clinic 1987; Transplant Surgery, Deaconess Hosp 1988; **Fac Appt:** Prof S, Vanderbilt Univ

America's Top Doctors® 11th Edition

Richards, William O MD [S] - **Spec Exp:** Laparoscopic Surgery; Obesity/Bariatric Surgery; Esophageal Disorders; Gastrointestinal Surgery; **Hospital:** Univ of S AL Med Ctr; **Address:** Univ S Alabama Dept Surgery, 2451 Fillingim St, Ste 101, Mobile, AL 36617; **Phone:** 251-445-8282; **Board Cert:** Surgery 2004; **Med School:** Univ MD Sch Med 1979; **Resid:** Surgery, Univ Maryland Med Ctr 1984; **Fellow:** Gastrointestinal Surgery, Emory Univ 1985; Vanderbilt Univ 1987; **Fac Appt:** Prof S, Univ S Ala Coll Med

Roh, Mark S MD [S] - **Spec Exp:** Liver Cancer; Cancer Surgery; **Hospital:** MD Anderson Cancer Ctr-Orlando; **Address:** 1400 S Orange Ave, MP 760, Orlando, FL 32806; **Phone:** 321-841-5134; **Board Cert:** Surgery 2006; **Med School:** Ohio State Univ 1979; **Resid:** Surgery, Univ Pittsburgh Med Ctr 1982; Surgery, Univ Pittsburgh Med Ctr 1986; **Fellow:** Surgical Oncology, Meml Sloan-Kettering Cancer Ctr 1984; Surgical Oncology, Meml Sloan-Kettering Cancer Ctr 1987; **Fac Appt:** Prof S, Drexel Univ Coll Med

Rosemurgy, Alexander S MD [S] - **Spec Exp:** Pancreatic Cancer; Gastrointestinal Surgery; Minimally Invasive Surgery; Portal Hypertension; **Hospital:** Tampa Genl Hosp; **Address:** Digestive Disorders Ctr, Tampa General Hospital, 2 Columbia Drive, rm F145, Tampa, FL 33601; **Phone:** 813-844-7393; **Board Cert:** Surgery 2005; **Med School:** Univ Mich Med Sch 1979; **Resid:** Surgery, Univ Chicago Hosps 1984; **Fac Appt:** Prof S, Univ S Fla Coll Med

Salo, Jonathan C MD [S] - **Spec Exp:** Gastrointestinal Cancer; Esophageal Cancer; **Hospital:** Carolinas Med Ctr; **Address:** Blumenthal Cancer Center, PO Box 32861, Charlotte, NC 28203; **Phone:** 704-355-2884; **Board Cert:** Surgery 2005; **Med School:** UCSF 1981; **Resid:** Surgery, UCSF Med Ctr 1993; **Fellow:** Surgical Oncology, Natl Cancer Inst 1991; Surgical Oncology, Meml Sloan-Kettering Cancer Ctr 1998; **Fac Appt:** Asst Prof S, Univ NC Sch Med

Schirmer, Bruce D MD [S] - **Spec Exp:** Laparoscopic Surgery; Gastrointestinal Surgery; Pancreatic Surgery; Liver Surgery; **Hospital:** Univ of Virginia Health Sys; **Address:** Univ VA Hlth Sys, Dept Surgery, PO Box 800709, Charlottesville, VA 22908; **Phone:** 434-924-2104; **Board Cert:** Surgery 2005; **Med School:** Duke Univ 1978; **Resid:** Surgery, Duke Univ Med Ctr 1985; **Fac Appt:** Prof S, Univ VA Sch Med

Sharp, Kenneth MD [S] - **Spec Exp:** Gastrointestinal Surgery; Esophageal Disorders; Laparoscopic Surgery; Pancreatic Surgery; **Hospital:** Vanderbilt Univ Med Ctr (page 76); **Address:** Vanderbilt Univ Med Ctr, Div Gen Surgery, D-5203 Med Ctr North, Nashville, TN 37232-2577; **Phone:** 615-322-0259; **Board Cert:** Surgery 2003; **Med School:** Johns Hopkins Univ 1977; **Resid:** Surgery, Johns Hopkins Univ Med Ctr 1984; **Fellow:** Hepatobiliary Surgery, Loch Raven VA Hosp 1981; Surgery, John Radcliffe Hosp 1982; **Fac Appt:** Prof S, Vanderbilt Univ

Shen, Perry MD [S] - **Spec Exp:** Liver & Biliary Cancer; Pancreatic Cancer; Gastrointestinal Cancer; Melanoma; **Hospital:** Wake Forest Univ Baptist Med Ctr; **Address:** Wake Forest Univ Baptist Med Ctr, Dept Surgery, Medical Center Blvd Fl 5, Winston-Salem, NC 27157; **Phone:** 336-716-0545; **Board Cert:** Surgery 2008; **Med School:** USC Sch Med 1992; **Resid:** Surgery, LAC-USC Med Ctr 1998; **Fellow:** Surgical Oncology, John Wayne Cancer Inst 2000; **Fac Appt:** Assoc Prof S, Wake Forest Univ

Shibata, David MD [S] - **Spec Exp:** Colon & Rectal Cancer; Minimally Invasive Surgery; Laparoscopic Surgery; **Hospital:** H Lee Moffitt Cancer Ctr & Research Inst (page 59); **Address:** H. Lee Moffitt Cancer Center, Research Institute, 12902 Magnolia Drive, Tampa, FL 33612; **Phone:** 813-745-6898; **Board Cert:** Surgery 2008; **Med School:** McGill Univ 1991; **Resid:** Surgery, Deaconess Hosp 1994; Surgery, Beth Israel Med Ctr 1998; **Fellow:** Research, Harvard Univ Med Sch 1996; Surgical Oncology, Meml Sloan-Kettering Cancer Ctr 2000; **Fac Appt:** Assoc Prof Med, Univ S Fla Coll Med

Surgery

Slingluff Jr, Craig L MD [S] - **Spec Exp:** Melanoma; Immunotherapy; **Hospital:** Univ of Virginia Health Sys; **Address:** UVA Health System, Dept Surgery, PO Box 800709, Charlottesville, VA 22908; **Phone:** 434-924-1730; **Board Cert:** Surgery 2002; **Med School:** Univ VA Sch Med 1984; **Resid:** Surgery, Duke Univ Med Ctr 1991; **Fellow:** Surgical Research, Duke Univ Med Ctr 1992; **Fac Appt:** Prof S, Univ VA Sch Med

Solorzano, Carmen C MD [S] - **Spec Exp:** Endocrine Cancers; Minimally Invasive Surgery; Thyroid & Parathyroid Cancer & Surgery; Adrenal Cancer; **Hospital:** Vanderbilt Univ Med Ctr (page 76); **Address:** 2220 Pierce Ave PRB Bldg Fl 5 - Ste 97, Ave, Nashville, TN 37232; **Phone:** 615-322-2391; **Board Cert:** Surgery 2009; **Med School:** Univ Fla Coll Med 1993; **Resid:** Surgery, Univ Florida Affil Hosp 1999; **Fellow:** Surgical Oncology, UT MD Anderson Cancer Ctr 2002; **Fac Appt:** Assoc Prof S, Vanderbilt Univ

Sondak, Vernon K MD [S] - **Spec Exp:** Cancer Surgery; Melanoma; Sarcoma; **Hospital:** H Lee Moffitt Cancer Ctr & Research Inst (page 59); **Address:** H Lee Moffitt Cancer Ctr, Cutaneous Program, 12902 Magnolia Drive, Tampa, FL 33612; **Phone:** 813-745-1968; **Board Cert:** Surgery 2008; **Med School:** Boston Univ 1980; **Resid:** Surgery, UCLA Med Ctr 1987; **Fellow:** Surgical Oncology, UCLA Med Ctr 1984; **Fac Appt:** Prof S, Univ S Fla Coll Med

Staley, Charles A MD [S] - **Spec Exp:** Gastrointestinal Cancer & Rare Tumors; Pancreatic Cancer; Liver & Biliary Cancer; **Hospital:** Emory Univ Hosp; **Address:** Emory - Winship Cancer Inst, 1365 Clifton Rd NE, C Bldg Fl 2, Atlanta, GA 30322; **Phone:** 404-778-3307; **Board Cert:** Surgery 2001; **Med School:** Dartmouth Med Sch 1987; **Resid:** Surgery, Univ Pittsburgh Med Ctr 1992; **Fellow:** Surgical Oncology, MD Anderson Cancer Ctr 1995; **Fac Appt:** Prof S, Emory Univ

Stratta, Robert J MD [S] - **Spec Exp:** Transplant-Pancreas; Transplant-Kidney; Dialysis Access; **Hospital:** Wake Forest Univ Baptist Med Ctr; **Address:** Wake Forest Univ Baptist Med Ctr, Dept Surgery, Medical Center Blvd, Winston-Salem, NC 27157-1095; **Phone:** 336-716-6371; **Board Cert:** Surgery 2006; **Med School:** Univ Chicago-Pritzker Sch Med 1980; **Resid:** Surgery, Univ Utah Med Ctr 1986; **Fellow:** Transplant Surgery, Univ Wisc Hosps & Clins 1988; **Fac Appt:** Prof S, Wake Forest Univ

Sweeney, John F MD [S] - **Spec Exp:** Obesity/Bariatric Surgery; Laparoscopic Surgery; Gastroesophageal Reflux Disease (GERD); Minimally Invasive Surgery; **Hospital:** Emory Univ Hosp; **Address:** Emory Univ Dept Surgery, 1365 Clifton Rd NE, Ste A 33000, Atlanta, GA 30322; **Phone:** 404-778-3712; **Board Cert:** Surgery 2004; **Med School:** Rush Med Coll 1988; **Resid:** Surgery, Univ S Florida Affil Hosps 1995; **Fellow:** Surgical Research, Univ S Florida 1993; **Fac Appt:** Prof S, Emory Univ

Tyler, Douglas S MD [S] - **Spec Exp:** Pancreatic Cancer; Colon & Rectal Cancer; Rectal Cancer/Sphincter Preservation; Melanoma; **Hospital:** Duke Univ Hosp, Durham VA Med Ctr; **Address:** Duke University Med Ctr, Box 3118, Durham, NC 27710; **Phone:** 919-684-6858; **Board Cert:** Surgery 2010; **Med School:** Dartmouth Med Sch 1985; **Resid:** Surgery, Duke Univ Med Ctr 1992; **Fellow:** Surgical Oncology, MD Anderson Cancer Ctr 1994; **Fac Appt:** Prof S, Duke Univ

Tzakis, Andreas G MD [S] - **Spec Exp:** Transplant-Liver; Transplant-Bowel; **Hospital:** Jackson Meml Hosp (page 70); **Address:** 1801 NW 9th Ave, Miami, FL 33136; **Phone:** 305-355-5748; **Board Cert:** Surgery 2003; **Med School:** Greece 1974; **Resid:** Surgery, Mt Sinai Hosp 1979; Surgery, SUNY Stony Brook 1983; **Fellow:** Transplant Surgery, Univ Pittsburgh 1985; **Fac Appt:** Prof S, Univ Miami Sch Med

Urist, Marshall M MD [S] - **Spec Exp:** Cancer Surgery; Breast Cancer; Melanoma; **Hospital:** Univ of Ala Hosp at Birmingham; **Address:** Univ Alabama Sch Med, Dept Surgery, 1922 7th Ave S, Kracke Bldg, Ste 321, Birmingham, AL 35294; **Phone:** 205-934-3065; **Board Cert:** Surgery 2000; **Med School:** Univ Chicago-Pritzker Sch Med 1971; **Resid:** Surgery, Johns Hopkins Hosp 1978; **Fellow:** Surgical Oncology, UCLA Med Ctr 1976; **Fac Appt:** Prof S, Univ Alabama

Weber, Collin J MD [S] - **Spec Exp:** Endocrine Surgery; Thyroid & Parathyroid Surgery; Adrenal Surgery; Pancreatic Islet Cell Transplant; **Hospital:** Emory Univ Hosp; **Address:** Emory Univ Hosp, Dept Surgery, 1364 Clifton Rd NE, Atlanta, GA 30322; **Phone:** 404-778-4733; **Board Cert:** Surgery 2008; **Med School:** Columbia P&S 1971; **Resid:** Surgery, Columbia Presby Med Ctr 1978; **Fellow:** Research, Natl Inst Hlth 1975; **Fac Appt:** Prof S, Emory Univ

White Jr, Richard L MD [S] - **Spec Exp:** Breast Cancer; Melanoma; Sarcoma; Immunotherapy; **Hospital:** Carolinas Med Ctr; **Address:** Carolinas Medical Center, 1000 Blythe Blvd, Box 32861, Charlotte, NC 28203; **Phone:** 704-355-2884; **Board Cert:** Surgery 2002; **Med School:** Columbia P&S 1986; **Resid:** Surgery, Georgetown Univ Hosp 1992; **Fellow:** Surgical Oncology, NIH-Natl Cancer Inst 1995; **Fac Appt:** Clin Prof S, Univ NC Sch Med

Whitworth, Pat W MD [S] - **Spec Exp:** Breast Cancer; **Hospital:** Baptist Hosp - Nashville, Centennial Med Ctr; **Address:** 300 20th Ave N, Ste 401, Nashville, TN 37203; **Phone:** 615-620-5535; **Board Cert:** Surgery 2009; **Med School:** Univ Tenn Coll Med 1983; **Resid:** Surgery, Univ Louisville Med Ctr 1988; **Fellow:** Surgical Oncology, MD Anderson Cancer Ctr 1991; **Fac Appt:** Assoc Clin Prof S, Vanderbilt Univ

Wood, William C MD [S] - **Spec Exp:** Breast Cancer; **Hospital:** Emory Univ Hosp; **Address:** Winship Cancer Institute, 1365C Clifton Rd NE, Ste B206, Atlanta, GA 30322; **Phone:** 404-778-3301; **Board Cert:** Surgery 1974; **Med School:** Harvard Med Sch 1966; **Resid:** Surgery, Mass Genl Hosp 1968; Surgery, Mass Genl Hosp 1974; **Fellow:** Surgical Oncology, Natl Cancer Inst 1970; **Fac Appt:** Prof S, Emory Univ

Yeatman, Timothy J MD [S] - **Spec Exp:** Liver Cancer; **Hospital:** H Lee Moffitt Cancer Ctr & Research Inst (page 59); **Address:** H Lee Moffitt Cancer Ctr, 12902 Magnolia Drive, Tampa, FL 33612-9497; **Phone:** 813-979-7292; **Board Cert:** Surgery 2000; **Med School:** Emory Univ 1984; **Resid:** Surgery, Univ Florida 1990; **Fellow:** Surgical Oncology, MD Anderson Cancer Ctr 1992; **Fac Appt:** Prof S, Univ S Fla Coll Med

Midwest

Abecassis, Michael MD [S] - **Spec Exp:** Transplant-Liver; Transplant-Kidney; Pancreatic & Biliary Surgery; Liver Cancer; **Hospital:** Northwestern Meml Hosp; **Address:** Northwestern Med Faculty Fdn, 676 N St Clair St, Galter Pavilion Fl 19 - Ste 100, Chicago, IL 60611; **Phone:** 312-695-8900; **Board Cert:** Surgery 2009; **Med School:** Univ Toronto 1983; **Resid:** Surgery, Toronto Genl Hosp 1989; **Fellow:** Hepatopancreatobiliary Surgery, Toronto Genl Hosp 1990; Transplant Surgery, Univ Iowa Hosp 1991; **Fac Appt:** Prof S, Northwestern Univ-Feinberg Sch Med

Abouljoud, Marwan S MD [S] - **Spec Exp:** Transplant-Liver; Liver Cancer; Liver Surgery; **Hospital:** Henry Ford Hosp; **Address:** Henry Ford Hospital, 2799 W Grand Blvd, CFP2, Detroit, MI 48202; **Phone:** 313-916-2941; **Board Cert:** Surgery 2002; **Med School:** Lebanon 1985; **Resid:** Surgery, Univ of Mich igan Med Ctr 1988; Surgery, Henry Ford Hosp 1992; **Fellow:** Transplant Surgery, Univ Alabama 1994; Transplant Surgery, Baylor Univ Med Ctr 1996; **Fac Appt:** Prof S, Wayne State Univ

Surgery

Andreoni, Kenneth A MD [S] - **Spec Exp:** Transplant-Kidney-Adult & Pediatric; Transplant-Liver-Adult & Pediatric; Transplant-Pancreas; **Hospital:** Ohio St Univ Med Ctr, Nationwide Chldn's Hosp; **Address:** 395 W 12th Ave, Columbus, OH 43210; **Phone:** 614-293-8746; **Board Cert:** Surgery 2004; **Med School:** Yale Univ 1988; **Resid:** Surgery, Johns Hopkins Hosp; **Fellow:** Transplant Surgery, OSU Med Ctr 1998; **Fac Appt:** Assoc Prof S, Ohio State Univ

Angelos, Peter MD/PhD [S] - **Spec Exp:** Thyroid & Parathyroid Cancer & Surgery; Pheochromocytoma; Adrenal Tumors; Ethics; **Hospital:** Univ of Chicago Med Ctr; **Address:** 5841 S Maryland Ave, MS 4052, Chicago, IL 60637; **Phone:** 773-702-4429; **Board Cert:** Surgery 2004; **Med School:** Boston Univ 1989; **Resid:** Surgery, Northwestern Univ 1995; **Fellow:** Medical Ethics, Univ of Chicago Hosps 1992; Endocrine Surgery, Univ of Michigan Med Sch 1996; **Fac Appt:** Prof S, Univ Chicago-Pritzker Sch Med

Aranha, Gerard V MD [S] - **Spec Exp:** Pancreatic & Biliary Surgery; Stomach Cancer; Esophageal Cancer; **Hospital:** Loyola Univ Med Ctr, Edward Hines, Jr. VA Hosp; **Address:** 2160 S first Ave, Bldg 110, rm 3236, Maywood, IL 60153-3328; **Phone:** 708-327-2391; **Board Cert:** Surgery 2006; **Med School:** India 1969; **Resid:** Surgery, Loyola Univ Med Ctr 1975; **Fellow:** Surgical Oncology, Univ Minn Hosp 1977; **Fac Appt:** Prof S, Loyola Univ-Stritch Sch Med

Averbook, Bruce J MD [S] - **Spec Exp:** Melanoma; Cancer Surgery; Clinical Trials; **Hospital:** MetroHealth Med Ctr; **Address:** Metrohealth Medical Ctr, Surgical Oncology, 2500 Metrohealth Drive, rm C2110, Cleveland, OH 44109; **Phone:** 216-778-4795; **Board Cert:** Surgery 2000; **Med School:** Geo Wash Univ 1983; **Resid:** Surgery, UC Irvine Med Ctr 1990; **Fellow:** Surgical Oncology, NCI, NIH Surg Br 1993; **Fac Appt:** Assoc Prof S, Case West Res Univ

Becker, Yolanda T MD [S] - **Spec Exp:** Transplant Surgery; Transplant-Kidney; Transplant-Pancreas; Dialysis Access; **Hospital:** Univ of Chicago Med Ctr; **Address:** Univ Chicago Med Ctr-Surgery Dept, 5841 S Maryland Ave, MC 5026, Chicago, IL 60637; **Phone:** 773-702-6319; **Board Cert:** Surgery 2006; **Med School:** Johns Hopkins Univ 1990; **Resid:** Surgery, Vanderbilt Univ Med Ctr 1997; **Fellow:** Transplant Surgery, Univ Wisconsin Hosp 1999; **Fac Appt:** Prof S, Univ Chicago-Pritzker Sch Med

Benedetti, Enrico MD [S] - **Spec Exp:** Transplant-Liver; Transplant-Pancreas; Transplant-Kidney; Transplant-Bowel; **Hospital:** Univ of IL Med Ctr at Chicago; **Address:** Univ Illinois, Dept Surgery/Transplant, 840 S Wood St, rm 402, Chicago, IL 60612; **Phone:** 312-996-6771; **Board Cert:** Surgery 2003; **Med School:** Italy 1985; **Resid:** Surgery, Univ IL at Chicago Med Ctr 1993; **Fellow:** Transplant Surgery, Univ Minn Med Ctr 1994; **Fac Appt:** Prof S, Univ IL Coll Med

Brems, John J MD [S] - **Spec Exp:** Pancreatic Cancer; Liver Cancer; Transplant-Liver; Liver Disease; **Hospital:** Sherman Hosp; **Address:** 745 Fletcher Drive, Ste 302, Elgin, IL 60123; **Phone:** 847-695-6600; **Board Cert:** Surgery 2004; Surgical Critical Care 2000; **Med School:** St Louis Univ 1981; **Resid:** Surgery, St Louis Univ 1986; **Fellow:** Transplant Surgery, UCLA Med Ctr 1987; **Fac Appt:** Prof S, Loyola Univ-Stritch Sch Med

Brown, Charles K MD [S] - **Spec Exp:** Melanoma; Sarcoma; **Hospital:** CTCA at Midwestern Reg Med Ctr; **Address:** Cancer Treatments Ctrs America, 2520 Elishe Ave, Zion, IL 60099; **Phone:** 800-955-2822; **Board Cert:** Surgery 2000; **Med School:** Univ Fla Coll Med 1992; **Resid:** Surgery, Univ Arizona Med Ctr 1998; **Fellow:** Surgical Oncology, UPMC Med Ctr 1999; Surgical Oncology, Univ Chicago Med Ctr 2000

Brunt, L Michael MD [S] - **Spec Exp:** Minimally Invasive Surgery; Adrenal Tumors; Hernia; Hernia-Sports; **Hospital:** Barnes-Jewish Hosp; **Address:** Washington Univ Sch Med, Dept Surgery, 660 S Euclid Ave, Box 8109, St Louis, MO 63110; **Phone:** 314-454-7194 x2; **Board Cert:** Surgery 2006; **Med School:** Johns Hopkins Univ 1980; **Resid:** Surgery, Barnes Jewish Hosp 1987; **Fellow:** Surgery, Barnes Jewish Hosp 1984; **Fac Appt:** Prof S, Washington Univ, St Louis

Chand, Bipan MD [S] - **Spec Exp:** Obesity/Bariatric Surgery; Gastrointestinal Metabolic Surgery; Gastroesophageal Reflux Disease (GERD); Barrett's Esophagus; **Hospital:** Cleveland Clin (page 56); **Address:** Cleveland Clinic, 9500 Euclid Ave, MC M-61, Cleveland, OH 44195; **Phone:** 216-444-6668; **Board Cert:** Surgery 2003; **Med School:** Univ MO-Kansas City 1996; **Resid:** Surgery, Cleveland Clinic 2002; **Fellow:** Laparoscopic Surgery, Cleveland Clinic 2003

Chang, Alfred E MD [S] - **Spec Exp:** Cancer Surgery; Breast Cancer; Gastrointestinal Cancer; Melanoma; **Hospital:** Univ of Michigan Hosp; **Address:** 1500 E Medical Center Drive, 3302 Cancer Geriatric Ctr SPC 5932, Ann Arbor, MI 48109-5932; **Phone:** 734-936-4392; **Board Cert:** Surgery 2001; **Med School:** Harvard Med Sch 1974; **Resid:** Surgery, Duke Univ Med Ctr 1976; Surgery, Hosp Univ Penn 1982; **Fellow:** Surgical Oncology, Natl Cancer Inst 1979; **Fac Appt:** Prof S, Univ Mich Med Sch

Chapman, William C MD [S] - **Spec Exp:** Transplant-Liver-Adult & Pediatric; Liver Cancer; Liver & Biliary Surgery; **Hospital:** Barnes-Jewish Hosp, St. Louis Chldns Hosp; **Address:** Washington Univ Sch Med, 660 S Euclid Ave, Box 8109, St Louis, MO 63110; **Phone:** 314-362-7792; **Board Cert:** Surgery 2001; Surgical Critical Care 2001; **Med School:** Med Univ SC 1984; **Resid:** Surgery, Vanderbilt Univ Med Ctr 1991; **Fellow:** Hepatobiliary Surgery, Kings College Hosp 1992; **Fac Appt:** Prof S, Washington Univ, St Louis

Cronin II, David C MD/PhD [S] - **Spec Exp:** Transplant-Liver; Transplant Surgery-Pediatric; Liver & Biliary Surgery; Pancreatic Surgery; **Hospital:** Froedtert and Med Ctr of WI; **Address:** Div Transplant Surgery, 9200 W Wisconsin Ave, Ste 5700, Milwaukee, WI 53226; **Phone:** 414-955-6920; **Board Cert:** Surgery 2005; **Med School:** Mount Sinai Sch Med 1987; **Resid:** Surgery, Univ Chicago Hosps 1995; **Fellow:** Transplant Surgery, Univ Chicago Hosps 1997; Medical Ethics, Univ Chicago Hosps 2002; **Fac Appt:** Assoc Prof S, Univ Wisc

Crowe Jr, Joseph P MD [S] - **Spec Exp:** Breast Cancer; Tumor Surgery; **Hospital:** Cleveland Clin (page 56); **Address:** Cleveland Clinic Fdn, Dept Surg, 9500 Euclid Ave, Desk A10, Cleveland, OH 44195; **Phone:** 216-444-3024; **Board Cert:** Surgery 2004; **Med School:** Case West Res Univ 1978; **Resid:** Surgery, Univ Hosp-Case West Reserve 1983; **Fellow:** Surgical Oncology, Meml Sloan Kettering Cancer Ctr 1985

Deziel, Daniel J MD [S] - **Spec Exp:** Hepatobiliary Surgery; Pancreatic Surgery; Laparoscopic Surgery; **Hospital:** Rush Univ Med Ctr; **Address:** 1725 W Harrison St, Ste 810/818, Chicago, IL 60612; **Phone:** 312-942-6500; **Board Cert:** Surgery 2003; **Med School:** Univ Minn 1979; **Resid:** Surgery, Rush-Presby-St Luke's Med Ctr 1984; **Fellow:** Gastrointestinal Surgery, Lahey Clinic 1985; **Fac Appt:** Prof S, Rush Med Coll

Doherty, Gerard M MD [S] - **Spec Exp:** Endocrine Surgery; Adrenal Surgery; Laparoscopic Surgery; Thyroid Surgery; **Hospital:** Univ of Michigan Hosp; **Address:** 2920 Taubman Ctr, 1500 E Medical Ctr Drive, Ann Arbor, MI 48109-5331; **Phone:** 734-936-5818; **Board Cert:** Surgery 2003; **Med School:** Yale Univ 1986; **Resid:** Surgery, UCSF Med Ctr 1993; **Fellow:** Surgical Oncology, Natl Cancer Inst 1991; **Fac Appt:** Prof S, Univ Mich Med Sch

Donohue, John H MD [S] - **Spec Exp:** Gastrointestinal Cancer; Breast Cancer; Stomach Cancer; **Hospital:** Mayo Med Ctr & Clin - Rochester; **Address:** Mayo Clinic, Dept General Surgery, 200 First St SW, Rochester, MN 55905; **Phone:** 507-284-0362; **Board Cert:** Surgery 2005; **Med School:** Harvard Med Sch 1978; **Resid:** Surgery, UCSF Med Ctr 1981; Surgery, UCSF Med Ctr 1985; **Fellow:** Surgery, Natl Inst Hlth 1983; Surgical Oncology, Meml Sloan-Kettering Canc Ctr 1987; **Fac Appt:** Prof S, Mayo Med Sch

Dulchavsky, Scott A MD/PhD [S] - **Spec Exp:** Trauma; **Hospital:** Henry Ford Hosp; **Address:** Henry Ford Hospital, 2799 W Grand Blvd, CFP1, Detroit, MI 48202; **Phone:** 313-916-3152; **Board Cert:** Surgery 2007; Surgical Critical Care 1998; **Med School:** Wayne State Univ 1983; **Resid:** Surgery, Wayne State 1989; **Fac Appt:** Prof S, Wayne State Univ

Eberlein, Timothy J MD [S] - **Spec Exp:** Breast Cancer; Melanoma; Immunotherapy; **Hospital:** Barnes-Jewish Hosp, St. Louis Chldns Hosp; **Address:** Wash Univ School Med, Dept Surgery, 660 S Euclid Ave, Box 8109, St Louis, MO 63110-1093; **Phone:** 314-362-8020; **Board Cert:** Surgery 2006; **Med School:** Univ Pittsburgh 1977; **Resid:** Surgery, Peter Bent Brigham Hosp 1979; Surgery, Brigham-Womens Hosp 1985; **Fellow:** Immunology, Natl Inst Hlth 1982; **Fac Appt:** Prof S, Washington Univ, St Louis

Edwards, Michael J MD [S] - **Spec Exp:** Breast Cancer; Melanoma; **Hospital:** Univ Hosp - Cincinnati; **Address:** 234 Goodman St, ML 0772, Cincinnati, OH 45219; **Phone:** 513-584-8900; **Board Cert:** Surgery 2005; **Med School:** Emory Univ 1981; **Resid:** Surgery, Univ Louisville Hosp 1986; **Fellow:** Surgical Oncology, MD Anderson Cancer Ctr 1987; **Fac Appt:** Prof S, Univ Ark

Ellison, E Christopher MD [S] - **Spec Exp:** Biliary Surgery; Biliary Cancer; Pancreatic Cancer; **Hospital:** Ohio St Univ Med Ctr; **Address:** 1654 Upham Drive, Ste 327 Means Hall, Columbus, OH 43210-1236; **Phone:** 614-293-4499; **Board Cert:** Surgery 2001; **Med School:** Univ Wisc 1976; **Resid:** Surgery, Ohio State Univ 1981; **Fac Appt:** Prof S, Ohio State Univ

Evans, Douglas B MD [S] - **Spec Exp:** Pancreatic Cancer; Thyroid Cancer; Endocrine Cancers; **Hospital:** Froedtert and Med Ctr of WI; **Address:** Medical Coll Wisconsin, Dept Surgery, 9200 W Wisconsin Ave, Ste 3510, Milwaukee, WI 53226-6533; **Phone:** 414-805-5706; **Board Cert:** Surgery 2008; **Med School:** Boston Univ 1983; **Resid:** Surgery, Dartmouth-Hitchcock Med Ctr 1988; **Fellow:** Surgical Oncology, MD Anderson Cancer Ctr 1990; **Fac Appt:** Prof S, Med Coll Wisc

Farley, David R MD [S] - **Spec Exp:** Endocrine Surgery; Hepatobiliary Surgery; Laparoscopic Surgery; Hernia; **Hospital:** Mayo Med Ctr & Clin - Rochester; **Address:** Mayo Clinic, 200 First St SW, Mayo West 12, Rochester, MN 55905; **Phone:** 507-284-2644; **Board Cert:** Surgery 2002; **Med School:** Univ Wisc 1988; **Resid:** Surgery, Mayo Clin 1994; **Fellow:** Endocrinology, Mayo Clin 1995; **Fac Appt:** Assoc Prof S, Mayo Med Sch

Farrar, William B MD [S] - **Spec Exp:** Breast Cancer; Thyroid Cancer; **Hospital:** Arthur G James Cancer Hosp & Research Inst, Ohio St Univ Med Ctr; **Address:** 410 W 10th Ave, N924 Doan Hall, Columbus, OH 43210-1240; **Phone:** 614-293-8890; **Board Cert:** Surgery 2000; **Med School:** Univ VA Sch Med 1975; **Resid:** Surgery, Ohio State Univ Hosps 1980; **Fellow:** Surgical Oncology, Meml Sloan-Kettering Cancer Ctr 1982; **Fac Appt:** Prof S, Ohio State Univ

Frantzides, Constantine T MD/PhD [S] - **Spec Exp:** Minimally Invasive Surgery; Laparoscopic Surgery; Obesity/Bariatric Surgery; Laparoscopic Abdominal Surgery; **Hospital:** St. Francis Hosp - Evanston, Evanston/North Shore Univ Hlth Sys; **Address:** Chicago Inst Minimally Invasive Surg, 4905 Old Orchard Ctr, Ste 409, Skokie, IL 60077; **Phone:** 847-676-2200; **Med School:** Greece 1976; **Resid:** Surgery, Athens Univ Affil Hosp 1982; **Fellow:** Surgery, Queen Mary's Hosp 1978; Surgery, Med Coll Wisc 1985; **Fac Appt:** Prof S, Univ IL Coll Med

Franz, Michael G MD [S] - **Spec Exp:** Hernia; Minimally Invasive Surgery; Abdominal Wall Reconstruction; Wound Healing/Care; **Hospital:** Univ of Michigan Hosp; **Address:** University of Michigan Health Systems, 2920 Taubman Health Care Center, 1500 E Medical Ctr Drive, Ann Arbor, MI 48109; **Phone:** 734-936-5738; **Board Cert:** Surgery 2008; **Med School:** Univ Fla Coll Med 1989; **Resid:** Surgery, Tampa General Hosp 1995; Research, Univ of S Florida; **Fellow:** Surgery, Moffitt Cancer Ctr 1997; **Fac Appt:** Assoc Prof S, Univ Mich Med Sch

Fung, John J MD/PhD [S] - **Spec Exp:** Transplant-Liver; Transplant-Kidney; Liver & Biliary Cancer; **Hospital:** Cleveland Clin (page 56), Euclid Hosp; **Address:** Cleveland Clinic, Dept Surgery, 9500 Euclid Ave, Desk A80, Cleveland, OH 44195-0001; **Phone:** 216-444-3776; **Board Cert:** Surgery 2008; **Med School:** Univ Chicago-Pritzker Sch Med 1982; **Resid:** Surgery, Strong Memorial Hosp 1988; **Fellow:** Transplant Surgery, Univ Pittsburgh 1986; **Fac Appt:** Prof S, Cleveland Cl Coll Med/Case West Res

Gamelli, Richard L MD [S] - **Spec Exp:** Burn Care; Trauma/Critical Care; **Hospital:** Loyola Univ Med Ctr; **Address:** 2160 S First Ave Bldg 103 - rm 1175, Maywood, IL 60153; **Phone:** 708-216-4444; **Board Cert:** Surgery 2009; **Med School:** Univ VT Coll Med 1974; **Resid:** Surgery, Vermont Med Ctr Hosp 1979; **Fac Appt:** Prof S, Loyola Univ-Stritch Sch Med

Goulet Jr, Robert J MD [S] - **Spec Exp:** Breast Cancer; Breast Surgery; **Hospital:** Commun Hosp E - Indianapolis; **Address:** Community Hospital Breast Care, 1400 N Ritter Ave, Ste 485, Indianapolis, IN 46219; **Phone:** 317-355-2727; **Board Cert:** Surgery 2006; **Med School:** SUNY Downstate 1979; **Resid:** Surgery, SUNY-Downstate Med Ctr 1986; **Fellow:** Surgical Research, SUNY-Downstate Med Ctr 1983

Grant, Clive S S MD [S] - **Spec Exp:** Thyroid & Parathyroid Cancer & Surgery; Adrenal Tumors; Breast Cancer; **Hospital:** Mayo Med Ctr & Clin - Rochester; **Address:** Mayo Clinic, Dept Surgery, 200 First St SW, Rochester, MN 55905-0001; **Phone:** 507-284-2644; **Board Cert:** Surgery 2001; **Med School:** Univ Colorado 1975; **Resid:** Surgery, Mayo Clinic 1980; **Fac Appt:** Prof S, Mayo Med Sch

Gruber, Scott A MD/PhD [S] - **Spec Exp:** Transplant-Kidney; Transplant-Pancreas; **Hospital:** John D. Dingell VA Med Ctr, Detroit, Harper Univ Hosp; **Address:** 4646 John R St, Detroit, MI 48201; **Phone:** 313-576-3327; **Board Cert:** Surgery 2001; **Med School:** SUNY Downstate 1983; **Resid:** Surgery, Univ Minnesota Med Ctr 1986; **Fellow:** Surgery, Univ Minnesota Med Ctr 1989; Transplant Surgery, Univ Minnesota Med Ctr 1993; **Fac Appt:** Prof S, Wayne State Univ

Hansen, Nora M MD [S] - **Spec Exp:** Sentinel Node Surgery; Breast Cancer-High Risk Women; Breast Cancer Risk Assessment; **Hospital:** Northwestern Meml Hosp; **Address:** Northwestern Meml Hosp, Surgical Onc, 675 N St Clair, Galter 21-700, Chicago, IL 60611; **Phone:** 312-695-1156; **Board Cert:** Surgery 2006; **Med School:** NY Med Coll 1988; **Resid:** Surgery, Univ Chicago Hosps 1995; **Fellow:** Surgical Oncology, Univ Chicago Hosps 1996; **Fac Appt:** Assoc Prof S, Northwestern Univ

Hering, Bernhard J MD [S] - **Spec Exp:** Pancreatic Islet Cell Transplant; Diabetes; **Hospital:** Univ Minn Med Ctr, Fairview - Riverside Campus; **Address:** University of Minnesotta, Dept Surgery, MMC 280, 420 Delaware St SE, Minneapolis, MN 55455; **Phone:** 612-626-5697; **Med School:** Germany 1983; **Resid:** Research, Islet Transplant lab, Justus Liebig Univ 1986; Internal Medicine, Justus Liebig Univ 1995; **Fellow:** Endocrinology, Justus Liebig Univ 1996; **Fac Appt:** Prof S, Univ Minn

Hinshaw, Daniel B MD [S] - **Spec Exp:** Palliative Care; **Hospital:** VA Ann Arbor Healthcare Sys, Univ of Michigan Hosp; **Address:** VA Medical Ctr, 2215 Fuller Rd, rm 530, MS 112, Ann Arbor, MI 48105; **Phone:** 734-769-7100 x5939; **Board Cert:** Surgery 2003; Hospice & Palliative Medicine 2008; **Med School:** Loma Linda Univ 1978; **Resid:** Surgery, Loma Linda U Med Ctr 1983; **Fellow:** Immunology, Scripps Clinic Rsch Fdn 1985; Cleveland Clin 2001; **Fac Appt:** Clin Prof S, Univ Mich Med Sch

Howe, James R MD [S] - **Spec Exp:** Endocrine Surgery; Gastrointestinal Cancer; Colon & Rectal Cancer; **Hospital:** Univ Iowa Hosp & Clinics; **Address:** 200 Hawkins Drive JCP Bldg - rm 4645, Iowa City, IA 52242-1086; **Phone:** 319-356-1727; **Board Cert:** Surgery 2006; **Med School:** Univ VT Coll Med 1987; **Resid:** Surgery, Barnes Hosp-Wash Univ 1994; **Fellow:** Research, Wash Univ-NCI 1991; Surgical Oncology, Meml Sloan Kettering Cancer Ctr 1996; **Fac Appt:** Prof S, Univ Iowa Coll Med

Ikramuddin, Sayeed MD [S] - **Spec Exp:** Minimally Invasive Surgery; Obesity/Bariatric Surgery; **Hospital:** Univ Minn Med Ctr, Fairview - Riverside Campus; **Address:** 516 Delaware St SE, Obesity and Bariatric Weight Mgmt, P Wagenstein Bldg Fl 1, Clinic 1E-MMC88, Minneapolis, MN 55455; **Phone:** 612-625-8446; **Board Cert:** Surgery 2007; **Med School:** Albany Med Coll 1990; **Resid:** Surgery, SUNY Hlth Sciences Ctr 1992; Surgery, SUNY Hlth Sciences Ctr 1996; **Fellow:** Research, SUNY Hlth Sciences Ctr 1993; Laparoscopic Surgery, Ohio State Univ Affil Hosp 1997; **Fac Appt:** Assoc Prof S, Univ Minn

Johnson Miller, Denise L MD [S] - **Spec Exp:** Breast Cancer; Breast Cancer-High Risk Women; Melanoma; **Hospital:** Franciscan St. Francis Hlth-Indianapolis; **Address:** St Francis Breast Specialists, 5255 E Stop 11 Rd, Ste 250, Indianapolis, IN 46237; **Phone:** 317-781-7391; **Board Cert:** Surgery 2001; **Med School:** Washington Univ, St Louis 1978; **Resid:** Immunology, Univ Texas SW Med Ctr 1982; Surgery, Univ Illinois Med Ctr 1986; **Fellow:** Surgical Oncology, City of Hope Med Ctr 1989

Kagan, Richard J MD [S] - **Spec Exp:** Burn Care; **Hospital:** Cincinnati Shriners Hosp, Univ Hosp - Cincinnati; **Address:** Cincinnati Shriners Hosp, 3229 Burnet Ave, Cincinnati, OH 45229; **Phone:** 513-872-6210; **Board Cert:** Surgery 2007; **Med School:** St Louis Univ 1974; **Resid:** Surgery, Univ IL Hosp 1980; **Fac Appt:** Prof S, Univ Cincinnati

Kaufman, Howard L MD [S] - **Spec Exp:** Cancer Surgery; Vaccine Therapy; Melanoma; Immunotherapy; **Hospital:** Rush Univ Med Ctr; **Address:** 1725 W Harrison St, Ste 845, Chicago, IL 60612-3244; **Phone:** 312-942-0600; **Board Cert:** Surgery 2007; **Med School:** Loyola Univ-Stritch Sch Med 1986; **Resid:** Surgery, Boston Univ Hosp 1995; **Fellow:** Surgical Oncology, Natl Cancer Inst 1996; **Fac Appt:** Prof S, Loyola Univ-Stritch Sch Med

Kendrick, Michael L MD [S] - **Spec Exp:** Pancreatic Cancer; Liver Cancer; Hepatobiliary Surgery; Laparoscopic Surgery; **Hospital:** Mayo Med Ctr & Clin - Rochester; **Address:** Mayo Clinic Atten: Dept of Surgery, 200 First St SW, Rochester, MN 55905; **Phone:** 507-284-2511; **Board Cert:** Surgery 2004; **Med School:** Geo Wash Univ 1997; **Resid:** Surgery, Mayo Clinic 2003; **Fellow:** Hepatopancreatobiliary Surgery, Mayo Clinic 2004; Laparoscopic Surgery, Mt Sinai Med Ctr 2005; **Fac Appt:** Assoc Prof S, Mayo Med Sch

Kim, Julian A MD [S] - **Spec Exp:** Melanoma; Breast Cancer; Gastrointestinal Cancer; Immunotherapy; **Hospital:** Univ Hosps Case Med Ctr (page 74); **Address:** 11100 Euclid Ave, LKS 5047, Cleveland, OH 44106-1716; **Phone:** 216-844-8247; **Board Cert:** Surgery 2002; **Med School:** Med Univ Ohio at Toledo 1986; **Resid:** Surgery, Univ Maryland Hosps 1991; **Fellow:** Surgical Oncology, Arthur James Cancer Hosp & Rsch Inst 1993; Immunotherapy, Ohio State Univ Comp Cancer Ctr 1994; **Fac Appt:** Assoc Prof S, Case West Res Univ

Leeming, Rosemary A MD [S] - **Spec Exp:** Breast Cancer & Surgery; Breast Disease; Clinical Trials; **Hospital:** Univ Hosps Case Med Ctr (page 74); **Address:** 3909 Orange Pl, Ste 4400, Orange Village, OH 44122; **Phone:** 216-591-1909; **Board Cert:** Surgery 2009; **Med School:** Hahnemann Univ 1983; **Resid:** Surgery, Mt Sinai Med Ctr 1989; **Fellow:** Breast Disease, Univ Pitts-Shadyside Hosp 1989; **Fac Appt:** Asst Prof S, Case West Res Univ

Mahvi, David M MD [S] - **Spec Exp:** Gastrointestinal Cancer & Surgery; Liver Cancer; Pancreatic Cancer; **Hospital:** Northwestern Meml Hosp; **Address:** NMH/ Arkes Family Pavilion, Ste 650, 676 N St Clair, Chicago, IL 60611; **Phone:** 312-695-1419; **Board Cert:** Surgery 2007; **Med School:** Med Univ SC 1981; **Resid:** Surgery, Duke Univ Med Ctr 1989; **Fac Appt:** Prof S, Northwestern Univ

Mamounas, Eleftherios P MD [S] - **Spec Exp:** Breast Cancer; **Hospital:** Aultman Hosp; **Address:** Aultman Cancer Ctr, 2600 6th St SW, Canton, OH 44710; **Phone:** 330-363-6281; **Board Cert:** Surgery 2009; **Med School:** Greece 1983; **Resid:** Surgery, McKeesport Hosp 1989; **Fellow:** Clinical Oncology, Univ Pittsburgh 1991; Surgical Oncology, Roswell Park Cancer Inst 1992; **Fac Appt:** Prof S, NE Ohio Univ

Marks, Jeffrey M MD [S] - **Spec Exp:** Gastrointestinal Surgery; Endoscopy; Laparoscopic Surgery; Natural Orifice Surgery (NOTES); **Hospital:** Univ Hosps Case Med Ctr (page 74); **Address:** Univ Hospitals Case Medical Ctr, Dept Surgery, 11100 Euclid Ave, Cleveland, OH 44106; **Phone:** 216-844-7874; **Board Cert:** Surgery 2001; **Med School:** Tufts Univ 1987; **Resid:** Surgery, Mt Sinai Hosp 1992; **Fellow:** Endoscopy, Mt Sinai Hosp 1992; **Fac Appt:** Assoc Prof S, Case West Res Univ

Matas, Arthur J MD [S] - **Spec Exp:** Transplant-Kidney; **Hospital:** Univ Minn Med Ctr, Fairview - Riverside Campus; **Address:** Univ Minn Med Ctr-Dept Surgery, 420 Delaware St SE, MMC 328, Minneapolis, MN 55455; **Phone:** 612-625-6460; **Board Cert:** Surgery 2000; **Med School:** Univ Manitoba 1972; **Resid:** Surgery, Univ Minnesota Hosps 1979; **Fellow:** Transplant Surgery, Univ Minnesota Hosps 1980; **Fac Appt:** Prof S, Univ Minn

Matthews, Jeffrey MD [S] - **Spec Exp:** Gastrointestinal Surgery; Pancreatic Surgery; Liver & Biliary Surgery; **Hospital:** Univ of Chicago Med Ctr; **Address:** 5841 S Maryland Ave, Ste 0220, MC 5029, Chicago, IL 60637; **Phone:** 773-702-0881; **Board Cert:** Surgery 2001; **Med School:** Harvard Med Sch 1985; **Resid:** Surgery, Beth Israel Hosp 1990; **Fellow:** Hepatobiliary Surgery, Univ Bern 1989; **Fac Appt:** Prof S, Univ Chicago-Pritzker Sch Med

McHenry, Christopher R MD [S] - **Spec Exp:** Adrenal Surgery; Thyroid Surgery; Parathyroid Surgery; **Hospital:** MetroHealth Med Ctr; **Address:** MetroHealth Medical Ctr, Dept Surgery, 2500 Metro Health Drive, Cleveland, OH 44109-1998; **Phone:** 216-778-4753; **Board Cert:** Surgery 2009; **Med School:** NE Ohio Univ 1984; **Resid:** Surgery, Loyola Univ Med Ctr 1989; **Fellow:** Endocrinology, Univ Toronto Med Ctr 1990; Head and Neck Surgery, Univ Toronto Med Ctr 1990; **Fac Appt:** Prof S, Case West Res Univ

Melvin, W Scott MD [S] - **Spec Exp:** Liver & Biliary Surgery; Pancreatic Cancer; Laparoscopic Surgery; **Hospital:** Ohio St Univ Med Ctr; **Address:** 410 W 10th Ave, rm N729, North Doan Hall, Columbus, OH 43210; **Phone:** 614-293-4499; **Board Cert:** Surgery 2002; **Med School:** Med Coll OH 1987; **Resid:** Surgery, Univ Maryland 1992; **Fellow:** Gastrointestinal Surgery, Grant Med Ctr 1993; **Fac Appt:** Prof S, Ohio State Univ

Millis, J Michael MD [S] - **Spec Exp:** Transplant-Liver-Adult & Pediatric; Liver Cancer; Transplant-Pancreas; Liver Disease; **Hospital:** Univ of Chicago Med Ctr; **Address:** 5841 S Maryland Ave, MS 5027, Chicago, IL 60637; **Phone:** 773-702-6319; **Board Cert:** Surgery 2001; Surgical Critical Care 2001; **Med School:** Univ Tenn Coll Med 1985; **Resid:** Surgery, UCLA Med Ctr 1992; **Fellow:** Transplant Surgery, UCLA Med Ctr 1994; **Fac Appt:** Prof S, Univ Chicago-Pritzker Sch Med

Moley, Jeffrey F MD [S] - **Spec Exp:** Thyroid Cancer & Surgery; Endocrine Cancers; Melanoma; **Hospital:** Barnes-Jewish Hosp; **Address:** Washington Univ School Med, Dept Surgery, 660 S Euclid Ave, Box 8109, St Louis, MO 63110; **Phone:** 314-362-2280; **Board Cert:** Surgery 2005; **Med School:** Columbia P&S 1980; **Resid:** Surgery, Yale-New Haven Hosp 1985; **Fellow:** Surgical Oncology, National Cancer Inst 1987; **Fac Appt:** Prof S, Washington Univ, St Louis

Nagorney, David M MD [S] - **Spec Exp:** Pancreatic Cancer; Hepatobiliary Surgery; Gastrointestinal Cancer; **Hospital:** Mayo Med Ctr & Clin - Rochester; **Address:** Mayo Clin, Dept Surgery, 200 1st St SW, Mayo E12, Rochester, MN 55905; **Phone:** 507-284-0362; **Board Cert:** Surgery 2001; **Med School:** Univ Kansas 1975; **Resid:** Surgery, Mayo Clin 1982; **Fellow:** Hepatobiliary Surgery, Hammersmith Hosp 1985; **Fac Appt:** Prof S, Mayo Med Sch

Nathanson, S David MD [S] - **Spec Exp:** Breast Cancer; Breast Cancer Risk Assessment; Melanoma; Sarcoma; **Hospital:** Henry Ford Hosp, Henry Ford- W Bloomfield Hosp; **Address:** 2799 W Grand Blvd, Detroit, MI 48202; **Phone:** 313-916-2917; **Board Cert:** Surgery 2002; **Med School:** South Africa 1966; **Resid:** Surgery, Univ Witwaterstrand 1974; Surgical Oncology, UCLA Med Ctr 1980; **Fellow:** Surgery, UC Davis 1982; **Fac Appt:** Prof S, Case West Res Univ

Newman, Lisa A MD [S] - **Spec Exp:** Breast Cancer; **Hospital:** Univ of Michigan Hosp; **Address:** Univ Michigan Cancer Center, 1500 E Medical Center Drive, rm 3308-CGC, Ann Arbor, MI 48109-5932; **Phone:** 734-936-8771; **Board Cert:** Surgery 2001; **Med School:** SUNY Downstate 1985; **Resid:** Surgery, Downstate Med Ctr 1990; **Fac Appt:** Assoc Prof S, Univ Mich Med Sch

Oberholzer, Jose MD [S] - **Spec Exp:** Diabetes; Transplant-Pancreas; Pancreatic Islet Cell Transplant; Hepatobiliary Surgery; **Hospital:** Univ of IL Med Ctr at Chicago, Adv Luth Genl Hosp; **Address:** Univ Illinois Med Ctr at Chicago, Div Transplantation, 840 S Wood St, Ste 402, MC 958, Chicago, IL 60612; **Phone:** 312-996-6771; **Med School:** Switzerland 1992; **Resid:** Surgery, Triemli Hosp 1996; Surgery, Univ Geneva Hosp 1998; **Fellow:** Transplant Surgery, Univ Geneva Hosp 2002; Hepatopancreatobiliary Surgery, Univ Alberta Hosp 2003; **Fac Appt:** Assoc Prof S, Univ IL Coll Med

Onders, Raymond P MD [S] - **Spec Exp:** Laparoscopic Surgery; Diaphragm Pacing via Laparoscopy; Gastrointestinal Cancer; **Hospital:** Univ Hosps Case Med Ctr (page 74); **Address:** 11100 Euclid Ave, MS LKS 5047, Cleveland, OH 44106-5047; **Phone:** 216-844-5797; **Board Cert:** Surgery 2001; **Med School:** NE Ohio Univ 1988; **Resid:** Surgery, Case Western Reserve Univ 1993; **Fac Appt:** Assoc Prof S, NE Ohio Univ

Ponsky, Jeffrey L MD [S] - **Spec Exp:** Minimally Invasive Surgery; Gastrointestinal Surgery; Endoscopy; **Hospital:** Univ Hosps Case Med Ctr (page 74); **Address:** Univ Hosps Cleveland, Dept Surgery, 11100 Euclid Ave, Cleveland, OH 44106; **Phone:** 216-844-3209; **Board Cert:** Surgery 2007; **Med School:** Case West Res Univ 1971; **Resid:** Surgery, Univ Hosps 1976; **Fac Appt:** Prof S, Case West Res Univ

Posner, Mitchell C MD [S] - **Spec Exp:** Pancreatic Cancer; Gastrointestinal Cancer; Esophageal Cancer; **Hospital:** Univ of Chicago Med Ctr; **Address:** Univ Chicago Medical Center, 5841 S Maryland Ave, Ste G209, MC 5094, Chicago, IL 60637-1447; **Phone:** 773-834-4007; **Board Cert:** Surgery 2006; **Med School:** SUNY Buffalo 1981; **Resid:** Surgery, Univ Colorado Med Ctr 1986; **Fellow:** Surgical Oncology, Meml Sloan Kettering Cancer Ctr 1988; **Fac Appt:** Prof S, Univ Chicago-Pritzker Sch Med

Prinz, Richard A MD [S] - **Spec Exp:** Adrenal Surgery; Thyroid & Parathyroid Surgery; Pancreatic & Biliary Surgery; Laparoscopic Surgery; **Hospital:** Evanston/North Shore Univ Hlth Sys, Highland Park/North Shore Univ Hlth Syst; **Address:** North Shore Univ Hlth System, 1000 Central St, Ste 800, Evanston, IL 60201; **Phone:** 847-570-1700; **Board Cert:** Surgery 2007; **Med School:** Loyola Univ-Stritch Sch Med 1972; **Resid:** Surgery, Barnes Hosp 1974; Surgery, Loyola Univ Hosp 1977; **Fellow:** Endocrine Surgery, Hammersmith Hosp 1980; **Fac Appt:** Prof S, Univ Chicago-Pritzker Sch Med

Renz, John MD/PhD [S] - **Spec Exp:** Transplant-Liver; Transplant-Liver-Adult & Pediatric; Transplant Surgery; **Hospital:** Univ of Chicago Med Ctr; **Address:** Univ Chicago Med Ctr- Surgery Dept, 5841 S Maryland Ave, MC 5027, Chicago, IL 60637; **Phone:** 773-702-4500; **Board Cert:** Surgery 2003; **Med School:** Jefferson Med Coll 1992; **Resid:** Surgery, UCSF Med Ctr 1999; **Fellow:** Transplant Surgery, UCLA Med Ctr 2002; **Fac Appt:** Prof S, Univ Chicago-Pritzker Sch Med

Rosen, Charles B MD [S] - **Spec Exp:** Transplant-Liver; Transplant-Bile Duct; **Hospital:** Mayo Med Ctr & Clin - Rochester; **Address:** Dept Surg-Div Transplantation, 200 First St SW, Charlton 10A, Rochester, MN 55905-0001; **Phone:** 507-266-6640; **Board Cert:** Surgery 1999; **Med School:** Mayo Med Sch 1984; **Resid:** Surgery, Mayo Clin 1989; **Fellow:** Transplant Surgery, Mayo Clin 1991; **Fac Appt:** Prof S, Mayo Med Sch

Rosen, Michael J MD [S] - **Spec Exp:** Hernia; Gastrointestinal Surgery; Minimally Invasive Surgery; **Hospital:** Univ Hosps Case Med Ctr (page 74); **Address:** Univ Hosp Case Med Ctr, 11100 Euclid Ave, LKS5047, Cleveland, OH 44106; **Phone:** 216-844-2763; **Board Cert:** Surgery 2005; **Med School:** USC-Keck School of Medicine 1997; **Resid:** Surgery, Mass Gen Hosp 2004; **Fellow:** Minimally Invasive Surgery, Cleveland Clinic 2002; Laparoscopic Surgery, Carolinas Med Ctr 2005; **Fac Appt:** Asst Prof S, Case West Res Univ

Saha, Sukamal MD [S] - **Spec Exp:** Sentinel Node Surgery; Colon Cancer; Head & Neck Cancer & Surgery; **Hospital:** McLaren Reg Med Ctr, Genesys Reg Med Ctr - St Joseph Campus; **Address:** 3500 Calkins Rd, Ste A, Flint, MI 48532; **Phone:** 810-230-9600 x500; **Board Cert:** Surgery 2000; **Med School:** India 1977; **Resid:** Surgery, Hahnemann Univ Hosp 1985; Surgery, Easton Hosp 1987; **Fellow:** Surgical Oncology, Tulane Univ Med Ctr 1989; Head and Neck Surgery, Roswell Park Meml Hosp 1990; **Fac Appt:** Asst Prof S, Mich State Univ

Sarr, Michael G MD [S] - **Spec Exp:** Pancreatic Cancer; Gastrointestinal Cancer; Obesity/Bariatric Surgery; Gastrointestinal Motility Disorders; **Hospital:** Mayo Med Ctr & Clin - Rochester; **Address:** Mayo Clinic, 200 First St SW, Dept Surg, Desk West 12A, Rochester, MN 55905; **Phone:** 507-284-0362; **Board Cert:** Surgery 2001; **Med School:** Johns Hopkins Univ 1976; **Resid:** Surgery, Johns Hopkins Hosp 1982; **Fellow:** Surgery, Mayo Clinic 1984; Surgery, Johns Hopkins Hosp 1985; **Fac Appt:** Prof S, Mayo Med Sch

Schauer, Philip MD [S] - **Spec Exp:** Obesity/Bariatric Surgery; Minimally Invasive Surgery; **Hospital:** Cleveland Clin (page 56); **Address:** Cleveland Clinic, 9500 Euclid Ave, MC M61, Cleveland, OH 44195; **Phone:** 216-444-4794; **Board Cert:** Surgery 2004; **Med School:** Baylor Coll Med 1986; **Resid:** Surgery, Univ Texas Med Ctr 1991; **Fellow:** Laparoscopic Surgery, Duke Univ Med Ctr 1992; **Fac Appt:** Prof S, Cleveland Cl Coll Med/Case West Res

Schulak, James A MD [S] - **Spec Exp:** Transplant-Kidney-Adult & Pediatric; Transplant-Pancreas & Liver; Pancreatic Surgery; **Hospital:** Univ Hosps Case Med Ctr (page 74); **Address:** Univ Hosps of Cleveland, Dept Surgery, 11100 Euclid Ave, MS 5047, Cleveland, OH 44106-5407; **Phone:** 216-844-0307; **Board Cert:** Surgery 2010; **Med School:** Univ Chicago-Pritzker Sch Med 1974; **Resid:** Surgery, Univ Chicago Hosp 1980; **Fellow:** Transplant Surgery, Univ Chicago Hosp 1981; **Fac Appt:** Prof S, Case West Res Univ

Schwartzentruber, Douglas J MD [S] - **Spec Exp:** Cancer Surgery; Melanoma; Kidney Cancer; **Hospital:** Indiana Univ Hlth Goshen Hosp; **Address:** Cancer Ctr at Goshen Health System, 200 High Park Ave, Goshen, IN 46526; **Phone:** 574-535-2888; **Board Cert:** Surgery 2008; **Med School:** Indiana Univ 1982; **Resid:** Surgery, Indiana Univ Med Ctr 1987; **Fellow:** Surgical Oncology, Natl Cancer Inst 1990; **Fac Appt:** Assoc Clin Prof S, Indiana Univ

Scott-Conner, Carol E H MD/PhD [S] - **Spec Exp:** Breast Cancer; Cancer Surgery; Laparoscopic Surgery; **Hospital:** Univ Iowa Hosp & Clinics, Iowa City VA Hlth Care Sys; **Address:** Univ Iowa, Dept Surg, 200 Hawkins Drive, 4622 JCP, Iowa City, IA 52242-1086; **Phone:** 319-356-0330; **Board Cert:** Surgery 2000; Surgical Critical Care 1998; **Med School:** NYU Sch Med 1976; **Resid:** Surgery, NYU Med Ctr 1981; **Fac Appt:** Prof S, Univ Iowa Coll Med

Shenk, Robert R MD [S] - **Spec Exp:** Breast Cancer; Melanoma; Pancreatic Cancer; Stomach Cancer; **Hospital:** Univ Hosps Case Med Ctr (page 74); **Address:** Univ Hosp Case Med Ctr, 11100 Euclid Ave, Dept General Surgery, Cleveland, OH 44106; **Phone:** 216-844-3026; **Board Cert:** Surgery 2004; **Med School:** Case West Res Univ 1978; **Resid:** Surgery, Univ Hosp 1985; Immunology, Natl Cancer Inst 1982; **Fellow:** Surgical Oncology, Anderson Hosp 1987; **Fac Appt:** Assoc Prof S, Case West Res Univ

Sielaff, Timothy D MD/PhD [S] - **Spec Exp:** Liver Cancer; Pancreatic Cancer; Gallbladder & Biliary Cancer; **Hospital:** Abbott - Northwestern Hosp; **Address:** Virginia Piper Cancer Inst, Liver and Pancreas Clinic, 800 E 28th St, Minneapolis, MN 55407; **Phone:** 612-863-7553; **Board Cert:** Surgery 2008; **Med School:** Med Coll VA 1989; **Resid:** Surgery, Univ Minn Hosps 1997; **Fellow:** Transplant Surgery, Univ Toronto Affil Hosp 1998; **Fac Appt:** Assoc Prof S, Univ Minn

Simeone, Diane M MD [S] - **Spec Exp:** Pancreatic Cancer; Cancer Surgery; **Hospital:** Univ of Michigan Hosp; **Address:** Univ Michigan Hlth Sys, 1500 E Med Ctr Drive, 2210B Taubman Center SPC 5343, Ann Arbor, MI 48109-5343; **Phone:** 734-615-1600; **Board Cert:** Surgery 2005; **Med School:** Duke Univ 1988; **Resid:** Surgery, Univ Mich Med Ctr 1995; **Fac Appt:** Prof S, Univ Mich Med Sch

Siperstein, Allan E MD [S] - **Spec Exp:** Laparoscopic Surgery; Endocrine Tumors; Thyroid & Parathyroid Cancer & Surgery; **Hospital:** Cleveland Clin (page 56); **Address:** Cleveland Clinic, Dept Endocrine Surg, 9500 Euclid Ave, MC F20, Cleveland, OH 44195; **Phone:** 216-444-5664; **Board Cert:** Surgery 2007; **Med School:** Univ Tex SW, Dallas 1983; **Resid:** Surgery, UCSF Med Ctr 1990; **Fellow:** Research, UCSF Med Ctr 1988

Soper, Nathaniel MD [S] - **Spec Exp:** Laparoscopic Surgery; Gastroesophageal Reflux Disease (GERD); Biliary Surgery; **Hospital:** Northwestern Meml Hosp; **Address:** Northwestern Meml Hosp, Dept Surg, 675 NE St Clair, Galter Bldg Fl 17 - rm 250, Chicago, IL 60611; **Phone:** 312-695-8918; **Board Cert:** Surgery 2005; **Med School:** Univ Iowa Coll Med 1980; **Resid:** Surgery, Univ Utah Hosps 1986; **Fellow:** Digestive Dis, Mayo Clinic 1988; **Fac Appt:** Prof S, Northwestern Univ

Stahl, Donna L MD [S] - **Spec Exp:** Breast Cancer; Breast Surgery; **Hospital:** Jewish Hosp - Kenwood - Cincinnati; **Address:** 4750 E Galbraith Rd, Ste 112, Cincinnati, OH 45236; **Phone:** 513-686-3109; **Board Cert:** Surgery 2000; **Med School:** Univ Iowa Coll Med 1971; **Resid:** Surgery, Univ Cincinnati Hosps 1978

Staren, Edgar MD/PhD [S] - **Spec Exp:** Breast Cancer; Endocrine Cancers; Liver Cancer; **Hospital:** CTCA at Midwestern Reg Med Ctr; **Address:** Cancer Treatment Ctrs America, 2610 Sheridan Rd, Zion, IL 60099; **Phone:** 847-731-5805; **Board Cert:** Surgery 2006; **Med School:** Loyola Univ-Stritch Sch Med 1982; **Resid:** Surgery, Rush-Presby-St Lukes Med Ctr 1987; **Fellow:** Surgical Oncology, Rush-Presby-St Lukes Med Ctr 1988

Talamonti, Mark S MD [S] - **Spec Exp:** Pancreatic Cancer; Liver Cancer; Gastrointestinal Cancer & Surgery; Melanoma; **Hospital:** Evanston/North Shore Univ Hlth Sys, Highland Park/North Shore Univ Hlth Syst; **Address:** North Shore Univ Health System, 2560 Ridge Ave, Evanston, IL 60201; **Phone:** 847-570-1700; **Board Cert:** Surgery 2009; **Med School:** Northwestern Univ 1983; **Resid:** Surgery, Northwestern Meml Hosp 1989; **Fellow:** Surgical Oncology, MD Anderson Cancer Ctr 1991; **Fac Appt:** Clin Prof S, Univ Chicago-Pritzker Sch Med

Thistlethwaite, J Richard MD/PhD [S] - **Spec Exp:** Transplant-Kidney; Transplant-Pancreas; Transplant-Liver; Transplant Surgery-Pediatric; **Hospital:** Univ of Chicago Med Ctr; **Address:** 5841 S Maryland Ave, rm J-517, MC 5026, Chicago, IL 60637; **Phone:** 773-702-6104; **Board Cert:** Surgery 2008; **Med School:** Duke Univ 1977; **Resid:** Surgery, Mass Genl Hosp 1983; **Fellow:** Surgical Oncology, Natl Inst Hlth 1981; Transplant Surgery, Mass Genl Hosp 1984; **Fac Appt:** Prof S, Univ Chicago-Pritzker Sch Med

Tuttle, Todd M MD [S] - **Spec Exp:** Breast Cancer; Minimally Invasive Surgery; Cancer Surgery; **Hospital:** Univ Minn Med Ctr, Fairview - Riverside Campus; **Address:** Univ Minn, Dept Surgery, 420 Delaware St SE, MMC 195, Minneapolis, MN 55455; **Phone:** 612-625-2991; **Board Cert:** Surgery 2004; **Med School:** Johns Hopkins Univ 1988; **Resid:** Surgery, Med Coll Virginia Hosps 1994; **Fellow:** Surgical Oncology, MD Anderson Cancer Ctr 1996; **Fac Appt:** Assoc Prof S

Vickers, Selwyn M MD [S] - **Spec Exp:** Pancreatic Cancer; Liver Cancer; Gastrointestinal Surgery; **Hospital:** Univ Minn Med Ctr, Fairview - Riverside Campus; **Address:** University of Minnesota, 420 Delaware St SE, Phillips Wangensteen Bldg, MMC 195, Minneapolis, MN 55455; **Phone:** 612-626-1999; **Board Cert:** Surgery 2003; **Med School:** Johns Hopkins Univ 1986; **Resid:** Surgery, Johns Hopkins Hosp 1992; **Fellow:** NIH-Dept Aging 1987; **Fac Appt:** Prof S, Johns Hopkins Univ

Wakefield, Thomas MD [S] - **Spec Exp:** Thrombotic Disorders; Bleeding/Coagulation Disorders; Pulmonary Embolism; **Hospital:** Univ of Michigan Hosp, VA Ann Arbor Healthcare Sys; **Address:** Univ Mich, Dept Surg, Div Vasc Surg, 1500 E Med Ctr Drive, CVC5463 SPC5867, Ann Arbor, MI 48109; **Phone:** 734-936-5820; **Board Cert:** Surgery 2002; Vascular Surgery 2005; Surgical Critical Care 2000; **Med School:** Med Coll OH 1978; **Resid:** Surgery, Univ Mich Med Ctr 1984; **Fellow:** Peripheral Vascular Surgery, Univ Mich Med Ctr 1986; **Fac Appt:** Prof S, Univ Mich Med Sch

Walker, Alonzo P MD [S] - **Spec Exp:** Breast Cancer; **Hospital:** Froedtert and Med Ctr of WI; **Address:** Dept Surgery, 9200 W Wisconsin Ave, Milwaukee, WI 53226-3522; **Phone:** 414-805-5737; **Board Cert:** Surgery 2004; **Med School:** Univ Fla Coll Med 1976; **Resid:** Surgery, Univ Maryland Hosps 1983; **Fac Appt:** Prof S, Med Coll Wisc

Walsh, R Matthew MD [S] - **Spec Exp:** Pancreatic Cancer; Gastrointestinal Surgery; Hepatobiliary Surgery; **Hospital:** Cleveland Clin (page 56); **Address:** Cleveland Clin, Dept Surgery, 9500 Euclid Ave, Desk A100, Cleveland, OH 44195; **Phone:** 216-445-7576; **Board Cert:** Surgery 1999; **Med School:** Med Coll Wisc 1985; **Resid:** Surgery, Loyola Univ Hosp 1990; **Fellow:** Endoscopy, Mass General Hosp 1991; Hepatopancreatobiliary Surgery, Cleveland Clinic; **Fac Appt:** Assoc Prof S, Cleveland Cl Coll Med/Case West Res

Weber, Sharon M MD [S] - **Spec Exp:** Liver Cancer; Pancreatic & Biliary Surgery; Colon & Rectal Cancer; Sarcoma; **Hospital:** Univ WI Hosp & Clins, Wm S Middleton Mem Vet Hosp-Madison; **Address:** 600 Highland Ave, Madison, WI 53792; **Phone:** 608-265-0500; **Board Cert:** Surgery 2009; **Med School:** Med Coll Wisc 1993; **Resid:** Surgery, Univ Wisc Med Ctr 1999; **Fellow:** Tumor Immunology, Univ Wisc Med Ctr 1997; Hepatobiliary Surgery, Meml Sloan Kettering Cancer Ctr 2001; **Fac Appt:** Assoc Prof S, Univ Wisc

Weigel, Ronald J MD/PhD [S] - **Spec Exp:** Breast Cancer; Endocrine Surgery; **Hospital:** Univ Iowa Hosp & Clinics; **Address:** Univ Iowa Carver Coll Med-Dept Surgery, 200 Hawkins Drive, 1516 JCP, Iowa City, IA 52242; **Phone:** 319-356-4200; **Board Cert:** Surgery 2001; **Med School:** Yale Univ 1986; **Resid:** Surgery, Duke Univ Med Ctr 1992; **Fellow:** Immunology, Duke Univ Med Ctr; **Fac Appt:** Prof S, Univ Iowa Coll Med

Surgery

Weigelt, John A MD [S] - **Spec Exp:** Trauma; Critical Care; **Hospital:** Froedtert and Med Ctr of WI; **Address:** Froedtert Hospital, Dept Surgery, 9200 W Wisconsin Ave, rm 295B, Milwaukee, WI 53226; **Phone:** 414-805-8636; **Board Cert:** Surgery 2010; Surgical Critical Care 2006; **Med School:** Med Coll Wisc 1974; **Resid:** Surgery, U Tex SW Hosps 1979; **Fac Appt:** Prof S, Univ Wisc

Wiebke, Eric A MD [S] - **Spec Exp:** Gastrointestinal Cancer & Surgery; Laparoscopic Surgery; Gastrointestinal Motility Disorders; **Hospital:** IU Health University Hosp; **Address:** Indiana Univ Dept Surgery, 545 Barnhill Drive, Emerson Hall 509, Indianapolis, IN 46202; **Phone:** 317-274-4990; **Board Cert:** Surgery 2010; Surgical Critical Care 2002; **Med School:** Vanderbilt Univ 1983; **Resid:** Surgery, Johns Hopkins Hosp 1989; **Fellow:** Surgical Oncology, Natl Cancer Inst/NIH 1987; **Fac Appt:** Prof S, Indiana Univ

Witt, Thomas R MD [S] - **Spec Exp:** Breast Cancer; Breast Disease; **Hospital:** Rush Univ Med Ctr; **Address:** Surgical Oncology Group, 1725 W Harrison St, Ste 409, Chicago, IL 60612-3828; **Phone:** 312-942-2302; **Board Cert:** Surgery 2000; **Med School:** Northwestern Univ 1975; **Resid:** Surgery, Rush Presby-St Lukes Med Ctr 1980; **Fellow:** Surgical Oncology, Meml Sloan Kettering Cancer Ctr 1982; **Fac Appt:** Assoc Prof S, Rush Med Coll

Great Plains and Mountains

Edney, James A MD [S] - **Spec Exp:** Breast Cancer; Thyroid & Parathyroid Cancer & Surgery; Cancer Surgery; Melanoma; **Hospital:** Nebraska Med Ctr; **Address:** Univ Nebraska Med Ctr, Dept Surgery, 984030 Nebraska Medical Ctr, Omaha, NE 68198-4030; **Phone:** 402-559-7272; **Board Cert:** Surgery 2000; **Med School:** Univ Nebr Coll Med 1975; **Resid:** Surgery, Univ Nebraska Med Ctr 1980; **Fellow:** Surgical Oncology, Univ Colorado Med Ctr 1981; **Fac Appt:** Prof S, Univ Nebr Coll Med

Finlayson, Christina A MD [S] - **Spec Exp:** Breast Cancer; Breast Disease; **Hospital:** Univ of CO Hosp - Anschutz Inpatient Pav; **Address:** 12631 E 17th Ave, P.O. Box 6511, Auora, CO 80045; **Phone:** 303-724-2728; **Board Cert:** Surgery 2004; **Med School:** Univ Utah 1989; **Resid:** Surgery, Univ Colorado Hlth Sci Ctr 1994; **Fellow:** Surgical Oncology, Fox Chase Cancer Ctr 1996; **Fac Appt:** Prof S, Univ Colorado

Fitzgibbons Jr, Robert J MD [S] - **Spec Exp:** Abdominal Wall Reconstruction; Minimally Invasive Surgery; Gastrointestinal Surgery; Hernia; **Hospital:** Creighton Univ Med Ctr, Bergan Mercy Med Ctr-Alegant Hlth; **Address:** Creighton Univ, Dept Surgery, 601 N 30th St, Ste 3700, Omaha, NE 68131-2100; **Phone:** 402-280-4503; **Board Cert:** Surgery 2002; **Med School:** Creighton Univ 1974; **Resid:** Surgery, Charity Hosp/LA State Univ 1979; **Fellow:** Surgical Oncology, Lahey Clin 1980; **Fac Appt:** Prof S, Creighton Univ

Loggie, Brian MD [S] - **Spec Exp:** Cancer Surgery; Mesothelioma; Solid Tumors; Melanoma; **Hospital:** Creighton Univ Med Ctr; **Address:** 601 N 30th St, Ste 2803, Omaha, NE 68131; **Phone:** 402-280-4100; **Board Cert:** Surgery 1998; **Med School:** McGill Univ 1979; **Resid:** Surgery, Montreal Genl Hosp 1986; **Fellow:** Surgical Oncology, Univ Illinois 1988; **Fac Appt:** Prof S, Creighton Univ

McIntyre Jr, Robert C MD [S] - **Spec Exp:** Endocrine Surgery; Trauma; Critical Care; **Hospital:** Univ of CO Hosp - Anschutz Inpatient Pav, Chldn's Hosp - Aurora (CO); **Address:** Univ Colorado at Denver & Hlth Sci Ctr, 12631 E 17th Ave, MS C313, Aurora, CO 80045; **Phone:** 303-724-2724; **Board Cert:** Surgery 2002; Surgical Critical Care 2003; **Med School:** Tulane Univ 1987; **Resid:** Surgery, Univ Colorado 1992; **Fac Appt:** Prof S, Univ Colorado

Mistry, Bhargav M MD [S] - **Spec Exp:** Transplant-Kidney; Transplant-Liver; Transplant-Pancreas; Trauma/Critical Care; **Hospital:** Sanford Med Ctr Fargo; **Address:** MeritCare Broadway Hlth Ctr, Transplantation Surgery, 736 Broadway N, Fargo, ND 58122; **Phone:** 701-234-3400; **Board Cert:** Surgery 2009; Surgical Critical Care 2009; **Med School:** India 1984; **Resid:** Surgery, St Louis Univ Med Ctr 2000; **Fellow:** Surgical Critical Care, St Louis Univ 1995; Transplant Surgery, St Louis Univ 1998; **Fac Appt:** Assoc Clin Prof S, Univ ND Sch Med

Moore, Ernest E MD [S] - **Spec Exp:** Liver Trauma; Aortic Injuries; Thoracic Aortic Surgery; Pelvic Surgery; **Hospital:** Denver Health Med Ctr, Yampa Valley Med Ctr; **Address:** Denver Hlth Med Ctr, 777 Bannock St, Denver, CO 80204-4597; **Phone:** 303-436-6558; **Board Cert:** Surgery 2006; Surgical Critical Care 2006; **Med School:** Univ Pittsburgh 1972; **Resid:** Surgery, Univ VT Med Ctr 1976; **Fac Appt:** Prof S, Univ Colorado

Mulvihill, Sean J MD [S] - **Spec Exp:** Gastrointestinal Surgery; Liver & Biliary Cancer; Pancreatic Cancer; **Hospital:** Univ Utah Hlth Care; **Address:** Univ Utah, Dept Surgery, 30 N 1900 E, rm 3B110, Salt Lake City, UT 84132; **Phone:** 801-581-7304; **Board Cert:** Surgery 2008; **Med School:** USC Sch Med 1981; **Resid:** Surgery, UCLA Med Ctr 1987; **Fac Appt:** Prof S, Univ Utah

Nelson, Edward W MD [S] - **Spec Exp:** Breast Cancer; **Hospital:** Univ Utah Hlth Care; **Address:** Univ Utah Med Ctr, Div Genl Surgery, 30 N 1900 E, rm 3B322, Salt Lake City, UT 84132; **Phone:** 801-581-7738; **Board Cert:** Surgery 2008; **Med School:** Univ Utah 1974; **Resid:** Surgery, Univ Utah Med Ctr 1979; **Fac Appt:** Prof S, Univ Utah

Petelin, Joseph B MD [S] - **Spec Exp:** Laparoscopic Abdominal Surgery; **Hospital:** Shawnee Mission Med Ctr; **Address:** 9119 W 74th St, Ste 255, Shawnee Mission, KS 66204; **Phone:** 913-432-5420; **Board Cert:** Surgery 2010; **Med School:** Univ Kansas 1976; **Resid:** Surgery, Univ Kansas 1981; **Fac Appt:** Assoc Clin Prof S, Univ Kansas

Saffle, Jeffrey MD [S] - **Spec Exp:** Burn Care; Wound Healing/Care; **Hospital:** Univ Utah Hlth Care; **Address:** Dept Surgery, 30 N 1900 E, rm 3B306, Salt Lake City, UT 84132; **Phone:** 801-581-3595; **Board Cert:** Surgery 2002; Surgical Critical Care 2007; **Med School:** Univ Chicago-Pritzker Sch Med 1976; **Resid:** Surgery, Univ Utah Med Ctr 1982; **Fellow:** Burn Surgery, Univ Utah Med Ctr 1980; **Fac Appt:** Prof S, Univ Utah

Sasson, Aaron R MD [S] - **Spec Exp:** Gastrointestinal Cancer; Pancreatic Cancer; Liver Cancer; Neuroendocrine Tumors; **Hospital:** Nebraska Med Ctr; **Address:** 984030 Univ Nebraska Med Ctr, Omaha, NE 68198-4030; **Phone:** 402-559-8941; **Board Cert:** Surgery 2000; **Med School:** UMDNJ-NJ Med Sch, Newark 1993; **Resid:** Surgery, UCSD Med Ctr 1999; **Fellow:** Surgical Oncology, Fox Chase Cancer Ctr 2001; **Fac Appt:** Assoc Prof S, Univ Nebr Coll Med

Sauter, Edward R MD/PhD [S] - **Spec Exp:** Breast Cancer; Breast Cancer Risk Assessment; Clinical Trials; **Hospital:** Fargo VA Med Ctr, Sanford Med Ctr Fargo; **Address:** Univ North Dakota Dept Surgery, 501 N Columbia Rd, MS 9037, Grand Forks, ND 58202; **Phone:** 701-777-4862; **Board Cert:** Surgery 2000; **Med School:** Louisiana State U, New Orleans 1986; **Resid:** Surgery, Ochsner Fdn Hosp 1991; **Fellow:** Surgical Oncology, Fox Chase Cancer Ctr 1993; **Fac Appt:** Prof S, Univ ND Sch Med

Traynor, Michael D MD [S] - **Spec Exp:** Endocrine Surgery; Thyroid & Parathyroid Surgery; Vascular Surgery; **Hospital:** Sanford Med Ctr Fargo; **Address:** MeritCare Broadway Health Ctr, 737 North Broadway, Fargo, ND 58122; **Phone:** 701-234-2251; **Board Cert:** Surgery 1986; **Med School:** Univ ND Sch Med 1986; **Resid:** Surgery, Mayo Clinic 1991; **Fac Appt:** Clin Prof S, Univ ND Sch Med

Surgery

Southwest

Ames, Frederick C MD [S] - **Spec Exp:** Breast Cancer; **Hospital:** UT MD Anderson Cancer Ctr; **Address:** MD Anderson Cancer Ctr, Dept Surgery, 1515 Holcombe Blvd, Unit 444, Houston, TX 77030-4009; **Phone:** 713-792-6929; **Board Cert:** Surgery 1975; **Med School:** Univ Tex Med Br, Galveston 1969; **Resid:** Surgery, Univ Texas Med Branch 1971; Surgery, St Joseph Hosp 1974; **Fellow:** Surgical Oncology, MD Anderson Cancer Ctr 1975; **Fac Appt:** Prof S, Univ Tex, Houston

Babiera, Gildy V MD [S] - **Spec Exp:** Breast Cancer; **Hospital:** UT MD Anderson Cancer Ctr; **Address:** MD Anderson Cancer Ctr, Dept Surgical Oncology, Unit 444, PO Box 301402, Houston, TX 77230-1402; **Phone:** 713-792-2121; **Board Cert:** Surgery 2007; **Med School:** NY Med Coll 1991; **Resid:** Surgery, NYU Med Ctr 1995; Surgery, NYU Med Ctr 1997; **Fellow:** Surgical Oncology, MD Anderson Cancer Ctr 1996; **Fac Appt:** Assoc Prof Surg & Onc, Univ Tex, Houston

Beitsch, Peter D MD [S] - **Spec Exp:** Breast Cancer; **Hospital:** Med City Dallas Hosp; **Address:** 7777 Forrest Ln, C Bldg, Ste 760, Dallas, TX 75230; **Phone:** 972-566-8039; **Board Cert:** Surgery 2002; **Med School:** Univ Tex SW, Dallas 1986; **Resid:** Surgery, Univ TX SW Med Ctr 1993; **Fellow:** Surgical Oncology, MD Anderson Cancer Ctr 1990; Surgical Oncology, John Wayne Cancer Inst 1994

Bellows, Charles F MD [S] - **Spec Exp:** Gastrointestinal Surgery; Minimally Invasive Surgery; Hernia-Complex; Abdominal Wall Reconstruction; **Hospital:** Tulane Med Ctr; **Address:** Tulane Univ Dept Surgery, 1430 Tulane Ave, New Orleans, LA 70112; **Phone:** 504-988-3589; **Board Cert:** Surgery 2002; **Med School:** Med Coll PA 1995; **Resid:** Surgery, Tulane Univ Hosp 2001; **Fellow:** Surgical Research, Tulane 1998; **Fac Appt:** Assoc Prof S, Tulane Univ

Bentley, Frederick R MD [S] - **Spec Exp:** Transplant-Kidney; Colon Cancer; **Hospital:** UAMS Med Ctr; **Address:** 4301 W Markham St, Slot 520, Little Rock, AR 72205; **Phone:** 501-526-7053; **Board Cert:** Surgery 2006; **Med School:** Louisiana State U, New Orleans 1977; **Resid:** Surgery, LSU Med Ctr 1983; **Fellow:** Research, Univ Minnesota Affil Hosp 1982; Transplant Surgery, Univ Minnesota Affil Hosp 1984; **Fac Appt:** Assoc Prof S, Univ Louisville Sch Med

Bolton, John S MD [S] - **Spec Exp:** Cancer Surgery; Esophageal Cancer; Pancreatic Cancer; Liver Cancer; **Hospital:** Ochsner Med Ctr-New Orleans; **Address:** Ochsner Clin, Dept Surg, 1514 Jefferson Hwy, New Orleans, LA 70121; **Phone:** 504-842-4072; **Board Cert:** Surgery 2002; **Med School:** Louisiana State U, New Orleans 1976; **Resid:** Surgery, Charity Hosp 1981; **Fellow:** Hepatopancreatobiliary Surgery, Lahey Clinic 1980; Surgical Oncology, Meml Sloan Kettering Cancer Ctr 1982; **Fac Appt:** Asst Clin Prof S, Louisiana State U, New Orleans

Brunicardi, F Charles MD [S] - **Spec Exp:** Pancreatic Islet Cell Transplant; Pancreatic Cancer; Gastroesophageal Reflux Disease (GERD); **Hospital:** St. Luke's Episcopal Hosp-Houston; **Address:** 6620 Main St, Ste 1475, Houston, TX 77030; **Phone:** 713-798-8070; **Board Cert:** Surgery 2009; **Med School:** UMDNJ-Rutgers Med Sch 1980; **Resid:** Surgery, SUNY Brooklyn Hlth Sci Ctr 1989; **Fellow:** Pancreatic Physiology, SUNY Brooklyn Hlth Sci Ctr 1986; **Fac Appt:** Prof S, Baylor Coll Med

Curley, Steven A MD [S] - **Spec Exp:** Colon & Rectal Cancer; Liver Cancer; Hepatobiliary Surgery; **Hospital:** UT MD Anderson Cancer Ctr; **Address:** MD Anderson Cancer Ctr, Dept Surg Oncology, 1515 Holcome Blvd, Unit 1484, Houston, TX 77230-1402; **Phone:** 713-792-2022; **Board Cert:** Surgery 2008; **Med School:** Univ Tex, Houston 1982; **Resid:** Surgery, Univ New Mexico Hosps 1988; **Fellow:** Surgical Oncology, MD Anderson Cancer Ctr 1990; **Fac Appt:** Prof S, Univ Tex, Houston

Demarest III, Gerald B MD [S] - **Spec Exp:** Trauma; Burn Care; **Hospital:** Univ Hosp - New Mexico; **Address:** Univ New Mexico Surgical Clin, 2211 Lomas Blvd NE, Albuquerque, NM 87106; **Phone:** 505-272-2336; **Board Cert:** Surgery 2008; Surgical Critical Care 2005; **Med School:** Columbia P&S 1973; **Resid:** Surgery, Univ Washington Med Ctr 1978; **Fellow:** Burn Surgery, Harborview Med Ctr 1979; Harborview Med Ctr 1980; **Fac Appt:** Assoc Prof S, Univ New Mexico

Dooley, William C MD [S] - **Spec Exp:** Breast Cancer; Tumors-Rare & Multiple; Sarcoma; Melanoma; **Hospital:** OU Med Ctr, St. Anthony Hosp -Oklahoma City; **Address:** 825 NE 10th St, Ste 4500, Oklahoma City, OK 73104; **Phone:** 405-271-7867; **Board Cert:** Surgery 2011; **Med School:** Vanderbilt Univ 1982; **Resid:** Surgery, Johns Hopkins Hosp 1987; Surgical Oncology, Oxford Univ 1986; **Fellow:** Surgical Oncology, Johns Hopkins 1988; **Fac Appt:** Prof S, Univ Okla Coll Med

Ellis, Lee M MD [S] - **Spec Exp:** Colon & Rectal Cancer; Metastatic Cancer; Peritoneal Carcinomatosis; **Hospital:** UT MD Anderson Cancer Ctr; **Address:** MD Anderson Cancer Ctr, Dept Surgery & Cancer Biology, 1515 Holcombe Blvd, Box 173, Houston, TX 77030; **Phone:** 713-792-6926; **Board Cert:** Surgery 2009; **Med School:** Univ VA Sch Med 1983; **Resid:** Surgery, Univ Fla-Shands Hosp 1990; **Fellow:** Surgical Oncology, MD Anderson Cancer Ctr 1992; **Fac Appt:** Prof S, Univ Tex, Houston

Euhus, David M MD [S] - **Spec Exp:** Breast Cancer; **Hospital:** UT Southwestern Med Ctr at Dallas; **Address:** Univ Texas SW Med Ctr - Div Surg Oncology, 5323 Harry Hines Blvd, MC 9155, Dallas, TX 75390; **Phone:** 214-648-6467; **Board Cert:** Surgery 2001; **Med School:** St Louis Univ 1984; **Resid:** Surgery, UCLA Med Ctr 1991; **Fellow:** Surgical Oncology, UCLA Med Ctr 1988; Breast Disease, Queens Med Ctr 1990; **Fac Appt:** Prof S, Univ Tex SW, Dallas

Feig, Barry W MD [S] - **Spec Exp:** Gastrointestinal Cancer; Sarcoma; Breast Cancer; **Hospital:** UT MD Anderson Cancer Ctr; **Address:** UT MD Anderson Cancer Ctr, Dept Surg Onc, 1400 Pressler St, Unit 1484, Houston, TX 77030; **Phone:** 713-792-2022; **Board Cert:** Surgery 2008; **Med School:** SUNY Upstate Med Univ 1984; **Resid:** Surgery, Northwestern Univ Med Ctr 1990; **Fellow:** Trauma, Univ Minnesota Affil Hosp 1991; Surgical Oncology, UT MD Anderson Cancer Ctr 1994; **Fac Appt:** Prof S, Univ Tex, Houston

Fisher, William E MD [S] - **Spec Exp:** Pancreatic Cancer; **Hospital:** St. Luke's Episcopal Hosp-Houston; **Address:** 6620 Main St, Ste 1475, Houston, TX 77030; **Phone:** 713-798-8070; **Board Cert:** Surgery 2006; **Med School:** Univ Cincinnati 1990; **Resid:** Surgery, Ohio State U Hosps 1996; **Fellow:** Cancer Research, Ohio State U Hosps 1998; **Fac Appt:** Prof S, Baylor Coll Med

Franklin, Morris E MD [S] - **Spec Exp:** Laparoscopic Abdominal Surgery; Colon & Rectal Surgery; **Hospital:** Southeast Baptist Hosp, Baptist Med Ctr - San Antonio; **Address:** 4242 E Southcross Blvd, Ste 1, San Antonio, TX 78222; **Phone:** 210-333-7510; **Board Cert:** Surgery 1973; **Med School:** Univ Tex SW, Dallas 1967; **Resid:** Surgery, Bexar Co Hosp 1972; **Fac Appt:** Clin Prof S, Univ Tex, San Antonio

Friese, Randall S MD [S] - **Spec Exp:** Trauma; Critical Care; **Hospital:** Univ Med Ctr - Tucson; **Address:** University Med Ctr - Trauma, 1501 N Campbell Ave, rm 5411, PO Box 245063, Tucson, AZ 85724; **Phone:** 520-694-6144; **Board Cert:** Surgery 2005; Surgical Critical Care 2002; **Med School:** Univ MD Sch Med 1990; **Resid:** Surgery, Univ Colorado Affil Hosp 1997; **Fellow:** Trauma/Critical Care, Univ Texas SW Med Ctr 2002; **Fac Appt:** Assoc Prof S, Univ Ariz Coll Med

Grant, Michael D MD [S] - **Spec Exp:** Breast Cancer; Breast Surgery; **Hospital:** Baylor Univ Medical Ctr-Dallas; **Address:** 3900 Junius St, Ste 220, Baylor Med Pavillion, Dallas, TX 75246; **Phone:** 214-826-7300; **Board Cert:** Surgery 2001; **Med School:** Univ Tex, Houston 1987; **Resid:** Surgery, Baylor Univ Med Ctr 1992; **Fellow:** Breast Cancer, Baylor Univ Med Ctr 1993

Surgery

Gray, Richard J MD [S] - **Spec Exp:** Breast Cancer; Melanoma; **Hospital:** Mayo Clinic - Phoenix, Mayo Clinic - Scottsdale; **Address:** Mayo Clinic, 5777 E Mayo Blvd, Phoenix, AZ 85054; **Phone:** 480-342-2849; **Board Cert:** Surgery 2001; **Med School:** Mich State Univ 1995; **Resid:** Surgery, Mayo Clinic 2000; **Fellow:** Surgical Oncology, H Lee Moffitt Cancer Ctr 2001; **Fac Appt:** Assoc Prof S, Mayo Med Sch

Griswold, John A MD [S] - **Spec Exp:** Burn Care; **Hospital:** Univ Med Ctr-Lubbock; **Address:** Dept Surgery, 3601 4th St, MS 9905, Lubbock, TX 79430; **Phone:** 806-743-2373; **Board Cert:** Surgery 2009; Surgical Critical Care 2000; **Med School:** Creighton Univ 1981; **Resid:** Surgery, Texas Tech Univ Hlth Scis Ctr 1986; **Fellow:** Burn Surgery, Univ Washington 1988

Halff, Glenn A MD [S] - **Spec Exp:** Transplant-Liver; Liver Surgery; **Hospital:** Univ Hlth Syst-San Antonio, Christus Santa Rosa Children's Hosp; **Address:** Univ Transplant Center, 7703 Floyd Curl Drive, MC 785, San Antonio, TX 78229; **Phone:** 210-567-5771; **Board Cert:** Surgery 2007; Surgical Critical Care 2000; **Med School:** Univ Tex, Houston 1983; **Resid:** Surgery, NYU Med Ctr 1987; **Fellow:** Transplant Surgery, Univ Pittsburgh 1989; **Fac Appt:** Assoc Prof S, Univ Tex, San Antonio

Holcomb, John B MD [S] - **Spec Exp:** Trauma; **Hospital:** Meml Hermann Hosp - Texas Med Ctr; **Address:** Univ Texas Dept Surgery, 6431 Fannin St, MSB 4.170, Houston, TX 77030; **Phone:** 713-500-7218; **Board Cert:** Surgery 2002; Surgical Critical Care 2004; **Med School:** Univ Ark 1985; **Resid:** Surgery, Wm Beaumont AMC 1991; **Fellow:** Surgical Critical Care, Univ Texas 2002; **Fac Appt:** Prof S, Univ Tex, Houston

Hollingsworth, Alan B MD [S] - **Spec Exp:** Breast Cancer; **Hospital:** Mercy Hlth Ctr - Oklahoma City; **Address:** Mercy Women's Ctr, Medical Director, 4300 McAuley Blvd, Oklahoma City, OK 73120; **Phone:** 405-936-5455; **Board Cert:** Surgery 2009; **Med School:** Univ Okla Coll Med 1975; **Resid:** Surgery, Univ Oklahoma Hlth Sci Ctr 1980; **Fellow:** Anatomic Pathology, UCLA Med Ctr 1978; **Fac Appt:** Prof S, Univ Okla Coll Med

Hunt, John L MD [S] - **Spec Exp:** Trauma; Burn Care; **Hospital:** UT Southwestern Med Ctr at Dallas; **Address:** Dept Surgery, 5323 Harry Hines Blvd, MC 9158, Dallas, TX 75390-9158; **Phone:** 214-648-2152; **Board Cert:** Surgery 1972; Surgical Critical Care 1996; **Med School:** Univ Cincinnati 1964; **Resid:** Surgery, Cincinnati Genl Hosp 1971; **Fac Appt:** Prof S, Univ Tex SW, Dallas

Hunt, Kelly K MD [S] - **Spec Exp:** Breast Cancer; Sarcoma-Soft Tissue; Gene Therapy; **Hospital:** UT MD Anderson Cancer Ctr; **Address:** MD Anderson Cancer Ctr, 1400 Pressler St, Unit 1484, Houston, TX 77030-4000; **Phone:** 713-792-7216; **Board Cert:** Surgery 2001; **Med School:** Univ Tenn Coll Med 1986; **Resid:** Surgery, UCLA Med Ctr 1993; **Fellow:** Surgical Oncology, MD Anderson Cancer Ctr 1996; **Fac Appt:** Prof Surg & Onc, Univ Tex, Houston

Jackson, Gilchrist MD [S] - **Spec Exp:** Thyroid & Parathyroid Surgery; Head & Neck Cancer & Surgery; Endocrine Tumors; Gastrointestinal Cancer & Surgery; **Hospital:** St. Luke's Episcopal Hosp-Houston, Woman's Hosp TX; **Address:** 2727 W Holcombe Blvd Fl 3-A, Houston, TX 77025; **Phone:** 713-442-1132; **Board Cert:** Surgery 2008; **Med School:** Univ Louisville Sch Med 1974; **Resid:** Surgery, Parkland Hosp 1979; **Fellow:** Surgical Oncology, MD Anderson Hosp 1980; **Fac Appt:** Assoc Clin Prof S, Baylor Coll Med

Jayaseelan, Nirmal S MD [S] - **Spec Exp:** Obesity/Bariatric Surgery; **Hospital:** Med City Dallas Hosp; **Address:** 7777 Forest Ln C Bldg - Ste 670, Dallas, TX 75230; **Phone:** 972-566-2263; **Board Cert:** Surgery 2002; **Med School:** Texas Tech Univ 1994; **Resid:** Surgery, Emanuel Hosp 1999

Kim, Lawrence Thomas MD [S] - **Spec Exp:** Endocrine Surgery; Thyroid Cancer; Parathyroid Disease; **Hospital:** UAMS Med Ctr; **Address:** 4301 W Markham, Slot# 721-2, Little Rock, AR 72205; **Phone:** 501-686-8211; **Board Cert:** Surgery 2005; **Med School:** Univ Tex SW, Dallas 1987; **Resid:** Surgery, South Western Med Ctr 1994; **Fellow:** Research, South Western Med Ctr 1991; Research, Natl Inst Health 1996; **Fac Appt:** Prof S, Univ Ark

Klimberg, Vicki S MD [S] - **Spec Exp:** Breast Cancer; Radiofrequency Tumor Ablation; Sentinel Node Surgery; **Hospital:** UAMS Med Ctr; **Address:** Univ Arkansas Medical Sciences, 4301 W Markham, MS 725, Little Rock, AR 72205-7199; **Phone:** 501-686-5669; **Board Cert:** Surgery 1999; **Med School:** Univ Fla Coll Med 1984; **Resid:** Surgery, Univ Fla Med Ctr 1989; **Fellow:** Clinical Oncology, Univ Fla 1990; Breast Disease, Univ Arkansas for Med Scis 1991; **Fac Appt:** Prof S, Univ Ark

Krouse, Robert S MD [S] - **Spec Exp:** Cancer Surgery; Gastrointestinal Cancer; Palliative Care; **Hospital:** Southern AZ VA Health Care Sys - Tucson; **Address:** Southern AZ VA Hosp Care System, Surg Care Line, 2-112, 3601 S 6th Ave, Tucson, AZ 85723; **Phone:** 520-792-1450 x6145; **Board Cert:** Surgery 2007; **Med School:** Hahnemann Univ 1991; **Resid:** Surgery, Univ Hawaii Integrated Surg Prog 1993; Immunotherapy, Natl Cancer Inst 1994; **Fellow:** Surgery, W Virginia Univ Sch Med 1997; Surgical Oncology, City of Hope Natl Med Ctr 2000; **Fac Appt:** Asst Prof S, Univ Ariz Coll Med

Kuhn, Joseph A MD [S] - **Spec Exp:** Liver Cancer; Peritoneal Carcinomatosis; Melanoma; Thyroid Cancer; **Hospital:** Baylor Univ Medical Ctr-Dallas; **Address:** 7777 Forest Lane St, Ste C-410, Dallas, TX 75230; **Phone:** 214-823-5000; **Board Cert:** Surgery 2009; Surgical Critical Care 2003; **Med School:** Univ Tex Med Br, Galveston 1984; **Resid:** Surgery, Baylor Univ Med Ctr 1989; **Fellow:** Surgical Oncology, City Hosp Natl Med Ctr 1992

Lee, Jeffrey E MD [S] - **Spec Exp:** Melanoma; Pancreatic Cancer; Endocrine Tumors; **Hospital:** UT MD Anderson Cancer Ctr; **Address:** UT MD Anderson Cancer Ctr, 1400 Holcombe Blvd, Unit 444 Fl 12, Houston, TX 77030-4009; **Phone:** 713-792-7218; **Board Cert:** Surgery 1999; **Med School:** Stanford Univ 1984; **Resid:** Surgery, Stanford Univ Hosp 1987; Surgery, Stanford Univ Hosp 1991; **Fellow:** Immunology, Stanford Univ Sch Med 1989; Surgical Oncology, Univ Tex-MD Anderson Cancer Ctr 1993; **Fac Appt:** Prof S, Univ Tex, Houston

Leitch, A Marilyn MD [S] - **Spec Exp:** Breast Cancer & Surgery; Melanoma; Sarcoma; **Hospital:** UT Southwestern Med Ctr at Dallas; **Address:** UT Southwestern Med Ctr - Dept Surgery, 5323 Harry Hines Blvd, Dallas, TX 75390-9155; **Phone:** 214-648-3039; **Board Cert:** Surgery 2003; **Med School:** Univ Tex SW, Dallas 1978; **Resid:** Surgery, UCLA Med Ctr 1984; **Fellow:** Surgical Oncology, MD Anderson Cancer Ctr 1985; **Fac Appt:** Prof S, Univ Tex SW, Dallas

Lentz, Christopher W MD [S] - **Spec Exp:** Burn Care; Trauma; Critical Care; Wound Healing/Care; **Hospital:** Univ Hosp - New Mexico; **Address:** 1 University of New Mexico, MSC10 5610, Albuquerque, NM 87131-0001; **Phone:** 505-272-2336; **Board Cert:** Surgery 2005; Surgical Critical Care 2006; **Med School:** Wayne State Univ 1988; **Resid:** Surgery, Med Coll Wisc 1994; **Fellow:** Surgical Critical Care, Shriners Burns Inst 1991; Burn Surgery, Univ N Carolina Med Ctr 1996; **Fac Appt:** Assoc Prof S, Univ Rochester

Li, Benjamin D L MD [S] - **Spec Exp:** Gastrointestinal Cancer; Sarcoma; Breast Cancer; **Hospital:** Louisiana State Univ Hosp, Willis-Knighton Med Ctr; **Address:** LSU Hlth Scis Ctr, Dept Surgery, 1501 Kings Hwy, Shreveport, LA 71130; **Phone:** 318-675-6100; **Board Cert:** Surgery 2002; **Med School:** Yale Univ 1986; **Resid:** Surgery, Northwestern Univ-McGraw Med Ctr 1992; **Fellow:** Surgical Oncology, Roswell Park Cancer Inst 1995; **Fac Appt:** Prof S, Louisiana State U, New Orleans

Livingston, Edward H MD [S] - **Spec Exp:** Gastrointestinal Surgery; Endocrine Surgery; Obesity/Bariatric Surgery; Hernia-Complex; **Hospital:** UT Southwestern Med Ctr at Dallas; **Address:** 1801 Inwood Rd Fl 7 - Ste 100, Dallas, TX 75390-9156; **Phone:** 214-648-7956; **Board Cert:** Surgery 2003; **Med School:** UCLA 1985; **Resid:** Surgery, UCLA Med Ctr 1992; **Fac Appt:** Prof S, Univ Tex SW, Dallas

Mansfield, Paul F MD [S] - **Spec Exp:** Appendix Cancer; Stomach Cancer; Colon Cancer; Melanoma; **Hospital:** UT MD Anderson Cancer Ctr; **Address:** UT MD Anderson Cancer Ctr, 1400 Pressler St, Ste FCT18.5000, Unit 1485, Houston, TX 77030; **Phone:** 713-794-5499; **Board Cert:** Surgery 2006; **Med School:** Jefferson Med Coll 1983; **Resid:** Surgery, Pennsylvania Hosp 1988; **Fellow:** Surgical Oncology, MD Anderson Cancer Ctr 1991; **Fac Appt:** Prof Surg & Onc, Univ Tex, Houston

McCabe, Daniel P MD [S] - **Spec Exp:** Cancer Surgery; **Hospital:** Tucson Med Ctr; **Address:** Southwestern Surgical Assoc, 1951 N Wilmot Rd Bldg 2, Tucson, AZ 85712; **Phone:** 520-795-5845; **Board Cert:** Surgery 2002; **Med School:** Creighton Univ 1979; **Resid:** Surgery, St Joseph Hosp 1982; Surgery, Baystate Med Ctr 1984; **Fellow:** Surgical Oncology, James Cancer Ctr/Ohio State 1986; **Fac Appt:** Asst Clin Prof S, Univ Ariz Coll Med

Meric-Bernstam, Funda MD [S] - **Spec Exp:** Breast Cancer & Surgery; Clinical Trials; **Hospital:** UT MD Anderson Cancer Ctr; **Address:** UT MD Anderson Cancer Center, 1400 Pressler St, Unit 1484, Houston, TX 77030; **Phone:** 713-563-6104; **Board Cert:** Surgery 2007; **Med School:** Yale Univ 1991; **Resid:** Surgery, Univ Mich Med Ctr 1998; **Fellow:** Surgical Oncology, UT MD Anderson Cancer Ctr 2001; **Fac Appt:** Prof Surg & Onc, Univ Tex, Houston

Pisters, Peter MD [S] - **Spec Exp:** Pancreatic Cancer; Sarcoma-Soft Tissue; Gastrointestinal Cancer; **Hospital:** UT MD Anderson Cancer Ctr; **Address:** MD Anderson Cancer Ctr, 1515 Holcombe Blvd, Unit 1484, Houston, TX 77230-1402; **Phone:** 713-792-2022; **Board Cert:** Surgery 2001; **Med School:** Univ Western Ontario 1985; **Resid:** Surgery, NYU/Bellevue Hosp 1992; **Fellow:** Surgical Research, Meml Sloan-Kettering Cancer Ctr 1989; Surgical Oncology, Meml Sloan-Kettering Cancer Ctr 1994; **Fac Appt:** Prof S, Univ Tex, Houston

Pockaj, Barbara A MD [S] - **Spec Exp:** Melanoma; Breast Cancer; Stomach Cancer; Clinical Trials; **Hospital:** Mayo Clinic - Scottsdale; **Address:** Mayo Clinic, Dept Surgery, 5777 E Mayo Blvd, Phoenix, AZ 85054; **Phone:** 480-342-2849; **Board Cert:** Surgery 2005; **Med School:** Vanderbilt Univ 1987; **Resid:** Surgery, Case Western Res Univ Affil Hosps 1995; **Fellow:** Surgical Oncology, Natl Inst Hlth 1992; **Fac Appt:** Assoc Prof S, Mayo Med Sch

Pollock, Raphael E MD/PhD [S] - **Spec Exp:** Sarcoma; **Hospital:** UT MD Anderson Cancer Ctr; **Address:** MD Anderson Cancer Ctr, Dept Surg Oncology, 1515 Holcombe Blvd, Unit 1447, Houston, TX 77030; **Phone:** 713-792-6928; **Board Cert:** Surgery 2003; **Med School:** St Louis Univ 1977; **Resid:** Surgery, Univ Chicago 1979; Surgery, Rush Presby-St Lukes Hosp 1982; **Fellow:** Surgical Oncology, MD Anderson Cancer Ctr 1984; **Fac Appt:** Prof S, Univ Tex, Houston

Postier, Russell G MD [S] - **Spec Exp:** Cancer Surgery; Pancreatic Cancer; Biliary Surgery; Gastrointestinal Surgery; **Hospital:** OU Med Ctr; **Address:** OU Physicians, Dept Surgery, 825 NE 10th St, Ste 4500, Oklahoma City, OK 73104; **Phone:** 405-271-1400; **Board Cert:** Surgery 2000; **Med School:** Univ Okla Coll Med 1975; **Resid:** Surgery, Johns Hopkins Hosp 1981; **Fac Appt:** Prof S, Univ Okla Coll Med

Rege, Robert V MD [S] - **Spec Exp:** Gastrointestinal Surgery; Laparoscopic Surgery; Hernia; **Hospital:** UT Southwestern Med Ctr at Dallas; **Address:** GI Endocrine Surgery, Dept Surgery, 5323 Harry Hines Blvd, Dallas, TX 75390; **Phone:** 214-648-3050; **Board Cert:** Surgery 2000; **Med School:** Penn State Coll Med 1975; **Resid:** Surgery, Milton S. Hershey Med Ctr 1976; Surgery, Milton S. Hershey Med Ctr 1982; **Fellow:** Research, Gastrointestinal Research Fel 1983; **Fac Appt:** Prof S, Univ Tex SW, Dallas

Rhee, Peter M MD [S] - **Spec Exp:** Trauma; Critical Care; **Hospital:** Univ Med Ctr - Tucson; **Address:** University Medical Ctr-Trauma, 1501 N Campbell Ave, rm 5411, PO Box 245063, Tucson, AZ 85274; **Phone:** 520-626-5056; **Board Cert:** Surgery 2002; Surgical Critical Care 2006; **Med School:** Uniformed Srvs Univ, Bethesda 1987; **Resid:** Surgery, UC Irvine Med Ctr 1992; **Fellow:** Trauma, Harborview Med Ctr 1995; **Fac Appt:** Prof S, Univ Ariz Coll Med

Ross, Merrick I MD [S] - **Spec Exp:** Sentinel Node Surgery; Breast Cancer; Melanoma; **Hospital:** UT MD Anderson Cancer Ctr; **Address:** UT MD Anderson Cancer Ctr, Dept Surg Onc, 1515 Holcombe Blvd, Unit 1484, Houston, TX 77030; **Phone:** 713-792-2022; **Board Cert:** Surgery 2007; **Med School:** Univ IL Coll Med 1980; **Resid:** Surgery, Univ Illinois Hosp & Clin 1982; Surgery, Univ Illinois Hosp & Clin 1987; **Fellow:** Research, Scripps Clin & Rsch 1984; Surgical Oncology, Univ TX-MD Anderson Cancer Ctr 1989; **Fac Appt:** Prof S, Univ Tex, Houston

Schlinkert, Richard T MD [S] - **Spec Exp:** Endocrine Surgery; Laparoscopic Surgery; Gastrointestinal Surgery; Adrenal Surgery; **Hospital:** Mayo Clinic - Phoenix; **Address:** Mayo Clin, Dept Surgery, 5779 E Mayo Blvd, Phoenix, AZ 85054; **Phone:** 480-342-1051; **Board Cert:** Surgery 2006; **Med School:** Med Coll OH 1981; **Resid:** Surgery, Mayo Clinic 1986; **Fellow:** Hepatobiliary Surgery, Royal Infirmary 1987; **Fac Appt:** Prof S, Mayo Med Sch

Skibber, John M MD [S] - **Spec Exp:** Rectal Cancer/Sphincter Preservation; Colon & Rectal Cancer-Familial Polyposis; **Hospital:** UT MD Anderson Cancer Ctr; **Address:** 1400 Pressler St, PO Box 301402, Unit 1484, Houston, TX 77230-1402; **Phone:** 713-792-5165; **Board Cert:** Surgery 2009; **Med School:** Jefferson Med Coll 1981; **Resid:** Surgery, NYU Med Ctr 1989; **Fellow:** Surgical Oncology, UT MD Anderson Cancer Ctr 1991; **Fac Appt:** Prof S, Univ Tex, Houston

Stewart, Ronald M MD [S] - **Spec Exp:** Trauma; **Hospital:** Univ Hlth Syst-San Antonio; **Address:** Univ Tex Hlth Sci Ctr, Dept Surg-Trauma, 7703 Floyd Curl Drive, MC 7740, San Antonio, TX 78229-3900; **Phone:** 210-567-3623; **Board Cert:** Surgery 2009; Surgical Critical Care 2002; **Med School:** Univ Tex, San Antonio 1985; **Resid:** Surgery, Univ Tex Hlth Sci Ctr 1991; **Fellow:** Trauma, Univ Tenn Coll Med 1993; **Fac Appt:** Assoc Prof S, Univ Tex, San Antonio

Stolier, Alan J MD [S] - **Spec Exp:** Breast Cancer; **Hospital:** Ochsner Baptist Med Ctr; **Address:** 2525 Severn Ave, Metairie, LA 70002; **Phone:** 504-832-4200; **Board Cert:** Surgery 2006; **Med School:** Louisiana State U, New Orleans 1970; **Resid:** Surgery, Charity Hosp 1974; **Fellow:** Surgical Oncology, MD Anderson Hosp 1976; **Fac Appt:** Clin Prof S, Tulane Univ

Vauthey, Jean Nicholas MD [S] - **Spec Exp:** Hepatobiliary Surgery; Liver Cancer; Gallbladder & Biliary Cancer; **Hospital:** UT MD Anderson Cancer Ctr; **Address:** UT MD Anderson Cancer Ctr -Surg Oncology, 1515 Holcombe Blvd, Unit 1484, Houston, TX 77030; **Phone:** 713-792-2022; **Board Cert:** Surgery 2000; **Med School:** Switzerland 1979; **Resid:** Surgery, Ochsner Med Fdn 1989; **Fellow:** Hepatobiliary Surgery, Med Fac Univ Bern 1991; Surgical Oncology, Meml Sloan-Kettering Cancer Ctr 1993; **Fac Appt:** Prof S, Univ Tex, Houston

Woltering, Eugene MD [S] - **Spec Exp:** Carcinoid Tumors; **Hospital:** Ochsner Med Ctr-New Orleans; **Address:** 200 W Esplanade, Ste 200, Kenner, LA 70062; **Phone:** 504-464-8500; **Board Cert:** Surgery 2002; **Med School:** Ohio State Univ 1975; **Resid:** Surgery, Vanderbilt Med Ctr 1982; Surgical Oncology, Natl Inst Hlth 1979; **Fellow:** Surgical Oncology, Ohio State Univ 1984; **Fac Appt:** Prof S, Louisiana State U, New Orleans

Surgery

Wood, R Patrick MD [S] - **Spec Exp:** Liver Cancer; Liver Surgery; **Hospital:** St. Luke's Episcopal Hosp-Houston; **Address:** 6624 Fannin St, Ste 1200, Houston, TX 77030; **Phone:** 713-795-8994; **Board Cert:** Surgery 2004; **Med School:** Univ Rochester 1979; **Resid:** Surgery, NYU/Bellevue Hosp Ctr 1984; **Fellow:** Transplant Surgery, Univ Pittsburgh 1985; **Fac Appt:** Clin Prof S, Univ Tex, Houston

Zannis, Victor J MD [S] - **Spec Exp:** Breast Cancer; **Hospital:** Phoenix Baptist Hosp & Med Ctr, J C Lincoln Hosp - North Mountain; **Address:** 2525 W Greenway Rd, Ste 130, Phoenix, AZ 85023; **Phone:** 602-942-8000; **Board Cert:** Surgery 2000; **Med School:** UCLA 1976; **Resid:** Surgery, Maricopa Med Ctr 1982

West Coast and Pacific

Anderson, Benjamin O MD [S] - **Spec Exp:** Breast Cancer & Surgery; **Hospital:** Univ Wash Med Ctr; **Address:** Univ Washington Dept Surgery, 1959 NE Pacific St, Box 356410, 1959 NE Pacific St, Box 356410, Seattle, WA 98195-6410; **Phone:** 206-288-6806; **Board Cert:** Surgery 2002; **Med School:** Albert Einstein Coll Med 1985; **Resid:** Surgery, Univ Colorado Affil Hosp 1992; **Fellow:** Surgical Oncology, Meml Sloan Kettering Cancer Ctr 1994; **Fac Appt:** Prof S, Univ Wash

Ascher, Nancy L MD/PhD [S] - **Spec Exp:** Transplant-Liver; Transplant-Kidney; **Hospital:** UCSF Med Ctr; **Address:** 513 Parnassus Ave, Box 0104, San Francisco, CA 94143-0104; **Phone:** 415-476-1236; **Board Cert:** Surgery 2002; **Med School:** Univ Mich Med Sch 1974; **Resid:** Surgery, Univ Minn Hosp 1981; **Fellow:** Transplant Surgery, Univ Minn Hosp 1982; **Fac Appt:** Prof S, UCSF

Bilchik, Anton J MD/PhD [S] - **Spec Exp:** Gastrointestinal Cancer; Laparoscopic Surgery; **Hospital:** St. John's Hlth Ctr, Santa Monica, Cedars-Sinai Med Ctr; **Address:** 2336 Santa Monica Blvd, Ste 206, Santa Monica, CA 90404; **Phone:** 310-696-0716; **Board Cert:** Surgery 2004; **Med School:** South Africa 1985; **Resid:** Surgery, UCLA Med Ctr 1996; **Fellow:** John Wayne Cancer Inst. 1998; **Fac Appt:** Asst Clin Prof S, UCLA

Billingsley, Kevin MD [S] - **Spec Exp:** Cancer Surgery; Liver Tumors; Hepatobiliary Surgery; Pancreatic Surgery; **Hospital:** OR Hlth & Sci Univ; **Address:** Surgical Oncology Div, 3181 SW Sam Jackson Park Rd, MC L619, Portland, OR 97239; **Phone:** 503-494-5501; **Board Cert:** Surgery 2007; **Med School:** Johns Hopkins Univ 1989; **Resid:** Surgery, Oregon Hlth Science Univ 1996; **Fellow:** Surgical Oncology, Natl Cancer Inst 1994; Surgical Oncology, Meml Sloan Kettering Cancer Ctr 1998; **Fac Appt:** Assoc Prof S, Oregon Hlth & Sci Univ

Bouvet, Michael MD [S] - **Spec Exp:** Endocrine Surgery; Pancreatic Cancer; Biliary Cancer; **Hospital:** UCSD Med Ctr; **Address:** UCSD Moores Cancer Ctr, 3855 Health Science Drive, La Jolla, CA 92093-0987; **Phone:** 858-822-6191; **Board Cert:** Surgery 2004; **Med School:** Univ Wash 1989; **Resid:** Surgery, UCSD Med Ctr 1995; **Fellow:** Surgical Oncology, MD Anderson Cancer Ctr 1998; **Fac Appt:** Assoc Prof S, UCSD

Busuttil, Ronald W MD/PhD [S] - **Spec Exp:** Transplant-Liver; Liver Cancer; **Hospital:** UCLA Ronald Reagan Med Ctr; **Address:** 757 WestWood Plaza, Ste 8236, Los Angeles, CA 90095-7430; **Phone:** 310-825-5318; **Board Cert:** Surgery 2007; **Med School:** Tulane Univ 1971; **Resid:** Surgery, UCLA Med Ctr 1976; **Fellow:** Surgery, UCLA Med Ctr 1975; **Fac Appt:** Prof S, UCLA

Butler, John A MD [S] - **Spec Exp:** Breast Cancer; Thyroid Cancer; Adrenal Tumors; Small Bowel Cancer; **Hospital:** UC Irvine Med Ctr; **Address:** UC-Irvine Medical Ctr-Zot 5376, 101 City Drive S, Rte 81 Bldg 56 - Ste 256, Orange, CA 92868-3298; **Phone:** 714-456-8030; **Board Cert:** Surgery 2003; **Med School:** Loyola Univ-Stritch Sch Med 1976; **Resid:** Surgery, LAC-USC Med Ctr 1982; Surgery, Harbor-UCLA Med Ctr 1982; **Fellow:** Surgical Oncology, Meml Sloan-Kettering Cancer Ctr 1984; **Fac Appt:** Prof S, UC Irvine

Byrd, David MD [S] - **Spec Exp:** Cancer Surgery; Tumor Surgery; Melanoma; Breast Cancer & Surgery; **Hospital:** Univ Wash Med Ctr; **Address:** Univ Washington Med Ctr, Dept Surgical Specialites Center, 1959 NE Pacific St, Box 356165, Seattle, WA 98195; **Phone:** 206-598-4477; **Board Cert:** Surgery 2008; **Med School:** Tulane Univ 1982; **Resid:** Surgery, Univ Wash Med Ctr 1987; **Fellow:** Surgical Oncology, Univ Tex-MD Anderson Cancer Ctr 1992; **Fac Appt:** Assoc Prof S, Univ Wash

Chang, Helena MD [S] - **Spec Exp:** Breast Cancer; Cancer Surgery; **Hospital:** UCLA Ronald Reagan Med Ctr; **Address:** 200 UCLA Medical Plaza Drive, Ste B265-1, Revlon Breast Clinic, Los Angeles, CA 90095-7028; **Phone:** 310-825-2144; **Board Cert:** Surgery 1997; **Med School:** Temple Univ 1981; **Resid:** Surgery, Episcopal Hosp 1986; **Fellow:** Cellular Molecular Biology, Temple Univ 1977; Surgical Oncology, Meml Sloan-Kettering Cancer Ctr 1988; **Fac Appt:** Prof S, UCLA

Clark, Orlo H MD [S] - **Spec Exp:** Thyroid Cancer & Surgery; Neuroendocrine Tumors; Parathyroid Cancer; **Hospital:** UCSF - Mt Zion Med Ctr, UCSF Med Ctr; **Address:** UCSF Mt Zion Med Ctr, 1600 Divisadero St, C-347, Box 1674, San Francisco, CA 94115-1926; **Phone:** 415-353-7687; **Board Cert:** Surgery 1974; **Med School:** Cornell Univ-Weill Med Coll 1967; **Resid:** Surgery, UCSF Med Ctr 1970; Surgery, UCSF Med Ctr 1973; **Fellow:** Surgery, Royal Med Sch London 1971; **Fac Appt:** Prof S, UCSF

Colquhoun, Steven D MD [S] - **Spec Exp:** Liver Cancer; Transplant-Liver; Pancreatic Cancer; Hepatobiliary Surgery; **Hospital:** Cedars-Sinai Med Ctr; **Address:** Cedars-Sinai Med Center, 8635 W 3rd St, Ste 590-W, Los Angeles, CA 90048; **Phone:** 310-423-2641; **Board Cert:** Surgery 2003; Surgical Critical Care 2008; **Med School:** Loyola Univ-Stritch Sch Med 1984; **Resid:** Surgery, UCLA Med Ctr 1990; **Fellow:** Surgical Oncology, UCLA Med Ctr 1993; Transplant Surgery, UCLA Med Ctr 1994; **Fac Appt:** Assoc Clin Prof S, UCLA

Crookes, Peter F MD [S] - **Spec Exp:** Obesity/Bariatric Surgery; Laparoscopic Surgery; Gastroesophageal Reflux Disease (GERD); Esophageal Disorders; **Hospital:** Keck Med Ctr of USC (page 75); **Address:** USC Healthcare Consultation Ctr, Ste 514, 1510 San Pablo St, Los Angeles, CA 90033-4612; **Phone:** 323-442-6236; **Med School:** Ireland 1978; **Resid:** Surgery, Royal Victoria Hosp 1989; Surgery, St Vincent's Hosp 1990; **Fellow:** Research, Creighton Univ 1992; Research, Univ SC 1994; **Fac Appt:** Assoc Prof S, Univ SC Sch Med

Dixon, Sherwood M MD [S] - **Spec Exp:** Wound Healing/Care; **Hospital:** Northern Nevada Med Ctr; **Address:** 1500 E 2nd St, Ste 206, Reno, NV 89502; **Phone:** 775-789-7000; **Board Cert:** Surgery 2000; **Med School:** Univ Alabama 1976; **Resid:** Surgery, UC Davis Med Ctr 1981; **Fellow:** Vascular Surgery, UCLA Ctr Hlth Scis 1982

Duh, Quan-Yang MD [S] - **Spec Exp:** Endocrine Surgery; Thyroid & Parathyroid Cancer & Surgery; Adrenal Tumors; Minimally Invasive Surgery; **Hospital:** UCSF Med Ctr, VA Med Ctr - San Francisco; **Address:** UCSF Medical Ctr, 1600 Divisadero St, Box 1926, San Francisco, CA 94115; **Phone:** 415-353-7687; **Board Cert:** Surgery 2007; **Med School:** UCSF 1981; **Resid:** Surgery, UCSF Med Ctr 1988; **Fellow:** Endocrine Surgery, UCSF Med Ctr 1987; **Fac Appt:** Prof S, UCSF

Easter, David W MD [S] - **Spec Exp:** Breast Cancer; Gastrointestinal Cancer; **Hospital:** VA San Diego Hlthcre Sys; **Address:** VA San Diego Healthcare Sys, 3350 La Jolla Village Drive, San Diego, CA 92161; **Phone:** 858-552-8585; **Board Cert:** Surgery 2000; **Med School:** Yale Univ 1983; **Resid:** Surgery, UCSD Med Ctr 1989; **Fellow:** Surgical Oncology, Ninewells, Dundee 1990; **Fac Appt:** Clin Prof S, UCSD

Eilber, Frederick R MD [S] - **Spec Exp:** Tumor Surgery; Sarcoma; **Hospital:** UCLA Ronald Reagan Med Ctr; **Address:** 10833 Le Conte Ave CHS Bldg - rm 54-140, Los Angeles, CA 90095; **Phone:** 310-825-7086; **Board Cert:** Surgery 1973; **Med School:** Univ Mich Med Sch 1965; **Resid:** Surgery, Univ Maryland Hosp 1972; **Fellow:** Surgery, Univ Tex-MD Anderson Hosp 1973; **Fac Appt:** Prof S, UCLA

Ellenhorn, Joshua DI MD [S] - **Spec Exp:** Gastrointestinal Cancer; Pancreatic Surgery; Cancer Surgery; **Hospital:** City of Hope Natl Med Ctr, Huntington Memorial Hosp; **Address:** 1500 E Duarte Rd, Duarte, CA 91010; **Phone:** 626-471-7100; **Board Cert:** Surgery 2000; **Med School:** Boston Univ 1984; **Resid:** Surgery, Univ Cincinnati Hosp 1991; **Fellow:** Surgical Oncology, Meml Sloan-Kettering Cancer Ctr 1993; **Fac Appt:** Prof S

Esquivel, Carlos O MD [S] - **Spec Exp:** Transplant-Liver-Adult & Pediatric; Transplant-Pancreas; Transplant-Kidney; **Hospital:** Stanford Univ Hosp & Clinics, Lucile Packard Chldn's Hosp; **Address:** 750 Welch Rd, Ste 319, Palo Alto, CA 94304; **Phone:** 650-498-5689; **Board Cert:** Surgery 2003; Surgical Critical Care 1999; **Med School:** Costa Rica 1975; **Resid:** Surgery, UC-Davis Med Ctr 1984; **Fellow:** Transplant Surgery, Univ Pittsburgh 1985; **Fac Appt:** Prof S, Stanford Univ

Esserman, Laura J MD [S] - **Spec Exp:** Breast Cancer; **Hospital:** UCSF - Mt Zion Med Ctr, UCSF Med Ctr; **Address:** UCSF-Helen Diller Family Comp Cancer Ctr, 1600 Divisadero St Fl 2, Box 1710, San Francisco, CA 94115; **Phone:** 415-353-7070; **Board Cert:** Surgery 2001; **Med School:** Stanford Univ 1983; **Resid:** Surgery, Stanford Univ Med Ctr 1991; **Fellow:** Oncology, Stanford Univ Med Ctr 1988; **Fac Appt:** Assoc Prof S, UCSF

Essner, Richard MD [S] - **Spec Exp:** Sentinel Node Surgery; Melanoma; Gastrointestinal Surgery; **Hospital:** St. John's Hlth Ctr, Santa Monica; **Address:** 2336 Santa Monica Blvd, Ste 206, Santa Monica, CA 90404-2302; **Phone:** 310-696-0716; **Board Cert:** Surgery 2002; **Med School:** Emory Univ 1985; **Resid:** Surgery, Univ NC Hosps 1992; **Fac Appt:** Asst Clin Prof S, USC Sch Med

Fisher, Jonathan S MD [S] - **Spec Exp:** Transplant-Kidney; Transplant-Liver; Transplant-Pancreas; Pancreatic Islet Cell Transplant; **Hospital:** Scripps Green Hosp; **Address:** Scripps Clinic Torrey Pines, 10666 N Torrey Pines Rd, MC 200N, La Jolla, CA 92037; **Phone:** 858-554-4310; **Board Cert:** Surgery 2002; **Med School:** Columbia P&S 1994; **Resid:** Surgery, Univ Chicago Hosps 2001; **Fellow:** Transplant Surgery, Univ Tennessee 2003

Giuliano, Armando E MD [S] - **Spec Exp:** Breast Cancer; Sentinel Node Surgery; Thyroid & Parathyroid Surgery; **Hospital:** Cedars-Sinai Med Ctr; **Address:** Saul & Joyce Brandman Breast Ctr, 310 N San Vincente Blvd, Los Angeles, CA 90048; **Phone:** 310-423-9331 x0; **Board Cert:** Surgery 2009; **Med School:** Univ Chicago-Pritzker Sch Med 1973; **Resid:** Surgery, UCSF Med Ctr 1980; **Fellow:** Surgical Oncology, UCLA Med Ctr 1978; **Fac Appt:** Prof S, UCLA

Goodnight, James E MD [S] - **Spec Exp:** Melanoma; Breast Cancer; Bone & Soft Tissue Tumors; **Hospital:** UC Davis Med Ctr; **Address:** 4501 X St, Sacramento, CA 95817; **Phone:** 916-734-5959; **Board Cert:** Surgery 2007; **Med School:** Baylor Coll Med 1968; **Resid:** Surgery, Univ Utah Hosp 1976; **Fellow:** Surgical Oncology, UCLA Med Ctr 1978; **Fac Appt:** Prof S, UC Davis

Goodson III, William H MD [S] - **Spec Exp:** Breast Cancer; Breast Disease; **Hospital:** CA Pacific Med Ctr-Pacific Campus, UCSF - Mt Zion Med Ctr; **Address:** 2100 Webster St, Ste 401, San Francisco, CA 94115-2378; **Phone:** 415-923-3925; **Board Cert:** Surgery 2006; **Med School:** Harvard Med Sch 1971; **Resid:** Surgery, Univ Hosps 1976; Surgery, Childrens Hosp 1977

Gower, Roland E MD [S] - **Spec Exp:** Breast Surgery; Biliary Surgery; Thyroid Surgery; **Hospital:** Providence Alaska Med Ctr, Alaska Regl Hosp; **Address:** 2841 De Barr Rd, Ste 41, Anchorage, AK 99508-2973; **Phone:** 907-279-3564; **Board Cert:** Surgery 2008; **Med School:** Vanderbilt Univ 1971; **Resid:** Surgery, Kansas Med Ctr 1975

Greenhalgh, David G MD [S] - **Spec Exp:** Burn Care; Nutrition; Wound Healing/Care; **Hospital:** Northern CA Shriners Hosp, UC Davis Med Ctr; **Address:** Shriners Hosp Chldn, 2425 Stockton Blvd, Sacramento, CA 95817; **Phone:** 916-453-2050; **Board Cert:** Surgery 2005; Surgical Critical Care 2008; **Med School:** SUNY Upstate Med Univ 1981; **Resid:** Surgery, MC Hosp of VT 1986; **Fellow:** Burn Surgery, Univ Wash Hosp 1989; **Fac Appt:** Prof S, UC Davis

Hemming, Alan W MD [S] - **Spec Exp:** Liver Cancer; Transplant-Liver; Hepatobiliary Surgery; Pancreatic Cancer; **Hospital:** UCSD Med Ctr, Rady Children's Hosp - San Diego; **Address:** UC San Diego Center for Hepatobiliary Disease and Transplantation, 200 W Arbor Drive, Fl 2nd, Ste 2, rm 280, MS 8401, Ste 2, rm 280, San Diego, CA 92103-8401; **Phone:** 619-543-5870; **Board Cert:** Surgery 2004; **Med School:** Univ British Columbia Fac Med 1987; **Resid:** Surgery, Univ British Columbia Med Ctr 1994; **Fellow:** Transplant Surgery, Univ Toronto/Hosp for Sick Children 1995; Hepatobiliary Surgery, Univ Toronto 1996; **Fac Appt:** Prof S, UCSD

Horvath, Karen MD [S] - **Spec Exp:** Colon & Rectal Surgery; Gastrointestinal Surgery; Minimally Invasive Surgery; **Hospital:** Univ Wash Med Ctr; **Address:** 1959 NE Pacific St, Box 356165, Seattle, WA 98195; **Phone:** 206-598-4477; **Board Cert:** Surgery 2007; **Med School:** NY Med Coll 1990; **Resid:** Surgery, NY Presby Hosp/Columbia 1997; **Fellow:** Surgical Critical Care, Mt Sinai Hosp 1994; Laparoscopic Surgery, Oregon Hlth Sci Ctr 1998; **Fac Appt:** Assoc Prof S, Univ Wash

Hunter, John G MD [S] - **Spec Exp:** Gastrointestinal Surgery; Laparoscopic Abdominal Surgery; Gastroesophageal Reflux Disease (GERD); Esophageal Surgery; **Hospital:** OR Hlth & Sci Univ; **Address:** Digestive Hlth Ctr, 3303 SW Bond Ave, MC CH6D, Portland, OR 97239; **Phone:** 503-494-4373; **Board Cert:** Surgery 2006; **Med School:** Univ Pennsylvania 1981; **Resid:** Surgery, Univ Utah Med Ctr 1987; **Fellow:** Gastrointestinal Surgery, Mass Genl Hosp 1988; Endoscopy, Univ West Ontario 1989; **Fac Appt:** Assoc Prof S, Oregon Hlth & Sci Univ

Karlan, Scott R MD [S] - **Spec Exp:** Breast Cancer & Surgery; **Hospital:** Cedars-Sinai Med Ctr; **Address:** 310 N San Vicente Blvd Fl 3, Los Angeles, CA 90048; **Phone:** 310-423-9331; **Board Cert:** Surgery 2005; **Med School:** Harvard Med Sch 1982; **Resid:** Surgery, Yale-New Haven Hosp 1987; **Fac Appt:** Clin Prof S, UCLA

Kaufman, Cary S MD [S] - **Spec Exp:** Breast Cancer & Surgery; Breast Disease; **Hospital:** St. Joseph Hosp - Bellingham; **Address:** 2940 Squalicum Pkwy, Ste 101, Bellingham, WA 98225; **Phone:** 360-671-9877; **Board Cert:** Surgery 2000; **Med School:** UCLA 1973; **Resid:** Surgery, Univ Wash Med Ctr 1975; Surgery, Harbor-UCLA Med Ctr 1979; **Fac Appt:** Asst Clin Prof S, Univ Wash

Kirgan, Daniel MD [S] - **Spec Exp:** Cancer Surgery; Breast Cancer & Surgery; **Hospital:** Univ Med Ctr - Las Vegas; **Address:** 1707 W Charleston Blvd, Ste 160, Las Vegas, NV 89102; **Phone:** 702-671-5150; **Board Cert:** Surgery 2004; **Med School:** Geo Wash Univ 1986; **Resid:** Surgery, Univ Med Ctr 1992; **Fellow:** Surgical Oncology, John Wayne Cancer Inst 1994; **Fac Appt:** Assoc Prof S, Univ Nevada

Klein, Andrew S MD [S] - **Spec Exp:** Transplant-Liver; Liver Cancer; Liver Failure; **Hospital:** Cedars-Sinai Med Ctr; **Address:** Liver & Transplant Ctr at Cedars-Sinai, 8635 W Third St, Ste 590W, Los Angeles, CA 90048; **Phone:** 310-423-2641; **Board Cert:** Surgery 2007; **Med School:** Johns Hopkins Univ 1979; **Resid:** Surgery, Johns Hopkins Hosp 1982; Surgery, Johns Hopkins Hosp 1986; **Fellow:** Transplant Surgery, UCLA-CHS 1988; **Fac Appt:** Clin Prof S, UCLA

Knudson, Mary Margaret MD [S] - **Spec Exp:** Breast Cancer; Trauma; **Hospital:** UCSF Med Ctr, San Francisco Genl Hosp; **Address:** 1001 Potrero Ave, Ste 3A, San Francisco, CA 94110; **Phone:** 415-206-4623; **Board Cert:** Surgery 2002; Surgical Critical Care 2008; **Med School:** Univ Mich Med Sch 1976; **Resid:** Surgery, Beth Israel Hosp 1979; Surgery, Univ Mich Med Ctr 1982; **Fellow:** Pediatric Surgery, Stanford Univ Hosps 1983; **Fac Appt:** Assoc Prof S, UCSF

Lowy, Andrew M MD [S] - **Spec Exp:** Pancreatic Cancer; Gastrointestinal Cancer; Peritoneal Carcinomatosis; Clinical Trials; **Hospital:** UCSD Med Ctr; **Address:** Moores UCSD Cancer Ctr, 3855 Health Sciences Drive, La Jolla, CA 92093-0987; **Phone:** 858-822-2124; **Board Cert:** Surgery 2003; **Med School:** Cornell Univ-Weill Med Coll 1988; **Resid:** Surgery, NY-Cornell Med Ctr 1996; **Fellow:** Surgical Oncology, MD Anderson Cancer Ctr 1996; **Fac Appt:** Prof S, UCSD

Moossa, AR MD [S] - **Spec Exp:** Pancreatic Cancer; Gastrointestinal Cancer; Hepatobiliary Surgery; **Hospital:** UCSD Med Ctr; **Address:** 9300 Campus Point Drive, La Jolla, CA 92037; **Phone:** 858-657-6113; **Med School:** England, UK 1965; **Resid:** Surgery, Liverpool Univ Hosps 1970; **Fellow:** Surgical Oncology, Johns Hopkins Hosp 1972; **Fac Appt:** Prof S, UCSD

Morton, John MD [S] - **Spec Exp:** Obesity/Bariatric Surgery; Minimally Invasive Surgery; **Hospital:** Stanford Univ Hosp & Clinics; **Address:** Surgical Specialties, 300 Pasteur Drive, rm H3680, Stanford, CA 94305-5655; **Phone:** 650-725-9777; **Board Cert:** Surgery 2002; **Med School:** Tulane Univ 1993; **Resid:** Surgery, Tulane Univ Hosp 1999; Surgery, Swedish Med Ctr 2001; **Fellow:** Laparoscopic Surgery, Univ N Carolina Affil Hosp 2003; **Fac Appt:** Assoc Prof S, Stanford Univ

Nakakura, Eric MD/PhD [S] - **Spec Exp:** Pancreatic Cancer; Liver Cancer; Gastrointestinal Cancer; Sarcoma; **Hospital:** UCSF Med Ctr; **Address:** 1600 Divisadero St Fl 4, Box 1705, San Francisco, CA 94115; **Phone:** 415-353-9888; **Board Cert:** Surgery 2004; **Med School:** Stanford Univ 1995; **Resid:** Surgery, Johns Hopkins Hosp 2000; **Fellow:** Surgical Oncology, Johns Hopkins Hosp 2004; **Fac Appt:** Asst Prof S, UCSF

Nguyen, Ninh T MD [S] - **Spec Exp:** Laparoscopic Surgery; Obesity/Bariatric Surgery; Gastrointestinal Cancer & Surgery; **Hospital:** UC Irvine Med Ctr; **Address:** Div Gastrointestinal Surgery, 333 City Blvd W, Ste 850, Orange, CA 92868; **Phone:** 714-456-8598; **Board Cert:** Surgery 2006; **Med School:** Univ Tex, San Antonio 1990; **Resid:** Surgery, Mt Sinai Med Ctr 1995; **Fellow:** Surgical Oncology, Univ Pittsburgh Med Ctr 1997; Laparoscopic Surgery, Univ Pittsburgh Med Ctr 1998; **Fac Appt:** Assoc Prof S, UC Irvine

Nissen, Nicholas N MD [S] - **Spec Exp:** Liver Cancer; Transplant-Liver; Pancreatic Cancer; Minimally Invasive Surgery; **Hospital:** Cedars-Sinai Med Ctr; **Address:** Cedars-Sinai Medical Center, 8635 W 3rd St, Ste 590-W, Los Angeles, CA 90048; **Phone:** 310-423-2641; **Board Cert:** Surgery 1999; Surgical Critical Care 1999; **Med School:** Univ Minn 1991; **Resid:** Surgery, Loyola Univ Med Ctr 1998; **Fellow:** Surgical Critical Care, Univ Pittsburgh Med Ctr 1999; Hepatobiliary Surgery, UCLA Med Ctr 2001

Norton, Jeffrey A MD [S] - **Spec Exp:** Pancreatic Cancer; Gastrointestinal Cancer & Surgery; Endocrine Surgery; **Hospital:** Stanford Univ Hosp & Clinics; **Address:** 875 Blake Wilbur Drive, Clin F, Stanford, CA 94305; **Phone:** 650-723-5461; **Board Cert:** Surgery 2001; **Med School:** SUNY Upstate Med Univ 1973; **Resid:** Surgery, Duke Univ Med Ctr 1982; **Fellow:** Research, Natl Cancer Inst 1989; **Fac Appt:** Prof S, Stanford Univ

Paz, Isaac Benjamin MD [S] - **Spec Exp:** Breast Cancer; Esophageal Cancer; **Hospital:** City of Hope Natl Med Ctr; **Address:** 1500 E Duarte Rd, Duarte, CA 91010; **Phone:** 626-256-4673 x67100; **Board Cert:** Surgery 2000; **Med School:** Chile 1981; **Resid:** Surgery, Univ Catolica de Chile 1985; Surgery, Univ Arizona 1990; **Fellow:** Surgical Oncology, City of Hope Med Ctr 1993

Pellegrini, Carlos MD [S] - **Spec Exp:** Esophageal Cancer; Esophageal Surgery; Barrett's Esophagus; Gastrointestinal Cancer & Surgery; **Hospital:** Univ Wash Med Ctr; **Address:** Univ Washington Medical Ctr, Dept Surgery, 1959 NE Pacific St, Box 356165, Seattle, WA 98195; **Phone:** 206-598-4547; **Board Cert:** Surgery 1998; **Med School:** Argentina 1971; **Resid:** Surgery, Granadero Hosp 1975; Surgery, Univ Chicago Hosps 1979; **Fac Appt:** Prof S, Univ Wash

Perkins, James D MD [S] - **Spec Exp:** Transplant-Pancreas; Transplant-Liver; Transplant-Kidney; **Hospital:** Univ Wash Med Ctr, Seattle Chldns Hosp; **Address:** Univ Wash Med Ctr, Dept Surg, 1959 NE Pacific St, Box 356410, Seattle, WA 98195; **Phone:** 206-543-3825; **Board Cert:** Surgery 2004; **Med School:** Univ Ark 1979; **Resid:** Surgery, St Francis Regl Med Ctr 1984; **Fellow:** Transplant Surgery, Mayo Grad Sch 1985; **Fac Appt:** Prof S, Univ Wash

Peterson, Laura D MD [S] - **Spec Exp:** Breast Cancer; Breast Surgery; **Hospital:** Kapiolani Med Ctr for Women & Chldn, Straub Clinic & Hosp; **Address:** Kapi'olani Womens Ctr, 1907 S Beretania St, Ste 501, Honolulu, HI 96826; **Phone:** 808-949-3444; **Board Cert:** Surgery 2004; **Med School:** UCSD 1998; **Resid:** Surgery, Univ Hawaii Affil Hosp 2004; **Fellow:** Minimally Invasive Surgery, Kaiser Permanente 2005; Surgical Oncology, Kaiser Permanente 2005

Phillips, Edward H MD [S] - **Spec Exp:** Laparoscopic Surgery; Obesity/Bariatric Surgery; **Hospital:** Cedars-Sinai Med Ctr; **Address:** 8635 W 3rd St, Ste 795 West, Los Angeles, CA 90048-6101; **Phone:** 310-423-8350; **Board Cert:** Surgery 2008; **Med School:** USC Sch Med 1973; **Resid:** Surgery, USC Medical Ctr 1978; Vascular Surgery, Los Angeles Co-USC Medical Ctr 1979; **Fac Appt:** Assoc Clin Prof S, USC Sch Med

Posselt, Andrew M MD/PhD [S] - **Spec Exp:** Obesity/Bariatric Surgery; Pancreatic Islet Cell Transplant; Transplant-Liver; Transplant-Pancreas; **Hospital:** UCSF Med Ctr; **Address:** UCSF Medical Ctr, Dept Surgery, 505 Parnassus Ave, M884, San Francisco, CA 94143; **Phone:** 415-353-1888; **Board Cert:** Surgery 2002; **Med School:** Univ Pennsylvania 1993; **Resid:** Internal Medicine, UCSF Med Ctr 1996; Surgery, UCSF Med Ctr 2001; **Fellow:** Transplant Surgery, UCSF Med Ctr 2002; **Fac Appt:** Asst Prof S, UCSF

Potenza, Bruce M MD [S] - **Spec Exp:** Burn Care; Critical Care; **Hospital:** UCSD Med Ctr; **Address:** UCSD Med Ctr, 200 W Arbor Drive, MC 8896, San Diego, CA 92103-8896; **Phone:** 619-543-6001; **Board Cert:** Surgery 2004; Internal Medicine 1988; Surgical Critical Care 2006; Critical Care Medicine 2006; **Med School:** Loyola Univ-Stritch Sch Med 1983; **Resid:** Internal Medicine, Good Samaritan Med Ctr 1987; Surgery, SUNY Syracuse Med Ctr 1993; **Fac Appt:** Clin Prof S, UCSD

Rassman, William R MD [S] - **Spec Exp:** Hair Restoration/Transplant; **Address:** 2080 Century Park East, Ste 607, Los Angeles, CA 90067; **Phone:** 310-553-9113; **Board Cert:** Surgery 1975; **Med School:** Med Coll VA 1966; **Resid:** Surgery, New York Hos -Cornell 1969; Surgery, Dartmouth Med Ctr 1973

Reber, Howard A MD [S] - **Spec Exp:** Pancreatic Cancer; Pancreatic Surgery; Gastrointestinal Cancer; **Hospital:** UCLA Ronald Reagan Med Ctr; **Address:** UCLA General Surgery, 10833 Le Cone Ave CHS Bldg - rm 72-215, Los Angeles, CA 90095; **Phone:** 310-794-7788; **Board Cert:** Surgery 1971; **Med School:** Univ Pennsylvania 1964; **Resid:** Surgery, Hosp Univ Penn 1970; **Fac Appt:** Prof S, UCLA

Roberts, John Paul MD [S] - **Spec Exp:** Transplant-Liver; **Hospital:** UCSF Med Ctr; **Address:** UCSF Medical Ctr, Div Transplant Surgery, 505 Parnassus Ave, rm M896, Box 0780, San Francisco, CA 94143-0780; **Phone:** 415-353-1888; **Board Cert:** Surgery 2006; **Med School:** UCSD 1980; **Resid:** Surgery, Univ Wash 1983; Surgery, Univ Wash 1987; **Fellow:** Surgery, Cornell-New York Hosp 1986; Transplant Surgery, Univ Minn Med Ctr 1988; **Fac Appt:** Prof S, UCSF

Rogers, Stanley J MD [S] - **Spec Exp:** Minimally Invasive Surgery; Gastrointestinal Surgery; Obesity/Bariatric Surgery; **Hospital:** UCSF Med Ctr, San Francisco Genl Hosp; **Address:** UCSF Med Ctr, Dept Surgery, 400 Parnassus Ave, Ste 665, Campus Box 0338, San Francisco, CA 94143; **Phone:** 415-353-2161; **Board Cert:** Surgery 2006; **Med School:** Univ Utah 1991; **Resid:** Surgery, UCSF Med Ctr 1997; **Fac Appt:** Assoc Prof S, UCSF

Satava, Richard M MD [S] - **Spec Exp:** Laparoscopic Abdominal Surgery; Gastrointestinal Surgery; **Hospital:** Univ Wash Med Ctr; **Address:** Univ Washington Med Ctr, Dept Surgery, 1959 NE Pacific St, Box 356410, Seattle, WA 98195; **Phone:** 206-685-0052; **Board Cert:** Surgery 2000; **Med School:** Hahnemann Univ 1968; **Resid:** Surgery, Mayo Clinic 1974; **Fellow:** Research, Mayo Clinic 1972

Schaffer, Randolph L MD [S] - **Spec Exp:** Transplant-Liver; Transplant-Kidney; Transplant-Pancreas; **Hospital:** Scripps Green Hosp; **Address:** Scripps Clinic Torrey Pines, 10666 N Torrey Pines Rd, MC 200N, La Jolla, CA 92037; **Phone:** 858-544-4310; **Board Cert:** Surgery 2002; **Med School:** Baylor Coll Med 1995; **Resid:** Surgery, Baylor Affil Hosp 2001; **Fellow:** Transplant Surgery, Univ Chicago 2003

Selby, Robert R MD [S] - **Spec Exp:** Liver & Biliary Surgery; Liver Cancer; **Hospital:** Keck Med Ctr of USC (page 75); **Address:** 1510 San Pablo St, Ste 514, Los Angeles, CA 90033-4612; **Phone:** 323-442-7172; **Board Cert:** Surgery 2008; Surgical Critical Care 2001; **Med School:** Univ MO-Columbia Sch Med 1979; **Resid:** Internal Medicine, Good Samaritan Hosp 1981; Surgery, Good Samaritan Hosp 1986; **Fellow:** Transplant Surgery, Presby Univ Hosp 1988; **Fac Appt:** Prof S, USC Sch Med

Sener, Stephen F MD [S] - **Spec Exp:** Breast Cancer; Lymphedema; Thyroid Cancer; Melanoma; **Hospital:** Keck Med Ctr of USC (page 75); **Address:** USC Norris Comprehensive Cancer Ctr, 1441 Eastlake Ave, Ste 7415, Los Angeles, CA 90033; **Phone:** 323-865-3535; **Board Cert:** Surgery 2001; **Med School:** Northwestern Univ 1977; **Resid:** Surgery, Northwestern Univ 1982; **Fellow:** Surgery, Meml Sloan Kettering Cancer Ctr 1984; **Fac Appt:** Prof S, USC-Keck School of Medicine

Silverstein, Melvin J MD [S] - **Spec Exp:** Breast Cancer; **Hospital:** Hoag Meml Hosp Presby; **Address:** 1 Hoag Drive, Breast Care Ctr, Newport Beach, CA 92658; **Phone:** 949-764-8281; **Board Cert:** Surgery 1971; **Med School:** Albany Med Coll 1965; **Resid:** Surgery, Boston City Hosp-Tufts Univ 1970; **Fellow:** Surgical Oncology, UCLA Med Ctr 1975

Sinanan, Mika N MD [S] - **Spec Exp:** Gastrointestinal Surgery; Gastrointestinal Cancer; Liver & Biliary Cancer; Laparoscopic Surgery; **Hospital:** Univ Wash Med Ctr; **Address:** Univ Washington, Dept Surgery, 1959 NE Pacific St, Box 356165, Seattle, WA 98195-6410; **Phone:** 206-598-4477; **Board Cert:** Surgery 2008; **Med School:** Johns Hopkins Univ 1980; **Resid:** Surgery, Univ Washington Hosp 1988; **Fellow:** Gastrointestinal Surgery, Univ Brit Columbia Med Ctr 1986; **Fac Appt:** Prof S, Univ Wash

Swanstrom, Lee L MD [S] - **Spec Exp:** Esophageal Surgery; Esophageal Disorders; Minimally Invasive Surgery; Gastrointestinal Motility Disorders; **Hospital:** Providence Portland Med Ctr, Legacy Good Samaritan Med Ctr; **Address:** 1040 NW 22nd Ave, Ste 560, Portland, OR 97210; **Phone:** 503-281-0561; **Board Cert:** Surgery 2009; **Med School:** Creighton Univ 1983; **Resid:** Surgery, Emanuel Hosp 1988; **Fac Appt:** Clin Prof S, Oregon Hlth & Sci Univ

Trisal, Vijay MD [S] - **Spec Exp:** Skin Cancer; **Hospital:** City of Hope Natl Med Ctr; **Address:** City of Hope Med Ctr, Dept Surgery, 1500 E Duarte Rd, Duarte, CA 91010; **Phone:** 626-256-4673 x67100; **Board Cert:** Surgery 2003; **Med School:** India 1993; **Resid:** Surgery, Providence Hosp & Med Ctrs 2002; **Fellow:** Surgical Oncology, City of Hope Natl Med Ctr 2004

Vetto, John MD [S] - **Spec Exp:** Cancer Surgery; **Hospital:** OR Hlth & Sci Univ; **Address:** 3181 SW Sam Jackson Park Rd, MC L619, Portland, OR 97239; **Phone:** 503-494-5501; **Board Cert:** Surgery 2009; **Med School:** Oregon Hlth & Sci Univ 1982; **Resid:** Surgery, Brigham & Women's Hosp 1984; Surgery, UCLA Med Ctr 1989; **Fellow:** Surgical Oncology, Natl Cancer Inst 1986; Surgical Oncology, Meml Sloan Kettering Cancer Ctr 1991; **Fac Appt:** Assoc Prof S, Oregon Hlth & Sci Univ

Wagman, Lawrence D MD [S] - **Spec Exp:** Liver Cancer; Gastrointestinal Cancer; Breast Cancer; Liver Surgery; **Hospital:** St. Joseph's Hosp - Orange, City of Hope Natl Med Ctr; **Address:** 1010 W La Veta Ave, Fl 4, Ste 470, Orange, CA 92868; **Phone:** 714-835-8300; **Board Cert:** Surgery 2004; **Med School:** Columbia P&S 1978; **Resid:** Surgery, Med Coll Virginia Hosp 1985; **Fellow:** Surgical Oncology, NIH/NCI 1982; **Fac Appt:** Assoc Clin Prof S, UCSD

Wallace, Anne Marie MD [S] - **Spec Exp:** Breast Cancer; Breast Reconstruction; Melanoma; **Hospital:** UCSD Med Ctr; **Address:** UCSD Moores Cancer Ctr, 3855 Health Sciences Drive #0987, La Jolla, CA 92093; **Phone:** 858-822-6193; **Board Cert:** Surgery 2001; Plastic Surgery 2005; **Med School:** Creighton Univ 1987; **Resid:** Surgery, Washington Hosp Ctr 1992; Plastic Surgery, UCSD Med Ctr 1994; **Fellow:** Surgical Breast Oncology, MD Anderson Cancer Ctr 1995; **Fac Appt:** Clin Prof S, UCSD

Wapnir, Irene L MD [S] - **Spec Exp:** Breast Surgery; Breast Cancer; **Hospital:** Stanford Univ Hosp & Clinics; **Address:** Stanford Univ Medical Ctr, 300 Pasteur Drive, rm H3625, Palo Alto, CA 94305; **Phone:** 650-736-1353; **Board Cert:** Surgery 2008; **Med School:** Mexico 1980; **Resid:** Surgery, Lincoln Hosp 1985; **Fellow:** Breast Disease, RW Johnson Univ Med Ctr 1986; **Fac Appt:** Assoc Prof S, Stanford Univ

Warren, Robert Samuel MD [S] - **Spec Exp:** Liver Cancer; **Hospital:** UCSF Med Ctr; **Address:** UCSF Comprehensive Cancer Center, 1600 Divisadero St Fl 4, San Francisco, CA 94115; **Phone:** 415-353-9846; **Med School:** Univ Minn 1980; **Resid:** Surgery, Univ Minn Hosps 1988; **Fellow:** Surgical Oncology, Meml Sloan-Kettering Cancer Ctr 1986; **Fac Appt:** Prof S, UCSF

Yeung, Raymond S W MD [S] - **Spec Exp:** Liver & Biliary Cancer; Liver Cancer; Melanoma; Breast Cancer; **Hospital:** Univ Wash Med Ctr; **Address:** Univ of Washington, Dept Surgery, 1959 NE Pacific St, Box 356165, Seattle, WA 98195; **Phone:** 206-598-4477; **Board Cert:** Surgery 2009; **Med School:** Univ Toronto 1982; **Resid:** Surgery, University of Toronto 1987; **Fellow:** Surgical Oncology, Fox Chase Cancer Ctr 1992; **Fac Appt:** Prof S, Univ Wash

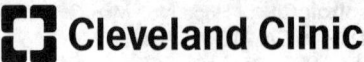

Cleveland Clinic

Every life deserves world class care.

General Surgery

Cleveland Clinic's Digestive Disease Institute (DDI) is one of the largest digestive programs in the country and is ranked No. 2 in the nation by *U.S.News & World Report*. DDI is the first to fully integrate its departments of Colorectal Surgery, Gastroenterology & Hepatology, General Surgery and Nutrition. Combining these disciplines in one location facilitates unprecedented patient care, multidisciplinary education and collaborative research. In 2010, DDI physicians performed more than 27,000 surgical cases and 38,000 endoscopic cases. Transplant surgeons completed more than 170 digestive disease-related organ transplants, including liver, pancreas and intestinal transplantation, achieving outstanding outcomes.

Highlights of the Department of General Surgery:

- Our hepato-pancreato-biliary surgeons have advanced the field of laparoscopic pancreatic surgery in areas including robotic Whipple surgery
- Cleveland Clinic is one of only a few programs in the country to offer Hyperthermic (or Heated) Intraoperative Peritoneal Chemotherapy to treat cancers that have spread to the lining of the abdominal cavity.
- Our Hernia Center performs more than 1,700 hernia repairs annually at 16 locations, from the routine to the most complex cases.
- The Acute Care Surgery program has a dedicated operating room 24/7 for emergent cases.
- Our Liver Tumor Clinic cares for patients with benign and cancerous liver tumors with treatment aimed at preserving liver function and quality of life.
- Our Pancreas Clinic is one of the few centers in the nation specializing in multidisciplinary, patient-centered treatments and frontline research for complicated acute pancreatitis, chronic pancreatitis, pancreatic cancer and pancreatic-biliary disorders.

Cleveland Clinic
Digestive Disease Institute
9500 Euclid Avenue
Cleveland, OH 44195

clevelandclinic.org/
surgerytopdocs

Offering Same-Day Appointments
Call 800.274.2009.

Treatment Guides

Cleveland Clinic has developed comprehensive treatment guides for many diseases and conditions. To download our free treatment guides, visit clevelandclinic.org/treatmentguides.

Online Medical Second Opinion

Cleveland Clinic's My**Consult** Online Medical Second Opinion program securely connects patients to our physician specialists for more than 1,000 life-changing or life-threatening diagnoses all by the click of a mouse. To learn more, log onto eclevelandclinic.org/myconsult or call 800.223.2273, ext. 43223.

Special Assistance for Out-of-State Patients

Cleveland Clinic Global Patient Services offers a complimentary Medical Concierge service for patients who travel from outside of Ohio. Call 800.223.2273, ext. 55580 or email medicalconcierge@ccf.org.

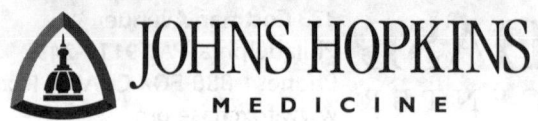

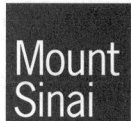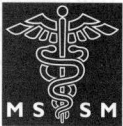

THE MOUNT SINAI MEDICAL CENTER
DEPARTMENT OF SURGERY
One Gustave L. Levy Place
Fifth Avenue and 100th Street
New York, NY 10029-6574
Physician Referral: 1-800-MD-SINAI (637-4624)
www.mountsinai.org/surgery

**MOUNT SINAI
SCHOOL OF
MEDICINE**

THE DEPARTMENT OF SURGERY continues to build upon the legacy of those who have gone before, caring for the very sickest of patients while developing new therapies and training tomorrow's physicians to save and enhance lives. Patients today are experiencing less pain, shorter hospital stays, and faster recovery times than was ever imaginable just 20 years ago.

Bariatric Surgery – The latest minimally invasive techniques are used to perform laparoscopic gastric bypass, lap band placement, duodenal switch, and sleeve gastrectomy.

Colon and Rectal Surgery – Leaders in the treatment of gastrointestinal disorders, our surgeons care for a wide range of diseases, including: inflammatory bowel disease (Crohn's disease and ulcerative colitis), diverticulitis, and colon and rectal cancers. We offer many important procedures not commonly available.

General Surgery – Treatment is individualized based on the patient's condition, with options from advanced laparoscopic procedures to complex operations.

Laparoscopic and Minimally Invasive Surgery – Mount Sinai surgeons rank as some of the world's most respected and innovative surgeons, performing more laparoscopic procedures than surgeons at any other hospital in New York.

Metabolic, Endocrine and Minimally Invasive Surgery – This division was formed to serve as the backbone for several disease-specific multidisciplinary programs. Ours is a truly novel metabolic surgery program that brings together traditional endocrine, bariatric and laparoscopic techniques to treat diseases of metabolism.

Pediatric Surgery – Surgeries involving children can be met with even more apprehension than those for adults. Fortunately, Mount Sinai surgeons offer a full range of pediatric surgical procedures in a family-focused, child-sensitive environment.

Plastic and Reconstructive Surgery – Surgical care from aesthetic to complex reconstruction is offered for benign and malignant disease, as well as for deformities that are either congenital or acquired. The aim is to restore function and correct deformities caused by birth defects, aging, accident, or illness.

Surgical Oncology – Patients are seen promptly and are cared for by a team of medical and surgical experts, enabling them to benefit from the opinions of dozens of nationally renowned doctors.

Vascular Surgery – A recognized world leader in the development of new techniques for the treatment of aortic aneurysms, Mount Sinai continues to perform extensive research to advance the field of vascular surgery. A wide array of advanced patient services are available, ensuring that conditions are managed successfully.

TOP-RANKING MINIMALLY INVASIVE SURGEONS
In surveys of leading minimally invasive surgeons in a variety of specialties, Mount Sinai's physicians are consistently at the top of the list in surgery of the colon and rectum, liver and bile ducts, thyroid, hernia, chest, and blood vessels.

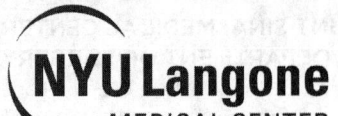

MINIMALLY INVASIVE SURGERY

NYU Langone Medical Center has been at the forefront of minimally invasive surgery for more than 20 years, treating conditions from heart disease and prostate cancer to obesity and fetal abnormalities in utero.

Robotic Surgery

NYU Langone Medical Center was the first hospital in New York City to use the minimally invasive da Vinci Si HD robotic surgical system which allows a 40 percent higher definition view of the surgical field. The device also enables physicians to import and display medical test results from any computer or diagnostic medical device.

Laparoscopic Surgery

Surgeons at NYU Langone Medical Center use laparoscopic techniques to manage kidney cancers, remove adrenal glands, perform renal biopsies, remove renal cysts and perform innovative urinary reconstruction. Kidney donations can also be performed laparoscopically.

Cardiac Surgery

Since 1996, over 5,000 minimally invasive heart surgery procedures have been performed by our cardiac surgeons. Most patients are candidates for minimally invasive procedures.

Thoracic Surgery

We offer a minimally invasive thoracic surgery program, incorporating video-assisted techniques along with the newest methods for post-operative pain relief.

Neurosurgical Technology

NYU Langone Medical Center was the first hospital in the Northeast with the highly advanced Leksell Gamma Knife, allowing neurosurgeons to remove deep-seated tumors, vascular malformations and other disease sites with outstanding results. Assisted by three-dimensional MRI technology, the Leksell Gamma Knife bombards its target with precise doses of radiation, while preserving healthy tissue.

Gynecologic Surgery

Minimally invasive gynecological surgery, including surgery for endometriosis and laparoscopic hysterectomy, are routinely performed at NYU Langone Medical Center.

Varicose Veins

Our physicians pioneered two minimally invasive procedures that do not require surgical incisions to treat varicose veins. They are endovascular closure, which uses radio heat waves to close down inadequate valves, and scope-based varicose vein treatment which allows veins to be removed without an open incision.

PENN ROBOTIC SURGERY

For more than 200 years, Penn has expanded the frontiers of medicine. Today, surgeons at Penn Medicine are leading the way in robotic-assisted surgery.

A Leading Program in the United States

Penn is home to eight daVinci® Surgical Systems making it one of the largest robotic-assisted surgical programs in the United States. The equipment has been used for some time in urologic/prostate procedures, cardiac surgery, gastrointestinal and gynecological operations.

In addition, Penn surgeons have pioneered new procedures in head and neck surgery using the robotic-assisted technology. Penn was the first medical center in the world with an approved study to perform this surgery and many patients have benefited from transoral robotic surgery (TORS).

Benefits of Robotic Surgery

The advantages of robotic-assisted surgery include a tremendous enhancement in the surgeon's control of the instruments and the ability to perform more intricate procedures.

For patients, the benefits of robotic-assisted surgery may include:
- Less post-operative pain
- Less risk of infection
- Less anesthesia
- Less blood loss
- Shorter hospital stay
- Faster and more complete recovery
- Quicker return to normal daily activities

Experience Makes the Difference

Because of its many benefits, robotic-assisted surgery has gained increased popularity among the medical community in recent years. But technology is only as good as the hands that control it. Robotic technology is meant to be operated by skilled and experienced surgeons. The robotic surgery program at Penn is staffed by surgeons who far exceed the recommended level of experience required for its use. In addition, Penn is one of the largest, state-of-the-art surgical training centers in the country.

As the medical community embraces robotic-assisted surgery, our researchers, nurses, and surgeons remain at the forefront of this field by relentlessly advancing the application of this technology as well as educating the next generation of surgeons who will use it. The result is that Penn is the first place surgeons turn to learn the technology of tomorrow and the first place you should turn for answers.

Robotic Surgery Available at Penn:

- **Cancer:** Head and Neck, Throat, Mouth and Tongue, Prostate, Kidney, Heart, Uterus, Cervix

- **Colon & Rectal Surgery:** Abdominal Perineal Resection; Proctocolectomy with IPAA and Temporary Loop Ileostomy; Right Colectomy; Sigmoid Resection with Rectoplexy

- **Gastrointestinal:** Bariatric LAP-BAND® and Sleeve Gastrectomy, Anti-reflux, Motility Disorders

- **Gynecology:** Pelvic Floor Reconstruction, Hysterectomy, Fibroid Removal, Myomectomy, Tubal Anastomosis

- **Heart:** Coronary Bypass, Mitral Valve Repair, Atrial Septal Defect Closure, Tumor Resection

- **Otorhinolaryngology—Head and Neck Surgery:** TORS; Thyroidectomy; Tongue, Palate and Tonsil Surgery; Sleep Apnea

- **Thoracic:** Lobectomy; Thymectomy; Resection of Esophageal and Mediastinal Masses, Tumors and Cysts

- **Urology:** Prostatectomy, Nephrectomy, Pelvic Reconstruction

Hospital of the University of Pennsylvania | Penn Presbyterian Medical Center | Pennsylvania Hospital

UHealth
UNIVERSITY OF MIAMI HEALTH SYSTEM
The DeWitt Daughtry Department of Surgery

UNIVERSITY OF MIAMI
MILLER SCHOOL
of MEDICINE

COMPREHENSIVE SURGERY

The University of Miami Miller School of Medicine Department of Surgery is recognized for its outstanding and innovative surgical expertise and leading research programs. We are leaders in medical breakthroughs providing patients with definitive diagnosis and treatment with a complete spectrum of leading-edge surgical interventions. Our faculty and hospitals are nationally and internationally renowned in clinical, educational and research expertise. We are committed to providing the highest-quality clinical care with compassion, world-class medical education and cutting-edge research.

AREAS OF EXCELLENCE

The University of Miami/Jackson Memorial Burn Center: Nicholas Namias, M.D., Louis R. Pizano, M.D., MBA, Carl I. Schulman M.D., MPH
To make an appointment please call 305.585.1192

The Division of Cardiothoracic Surgery: Tammy M. Baxter, M.D., Rogerio G. Carrillo, M.D., Didier De Canniere, M.D., Ph.D., Andres Medina, M.D., Dao M. Nguyen, M.D., Anthony L. Panos, M.D., Si Pham, M.D., F.A.C.S, F.A.H.A, Marco Ricci, M.D., Ph.D, Elliot R. Rosenkranz, M.D., Tomas A. Salerno, M.D., James F. Symes, M.D., Richard J. Thurer, M.D., Donald B. Williams, M.D.
To make an appointment please call 305.585.5271

The Division of Colon & Rectal Surgery: Heidi Bahna, M.D., Floriano Marchetti, M.D., Laurence R. Sands, M.D., MBA,
To make and appointment please call 305.243.9110

The Division of Endocrine Surgery: John I. Lew, M.D. Steven E. Rodgers, M.D., Ph.D.
To make an appointment please call 305.243.4211

The Division of General Surgery: Robert A. Kozol, M.D., Joe U Levi, M.D., John I. Lew, M.D., Danny Sleeman, M.D.
To make an appointment please call 305.243.4211

Miami Transplant Institute Heart & Lung Transplantation: Si M. Pham, M.D., Elliot R. Rosenkranz, M.D., Anthony L. Panos, M.D., Marco Ricci, M.D., Ph.D
To make an appointment please call 305.355.5000

Miami Transplant Institute Kidney & Pancreas Transplantation: George W. Burke III, M.D., F.A.C.S., Gaetano Ciancio, M.D., M.B.A, F.A.C.S, Linda Chen, M.D., Junichiro Sageshima, M.D.
To make an appointment please call 305.355.5000

Miami Transplant Institute Liver & Gastrointestinal Transplantation: Andreas G. Tzakis, M.D., Ph.D., David Levi, M.D., Seigo Nishida, M.D., Ph.D, Gennaro Selvaggi, M.D., Akin Tekin, M.D.
To make an appointment please call 305.355.5000

The Division of Laparoendoscopic and Bariatric Surgery: Nestor de la Cruz-Munoz, M.D., Jose M. Martinez, M.D., Alberto R. Iglesias, M.D., Leonardo J. Henriquez, M.D.
To make an appointment please call 305-243-2424

The Division of Oral Maxillofacial Surgery & Dentistry Gabriela Albota, DDS, Daniel Atallah, DDS, Odile M. Carro, DM.D, Leo S. Dorado, DDS, Jesus A. Gomez, DDS, Robert E. Marx, DDS, Michael Peleg, DDS, Yoh Sawatari, DDS, Maritza Vega, DDS
To make an appointment please call 305.689.6725

The Division of Pediatric & Adolescent Surgery: Holly L. Neville, M.D., Eduardo A. Perez, M.D., Juan E. Sola, M.D.
To make an appointment please call 305-243-2247

The Division of Plastic, Aesthetic & Reconstructive Surgery: Wrood M. Kassira, M.D., Haaris S. Mir, M.D., John C. Oeltjen, M.D., Zubin J. Panthaki, M.D., Christopher J. Salgado, M.D., Seth R. Thaller, M.D., Morad Askari, M.D.
To make an appointment please call 305-243-7500

The Division of Surgical Oncology: Eli Avisar, M.D., Dido Franceschi, M.D., Alan S. Livingstone, M.D., Frederick L. Moffat, M.D., Mecker G. Moller, M.D., Steven E. Rodgers, M.D., Ph.D., Seth A. Spector, M.D.
To make an appointment please call 305-243-4902

The Division of Vascular & Endovascular Surgery: Arash Bornak, M.D., Lee J. Goldstein, M.D., Jorge Rey M.D., Handel Robinson, M.D., Marwan R. Tabbara, M.D., Omaida C. Velazquez, M.D.,
To make and appointment please call 305.585.5284

For more information on the Department of Surgery please visit our website: www.surgery.med.miami.edu

UHealth: Top-ranked doctors and hospitals providing the finest health care at more than 30 locations throughout South Florida.

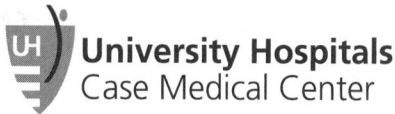

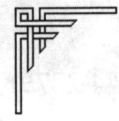

The Best in American Medicine
www.CastleConnolly.com

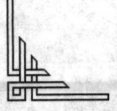
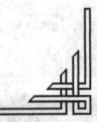

Thoracic Surgery

A thoracic surgeon provides the operative, perioperative care and critical care of patients with pathologic conditions within the chest. Included is the surgical care of coronary artery disease, cancers of the lung, esophagus and chest wall, abnormalities of the trachea, abnormalities of the great vessels and heart valves, congenital anomalies, tumors of the mediastinum and diseases of the diaphragm. The management of the airway and injuries of the chest is within the scope of the specialty.

Thoracic surgeons have the knowledge, experience and technical skills to accurately diagnose, operate upon safely and effectively manage patients with thoracic diseases of the chest. This requires substantial knowledge of cardiorespiratory physiology and oncology, as well as capability in the use of heart assist devices, management of abnormal heart rhythms and drainage of the chest cavity, respiratory support systems, endoscopy and invasive and noninvasive diagnostic techniques.

Training Required: Seven to eight years

THORACIC SURGERY

New England

Akins, Cary W MD [TS] - **Spec Exp:** Heart Valve Surgery; Coronary Artery Surgery; Aneurysm-Thoracic Aortic; **Hospital:** Mass Genl Hosp; **Address:** Mass Genl Hosp, Dept Surgery, 55 Fruit St White Bldg - Ste 503, Boston, MA 02114; **Phone:** 617-726-8218; **Board Cert:** Thoracic Surgery 2005; **Med School:** Harvard Med Sch 1970; **Resid:** Cardiovascular Surgery, Mass Genl Hosp 1975; **Fac Appt:** Clin Prof S, Harvard Med Sch

Bolman III, Ralph Morton MD [TS] - **Spec Exp:** Heart Failure & Ventricular Containment; Ventricular Assist Device (LVAD); Mitral Valve Surgery; Aneurysm; **Hospital:** Brigham and Women's Hosp (page 57); **Address:** Brigham & Womens Hosp, Dept Cardiac Surg, 75 Francis St, rm CA211, Boston, MA 02115; **Phone:** 617-732-7678; **Board Cert:** Thoracic Surgery 2004; **Med School:** St Louis Univ 1973; **Resid:** Surgery, Duke Univ Med Ctr 1980; **Fellow:** Thoracic Surgery, Univ Minn Hosp 1982; **Fac Appt:** Prof S, Harvard Med Sch

Brinckerhoff, Laurence H MD [TS] - **Spec Exp:** Lung Cancer; Esophageal Cancer; Minimally Invasive Thoracic Surgery; **Hospital:** Tufts Med Ctr; **Address:** Tufts Dept Thoracic Surgery, 750 Washington St, Box 5589, Boston, MA 02111; **Phone:** 617-636-5589; **Board Cert:** Surgery 2002; Thoracic Surgery 2006; **Med School:** Dartmouth Med Sch 1994; **Resid:** Surgery, Univ Virginia Med Ctr 2001; **Fellow:** Cardiothoracic Surgery, Univ Colorado Hlth Sci Ctr 2004

Bueno, Raphael MD [TS] - **Spec Exp:** Lung Cancer; Minimally Invasive Thoracic Surgery; Minimally Invasive Esophageal Surgery; Endoscopic Surgery; **Hospital:** Brigham and Women's Hosp (page 57), Dana-Farber Cancer Inst (page 57); **Address:** Brigham and Women's Hospital, Division of Thoracic Surgery Clin, 75 Francis St, Boston, MA 02115; **Phone:** 617-732-6824; **Board Cert:** Thoracic Surgery 2006; Surgery 2002; Surgical Critical Care 2003; **Med School:** Harvard Med Sch 1985; **Resid:** Surgery, Brigham & Women's Hosp 1992; **Fellow:** Surgical Critical Care, Brigham & Women's Hosp 1993; Thoracic Surgery, Mass Genl Hosp 1995; **Fac Appt:** Assoc Prof S, Harvard Med Sch

Del-Nido, Pedro J MD [TS] - **Spec Exp:** Heart Valve Surgery-Pediatric; Congenital Heart Disease; Minimally Invasive Surgery; Robotic Surgery; **Hospital:** Children's Hospital - Boston; **Address:** Children's Hospital Boston, Dept Cardiac Surgery, 300 Longwood Ave, Bader 273, Boston, MA 02115; **Phone:** 617-355-8290; **Board Cert:** Surgery 2006; Thoracic Surgery 2004; **Med School:** Univ Wisc 1977; **Resid:** Surgery, Boston Univ Med Ctr 1982; Thoracic Surgery, Toronto Genl Hosp 1985; **Fellow:** Pediatric Cardiothoracic Surgery, Hosp Sick Children 1986; **Fac Appt:** Prof S, Harvard Med Sch

Elefteriades, John MD [TS] - **Spec Exp:** Aneurysm-Thoracic Aortic; Transplant-Heart; Ventricular Assist Device (LVAD); **Hospital:** Yale-New Haven Hosp, Yale Med Group; **Address:** Yale Sch of Medicine, Dept Cardiothoracic Surgery, PO Box 208039, New Haven, CT 06520; **Phone:** 203-785-2705; **Board Cert:** Thoracic Surgery 2004; **Med School:** Yale Univ 1976; **Resid:** Surgery, Yale-New Haven Hosp 1981; Cardiothoracic Surgery, Yale-New Haven Hosp 1983; **Fellow:** Cardiothoracic Surgery, Yale-New Haven Hosp 1983; **Fac Appt:** Prof S, Yale Univ

Fernando, Hiran C MD [TS] - **Spec Exp:** Esophageal Cancer; Lung Cancer; Esophageal Disorders; Minimally Invasive Thoracic Surgery; **Hospital:** Boston Med Ctr; **Address:** Boston Med Ctr Thoracic Surgery, 88 E Newton St, Robinson B402, Boston, MA 02118; **Phone:** 617-638-5600; **Board Cert:** Surgery 2005; Thoracic Surgery 2009; **Med School:** England, UK 1986; **Resid:** Surgery, Harbor/UCLA Med Ctr 1993; Thoracic Surgery, UC Davis Med Ctr 1998; **Fellow:** Minimally Invasive Surgery, Univ Pittsburgh 2001; **Fac Appt:** Assoc Prof TS, Boston Univ

Gaissert, Henning A MD [TS] - **Spec Exp:** Esophageal Cancer; Tracheal Surgery; Lung Cancer; Thymoma; **Hospital:** Mass Genl Hosp, Newton - Wellesley Hosp; **Address:** Mass Genl Hosp, 55 Fruit St, BLK 1570, Boston, MA 02114; **Phone:** 617-726-5341; **Board Cert:** Surgery 2011; Thoracic Surgery 2004; **Med School:** Germany 1984; **Resid:** Surgery, Mass Genl Hosp 1989; Surgery, Barnes Jewish Hosp 1991; **Fellow:** Research, Harvard Med Sch 1993; Cardiothoracic Surgery, Barnes Jewish Hosp 1996; **Fac Appt:** Assoc Prof S, Harvard Med Sch

Hashim, Sabet W MD [TS] - **Spec Exp:** Mitral Valve Surgery; Heart Valve Surgery; Maze Procedure for Atrial Fibrillation; **Hospital:** Yale-New Haven Hosp, Yale Med Group; **Address:** Yale Univ Cardiothoracic Surgery, 330 Cedar St, Ste BB204, PB Box 208039, New Haven, CT 06520-8039; **Phone:** 203-785-6214; **Board Cert:** Thoracic Surgery 2001; **Med School:** Lebanon 1975; **Resid:** Surgery, St Lukes Roosevely Hosp 1979; Cardiothoracic Surgery, Yale-New Haven Hosp 1981

Kopf, Gary S MD [TS] - **Spec Exp:** Cardiac Surgery; Pediatric Cardiothoracic Surgery; Congenital Heart Disease; **Hospital:** Yale-New Haven Hosp, Yale Med Group; **Address:** Yale Univ Sch Med, Dept of Surgery, Box 208039, New Haven, CT 06520-8039; **Phone:** 203-785-2702; **Board Cert:** Thoracic Surgery 2000; **Med School:** Harvard Med Sch 1970; **Resid:** Surgery, Peter Bent Brigham Hosp 1977; Cardiothoracic Surgery, Chldns Hosp Med Ctr 1980; **Fellow:** Cardiothoracic Surgery, Peter Bent Brigham Hosp 1980; **Fac Appt:** Prof S, Yale Univ

Lazar, Harold L MD [TS] - **Spec Exp:** Aortic Surgery; Coronary Artery Surgery; Heart Valve Surgery; Esophageal Surgery; **Hospital:** Boston Med Ctr; **Address:** Boston Med Ctr, 88 E Newton St Robinson Bldg - Ste B-402, Boston, MA 02118; **Phone:** 617-638-7350; **Board Cert:** Thoracic Surgery 2003; Surgery 2001; **Med School:** Boston Univ 1974; **Resid:** Surgery, Univ Michigan Med Ctr 1981; Cardiothoracic Surgery, Columbia-Presbyterian Med Ctr 1983; **Fellow:** Cardiovascular Research, UCLA Med Ctr 1979; **Fac Appt:** Prof TS, Boston Univ

Mathisen, Douglas MD [TS] - **Spec Exp:** Tracheal Surgery; Lung Cancer; Esophageal Cancer; **Hospital:** Mass Genl Hosp, Newton - Wellesley Hosp; **Address:** Mass Genl Hosp, Thoracic Surgery, 55 Fruit St, Blake 1570, Boston, MA 02114; **Phone:** 617-726-6826; **Board Cert:** Thoracic Surgery 2002; **Med School:** Univ IL Coll Med 1974; **Resid:** Surgery, Mass Genl Hosp 1981; Thoracic Surgery, Mass Genl Hosp 1982; **Fellow:** Surgical Oncology, Natl Cancer Inst 1979; **Fac Appt:** Prof S, Harvard Med Sch

Mayer Jr, John E MD [TS] - **Spec Exp:** Pediatric Cardiothoracic Surgery; Cardiovascular Surgery; Transplant-Heart; **Hospital:** Children's Hospital - Boston; **Address:** Chldns Hosp, Dept Cardiac Surg, 300 Longwood Ave, Bader 273, Boston, MA 02115; **Phone:** 617-355-8258; **Board Cert:** Thoracic Surgery 2001; **Med School:** Yale Univ 1972; **Resid:** Surgery, Univ Minn Med Ctr 1979; **Fellow:** Cardiothoracic Surgery, Univ Minn Med Ctr 1981; **Fac Appt:** Prof S, Harvard Med Sch

Nugent, William C MD [TS] - **Spec Exp:** Thoracic Cancers; Hyperhidrosis-Palmar; **Hospital:** Dartmouth - Hitchcock Med Ctr; **Address:** Dartmouth-Hitchcock Med Ctr, Dept Cardiothoracic Surgery, 1 Medical Center Drive, Lebanon, NH 03756; **Phone:** 603-650-8572; **Board Cert:** Thoracic Surgery 2002; **Med School:** Albany Med Coll 1975; **Resid:** Surgery, Beth Israel Hosp 1980; Thoracic Surgery, Univ Michigan Med Ctr 1983; **Fellow:** Cardiothoracic Surgery, Mass Genl Hosp 1981; **Fac Appt:** Prof S, Dartmouth Med Sch

Rastegar, Hassan MD [TS] - **Spec Exp:** Cardiac Surgery-Adult; Heart Valve Surgery; Minimally Invasive Cardiac Surgery; **Hospital:** Tufts Med Ctr; **Address:** 800 Washington St, Box 266, Boston, MA 02111; **Phone:** 617-636-5528; **Board Cert:** Thoracic Surgery 2003; **Med School:** Iran 1974; **Resid:** Surgery, Hosp Univ Penn 1980; Cardiothoracic Surgery, Northwestern Univ 1982; **Fac Appt:** Prof S, Tufts Univ

Sellke, Frank W MD [TS] - **Spec Exp:** Heart Valve Surgery; Angiogenesis; Coronary Artery Surgery; Aortic Surgery; **Hospital:** Rhode Island Hosp, Miriam Hosp; **Address:** Rhode Island Hosp, 2 Dudley St, MOC, Ste 360, Providence, RI 02905; **Phone:** 401-274-7546; **Board Cert:** Surgery 2005; Thoracic Surgery 2009; **Med School:** Indiana Univ 1981; **Resid:** Surgery, Akron City Hosp 1987; Cardiothoracic Surgery, Univ Iowa Hosps & Clinics 1990; **Fac Appt:** Prof S, Brown Univ

Singh, Arun K MD [TS] - **Spec Exp:** Cardiac Surgery; **Hospital:** Rhode Island Hosp; **Address:** University Cardiovascular Surgical, 2 Dudley St, Ste 360, Providence, RI 02905-3248; **Phone:** 401-274-7546; **Board Cert:** Surgery 1973; Thoracic Surgery 1975; **Med School:** India 1967; **Resid:** Surgery, Columbia Presby Med Ctr 1972; Cardiothoracic Surgery, Rhode Island Hosp 1974; **Fellow:** Cardiac Surgery, Hosp Sick Chldn 1975; **Fac Appt:** Clin Prof S, Brown Univ

Sugarbaker, David J MD [TS] - **Spec Exp:** Mesothelioma; Transplant-Lung; Esophageal Cancer; **Hospital:** Brigham and Women's Hosp (page 57), Dana-Farber Cancer Inst (page 57); **Address:** Brigham & Women's Hosp, 75 Francis St, Division of Thoracic Surgery, Boston, MA 02115-6110; **Phone:** 617-732-6824; **Board Cert:** Thoracic Surgery 1999; **Med School:** Cornell Univ-Weill Med Coll 1979; **Resid:** Surgery, Brigham & Women's Hosp 1982; Surgery, Brigham & Women's Hosp 1986; **Fellow:** Thoracic Surgery, Toronto Genl Hosp 1988; **Fac Appt:** Prof S, Harvard Med Sch

Swanson, Scott J MD [TS] - **Spec Exp:** Lung Cancer; Video Assisted Thoracic Surgery (VATS); Esophageal Cancer; **Hospital:** Brigham and Women's Hosp (page 57), Dana-Farber Cancer Inst (page 57); **Address:** Div Thoracic Surgery, Brigham & Women's Hosp, 75 Francis St, Boston, MA 02115; **Phone:** 617-525-7532; **Board Cert:** Surgery 2003; Thoracic Surgery 2006; **Med School:** Harvard Med Sch 1985; **Resid:** Surgery, Brigham & Womens Hosp 1990; **Fellow:** Cardiothoracic Surgery, Brigham & Womens Hosp 1994

Vander Salm, Thomas MD [TS] - **Spec Exp:** Heart Valve Surgery-Mitral; Cardiovascular Surgery; **Hospital:** N Shore Med Ctr - Salem Hosp; **Address:** Salem Hosp, Div Cardiac Surgery, 81 Highland Ave, Axelrod Fl 5th, Salem, MA 01970; **Phone:** 978-354-2500; **Board Cert:** Surgery 1974; Thoracic Surgery 2006; **Med School:** Johns Hopkins Univ 1966; **Resid:** Surgery, Mass Genl Hosp 1968; Thoracic Surgery, Johns Hopkins Hosp 1969; **Fac Appt:** Prof S, Univ Mass Sch Med

Vlahakes, Gus J MD [TS] - **Spec Exp:** Cardiac Surgery; Transplant-Heart; Maze Procedure for Atrial Fibrillation; **Hospital:** Mass Genl Hosp; **Address:** Mass Genl Hosp, 55 Fruit St, Ste COX 652, Boston, MA 02114; **Phone:** 617-726-1861; **Board Cert:** Surgery 2002; Surgical Critical Care 2000; Thoracic Surgery 2005; **Med School:** Harvard Med Sch 1975; **Resid:** Surgery, Mass Genl Hosp 1983; Cardiothoracic Surgery, Mass Genl Hosp 1985; **Fellow:** Pediatric Cardiac Surgery, Chldns Hosp 1985; **Fac Appt:** Prof S, Harvard Med Sch

Wain, John MD [TS] - **Spec Exp:** Transplant-Lung; Lung Cancer; Esophageal Cancer; **Hospital:** Mass Genl Hosp; **Address:** Mass Genl Hosp, Div Thoracic Surgery, 55 Fruit St, Blake 1570, Boston, MA 02114; **Phone:** 617-726-5200; **Board Cert:** Thoracic Surgery 2000; **Med School:** Jefferson Med Coll 1980; **Resid:** Surgery, Mass Genl Hosp 1985; **Fellow:** Cardiothoracic Surgery, Mass Genl Hosp 1988; **Fac Appt:** Asst Prof TS, Harvard Med Sch

Warner, Kenneth G MD [TS] - **Spec Exp:** Cardiac Surgery-Adult & Pediatric; Congenital Heart Surgery; Heart Valve Surgery; Aortic Surgery; **Hospital:** Tufts Med Ctr; **Address:** 800 Washington St, Ste 266, Boston, MA 02111-1526; **Phone:** 617-636-0033; **Board Cert:** Surgery 2007; Thoracic Surgery 2009; Surgical Critical Care 2001; **Med School:** Univ Mich Med Sch 1982; **Resid:** Surgery, Brigham & Women's Hosp 1984; Cardiothoracic Surgery, Brigham & Women's Hosp 1990; **Fellow:** Research, West Roxbury VA Hosp 1986; **Fac Appt:** Assoc Prof S, Tufts Univ

Wright, Cameron D MD [TS] - **Spec Exp:** Lung Cancer; Esophageal Cancer; Tracheal Surgery; **Hospital:** Mass Genl Hosp; **Address:** Mass Genl Hosp, Div Thoracic Surg, 55 Fruit St, Blake 1570, Boston, MA 02114; **Phone:** 617-726-5801; **Board Cert:** Surgery 2006; Thoracic Surgery 2007; **Med School:** Univ Mich Med Sch 1980; **Resid:** Surgery, Mass Genl Hosp 1986; Thoracic Surgery, Mass Genl Hosp 1988; **Fac Appt:** Assoc Prof S, Harvard Med Sch

Mid Atlantic

Acker, Michael A MD [TS] - **Spec Exp:** Transplant-Heart; Ventricular Assist Device (LVAD); Coronary Artery Surgery; Heart Valve Surgery; **Hospital:** Hosp Univ Penn - UPHS (page 68); **Address:** 3400 Spruce St, 6 Silverstein, Philadelphia, PA 19104-4227; **Phone:** 215-349-8305; **Board Cert:** Surgery 2001; Thoracic Surgery 2001; **Med School:** Brown Univ 1981; **Resid:** Surgery, Hosp Univ Penn 1988; Cardiothoracic Surgery, Johns Hopkins Hosp 1991; **Fac Appt:** Prof S, Univ Pennsylvania

Adams, David H MD [TS] - **Spec Exp:** Mitral Valve Surgery; Heart Valve Surgery; Minimally Invasive Cardiac Surgery; Coronary Artery Surgery; **Hospital:** Mount Sinai Med Ctr (page 63); **Address:** The Mount Sinai Medical Center, Cardiothoracic Surgery, 1190 Fifth Ave, Box 1028, New York, NY 10029; **Phone:** 212-659-6820; **Board Cert:** Thoracic Surgery 2003; **Med School:** Duke Univ 1983; **Resid:** Surgery, Brigham & Women's Hosp 1988; Thoracic Surgery, Brigham & Women's Hosp 1990; **Fac Appt:** Prof TS, Mount Sinai Sch Med

Altorki, Nasser MD [TS] - **Spec Exp:** Esophageal Cancer; Lung Cancer; Thoracic Cancers; Vaccine Therapy; **Hospital:** NY-Presby/Weill Cornell Med Ctr, NY (page 65); **Address:** 525 E 68th St, M-404, New York, NY 10065; **Phone:** 212-746-5156; **Board Cert:** Surgery 2006; Thoracic Surgery 2007; **Med School:** Egypt 1978; **Resid:** Surgery, Univ Chicago Hosps 1985; **Fellow:** Cardiothoracic Surgery, Univ Chicago Hosps 1987; **Fac Appt:** Prof S, Cornell Univ-Weill Med Coll

Argenziano, Michael MD [TS] - **Spec Exp:** Robotic Cardiac Surgery; Coronary Artery Surgery; Maze Procedure for Atrial Fibrillation; **Hospital:** NY-Presby/Columbia Univ Med Ctr, NY (page 65); **Address:** NY Presby Med Ctr, Milstein Bldg, 177 Fort Washington Ave, rm 7-435, New York, NY 10032; **Phone:** 212-305-5888; **Board Cert:** Thoracic Surgery 2002; **Med School:** Columbia P&S 1992; **Resid:** Surgery, Columbia Presby Med Ctr 1998; **Fellow:** Cardiothoracic Surgery, Columbia Presby Med Ctr 1999; **Fac Appt:** Asst Prof S, Columbia P&S

Bains, Manjit MD [TS] - **Spec Exp:** Cardiothoracic Surgery; Esophageal Cancer; Lung Cancer; **Hospital:** Meml Sloan-Kettering Cancer Ctr; **Address:** 1275 York Ave, rm C681, New York, NY 10065; **Phone:** 212-639-7450; **Board Cert:** Surgery 1971; Thoracic Surgery 1972; **Med School:** India 1963; **Resid:** Surgery, Rochester Genl Hosp 1970; **Fellow:** Thoracic Surgery, Sloan Kettering Cancer Ctr 1972; **Fac Appt:** Clin Prof S, Cornell Univ-Weill Med Coll

Battafarano, Richard J MD [TS] - **Spec Exp:** Lung Cancer; Barrett's Esophagus; Esophageal Surgery; Mesothelioma; **Hospital:** Univ of MD Med Ctr; **Address:** Univ MD Med Ctr, Greenebaum Cancer Ctr-Dept Thoracic Surgery, 29 S Greene St, Ste 504, Baltimore, MD 21201; **Phone:** 410-328-6366; **Board Cert:** Surgery 2008; Thoracic Surgery 2000; **Med School:** Hahnemann Univ 1988; **Resid:** Surgery, Univ Minn Hosp & Clin 1997; **Fellow:** Thoracic Surgery, Meml Sloan Kettering Cancer Ctr 1999; **Fac Appt:** Assoc Prof S, Univ MD Sch Med

Bavaria, Joseph E MD [TS] - **Spec Exp:** Aortic Surgery; Transplant-Lung; Heart Valve Surgery; **Hospital:** Hosp Univ Penn - UPHS (page 68); **Address:** Hosp Univ Pennsylvania, 3400 Spruce St, 6 Silverstein, Philadelphia, PA 19104; **Phone:** 215-662-2017; **Board Cert:** Thoracic Surgery 2001; **Med School:** Tulane Univ 1983; **Resid:** Surgery, Hosp Univ Penn 1990; Cardiothoracic Surgery, Hosp Univ Penn/Children's Hosp 1992; **Fac Appt:** Prof S, Univ Pennsylvania

Chen, Jonathan M MD [TS] - Spec Exp: Pediatric Cardiothoracic Surgery; Arrhythmias; Congenital Heart Disease; **Hospital:** Morgan Stanley Children's Hosp of NY-Presby, NY (page 65), NY-Presby/Columbia Univ Med Ctr, NY (page 65); **Address:** NY Presbyterian-Weill Cornell Med Ctr, 525 E 68th St, Box 110, New York, NY 10065; **Phone:** 212-746-5014; **Board Cert:** Surgery 2001; Thoracic Surgery 2003; **Med School:** Columbia P&S 1994; **Resid:** Surgery, NY Columbia Presby Hosp 2000; **Fellow:** Cardiothoracic Surgery, NY Columbia Presby Hosp 2001; **Fac Appt:** Asst Prof S, Columbia P&S

Cohen, Neri M MD/PhD [TS] - Spec Exp: Hyperhidrosis; Minimally Invasive Surgery; Radiofrequency Tumor Ablation; **Hospital:** Greater Baltimore Med Ctr; **Address:** Greater Baltimore Thoracic Surgery, 6569 N Charles St, Ste 701, Baltimore, MD 21204; **Phone:** 443-849-3470; **Board Cert:** Surgery 2009; Thoracic Surgery 2008; **Med School:** Univ MD Sch Med 1989; **Resid:** Surgery, Med Coll Virginia Hosp 1996; **Fellow:** Cardiothoracic Surgery, Med Coll Virginia 1997; Thoracic Surgery, Cleveland Clinic 1998

Conte Jr, John V MD [TS] - Spec Exp: Transplant-Heart; Transplant-Lung; Cardiac Surgery-Adult; Coronary Artery Surgery; **Hospital:** Johns Hopkins Hosp (page 61); **Address:** 600 N Wolfe St, Blalock 618, Baltimore, MD 21287-4618; **Phone:** 410-955-2800; **Board Cert:** Thoracic Surgery 2007; **Med School:** Georgetown Univ 1986; **Resid:** Surgery, Georgetown Univ Med Ctr 1992; Thoracic Surgery, Stanford Univ Med Ctr 1995; **Fac Appt:** Prof S, Johns Hopkins Univ

Cooper, Joel D MD [TS] - Spec Exp: Transplant-Lung; Emphysema-Lung Volume Reduction; Lung Surgery; **Hospital:** Hosp Univ Penn - UPHS (page 68); **Address:** Hosp Univ Penn, 3400 Spruce St, 6 White, Philadelphia, PA 19104; **Phone:** 215-662-2022; **Board Cert:** Surgery 1971; Thoracic Surgery 1972; **Med School:** Harvard Med Sch 1964; **Resid:** Surgery, Mass Genl Hosp 1968; Thoracic Surgery, Frenchay Hosp; **Fellow:** Research, Hammersmith Hosp; Thoracic Surgery, Mass Genl Hosp; **Fac Appt:** Prof S, Univ Pennsylvania

Demmy, Todd L MD [TS] - Spec Exp: Lung Cancer; Thoracic Cancers; Esophageal Cancer; Minimally Invasive Thoracic Surgery; **Hospital:** Roswell Park Cancer Inst, Buffalo General Hosp; **Address:** Roswell Park Cancer Inst, Dept Thoracic Surgery, Elm & Carlton Sts, Buffalo, NY 14263; **Phone:** 716-845-5873; **Board Cert:** Surgery 2008; Thoracic Surgery 2010; Surgical Critical Care 2010; **Med School:** Jefferson Med Coll 1983; **Resid:** Surgery, Baylor Univ Medical Ctr 1988; Thoracic Surgery, Allegheny Genl Hosp 1991; **Fac Appt:** Assoc Prof S, SUNY Buffalo

DeRose Jr, Joseph J MD [TS] - Spec Exp: Robotic Cardiac Surgery; Minimally Invasive Cardiac Surgery; Mitral Valve Surgery; **Hospital:** Montefiore Med Ctr - Div. Weiler, Montefiore Med Ctr - Div. Moses; **Address:** Montefiore-Weiler Medical Ctr, Dept Cardiothoracic Surgery, 1575 Blondell Ave, Ste 125, Bronx, NY 10461; **Phone:** 718-405-8371; **Board Cert:** Thoracic Surgery 2002; **Med School:** Columbia P&S 1993; **Resid:** Surgery, Columbia Presby Med Ctr 1995; **Fellow:** Cardiothoracic Surgery, Columbia Presby Med Ctr 1999; **Fac Appt:** Assoc Prof TS, Albert Einstein Coll Med

Diehl, James T MD [TS] - Spec Exp: Cardiac Surgery-Adult; Aortic Surgery; Heart Valve Surgery-Aortic; Heart Valve Surgery-Mitral; **Hospital:** Thomas Jefferson Univ Hosp, Albert Einstein Med Ctr; **Address:** 1025 Walnut St, Ste 607, Philadelphia, PA 19107; **Phone:** 215-955-6996; **Board Cert:** Thoracic Surgery 2004; **Med School:** Albert Einstein Coll Med 1978; **Resid:** Surgery, Cleveland Clinic 1984; Cardiothoracic Surgery, Univ Toronto Med Ctr 1986; **Fac Appt:** Prof S, Thomas Jefferson Univ

Downey, Robert MD [TS] - Spec Exp: Lung Cancer; Thoracic Cancers; **Hospital:** Meml Sloan-Kettering Cancer Ctr; **Address:** 1275 York Avenue, New York, NY 10065; **Phone:** 800-525-2225; **Board Cert:** Surgery 2002; Thoracic Surgery 2005; Thoracic Surgery 2005; **Med School:** Columbia P&S 1985; **Resid:** Surgery, Columbia-Presby Med Ctr 1991; **Fellow:** Thoracic Surgery, Mayo Clinic 1992; Thoracic Surgery, Columbia-Presby Med Ctr 1994

Edwards, Niloo M MD [TS] - **Spec Exp:** Transplant-Heart; Cardiac Surgery-Geriatric; **Hospital:** St. Peter's Hosp - Albany; **Address:** 319 S Manning Blvd, Ste 110, Albany, NY 12208; **Phone:** 518-525-2525; **Board Cert:** Surgery 2004; Thoracic Surgery 2006; **Med School:** Columbia P&S 1986; **Resid:** Surgery, Strong Meml Hosp 1992; **Fellow:** Cardiothoracic Surgery, Columbia-Presby Med Ctr 1996; **Fac Appt:** Assoc Prof TS, Univ Wisc

Filsoufi, Farzan MD [TS] - **Spec Exp:** Mitral Valve Surgery; Minimally Invasive Heart Valve Surgery; Heart Valve Surgery; Robotic Cardiac Surgery; **Hospital:** Mount Sinai Med Ctr (page 63), Elmhurst Hosp Ctr; **Address:** Mt Sinai Med Ctr, Dept Cardiothoracic Surg, 1190 5th Ave, Box 1028, New York, NY 10029; **Phone:** 212-659-6813; **Med School:** France 1991; **Resid:** Surgery, Univ Paris Hosps 1994; Thoracic Surgery, Hospital Broussais/U of Paris 1995; **Fellow:** Cardiothoracic Surgery, Hospital Broussais/U of Paris 1996; Heart Valve Surgery, Brigham & Women's Hosp 2000; **Fac Appt:** Prof TS, Mount Sinai Sch Med

Flores, Raja M MD [TS] - **Spec Exp:** Mesothelioma; Lung Cancer; Video Assisted Thoracic Surgery (VATS); Esophageal Cancer; **Hospital:** Mount Sinai Med Ctr (page 63); **Address:** Chief, Div Thoracic Surgery, Mount Sinai Med Ctr, 1190 Fifth Ave, New York, NY 10029; **Phone:** 212-241-9466; **Board Cert:** Surgery 1999; Thoracic Surgery 2001; **Med School:** Albert Einstein Coll Med 1992; **Resid:** Surgery, Columbia Presby Med Ctr 1997; **Fellow:** Thoracic Surgery, Brigham & Womens Hosp/Dana Faber Cancer Inst 2000; **Fac Appt:** Assoc Prof TS, Cornell Univ-Weill Med Coll

Friedberg, Joseph MD [TS] - **Spec Exp:** Mesothelioma; Pleural Disease; Lung Cancer; Thoracic Cancers; **Hospital:** Penn Presby Med Ctr - UPHS (page 68), Hosp Univ Penn - UPHS (page 68); **Address:** Penn-Presbyterian Medical Ctr, 51 N 39th St, rm W250, Philadelphia, PA 19104; **Phone:** 215-662-9195; **Board Cert:** Surgery 2006; Thoracic Surgery 2006; **Med School:** Harvard Med Sch 1986; **Resid:** Surgery, Mass General Hosp 1994; **Fellow:** Cardiothoracic Surgery, Brigham & Womens Hosp 1996; **Fac Appt:** Assoc Prof TS, Univ Pennsylvania

Furukawa, Satoshi MD [TS] - **Spec Exp:** Transplant-Heart & Lung; Cardiac Surgery-High Risk; Heart Valve Surgery; Minimally Invasive Cardiac Surgery; **Hospital:** Temple Univ Hosp; **Address:** 3401 N Broad St, Ste 300, Philadelphia, PA 19140; **Phone:** 215-707-3601; **Board Cert:** Surgery 2003; Thoracic Surgery 2005; **Med School:** Univ Pennsylvania 1984; **Resid:** Surgery, Hosp Univ Penn 1991; Thoracic Surgery, Hosp Univ Penn 1993; **Fac Appt:** Prof TS, Temple Univ

Galloway, Aubrey MD [TS] - **Spec Exp:** Minimally Invasive Heart Valve Surgery; Mitral Valve Surgery; Aneurysm-Thoracic Aortic; Robotic Surgery; **Hospital:** NYU Langone Med Ctr (page 66); **Address:** 530 1st Ave, Ste 9V, New York, NY 10016-6402; **Phone:** 212-263-7185; **Board Cert:** Thoracic Surgery 2006; **Med School:** Tulane Univ 1978; **Resid:** Surgery, Univ Colo Hlth Sci Ctr 1983; Cardiovascular Surgery, NYU Med Ctr 1985; **Fellow:** Research, Boston Chldns Hosp 1981; Cardiothoracic Surgery, NYU Med Ctr 1985; **Fac Appt:** Prof TS, NYU Sch Med

Gaynor, J. William MD [TS] - **Spec Exp:** Pediatric Cardiothoracic Surgery; Congenital Heart Surgery; Transplant-Heart; **Hospital:** Chldns Hosp of Philadelphia; **Address:** CHOP, Div of Cardiothoracic Surgery, Main Bldg - rm 8527, 34th St & Civic Ctr Blvd, Philadelphia, PA 19104; **Phone:** 215-590-2708; **Board Cert:** Thoracic Surgery 2004; Congenital Cardiac Surgery 2009; **Med School:** Med Univ SC 1982; **Resid:** Surgery, Parkland Meml Hosp; Thoracic Surgery, Duke Univ Med Ctr; **Fellow:** Congenital Heart Surgery, Hosp for Sick Childn; **Fac Appt:** Assoc Prof TS, Univ Pennsylvania

Gharagozloo, Farid MD [TS] - **Spec Exp:** Video Assisted Thoracic Surgery (VATS); Lung Cancer; **Hospital:** G Washington Univ Hosp, Harbor Hosp; **Address:** 2175 K St NW, Ste 300, Washington, DC 20037; **Phone:** 202-775-8600; **Board Cert:** Thoracic Surgery 2001; **Med School:** Johns Hopkins Univ 1983; **Resid:** Surgery, Mayo Clinic 1989; Research, Harvard Med Sch 1986; **Fellow:** Cardiothoracic Surgery, Mayo Clinic 1992; **Fac Appt:** Prof S, Geo Wash Univ

Ginsburg, Mark MD [TS] - **Spec Exp:** Lung Cancer; Transplant-Lung; Emphysema-Lung Volume Reduction; **Hospital:** NY-Presby/Columbia Univ Med Ctr, NY (page 65), Good Samaritan Hosp - Suffern; **Address:** 161 Ft Washington Ave Fl 3 - Ste 301, New York, NY 10032; **Phone:** 212-305-3408; **Board Cert:** Surgery 2006; Thoracic Surgery 2005; **Med School:** Tufts Univ 1980; **Resid:** Surgery, Strong Meml Hosp 1985; **Fellow:** Thoracic Surgery, Strong Meml Hosp 1987; **Fac Appt:** Asst Clin Prof S, Columbia P&S

Girardi, Leonard N MD [TS] - **Spec Exp:** Aneurysm-Aortic; Cardiac Surgery; Marfan's Syndrome; Cardiothoracic Surgery; **Hospital:** NY-Presby/Weill Cornell Med Ctr, NY (page 65); **Address:** 525 E 68th St, Ste M404, New York, NY 10065; **Phone:** 212-746-5194; **Board Cert:** Surgery 2005; Thoracic Surgery 2007; **Med School:** Cornell Univ-Weill Med Coll 1989; **Resid:** Surgery, NY Presby-Cornell Med Ctr 1994; **Fellow:** Cardiothoracic Surgery, NY Presby Hosp 1996; Cardiothoracic Surgery, Baylor Coll Med 1997; **Fac Appt:** Assoc Prof TS, Cornell Univ-Weill Med Coll

Graver, L Michael MD [TS] - **Spec Exp:** Minimally Invasive Heart Valve Surgery; Coronary Artery Surgery; Aortic Surgery; **Hospital:** Long Island Jewish Med Ctr, N Shore Univ Hosp; **Address:** 270-05 76th Ave, Ste O-4000, Long Island Jewish Medical Center, New Hyde Park, NY 11040-1433; **Phone:** 718-470-7460; **Board Cert:** Surgery 2003; Thoracic Surgery 2004; **Med School:** Albany Med Coll 1977; **Resid:** Surgery, St Luke's-Roosevelt Hosp Ctr 1982; Cardiovascular Surgery, Deaconness Hosp 1983; **Fellow:** Cardiovascular Pathology, NY Hosp-Cornell Med Ctr 1985; **Fac Appt:** Prof TS, Albert Einstein Coll Med

Griepp, Randall B MD [TS] - **Spec Exp:** Aneurysm-Abdominal Aortic; Aneurysm-Thoracic Aortic; **Hospital:** Mount Sinai Med Ctr (page 63); **Address:** Mt Sinai Med Ctr, Dept Cardiothoracic Surgery, 1190 5th Ave, New York, NY 10029; **Phone:** 212-659-9495; **Board Cert:** Thoracic Surgery 2007; **Med School:** Stanford Univ 1967; **Resid:** Surgery, Stanford Univ Hosp 1973; **Fellow:** Cardiothoracic Surgery, Stanford Univ Hosp 1972; **Fac Appt:** Prof TS, Mount Sinai Sch Med

Griffith, Bartley MD [TS] - **Spec Exp:** Transplant-Heart & Lung; Aneurysm-Aortic; Heart Valve Surgery; **Hospital:** Univ of MD Med Ctr; **Address:** Univ Maryland, Div Cardiac Surg, N4W94, 22 S Greene St, Baltimore, MD 21201; **Phone:** 410-328-3822; **Board Cert:** Thoracic Surgery 2001; **Med School:** Jefferson Med Coll 1974; **Resid:** Surgery, Univ Hlth Ctr Hosps 1979; Thoracic Surgery, Univ Hlth Ctr Hosps 1981; **Fellow:** Research, Univ Hlth Ctr Hosps 1978; **Fac Appt:** Prof S, Univ MD Sch Med

Grossi, Eugene A MD [TS] - **Spec Exp:** Minimally Invasive Cardiac Surgery; Mitral Valve Surgery; Cardiac Tumors, Myxomas; **Hospital:** NYU Langone Med Ctr (page 66); **Address:** NYU Langone Med Ctr, 530 1st Ave, Ste 9V, New York, NY 10016-6402; **Phone:** 212-263-7452; **Board Cert:** Thoracic Surgery 2002; **Med School:** Columbia P&S 1981; **Resid:** Surgery, NYU Med Ctr 1987; Thoracic Surgery, NYU Med Ctr 1991; **Fac Appt:** Prof S, NYU Sch Med

Hargrove III, W Clark MD [TS] - **Spec Exp:** Mitral Valve Robotic Surgery; Heart Valve Surgery; Minimally Invasive Cardiac Surgery; **Hospital:** Penn Presby Med Ctr - UPHS (page 68); **Address:** Philadelphia Heart Inst Bldg, 51 N 39th St, Ste 2A, Philadelphia, PA 19104; **Phone:** 215-662-9595; **Board Cert:** Thoracic Surgery 2004; **Med School:** Wake Forest Univ 1973; **Resid:** Surgery, Hosp Univ Penn 1979; Cardiothoracic Surgery, Hosp Univ Penn 1984; **Fellow:** Vascular Surgery, Hosp Univ Penn 1981; **Fac Appt:** Clin Prof S, Univ Pennsylvania

Heitmiller, Richard F MD [TS] - **Spec Exp:** Esophageal Surgery; Esophageal Cancer; Lung Cancer; **Hospital:** Union Meml Hosp-Baltimore; **Address:** 3333 N Calvert St, Ste 610, Baltimore, MD 21218; **Phone:** 410-554-2063; **Board Cert:** Therapeutic Radiology 2008; **Med School:** Johns Hopkins Univ 1979; **Resid:** Surgery, Mass Genl Hosp 1985; **Fellow:** Thoracic Surgery, Mass Genl Hosp 1987; **Fac Appt:** Assoc Prof Surg & Onc, Johns Hopkins Univ

Horvath, Keith MD [TS] - **Spec Exp:** Minimally Invasive Cardiac Surgery; Heart Valve Surgery; Heart Laser Revascularization; **Hospital:** Suburban Hosp, Johns Hopkins Hosp (page 61); **Address:** Suburban Hospital, 8600 Old Georgetown Rd, Bethesda, MD 20814; **Phone:** 301-896-7610; **Board Cert:** Thoracic Surgery 2005; **Med School:** Univ Chicago-Pritzker Sch Med 1987; **Resid:** Surgery, Brigham & Women's Hosp 1994; Brigham & Women's Hosp 1996; **Fellow:** Research, Mass Genl Hosp 1991; **Fac Appt:** Assoc Prof S, Northwestern Univ

Isom, O Wayne MD [TS] - **Spec Exp:** Cardiac Surgery; Coronary Artery Surgery; Heart Valve Surgery; **Hospital:** NY-Presby/Weill Cornell Med Ctr, NY (page 65), NY Hosp Queens; **Address:** 525 E 68th St, rm M-404, New York, NY 10065; **Phone:** 212-746-5151; **Board Cert:** Surgery 1971; Thoracic Surgery 1972; **Med School:** Univ Tex, Houston 1965; **Resid:** Surgery, Parkland Meml Hosp 1970; **Fellow:** Thoracic Surgery, NYU Med Ctr 1972; **Fac Appt:** Prof TS, Cornell Univ-Weill Med Coll

Jonas, Richard A MD [TS] - **Spec Exp:** Pediatric Cardiothoracic Surgery; Congenital Heart Surgery; **Hospital:** Chldns Natl Med Ctr, Georgetown Univ Hosp; **Address:** 111 Michigan Ave NW, Washington, DC 20010; **Phone:** 202-476-2811; **Med School:** Australia 1974; **Resid:** Surgery, Royal Melbourne Hosp 1979; Thoracic Surgery, Green Lane Hosp 1982; **Fellow:** Thoracic Surgery, Brigham & Women's Hosp 1984; **Fac Appt:** Prof S, Geo Wash Univ

Kaiser, Larry R MD [TS] - **Spec Exp:** Lung Cancer; Esophageal Cancer; Mediastinal Tumors; Myasthenia Gravis; **Hospital:** Temple Univ Hosp; **Address:** 3500 N Broad St, MERB Bldg - Fl 11, PO Box 20036, Philadelphia, PA 19140; **Phone:** 215-707-8773; **Board Cert:** Surgery 2005; Thoracic Surgery 2006; **Med School:** Tulane Univ 1977; **Resid:** Surgery, UCLA Med Ctr 1983; Cardiothoracic Surgery, Univ Toronto Hosps 1985; **Fellow:** Surgical Oncology, UCLA Med Ctr 1981; **Fac Appt:** Prof TS, Temple Univ

Kanda, Louis T MD [TS] - **Spec Exp:** Heart Valve Surgery; **Hospital:** Washington Hosp Ctr; **Address:** 110 Irving St NW, Ste 1041, Washington, DC 20010; **Phone:** 202-877-5039; **Board Cert:** Thoracic Surgery 2002; **Med School:** Geo Wash Univ 1970; **Resid:** Surgery, Washington Hosp Ctr 1975; **Fellow:** Cardiothoracic Surgery, Cleveland Clin Fdn 1980; **Fac Appt:** Asst Prof S, Howard Univ

Katz, Nevin M MD [TS] - **Spec Exp:** Coronary Artery Surgery; Heart Valve Surgery; Aortic Surgery; Congenital Heart Disease-Adult; **Hospital:** Johns Hopkins Hosp (page 61), G Washington Univ Hosp; **Address:** 600 N Wolfe St, Blalock 618, Baltimore, MD 21287-4618; **Phone:** 202-775-8600; **Board Cert:** Thoracic Surgery 2000; **Med School:** Case West Res Univ 1971; **Resid:** Surgery, Mass Genl Hosp 1976; Cardiothoracic Surgery, Univ Alabama Hosp 1980; **Fellow:** Cardiovascular Surgery, Univ Alabama 1978; **Fac Appt:** Clin Prof S, Geo Wash Univ

Keenan, Robert J MD [TS] - **Spec Exp:** Lung Cancer; Esophageal Cancer; Mediastinal Tumors; Emphysema-Lung Volume Reduction; **Hospital:** Allegheny General Hosp, West Penn Hosp-Forbes Campus; **Address:** Allegheny General Hospital, 320 E North Ave, Pittsburgh, PA 15212; **Phone:** 412-359-6137; **Board Cert:** Surgery 2010; **Med School:** Canada 1984; **Resid:** Surgery, Univ Toronto Med Ctr 1989; **Fellow:** Thoracic Surgery, Univ Pittsburgh Med Ctr 1990; Thoracic Surgery, Univ Toronto Med Ctr 1992; **Fac Appt:** Prof TS, Drexel Univ Coll Med

Keller, Steven M MD [TS] - **Spec Exp:** Lung Cancer; Esophageal Cancer; Mediastinal Tumors; Hyperhidrosis-Palmar; **Hospital:** Montefiore Med Ctr - Div. Moses, Montefiore Med Ctr - Div. Weiler; **Address:** 1575 Blondell St, Ste 125, Bronx, NY 10461; **Phone:** 718-405-8378; **Board Cert:** Thoracic Surgery 2007; **Med School:** Albany Med Coll 1977; **Resid:** Surgery, Mount Sinai Hosp 1985; Thoracic Surgery, Mem Sloan Kettering Cancer Ctr 1987; **Fellow:** Surgical Oncology, NIH/National Cancer Inst 1983; **Fac Appt:** Prof TS, Albert Einstein Coll Med

Kiev, Jonathan MD [TS] - **Spec Exp:** Chest Wall Tumors; Esophageal Cancer; Lung Cancer; **Hospital:** Anne Arundel Med Ctr; **Address:** Annapolis Thoracic Surgery, 2002 Medical Pkwy, Ste 660, Annapolis, MD 21401; **Phone:** 877-503-2609; **Board Cert:** Surgery 2005; Thoracic Surgery 2002; **Med School:** Tulane Univ 1989; **Resid:** Surgery, Hahnemann Univ Hosp 1996; Cardiothoracic Surgery, Loma Linda Univ 2000; **Fellow:** Thoracic Surgery, Univ Pittsburgh 2001; Thoracic Surgery, Mayo Clinic 2001

Kormos, Robert MD [TS] - **Spec Exp:** Transplant-Heart; Artificial Heart Devices; **Hospital:** UPMC Presby, Pittsburgh; **Address:** UPMC Presbyterian Hosp, 200 Lothrop St, Ste C700, Pittsburgh, PA 15213; **Phone:** 412-648-6259; **Med School:** Univ Western Ontario 1976; **Resid:** Surgery, Toronto Western Hosp 1978; Cardiothoracic Surgery, Toronto Genl Hosp/Hosp for Sick Chldn 1982; **Fellow:** Transplant Surgery, Univ Pittsburgh Med Ctr 1987; **Fac Appt:** Prof S, Univ Pittsburgh

Krasna, Mark MD [TS] - **Spec Exp:** Esophageal Cancer; Lung Cancer; Hyperhidrosis-Palmar; **Hospital:** St. Joseph Med Ctr, Univ of MD Med Ctr; **Address:** 7501 Osler Drive, Odea Bldg, Ste 104, Towson, MD 21204; **Phone:** 410-427-2220; **Board Cert:** Thoracic Surgery 2000; **Med School:** Israel 1982; **Resid:** Surgery, UMDNJ-Rutgers Med Sch 1988; **Fellow:** Cardiothoracic Surgery, New England Deaconess-Harvard 1990; **Fac Appt:** Prof S, Univ MD Sch Med

Krellenstein, Daniel J MD [TS] - **Spec Exp:** Lung Cancer; Minimally Invasive Thoracic Surgery; Asbestos-related Lung Disease; **Hospital:** Mount Sinai Med Ctr (page 63), Lenox Hill Hosp; **Address:** 16 E 98th St, Ste 1F, New York, NY 10029-6545; **Phone:** 212-423-9311; **Board Cert:** Surgery 1974; Thoracic Surgery 2006; **Med School:** SUNY Buffalo 1964; **Resid:** Surgery, SUNY Downstate Med Ctr 1972; **Fac Appt:** Assoc Clin Prof TS, Mount Sinai Sch Med

Krieger, Karl H MD [TS] - **Spec Exp:** Heart Valve Surgery; Coronary Artery Surgery; Cardiac Surgery-Adult; **Hospital:** NY-Presby/Weill Cornell Med Ctr, NY (page 65), NY Hosp Queens; **Address:** Cardiothoracic Surgery Dept, 525 E 68th St, Ste M404, New York, NY 10065; **Phone:** 212-746-5152; **Board Cert:** Thoracic Surgery 2004; **Med School:** Johns Hopkins Univ 1975; **Resid:** Surgery, Johns Hopkins 1976; Bellevue Hosp 1979; **Fellow:** Thoracic Surgery, NYU Med Ctr 1981; **Fac Appt:** Prof S, Cornell Univ-Weill Med Coll

Kucharczuk, John C MD [TS] - **Spec Exp:** Lung Cancer; Esophageal Cancer; Mesothelioma; Mediastinal Tumors; **Hospital:** Hosp Univ Penn - UPHS (page 68); **Address:** Penn Surgery, 3400 Spruce St, 6 White Bldg, Philadelphia, PA 19104; **Phone:** 215-662-4988; **Board Cert:** Surgery 2008; Thoracic Surgery 2002; **Med School:** Univ Pennsylvania 1992; **Resid:** Surgery, Hosp Univ Penn 1999; **Fellow:** Cardiothoracic Surgery, Hosp Univ Penn 2001; **Fac Appt:** Assoc Prof S, Univ Pennsylvania

Landreneau, Rodney MD [TS] - **Spec Exp:** Lung Cancer; Esophageal Cancer; Gastroesophageal Reflux Disease (GERD); **Hospital:** UPMC Passavant-McCandless, UPMC St Margaret; **Address:** 5200 Centre Ave, Ste 715, Pittsburgh, PA 15232; **Phone:** 412-623-2025; **Board Cert:** Thoracic Surgery 1994; **Med School:** Louisiana State U, New Orleans 1965; **Resid:** Surgery, Parkland Meml Hosp 1983; **Fellow:** Cardiothoracic Surgery, Univ Mich Med Ctr 1985; **Fac Appt:** Prof S, Univ Pittsburgh

Lang, Samuel J MD [TS] - **Spec Exp:** Minimally Invasive Cardiac Surgery; Heart Valve Surgery; Cardiothoracic Surgery; **Hospital:** NY Hosp Queens; **Address:** 56-45 Main St, rm 387, Flushing, NY 11355; **Phone:** 718-670-1137; **Board Cert:** Thoracic Surgery 2006; **Med School:** Univ Alabama 1978; **Resid:** Surgery, UCLA Med Ctr 1982; Thoracic Surgery, NYU Med Ctr 1983; **Fellow:** Cardiothoracic Surgery, UCLA Med Ctr 1985; Pediatric Cardiac Surgery, Hosp for Sick Chldn 1986

Lansman, Steven L MD/PhD [TS] - **Spec Exp:** Coronary Artery Surgery; Heart Valve Surgery; Ventricular Assist Device (LVAD); Transplant-Heart; **Hospital:** Westchester Med Ctr; **Address:** Westchester Medical Ctr, 100 Woods Rd, Macy Pavilion, rm 114W, Valhalla, NY 10595; **Phone:** 914-493-8793; **Board Cert:** Thoracic Surgery 2004; **Med School:** SUNY Hlth Sci Ctr 1977; **Resid:** Surgery, Montefiore Med Ctr 1982; **Fellow:** Thoracic Surgery, Univ Hosp 1984; **Fac Appt:** Prof S, NY Med Coll

Lazzaro, Richard MD [TS] - **Spec Exp:** Minimally Invasive Surgery; Obesity/Bariatric Surgery; Cardiac Surgery; **Hospital:** New York Methodist Hosp; **Address:** New York Methodist Hospital, 506 Sixth St, Brooklyn, NY 11215; **Phone:** 718-780-7700; **Board Cert:** Surgery 2006; Thoracic Surgery 2007; **Med School:** Albany Med Coll 1988; **Resid:** Surgery, North Shore Univ Hosp 1994; **Fellow:** Cardiothoracic Surgery, SUNY Downstate Med Ctr 1997; Thoracic Surgery, Univ Pittsburgh Med Ctr 1998; **Fac Appt:** Assoc Prof S, SUNY Downstate

Loulmet, Didier F MD [TS] - **Spec Exp:** Heart Valve Surgery; Robotic Cardiac Surgery; Minimally Invasive Cardiac Surgery; Aneurysm-Aortic; **Hospital:** NYU Langone Med Ctr (page 66); **Address:** NYU Medical Ctr, Cardiothoracic Surgery, 530 1st Ave, Ste 9V, New York, NY 10016; **Phone:** 212-263-2329; **Med School:** France 1984; **Resid:** Cardiothoracic Surgery, Paris Univ Hosp 1990; Cardiothoracic Surgery, Brigham & Women's Hosp 1991; **Fellow:** Pediatric Cardiac Surgery, Children's Hosp 1992; **Fac Appt:** Assoc Prof TS, NYU Sch Med

Magovern Jr, George J MD [TS] - **Spec Exp:** Cardiac Surgery; Ventricular Assist Device (LVAD); **Hospital:** Allegheny General Hosp; **Address:** Cardiovascular Surgery Ctr, CVI-1, 320 E North Ave, NW Wing-Snyder Pavilion, Allegheny Genl Hosp, Pittsburgh, PA 15212; **Phone:** 412-359-8820; **Board Cert:** Thoracic Surgery 2005; **Med School:** Univ Pittsburgh 1978; **Resid:** Surgery, Johns Hopkins Hosp 1981; Cardiovascular Surgery, Johns Hopkins Hosp 1985; **Fac Appt:** Prof S, Drexel Univ Coll Med

Marshall, Margaret Blair MD [TS] - **Spec Exp:** Lung Cancer; Esophageal Cancer; Thymoma; Chest Wall Tumors; **Hospital:** Georgetown Univ Hosp, Sibley Mem Hosp; **Address:** Georgetown Univ Hosp, 3800 Reservoir Rd NW, 4PHC, Washington, DC 20007; **Phone:** 202-444-5045; **Board Cert:** Surgery 2009; Thoracic Surgery 2002; **Med School:** Georgetown Univ 1991; **Resid:** Surgery, Georgetown Univ Med Ctr 1995; Cardiothoracic Surgery, Hosp Univ Penn 2001; **Fellow:** Research, Chldn's Hosp 1998; **Fac Appt:** Assoc Prof S, Georgetown Univ

Morris, Rohinton J MD [TS] - **Spec Exp:** Transplant-Heart; Ventricular Assist Device (LVAD); Coronary Artery Surgery; **Hospital:** Abington Mem Hosp; **Address:** Abington Memorial Hospital, Toll Bldg Fl 5, 1200 Old York Rd, Abington, PA 19001; **Phone:** 215-481-4200; **Board Cert:** Thoracic Surgery 2003; **Med School:** Hahnemann Univ 1984; **Resid:** Surgery, Hahnemann Univ Hosp 1989; Thoracic Surgery, Hahnemann Univ Hosp 1992; **Fac Appt:** Assoc Clin Prof S, Univ Pennsylvania

Naka, Yoshifumi MD/PhD [TS] - **Spec Exp:** Transplant-Heart & Lung; Ventricular Assist Device (LVAD); Heart Failure & Ventricular Containment; Mitral Valve Surgery; **Hospital:** NY-Presby/Columbia Univ Med Ctr, NY (page 65); **Address:** 177 Fort Washington Ave, MHB 7-435, New York, NY 10032; **Phone:** 212-305-0828; **Med School:** Japan 1984; **Resid:** Surgery, Osaka Police Hosp 1991; **Fellow:** Cardiovascular Surgery, Osaka Police Hosp 1993; Cardiothoracic Surgery, Columbia Univ Med Ctr 1998; **Fac Appt:** Asst Prof S, Columbia P&S

Oz, Mehmet C MD [TS] - **Spec Exp:** Transplant-Heart; Heart Valve Surgery; Minimally Invasive Cardiac Surgery; **Hospital:** NY-Presby/Columbia Univ Med Ctr, NY (page 65); **Address:** NY Presby Hosp, Dept Cardiothoracic Surg, 177 Ft Washington Ave, MHB- Rm 7, GN435, New York, NY 10032; **Phone:** 212-305-4434; **Board Cert:** Thoracic Surgery 2003; **Med School:** Univ Pennsylvania 1986; **Resid:** Surgery, Columbia Presby Med Ctr 1991; **Fellow:** Cardiothoracic Surgery, Columbia Presby Med Ctr 1993; **Fac Appt:** Prof S, Columbia P&S

Pass, Harvey MD [TS] - **Spec Exp:** Lung Cancer; Mesothelioma; Clinical Trials; **Hospital:** NYU Langone Med Ctr (page 66); **Address:** NYU Cancer Ctr, 160 E 34th St Fl 8, New York, NY 10016; **Phone:** 212-731-5414; **Board Cert:** Thoracic Surgery 2001; **Med School:** Duke Univ 1973; **Resid:** Surgery, Duke Univ Med Ctr 1975; Surgery, Univ Miss Med Ctr 1980; **Fellow:** Cardiothoracic Surgery, MUSC Med Ctr 1982; **Fac Appt:** Prof S, NYU Sch Med

Pierson III, Richard N MD [TS] - **Spec Exp:** Transplant-Lung; Lung Cancer; Transplant-Heart; **Hospital:** Univ of MD Med Ctr; **Address:** Univ Md Med Ctr, Dept Cardiothoracic Surg, 22 S Greene St, rm N4W94, Baltimore, MD 21201; **Phone:** 410-328-5842; **Board Cert:** Surgery 2000; Thoracic Surgery 2002; **Med School:** Columbia P&S 1983; **Resid:** Surgery, Univ Mich Med Ctr 1990; **Fellow:** Cardiothoracic Surgery, Mass Genl Hosp 1992; **Fac Appt:** Assoc Prof TS, Univ MD Sch Med

Pochettino, Alberto MD [TS] - **Spec Exp:** Aneurysm-Thoracic Aortic; Transplant-Lung; Left Ventricular Assist Device (LVAD); Heart Valve Surgery; **Hospital:** Hosp Univ Penn - UPHS (page 68); **Address:** Dept Thoracic Surgery, 3400 Spruce St, 6 Silverstein Pavillion, Philadelphia, PA 19104; **Phone:** 215-662-2957; **Board Cert:** Surgery 2005; Thoracic Surgery 2005; **Med School:** Northwestern Univ 1987; **Resid:** Surgery, SUNY-Upstate Med Ctr 1992; Thoracic Surgery, Hosp Univ Penn 1994; **Fac Appt:** Assoc Prof TS, Univ Pennsylvania

Rosengart, Todd MD [TS] - **Spec Exp:** Transfusion Free Surgery; Gene Therapy-Cardiac Angiogenesis; Minimally Invasive Surgery; Cardiac Surgery; **Hospital:** Stony Brook Univ Med Ctr; **Address:** Stonybrook Univ Hosp, Health Sci Ctr, Cardiothoracic Surgery, HSC-T19, rm 020, Stonybrook, NY 11794-0001; **Phone:** 631-444-7875; **Board Cert:** Surgery 1999; Thoracic Surgery 2001; **Med School:** Northwestern Univ 1983; **Resid:** Surgery, NYU Med Ctr 1985; Surgery, NYU Med Ctr 1989; **Fellow:** Thoracic Surgery, Natl Inst Hlth 1987; Cardiothoracic Surgery, NY-Cornell Med Ctr 1991; **Fac Appt:** Prof S, SUNY Stony Brook

Samuels, Louis MD [TS] - **Spec Exp:** Transplant-Heart; Artificial Heart Devices; Ventricular Assist Device (LVAD); **Hospital:** Lankenau Hosp; **Address:** 100 E Lancaster Ave, 280 Lankenau Medical Science Bldg, Wynnwood, PA 19096; **Phone:** 610-896-9255; **Board Cert:** Thoracic Surgery 2005; **Med School:** Hahnemann Univ 1987; **Resid:** Surgery, Hahnemann Hosp 1992; Thoracic Surgery, Hahnemann Hosp 1995; **Fac Appt:** Prof S, Hahnemann Univ

Scott, Walter J MD [TS] - **Spec Exp:** Lung Cancer; Esophageal Cancer; Mediastinal Tumors; Video Assisted Thoracic Surgery (VATS); **Hospital:** Fox Chase Cancer Ctr (page 58); **Address:** Fox Chase Cancer Ctr, 333 Cottman Ave, rm C308, Philadelphia, PA 19111; **Phone:** 215-214-1427; **Board Cert:** Thoracic Surgery 1998; **Med School:** Univ Chicago-Pritzker Sch Med 1981; **Resid:** Surgery, Univ Chicago Med Ctr 1987; **Fellow:** Cardiothoracic Surgery, Univ Chicago Med Ctr 1989

Smith, Craig R MD [TS] - **Spec Exp:** Mitral Valve Surgery; Transplant-Heart; Minimally Invasive Cardiac Surgery; Robotic Cardiac Surgery; **Hospital:** NY-Presby/Columbia Univ Med Ctr, NY (page 65); **Address:** Columbia Presbyterian Med Ctr, 177 Fort Washington Ave, Ste 7-435, New York, NY 10032; **Phone:** 212-305-8312; **Board Cert:** Thoracic Surgery 2004; **Med School:** Case West Res Univ 1977; **Resid:** Surgery, Strong Meml Hosp 1982; **Fellow:** Cardiothoracic Surgery, Columbia Presby Med Ctr 1984; **Fac Appt:** Prof S, Columbia P&S

Soberman, Mark S MD [TS] - **Spec Exp:** Thoracic Cancers; Lung Cancer; Esophageal Cancer; Esophageal Surgery; **Hospital:** Washington Hosp Ctr; **Address:** 110 Irving St NW, rm 1218, Unit 1F, Washington, DC 20010; **Phone:** 202-877-8115; **Board Cert:** Thoracic Surgery 2003; **Med School:** Emory Univ 1983; **Resid:** Surgery, Emory Univ 1986; **Fellow:** Cardiothoracic Surgery, George Washington Univ 1992; Thoracic Surgery, Cleveland Clinic Fdn 1993

Sonett, Joshua R MD [TS] - **Spec Exp:** Minimally Invasive Thoracic Surgery; Transplant-Lung; Thoracic Cancers; Emphysema-Lung Volume Reduction; **Hospital:** NY-Presby/Columbia Univ Med Ctr, NY (page 65); **Address:** 161 Fort Washington Ave, Ste 301, New York, NY 10032; **Phone:** 212-305-8086; **Board Cert:** Surgery 2004; Thoracic Surgery 2007; **Med School:** E Carolina Univ 1988; **Resid:** Surgery, Univ Mass Med Ctr 1993; **Fellow:** Cardiothoracic Surgery, Univ Pittsburgh Med Ctr 1994; Thoracic Surgery, Meml Sloan Kettering Cancer Ctr; **Fac Appt:** Assoc Prof S, Columbia P&S

Spray, Thomas L MD [TS] - **Spec Exp:** Cardiac Surgery-Adult & Pediatric; Transplant-Heart & Lung; Neonatal & Infant Cardiac Surgery; Congenital Heart Disease-Adult; **Hospital:** Chldns Hosp of Philadelphia, Hosp Univ Penn - UPHS (page 68); **Address:** Childrens Hosp, Div Cardiothoracic Surg, 34th St & Civic Ctr Blvd, Ste 12NW10, Philadelphia, PA 19104; **Phone:** 215-590-2708; **Board Cert:** Thoracic Surgery 2004; Congenital Cardiac Surgery 2009; **Med School:** Duke Univ 1973; **Resid:** Surgery, Duke Univ Med Ctr 1975; Cardiothoracic Surgery, Duke Univ Med Ctr 1983; **Fac Appt:** Prof S, Univ Pennsylvania

Stewart, Allan MD [TS] - **Spec Exp:** Heart Valve Surgery-Aortic; Aneurysm-Aortic; Aortic Surgery; **Hospital:** NY-Presby/Columbia Univ Med Ctr, NY (page 65); **Address:** 177 Fort Washington Ave, Milstein Hosp Bldg Fl 7 - rm 435, New York, NY 10030; **Phone:** 212-305-4980; **Board Cert:** Surgery 2003; Thoracic Surgery 2006; **Med School:** UMDNJ-NJ Med Sch, Newark 1995; **Resid:** Surgery, Univ PA Hlth Sys 2002; **Fellow:** Thoracic Surgery, NY Presby Hosp 2004; **Fac Appt:** Asst Prof TS, Columbia P&S

Strong III, Michael D MD [TS] - **Spec Exp:** Coronary Artery Surgery; Heart Valve Surgery; Thoracic Aortic Surgery; **Hospital:** Hahnemann Univ Hosp; **Address:** Div Cardiothoracic Surgery, 245 N 15th St, N Tower Bldg Fl 7 - Ste 744, Philadelphia, PA 19102; **Phone:** 215-762-7802; **Board Cert:** Surgery 1974; Thoracic Surgery 2006; **Med School:** Jefferson Med Coll 1966; **Resid:** Surgery, Jefferson Hosp 1973; Thoracic Surgery, Temple Univ Hosp 1975; **Fac Appt:** Prof TS, Drexel Univ Coll Med

Swistel, Daniel MD [TS] - **Spec Exp:** Coronary Artery Surgery; Minimally Invasive Surgery; Heart Valve Surgery; Hypertrophic Cardiomyopathy; **Hospital:** St. Luke's - Roosevelt Hosp Ctr - St Luke's Hosp (page 55); **Address:** 1090 Amsterdam Ave, Ste 8B, New York, NY 10025; **Phone:** 212-523-4088; **Board Cert:** Thoracic Surgery 2006; **Med School:** UMDNJ-RW Johnson Med Sch 1979; **Resid:** Surgery, St Lukes-Roosevelt Hosp 1984; Cardiothoracic Surgery, Montefiore Med Ctr 1986; **Fac Appt:** Assoc Clin Prof TS, Columbia P&S

Tortolani, Anthony J MD [TS] - **Spec Exp:** Transfusion Free Surgery; Heart Valve Surgery; Coronary Artery Surgery; **Hospital:** New York Methodist Hosp, NY-Presby/Weill Cornell Med Ctr, NY (page 65); **Address:** New York Methodist Hosp, Dept Surgery, 506 6th St Fl 6, Brooklyn, NY 11215; **Phone:** 718-780-5990; **Board Cert:** Surgery 1975; Thoracic Surgery 1999; **Med School:** Geo Wash Univ 1969; **Resid:** Surgery, N Shore Univ Hosp 1974; **Fellow:** Cardiothoracic Surgery, NYU Med Ctr 1978; **Fac Appt:** Assoc Prof S, Cornell Univ-Weill Med Coll

Toyoda, Yoshiya MD/PhD [TS] - **Spec Exp:** Cardiothoracic Surgery; Transplant-Heart; Heart Valve Surgery; Coronary Artery Surgery; **Hospital:** UPMC Presby, Pittsburgh; **Address:** UPMC Presby, 200 Lothrop St, Ste C900, Pittsburgh, PA 15213; **Phone:** 412-692-2779; **Med School:** Japan 1990; **Resid:** Surgery, Kobe Univ Hosp 1994; Cardiothoracic Surgery, Kove Univ Hosp 1997; **Fellow:** Cardiothoracic Research, Harvard Med School 2001; Cardiovascular Surgery, Havard Univ Affil Hosp 2004; **Fac Appt:** Assoc Prof S, Univ Pittsburgh

Thoracic Surgery

Tranbaugh, Robert MD [TS] - **Spec Exp:** Coronary Artery Surgery; Heart Valve Surgery; Aneurysm-Thoracic Aortic; **Hospital:** Beth Israel Med Ctr - Petrie Division (page 55); **Address:** 317 E 17th St Fl 11, New York, NY 10003; **Phone:** 212-420-2584; **Board Cert:** Thoracic Surgery 2004; **Med School:** Univ Pennsylvania 1976; **Resid:** Surgery, UCSF Med Ctr 1983; Cardiothoracic Surgery, UCSF Med Ctr 1985; **Fac Appt:** Assoc Prof TS, Albert Einstein Coll Med

Watson, Thomas J MD [TS] - **Spec Exp:** Esophageal Cancer; Gastroesophageal Reflux Disease (GERD); Lung Cancer; **Hospital:** Univ of Rochester Strong Meml Hosp, Highland Hosp of Rochester; **Address:** 601 Elmwood Ave, Box SURG, Rochester, NY 14642; **Phone:** 585-275-1509; **Board Cert:** Thoracic Surgery 2007; Surgery 2003; **Med School:** Univ SC Sch Med 1988; **Resid:** Surgery, LAC-USC Med Ctr 1993; Cardiothoracic Surgery, LAC-USC Med Ctr 1996; **Fellow:** Esophageal Surgery, LAC-USC Med Ctr 1994; **Fac Appt:** Assoc Prof S, Univ Rochester

Weksler, Benny MD [TS] - **Spec Exp:** Thoracic Cancers; Lung Cancer; Esophageal Cancer; Minimally Invasive Thoracic Surgery; **Hospital:** UPMC Presby, Pittsburgh; **Address:** university of Pittsburgh Medical Center, 200 Lothrop St, PUH Bldg - Fl C800, Pittsburgh, PA 15213; **Phone:** 412-648-6271; **Board Cert:** Surgery 2007; Thoracic Surgery 2007; **Med School:** Brazil 1987; **Resid:** Surgery, NY Med Coll/ Lincoln Med Ctr 1991; Research, NY Med Coll/Lincoln Med Ctr 1995; **Fellow:** Cardiothoracic Surgery, Meml Sloan Kettering Cancer Ctr 1997; Minimally Invasive Surgery, Univ Pittsburgh Med Ctr 2008; **Fac Appt:** Assoc Prof TS, Univ Pittsburgh

Williams, Mathew R MD [TS] - **Spec Exp:** Interventional Cardiology; Heart Valve Surgery; **Hospital:** NY-Presby/Columbia Univ Med Ctr, NY (page 65); **Address:** Milstein Hospital Bldg Fl 7 - rm 435, 177 Fort Washington Ave, New York, NY 10032; **Phone:** 212-305-9320; **Board Cert:** Thoracic Surgery 2007; **Med School:** Columbia P&S 1996; **Resid:** Surgery, UCLA Med Ctr 1998; Surgery, NY Presby Hosp/Columbia 2003; **Fellow:** Cardiothoracic Surgery, NY Presby Hosp/Columbia 2005; Interventional Cardiology, NY Presby Hosp/Columbia 2006; **Fac Appt:** Asst Prof S, Columbia P&S

Woo, Y Joseph MD [TS] - **Spec Exp:** Minimally Invasive Cardiac Surgery; Robotic Cardiac Surgery; Aneurysm-Abdominal & Thoracic Aortic; Mitral Valve Robotic Surgery; **Hospital:** Hosp Univ Penn - UPHS (page 68); **Address:** Penn Cardiac Care, 6 Silverstein Bldg, 3400 Spruce St, Philadelphia, PA 19104; **Phone:** 215-662-2956; **Board Cert:** Surgery 2009; Thoracic Surgery 2010; **Med School:** Univ Pennsylvania 1992; **Resid:** Surgery, Hosp Univ Penn 1998; Thoracic Surgery, Hosp Univ Penn 2001; **Fac Appt:** Assoc Prof S, Univ Pennsylvania

Yang, Stephen C MD [TS] - **Spec Exp:** Mesothelioma; Lung Cancer; Esophageal Cancer; Robotic Surgery; **Hospital:** Johns Hopkins Hosp (page 61), Johns Hopkins Bayview Med Ctr (page 61); **Address:** Johns Hopkins Hosp, 600 N Wolfe St Blalock Bldg - rm 240, Baltimore, MD 21287; **Phone:** 410-933-1233; **Board Cert:** Surgery 2003; Thoracic Surgery 2005; **Med School:** Med Coll VA 1984; **Resid:** Surgery, Univ Tex Hlth Sci Ctr 1990; **Fellow:** Thoracic Surgery, MD Anderson Cancer Ctr 1992; Cardiothoracic Surgery, Med Coll Virginia 1994; **Fac Appt:** Assoc Prof TS, Johns Hopkins Univ

Southeast

Bichell, David P MD [TS] - **Spec Exp:** Cardiac Surgery-Neonatal; Cardiac Surgery-Pediatric; Congenital Heart Surgery; Minimally Invasive Cardiac Surgery; **Hospital:** Vanderbilt Monroe Carrell Jr. Chldn's Hosp (page 76), Vanderbilt Univ Med Ctr (page 76); **Address:** Vanderbilt Childrens Hosp, Div Pediatric Cardiac Surgery, 2200 Childrens Way, 5247 DOT, Nashville, TN 37232-9292; **Phone:** 615-343-6525; **Board Cert:** Thoracic Surgery 2006; **Med School:** Columbia P&S 1987; **Resid:** Surgery, Barnes Jewish Hosp 1994; Cardiothoracic Surgery, Brigham & Womens Hosp/Chldns Hosp 1996; **Fellow:** Cardiac Surgery, Brigham & Womens Hosp 1997; **Fac Appt:** Prof TS, Vanderbilt Univ

Bridges Jr, Charles R MD [TS] - **Spec Exp:** Minimally Invasive Cardiac Surgery; Maze Procedure for Atrial Fibrillation; Aneurysm-Aortic; Heart Valve Surgery; **Hospital:** Carolinas Med Ctr-Univ; **Address:** Sanger Heart & Vascular Inst, 1001 Blythe Blvd, Charlotte, NC 28203; **Phone:** 704-373-0212; **Board Cert:** Surgery 2003; Thoracic Surgery 2004; **Med School:** Harvard Med Sch 1981; **Resid:** Internal Medicine, Brigham & Women's Hosp 1984; Surgery, Hosp Univ Penn 1991; **Fellow:** Cardiothoracic Surgery, Hosp Univ Penn 1993; **Fac Appt:** Prof S, Univ Pennsylvania

Burke, Redmond B MD [TS] - **Spec Exp:** Pediatric Cardiac Surgery; Congenital Heart Surgery; **Hospital:** Miami Children's Hosp; **Address:** 3200 SW 60th Ct, Ste 102, Miami Children's Hosp, Miami, FL 33155; **Phone:** 305-663-8401; **Board Cert:** Thoracic Surgery 2001; Surgery 2002; **Med School:** Harvard Med Sch 1984; **Resid:** Surgery, Brigham & Women's Hosp 1989; **Fellow:** Research, Brigham & Women's Hosp 1990; Cardiothoracic Surgery, Brigham & Women's Hosp 1992

Byrne, John G MD [TS] - **Spec Exp:** Cardiothoracic Surgery; Heart Failure; Heart Valve Surgery; Transplant-Heart; **Hospital:** Vanderbilt Univ Med Ctr (page 76); **Address:** Vanderbilt Heart Inst, 1512 21 Ave S, Ste 5209, MCE-North Tower, Nashville, TN 37232-8802; **Phone:** 615-343-9195; **Board Cert:** Thoracic Surgery 2008; **Med School:** Boston Univ 1987; **Resid:** Surgery, Univ Illinois Affil Hosp 1995; Thoracic Surgery, Brigham & Women's Hosp 1997; **Fellow:** Cardiothoracic Research, Harvard Med School 1992; **Fac Appt:** Prof S, Vanderbilt Univ

Cerfolio, Robert J MD [TS] - **Spec Exp:** Lung Cancer; Tracheal Surgery; Chest Wall Tumors; Esophageal Cancer; **Hospital:** Univ of Ala Hosp at Birmingham; **Address:** 703 19th St S, Ste 739, Zigler Rsch Bldg, Birmingham, AL 35294-0007; **Phone:** 205-934-5937; **Board Cert:** Surgery 2003; Thoracic Surgery 2006; **Med School:** Univ Rochester 1988; **Resid:** Surgery, Cornell-NY Hosp 1990; Surgery, Mayo Clinic 1993; **Fellow:** Cardiothoracic Surgery, Mayo Clinic 1996; **Fac Appt:** Prof TS, Univ Alabama

Chitwood Jr, W Randolph MD [TS] - **Spec Exp:** Robotic Cardiac Surgery; Minimally Invasive Cardiac Surgery; Heart Valve Surgery; Mitral Valve Surgery; **Hospital:** Univ Hlth Sys-Pitt Co Meml Hosp; **Address:** E Carolina Heart Inst @ ECU, 115 Heart Drive, rm 3107, Greenville, NC 27834; **Phone:** 252-744-4536; **Board Cert:** Thoracic Surgery 2005; **Med School:** Univ VA Sch Med 1974; **Resid:** Surgery, Duke Univ Med Ctr 1983; **Fellow:** Cardiovascular Surgery, Duke Univ Med Ctr 1984; **Fac Appt:** Prof S, E Carolina Univ

Christian, Karla G MD [TS] - **Spec Exp:** Congenital Heart Surgery; Transplant-Heart-Pediatric; Cardiac Surgery-Adult & Pediatric; **Hospital:** Vanderbilt Monroe Carrell Jr. Chldn's Hosp (page 76), Vanderbilt Univ Med Ctr (page 76); **Address:** Vanderbilt Chldns Hosp, Cardiac Surgery, 2200 Childrens Way, 5247 Doctors Office Tower, Nashville, TN 37232-9292; **Phone:** 615-343-6525; **Board Cert:** Surgery 2001; Thoracic Surgery 2003; **Med School:** Univ Wash 1985; **Resid:** Surgery, Univ Washington Med Ctr 1987; Surgery, Vanderbilt Univ Med Ctr 1991; **Fellow:** Cardiothoracic Surgery, Vanderbilt Univ Med Ctr 1994; **Fac Appt:** Assoc Prof S, Vanderbilt Univ

D'Amico, Thomas MD [TS] - **Spec Exp:** Lung Cancer; Esophageal Cancer; **Hospital:** Duke Univ Hosp; **Address:** Duke Univ Med Ctr, Dept Thoracic Surg, Box 3496, Durham, NC 27710; **Phone:** 919-684-4891; **Board Cert:** Surgery 2004; Thoracic Surgery 2006; **Med School:** Columbia P&S 1987; **Resid:** Surgery, Duke Univ Med Ctr 1989; Cardiothoracic Surgery, Duke Univ Med Ctr 1996; **Fellow:** Thoracic Oncology, Meml Sloan Kettering Cancer Ctr; **Fac Appt:** Assoc Prof S, Duke Univ

Dabal, Robert Joseph MD [TS] - **Spec Exp:** Pediatric Cardiac Surgery; Neonatal & Infant Cardiac Surgery; **Hospital:** Univ of Ala Hosp at Birmingham, Children's Hospital - Birmingham; **Address:** 712 Tinsley Harris Towers, 1900 University Blvd, Birmingham, AL 35294; **Phone:** 205-935-2419; **Board Cert:** Surgery 2002; Thoracic Surgery 2004; **Med School:** Duke Univ 1995; **Resid:** Surgery, NY Presby Hosp/Columbia 2000; Thoracic Surgery, Univ Washington Med Ctr 2003; **Fellow:** Pediatric Cardiothoracic Surgery, Chldn's Hosp 2004; Pediatric Cardiothoracic Surgery, Chldn's Hosp 2005; **Fac Appt:** Asst Prof S, Univ Alabama

Drinkwater Jr, Davis C MD [TS] - **Spec Exp:** Cardiac Surgery-Adult & Pediatric; Heart Valve Surgery; Congenital Heart Surgery; **Hospital:** Centennial Med Ctr, Vanderbilt Monroe Carrell Jr. Chldn's Hosp (page 76); **Address:** 2400 Patterson St, Ste 400, Nashville, TN 37203; **Phone:** 615-342-5812; **Board Cert:** Thoracic Surgery 2005; **Med School:** Univ VT Coll Med 1976; **Resid:** Surgery, McGill Univ 1981; Cardiothoracic Surgery, McGill Univ 1983; **Fellow:** Cardiothoracic Surgery, Childrens Hosp 1984; **Fac Appt:** Clin Prof TS, Vanderbilt Univ

Feins, Richard H MD [TS] - **Spec Exp:** Thoracic Cancers; Lung Cancer; Robotic Surgery; Esophageal Surgery; **Hospital:** NC Memorial Hosp - UNC; **Address:** UNC Dept Surgery, Div Cardiothoracic Surgery, 3040 Burnett-Womack Bldg, CB#7065, Chapel Hill, NC 27599-7065; **Phone:** 919-966-3383; **Board Cert:** Thoracic Surgery 2003; **Med School:** Univ VT Coll Med 1973; **Resid:** Surgery, Strong Meml Hosp 1980; Cardiothoracic Surgery, Univ Rochester Affil Hosp 1982; **Fac Appt:** Prof S, Univ NC Sch Med

Glassford Jr, David M MD [TS] - **Spec Exp:** Cardiothoracic Surgery; **Hospital:** Saint Thomas Hosp - Nashville; **Address:** Cardiovascular Surgery Assocs, 4230 Harding Rd, Ste 202, Nashville, TN 37205; **Phone:** 615-385-4781; **Board Cert:** Thoracic Surgery 2007; Surgical Critical Care 1999; **Med School:** Univ Tex Med Br, Galveston 1970; **Resid:** Surgery, Univ Texas Med Br 1975; Thoracic Surgery, Ochsner Clinic 1977; **Fac Appt:** Asst Clin Prof TS, Vanderbilt Univ

Guyton, Robert A MD [TS] - **Spec Exp:** Coronary Artery Surgery; Minimally Invasive Cardiac Surgery; Heart Valve Surgery; Heart Valve-Percutaneous; **Hospital:** Emory Univ Hosp Midtown, Emory Univ Hosp; **Address:** Emory Dept Cardiothoracic Surgery, 550 Peachtree St Fl 6 MOT, Atlanta, GA 30308; **Phone:** 404-686-2513; **Board Cert:** Thoracic Surgery 2010; **Med School:** Harvard Med Sch 1971; **Resid:** Surgery, Mass Genl Hosp 1975; **Fellow:** Thoracic Surgery, National Heart Lung Inst 1975; **Fac Appt:** Prof S, Emory Univ

Harpole Jr, David H MD [TS] - **Spec Exp:** Lung Cancer; Mesothelioma; Esophageal Cancer; **Hospital:** Duke Univ Hosp; **Address:** 3627 DUMC, Durham, NC 27705; **Phone:** 919-668-8413; **Board Cert:** Surgery 2002; Thoracic Surgery 2003; **Med School:** Univ VA Sch Med 1984; **Resid:** Surgery, Duke Univ Med Ctr 1991; **Fellow:** Thoracic Surgery, Duke Univ Med Ctr 1993; **Fac Appt:** Prof S, Duke Univ

Jones, David R MD [TS] - **Spec Exp:** Lung Cancer; Esophageal Cancer; Minimally Invasive Thoracic Surgery; **Hospital:** Univ of Virginia Health Sys; **Address:** Univ Virginnia Hlth Sys, Dept Surgery, PO Box 800679, Charlottesville, VA 22908; **Phone:** 434-243-6443; **Board Cert:** Surgery 2005; Thoracic Surgery 2007; **Med School:** W VA Univ 1989; **Resid:** Surgery, West Va Univ 1995; **Fellow:** Thoracic Surgery, Univ North Carolina 1998; **Fac Appt:** Assoc Prof S, Univ VA Sch Med

Kanter, Kirk R MD [TS] - **Spec Exp:** Pediatric Cardiac Surgery; Transplant-Heart-Pediatric; Transplant-Lung-Pediatric; **Hospital:** Chldns Hlthcare Atlanta @ Egleston, Emory Univ Hosp; **Address:** Childrens Hlthcare Atlanta at Egleston, Pediatric Cardiothoracic Surgery, 1405 Clifton Rd NE Fl 2, Atlanta, GA 30322; **Phone:** 404-785-6330; **Board Cert:** Thoracic Surgery 2008; Congenital Cardiac Surgery 2009; **Med School:** Albany Med Coll 1976; **Resid:** Surgery, Johns Hopkins Hosp 1982; Thoracic Surgery, Johns Hopkins Hosp 1984; **Fellow:** Pediatric Cardiac Surgery, Brompton/Harefield Hosps 1985; **Fac Appt:** Prof S, Emory Univ

Kiernan, Paul D MD [TS] - **Spec Exp:** Lung Cancer; Esophageal Cancer; Mediastinal Tumors; **Hospital:** Inova Fairfax Hosp, Inova Alexandria Hosp; **Address:** 2921 Telestar Court Fl 2, Falls Church, VA 22042; **Phone:** 703-280-5858; **Board Cert:** Thoracic Surgery 2002; **Med School:** Georgetown Univ 1974; **Resid:** Surgery, Mayo Clinic 1979; Cardiothoracic Surgery, Mayo Clinic 1981; **Fellow:** Vascular Surgery, Mayo Clinic 1982; **Fac Appt:** Assoc Clin Prof S, Georgetown Univ

Kirklin, James K MD [TS] - **Spec Exp:** Transplant-Heart-Adult & Pediatric; Cardiac Surgery-Adult & Pediatric; Transplant-Heart & Lung; **Hospital:** Univ of Ala Hosp at Birmingham; **Address:** UAB CardioThoracic Surgery, 1900 University Blvd, THT 760, Birmingham, AL 35294; **Phone:** 205-934-3368; **Board Cert:** Thoracic Surgery 2000; **Med School:** Harvard Med Sch 1973; **Resid:** Surgery, Mass Genl Hosp 1977; Cardiothoracic Surgery, Mass Genl Hosp 1979; **Fellow:** Cardiothoracic Surgery, Chidren's Hosp Med Ctr 1979; **Fac Appt:** Prof S, Univ Alabama

Kron, Irving L MD [TS] - **Spec Exp:** Coronary Artery Surgery; Transplant-Heart; **Hospital:** Univ of Virginia Health Sys; **Address:** Univ VA Hlth Sys, Div Cardiovascular Surg, PO Box 800679, Charlottesville, VA 22908; **Phone:** 434-924-2158; **Board Cert:** Surgery 1999; Thoracic Surgery 2001; Vascular Surgery 2006; **Med School:** Med Coll Wisc 1975; **Resid:** Surgery, Maine Med Ctr 1980; **Fellow:** Cardiothoracic Surgery, Univ Virginia Med Ctr 1982; **Fac Appt:** Prof S, Univ VA Sch Med

Lau, Christine L MD [TS] - **Spec Exp:** Lung Cancer; Transplant-Lung; Esophageal Cancer; **Hospital:** Univ of Virginia Health Sys; **Address:** Univ VA Hlth System, Div Thoracic & Cardiovascular Surg, P.O. Box 800679, Charlottesville, VA 22908; **Phone:** 434-924-8016; **Board Cert:** Surgery 2003; Thoracic Surgery 2007; **Med School:** Dartmouth Med Sch 1995; **Resid:** Surgery, Duke Affil Hosp; **Fellow:** Cardiothoracic Surgery, Washington Univ Affil Hosps 2005; **Fac Appt:** Assoc Prof S, Univ VA Sch Med

Martin, Tomas D MD [TS] - **Spec Exp:** Cardiothoracic Surgery; Aortic Surgery; Aneurysm-Abdominal Aortic; **Hospital:** Shands at Univ of FL; **Address:** TCV Surgery, PO Box 100129, Gainesville, FL 32610-0129; **Phone:** 352-273-5505; **Board Cert:** Thoracic Surgery 2008; **Med School:** Univ Tex, Houston 1981; **Resid:** Surgery, Baylor Coll Med 1986; Vascular Surgery, Baylor Coll Med 1987; **Fellow:** Cardiothoracic Surgery, Shands/Univ Florida 1989; **Fac Appt:** Assoc Prof S, Univ Fla Coll Med

Mill, Michael R MD [TS] - **Spec Exp:** Pediatric Cardiac Surgery; Transplant-Heart-Adult & Pediatric; Transplant-Heart & Lung; Heart Valve Surgery; **Hospital:** NC Memorial Hosp - UNC; **Address:** UNC Sch Med, Cardiothoracic Surgery, 3040 Burnett Womack Bldg, CB.7065, Chapel Hill, NC 27599-7965; **Phone:** 919-966-3381; **Board Cert:** Thoracic Surgery 2009; **Med School:** Univ Colorado 1980; **Resid:** Surgery, Univ Colorado Hlth Sci Ctr 1985; **Fellow:** Cardiothoracic Surgery, Stanford Univ Med Ctr 1987; Transplant Surgery, Stanford Univ Med Ctr 1988; **Fac Appt:** Prof S, Univ NC Sch Med

Miller, Daniel L MD [TS] - **Spec Exp:** Esophageal Cancer; Lung Cancer; Mesothelioma; Emphysema-Lung Volume Reduction; **Hospital:** Emory Univ Hosp, Emory Univ Hosp Midtown; **Address:** The Emory Clinic, 1365A Clifton Rd NE, Ste 2219, Atlanta, GA 30322; **Phone:** 404-778-3755; **Board Cert:** Thoracic Surgery 2005; Surgery 2001; **Med School:** Univ KY Coll Med 1985; **Resid:** Surgery, Georgetown Univ Hosp 1991; **Fellow:** Cardiothoracic Surgery, Mayo Clinic 1994; **Fac Appt:** Prof S, Emory Univ

Mullett, Timothy W MD [TS] - **Spec Exp:** Lung Cancer; Transplant-Heart & Lung; Cardiac Surgery-Adult & Pediatric; Esophageal Surgery; **Hospital:** Univ of Kentucky Albert B. Chandler Hosp; **Address:** Charles T. Wethington Bld, 900 S Limestone St, rm 326, Lexington, KY 40536; **Phone:** 859-323-6494; **Board Cert:** Thoracic Surgery 2007; Surgery 2005; **Med School:** Univ Fla Coll Med 1987; **Resid:** Surgery, Shands/Univ of FL 1993; **Fellow:** Pediatric Surgery, Shands/Univ of FL 1994; Cardiothoracic Surgery, Shands/Univ of FL 1995; **Fac Appt:** Assoc Prof S, Univ KY Coll Med

Murphy, Douglas A MD [TS] - **Spec Exp:** Robotic Surgery; Minimally Invasive Cardiac Surgery; Heart Valve Surgery; Mitral Valve Robotic Surgery; **Hospital:** St. Joseph's Hosp - Atlanta, NE Georgia Med Ctr; **Address:** 5665 Peachtree Dunwoody Rd NE, Ste 200, Atlanta, GA 30342; **Phone:** 404-252-6104; **Board Cert:** Internal Medicine 1978; Thoracic Surgery 2004; **Med School:** Univ Pennsylvania 1975; **Resid:** Internal Medicine, Mass Genl Hosp 1977; Surgery, Mass Genl Hosp 1981; **Fellow:** Thoracic Surgery, Emory Univ Affil Hosp 1983; **Fac Appt:** Prof TS, Emory Univ

Nesbitt, Jonathan C MD [TS] - **Spec Exp:** Lung Cancer; Esophageal Cancer; Chest Diseases-Benign; Minimally Invasive Thoracic Surgery; **Hospital:** Vanderbilt Univ Med Ctr (page 76), Saint Thomas Hosp - Nashville; **Address:** Vanderbilt-Ingram Cancer Center, 1301 Medical Center Drive, Ste 1710, Nashville, TN 37232; **Phone:** 615-322-0064; **Board Cert:** Thoracic Surgery 2009; **Med School:** Georgetown Univ 1981; **Resid:** Surgery, Vanderbilt Univ Med Ctr 1987; Cardiothoracic Surgery, Albany Med Ctr 1989; **Fac Appt:** Assoc Prof TS, Vanderbilt Univ

Nguyen, Dao M MD [TS] - **Spec Exp:** Thoracic Cancers; Lung Cancer; **Hospital:** Univ of Miami Hosp (page 72); **Address:** PO Box 016960 (R-114), Miami, FL 33136; **Phone:** 305-585-5271; **Board Cert:** Thoracic Surgery 2005; **Med School:** McGill Univ 1986; **Resid:** Surgery, McGill Univ Affil Hosp 1992; Thoracic Surgery, McGill Univ Affil Hosp 1994; **Fellow:** Thoracic Oncology, MD Anderson Cancer Ctr 1996; **Fac Appt:** Prof S, Univ Miami Sch Med

Ninan, Mathew MD [TS] - **Spec Exp:** Lung Cancer; Transplant-Lung; Esophageal Cancer; **Hospital:** Centennial Med Ctr; **Address:** 2410 Patterson St, Ste 212, Nashville, TN 37203; **Phone:** 615-342-7345; **Med School:** India 1988; **Resid:** Surgery, Univ London Affil Hosp 1994; **Fellow:** Cardiothoracic Surgery, Univ Pittsburgh Affil Hosp 1998; **Fac Appt:** Assoc Prof TS, Vanderbilt Univ

Oaks, Timothy E MD [TS] - **Spec Exp:** Transplant-Heart; Cardiovascular Surgery-Complex; Lung Cancer; **Hospital:** Wake Forest Univ Baptist Med Ctr; **Address:** Wake Forest Baptist Med Ctr, Dept Cardiothoracic Surgery, Medical Center Blvd, Winston-Salem, NC 27157; **Phone:** 336-716-9800; **Board Cert:** Thoracic Surgery 2001; **Med School:** Penn State Coll Med 1984; **Resid:** Surgery, Penn State-Hershey Med Ctr 1990; **Fellow:** Cardiothoracic Surgery, Penn State-Hershey Med Ctr 1992; Cardiothoracic Surgery, Papworth Hosp 1993; **Fac Appt:** Assoc Prof TS, Wake Forest Univ

Panos, Anthony MD [TS] - **Spec Exp:** Cardiac Surgery-Adult; Transplant-Heart; Minimally Invasive Cardiac Surgery; **Hospital:** Jackson Meml Hosp (page 70); **Address:** Jackson Meml Hosp (R114), 1611 NW 12th Ave, ET3072, Miami, FL 33136; **Phone:** 305-585-5271; **Board Cert:** Thoracic Surgery 2004; **Med School:** Univ Toronto 1980; **Resid:** Surgery, Univ Toronto Affil Hosp 1987; Cardiovascular Surgery, Univ Toronto Affil Hosp 1990; **Fellow:** Thoracic Surgery, Toronto Genl Hosp 1985; Cardiovascular Surgery, St Michaels Hosp 1990; **Fac Appt:** Prof S, Univ Miami Sch Med

Philpott, Jonathan M MD [TS] - **Spec Exp:** Cardiac Surgery; Atrial Fibrillation; Clinical Trials; **Hospital:** Sentara Norfolk Genl Hosp; **Address:** Mid-Atlantic Cardiothoracic Surgeons, Sentara Heart Hospital Fl 6, 600 Gresham Drive, Ste 8600, Norfolk, VA 23507; **Phone:** 757-388-6005; **Board Cert:** Surgery 2001; Surgical Critical Care 2002; Thoracic Surgery 2005; **Med School:** Eastern VA Med Sch 1994; **Resid:** Surgery, E Carolina Univ Affil Hosp 2000; **Fellow:** Thoracic Surgery, Hosp Univ Penn 2002; Med Coll VA-West Hosp 2004

Putnam Jr, Joe B MD [TS] - **Spec Exp:** Lung Cancer; Esophageal Cancer; Sarcoma-Soft Tissue; **Hospital:** Vanderbilt Univ Med Ctr (page 76), TN Valley Healthcare Sys-Nashville; **Address:** Vanderbilt Univ Med Ctr - Thoracic Surgery, 609 Oxford House, 1313 21st Ave S, Nashville, TN 37232-4682; **Phone:** 615-343-9202; **Board Cert:** Thoracic Surgery 2007; **Med School:** Univ NC Sch Med 1979; **Resid:** Surgery, Univ Rochester 1986; Thoracic Surgery, Univ Mich Med Ctr 1988; **Fellow:** Surgical Oncology, NCI/NIH-Surg Branch 1984; **Fac Appt:** Prof TS, Vanderbilt Univ

Quintessenza, James A MD [TS] - **Spec Exp:** Transplant-Heart; Coronary Artery Surgery; Cardiovascular Surgery; **Hospital:** All Children's Hosp; **Address:** 625 6th Ave S, Ste 475, St Petersburg, FL 33701; **Phone:** 727-822-6666; **Board Cert:** Thoracic Surgery 2007; **Med School:** Univ Fla Coll Med 1981; **Resid:** Surgery, Univ Florida Hosps 1986; **Fellow:** Thoracic Surgery, UCSD Medical Ctr 1988; **Fac Appt:** Assoc Clin Prof S, Univ S Fla Coll Med

Reed, Carolyn E MD [TS] - **Spec Exp:** Esophageal Cancer; Lung Cancer; **Hospital:** MUSC Med Ctr; **Address:** 25 Coourteney Drive, Ste 7018, MSC 295, Charleston, SC 29425; **Phone:** 843-876-4845; **Board Cert:** Thoracic Surgery 2004; **Med School:** Univ Rochester 1977; **Resid:** Surgery, NY Hosp 1982; Thoracic Surgery, NY Hosp 1985; **Fellow:** Surgical Oncology, Meml Sloan Kettering Cancer Ctr 1983; **Fac Appt:** Prof S, Med Univ SC

Robinson, Lary A MD [TS] - **Spec Exp:** Lung Cancer; Mesothelioma; **Hospital:** H Lee Moffitt Cancer Ctr & Research Inst (page 59), Tampa Genl Hosp; **Address:** H Lee Moffitt Cancer Ctr, Div Thoracic Oncology, 12902 Magnolia Drive, Tampa, FL 33612-9497; **Phone:** 813-745-7282; **Board Cert:** Thoracic Surgery 2003; Surgery 2002; Surgical Critical Care 2000; **Med School:** Washington Univ, St Louis 1972; **Resid:** Surgery, Duke Univ Med Ctr 1974; Thoracic Surgery, Duke Univ Med Ctr 1981; **Fellow:** Cardiothoracic Surgery, St Thomas Hosp 1982; Cardiothoracic Surgery, Duke Univ Med Ctr 1983; **Fac Appt:** Prof S, Univ S Fla Coll Med

Rosenkranz, Eliot Robert MD [TS] - **Spec Exp:** Pediatric Cardiac Surgery; Transplant-Heart-Pediatric; Cardiac Surgery-Neonatal; Congenital Heart Surgery; **Hospital:** Jackson Meml Hosp (page 70), Univ of Miami Hosp (page 72); **Address:** Jackson Meml Hosp (R114), 1611 NW 12th Ave, ET3072, Miami, FL 33136-1005; **Phone:** 305-585-5271; **Board Cert:** Thoracic Surgery 2008; **Med School:** UCSD 1979; **Resid:** Surgery, UCLA Med Ctr 1985; **Fellow:** Cardiothoracic Surgery, UCLA Med Ctr 1987; **Fac Appt:** Prof S, Univ Miami Sch Med

Salerno, Tomas A MD [TS] - **Spec Exp:** Cardiothoracic Surgery; Heart Valve Surgery; Aortic Surgery; Coronary Artery Surgery; **Hospital:** Jackson Meml Hosp (page 70), Univ of Miami Hosp (page 72); **Address:** Jackson Meml Hosp (R114), 1611 NW 12th Ave, ET3072, Miami, FL 33136; **Phone:** 305-585-5271; **Board Cert:** Thoracic Surgery 2008; **Med School:** McGill Univ 1971; **Resid:** Surgery, Royal Victoria Hosp 1975; Cardiothoracic Surgery, Royal Victoria Hosp 1977; **Fac Appt:** Prof S, Univ Miami Sch Med

Slaughter, Mark S MD [TS] - **Spec Exp:** Ventricular Assist Device (LVAD); Mitral Valve Surgery; Transplant-Heart; **Hospital:** Jewish Hosp; **Address:** 201 Abraham Flexner Way, Ste 1200, Louisville, KY 40202; **Phone:** 502-583-8383; **Board Cert:** Surgery 2002; Thoracic Surgery 2003; **Med School:** Indiana Univ 1986; **Resid:** Surgery, Northwestern Meml Hosp 1992; **Fellow:** Thoracic Surgery, Univ Minnesota Affil Hosp 1994

Smith, Peter K MD [TS] - **Spec Exp:** Coronary Artery Surgery; Heart Valve Surgery; **Hospital:** Duke Univ Hosp, Durham VA Med Ctr; **Address:** Duke Univ Med Ctr, 200 Trent Drive, Box 3442, Durham, NC 27710; **Phone:** 919-684-2890; **Board Cert:** Thoracic Surgery 2007; **Med School:** Duke Univ 1977; **Resid:** Surgery, Duke Univ Med Ctr 1984; Thoracic Surgery, Duke Univ Med Ctr 1987; **Fac Appt:** Prof S, Duke Univ

Staples, Edward D MD [TS] - **Spec Exp:** Transplant-Heart & Lung; Ventricular Assist Device (LVAD); **Hospital:** Malcolm Randall VA Med Ctr, Shands at Univ of FL; **Address:** 1601 SW Archer Rd, Gainesville, FL 32610; **Phone:** 352-273-5507; **Board Cert:** Thoracic Surgery 2004; Surgical Critical Care 2002; **Med School:** Univ S Fla Coll Med 1977; **Resid:** Surgery, Med Coll Va 1979; Surgery, Univ Hosp 1982; **Fellow:** Cardiothoracic Surgery, Univ Florida Affil Hosp 1984; **Fac Appt:** Assoc Prof S, Univ Fla Coll Med

Thoracic Surgery

Stowe, Cary MD [TS] - **Spec Exp:** Aortic Surgery; **Hospital:** Indian River Med Ctr; **Address:** 1040 37th Pl, Ste 101, Vero Beach, FL 32960; **Phone:** 772-563-4580; **Board Cert:** Thoracic Surgery 2008; Vascular Surgery 2008; **Med School:** Univ Alabama 1978; **Resid:** Surgery, Barnes Hosp 1982; **Fellow:** Vascular Surgery, Baylor Coll Med 1983; Cardiothoracic Surgery, Emory Univ Sch Med 1994

Tedder, Mark MD [TS] - **Spec Exp:** Transplant-Heart; Cardiac Surgery; Artificial Heart Devices; **Hospital:** Saint Thomas Hosp - Nashville; **Address:** Cardiovascular Surgery Assocs, 4230 Harding Rd, Ste 202, Nashville, TN 37205; **Phone:** 615-385-4781; **Board Cert:** Thoracic Surgery 2007; **Med School:** Duke Univ 1988; **Resid:** Surgery, Duke Univ Med Ctr 1995; Cardiothoracic Surgery, Duke Univ Med Ctr 1997

Ungerleider, Ross M MD [TS] - **Spec Exp:** Pediatric Cardiac Surgery; Cardiac Surgery; Congenital Heart Surgery; **Hospital:** Wake Forest Univ Baptist Med Ctr; **Address:** Dept of Cardiothoracic Surgery, Medical Ctr Blvd, Winston-Salem, NC 27157-1096; **Phone:** 336-716-2124; **Board Cert:** Thoracic Surgery 2007; Congenital Cardiac Surgery 2009; **Med School:** Rush Med Coll 1977; **Resid:** Surgery, Duke Univ Med Ctr 1987; **Fellow:** Cardiothoracic Surgery, Duke Univ Med Ctr 1989; Pediatric Cardiac Surgery, UCSF Med Ctr; **Fac Appt:** Prof

Weiman, Darryl S MD [TS] - **Spec Exp:** Cardiothoracic Surgery; Lung Cancer; **Hospital:** VA Med Ctr - Memphis; **Address:** VA Med Ctr, 1030 Jefferson Ave Fl 3, Dept Surgery, Memphis, TN 38104; **Phone:** 901-577-7352; **Board Cert:** Thoracic Surgery 2000; Surgery 2002; **Med School:** St Louis Univ 1978; **Resid:** Surgery, Univ Chicago Pritzker Sch Med 1983; Thoracic Surgery, Univ Chicago Pritzker Sch Med 1984; **Fellow:** Cardiothoracic Surgery, Long Island Jewish Hosp 1991; **Fac Appt:** Prof S, Univ Tenn Coll Med

Zwischenberger, Joseph B MD [TS] - **Spec Exp:** Thoracic Cancers; Lung Cancer; Esophageal Cancer; Respiratory Failure; **Hospital:** Univ of Kentucky Albert B. Chandler Hosp; **Address:** MN264 A B Chandler Med Ctr, 800 Rose St, Lexington, KY 40536; **Phone:** 859-257-1000; **Board Cert:** Surgery 2002; Thoracic Surgery 2005; Surgical Critical Care 1996; **Med School:** Univ KY Coll Med 1977; **Resid:** Surgery, Univ Michigan Hosp 1984; Cardiothoracic Surgery, Univ Michigan Hosp 1985; **Fellow:** Cardiac Surgery, Natl Inst Hlth 1981; **Fac Appt:** Prof S, Univ KY Coll Med

Midwest

Alexander Jr, John C MD [TS] - **Spec Exp:** Minimally Invasive Cardiac Surgery; Mitral Valve Surgery; Arrhythmias; **Hospital:** Evanston/North Shore Univ Hlth Sys; **Address:** Evanston Hosp, Cardiothoracic Surgery, 2650 Ridge Ave Walgreens Bldg - Ste 3507, Evanston, IL 60201; **Phone:** 847-570-2868; **Board Cert:** Thoracic Surgery 2001; **Med School:** Duke Univ 1972; **Resid:** Surgery, Duke Univ Med Ctr 1979; **Fellow:** Cardiothoracic Surgery, Duke Univ Med Ctr 1980; **Fac Appt:** Prof S, Northwestern Univ-Feinberg Sch Med

Backer, Carl L MD [TS] - **Spec Exp:** Pediatric Cardiothoracic Surgery; Transplant-Heart; Tracheal Surgery; Congenital Heart Disease-Adult; **Hospital:** Children's Mem Hosp -Chicago, Northwestern Meml Hosp; **Address:** 2300 Childrens Plaza, MC 22, Chicago, IL 60614-3318; **Phone:** 773-880-4378; **Board Cert:** Thoracic Surgery 2007; Congenital Cardiac Surgery 2009; **Med School:** Mayo Med Sch 1980; **Resid:** Surgery, Northwestern Meml Hosp 1985; **Fellow:** Cardiothoracic Surgery, Northwestern Meml Hosp 1987; Pediatric Cardiac Surgery, Chldns Meml Hosp 1988; **Fac Appt:** Prof S, Northwestern Univ

Bakhos, Mamdouh MD [TS] - **Spec Exp:** Mitral Valve Surgery; Minimally Invasive Cardiac Surgery; Transplant-Heart & Lung; **Hospital:** Loyola Univ Med Ctr, Adv Good Samaritan Hosp; **Address:** Loyola Univ, Dept Cardiothoracic Surgery, 2160 S First Ave, Bldg 110 - rm 6240, Maywood, IL 60153; **Phone:** 708-327-2503; **Board Cert:** Thoracic Surgery 2007; **Med School:** Syria 1971; **Resid:** Surgery, Huron Road Hosp 1976; **Fellow:** Thoracic Surgery, Loyola Univ Med Ctr 1978; **Fac Appt:** Prof TS, Loyola Univ-Stritch Sch Med

Brown, John W MD [TS] - **Spec Exp:** Cardiac Surgery-Neonatal & Pediatric; Transplant-Heart; Heart Valve Surgery; Congenital Heart Disease; **Hospital:** Riley Hosp for Children, IU Health University Hosp; **Address:** Indiana Univ Dept Surgery, 545 Barnhill Drive, EH 215, Indianapolis, IN 46202-5112; **Phone:** 317-274-7150; **Board Cert:** Thoracic Surgery 2007; **Med School:** Indiana Univ 1970; **Resid:** Surgery, Univ Mich Med Ctr 1976; Cardiothoracic Surgery, Univ Mich Med Ctr 1978; **Fellow:** Cardiovascular Surgery, Natl Heart Lung-Blood Inst 1974; **Fac Appt:** Prof S, Indiana Univ

Brunsting III, Louis A MD [TS] - **Spec Exp:** Robotic Cardiac Surgery; **Hospital:** Centennial Med Ctr, Baptist Hosp - Nashville; **Address:** St Vincent's Med Ctr, 2222 Cherry St, Med Bldg 2 - Ste 1250, Toledo, OH 43608; **Phone:** 419-251-3180; **Board Cert:** Thoracic Surgery 2001; **Med School:** UCSD 1983; **Resid:** Surgery, Univ Rochester 1985; Surgery, Univ Rochester 1989; **Fellow:** Surgery, Duke Univ 1987; Thoracic Surgery, Duke Univ 1991

Damiano Jr, Ralph J MD [TS] - **Spec Exp:** Minimally Invasive Cardiac Surgery; Coronary Artery Surgery; Endoscopic Surgery; **Hospital:** Barnes-Jewish Hosp; **Address:** 660 S Euclid Ave, Campus Box 8234, St Louis, MO 63110; **Phone:** 314-362-7327; **Board Cert:** Thoracic Surgery 2002; **Med School:** Duke Univ 1980; **Resid:** Surgery, Duke Univ Med Ctr 1988; **Fellow:** Cardiothoracic Surgery, Duke Univ Med Ctr 1989; **Fac Appt:** Prof S, Washington Univ, St Louis

DeCamp Jr, Malcolm M MD [TS] - **Spec Exp:** Lung Surgery; Esophageal Surgery; Emphysema-Lung Volume Reduction; **Hospital:** Northwestern Meml Hosp; **Address:** Northwestern Div Thoracic Surgery, 676 N St Clair St, Ste 650, Chicago, IL 60611; **Phone:** 312-695-4630; **Board Cert:** Surgery 2001; Thoracic Surgery 2003; **Med School:** Univ Louisville Sch Med 1983; **Resid:** Surgery, Brighams & Womens Hosp 1986; Surgery, Brighams & Womens Hosp 1990; **Fellow:** Cardiac Surgery, Brighams & Womens Hosp 1993; **Fac Appt:** Prof S, Northwestern Univ

Delius, Ralph MD [TS] - **Spec Exp:** Pediatric Cardiac Surgery; Congenital Heart Surgery; **Hospital:** Chldns Hosp of Michigan; **Address:** Chldns Hosp of Michigan, 3901 Beaubien Blvd, Detroit, MI 48201; **Phone:** 313-745-5538; **Board Cert:** Surgery 2001; Thoracic Surgery 2005; **Med School:** UC Davis 1984; **Resid:** Surgery, Univ Michigan Hosp 1989; Cardiothoracic Surgery, Univ Iowa Hosp 1994; **Fellow:** Cardiothoracic Surgery, Univ Michigan Hosp 1990; Cardiac Surgery, Mass Genl Hosp 1992; **Fac Appt:** Assoc Prof S, Wayne State Univ

Deschamps, Claude MD [TS] - **Spec Exp:** Gastroesophageal Reflux Disease (GERD); Esophageal Cancer; Lung Cancer; **Hospital:** St. Mary's Hosp - Rochester MN (Mayo); **Address:** Mayo Clinic, Div Thoracic Surgery, 200 First St SW, Rochester, MN 55905; **Phone:** 507-284-8462; **Board Cert:** Surgery 2004; **Med School:** Univ Montreal 1979; **Resid:** Surgery, Univ Montreal Hosps 1984; Thoracic Surgery, Univ Montreal Hosps 1985; **Fellow:** Thoracic Surgery, Mayo Clinic 1987; **Fac Appt:** Prof S, Mayo Med Sch

Durham, Samuel J MD [TS] - **Spec Exp:** Cardiothoracic Surgery; **Hospital:** Lakeland Specialty Hosp; **Address:** Lakeshore Cardiothoracic Surgery, 2500 Niles Rd, Ste 6, St Joseph, MI 49085; **Phone:** 269-408-1660; **Board Cert:** Surgery 2001; Thoracic Surgery 2003; **Med School:** Harvard Med Sch 1983; **Resid:** Surgery, Univ Pittsburgh Med Ctr 1987; Thoracic Surgery, Univ Pittsburgh Med Ctr 1988; **Fellow:** Pediatric Surgery, Chldren's Hosp 1993; **Fac Appt:** Prof S, Ohio State Univ

Thoracic Surgery

Ferguson, Mark K MD [TS] - **Spec Exp:** Lung Cancer; Esophageal Cancer; Barrett's Esophagus; Minimally Invasive Surgery; **Hospital:** Univ of Chicago Med Ctr; **Address:** Univ Chicago Medical Ctr, 5841 S Maryland Ave, MC 5035, Chicago, IL 60637; **Phone:** 773-702-3551; **Board Cert:** Thoracic Surgery 2003; **Med School:** Univ Chicago-Pritzker Sch Med 1977; **Resid:** Surgery, Univ Chicago Hosps 1982; **Fellow:** Cardiothoracic Surgery, Univ Chicago Hosps 1984; **Fac Appt:** Prof S, Univ Chicago-Pritzker Sch Med

Galantowicz, Mark E MD [TS] - **Spec Exp:** Cardiothoracic Surgery; **Hospital:** Nationwide Chldn's Hosp; **Address:** 700 Children's Drive, Nationwide Chldns Hosp, Columbus, OH 43205; **Phone:** 614-722-3101; **Board Cert:** Thoracic Surgery 2004; **Med School:** Cornell Univ 1987; **Resid:** Surgery, Columbia-Presby Med Ctr 1993; **Fellow:** Cardiothoracic Surgery, Columbia-Presby Med Ctr 1995; **Fac Appt:** Assoc Prof S, Ohio State Univ

Gandy, Kimberly MD/PhD [TS] - **Spec Exp:** Pediatric Cardiac Surgery; Transplant-Heart-Pediatric; Neonatal & Infant Cardiac Surgery; **Hospital:** Chldns Mercy Hosps & Clinics; **Address:** Chldn's Mercy Hosp, 2401 Gillham Rd, Kansas City, MO 64108; **Phone:** 816-234-3580; **Board Cert:** Surgery 2001; Thoracic Surgery 2006; **Med School:** Northwestern Univ 1990; **Resid:** Surgery, Duke Univ Med Ctr 2000; Cardiovascular Surgery, Duke Univ Med Ctr 2003; **Fellow:** Cardiothoracic Research, Stanford Univ Affil Hosp 1995; Pediatric Cardiac Surgery, Stanford Univ Affil Hosp 2005; **Fac Appt:** Assoc Prof Ped, Univ MO-Kansas City

Howington, John A MD [TS] - **Spec Exp:** Lung Cancer; Esophageal Cancer; Thymoma; Minimally Invasive Thoracic Surgery; **Hospital:** Evanston/North Shore Univ Hlth Sys, Highland Park/North Shore Univ Hlth Syst; **Address:** Evanston NorthShore Health System, 2650 Ridge Ave, Walgreen Bldg - Ste 3507, Evanston, IL 60201; **Phone:** 847-570-2868; **Board Cert:** Thoracic Surgery 2006; Surgery 2004; **Med School:** Univ Tenn Coll Med 1989; **Resid:** Surgery, Truman Med Ctr 1994; **Fellow:** Cardiothoracic Surgery, Vanderbilt Univ Med Ctr 1997; **Fac Appt:** Assoc Prof S, Northwestern Univ

Huddleston, Charles B MD [TS] - **Spec Exp:** Transplant-Lung-Pediatric; Transplant-Heart-Pediatric; Hypoplastic Left Heart Syndrome; **Hospital:** St. Louis Chldns Hosp, Barnes-Jewish Hosp; **Address:** St Louis Children's Hospital, One Children's Pl, Ste 5 South 50, St Louis, MO 63110; **Phone:** 314-454-6165; **Board Cert:** Thoracic Surgery 2007; **Med School:** Vanderbilt Univ 1978; **Resid:** Surgery, Vanderbilt Univ Hosp 1986; Cardiothoracic Surgery, Vanderbilt Univ Hosp 1988; **Fellow:** Pediatric Cardiothoracic Surgery, Hosp for Sick Chldn 1989; **Fac Appt:** Prof S, Washington Univ, St Louis

Iannettoni, Mark D MD [TS] - **Spec Exp:** Transplant-Lung; Lung Cancer; Esophageal Surgery; **Hospital:** Univ Iowa Hosp & Clinics; **Address:** Univ Iowa Hosp & Clinics, 200 Hawkins Drive, rm SE514GH, Iowa City, IA 52242; **Phone:** 319-356-1133; **Board Cert:** Surgery 2002; Thoracic Surgery 2002; **Med School:** SUNY Upstate Med Univ 1985; **Resid:** Surgery, SUNY Upstate Med Ctr 1991; Thoracic Surgery, Univ Mich Med Ctr 1993; **Fellow:** Thoracic Surgery, Univ Mich Med Sch 1994

Ilbawi, Michel N MD [TS] - **Spec Exp:** Pediatric Cardiac Surgery; Congenital Anomalies; **Hospital:** Adv Christ Med Ctr, Univ of IL Med Ctr at Chicago; **Address:** Hope Chldns Hosp at Adv Christ Med Ctr, 4440 W 95th St, Oak Lawn, IL 60453; **Phone:** 708-684-3029; **Board Cert:** Thoracic Surgery 2007; Congenital Cardiac Surgery 2009; **Med School:** Lebanon 1971; **Resid:** Surgery, American Univ Hosp 1975; Thoracic Surgery, Univ Hosps 1977; **Fellow:** Thoracic Surgery, Chldns Meml Hosp 1978; **Fac Appt:** Clin Prof S, Univ IL Coll Med

Jeevanandam, Valluvan MD [TS] - **Spec Exp:** Minimally Invasive Heart Valve Surgery; Transplant-Heart; Artificial Heart Devices; **Hospital:** Univ of Chicago Med Ctr; **Address:** 5841 S Maryland Ave, MC 5040, Chicago, IL 60637-1483; **Phone:** 773-702-2500; **Board Cert:** Thoracic Surgery 2002; **Med School:** Columbia P&S 1984; **Resid:** Surgery, Columbia-Presby Med Ctr 1989; **Fellow:** Cardiothoracic Surgery, Columbia-Presby Med Ctr 1991; **Fac Appt:** Prof S, Univ Chicago-Pritzker Sch Med

Joyce, Lyle MD/PhD [TS] - **Spec Exp:** Cardiac Surgery-Adult; Minimally Invasive Cardiac Surgery; Heart Valve Surgery; **Hospital:** Mayo Med Ctr & Clin - Rochester; **Address:** 200 1st St SW, Rochester, MN 55905; **Phone:** 507-255-2000; **Board Cert:** Thoracic Surgery 2003; **Med School:** Baylor Coll Med 1973; **Resid:** Surgery, Univ Minnesota Hosp 1980; Cardiothoracic Surgery, Univ Utah Affil Hosp 1982; **Fac Appt:** Prof S, Mayo Med Sch

Liao, Kenneth K MD [TS] - **Spec Exp:** Minimally Invasive Surgery; Transplant-Heart; Transplant-Lung; Aneurysm-Thoracic Aortic; **Hospital:** Univ Minn Med Ctr, Fairview - Riverside Campus; **Address:** Univ Minnesota- Dept Surgery, 420 Delaware St SE, MMC 207, Minneapolis, MN 55455; **Phone:** 612-625-1400; **Board Cert:** Surgery 2002; Thoracic Surgery 2003; **Med School:** China 1989; **Resid:** Surgery, Brookdale Univ Hosp 1999; Cardiothoracic Surgery, Univ MN Hosp 2002; **Fellow:** Research, Albert Einstein Coll Med 1994; **Fac Appt:** Assoc Prof S, Univ Minn

Love, Robert B MD [TS] - **Spec Exp:** Transplant-Heart & Lung; Lung Cancer; Esophageal Cancer; Heart Valve Surgery; **Hospital:** Loyola Univ Med Ctr; **Address:** Loyola Univ Med Ctr, 2160 S First Ave Bldg 110 - rm 6243, Maywood, IL 60153; **Phone:** 708-327-2488; **Board Cert:** Surgery 2007; Thoracic Surgery 2000; Surgical Critical Care 2001; **Med School:** Rush Med Coll 1982; **Resid:** Surgery, Univ of Wisconsin Hosp 1988; Thoracic Surgery, Gloucestershire Royal Hosp 1989; **Fellow:** Cardiothoracic Surgery, Univ of Wisconsin Hosp 1991; **Fac Appt:** Prof TS, Loyola Univ-Stritch Sch Med

Lytle, Bruce W MD [TS] - **Spec Exp:** Heart Valve Surgery; Coronary Artery Surgery; Aortic Surgery; **Hospital:** Cleveland Clin (page 56); **Address:** Cleveland Clinic, Dept Thoracic Surgery, 9500 Euclid Ave, MC J4-1, Cleveland, OH 44195; **Phone:** 216-444-6962; **Board Cert:** Thoracic Surgery 2007; **Med School:** Harvard Med Sch 1971; **Resid:** Surgery, Mass Genl Hsop 1975; Surgery, Shotley Bridge Hosp 1976; **Fellow:** Thoracic Surgery, Mass Genl Hosp 1979; **Fac Appt:** Prof TS, Cleveland Cl Coll Med/Case West Res

Maddaus, Michael A MD [TS] - **Spec Exp:** Esophageal Cancer; Lung Cancer; Minimally Invasive Thoracic Surgery; **Hospital:** Abbott - Northwestern Hosp; **Address:** Univ Minn Med Ctr, Div Thoracic Surgery, 420 Delaware St SE, MMC 207, Minneapolis, MN 55455; **Phone:** 612-624-9461; **Board Cert:** Surgery 2000; Thoracic Surgery 2003; **Med School:** Univ Minn 1982; **Resid:** Surgery, Univ Minn Affil Hosp 1990; Thoracic Surgery, Univ Toronto Affil Hosp 1991; **Fellow:** Cardiac Surgery, St Michael's Hosp/Hosp Sick Chldn 1992; Thoracic Oncology, Meml Sloan Kettering Cancer Ctr 1992; **Fac Appt:** Prof S, Univ Minn

Mason, David P MD [TS] - **Spec Exp:** Minimally Invasive Thoracic Surgery; Lung Cancer; Mesothelioma; Transplant-Lung; **Hospital:** Cleveland Clin (page 56); **Address:** Cleveland Clinic, 9500 Euclid Ave, MC J41, Cleveland, OH 44195; **Phone:** 216-444-4053; **Board Cert:** Surgery 2002; Thoracic Surgery 2004; **Med School:** Columbia P&S 1994; **Resid:** Surgery, Brigham & Womens Hosp 2001; **Fellow:** Vascular Surgery, Univ Washington 1999; Thoracic Surgery, Brigham & Womens Hosp 2003

Mavroudis, Constantine MD [TS] - **Spec Exp:** Pediatric Cardiac Surgery; Congenital Heart Disease; Transplant-Heart & Lung; **Hospital:** Cleveland Clin (page 56); **Address:** 9500 Euclid Ave, Pediatric Cardiology, M41, Cleveland, OH 44195; **Phone:** 216-636-5288; **Board Cert:** Surgery 2000; Thoracic Surgery 2000; **Med School:** Univ VA Sch Med 1973; **Resid:** Surgery, UCSF Med Ctr 1979; **Fellow:** Thoracic Surgery, UCSF Med Ctr 1977; **Fac Appt:** Prof S, Northwestern Univ

McCarthy, Patrick M MD [TS] - **Spec Exp:** Heart Valve Surgery; Coronary Artery Surgery; Ventricular Assist Device (LVAD); **Hospital:** Northwestern Meml Hosp; **Address:** Bluhm Cardiovascular Inst, 675 N St Clair St, Galter 19-100, Chicago, IL 60611-2968; **Phone:** 312-695-4965; **Board Cert:** Thoracic Surgery 2008; **Med School:** Loyola Univ-Stritch Sch Med 1980; **Resid:** Surgery, Mayo Clinic 1985; Thoracic Surgery, Mayo Clinic 1988; **Fellow:** Cardiopulmonary Transplant Surgery, Stanford Univ 1989; **Fac Appt:** Prof S, Northwestern Univ

Meyers, Bryan MD [TS] - **Spec Exp:** Lung Cancer; Esophageal Cancer; Transplant-Lung; Emphysema-Lung Volume Reduction; **Hospital:** Barnes-Jewish Hosp, Barnes-Jewish West County Hosp; **Address:** 4921 Parkview Pl, Ste 8B, St Louis, MO 63110; **Phone:** 314-362-8598; **Board Cert:** Thoracic Surgery 2007; **Med School:** Univ Chicago-Pritzker Sch Med 1986; **Resid:** Surgery, Mass Genl Hosp 1996; **Fellow:** Cardiothoracic Surgery, Barnes Hosp-Wash Univ 1998; **Fac Appt:** Assoc Prof S, Washington Univ, St Louis

Moon, Marc R MD [TS] - **Spec Exp:** Aneurysm-Thoracic Aortic; Cardiothoracic Surgery; Mitral Valve Surgery; **Hospital:** Barnes-Jewish Hosp; **Address:** Barnes Jewish Hospital, Queeny Tower, One Barnes Jewish Hospital Plaza, Ste 3108, St Louis, MO 63110-1094; **Phone:** 314-362-0993; **Board Cert:** Surgery 2005; Thoracic Surgery 2008; **Med School:** Wayne State Univ 1988; **Resid:** Surgery, Med Coll Wisconsin 1995; Thoracic Surgery, Stanford U Med Ctr 1996; **Fac Appt:** Prof S, Washington Univ, St Louis

Naunheim, Keith S MD [TS] - **Spec Exp:** Lung Cancer; Esophageal Cancer; Chest Wall Tumors; Video Assisted Thoracic Surgery (VATS); **Hospital:** St. Louis Univ Hosp, SSM St Mary's Hlth Ctr - St Louis; **Address:** 3655 Vista Ave Fl 1, St Louis, MO 63110; **Phone:** 314-577-8360; **Board Cert:** Thoracic Surgery 2004; **Med School:** Univ Chicago-Pritzker Sch Med 1978; **Resid:** Surgery, Univ Chicago Hosp 1983; **Fellow:** Cardiothoracic Surgery, Univ Chicago Hosp 1985; **Fac Appt:** Prof TS, St Louis Univ

Orringer, Mark B MD [TS] - **Spec Exp:** Esophageal Cancer; Lung Cancer; Mediastinal Tumors; Lung Cancer; **Hospital:** Univ of Michigan Hosp; **Address:** Univ Mich, Taubman Ctr, 1500 E Medical Center Drive, 2120 TC, SPC 5344, Ann Arbor, MI 48109; **Phone:** 734-936-4975; **Board Cert:** Surgery 1973; Thoracic Surgery 1974; **Med School:** Univ Pittsburgh 1967; **Resid:** Thoracic Surgery, Johns Hopkins Hosp 1973; **Fac Appt:** Prof S, Univ Mich Med Sch

Pagani, Francis D MD/PhD [TS] - **Spec Exp:** Transplant-Heart; Coronary Artery Surgery; Left Ventricular Assist Device (LVAD); **Hospital:** Univ of Michigan Hosp; **Address:** Univ Mich Med Ctr, 5144 Cardiovascular Ctr, 1500 E Med Ctr Drive, SPC 5864, Ann Arbor, MI 48109-5864; **Phone:** 734-647-2894; **Board Cert:** Surgery 2002; Thoracic Surgery 2004; **Med School:** Georgetown Univ 1986; **Resid:** Surgery, Georgetown Univ Med Ctr 1993; Thoracic Surgery, Univ Mich Hosp 1995; **Fellow:** Research, Univ Mass Med Ctr 1990; **Fac Appt:** Prof S, Univ Mich Med Sch

Patterson, G Alexander MD [TS] - **Spec Exp:** Lung Cancer; Esophageal Cancer; Transplant-Lung; Transplant-Heart & Lung; **Hospital:** Barnes-Jewish Hosp; **Address:** 660 S Euclid Ave, Box 8234, St Louis, MO 63110; **Phone:** 314-362-6025; **Board Cert:** Surgery 1978; Thoracic Surgery 1981; Vascular Surgery 1982; **Med School:** Canada 1974; **Resid:** Surgery, Queens Univ Med Ctr 1978; Vascular Surgery, Univ Toronto Med Ctr 1979; **Fellow:** Research, Toronto Genl Hosp 1981; Surgical Critical Care, Johns Hopkins Hosp 1982; **Fac Appt:** Prof S, Washington Univ, St Louis

Rice, Thomas W MD [TS] - **Spec Exp:** Esophageal Surgery; Minimally Invasive Thoracic Surgery; Lung Cancer; **Hospital:** Cleveland Clin (page 56); **Address:** Cleveland Clinic, 9500 Euclid Ave, Desk J4-1, Cleveland, OH 44195; **Phone:** 216-444-1921; **Board Cert:** Surgery 2004; Thoracic Surgery 2005; **Med School:** Univ Toronto 1978; **Resid:** Surgery, Univ Toronto Med Ctr 1983; Thoracic Surgery, Univ Toronto Med Ctr 1986; **Fellow:** Pulmonary Disease, UCSF Med Ctr 1984; **Fac Appt:** Prof S, Cleveland Cl Coll Med/Case West Res

Schaff, Hartzell MD [TS] - **Spec Exp:** Heart Valve Surgery; Congenital Heart Disease; Maze Procedure for Atrial Fibrillation; **Hospital:** St. Mary's Hosp - Rochester MN (Mayo); **Address:** Mayo Clin, Div Cardiovasc Surg, 200 First St SW, Rochester, MN 55905-0001; **Phone:** 507-255-7068; **Board Cert:** Thoracic Surgery 2010; **Med School:** Univ Okla Coll Med 1973; **Resid:** Surgery, Johns Hopkins Hosp 1978; Thoracic Surgery, Johns Hopkins Hosp 1980; **Fellow:** Surgery, Johns Hopkins Hosp 1976; **Fac Appt:** Prof S, Mayo Med Sch

Smedira, Nicholas MD [TS] - **Spec Exp:** Transplant-Heart; Transplant-Lung; Ventricular Assist Device (LVAD); Aortic Surgery; **Hospital:** Cleveland Clin (page 56); **Address:** Cleveland Clin, Dept Cardiothoracic Surg, 9500 Euclid Ave, Desk J4-1, Cleveland, OH 44195; **Phone:** 216-445-7052; **Board Cert:** Thoracic Surgery 2003; **Med School:** Univ Rochester 1984; **Resid:** Surgery, UCSF Med Ctr 1991; Thoracic Surgery, UCSF Med Ctr 1994; **Fellow:** Cardiothoracic Surgery, UCSF Med Ctr 1994

Smith, John Michael MD [TS] - **Spec Exp:** Mitral Valve Robotic Surgery; **Hospital:** Good Samaritan Hosp - Cincinnati; **Address:** 4030 Smith Rd, Ste 300, Cincinnati, OH 45209; **Phone:** 513-421-3494; **Board Cert:** Surgery 2003; Thoracic Surgery 2006; **Med School:** Univ Louisville Sch Med 1989; **Resid:** Surgery, Good Samaritan Hosp 1994; **Fellow:** Cardiothoracic Surgery, Yale Univ Hosp 1996

Stuart, Richard MD [TS] - **Spec Exp:** Cardiac Surgery; Cardiothoracic Surgery; Robotic Cardiac Surgery; **Hospital:** St. Luke's Hosp of Kansas City, N Kansas City Hosp; **Address:** 4320 Wornall Rd Bldg 2 - Ste 50, Kansas City, MO 64111; **Phone:** 816-931-3312; **Board Cert:** Thoracic Surgery 1999; Surgical Critical Care 2003; **Med School:** Johns Hopkins Univ 1981; **Resid:** Surgery, Johns Hopkins Hosp 1986; **Fellow:** Cardiothoracic Surgery, Johns Hopkins Hosp 1989; **Fac Appt:** Clin Prof TS, Univ MO-Kansas City

Svensson, Lars G MD/PhD [TS] - **Spec Exp:** Aortic Surgery; Heart Valve Surgery; Heart Valve-Percutaneous; Marfan's Syndrome; **Hospital:** Cleveland Clin (page 56); **Address:** Cleveland Clinic, 9500 Euclid Ave, MC J4-1, Cleveland, OH 44195; **Phone:** 216-445-4813; **Med School:** South Africa 1978; **Resid:** Surgery, Johannesburg Hosp 1986; Cardiothoracic Surgery, Baylor Coll of Med 1991; **Fellow:** Cardiovascular Surgery, Cleveland Clinic 1987; Cardiovascular Surgery, Baylor Coll of Med 1989; **Fac Appt:** Prof S, Case West Res Univ

Turrentine, Mark W MD [TS] - **Spec Exp:** Cardiac Surgery-Pediatric; Transplant-Heart; Transplant-Lung; Congenital Heart Disease; **Hospital:** Riley Hosp for Children, IU Health University Hosp; **Address:** Indiana Univ Dept Surgery, 545 Barnhill Drive, EH 215, Indianapolis, IN 46202; **Phone:** 317-274-1121; **Board Cert:** Thoracic Surgery 2002; **Med School:** Univ Kansas 1983; **Resid:** Surgery, Univ Kansas Med Ctr 1988; Cardiothoracic Surgery, Indiana Univ Med Ctr 1991; **Fellow:** Cardiothoracic Surgery, Texas Heart Inst 1986; Transplant Surgery, Indiana Univ Med Ctr 1989; **Fac Appt:** Prof S, Indiana Univ

Vigneswaran, Wickii MD [TS] - **Spec Exp:** Transplant-Lung; Thoracic Cancers; Mesothelioma; Hyperhidrosis-Palmar; **Hospital:** Univ of Chicago Med Ctr; **Address:** Univ Chicago Hosps, Lung Transplant Div, 5841 S Maryland Ave, MC 5040, Chicago, IL 60637; **Phone:** 773-795-1267; **Med School:** Sri Lanka 1978; **Resid:** Surgery, Royal Coll Surgeons 1983; Cardiothoracic Surgery, Royal Coll Surgeons 1990; **Fellow:** Cardiothoracic Transplant Surg, Mayo Clin 1994; **Fac Appt:** Prof S, Univ Chicago-Pritzker Sch Med

Walters, Henry L MD [TS] - **Spec Exp:** Pediatric Cardiac Surgery; Transplant-Heart-Pediatric; Cardiac Surgery-Neonatal; **Hospital:** Chldns Hosp of Michigan; **Address:** Chldns Hosp of Michigan, 3901 Beaubien Blvd, Detroit, MI 48201; **Phone:** 313-745-5538; **Board Cert:** Thoracic Surgery 2009; Congenital Cardiac Surgery 2009; **Med School:** Baylor Coll Med 1982; **Resid:** Surgery, Mass Genl Hosp 1988; **Fellow:** Pediatric Cardiothoracic Surgery, UAB Med Ctr 1992; **Fac Appt:** Prof S, Wayne State Univ

Thoracic Surgery

Weigel, Tracey MD [TS] - **Spec Exp:** Esophageal Cancer; Lung Cancer; Mesothelioma; Graves' Disease; **Hospital:** Univ WI Hosp & Clins; **Address:** Univ Wisconsin Hosp - Thoracic Surg, 600 Highland Ave, H4/316 CSS, Madison, WI 53792-7375; **Phone:** 608-265-0499; **Board Cert:** Surgery 2003; Thoracic Surgery 2006; **Med School:** Univ Rochester 1986; **Resid:** Surgery, Rhode Island Hosp 1993; **Fellow:** Surgical Oncology, Meml Sloan Kettering Cancer Ctr 1995; Cardiothoracic Surgery, Univ Wisconsin 1996; **Fac Appt:** Assoc Prof S, Univ Wisc

Ziemer, Gerhard MD/PhD [TS] - **Spec Exp:** Pediatric Cardiac Surgery; Neonatal & Infanct Cardiac Surgery; Congenital Heart Disease; **Hospital:** Univ of Chicago Med Ctr; **Address:** Univ Chicago-Pediatric Cardiac Surgery, 5841 S Maryland Ave, MC 5040, Chicago, IL 60637; **Phone:** 773-702-2500; **Med School:** Germany 1978; **Resid:** Surgery, Hannover Med School Affil Hosp 1984; Cardiothoracic Surgery, Chldn's Hosp 1986; **Fellow:** Cardiothoracic Surgery, Hannover Med Schol Affil Hosp 1988; **Fac Appt:** Prof S, Univ Chicago-Pritzker Sch Med

Great Plains and Mountains

Bull, David A MD [TS] - **Spec Exp:** Cardiothoracic Surgery; Esophageal Cancer; **Hospital:** Univ Utah Hlth Care; **Address:** Univ Utah, Dept Cardiothoracic Surgery, 30 N 1900 East, Ste 3C127, Salt Lake City, UT 84132; **Phone:** 801-581-5311; **Board Cert:** Surgery 2008; Surgical Critical Care 1999; Vascular Surgery 2003; Thoracic Surgery 2004; **Med School:** UCSF 1985; **Resid:** Surgery, UCSF Medical Ctr 1987; Surgery, Univ Arizona Hosps 1990; **Fellow:** Vascular Surgery, Univ Arizona Hosps 1992; Cardiothoracic Surgery, Univ Arizona Hosps 1994; **Fac Appt:** Assoc Prof TS, Univ Utah

Campbell, David N MD [TS] - **Spec Exp:** Pediatric Cardiothoracic Surgery; Transplant-Heart-Pediatric; Transplant-Lung; Congenital Heart Surgery; **Hospital:** Chldn's Hosp - Aurora (CO), Univ of CO Hosp - Anschutz Inpatient Pav; **Address:** Childrens Hosp Cardiothoracic Surgery, 13123 E 16th Ave, B-200, Aurora, CO 80045; **Phone:** 720-777-6624; **Board Cert:** Surgery 1999; Thoracic Surgery 2010; Surgical Critical Care 2000; Congenital Cardiac Surgery 2009; **Med School:** Rush Med Coll 1974; **Resid:** Surgery, Univ Colo Med Ctr 1980; Cardiothoracic Surgery, Univ Colo Med Ctr 1979; **Fellow:** Cardiothoracic Surgery, Childrens Hosp 1980; **Fac Appt:** Prof S, Univ Colorado

Fullerton, David A MD [TS] - **Spec Exp:** Maze Procedure for Atrial Fibrillation; Ross Procedure for Aortic Valve Disease; Mitral Valve Surgery; Transplant-Heart & Lung; **Hospital:** Univ of CO Hosp - Anschutz Inpatient Pav, VA Eastern CO Health Care Sys-Denver; **Address:** Univ of Colorado, Cardiothoracic Surgery, 12631 E 17th Ave, rm 6602, MS C310, Aurora, CO 80045; **Phone:** 303-724-2798; **Board Cert:** Surgery 2007; Surgical Critical Care 2001; Thoracic Surgery 2001; **Med School:** Univ MO-Columbia Sch Med 1981; **Resid:** Surgery, Univ Wash Med Ctr 1987; Thoracic Surgery, Univ Colorado Hosp 1990; **Fac Appt:** Prof S, Univ Colorado

Karwande, Shreekanth V MD [TS] - **Spec Exp:** Thoracic Cancers; Lung Cancer; Cardiac Surgery; **Hospital:** St. Mark's Hosp - Salt Lake City; **Address:** MountainStar Cardiovascular Surgery, 1160 E 3900 St S, Ste 3500, Salt Lake City, UT 84124; **Phone:** 801-743-4750; **Board Cert:** Thoracic Surgery 2003; **Med School:** India 1973; **Resid:** Surgery, Erie Co Med Ctr 1981; Cardiothoracic Surgery, NY Hosp 1985; **Fellow:** Cardiothoracic Surgery, Meml Sloan Kettering Cancer Ctr

Mitchell, John D MD [TS] - **Spec Exp:** Lung Cancer; Esophageal Surgery; Transplant-Lung; Hyperhidrosis-Palmar; **Hospital:** Univ of CO Hosp - Anschutz Inpatient Pav, VA Eastern CO Health Care Sys-Denver; **Address:** Univ Colorado, Dept Cardiothoracic Surg, 12631 E 17th Ave, MS C310, Aurora, CO 80045; **Phone:** 303-724-2800; **Board Cert:** Surgery 2005; Thoracic Surgery 2007; **Med School:** Univ Mich Med Sch 1987; **Resid:** Surgery, Mass Genl Hosp 1994; Cardiothoracic Surgery, Mass Genl Hosp 1996; **Fac Appt:** Assoc Prof TS, Univ Colorado

Mitchell, Max B MD [TS] - **Spec Exp:** Congenital Heart Surgery; Heart Valve Surgery; Pediatric Cardiac Surgery; Transplant-Lung; **Hospital:** Chldn's Hosp - Aurora (CO), Univ of CO Hosp - Anschutz Inpatient Pav; **Address:** Childrens Hosp Cardiothoracic Surgery, 13123 E 16th Ave, B-200, Aurora, CO 80045; **Phone:** 720-777-6624; **Board Cert:** Surgery 2004; Thoracic Surgery 2007; Congenital Cardiac Surgery 2009; **Med School:** Geo Wash Univ 1988; **Resid:** Surgery, Univ Colorado Affil Hosp 1995; Cardiovascular Surgery, Univ Colorado Affil Hosp 1998; **Fellow:** Pediatric Cardiac Surgery, Royal Childrens Hosp 1999; **Fac Appt:** Assoc Prof S, Univ Colorado

Southwest

Aklog, Lishan MD [TS] - **Spec Exp:** Mitral Valve Surgery; Minimally Invasive Cardiac Surgery; Coronary Artery Surgery; Heart Failure; **Hospital:** St. Joseph's Hosp & Med Ctr - Phoenix; **Address:** Heart and Lung Inst at St Josephs, 500 W Thomas Rd, Ste 500, Phoenix, AZ 85013-4224; **Phone:** 602-406-4000; **Board Cert:** Thoracic Surgery 2000; **Med School:** Harvard Med Sch 1989; **Resid:** Surgery, Brigham & Womens Hosp 1996; **Fellow:** Cardiothoracic Surgery, Brigham & Womens Hosp 1998; Cardiac Surgery, Harefield Hosp 1999

Calhoon, John H MD [TS] - **Spec Exp:** Transplant-Heart & Lung; Congenital Heart Surgery; Cardiac Surgery-Adult & Pediatric; **Hospital:** Univ Hlth Syst-San Antonio, Christus Santa Rosa Children's Hosp; **Address:** UTHSCSA, Dept Thoracic Surg, 7703 Floyd Curl Drive, MC 7841, San Antonio, TX 78229-3901; **Phone:** 210-567-2878; **Board Cert:** Surgery 2004; Thoracic Surgery 2007; **Med School:** Baylor Coll Med 1981; **Resid:** Surgery, Univ Hosp/Univ Texas HSC 1986; Univ Hosp/Univ Texas HSC 1988; **Fellow:** Pediatric Cardiac Surgery, Chldns Hosp/Harvard 1989; **Fac Appt:** Prof TS, Univ Tex, San Antonio

Coselli, Joseph S MD [TS] - **Spec Exp:** Aneurysm-Abdominal & Thoracic Aortic; Marfan's Syndrome; Aortic Surgery; **Hospital:** St. Luke's Episcopal Hosp-Houston; **Address:** 6770 Bertner St, Ste C350, Houston, TX 77030; **Phone:** 832-355-9910; **Board Cert:** Thoracic Surgery 2004; **Med School:** Univ Tex Med Br, Galveston 1977; **Resid:** Surgery, Baylor Coll Med 1982; Thoracic Surgery, Baylor Coll Med 1984; **Fac Appt:** Assoc Prof S, Baylor Coll Med

Diethrich, Edward B MD [TS] - **Spec Exp:** Vascular Surgery; Endovascular Surgery; Cardiovascular Surgery; **Hospital:** Arizona Heart Hosp; **Address:** Arizona Heart Inst, 2632 N 20th St, Phoenix, AZ 85006-1339; **Phone:** 602-266-2200; **Board Cert:** Thoracic Surgery 1967; Surgery 1966; **Med School:** Univ Mich Med Sch 1960; **Resid:** Surgery, St Joseph Mercy Hosp 1964; **Fellow:** Cardiothoracic Surgery, Baylor Coll Med 1966; **Fac Appt:** Prof TS, Univ Ariz Coll Med

Echeverri, Luis G MD [TS] - **Spec Exp:** Cardiac Surgery; Aortic Surgery; Transplant-Heart; **Hospital:** St. Luke's Episcopal Hosp-Houston; **Address:** 7737 SW Freeway, Ste 201, Houston, TX 77074; **Phone:** 713-776-3402; **Board Cert:** Surgery 2007; Thoracic Surgery 2010; **Med School:** Colombia 1982; **Resid:** Surgery, Univ Texas Med Ctr 1996; Cardiothoracic Surgery, Univ Arizona 2001; **Fellow:** Transplant Surgery, Univ Pittsburgh 1993; Cardiovascular Surgery, Texas Heart Inst 1998

Forbess, Joseph M MD [TS] - **Spec Exp:** Pediatric Cardiothoracic Surgery; Heart Valve Surgery-Pediatric; **Hospital:** Chldns Med Ctr of Dallas, UT Southwestern Med Ctr at Dallas; **Address:** Univ Texas SW Med Ctr, Div Ped Cardiothor Surg, 1935 Medical District Drive, MC C3211, Dallas, TX 75235; **Phone:** 214-456-5000; **Board Cert:** Surgery 2008; **Med School:** Harvard Med Sch 1990; **Resid:** Surgery, Duke Univ Med Ctr 1997; Cardiothoracic Surgery, Duke Univ Med Ctr 1999; **Fellow:** Cardiac Surgery, Childrens Hosp 1994; **Fac Appt:** Assoc Prof TS, Univ Tex SW, Dallas

Fraser, Charles D MD [TS] - **Spec Exp:** Pediatric Cardiothoracic Surgery; Congenital Heart Surgery; **Hospital:** Texas Chldns Hosp; **Address:** Texas Chldns Hosp-Heart Ctr, 6621 Fannin St, MC 19-345H, Houston, TX 77030-2399; **Phone:** 832-826-2030; **Board Cert:** Surgery 2010; Thoracic Surgery 2002; Congenital Cardiac Surgery 2009; **Med School:** Univ Tex Med Br, Galveston 1984; **Resid:** Surgery, Johns Hopkins Hosp 1990; Cardiovascular Surgery, Johns Hopkins Hosp 1993; **Fac Appt:** Prof S, Baylor Coll Med

Frazier, O Howard MD [TS] - **Spec Exp:** Transplant-Heart; Lung Surgery; Artificial Heart Devices; **Hospital:** St. Luke's Episcopal Hosp-Houston; **Address:** Surgical Assocs - Texas Heart Institute, PO Box 20345, MC 2-114A, Houston, TX 77030; **Phone:** 832-355-4900; **Board Cert:** Surgery 1975; Thoracic Surgery 2005; **Med School:** Baylor Coll Med 1967; **Resid:** Surgery, Baylor Affil Hosp 1974; Thoracic Surgery, Texas Heart Inst 1976; **Fac Appt:** Prof S, Univ Tex, Houston

Harrell Jr, James E MD [TS] - **Spec Exp:** Transplant-Heart; Cardiac Surgery-Pediatric; **Hospital:** Covenant Children's Hosp; **Address:** 3606 21st St, Ste 103, Lubbock, TX 79410; **Phone:** 806-725-4425; **Board Cert:** Surgery 2006; Thoracic Surgery 2006; **Med School:** Baylor Coll Med 1978; **Resid:** Surgery, Univ Tex Hlth Scis Ctr 1984; Thoracic Surgery, Baylor Coll Med 1986; **Fellow:** Cardiovascular Surgery, Hosp Sick Chldn 1987

Jessen, Michael Erik MD [TS] - **Spec Exp:** Cardiac Surgery; Transplant-Heart; Aneurysm-Aortic; Heart Valve Surgery; **Hospital:** UT Southwestern Med Ctr at Dallas, Baylor Univ Medical Ctr-Dallas; **Address:** 5323 Harry Hines Blvd, MC 8879, Dallas, TX 75390-8879; **Phone:** 214-645-7721; **Board Cert:** Surgery 2007; Thoracic Surgery 2000; **Med School:** Univ Manitoba 1981; **Resid:** Surgery, Univ Manitoba 1986; Thoracic Surgery, Duke Univ Med Ctr 1990; **Fellow:** Research, Duke Univ Med Ctr 1988; **Fac Appt:** Prof TS, Univ Tex SW, Dallas

Johnson, Scott B MD [TS] - **Spec Exp:** Thoracic Cancers; **Hospital:** Univ Hlth Syst-San Antonio; **Address:** UT Hlth-San Antonio, Cardiac Surgery, 7703 Floyd Curl Drive, MSC7841, San Antonio, TX 78229; **Phone:** 210-567-5615; **Board Cert:** Surgery 2000; Surgical Critical Care 2001; Thoracic Surgery 2004; **Med School:** Univ New Mexico 1987; **Resid:** Surgery, LAC-USC Hosp 1992; Surgery, UTHSC V Hosp 1995; **Fellow:** Cardiothoracic Surgery, LAC-USC Hosp 1993

Kernstine, Kemp H MD/PhD [TS] - **Spec Exp:** Lung Cancer; Esophageal Cancer; Tracheal Surgery; Esophageal Surgery; **Hospital:** UT Southwestern Med Ctr at Dallas; **Address:** U Texas SW Med Ctr, Cardiothoracic Surgery, 5323 Harry Hines Blvd Fl 9, Ste HA09.134, Dallas, TX 75390-8879; **Phone:** 214-645-7748; **Board Cert:** Thoracic Surgery 2004; Surgery 2001; **Med School:** Duke Univ 1982; **Resid:** Surgery, Univ Minn Med Ctr 1988; **Fellow:** Cardiothoracic Surgery, Brigham & Women's Hosp 1994; **Fac Appt:** Prof TS, Univ Tex SW, Dallas

Lanza, Louis MD [TS] - **Spec Exp:** Lung Cancer; Cardiac Surgery; **Hospital:** Mayo Clinic - Scottsdale; **Address:** Mayo Clinic Hosp, 5779 E Mayo Blvd MCSB Bldg Fl 1, Phoenix, AZ 85054; **Phone:** 480-342-2270; **Board Cert:** Thoracic Surgery 2002; **Med School:** Loyola Univ-Stritch Sch Med 1981; **Resid:** Surgery, Univ Michigan Med Ctr 1988; Cardiovascular Surgery, Texas Heart Inst 1991; **Fellow:** Surgical Oncology, Natl Cancer Inst 1986; Thoracic Oncology, MD Anderson Cancer Ctr 1989

Mack, Michael J MD [TS] - **Spec Exp:** Transplant-Heart & Lung; Cardiac Surgery; Minimally Invasive Surgery; **Hospital:** Med City Dallas Hosp, Med Ctr of Plano; **Address:** 4708 Alliance Blvd, Pavilion 1, Ste 700, Plano, TX 75093; **Phone:** 972-596-6676; **Board Cert:** Internal Medicine 1976; Thoracic Surgery 2001; **Med School:** St Louis Univ 1973; **Resid:** Internal Medicine, Univ MN Hosp 1976; Surgery, Parkland Hosp 1980; **Fellow:** Thoracic Surgery, Parkland Hosp 1982

Ott, David A MD [TS] - **Spec Exp:** Heart Valve Surgery; Coronary Artery Surgery; Aneurysm-Abdominal Aortic; Carotid Artery Surgery; **Hospital:** St. Luke's Episcopal Hosp-Houston; **Address:** 1101 Bates St, Ste P-514, Houston, TX 77030-2607; **Phone:** 832-355-4900; **Board Cert:** Thoracic Surgery 2008; **Med School:** Baylor Coll Med 1972; **Resid:** Surgery, Baylor Coll Med 1976; Cardiothoracic Surgery, Tex Heart Inst 1978; **Fac Appt:** Clin Prof S, Baylor Coll Med

Reardon, Michael J MD [TS] - **Spec Exp:** Cardiac Tumors/Cancer; Heart Valve Surgery-Aortic; **Hospital:** Methodist Hosp - Houston, UT MD Anderson Cancer Ctr; **Address:** 6550 Fannin St, Ste 1401, Houston, TX 77030; **Phone:** 713-441-5200; **Board Cert:** Thoracic Surgery 2006; **Med School:** Baylor Coll Med 1978; **Resid:** Surgery, Baylor Affil Hosps 1983; Thoracic Surgery, Texas Heart Inst 1985; **Fac Appt:** Prof TS, Cornell Univ-Weill Med Coll

Rice, David C MD [TS] - **Spec Exp:** Mesothelioma; Thoracic Cancers; Minimally Invasive Surgery; **Hospital:** UT MD Anderson Cancer Ctr; **Address:** MD Anderson Cancer Ctr, 1515 Holcombe Blvd, Box 1489, Houston, TX 77030; **Phone:** 713-794-1477; **Board Cert:** Surgery 2002; Thoracic Surgery 2004; **Med School:** Ireland 1991; **Resid:** Surgery, Mayo Clinic 1998; Cardiothoracic Surgery, Baylor Affil Hosps 2001; **Fellow:** Thoracic Surgery, Mayo Clinic 1999

Roth, Jack MD [TS] - **Spec Exp:** Esophageal Cancer; Lung Cancer; Gene Therapy; **Hospital:** UT MD Anderson Cancer Ctr; **Address:** Dept Thoracic & Cardiovasc Surg, 1515 Holcombe Blvd, Unit 1489, Houston, TX 77030-4000; **Phone:** 713-792-7664; **Board Cert:** Thoracic Surgery 2002; **Med School:** Johns Hopkins Univ 1971; **Resid:** Surgery, Johns Hopkins Hosp 1973; Thoracic Surgery, UCLA Ctr Hlth Sci 1979; **Fellow:** Surgical Oncology, UCLA Div Surg Onc 1975; **Fac Appt:** Prof TS, Univ Tex, Houston

Safi, Hazim J MD [TS] - **Spec Exp:** Aneurysm-Abdominal Aortic; **Hospital:** Meml Hermann Hosp - Texas Med Ctr; **Address:** UT, Dept Cardiothoracic & Vascular Surg, 6400 Fannin St, Ste 2850, Houston, TX 77030; **Phone:** 713-500-5304; **Board Cert:** Vascular Surgery 2005; Thoracic Surgery 2007; **Med School:** Iraq 1970; **Resid:** Surgery, Baylor Coll Med 1980; Radiation Oncology, Baylor Coll Med 1981; **Fellow:** Thoracic Surgery, Baylor Coll Med 1983; **Fac Appt:** Assoc Prof S, Univ Tex, Houston

Smythe, W Roy MD [TS] - **Spec Exp:** Lung Cancer; Mesothelioma; **Hospital:** Scott & White Mem Hosp; **Address:** 2401 S 31st St, Temple, TX 76508; **Phone:** 254-724-2334; **Board Cert:** Thoracic Surgery 2000; **Med School:** Texas A&M Univ 1989; **Resid:** Surgery, Hosp Univ Penn 1996; **Fellow:** Cardiothoracic Surgery, Hosp Univ Penn 1998; Surgical Oncology, Am Cancer Soc 1996; **Fac Appt:** Asst Prof S, Univ Tex, Houston

Swisher, Stephen G MD [TS] - **Spec Exp:** Esophageal Cancer; Lung Cancer; Mesothelioma; Thoracic Cancers; **Hospital:** UT MD Anderson Cancer Ctr; **Address:** Dept of Thoracic & Cardiovasc Surg, 1515 Holcombe Blvd, Unit 1489, Houston, TX 77030; **Phone:** 713-792-8659; **Board Cert:** Surgery 2002; Thoracic Surgery 2006; **Med School:** UCSD 1986; **Resid:** Surgery, UCLA Med Ctr 1993; **Fellow:** Surgical Oncology, UCLA Med Ctr 1990; Cardiothoracic Surgery, MD Anderson Canc Ctr 1996; **Fac Appt:** Prof TS, Univ Tex, Houston

Turner, William F MD [TS] - **Spec Exp:** Coronary Artery Surgery; Cardiac Surgery; **Hospital:** E TX Med Ctr-Tyler, Trinity Mother Frances Hosp; **Address:** 619 S Fleichel St, Ste 207, Tyler, TX 75701; **Phone:** 903-593-0900; **Board Cert:** Thoracic Surgery 2008; **Med School:** Baylor Coll Med 1981; **Resid:** Surgery, Baylor Coll Med 1987; Thoracic Surgery, Baylor Coll Med 1989

Walsh, Garrett MD [TS] - **Spec Exp:** Esophageal Cancer; **Hospital:** UT MD Anderson Cancer Ctr; **Address:** 1515 Holcombe Blvd, Unit 1489, Houston, TX 77030; **Phone:** 713-792-6849; **Board Cert:** Surgery 2009; Thoracic Surgery 2009; **Med School:** Queens Univ 1983; **Resid:** Surgery, Royal Victoria Hosp-McGill 1988; Cardiovascular Surgery, McGill Univ 1990

Thoracic Surgery

West Coast and Pacific

Aldea, Gabriel S MD [TS] - **Spec Exp:** Thoracic Aortic Surgery; Heart Valve Surgery; Minimally Invasive Cardiac Surgery; **Hospital:** Univ Wash Med Ctr; **Address:** Univ Washington-Cardiothoracic Surgery, 1959 NE Pacific St, Box 356310, Seattle, WA 98195-6310; **Phone:** 206-221-3166; **Board Cert:** Thoracic Surgery 2010; **Med School:** Columbia P&S 1981; **Resid:** Surgery, NY Presby Hosp/Cornell 1986; Cardiothoracic Surgery, NY Presby Hosp/Cornell 1990; **Fellow:** Research, UCSF Affil Rsch Inst 1988; **Fac Appt:** Prof TS, Univ Wash

Bailey, Leonard L MD [TS] - **Spec Exp:** Cardiac Surgery-Pediatric; Congenital Heart Surgery; Transplant-Heart-Pediatric; **Hospital:** Loma Linda Chldns Hosp; **Address:** 11234 Anderson St, rm 1617, Loma Linda, CA 92354; **Phone:** 909-558-4200; **Board Cert:** Surgery 1975; Thoracic Surgery 2006; **Med School:** Loma Linda Univ 1969; **Resid:** Surgery, Loma Linda Univ Med Ctr 1973; Thoracic Surgery, Loma Linda Univ Med Ctr 1974; **Fellow:** Cardiovascular Surgery, Hosp Sick Chldn 1975; **Fac Appt:** Prof S, Loma Linda Univ

Boyd, Walter Douglas MD [TS] - **Spec Exp:** Robotic Cardiac Surgery; Minimally Invasive Cardiac Surgery; Stem Cell Therapy & Biosurgery; Coronary Artery Surgery; **Hospital:** UC Davis Med Ctr; **Address:** 2221 Stockton Blvd, Cypres Bldg - rm 2122, Sacramento, CA 95817; **Phone:** 916-734-3861; **Med School:** Univ Ottawa 1984; **Resid:** Surgery, Ottawa Civic Hospital 1990; Cardiothoracic Surgery, Ottowa Civic Hospital 1992; **Fellow:** Transplantation/Mechanical Assist Devices, Ottawa Heart Inst 1995; **Fac Appt:** Prof S, UC Davis

Cameron, Robert Brian MD [TS] - **Spec Exp:** Lung Cancer; Mesothelioma; **Hospital:** UCLA Ronald Reagan Med Ctr; **Address:** UCLA Medical Ctr-Dept of Thoracic Surg, 10833 Le Conte Ave, rm 64-128CHS, Los Angeles, CA 90095; **Phone:** 310-470-8980; **Board Cert:** Surgery 2002; Thoracic Surgery 2005; **Med School:** UCLA 1984; **Resid:** Surgery, UCLA Hosp & Clinic 1992; **Fellow:** Surgical Oncology, National Inst Health 1989; Cardiothoracic Surgery, NY Hosp/Cornell 1994

Cohen, Gordon MD/PhD [TS] - **Spec Exp:** Pediatric Cardiothoracic Surgery; Neonatal Surgery; Transplant-Heart-Pediatric; Heart Failure; **Hospital:** Seattle Chldns Hosp; **Address:** Seattle Children's, Thoracic Surgery Dept, 4800 Sand Point Way NE, MS G0035, Seattle, WA 98105; **Phone:** 206-987-2198; **Board Cert:** Surgery 1999; Thoracic Surgery 2001; **Med School:** Tulane Univ 1989; **Resid:** Surgery, UCLA Med Ctr 1996; Cardiothoracic Surgery, Univ Washington Med Ctr 1998; **Fellow:** Pediatric Cardiac Surgery, Great Ormond St Hosp for Chldn 1999; **Fac Appt:** Prof TS, Univ Wash

Cohen, Robbin G MD [TS] - **Spec Exp:** Minimally Invasive Surgery; Heart Valve Surgery; Thoracic Aortic Surgery; **Hospital:** Keck Med Ctr of USC (page 75), Huntington Memorial Hosp; **Address:** 1520 San Pueblo St, Ste 4300, Los Angeles, CA 90033; **Phone:** 323-442-5850; **Board Cert:** Thoracic Surgery 2008; **Med School:** Univ Colorado 1980; **Resid:** Surgery, Stanford Univ Med Ctr 1986; **Fellow:** Cardiothoracic Surgery, Stanford Univ Med Ctr 1989; **Fac Appt:** Assoc Prof TS, USC Sch Med

Dang, Michael H MD [TS] - **Spec Exp:** Cardiac Surgery; Peripheral Vascular Disease; Transplant-Heart; **Hospital:** Queen's Med Ctr - Honolulu; **Address:** Queens Heart Physicians Practice, 550 S Beretania St, Ste 300, Honolulu, HI 96813; **Phone:** 808-545-8900; **Board Cert:** Thoracic Surgery 2002; **Med School:** Univ Colorado 1968; **Resid:** Surgery, Baylor Univ Med Ctr 1976; Thoracic Surgery, Baylor Univ Med Ctr 1978

De Meester, Tom R MD [TS] - **Spec Exp:** Stomach Cancer; Esophageal Cancer; Lung Cancer; Tracheal Surgery; **Hospital:** Keck Med Ctr of USC (page 75); **Address:** 1510 San Pablo St, Ste 514, Los Angeles, CA 90033; **Phone:** 323-442-5925; **Board Cert:** Surgery 1971; Thoracic Surgery 1971; **Med School:** Univ Mich Med Sch 1963; **Resid:** Surgery, Johns Hopkins Hosp 1966; **Fellow:** Thoracic Surgery, Johns Hopkins Hosp 1968; **Fac Appt:** Prof S, USC Sch Med

DeFilippi, Vincent J MD [TS] - **Spec Exp:** Minimally Invasive Cardiac Surgery; Mitral Valve Surgery; Maze Procedure for Atrial Fibrillation; Robotic Cardiac Surgery; **Hospital:** Salinas Valley Meml Hlthcare Systs, Stanford Univ Hosp & Clinics; **Address:** Stanford Univ at Salinas Valley, Cardiac Surgery Program, 212 San Jose St, Ste 301, Salinas, CA 93901; **Phone:** 831-759-3289; **Board Cert:** Thoracic Surgery 2005; **Med School:** Columbia P&S 1988; **Resid:** Surgery, Univ Chicago Hosps 1994; **Fellow:** Cardiothoracic Surgery, New York Hosp/Meml Sloan Kettering Cancer Ctr 1995; **Fac Appt:** Assoc Clin Prof TS, Stanford Univ

Fontana, Gregory MD [TS] - **Spec Exp:** Minimally Invasive Surgery; Cardiac Surgery-Pediatric; Mitral Valve Surgery; Coronary Artery Surgery; **Hospital:** Cedars-Sinai Med Ctr; **Address:** 8700 Beverly Blvd, North Twr, rm 6215, Los Angeles, CA 90048-1804; **Phone:** 310-423-1874; **Board Cert:** Thoracic Surgery 2004; **Med School:** UCLA 1984; **Resid:** Surgery, Duke Univ Med Ctr 1990; Thoracic Surgery, Duke Univ Med Ctr 1993; **Fellow:** Pediatric Cardiac Surgery, UCLA Med Ctr; Pediatric Cardiac Surgery, Chldns Hosp; **Fac Appt:** Clin Prof S, UCLA

Grannis Jr, Frederic W MD [TS] - **Spec Exp:** Lung Cancer; Tobacco Abuse; Thoracic Cancers; Palliative Care; **Hospital:** City of Hope Natl Med Ctr, Methodist Hosp - Southern California; **Address:** Thor Surg-City of Hope Natl Med Ctr, 1500 E Duarte Rd, Duarte, CA 91010; **Phone:** 626-359-8111 x62669; **Board Cert:** Surgery 1975; Thoracic Surgery 2000; **Med School:** NY Med Coll 1969; **Resid:** Surgery, Mayo Clinic 1974; Thoracic Surgery, Mayo Clinic 1977; **Fac Appt:** Assoc Prof TS, UCSD

Gundry, Steven MD [TS] - **Spec Exp:** Cardiac Surgery-Adult & Pediatric; Cardiac Surgery-High Risk; Nutrition in Heart Disease; **Hospital:** Desert Regl Med Ctr; **Address:** International Heart & Lung Inst, 555 Tachevah Drive, 3W - Ste 103, Palm Springs, CA 92262; **Phone:** 760-323-5553; **Board Cert:** Thoracic Surgery 2005; **Med School:** Med Coll GA 1977; **Resid:** Surgery, Univ Michigan Hosps 1983; Thoracic Surgery, Univ Michigan Hosps 1985; **Fellow:** Pediatric Cardiac Surgery, Hosp-Sick Chldn 1986; **Fac Appt:** Clin Prof S, Loma Linda Univ

Handy Jr, John R MD [TS] - **Spec Exp:** Lung Cancer; Esophageal Cancer; Mesothelioma; Chest Wall Tumors; **Hospital:** Providence Portland Med Ctr; **Address:** Oregon Clinic-Cardiothoracic Surgery, 1111 NE 99th Ave, Ste 201, Portland, OR 97220; **Phone:** 503-963-3030; **Board Cert:** Surgery 1999; Thoracic Surgery 2001; **Med School:** Duke Univ 1983; **Resid:** Surgery, Brown Univ Hosp 1990; **Fellow:** Cardiothoracic Surgery, MUSC Med Ctr 1993

Hanley, Frank L MD [TS] - **Spec Exp:** Pediatric Thoracic Surgery; **Hospital:** Lucile Packard Chldn's Hosp, Chldns Hosp - Oakland; **Address:** 300 Pasteur Drive, FALK CVRB, MC 5407, Stanford, CA 94305-5407; **Phone:** 650-723-0190; **Board Cert:** Thoracic Surgery 2002; **Med School:** Tufts Univ 1978; **Resid:** Surgery, UCSF Med Ctr 1981; Cardiothoracic Surgery, UCSF Med Ctr 1988; **Fellow:** Research, UCSF Sch Med 1984; **Fac Appt:** Prof S, UCSF

Harken, Alden H MD [TS] - **Spec Exp:** Arrhythmias; Cardiac Surgery; Coronary Artery Surgery; **Hospital:** Alameda County Med Ctr-Highland Campus, UCSF Med Ctr; **Address:** UCSF East Bay Surgical Program, 1411 E 31st St, Oakland, CA 94602; **Phone:** 510-437-4091; **Board Cert:** Surgery 1990; Thoracic Surgery 2006; **Med School:** Case West Res Univ 1967; **Resid:** Surgery, Peter Bent Brigham Hosp 1970; Thoracic Surgery, Peter Bent Brigham Hosp 1973; **Fellow:** Cardiovascular Surgery, Boston Chldns Hosp 1971; **Fac Appt:** Prof S, UCSF

Jablons, David M MD [TS] - **Spec Exp:** Lung Cancer; Mesothelioma; Esophageal Surgery; **Hospital:** UCSF - Mt Zion Med Ctr; **Address:** UCSF Thoracic Surgery, 1600 Divisadero St Fl 4, San Francisco, CA 94115; **Phone:** 415-885-3882; **Board Cert:** Thoracic Surgery 2002; **Med School:** Albany Med Coll 1984; **Resid:** Surgery, New Eng Med Ctr-Tufts Univ 1986; Surgery, New Eng Med Ctr-Tufts Univ 1991; **Fellow:** Surgical Oncology, Natl Cancer Inst-NIH 1989; Cardiothoracic Surgery, New York Hosp-Cornell 1993; **Fac Appt:** Prof S, UCSF

Thoracic Surgery

Jamieson, Stuart W MD [TS] - **Spec Exp:** Pulmonary Embolism; Transplant-Heart & Lung; **Hospital:** UCSD Med Ctr; **Address:** UCSD Med Ctr, Div CTS, 200 W Arbor Drive, MC 8892, San Diego, CA 92103-8892; **Phone:** 619-543-7777; **Med School:** England, UK 1971; **Resid:** Surgery 1975; **Fellow:** Cardiothoracic Surgery 1977; Cardiothoracic Surgery, Stanford Univ/American Heart Assoc 1980; **Fac Appt:** Prof S, UCSD

Laks, Hillel MD [TS] - **Spec Exp:** Congenital Heart Disease; Transplant-Heart; **Hospital:** UCLA Ronald Reagan Med Ctr; **Address:** UCLA Med Ctr, 10833 Le Conte Ave CHS Bldg, rm 62-215, Los Angeles, CA 90095-1741; **Phone:** 310-206-1837; **Board Cert:** Surgery 1975; Thoracic Surgery 2006; **Med School:** Africa 1965; **Resid:** Surgery, Peter Bent Brigham Hosp 1969; Thoracic Surgery, Peter Bent Brigham Hosp 1973; **Fac Appt:** Prof S, UCLA

Lamberti Jr, John J MD [TS] - **Spec Exp:** Pediatric Cardiac Surgery; Heart Valve Surgery; Congenital Heart Surgery; **Hospital:** Rady Children's Hosp - San Diego, UCSD Med Ctr; **Address:** 3030 Children's Way, Ste 202, MC 5078, San Diego, CA 92123-4227; **Phone:** 858-966-8030; **Board Cert:** Surgery 1973; Thoracic Surgery 1975; **Med School:** Univ Pittsburgh 1967; **Resid:** Surgery, Peter Bent Brigham Hosp 1972; Thoracic Surgery, Peter Bent Brigham Hosp 1973; **Fellow:** Pediatric Cardiac Surgery, Chldns Hosp 1974; **Fac Appt:** Prof S, UCSD

Merrick, Scot H MD [TS] - **Spec Exp:** Cardiac Surgery-Adult; Heart Valve Surgery; Coronary Revascularization; Congenital Heart Disease; **Hospital:** UCSF Med Ctr; **Address:** UCSF Med Ctr, Div Cardiothoracic Surg, 500 Parnassus Ave, Ste MU405, San Francisco, CA 94143-0118; **Phone:** 415-353-1606; **Board Cert:** Thoracic Surgery 2008; **Med School:** Univ Wash 1980; **Resid:** Surgery, UCSF Med Ctr 1985; **Fellow:** Cardiothoracic Surgery, UCSF Med Ctr 1987; **Fac Appt:** Assoc Prof S, UCSF

Miller, D Craig MD [TS] - **Spec Exp:** Thoracic Aortic Surgery; Heart Valve Surgery; Endovascular Stent Grafts; **Hospital:** Stanford Univ Hosp & Clinics; **Address:** Stanford Cardiothoracic Surgery, 300 Pasteur Drive, Falk Research Bldg, Stanford, CA 94305-5407; **Phone:** 650-725-3826; **Board Cert:** Thoracic Surgery 2008; **Med School:** Stanford Univ 1972; **Resid:** Thoracic Surgery, Standford Univ Med Ctr 1978; **Fac Appt:** Prof TS, Stanford Univ

Reitz, Bruce A MD [TS] - **Spec Exp:** Transplant-Heart & Lung; Heart Valve Surgery; Congenital Heart Surgery; **Hospital:** Stanford Univ Hosp & Clinics, El Camino Hosp; **Address:** Stanford Dept Cardiothoracic Surgery, 300 Pasteur Drive, Falk Rsch Bldg CV 297, Stanford, CA 94305-5407; **Phone:** 650-725-4497; **Board Cert:** Thoracic Surgery 1999; **Med School:** Yale Univ 1970; **Resid:** Surgery, Stanford Univ Hosp 1972; Cardiothoracic Surgery, Stanford Univ Hosp 1978; **Fellow:** Cardiac Surgery, Natl Heart Inst 1974; **Fac Appt:** Prof Emeritus TS, Stanford Univ

Robbins, Robert C MD [TS] - **Spec Exp:** Transplant-Heart; Transplant-Lung; Cardiothoracic Surgery; **Hospital:** Stanford Univ Hosp & Clinics; **Address:** Stanford Cardiothoracic Surgery, 300 Pasteur Drive, Falk Research Bldg, 2nd Fl, Stanford, CA 94305-5407; **Phone:** 650-725-3828; **Board Cert:** Thoracic Surgery 2002; Surgery 2002; **Med School:** Univ Miss 1983; **Resid:** Surgery, Univ Miss Med Ctr 1988; **Fellow:** Thoracic Surgery, Stanford Univ Med Ctr 1991; **Fac Appt:** Prof TS, Stanford Univ

Shemin, Richard MD [TS] - **Spec Exp:** Minimally Invasive Cardiac Surgery; Heart Valve Surgery; Aneurysm-Thoracic Aortic; **Hospital:** UCLA Ronald Reagan Med Ctr; **Address:** 757 Westwood Plaza, Ste 8501E, Los Angeles, CA 90095; **Phone:** 310-206-8232; **Board Cert:** Thoracic Surgery 2002; **Med School:** Boston Univ 1974; **Resid:** Surgery, PB Brigham Hosp 1980; NYU Med Ctr 1982; **Fellow:** Cardiac Surgery, Natl Inst Hlth 1978; **Fac Appt:** Prof TS, UCLA-David Geffen Sch Med

Shrager, Joseph B MD [TS] - **Spec Exp:** Lung Cancer; Thymoma; Emphysema-Lung Volume Reduction; Chest Wall Tumors; **Hospital:** Stanford Univ Hosp & Clinics, VA Hlth Care Sys - Palo Alto; **Address:** Stanford Univ Medical Ctr, Falk Bldg, 300 Pasteur, Fl 2, rm CV207, Stanford, CA 94305-5407; **Phone:** 650-721-2086; **Board Cert:** Thoracic Surgery 2008; Surgery 2009; **Med School:** Harvard Med Sch 1988; **Resid:** Surgery, Hosp Univ Penn 1995; Thoracic Surgery, Mass Genl Hosp 1997; **Fac Appt:** Prof TS, Stanford Univ

Starnes, Vaughn A MD [TS] - **Spec Exp:** Transplant-Heart & Lung; Heart Valve Surgery; Ross Procedure for Aortic Valve Disease; Robotic Cardiac Surgery; **Hospital:** Keck Med Ctr of USC (page 75), Huntington Memorial Hosp; **Address:** USC Cardiothoracic Surgery, 1520 San Pablo St, Ste 4300, Los Angeles, CA 90033; **Phone:** 323-442-5849; **Board Cert:** Thoracic Surgery 2007; **Med School:** Univ NC Sch Med 1977; **Resid:** Surgery, Vanderbilt Univ Hosp 1984; Cardiovascular Surgery, Stanford Unv Hosp 1986; **Fellow:** Cardiothoracic Transplant Surg, Stanford Unv Hosp 1987; Pediatric Cardiac Surgery, Univ NC Hosp; **Fac Appt:** Prof TS, USC Sch Med

Thistlethwaite, Patricia A MD/PhD [TS] - **Spec Exp:** Cardiac Surgery; Lung Cancer; Cardiothoracic Surgery; **Hospital:** UCSD Med Ctr; **Address:** UCSD Med Ctr, Div CTS, 200 W Arbor Drive, MC 8892, San Diego, CA 92103; **Phone:** 619-543-7777; **Board Cert:** Surgery 2005; Thoracic Surgery 2007; **Med School:** Harvard Med Sch 1989; **Resid:** Surgery, Mass Genl Hosp 1994; **Fellow:** Cardiothoracic Surgery, Univ Pittsburgh Med Ctr 1997; **Fac Appt:** Prof S, UCSD

Trento, Alfredo MD [TS] - **Spec Exp:** Transplant-Heart; Cardiac Surgery; Pediatric Cardiac Surgery; Coronary Artery Surgery; **Hospital:** Cedars-Sinai Med Ctr; **Address:** Cedars-Sinai Med Ctr, Dept Thoracic Surg, 8700 Beverly Blvd, North Tower, Ste 6215, Los Angeles, CA 90048; **Phone:** 310-423-3851; **Board Cert:** Thoracic Surgery 2005; **Med School:** Italy 1975; **Resid:** Surgery, Univ Mass Med Ctr 1982; Thoracic Surgery, Univ Pittsburgh Med Ctr 1985; **Fellow:** Cardiothoracic Surgery, Univ Mass Med Ctr 1982; **Fac Appt:** Prof S, UCLA

Vallieres, Eric MD [TS] - **Spec Exp:** Lung Cancer; Mesothelioma; Mediastinal Tumors; Thoracic Cancers; **Hospital:** Swedish Med Ctr-First Hill-Seattle; **Address:** 1101 Madison St, Ste 850, Seattle, WA 98104; **Phone:** 206-215-6800; **Board Cert:** Surgery 1988; Thoracic Surgery 1990; **Med School:** Canada 1982; **Resid:** Surgery, Univ Toronto Affil Hosp 1988; Thoracic Surgery, Univ Toronto Affil Hosp 1989; **Fellow:** Cardiovascular Surgery, Univ Montreal 1990

Verrier, Edward D MD [TS] - **Spec Exp:** Coronary Artery Surgery; Heart Valve Surgery; **Hospital:** Univ Wash Med Ctr, Northwest Hosp - Seattle; **Address:** University Washington Medical Ctr, 1959 NE Pacific St, Ste AA115, Box 356310, Seattle, WA 98195-6310; **Phone:** 206-598-3636; **Board Cert:** Thoracic Surgery 2003; **Med School:** Tufts Univ 1974; **Resid:** Surgery, UCSF Med Ctr 1982; Thoracic Surgery, UCSF Med Ctr 1984; **Fellow:** Cardiac Surgery, UCSF Med Ctr 1980; **Fac Appt:** Prof TS, Univ Wash

Wells, Winfield J MD [TS] - **Spec Exp:** Tracheal Surgery-Pediatric; Congenital Heart Surgery; **Hospital:** Chldns Hosp - Los Angeles; **Address:** Chlds Hosp, Div Cardiothoracic Surgery, 4650 Sunset Blvd, MS 66, Los Angeles, CA 90027; **Phone:** 323-361-4148; **Board Cert:** Thoracic Surgery 2007; **Med School:** USC Sch Med 1970; **Resid:** Surgery, Columbia-Presby Med Ctr 1976; **Fac Appt:** Assoc Prof S, USC Sch Med

Whyte, Richard MD [TS] - **Spec Exp:** Lung Cancer; Esophageal Cancer; Chest Wall Tumors; **Hospital:** Stanford Univ Hosp & Clinics; **Address:** Stanford Univ Sch Med, Div Thor Surg, 300 Pasteur Dr, Bldg CVRB - rm 205, Stanford, CA 94305-5407; **Phone:** 650-723-6649; **Board Cert:** Surgery 2001; Thoracic Surgery 2003; **Med School:** Univ Pittsburgh 1983; **Resid:** Surgery, Mass Genl Hosp 1990; Thoracic Surgery, Univ Michigan Hosp 1992; **Fac Appt:** Prof TS, Stanford Univ

Thoracic Surgery

Wood, Douglas E MD [TS] - **Spec Exp:** Lung Cancer; Esophageal Cancer; Tracheal Surgery; Mesothelioma; **Hospital:** Univ Wash Med Ctr, Northwest Hosp - Seattle; **Address:** Univ Washington, Div Cardiothoracic Surg, 1959 NE Pacific St, rm AA-115, MS 356310, AA Bldg, rm 115, Box 356310, Seattle, WA 98195-6310; **Phone:** 206-685-3228; **Board Cert:** Surgery 2009; Thoracic Surgery 2001; **Med School:** Harvard Med Sch 1983; **Resid:** Surgery, Mass Genl Hosp 1989; Thoracic Surgery, Mass Genl Hosp 1991; **Fellow:** Surgical Critical Care, Mass Genl Hosp 1991; **Fac Appt:** Prof TS, Univ Wash

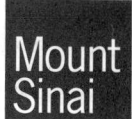
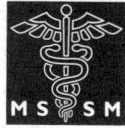

MOUNT SINAI
SCHOOL OF
MEDICINE

THE MOUNT SINAI MEDICAL CENTER
THORACIC SURGERY
One Gustave L. Levy Place
Fifth Avenue and 100th Street
New York, NY 10029-6574
Physician Referral: 1-800-MD-SINAI (637-4624)
www.mountsinai.org/thoracicsurgery

THORACIC SURGERY at The Mount Sinai Medical Center is known for its state-of-the-art surgery, multidisciplinary team approach to treatment, and commitment to compassionate patient care. Protocol-driven therapy ensures that Mount Sinai patients are given access to many clinical trials.

The Division of Thoracic Surgery at Mount Sinai engages in multidisciplinary collaboration, partnering with medical oncology, radiation oncology, pulmonary medicine, diagnostic and interventional radiology, gastroenterology, neurology, and anesthesiology, so patients can benefit from the insights of multiple experts across different specialties. This coordination among teams ensures seamless delivery of high-quality care to patients.

With an integrated approach to clinical care and research, our team of dedicated thoracic surgeons are experts in the treatment of all primary cancers of the chest, lung, esophagus, mediastinum, and airway, and all metastatic tumors of the chest. We also diagnose and treat patients who are affected by benign esophageal disorders such as gastroesophageal reflux disease, achalasia, and motility disorders.

Minimally Invasive Care: Minimally invasive interventions are preferred whenever possible, allowing less tissue damage, faster recovery time, and less scarring than open surgery. Mount Sinai's Division of Thoracic Surgery offers state-of-the-art assessment and treatment approaches, including thoroscopy, rigid and flexible bronchoscopy, and endoscopic laser resection in the diagnosis and management of thoracic conditions. The division has led the national trials for VATS (video-assisted thoracoscopic surgery) lobectomy, a procedure using three small incisions, which is now the surgical approach of choice, particularly for patients with early-stage lung cancer.

Personalized and Targeted Therapy: A unique part of our division is the integration and application of groundbreaking scientific research into the clinical care of our patients. These research efforts are being carried out in the Thoracic Surgery Translational Laboratory. Mount Sinai's thoracic surgeons and physician-scientists are conducting state-of-the-art translational thoracic research, including genomic analysis of tumors to better understand and predict behavior, in order to develop more directed, personalized, therapeutic approaches to treatment with novel targeted therapies.

Lung and Esophageal Cancer: Mount Sinai is New York City's leading center for comprehensive screening for lung and esophageal cancer, including CT scans for early detection, advanced endoscopic techniques, PET scans, and innovative MRI technology with ultrasensitive resolution. Our team is unique in our abilities to screen for cancers in people at risk, treat early cancers less invasively, and provide the most advanced protocol driven treatments available. Our approach to lung cancer care focuses on patients first, providing not only VATS and advanced minimally invasive techniques, but also an ability to treat advanced and challenging cases that require skills and expertise found in few other medical centers.

Mesothelioma: Irving J. Selikoff, MD, was the first to determine the association between mesothelioma and asbestos exposure. His tireless research efforts at Mount Sinai led to the Selikoff Center for Occupational and Environmental Medicine. This tradition of cutting-edge developments continues with Raja M. Flores' work using different modalities in the treatment of mesothelioma, such as the extrapleural pneumonectomy and pleurectomy (decortication) procedures. The Division of Thoracic Surgery is also currently involved in several ongoing studies with the goal of discovering new treatments for mesothelioma.

LEADING SURGEONS, PIONEERING RESEARCH

Led by Raja M. Flores, the Division of Thoracic Surgery is internationally recognized as a leader in thoracic surgery drawing patients from across the globe to seek our expertise.

Dr. Flores is a recognized leader in the treatment of mesothelioma and one of the first physicians in the world to use robotic surgery to treat lung and esophageal cancer. Dr. Flores established VATS lobectomy as the gold standard in the surgical treatment of lung cancer. He is one of the foremost educators of other surgeons about the VATS lobectomy.

Our award-winning physicians have consistently contributed to the evolution of this field through their efforts to bring about new technologies and therapies.

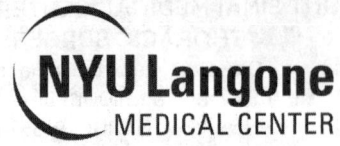

550 First Avenue *(at 31st Street)*
New York, NY 10016
www.NYULMC.org
Physician Referral: **888-7-NYU-MED** *(888-769-8633)*

THORACIC SURGERY

About the Division of Thoracic Surgery

Thoracic Surgeons at NYU Langone Medical Center offer the most advanced diagnosis and treatment options available to patients for either benign or malignant lesions of the lung, esophagus, mediastinum and chest wall. All thoracic attending surgeons at the Medical Center are experts in minimally invasive, video-assisted thoracic surgery which minimizes patient discomfort and shortens recuperation time. We specialize in the following areas:

Airway Stenting

Patients experiencing trouble breathing may require stenting to maintain an open airway (windpipe). Treatment of primary and metastatic lung cancer often requires the use of hollow tubes (stents) to maintain an unobstructed airway. At NYU Langone, stent placement is performed in the operating room by an experienced team that includes a surgeon, anesthesiologist and nursing staff. The procedure can be performed through either rigid or flexible bronchoscopy using temporary (plastic) or more permanent (metal) stents. Post-operative patients are carefully monitored by a multidisciplinary team to ensure their comfort and care.

Minimally Invasive Thoracic Surgery

The Division of Thoracic Surgery offers a minimally invasive surgery program, incorporating both video-assisted and "open chest" techniques along with the newest methods for post-operative pain relief. The use of video-assisted equipment allows for a smaller incision without spreading the rib spaces, leading to greater patient comfort, a shorter recovery time and decreased length of stay for patients. Procedures offered include video-assisted thoracoscopy for biopsy with or without removal of a portion of the lungs, as well as repair of hiatal hernias and minimally invasive esophagectomy.

Pioneering Treatments

NYU Langone Medical Center continues to pioneer new treatments for the early detection of airway malignancies, diagnosis and treatment strategies for endobronchial abnormalities, investigation of non-surgical techniques for destruction of lung cancer nodules, and the use of stents (including replaceable stents) to relieve blockages of the windpipe and esophagus.

Research

NYU Langone is committed to state-of-the-art surgical management and development of novel treatment strategies through clinical trials. We also leverage the resources of the New York Thoracic Surgery Laboratory at Bellevue Hospital Center to search for genes and proteins in malignancies of the chest in order to develop novel targeted therapies.

Urology

A urologist manages benign and malignant medical and surgical disorders of the genitourinary system and the adrenal gland. This specialist has comprehensive knowledge of, and skills in, endoscopic, percutaneous and open surgery of congenital and acquired conditions of the urinary and reproductive systems and their contiguous structures.

Training Required: Five years

UROLOGY

New England

Albertsen, Peter C MD [U] - **Spec Exp:** Prostate Cancer; **Hospital:** Univ of Conn Hlth Ctr, John Dempsey Hosp; **Address:** 263 Farmington Ave, Dowling South Fl 2 - Ste 220, Farmington, CT 06030; **Phone:** 860-679-4100; **Board Cert:** Urology 2004; **Med School:** Columbia P&S 1978; **Resid:** Surgery, New England Deaconess Hosp 1980; Urology, Johns Hopkins Hospital 1984; **Fellow:** Preventive Medicine, Univ WI Affil Hosp 1990; **Fac Appt:** Prof U, Univ Conn

Bauer, Stuart B MD [U] - **Spec Exp:** Pediatric Urology; Neuro-Urology; Neurogenic Bladder; **Hospital:** Children's Hospital - Boston; **Address:** Chldns Hosp, Hunnewell-3, 300 Longwood Ave, Boston, MA 02115-6264; **Phone:** 617-355-7796; **Board Cert:** Urology 1977; **Med School:** Univ Rochester 1968; **Resid:** Urology, Tufts New Engl Med Ctr 1975; **Fac Appt:** Prof U, Harvard Med Sch

Caldamone, Anthony A MD [U] - **Spec Exp:** Pediatric Urology; **Hospital:** Rhode Island Hosp; **Address:** 2 Dudley St, Ste 185, Providence, RI 02905; **Phone:** 401-421-0710; **Board Cert:** Urology 1983; Pediatric Urology 2008; **Med School:** Brown Univ 1975; **Resid:** Urology, Strong Meml Hosp 1981; **Fellow:** Pediatric Urology, Childrens Hosp 1982; **Fac Appt:** Prof U, Brown Univ

Colberg, John W MD [U] - **Spec Exp:** Prostate Cancer; Bladder Cancer; Kidney Cancer; Testicular Cancer; **Hospital:** Yale-New Haven Hosp, Yale Med Group; **Address:** Yale Urology Group, 800 Howard Ave Fl 3, New Haven, CT 06519; **Phone:** 203-785-2815; **Board Cert:** Urology 2001; **Med School:** Washington Univ, St Louis 1985; **Resid:** Surgery, Yale-New Haven Hosp 1987; Urology, Yale-New Haven Hosp 1990; **Fac Appt:** Assoc Prof U, Yale Univ

Foster Jr, Harris E MD [U] - **Spec Exp:** Incontinence; Urodynamics; Voiding Dysfunction; Urology-Female; **Hospital:** Yale-New Haven Hosp, Yale Med Group; **Address:** Yale Urology Grp, 800 Howard Ave Fl 3, New Haven, CT 06520-8062; **Phone:** 203-200-4822; **Board Cert:** Urology 2003; **Med School:** Univ Miami Sch Med 1987; **Resid:** Surgery, Univ Michigan Med Ctr 1989; Urology, Univ Michigan Med Ctr 1992; **Fac Appt:** Prof U, Yale Univ

Gomery, Pablo MD [U] - **Spec Exp:** Neuro-Urology; Erectile Dysfunction; Voiding Dysfunction; Infertility-Male; **Hospital:** Mass Genl Hosp, Spaulding Rehab Hosp; **Address:** Mass Genl Hosp-Dept Urology, 55 Fruit St, GRB 1102, Boston, MA 02114; **Phone:** 617-726-8482; **Board Cert:** Urology 2000; **Med School:** Albert Einstein Coll Med 1974; **Resid:** Surgery, New England Deaconess Hosp 1977; Urology, Mass General Hosp 1980

Heney, Niall M MD [U] - **Spec Exp:** Urologic Cancer; Prostate Cancer; **Hospital:** Mass Genl Hosp; **Address:** Mass Genl Hosp, Dept Urology, 55 Fruit St, GRB 1102, Boston, MA 02114; **Phone:** 617-726-3011; **Board Cert:** Urology 1977; **Med School:** Ireland 1965; **Resid:** Urology, Regional Hosp 1972; Urology, Mass Genl Hosp 1976; **Fac Appt:** Prof U, Harvard Med Sch

Janeiro Jr, John J MD [U] - **Spec Exp:** Urologic Cancer; Kidney Stones; Vasectomy Reversal; **Hospital:** Southern NH Med Ctr, St. Joseph Hosp & Trauma Ctr; **Address:** Urology Center Southern New Hampshire, 17 Riverside St, Ste 201, Nashua, NH 03062; **Phone:** 603-883-1550; **Board Cert:** Urology 2008; **Med School:** Univ Mass Sch Med 1982; **Resid:** Urology, Lahey Clinic 1987; **Fellow:** Pediatric Urology, Childrens Hosp 1989

Libertino, John A MD [U] - **Spec Exp:** Kidney Cancer; Prostate Cancer; Adrenal Tumors; **Hospital:** Lahey Clin; **Address:** Lahey Clinic, Dept Urology, 41 Mall Rd, Burlington, MA 01805-0001; **Phone:** 781-744-2511; **Board Cert:** Urology 1973; **Med School:** Georgetown Univ 1965; **Resid:** Surgery, Strong Meml Hosp 1967; Urology, Yale-New Haven Hosp 1970; **Fellow:** Urology, Yale-New Haven Hosp 1969; **Fac Appt:** Prof S, Harvard Med Sch

Loughlin, Kevin R MD [U] - **Spec Exp:** Prostate Cancer; Bladder Cancer; Penile Cancer; Incontinence-Female; **Hospital:** Brigham and Women's Hosp (page 57), Dana-Farber Cancer Inst (page 57); **Address:** Brigham & Women's Hosp, Div Urology, 45 Francis St, ASB2-3, Boston, MA 02115; **Phone:** 617-732-6325; **Board Cert:** Urology 2004; **Med School:** NY Med Coll 1975; **Resid:** Pediatrics, New York Hosp 1978; Surgery, Bellevue Hosp Ctr 1979; **Fellow:** Urology, Brigham & Women's Hosp 1983; Urologic Oncology, Meml Sloan Kettering Cancer Ctr 1983; **Fac Appt:** Prof S, Harvard Med Sch

McDougal, W Scott MD [U] - **Spec Exp:** Penile Cancer; Prostate Cancer; Bladder Cancer; Urologic Cancer; **Hospital:** Mass Genl Hosp; **Address:** Mass Genl Hosp, 55 Fruit St GRB Bldg - rm 1102, Boston, MA 02114; **Phone:** 617-726-3010; **Board Cert:** Surgery 1975; Urology 1992; **Med School:** Cornell Univ-Weill Med Coll 1968; **Resid:** Surgery, Univ Hosps Cleveland 1975; Urology, Univ Hosps Cleveland 1975; **Fellow:** Physiology, Yale Med Sch 1972; **Fac Appt:** Prof U, Harvard Med Sch

McGovern, Francis J MD [U] - **Spec Exp:** Prostate Cancer; Urologic Cancer; **Hospital:** Mass Genl Hosp; **Address:** One Hawthorne Pl, Ste 109, Boston, MA 02114; **Phone:** 617-726-3560; **Board Cert:** Urology 2009; **Med School:** Case West Res Univ 1983; **Resid:** Urology, Mass Genl Hosp 1989

Merguerian, Paul A MD [U] - **Spec Exp:** Pediatric Urology; Bladder Exstrophy; Genital Reconstruction; Minimally Invasive Surgery; **Hospital:** Dartmouth - Hitchcock Med Ctr; **Address:** Darthmouth-Hirchcock Med Ctr, Dept Pediatric Surgery, 1 Med Ctr Drive, Lebanon, NH 03756; **Phone:** 603-653-9882; **Board Cert:** Urology 2008; Pediatric Urology 2008; **Med School:** Israel 1980; **Resid:** Surgery, Univ Rochester Med Ctr 1984; Urology, Univ Rochester Med Ctr 1988; **Fellow:** Pediatric Urology, Hosp for Sick Chldn 1990; **Fac Appt:** Prof S, Dartmouth Med Sch

O'Leary, Michael P MD [U] - **Spec Exp:** Sexual Dysfunction; Kidney Stones; Prostate Disease; **Hospital:** Brigham and Women's Hosp (page 57), Dana-Farber Cancer Inst (page 57); **Address:** Brigham & Women's Hosp, Div Urology, 45 Francis St, ASBII-3, Boston, MA 02115; **Phone:** 617-732-6325; **Board Cert:** Urology 2010; **Med School:** Geo Wash Univ 1980; **Resid:** Urology, Tufts New Eng Med Ctr 1982; Urology, Mass Genl Hosp 1986; **Fellow:** Urology, UCSF Med Ctr 1989; **Fac Appt:** Assoc Prof S, Harvard Med Sch

Oates, Robert D MD [U] - **Spec Exp:** Infertility-Male; Vasectomy Reversal; Reproductive Genetics; Congenital Absence of Vas Deferens; **Hospital:** Boston Med Ctr; **Address:** Boston Univ Med Ctr, Dept Urology, 725 Albany St Sharpiro Bldg - Ste 3B, Boston, MA 02118-2334; **Phone:** 617-638-8485; **Board Cert:** Urology 2010; **Med School:** Boston Univ 1982; **Resid:** Surgery, Boston Univ Hosp 1984; Urology, Boston Univ Hosp 1987; **Fellow:** Reproductive Medicine, Baylor Coll Med 1988; **Fac Appt:** Prof U, Boston Univ

Olumi, Aria F MD [U] - **Spec Exp:** Prostate Cancer; Testicular Cancer; Kidney Cancer; Bladder Cancer; **Hospital:** Mass Genl Hosp; **Address:** Mass General Urology Associates, 55 Fruit St, Yawkey Bldg, Ste 7E, Boston, MA 02114; **Phone:** 617-643-0237; **Board Cert:** Urology 2002; **Med School:** Univ SC Sch Med 1992; **Resid:** Surgery, Brigham & Women's Hosp 1994; Urology, Brigham & Women's Hosp 2000; **Fellow:** Research, UCSF Affil Hosp 1998; **Fac Appt:** Assoc Prof S, Harvard Med Sch

Urology

Richie, Jerome P MD [U] - **Spec Exp:** Prostate Cancer; Testicular Cancer; Kidney Cancer; **Hospital:** Brigham and Women's Hosp (page 57), Dana-Farber Cancer Inst (page 57); **Address:** Brigham & Womens Hosp, 45 Francis St, Ste ASB2, Boston, MA 02115; **Phone:** 617-732-6227; **Board Cert:** Urology 1977; **Med School:** Univ Tex Med Br, Galveston 1969; **Resid:** Surgery, UCLA Med Ctr 1971; Urology, UCLA Med Ctr 1975; **Fac Appt:** Prof S, Harvard Med Sch

Sanda, Martin G MD [U] - **Spec Exp:** Prostate Cancer; Bladder Cancer; Kidney Cancer; Urologic Cancer; **Hospital:** Beth Israel Deaconess Med Ctr - Boston; **Address:** Beth Israel Deaconess Medical Ctr, 330 Brookline Ave, Rabb 440, Boston, MA 02115; **Phone:** 617-735-2100; **Board Cert:** Urology 2007; **Med School:** Columbia P&S 1987; **Resid:** Surgery, Med Coll Virginia 1989; Urology, Johns Hopkins Hosp 1994; **Fellow:** Surgical Oncology, Natl Cancer Inst 1991; **Fac Appt:** Assoc Prof U, Harvard Med Sch

Sigman, Mark MD [U] - **Spec Exp:** Infertility-Male; Vasectomy Reversal; **Hospital:** Rhode Island Hosp; **Address:** 2 Dudley St, Ste 175, Providence, RI 02905-3247; **Phone:** 401-421-0710; **Board Cert:** Urology 2010; **Med School:** Univ Conn 1981; **Resid:** Surgery, Univ VA 1983; Urology, Univ VA 1987; **Fellow:** Male Reproduction, Baylor Coll Med 1989; **Fac Appt:** Assoc Prof U, Brown Univ

Singh, Dinesh MD [U] - **Spec Exp:** Laparoscopic Surgery; Robotic Surgery; Kidney Cancer; Prostate Cancer; **Hospital:** Yale Med Group; **Address:** Yale Urologic Group, Yale Physicians Bldg, 800 Howard Ave Fl 3, New Haven, CT 06519; **Phone:** 203-785-2815; **Board Cert:** Urology 2006; **Med School:** Columbia P&S 1997; **Resid:** Surgery, Brigham & Women's Hosp 1999; Urology, Harvard Med Sch Affil Hosp 2003; **Fellow:** Research, Dana Farber Cancer Inst 2001; Laparoscopic Surgery, Cleveland Clin 2004; **Fac Appt:** Asst Prof U, Yale Univ

Weiss, Robert M MD [U] - **Spec Exp:** Pediatric Urology; Testicular Cancer; Penile Cancer; Bladder Cancer; **Hospital:** Yale-New Haven Hosp, Yale Med Group; **Address:** Yale Univ Sch Med, Dept Urology, 800 Howard Ave, Box 208041, New Haven, CT 06520-8041; **Phone:** 203-785-2815; **Board Cert:** Urology 1970; **Med School:** SUNY Downstate 1960; **Resid:** Surgery, Beth Israel Hosp 1962; Urology, Columbia Presby Hosp 1967; **Fellow:** Pharmacology, Columbia Presby Hosp 1965; **Fac Appt:** Prof U, Yale Univ

Mid Atlantic

Albala, David M MD [U] - **Spec Exp:** Prostate Cancer/Robotic Surgery; Kidney Stones; Laparoscopic Surgery; **Hospital:** Crouse Hosp, St. Joseph's Hosp Hlth Ctr; **Address:** Associated Medical Professionals, 1226 E Water St, Syracuse, NY 13210; **Phone:** 315-478-4185; **Board Cert:** Urology 2002; **Med School:** Mich State Univ 1983; **Resid:** Surgery, Dartmouth-Hitchcock Med Ctr 1985; Urology, Dartmouth-Hitchcock Med Ctr 1990; **Fellow:** Endourology, Wash Univ Med Ctr 1991

Alexander, Richard B MD [U] - **Spec Exp:** Prostate Disease; Prostate Cancer; **Hospital:** Univ of MD Med Ctr; **Address:** 419 W Redwood St, Ste 320, Baltimore, MD 21201; **Phone:** 410-328-5109; **Board Cert:** Urology 1999; **Med School:** Johns Hopkins Univ 1981; **Resid:** Surgery, Vanderbilt Univ Affl Hosps 1983; Urology, Johns Hopkins Hosp 1988; **Fellow:** Cancer Immunology, Natl Cancer Inst 1989; **Fac Appt:** Prof U, Univ MD Sch Med

Bagley, Demetrius H MD [U] - **Spec Exp:** Endourology; Kidney Stones; Kidney Cancer; Ureter & Renal Pelvis Cancer; **Hospital:** Thomas Jefferson Univ Hosp; **Address:** 833 Chestnut St, Fl 7, Ste 703, Philadelphia, PA 19107; **Phone:** 215-955-1000; **Board Cert:** Urology 1981; **Med School:** Johns Hopkins Univ 1970; **Resid:** Surgery, Yale-New Haven Hosp 1972; Urology, Yale-New Haven Hosp 1979; **Fellow:** Surgery, NCI-USPHS 1975; **Fac Appt:** Prof U, Thomas Jefferson Univ

Bar-Chama, Natan MD [U] - **Spec Exp:** Infertility-Male; Erectile Dysfunction; Vasectomy Reversal; Varicocele Microsurgery; **Hospital:** Mount Sinai Med Ctr (page 63); **Address:** Center for Male Reproductive Health, 635 Madison Ave, New York, NY 10022; **Phone:** 212-756-5777; **Board Cert:** Urology 2006; **Med School:** Albert Einstein Coll Med 1987; **Resid:** Urology, Montefiore Med Ctr 1993; **Fellow:** Male Infertility, Baylor Coll Med 1994; **Fac Appt:** Assoc Prof U, Mount Sinai Sch Med

Benson, Mitchell C MD [U] - **Spec Exp:** Prostate Cancer/Robotic Surgery; Bladder Cancer; Kidney Cancer; Continent Urinary Diversions; **Hospital:** NY-Presby/Columbia Univ Med Ctr, NY (page 65); **Address:** NY Presby Hosp-Columbia, Dept Urology, 161 Ft Washington Ave Fl 11 - rm 1102, New York, NY 10032-3713; **Phone:** 212-305-5201; **Board Cert:** Urology 1984; **Med School:** Columbia P&S 1977; **Resid:** Surgery, Mount Sinai Med Ctr 1979; Urology, Columbia-Presby Hosp 1982; **Fellow:** Oncology, Johns Hopkins Hosp 1984; **Fac Appt:** Prof U, Columbia P&S

Blaivas, Jerry G MD [U] - **Spec Exp:** Uro-Gynecology; Urology-Female; Neurogenic Bladder; Incontinence after Prostate Cancer; **Hospital:** NY-Presby/Weill Cornell Med Ctr, NY (page 65), Lenox Hill Hosp; **Address:** 445 E 77th St, New York, NY 10075; **Phone:** 212-772-3900; **Board Cert:** Urology 1978; **Med School:** Tufts Univ 1968; **Resid:** Surgery, Boston Med Ctr 1971; Urology, New England Med Ctr 1976; **Fac Appt:** Clin Prof U, Cornell Univ-Weill Med Coll

Burnett II, Arthur L MD [U] - **Spec Exp:** Prostate Cancer; Erectile Dysfunction; **Hospital:** Johns Hopkins Hosp (page 61); **Address:** 600 N Wolfe St, Marburg Bldg, Ste 407, Baltimore, MD 21287; **Phone:** 410-955-6100; **Board Cert:** Urology 2007; **Med School:** Johns Hopkins Univ 1988; **Resid:** Surgery, Johns Hopkins Hosp 1990; Urology, Johns Hopkins Hosp 1994; **Fac Appt:** Prof U, Johns Hopkins Univ

Canning, Douglas MD [U] - **Spec Exp:** Pediatric Urology; Hypospadias; **Hospital:** Chldns Hosp of Philadelphia; **Address:** Childrens Hosp, Div Urology, 34th St & Civic Center Blvd, Wood Bldg, 3rd Fl, Philadelphia, PA 19104; **Phone:** 215-590-2754; **Board Cert:** Urology 2008; Pediatric Urology 2008; **Med School:** Dartmouth Med Sch 1982; **Resid:** Urology, Naval Hosp 1987; **Fellow:** Pediatric Urology, Johns Hopkins Hosp 1988; **Fac Appt:** Prof U, Univ Pennsylvania

Carter, H Ballentine MD [U] - **Spec Exp:** Prostate Cancer; **Hospital:** Johns Hopkins Hosp (page 61); **Address:** Brady Urological Inst, Johns Hopkins Hosp, 600 N Wolfe St Marburg Bldg - rm 143, Baltimore, MD 21287; **Phone:** 410-955-6100; **Board Cert:** Urology 1999; **Med School:** Med Univ SC 1981; **Resid:** Surgery, New York Hosp 1983; Urology, New York Hosp 1987; **Fellow:** Research, Johns Hopkins Hosp 1989; **Fac Appt:** Prof U, Johns Hopkins Univ

Chen, David Y T MD [U] - **Spec Exp:** Kidney Cancer; Prostate Cancer; Robotic Surgery; Bladder Cancer; **Hospital:** Fox Chase Cancer Ctr (page 58); **Address:** Fox Chase Cancer Ctr, 8 Huntingdon Pike Fl 3 Urology, Rockledge, PA 19046; **Phone:** 215-728-1111; **Board Cert:** Urology 2006; **Med School:** Cornell Univ 1997; **Resid:** Urology, NY Presby/Cornell Hosp; **Fellow:** NIH/Howard Hughes Med Inst; Urologic Oncology, NY Presby/Cornell Hosp

Cohen, Jeffrey K MD [U] - **Spec Exp:** Urologic Cancer; Prostate Cancer; **Hospital:** Allegheny General Hosp; **Address:** Triangle Urological Group, 1307 Federal St, Ste 300, Pittsburgh, PA 15212-1757; **Phone:** 412-281-1757; **Board Cert:** Urology 2005; **Med School:** SUNY Upstate Med Univ 1979; **Resid:** Surgery, Case Western Reserve Univ Hosp 1981; Urology, Case Western Reserve Univ Hosp 1984; **Fellow:** Urologic Oncology, MD Anderson Cancer Ctr 1985; **Fac Appt:** Assoc Prof U, Drexel Univ Coll Med

Urology

Docimo, Steven G MD [U] - **Spec Exp:** Pediatric Urology; Minimally Invasive Surgery; Bladder Reconstruction; Voiding Dysfunction; **Hospital:** Chldns Hosp of Pittsburgh - UPMC; **Address:** Executive Suites Children's Hosp of Pittsburgh, Children's Hosp Drive, Pittsburgh, PA 15224; **Phone:** 412-692-7932; **Board Cert:** Urology 2008; Pediatric Urology 2008; **Med School:** Johns Hopkins Univ 1984; **Resid:** Surgery, Georgetown Univ Med Ctr 1986; Urology, Brigham & Womens Hosp 1990; **Fellow:** Pediatric Urology, Johns Hopkins 1994; Research, Childrens Hosp 1988; **Fac Appt:** Prof U, Univ Pittsburgh

Droller, Michael J MD [U] - **Spec Exp:** Urologic Cancer; Bladder Cancer; Prostate Cancer; Kidney Cancer; **Hospital:** Mount Sinai Med Ctr (page 63); **Address:** 5 E 98th St Fl 6, Box 1272, New York, NY 10029-6501; **Phone:** 212-241-3868; **Board Cert:** Urology 2001; **Med School:** Harvard Med Sch 1968; **Resid:** Surgery, Peter Bent Brigham Hosp 1970; Urology, Stanford Univ Med Ctr 1976; **Fellow:** Immunology, Univ Stockholm 1977; **Fac Appt:** Prof U, Mount Sinai Sch Med

Fisch, Harry MD [U] - **Spec Exp:** Infertility-Male; Microsurgery; Vasectomy Reversal; **Hospital:** NY-Presby/Weill Cornell Med Ctr, NY (page 65), Lenox Hill Hosp; **Address:** 944 Park Ave, Ste 1C, New York, NY 10028; **Phone:** 212-879-0800; **Board Cert:** Urology 1999; **Med School:** Mount Sinai Sch Med 1983; **Resid:** Surgery, Montefiore Med Ctr 1985; Urology, Montefiore Med Ctr 1989; **Fac Appt:** Prof U, Columbia P&S

Gearhart, John P MD [U] - **Spec Exp:** Pediatric Urology; **Hospital:** Johns Hopkins Hosp (page 61); **Address:** Johns Hopkins Hospital, Brady Urological Institute, 600 N Wolfe St Marburg Bldg - Ste 146, Baltimore, MD 21287-2101; **Phone:** 410-955-5358; **Board Cert:** Urology 1982; **Med School:** Univ Louisville Sch Med 1975; **Resid:** Urology, Med Coll Georgia Hosp 1980; **Fellow:** Pediatric Urology, Alder Hey Chldns Hosp 1981; Pediatric Urology, Johns Hopkins Hosp 1985; **Fac Appt:** Prof U, Johns Hopkins Univ

Glassberg, Kenneth MD [U] - **Spec Exp:** Pediatric Urology; Genital Reconstruction; Varicocele in Adolescents; **Hospital:** Morgan Stanley Children's Hosp of NY-Presby, NY (page 65); **Address:** Morgan Stanley Chlds Hosp of NY-Presby, 3959 Broadway, rm 1117, New York, NY 10032; **Phone:** 212-305-9918; **Board Cert:** Urology 1977; Pediatric Urology 2009; **Med School:** SUNY Downstate 1968; **Resid:** Surgery, Montefiore Hosp Med Ctr 1972; Urology, Univ Hosp 1975; **Fellow:** Pediatric Urology, Adler Hey Chldns Hosp 1976; Pediatric Urology, Hosp For Sick Chldn 1976; **Fac Appt:** Prof U, Columbia P&S

Goldstein, Marc MD [U] - **Spec Exp:** Infertility-Male; Vasectomy Reversal; Varicocele Microsurgery; Erectile Dysfunction; **Hospital:** NY-Presby/Weill Cornell Med Ctr, NY (page 65); **Address:** Cornell Inst for Reproductive Med, 525 E 68th St, Box 580, New York, NY 10021-4870; **Phone:** 212-746-5470; **Board Cert:** Urology 1982; **Med School:** SUNY Downstate 1972; **Resid:** Surgery, Columbia-Presby Med Ctr 1974; Urology, SUNY Downstate Med Ctr 1980; **Fellow:** Microsurgery, Rockefeller Univ 1982; **Fac Appt:** Prof U, Cornell Univ-Weill Med Coll

Gomella, Leonard G MD [U] - **Spec Exp:** Prostate Cancer; Minimally Invasive Urologic Surgery; Urologic Cancer; **Hospital:** Thomas Jefferson Univ Hosp; **Address:** Thomas Jefferson Univ, 833 Chestnut St Fl 7 - Ste 703, Philadelphia, PA 19107-5001; **Phone:** 215-955-1000; **Board Cert:** Urology 2008; **Med School:** Univ KY Coll Med 1980; **Resid:** Surgery, Univ Kentucky Med Ctr 1982; Urology, Univ Kentucky Med Ctr 1986; **Fellow:** Urologic Oncology, Natl Cancer Inst 1988; **Fac Appt:** Prof U, Jefferson Med Coll

Grasso, Michael MD [U] - **Spec Exp:** Urologic Cancer; Laparoscopic Surgery; Kidney Stones; Testicular Cancer; **Hospital:** Lenox Hill Hosp, Westchester Med Ctr; **Address:** 100 E 77 th St, East Bldg - Fl 4th, Dept Urology - Cronin 205, New York, NY 10075; **Phone:** 212-434-6300; **Board Cert:** Urology 2004; **Med School:** Jefferson Med Coll 1986; **Resid:** Surgery, Jefferson Univ Hosp 1988; Urology, Jefferson Univ Hosp 1992; **Fac Appt:** Prof U, NY Med Coll

Greenberg, Richard E MD [U] - **Spec Exp:** Prostate Cancer; Bladder Cancer; Kidney Cancer; Prostate Cancer/Robotic Surgery; **Hospital:** Fox Chase Cancer Ctr (page 58), Abington Mem Hosp; **Address:** Fox Chase Cancer Ctr, Div Urol-Dept Surg, 333 Cottman Ave, Ste H3 - rm H3-116, Philadelphia, PA 19111; **Phone:** 215-728-5341; **Board Cert:** Urology 2004; **Med School:** Cornell Univ-Weill Med Coll 1976; **Resid:** Surgery, New York Hosp 1979; Urology, New York Hosp 1983; **Fac Appt:** Prof U, Temple Univ

Greenfield, Saul P MD [U] - **Spec Exp:** Pediatric Urology; Urinary Tract Infections; Neurogenic Bladder; Reconstructive Urologic Surgery; **Hospital:** Women's & Chldn's Hosp of Buffalo, The; **Address:** CHOB- Dept Pediatric Urology, 219 Bryant St, Buffalo, NY 14222; **Phone:** 716-878-7393; **Board Cert:** Urology 1984; Pediatric Urology 2008; **Med School:** Univ Pennsylvania 1977; **Resid:** Surgery, NYU Med Ctr 1979; Urology, Columbia-Presby Med Ctr 1982; **Fellow:** Pediatric Urology, Chldns Hosp Buffalo 1984; **Fac Appt:** Clin Prof U, SUNY Buffalo

Gribetz, Michael MD [U] - **Spec Exp:** Prostate Disease; Urology-Female; Sexual Dysfunction; Kidney Stones; **Hospital:** Mount Sinai Med Ctr (page 63); **Address:** 1155 Park Ave, New York, NY 10128-1209; **Phone:** 212-831-1300; **Board Cert:** Urology 1980; **Med School:** Albert Einstein Coll Med 1973; **Resid:** Surgery, Montefiore Med Ctr 1975; Urology, Mt Sinai Hosp 1978; **Fac Appt:** Asst Clin Prof U, Mount Sinai Sch Med

Hall, Simon J MD [U] - **Spec Exp:** Urologic Cancer; Minimally Invasive Urologic Surgery; Continent Urinary Diversions; Prostate Cancer; **Hospital:** Mount Sinai Med Ctr (page 63); **Address:** Mount Sinai Medical Ctr, 5 98th St, Box 1272, New York, NY 10029; **Phone:** 212-241-4812; **Board Cert:** Urology 2009; **Med School:** Columbia P&S 1988; **Resid:** Surgery, Mt Sinai Med Ctr 1990; Urology, Boston Univ 1994; **Fellow:** Urology, Baylor Coll Med 1996; **Fac Appt:** Assoc Prof U, Mount Sinai Sch Med

Hensle, Terry MD [U] - **Spec Exp:** Pediatric Urology; Hypospadias; Urinary Reconstruction; Wilms' Tumor; **Hospital:** Hackensack Univ Med Ctr; **Address:** 699 Teaneck Rd, Ste 103, Teaneck, NJ 07616; **Phone:** 201-645-3362; **Board Cert:** Urology 1978; **Med School:** Cornell Univ-Weill Med Coll 1968; **Resid:** Surgery, Boston City Hosp 1973; Urology, Mass Genl Hosp 1976; **Fellow:** Pediatric Urology, Mass Genl Hosp 1977; Pediatric Urology, Great Ormond St Hosp 1978; **Fac Appt:** Prof U, Columbia P&S

Herr, Harry W MD [U] - **Spec Exp:** Bladder Cancer; Prostate Cancer; Testicular Cancer; **Hospital:** Meml Sloan-Kettering Cancer Ctr, NY-Presby/Weill Cornell Med Ctr, NY (page 65); **Address:** 1275 York Avenue, New York, NY 10065; **Phone:** 800-525-2225; **Board Cert:** Urology 1976; **Med School:** UCSF 1969; **Resid:** Urology, UC Irvine Med Ctr 1974; **Fellow:** Urology, Meml Sloan Kettering Cancer Ctr 1976; **Fac Appt:** Assoc Prof S, Cornell Univ-Weill Med Coll

Hrebinko Jr, Ronald L MD [U] - **Spec Exp:** Urologic Cancer; Kidney Cancer; Bladder Cancer; Testicular Cancer; **Hospital:** UPMC Presby, Pittsburgh; **Address:** Univ Pittsburgh Dept of Urology, Shadyside Med Bldg, Ste 209, 5200 Centre Ave, Pittsburgh, PA 15232; **Phone:** 412-605-3022; **Board Cert:** Urology 2004; **Med School:** Univ Pittsburgh 1986; **Resid:** Urology, Univ Pittsburgh Med Ctr 1992; **Fellow:** Urologic Oncology, Roswell Park Cancer Ctr 1993; **Fac Appt:** Assoc Prof U, Univ Pittsburgh

Jackman, Stephen V MD [U] - **Spec Exp:** Prostate Cancer/Robotic Surgery; Laparoscopic Surgery; Kidney Stones; **Hospital:** UPMC Shadyside, UPMC Presby, Pittsburgh; **Address:** 3471 Fifth Ave, Ste 700, Univ Pittsburgh Med Ctr, Dept Urology, Pittsburgh, PA 15213; **Phone:** 412-692-4095; **Board Cert:** Urology 2002; **Med School:** Yale Univ 1994; **Resid:** Urology, Johns Hopkins Hosp 2000; **Fac Appt:** Assoc Prof U, Univ Pittsburgh

Urology

Kaplan, Steven A MD [U] - **Spec Exp:** Urodynamics; Voiding Dysfunction; Incontinence after Prostate Cancer; Incontinence; **Hospital:** NY-Presby/Weill Cornell Med Ctr, NY (page 65); **Address:** NY Presbyterian-Weill Cornell Med Ctr, 525 E 68th St, rm F9West, New York, NY 10021-4870; **Phone:** 212-746-4811; **Board Cert:** Urology 2001; **Med School:** Mount Sinai Sch Med 1982; **Resid:** Surgery, Mount Sinai Hosp 1984; Urology, Columbia Presby Med Ctr 1988; **Fellow:** Urology, Columbia Presby Med Ctr 1990; **Fac Appt:** Prof U, Cornell Univ-Weill Med Coll

Katz, Aaron E MD [U] - **Spec Exp:** Prostate Cancer-Cryosurgery; Kidney Cancer-Cryosurgery; Complementary Medicine; Nutrition & Cancer Prevention; **Hospital:** NY-Presby/Columbia Univ Med Ctr, NY (page 65); **Address:** NY Presby Med Ctr, Herbert Irving Pav, 161 Ft Washington Ave Fl 11, New York, NY 10032; **Phone:** 212-305-6408; **Board Cert:** Urology 2006; **Med School:** NY Med Coll 1986; **Resid:** Urology, Maimonides Med Ctr 1992; **Fellow:** Urologic Oncology, Columbia Presby Med Ctr 1993; **Fac Appt:** Assoc Clin Prof U, Columbia P&S

Kavoussi, Louis R MD [U] - **Spec Exp:** Laparoscopic Surgery; Urologic Cancer; Prostate Cancer; Kidney Cancer; **Hospital:** Long Island Jewish Med Ctr, N Shore Univ Hosp; **Address:** 450 Lakeville Rd, Ste M-41, New Hyde Park, NY 11040; **Phone:** 516-734-8558; **Board Cert:** Urology 2009; **Med School:** SUNY Buffalo 1983; **Resid:** Surgery, Barnes Jewish Hosp 1985; Urology, Barnes Jewish Hosp 1989; **Fac Appt:** Prof U, NYU Sch Med

Kirschenbaum, Alexander M MD [U] - **Spec Exp:** Prostate Cancer; Bladder Cancer; Kidney Cancer; **Hospital:** Mount Sinai Med Ctr (page 63); **Address:** 58A E 79th St, New York, NY 10021; **Phone:** 646-422-0926; **Board Cert:** Urology 2006; **Med School:** Mount Sinai Sch Med 1980; **Resid:** Surgery, Mt Sinai Hosp 1982; Urology, Mt Sinai Hosp 1985; **Fellow:** Urologic Oncology, Mt Sinai Hosp 1987; **Fac Appt:** Assoc Prof U, Mount Sinai Sch Med

Lanteri, Vincent J MD [U] - **Spec Exp:** Prostate Cancer/Robotic Surgery; Urologic Cancer; Minimally Invasive Urologic Surgery; **Hospital:** Hackensack Univ Med Ctr, Monmouth Med Ctr; **Address:** 255 W Spring Valley Ave, Ste 101, Maywood, NJ 07607; **Phone:** 201-487-8866; **Board Cert:** Urology 1982; **Med School:** Mexico 1974; **Resid:** Surgery, UMDNJ Med Ctr 1977; Urology, UMDNJ Med Ctr 1980; **Fellow:** Urologic Oncology, Roswell Park Cancer Inst 1981

Lepor, Herbert MD [U] - **Spec Exp:** Prostate Cancer; **Hospital:** NYU Langone Med Ctr (page 66); **Address:** 150 E 32nd St Fl 2, New York, NY 10016; **Phone:** 646-825-6327; **Board Cert:** Urology 2006; **Med School:** Johns Hopkins Univ 1975; **Resid:** Urology, Johns Hopkins Hosp 1986; **Fac Appt:** Prof U, NYU Sch Med

Linsenmeyer, Todd A MD [U] - **Spec Exp:** Infertility-Male in Spinal Cord Injury; Voiding Dysfunction/Spinal Cord Injury; Urodynamics in Spinal Cord Injury; **Hospital:** Kessler Inst for Rehab - W Orange; **Address:** Kessler Inst Rehab, 1199 Pleasant Valley Way, West Orange, NJ 07052; **Phone:** 973-731-3900 x2274; **Board Cert:** Urology 2005; Physical Medicine & Rehabilitation 1990; Spinal Cord Injury Medicine 2002; **Med School:** Univ Hawaii JA Burns Sch Med 1979; **Resid:** Urology, Tripler AMC 1984; **Fellow:** Physical Medicine & Rehabilitation, Stanford Univ Hosp 1989; **Fac Appt:** Assoc Prof S, UMDNJ-NJ Med Sch, Newark

Loo, Marcus Hsieu-Hong MD [U] - **Spec Exp:** Prostate Disease; Kidney Stones; Voiding Dysfunction; Prostate Cancer; **Hospital:** NY-Presby/Weill Cornell Med Ctr, NY (page 65); **Address:** 254 Canal St, Ste 3001, New York, NY 10013-3501; **Phone:** 212-925-8388; **Board Cert:** Urology 2008; **Med School:** Cornell Univ-Weill Med Coll 1981; **Resid:** Surgery, NY Hosp-Cornell Med Ctr 1983; Urology, NY Hosp-Cornell Med Ctr 1988; **Fellow:** Urology, NY Hosp-Cornell Med Ctr 1984; **Fac Appt:** Clin Prof U, Cornell Univ-Weill Med Coll

Lowe, Franklin MD [U] - **Spec Exp:** Prostate Disease; Complementary Medicine; Prostate Cancer; **Hospital:** St. Luke's - Roosevelt Hosp Ctr - Roosevelt Div (page 55), NY-Presby/Columbia Univ Med Ctr, NY (page 65); **Address:** 425 W 59th St, Ste 3A, New York, NY 10019-1104; **Phone:** 212-523-7790; **Board Cert:** Urology 2006; **Med School:** Columbia P&S 1979; **Resid:** Surgery, Johns Hopkins Hosp 1981; Urology, Johns Hopkins Hosp 1984; **Fac Appt:** Clin Prof U, Columbia P&S

Malkowicz, S Bruce MD [U] - **Spec Exp:** Prostate Cancer; Bladder Cancer; Kidney Cancer; Gene Therapy; **Hospital:** Hosp Univ Penn - UPHS (page 68); **Address:** 3400 Civic Blvd Perelman Bldg Fl 3W, Philadelphia, PA 19104; **Phone:** 215-662-2891 x7330; **Board Cert:** Urology 2009; **Med School:** Univ Pennsylvania 1981; **Resid:** Surgery, Hosp Univ Penn 1983; Urology, Hosp Univ Penn 1987; **Fellow:** Urologic Oncology, USC Med Ctr 1998; Urologic Oncology, Hosp Univ Penn/Wistar Inst 1990; **Fac Appt:** Prof U, Univ Pennsylvania

McCullough, Andrew R MD [U] - **Spec Exp:** Erectile Dysfunction; Infertility-Male; Prostate Cancer; **Hospital:** Albany Med Ctr; **Address:** The Urological Inst of Northeastern NY, South Clinical Campus, 23 Hackett Blvd, Albany, NY 12208; **Phone:** 518-262-3341; **Board Cert:** Urology 2005; **Med School:** Univ MD Sch Med 1978; **Resid:** Urology, Johns Hopkins Hosp 1983; **Fellow:** Urologic Oncology, Johns Hopkins Hosp 1984; **Fac Appt:** Assoc Prof U, Albany Med Coll

Mohler, James L MD [U] - **Spec Exp:** Prostate Cancer; **Hospital:** Roswell Park Cancer Inst; **Address:** RPCI Dept Urology, Elm & Carlton Streets, Buffalo, NY 14263; **Phone:** 716-845-3159; **Board Cert:** Urology 2007; **Med School:** Med Coll GA 1980; **Resid:** Surgery, Univ Kentucky Med Ctr 1982; Urology, Univ Kentucky Med Ctr 1985; **Fellow:** Urologic Oncology, Johns Hopkins Hosp 1987; **Fac Appt:** Prof U, SUNY Buffalo

Mostwin, Jacek L MD/PhD [U] - **Spec Exp:** Prostate Cancer; **Hospital:** Johns Hopkins Hosp (page 61); **Address:** Johns Hopkins Hosp, 600 N Wolfe St Park 207 Bldg, Baltimore, MD 21287; **Phone:** 410-955-6100; **Board Cert:** Urology 2007; **Med School:** Univ MD Sch Med 1975; **Resid:** Surgery, Univ Michigan Med Ctr 1978; Urology, Johns Hopkins Hosp 1983; **Fac Appt:** Prof U, Johns Hopkins Univ

Mulhall, John P MD [U] - **Spec Exp:** Erectile Dysfunction; Peyronie's Disease; Penile Prostheses; Infertility-Male; **Hospital:** Meml Sloan-Kettering Cancer Ctr; **Address:** Prostate Ctr at Meml Sloan Kettering, 353 E 68th St Fl 5, New York, NY 10021; **Phone:** 646-422-4359; **Board Cert:** Urology 2008; **Med School:** Ireland 1985; **Resid:** Urology, Univ Conn Health Ctr 1995; **Fellow:** Urology, Boston Univ Med Ctr 1996; **Fac Appt:** Assoc Prof U, Cornell Univ-Weill Med Coll

Nagler, Harris M MD [U] - **Spec Exp:** Vasectomy Reversal; Infertility-Male; Varicocele Microsurgery; Erectile Dysfunction; **Hospital:** Beth Israel Med Ctr - Petrie Division (page 55); **Address:** Beth Israel Med Ctr, Dept Urology, 10 Union Square E, Ste 3A, New York, NY 10003-3314; **Phone:** 212-844-8700; **Board Cert:** Urology 1982; **Med School:** Temple Univ 1975; **Resid:** Urology, Columbia Presby Med Ctr 1980; **Fellow:** Reproductive Medicine, Columbia Presby Med Ctr 1981; **Fac Appt:** Prof U, Albert Einstein Coll Med

Naslund, Michael MD [U] - **Spec Exp:** Prostate Cancer; Prostate Disease; **Hospital:** Univ of MD Med Ctr; **Address:** Maryland Prostate Ctr, 419 W Redwood St, Ste 320, Baltimore, MD 21201; **Phone:** 410-328-0800; **Board Cert:** Urology 2008; **Med School:** Johns Hopkins Univ 1981; **Resid:** Surgery, Johns Hopkins Hosp 1983; Urology, Johns Hopkins Hosp 1987; **Fac Appt:** Prof U, Univ MD Sch Med

Nelson, Joel B MD [U] - **Spec Exp:** Prostate Cancer; **Hospital:** UPMC Shadyside; **Address:** UPMC Shadyside Med Ctr, 5200 Centre Ave, Ste 209, Pittsburgh, PA 15232-1312; **Phone:** 412-605-3013; **Board Cert:** Urology 2008; **Med School:** Northwestern Univ 1988; **Resid:** Surgery, Northwestern MemL Hosp 1990; Urology, Northwestern Meml Hosp 1994; **Fellow:** Urology, Johns Hopkins Hosp; **Fac Appt:** Prof U, Univ Pittsburgh

Urology

Nitti, Victor MD [U] - **Spec Exp:** Urology-Female; Incontinence-Male & Female; Urodynamics; Voiding Dysfunction; **Hospital:** NYU Langone Med Ctr (page 66); **Address:** NYU Urology Assocs, 150 E 32nd St, 2nd Fl, New York, NY 10016; **Phone:** 646-825-6324; **Board Cert:** Urology 2002; **Med School:** UMDNJ-NJ Med Sch, Newark 1985; **Resid:** Surgery, Univ Hosp 1987; Urology, Univ Hosp 1991; **Fellow:** Female Urology, UCLA 1992; **Fac Appt:** Prof U, NYU Sch Med

Partin, Alan W MD/PhD [U] - **Spec Exp:** Prostate Cancer; Prostate Disease; **Hospital:** Johns Hopkins Hosp (page 61); **Address:** Johns Hopkins Hosp, 600 N Wolfe St Marburg Bldg - rm 134, Baltimore, MD 21287-2101; **Phone:** 410-955-6100; **Board Cert:** Urology 2007; **Med School:** Johns Hopkins Univ 1989; **Resid:** Surgery, Johns Hopkins Hosp 1991; Urology, Johns Hopkins Hosp 1996; **Fac Appt:** Prof U, Johns Hopkins Univ

Poppas, Dix P MD [U] - **Spec Exp:** Genital Reconstruction-Pediatric; Robotic Surgery-Pediatric; Minimally Invasive Surgery-Pediatric; Pediatric Urology; **Hospital:** NY-Presby/Weill Cornell Med Ctr, NY (page 65); **Address:** Inst for Pediatric Urology, NY Presby Hosp-Weill Cornell, 525 E 68th St, Box 94, New York, NY 10065; **Phone:** 212-746-5337; **Board Cert:** Urology 1999; Pediatric Urology 2008; **Med School:** Eastern VA Med Sch 1988; **Resid:** Urology, NY Hosp-Cornell Med Ctr 1994; **Fellow:** Pediatric Urology, Chldns Hosp Harvard Med Sch 1996; **Fac Appt:** Prof U, Cornell Univ-Weill Med Coll

Rushton Jr, H Gil MD [U] - **Spec Exp:** Pediatric Urology; Fetal Urology; Hypospadias; Hydronephrosis; **Hospital:** Chldns Natl Med Ctr; **Address:** Dept Urology, 111 Michigan Ave NW, Ste 400-W, Washington, DC 20010; **Phone:** 202-476-5042; **Board Cert:** Urology 2004; Pediatric Urology 2009; **Med School:** Univ SC Sch Med 1978; **Resid:** Urology, Univ SC Med Ctr 1983; **Fellow:** Pediatric Urology, Hosp Sick Chldn 1984; Pediatric Urology, Emory Chldns Hosp 1986; **Fac Appt:** Prof U, Geo Wash Univ

Sadeghi-Nejad, Hossein MD [U] - **Spec Exp:** Infertility-Male; Erectile Dysfunction; Penile Prostheses; Peyronie's Disease; **Hospital:** Hackensack Univ Med Ctr, Univ Hosp-UMDNJ—Newark; **Address:** Hackensack Univ Medical Ctr, 20 Prospect Ave, Ste 711, Hackensack, NJ 07601; **Phone:** 201-342-7977; **Board Cert:** Urology 2009; **Med School:** McGill Univ 1989; **Resid:** Surgery, UCSF Med Ctr 1991; Urology, Boston Univ Med Ctr 1996; **Fellow:** Microsurgery, Boston Univ Med Ctr 1997; Reproductive Medicine, Boston Univ Med Ctr 1997; **Fac Appt:** Prof U, UMDNJ-NJ Med Sch, Newark

Samadi, David B MD [U] - **Spec Exp:** Prostate Cancer/Robotic Surgery; Kidney Cancer; Bladder Cancer; Urologic Cancer; **Hospital:** Mount Sinai Med Ctr (page 63); **Address:** 625 Madison Ave Fl 2, New York, NY 10022; **Phone:** 212-241-8779; **Board Cert:** Urology 2004; **Med School:** SUNY Stony Brook 1994; **Resid:** Surgery, Montefiore Med Ctr 1996; Urology, Montefiore Med Ctr 2000; **Fellow:** Urologic Oncology, Meml Sloan Kettering Cancer Ctr 2001; Laparoscopic Surgery, Henri Mondor Hosp 2003; **Fac Appt:** Asst Prof U, Mount Sinai Sch Med

Sawczuk, Ihor S MD [U] - **Spec Exp:** Bladder Cancer; Kidney Cancer; Prostate Cancer/Robotic Surgery; Bladder Reconstruction; **Hospital:** Hackensack Univ Med Ctr, NY-Presby/Columbia Univ Med Ctr, NY (page 65); **Address:** Hackensack Univ Med Ctr, 360 Essex St, Ste 403, Hackensack, NJ 07601; **Phone:** 201-336-8090; **Board Cert:** Urology 2005; **Med School:** Med Coll PA Hahnemann 1979; **Resid:** Surgery, St Vincents Hosp 1981; Urology, Columbia-Presby Med Ctr 1984; **Fellow:** Urologic Oncology, Columbia-Presby Med Ctr 1986; **Fac Appt:** Prof U, Columbia P&S

Scardino, Peter T MD [U] - **Spec Exp:** Prostate Cancer; Bladder Cancer; Urologic Cancer; Urinary Reconstruction; **Hospital:** Meml Sloan-Kettering Cancer Ctr; **Address:** 1275 York Avenue, New York, NY 10065; **Phone:** 646-422-4329; **Board Cert:** Urology 1981; **Med School:** Duke Univ 1971; **Resid:** Surgery, Mass Genl Hosp 1973; Urology, UCLA Med Ctr 1979; **Fellow:** Urology, Natl Cancer Inst 1976; **Fac Appt:** Prof U, Cornell Univ-Weill Med Coll

Scherr, Douglas S MD [U] - **Spec Exp:** Prostate Cancer/Robotic Surgery; Bladder Cancer; Robotic Surgery; Testicular Cancer; **Hospital:** NY-Presby/Weill Cornell Med Ctr, NY (page 65); **Address:** NY Cornell Medical Ctr, Dept Urology, 525 E 68th St Starr 900, New York, NY 10021; **Phone:** 212-746-5788; **Board Cert:** Urology 2003; **Med School:** Geo Wash Univ 1994; **Resid:** Urology, NY Hosp-Cornell Med Ctr 1999; **Fellow:** Urologic Oncology, Meml Sloan-Kettering Canc Ctr 2002; **Fac Appt:** Assoc Prof U, Cornell Univ-Weill Med Coll

Schlegel, Peter N MD [U] - **Spec Exp:** Prostate Cancer; Infertility-Male; **Hospital:** NY-Presby/Weill Cornell Med Ctr, NY (page 65), Hosp For Special Surgery (page 60); **Address:** 525 E 68th St, Starr Bldg - Fl 9th - Ste 900, New York, NY 10021-4870; **Phone:** 212-746-5491; **Board Cert:** Urology 2001; **Med School:** Univ Mass Sch Med 1983; **Resid:** Surgery, Johns Hopkins Hosp 1985; Urology, Johns Hopkins Hosp 1989; **Fellow:** Medical Oncology, Johns Hopkins Hosp 1987; Male Reproduction, NY Hosp-Cornell Med Ctr 1991; **Fac Appt:** Prof U, Cornell Univ-Weill Med Coll

Schoenberg, Mark P MD [U] - **Spec Exp:** Bladder Cancer; Urinary Reconstruction; **Hospital:** Johns Hopkins Hosp (page 61); **Address:** Johns Hopkins Hosp, 150 Marburg Bldg, 600 N Wolfe St, Baltimore, MD 21287; **Phone:** 410-955-6100; **Board Cert:** Urology 2005; **Med School:** Univ Tex, Houston 1986; **Resid:** Surgery, Hosp U Penn 1988; Urologic Surgery, Hosp U Penn 1992; **Fellow:** Urologic Oncology, Brady Inst/Johns Hopkins 1994; **Fac Appt:** Prof U, Johns Hopkins Univ

Seftel, Allen D MD [U] - **Spec Exp:** Sexual Dysfunction; Infertility-Male; Prostate Disease; Peyronie's Disease; **Hospital:** Cooper Univ Hosp; **Address:** Cooper Univ Hosp, 3 Cooper Plaza, Ste 411, Camden, NJ 08103; **Phone:** 856-963-3577; **Board Cert:** Urology 2003; **Med School:** SUNY Downstate 1984; **Resid:** Urology, SUNY Downstate Med Ctr 1987; Urology, Univ Hosps-Case West Res 1990; **Fellow:** Reproductive Medicine, Boston Univ Med Ctr 1992; **Fac Appt:** Prof U

Shabsigh, Ridwan MD [U] - **Spec Exp:** Erectile Dysfunction; Hypogonadism; Clinical Trials; **Hospital:** Maimonides Med Ctr (page 62), NY-Presby/Columbia Univ Med Ctr, NY (page 65); **Address:** 3121 Ocean Ave, Brooklyn, NY 11235; **Phone:** 718-283-7746; **Board Cert:** Urology 2000; **Med School:** Syria 1976; **Resid:** Urology, Seepark Hosp 1983; Urology, Baylor Affil Hsop 1990; **Fellow:** Urology, Baylor Affil Hosp 1987; **Fac Appt:** Clin Prof U, Columbia P&S

Sheinfeld, Joel MD [U] - **Spec Exp:** Testicular Cancer; Bladder Cancer; Fertility Preservation in Cancer; **Hospital:** Meml Sloan-Kettering Cancer Ctr; **Address:** 353 E 68th St, New York, NY 10065; **Phone:** 646-422-4311; **Board Cert:** Urology 2009; **Med School:** Univ Fla Coll Med 1981; **Resid:** Urology, Strong Meml Hosp 1986; **Fellow:** Urologic Oncology, Meml Sloan Kettering Cancer Ctr 1989; **Fac Appt:** Assoc Prof U, Cornell Univ-Weill Med Coll

Shenot, Patrick J MD [U] - **Spec Exp:** Voiding Dysfunction/Spinal Cord Injury; Voiding Dysfunction; Genitourinary Disorders; Incontinence; **Hospital:** Thomas Jefferson Univ Hosp, Magee Rehab Hosp; **Address:** 833 Chestnut St E Fl 7 - Ste 703, Philadelphia, PA 19107; **Phone:** 215-955-1000; **Board Cert:** Urology 2010; **Med School:** SUNY Stony Brook 1991; **Resid:** Surgery, Thos Jefferson Univ Hosp 1993; Urology, Thos Jefferson Univ Hosp 1997; **Fac Appt:** Asst Prof U, Thomas Jefferson Univ

Siegelbaum, Marc MD [U] - **Spec Exp:** Prostate Cancer/Robotic Surgery; Laparoscopic Surgery; Kidney Cancer; Pediatric Urology; **Hospital:** St. Joseph Med Ctr; **Address:** Chesapeake Urology Assocs, 7505 Osler Drive, Ste 506, Towson, MD 21204; **Phone:** 410-296-0167; **Board Cert:** Urology 2009; **Med School:** Univ MD Sch Med 1982; **Resid:** Surgery, Sinai Hosp 1989; Urology, Temple Univ Hlth Sci Ctr 1991

Snyder III, Howard M MD [U] - **Spec Exp:** Pediatric Urology-Non Surgical Only; **Hospital:** Chldns Hosp of Philadelphia, Hosp Univ Penn - UPHS (page 68); **Address:** Chldrns Hosp, Dept Ped Urology, 34th St & Civic Ctr Blvd, Wood Bldg, Fl 3, Philadelphia, PA 19104; **Phone:** 215-590-2767; **Board Cert:** Surgery 2003; Urology 1982; Pediatric Surgery 1995; Pediatric Urology 2008; **Med School:** Harvard Med Sch 1969; **Resid:** Surgery, Peter Bent Brigham Hosp 1973; Pediatric Surgery, Boston Chldns Hosp Med Ctr 1974; **Fellow:** Urology, Peter Bent Brigham Hosp 1980; **Fac Appt:** Prof Emeritus S, Univ Pennsylvania

Sosa, R Ernest MD [U] - **Spec Exp:** Kidney Stones; Laparoscopic Surgery; Adrenal Surgery; **Hospital:** Lenox Hill Hosp, NY-Presby/Weill Cornell Med Ctr, NY (page 65); **Address:** 880 5th Ave, New York, NY 10021; **Phone:** 212-570-6800; **Board Cert:** Urology 2006; **Med School:** Cornell Univ-Weill Med Coll 1978; **Resid:** Surgery, New York Hosp 1980; Urology, New York Hosp 1984; **Fellow:** Renal Physiology, New York Hosp-Cornell 1986; **Fac Appt:** Assoc Clin Prof U, Cornell Univ-Weill Med Coll

Taneja, Samir S MD [U] - **Spec Exp:** Prostate Cancer; Kidney Cancer; Bladder Cancer; **Hospital:** NYU Langone Med Ctr (page 66); **Address:** NYU Urology Associates, 150 E 32nd St Fl 2, New York, NY 10016-6024; **Phone:** 646-825-6321; **Board Cert:** Urology 2009; **Med School:** Northwestern Univ 1990; **Resid:** Urology, UCLA Med Ctr 1996; **Fellow:** Urologic Oncology, NYU Med Ctr 1998; **Fac Appt:** Assoc Prof U, NYU Sch Med

Tewari, Ashutosh MD [U] - **Spec Exp:** Prostate Cancer/Robotic Surgery; **Hospital:** NY-Presby/Weill Cornell Med Ctr, NY (page 65); **Address:** Weill Cornell Brady Urologic Health Ct, 525 E 68th St, Starr 900, New York, NY 10021; **Phone:** 212-746-5638; **Board Cert:** Urology 2006; **Med School:** India 1984; **Resid:** Surgery, GSVM Medical College 1990; Urology, Henry Ford Hosp 2003; **Fellow:** Transplant Surgery, Liverpool Univ Med Ctr 1993; Urologic Oncology, Shands Healthcare 1995; **Fac Appt:** Assoc Prof U, Cornell Univ-Weill Med Coll

Trabulsi, Edouard J MD [U] - **Spec Exp:** Minimally Invasive Urologic Surgery; Urologic Cancer; Prostate Cancer; **Hospital:** Thomas Jefferson Univ Hosp; **Address:** 833 Chesnut St, Ste 703, Philadelphia, PA 19107; **Phone:** 215-955-1000; **Board Cert:** Urology 2005; **Med School:** SUNY Buffalo 1995; **Resid:** Surgery, Thomas Jefferson Univ Hosp 1997; Urology, Thomas Jefferson Univ Hosp 2001; **Fellow:** Urologic Oncology, Meml Sloan Kettering Cancer Ctr 2003; **Fac Appt:** Assoc Prof U, Thomas Jefferson Univ

Uzzo, Robert MD [U] - **Spec Exp:** Bladder Cancer; Prostate Cancer; Robotic Surgery; Minimally Invasive Urologic Surgery; **Hospital:** Fox Chase Cancer Ctr (page 58); **Address:** Fox Chase Cancer Ctr, 333 Cottman Ave, Philadelphia, PA 19111; **Phone:** 215-728-3501; **Board Cert:** Urology 2009; **Med School:** Cornell Univ-Weill Med Coll 1991; **Resid:** Surgery, New York Hosp-Cornell Med Ctr 1993; Urology, New York Hosp-Cornell Med Ctr 1997; **Fellow:** Urologic Oncology, Cleveland Clinic 1999; Renal Transplant, Cleveland Clinic 2000; **Fac Appt:** Assoc Prof S, Temple Univ

Van Arsdalen, Keith N MD [U] - **Spec Exp:** Infertility-Male; Varicocele Microsurgery; Urologic Cancer; Vasectomy Reversal; **Hospital:** Hosp Univ Penn - UPHS (page 68), Chldns Hosp of Philadelphia; **Address:** Hosp Univ Penn, Div Urology, 3400 Civic Ctr Blvd, Perelman Center Fl 3W, Philadelphia, PA 19104-4283; **Phone:** 215-662-2891; **Board Cert:** Urology 1984; **Med School:** Med Coll VA 1977; **Resid:** Surgery, Univ Maryland Hosp 1979; Urology, Med Coll Virginia 1982; **Fellow:** Urodynamics, Hosp Univ Penn 1983; **Fac Appt:** Prof U, Univ Pennsylvania

Vapnek, Jonathan M MD [U] - **Spec Exp:** Incontinence; Urology-Female; Neurogenic Bladder; Urodynamics; **Hospital:** Mount Sinai Med Ctr (page 63); **Address:** 229 E 79th St, Ste 1A, New York, NY 10075; **Phone:** 212-717-9500; **Board Cert:** Urology 2005; **Med School:** UCSD 1986; **Resid:** Surgery, UCSD Med Ctr 1988; Urology, UCSF Med Ctr 1992; **Fellow:** Neurourology, UC Davis Med Ctr 1993; **Fac Appt:** Assoc Clin Prof U, Mount Sinai Sch Med

Verghese, Mohan MD [U] - **Spec Exp:** Urologic Cancer; **Hospital:** Washington Hosp Ctr; **Address:** 110 Irving St NW, Ste 3B19, Washington, DC 20010; **Phone:** 202-877-3968; **Board Cert:** Urology 2005; **Med School:** India 1976; **Resid:** Surgery, Bay State Med Ctr 1980; Urology, Washington Hosp Ctr 1984; **Fellow:** Urologic Oncology, Roswell Park Meml Inst 1992

Walsh, Patrick MD [U] - **Spec Exp:** Prostate Cancer; **Hospital:** Johns Hopkins Hosp (page 61); **Address:** Brady Urological Inst, 600 N Wolfe St, Park 224, Baltimore, MD 21287-2101; **Phone:** 410-955-6100; **Board Cert:** Urology 1975; **Med School:** Case West Res Univ 1964; **Resid:** Surgery, Peter Bent Brigham Hosp/Childrens Hosp 1967; Urology, UCLA Med Ctr 1971; **Fellow:** Endocrinology, Harbor Genl Hosp 1970; **Fac Appt:** Prof U, Johns Hopkins Univ

Wein, Alan J MD [U] - **Spec Exp:** Neuro-Urology; Prostate Cancer; Testicular Cancer; Bladder Cancer; **Hospital:** Hosp Univ Penn - UPHS (page 68), Pennsylvania Hosp-UPHS (page 68); **Address:** Univ Penn Hlth Sys, Div Uro, Penn Med, 34th & Civic Ctr Blvd, Perelman Ctr, West Pavilion, Fl 3, Philadelphia, PA 19104-4283; **Phone:** 215-662-2891; **Board Cert:** Urology 1995; **Med School:** Univ Pennsylvania 1966; **Resid:** Surgery, Hosp Univ Penn 1968; Urology, Hosp Univ Penn 1972; **Fellow:** Urology, Hosp Univ Penn 1969; **Fac Appt:** Prof U, Univ Pennsylvania

Weiss, Robert E MD [U] - **Spec Exp:** Bladder Cancer; Kidney Cancer; Testicular Cancer; Robotic Surgery; **Hospital:** Robert Wood Johnson Univ Hosp - New Brunswick, Univ Med Ctr - Princeton; **Address:** 1 Robert Wood Johnson Pl Ste MB588, New Brunswick, NJ 08901-1928; **Phone:** 732-235-9843; **Board Cert:** Urology 2004; **Med School:** NYU Sch Med 1985; **Resid:** Surgery, Mount Sinai Med Ctr 1987; Urology, Mount Sinai Med Ctr 1991; **Fellow:** Urologic Oncology, Meml Sloan Kettering Cancer Ctr 1994; **Fac Appt:** Assoc Prof U, UMDNJ-RW Johnson Med Sch

Yu, George W MD [U] - **Spec Exp:** Nutrition & Disease Prevention/Control; Nutrition & Cancer Prevention/Control; **Hospital:** G Washington Univ Hosp, Anne Arundel Med Ctr; **Address:** 122 Defense Hwy, Ste 224, Annapolis, MD 21401; **Phone:** 410-897-0540; **Board Cert:** Urology 1981; **Med School:** Tufts Univ 1973; **Resid:** Surgery, Brigham & Women's Hosp 1976; Urology, Johns Hopkins Hosp 1981; **Fac Appt:** Prof U, Geo Wash Univ

Southeast

Assimos, Dean G MD [U] - **Spec Exp:** Kidney Stones; Reconstructive Urologic Surgery; Minimally Invasive Urologic Surgery; **Hospital:** Wake Forest Univ Baptist Med Ctr; **Address:** Wake Forest Univ Baptist Med Ctr, Dept Urology, 140 Charlois Blvd, Winston-Salem, NC 27103; **Phone:** 336-716-4131; **Board Cert:** Urology 2003; **Med School:** Loyola Univ-Stritch Sch Med 1977; **Resid:** Surgery, Northwestern Univ Hosp 1979; Urology, Northwestern Univ Hosp 1983; **Fellow:** Urology, Bowman Gray Sch Med 1984; **Fac Appt:** Prof S, Wake Forest Univ

Atala, Anthony MD [U] - **Spec Exp:** Pediatric Urology; Reconstructive Surgery; Hernia; Hypospadias; **Hospital:** Wake Forest Univ Baptist Med Ctr; **Address:** Wake Forest Univ Baptist Med Ctr, Dept Urology, 140 Charlois Blvd, Winston-Salem, NC 27103; **Phone:** 336-716-4131; **Board Cert:** Urology 2004; Pediatric Urology 2008; **Med School:** Univ Louisville Sch Med 1985; **Resid:** Surgery, Univ Louisville Hosp 1987; Urology, Univ Louisville Hosp 1990; **Fellow:** Research, Childrens Hosp/Harvard 1991; Pediatric Urology, Childrens Hosp/Harvard 1992; **Fac Appt:** Prof U, Wake Forest Univ

Balaji, K C MD [U] - **Spec Exp:** Prostate Cancer; Urologic Cancer; Robotic Surgery; Minimally Invasive Surgery; **Hospital:** Wake Forest Univ Baptist Med Ctr; **Address:** Wake Forest Univ School of Medicine, Urology Clinic, 140 Charlois Blvd, Winston-Salem, NC 27103; **Phone:** 336-716-4131; **Board Cert:** Urology 2009; **Med School:** India 1986; **Resid:** Surgery, Lebanon Hosp Ctr 1993; Urology, Univ Massachusetts Med Ctr 1997; **Fellow:** Urologic Oncology, Meml Sloan Kettering 1999; **Fac Appt:** Prof U, Wake Forest Univ

Urology

Beall, Michael E MD [U] - **Spec Exp:** Prostate Cancer; Testicular Cancer; Vasectomy Reversal; **Hospital:** Inova Fairfax Hosp, Reston Hosp Ctr; **Address:** 8503 Arlington Blvd, Ste 310, Fairfax, VA 22031; **Phone:** 703-208-4200; **Board Cert:** Urology 1979; **Med School:** Geo Wash Univ 1972; **Resid:** Urology, Geo Wash Univ Hosp 1977; **Fac Appt:** Assoc Clin Prof U, Geo Wash Univ

Brock III, John W MD [U] - **Spec Exp:** Pediatric Urology; Reconstructive Surgery; Bladder Exstrophy; Spina Bifida; **Hospital:** Vanderbilt Monroe Carrell Jr. Chldn's Hosp (page 76); **Address:** Vanderbilt Chldns Hosp, Div Ped Urology, 2200 Childrens Way, 4102 DOT, Nashville, TN 37232-9820; **Phone:** 615-936-1060; **Board Cert:** Urology 2004; Pediatric Urology 2008; **Med School:** Med Coll GA 1978; **Resid:** Urology, Vanderbilt Univ Med Ctr 1983; **Fac Appt:** Prof U, Vanderbilt Univ

Broderick, Gregory MD [U] - **Spec Exp:** Erectile Dysfunction; Voiding Dysfunction; Peyronie's Disease; **Hospital:** Mayo - Jacksonville; **Address:** Mayo Clinic, Dept Urology, 4500 San Pablo Rd, Jacksonville, FL 32224; **Phone:** 904-953-7330; **Board Cert:** Urology 2002; **Med School:** UCSF 1983; **Resid:** Surgery, UCSF Med Ctr 1985; Urology, UCSF Med Ctr 1988; **Fellow:** Neurourology, UC Davis Med Ctr 1990; **Fac Appt:** Prof U, Mayo Med Sch

Busby, J Erik MD [U] - **Spec Exp:** Prostate Cancer; Robotic Surgery; **Hospital:** Univ of Ala Hosp at Birmingham; **Address:** 1530 3rd Ave S, SOT 1105, Birmingham, AL 35294; **Phone:** 205-996-8765; **Board Cert:** Urology 2009; **Med School:** Med Univ SC 1998; **Resid:** Urology, UC Davis Hlth Ctr 2004; **Fellow:** Urologic Oncology, UT MD Anderson Cancer Ctr 2007; **Fac Appt:** Asst Prof S, Univ Alabama

Carson III, Culley C MD [U] - **Spec Exp:** Erectile Dysfunction; Kidney Stones; Peyronie's Disease; **Hospital:** NC Memorial Hosp - UNC; **Address:** Univ North Carolina, Dept Urology, 2113 Physicians Office Bldg, Chapel Hill, NC 27599-7235; **Phone:** 919-966-2571; **Board Cert:** Urology 1980; **Med School:** Geo Wash Univ 1971; **Resid:** Surgery, Dartmouth-Hitchcock Med Ctr 1973; Urology, Mayo Clinic 1978; **Fac Appt:** Prof U, Univ NC Sch Med

Chang, Sam S MD [U] - **Spec Exp:** Urologic Cancer; Prostate Cancer; Bladder Cancer; Kidney Cancer; **Hospital:** Vanderbilt Univ Med Ctr (page 76); **Address:** A1302 Vanderbilt University Med Ctr N, Nashville, TN 37232-2765; **Phone:** 615-322-2101; **Board Cert:** Urology 2010; **Med School:** Vanderbilt Univ 1992; **Resid:** Urology, Vanderbilt Univ Med Ctr 1998; **Fellow:** Urologic Oncology, Meml Sloan Kettering Cancer Ctr 1999; **Fac Appt:** Prof U, Vanderbilt Univ

Ciancio, Gaetano MD [U] - **Spec Exp:** Transplant-Kidney; Transplant-Pancreas; Kidney Cancer; **Hospital:** Jackson Meml Hosp (page 70), Univ of Miami Hosp (page 72); **Address:** Highland Professional Bldg, 1801 NW 9th Ave Fl 5, Miami, FL 33136; **Phone:** 305-355-5111; **Board Cert:** Urology 2005; **Med School:** Venezuela 1982; **Resid:** Surgery, Univ Miami/Jackson Meml Hosp 1989; Urology, Univ Miami/Jackson Meml Hosp 1993; **Fellow:** Transplant Surgery, Univ Miami/Jackson Meml Hosp 1995; **Fac Appt:** Prof U, Univ Miami Sch Med

Cookson, Michael S MD [U] - **Spec Exp:** Urologic Cancer; Bladder Cancer; Prostate Cancer; Testicular Cancer; **Hospital:** Vanderbilt Univ Med Ctr (page 76), Saint Thomas Hosp - Nashville; **Address:** Vanderbilt Univ Med Ctr, Urol Surg A1302 MCN, Nashville, TN 37232-2765; **Phone:** 615-322-2101; **Board Cert:** Urology 2006; **Med School:** Univ Okla Coll Med 1988; **Resid:** Urology, UTSA Med Ctr 1994; **Fellow:** Urologic Oncology, Meml Sloan-Kettering Cancer Ctr 1996; **Fac Appt:** Prof U, Vanderbilt Univ

El-Galley, Rizk MD [U] - **Spec Exp:** Urologic Cancer; Laparoscopic Surgery; Bladder Cancer; Hydrocele; **Hospital:** Univ of Ala Hosp at Birmingham; **Address:** UAB Hosp FOT-1105, 1530 3rd Ave S, Birmingham, AL 35294-3411; **Phone:** 205-996-8765; **Board Cert:** Urology 2003; **Med School:** Egypt 1983; **Resid:** Urology, Emory Univ Hosp 1999; **Fac Appt:** Asst Prof U, Univ Alabama

Fraser Jr, Lionel B MD [U] - **Spec Exp:** Prostate Cancer; Incontinence after Prostate Cancer; Erectile Dysfunction; **Hospital:** Baptist Med Ctr-Jackson; **Address:** Metropolitan Urology, St Dominics West Med Tower, 971 Lakeland Drive, Ste 360, Jackson, MS 39216; **Phone:** 601-982-0982; **Board Cert:** Urology 2005; **Med School:** Univ Mich Med Sch 1977; **Resid:** Surgery, New England Deaconness Hosp 1979; **Fellow:** Urology, Brigham & Womens Hosp 1983

Greene, Graham MD [U] - **Spec Exp:** Urologic Cancer; **Hospital:** Lakeland Regl Med Ctr; **Address:** Lakeland Regl Cancer Ctr, 3525 Lakeland Hills Blvd, Lakeland, FL 33805; **Phone:** 863-603-6565; **Board Cert:** Urology 2007; **Med School:** Dalhousie Univ 1989; **Resid:** Urology, Victoria Genl Hosp 1994; **Fellow:** Urologic Oncology, M.D. Anderson Cancer Ctr 1997; **Fac Appt:** Assoc Prof

Hemal, Ashok K MD [U] - **Spec Exp:** Urologic Cancer; Robotic Surgery; Reconstructive Urologic Surgery; Laparoscopic Surgery; **Hospital:** Wake Forest Univ Baptist Med Ctr; **Address:** Department of Urology, Medical Center Blvd, Winston-Salem, NC 27157; **Phone:** 336-716-5702; **Med School:** India 1981; **Resid:** Surgery, G R Med College 1985; Urology, Post Grad Inst Med Ed & Rsch 1988; **Fellow:** Robotic Surgery, Henry Ford Hosp; **Fac Appt:** Prof U, Wake Forest Univ

Irby III, Pierce B MD [U] - **Spec Exp:** Kidney Stones; Minimally Invasive Surgery; Vasectomy; **Hospital:** Carolinas Med Ctr, Presby Hosp - Charlotte; **Address:** McKay Urology, 1023 Edgehill Rd S, Charlotte, NC 28207; **Phone:** 704-355-8686; **Board Cert:** Urology 2003; **Med School:** Uniformed Srvs Univ, Bethesda 1983; **Resid:** Urology, Letterman Army Med Ctr 1990; **Fellow:** Endourology, UCSF Med Ctr 1992; **Fac Appt:** Assoc Clin Prof U, Univ NC Sch Med

Joseph, David B MD [U] - **Spec Exp:** Pediatric Urology; Urodynamics; Neuro-Urology; **Hospital:** Children's Hospital - Birmingham, Univ of Ala Hosp at Birmingham; **Address:** Childrens Hospital, Dept Urology, 1600 7th Ave S, ACC-Ste 318, Birmingham, AL 35233; **Phone:** 205-939-9840; **Board Cert:** Urology 2005; Pediatric Urology 2008; **Med School:** Univ Wisc 1980; **Resid:** Urology, Univ Wisconsin Med Ctr 1985; **Fellow:** Pediatric Urology, Boston Childrens Hosp 1986; **Fac Appt:** Prof U, Univ Alabama

Keane, Thomas E MD [U] - **Spec Exp:** Urologic Cancer; Genitourinary Cancer; Prostate Cancer; Clinical Trials; **Hospital:** MUSC Med Ctr; **Address:** MUSC-Urology Dept, 96 Jonathan Lucas St, Ste CSB644, Charleston, SC 29425; **Phone:** 843-792-1666; **Board Cert:** Urology 2003; **Med School:** Ireland 1981; **Resid:** Urology, St Vincents Hosp 1986; Urology, N Tees Gen Hosp 1988; **Fellow:** Urology, Duke Univ Med Ctr 1993; **Fac Appt:** Prof U, Univ SC Sch Med

Kennelly, Michael J MD [U] - **Spec Exp:** Incontinence; Voiding Dysfunction; Pelvic Organ Prolapse Repair; Neurogenic Bladder; **Hospital:** Carolinas Med Ctr, Presby Hosp - Charlotte; **Address:** 1023 Edgehill Rd S, Charlotte, NC 28207; **Phone:** 704-355-8686; **Board Cert:** Urology 2005; **Med School:** Univ Cincinnati 1989; **Resid:** Urology, Univ Mich Med Ctr 1994; **Fellow:** Neurology, Univ Tex Hlth Sci Ctr 1995; **Fac Appt:** Clin Prof U, Univ NC Sch Med

Kim, Edward D MD [U] - **Spec Exp:** Infertility-Male; Prostate Cancer; Bladder Cancer; **Hospital:** Univ of Tennesee Med Ctr; **Address:** University Urology, 1928 Alcoa Hwy, Med Office B Bldg - Ste 222, Knoxville, TN 37920; **Phone:** 865-305-9254; **Board Cert:** Urology 2007; **Med School:** Northwestern Univ 1989; **Resid:** Urology, Northwestern Meml Hosp 1995; **Fellow:** Baylor Coll Med 1996; **Fac Appt:** Assoc Prof U, Univ Tenn Coll Med

Lloyd, L Keith MD [U] - **Spec Exp:** Erectile Dysfunction; Incontinence; Interstitial Cystitis; Neurogenic Bladder; **Hospital:** Univ of Ala Hosp at Birmingham; **Address:** UAB Urology, 1530 3rd Ave S, FOT 1105, Birmingham, AL 35294-3400; **Phone:** 205-975-0088; **Board Cert:** Urology 1976; **Med School:** Tulane Univ 1966; **Resid:** Urology, Tulane Univ Hosp 1974; **Fac Appt:** Prof U, Univ Alabama

Lockhart, Jorge L MD [U] - **Spec Exp:** Voiding Dysfunction; Bladder Cancer; Incontinence; Urinary Reconstruction; **Hospital:** Tampa Genl Hosp, H Lee Moffitt Cancer Ctr & Research Inst (page 59); **Address:** USF Dept Urology, 2 Tampa General Circle Fl 7, Tampa, FL 33606; **Phone:** 813-250-2213; **Board Cert:** Urology 1980; **Med School:** Uruguay 1973; **Resid:** Urology, Duke Univ Med Ctr 1977; **Fellow:** Urodynamics, Duke Univ Med Ctr 1978; **Fac Appt:** Prof S, Univ S Fla Coll Med

Lynne, Charles M MD [U] - **Spec Exp:** Infertility-Male in Spinal Cord Injury; Voiding Dysfunction/Spinal Cord Injury; Urodynamics; **Hospital:** Jackson Meml Hosp (page 70), Univ of Miami Hosp (page 72); **Address:** Professional Arts Ctr, 1150 NW 14 St, Ste 309, Miami, FL 33101; **Phone:** 305-243-6590; **Board Cert:** Urology 1974; **Med School:** Univ Miami Sch Med 1964; **Resid:** Urology, Univ Miami Affil Hosps 1971; **Fac Appt:** Prof U, Univ Miami Sch Med

Marshall, Fray F MD [U] - **Spec Exp:** Prostate Cancer; **Hospital:** Emory Univ Hosp; **Address:** Emory Urology, 1365 Clifton Rd NE B Bldg - Ste 1400, Atlanta, GA 30322; **Phone:** 404-778-4898; **Board Cert:** Urology 1977; **Med School:** Univ VA Sch Med 1969; **Resid:** Surgery, Univ Mich Hosps 1972; Urology, Mass Genl Hosp 1975; **Fac Appt:** Prof U, Emory Univ

McConnell, John D MD [U] - **Spec Exp:** Prostate Cancer; **Hospital:** Wake Forest Univ Baptist Med Ctr; **Address:** Wake Forest Univ Baptist Med Ctr, Medical Center Blvd, Winston-Salem, NC 27157; **Phone:** 336-716-3408; **Board Cert:** Urology 2004; **Med School:** Loyola Univ-Stritch Sch Med 1978; **Resid:** Surgery, Parkland Hosp 1980; Urology, Parkland Hosp 1984; **Fac Appt:** Prof U, Wake Forest Univ

Milam, Douglas F MD [U] - **Spec Exp:** Urodynamics; Voiding Dysfunction; Sexual Dysfunction; **Hospital:** Vanderbilt Univ Med Ctr (page 76); **Address:** Vanderbilt Dept Urologic Surgery, 1301 Med Ctr Drive N, Ste A-1302, Nashville, TN 37232-2765; **Phone:** 615-322-2880; **Board Cert:** Urology 2003; **Med School:** W VA Univ 1986; **Resid:** Surgery, Univ Utah Hosps 1988; Urology, Univ Utah Hosps 1991; **Fac Appt:** Assoc Prof U, Vanderbilt Univ

Miller, Scott D MD [U] - **Spec Exp:** Robotic Surgery; Prostate Cancer/Robotic Surgery; Minimally Invasive Urologic Surgery; Reconstructive Surgery; **Hospital:** Northside Hosp, St. Joseph's Hosp - Atlanta; **Address:** Georgia Urology, 5670 Peachtree Dunwoody Rd, Ste 1250, Atlanta, GA 30342; **Phone:** 404-256-1844; **Board Cert:** Urology 2005; **Med School:** Med Coll GA 1990; **Resid:** Urology, Univ Kentucky Med Ctr 1995

Moul, Judd W MD [U] - **Spec Exp:** Prostate Cancer; Testicular Cancer; Minimally Invasive Urologic Surgery; Clinical Trials; **Hospital:** Duke Univ Hosp, Durham VA Med Ctr; **Address:** Duke Univ Med Ctr, Duke South Bldg - rm 1573, Box 3707, Durham, NC 27710; **Phone:** 919-668-8108; **Board Cert:** Urology 2008; **Med School:** Jefferson Med Coll 1982; **Resid:** Urology, Walter Reed Army Med Ctr 1987; **Fellow:** Urologic Oncology, Duke Univ Med Ctr 1989; **Fac Appt:** Prof S, Duke Univ

Patel, Vipul R MD [U] - **Spec Exp:** Prostate Cancer/Robotic Surgery; Kidney Cancer; **Hospital:** Florida Hosp Celebration Hlth; **Address:** 410 Celebration Pl, Ste 200, Celebration, FL 34747; **Phone:** 407-303-4673; **Board Cert:** Urology 2004; **Med School:** Baylor Coll Med 1995; **Resid:** Urology, Univ Miami; **Fellow:** Urologic Laparoscopic Surg-Endourology, Univ Miami

Patterson, Anthony L MD [U] - **Spec Exp:** Laparoscopic Surgery; Kidney Stones; **Hospital:** Univ of Tennesee Med Ctr; **Address:** UT Medical Group, 7945 Wolf River Blvd, Ste 350, Germantown, TN 38138-1733; **Phone:** 901-347-8350; **Board Cert:** Urology 2007; **Med School:** Univ Tenn Coll Med 1982; **Resid:** Surgery, Univ Tenn Med Ctr 1984; Urology, Univ Tenn Med Ctr 1987; **Fac Appt:** Assoc Prof U, Univ Tenn Coll Med

Penson, David F MD [U] - **Spec Exp:** Prostate Disease; Urologic Cancer; Bladder Cancer; Erectile Dysfunction; **Hospital:** Vanderbilt Univ Med Ctr (page 76); **Address:** 2525 West End Ave, Ste 600, Nashville, TN 37203-1738; **Phone:** 615-322-2880; **Board Cert:** Urology 2009; **Med School:** Boston Univ 1991; **Resid:** Urology, UCLA Med Ctr 1997; **Fellow:** Urologic Oncology, Yale-New Haven Hosp 1999; **Fac Appt:** Prof U, Vanderbilt Univ

Pope IV, John C MD [U] - **Spec Exp:** Pediatric Urology; Kidney Stones; **Hospital:** Vanderbilt Monroe Carrell Jr. Chldn's Hosp (page 76); **Address:** 2200 Children's Way, Ste 4102 DOT, Nashville, TN 37232; **Phone:** 615-936-1060; **Board Cert:** Urology 2008; Pediatric Urology 2008; **Med School:** Univ Tenn Coll Med 1989; **Resid:** Surgery, Vanderbilt Univ Med Ctr 1991; Urology, Vanderbilt Univ Med Ctr 1995; **Fellow:** Pediatric Urology, Indiana Univ Med Ctr 1997; **Fac Appt:** Assoc Prof U, Vanderbilt Univ

Pow-Sang, Julio M MD [U] - **Spec Exp:** Prostate Cancer; **Hospital:** H Lee Moffitt Cancer Ctr & Research Inst (page 59); **Address:** H Lee Moffitt Cancer Ctr, GU Clinic, 12902 Magnolia Drive, Tampa, FL 33612-9416; **Phone:** 813-972-8418; **Board Cert:** Urology 1999; **Med School:** Mexico 1978; **Resid:** Surgery, Univ Miami Sch Med 1983; Urology, Univ Miami Sch Med 1986; **Fellow:** Urologic Oncology, Univ Fla Coll Med 1987; **Fac Appt:** Prof S, Univ S Fla Coll Med

Preminger, Glenn M MD [U] - **Spec Exp:** Kidney Stones; **Hospital:** Duke Univ Hosp; **Address:** Duke Univ Med Ctr, Div Urologic Surgery, rm 1587, Box 3167, White Zone Duke S, Durham, NC 27710; **Phone:** 919-681-5506; **Board Cert:** Urology 2003; **Med School:** NY Med Coll 1977; **Resid:** Surgery, N Carolina Meml Hosp 1979; Urology, N Carolina Meml Hosp 1983; **Fellow:** Urology, Univ Texas SW Med Ctr 1985; **Fac Appt:** Prof U, Duke Univ

Pruthi, Raj S MD [U] - **Spec Exp:** Urologic Cancer; Robotic Surgery; **Hospital:** NC Memorial Hosp - UNC; **Address:** UNC Dept Surgery, Urologic Surgery, 2113 POB, rm CB 7235, 170 Manning Drive, Chapel Hill, NC 27514; **Phone:** 919-966-2571; **Board Cert:** Urology 2002; **Med School:** Duke Univ 1992; **Resid:** Surgery, Stanford Univ Hosp 1993; Urology, Stanford Univ Hosp 1998; **Fac Appt:** Assoc Prof U, Univ NC Sch Med

Robertson, Cary N MD [U] - **Spec Exp:** Prostate Cancer; Kidney Cancer; High Intensity Focused Ultrasound(HIFU); Testicular Cancer; **Hospital:** Duke Univ Hosp; **Address:** Duke Univ Med Ctr, rm 1108, Box 3833, Green Zone Duke South, Durham, NC 27710; **Phone:** 919-684-2446; **Board Cert:** Urology 2006; **Med School:** Tulane Univ 1977; **Resid:** Urology, Duke Univ Med Ctr 1985; **Fellow:** Urologic Oncology, Natl Inst Hlth 1987; **Fac Appt:** Assoc Prof U, Duke Univ

Rowland, Randall MD [U] - **Spec Exp:** Urologic Cancer; **Hospital:** Univ of Kentucky Albert B. Chandler Hosp; **Address:** Univ Kentucky Med Ctr, Div Urology, 800 Rose St, rm MS283, Lexington, KY 40536-0001; **Phone:** 859-323-6677; **Board Cert:** Urology 1980; **Med School:** Northwestern Univ 1972; **Resid:** Urology, Northwestern Meml Hosp 1978; **Fellow:** Urology, Northwestern Meml Hosp 1977; **Fac Appt:** Prof U, Univ KY Coll Med

Sanders, William Holt MD [U] - **Spec Exp:** Prostate Cancer; Kidney Stones; Kidney Cancer; **Hospital:** Northside Hosp; **Address:** 980 Johnson Ferry Rd NE, Ste 490, Atlanta, GA 30342-1767; **Phone:** 404-257-0133; **Board Cert:** Urology 2006; **Med School:** Emory Univ 1988; **Resid:** Surgery, Emory Affil Hosp 1990; Urology, Yale-New Haven Hosp 1993; **Fellow:** Urologic Oncology, Emory Univ Hosp 1994

Shaban, Stephen F MD [U] - **Spec Exp:** Infertility-Male; Congenital Absence of Vas Deferens; **Hospital:** Rex HlthCare, WakeMed-Raleigh Campus; **Address:** 2800 Blue Ridge Rd, Ste 405, Raleigh, NC 27607; **Phone:** 919-851-5482; **Board Cert:** Urology 2004; **Med School:** Mount Sinai Sch Med 1982; **Resid:** Urology, Univ S Fla 1987; **Fellow:** Male Reproduction, Baylor Coll Med 1988; **Fac Appt:** Prof U, Univ NC Sch Med

Urology

Smith, Joseph A MD [U] - **Spec Exp:** Prostate Cancer/Robotic Surgery; Bladder Cancer; Kidney Cancer; **Hospital:** Vanderbilt Univ Med Ctr (page 76); **Address:** Vanderbilt Univ Med Ctr, Dept Urology, A-1302 Medical Center North, Nashville, TN 37232-2765; **Phone:** 615-343-0234; **Board Cert:** Urology 2000; **Med School:** Univ Tenn Coll Med 1974; **Resid:** Surgery, Parkland Meml Hosp 1976; Urology, Univ Utah 1979; **Fellow:** Urologic Oncology, Meml Sloan Kettering Cancer Ctr 1980; **Fac Appt:** Prof U, Vanderbilt Univ

Soloway, Mark S MD [U] - **Spec Exp:** Bladder Cancer; Kidney Cancer; Prostate Cancer; Urologic Pathology; **Hospital:** Jackson Meml Hosp (page 70), Univ of Miami Hosp & Clins/Sylvester Comp Canc Ctr (page 73); **Address:** 1150 NW 14th St, Ste 309, Miami, FL 33136; **Phone:** 305-243-6596; **Board Cert:** Urology 1977; **Med School:** Case West Res Univ 1968; **Resid:** Surgery, Univ Hosps 1970; Urology, Univ Hosps 1975; **Fellow:** Surgery, Natl Cancer Inst 1972; **Fac Appt:** Prof U, Univ Miami Sch Med

Steers, William D MD [U] - **Spec Exp:** Incontinence; Erectile Dysfunction; Prostate Cancer/Robotic Surgery; **Hospital:** Univ of Virginia Health Sys; **Address:** UVA Hlth System, Dept Urology, PO Box 800422, Charlottesville, VA 22908-0422; **Phone:** 434-924-9107; **Board Cert:** Urology 1999; **Med School:** Med Coll OH 1980; **Resid:** Urology, Univ Tex Hlth Sci Ctr 1986; **Fellow:** Neurology, Univ Pittsburgh Med Ctr 1988; **Fac Appt:** Prof U, Univ VA Sch Med

Strup, Stephen E MD [U] - **Spec Exp:** Urologic Cancer; Minimally Invasive Urologic Surgery; Robotic Surgery; **Hospital:** Univ of Kentucky Albert B. Chandler Hosp; **Address:** MS-283 Chandler Med Ctr, 800 Rose St, Lexington, KY 40536; **Phone:** 859-323-6679; **Board Cert:** Urology 2007; **Med School:** Indiana Univ 1988; **Resid:** Urology, Thomas Jefferson Univ Hosp 1994; **Fellow:** Urologic Oncology, National Cancer Inst 1996; **Fac Appt:** Prof S, Univ KY Coll Med

Su, Li-Ming MD [U] - **Spec Exp:** Prostate Cancer; Bladder Cancer; Testicular Cancer; **Hospital:** Shands at Univ of FL; **Address:** Shands at Univ Florida, Dept Urology, 1600 SW Archer St, Gainesville, FL 32610; **Phone:** 352-265-8282; **Board Cert:** Urology 2003; **Med School:** Cornell Univ-Weill Med Coll 1994; **Resid:** Surgery, NY Presby-Cornell Med Ctr 1996; Urology, NY Presby-Cornell Med Ctr 2000; **Fellow:** Robotic Surgery, Johns Hopkins Hosp 2001; **Fac Appt:** Prof U, Univ Fla Coll Med

Sutherland, Richard W MD [U] - **Spec Exp:** Pediatric Urology; **Hospital:** NC Memorial Hosp - UNC; **Address:** UNC-Chapel Hill, Div Urologic Surgery, 2113 POB Bldg, 170 Manning Drive, CB 7235, Chapel Hill, NC 27599-7235; **Phone:** 919-966-2573; **Board Cert:** Urology 2007; Pediatric Urology 2008; **Med School:** Oregon Hlth & Sci Univ 1989; **Resid:** Urology, Albany Med Ctr 1994; **Fellow:** Pediatric Urology, Baylor Coll Med 1996; **Fac Appt:** Assoc Prof U, Univ NC Sch Med

Teigland, Chris M MD [U] - **Spec Exp:** Prostate Cancer/Robotic Surgery; Kidney Cancer; Laparoscopic Surgery; **Hospital:** Carolinas Med Ctr; **Address:** Mckay Urology, 1023 Edgehill Rd S, Charlotte, NC 28207; **Phone:** 704-355-8686; **Board Cert:** Urology 2007; **Med School:** Duke Univ 1980; **Resid:** Surgery, Univ Utah Affil Hosps 1982; Urology, Univ Texas SW Med Ctr 1987; **Fac Appt:** Clin Prof S, Univ NC Sch Med

Terris, Martha K MD [U] - **Spec Exp:** Prostate Cancer; Brachytherapy; Urologic Cancer; Bladder Cancer; **Hospital:** Charlie Norwood VA Med Ctr - Augusta, Med Coll of GA Hosp and Clin (MCG Health Inc); **Address:** Charlie Norwood VA Medical Center, 1 Freedom Way, Augusta, GA 30904; **Phone:** 706-733-0188; **Board Cert:** Urology 2007; **Med School:** Univ Miss 1986; **Resid:** Surgery, Duke Univ Med Ctr 1988; Urology, Stanford Univ Med Ctr 1995; **Fellow:** Ultrasound, Stanford Univ 1991; **Fac Appt:** Prof S, Med Coll GA

Wallen, Eric M MD [U] - **Spec Exp:** Laparoscopic Surgery; Prostate Cancer; Urologic Cancer; Robotic Surgery; **Hospital:** NC Memorial Hosp - UNC; **Address:** Div of Urologic Surgery, CB 7235, 2113 Physicians Office Bldg, 170 Manning Drive, Chapel Hill, NC 27599-7235; **Phone:** 919-966-8802; **Board Cert:** Urology 2002; **Med School:** UCLA 1994; **Resid:** Surgery, Stanford Univ Med Ctr 1996; Urology, Stanford Univ Med Ctr 2000; **Fac Appt:** Assoc Prof S, Univ NC Sch Med

Webster, George D MD [U] - **Spec Exp:** Reconstructive Urologic Surgery; Urology-Female; Urodynamics; Incontinence-Male & Female; **Hospital:** Duke Univ Hosp; **Address:** Duke Univ Med Ctr, Box 3146, Durham, NC 27710; **Phone:** 919-684-2516; **Board Cert:** Urology 1981; **Med School:** England, UK 1968; **Resid:** Surgery, Harare Hosp 1972; Urology, Inst Urology 1974; **Fellow:** Urology, Duke Univ Med Ctr 1978; **Fac Appt:** Prof U, Duke Univ

Winfield, Howard N MD [U] - **Spec Exp:** Kidney Stones; Laparoscopic Surgery; Robotic Surgery; **Hospital:** DCH Reg Med Ctr; **Address:** W Alabama Urology Assoc, DCH Med Towers, Suite 908, 701 Univ Blvd E, Tuscaloosa, AL 35401; **Phone:** 205-344-9393; **Board Cert:** Urology 2008; **Med School:** McGill Univ 1978; **Resid:** Urology, McGill Univ Tchg Hosp 1984; **Fellow:** Endourology, Washington Univ 1985; Endourology, UCLA 1986; **Fac Appt:** , Univ Iowa Coll Med

Midwest

Andriole, Gerald L MD [U] - **Spec Exp:** Urologic Cancer; Prostate Cancer; Laparoscopic Surgery; **Hospital:** Barnes-Jewish Hosp; **Address:** 4960 Children's Place, Campus Box 8242, St Louis, MO 63110; **Phone:** 314-362-8212; **Board Cert:** Urology 2003; **Med School:** Jefferson Med Coll 1978; **Resid:** Surgery, Strong Meml Hosp 1980; Urology, Brigham & Womens Hosp 1983; **Fellow:** Urologic Oncology, NCI/NIH 1985; **Fac Appt:** Prof U, Washington Univ, St Louis

Bahnson, Robert MD [U] - **Spec Exp:** Prostate Cancer; Bladder Cancer; Continent Urinary Diversions; **Hospital:** Ohio St Univ Med Ctr, Arthur G James Cancer Hosp & Research Inst; **Address:** 456 West 10th Avenue, Dept of Urology, 3142 Cramblett Med Ctr, Columbus, OH 43210-1228; **Phone:** 614-293-3646; **Board Cert:** Urology 2006; **Med School:** Tufts Univ 1979; **Resid:** Surgery, Northwestern Univ 1981; Urology, Northwestern Univ 1985; **Fellow:** Urology, Northwestern Univ 1984; Research, Univ Pittsburgh 1991; **Fac Appt:** Prof U, Ohio State Univ

Bloom, David A MD [U] - **Spec Exp:** Pediatric Urology; Voiding Dysfunction; Genitourinary Reconstruction; Spina Bifida; **Hospital:** Univ of Michigan Hosp; **Address:** Univ Mich, Dept Urology, 1500 E Med Ctr Dr, 3875 Taubman Ctr, Ann Arbor, MI 48109-5330; **Phone:** 734-232-4943; **Board Cert:** Urology 1982; Pediatric Urology 2008; **Med School:** SUNY Buffalo 1971; **Resid:** Surgery, UCLA Med Ctr 1976; Urology, UCLA Med Ctr 1980; **Fellow:** Pediatric Urology, Inst Urol-St Peters Hosp 1978; **Fac Appt:** Prof U, Univ Mich Med Sch

Bodner, Donald MD [U] - **Spec Exp:** Neuro-Urology; Spinal Cord Injury; **Hospital:** Univ Hosps Case Med Ctr (page 74); **Address:** Urologic Institute, 11100 Euclid Ave, Cleveland, OH 44106; **Phone:** 216-844-5503; **Board Cert:** Urology 2004; **Med School:** Indiana Univ 1979; **Resid:** Surgery, Case Western Reserve Univ Affil Hosp 1981; Urology, Case Western Reserve Univ Affil Hosp 1984

Brendler, Charles B MD [U] - **Spec Exp:** Prostate Cancer; **Hospital:** Evanston/North Shore Univ Hlth Sys; **Address:** NorthShore Dept Urology, 2650 Ridge Ave Walgreen Bldg - Ste 2507, Evanston, IL 60201; **Phone:** 847-657-5730; **Board Cert:** Urology 1981; **Med School:** Univ VA Sch Med 1974; **Resid:** Surgery, Duke Univ Med Ctr 1976; Urology, Duke Univ Med Ctr 1979; **Fellow:** Urologic Oncology, Univ Hosp Wales 1980; Urologic Oncology, Johns Hopkins Hosp 1982; **Fac Appt:** Prof U, Northwestern Univ-Feinberg Sch Med

Bushman, Wade MD [U] - **Spec Exp:** Neuro-Urology; Urodynamics; Urology-Female; **Hospital:** Univ WI Hosp & Clins; **Address:** Dept Urology, 600 Highland Ave, C52, Madison, WI 53792-3236; **Phone:** 608-263-4757; **Board Cert:** Urology 2006; **Med School:** Univ Chicago-Pritzker Sch Med 1986; **Resid:** Urology, Univ VA Med Ctr 1992; **Fac Appt:** Assoc Prof U, Univ Wisc

Cain, Mark P MD [U] - **Spec Exp:** Pediatric Urology; Hydronephrosis-Prenatal; Genitourinary Reconstruction; Incontinence; **Hospital:** Riley Hosp for Children, Peyton Manning Children's Hosp at St. Vincent; **Address:** IU Health Physicians-Pediatric Urology, 705 Riley Hospital Drive, rm 1210, Indianapolis, IN 46202; **Phone:** 317-944-8896; **Board Cert:** Urology 2008; Pediatric Urology 2008; **Med School:** Oregon Hlth & Sci Univ 1987; **Resid:** Surgery, Albany Med Ctr 1989; Urology, Albany Med Ctr 1992; **Fellow:** Pediatric Urology, Mayo Clinic 1994; **Fac Appt:** Prof U, Indiana Univ

Campbell, Steven C MD/PhD [U] - **Spec Exp:** Kidney Cancer; Prostate Cancer; Bladder Cancer; **Hospital:** Cleveland Clin (page 56); **Address:** Cleveland Clinic, Glickman Urological Inst, 9500 Euclid Ave, MS Q10-1, Cleveland, OH 44195; **Phone:** 216-444-5595; **Board Cert:** Urology 2008; **Med School:** Univ Chicago-Pritzker Sch Med 1989; **Resid:** Urology, Cleveland Clinic 1995; **Fellow:** Urology, Meml Sloan Kettering Cancer Ctr 1996; **Fac Appt:** Prof S, Cleveland Cl Coll Med/Case West Res

Catalona, William J MD [U] - **Spec Exp:** Prostate Cancer; Prostate Disease; **Hospital:** Northwestern Meml Hosp; **Address:** Northwestern Med Faculty Foundation, 675 N St Clair St, Ste 20-150, Chicago, IL 60611; **Phone:** 312-695-6126; **Board Cert:** Urology 1978; **Med School:** Yale Univ 1968; **Resid:** Surgery, UCSF Med Ctr 1970; Urology, Johns Hopkins Hosp 1976; **Fellow:** Surgical Oncology, Natl Cancer Inst 1972; **Fac Appt:** Prof U, Northwestern Univ

Chancellor, Michael B MD [U] - **Spec Exp:** Incontinence-Female; Urology-Female; Neuro-Urology; **Hospital:** Beaumont Hosp-Royal Oak; **Address:** William Beaumont Hosp, Urology, 3535 W 13 Mile Rd, Ste 438, Royal Oak, MI 48073; **Phone:** 248-551-3519; **Board Cert:** Urology 2010; **Med School:** Med Coll Wisc 1983; **Resid:** Surgery, Univ Michigan 1985; Urology, Univ Michigan 1988; **Fellow:** Neurourology, Columbia-Presby Med Ctr 1990; **Fac Appt:** Prof U, Univ Mich Med Sch

Coplen, Douglas E MD [U] - **Spec Exp:** Pediatric Urology; Urologic Cancer-Pediatric; Testicular Cancer-Pediatric; Fetal Urology; **Hospital:** St. Louis Chldns Hosp; **Address:** St Louis Children's Hosp, 4990 Children's Pl, Northwest Tower, Ste 1120, St Louis, MO 63110; **Phone:** 314-454-6034; **Board Cert:** Urology 2005; Pediatric Urology 2008; **Med School:** Indiana Univ 1985; **Resid:** Urology, Barnes Jewish Hosp 1992; **Fellow:** Pediatric Urology, Childrens Hosp 1994; **Fac Appt:** Asst Prof S, Washington Univ, St Louis

Donovan Jr, James F MD [U] - **Spec Exp:** Prostate Cancer/Robotic Surgery; Infertility-Male; Erectile Dysfunction; Kidney Cancer; **Hospital:** Univ Hosp - Cincinnati, Christ Hosp, The - Cincinnati; **Address:** Univ Cincinnati Med Ctr, Medical Arts Bldg, 222 Piedmont Ave, Ste 7000, Cincinnati, OH 45219; **Phone:** 513-475-8787; **Board Cert:** Urology 2009; **Med School:** Northwestern Univ 1978; **Resid:** Surgery, Northwestern Meml Hosp 1982; Urology, Northwestern Meml Hosp 1986; **Fellow:** Male Infertility, Baylor Coll Med 1986; **Fac Appt:** Prof U, Univ Cincinnati

Elder, Jack S MD [U] - **Spec Exp:** Pediatric Urology; Hypospadias; Urinary Reconstruction; Robotic Surgery; **Hospital:** Henry Ford Hosp, Chldns Hosp of Michigan; **Address:** Henry Ford Hosp, 2799 W Grand Blvd Fl K-9, Detroit, MI 48202; **Phone:** 313-916-2626; **Board Cert:** Urology 1984; **Med School:** Univ Okla Coll Med 1976; **Resid:** Surgery, Yale-New Haven Hosp 1978; Urology, Johns Hopkins Hosp 1982; **Fellow:** Pediatric Urology, Johns Hopkins Hosp 1982; Pediatric Urology, Chldns Hosp 1986; **Fac Appt:** Prof U, Case West Res Univ

Firlit, Casimir MD/PhD [U] - **Spec Exp:** Pediatric Urology; Genitourinary Reconstruction; Transplant-Kidney-Pediatric; **Hospital:** Cardinal Glennon Mem Children's Hosp; **Address:** Cardinal Glennon Chlds Hosp, 1465 S Grand Blvd Fl 5, Glennon Hall, St Louis, MO 63104; **Phone:** 314-577-5334; **Board Cert:** Urology 1975; **Med School:** Loyola Univ-Stritch Sch Med 1965; **Resid:** Surgery, Hines VA Hosp 1970; Urology, Hines VA Hosp 1973; **Fellow:** Pediatric Urology, Chldns Meml Hosp 1974; **Fac Appt:** Prof U, Univ MO-Columbia Sch Med

Flanigan, Robert C MD [U] - **Spec Exp:** Urologic Cancer; Prostate Cancer; Kidney Cancer; Bladder Cancer; **Hospital:** Loyola Univ Med Ctr; **Address:** Loyola Univ Med-Fahey Bldg, 2160 S First Ave, rm 267, Maywood, IL 60153; **Phone:** 708-216-5100; **Board Cert:** Urology 2001; **Med School:** Case West Res Univ 1972; **Resid:** Surgery, Case West Univ Med Ctr 1978; Urology, Case West Univ Med Ctr 1978; **Fac Appt:** Prof U, Loyola Univ-Stritch Sch Med

Foster, Richard S MD [U] - **Spec Exp:** Testicular Cancer; Reconstructive Surgery; **Hospital:** IU Health University Hosp; **Address:** Indiana Univ Dept Urology, 535 Barnhill Drive, Ste 420, Indianapolis, IN 46202; **Phone:** 317-274-3458; **Board Cert:** Urology 2008; **Med School:** Indiana Univ 1980; **Resid:** Urology, Indiana Univ Hosp 1986; **Fac Appt:** Prof U, Indiana Univ

Gluckman, Gordon R MD [U] - **Spec Exp:** Prostate Cancer; Kidney Cancer; Minimally Invasive Urologic Surgery; Robotic Surgery; **Hospital:** Adv Luth Genl Hosp, Resurrection Med Ctr; **Address:** Northwest Suburban Urologists, 900 Rand Rd, Ste 120, Des Plaines, IL 60016; **Phone:** 847-823-3185; **Board Cert:** Urology 2006; **Med School:** Northwestern Univ 1989; **Resid:** Surgery, UCSF Med Ctr 1991; Urology, UCSF Med Ctr 1995; **Fac Appt:** Asst Clin Prof S, Ros Franklin Univ/Chicago Med Sch

Gujral, Saroj MD [U] - **Spec Exp:** Urologic Cancer; Urology-Female; **Hospital:** Albert Lea Med Ctr-Mayo Hlth Sys; **Address:** 404 W Fountain St, Albert Lea, MN 56007; **Phone:** 507-379-2130; **Board Cert:** Urology 1979; **Med School:** India 1970; **Resid:** Urology, Suburban Hosp 1978; Urology, Dalhousie Univ Med Ctrs

Jones, J Stephen MD [U] - **Spec Exp:** Prostate Cancer; **Hospital:** Cleveland Clin (page 56); **Address:** 26900 Cedar Rd, Ste 306 South, Beachwood, OH 44122; **Phone:** 216-839-3666; **Board Cert:** Urology 2002; **Med School:** Univ Ark 1986; **Resid:** Urology, Vanderbilt Univ Med Ctr 1993; **Fac Appt:** Prof S, Cleveland Cl Coll Med/Case West Res

Kaefer, Martin MD [U] - **Spec Exp:** Pediatric Urology; Reconstructive Surgery; Genitourinary Congenital Anomalies; Hydronephrosis-Prenatal; **Hospital:** Riley Hosp for Children, Franciscan St. Francis Hlth-Indianapolis; **Address:** IU Health - Pediatric Urology, 705 Riley Hospital Drive, rm 1210, Indianapolis, IN 46202; **Phone:** 317-944-8896; **Board Cert:** Urology 2000; Pediatric Urology 2008; **Med School:** Northwestern Univ 1989; **Resid:** Surgery, Indiana Univ Med Ctr 1991; Urology, Indiana Univ Med Ctr 1995; **Fellow:** Pediatric Urology, Childrens Hosp 1998; **Fac Appt:** Prof U, Indiana Univ

Kaouk, Jihad MD [U] - **Spec Exp:** Minimally Invasive Urologic Surgery; Robotic Surgery; Kidney Cancer; Bladder Cancer; **Hospital:** Cleveland Clin (page 56); **Address:** Cleveland Clinic, 9500 Euclid Ave, MC Q10, Cleveland, OH 44195; **Phone:** 216-444-2976; **Med School:** Lebanon 1993; **Resid:** Surgery, Amer Univ of Beirut Med Ctr 1996; Urology, Amer Univ of Beirut Med Ctr 1999; **Fellow:** Minimally Invasive Surgery, Cleveland Clinic 2001; Laparoscopic Surgery, Cleveland Clinic 2002; **Fac Appt:** Assoc Prof S, Cleveland Cl Coll Med/Case West Res

Kass, Evan J MD [U] - **Spec Exp:** Pediatric Urology; Hydronephrosis; Hypospadias; Varicocele in Adolescents; **Hospital:** Beaumont Hosp-Royal Oak; **Address:** 2221 Livernois, Ste 103, Troy, MI 48084; **Phone:** 248-519-0305; **Board Cert:** Urology 1978; Pediatric Urology 2009; **Med School:** SUNY Downstate 1968; **Resid:** Urology, Univ Mich Hosp 1976; **Fellow:** Pediatric Urology, Hosp for Sick Chldn 1978; **Fac Appt:** Assoc Prof U, Wayne State Univ

Urology

Kibel, Adam S MD [U] - **Spec Exp:** Prostate Cancer; Bladder Cancer; Kidney Cancer; Minimally Invasive Surgery; **Hospital:** Barnes-Jewish Hosp, Barnes-Jewish West County Hosp; **Address:** 4960 Chldns Pkwy, Wohl Hosp Bldg Fl 2, Box 82, St Louis, MO 63110-1000; **Phone:** 314-362-8295; **Board Cert:** Urology 2009; **Med School:** Cornell Univ-Weill Med Coll 1991; **Resid:** Urology, Brigham & Women's Hosp 1996; **Fellow:** Urologic Oncology, Johns Hopkins Hosp 1999; **Fac Appt:** Prof U, Washington Univ, St Louis

Klein, Eric A MD [U] - **Spec Exp:** Urologic Cancer; Testicular Cancer; Kidney Cancer; Prostate Cancer; **Hospital:** Cleveland Clin (page 56); **Address:** 9500 Euclid Ave, MS Q-10, Glickman Urologic and Kidney Institute, Cleveland, OH 44195-0001; **Phone:** 216-444-5591; **Board Cert:** Urology 2008; **Med School:** Univ Pittsburgh 1981; **Resid:** Urology, Cleveland Clinic Fdn 1986; **Fellow:** Urologic Oncology, Meml Sloan Kettering Canc Ctr 1989; **Fac Appt:** Prof S, Cleveland Cl Coll Med/Case West Res

Klutke, Carl G MD [U] - **Spec Exp:** Urology-Female; Incontinence; Urodynamics; **Hospital:** Barnes-Jewish Hosp; **Address:** 1040 N Mason Rd Bldg 1 - Ste 122, St Louis, MO 63141; **Phone:** 314-996-8060; **Board Cert:** Urology 2009; **Med School:** Univ Mich Med Sch 1983; **Resid:** Surgery, Henry Ford Hosp 1985; Urology, Henry Ford Hosp 1988; **Fellow:** Female Urology, UCLA Med Ctr 1989; **Fac Appt:** Assoc Prof S, Washington Univ, St Louis

Koch, Michael O MD [U] - **Spec Exp:** Prostate Cancer; Bladder Cancer; Robotic Surgery; Reconstructive Urologic Surgery; **Hospital:** IU Health University Hosp; **Address:** IU Health Physicians, Dept Urology, 535 Barnhill Drive, Ste 420, Indianapolis, IN 46202; **Phone:** 317-274-7338; **Board Cert:** Urology 2007; **Med School:** Dartmouth Med Sch 1981; **Resid:** Surgery, Dartmouth-Hitchcock Med Ctr 1983; Urology, Vanderbilt Univ Med Ctr 1987; **Fellow:** Surgical Research, Dartmouth Med Sch 1984; **Fac Appt:** Prof U, Indiana Univ

Koff, Stephen A MD [U] - **Spec Exp:** Pediatric Urology; **Hospital:** Nationwide Chldn's Hosp; **Address:** Nationwide Chldns Hosp-Dept Urology, 555 S 18th St, Ste 6D, Columbus, OH 43205; **Phone:** 614-722-3114; **Board Cert:** Urology 1978; **Med School:** Duke Univ 1969; **Resid:** Internal Medicine, New York Hosp 1971; Urology, Univ Mich Med Ctr 1975; **Fellow:** Pediatric Urology, Alder Hey Chldns Hosp 1977; **Fac Appt:** Prof U, Ohio State Univ

Kozlowski, James M MD [U] - **Spec Exp:** Prostate Cancer; Continent Urinary Diversions; Laparoscopic Surgery; **Hospital:** Northwestern Meml Hosp, Jesse Brown VA Med Ctr; **Address:** 675 N St Clair St, Galter 20-150, Chicago, IL 60611; **Phone:** 312-695-8146; **Board Cert:** Surgery 2004; Urology 1983; **Med School:** Northwestern Univ 1975; **Resid:** Surgery, McGaw Med Ctr 1979; Urology, McGaw Med Ctr 1982; **Fellow:** Research, NCI-Frederick Cancer Rsch 1984; **Fac Appt:** Assoc Prof U, Northwestern Univ

Lee, Cheryl T MD [U] - **Spec Exp:** Urologic Cancer; Bladder Cancer; **Hospital:** Univ of Michigan Hosp; **Address:** Univ of Michigan Cancer Ctr, 1500 E Medical Ctr Drive, Reception D LB1-229, Ann Arbor, MI 48109; **Phone:** 734-647-8903; **Board Cert:** Urology 2002; **Med School:** Albany Med Coll 1991; **Resid:** Urology, Albany Med Ctr; **Fellow:** Urologic Oncology, Meml Sloan Kettering Cancer Ctr 2000; **Fac Appt:** Assoc Prof U, Univ Mich Med Sch

Levine, Laurence A MD [U] - **Spec Exp:** Erectile Dysfunction; Infertility-Male; Peyronie's Disease; Prostate Cancer; **Hospital:** Rush Univ Med Ctr; **Address:** 1725 W Harrison St, Ste 352, Chicago, IL 60612; **Phone:** 312-563-5000; **Board Cert:** Urology 2009; **Med School:** Univ Colorado 1980; **Resid:** Surgery, Tufts-New Eng Med Ctr 1982; Urology, Brigham & Women's Hosp 1987; **Fac Appt:** Prof U, Rush Med Coll

McGuire, Edward J MD [U] - **Spec Exp:** Incontinence; Urology-Female; Neurogenic Bladder; Uro-Gynecology; **Hospital:** Univ of Michigan Hosp; **Address:** Univ Mich Med Ctr, Dept Urology, 1500 E Med Ctr Drive, 3875 Taubman, Ann Arbor, MI 48109-5330; **Phone:** 734-232-4943; **Board Cert:** Urology 1975; **Med School:** Wayne State Univ 1965; **Resid:** Surgery, Yale-New Haven Hosp 1969; Urology, Yale-New Haven Hosp 1972; **Fac Appt:** Prof U, Univ Mich Med Sch

McVary, Kevin T MD [U] - **Spec Exp:** Prostate Cancer; Erectile Dysfunction; Prostate Disease; Minimally Invasive Surgery; **Hospital:** Northwestern Meml Hosp; **Address:** 675 N St Clair St, Galter 20-150, Chicago, IL 60611-4813; **Phone:** 312-695-8146; **Board Cert:** Urology 2010; **Med School:** Northwestern Univ 1983; **Resid:** Surgery, Northwestern Meml Hosp 1985; Urology, Northwestern Meml Hosp 1988; **Fellow:** Research, Northwestern Meml Hosp; **Fac Appt:** Prof U, Northwestern Univ

Menon, Mani MD [U] - **Spec Exp:** Prostate Cancer/Robotic Surgery; Transplant-Kidney; Urologic Cancer; **Hospital:** Henry Ford Hosp; **Address:** Henry Ford Hosp - Vattikuti Urology Inst, 2799 W Grand Bvd, Clinic Bldg - K-9, Detroit, MI 48202; **Phone:** 313-916-2066; **Board Cert:** Urology 1982; **Med School:** India 1969; **Resid:** Urology, Bryn Mawr Hosp 1974; Urology, Johns Hopkins Hosp 1980; **Fellow:** Transplant Surgery, Johns Hopkins Univ 1977; **Fac Appt:** Prof S, Univ Mass Sch Med

Mesrobian, Hrair-George O MD [U] - **Spec Exp:** Pediatric Urology; **Hospital:** Chldns Hosp - Wisconsin; **Address:** 999 N 92nd St, Ste 330, Milwaukee, WI 53226; **Phone:** 414-266-3794; **Board Cert:** Urology 2005; Pediatric Urology 2008; **Med School:** Lebanon 1978; **Resid:** Surgery, SUNY Upstate Med Ctr 1980; Urology, UCSF Med Ctr 1983; **Fellow:** Pediatric Urology, Mayo Clinic 1984; **Fac Appt:** Prof U, Med Coll Wisc

Mitchell, Michael E MD [U] - **Spec Exp:** Genitourinary Congenital Anomalies; Pediatric Urology; Bladder Reconstruction; Bladder Exstrophy; **Hospital:** Chldns Hosp - Wisconsin, Froedtert and Med Ctr of WI; **Address:** Children's Hospital of Wisconsin, 999 N 92nd St, Ste 330, Milwaukee, WI 53226; **Phone:** 414-266-3794; **Board Cert:** Urology 2000; **Med School:** Harvard Med Sch 1969; **Resid:** Surgery, Peter Bent Brigham Hosp 1974; Urology, Mass Genl Hosp 1977; **Fellow:** Pediatric Urology, Mass Genl Hosp 1978; **Fac Appt:** Prof U, Univ Wisc

Montague, Drogo K MD [U] - **Spec Exp:** Erectile Dysfunction; Genitourinary Prosthetics; Incontinence; Peyronie's Disease; **Hospital:** Cleveland Clin (page 56); **Address:** Glickman Urological & Kidney Inst, Cleveland Clinic, 9500 Euclid Ave, Q10-1, Cleveland, OH 44195-5041; **Phone:** 216-444-5600; **Board Cert:** Urology 1995; **Med School:** Univ Mich Med Sch 1968; **Resid:** Surgery, Cleveland Clinic 1970; Urology, Cleveland Clinic 1973; **Fac Appt:** Prof U, Cleveland Cl Coll Med/Case West Res

Montie, James MD [U] - **Spec Exp:** Bladder Cancer; Prostate Cancer; Genitourinary Cancer; **Hospital:** Univ of Michigan Hosp; **Address:** UMH Cancer Ctr, Team 3, Reception D, Level B1-229, 1500 E Med Ctr Drive, Ann Arbor, MI 48109-5913; **Phone:** 734-647-8903; **Board Cert:** Urology 1978; **Med School:** Univ Mich Med Sch 1971; **Resid:** Urology, Cleveland Clinic Fdn 1976; **Fellow:** Urologic Oncology, Meml Sloan-Kettering Cancer Ctr 1979; **Fac Appt:** Prof U, Univ Mich Med Sch

Nehra, Ajay MD [U] - **Spec Exp:** Erectile Dysfunction; **Hospital:** Mayo Med Ctr & Clin - Rochester; **Address:** Mayo Clinic-Dept of Urology, 200 First St SW, Rochester, MN 55905; **Phone:** 507-266-4446; **Board Cert:** Urology 2006; **Med School:** India 1984; **Resid:** Surgery, Boston Univ Sch Med 1987; Urology, Maimonides Med Ctr 1993; **Fellow:** Female Urology, Boston Univ Sch Med 1989; Male Infertility, Boston Univ Sch Med 1995; **Fac Appt:** Prof U, Mayo Med Sch

Urology

O'Donnell, Michael A MD [U] - **Spec Exp:** Bladder Cancer; Immunotherapy; Urologic Cancer; Ureter & Renal Pelvis Cancer; **Hospital:** Univ Iowa Hosp & Clinics; **Address:** 200 Hawkins Drive RCP Bldg Fl 3, Iowa City, IA 52242-1089; **Phone:** 319-384-6040; **Board Cert:** Urology 2005; **Med School:** Duke Univ 1984; **Resid:** Surgery, Brigham & Womens Hosp 1987; Urology, Brigham & Womens Hosp 1991; **Fellow:** Urology, Brigham & Womens Hosp 1993; **Fac Appt:** Prof U, Univ Iowa Coll Med

Ohl, Dana MD [U] - **Spec Exp:** Infertility-Male; Erectile Dysfunction; **Hospital:** Univ of Michigan Hosp; **Address:** Univ Mich Med Ctr, Dept Urology, 1500 E Med Ctr Drive, 3875 Taubman, Ann Arbor, MI 48109-5330; **Phone:** 734-232-4943; **Board Cert:** Urology 2008; **Med School:** Univ Mich Med Sch 1982; **Resid:** Urology, Univ Mich Hosps 1987; **Fac Appt:** Prof U, Univ Mich Med Sch

Rink, Richard C MD [U] - **Spec Exp:** Pediatric Urology; Reconstructive Urologic Surgery; Genital Reconstruction; Neurogenic Bladder; **Hospital:** Riley Hosp for Children, IU Health University Hosp; **Address:** IU Health - Pediatric Urology, 705 Riley Hospital Drive, Ste 1210, Indianapolis, IN 46202; **Phone:** 317-944-8896; **Board Cert:** Urology 2008; Pediatric Urology 2008; **Med School:** Indiana Univ 1978; **Resid:** Surgery, Emory Univ Med Ctr 1980; Urology, Indiana Univ Med Ctr 1984; **Fellow:** Pediatric Urology, Chldns Hosp-Harvard 1985; **Fac Appt:** Prof U, Indiana Univ

Ross, Lawrence S MD [U] - **Spec Exp:** Infertility-Male; Erectile Dysfunction; Prostate Disease; **Hospital:** Univ of IL Med Ctr at Chicago; **Address:** Univ Ctr fo Urology, 60 E Delaware Pl, Ste 1420, Chicago, IL 60611; **Phone:** 312-440-5127; **Board Cert:** Urology 1974; **Med School:** Univ Chicago-Pritzker Sch Med 1965; **Resid:** Urology, Michael Reese Hosp 1970; **Fac Appt:** Prof U, Univ IL Coll Med

Sandlow, Jay I MD [U] - **Spec Exp:** Infertility-Male; Varicocele Microsurgery; Vasectomy & Vasectomy Reversal; **Hospital:** Froedtert and Med Ctr of WI, St. Joseph's Hosp; **Address:** Med Coll of WI, Urology Dept, 9200 W Wisconsin Ave, Milwaukee, WI 53226-3522; **Phone:** 414-805-0805; **Board Cert:** Urology 2005; **Med School:** Rush Med Coll 1987; **Resid:** Urology, Univ Iowa Hosps 1993; **Fellow:** Infertility, Univ Iowa Hosps 1995; **Fac Appt:** Prof U, Med Coll Wisc

Schaeffer, Anthony MD [U] - **Spec Exp:** Interstitial Cystitis; Incontinence after Prostate Cancer; Urology-Female; Urinary Tract Infections; **Hospital:** Northwestern Meml Hosp; **Address:** 675 N St Clair St, Galter 20-150, Chicago, IL 60611; **Phone:** 312-695-8146; **Board Cert:** Urology 1978; **Med School:** Northwestern Univ 1968; **Resid:** Surgery, Northwestern Meml Hosp 1970; Urology, Stanford Med Ctr 1976; **Fac Appt:** Prof U, Northwestern Univ

See, William A MD [U] - **Spec Exp:** Prostate Cancer; Bladder Cancer; Testicular Cancer; **Hospital:** Froedtert and Med Ctr of WI; **Address:** Med Coll Wisconsin, Dept Urology, 9200 W Wisconsin Ave, Milwaukee, WI 53226; **Phone:** 414-805-0805; **Board Cert:** Urology 2008; **Med School:** Univ Chicago-Pritzker Sch Med 1982; **Resid:** Urology, Univ Washington 1988; **Fellow:** Research, Natl Kidney Fdn/Univ Wash 1986; Research, Amer Fdn for Urol Dis/Univ Iowa 1990; **Fac Appt:** Prof U, Med Coll Wisc

Silber, Sherman J MD [U] - **Spec Exp:** Infertility-Male; Vasectomy Reversal; Infertility-IVF; Transplant-Ovarian Tissue; **Hospital:** St. Luke's Hosp - Chesterfield, MO; **Address:** 224 S Woods Mill Rd, Ste 730, St Louis, MO 63017-3451; **Phone:** 314-576-1400; **Board Cert:** Urology 1977; **Med School:** Univ Mich Med Sch 1966; **Resid:** Internal Medicine, PH Service Comm Corps 1969; Urology, Univ Michigan 1973; **Fellow:** Microsurgery, Univ Melbourne 1974

Steinberg, Gary D MD [U] - **Spec Exp:** Bladder Cancer; Kidney Cancer; Prostate Cancer; **Hospital:** Univ of Chicago Med Ctr; **Address:** 5841 S Maryland Ave, rm J653, Chicago, IL 60637-1447; **Phone:** 773-702-3080; **Board Cert:** Urology 2003; **Med School:** Univ Chicago-Pritzker Sch Med 1985; **Resid:** Surgery, Johns Hopkins Hosp 1987; Urology, Brady Urol Inst/Johns Hopkins 1991; **Fellow:** Oncology, Johns Hopkins Hosp 1989; **Fac Appt:** Prof U, Univ Chicago-Pritzker Sch Med

Sundaram, Chandru P MD [U] - **Spec Exp:** Kidney Cancer; Prostate Cancer; Adrenal Tumors; Robotic Surgery; **Hospital:** IU Health University Hosp; **Address:** Indiana Univ, Dept Urology, 535 Barnhill Drive, Ste 420, Indianapolis, IN 46202; **Phone:** 317-278-3098; **Board Cert:** Urology 2009; **Med School:** India 1985; **Resid:** Urology, Univ Minn Med Ctr 1997; **Fellow:** Endourology, Beth Israel Deaconess Med Ctr/Harvard Med Sch 1998; **Fac Appt:** Prof U, Indiana Univ

Wong, Carson MD [U] - **Spec Exp:** Laparoscopic Surgery; Endourology; Prostate Cancer/Robotic Surgery; Urinary Reconstruction; **Address:** 6900 Pearl Rd Fl 2, SouthWest Urology, Inc, Middleburgh Heights, OH 44130; **Phone:** 440-845-0414; **Board Cert:** Urology 2003; **Med School:** Univ Western Ontario 1995; **Resid:** Urology, McGill Univ Affil Hosps 1999; **Fellow:** Urologic Surgery, Univ Miami 2001; **Fac Appt:** U

Wood, David P MD [U] - **Spec Exp:** Genitourinary Cancer; Bladder Cancer; Prostate Cancer; Robotic Surgery; **Hospital:** Univ of Michigan Hosp; **Address:** UMH Cancer Ctr, Team 3, Reception D, Level B1-229, 1500 E Medical Center Drive, Ann Arbor, MI 48109-5913; **Phone:** 734-647-8903; **Board Cert:** Urology 2002; **Med School:** Univ Mich Med Sch 1983; **Resid:** Urology, Cleveland Clinic 1988; **Fellow:** Urologic Oncology, Meml Sloan-Kettering Cancer Ctr 1991; **Fac Appt:** Prof U, Univ Mich Med Sch

Zippe, Craig D MD [U] - **Spec Exp:** Prostate Cancer; Bladder Cancer; Kidney Cancer; **Hospital:** Univ Hosps Case Med Ctr (page 74), UH Richmond Med Ctr (page 74); **Address:** University Hospitals - Case Medical Ctr, 88 Center Rd, Ste 360, Bedford, OH 44146; **Phone:** 440-232-8955; **Board Cert:** Urology 2007; **Med School:** Rush Med Coll 1980; **Resid:** Surgery, Duke Univ Med Ctr 1983; Urology, Columbia Presby Med Ctr 1989; **Fellow:** Cancer Research, Rhode Island Hosp 1985; Urologic Oncology, Meml Sloan Kettering Cancer Ctr 1992; **Fac Appt:** Clin Prof U, Case West Res Univ

Great Plains and Mountains

Cartwright, Patrick C MD [U] - **Spec Exp:** Pediatric Urology; **Hospital:** Primary Children's Med Ctr, Univ Utah Hlth Care; **Address:** Primary Childrens Med Ctr, 100 N Mario Capecchi Drive, Ste 2200, Salt Lake City, UT 84113-1100; **Phone:** 801-662-5555; **Board Cert:** Urology 2010; Pediatric Urology 2010; **Med School:** Univ Tex SW, Dallas 1984; **Resid:** Urology, Univ Utah Affil Hosp 1989; **Fellow:** Pediatric Urology, Chldns Hosp 1990; **Fac Appt:** Prof S, Univ Utah

Childs, Stacy J MD [U] - **Spec Exp:** Voiding Dysfunction; Erectile Dysfunction; Prostate Cancer; Bladder Cancer; **Hospital:** Yampa Valley Med Ctr, Memorial Hosp - Craig; **Address:** 501 Anglers Drive, Ste 202, Steamboat Springs, CO 80487-8841; **Phone:** 970-871-9710; **Board Cert:** Urology 1979; **Med School:** Louisiana State U, New Orleans 1972; **Resid:** Urology, Carraway Meth Med Ctr 1977; **Fac Appt:** Clin Prof U, Univ Colorado

Crawford, E David MD [U] - **Spec Exp:** Prostate Cancer; Testicular Cancer; Bladder Cancer; **Hospital:** Univ of CO Hosp - Anschutz Inpatient Pav; **Address:** Urologic Oncology, MS F710, 1665 Aurora Ct, rm 1004, MS F-710, Aurora, CO 80045; **Phone:** 720-848-0170; **Board Cert:** Urology 1980; **Med School:** Univ Cincinnati 1973; **Resid:** Urology, Good Samaritan Hosp 1977; **Fellow:** Genitourinary Surgery, UCLA Med Ctr 1978; **Fac Appt:** Prof U, Univ Colorado

Urology

Davis, Bradley E MD [U] - **Spec Exp:** Urologic Cancer; Bladder Cancer; Reconstructive Surgery; Prostate Cancer; **Hospital:** Overland Pk Regl Med Ctr, St. Luke's Hosp of Kansas City; **Address:** Urologic Surgery Assocs, 10550 Quivira Rd, Ste 105, Overland Park, KS 66215; **Phone:** 913-438-3833; **Board Cert:** Urology 2004; **Med School:** Univ Kansas 1986; **Resid:** Surgery, St Lukes Hosp 1991; Urology, Univ Kansas Med Ctr 1991; **Fellow:** Urologic Oncology, Meml Sloan-Kettering Cancer Ctr 1993; **Fac Appt:** Asst Clin Prof U, Univ Kansas

Griebling, Tomas L MD [U] - **Spec Exp:** Urology-Geriatric; Urology-Female; Incontinence; Reconstructive Surgery; **Hospital:** Univ of Kansas Hosp; **Address:** Univ Kansas Hosp-Urology Dept, 3901 Rainbow Blvd, MS 3106, Kansas City, KS 66160; **Phone:** 913-588-6147; **Board Cert:** Urology 2009; **Med School:** Univ Iowa Coll Med 1991; **Resid:** Urology, Univ Iowa Affil Hosp 1998; **Fellow:** Reconstructive Surgery, Univ Iowa Affil Hosp 2001; **Fac Appt:** Prof U, Univ Kansas

Lugg, James A MD [U] - **Spec Exp:** Prostate Cancer; Laparoscopic Surgery; Incontinence after Prostate Cancer; **Hospital:** Cheyenne Regl Med Ctr, Univ of CO Hosp - Anschutz Inpatient Pav; **Address:** 2301 House Ave, Ste 502, Cheyenne, WY 82001; **Phone:** 307-635-4131; **Board Cert:** Urology 2008; **Med School:** Northwestern Univ 1990; **Resid:** Urology, UCLA Med Ctr 1995; **Fac Appt:** Asst Prof U, Univ Colorado

Thrasher, J Brantley MD [U] - **Spec Exp:** Prostate Cancer; Reconstructive Urologic Surgery; **Hospital:** Univ of Kansas Hosp; **Address:** 3901 Rainbow Blvd, MS 3016, Kansas City, KS 66160; **Phone:** 913-588-6146; **Board Cert:** Urology 2003; **Med School:** Med Univ SC 1986; **Resid:** Urology, Fitzsimons Army Med Ctr 1992; **Fellow:** Urologic Oncology, Duke Univ Med Ctr 1994; **Fac Appt:** Prof U, Univ Kansas

Southwest

Andrews, Paul E MD [U] - **Spec Exp:** Urologic Cancer; Minimally Invasive Urologic Surgery; Robotic Surgery; **Hospital:** Mayo Clinic - Phoenix; **Address:** Mayo Clinic-Urology, 5779 E Mayo Blvd, Phoenix, AZ 85054; **Phone:** 480-342-2951; **Board Cert:** Urology 2003; **Med School:** Texas Tech Univ 1987; **Resid:** Urology, Mayo Clinic 1993; **Fac Appt:** Prof U, Mayo Med Sch

Bans, Larry L MD [U] - **Spec Exp:** Prostate Cancer; Prostate Disease; **Hospital:** Banner Good Samaritan Regl Med Ctr - Phoenix; **Address:** Prostate Solutions of Arizona, 2525 E Arizona Biltmore Cir, Ste C236, Phoenix, AZ 85016; **Phone:** 602-426-9772; **Board Cert:** Urology 2004; **Med School:** Cornell Univ-Weill Med Coll 1978; **Resid:** Urology, Ind Univ Med Ctr 1983

Bardot, Stephen F MD [U] - **Spec Exp:** Urologic Cancer; Prostate Cancer; **Hospital:** Ochsner Med Ctr-New Orleans; **Address:** Ochsner Clinic, 1514 Jefferson Hwy Fl 4, Atrium 4 West, Dept Urology, New Orleans, LA 70121-2483; **Phone:** 504-842-4083; **Board Cert:** Urology 2002; **Med School:** Univ Kansas 1985; **Resid:** Surgery, St Luke's Hosp 1987; Urology, Kansas City Univ Med Ctr 1990; **Fellow:** Urologic Oncology, Cleveland Clinic 1991

Basler, Joseph W MD [U] - **Spec Exp:** Prostate Cancer; Urologic Cancer; Kidney Stones; **Hospital:** Audie L Murphy Meml Vets Hosp - San Antonio; **Address:** 7703 Floyd Curl Dr, MC-7845, San Antonio, TX 78229-3900; **Phone:** 210-567-5640; **Board Cert:** Urology 2001; **Med School:** Univ MO-Columbia Sch Med 1984; **Resid:** Surgery, Univ Missouri Affil Hosp 1986; Urology, Barnes Hosp/Wash Univ 1990; **Fac Appt:** Prof U, Univ Tex, San Antonio

Boone, Timothy B MD/PhD [U] - **Spec Exp:** Neuro-Urology; Urinary Reconstruction; Incontinence; **Hospital:** Methodist Hosp - Houston, St. Luke's Episcopal Hosp-Houston; **Address:** Scurlock Tower, 6560 Fannin, Ste 2100, Houston, TX 77030-2769; **Phone:** 713-441-6455; **Board Cert:** Urology 2004; **Med School:** Univ Tex, Houston 1985; **Resid:** Surgery, Univ Tex SW Med Ctr 1987; Urology, Univ Tex SW Med Ctr 1991; **Fac Appt:** Prof U, Cornell Univ-Weill Med Coll

Buch, Jeffrey Phillip MD [U] - **Spec Exp:** Vasectomy Reversal; Infertility-Male; Sexual Dysfunction; **Hospital:** Baylor Univ Medical Ctr-Dallas; **Address:** Legacy Male Health Institute, 5616 Warren Pkwy, Ste 101, Frisco, TX 75034; **Phone:** 972-612-7131; **Board Cert:** Urology 2005; **Med School:** Univ Mich Med Sch 1980; **Resid:** Surgery, Albany Med Ctr 1982; Urology, Albany Med Ctr 1985; **Fellow:** Male Infertility, Baylor Coll Med 1987; Microsurgery, Baylor Coll Med 1987; **Fac Appt:** Assoc Clin Prof U, Univ Tex SW, Dallas

Culkin, Daniel J MD [U] - **Spec Exp:** Voiding Dysfunction; Interstitial Cystitis; Urologic Cancer; Laparoscopic Surgery; **Hospital:** OU Med Ctr; **Address:** OU Medical Ctr, Dept Urology, 825 NE 10th St, Ste 5400, Oklahoma City, OK 73104; **Phone:** 405-271-6452; **Board Cert:** Urology 2006; **Med School:** Creighton Univ 1979; **Resid:** Surgery, Loyola Univ Med Ctr 1981; Urology, Loyola Univ Med Ctr 1983; **Fellow:** Neurourology, Loyola Univ Med Ctr 1984; **Fac Appt:** Prof U, Univ Okla Coll Med

Ellis, David S MD [U] - **Spec Exp:** Prostate Cancer-Cryosurgery; **Hospital:** Arlington Meml Hosp; **Address:** Urology Assocs of N Texas (UANT), Arlington-North, 1001 Waldrop Drive, Ste 708, Arlington, TX 76012; **Phone:** 817-312-8181; **Board Cert:** Urology 2000; **Med School:** Univ Tex, Houston 1982; **Resid:** Urology, Univ Texas Med Ctr 1988

Ewalt, David H MD [U] - **Spec Exp:** Pediatric Urology; Hypospadias; Urinary Reconstruction; Neurogenic Bladder; **Hospital:** Chldns Med Ctr of Dallas, Med City Dallas Hosp; **Address:** 8315 Walnut Hill Lane, Ste 205, Dallas, TX 75231; **Phone:** 214-750-0808; **Board Cert:** Urology 2003; Pediatric Urology 2008; **Med School:** Univ Tex SW, Dallas 1984; **Resid:** Urology, Univ Texas SW Affil Hosps 1990; **Fellow:** Pediatric Urology, Chldns Hosp 1992

Gonzales, Edmond T MD [U] - **Spec Exp:** Pediatric Urology; **Hospital:** Texas Chldns Hosp; **Address:** Clinical Care Center, 6701 Fannin St, Ste 660, Houston, TX 77030; **Phone:** 832-822-3160; **Board Cert:** Urology 1975; Pediatric Urology 2008; **Med School:** Tulane Univ 1965; **Resid:** Surgery, Duke Univ Med Ctr 1968; Urology, Duke Univ Med Ctr 1972; **Fellow:** Pediatric Urology, Childrens Hosp; **Fac Appt:** Prof U, Baylor Coll Med

Grossman, H Barton MD [U] - **Spec Exp:** Bladder Cancer; **Hospital:** UT MD Anderson Cancer Ctr; **Address:** MD Anderson Cancer Ctr, Dept Urology, 1373, 1515 Holcombe Blvd, Houston, TX 77030-4009; **Phone:** 713-792-3250; **Board Cert:** Urology 1979; **Med School:** Temple Univ 1970; **Resid:** Surgery, St Joseph Mercy Hosp 1974; Urology, Univ Michigan Med Ctr 1977; **Fellow:** Urologic Oncology, Meml Sloan Kettering Cancer Ctr 1979; **Fac Appt:** Clin Prof U, Univ Tex, Houston

Hellstrom, Wayne J MD [U] - **Spec Exp:** Infertility-Male; Erectile Dysfunction; Peyronie's Disease; Penile Prostheses; **Hospital:** Tulane Med Ctr; **Address:** Tulane Urology, 1415 Tulane Ave Fl 3, New Orleans, LA 70112; **Phone:** 504-988-5271; **Board Cert:** Urology 2007; **Med School:** McGill Univ 1981; **Resid:** Surgery, Montreal Genl/Royal Vistoria Hosp 1983; Urology, UCSF Med Ctr 1985; **Fellow:** Andrology, UC Davis Med Ctr 1988; **Fac Appt:** Prof U, Tulane Univ

Kadmon, Dov MD [U] - **Spec Exp:** Prostate Cancer; **Hospital:** St. Luke's Episcopal Hosp-Houston, Methodist Hosp - Houston; **Address:** Baylor Dept Urology, 6620 Main St, Ste 1325, Houston, TX 77030; **Phone:** 713-798-4001; **Board Cert:** Urology 1984; **Med School:** Israel 1970; **Resid:** Surgery, Barnes Jewish Hosp 1977; Urology, Barnes Jewish Hosp 1980; **Fellow:** Urology, Barnes Jewish Hosp 1982; **Fac Appt:** Prof U, Baylor Coll Med

Lerner, Seth P MD [U] - **Spec Exp:** Bladder Cancer; Testicular Cancer; Urinary Reconstruction; **Hospital:** St. Luke's Episcopal Hosp-Houston, Methodist Hosp - Houston; **Address:** 6620 Main St, Ste 1325, Houston, TX 77030; **Phone:** 713-798-6841; **Board Cert:** Urology 2002; **Med School:** Baylor Coll Med 1984; **Resid:** Surgery, Virginia Mason Hosp 1986; Urology, Baylor Coll Med 1990; **Fellow:** Urologic Oncology, LAC-USC Med Ctr 1992; **Fac Appt:** Prof U, Baylor Coll Med

Urology

Lipshultz, Larry MD [U] - **Spec Exp:** Infertility-Male; Microsurgery; Erectile Dysfunction; Infertility-IVF; **Hospital:** St. Luke's Episcopal Hosp-Houston, Methodist Hosp - Houston; **Address:** 6224 Fannin St, O'Quinn Medical Twr, Ste 1700, Houston, TX 77030-2706; **Phone:** 713-798-4001; **Board Cert:** Urology 1977; **Med School:** Univ Pennsylvania 1968; **Resid:** Urology, Hosp Univ Penn 1971; **Fellow:** Reproductive Medicine, Univ Tex Med Sch Affil Hosp 1977; **Fac Appt:** Prof U, Baylor Coll Med

Miles, Brian J MD [U] - **Spec Exp:** Prostate Cancer; Urologic Cancer; Gene Therapy; **Hospital:** Methodist Hosp - Houston, St. Luke's Episcopal Hosp-Houston; **Address:** 6560 Fannin St, Ste 2100, Houston, TX 77030; **Phone:** 713-441-6455; **Board Cert:** Urology 1984; **Med School:** Univ Mich Med Sch 1974; **Resid:** Urology, Walter Reed Army Med Ctr 1982; **Fac Appt:** Clin Prof U, Baylor Coll Med

Pisters, Louis L MD [U] - **Spec Exp:** Prostate Cancer; Bladder Cancer; Genitourinary Cancer; Prostate Cancer/Robotic Surgery; **Hospital:** UT MD Anderson Cancer Ctr; **Address:** MD Anderson Cancer Ctr, 1515 Holcombe Blvd, Unit 1373, Houston, TX 77030; **Phone:** 713-792-3250; **Board Cert:** Urology 2003; **Med School:** Univ Western Ontario 1986; **Resid:** Urology, Shands Hosp/UNIV Florida 1991; **Fellow:** Urologic Oncology, MD Anderson Cancer Ctr 1993; **Fac Appt:** Assoc Prof U, Univ Tex, Houston

Roehrborn, Claus Georg MD [U] - **Spec Exp:** Prostate Cancer; Prostate Disease; Voiding Dysfunction; **Hospital:** UT Southwestern Med Ctr at Dallas, Parkland Hlth & Hosp Sys; **Address:** Professor and Chairman, Department of Urology at UT Southwestern Medical Center in Dallas, 5323 Harry Hines Blvd, Moss (J) Bldg Fl 8 - Ste 148, Dallas, TX 75390-9110; **Phone:** 214-645-8765; **Board Cert:** Urology 2004; **Med School:** Germany 1980; **Resid:** Surgery, W Germany Army Hosp 1982; Urology, UT SW Med Ctr 1989; **Fellow:** Urology, Am Fdn Urol Dis 1991; **Fac Appt:** Prof U, Univ Tex SW, Dallas

Sagalowsky, Arthur I MD [U] - **Spec Exp:** Urologic Cancer; Transplant-Kidney; Testicular Cancer; Continent Urinary Diversions; **Hospital:** UT Southwestern Med Ctr at Dallas; **Address:** UT SW Med Ctr, Dept Urology, 5323 Harry Hines Blvd, J8.130, Dallas, TX 75390-9110; **Phone:** 214-648-3976; **Board Cert:** Urology 1980; **Med School:** Indiana Univ 1973; **Resid:** Surgery, Indiana Univ Hosps 1975; Urology, Indiana Univ Hosps 1978; **Fellow:** Clinical Pharmacology, Univ Tex SW Med Ctr 1980; **Fac Appt:** Prof U, Univ Tex SW, Dallas

Slawin, Kevin Mark MD [U] - **Spec Exp:** Prostate Cancer; Prostate Cancer/Robotic Surgery; Prostate Disease; **Hospital:** Meml Hermann Hosp - Texas Med Ctr, Methodist Hosp - Houston; **Address:** Vanguard Urologic Inst, Meml Hermann Med Plaza, 6400 Fannin, Ste 2300, Houston, TX 77030; **Phone:** 713-366-7847; **Board Cert:** Urology 2005; **Med School:** Columbia P&S 1986; **Resid:** Surgery, Mt Sinai Med Ctr 1988; Urology, Columbia-Presby Hosp 1992; **Fellow:** Urologic Oncology, Am Fdn Urol Dis/Baylor Coll Med 1994; **Fac Appt:** Clin Prof U, Baylor Coll Med

Strand, William R MD [U] - **Spec Exp:** Pediatric Urology; Laparoscopic Surgery; Hypospadias; Reconstructive Surgery; **Hospital:** Chldns Med Ctr of Dallas; **Address:** 4001 W 15th St Bldg 3 - Ste 300, Plano, TX 75093; **Phone:** 214-750-0808 x5400; **Board Cert:** Urology 2001; Pediatric Urology 2008; **Med School:** Mayo Med Sch 1983; **Resid:** Surgery, Naval Med Ctr 1984; Urology, Natl Naval Med Ctr 1988; **Fellow:** Pediatric Urology, Chldns Med Ctr of Dallas; **Fac Appt:** Assoc Prof U, Univ Tex SW, Dallas

Swanson, David A MD [U] - **Spec Exp:** Kidney Cancer; Prostate Cancer; Testicular Cancer; **Hospital:** UT MD Anderson Cancer Ctr; **Address:** UT MD Anderson Canc Ctr, Dept Urol, 1515 Holcombe Blvd , Unit 1373, Houston, TX 77030-4009; **Phone:** 713-792-3250; **Board Cert:** Urology 1977; **Med School:** Univ Pennsylvania 1967; **Resid:** Surgery, Harbor Genl Hosp 1969; Urology, UC Davis Med Ctr 1975; **Fellow:** Urologic Oncology, Univ Tex-MD Anderson Hosp 1978

Thompson Jr, Ian M MD [U] - **Spec Exp:** Prostate Cancer; Prostate Disease; **Hospital:** Univ Hlth Syst-San Antonio; **Address:** Univ Tex Hlth Scis Ctr, Dept Urol, 8300 Floyd Curl Drive, San Antonio, TX 78229; **Phone:** 210-567-5643; **Board Cert:** Urology 2005; **Med School:** Tulane Univ 1980; **Resid:** Urology, Brooke Army Med Ctr 1985; **Fellow:** Medical Oncology, Meml Sloan-Kettering Canc Ctr 1988; **Fac Appt:** Prof S, Univ Tex, San Antonio

Woo, Howard H MD [U] - **Spec Exp:** Pain-Pelvic; Voiding Dysfunction; Incontinence; Urology-Female; **Hospital:** Ochsner Med Ctr-New Orleans; **Address:** Ochsner Clinic, Dept Urology, 1514 Jefferson Hwy, New Orleans, LA 70121; **Phone:** 504-842-4083; **Board Cert:** Urology 2006; **Med School:** Med Coll Wisc 1989; **Resid:** Surgery, UC Irvine Med Ctr 1991; Urology, Univ Colorado Affil Hosp 1995

West Coast and Pacific

Ahlering, Thomas E MD [U] - **Spec Exp:** Prostate Cancer/Robotic Surgery; **Hospital:** UC Irvine Med Ctr, VA Long Beach Hlthcare Sys; **Address:** UC Irvine Med Ctr, 333 City Blvd W, Ste 2100, Orange, CA 92868; **Phone:** 714-456-6068; **Board Cert:** Urology 2005; **Med School:** St Louis Univ 1979; **Resid:** Urology, LAC-USC Med Ctr 1984; **Fellow:** Urologic Oncology, USC-Norris Comp Cancer Ctr 1986; **Fac Appt:** Prof U, UC Irvine

Amling, Christopher L MD [U] - **Spec Exp:** Prostate Cancer/Robotic Surgery; Kidney Cancer; Bladder Cancer; Testicular Cancer; **Hospital:** OR Hlth & Sci Univ; **Address:** 3303 SW Bond Ave, MC CH10U, Portland, OR 97239; **Phone:** 503-346-1500; **Board Cert:** Urology 2008; **Med School:** Oregon Hlth & Sci Univ 1985; **Resid:** Urology, Duke Univ Med Ctr 1996; **Fellow:** Urologic Oncology, Mayo Clinic 1997; **Fac Appt:** Prof U, Univ Alabama

Baskin, Laurence S MD [U] - **Spec Exp:** Pediatric Urology; Hypospadias; **Hospital:** UCSF Med Ctr; **Address:** Urology Faculty Practice, 400 Parnassus Ave, Ste A-610, Box 0330, San Francisco, CA 94143-0330; **Phone:** 415-353-2200; **Board Cert:** Urology 2008; Pediatric Urology 2008; **Med School:** UCLA 1986; **Resid:** Urology, UCSF Med Ctr 1991; **Fellow:** Pediatric Urology, Childrens Hosp 1993; **Fac Appt:** Prof U, UCSF

Belldegrun, Arie S MD [U] - **Spec Exp:** Urologic Cancer; Gene Therapy; **Hospital:** UCLA Ronald Reagan Med Ctr; **Address:** 924 Westwood Blvd, Ste 1050, Los Angeles, CA 90024; **Phone:** 310-206-1434; **Board Cert:** Urology 1999; **Med School:** Israel 1974; **Resid:** Urology, Brigham and Women's Hosp 1985; **Fellow:** Urologic Oncology, Natl Cancer Inst, NIH 1988; **Fac Appt:** Prof U, UCLA

Boyd, Stuart D MD [U] - **Spec Exp:** Incontinence; Erectile Dysfunction; Urologic Cancer; **Hospital:** USC Norris Cancer Hosp (page 75), Keck Med Ctr of USC (page 75); **Address:** 1441 Eastlake Ave, Ste 7416, Los Angeles, CA 90089-9178; **Phone:** 323-865-3704; **Board Cert:** Urology 1984; **Med School:** UCLA 1975; **Resid:** Urology, UCLA Med Ctr 1982; **Fac Appt:** Prof U, USC Sch Med

Carroll, Peter R MD [U] - **Spec Exp:** Testicular Cancer; Prostate Cancer; Bladder Cancer; Bladder Reconstruction; **Hospital:** UCSF - Mt Zion Med Ctr; **Address:** UCSF Urologic Oncology Practice, 1600 Divisadero St Fl 3, San Francisco, CA 94115-1711; **Phone:** 415-353-7171; **Board Cert:** Urology 2006; **Med School:** Georgetown Univ 1979; **Resid:** Surgery, UCSF Med Ctr 1984; **Fellow:** Urology, Meml Sloan Kettering Cancer Ctr 1986; **Fac Appt:** Prof U, UCSF

Clayman, Ralph V MD [U] - **Spec Exp:** Kidney Stones; Kidney Cancer; Laparoscopic Surgery; Robotic Surgery; **Hospital:** UC Irvine Med Ctr; **Address:** UCI Med Ctr, Dept Urology, 333 City Blvd W, Ste 2100, Orange, CA 92868; **Phone:** 714-456-3330; **Board Cert:** Urology 2007; **Med School:** UCSD 1973; **Resid:** Urology, Univ Minn Med Ctr 1979; **Fac Appt:** Prof U, UC Irvine

Dalkin, Bruce MD [U] - **Spec Exp:** Urologic Cancer; Prostate Cancer; Bladder Cancer; Testicular Cancer; **Hospital:** Univ Wash Med Ctr; **Address:** Univ Washington-Dept Urology, 1959 NE Pacific St, Box 356510, Seattle, WA 98195; **Phone:** 206-598-4294; **Board Cert:** Urology 2002; **Med School:** Northwestern Univ 1985; **Resid:** Urology, Northwestern Meml Hosp 1991; **Fac Appt:** Prof U, Univ Wash

Daneshmand, Siamak MD [U] - **Spec Exp:** Bladder Cancer; Prostate Cancer; Kidney Cancer; Testicular Cancer; **Hospital:** Keck Med Ctr of USC (page 75); **Address:** 1441 Eastlake Ave, Ste 7416, Los Angeles, CA 90089; **Phone:** 323-865-3700; **Board Cert:** Urology 2006; **Med School:** UC Davis 1996; **Resid:** Surgery, USC Med Ctr 1998; Urology, USC Med Ctr 2002; **Fellow:** Urologic Oncology, USC/Norris Comprehensive Cancer Ctr 2004; **Fac Appt:** Assoc Prof U, USC Sch Med

Danoff, Dudley S MD [U] - **Spec Exp:** Prostate Cancer; Bladder Cancer; Erectile Dysfunction; **Hospital:** Cedars-Sinai Med Ctr; **Address:** 8635 W 3rd St, Ste 1 West, Los Angeles, CA 90048; **Phone:** 310-854-9898; **Board Cert:** Urology 1974; **Med School:** Yale Univ 1963; **Resid:** Urology, Yale-New Haven Hosp 1965; Urology, Columbia-Presby Med Ctr 1969

DeKernion, Jean B MD [U] - **Spec Exp:** Urologic Cancer; Kidney Cancer; Prostate Cancer; Prostate Disease; **Hospital:** UCLA Ronald Reagan Med Ctr; **Address:** UCLA Medical Plaza Drive, rm 140, Los Angeles, CA 90095-1738; **Phone:** 310-206-6453; **Board Cert:** Surgery 1973; Urology 1975; **Med School:** Louisiana State U, New Orleans 1965; **Resid:** Surgery, Univ Hosps-Case West Res 1967; Urology, Univ Hosps-Case West Res 1973; **Fellow:** Urologic Oncology, Natl Cancer Inst 1969; **Fac Appt:** Prof U, UCLA

Ellis, William J MD [U] - **Spec Exp:** Prostate Cancer; Prostate Disease; Kidney Cancer; **Hospital:** Univ Wash Med Ctr; **Address:** Univ Wash Med Ctr, Dept Urology, 1959 NE Pacific St, Box 356510, Seattle, WA 98195; **Phone:** 206-598-4294; **Board Cert:** Urology 2001; **Med School:** Johns Hopkins Univ 1985; **Resid:** Surgery, Northwestern Meml Hosp 1987; Urology, Northwestern Meml Hosp 1991; **Fac Appt:** Assoc Prof U, Univ Wash

Fuchs, Eugene F MD [U] - **Spec Exp:** Infertility-Male; Kidney Stones; Vasectomy Reversal; **Hospital:** OR Hlth & Sci Univ; **Address:** Dept of Urology, MC CH1OU, 3303 SW Bond Ave, Portland, OR 97239; **Phone:** 503-346-1500; **Board Cert:** Urology 1977; **Med School:** Univ VT Coll Med 1970; **Resid:** Urology, Univ Oregon Hosp 1975; **Fac Appt:** Prof U, Oregon Hlth & Sci Univ

Gill, Harcharan Singh MD [U] - **Spec Exp:** Urologic Cancer; Prostate Cancer; Prostate Disease; **Hospital:** Stanford Univ Hosp & Clinics; **Address:** 875 Blake Wilbur Drive, rm 2218, Stanford, CA 94305-5826; **Phone:** 650-725-5544; **Board Cert:** Urology 2004; **Med School:** Kenya 1977; **Resid:** Urology, Inst of Urology; Urology, Univ Hosp Penn 1991; **Fellow:** Urology, Univ Hosp Penn 1986; **Fac Appt:** Prof U, Stanford Univ

Gill, Inderbir Singh MD [U] - **Spec Exp:** Prostate Cancer; Kidney Cancer; Urologic Cancer; Minimally Invasive Urologic Surgery; **Hospital:** USC Norris Cancer Hosp (page 75); **Address:** USC/Norris Cancer Ctr, Dept Urology, 1441 Eastlake Ave, Ste 7416, Los Angeles, CA 90089; **Phone:** 323-865-3700; **Board Cert:** Urology 2008; **Med School:** India 1980; **Resid:** Surgery, Dayanand Med Coll & Hosp; Urology, Univ Kentucky Hosp 1993; **Fac Appt:** Prof U, Univ SC Sch Med

Ginsberg, David A MD [U] - **Spec Exp:** Incontinence; Urinary Reconstruction; Neuro-Urology; Neurogenic Bladder; **Hospital:** Keck Med Ctr of USC (page 75); **Address:** USC-Norris Cancer Ctr, 1441 Eastlake Ave, Ste 7416, Los Angeles, CA 90089; **Phone:** 323-865-3703; **Board Cert:** Urology 2008; **Med School:** USC Sch Med 1990; **Resid:** Surgery, LAC-USC Med Ctr 1992; Urology, LAc-USC Med Ctr 1996; **Fellow:** Reconstructive Surgery, UCLA Med Ctr 1997; **Fac Appt:** Assoc Clin Prof U, USC-Keck School of Medicine

Goldstein, Irwin MD [U] - **Spec Exp:** Sexual Dysfunction-Male & Female; Vulvar Pain; Erectile Dysfunction; Penile Microvascular Bypass Surgery; **Hospital:** Alvarado Hosp & Med Ctr; **Address:** Ctr for Sexual Medicine, 6719 Alvarado Rd, Ste 108, San Diego, CA 92120; **Phone:** 619-265-8865; **Board Cert:** Urology 1982; **Med School:** McGill Univ 1975; **Resid:** Surgery, Boston Univ Med Ctr; Urology, Boston Univ Med Ctr 1980; **Fellow:** Urology, Boston Univ Med Ctr; **Fac Appt:** Prof U, Univ SD Sch Med

Holden, Stuart MD [U] - **Spec Exp:** Kidney Cancer; **Hospital:** Cedars-Sinai Med Ctr; **Address:** 8635 W 3rd St, Ste 1 W, Los Angeles, CA 90048; **Phone:** 310-854-9898; **Board Cert:** Urology 1977; **Med School:** Cornell Univ-Weill Med Coll 1968; **Resid:** Surgery, NY Hosp-Cornell 1970; Urology, Emory Univ Hosp 1975; **Fellow:** Urology, Meml Sloan Kettering Cancer Ctr 1978

Kawachi, Mark H MD [U] - **Spec Exp:** Prostate Cancer/Robotic Surgery; Minimally Invasive Urologic Surgery; **Hospital:** City of Hope Natl Med Ctr; **Address:** Div Urologic Oncology, 1500 E Duarte Rd, Duarte, CA 91010-3012; **Phone:** 626-359-8111 x62655; **Board Cert:** Urology 2004; **Med School:** USC Sch Med 1979; **Resid:** Urology, USC Med Ctr 1984

Lange, Paul H MD [U] - **Spec Exp:** Prostate Cancer; **Hospital:** Univ Wash Med Ctr; **Address:** Univ Wash Med Ctr, Dept Urology, 1959 NE Pacific St, Box 356510, Seattle, WA 98195; **Phone:** 206-598-4294; **Board Cert:** Urology 2006; **Med School:** Washington Univ, St Louis 1967; **Resid:** Surgery, Duke Univ Med Ctr 1972; Urology, Univ Minn Med Ctr 1975; **Fellow:** Immunology, Univ Minn Med Ctr 1973; Research, Natl Inst Hlth 1970; **Fac Appt:** Prof U, Univ Wash

Lieskovsky, Gary MD [U] - **Spec Exp:** Prostate Cancer; **Hospital:** USC Norris Cancer Hosp (page 75), Keck Med Ctr of USC (page 75); **Address:** 1441 Eastlake Ave, Ste 7416, Los Angeles, CA 90089-0112; **Phone:** 323-865-3702; **Board Cert:** Urology 1980; **Med School:** Canada 1973; **Resid:** Urology, Univ Alberta Hosp 1978; **Fellow:** Urology, UCLA Med Ctr 1980; **Fac Appt:** Prof U, USC Sch Med

Lin, Daniel W MD [U] - **Spec Exp:** Bladder Cancer; **Hospital:** Univ Wash Med Ctr; **Address:** Urology Clinic at UWMC, 1959 NE Pacific St, Ste SP1266, Box 356158, Seattle, WA 98195; **Phone:** 206-598-4294; **Board Cert:** Urology 2003; **Med School:** Vanderbilt Univ 1994; **Resid:** Urology, Univ WA Med Ctr 2000; **Fellow:** Urologic Oncology, Meml Sloan-Kettering Canc Ctr 2001; **Fac Appt:** Assoc Prof U, Univ Wash

Marsh, Christopher L MD [U] - **Spec Exp:** Transplant-Kidney; Transplant-Pancreas; Transplant-Liver; Adrenal Surgery; **Hospital:** Scripps Green Hosp; **Address:** Scripps Clinic, 10666 N Torrey Pines Rd, MC N200, La Jolla, CA 92037; **Phone:** 858-554-4310; **Board Cert:** Urology 2006; **Med School:** Loma Linda Univ 1980; **Resid:** Urology, Loma Linda Univ Med Ctr 1986; **Fellow:** Transplant Surgery, Mayo Clinic 1987

McAninch, Jack W MD [U] - **Spec Exp:** Genitourinary Trauma; Genitourinary Reconstruction; **Hospital:** UCSF Med Ctr, San Francisco Genl Hosp; **Address:** San Francisco Genl Hosp, Dept Urology, 1001 Potrero Ave, Ste 3A20, San Francisco, CA 94110; **Phone:** 415-476-3372; **Board Cert:** Urology 1995; **Med School:** Univ Tex Med Br, Galveston 1964; **Resid:** Surgery, Darnall Army Hosp 1966; Urology, Letterman AMC 1969; **Fac Appt:** Prof U, UCSF

McClure, Robert D MD [U] - **Spec Exp:** Infertility-Male; **Hospital:** Virginia Mason Med Ctr; **Address:** Virginia Mason Med Ctr, 1100 9th Ave Buck Bldg, MS C7URO, Seattle, WA 98101; **Phone:** 206-223-6179; **Board Cert:** Urology 1979; **Med School:** Canada 1968; **Resid:** Urology, McGill Univ Hosp 1975; **Fellow:** Endocrinology, Univ Washington Med Ctr 1977

Payne, Christopher K MD [U] - **Spec Exp:** Interstitial Cystitis; Pelvic Organ Prolapse Repair; Incontinence; Neurogenic Bladder; **Hospital:** Stanford Univ Hosp & Clinics; **Address:** Stanford Univ, Dept Urology, 300 Pasteur Drive, rm S-287, Stanford, CA 94305-5118; **Phone:** 650-723-3391; **Board Cert:** Urology 2004; **Med School:** Vanderbilt Univ 1986; **Resid:** Urology, Hosp Univ Penn 1992; **Fellow:** Urology, UCLA Med Ctr 1993; **Fac Appt:** Prof U, Stanford Univ

Porter, Christopher R MD [U] - **Spec Exp:** Urologic Cancer; Prostate Cancer; Testicular Cancer; Robotic Surgery; **Hospital:** Virginia Mason Med Ctr; **Address:** Virginia Mason Med Ctr, 1100 9th Ave, MS C7-URO, Seattle, WA 98101; **Phone:** 206-341-0560; **Board Cert:** Urology 2009; **Med School:** Rush Med Coll 1990; **Resid:** Urology, Brown Univ Affil Hosp 1997; **Fellow:** Urologic Oncology, Meml Sloan Kettering Canc Ctr 1999; **Fac Appt:** Assoc Clin Prof U, Univ Wash

Presti Jr, Joseph C MD [U] - **Spec Exp:** Prostate Cancer; Bladder Cancer; Kidney Cancer; Testicular Cancer; **Hospital:** Stanford Univ Hosp & Clinics; **Address:** Stanford Cancer Ctr, 875 Blake Wilbur Dr MC 5826, Palo Alto, CA 94305-5826; **Phone:** 650-725-5544; **Board Cert:** Urology 2002; **Med School:** UC Irvine 1984; **Resid:** Surgery, UCSF Med Ctr 1986; Urology, UCSF Med Ctr 1989; **Fellow:** Urologic Oncology, Meml Sloan-Kettering Cancer Ctr 1992; **Fac Appt:** Prof U, Stanford Univ

Rajfer, Jacob MD [U] - **Spec Exp:** Erectile Dysfunction; Prostate Disease; Infertility-Male; **Hospital:** LAC - Harbor - UCLA Med Ctr, UCLA Ronald Reagan Med Ctr; **Address:** 21840 S Normandy Ave, Ste 600, Torrance, CA 90502; **Phone:** 310-222-5189; **Board Cert:** Urology 1980; **Med School:** Northwestern Univ 1972; **Resid:** Surgery, St Josephs Hosp 1974; Urology, Johns Hopkins Hosp 1978; **Fellow:** Research, Johns Hopkins Hosp 1976; **Fac Appt:** Prof U, UCLA

Raz, Shlomo MD [U] - **Spec Exp:** Incontinence-Female; Urology-Female; **Hospital:** UCLA Ronald Reagan Med Ctr; **Address:** 200 Med Plaza, Ste 140, Los Angeles, CA 90095; **Phone:** 310-794-0206; **Board Cert:** Urology 1979; **Med School:** Uruguay 1962; **Resid:** Surgery, Hadassah Univ Hosp 1973; **Fellow:** Urology, UCLA Med Ctr 1975; **Fac Appt:** Prof U, UCLA

Sharlip, Ira D MD [U] - **Spec Exp:** Vasectomy Reversal; Erectile Dysfunction; Infertility-Male; **Hospital:** CA Pacific Med Ctr-Pacific Campus, UCSF Med Ctr; **Address:** 2100 Webster St, Ste 222, San Francisco, CA 94115-2376; **Phone:** 415-202-0250; **Board Cert:** Internal Medicine 1972; Urology 1977; **Med School:** Univ Pennsylvania 1965; **Resid:** Internal Medicine, Hosp Univ Penn 1967; Urology, UCSF Med Ctr 1975; **Fellow:** Urology, Middlesex Hosp 1976; **Fac Appt:** Clin Prof U, UCSF

Shortliffe, Linda M MD [U] - **Spec Exp:** Pediatric Urology; Hypospadias; Hydronephrosis; **Hospital:** Lucile Packard Chldn's Hosp, Stanford Univ Hosp & Clinics; **Address:** 300 Pasteur Drive, rm S287, Stanford Univ, Dept of Urology, Stanford, CA 94305-5118; **Phone:** 650-724-7608; **Board Cert:** Urology 2002; Pediatric Urology 2008; **Med School:** Stanford Univ 1975; **Resid:** Surgery, Tufts-New England Med Ctr 1977; Urology, Stanford Univ Med Ctr 1981; **Fellow:** Pediatric Urology, Childrens Hosp 1987; **Fac Appt:** Prof U, Stanford Univ

Skinner, Eila C MD [U] - **Spec Exp:** Urologic Cancer; Genitourinary Disorders-Geriatric; Urinary Reconstruction; **Hospital:** USC Norris Cancer Hosp (page 75), Keck Med Ctr of USC (page 75); **Address:** USC-Keck Sch Med, Dept Urology, 1441 Eastlake Ave, Ste 7416, Los Angeles, CA 90089; **Phone:** 323-865-3707; **Board Cert:** Urology 2001; **Med School:** USC Sch Med 1983; **Resid:** Urology, LAC-USC Med Ctr 1988; **Fellow:** Urologic Oncology, LAC-USC Med Ctr 1990; **Fac Appt:** Assoc Prof U, USC Sch Med

Stoller, Marshall L MD [U] - **Spec Exp:** Laparoscopic Surgery; Kidney Stones; **Hospital:** UCSF Med Ctr; **Address:** 400 Parnassus Ave, A-610, San Francisco, CA 94145-0738; **Phone:** 415-353-2200; **Board Cert:** Urology 2009; **Med School:** Baylor Coll Med 1981; **Resid:** Surgery, UCSF Med Ctr 1983; Urology, UCSF Med Ctr 1987; **Fellow:** Urology, Prince Henry Hosp 1986; **Fac Appt:** Prof U, UCSF

Stone, Anthony R MD [U] - **Spec Exp:** Urology-Female; Voiding Dysfunction; **Hospital:** UC Davis Med Ctr; **Address:** UC Davis Medical Group, 4860 Y St, Ste 3500, Sacramento, CA 95817-2214; **Phone:** 916-734-2222; **Board Cert:** Urology 2006; **Med School:** Scotland, UK 1972; **Resid:** Surgery, Stobhill Hosp 1978; Urology, Cardiff Royal Infirm 1983; **Fellow:** Urodynamics, Duke Univ Med Ctr 1986; **Fac Appt:** Prof U, UC Davis

Takayama, Thomas K MD [U] - **Spec Exp:** Urologic Cancer; Prostate Cancer; Robotic Surgery; Laparoscopic Surgery; **Hospital:** Overlake Hosp Med Ctr; **Address:** Bellevue Urology Associates, 1135 116th Ave NE, Ste 620, Bellevue, WA 98004; **Phone:** 425-454-8016; **Board Cert:** Urology 2007; **Med School:** Tufts Univ 1985; **Resid:** Surgery, UMass Med Ctr 1987; Urology, Univ Washington Med Ctr 1993; **Fellow:** Urologic Oncology, Univ Washington Med Ctr 1996; **Fac Appt:** Assoc Prof U, Univ Wash

Turek, Paul J MD [U] - **Spec Exp:** Infertility-Male; Varicocele Microsurgery; Fertility Preservation in Cancer; Erectile Dysfunction; **Address:** 55 Francisco St, Ste 300, San Francisco, CA 94133; **Phone:** 415-392-3200; **Board Cert:** Urology 2005; **Med School:** Stanford Univ 1987; **Resid:** Surgery, Hosp Univ Penn 1989; Urology, Hosp Univ Penn 1993; **Fellow:** Microsurgery, Baylor Coll Med 1994; **Fac Appt:** Prof U, UCSF

Wilson, Timothy G MD [U] - **Spec Exp:** Prostate Cancer/Robotic Surgery; Minimally Invasive Urologic Surgery; Urinary Reconstruction; **Hospital:** City of Hope Natl Med Ctr; **Address:** Div Urologic Oncology, 1500 E Duarte Rd, Duarte, CA 91010; **Phone:** 626-359-8111 x62655; **Board Cert:** Urology 2001; **Med School:** Oregon Hlth & Sci Univ 1984; **Resid:** Urology, USC Med Ctr 1990; **Fellow:** Urologic Oncology, City Hosp Natl Med Ctr 1991; **Fac Appt:** Assoc Clin Prof U, USC Sch Med

◻️ Cleveland Clinic

Every life deserves world class care.

Urology

With nearly 70 physicians and scientists, Cleveland Clinic Glickman Urological & Kidney Institute's urology program is one of the world's largest and most comprehensive, and has been ranked as one of the top two programs by *U.S.News & World Report* since 2000.

Urologic Cancer Treatment: More than 1,000 prostate cancer patients treated annually utilizing a variety of surgical techniques, including robotic prostatectomy. We have the most experience in partial nephrectomy, with more than 3,000 performed to date and more than 1,200 performed using minimally invasive techniques.

Kidney Transplantation: Since the first kidney transplant at Cleveland Clinic in 1963, the program has performed more than 3,000 kidney transplants. Our surgeons pioneered the technique for removing donor kidneys through a single incision in the belly button.

Female Pelvic Health and Reconstructive Surgery: We treat women with genitourinary disorders, including urinary incontinence and pelvic organ prolapse.

Genitourinary Reconstruction: Our staff performs complex urethral reconstruction for stricture diseases using plastic surgery principles and completes about 60 procedures and 150 prosthetic surgeries annually.

Benign Prostatic Hyperplasia: Minimally invasive treatment options, including laser, microwave and radiofrequency therapies. Many of these options are performed on an outpatient basis with minimal catheterization.

Male Infertility: Comprehensive, individualized evaluation and treatment using state-of-the-art diagnostic procedures and microsurgical techniques.

Endourology and Stone Disease: More than 3,000 patients treated and a success rate of greater than 90 percent with shock wave lithotripsy. Percutaneous kidney stone surgery available for more complicated stone disease. On average, 900 procedures are performed each year.

Cleveland Clinic
Glickman Urological &
Kidney Institute
9500 Euclid Avenue
Cleveland, OH 44195

clevelandclinic.org/
urologytopdocs

Offering Same-Day Appointments
Call 800.274.2009.

Treatment Guides

Cleveland Clinic has developed comprehensive treatment guides for many diseases and conditions. To download our free treatment guides, visit clevelandclinic.org/treatmentguides.

Online Medical Second Opinion

Cleveland Clinic's My**Consult** Online Medical Second Opinion program securely connects patients to our physician specialists for more than 1,000 life-changing or life-threatening diagnoses all by the click of a mouse. To learn more, log onto eclevelandclinic.org/myconsult or call 800.223.2273, ext. 43223.

Special Assistance for Out-of-State Patients

Cleveland Clinic Global Patient Services offers a complimentary Medical Concierge service for patients who travel from outside of Ohio. Call 800.223.2273, ext. 55580 or email medicalconcierge@ccf.org.

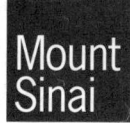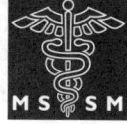

THE MOUNT SINAI MEDICAL CENTER
UROLOGY
One Gustave L. Levy Place
Fifth Avenue and 100th Street
New York, NY 10029-6574
Physician Referral: 1-800-MD-SINAI (637-4624)
www.mountsinai.org/urology

Mount Sinai

MSSM

MOUNT SINAI
SCHOOL OF
MEDICINE

UROLOGY

The Milton and Carroll Petrie Department of Urology at The Mount Sinai Medical Center offers the latest technologic advances for the diagnosis and treatment of urologic diseases and conditions while supporting a translational and clinical research program.

Prostate Cancer: The Department of Urology's Barbara and Maurice Deane Center for Prostate Health and Research offers an extensive range of surgical and radiation treatments for the management of localized prostate cancer. The Robotics Prostatectomy program is one of the world's busiest. Our research has assisted in the development of innovative therapies, including the recently FDA-approved vaccine for prostate cancer, *Provenge*.

Bladder Cancer: As recognized leaders in the assessment and treatment of all forms of bladder cancer, Mount Sinai urologic oncologists are successfully using tumor markers and new diagnostic techniques. Our surgeons employ robotic and laparoscopic surgery to perform cystectomies (removal of bladder) resulting in minimal impact on quality of life.

Kidney Cancer: Mount Sinai specialists helped pioneer robotic partial nephrectomy for the treatment of small kidney cancers. Other minimally invasive options such as cryoablation (freezing) or radiofrequency ablation (heating) are offered as a means to treat small cancers while preserving maximum kidney function.

Benign Prostatic Hyperplasia (BPH): The Deane Center offers the latest minimally invasive technologies and treatments for BPH, including Holium Laser Enucleation, Greenlight ™ Laser Photoselective Vaporization of the Prostate and bipolar cautery vaporization (Button TURP) in addition to TURP for symptoms of an enlarged prostate. Many of these procedures can be performed on an ambulatory basis.

Reconstructive Urology, Female Urology and Voiding Dysfunction: The Department of Urology provides comprehensive resources for the evaluation and treatment of urinary incontinence, neuro-urologic problems (e.g., spinal cord injury, multiple sclerosis) and pelvic pain syndrome for both men and women. Our specialists are among the few in the country with advanced training in urethral reconstruction. A state-of-the-art Continence Center provides the convenience of on-site diagnosis and treatment.

Erectile Dysfunction and Infertility: The Mount Sinai Sexual Health Program uses the most advanced techniques available to evaluate the causes of erectile dysfunction. Treatment options are extensive and effective. Importantly, patients and their partners receive the guidance they need to make the appropriate personal decision regarding treatment.

THE BARBARA AND MAURICE DEANE PROSTATE HEALTH AND RESEARCH CENTER offers a multidisciplinary approach for the assessment and treatment of all aspects of prostate disease, including cancer, benign enlargement, and inflammation. The Center strives to empower the patient and his family, as well as help them to better understand various prostate conditions so they can choose the most appropriate treatment for lasting benefits.

Mount Sinai offers a comprehensive **Minimally Invasive Urologic Surgery Program** and is a recognized leader in the greater New York area for performing complex and laparoscopic procedures to treat urologic cancers. Areas of focus also include the treatment and management of stone disease and reconstructive procedures for various urologic cancers and anatomic abnormalities.

Kidney Stones: Mount Sinai's specialists utilize minimally invasive procedures to treat kidney stones, including laser and ultrasonic lithotripsy techniques. Medical and surgical care is highly customized based on type of stone and stone burden.

Infertility: Mount Sinai's state-of-the-art use of medications, in vitro fertilization techniques and microsurgical repairs have resulted in high success rates.

Pediatric Urology: Mount Sinai excels in treating urologic problems in newborns, infants, children, and adolescents. The Division of Pediatric Urology offers the latest minimally invasive treatments, including robotic assisted surgery for major reconstructive procedures.

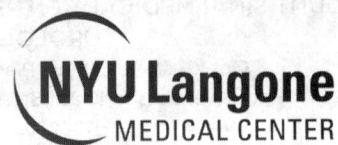

UROLOGY

Urologists at NYU Langone Medical Center continue to pioneer in the surgical and medical treatment of urological disease and are recognized as a top urology program in the country by U.S. News and World Report.

Smilow Comprehensive Prostate Cancer Center
As part of the NCI-designated NYU Cancer Institute, the Center offers care by a team of uro-oncologic surgeons, radiation oncologists, oncologists, naturopathic doctors and radiologists.

Benign Prostatic Diseases
Innovative medical and surgical therapies for benign prostatic disease (as well as for prostatitis (the inflammation of the prostate gland), are offered.

Urological Diseases Center of Excellence
We are focused on discovering novel treatments for bladder and prostate cancer, while exploring how cancer markers can be used to determine how cancer treatments are working.

Female Urology and Incontinence
NYU Langone specializes in urological problems unique to women, including recurrent urinary tract infections, pelvic pain, prolapse and sexual dysfunction.

Latest Minimally Invasive Treatments
The Smilow Comprehensive Prostate Cancer Center, offers advances in prostate imaging and computer biopsy are providing valuable information about tumor location and growth to enable targeted treatment.

Male Sexual Health
Working in collaboration with NYU Langone's Fertility Center, urologists use the latest techniques to enable infertile couples to have children. Treatment is also offered to men suffering from erectile dysfunction and low testosterone.

Pediatric Urology and Reconstructive Surgery
Pediatric urologists focus on urinary system disorders in children from birth to early adults.

Robotic Urological Surgery
The Department's robotic surgery program includes prostate and kidney cancers, as well as female incontinence and urinary tract reconstruction.

Urologic Oncology
Because cancer treatment often requires a collaborative approach, urologists work closely with their colleagues at the NYU Cancer Institute to tailor treatments for each patient.

Vascular Surgery

a subspecialty of Surgery

A surgeon with expertise in the management of surgical disorders of the blood vessels, excluding the intercranial vessels or the heart.

Training Required: Five years in surgery *plus* additional training and examination.

Vascular Surgery

New England

Belkin, Michael MD [VascS] - **Spec Exp:** Aneurysm; Arterial Bypass Surgery; Carotid Artery Surgery; **Hospital:** Brigham and Women's Hosp (page 57), Faulkner Hosp; **Address:** Brigham & Women's Hosp, Dept Vasc Surg, 75 Francis St Shapiro Bldg Fl 5, Boston, MA 02115; **Phone:** 857-307-1920; **Board Cert:** Vascular Surgery 2009; **Med School:** Univ Conn 1982; **Resid:** Surgery, Hartford Hosp 1987; **Fellow:** Vascular Surgery, Brigham & Women's Hosp 1989; **Fac Appt:** Assoc Prof S, Harvard Med Sch

Brewster, David C MD [VascS] - **Spec Exp:** Aneurysm-Abdominal Aortic; Endovascular Surgery; Angioplasty & Stent Placement; **Hospital:** Mass Genl Hosp, Newton - Wellesley Hosp; **Address:** Massachusetts General Hospital, 15 Parkman St, WAC 440, Boston, MA 02114; **Phone:** 617-726-3567; **Board Cert:** Surgery 1975; Vascular Surgery 2003; **Med School:** Columbia P&S 1967; **Resid:** Surgery, Mass Genl Hosp 1975; **Fellow:** Vascular Surgery, Mass Genl Hosp 1976; **Fac Appt:** Clin Prof S, Harvard Med Sch

Cambria, Richard P MD [VascS] - **Spec Exp:** Aneurysm-Abdominal Aortic; Cerebrovascular Disease; Renovascular Disease; Aortic Reconstruction; **Hospital:** Mass Genl Hosp, Newton - Wellesley Hosp; **Address:** Mass Genl Hosp, Dept Vascular Surgery, 15 Parkman St, WAC 440, Boston, MA 02114; **Phone:** 617-726-8278; **Board Cert:** Vascular Surgery 2006; **Med School:** Columbia P&S 1977; **Resid:** Surgery, Mass Genl Hosp 1978; **Fellow:** Vascular Surgery, Mass Genl Hosp 1984; **Fac Appt:** Prof S, Harvard Med Sch

Chaikof, Elliot L MD/PhD [VascS] - **Spec Exp:** Aneurysm-Aortic; Carotid Artery Disease; Peripheral Vascular Disease; Endovascular Surgery; **Hospital:** Beth Israel Deaconess Med Ctr - Boston; **Address:** BIDMC, Div Vascular Surgery, 110 Francis St NE, Ste 5B, Boston, MA 02215; **Phone:** 617-632-9959; **Board Cert:** Surgery 2002; Vascular Surgery 2003; **Med School:** Johns Hopkins Univ 1982; **Resid:** Surgery, Mass Genl Hosp 1985; Surgery, Mass Genl Hosp 1991; **Fellow:** Vascular Surgery, Emory Univ 1992; **Fac Appt:** Prof S, Harvard Med Sch

Cronenwett, Jack MD [VascS] - **Spec Exp:** Peripheral Vascular Disease; Aneurysm-Abdominal Aortic; Carotid Artery Surgery; **Hospital:** Dartmouth - Hitchcock Med Ctr, Mary Hitchcock Mem Hosp; **Address:** Dartmouth-Hitchcock Med Ctr, Sect Vascular Surgery, One Medical Center Drive, Lebanon, NH 03756; **Phone:** 603-650-8670; **Board Cert:** Vascular Surgery 2003; **Med School:** Stanford Univ 1973; **Resid:** Surgery, Univ Mich Hosp 1979; **Fellow:** Vascular Surgery, Univ Tenn Hosp 1980; **Fac Appt:** Prof S, Dartmouth Med Sch

Gusberg, Richard J MD [VascS] - **Spec Exp:** Endovascular Surgery; Aneurysm-Aortic; Renovascular Disease; **Hospital:** Yale-New Haven Hosp, VA Conn Hlthcre Sys-W Haven Campus; **Address:** Yale Univ School of Med-Dept Surgery, 333 Cedar St, Box 208062, BB 204, New Haven, CT 06520-8062; **Phone:** 203-785-6217; **Board Cert:** Vascular Surgery 2008; **Med School:** Columbia P&S 1970; **Resid:** Surgery, Columbia-Presby Med Ctr 1975; **Fellow:** Vascular Surgery, Columbia-Presby Med Ctr 1976; **Fac Appt:** Prof S, Yale Univ

Iafrati, Mark D MD [VascS] - **Spec Exp:** Endovascular Surgery; Minimally Invasive Vascular Surgery; Wound Healing/Care; Vein Disorders; **Hospital:** Tufts Med Ctr, Morton Hosp & Med Ctr; **Address:** 800 Washington St, Box 259, Boston, MA 02111; **Phone:** 617-636-5019; **Board Cert:** Surgery 2005; Vascular Surgery 2005; **Med School:** Tufts Univ 1989; **Resid:** Surgery, Tufts New England Med Ctr 1995; **Fellow:** Vascular Surgery, Tufts New England Med Ctr 1997; **Fac Appt:** Asst Prof S, Tufts Univ

Kwolek, Christopher J MD [VascS] - **Spec Exp:** Aneurysm-Abdominal & Thoracic Aortic; Endovascular Surgery; Carotid Artery Stent Placement; **Hospital:** Mass Genl Hosp, Newton - Wellesley Hosp; **Address:** 15 Parkman St, Wang Bldg Fl 4, Boston, MA 02114; **Phone:** 617-724-6101; **Board Cert:** Surgery 2003; Vascular Surgery 2006; **Med School:** UCSF 1987; **Resid:** Surgery, New England Deaconess Hosp 1993; Vascular Surgery, Mass Genl Hosp 1995; **Fellow:** Endovascular Surgery, Arizona Heart Inst 1999; **Fac Appt:** Assoc Prof VascS, Harvard Med Sch

LaMuraglia, Glenn M MD [VascS] - **Spec Exp:** Carotid Body Tumors; Aneurysm-Aortic; Endovascular Surgery; Vascular Disease; **Hospital:** Mass Genl Hosp; **Address:** Mass Gen Hosp, Vascular Surgery, 55 Fruit St, Boston, MA 02114; **Phone:** 617-726-6997; **Board Cert:** Surgery 2004; Vascular Surgery 2007; **Med School:** Harvard Med Sch 1979; **Resid:** Surgery, Mass Genl Hosp 1985; Vascular Surgery, Mass Genl Hosp 1986; **Fac Appt:** Assoc Prof S, Harvard Med Sch

Mackey, William C MD [VascS] - **Spec Exp:** Carotid Artery Surgery; Aneurysm-Abdominal Aortic; Lower Limb Arterial Disease; **Hospital:** Tufts Med Ctr; **Address:** Tufts Med Ctr, 800 Washington St, Box 1035, Boston, MA 02111; **Phone:** 617-636-5927; **Board Cert:** Surgery 2002; Vascular Surgery 2004; Surgical Critical Care 2007; **Med School:** Duke Univ 1977; **Resid:** Surgery, New York Hosp 1982; **Fellow:** Vascular Surgery, Tufts-New Eng Med Ctr 1984; **Fac Appt:** Prof S, Tufts Univ

Pomposelli, Frank B MD [VascS] - **Spec Exp:** Diabetic Leg/Foot; Aortic Surgery; Carotid Artery Disease; Endovascular Surgery; **Hospital:** Beth Israel Deaconess Med Ctr - Boston, New England Bapt Hosp; **Address:** Beth Israel Deac Med Ctr, 110 Francis St, Ste 5B, Boston, MA 02215-5566; **Phone:** 617-632-9847; **Board Cert:** Vascular Surgery 2008; **Med School:** Boston Univ 1979; **Resid:** Surgery, New England Deaconess Hosp 1986; **Fellow:** Peripheral Vascular Surgery, NYU Med Ctr 1987; **Fac Appt:** Assoc Prof S, Harvard Med Sch

Sumpio, Bauer E MD/PhD [VascS] - **Spec Exp:** Diabetic Leg/Foot; Endovascular Surgery; **Hospital:** Yale-New Haven Hosp, Yale Med Group; **Address:** Yale Univ School Medicine, Dept Surgery, 333 Cedar St, Box 208062, BB 204, New Haven, CT 06520; **Phone:** 203-785-6217; **Board Cert:** Vascular Surgery 2009; Surgery 2009; **Med School:** Cornell Univ-Weill Med Coll 1980; **Resid:** Surgery, Yale-New Haven Hosp 1986; **Fellow:** Vascular Surgery, Univ N Carolina Hosp 1987; **Fac Appt:** Prof S, Yale Univ

Mid Atlantic

Adelman, Mark MD [VascS] - **Spec Exp:** Carotid Artery Surgery; Aneurysm-Abdominal Aortic; Vein Disorders; Endovascular Surgery; **Hospital:** NYU Langone Med Ctr (page 66), Bellevue Hosp Ctr; **Address:** 530 1st Ave, Ste 6F, New York, NY 10016-6402; **Phone:** 212-263-7311; **Board Cert:** Surgery 1999; Vascular Surgery 2001; **Med School:** NYU Sch Med 1985; **Resid:** Surgery, NYU Med Ctr 1990; **Fellow:** Vascular Surgery, NYU Med Ctr 1991; **Fac Appt:** Prof VascS, NYU Sch Med

Ascher, Enrico MD [VascS] - **Spec Exp:** Endovascular Surgery; Carotid Artery Surgery; Limb Sparing Surgery; Aneurysm; **Hospital:** Maimonides Med Ctr (page 62), Mount Sinai Med Ctr (page 63); **Address:** 903 49th St, Brooklyn, NY 11219; **Phone:** 718-283-7957; **Board Cert:** Vascular Surgery 2004; **Med School:** Brazil 1974; **Resid:** Surgery, NY Med Coll 1981; **Fellow:** Vascular Surgery, Montefiore Med Ctr 1982; **Fac Appt:** Prof S, SUNY Downstate

Vascular Surgery

Atnip, Robert G MD [VascS] - **Spec Exp:** Aneurysm-Abdominal Aortic; Peripheral Vascular Disease; Carotid Artery Disease; Endovascular Surgery; **Hospital:** Penn State Milton S Hershey Med Ctr; **Address:** Hershey Med Ctr Vascular Surgery, 500 University Drive, Hershey, PA 17033; **Phone:** 717-531-4554; **Board Cert:** Surgery 2005; Vascular Surgery 2007; Surgical Critical Care 2010; **Med School:** Univ Alabama 1978; **Resid:** Surgery, Mass Genl Hosp 1984; **Fellow:** Vascular Surgery, Mass Genl Hosp 1985; **Fac Appt:** Prof S

Benckart, Daniel MD [VascS] - **Hospital:** Allegheny General Hosp; **Address:** Allegheny Cardiovascular Inst, 1, 320 E North Ave, Pittsburgh, PA 15212; **Phone:** 412-359-8820; **Board Cert:** Thoracic Surgery 2004; Surgery 2003; Vascular Surgery 1999; **Med School:** Georgetown Univ 1977; **Resid:** Surgery, Vanderbilt Affil Hosp 1982; **Fellow:** Vascular Thoracic Surgery, NYU Med Ctr 1985; **Fac Appt:** Assoc Prof TS, Drexel Univ Coll Med

Benvenisty, Alan I MD [VascS] - **Spec Exp:** Renovascular Disease; Aneurysm-Aortic; Endovascular Surgery; Minimally Invasive Vascular Surgery; **Hospital:** St. Luke's - Roosevelt Hosp Ctr - St Luke's Hosp (page 55), St. Luke's - Roosevelt Hosp Ctr - Roosevelt Div (page 55); **Address:** 1090 Amsterdam Ave Fl 12, New York, NY 10025; **Phone:** 212-523-4706; **Board Cert:** Surgery 2004; Vascular Surgery 2009; **Med School:** Columbia P&S 1978; **Resid:** Surgery, Columbia-Presby Med Ctr 1983; **Fellow:** Vascular Surgery, Columbia-Presby Med Ctr 1984; Transplant Surgery, Columbia-Presby Med Ctr 1984; **Fac Appt:** Clin Prof S, Columbia P&S

Brener, Bruce J MD [VascS] - **Spec Exp:** Endovascular Surgery; Minimally Invasive Vascular Surgery; Carotid Artery Surgery; Aneurysm-Aortic; **Hospital:** Newark Beth Israel Med Ctr, Saint Barnabas Med Ctr; **Address:** 200 South Orange Ave, Livingston, NJ 07039; **Phone:** 973-322-7233; **Board Cert:** Surgery 1972; Vascular Surgery 2005; **Med School:** Harvard Med Sch 1966; **Resid:** Surgery, Chldns Hosp Med Ctr 1968; Surgery, Peter Bent Brigham Hosp 1972; **Fellow:** Vascular Surgery, Mass Genl Hosp 1973; **Fac Appt:** Assoc Clin Prof S, Columbia P&S

Calligaro, Keith D MD [VascS] - **Spec Exp:** Aneurysm-Abdominal & Thoracic Aortic; Carotid Artery Disease; Renal Artery Stenosis; **Hospital:** Pennsylvania Hosp-UPHS (page 68); **Address:** 700 Spruce St, Ste 101, Philadelphia, PA 19106; **Phone:** 215-829-5000; **Board Cert:** Vascular Surgery 2008; **Med School:** UMDNJ-Rutgers Med Sch 1982; **Resid:** Surgery, St Barnabas Med Ctr 1984; Surgery, Univ Hlth Scis/Chicago Med Sch 1987; **Fellow:** Vascular Surgery, Montefiore Med Ctr 1989; **Fac Appt:** Clin Prof S, Univ Pennsylvania

Carpenter, Jeffrey P MD [VascS] - **Spec Exp:** Aneurysm-Abdominal & Thoracic Aortic; Carotid Artery Surgery; Endovascular Surgery; Peripheral Vascular Disease; **Hospital:** Cooper Univ Hosp; **Address:** 3 Cooper Plaza, Ste 411, Camden, NJ 08104; **Phone:** 856-325-6516; **Board Cert:** Surgery 2001; Vascular Surgery 2001; **Med School:** Yale Univ 1986; **Resid:** Surgery, Hosp Univ Penn 1991; **Fellow:** Vascular Surgery, Hosp Univ Penn 1992; **Fac Appt:** Prof S

Criado, Frank J MD [VascS] - **Spec Exp:** Endovascular Surgery; Aneurysm-Abdominal & Thoracic Aortic; Carotid Artery Stent Placement; **Hospital:** Union Meml Hosp-Baltimore; **Address:** 3333 N Calvert St, Ste 570, Baltimore, MD 21218; **Phone:** 410-554-6400; **Board Cert:** Vascular Surgery 2008; **Med School:** Uruguay 1974; **Resid:** Surgery, Union Meml Hosp 1980; Vascular Surgery, Union Meml Hosp 1985; **Fellow:** Cardiovascular Surgery, Baylor Univ Med Ctr 1981

D'Ayala, Marcus D MD [VascS] - **Spec Exp:** Endovascular Surgery; Aneurysm-Abdominal Aortic; **Hospital:** New York Methodist Hosp; **Address:** NY Methodist Hospital, Dept Surgery, 506 Sixth St, Brooklyn, NY 11215; **Phone:** 718-780-3288; **Board Cert:** Surgery 2008; Vascular Surgery 2009; **Med School:** Univ Wisc 1992; **Resid:** Surgery, Montefiore Med Ctr 1997; **Fellow:** Vascular Surgery, Mt Sinai Med Ctr 1998; **Fac Appt:** Asst Prof S, Mount Sinai Sch Med

Darling III, R Clement MD [VascS] - **Spec Exp:** Aneurysm-Abdominal & Thoracic Aortic; Arterial Bypass Surgery; Carotid Artery Surgery; **Hospital:** Albany Med Ctr, St. Peter's Hosp - Albany; **Address:** Albany Med Ctr, Vascular Inst, 43 New Scotland Ave, MC 157, Albany, NY 12208; **Phone:** 518-262-5640; **Board Cert:** Surgery 1999; Vascular Surgery 2002; **Med School:** Univ Cincinnati 1984; **Resid:** Surgery, Beth Israel Deaconess Hosp 1989; **Fellow:** Vascular Surgery, Albany Med Ctr 1991; **Fac Appt:** Prof S, Albany Med Coll

Dougherty, Matthew J MD [VascS] - **Spec Exp:** Endovascular Stent Grafts; Aneurysm; **Hospital:** Pennsylvania Hosp-UPHS (page 68); **Address:** 700 Spruce St, Ste 101, Philadelphia, PA 19106; **Phone:** 215-829-5000; **Board Cert:** Vascular Surgery 2001; Surgery 1999; **Med School:** Harvard Med Sch 1984; **Resid:** Surgery, Mass Genl Hosp 1990; **Fellow:** Vascular Surgery, Mayo Clinic 1992; **Fac Appt:** Assoc Clin Prof S, Univ Pennsylvania

Fairman, Ronald M MD [VascS] - **Spec Exp:** Aneurysm-Aortic; Peripheral Vascular Disease; Carotid Artery Surgery; Aneurysm-Abdominal & Thoracic Aortic; **Hospital:** Hosp Univ Penn - UPHS (page 68); **Address:** Perelman Ctr for Advanced Medicine, 3400 Civic Ctr Blvd Fl 2-East, Philadelphia, PA 19104; **Phone:** 215-615-4949; **Board Cert:** Vascular Surgery 2010; **Med School:** Thomas Jefferson Univ 1977; **Resid:** Surgery, Hosp U Penn 1983; **Fellow:** Vascular Surgery, Hosp U Penn 1984; **Fac Appt:** Prof S, Univ Pennsylvania

Fantini, Gary A MD [VascS] - **Spec Exp:** Spinal Access Surgery; Thoracic Outlet Syndrome; **Hospital:** Hosp For Special Surgery (page 60), NY-Presby/Weill Cornell Med Ctr, NY (page 65); **Address:** 635 Madison Ave, New York, NY 10022; **Phone:** 212-317-4550; **Board Cert:** Surgery 2007; Vascular Surgery 2009; **Med School:** Albert Einstein Coll Med 1983; **Resid:** Surgery, NY Hosp-Cornell Med Ctr 1989; **Fellow:** Vascular Surgery, UCSF Med Ctr 1990; **Fac Appt:** Assoc Prof S, Cornell Univ-Weill Med Coll

Faries, Peter MD [VascS] - **Spec Exp:** Aneurysm-Abdominal Aortic; Peripheral Vascular Disease; Renovascular Disease; Carotid Artery Surgery; **Hospital:** Mount Sinai Med Ctr (page 63); **Address:** 5 E 98th St, Ste 415, New York, NY 10029; **Phone:** 212-241-5386; **Board Cert:** Surgery 2008; Vascular Surgery 2009; **Med School:** Univ Pennsylvania 1992; **Resid:** Surgery, Montefiore Med Ctr 1998; **Fellow:** Vascular Surgery, Beth Israel Deaconess Med Ctr 2000; **Fac Appt:** Prof S, Mount Sinai Sch Med

Freischlag, Julie A MD [VascS] - **Spec Exp:** Aneurysm-Aortic; Carotid Artery Disease; Thoracic Outlet Syndrome; **Hospital:** Johns Hopkins Hosp (page 61); **Address:** Johns Hopkins Hosp, Dept Surg, 720 Rutland Ave, Ross Bldg-759, Baltimore, MD 21205; **Phone:** 443-287-3497; **Board Cert:** Surgery 2005; Vascular Surgery 2005; **Med School:** Rush Med Coll 1980; **Resid:** Surgery, UCLA Medical Ctr 1986; **Fellow:** Vascular Surgery, UCLA Medical Ctr 1987; **Fac Appt:** Prof S, Johns Hopkins Univ

Golden, Michael A MD [VascS] - **Spec Exp:** Aneurysm; Endovascular Surgery; **Hospital:** Penn Presby Med Ctr - UPHS (page 68); **Address:** Penn Presbyterian, Vascular Surgery, 51 N 39th & Market St, 266 Wright Saunders Bldg, Philadelphia, PA 19104; **Phone:** 215-662-9660; **Board Cert:** Surgery 2007; Vascular Surgery 2010; **Med School:** Univ Pennsylvania 1981; **Resid:** Surgery, Brigham & Women's Hosp 1987; **Fellow:** Vascular Surgery, Brigham & Women's Hosp 1990; **Fac Appt:** Assoc Prof S, Univ Pennsylvania

Green, Richard M MD [VascS] - **Spec Exp:** Aneurysm-Abdominal Aortic; Carotid Artery Surgery; Percutaneous Vascular Interventions; **Hospital:** Lenox Hill Hosp; **Address:** 130 E 77th St, Fl 13, New York, NY 10075; **Phone:** 212-434-3420; **Board Cert:** Vascular Surgery 2003; **Med School:** Univ Rochester 1970; **Resid:** Surgery, Strong Meml Hosp 1976

Vascular Surgery

Harrington, Elizabeth MD [VascS] - **Spec Exp:** Carotid Artery Surgery; Aneurysm-Aortic; Arterial Bypass Surgery-Leg; **Hospital:** Mount Sinai Med Ctr (page 63); **Address:** 2 E 93rd St, New York, NY 10128; **Phone:** 212-876-7400; **Board Cert:** Surgery 2009; Vascular Surgery 2006; **Med School:** NY Med Coll 1975; **Resid:** Surgery, Mt Sinai Hosp 1980; **Fellow:** Vascular Surgery, Mt Sinai Hosp 1981; **Fac Appt:** Assoc Prof VascS, Mount Sinai Sch Med

Makaroun, Michel S MD [VascS] - **Spec Exp:** Endovascular Surgery; Aneurysm; Carotid Artery Disease; Peripheral Vascular Disease; **Hospital:** UPMC Shadyside, UPMC Presby, Pittsburgh; **Address:** 200 Lothrop St, PUH Bldg - Fl 10 - Ste A-1011, Pittsburgh, PA 15213; **Phone:** 412-802-3333; **Board Cert:** Surgery 2004; Vascular Surgery 2009; **Med School:** Lebanon 1978; **Resid:** Surgery, American Univ Hosp 1980; Surgery, Univ Pittsburgh Med Ctr 1985; **Fac Appt:** Prof S, Univ Pittsburgh

Marin, Michael L MD [VascS] - **Spec Exp:** Aneurysm-Aortic; Carotid Artery Surgery; Limb Sparing Surgery; Endovascular Surgery; **Hospital:** Mount Sinai Med Ctr (page 63); **Address:** Mount Sinai Medical Ctr, 5 E 98th St, Box 1273, New York, NY 10029; **Phone:** 212-241-5315; **Board Cert:** Surgery 1999; **Med School:** Mount Sinai Sch Med 1984; **Resid:** Surgery, Columbia-Presby Med Ctr 1990; **Fellow:** Transplant Surgery, Columbia-Presby Med Ctr 1988; Vascular Surgery, Montefiore Med Ctr 1992; **Fac Appt:** Prof S, Mount Sinai Sch Med

Neville Jr, Richard F MD [VascS] - **Spec Exp:** Endovascular Surgery; Wound Healing/Care; **Hospital:** G Washington Univ Hosp, Inova Mt Vernon Hosp; **Address:** GWU Med Faculty Assocs, 2150 Pennsylvania Ave NW, Ste 6B412, Washington, DC 20037; **Phone:** 202-741-3210; **Board Cert:** Surgery 2000; Vascular Surgery 2002; **Med School:** Univ MD Sch Med 1983; **Resid:** Surgery, Georgetown Univ Hosp 1988; **Fellow:** Vascular Surgery, UMDNJ Affil Hosp 1991; **Fac Appt:** Assoc Prof S, Georgetown Univ

Perler, Bruce MD [VascS] - **Spec Exp:** Carotid Artery Surgery; Aneurysm; Arterial Bypass Surgery-Leg; **Hospital:** Johns Hopkins Hosp (page 61), Johns Hopkins Bayview Med Ctr (page 61); **Address:** Johns Hopkins Hosp, Dept Surgery, 600 N Wolfe St Harvey 611 Bldg, Baltimore, MD 21287-8611; **Phone:** 410-955-2618; **Board Cert:** Vascular Surgery 2008; **Med School:** Duke Univ 1976; **Resid:** Surgery, Mass Genl Hosp 1981; **Fellow:** Vascular Surgery, Mass Genl Hosp 1982; **Fac Appt:** Prof S, Johns Hopkins Univ

Ricotta, John MD [VascS] - **Spec Exp:** Aneurysm; Carotid Artery Surgery; Vein Disorders; **Hospital:** Washington Hosp Ctr; **Address:** Washington Hospital Ctr, Dept Surgery, 110 Irving St NW, rm G253, Washington, DC 20010; **Phone:** 202-877-0725; **Board Cert:** Surgery 2004; Vascular Surgery 2003; **Med School:** Johns Hopkins Univ 1973; **Resid:** Surgery, Johns Hopkins Hosp 1977; **Fellow:** Vascular Surgery, Johns Hopkins Hosp 1979; **Fac Appt:** Prof S

Riles, Thomas MD [VascS] - **Spec Exp:** Aneurysm-Abdominal Aortic; Carotid Artery Surgery; **Hospital:** NYU Langone Med Ctr (page 66); **Address:** NYU Med Ctr, Univ Vascular Assoc, 530 1st Ave, HCC-6D, New York, NY 10016; **Phone:** 212-263-6360; **Board Cert:** Vascular Surgery 2003; **Med School:** Baylor Coll Med 1969; **Resid:** Surgery, NYU Med Ctr 1976; **Fellow:** Vascular Surgery, NYU Med Ctr 1977; **Fac Appt:** Prof S, NYU Sch Med

Schneider, Darren B MD [VascS] - **Spec Exp:** Endovascular Surgery; Minimally Invasive Vascular Surgery; Aneurysm-Aortic; Peripheral Vascular Disease; **Hospital:** NY-Presby/Weill Cornell Med Ctr, NY (page 65); **Address:** Weill Cornell Dept Vascular Surgery, 525 E 68th St, New York, NY 10021; **Phone:** 212-746-5192; **Board Cert:** Surgery 2001; Vascular Surgery 2003; **Med School:** UCSD 1992; **Resid:** Surgery, UCSF Med Ctr 2000; **Fellow:** Interventional Radiology, UCSF Med Ctr 2001; Vascular Surgery, UCSF Med Ctr 2002; **Fac Appt:** Asst Prof S, Cornell Univ-Weill Med Coll

Todd, George MD [VascS] - **Spec Exp:** Minimally Invasive Vascular Surgery; Aneurysm-Abdominal Aortic; Carotid Artery Surgery; **Hospital:** St. Luke's - Roosevelt Hosp Ctr - Roosevelt Div (page 55); **Address:** St Luke's-Roosevelt Hosp Ctr, Dept Surg, 1000 10th Ave, rm 5G77, New York, NY 10019; **Phone:** 212-523-7481; **Board Cert:** Surgery 2010; Vascular Surgery 2006; **Med School:** Penn State Coll Med 1974; **Resid:** Surgery, Columbia-Presby Med Ctr 1979; **Fellow:** Vascular Surgery, Columbia-Presby Med Ctr 1980; **Fac Appt:** Prof S, Columbia P&S

Southeast

Bandyk, Dennis F MD [VascS] - **Spec Exp:** Endovascular Stent Grafts; Lower Limb Arterial Disease; Thoracic Outlet Syndrome; **Hospital:** Tampa Genl Hosp; **Address:** USF Physicians Group, 2 Tampa General Circle, Ste 7001, Tampa, FL 33606; **Phone:** 813-259-0921; **Board Cert:** Surgery 2000; Vascular Surgery 2001; **Med School:** Univ Mich Med Sch 1975; **Resid:** Surgery, Univ Wash Hosp 1980; **Fellow:** Vascular Surgery, Univ Wash Hosp 1981; **Fac Appt:** Prof S, Univ S Fla Coll Med

Brophy, Colleen M MD [VascS] - **Spec Exp:** Aneurysm; Carotid Artery Surgery; Peripheral Vascular Disease; **Hospital:** VA Tennessee Valley Healthcare System-Alvin C. Yor, Vanderbilt Univ Med Ctr (page 76); **Address:** Vanderbilt U Med Ctr, Vascular Surgery, D-5237 Medical Ctr North, Nashville, TN 37232-2735; **Phone:** 615-322-2343; **Board Cert:** Surgery 2009; Vascular Surgery 2009; **Med School:** Univ Utah 1983; **Resid:** Surgery, Yale-New Haven Hosp 1988; **Fellow:** Vascular Surgery, New England Med Ctr 1990; **Fac Appt:** Prof S, Vanderbilt Univ

Cherry Jr, Kenneth J MD [VascS] - **Spec Exp:** Vascular Reconstruction; Aortic Graft Infections; **Hospital:** Univ of Virginia Health Sys; **Address:** Univ Virginia Health System, PO Box 800679, Charlottesville, VA 22908-0679; **Phone:** 434-243-7052; **Board Cert:** Vascular Surgery 2004; **Med School:** Univ VA Sch Med 1974; **Resid:** Surgery, Univ Virginia Hosp 1980; Vascular Surgery, UCSF Med Ctr 1981; **Fac Appt:** Prof S, Univ VA Sch Med

Dattilo, Jeffery MD [VascS] - **Hospital:** Vanderbilt Univ Med Ctr (page 76), VA Tennessee Valley Healthcare System-Alvin C. Yor; **Address:** Division of Vascular Surgery, Vanderbilt University Medical Center, D-5237 Medical Center North, Nashville, TN 37232-2735; **Phone:** 615-322-2343; **Board Cert:** Surgery 2002; Vascular Surgery 2005; **Med School:** E Carolina Univ 1993; **Resid:** Surgery, Medical College of Virginia Hosp 2000; **Fellow:** Vascular Surgery, Mass Genl Hosp 2002; **Fac Appt:** Assoc Prof S, Vanderbilt Univ

Flynn, Timothy C MD [VascS] - **Spec Exp:** Peripheral Vascular Disease; Aortic Graft Infections; **Hospital:** Shands at Univ of FL; **Address:** Shands Hlthcare Univ Florida, PO Box 100129, Gainesville, FL 32610-0286; **Phone:** 352-265-0152; **Board Cert:** Surgery 1999; Vascular Surgery 2008; Surgical Critical Care 1998; **Med School:** Baylor Coll Med 1974; **Resid:** Surgery, Univ Texas 1980; **Fac Appt:** Prof S, Univ Fla Coll Med

Hakaim, Albert G MD [VascS] - **Spec Exp:** Aneurysm-Abdominal Aortic; Endovascular Surgery; **Hospital:** Mayo - Jacksonville; **Address:** Mayo Clinic, Dept Vascular Surgery, 4500 San Pablo Rd, Ste 323N, Jacksonville, FL 32224; **Phone:** 904-953-2077; **Board Cert:** Surgery 2002; Vascular Surgery 2003; **Med School:** Ohio State Univ 1984; **Resid:** Surgery, Cleveland Clinic 1989; **Fellow:** Transplant Surgery, Boston Univ Hosp 1991; Vascular Surgery, Cleveland Clinic 1992; **Fac Appt:** Assoc Prof S, Mayo Med Sch

Vascular Surgery

Hallett Jr, John W MD [VascS] - **Spec Exp:** Aneurysm-Abdominal Aortic; Carotid Artery Surgery; Thoracic Outlet Syndrome; **Hospital:** Roper Hosp; **Address:** Roper St Francis Heart & Vascular Ctr, 316 Calhoun St, Charleston, SC 29401; **Phone:** 843-720-5665; **Board Cert:** Surgery 1999; Vascular Surgery 2003; **Med School:** Duke Univ 1973; **Resid:** Surgery, Wilford Hall USAF Med Ctr 1978; **Fellow:** Vascular Surgery, Mass Genl Hosp-Harvard Med Sch 1979; **Fac Appt:** Assoc Clin Prof VascS, Med Univ SC

Hansen, Kimberley J MD [VascS] - **Spec Exp:** Aortic & Visceral Artery Surgery; Renovascular Disease; Carotid Artery Surgery; **Hospital:** Wake Forest Univ Baptist Med Ctr, Forsyth Med Ctr; **Address:** Dept Vascular & Endovascular Surgery, Wake Forest Univ Baptist Med Ctr, Medical Center Blvd, Winston-Salem, NC 27157-1095; **Phone:** 336-716-4151; **Board Cert:** Surgery 2006; Vascular Surgery 2008; Surgical Critical Care 2001; **Med School:** Univ Alabama 1980; **Resid:** Surgery, NC Baptist Hosp/WFU Sch MEd 1986; **Fellow:** Vascular Surgery, UCSF Med Ctr 1987; **Fac Appt:** Prof S, Wake Forest Univ

McCann, Richard L MD [VascS] - **Spec Exp:** Endovascular Surgery; **Hospital:** Duke Univ Hosp; **Address:** Duke Univ Med Ctr, Box 2990, Durham, NC 27710; **Phone:** 919-681-2406; **Board Cert:** Surgery 2003; Vascular Surgery 2006; **Med School:** Cornell Univ-Weill Med Coll 1974; **Resid:** Surgery, Duke Univ Med Ctr 1983; **Fac Appt:** Prof S, Duke Univ

Mitchell, Marc E MD [VascS] - **Spec Exp:** Renal Artery Stenosis; Carotid Artery Surgery; Aneurysm-Aortic; Peripheral Vascular Disease; **Hospital:** Univ Mississippi Med Ctr; **Address:** Univ Mississippi Med Ctr, Dept Surgery, 2500 N State St, Jackson, MS 39216; **Phone:** 601-984-5105; **Board Cert:** Surgery 2010; Surgical Critical Care 2005; Vascular Surgery 2007; **Med School:** Georgetown Univ 1984; **Resid:** Surgery, UCSF Med Ctr 1986; Surgery, Univ Mississippi Med Ctr 1991; **Fellow:** Cardiac Surgery, NIH 1998; Vascular Surgery, Univ Penn 1997; **Fac Appt:** Prof S, Univ Miss

Naslund, Thomas C MD [VascS] - **Spec Exp:** Endovascular Surgery; Aneurysm-Aortic; **Hospital:** Vanderbilt Univ Med Ctr (page 76); **Address:** Vanderbilt Univ Med Ctr, Div Vasc Surg, 1161 21st Ave S, D-5237 MCN, Nashville, TN 37232-2735; **Phone:** 615-322-2343; **Board Cert:** Vascular Surgery 2000; Surgery 1999; **Med School:** Vanderbilt Univ 1984; **Resid:** Surgery, Vanderbilt Univ Med Ctr 1990; **Fellow:** Vascular Surgery, Ochsner Med Fdn 1992; **Fac Appt:** Prof S, Vanderbilt Univ

Rosenthal, David MD [VascS] - **Spec Exp:** Stroke; Aneurysm; Endovascular Surgery; **Hospital:** Atlanta Med Ctr, Piedmont Hosp; **Address:** Atlanta Vascular Specialists, 315 Boulevard NE, Ste 412, Atlanta, GA 30312; **Phone:** 404-524-0095; **Board Cert:** Vascular Surgery 2003; **Med School:** SUNY Downstate 1973; **Resid:** Surgery, Tufts-New Eng Med Ctr 1977; **Fellow:** Vascular Surgery, Tufts-New Eng Med Ctr 1978; **Fac Appt:** Clin Prof S, Med Coll GA

Sivina, Manuel MD [VascS] - **Hospital:** Mount Sinai Med Ctr - Miami; **Address:** Mount Sinai Med Ctr, 4300 Alton Rd, Ste 2240, Miami Beach, FL 33140; **Phone:** 305-674-2760; **Board Cert:** Surgery 2000; **Med School:** Peru 1969; **Resid:** Surgery, Mt Sinai Med Ctr 1975; **Fellow:** Vascular Surgery, Mt Sinai Med Ctr 1976

Midwest

Alexander, J Jeffrey MD [VascS] - **Spec Exp:** Peripheral Vascular Disease; Carotid Artery Disease; Dialysis Access; **Hospital:** MetroHealth Med Ctr; **Address:** Metrohealth Med Ctr, Heart & Vascular Dept, 2500 Metrohealth Drive, Ste H328, Cleveland, OH 44109-1928; **Phone:** 216-778-4811; **Board Cert:** Surgery 2002; Vascular Surgery 2006; **Med School:** Univ Pittsburgh 1978; **Resid:** Surgery, Univ Chicago Hosps 1983; **Fellow:** Vascular Surgery, Univ Chicago Hosps 1984; **Fac Appt:** Assoc Prof S, Case West Res Univ

Berguer, Ramon MD/PhD [VascS] - **Spec Exp:** Cerebrovascular Disease; Aortic & Visceral Artery Surgery; **Hospital:** Univ of Michigan Hosp; **Address:** Univ Michigan Hlth Sys, 1500 E Med Ctr Dr, SPC5856, Ann Arbor, MI 48109; **Phone:** 734-936-8247; **Board Cert:** Surgery 1970; Vascular Surgery 2003; **Med School:** Spain 1963; **Resid:** Surgery, Henry Ford Hosp 1969; **Fellow:** Vascular Surgery, Henry Ford Hosp 1970; Vascular Surgery, Kings College Hosp; **Fac Appt:** Prof S, Univ Mich Med Sch

Clair, Daniel G MD [VascS] - **Spec Exp:** Carotid Artery Surgery; Aneurysm-Abdominal & Thoracic Aortic; Peripheral Vascular Disease; Endovascular Stent Grafts; **Hospital:** Cleveland Clin (page 56); **Address:** Cleveland Clinic, Dept Vascular Surgery, 9500 Euclid Ave, MC H32, Cleveland, OH 44195; **Phone:** 216-444-3857; **Board Cert:** Surgery 2003; Vascular Surgery 2004; **Med School:** Univ VA Sch Med 1986; **Resid:** Surgery, Brigham & Women's Hosp 1992; **Fellow:** Oncology, Brigham & Women's Hosp 1991; Vascular Surgery, Brigham & Women's Hosp 1994

Comerota, Anthony J MD [VascS] - **Spec Exp:** Carotid Artery Disease; Gene Therapy; Aneurysm-Aortic; Peripheral Vascular Disease; **Hospital:** Toledo Hosp; **Address:** Jobst Vascular Ctr, 2109 Hughes Drive, Ste 400, Toledo, OH 43606; **Phone:** 419-291-2088; **Board Cert:** Surgery 1999; Vascular Surgery 2003; **Med School:** Temple Univ 1974; **Resid:** Surgery, Temple Univ Hosp 1978; **Fellow:** Vascular Surgery, Good Samaritan Hosp 1981; **Fac Appt:** Clin Prof S, Univ Mich Med Sch

Dalsing, Michael C MD [VascS] - **Spec Exp:** Peripheral Vascular Disease; Carotid Artery Disease; Aortic Reconstruction; Percutaneous Vascular Interventions; **Hospital:** IU Health Methodist Hosp, IU Health University Hosp; **Address:** University Vascular Surgery, 1801 N Senate Blvd, MPC2-3500, Indianapolis, IN 46202; **Phone:** 317-962-0280; **Board Cert:** Surgery 2002; Vascular Surgery 2003; Surgical Critical Care 2001; **Med School:** Med Coll Wisc 1978; **Resid:** Surgery, Indiana Univ Med Ctr 1983; **Fellow:** Vascular Surgery, Northwestern Univ Med Ctr 1984; **Fac Appt:** Prof S, Indiana Univ

Gloviczki, Peter MD [VascS] - **Spec Exp:** Aneurysm-Abdominal Aortic; Lower Limb Arterial Disease; Vein Disorders; **Hospital:** Mayo Med Ctr & Clin - Rochester; **Address:** Mayo Clin, Div Vasc Surg, 200 First St SW, Rochester, MN 55905-0001; **Phone:** 507-284-4652; **Board Cert:** Surgery 1998; Vascular Surgery 2008; **Med School:** Hungary 1972; **Resid:** Vascular Surgery, Semmelweis Med Sch 1980; Surgery, Mayo Clin 1987; **Fellow:** Vascular Surgery, Mayo Clin 1983; **Fac Appt:** Prof S, Mayo Med Sch

Greisler, Howard MD [VascS] - **Spec Exp:** Peripheral Vascular Disease; Aneurysm; Carotid Artery Disease; **Hospital:** Edward Hines, Jr. VA Hosp; **Address:** VA Hospital, 5000 S 5th Ave, Rte 112, Hines, IL 60141; **Phone:** 708-202-2036; **Board Cert:** Vascular Surgery 2003; **Med School:** Penn State Coll Med 1975; **Resid:** Surgery, Columbia Presby Med Ctr 1980; **Fellow:** Vascular Surgery, Columbia Presby Med Ctr 1981; **Fac Appt:** Prof S, Loyola Univ-Stritch Sch Med

Hodgson, Kim John MD [VascS] - **Spec Exp:** Aneurysm; Carotid Artery Surgery; Endovascular Surgery; **Hospital:** St. John's Hosp - Springfield, Memorial Med Ctr-Springfield; **Address:** PO Box 19638, Springfield, IL 62794-9638; **Phone:** 217-545-5555; **Board Cert:** Vascular Surgery 2005; **Med School:** Univ Pennsylvania 1981; **Resid:** Surgery, Albany Med Ctr 1986; **Fellow:** Vascular Surgery, Southern Ill Univ 1987; **Fac Appt:** Prof VascS, Southern IL Univ

Kazmers, Andris MD [VascS] - **Spec Exp:** Aneurysm-Abdominal & Thoracic Aortic; Carotid Artery Stent Placement; Angioplasty & Stent Placement; Endovascular Surgery; **Hospital:** Northern Michigan Hosp; **Address:** Petoskey Surgeons, 521 Monroe St, Petoskey, MI 49770; **Phone:** 231-487-1900; **Board Cert:** Vascular Surgery 2005; Surgery 2000; Surgical Critical Care 2000; **Med School:** Wayne State Univ 1976; **Resid:** Surgery, Univ Michigan Hosps 1982; **Fellow:** Vascular Surgery, Univ Michigan Hosps 1984

Vascular Surgery

Kent, Kenneth C MD [VascS] - **Spec Exp:** Carotid Artery Surgery; Aneurysm-Abdominal Aortic; Lower Limb Arterial Disease; **Hospital:** Univ WI Hosp & Clins, Meriter Hosp; **Address:** UW Hosp, 600 Highland Ave, Ste H4/710, Madison, WI 53792-7375; **Phone:** 608-265-8854; **Board Cert:** Surgery 2007; Vascular Surgery 2008; **Med School:** UCSF 1981; **Resid:** Surgery, UCSF Med Ctr 1986; **Fellow:** Vascular Surgery, Brigham & Women's Hosp 1988; **Fac Appt:** Prof S, Univ Wisc

McLafferty, Robert B MD [VascS] - **Spec Exp:** Minimally Invasive Vascular Surgery; Endovascular Stent Grafts; Carotid Artery Stent Placement; Aneurysm; **Hospital:** Memorial Med Ctr-Springfield, St. John's Hosp - Springfield; **Address:** PO Box 19680, Springfield, IL 62794-9680; **Phone:** 217-545-5555; **Board Cert:** Surgery 2005; Vascular Surgery 2007; **Med School:** Univ VT Coll Med 1990; **Resid:** Surgery, Oregon Hlth Sci Ctr 1996; **Fellow:** Vascular Surgery, Oregon Hlth Sci Ctr 1998; **Fac Appt:** Prof VascS, Southern IL Univ

Pearce, William H MD [VascS] - **Spec Exp:** Aneurysm-Abdominal Aortic; Stroke; Peripheral Vascular Disease; **Hospital:** Northwestern Meml Hosp, Northwestern Lake Forest Hosp; **Address:** Galter Pavilion, 675 N St Clair St, Ste 19-100, Chicago, IL 60611-2647; **Phone:** 312-695-2714; **Board Cert:** Surgery 2010; Vascular Surgery 2003; **Med School:** Univ Colorado 1975; **Resid:** Surgery, Univ Co Hlth Sci Ctr 1981; **Fellow:** Vascular Surgery, Northwestern Meml Hosp 1982; **Fac Appt:** Prof S, Northwestern Univ

Sanchez, Luis A MD [VascS] - **Spec Exp:** Aneurysm-Abdominal & Thoracic Aortic; Endovascular Stent Grafts; Peripheral Vascular Disease; **Hospital:** Barnes-Jewish Hosp, Barnes-Jewish West County Hosp; **Address:** Washington Univ School Medicine, 660 S Euclid Ave, Box 8109-Surgery, St Louis, MO 63110; **Phone:** 314-362-7408; **Board Cert:** Surgery 2004; Vascular Surgery 2003; **Med School:** Harvard Med Sch 1987; **Resid:** Surgery, Montefiore Med Ctr 1992; **Fellow:** Vascular Surgery, Montefiore Med Ctr 1994; **Fac Appt:** Prof VascS, Washington Univ, St Louis

Shepard, Alexander D MD [VascS] - **Spec Exp:** Aneurysm-Aortic; Aortic Reconstruction; Vascular Surgery-Secondary; **Hospital:** Henry Ford Hosp; **Address:** 2799 W Grand Blvd, Detroit, MI 48202-2608; **Phone:** 313-916-3155; **Board Cert:** Surgery 2001; Vascular Surgery 2005; **Med School:** Johns Hopkins Univ 1976; **Resid:** Surgery, Johns Hopkins Hosp 1982; **Fellow:** Vascular Surgery, New England Med Ctr 1985; **Fac Appt:** Prof S, Wayne State Univ

Sicard, Gregorio A MD [VascS] - **Spec Exp:** Aneurysm-Abdominal Aortic; **Hospital:** Barnes-Jewish Hosp; **Address:** Wash Univ Vascular Surgery, 660 S Euclid Ave, Box 8109, St Louis, MO 63110; **Phone:** 314-362-7841; **Board Cert:** Vascular Surgery 2002; **Med School:** Univ Puerto Rico 1972; **Resid:** Surgery, Barnes Hosp 1977; **Fellow:** Transplant Surgery, Wash Univ Hosp 1978; **Fac Appt:** Prof S, Washington Univ, St Louis

Stanley, James C MD [VascS] - **Spec Exp:** Peripheral Vascular Disease; Renovascular Disease; Aneurysm; **Hospital:** Univ of Michigan Hosp; **Address:** Univ Mich, Dept Vascular Surgery, 1500 E Med Ctr Drive, CVC5167 SPC5167, Ann Arbor, MI 48109-5867; **Phone:** 734-936-5820; **Board Cert:** Surgery 1973; Vascular Surgery 2001; **Med School:** Univ Mich Med Sch 1964; **Resid:** Surgery, Univ Mich Med Ctr 1972; **Fac Appt:** Prof S, Univ Mich Med Sch

Great Plains and Mountains

Annest, Stephen J MD [VascS] - **Spec Exp:** Thoracic Outlet Syndrome; **Hospital:** Presby - St Luke's Med Ctr, Exempla Saint Jos. Hosp.-Denver; **Address:** Vascular Inst of The Rockies, 1601 E 19th Ave, Ste 3950, Denver, CO 80218; **Phone:** 303-539-0736; **Board Cert:** Surgery 2000; Vascular Surgery 2005; **Med School:** Univ Wash 1975; **Resid:** Surgery, Albany Med Ctr 1981; **Fellow:** Trauma, Albany Med Ctr 1980; Vascular Surgery, Baylor Univ Med Ctr 1982

Cooper, Michael A MD [VascS] - **Spec Exp:** Peripheral Vascular Disease; **Hospital:** Rose Med Ctr; **Address:** Colorado Cardiovascular Surgical Assocs, 4600 E Hale Pkwy, Ste 460, Denver, CO 80220; **Phone:** 303-388-7265; **Board Cert:** Surgery 2008; Vascular Surgery 2001; **Med School:** Univ Nebr Coll Med 1984; **Resid:** Surgery, Univ Kansas Med Ctr 1989; **Fellow:** Vascular Surgery, LSU Med Ctr 1992

Howard, Thomas C MD [VascS] - **Spec Exp:** Aortic Surgery; Aneurysm-Aortic; Carotid Artery Surgery; Lower Limb Arterial Disease; **Hospital:** Nebraska Med Ctr; **Address:** Surgery Ctr of the Heartland, 4242 Farnam St, Ste 490, Omaha, NE 68131; **Phone:** 402-552-3015; **Board Cert:** Surgery 1975; Vascular Surgery 2002; **Med School:** Yale Univ 1969; **Resid:** Surgery, Yale-New Haven Hosp 1974; **Fac Appt:** Assoc Prof S, Univ Nebr Coll Med

Southwest

Eidt, John F MD [VascS] - **Spec Exp:** Aneurysm-Abdominal Aortic; Carotid Artery Stent Placement; Endovascular Surgery; Peripheral Vascular Disease; **Hospital:** UAMS Med Ctr; **Address:** 4301 W Markham St, Slot 520-2, Little Rock, AR 72205; **Phone:** 501-686-6176; **Board Cert:** Surgery 2004; Vascular Surgery 2006; **Med School:** Univ Tex SW, Dallas 1981; **Resid:** Surgery, Brigham-Womens Hosp 1986; **Fellow:** Vascular Surgery, Univ Tex SW Med Ctr 1988; **Fac Appt:** Prof S, Univ Ark

Fowl, Richard J MD [VascS] - **Spec Exp:** Aneurysm-Aortic; Carotid Artery Surgery; Arterial Bypass Surgery-Leg; Endovascular Surgery; **Hospital:** Mayo Clinic - Phoenix; **Address:** Mayo Clinic, Dept Vascular Surgery, 5779 E Mayo Blvd, Phoenix, AZ 85054; **Phone:** 480-342-2868; **Board Cert:** Surgery 2002; Vascular Surgery 2004; **Med School:** Rush Med Coll 1978; **Resid:** Surgery, MCV Affil Hosp 1980; Surgery, Univ Iowa Med Ctr 1983; **Fellow:** Vascular Surgery, Mayo Clinic 1985; Endovascular Surgery, Cornell-Weill Med Coll 2004; **Fac Appt:** Prof S, Mayo Med Sch

Hollier, Larry H MD [VascS] - **Spec Exp:** Aortic Surgery; Carotid Artery Surgery; Endovascular Surgery; Aneurysm; **Hospital:** West Jefferson Med Ctr, LSU Interim Public Hosp; **Address:** 433 Bolivar St, Ste 815, New Orleans, LA 70112; **Phone:** 504-568-4800; **Board Cert:** Surgery 2007; Vascular Surgery 2001; **Med School:** Louisiana State U, New Orleans 1968; **Resid:** Surgery, Charity Hosp 1973; **Fellow:** Vascular Surgery, Baylor Med Ctr 1974; **Fac Appt:** Prof S, Louisiana State U, New Orleans

Kougias, Panagiotis MD [VascS] - **Spec Exp:** Vascular Reconstruction; Carotid Artery Surgery; Stroke; Endovascular Surgery; **Hospital:** St. Luke's Episcopal Hosp-Houston; **Address:** 2002 Holcombe Blvd, MEDVAMC (112), Houston, TX 77030; **Phone:** 713-794-7524; **Board Cert:** Surgery 2005; Vascular Surgery 2007; **Med School:** Greece 1992; **Resid:** Surgery, East Tennessee State Univ 2004; **Fellow:** Vascular Surgery, Baylor Coll Med 2006; **Fac Appt:** Asst Prof VascS, Baylor Coll Med

Lumsden, Alan B MD [VascS] - **Spec Exp:** Aortic Stent Grafts; Minimally Invasive Surgery; Vein Disorders; **Hospital:** Methodist Hosp - Houston; **Address:** 6550 Fannin St, Ste 1401, Smith Tower, Houston, TX 77030; **Phone:** 713-441-5200; **Board Cert:** Vascular Surgery 2002; **Med School:** Scotland, UK 1981; **Resid:** Surgery, Emory Univ Hosp 1987; **Fellow:** Vascular Surgery, Emory Univ Hosp 1989; **Fac Appt:** Prof VascS, Baylor Coll Med

Money, Samuel R MD [VascS] - **Spec Exp:** Aneurysm-Abdominal Aortic; Arterial Bypass Surgery-Leg; Endovascular Surgery; Aneurysm; **Hospital:** Mayo Clinic - Phoenix; **Address:** Mayo Clinic, Dept Vascular Surgery, 5779 E Mayo Blvd, Phoenix, AZ 85054; **Phone:** 480-342-2868; **Board Cert:** Surgery 2000; Vascular Surgery 2002; **Med School:** SUNY Downstate 1983; **Resid:** Surgery, Kings Co Med Ctr 1990; **Fellow:** Vascular Surgery, Ochsner Clinic 1993; **Fac Appt:** Prof S, Mayo Med Sch

Vascular Surgery

West Coast and Pacific

Ahn, Sam S MD [VascS] - **Spec Exp:** Minimally Invasive Vascular Surgery; Endovascular Surgery; Thoracic Outlet Syndrome; Hyperhidrosis; **Hospital:** UCLA Ronald Reagan Med Ctr, St. John's Hlth Ctr, Santa Monica; **Address:** 1082 Glendon Ave, Los Angeles, CA 90024; **Phone:** 310-209-2011; **Board Cert:** Surgery 2004; Vascular Surgery 2008; **Med School:** Univ Tex SW, Dallas 1978; **Resid:** Surgery, UCLA Med Ctr 1984; **Fellow:** Vascular Surgery, UCLA Med Ctr 1986; **Fac Appt:** Prof S, UCLA

Flanigan, D Preston MD [VascS] - **Spec Exp:** Carotid Artery Disease; Aneurysm; Vein Disorders; Minimally Invasive Surgery; **Hospital:** St. Joseph's Hosp - Orange; **Address:** 1140 W LaVeta Ave, Ste 850, Orange, CA 92868; **Phone:** 714-560-4450; **Board Cert:** Vascular Surgery 2002; **Med School:** Jefferson Med Coll 1972; **Resid:** Surgery, St Joseph-Mercy Hosp 1977; **Fellow:** Vascular Surgery, Northwest Med Ctr 1978; **Fac Appt:** Clin Prof S, UC Irvine

Gewertz, Bruce MD [VascS] - **Spec Exp:** Carotid Artery Surgery; Peripheral Vascular Disease; Aneurysm-Aortic; Renovascular Disease; **Hospital:** Cedars-Sinai Med Ctr; **Address:** 8700 Beverly Blvd, N Tower, Ste 8215, Los Angeles, CA 90048; **Phone:** 310-423-5884; **Board Cert:** Vascular Surgery 2002; **Med School:** Jefferson Med Coll 1972; **Resid:** Surgery, Univ Mich Hosp 1977; **Fac Appt:** Prof S, UCLA

Pevec, William C MD [VascS] - **Spec Exp:** Vascular Disease; Aortic Reconstruction; Endovascular Surgery; **Hospital:** UC Davis Med Ctr; **Address:** UC Davis Vascular Center, 4860 Y St, Ste 2100, Sacramento, CA 95817; **Phone:** 916-734-3524; **Board Cert:** Surgery 1999; Vascular Surgery 2001; **Med School:** Univ Cincinnati 1984; **Resid:** Surgery, Univ Pittsburgh Med Ctr 1990; **Fellow:** Vascular Surgery, Mass Genl Hosp 1992; **Fac Appt:** Prof VascS, UC Davis

Sobel, Michael MD [VascS] - **Spec Exp:** Vein Disorders; **Hospital:** Univ Wash Med Ctr, VA Puget Sound Hlth Care Sys; **Address:** East Side Specialty Center, 1700 116th Ave NE, Bellevue, WA 98004; **Phone:** 425-646-7777; **Board Cert:** Surgery 2002; Vascular Surgery 2008; **Med School:** Albert Einstein Coll Med 1975; **Resid:** Surgery, Beth Israel Hosp 1982; **Fellow:** Vascular Surgery, NYU Med Ctr 1983; **Fac Appt:** Prof VascS, Univ Wash

White, Rodney A MD [VascS] - **Spec Exp:** Endovascular Surgery; Aneurysm; Carotid Artery Surgery; Aortic Surgery-Complex; **Hospital:** LAC - Harbor - UCLA Med Ctr; **Address:** Harbor-UCLA Med Ctr, 1000 W Carson St, Box 11, Torrance, CA 90502; **Phone:** 310-222-2704; **Board Cert:** Surgery 1998; Vascular Surgery 2006; **Med School:** SUNY Upstate Med Univ 1974; **Resid:** Surgery, LAC-Harbor-UCLA Med Ctr 1979; **Fellow:** Vascular Surgery, LAC-Harbor-UCLA Med Ctr 1980; **Fac Appt:** Prof S, UCLA

Zarins, Christopher K MD [VascS] - **Spec Exp:** Carotid Artery Surgery; Aneurysm-Abdominal Aortic; Endovascular Surgery; **Hospital:** Stanford Univ Hosp & Clinics, El Camino Hosp; **Address:** Stanford Univ Vascular Surgery, 300 Pasteur Drive, rm H-3600, Stanford, CA 94305-5642; **Phone:** 650-725-5227; **Board Cert:** Surgery 1975; Vascular Surgery 2002; **Med School:** Johns Hopkins Univ 1968; **Resid:** Surgery, Univ Michigan Hosp 1974; **Fellow:** Surgery, Johns Hopkins Hosp 1972; **Fac Appt:** Prof Emeritus S, Stanford Univ

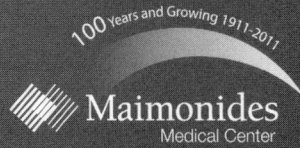

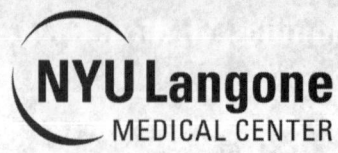

VASCULAR SURGERY

Staffed by one of the largest vascular surgery teams in the country, NYU Langone Medical Center emphasizes both expert patient care and minimally invasive therapies. Physicians have extensive experience performing the most advanced procedures, including stents and angioplasty for carotid artery disease, aortic aneurysms and blockages in arteries throughout the body. In addition to its expertise in arterial disease, NYU Langone is proud to offer one of the few academic Vein Centers in the United States. We specialize in the following areas:

Aortic Pathology

The Medical Center offers minimally invasive surgical solutions as well as treatments for complex aortic problems. Patients usually require no blood transfusions and are able to leave the hospital one or two days after surgery. We are also a training center for endovascular management of abdominal and thoracic aneurysms.

Carotid Artery Disease

NYU Langone remains a leader in both the screening for carotid disease and the prevention of stroke in patients being treated for carotid artery occlusive disease. Our physicians helped pioneer carotid endarterectomy as an open surgical procedure, and played a pivotal role in the development of the carotid stenting procedure.

Peripheral Arterial Disease

Vascular surgeons at the Medical Center draw on a wealth of experience in treating peripheral arterial disease (PAD). The team specializes in new and innovative technologies such as laser and "Silverhawk" atherectomy procedures, as well as cryoplasty. Additionally, we offer drug-eluting stents, which are coated with special medicines to prevent scar formation and re-occlusion of the stent.

Vascular Screenings

Our physicians are committed to improving public awareness and understanding of vascular disease through preventative screenings. The disease is among the leading causes of death in the U.S., yet is generally asymptomatic until a stroke or aneurysm occurs. Effective screening techniques at the Medical Center include ultrasound scans of the aorta, ultrasound scans of the carotid arteries, and blood pressure measurements.

Venous Disease

The Vein Center at NYU Langone is considered an authority in the minimally invasive treatment of venous disease. The Center treats patients with all forms of venous pathology, from venous insufficiency and varicose veins to occlusive disease and deep vein thrombosis.

Appendices

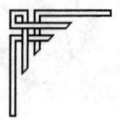

The Best in American Medicine
www.CastleConnolly.com

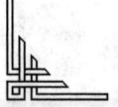
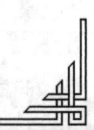

APPENDIX A:
Medical Boards

Introduction to ABMS and Osteopathic Specialties

The following pages contain descriptions of the "official" medical specialties, approved by the American Board of Medical Specialists (for M.D.s) or by the American Osteopathic Association (for D.O.s). These are important because they are the only specialties recognized by the official governing boards. There may be physicians who call themselves one kind of specialist or another, but they may not be certified by the "official" boards. There are, in fact, over 100 such "self-designated" boards, some simply groups of physicians interested in a given area of medicine with no qualifications for membership to other groups with very specific qualifications for membership.

It is important for the medical consumer to seek out physicians certified by the ABMS or AOA to assure their doctor has had the appropriate training and passed the board certification exam.

ABMS

The ABMS is an organization of ABMS Approved medical specialty boards. The mission of the ABMS is to maintain and improve the quality of medical care by assisting the Member Boards in their efforts to develop and utilize professional and educational standards for the evaluation and certification of physician specialists. The intent of certification of physicians is to provide assurance to the public that a physician specialist certified by a Member Board of the ABMS has successfully completed an approved educational program and evaluation process which includes an examination designed to assess the knowledge, skills, and experience required to provide quality patient care in that specialty. The ABMS serves to coordinate the activities of its Member Boards and to provide information to the public, the government, the profession and its Members concerning issues involving specialization and certification in medicine.

Following is a list of the addresses of the various medical specialty boards approved by the ABMS. Note that there are 24 board organizations for 25 medical specialties. Psychiatry and Neurology share the same board.

To find out if a physician is certified, consumers can call the individual boards which may charge a fee for the information, or they can contact the ABMS at (866) 275-2267 (no fee) or www.abms.org.

Appendix A: Medical Boards

American Board of Allergy and Immunology
111 S Independence Mall E, Ste 701
Philadelphia, PA 19106
(215) 592-9466, (866) 264-5568

General Certification in Allergy and Immunology. Certifications awarded since 1989 are valid for 10 years. For those certified prior to 1989 there is no recertification requirement.

American Board of Anesthesiology
4208 Six Forks Rd, Ste 900
Raleigh, NC 27609-5735
(919) 745-2200

General Certification in Anesthesiology; with Special and Added Qualifications in Critical Care Medicine, Hospice & Palliative Medicine, Pain Medicine, Pediatric Anesthesiology and Sleep Medicine. Certifications awarded since 2000 are valid for 10 years.

American Board of Colon and Rectal Surgery
20600 Eureka Road, Suite 600
Taylor, MI 48180
(734) 282-9400

General Certification is in Colon and Rectal Surgery. Certifications awarded since 1990 are valid for 10 years.

American Board of Dermatology
Henry Ford Health System
1 Ford Place
Detroit, MI 48202-3450
(313) 874-1088

General Certification in Dermatology; with Special Qualifications Dermatopathology, and Pediatric Dermatology. Certifications awarded since 1991 valid for 10 years.

American Board of Emergency Medicine
3000 Coolidge Road
East Lansing, MI 48823-6319
(517) 332-4800

General Certification in Emergency Medicine; with Special and Added Qualifications in Critical Care Medicine, Emergency Medical Services, Hospice & Palliative Medicine, Medical Toxicology, Pediatric Emergency Medicine, Sports Medicine and Undersea and Hyperbaric Medicine. Certifications awarded since 1980 are valid for 10 years

American Board of Family Medicine
   1648 McGranthiana Pkwy, FL 5
   Lexington, KY 40511
   (859) 269-5626, (888) 995-5700

   General Certification in Family Practice; with Added Qualifications in Adolescent
   Medicine, Geriatric Medicine, Hospice & Palliative Medicine, Sleep Medicine and Sports
   Medicine. Certifications awarded since 1970 are valid for 7 years.

American Board of Internal Medicine
   510 Walnut Street, Suite 1700
   Philadelphia, PA 19106-3699
   (215) 446-3500, (800) 441-ABIM

   General Certification in Internal Medicine; with Special Qualifications in Cardiovascular
   Disease, Endocrinology, Diabetes and Metabolism, Gastroenterology, Hematology,
   Infectious Disease, Medical Oncology, Nephrology, Pulmonary Disease, and
   Rheumatology; and Added Qualifications in Advanced Heart Failure & Transplant
   Cardiology, Adolescent Medicine, Clinical Cardiac Electrophysiology, Critical Care
   Medicine, Geriatric Medicine, Hospice and Palliative Medicine, Interventional
   Cardiology, Sleep Medicine, Sports Medicine and Transplant Hepatology. Certifications
   awarded since 1990 are valid for 10 years.

American Board of Medical Genetics
   9650 Rockville Pike
   Bethesda, MD 20814-3998
   (301) 634-7315

   General Certification in Clinical Genetics (MD), Clinical Biochemical Genetics, Clinical
   Cytogenetics and Clinical Molecular Genetics; with Added Qualifications in Medical
   Biochemical Genetics and Molecular Genetic Pathology. Certifications awarded since
   2002 are valid for 2 years.

American Board of Neurological Surgery
   6550 Fannin Street, Suite 2139
   Houston, TX 77030-2701
   (713) 441-6015

   General Certification in Neurological Surgery. Certifications awarded since 1999 are
   valid for 10 years.

American Board of Nuclear Medicine
4555 Forest Park Boulevard, Suite 119
St. Louis, MO 63108
(314) 367-2225

General Certification in Nuclear Medicine. Certifications awarded since 1992 are valid for 10 years.

American Board of Obstetrics and Gynecology
2915 Vine Street, Suite 300
Dallas, TX 75204
(214) 871-1619

General Certification in Obstetrics and Gynecology; with Special Qualifications in Gynecologic Oncology, Maternal and Fetal Medicine, Reproductive Endocrinology/Infertility; and Added Qualifications in Critical Care Medicine, Female Pelvic Medicine and Reconstructive Surgery, and Hospice & Palliative Medicine. Certifications awarded since 1986 are valid for 6 years.

American Board of Ophthalmology
111 Presidential Boulevard, Suite 241
Bala Cynwyd, PA 19004-1075
(610) 664-1175

Certifications Awarded since 1992 are valid for 10 years. For those certified prior to 1992, there is no recertification requirement.

American Board of Orthopaedic Surgery
400 Silver Cedar Court
Chapel Hill, NC 27514
(919) 929-7103

General Certification in Orthopaedic Surgery; with Added Qualification in Hand Surgery; with Added Qualifications in Hand Surgery and Orthopaedic Sports Medicine. Certifications awarded since 1986 are valid for 10 years.

American Board of Otolaryngology
5615 Kirby Drive, Suite 600
Houston, TX 77005
(713) 850-0399

General Certification in Otolaryngology; with Added Qualifications in Neurotology, Pediatric Otolaryngology, Plastic Surgery within the Head and Neck and Sleep Medicine. Certifications awarded since 2002 are valid for10 years.

American Board of Pathology
P.O. Box 25915
Tampa, FL 33622-5915
(813) 286-2444

General Certification in Anatomic and Clinical Pathology, Anatomic Pathology and
Clinical Pathology; with Special Qualifications in Blood Banking/Transfusion Medicine,
Chemical Pathology, Clinical Informatics, Dermatopathology, Forensic Pathology,
Hematology, Medical Microbiology, Molecular Genetic Pathology, Neuropathology and
Pediatric Pathology; and Added Qualifications in Cytopathology. Certifications awarded
since 1997 are valid for 10 years.

American Board of Pediatrics
111 Silver Cedar Court
Chapel Hill, NC 27514-1651
(919) 929-0461

General Certification in Pediatrics; with Special Qualifications in Adolescent Medicine,
Developmental-Behavioral Pediatrics, Neonatal-Perinatal Medicine, Pediatric Cardiology,
Pediatric Critical Care Medicine, Pediatric Emergency Medicine, Pediatric
Endocrinology, Pediatric Gastroenterology, Pediatric Hematology-Oncology, Pediatric
Infectious Diseases, Pediatric Nephrology, Pediatric Pulmonology, and Pediatric
Rheumatology; and Added Qualifications in Child Abuse Pediatrics, Medical Toxicology,
Neurodevelopmental Disabilities, Pediatric Transplant Hepatology, Sleep Medicine and
Sports Medicine. Certifications awarded since 1988 valid for 7 years.

American Board of Physical Medicine and Rehabilitation
3015 Allegro Park Lane, S.W.
Rochester, MN 55902-4139
(507) 282-1776

General Certification in Physical Medicine and Rehabilitation; with Special
Qualifications in Brain Injury Medicine, Hospice & Palliative Medicine, Neuromuscular
Medicine, Pain Medicine, Pediatric Rehabilitation Medicine, Spinal Cord Injury
Medicine and Sports Medicine. Certifications awarded since 1993 are valid for 10 years.

American Board of Plastic Surgery
Seven Penn Center, Suite 400
1635 Market Street
Philadelphia, PA 19103
(215) 587-9322

General Certification in Plastic Surgery; with Added Qualifications in Hand Surgery and
Plastic Surgery within the Head & Neck. Certifications awarded since 1995 are valid for
a 10-year period.

American Board of Preventive Medicine
  111 W Jackson, Ste 1110
  Chicago, IL 60604
  (312) 939-ABPM [2276]

General Certification in Aerospace Medicine, Occupational Medicine and Public Health and General Preventive Medicine; with Added Qualifications in Clinical Informatics, Undersea and Hyperbaric Medicine and Medical Toxicology. Certifications awarded since 1997 are valid for 10 years.

American Board of Psychiatry and Neurology
  2150 E Lake Cook Rd, Ste 900
  Buffalo Grove, IL 60089
  (849) 229-6500

General Certification in Psychiatry, Neurology and Neurology with Special Qualification in Child Neurology; with Special Qualifications in Child and Adolescent Psychiatry, Epilepsy, Hospice & Palliative Medicine, Pain Medicine and Sleep Medicine; and Added Qualifications in Addiction Psychiatry, Brain Injury Medicine, Clinical Neurophysiology, Forensic Psychiatry, Geriatric Psychiatry, Neurodevelopmental Disabilities, Neuromuscular Medicine, Psychosomatic Medicine and Vascular Neurology . Certifications awarded since 1994 are valid for 10 years.

American Board of Radiology
  5441 E. Williams Boulevard, Suite 200
  Tucson, AZ 85711
  (520) 790-2900

General Certification in Diagnostic Radiology, Medical Physics and Radiation Oncology; with Special Competency in Nuclear Radiology; and Added Qualifications in Hospice & Palliative Medicine, Neuroradiology, Nuclear Radiology, Pediatric Radiology and Vascular and Interventional Radiology. Radiological Physics is a non-clinical certification. Certificates are valid for 10 years.

American Board of Surgery
  1617 John F. Kennedy Boulevard, Suite 860
  Philadelphia, PA 19103-1847
  (215) 568-4000

General Certification in Surgery and Vascular Surgery; with Special Qualifications in Pediatric Surgery and Surgery of the Hand; and Added Qualifications in Complex Surgical Oncology, Hospice & Palliative Medicine and Surgical Critical Care. Certifications awarded since 1976 are valid for 10 years.

American Board of Thoracic Surgery
633 North St. Clair Street, Suite 2320
Chicago, IL 60611
(312 202-5900

General Certification in Thoracic Surgery; with Special Qualifications in Congenital
Cardiac Surgey. Certifications awarded since 1976 are valid for 10 years and Added
Qualifications in Congenital Cardiac Surgery.

American Board of Urology
600 Peter Jefferson Pkwy, Ste 150
Charlottesville, VA 22911
(434) 979-0266

General Certification in Urology; with Special Qualifications in Pediatric Urology and
Female Pelvic Medicine & Reconstructive Surgery. Certifications awarded as of 1985 are
valid for 10 years with Special Qualifications in Pediatric Urology.

Osteopathic

The American Osteopathic Association (AOA) is a member association
representing more than 78,000 osteopathic physicians (D.O.s). The AOA serves as
the primary certifying body for D.O.s, and is the accrediting agency for all
osetopathic medical colleges and health care facilities. The AOA's mission is to
advance the philosophy and practice of osteopathic medicine by promoting
excellence in education, research, and the delivery of quality, cost-effective
healthcare within a distinct, unified profession. American Osteopathic Association
142 E Ontario Street Chicago, IL 60611.

Consumers may call the American Osteopathic Association at (800) 621-1773 or
visit the website, www.osteopathic.org, for general certification information.

American Osteopathic Board of Anesthesiology

General certification in Anesthesiology; with Added Qualifications in Critical Care
Medicine, and Pain Management. Certifications awarded since 2004 are valid for 10
years. For those certified prior to 2004 there is no recertification requirement.

American Osteopathic Board of Dermatology

General certification in Dermatology; with Added Qualifications in Dermatopathology
and MOHS-Micrographic Surgery. Certifications awarded since 2004 are valid for 10
years.

Appendix A: Medical Boards

American Osteopathic Board of Emergency Medicine

General certification in Emergency Medicine; with Added Qualifications in Emergency Medical Services, Medical Toxicology, and Sports Medicine. Certifications awarded since 1994 are valid for 10 years.

American Osteopathic Board of Family Physicians

General certification in Family Practice and Osteopathic Manipulative Treatment (OMT); with Added Qualifications in Adolescent Medicine, Geriatric Medicine, Sports Medicine, Hospice & Palliative Medicine, Sleep Medicine and Undersea & Hyperbaric Medicine. Certifications awarded since March 1,1997 are valid for 8 years.

American Osteopathic Board of Internal Medicine

General certification in Internal Medicine; with Special Qualifications in Allergy/Immunology, Cardiology, Endocrinology, Gastroenterology, Hematology, Infectious Disease, Nephrology, Oncology, Pulmonary Disease, Rheumatology; with Added Qualifications in Addiction Medicine, Critical Care Medicine, Clinical Cardiac Electrophysiology, Geriatric Medicine, Hospice & Palliative Medicine, Interventional Cardiology, Sleep Medicine, Sports Medicine and Undersea & Hyperbaric Medicine. Certifications awarded since 1993 are valid for 10 years.

American Osteopathic Board of Neurology and Psychiatry

General certification in Neurology and Psychiatry; with Special Qualifications in Child/Adolescent Psychiatry and Child/Adolescent Neurology; with Added Qualifications in Addiction Medicine, Geriatric Psychiatry, Hospice & Palliative Medicine, Neurophysiology and Sleep Medicine. Certifications awarded since 1995 are valid for 10 years.

American Osteopathic Board of Neuromusculoskeletal Medicine

(Formerly American Osteopathic Board of Special Proficiency in Osteopathic Manipulative Medicine)

General certification in Neuromusculoskeletal Medicine & Osteopathic Manipulative Medicine with Added Qualifications in Sports Medicine. Certifications awarded since 1995 are valid for 10 years. For those certified prior to 1995 there is no recertification requirement.

American Osteopathic Board of Nuclear Medicine

General certification in Nuclear Medicine. Certifications awarded since 1995 are valid for 10 years

American Osteopathic Board of Obstetrics and Gynecology

General certification in Obstetrics and Gynecology; with Special Qualifications in Gynecologic Oncology; Maternal and Fetal Medicine and Reproductive Endocrinology. Certifications awarded since June, 2002 are valid for 6 years.

American Osteopathic Board of Ophthalmology and Otolaryngology

General certification in Ophthalmology, Otolaryngolgy and Otolaryngology/Facial Plastic Surgery; with Added Qualifications in Otolaryngic Allergy and Sleep Medicine. Certifications awarded in Ophthalmology since 2000 are valid for 10 years. For those certified prior to 2000 there is no recertification requirement. Certifications awarded in Otolaryngology and/or Otolaryngology/Facial Plastic Surgery since 2002 are valid for 10 years.

American Osteopathic Board of Orthopaedic Surgery

General certification in Orthopaedic Surgery; with Added Qualifications in Hand Surgery. Certifications awarded since 1994 are valid for 10 years.

American Osteopathic Board of Pathology

General certification in Laboratory Medicine, Anatomic Pathology and Anatomic Pathology and Laboratory Medicine; with Special Qualifications in Forensic Pathology; and with Added Qualifications in Dermatopathology. Certifications awarded since 1995 are valid for 10 years.

American Osteopathic Board of Pediatrics

General certification in Pediatrics with Special Qualifications in Adolescent and Young Adult Medicine, Neonatology, Pediatric Allergy/Immunology and Pediatric Endocrinology; with Added Qualifications in Sports Medicine. Certifications awarded since 1995 are valid for 7 years.

American Osteopathic Board of Physical Medicine and Rehabilitation Medicine

General certification in Physical Medicine and Rehabilitation; with Added Qualifications in Hospice & Palliative Medicine and Sports Medicine. Certifications awarded since 2004 are valid for 10 years.

American Osteopathic Board of Preventive Medicine

General certification in Preventive Medicine/Aerospace Medicine, Preventive Medicine/Occupational-Environmental Medicine and Preventive Medicine/Public Health; with Added Qualifications in Occupational Medicine and Undersea & Hyperbaric Medicine. Certifications awarded since 1994 are valid for 10 years.

American Osteopathic Board of Proctology

General certification in Proctology. Certifications awarded since 2004 are valid for 10 years.

Appendix A: Medical Boards

American Osteopathic Board of Radiology

General certification in Diagnostic Radiology and Radiation Oncology; with Added Qualifications in Angiography and Interventional Radiology, Diagnostic Ultrasound and Pediatric Radiology. Certifications awarded since 2002 are valid for 10 years.

American Osteopathic Board of Surgery

General certification in Surgery, Neurological Surgery, Plastic and Reconstructive Surgery, Thoracic Cardiovascular Surgery, Urological Surgery and General Vascular Surgery; with Added Qualifications in Surgical Critical Care. Certifications awarded since 1997 are valid for 10 years.

Appendix B:
Self-Designated Medical Specialties

This list of self-designated medical specialty groups was obtained from the American Board of Medical Specialties. However, it is important to point out that these groups are not recognized by the ABMS, the governing board for the recognized twenty-four medical specialty boards (listed in Appendix A).

The organizations listed below range from highly organized groups that are attempting to formalize training and certification in their field to informal groups interested in a particular aspect of medicine.

If you wish to obtain information from any of these groups you will have to do some detective work. Because so many are informal, the location, phone and mailing addresses change frequently, depending upon the person who is functioning as secretary or administrator.

The best way to track down one of these groups is to consult the doctor listings to find a doctor who has expressed a special interest in that field, and call his or her office. You might also call a nearby academic health center in the area to see if they have a faculty or staff member known to be involved in that particular medical interest. If that fails, take the same approach with your community hospital.

A

Abdominal Surgeons

Acupuncture Medicine

Addiction Medicine

Addictionology

Adolescent Psychiatry

Aesthetic Plastic Surgery

Alcoholism and Other Drug
    Dependencies (AMSAODD)

Algology (Chronic Pain)

Alternative Medicine

Ambulatory Anesthesia

Ambulatory Foot Surgery

Anesthesia

Arthroscopic Surgery

Arthroscopy (Board of North America)

B

Bariatric Medicine

Bionic Psychology

Bloodless Medicine & Surgery

C

Chelation Therapy

Chemical Dependence

Clinical Chemistry

Clinical Ecology

Clinical Medicine and Surgery

Clinical Neurology

Clinical Neurophysiology

Clinical Neurosurgery

Clinical Nutrition

Clinical Orthopaedic Surgery

Clinical Pharmacology

Clinical Polysomnography

Clinical Psychiatry

Clinical Psychology

Clinical Toxicology

Cosmetic Plastic Surgery

Cosmetic Surgery

Council of Non-Board Certified Physicians

Critical Care in Medicine & Surgery

D

Disability Analysis

Disability Evaluating Physicians

E

Electrodiagnostic Medicine

Electroencephalography

Electromyography & Electrodiagnosis

Environmental Medicine

Epidemiology (College)

Eye Surgery

F

Facial Cosmetic Surgery

Facial Plastic & Reconstructive Surgery

Family Practice, Certification

Forensic Examiners

Forensic Psychiatry

Forensic Toxicology

H

Hand Surgery

Head, Facial & Neck Pain & TMJ Orthopaedics

Health Physics

Homeopathic Physicians

Homeotherapeutics

Hypnotic Anesthesiology, National Board for

I

Independent Medical Examiners

Industrial Medicine & Surgery

Insurance Medicine

International Cosmetic & Plastic
    Facial Reconstructive Standards

Interventional Radiology

L

Laser Surgery
Law in Medicine
Longevity Medicine/Surgery

M

Malpractice Physicians
Maxillofacial Surgeons
Medical Accreditation (American Federation for)
Medical Hypnosis
Medical Laboratory Immunology
Medical-Legal Analysis of Medicine & Surgery
Medical Legal & Workers
    Comp. Medicine & Surgery
Medical-Legal Consultants
Medical Management
Medical Microbiology
Medical Preventics (Academy)
Medical Psychotherapists
Medical Toxicology
Microbiology (Medical Microbiology)
Military Medicine
Mohs Micrographic Surgery &
    Cutaneous Oncology

N

Neuroimaging
Neurologic & Orthopaedic Dental
    Medicine and Surgery
Neurological & Orthopaedic Medicine
Neurological & Orthopaedic Surgery
Neurological Microsurgery
Neurology
Neuromuscular Thermography
Neuro-Orthopaedic Dental Medicine
Neuro-Orthopaedic Electrodiagnosis
Neuro-Orthopaedic Laser Surgery
Neuro-Orthopaedic Psychiatry
Neuro-Orthopaedic Thoracic Medicine
Neurorehabilitation
Nutrition

O

Orthopaedic Medicine
Orthopaedic Microneurosurgery
Otorhinolaryngology

P

Pain Management (American Academy of)
Pain Management Specialties
Pain Medicine
Palliative Medicine
Percutaneous Diskectomy
Plastic Esthetic Surgeons
Prison Medicine
Professional Disability Consultants Psychiatric
    Medicine
Psychiatry (American National Board of)
Psychoanalysis (American Examining
    Board in)
Psychological Medicine (International)

Q

Quality Assurance & Utilization Review

R

Radiology & Medical Imaging
Rheumatologic Surgery
Rheumatological & Reconstructive Medicine
Ringside Medicine & Surgery

S

Skin Specialists
Sleep Medicine (Polysomnography)
Spinal Cord Injury
Spinal Surgery
Sports Medicine
Sports Medicine/Surgery

T

Toxicology
Trauma Surgery
Traumatologic Medicine & Surgery
Tropical Medicine

U

Ultrasound Technology
Urologic Allied Health Professionals
Urological Surgery

W

Weight Reduction Medicine

APPENDIX C:
Hospital Listings

The following is an alphabetical listing of all hospitals that have at least one Castle Connolly Top Doctor in this guide. Institutions listed in **Bold** are profiled in this Guide in association with Castle Connolly's *Partnership for Excellence* program. The abbreviations as they appear in the listings are in italics below. Due to the many changes taking place in the hospital industry, the names on this list may have changed subsequent to publication of this guide.

Abbott - Northwestern Hospital		(612) 863-4000
Abbott - Northwestern Hosp		
800 E 28th St	Minneapolis, MN 55407	MIDWEST
Abington Memorial Hospital		(215) 576-2000
Abington Mem Hosp		
1200 Old York Rd	Abington, PA 19001	MID ATLANTIC
Adventist Hinsdale Hospital		(630) 856-9000
Adventist Hinsdale Hosp		
120 N Oak St	Hinsdale, IL 60521	MIDWEST
Advocate Christ Medical Center		(708) 684-8000
Adv Christ Med Ctr		
4440 W 95th St	Oak Lawn, IL 60453	MIDWEST
Advocate Good Samaritan Hospital		(630) 275-5900
Adv Good Samaritan Hosp		
3815 Highland Ave	Downers Grove, IL 60515	MIDWEST
Advocate Illinois Masonic Medical Center		(773) 975-1600
Adv Illinois Masonic Med Ctr		
836 W Wellington Ave	Chicago, IL 60657-5147	MIDWEST
Advocate Lutheran General Hospital		(847) 723-2210
Adv Luth Genl Hosp		
1775 West Dempster St	Park Ridge, IL 60068	MIDWEST
Akron Children's Hospital		(330) 543-1000
Akron Children's Hosp		
One Perkins Square	Akron, OH 44308	MIDWEST
Alameda County Medical Center-Highland Campus		(714) 437-4800
Alameda County Med Ctr-Highland Campus		
1411 East 31st	Oakland, CA 94602	WEST COAST AND PACIFIC

Albany Medical Center   (518) 262-3125
Albany Med Ctr
43 New Scotland Ave   Albany, NY 12208   MID ATLANTIC

Albert Einstein Medical Center   (215) 456-7890
Albert Einstein Med Ctr
5501 Old York Rd   Philadelphia, PA 19141   MID ATLANTIC

Albert Lea Medical Center-Mayo Health System   (507) 373-2384
Albert Lea Med Ctr-Mayo Hlth Sys
404 W Fountain St   Albert Lea, MN 56007   MIDWEST

Alegent Health - Immanuel Medical Center   (402) 572-2121
Alegent Hlth - Immanuel Med Ctr
6901 N 72nd St   Omaha, NE 68122   GREAT PLAINS AND MOUNTAINS

Alexian Brothers Medical Center   (847) 437-5500
Alexian Brothers Med Ctr
800 Biesterfield Rd   Elk Grove Village, IL 60007   MIDWEST

Alfred I duPont Hospital for Children   (302) 651-4000
Alfred I duPont Hosp for Children
1600 Rockland Rd, Box 269   Wilmington, DE 19889   MID ATLANTIC

All Children's Hospital   (727) 898-7451
All Children's Hosp
801 Sixth Street South   St. Petersburg, FL 33701   SOUTHEAST

Allegheny General Hospital   (412) 359-3131
Allegheny General Hosp
320 E. North Avenue   Pittsburgh, PA 15212   MID ATLANTIC

Alta Bates Summit Medical Center-Alta Bates Campus   (510) 204-4444
Alta Bates Summit Med Ctr-Alta Bates Campus
2450 Ashby Avenue   Berkeley, CA 94705   WEST COAST AND PACIFIC

Alvarado Hospital & Medical Center   (714) 287-3270
Alvarado Hosp & Med Ctr
6655 Alvarado Rd   San Diego, CA 92120   WEST COAST AND PACIFIC

Anne Arundel Medical Center   (443) 481-1000
Anne Arundel Med Ctr
64 Franklin Street   Annapolis, MD 21401   MID ATLANTIC

Arizona Heart Hospital   (602) 532-1000
Arizona Heart Hosp
1930 Thomas Rd   Phoenix, AZ 85016   SOUTHWEST

Arkansas Children's Hospital   (501) 364-1100
Arkansas Chldns Hosp
800 Marshall St   Little Rock, AR 72202   SOUTHWEST

Arlington Memorial Hospital   (817) 548-6100
Arlington Meml Hosp
800 W Randol Mill Rd   Arlington, TX 76012-2503   SOUTHWEST

Arthur G. James Cancer Hospital & Research Institute   (614) 293-3300
Arthur G James Cancer Hosp & Research Inst
300 West 10th Avenue   Columbus, OH 43210   MIDWEST

Atlanta Medical Center   (404) 265-4000
Atlanta Med Ctr
303 Parkway Dr. NE   Atlanta, GA 30312   SOUTHEAST

Atlanta VA Medical Center   (404) 321-6111
Atlanta VA Med Ctr
1670 Clairmont Rd   Decatur, GA 30033   SOUTHEAST

Audie L Murphy Memorial Veterans Hospital - San Antonio   (210) 617-5300
Audie L Murphy Meml Vets Hosp - San Antonio
7400 Merton Minter Blvd   San Antonio, TX 78229   SOUTHWEST

Aultman Hospital   (330) 452-9911
Aultman Hosp
2600 6th St SW   Canton, OH 44710-1799   MIDWEST

Austen Riggs Center   (413) 298-5511
Austen Riggs Ctr
25 Main Street or PO Box 962   Stockbridge, MA 01262-0962   NEW ENGLAND

Aventura Hosp & Medical Center   (305) 682-7000
Aventura Hosp & Med Ctr
20900 Biscayne Blvd   Aventura, FL 33180   SOUTHEAST

Banner Desert Medical Center   (480) 512-3000
Banner Desert Med Ctr
1400 S Dobson Rd   Mesa, AZ 85202   SOUTHWEST

Banner Good Samaritan Regional Medical Center - Phoenix   (602) 839-2000
Banner Good Samaritan Regl Med Ctr - Phoenix
1111 E McDowell Rd   Phoenix, AZ 85006   SOUTHWEST

Baptist Hospital - Nashville   (615) 284-5555
Baptist Hosp - Nashville
2000 Church St   Nashville, TN 37236   SOUTHEAST

Baptist Hospital - Pensacola   (850) 434-4011
Baptist Hosp - Pensacola
1000 W Moreno St   Pensacola, FL 32501   SOUTHEAST

Baptist Hospital of Miami   (786) 596-1960
Baptist Hosp of Miami
8900 N Kendall Dr   Miami, FL 33176   SOUTHEAST

Baptist Medical Center - San Antonio   (210) 297-7000
Baptist Med Ctr - San Antonio
111 Dallas St   San Antonio, TX 78205   SOUTHWEST

Baptist Medical Center-Jackson   (601) 968-1000
Baptist Med Ctr-Jackson
1225 N State St   Jackson, MS 39202   SOUTHEAST

Baptist Memorial Hospital-Memphis   (901) 226-5000
Baptist Memorial Hospital-Memphis
6019 Walnut Grove Rd   Memphis, TN 38120   SOUTHEAST

Barbara Ann Karmanos Cancer Institute   (800) 527-6266
Barbara Ann Karmanos Cancer Inst
4100 John R   Detroit, MI 48201   MIDWEST

Barnes-Jewish Hospital   (314) 747-3000
Barnes-Jewish Hosp
One Barnes-Jewish Hospital Plaza   St. Louis, MO 63110   MIDWEST

Barnes-Jewish West County Hospital   (314) 996-8000
Barnes-Jewish West County Hosp
12634 Olive Blvd   St. Louis, MO 63141   MIDWEST

Bascom Palmer Eye Institute   (305) 326-6000
Bascom Palmer Eye Inst
900 NW 17 St   Miami, FL 33136   SOUTHEAST

Baylor Clinic & Hospital-Houston   (713) 798-1000
Baylor Clinic & Hosp-Houston
6620 Main St   Houston, TX 77030   SOUTHWEST

Baylor Institute for Rehabilitation   (214) 826-7030
Baylor Inst for Rehabilitation
3505 Gaston Avenue   Dallas, TX 75246   SOUTHWEST

Baylor University Medical Center-Dallas   (214) 820-0111
Baylor Univ Medical Ctr-Dallas
3500 Gaston Avenue   Dallas, TX 75246   SOUTHWEST

Baystate Medical Center | (413) 794-0000
Baystate Med Ctr
759 Chestnut Street | Springfield, MA 01199 | NEW ENGLAND

Beaumont Hospital-Royal Oak | (248) 898-5000
Beaumont Hosp-Royal Oak
3601 W 13 Mile Rd | Royal Oak, MI 48073 | MIDWEST

Ben Taub General Hospital | (713) 873-2000
Ben Taub Genl Hosp
1504 Taub Loop | Houston, TX 77001 | SOUTHWEST

Beth Israel Deaconess Medical Center - Boston | (617) 667-7000
Beth Israel Deaconess Med Ctr - Boston
330 Brookline Ave | Boston, MA 02215 | NEW ENGLAND

Beth Israel Medical Center - Milton & Caroll Petrie Division | (212) 420-2000
Beth Israel Med Ctr - Petrie Division
First Avenue @ 16th Street | New York, NY 10003 | MID ATLANTIC

Bethesda North Hospital | (513) 745-1111
Bethesda North Hosp
10500 Montgomery Rd | Cincinnati, OH 45242-4415 | MIDWEST

Boca Raton Regional Hospital | (561) 955-7100
Boca Raton Regl Hosp
800 Meadows Road | Boca Raton, FL 33486 | SOUTHEAST

Bon Secours Mary Immaculate Hospital | (757) 886-6000
Bon Secours Mary Immaculate Hosp
2 Bernardine Dr | Newport News, VA 23602 | SOUTHEAST

Boston Medical Center | (617) 638-8000
Boston Med Ctr
1 Boston Medical Center Pl | Boston, MA 02118 | NEW ENGLAND

Boulder Community Hospital | (303) 440-2273
Boulder Community Hospital
1100 Balsam Ave, Box 9019 | Boulder, CO 80301 | GREAT PLAINS AND MOUNTAINS

Boys Town National Research Hospital | (402) 498-6511
Boys Town Natl Rsch Hosp
555 N 30th St | Omaha, NE 68101 | GREAT PLAINS AND MOUNTAINS

Brenner Children's Hospital | (336) 716-2011
Brenner Chldrn's Hosp
Medical Center Blvd | Winston-Salem, NC 27157-1015 | SOUTHEAST

Brigham and Women's Hospital (617) 732-5500
Brigham and Women's Hosp
75 Francis St   Boston, MA 02115   NEW ENGLAND

Brooklyn Hospital Center-Downtown (718) 250-8000
Brooklyn Hosp Ctr-Downtown
121 DeKalb Avenue   Brooklyn, NY 11201   MID ATLANTIC

Brookwood Medical Center   (205) 877-1000
Brookwood Med Ctr
2010 Brookwood Medical Ctr Drive   Birmingham, AL 35209-6804   SOUTHEAST

Broward General Medical Center   (954) 355-4400
Broward General Med Ctr
1600 S Andrews Ave   Fort Lauderdale, FL 33316   SOUTHEAST

Bryn Mawr Hospital   (610) 526-3000
Bryn Mawr Hosp
130 S Bryn Mawr Ave   Bryn Mawr, PA 19010-3143   MID ATLANTIC

Bucks Specialty Institute   (215) 633-3456
Bucks Specialty Inst
3300 Tillman Drive   Bensalem, PA 19020   MID ATLANTIC

Buffalo General Hospital   (716) 859-5600
Buffalo General Hosp
100 High Street   Buffalo, NY 14203   MID ATLANTIC

Burke Rehabilitation Hospital   (914) 597-2500
Burke Rehab Hosp
785 Mamaroneck Avenue   White Plains, NY 10605   MID ATLANTIC

Butler Hospital   (401) 455-6200
Butler Hosp
345 Blackstone Blvd   Providence, RI 02906   NEW ENGLAND

California Pacific Medical Center - California Campus   (415) 600-6000
CA Pacific Med Ctr - CA Campus
3700 California St   San Francisco, CA 94114   WEST COAST AND PACIFIC

California Pacific Medical Center - Davies Campus   (415) 565-6000
CA Pacific Med Ctr - Davies Campus
Castro & Duboce St   San Francisco, CA 94114   WEST COAST AND PACIFIC

California Pacific Medical Center-Pacific Campus   (415) 600-6000
CA Pacific Med Ctr-Pacific Campus
2333 Buchanan St, Box 7999   San Francisco, CA 94115   WEST COAST AND PACIFIC

Cape Cod Hospital		(508) 771-1800
Cape Cod Hosp		
27 Park St	Hyannis, MA 02601-5203	NEW ENGLAND

Carilion Roanoke Memorial Hospital		(540) 981-7000
Carilion Roanoke Meml Hosp		
1906 Belleview Ave, PO Box 13367	Roanoke, VA 24014	SOUTHEAST

Caritas St. Elizabeth's Medical Center-Boston		(617) 789-3000
Caritas St Elizabeth's Med Ctr-Boston		
736 Cambridge St	Boston, MA 02135	NEW ENGLAND

Carolinas Medical Center		(704) 355-2000
Carolinas Med Ctr		
1000 Blythe Blvd, PO Box 32861	Charlotte, NC 28203-5871	SOUTHEAST

Carolinas Medical Center-University		(704) 548-6000
Carolinas Med Ctr-Univ		
PO Box 560727	Charlotte, NC 28256	SOUTHEAST

Carolinas Specialty Hospital		(704) 379-6450
Carolinas Specialty Hosp		
2001 Vail Ave 7th Fl	Charlotte, NC 28207	SOUTHEAST

Cedars-Sinai Medical Center		(310) 423-3277
Cedars-Sinai Med Ctr		
8700 Beverly Boulevard	Los Angeles, CA 90048	WEST COAST AND PACIFIC

Centennial Medical Center		(615) 342-1000
Centennial Med Ctr		
2300 Patterson Street	Nashville, TN 37203	SOUTHEAST

Central Baptist Hospital		(859) 260-6592
Central Baptist Hosp		
1740 Nicholasville Rd	Lexington, KY 40503-1499	SOUTHEAST

Central DuPage Hospital		(630) 933-1600
Central DuPage Hosp		
25 N Winfield Rd	Winfield, IL 60190	MIDWEST

Chandler Regional Medical Center		(602) 963-4561
Chandler Regional Med Ctr		
475 S Dobson Rd	Chandler, AZ 85224-5695	SOUTHWEST

Charlie Norwood VA Medical Center - Augusta		(706) 733-0188
Charlie Norwood VA Med Ctr - Augusta		
One Freedom Way	Augusta, GA 30904	SOUTHEAST

Chelsea Community Hospital   (734) 475-1311
Chelsea Comm Hosp
775 S Main St   Chelsea, MI 48118   MIDWEST

Chestnut Hill Hospital   (212) 248-8200
Chestnut Hill Hosp
8835 Germantown Ave   Philadelphia, PA 19118   MID ATLANTIC

Cheyenne Regional Medical Center   (307) 634-2273
Cheyenne Regl Med Ctr
214 E 23rd St   Cheyenne, WY 82001   GREAT PLAINS AND MOUNTAINS

Children's Healthcare of Atlanta at Egleston   (404) 785-6000
Chldns Hlthcare Atlanta @ Egleston
1405 Clifton Rd NE   Atlanta, GA 30322   SOUTHEAST

Children's Healthcare of Atlanta at Scottish Rite   (404) 785-5252
Chldns Hlthcare Atlanta @ Scottish Rite
1001 Johnson Ferry Rd   Atlanta, GA 30342   SOUTHEAST

Children's Hospital - Aurora (Colorado)   (720) 777-1234
Chldn's Hosp - Aurora (CO)
13123 E 16th Ave   Aurora, CO 80045   GREAT PLAINS AND MOUNTAINS

Children's Hospital - Boston   (617) 355-6000
Children's Hospital - Boston
300 Longwood Avenue   Boston, MA 02115   NEW ENGLAND

Children's Hospital - DowntownDenver   (720) 777-1360
Children's Hosp - Denver
1830 Franklin St   Denver, CO 80218   GREAT PLAINS AND MOUNTAINS

Children's Hospital - Los Angeles   (323) 660-2450
Chldns Hosp - Los Angeles
4650 Sunset Blvd   Los Angeles, CA 90027   WEST COAST AND PACIFIC

Children's Hospital - New Orleans   (504) 899-9511
Children's Hospital - New Orleans
200 Henry Clay Ave   New Orleans, LA 70118   SOUTHWEST

Children's Hospital - Oakland   (510) 428-3000
Chldns Hosp - Oakland
747 52nd St   Oakland, CA 94609   WEST COAST AND PACIFIC

Children's Hospital - Omaha   (402) 955-5400
Children's Hosp - Omaha
8200 Dodge St   Omaha, NE 68114   GREAT PLAINS AND MOUNTAINS

Children's Hospital and Clinics - Minneapolis
Chldns Hosp and Clinics - Minneapolis
2525 Chicago Ave S   Minneapolis, MN 55404
(612) 813-6111
MIDWEST

Children's Hospital at OU Medical Center
Chldns Hosp OU Med Ctr
1200 N Everett Drive   Oklahoma City, OK 73104
(405) 271-5437
SOUTHWEST

Children's Hospital Central California
Chldns Hosp Central CA
9300 Valley Children's Pl   Madera, CA 93638
(559) 353-3000
WEST COAST AND PACIFIC

Children's Hospital of Alabama - Birmingham
Children's Hospital - Birmingham
1600 7th Ave South   Birmingham, AL 35233
(205) 939-9100
SOUTHEAST

Children's Hospital of Michigan
Chldns Hosp of Michigan
3901 Beaubian Blvd   Detroit, MI 48201
(313) 745-5437
MIDWEST

Children's Hospital of Orange County
Chldns Hosp Orange Co
455 South Main Street   Orange, CA 92868
(714) 997-3000
WEST COAST AND PACIFIC

Children's Hospital of Philadelphia
Chldns Hosp of Philadelphia
34th St & Civic Center Blvd   Philadelphia, PA 19104
(215) 590-1000
MID ATLANTIC

Children's Hospital of Pittsburgh - UPMC
Chldns Hosp of Pittsburgh - UPMC
4401 Penn Ave   Pittsburgh, PA 15224
(412) 692-5325
MID ATLANTIC

Children's Hospital of the King's Daughters
Chldns Hosp of King's Daughters
601 Children's Ln   Norfolk, VA 23507
(757) 668-7500
SOUTHEAST

Children's Hospital of Wisconsin
Chldns Hosp - Wisconsin
9000 W Wisconsin Ave   Milwaukee, WI 53226
(414) 266-2000
MIDWEST

Children's Medical Center of Dallas
Chldns Med Ctr of Dallas
1935 Motor St   Dallas, TX 75235
(214) 456-7000
SOUTHWEST

Children's Memorial Hospital- Chicago
Children's Mem Hosp -Chicago
2300 Children's Plaza   Chicago, IL 60614
(773) 880-4000
MIDWEST

Children's Mercy Hospitals & Clinics		(816) 234-3000
Chldns Mercy Hosps & Clinics		
2401 Gilham Rd	Kansas City, MO 64108	MIDWEST

Children's National Medical Center - DC		(202) 476-3000
Chldns Natl Med Ctr		
111 Michigan Ave NW	Washington, DC 20010	MID ATLANTIC

Christ Hospital, The - Cincinnati		(513) 585-2000
Christ Hosp, The - Cincinnati		
2139 Auburn Ave	Cincinnati, OH 45219	MIDWEST

Christiana Hospital		(302) 733-1000
Christiana Hospital		
4755 Ogletown-Stanton Rd, PO Box 6001	Newark, DE 19718-0001	MID ATLANTIC

Christus Santa Rosa Children's Hospital		(512) 228-2011
Christus Santa Rosa Children's Hosp		
333 N Santa Rosa St	San Antonio, TX 78207	SOUTHWEST

Christus Santa Rosa Medical Center Hospital		(210) 705-6300
Christus Santa Rosa Med Ctr Hosp		
2827 Babcock Rd	San Antonio, TX 78229-6098	SOUTHWEST

Christus St Vincent Regional Medical Center-Santa Fe		(505) 983-3361
Christus St Vincent Reg Med Ctr-Santa Fe		
455 St Michaels Dr	Santa Fe, NM 87504-2107	SOUTHWEST

CHRISTUS St. Frances Cabrini Hospital		(318) 487-1122
CHRISTUS St. Frances Cabrini Hosp		
3330 Masonic Dr	Alexandria, LA 71301	SOUTHWEST

Cincinnati Children's Hospital Medical Center		(513) 636-4200
Cincinnati Chldns Hosp Med Ctr		
3333 Burnet Ave	Cincinnati, OH 45229-3039	MIDWEST

Cincinnati Shriners Hospital		(513) 872-6000
Cincinnati Shriners Hosp		
3229 Burnet Ave	Cincinnati, OH 45229-3095	MIDWEST

City of Hope National Medical Center		(626) 256-4673
City of Hope Natl Med Ctr		
1500 E Duarte Rd	Duarte, CA 91010	WEST COAST AND PACIFIC

Clara Maass Medical Center		(973) 450-2000
Clara Maass Med Ctr		
One Clara Maass Drive	Belleville, NJ 07109	MID ATLANTIC

Cleveland Clinic		(216) 444-2200
Cleveland Clin		
9500 Euclid Avenue	Cleveland, OH 44195	MIDWEST
Cleveland Clinic Florida - Weston		(954) 659-5000
Cleveland Clin - Weston		
2950 Cleveland Clinic Blvd	Weston, FL 33331	SOUTHEAST
Columbia Hospital - West Palm Beach		(561) 842-6141
Columbia Hosp - W Palm Beach		
2201 45th St	West Palm Beach, FL 33407	SOUTHEAST
Columbia Medical Center - Plano		(972) 596-6800
Columbia Med Ctr - Plano		
3901 West 15th Street	Plano, TX 75075	SOUTHWEST
Columbus Regional Medical Center		(706) 571-1000
Columbus Regl Med Ctr		
710 Center St	Columbus, GA 31902	SOUTHEAST
Community Hospital East - Indianapolis		(317) 355-5411
Commun Hosp E - Indianapolis		
1500 N Ritter Ave	Indianapolis, IN 46219	MIDWEST
Community Hospital of Monterey Peninsula		(831) 624-5311
Comm Hosp of Monterey Pen		
23625 Holman Hwy	Monterey, CA 93940	WEST COAST AND PACIFIC
Community Memorial Hospital - Ventura		(805) 652-5011
Comm Meml Hosp - Ventura		
147 N Brent St	Ventura, CA 93003	WEST COAST AND PACIFIC
Concord Hospital		(603) 225-2711
Concord Hospital		
250 Pleasant St	Concord, NH 03301-2598	NEW ENGLAND
Connecticut Children's Medical Center		(860) 545-9000
CT Chldns Med Ctr		
282 Washington St	Hartford, CT 06106	NEW ENGLAND
Connecticut Mental Health Center		(203) 789-7092
Connecticut Mental Hlth Ctr		
34 Park St	New Haven, CT 06508-1842	NEW ENGLAND
Cook Children's Medical Center		(682) 885-4000
Cook Chldns Med Ctr		
801 7th Ave	Fort Worth, TX 76104-2796	SOUTHWEST

Cooper University Hospital		(856) 342-2000
Cooper Univ Hosp		
1 Cooper Plaza	Camden, NJ 08103	MID ATLANTIC

Covenant Children's Hospital		(806) 725-1011
Covenant Children's Hosp		
3610 21st St	Lubbock, TX 79410	SOUTHWEST

Covenant Medical Center		(319) 272-8000
Covenant Med Ctr		
3421 W 9th St	Waterloo, IA 50702-5499	MIDWEST

Creighton University Medical Center		(402) 449-4000
Creighton Univ Med Ctr		
601 N 30th St	Omaha, NE 68131-2197	GREAT PLAINS AND MOUNTAINS

Crouse Hospital		(315) 470-7111
Crouse Hosp		
736 Irving Ave	Syracuse, NY 13210-1607	MID ATLANTIC

Crozer - Chester Medical Center		(610) 447-2000
Crozer - Chester Med Ctr		
One Medical Center Boulevard	Upland, PA 19013	MID ATLANTIC

CTCA at Midwestern Regional Medical Center		(847) 872-4561
CTCA at Midwestern Reg Med Ctr		
2520 Elisha Ave	Zion, IL 60099	MIDWEST

Dana-Farber Cancer Institute		(617) 632-3000
Dana-Farber Cancer Inst		
44 Binney St	Boston, MA 02115	NEW ENGLAND

Dartmouth - Hitchcock Medical Center		(603) 650-5000
Dartmouth - Hitchcock Med Ctr		
1 Medical Center Dr	Lebanon, NH 03756-0002	NEW ENGLAND

DCH Regional Medical Center		(205) 759-7111
DCH Reg Med Ctr		
809 Univ Blvd E	Tuscaloosa, AL 35401-2029	SOUTHEAST

Dell Children's Medical Center of Central Texas		(512) 324-0000
Dell Children's Med Ctr of Central Texas		
4900 Mueller Blvd	Austin, TX 78723	SOUTHWEST

Denver Health Medical Center		(303) 436-6000
Denver Health Med Ctr		
777 Bannock St	Denver, CO 80204	GREAT PLAINS AND MOUNTAINS

Desert Regional Medical Center   (760) 323-6511
Desert Regl Med Ctr
1150 N Indian Canyon Dr   Palm Springs, CA 92262   WEST COAST AND PACIFIC

DMC Surgery Hospital   (248) 733-2200
DMC Surgery Hosp
30671 Stephenson Hwy   Madison Heights, MI 48071   MIDWEST

Doctors' Hospital   (305) 666-2111
Doctors' Hosp
5000 University Dr   Coral Gables, FL 33146   SOUTHEAST

Doernbecher Children's Hospital/Oregon Health Science University   (503) 494-8811
Doernbecher Chldns Hosp/OHSU
3181 SW Sam Jackson Park Rd   Portland, OR 97201   WEST COAST AND PACIFIC

Duke Health Raleigh Hospital   (919) 954-3000
Duke Health Raleigh
3400 Wake Forest Rd   Raleigh, NC 27609   SOUTHEAST

Duke University Hospital   (919) 684-8111
Duke Univ Hosp
2301 Erwin Rd, PO Box 3708   Durham, NC 27710   SOUTHEAST

Durham Regional Hospital   (919) 470-4000
Durham Regional Hosp
3643 N Roxboro Rd   Durham, NC 27704   SOUTHEAST

Durham VA Medical Center   (919) 286-0411
Durham VA Med Ctr
508 Fulton St   Durham, NC 27705   SOUTHEAST

East Jefferson General Hospital   (504) 454-4000
E Jefferson Genl Hosp
4200 Houma Blvd   Metairie, LA 70006-2973   SOUTHWEST

East Texas Medical Center-Tyler   (903) 597-0351
E TX Med Ctr-Tyler
1000 S Beckham Ave   Tyler, TX 75701   SOUTHWEST

Edward Hines, Jr. VA Hospital   (708) 202-3800
Edward Hines, Jr. VA Hosp
5000 South 5th Avenue   Hines, IL 60141   MIDWEST

Edward Hospital   (630) 355-0450
Edward Hosp
801 S Washington St   Naperville, IL 60540   MIDWEST

El Camino Hospital   (650) 940-7000
El Camino Hosp
2500 Grant Road   Mountain View, CA 94039   WEST COAST AND PACIFIC

Elliot Hospital   (603) 669-5300
Elliot Hosp
1 Elliot Way   Manchester, NH 03103   NEW ENGLAND

Elmhurst Hospital Center   (718) 334-4000
Elmhurst Hosp Ctr
79-01 Broadway   Elmhurst, NY 11373   MID ATLANTIC

Emory University Hospital   (404) 712-2000
Emory Univ Hosp
1364 Clifton Rd NE   Atlanta, GA 30322   SOUTHEAST

Emory University Hospital Midtown   (404) 686-4411
Emory Univ Hosp Midtown
550 Peachtree St NE   Atlanta, GA 30365   SOUTHEAST

Englewood Hospital & Medical Center   (201) 894-3000
Englewood Hosp & Med Ctr
350 Engle Street   Englewood, NJ 07631   MID ATLANTIC

Erie County Medical Center   (716) 898-3000
Erie County Med Ctr
462 Grider St   Buffalo, NY 14215   MID ATLANTIC

Erlanger Medical Center   (423) 778-7000
Erlanger Med Ctr
975 E 3rd St   Chattanooga, TN 37403   SOUTHEAST

Evanston/North Shore University Health System   (847) 570-2000
Evanston/North Shore Univ Hlth Sys
2650 Ridge Ave   Evanston, IL 60201   MIDWEST

Fairview Southdale Hospital   (952) 924-5000
Fairview Southdale Hosp
6401 France Ave S   Edina, MN 55435-2199   MIDWEST

Fargo VA Medical Center   (701) 239-3700
Fargo VA Med Ctr
2101 Elm St   Fargo, ND 58102   GREAT PLAINS AND MOUNTAINS

Fletcher Allen Health Care-Medical Center Campus   (802) 847-0000
Fletcher Allen Health Care- Med Ctr Campus
111 Colchester Ave   Burlington, VT 05401   NEW ENGLAND

Floating Hospital for Children at Tufts Medical Center, The   (617) 636-5000
Floating Hosp for Children at Tufts Med Ce
755 Washington St   Boston, MA 02111   NEW ENGLAND

Florida Hospital - Celebration Health   (407) 764-4000
Florida Hosp Celebration Hlth
400 Celebration Pl   Celebration, FL 34747   SOUTHEAST

Florida Hospital - Orlando   (407) 303-5600
Florida Hosp - Orlando
601 E Rollins St   Orlando, FL 32803   SOUTHEAST

Floyd Memorial Hospital & Health Services   (812) 944-7701
Floyd Meml Hosp & Hlth Svcs
1850 State St   New Albany, IN 47150-4997   MIDWEST

Forsyth Medical Center   (336) 718-5000
Forsyth Med Ctr
3333 Silas Creek Pkwy   Winston-Salem, NC 27103   SOUTHEAST

Four Winds Hospital   (914) 763-8151
Four Winds Hosp
800 Cross River Road   Katonah, NY 10536   MID ATLANTIC

Fox Chase Cancer Center   (215) 728-6900
Fox Chase Cancer Ctr
333 Cottman Avenue   Philadelphia, PA 19111   MID ATLANTIC

Franciscan St. Francis Health-Indianapolis   (317) 865-5000
Franciscan St. Francis Hlth-Indianapolis
8111 S Emerson Ave   Indianapolis, IN 46143   MIDWEST

Franklin Square Hospital   (443) 777-7000
Franklin Square Hosp
9000 Franklin Square Drive   Baltimore, MD 21237   MID ATLANTIC

Frazier Rehabilitation Institute   (502) 582-7400
Frazier Rehab Inst
220 Abraham Flexner Way   Louisville, KY 40202   SOUTHEAST

Froedtert and the Medical Center of Wisconsin   (414) 805-3666
Froedtert and Med Ctr of WI
9200 W Wisconsin Ave   Milwaukee, WI 53226   MIDWEST

Gaston Memorial Hospital   (704) 834-2000
Gaston Meml Hosp
2525 Court Dr   Gastonia, NC 28054   SOUTHEAST

George Washington University Hospital   (202) 715-4000
G Washington Univ Hosp
900 23rd St NW   Washington, DC 20037   MID ATLANTIC

Georgetown University Hospital   (202) 444-2000
Georgetown Univ Hosp
3800 Reservoir Rd NW   Washington, DC 20007   MID ATLANTIC

Glenbrook Hospital-NorthShore University Health System   (847) 657-5800
Glenbrook Hosp-NorthShore Univ Hlth Syst
2100 Pfingsten Rd   Glenview, IL 60025   MIDWEST

Glendale Memorial Hospital & Health Center   (818) 502-1900
Glendale Mem Hosp & Hlth Ctr
1420 S Central Ave   Glendale, CA 91204   WEST COAST AND PACIFIC

Good Samaritan Hosp - Cincinnati   (513) 872-1400
Good Samaritan Hosp - Cincinnati
375 Dixmyth Ave   Cincinnati, OH 45220   MIDWEST

Good Samaritan Hospital   (410) 532-8000
Good Samaritan Hosp
5601 Loch Raven Blvd   Baltimore, MD 21208   MID ATLANTIC

Good Samaritan Hospital - Los Angeles   (213) 977-2121
Good Samaritan Hosp - LA
1225 Wilshire Boulevard   Los Angeles, CA 90017   WEST COAST AND PACIFIC

Good Samaritan Medical Center - West Palm Beach   (561) 655-5511
Good Sam Med Ctr - W Palm Beach
1309 N Flagler Dr   West Palm Beach, FL 33401   SOUTHEAST

Gottlieb Memorial Hospital   (708) 681-3200
Gottlieb Meml Hosp
701 W North Ave   Melrose Park, IL 60160   MIDWEST

Grady Health System   (404) 616-1000
Grady Hlth Sys
80 Jesse Hill Jr SE   Atlanta, GA 30303   SOUTHEAST

Greater Baltimore Medical Center   (443) 849-2000
Greater Baltimore Med Ctr
6701 N Charles St   Baltimore, MD 21204   MID ATLANTIC

Greenwich Hospital   (203) 863-3000
Greenwich Hosp
Five Perryridge Road   Greenwich, CT 06830   NEW ENGLAND

H Lee Moffitt Cancer Center & Research Institute   (813) 745-4673
H Lee Moffitt Cancer Ctr & Research Inst
12902 Magnolia Drive   Tampa, FL 33612-9497   SOUTHEAST

Hackensack University Medical Center   (201) 996-2000
Hackensack Univ Med Ctr
30 Prospect Avenue   Hackensack, NJ 07601   MID ATLANTIC

Hahnemann University Hospital   (215) 762-7000
Hahnemann Univ Hosp
Broad & Vine St   Philadelphia, PA 19102   MID ATLANTIC

Harborview Medical Center   (206) 744-3000
Harborview Med Ctr
325 9th Ave   Seattle, WA 98104   WEST COAST AND PACIFIC

Harper University Hospital   (313) 745-8040
Harper Univ Hosp
3990 John R St   Detroit, MI 48201-2097   MIDWEST

Harrison Medical Center   (360) 377-3911
Harrison Med Ctr
2520 Cherry Ave   Bremerton, WA 98310   WEST COAST AND PACIFIC

Hartford Hospital   (860) 545-5000
Hartford Hosp
80 Seymour St, Box 5037, PO Box 5037   Hartford, CT 06102-5037   NEW ENGLAND

Healthsouth Lakeshore Rehabilitation Hospital   (205) 868-2000
Healthsouth Lakeshore Rehab Hosp
3800 Ridgeway   Birmingham, AL 35209   SOUTHEAST

Hennepin County Medical Center   (612) 873-3000
Hennepin Cnty Med Ctr
701 Park Ave S   Minneapolis, MN 55415   MIDWEST

Henrico Doctors Hospital   (804) 289-4500
Henrico Doctors Hosp
1602 Skipwith Road   Richmond, VA 23229   SOUTHEAST

Henry Ford Hospital   (313) 916-2600
Henry Ford Hosp
2799 W Grand Blvd   Detroit, MI 48202   MIDWEST

Henry Ford West Bloomfield Hospital   (248) 661-4100
Henry Ford- W Bloomfield Hosp
6777 W Maple Rd   West Bloomfield, MI 48322   MIDWEST

Henry Mayo Newhall Memorial Hospital   (805) 253-8000
Henry Mayo Newhall Memorial Hosp
23845 McBean Parkway   Valencia, CA 91355   WEST COAST AND PACIFIC

Highland Park/North Shore University Health System   (847) 432-8000
Highland Park/North Shore Univ Hlth Syst
718 Glenview Ave   Highland Park, IL 60035   MIDWEST

Hilton Head Regional Medical Center   (843) 681-6122
Hilton Head Reg Med Ctr
25 Hospital Ctr Blvd, PO Box 21117   Hartsville, SC 29925-1117   SOUTHEAST

Hoag Memorial Hospital Presbyterian   (949) 645-8600
Hoag Meml Hosp Presby
One Hoag Drive   Newport Beach, CA 92663   WEST COAST AND PACIFIC

Hollywood Presbyterian Medical Center   (213) 413-3000
Hollywood Presby Med Ctr
1300 N Vermont Ave   Los Angeles, CA 90027-6069   WEST COAST AND PACIFIC

Holy Cross Hospital - Fort Lauderdale   (954) 771-8000
Holy Cross Hosp - Fort Lauderdale
4725 N Federal Hwy   Fort Lauderdale, FL 33308   SOUTHEAST

Holy Cross Hospital - Silver Spring   (301) 754-7000
Holy Cross Hospital - Silver Spring
1500 Forest Glen Road   Silver Spring, MD 20910   MID ATLANTIC

Holy Name Medical Center   (201) 833-3000
Holy Name Med Ctr
718 Teaneck Road   Teaneck, NJ 07666-4281   MID ATLANTIC

Hospital for Special Surgery   (212) 606-1000
Hosp For Special Surgery
535 East 70th Street   New York, NY 10021   MID ATLANTIC

Hospital of Central CT at New Britain   (860) 224-5011
Hosp of Central CT at New Britain
100 Grand St   New Britain, CT 06050   NEW ENGLAND

Hospital of St Raphael   (203) 789-3000
Hosp of St Raphael
1450 Chapel Street   New Haven, CT 06511   NEW ENGLAND

Hospital of the University of Pennsylvania - UPHS   (215) 662-4000
Hosp Univ Penn - UPHS
3400 Spruce Street   Philadelphia, PA 19104   MID ATLANTIC

Howard University Hospital   (202) 865-6100
Howard Univ Hosp
2041 Georgia Ave NW   Washington, DC 20060   MID ATLANTIC

Hunter Holmes McGuire Veterans Affairs Medical Center - Richmond   (804) 675-5500
Hunter Holmes McGuire VA Med Ctr - Richmond
1201 Broad Rock Boulevard   Richmond, VA 23249   SOUTHEAST

Huntsville Hospital, The   (256) 517-8020
Huntsville Hosp, The
101 Sivley Rd   Huntsville, AL 35801-4470   SOUTHEAST

Hutzel Women's Hospital - Detroit   (313) 745-7555
Hutzel Hosp - Detroit
3980 John R. Blvd   Detroit, MI 48201-2018   MIDWEST

Indian River Medical Center   (772) 567-4311
Indian River Med Ctr
1000 36th St   Vero Beach, FL 32960   SOUTHEAST

Indiana University Health Goshen Hospital   (574) 533-2141
Indiana Univ Hlth Goshen Hosp
200 High Park Ave   Goshen, IN 46526   MIDWEST

Indiana University Health Methodist Hospital   (317) 962-2000
IU Health Methodist Hosp
I65 at 21st Street, Box 1367   Indianapolis, IN 46202   MIDWEST

Indiana University Health University Hospital   (317) 944-5000
IU Health University Hosp
550 N University Blvd   Indianapolis, IN 46202   MIDWEST

Ingalls Memorial Hospital   (708) 333-2300
Ingalls Meml Hosp
1 Ingalls Dr   Harvey, IL 60426   MIDWEST

Inova Fair Oaks Hospital   (703) 391-3600
Inova Fair Oaks Hosp
3600 Joseph Siewick Dr   Fairfax, VA 22033   SOUTHEAST

Inova Fairfax Hospital   (703) 776-4001
Inova Fairfax Hosp
3300 Gallows Road   Falls Church, VA 22042   SOUTHEAST

Inova Fairfax Hospital for Children   (703) 204-6777
Inova Fairfax Hosp for Chldn
3300 Gallows Rd   Fairfax, VA 22042   SOUTHEAST

Integris Baptist Medical Center - Oklahoma   (405) 949-3011
Integris Baptist Med Ctr - OK
3300 NW Expressway   Oklahoma City, OK 73112-9028   SOUTHWEST

Intermountain Medical Center   (801) 507-7000
Intermountain Med Ctr
5121 S Cottonwood St   Salt Lake City, UT 84107   GREAT PLAINS AND MOUNTAINS

Jackson Memorial Hospital   (305) 585-1111
Jackson Meml Hosp
1611 NW 12th Ave   Miami, FL 33136   SOUTHEAST

Jackson North Medical Center   (305) 651-1100
Jackson N Med Ctr
160 NW 170 St   North Miami Beach, FL 33169   SOUTHEAST

Jewish Hospital   (502) 587-4011
Jewish Hosp
200 Abraham Flexner Way   Louisville, KY 40202   SOUTHEAST

Jewish Hospital - Kenwood - Cincinnati   (513) 686-3000
Jewish Hosp - Kenwood - Cincinnati
4777 E Galbraith Rd   Cincinnati, OH 45236-2891   MIDWEST

JFK Medical Center - Atlantis   (561) 965-7300
JFK Med Ctr - Atlantis
5301 S Congress Ave   Atlantis, FL 33462   SOUTHEAST

JFK Medical Center - Edison   (732) 321-7000
JFK Med Ctr - Edison
65 James St   Edison, NJ 08818   MID ATLANTIC

Joe DiMaggio Children's Hospital   (954) 987-2000
Joe DiMaggio Chldns Hosp
3501 Johnson St   Hollywood, FL 33021   SOUTHEAST

John D. Dingell VA Medical Center, Detroit   (313) 562-1000
John D. Dingell VA Med Ctr, Detroit
4646 John R. Street   Detroit, MI 48201   MIDWEST

John M & Sally B Thornton Hospital
John M & Sally B Thornton Hosp
9300 Campus Point Drive   La Jolla, CA 92037   WEST COAST AND PACIFIC

John Sealy Hospital - (University of Texas Medical Branch Galveston)   (409) 747-1935
UTMB - John Sealy Hospital
301 University Blvd   Galveston, TX 77555   SOUTHWEST

Johns Hopkins Bayview Medical Center   (410) 550-0100
Johns Hopkins Bayview Med Ctr
4940 Eastern Avenue   Baltimore, MD 21224   MID ATLANTIC

Johns Hopkins Hospital   (410) 955-5000
Johns Hopkins Hosp
600 N Wolfe St   Baltimore, MD 21287   MID ATLANTIC

Kaiser Permanente Baldwin Park Medical Center   (626) 851-1011
Kaiser Permanente Baldwin Pk Med Ctr
1011 Baldwin Park Blvd   Baldwin Park, CA 91706   WEST COAST AND PACIFIC

Kaiser Permanente Oakland Medical Center   (510) 752-1000
Kaiser Permanente Oakland Med Ctr
280 West MacArthur Boulevard   Oakland, CA 94611   WEST COAST AND PACIFIC

Kaiser Permanente South San Francisco Medical Center   (650) 742-2000
Kaiser Permanente S San Francisco Med Ctr
1200 El Camino Real   South San Francisco, CA 94080   WEST COAST AND
                                                                        PACIFIC

Kaiser Permanente Woodland Hills Medical Center   (818) 719-2000
Kaiser Permanente Woodland Hills Med Ctr
5601 DeSoto Ave   Woodland Hills, CA 91365   WEST COAST AND PACIFIC

Kalispell Regional Medical Center   (406) 752-5111
Kalispell Regl Med Ctr
310 Sunnyview Ln   Kalispell, MT 59901   GREAT PLAINS AND MOUNTAINS

Kapiolani Medical Center for Women & Children   (808) 983-6000
Kapiolani Med Ctr for Women & Chldn
1319 Punahou St   Honolulu, HI 96826   WEST COAST AND PACIFIC

Keck Medical Center of USC   (323) 442-8500
Keck Med Ctr of USC
1500 San Pablo St   Los Angeles, CA 90033   WEST COAST AND PACIFIC

Kenmore Mercy Hospital   (845) 331-3131
Kenmore Mercy Hosp
2950 Elmwood Ave   Kenmore, NY 14217   MID ATLANTIC

Kennedy Krieger Institute   (443) 923-9200
Kennedy Krieger Inst
707 N Broadway   Baltimore, MD 21208   MID ATLANTIC

Kessler Institute for Rehabilitation - West Orange   (973) 243-6800
Kessler Inst for Rehab - W Orange
1199 Pleasant Valley Way   West Orange, NJ 07052-1499   MID ATLANTIC

Kootenai Medical Center   (208) 666-2000
Kootenai Med Ctr
2003 Lincoln Way   Coeur d'Alene, ID 83814   GREAT PLAINS AND MOUNTAINS

Kosair Children's Hospital   (502) 629-6000
Kosair Chldn's Hosp
231 E Chestnut St   Louisville, KY 40202   SOUTHEAST

La Grange Memorial Hospital   (708) 352-1200
La Grange Meml Hosp
5101 S Willow Springs Rd   La Grange, IL 60525   MIDWEST

LAC & USC Medical Center   (323) 266-2622
LAC & USC Med Ctr
1200 N State St   Los Angeles, CA 90033   WEST COAST AND PACIFIC

LAC - Harbor - UCLA Medical Center   (310) 222-2345
LAC - Harbor - UCLA Med Ctr
1000 W Carson St, Box 27 PO Box 2910   Torrance, CA 90509   WEST COAST AND PACIFIC

Lafayette General Medical Center   (337) 289-7991
Lafayette Genl Med Ctr
1214 Coolidge Blvd   Lafayette, LA 70503   SOUTHWEST

Lahey Clinic   (781) 744-5100
Lahey Clin
41 Mall Road   Burlington, MA 01805   NEW ENGLAND

Lakeland Regional Medical Center   (863) 687-1100
Lakeland Regl Med Ctr
1324 Lakeland Hills Blvd   Lakeland, FL 33805   SOUTHEAST

Lakeland Specialty Hospital   (269) 471-7761
Lakeland Specialty Hosp
6418 Deans Hill Rd   Berrien Cnter, MI 49102   MIDWEST

Lancaster General Hospital   (717) 290-5511
Lancaster Genl Hosp
555 N Duke St, PO Box 3555   Lancaster, PA 17604-3555   MID ATLANTIC

Lankenau Hospital   (610) 645-2000
Lankenau Hosp
100 Lancaster Ave   Wynnewood, PA 19096-3498   MID ATLANTIC

Lawrence & Memorial Hospital   (860) 442-0711
Lawrence & Meml Hosp
365 Montauk Ave   New London, CT 06320   NEW ENGLAND

LDS Hospital	(801) 408-1100
LDS Hosp	
8th Ave & C St	Salt Lake City, UT 84143 GREAT PLAINS AND MOUNTAINS

Le Bonheur Children's Medical Center	(901) 287-5437
Le Bonheur Chldns Med Ctr	
50 N Dunlap	Memphis, TN 38103-2893 SOUTHEAST

Lee Memorial Health Systems	(239) 334-5314
Lee Memorial Hlth Systems	
2776 Cleveland Ave	Fort Myers, FL 33901 SOUTHEAST

Legacy Emanuel Children's Hospital	(503) 413-2200
Legacy Emanuel Chldn's Hosp	
2801 Gantenbein Ave	Portland, OR 97227 WEST COAST AND PACIFIC

Legacy Good Samaritan Medical Center	(503) 413-7711
Legacy Good Samaritan Med Ctr	
1015 NW 22nd Ave	Portland, OR 97210-3025 WEST COAST AND PACIFIC

Lenox Hill Hospital	(212) 434-2000
Lenox Hill Hosp	
100 East 77th Street	New York, NY 10021 MID ATLANTIC

Lenox Hill Hospital (Manhattan Eye, Ear & Throat Hosp)	(212) 838-9200
Lenox Hill Hosp (Manh Eye, Ear & Throat Hosp)	
210 East 64th Street	New York, NY 10021 MID ATLANTIC

Loma Linda Children's Hospital	(909) 558-8000
Loma Linda Chldns Hosp	
11234 Anderson St	Loma Linda, CA 92354 WEST COAST AND PACIFIC

Loma Linda University Medical Center	(909) 558-4000
Loma Linda Univ Med Ctr	
11234 Anderson St	Loma Linda, CA 92354 WEST COAST AND PACIFIC

Long Beach Memorial Medical Center	(562) 933-2000
Long Beach Meml Med Ctr	
2801 Atlantic Ave	Long Beach, CA 90801 WEST COAST AND PACIFIC

Long Island Jewish Medical Center	(718) 470-7000
Long Island Jewish Med Ctr	
270-05 76th Avenue	New Hyde Park, NY 11040 MID ATLANTIC

Los Alamitos Medical Center	(562) 598-1311
Los Alamitos Med Ctr	
3751 Katella Ave	Los Alamitos, CA 90720 WEST COAST AND PACIFIC

Louisiana State University Hospital (318) 675-4239
Louisiana State Univ Hosp
1501 Kings Highway P.O. Box 33932   Shreveport, LA 71130   SOUTHWEST

Loyola University Medical Center (708) 216-9000
Loyola Univ Med Ctr
2160 S 1st Ave   Maywood, IL 60153   MIDWEST

LSU Interim Public Hospital (504) 903-3000
LSU Interim Public Hosp
2021 Perdido St   New Orleans, LA 70112   SOUTHWEST

Lucile Packard Children's Hospital (650) 497-8000
Lucile Packard Chldn's Hosp
725 Welch Rd   Palo Alto, CA 94304   WEST COAST AND PACIFIC

Lutheran Medical Center - Cleveland (216) 696-4300
Lutheran Med Ctr - Cleveland
1730 W 25th St   Cleveland, OH 44113   MIDWEST

Magee Rehabilitation Hospital (215) 587-3000
Magee Rehab Hosp
1513 Race St   Philadelphia, PA 19102-1177   MID ATLANTIC

Magee-Womens Hospital of UPMC (412) 641-1000
Magee-Womens Hosp - UPMC
300 Halket Street   Pittsburgh, PA 15213   MID ATLANTIC

Maimonides Medical Center (718) 283-6000
Maimonides Med Ctr
4802 Tenth Avenue   Brooklyn, NY 11219   MID ATLANTIC

Maine Medical Center (207) 662-0111
Maine Med Ctr
22 Bramhall St   Portland, ME 04102   NEW ENGLAND

Malcolm Randall VA Medical Center (352) 376-1611
Malcolm Randall VA Med Ctr
1601 SW Archer Rd   Gainesville, FL 32608   SOUTHEAST

Maple Grove Hospital (763) 581-1000
Maple Grove Hosp
9875 Hospital Dr   Maple Grove, MN 55369   MIDWEST

Marianjoy Rehabilitation Hospital (630) 462-4000
Marianjoy Rehab Hosp
26 W 171 Roosevelt Rd   Wheaton, IL 60187   MIDWEST

Marin General Hospital		(415) 925-7000
Marin Genl Hosp		
250 Bon Air Rd	Greenbrae, CA 94904	WEST COAST AND PACIFIC

Marina Del Rey Hospital		(310) 823-8911
Marina Del Rey Hosp		
4650 Lincoln Blvd	Marina Del Rey, CA 90292	WEST COAST AND PACIFIC

Mary Bridge Children's Hospital & Health Center		(253) 552-1400
Mary Bridge Chldns Hosp & Hlth Ctr		
317 Martin Luther King Jr Way	Tacoma, WA 98405	WEST COAST AND PACIFIC

Mary Shiels Hospital		(214) 443-3000
Mary Shiels Hosp		
3515 Howell St	Dallas, TX 75204	SOUTHWEST

Maryland General Hospital		(410) 225-8000
Maryland Genl Hosp		
827 Linden Ave	Baltimore, MD 21201	MID ATLANTIC

Massachusetts Eye and Ear Infirmary		(617) 523-7900
Mass Eye & Ear Infirmary		
243 Charles Street	Boston, MA 02114	NEW ENGLAND

Massachusetts General Hospital		(617) 726-2000
Mass Genl Hosp		
55 Fruit St	Boston, MA 02114	NEW ENGLAND

Massachusetts Mental Health Center		(617) 626-9300
MA Mental Hlth Ctr		
180 Morton St	Jamaica Plain, MA 02130	NEW ENGLAND

Mattel Children's Hospital at UCLA		(310) 825-9111
Mattel Chldns Hosp at UCLA		
10833 Le Conte Ave	Los Angeles, CA 90095	WEST COAST AND PACIFIC

Mayo Clinic - Jacksonville, FL		(904) 953-2000
Mayo - Jacksonville		
4500 San Pablo Road	Jacksonville, FL 32224	SOUTHEAST

Mayo Clinic - Phoenix		(480) 515-6296
Mayo Clinic - Phoenix		
5777 E Mayo Blvd	Phoenix, AZ 85054	SOUTHWEST

Mayo Clinic - Rochester, MN		(507) 284-2511
Mayo Med Ctr & Clin - Rochester		
200 First St SW	Rochester, MN 55905	MIDWEST

Mayo Clinic - Scottsdale		(480) 301-8000
Mayo Clinic - Scottsdale		
13400 E Shea Blvd	Scottsdale, AZ 85259	SOUTHWEST

McLaren Regional Medical Center		(810) 342-2000
McLaren Reg Med Ctr		
401 S. Ballenger Highway	Flint, MI 48532	MIDWEST

McLean Hospital		(617) 855-2000
McLean Hosp		
115 Mill St	Belmont, MA 02478	NEW ENGLAND

MD Anderson Cancer Center-Orlando		(407) 648-3800
MD Anderson Cancer Ctr-Orlando		
1400 S Orange Ave	Orlando, FL 32806	SOUTHEAST

Meadowlands Hospital Medical Center		(201) 392-3100
Meadowlands Hosp Med Ctr		
55 Meadowland Parkway	Secaucus, NJ 07096	MID ATLANTIC

Medical Center of Central Georgia		(478) 633-1000
Med Ctr of Central GA		
777 Hemlock Street	Macon, GA 31201	SOUTHEAST

Medical City Dallas Hospital		(972) 566-7000
Med City Dallas Hosp		
7777 Forest Ln	Dallas, TX 75230-2594	SOUTHWEST

Medical College of Georgia Hospital & Clinic (MCG Health Inc)		(706) 721-0211
Med Coll of GA Hosp and Clin (MCG Health Inc)		
1120 15th Street	Augusta, GA 30912	SOUTHEAST

Medical College of Virginia Hospitals		(804) 828-9000
Med Coll of VA Hosp		
1250 E Marshall St, Box 980510	Richmond, VA 23219	SOUTHEAST

Medical University of South Carolina Children's Hospital		(843) 792-1414
MUSC Chldns Hosp		
169 Ashley Ave	Charleston, SC 29425	SOUTHEAST

Medical University of South Carolina Medical Center		(843) 792-2300
MUSC Med Ctr		
171 Ashley Ave	Charleston, SC 29425	SOUTHEAST

Memorial Health University Medical Center - Savannah		(912) 350-8000
Meml Hlth Univ Med Ctr - Savannah		
4700 Waters Ave	Savannah, GA 31404	SOUTHEAST

Memorial Hermann Hospital - Texas Medical Center   (713) 704-4000
Meml Hermann Hosp - Texas Med Ctr
6411 Fannin   Houston, TX 77030   SOUTHWEST

Memorial Hermann Memorial City Hospital   (713) 242-3000
Meml Hermann Meml City Hosp
921 Gessner Ave   Houston, TX 77024-2412   SOUTHWEST

Memorial Medical Center-Springfield   (217) 788-3000
Memorial Med Ctr-Springfield
701 N First St   Springfield, IL 62781   MIDWEST

Memorial Regional Hospital   (954) 987-2000
Meml Regl Hosp
3501 Johnson Street   Hollywood, FL 33021   SOUTHEAST

Memorial Sloan-Kettering Cancer Center   (212) 639-2000
Meml Sloan-Kettering Cancer Ctr
1275 York Avenue   New York, NY 10021   MID ATLANTIC

Menninger Clinic   (800) 351-9058
Menninger Clinic
PO Box 809045   Houston, TX 77280   SOUTHWEST

Mercy General Hospital - Sacramento   (916) 453-4545
Mercy General Hosp - Sacramento
4001 J Street   Sacramento, CA 95819   WEST COAST AND PACIFIC

Mercy Gilbert Medical Center   (480) 728-8000
Mercy Gilbert Med Ctr
3555 S Val Vista Drive   Gilbert, AZ 85296   SOUTHWEST

Mercy Health Center - Oklahoma City   (405) 755-1515
Mercy Hlth Ctr - Oklahoma City
4300 W Memorial Dr   Oklahoma City, OK 73120   SOUTHWEST

Mercy Hospital   (305) 854-4400
Mercy Hosp
3663 S Miami Ave   Miami, FL 33133   SOUTHEAST

Mercy Hospital - Coon Rapids   (763) 236-6000
Mercy Hosp - Coon Rapids
4050 Coon Rapids Blvd   Coon Rapids, MN 55433-2522   MIDWEST

Mercy Hospital - Fairfield   (513) 870-7000
Mercy Hosp - Fairfield
3000 Mack Rd   Fairfield, OH 45014   MIDWEST

Mercy Medical Center - Baltimore (410) 332-9000
Mercy Med Ctr - Baltimore
301 St Paul Pl   Baltimore, MD 21202   MID ATLANTIC

Methodist Hospital System (713) 790-3311
Methodist Hosp - Houston
6565 Fannin St   Houston, TX 77030   SOUTHWEST

Methodist Hospital-Omaha (402) 354-4000
Methodist Hosp - Omaha
8303 Dodge St   Omaha, NE 68114   GREAT PLAINS AND MOUNTAINS

Methodist Hospital-San Antonio (210) 575-4000
Methodist Hosp-San Antonio
7700 Floyd Curl Dr   San Antonio, TX 78229   SOUTHWEST

Methodist University Hospital - Memphis (901) 516-7000
Methodist Univ Hosp - Memphis
1265 Union Ave   Memphis, TN 38104   SOUTHEAST

MetroHealth Medical Center (216) 778-7800
MetroHealth Med Ctr
2500 MetroHealth Drive   Cleveland, OH 44109-1998   MIDWEST

Miami Children's Hospital (305) 666-6511
Miami Children's Hosp
3100 SW 62nd Ave   Miami, FL 33155   SOUTHEAST

Michael E. DeBakey VA Medical Center - Houston (713) 791-1414
DeBakey VA Med Ctr-Houston
2002 Holcombe Blvd   Houston, TX 77030-1414   SOUTHWEST

Michigan State University-Sparrow Hospital (517) 364-1000
Mich State Univ-Sparrow Hos
1215 E Michigan Ave, MS 0   Lansing, MI 48912   MIDWEST

Milford Hospital (203) 876-4000
Milford Hosp
300 Seaside Ave   Milford, CT 06460   NEW ENGLAND

Millard Fillmore Gates Circle Hospital (716) 887-4600
Millard Fillmore Gates Cir Hosp
3 Gates Cir   Buffalo, NY 14209   MID ATLANTIC

Miriam Hospital (401) 793-2500
Miriam Hosp
164 Summit Avenue   Providence, RI 02906-2894   NEW ENGLAND

Missouri Baptist Medical Center   (314) 996-5000
Missouri Baptist Med Ctr
3015 N Ballas Rd   St Louis, MO 63131   MIDWEST

Mobile Infirmary Medical Center   (334) 431-2400
Mobile Infirmary Med Ctr
5 Mobile Infirmary Circle   Mobile, AL 36607-3513   SOUTHEAST

Montefiore Medical Center - Henry and Lucy Moses Division   (718) 920-4321
Montefiore Med Ctr - Div. Moses
111 East 210 Street   Bronx, NY 10467   MID ATLANTIC

Montefiore Medical Center - Jack D. Weiler Division   (718) 904-2000
Montefiore Med Ctr - Div. Weiler
1825 Eastchester Road   Bronx, NY 10461   MID ATLANTIC

Morgan Stanley Children's Hospital of NewYork-Presbyterian, NY   (212) 305-2500
Morgan Stanley Children's Hosp of NY-Presby, NY
622 W 168th St   New York, NY 10032   MID ATLANTIC

Morristown Medical Center   (973) 971-5000
Morristown Med Ctr
100 Madison Avenue   Morristown, NJ 07960-6095   MID ATLANTIC

Moss Rehab Hospital   (215) 663-6000
Moss Rehab Hosp
60 E Township Line Rd   Elkins Park, PA 19027   MID ATLANTIC

Mott Children's Hospital   (734) 936-4000
Mott Chldns Hosp
1500 E Medical Center Dr   Ann Arbor, MI 48109   MIDWEST

Mount Auburn Hospital   (617) 492-3500
Mount Auburn Hosp
330 Mount Auburn St   Cambridge, MA 02138   NEW ENGLAND

Mount Carmel West Hospital   (614) 234-5000
Mt Carmel W Hosp
793 W State St   Columbus, OH 43085   MIDWEST

Mount Clemens Regional Medical Center   (586) 493-8000
Mount Clemens Regional Med Ctr
1000 Harrington Blvd   Mount Clemens, MI 48043   MIDWEST

Mount Sinai Medical Center   (212) 241-6500
Mount Sinai Med Ctr
One Gustave L. Levy Pl   New York, NY 10029   MID ATLANTIC

Mount Sinai Medical Center - Miami   (305) 674-2121
Mount Sinai Med Ctr - Miami
4300 Alton Rd   Miami Beach, FL 33140   SOUTHEAST

Mountainview Hospital - Las Vegas   (702) 255-5074
Mountainview Hosp - Las Vegas
3100 N Tenaya Way   Las Vegas, NV 89128   WEST COAST AND PACIFIC

Munroe Regional Medical Center   (352) 351-7200
Munroe Regional Med Ctr
131 SW 15th Street   Ocala, FL 34474   SOUTHEAST

National Institutes of Health - Clinical Center   (301) 496-4000
Natl Inst of Hlth - Clin Ctr
10 Center Drive   Bethesda, MD 20892-0001   MID ATLANTIC

National Jewish Medical & Research Center   (303) 388-4461
Natl Jewish Med & Rsch Ctr
1400 Jackson St   Denver, CO 80206-2762   GREAT PLAINS AND MOUNTAINS

National Rehabilitation Hospital   (202) 877-1000
Natl Rehab Hosp
102 Irving St NW   Washington, DC 20010   MID ATLANTIC

Nationwide Children's Hospital   (614) 722-2000
Nationwide Chldn's Hosp
700 Children's Drive   Columbus, OH 43205   MIDWEST

Nebraska Medical Center   (402) 559-2000
Nebraska Med Ctr
4350 Dewey Ave   Omaha, NE 68198   GREAT PLAINS AND MOUNTAINS

Nebraska Methodist Hospital   (402) 354-4000
Nebraska Meth Hosp
8303 Dodge St   Omaha, NE 68114   GREAT PLAINS AND MOUNTAINS

Nemours Children's Clinic - Wilmington   (302) 651-6600
Nemours Chldns Clinic - Wilmington
1600 Rockland Rd   Wilmington, DE 19803   MID ATLANTIC

New England Baptist Hospital   (617) 754-5800
New England Bapt Hosp
125 Parker Hill Ave   Boston, MA 02120   NEW ENGLAND

New York Eye & Ear Infirmary   (212) 979-4000
New York Eye & Ear Infirm
310 East 14th Street   New York, NY 10003   MID ATLANTIC

New York Hospital Queens		(718) 670-1231
NY Hosp Queens		
56-45 Main Street	Flushing, NY 11355	MID ATLANTIC
New York Methodist Hospital		(718) 780-3000
New York Methodist Hosp		
506 Sixth Street	Brooklyn, NY 11215	MID ATLANTIC
New York State Psychiatric Institute		(212) 543-5000
NY State Psychiatric Inst		
1051 Riverside Dr	New York, NY 10032	MID ATLANTIC
Newark Beth Israel Medical Center		(973) 926-7000
Newark Beth Israel Med Ctr		
201 Lyons Ave	Newark, NJ 07112	MID ATLANTIC
Newton - Wellesley Hospital		(617) 243-6000
Newton - Wellesley Hosp		
2014 Washington St	Newton, MA 02462	NEW ENGLAND
NewYork-Presbyterian/Columbia University Medical Center, NY		(212) 305-2500
NY-Presby/Columbia Univ Med Ctr, NY		
622 W 168th St	New York, NY 10032	MID ATLANTIC
NewYork-Presbyterian/Weill Cornell Medical Center, NY		(212) 746-5454
NY-Presby/Weill Cornell Med Ctr, NY		
525 E 68th St	New York, NY 10021	MID ATLANTIC
NewYork-Presbyterian/Westchester Division, NY		(914) 682-9100
NY-Presby/Westchester Div, NY		
21 Bloomingdale Rd	White Plains, NY 10605	MID ATLANTIC
North Carolina Memorial Hospital - UNC		(919) 966-4131
NC Memorial Hosp - UNC		
101 Manning Drive, Box 7600	Chapel Hill, NC 27514	SOUTHEAST
North Oaks Medical Center		(985) 230-6601
North Oaks Med Ctr		
15790 Paul Vega MD Dr	Hammond, LA 70403	SOUTHWEST
North Shore Medical Center - Salem Hospital		(978) 741-1215
N Shore Med Ctr - Salem Hosp		
81 Highland Avenue	Salem, MA 01970	NEW ENGLAND
North Shore University Hospital		(516) 562-0100
N Shore Univ Hosp		
300 Community Dr	Manhasset, NY 11030	MID ATLANTIC

North Shore-LIJ Health System		(516) 465-2600
NS-LIJ Hlth Sys		
125 Community Drive	Great Neck, NY 11021	MID ATLANTIC

Northern California Shriners Hospital		(916) 453-2000
Northern CA Shriners Hosp		
2425 Stockton Blvd	Sacramento, CA 95817	WEST COAST AND PACIFIC

Northern Michigan Hospital		(231) 487-4000
Northern Michigan Hosp		
416 Connable Ave	Petoskey, MI 49770	MIDWEST

Northern Nevada Medical Center		(775) 531-7000
Northern Nevada Med Ctr		
2375 E Prater Way	Sparks, NV 89434-9644	WEST COAST AND PACIFIC

Northern Westchester Hospital		(914) 666-1200
Northern Westchester Hosp		
400 East Main Street	Mount Kisco, NY 10549	MID ATLANTIC

Northside Hospital - Atlanta		(404) 851-8000
Northside Hosp		
1000 Johnson Ferry Rd NE	Atlanta, GA 30342	SOUTHEAST

Northwest Hospital - Seattle		(206) 364-0500
Northwest Hosp - Seattle		
1550 N 115th St	Seattle, WA 98133-0806	WEST COAST AND PACIFIC

Northwest Medical Center		(954) 974-0400
Northwest Med Ctr		
2801 N State Rd 7	Margate, FL 33063	SOUTHEAST

Northwestern Memorial Hospital		(312) 926-2000
Northwestern Meml Hosp		
251 E Huron St	Chicago, IL 60611	MIDWEST

Norton Hospital		(502) 629-8000
Norton Hosp		
200 E Chestnut St	Louisville, KY 40202	SOUTHEAST

NYU Hospital for Joint Diseases		(212) 598-6000
NYU Hosp For Joint Diseases		
301 East 17th Street	New York, NY 10003	MID ATLANTIC

NYU Langone Medical Center		(212) 263-7300
NYU Langone Med Ctr		
550 First Avenue	New York, NY 10016	MID ATLANTIC

NYU Rusk Institute   (212) 263-2606
NYU Rusk Inst
400 East 34th Street   New York, NY 10016   MID ATLANTIC

Ochsner Baptist Medical Center   (504) 899-9311
Ochsner Baptist Med Ctr
2700 Napoleon Ave   New Orleans, LA 70115   SOUTHWEST

Ochsner Medical Center-Baton Rouge   (225) 752-2470
Ochsner Med Ctr-Baton Rouge
17000 Medical Center Drive   Baton Rouge, LA 70816   SOUTHWEST

Ochsner Medical Center-Kenner   (504) 468-8600
Ochsner Med Ctr-Kenner
180 W Esplanade Ave   Kenner, LA 70065-2467   SOUTHWEST

Ochsner Medical Center-New Orleans   (504) 842-3000
Ochsner Med Ctr-New Orleans
1514 Jefferson Hwy   New Orleans, LA 70121   SOUTHWEST

Ohio State University Medical Center   (614) 293-8000
Ohio St Univ Med Ctr
410 W 10th Avenue   Columbus, OH 43210   MIDWEST

Olathe Medical Center   (913) 791-4200
Olathe Med Ctr
20333 W 151st St   Olathe, KS 66061-5352   GREAT PLAINS AND MOUNTAINS

Olive View-UCLA Medical Center   (818) 364-1555
Olive View-UCLA Med Ctr
14445 Olive View Dr   Sylmar, CA 91342   WEST COAST AND PACIFIC

Olympia Medical Center   (323) 938-3161
Olympia Med Ctr
5900 W Olympic Blvd   Los Angeles, CA 90036   WEST COAST AND PACIFIC

Oregon Health & Science University   (503) 494-8311
OR Hlth & Sci Univ
3181 SW Sam Jackson Park Rd   Portland, OR 97239   WEST COAST AND PACIFIC

Orlando Regional Medical Center   (407) 841-5111
Orlando Regl Med Ctr
1414 Kuhl Ave   Orlando, FL 32806   SOUTHEAST

Orthopedic Specialty Hospital, The (TOSH)   (801) 314-4100
Ortho Spec Hosp, The (TOSH)
5848 Fashion Blvd   Salt Lake City, UT 84107   GREAT PLAINS AND MOUNTAINS

OSF Saint Francis Medical Center   (309) 655-2000
OSF Saint Francis Med Ctr
530 NE Glen Oak Ave   Peoria, IL 61637   MIDWEST

OU Medical Center   (405) 271-4700
OU Med Ctr
1200 Everett Dr, PO Box 26307   Oklahoma City, OK 73104-5098   SOUTHWEST

Our Lady of Lourdes Regional Medical Center - Lafayette   (337) 289-2000
Our Lady of Lourdes Reg Med Ctr - Lafayette
611 St. Landry St   Lafayette, LA 70506-4697   SOUTHWEST

Our Lady of the Lake Regional Medical Center   (225) 765-6565
Our Lady of the Lake Regl Med Ctr
5000 Hennessy Blvd   Baton Rouge, LA 70808-4398   SOUTHWEST

Overlake Hospital Medical Center   (425) 688-5000
Overlake Hosp Med Ctr
1035 116th Ave NE   Bellevue, WA 98004   WEST COAST AND PACIFIC

Overland Park Regional Medical Center   (913) 541-5000
Overland Pk Regl Med Ctr
10500 Quivira Rd   Overland Park, KS 66215   GREAT PLAINS AND MOUNTAINS

Palmetto Health Richland Memorial Hospital   (803) 434-7000
Palmetto Health Richland Mem Hosp
5 Richland Medical Park Drive   Columbia, SC 29203   SOUTHEAST

Park Nicollet Methodist Hospital - Minnesota   (952) 993-5000
Park Nicollet Methodist Hosp - Minnesota
6500 Excelsior Blvd   Minneapolis, MN 55426-4700   MIDWEST

Parkinson's Institute/Movement Disorders Treament Center, The   (408) 734-2800
Parkinson's Inst/Movement Disorders Trmt Ctr, The
675 Almanor Ave   Sunnyvale, CA 94085   WEST COAST AND PACIFIC

Parkland Health & Hospital System   (214) 590-8000
Parkland Hlth & Hosp Sys
5201 Harry Hines Blvd   Dallas, TX 75235   SOUTHWEST

Peninsula Medical Center   (650) 696-5400
Peninsula Med Ctr
1783 El Camino Real   Burlingame, CA 94010   WEST COAST AND PACIFIC

Penn Presbyterian Medical Center - UPHS   (215) 662-8000
Penn Presby Med Ctr - UPHS
51 N 39th St   Philadelphia, PA 19104   MID ATLANTIC

Penn State Children's Hospital   (717) 531-8521
Penn State Chldns Hosp
500 University Dr   Hershey, PA 17033   MID ATLANTIC

Penn State Milton S. Hershey Medical Center   (717) 531-8521
Penn State Milton S Hershey Med Ctr
500 University Drive   Hershey, PA 17033-0850   MID ATLANTIC

Pennsylvania Hospital - UPHS   (215) 829-3000
Pennsylvania Hosp-UPHS
800 Spruce St, Ste 240   Philadelphia, PA 19107   MID ATLANTIC

Penrose Hospital   (719) 776-5000
Penrose Hosp
2222 N Nevada   Colorado Springs, CO 80907   GREAT PLAINS AND MOUNTAINS

Peyton Manning Children's Hospital at St. Vincent   (317) 338-2345
Peyton Manning Children's Hosp at St. Vincent
2001 W 86th St   Indianapolis, IN 46260   MIDWEST

Philadelphia Shriners Hospital   (215) 430-4000
Philadelphia Shriners Hosp
3351 N Broad St   Philadelphia, PA 19140   MID ATLANTIC

Phillips Eye Institute   (612) 775-8800
Phillips Eye Inst
2215 Park Ave S   Minneapolis, MN 55404   MIDWEST

Phoenix Baptist Hospital & Medical Center   (602) 249-0212
Phoenix Baptist Hosp & Med Ctr
2000 West Bethany Home Rd   Phoenix, AZ 85015-2184   SOUTHWEST

Phoenix Children's Hospital   (602) 546-1000
Phoenix Children's Hosp
1919 E Thomas Rd   Phoenix, AZ 85106   SOUTHWEST

Physicians Regional Healthcare System-Pine Ridge   (239) 348-4000
Physicians Regl Hlthcare Med Ctr-Pine Ridge
6101 Pine Ridge Rd   Naples, FL 34119   SOUTHEAST

Piedmont Hospital   (404) 605-5000
Piedmont Hosp
1968 Peachtree Rd NW   Atlanta, GA 30309   SOUTHEAST

Porter Adventist Hospital   (303) 778-1955
Porter Adventist Hosp
2525 S Downing St   Denver, CO 80210   GREAT PLAINS AND MOUNTAINS

Portsmouth Regional Hospital (603) 436-5110
Portsmouth Regl Hosp
333 Borthwick Ave   Portsmouth, NH 03801-7002   NEW ENGLAND

Presbyterian - St Luke's Medical Center (303) 839-6000
Presby - St Luke's Med Ctr
1719 E 19th Ave   Denver, CO 80218   GREAT PLAINS AND MOUNTAINS

Presbyterian Hospital - Charlotte (704) 384-4000
Presby Hosp - Charlotte
200 Hawthorne Ln   Charlotte, NC 28204-2528   SOUTHEAST

Primary Children's Medical Center (801) 588-2000
Primary Children's Med Ctr
100 N Medical Drive   Salt Lake City, UT 84113   GREAT PLAINS AND MOUNTAINS

Providence Alaska Medical Center (907) 562-2211
Providence Alaska Med Ctr
3200 Providence Dr   Anchorage, AK 99508   WEST COAST AND PACIFIC

Providence Hospital - Southfield (248) 424-3000
Providence Hosp - Southfield
16001 W Nine Mile Rd   Southfield, MI 48075   MIDWEST

Providence Portland Medical Center (503) 215-1111
Providence Portland Med Ctr
4805 NE Glisan   Portland, OR 97213   WEST COAST AND PACIFIC

Providence Saint Joseph Medical Center (818) 843-5111
Providence St Joseph Med Ctr
501 S Buena Vista St   Burbank, CA 91505   WEST COAST AND PACIFIC

Providence St Vincent Medical Center (503) 216-1234
Providence St Vincent Med Ctr
9205 SW Barnes Rd   Portland, OR 97225   WEST COAST AND PACIFIC

Queen's Medical Center - Honolulu (808) 538-9011
Queen's Med Ctr - Honolulu
1301 Punchbowl Street   Honolulu, HI 96813   WEST COAST AND PACIFIC

Rady Children's Hospital - San Diego (858) 576-1700
Rady Children's Hosp - San Diego
3020 Children's Way   San Diego, CA 92123   WEST COAST AND PACIFIC

Rancho Los Amigos National Rehabilitation Center (562) 401-7111
Rancho Los Amigos Natl Rehab Ctr
7601 East Imperial Highway   Downey, CA 90242   WEST COAST AND PACIFIC

Regional Medical Center - Memphis | (901) 545-7100
Regional Med Ctr - Memphis
877 Jefferson Avenue | Memphis, TN 38103 | SOUTHEAST

Regions Hospital - St Paul | (651) 254-3456
Regions Hosp - St Paul
640 Jackson Street | St Paul, MN 55101 | MIDWEST

Rehabilitation Institute of Chicago | (312) 238-1000
Rehab Inst of Chicago
345 E. Superior Street | Chicago, IL 60611 | MIDWEST

Rehabilitation Institute of Michigan | (313) 745-1203
Rehab Inst of Mich
261 Mack Ave | Detroit, MI 48201 | MIDWEST

Rehabilitation Institute of St. Louis | (314) 658-3800
Rehab Inst St. Louis
4455 Duncan Ave | St. Louis, MO 63110 | MIDWEST

Renown Regional Medical Center | (775) 982-4100
Renown Reg Med Ctr
1155 Mill St | Reno, NV 89502 | WEST COAST AND PACIFIC

Resnick Neuropsychiatric Hospital at UCLA | (310) 825-0511
Resnick Neuropsychiatric Hosp at UCLA
760 Westwood Plaza | Los Angeles, CA 90095 | WEST COAST AND PACIFIC

Reston Hospital Center | (703) 689-9000
Reston Hosp Ctr
1850 Town Center Pkwy | Reston, VA 20190 | SOUTHEAST

Resurrection Health Care Saint Joseph Hospital | (773) 665-3000
Resurrection Hlth Care St Joseph Hosp
2900 N Lake Shore Dr | Chicago, IL 60657 | MIDWEST

Rex HealthCare | (919) 784-3100
Rex HlthCare
4420 Lake Boone Trail | Raleigh, NC 27607 | SOUTHEAST

Rhode Island Hospital | (401) 444-4000
Rhode Island Hosp
593 Eddy Street | Providence, RI 02903-4923 | NEW ENGLAND

Riddle Memorial Hospital | (610) 566-9400
Riddle Meml Hosp
1068 W Baltimore Pike | Media, PA 19063 | MID ATLANTIC

Riley Hospital for Children
Riley Hosp for Children
702 Barnhill Drive   Indianapolis, IN 46202   (317) 274-5000

MIDWEST

Riverside Community Hospital
Riverside Comm Hosp
4445 Magnolia Avenue   Riverside, CA 92502   (951) 788-3000

WEST COAST AND PACIFIC

Riverview Medical Center
Riverview Med Ctr
1 Riverview Plaza   Red Bank, NJ 07701   (732) 741-2700

MID ATLANTIC

Robert Wood Johnson University Hospital - New Brunswick
Robert Wood Johnson Univ Hosp - New Brunswick
1 Robert Wood Johnson Pl   New Brunswick, NJ 08903   (732) 828-3000

MID ATLANTIC

Rochester General Hospital
Rochester Genl Hosp
1425 Portland Avenue   Rochester, NY 14621   (585) 922-4000

MID ATLANTIC

Rochester Methodist Hospital
Rochester Methodist Hosp
201 W Center St   Rochester, MN 55905-3003   (507) 284-2511

MIDWEST

Rockefeller University
Rockefeller Univ
1230 York Avenue   New York, NY 10021   (212) 327-8000

MID ATLANTIC

Roger Williams Medical Center
Roger Williams Med Ctr
825 Chalkstone Avenue   Providence, RI 02908   (401) 456-2000

NEW ENGLAND

Roper Hospital
Roper Hosp
316 Calhoun St   Charleston, SC 29401   (843) 724-2000

SOUTHEAST

Rose Medical Center
Rose Med Ctr
4567 E 9th Ave   Denver, CO 80220-3941   (303) 320-2121

GREAT PLAINS AND MOUNTAINS

Roswell Park Cancer Institute
Roswell Park Cancer Inst
Elm and Carlton Streets   Buffalo, NY 14263   (716) 845-2300

MID ATLANTIC

Ruby Memorial - WVU Hospital
Ruby Memorial - WVU Hosp
1 Medical Center Drive   Morgantown, WV 26506   (304) 598-4000

MID ATLANTIC

Rush University Medical Center   (312) 942-5000
Rush Univ Med Ctr
1653 W Congress Pkwy   Chicago, IL 60612-3833   MIDWEST

Sacred Heart Medical Center   (541) 686-7300
Sacred Heart Med Ctr
1255 Hilyard St   Eugene, OR 97440-3700   WEST COAST AND PACIFIC

Saddleback Memorial Medical Center   (949) 837-4500
Saddleback Mem Med Ctr
24451 Health Center Drive   Laguna Hills, CA 92653   WEST COAST AND PACIFIC

Saint Barnabas Medical Center   (973) 322-5000
Saint Barnabas Med Ctr
94 Old Short Hills Rd   Livingston, NJ 07039-5672   MID ATLANTIC

Saint Francis Hospital - Memphis   (901) 765-1000
St. Francis Hosp - Memphis
5959 Park Ave   Memphis, TN 38119   SOUTHEAST

Saint John's Health Center   (310) 829-5511
St. John's Hlth Ctr, Santa Monica
1328 22nd St   Santa Monica, CA 90404   WEST COAST AND PACIFIC

Saint Joseph's Hospital - Atlanta   (404) 851-7001
St. Joseph's Hosp - Atlanta
5665 Peachtree Dunwoody Rd NE   Atlanta, GA 30342   SOUTHEAST

Saint Thomas Hospital - Nashville   (615) 222-2111
Saint Thomas Hosp - Nashville
4220 Harding Road   Nashville, TN 37205   SOUTHEAST

Salinas Valley Memorial Healthcare Systems   (831) 757-4333
Salinas Valley Meml Hlthcare Systs
450 E Romie Ln   Salinas, CA 93901   WEST COAST AND PACIFIC

Salt Lake Regional Medical Center   (801) 350-4111
Salt Lake Regional Med Ctr
1050 E South Temple   Salt Lake City, UT 84102   GREAT PLAINS AND MOUNTAINS

San Diego Hospice   (619) 688-1600
San Diego Hospice
4311 3rd Ave   San Diego, CA 92103-7499   WEST COAST AND PACIFIC

San Francisco General Hospital   (415) 206-8000
San Francisco Genl Hosp
1001 Potrero Avenue   San Francisco, CA 94110   WEST COAST AND PACIFIC

Sanford Medical Center Fargo		(701) 234-2000
Sanford Med Ctr Fargo		
801 Broadway Drive, PO Box MC	Fargo, ND 58122	GREAT PLAINS AND MOUNTAINS
Sanford USD Medical Center		(605) 333-1000
Sanford USD Med Ctr		
1305 W 18th St	Sioux Falls, SD 57717	GREAT PLAINS AND MOUNTAINS
Santa Barbara Cottage Hospital		(805) 682-7111
Santa Barbara Cottage Hosp		
Pueblo at Bath St	Santa Barbara, CA 93105	WEST COAST AND PACIFIC
Santa Clara Valley Medical Center		(408) 885-5000
Santa Clara Vly Med Ctr		
751 S Bascom Ave	San Jose, CA 95128	WEST COAST AND PACIFIC
Santa Monica - UCLA Medical Center and Orthopaedic Hospital		(310) 319-4000
Santa Monica - UCLA Med Ctr & Ortho Hosp		
1250 16th St	Santa Monica, CA 90404	WEST COAST AND PACIFIC
Sarasota Memorial Hospital		(941) 917-9000
Sarasota Meml Hosp		
1700 S Tamiami Trail	Sarasota, FL 34239	SOUTHEAST
Schwab Rehabilitation Hospital		(773) 522-2010
Schwab Rehab Hosp		
1401 S. California Boulevard	Chicago, IL 60608	MIDWEST
Scott & White Memorial Hospital		(254) 724-2111
Scott & White Mem Hosp		
2401 S 31st St	Temple, TX 76508-0001	SOUTHWEST
Scottsdale Healthcare - Osborn		(480) 675-4000
Scottsdale Hlthcare - Osborn		
7400 E Osborn Rd	Scottsdale, AZ 85251-6403	SOUTHWEST
Scottsdale Healthcare - Shea		(480) 860-3000
Scottsdale Hlthcare - Shea		
9000 E Shea Blvd	Scottsdale, AZ 85258-4514	SOUTHWEST
Scripps Green Hospital		(858) 455-9100
Scripps Green Hosp		
10666 N Torrey Pines Rd	La Jolla, CA 92037	WEST COAST AND PACIFIC
Scripps Memorial Hospital - La Jolla		(858) 457-4123
Scripps Meml Hosp - La Jolla		
9888 Genesee Ave	La Jolla, CA 92037	WEST COAST AND PACIFIC

Scripps Mercy Hospital & Medical Center   (619) 294-8111
Scripps Mercy Hosp & Med Ctr
4077 Fifth Ave   San Diego, CA 92103   WEST COAST AND PACIFIC

Seattle Children's Hospital   (206) 987-2000
Seattle Chldns Hosp
4800 Sand Point Way NE   Seattle, WA 98105   WEST COAST AND PACIFIC

Self Regional Healthcare   (864) 227-4111
Self Regional Healthcare
1325 Spring St   Greenwood, SC 29646   SOUTHEAST

Sentara Leigh Hospital   (757) 466-6000
Sentara Leigh Hosp
830 Kempsville Rd   Norfolk, VA 23502-3981   SOUTHEAST

Sentara Norfolk General Hospital   (757) 388-3000
Sentara Norfolk Genl Hosp
600 Gresham Dr   Norfolk, VA 23507   SOUTHEAST

Sentara Virginia Beach General Hospital   (757) 395-8000
Sentara VA Beach Genl Hosp
1060 First Colonial Rd   Virginia Beach, VA 23454   SOUTHEAST

Seton Medical Center   (512) 324-1000
Seton Med Ctr
1201 W 38th St   Austin, TX 78705   SOUTHWEST

Shady Grove Adventist Hospital   (301) 279-6000
Shady Grove Adven Hosp
9901 Medical Center Drive   Rockville, MD 20850   MID ATLANTIC

Shands at University of Florida   (352) 265-8000
Shands at Univ of FL
1600 SW Archer Rd   Gainesville, FL 32610   SOUTHEAST

Shands Jacksonville   (904) 244-0411
Shands Jacksonville
655 W 8th St   Jacksonville, FL 32209   SOUTHEAST

Shawnee Mission Medical Center   (913) 676-2000
Shawnee Mission Med Ctr
9100 W 74th St   Shawnee Mission, KS 66204   GREAT PLAINS AND MOUNTAINS

Shepherd Center - Atlanta   (404) 352-2020
Shepherd Ctr - Atlanta
2020 Peachtree Rd NW   Atlanta, GA 30309-1402   SOUTHEAST

Sheppard Pratt Health System   (410) 938-3000
Sheppard Pratt Hlth Sys
6501 N Charles St   Baltimore, MD 21285-6815   MID ATLANTIC

Sherman Hospital   (847) 742-9800
Sherman Hosp
934 Center St   Elgin, IL 60120   MIDWEST

Sibley Memorial Hospital   (202) 537-4000
Sibley Mem Hosp
5255 Loughboro Road NW   Washington, DC 20016   MID ATLANTIC

Silver Hill Hospital   (203) 966-3561
Silver Hill Hosp
208 Valley Rd   New Canaan, CT 06840-3899   NEW ENGLAND

Sinai Hospital - Baltimore   (410) 601-9000
Sinai Hosp - Baltimore
2401 W Belvedere Ave   Baltimore, MD 21215   MID ATLANTIC

Sinai-Grace Hospital   (313) 966-3300
Sinai-Grace Hosp
6071 W Outer Dr   Detroit, MI 48235   MIDWEST

Sky Ridge Medical Center   (720) 225-1000
Sky Ridge Med Ctr
10101 Ridge Gate Pkwy   Lone Tree, CO 80124   GREAT PLAINS AND MOUNTAINS

South Miami Hospital   (305) 661-4611
South Miami Hosp
6200 SW 73 St   South Miami, FL 33143   SOUTHEAST

South Nassau Communities Hospital   (516) 632-3000
South Nassau Comm Hosp
1 Healthy Way   Oceanside, NY 11572   MID ATLANTIC

Southampton Hospital   (631) 726-8200
Southampton Hosp
240 Meeting House Ln   Southampton, NY 11968   MID ATLANTIC

Southeast Baptist Hospital   (210) 297-3000
Southeast Baptist Hosp
4214 E Southcross Blvd   San Antonio, TX 78222   SOUTHWEST

Southern Arizona VA Health Care System - Tucson   (520) 792-1450
Southern AZ VA Health Care Sys - Tucson
3601 S 6th Avenue   Tucson, AZ 85723   SOUTHWEST

Southern Hills Hospital & Medical Center (702) 880-2100
Southern Hills Hosp & Med Ctr
9300 W Sunset Rd Las Vegas, NV 89148 WEST COAST AND PACIFIC

Southern New Hampshire Medical Center (603) 577-2000
Southern NH Med Ctr
8 Prospect St Nashua, NH 03061 NEW ENGLAND

Spaulding Rehabilitation Hospital (617) 573-7000
Spaulding Rehab Hosp
125 Nashua Street Boston, MA 02114 NEW ENGLAND

Spectrum Health - Blodgett Campus (616) 774-7444
Spectrum Hlth Blodgett Campus
1840 Wealthy St SE Grand Rapids, MI 49506 MIDWEST

Spectrum Health Butterworth Campus (616) 391-1774
Spectrum Hlth Butterworth Campus
100 Michigan St NE Grand Rapids, MI 49503 MIDWEST

SSM Cardinal Glennon Children's Hospital (314) 577-5600
Cardinal Glennon Mem Children's Hosp
1465 S Grand Blvd St Louis, MO 63104 MIDWEST

SSM St. Clare Health Ctr (636) 496-2000
SSM St. Clare Hlth Ctr
1015 Bowles Ave Fenton, MO 63026 MIDWEST

St. Alphonsus Regional Medical Center (208) 367-2121
St. Alphonsus Regl Med Ctr
1055 N Curtis Rd Boise, ID 83706-1370 GREAT PLAINS AND MOUNTAINS

St. Anthony Hospital - Oklahoma City (405) 272-7000
St. Anthony Hosp -Oklahoma City
1000 N Lee St Oklahoma City, OK 73102 SOUTHWEST

St. Anthony's Hospital - St Petersburg (727) 893-6814
St. Anthony's Hosp - St Petersburg
1200 7th Avenue North St Petersburg, FL 33705 SOUTHEAST

St. Christopher's Hospital for Children (215) 427-5000
St. Christopher's Hosp for Chldn
3601 A St Philadelphia, PA 19134 MID ATLANTIC

St. Elizabeth Healthcare-Edgewood (859) 301-2000
St. Elizabeth Hlthcare-Edgewood
1 Medical Village Dr Edgewood, KY 41017 SOUTHEAST

St. Francis Hospital & Medical Center   (860) 714-4000
St. Francis Hosp & Med Ctr
114 Woodland St   Hartford, CT 06105   NEW ENGLAND

St. Francis Hospital - Evanston   (847) 316-4000
St. Francis Hosp - Evanston
355 Ridge Ave   Evanston, IL 60202   MIDWEST

St. Francis Hospital - The Heart Center   (516) 562-6000
St. Francis Hosp - The Heart Ctr
100 Port Washington Boulevard   Roslyn, NY 11576   MID ATLANTIC

St. John's Hospital - Springfield   (217) 544-6464
St. John's Hosp - Springfield
800 E Carpenter St   Springfield, IL 62769   MIDWEST

St. John's Hospital-Maplewood MN   (651) 232-7000
St. John's Hosp-Maplewood MN
1575 Beam Ave   Maplewood, MN 55109   MIDWEST

St. John's Mercy Medical Center - St Louis   (314) 251-6000
St. John's Mercy Med Ctr - St Louis
615 S New Ballas Rd   St Louis, MO 63141   MIDWEST

St. Joseph Hospital   (773) 665-3000
St. Joseph Hosp
2900 N Lake Shore Drive   Chicago, IL 60657   MIDWEST

St. Joseph Hospital   (360) 734-5400
St. Joseph Hosp - Bellingham
2901 Squalicum Pkwy   Bellingham, WA 98225   WEST COAST AND PACIFIC

St. Joseph Hospital & Trauma Center   (603) 883-3414
St. Joseph Hosp & Trauma Ctr
172 Kinsley St   Nashua, NH 03060   NEW ENGLAND

St. Joseph Medical Center   (410) 337-1000
St. Joseph Med Ctr
7601 Osler Drive   Baltimore, MD 21208   MID ATLANTIC

St. Joseph Medical Center - Tacoma   (253) 627-4101
St. Joseph Med Ctr - Tacoma
1717 South J St   Tacoma, WA 98401   WEST COAST AND PACIFIC

St. Joseph Mercy Hospital - Ann Arbor   (734) 712-3456
St. Joseph Mercy Hosp - Ann Arbor
5301 E Huron River Dr, Box 992   Ann Arbor, MI 48106   MIDWEST

St. Joseph Mercy Oakland Hospital		(248) 858-3000
St. Joseph Mercy Oakland Hosp		
44405 Woodward Ave	Pontiac, MI 48341	MIDWEST

St. Joseph's Children's Hospital		(813) 554-8500
St. Josephs Chldns Hosp		
3001 W Dr Martin Luther King Jr Blvd	Tampa, FL 33607	SOUTHEAST

St. Joseph's Hospital & Medical Center - Phoenix		(602) 406-3000
St. Joseph's Hosp & Med Ctr - Phoenix		
350 W Thomas Rd	Phoenix, AZ 85013-4496	SOUTHWEST

St. Joseph's Hospital - Orange		(714) 633-9111
St. Joseph's Hosp - Orange		
1100 West Stewart Drive	Orange, CA 92868	WEST COAST AND PACIFIC

St. Joseph's Hospital - Tampa		(813) 870-4000
St. Joseph's Hosp - Tampa		
3001 W Martin Luther King Jr Blvd	Tampa, FL 33607	SOUTHEAST

St. Joseph's Hospital - Tucson		(520) 296-3211
St. Joseph's Hosp - Tucson		
350 N Wilmot Rd	Tucson, AZ 85711	SOUTHWEST

St. Joseph's Regional Medical Center - Paterson		(973) 754-2000
St. Joseph's Regl Med Ctr - Paterson		
703 Main St	Paterson, NJ 07503	MID ATLANTIC

St. Jude Children's Research Hospital		(901) 495-3300
St. Jude Children's Research Hosp		
262 Danny Thomas Pl	Memphis, TN 38105	SOUTHEAST

St. Louis Children's Hospital		(314) 454-6000
St. Louis Chldns Hosp		
One Children's Pl	St Louis, MO 63110	MIDWEST

St. Louis University Hospital		(314) 577-8000
St. Louis Univ Hosp		
3635 Vista at Grand Blvd	St Louis, MO 63110	MIDWEST

St. Luke's - Roosevelt Hospital Center - Roosevelt Division		(212) 523-4000
St. Luke's - Roosevelt Hosp Ctr - Roosevelt Div		
1000 Tenth Avenue	New York, NY 10019	MID ATLANTIC

St. Luke's - Roosevelt Hospital Center - St Luke's Hospital		(212) 523-4000
St. Luke's - Roosevelt Hosp Ctr - St Luke's Hosp		
1111 Amsterdam Ave	New York, NY 10025	MID ATLANTIC

St. Luke's Boise Medical Center (208) 381-2222
St. Luke's Boise Med Ctr
190 E Bannock St Boise, ID 83712 GREAT PLAINS AND MOUNTAINS

St. Luke's Episcopal Hospital-Houston (832) 355-1000
St. Luke's Episcopal Hosp-Houston
6720 Bertner Avenue, PO Box 20269 Houston, TX 77030 SOUTHWEST

St. Luke's Hospital - Allentown Campus (610) 770-8300
St. Luke's Hosp - Allentown
1736 Hamilton St Allentown, PA 18104 MID ATLANTIC

St. Luke's Hospital - Chesterfield, MO (314) 434-1500
St. Luke's Hosp - Chesterfield, MO
232 S Woods Mill Rd Chesterfield, MO 63017 MIDWEST

St. Luke's Hospital - Duluth (218) 249-5555
St. Luke's Hosp - Duluth
915 E 1st St Duluth, MN 55805-2193 MIDWEST

St. Luke's Hospital of Kansas City (816) 932-2000
St. Luke's Hosp of Kansas City
4401 Wornall Rd Kansas City, MO 64111 MIDWEST

St. Mark's Hospital - Salt Lake City (801) 268-7111
St. Mark's Hosp - Salt Lake City
1200 E. 3900 S Salt Lake City, UT 84124 GREAT PLAINS AND MOUNTAINS

St. Mary Medical Center - Long Beach (562) 491-9000
St. Mary Med Ctr - Long Beach
1050 Linden Ave Long Beach, CA 90813 WEST COAST AND PACIFIC

St. Mary's Hospital - Rochester, MN (Mayo Clinic) (507) 255-5123
St. Mary's Hosp - Rochester MN (Mayo)
1216 2nd St SW Rochester, MN 55902 MIDWEST

St. Mary's Medical Center - Huntington (304) 526-1234
St. Mary's Med Ctr - Huntington
2900 First Ave Huntington, WV 25702-1272 MID ATLANTIC

St. Mary's Medical Center - West Palm Beach (561) 844-6300
St. Mary's Med Ctr - W Palm Bch
901 45th St West Palm Beach, FL 33407 SOUTHEAST

St. Patrick Hospital & Health Sciences Center (406) 543-7271
St. Patrick Hospital - Missoula
500 W Broadway Missoula, MT 59802 GREAT PLAINS AND MOUNTAINS

St. Peter's Hospital - Albany   (518) 454-1550
St. Peter's Hosp - Albany
315 S Manning Blvd   Albany, NY 12208   MID ATLANTIC

St. Peter's University Hospital   (732) 745-8600
St. Peter's Univ Hosp
254 Easton Ave   New Brunswick, NJ 08901-1780   MID ATLANTIC

St. Rose Dominican Hospital - San Martin Campus   (702) 492-8000
St. Rose Dom Hosp-San Martin
8280 W Warm Springs Rd   Las Vegas, NV 89113   WEST COAST AND PACIFIC

St. Tammany Parish Hospital   (985) 898-4000
St. Tammany Parish Hosp
1202 S Tyler St   Covington, LA 70433   SOUTHWEST

St. Vincent Carmel Hospital   (317) 573-7000
St. Vincent Carmel Hosp
13500 N Meridian St   Carmel, IN 46032-1496   MIDWEST

St. Vincent Health System   (501) 552-3000
St. Vincent Health System
2 St. Vincent Cir   Little Rock, AR 72205   SOUTHWEST

St. Vincent Hospital - Green Bay   (920) 433-0111
St. Vincent Hosp - Green Bay
835 S Van Buren St, P.O. Box 13508   Green Bay, WI 54307-3508   MIDWEST

St. Vincent Indianapolis Hospital   (317) 338-2345
St. Vincent Indianapolis Hosp
2001 W 86th St   Indianapolis, IN 46260-1991   MIDWEST

St. Vincent Infirmary Medical Center & Doctors Hospital   (501) 552-3000
St. Vincent Med Ctr
2 St. Vincent Cir   Little Rock, AR 72205   SOUTHWEST

St. Vincent's Hospital - Birmingham   (205) 939-7000
St. Vincent's Hosp - Birmingham
810 St. Vincent's Drive or PO Box 12407   Birmingham, AL 35202-2407   SOUTHEAST

St. Vincent's Medical Center - Jacksonville   (904) 308-7300
St. Vincent's Med Ctr - Jacksonville
1800 Barrs St   Jacksonville, FL 32204   SOUTHEAST

St. Vincent's Medical Center - Los Angeles   (213) 484-7111
St. Vincent's Med Ctr - Los Angeles
2131 W 3rd St   Los Angeles, CA 90057   WEST COAST AND PACIFIC

Stamford Hospital (203) 276-1000
Stamford Hosp
30 Shelburne Rd @ W Broad St, Box 9317   Stamford, CT 06904   NEW ENGLAND

Stanford University Hospital & Clinics (650) 723-4000
Stanford Univ Hosp & Clinics
300 Pasteur Dr   Stanford, CA 94305   WEST COAST AND PACIFIC

Staten Island University Hospital - North (718) 226-9000
Staten Island Univ Hosp - North
475 Seaview Avenue   Staten Island, NY 10305   MID ATLANTIC

Steven and Alexandra Cohen Children's Medical Center of New York (718) 470-3000
Steven & Alexandra Cohen Chldn's Med Ctr of NY
269-01 76th Ave   New Hyde Park, NY 11040   MID ATLANTIC

Stony Brook University Medical Center (631) 444-4000
Stony Brook Univ Med Ctr
101 Nicolls Rd   Stony Brook, NY 11794-8410   MID ATLANTIC

Suburban Hospital (301) 896-3100
Suburban Hosp
8600 Old Georgetown Rd   Bethesda, MD 20814   MID ATLANTIC

Summerlin Hospital Medical Center (702) 233-7000
Summerlin Hosp Med Ctr
657 Town Center Drive   Las Vegas, NV 89144   WEST COAST AND PACIFIC

Sunnyview Hospital & Rehabilitation Center (518) 382-4500
Sunnyview Hosp & Rehab Ctr
1270 Belmont Ave   Schenectady, NY 12308-2198   MID ATLANTIC

Sunrise Hospital & Medical Center (702) 731-8000
Sunrise Hosp & Med Ctr
3186 Maryland Pkwy   Las Vegas, NV 89109   WEST COAST AND PACIFIC

SUNY Downstate Medical Center (University Hospital of Brooklyn) (718) 270-1000
SUNY Downstate Med Ctr
445 Lenox Rd   Brooklyn, NY 11203   MID ATLANTIC

SUNY Upstate Medical University Hospital (315) 464-5540
SUNY Upstate Med Univ Shos
750 E Adams Street   Syracuse, NY 13210   MID ATLANTIC

Swedish Covenant Hospital (773) 878-8200
Swedish Covenant Hosp
5145 N California Ave   Chicago, IL 60625   MIDWEST

Swedish Medical Center - Englewood
Swedish Med Ctr - Englewood
501 E Hamden Ave   Englewood, CO 80110   (303) 788-5000
GREAT PLAINS AND MOUNTAINS

Swedish Medical Center-First Hill Campus - Seattle
Swedish Med Ctr-First Hill-Seattle
747 Broadway   Seattle, WA 98122   (206) 386-6000
WEST COAST AND PACIFIC

Tampa General Hospital
Tampa Genl Hosp
1 Tampa General Cir, PO Box 1289   Tampa, FL 33601   (813) 844-7000
SOUTHEAST

Tanner Medical Center - Carrollton
Tanner Med Ctr
705 Dixie Street   Carrollton, GA 30117   (770) 836-9666
SOUTHEAST

Temple University Hospital
Temple Univ Hosp
3401 N Broad St   Philadelphia, PA 19140-5189   (215) 707-2000
MID ATLANTIC

Tennessee Valley Healthcare System - Nashville
TN Valley Healthcare Sys-Nashville
1310 24th Ave S   Nashville, TN 37212   (615) 327-4751
SOUTHEAST

Texas Children's Hospital
Texas Chldns Hosp
6621 Fannin St   Houston, TX 77030   (832) 824-1000
SOUTHWEST

Texas Health Presbyterian Hospital Dallas
TX Hlth Presby Hosp Dallas
8200 Walnut Hill Ln   Dallas, TX 75231   (214) 345-6789
SOUTHWEST

Texas Health Presbyterian Hospital Plano
TX Hlth Presby Hosp Plano
6200 West Parker Road   Plano, TX 75093   (972) 608-8000
SOUTHWEST

Texas Orthopedic Hospital
Texas Ortho Hosp
7401 S Main   Houston, TX 77030   (713) 799-8600
SOUTHWEST

Texas Scottish Rite Hospital for Children
Texas Scottish Rite Hosp for Chldn
2222 Welborn St   Dallas, TX 75219   (214) 559-5000
SOUTHWEST

Thomas Jefferson University Hospital
Thomas Jefferson Univ Hosp
111 S 11th St   Philadelphia, PA 19107   (215) 955-6000
MID ATLANTIC

TIRR-Institute for Rehabilitation & Research (713) 799-5000
TIRR-Inst for Rehab and Research
1333 Moursund   Houston, TX 77030   SOUTHWEST

Toledo Hospital   (419) 291-4000
Toledo Hosp
2142 N Cove Blvd   Toledo, OH 43606   MIDWEST

Touro Infirmary   (504) 897-7011
Touro Infirmary
1401 Foucher Street   New Orleans, LA 70115   SOUTHWEST

Tucson Medical Center   (520) 327-5461
Tucson Med Ctr
5301 E Grant Rd   Tucson, AZ 85733-2195   SOUTHWEST

Tufts Medical Center   (617) 636-5000
Tufts Med Ctr
750 Washington St   Boston, MA 02111   NEW ENGLAND

Tulane Medical Center   (504) 988-5800
Tulane Med Ctr
1415 Tulane Ave   New Orleans, LA 70112   SOUTHWEST

Tulane-Lakeside Hospital   (504) 780-8282
Tulane-Lakeside Hosp
4700 I-10 Service Rd   Metairie, LA 70001   SOUTHWEST

UAB Highlands Hospital   (205) 930-7000
UAB Highlands Hosp
1201 11th Ave S   Birmingham, AL 35205-5299   SOUTHEAST

UAB Spain Rehabilitation Center   (205) 934-3450
UAB Spain Rehab Ctr
1717 6th Ave S   Birmingham, AL 35249   SOUTHEAST

UCLA Ronald Reagan Medical Center   (310) 267-8000
UCLA Ronald Reagan Med Ctr
757 Westwood Plaza   Los Angeles, CA 90095   WEST COAST AND PACIFIC

UCSD Medical Center   (619) 543-6222
UCSD Med Ctr
200 W Arbor   San Diego, CA 92103   WEST COAST AND PACIFIC

UCSF - Mount Zion Medical Center   (415) 567-6600
UCSF - Mt Zion Med Ctr
1600 Divisadero St   San Francisco, CA 94115   WEST COAST AND PACIFIC

UCSF Medical Center   (415) 476-1000
UCSF Med Ctr
505 Parnassus Ave   San Francisco, CA 94143   WEST COAST AND PACIFIC

UMass Memorial Medical Center   (508) 334-1000
UMass Memorial Med Ctr
55 Lake Ave N   Worcester, MA 01655   NEW ENGLAND

UMass Memorial Medical Center - University Campus   (508) 334-1000
UMass Meml Med Ctr - Univ Campus
55 Lake Ave N   Worcester, MA 01655-0002   NEW ENGLAND

UMass Memorial Medical Center-Memorial Campus   (508) 334-1000
UMass Mem Med Ctr-Memorial Campus
119 Belmont St   Worcester, MA 01605   NEW ENGLAND

Union Memorial Hospital-Baltimore   (410) 554-2000
Union Meml Hosp-Baltimore
201 E University Pkwy   Baltimore, MD 21218   MID ATLANTIC

United Hospital   (651) 241-8000
United Hosp
333 N Smith Ave   St Paul, MN 55102   MIDWEST

University Community Hospital   (813) 971-6000
University Comm Hosp
3100 E Fletcher Avenue   Tampa, FL 33613   SOUTHEAST

University General Hospital   (713) 375-7000
Univ Genl Hosp-Houston
7501 Fannin St   Houston, TX 77054   SOUTHWEST

University Health System-San Antonio   (210) 358-4000
Univ Hlth Syst-San Antonio
4502 Medical Dr   San Antonio, TX 78229   SOUTHWEST

University Health Systems-Pitt County Memorial Hospital   (252) 847-4100
Univ Hlth Sys-Pitt Co Meml Hosp
2100 Stantonsburg Rd   Greenville, NC 27834   SOUTHEAST

University Hospital - Cincinnati   (513) 584-1000
Univ Hosp - Cincinnati
234 Goodman St   Cincinnati, OH 45219   MIDWEST

University Hospital - New Mexico   (505) 272-2111
Univ Hosp - New Mexico
2211 Lomas Blvd NE   Albuquerque, NM 87106   SOUTHWEST

University Hospital of Brooklyn at Long Island College Hospital (718) 780-1000
Univ Hosp of Bklyn at Long Island Coll Hosp
339 Hicks Street   Brooklyn, NY 11201   MID ATLANTIC

University Hospital-UMDNJ-Newark (973) 972-4300
Univ Hosp-UMDNJ—Newark
150 Bergen St   Newark, NJ 07103-2406   MID ATLANTIC

University Hospitals Case Medical Center (216) 844-8447
Univ Hosps Case Med Ctr
11100 Euclid Ave   Cleveland, OH 44106   MIDWEST

University Hospitals Rainbow Babies & Children's Hospital (216) 844-1000
UH Rainbow Babies & Chldns Hosp
11100 Euclid Ave   Cleveland, OH 44106   MIDWEST

University Medical Center at Princeton (609) 497-4000
Univ Med Ctr - Princeton
253 Witherspoon St   Princeton, NJ 08540   MID ATLANTIC

University Medical Center of Southern Nevada - Las Vegas (702) 383-2000
Univ Med Ctr - Las Vegas
1800 W Charleston Blvd   Las Vegas, NV 89102   WEST COAST AND PACIFIC

University Medical Center- Tucson (520) 694-0111
Univ Med Ctr - Tucson
1501 N Campbell Ave   Tucson, AZ 85724-5128   SOUTHWEST

University Medical Center-Lubbock (806) 775-8200
Univ Med Ctr-Lubbock
602 Indiana Ave   Lubbock, TX 79408   SOUTHWEST

University of Alabama Hospital at Birmingham (205) 934-4011
Univ of Ala Hosp at Birmingham
1802 6th Ave S   Birmingham, AL 35249-6544   SOUTHEAST

University of Arkansas for Medical Sciences Medical Center (501) 686-7000
UAMS Med Ctr
4301 W Markham St   Little Rock, AR 72205   SOUTHWEST

University of California - Davis Medical Center (916) 734-2011
UC Davis Med Ctr
2315 Stockton Blvd   Sacramento, CA 95817   WEST COAST AND PACIFIC

University of California - Irvine Medical Center (714) 456-7890
UC Irvine Med Ctr
101 The City Dr   Orange, CA 92868   WEST COAST AND PACIFIC

University of Chicago Comer Children's Hospital   (773) 702-1000
Univ Chicago-Comer Chldn's Hosp
5721 S Maryland Ave   Chicago, IL 60637   MIDWEST

University of Chicago Medical Center   (773) 702-1000
Univ of Chicago Med Ctr
5841 S Maryland Ave   Chicago, IL 60637   MIDWEST

University of Colorado Hospital-Anschutz Inpatient Pavilion   (720) 848-4011
Univ of CO Hosp - Anschutz Inpatient Pav
12605 E 16th Ave   Aurora, CO 80045   GREAT PLAINS AND MOUNTAINS

University of Connecticut Health Center - John Dempsey Hospital   (860) 679-2000
Univ of Conn Hlth Ctr, John Dempsey Hosp
263 Farmington Ave   Farmington, CT 06030   NEW ENGLAND

University of Illinois at Chicago Eye & Ear Infirmary   (312) 996-6500
Univ of IL at Chicago Eye & Ear Infirm
1855 W Taylor St   Chicago, IL 60612   MIDWEST

University of Illinois Medical Center at Chicago   (312) 355-4000
Univ of IL Med Ctr at Chicago
1740 W Taylor St, Ste 1400   Chicago, IL 60612   MIDWEST

University of Iowa Hospitals and Clinics   (319) 356-1616
Univ Iowa Hosp & Clinics
200 Hawkins Drive   Iowa City, IA 52242   MIDWEST

University of Kansas Hospital   (913) 588-5000
Univ of Kansas Hosp
3901 Rainbow Blvd   Kansas City, KS 66160   GREAT PLAINS AND MOUNTAINS

University of Kentucky Albert B. Chandler Hospital   (859) 323-5000
Univ of Kentucky Albert B. Chandler Hosp
800 Rose Street   Lexington, KY 40536   SOUTHEAST

University of Louisville Hospital   (502) 562-3000
Univ of Louisville Hosp
530 S Jackson St   Louisville, KY 40202   SOUTHEAST

University of Maryland Medical Center   (410) 328-8667
Univ of MD Med Ctr
22 S Greene St   Baltimore, MD 21201   MID ATLANTIC

University of Miami Hosp & Clinics/Sylvester Comprehensive Cancer Cntr   (305) 243-1000
Univ of Miami Hosp & Clins/Sylvester Comp Canc Ctr
1475 NW 12th Ave   Miami, FL 33136   SOUTHEAST

University of Miami Hospital (305) 325-5511
Univ of Miami Hosp
1400 NW 12 Ave Miami, FL 33136 SOUTHEAST

University of Michigan Hospital (734) 936-4000
Univ of Michigan Hosp
1500 E Medical Center Dr Ann Arbor, MI 48109 MIDWEST

University of Minnesota Medical Center, Fairview - Riverside Campus (612) 273-3000
Univ Minn Med Ctr, Fairview - Riverside Campus
2450 Riverside Ave S Minneapolis, MN 55454 MIDWEST

University of Mississippi Medical Center (601) 984-1000
Univ Mississippi Med Ctr
2500 N State St Jackson, MS 39216 SOUTHEAST

University of Missouri Hospital (573) 882-4141
Univ of Missouri Hosp
1 Hospital Dr Columbia, MO 65212 MIDWEST

University of Rochester Strong Memorial Hospital (585) 275-2100
Univ of Rochester Strong Meml Hosp
601 Elmwood Ave Rochester, NY 14642 MID ATLANTIC

University of South Alabama Medical Center (251) 471-7000
Univ of S AL Med Ctr
2451 Fillingim St Mobile, AL 36617 SOUTHEAST

University of Tennessee Medical Center (865) 305-9000
Univ of Tennesee Med Ctr
1924 Alcoa Hwy Knoxville, TN 37920 SOUTHEAST

University of Texas Health Science Center at Tyler (903) 877-3451
Univ of Texas Hlth Sci Ctr at Tyler
11937 US Hwy 271 Tyler, TX 75708 SOUTHWEST

University of Texas MD Anderson Cancer Center (713) 792-2121
UT MD Anderson Cancer Ctr
1515 Holcombe Blvd Houston, TX 77030-4095 SOUTHWEST

University of Texas Medical Branch at Galveston (409) 772-1011
UT Med Br at Galveston
301 University Blvd Galveston, TX 77555 SOUTHWEST

University of Toledo Medical Center (419) 383-4000
Univ of Toledo Med Ctr
3000 Arlington Ave Toledo, OH 43614 MIDWEST

University of Utah Health Care	(801) 581-2121
Univ Utah Hlth Care	
50 N Medical Dr	Salt Lake City, UT 84132 GREAT PLAINS AND MOUNTAINS

University of Virginia Health System	(434) 924-0211
Univ of Virginia Health Sys	
1215 Lee Street	Charlottesville, VA 22908-0001 SOUTHEAST

University of Washington Medical Center	(206) 598-3300
Univ Wash Med Ctr	
1959 NE Pacific St, PO Box 656355	Seattle, WA 98195 WEST COAST AND PACIFIC

University of Wisconsin Hospital & Clinics	(608) 263-6400
Univ WI Hosp & Clins	
600 Highland Avenue	Madison, WI 53792 MIDWEST

University Physicians Hospital at Kino	(520) 874-2000
University Physicians Hosp at Kino	
2800 E Ajo Way	Tucson, AZ 85713 SOUTHWEST

UPMC Hamot	(814) 877-6000
UPMC Hamot	
201 State Street	Erie, PA 16550-0001 MID ATLANTIC

UPMC Mercy	(412) 232-8111
UPMC Mercy, Pittsburgh	
1400 Locust Street	Pittsburgh, PA 15219 MID ATLANTIC

UPMC Montefiore	(412) 647-2345
UPMC Montefiore	
200 Lothrop St	Pittsburgh, PA 15213 MID ATLANTIC

UPMC Passavant-McCandless	(412) 367-6700
UPMC Passavant-McCandless	
9100 Babcock Blvd	Pittsburgh, PA 15237 MID ATLANTIC

UPMC Presbyterian	(412) 647-2345
UPMC Presby, Pittsburgh	
200 Lothrop St	Pittsburgh, PA 15213 MID ATLANTIC

UPMC Shadyside	(412) 623-2121
UPMC Shadyside	
5230 Centre Ave	Pittsburgh, PA 15232 MID ATLANTIC

UPMC South Side-Outpatient Center	(412) 488-5550
UPMC South Side-Out Pt Ctr	
2000 Mary St	Pittsburgh, PA 15203 MID ATLANTIC

UPMC St Margaret		(412) 784-4000
UPMC St Margaret		
815 Freeport Rd	Pittsburgh, PA 15215-3301	MID ATLANTIC
USC Norris Cancer Hospital		(323) 865-3000
USC Norris Cancer Hosp		
1441 Eastlake Ave	Los Angeles, CA 90033	WEST COAST AND PACIFIC
UT Southwestern Medical Center at Dallas		(214) 648-3111
UT Southwestern Med Ctr at Dallas		
5323 Harry Hines Blvd	Dallas, TX 75390	SOUTHWEST
VA Ann Arbor Healthcare System		(734) 769-7100
VA Ann Arbor Healthcare Sys		
2215 Fuller Rd	Ann Arbor, MI 48105	MIDWEST
VA Connecticut Healthcare System-West Haven Campus		(203) 932-5711
VA Conn Hlthcre Sys-W Haven Campus		
950 Campbell Ave	West Haven, CT 06516	NEW ENGLAND
VA Greater Los Angeles Healthcare System		(310) 478-3711
VA Greater Los Angeles Hthecare Sys		
11301 Wilshire Blvd	Los Angeles, CA 90073	WEST COAST AND PACIFIC
VA Health Care System - Palo Alto		(650) 493-5000
VA Hlth Care Sys - Palo Alto		
3801 Miranda Ave	Palo Alto, CA 94304	WEST COAST AND PACIFIC
VA Medical Center - Memphis		(901) 523-8990
VA Med Ctr - Memphis		
1030 Jefferson Ave	Memphis, TN 38104	SOUTHEAST
VA Medical Center - Portland		(503) 220-8262
VA Medical Center - Portland		
3710 SW US Veteran Hospital Rd, PO Box 1034 Portland, OR 97239		WEST COAST AND PACIFIC
VA Medical Center - San Francisco		(415) 221-4810
VA Med Ctr - San Francisco		
4150 Clement St	San Francisco, CA 94121	WEST COAST AND PACIFIC
VA Medical Center - Washington, DC		(202) 745-8000
VA Med Ctr - Washington		
50 Irving St NW	Washington, DC 20422	MID ATLANTIC
VA Puget Sound Health Care System		(206) 762-1010
VA Puget Sound Hlth Care Sys		
1660 S Columbian Way	Seattle, WA 98108	WEST COAST AND PACIFIC

VA San Diego Healthcare System   (858) 552-8585
VA San Diego Hlthcre Sys
3350 La Jolla Village Drive   San Diego, CA 92161   WEST COAST AND PACIFIC

VA Tennessee Valley Healthcare System-Alvin C. York Campus   (615) 867-6000
VA Tennessee Valley Healthcare System-Alvin C. Yor
3400 Lebanon Pike   Murfreesboro, TN 37129   SOUTHEAST

Vail Valley Medical Center   (970) 476-2451
Vail Valley Med Ctr
181 W Meadow Dr   Vail, CO 81657-5058   GREAT PLAINS AND MOUNTAINS

Valley Medical Center - Renton, WA   (425) 228-3450
Valley Med Ctr-Renton, WA
404 S 43 St   Renton, WA 98058-5010   WEST COAST AND PACIFIC

Vanderbilt Monroe Carrell Jr. Children's Hospital   (615) 936-1000
Vanderbilt Monroe Carrell Jr. Chldn's Hosp
2200 Children's Way   Nashville, TN 37232   SOUTHEAST

Vanderbilt University Medical Center   (615) 322-5000
Vanderbilt Univ Med Ctr
1211 Medical Center Drive   Nashville, TN 37232   SOUTHEAST

VCU Medical Center   (904) 828-9000
VCU Med Ctr
1250 E Marshall St, PO Box 980510   Richmond, VA 23298   SOUTHEAST

Virginia Hospital Center - Arlington   (703) 558-5000
Virginia Hosp Ctr - Arlington
1701 N George Mason Dr   Arlington, VA 22205-3698   SOUTHEAST

Virginia Mason Medical Center   (206) 223-6600
Virginia Mason Med Ctr
1100 Ninth Ave, Box 900   Seattle, WA 98111   WEST COAST AND PACIFIC

Wake Forest University Baptist Medical Center   (336) 716-2255
Wake Forest Univ Baptist Med Ctr
Medical Center Blvd   Winston-Salem, NC 27157-1015   SOUTHEAST

WakeMed Cary Hospital   (919) 350-2300
WakeMed Cary
1900 Kildaire Farm Rd   Cary, NC 27511-6616   SOUTHEAST

WakeMed-Raleigh Campus   (919) 350-8000
WakeMed-Raleigh Campus
3000 New Bern Ave   Raleigh, NC 27610   SOUTHEAST

Walter Reed National Military Medical Center		(301) 295-4611
Walter Reed Natl Military Med Ctr		
8901 Wisconsin Ave	Bethesda, MD 20889-5600	MID ATLANTIC
Washington Hospital Center		(202) 877-7000
Washington Hosp Ctr		
110 Irving St NW	Washington, DC 20010	MID ATLANTIC
Washington Hospital, The		(724) 225-7000
Washington Hosp, The		
155 Wilson Ave	Washington, PA 15301	MID ATLANTIC
Washington University Physicians		(314) 362-6828
Washington Univ Physicians		
4444 Forest Park Ave	St Louis, MO 63108	MIDWEST
WellStar Windy Hill Hospital		(770) 644-1000
WellStar Windy Hill Hosp		
2540 Windy Hill Road	Marietta, GA 30067	SOUTHEAST
Wesley Woods Geriatric Hospital		(404) 728-6200
Wesley Woods Ger Hosp		
1821 Clifton Rd	Atlanta, GA 30329	SOUTHEAST
West Jefferson Medical Center		(504) 347-5511
West Jefferson Med Ctr		
1101 Medical Ctr Blvd	Marrero, LA 70072	SOUTHWEST
Westchester Medical Center		(914) 493-7000
Westchester Med Ctr		
95 Grasslands Road	Valhalla, NY 10595	MID ATLANTIC
Western Maryland Hospital Center		(301) 745-4200
W MD Hosp Ctr		
1500 Pennsylvania Ave	Hagerstown, MD 21742	MID ATLANTIC
Western Pennsylvania Hospital		(412) 578-5000
Western Penn Hosp		
4800 Friendship Avenue	Pittsburgh, PA 15224	MID ATLANTIC
Western Psychiatric Institute and Clinic-UPMC		(412) 624-1000
Western Psych Inst & Clin-UPMC		
3811 O'Hara St	Pittsburgh, PA 15213	MID ATLANTIC
Wheaton Franciscan Healthcare-St Joseph		(414) 447-2000
Wheaton Franciscan Hlthcare-St Joseph-Milwaukee		
5000 W. Chambers Street	Milwaukee, WI 53210	MIDWEST

White River Junction VA Medical Center   (802) 295-9363
White River Junction VA Med Ctr
215 North Maine Street   White River Junction, VT 05009   NEW ENGLAND

Wills Eye Hospital   (215) 928-3000
Wills Eye Hosp
840 Walnut St   Philadelphia, PA 19107-5598   MID ATLANTIC

Wilmington Hospital   (302) 733-1000
Wilmington Hosp
501 W 14th St   Wilmington, DE 19801   MID ATLANTIC

Winthrop University Hospital   (516) 663-0333
Winthrop Univ Hosp
259 1st St   Mineola, NY 11501   MID ATLANTIC

Wolfson Children's Hospital   (904) 202-8000
Wolfson Chldns Hosp
800 Prudential Dr   Jacksonville, FL 32207   SOUTHEAST

Woman's Hospital of Texas   (713) 790-1234
Woman's Hosp TX
7600 Fannin St   Houston, TX 77054   SOUTHWEST

Women & Infants Hospital of Rhode Island   (401) 274-1100
Women & Infants Hosp of RI
101 Dudley Street   Providence, RI 02905   NEW ENGLAND

Women's and Children's Hospital of Buffalo, The   (716) 878-7000
Women's & Chldn's Hosp of Buffalo, The
219 Bryant St   Buffalo, NY 14222   MID ATLANTIC

Yakima Valley Memorial Hospital   (509) 575-8000
Yakima Valley Mem Hosp
2811 Tieton Dr   Yakima, WA 98902-3799   WEST COAST AND PACIFIC

Yale Medical Group
Yale Med Group
300 George St Fl 6   New Haven, CT 06511   NEW ENGLAND

Yale-New Haven Hospital   (203) 688-4242
Yale-New Haven Hosp
20 York St   New Haven, CT 06510   NEW ENGLAND

Yampa Valley Medical Center   (970) 879-1322
Yampa Valley Med Ctr
1024 Central Park Dr   Steamboat Springs, CO 80487   GREAT PLAINS AND MOUNTAINS

Zucker Hillside Hospital   (718) 470-8000
Zucker Hillside Hosp
75-59 263rd St   Glen Oaks, NY 11004   MID ATLANTIC

Appendix D:
Selected Resources

GENERAL RESOURCES

AMERICAN AMBULANCE ASSOCIATION (AAA)
The American Ambulance Association represents emergency and non-emergency medical transportation providers, advocating high quality pre-hospital care and keeping these providers aware of legislation and news that may affect them.

8400 West Park Drive, FL2
McLean, VA 22102

800-523-4447
703-610-9018
fax 703-610-0210
www.the-aaa.org/

AMERICA'S HEALTH INSURANCE PLANS (AHIP)
America's Health Insurance Plans is a national trade association representing nearly 1,300 member companies providing health benefits to more than 200 million Americans.

601 Pennsylvania Ave, NW
South Building Suite 500
Washington, DC 20004

202-778-3200
fax: 202-331-7487
www.ahip.org/

AMERICAN BOARD OF MEDICAL SPECIALTIES (ABMS)
The ABMS is the authoritative body for the recognition of medical specialties, coordinating 24 medical specialty boards (including 25 medical specialties) and providing information on the board certification of doctors.

222 N LaSalle, Ste 1500
Chicago, Illinois 60601

312-436-2600 or 866-ASK-ABMS
fax 847-328-3596
www.abms.org

AMERICAN HOSPITAL ASSOCIATION (AHA)
A national health advocacy organization, the AHA represents hospitals and healthcare networks in legislative and regulatory matters. In 1973 the AHA adopted the Patient Bill of Rights to help patients understand their rights and responsibilities.

155 N Wacker Drive
Chicago, IL 60606

800-424-4301 or 312-422-3000
fax 312-422-4796
www.aha.org/

325 7th St. NW
Washington, DC 20004

800-424-4301 or 202-638-1100
fax 202-626-2345

AMERICAN MEDICAL ASSOCIATION (AMA)

The AMA is an association that maintains information on physicians practicing throughout the nation. Healthcare consumers can use their database to check the location, licensing, education and specialty of many doctors in the United States.

515 North State Street
Chicago, IL 60610

800-621-8335
www.ama-assn.org/

CENTER FOR MEDICAL CONSUMERS

Provides volume and outcome data on certain medical procedures performed in New York state.

239 Thompson St.
New York, NY 10012

212-674-7105
fax 212-674-7100
centerformedicalconsumers@gmail.com
www.medicalconsumers.org

CENTERS FOR DISEASE CONTROL AND PREVENTION (CDC)

Part of the Department of Health and Human Services, the CDC's mission is to prevent and manage diseases and illnesses. Its Web site contains information on a range of illnesses and the research being pursued to manage them. It also provides free faxed reports on disease risk and prevention in various parts of the world.

Public Inquiries/MASO
Mailstop E11
1600 Clifton Road
Atlanta, GA 30333

800-CDC-INFO
TTY: 888-232-6348

toll free number for international travelers 877 FYI-TRIP or 404-639-3534
fax information service for international travelers 888-232-3299
www.cdc.gov/netinfo.htm

THE CENTERWATCH CLINICAL TRIALS LISTING SERVICE

Profiles centers conducting clinical research by therapeutic area and geographic region, including more than 41,000 international industry and government-sponsored clinical trials and new FDA approved drug therapies, as well as 5,200 clinical trials that are actively recruiting patients.

10 Winthrop Square
Fl 5
Boston, MA 02110

617-948-5100
fax 617-948-5101
www.centerwatch.com

INTERNATIONAL ASSOCIATION FOR MEDICAL ASSISTANCE TO TRAVELLERS (IAMAT)

IAMAT is a non-profit organization that disseminates information on health and sanitary conditions worldwide. Membership is free but donations are appreciated. Members will receive a membership card making them eligible to access English speaking physicians all over the world. The organization also provides information on immunization requirements, malaria, and other tropical diseases, and sanitary and climactic conditions around the world. For information, send request in writing.

1623 Military Road #279
Niagra Falls, New York 14304-1745

716-754-4883
www.iamat.org

JOINT COMMISSION ON ACCREDITATION OF HEALTHCARE ORGANIZATIONS

The Joint Commission (JCAHO) is an independent, not-for-profit organization, which evaluates the quality and safety of care for nearly 17,000 health care organizations. To maintain and earn accreditation, organizations must have an extensive on-site review by a team of JCAHO health care professionals, at least once every three years. JCAHO is governed by a board that includes physicians, nurses, and consumers. JCAHO sets the standards by which health care quality is measured in America and around the world.

One Renaissance Boulevard   630-792-5000
Oakbrook Terrace, IL 60181   fax 630-792-5005
                                             www.jcaho.org

MEDIC ALERT FOUNDATION

The Medic Alert Foundation (a non-profit organization) provides an "ID tag" engraved with personal medical facts, as well as a 24-hour emergency response center which can release additional personal medical details. Membership is $30/year (plus $9.95 initial setup fee) and members need to purchase the "ID tag" which sells for as low as $35.

2323 Colorado Avenue   888-633-4298
Turlock, CA 95382   Fax 209-669-2450
                                             www.medicalert.org

MEDLINE

One Medline Place   1-800-MEDLINE (800-633-5463)
Mundelein, Illinois 60060   fax 1-800-351-1512
                                             www.medline.com

A medical database including millions of medical references and abstracts from thousands of scientific and medical journals.

THE NATIONAL CANCER INSTITUTE (NCI)

Part of the NIH, the NCI sponsors cancer clinical trials at more than 100 sites in the United States. Trials are carried out in major medical research centers, such as teaching hospitals, as well as in community hospitals, specialized medical clinics and even in doctors' offices.

Clinical Studies Support Center (CSSC)   800-4-CANCER (800-422-6237)
6116 Executive Boulevard   www.nci.nih.gov
Bethesda, MD 20892-8322   www.cancer.gov
                                             cancergovstaff@mail.nih.gov

NATIONAL CENTER FOR COMPLEMENTARY AND ALTERNATIVE MEDICINE CLEARINGHOUSE (NCCAMC)

The NCCAMC facilitates the evaluation of alternative medical treatment modalities to help determine their effectiveness and bring alternative medicine into mainstream medicine. This agency does not provide referrals.

9000 Rockville Pike   888-644-6226
Bethesda, MD 20892   fax 866-464-3616
                                             www.nccam.nih.gov
                                             info@nccam.nih.gov

NATIONAL CONSUMERS LEAGUE (NCL)

NCL is a private, nonprofit consumer advocacy organization. NCL strives to investigate, educate, and advocate on a variety of issues including healthcare. Membership is $20 annually, but individuals can also write to the organization for a list of publications that non-members can purchase.

1701 K Street, NW, Suite 1200
Washington, DC 20006

202-835-3323
fax 202-835-0747
www.nclnet.org
info@nclnet.org

THE NATIONAL INSTITUTES OF HEALTH (NIH)

An organization operated by the U.S. government, the NIH operates its own hospital at which the care provided is usually related to clinical studies its researchers are undertaking. Information about the Warren G. Magnuson Clinical Center is also available.

Patient Recruitment Referral Center
9000 Rockville Pike
Bethesda, MD 20892

212-346-5500
www.nih.gov
www.clinicaltrials.gov
nihinfo@od.nih.gov

NATIONAL INSURANCE INFORMATION INSTITUTE

The National Insurance Information Institute Helpline advises consumers on how to choose an insurance company or broker. It also offers an analysis of life insurance and assists in insurance complaints.

110 William St
New York, NY 10038

800-411-1222 or 301-496-4000
www.iii.org

THE PATIENT ADVOCATE FOUNDATION

A national non-profit organization that provides consultation, referrals and case management to patients to ensure that they are not denied access to healthcare, insurance coverage, employment and public assistance programs during an illness. In particular, the organization maintains comprehensive information on cancer treatment options that are available to consumers through a separate Web site: www.oncology.com.

421 Butler Farm Rd
Hampton, VA 23666

800-532-5274
fax 757-873-8999
www.patientadvocate.org/
help@patientadvocate.org

PEOPLE'S MEDICAL SOCIETY

The People's Medical Society, a nonprofit organization, is focused on educating the healthcare consumer about healthcare issues and medical rights. Their Web site provides information on useful books and publications as well as the latest healthcare developments.

P.O. Box 868
Allentown, PA 18105

610-770-1670
fax 610-770-0607
cbi@peoplesmed.org

PERSONS UNITED LIMITING SUBSTANDARDS AND ERRORS IN HEALTHCARE (P.U.L.S.E.)
A support group for the survivors of medical malpractice and substandard healthcare, this nonprofit group also advocates patient education and patient-doctor communication.

PO Box 353
Wantagh NY 11793-0353

800-96-pulse (800-967-8573) or
516-579-4711
fax: 516-520-8105
www.PULSEamerica.org
www.PULSEofNY.com
pulse516@aol.com

Colorado Office

719-250-1286
PULSECOLO@YAHOO.COM

PUBLIC CITIZEN'S HEALTH AND RESEARCH GROUP
A non-profit organization, the Public Citizen's Group acts as a watchdog agency by advocating accountability and the open use of doctors' disciplinary backgrounds.

1600 20th Street NW
Washington, D.C. 20009

202-588-1000
www.citizen.org/hrg/

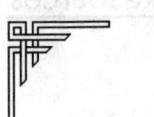

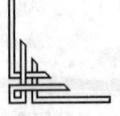
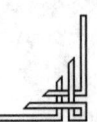

The Best in American Medicine
www.CastleConnolly.com

Appendix E:
Sources of Quality Data on Hospitals

U.S. NEWS AND WORLD REPORT

U.S. News & World Report has been the nation's leading source of information on hospital rankings since 1990. The Best Hospitals rankings evaluate medical centers on their competence in high-stakes situations. Their annual feature on Best Hospitals has become the standard in the field where rankings are concerned and is heavily anticipated and utilized by consumers and members of the health care profession. Castle Connolly teamed up with *U.S. News & World Report* in July 2011 to bring its listing of Top Doctors online to www.usnews.com/health in conjunction with the Top Hospitals rankings. There, consumers can search the full Castle Connolly database of nearly 30,000 Top Doctors across the nation.

WWW.WHYNOTTHEBEST.ORG

WhyNotTheBest.org was created and is maintained by The Commonwealth Fund, a private foundation working toward a high performance health system. It is a free resource for health care professionals and consumers interested in tracking performance on various measures of health care quality. It enables organizations to compare their performance against that of peer organizations, against a range of benchmarks and over a given period of time. Case studies and improvement tools spotlight successful improvement strategies of the nation's top performers. A regional map shows performance at the county, state and national levels. This site also includes process-of-care measures, patient satisfaction measures, readmission rates, mortality rates and average reimbursement rates. All of these performance measures are publicly reported on the Centers for Medicare and Medicaid Services website, Hospital Compare, and include data from nearly all U.S. hospitals.

THE LEAPFROG GROUP

The Leapfrog Group, http://www.leapfroggroup.org/cp, started in 1998 by a group of large employers. The Leapfrog Hospital Survey compares hospitals' performance on the national standards of safety, quality and efficiency - areas of healthcare that are most relevant to consumers. Hospitals that participate in The Leapfrog Hospital Survey achieve hospital-wide improvements that translate into saving millions of lives and cutting costs for hospitals and consumers. Leapfrog's survey results are later used to inform key employees on purchasing strategies.

HOSPITAL COMPARE

The Hospital Compare website was created through the efforts of the Centers for Medicare & Medicaid Services (CMS), an agency of the U.S. Department of Health and Human Services (DHHS), along with the Hospital Quality Alliance (HQA). The HQA was established to promote reporting on hospital quality of care. The HQA consists of organizations that represent consumers, hospitals, doctors and nurses, employers, accrediting organizations and Federal agencies. The information on this website can be used by patients requiring hospital care. This information helps the consumer and health care providers to compare the quality of care provided in participating hospitals. This information not only helps one to make good decisions about health care, but also encourages hospitals to improve the quality of the care that they provide to their communities. This website can be found at: http://www.hospitalcompare.hhs.gov/hospital-search.aspx or http://bit.ly/jdvCzW

Indices

Subject Index

A

B

C

D

E

F

G

H

I

L

Professional Reputation 13

Protocol 27-28, 30

R

Recertification 12, 50

Referral 3, 8, 14, 18, 35

Residency 2, 10-11, 16-17, 37, 49-50

S

Second Opinions 17-18

Selection Process 2

Self-Designated Medical Specialties 12

Side Effects 26-27, 32-33

Special Resources 25-26, 28, 30, 32, 34

Specialists 1-10, 12, 14-16, 18, 37, 41, 43, 49-51, 53

Specialties 3-6, 9-12, 14, 24, 38, 41-47, 49-51, 53

Standard Therapies 25

Subspecialties 1, 5-6, 10, 12-13, 15, 41-42, 49-50, 53

T

Therapeutic Approaches 1, 6, 25

Treatment Plan 21, 30

Treatment Studies 25, 30

Trust 19

U

United States Department of Health 33

United States Medical Licensing Exam 9

V

Veritas Medicine 26

W

Specialty & Special Expertise Index

This index lists the areas that the physicians listed in the Guide have identified as their "special expertise." They are specific elements of disease, procedures, techniques and treatments for which these physicians are best known and are referred patients. Each doctor's medical specialty is also included.

Spec	Name	St	Pg

A

Abdominal Imaging

Spec	Name	St	Pg
DR	Berland, L	AL	978
DR	Coakley, F	CA	982
DR	Federle, M	CA	983
DR	Fishman, E	MD	975
DR	Levy, A	DC	976
DR	Megibow, A	NY	976
DR	Sivit, C	OH	981
DR	Weinreb, J	CT	973
DR	Zagoria, R	NC	979

Abdominal Wall Reconstruction

Spec	Name	St	Pg
PlS	Kuzon, W	MI	863
PlS	Seyfer, A	MD	855
PlS	Stahl, R	CT	849
S	Bellows, C	LA	1082
S	Fitzgibbons, R	NE	1080
S	Franz, M	MI	1072

Abdominoplasty

Spec	Name	St	Pg
PlS	Erdmann, D	NC	859
PlS	Eriksson, E	MA	848
PlS	Gallico, G	MA	848
PlS	Hunstad, J	NC	860
PlS	Lesavoy, M	CA	873
PlS	Markowitz, B	CA	873
PlS	Matarasso, A	NY	854
PlS	Nahabedian, M	DC	854
PlS	Ness, J	MN	864
PlS	Pitman, G	NY	855
PlS	Singh, N	MD	856

Abuse/Neglect

Spec	Name	St	Pg
AM	Diaz, A	NY	80
ChAP	Zeanah, C	LA	908
Ger	Lachs, M	NY	263

Achalasia

Spec	Name	St	Pg
Ge	Ravich, W	MD	237
Ge	Vaezi, M	TN	242

Acne

Spec	Name	St	Pg
D	Barbosa, V	IL	193
D	Del Giudice, S	NH	182
D	Eichenfield, L	CA	198
D	James, W	PA	187
D	Lowitt, M	MD	187

Spec	Name	St	Pg
D	Lucky, A	OH	194

Acoustic Neuroma

Spec	Name	St	Pg
NS	Adler, J	CA	491
NS	Black, K	CA	492
NS	Eisenberg, H	MD	469
NS	Giannotta, S	CA	493
NS	Golfinos, J	NY	469
NS	Grubb, R	MO	484
NS	Gutin, P	NY	470
NS	Harsh, G	CA	493
NS	Judy, K	PA	471
NS	Martuza, R	MA	467
NS	Mayberg, M	WA	494
NS	Sisti, M	NY	474
NS	Stieg, P	NY	475
NS	Swaid, S	AL	481
NS	Thompson, B	MI	486
Oto	Arriaga, M	LA	680
Oto	Beatty, C	MN	672
Oto	Brackmann, D	CA	683
Oto	Driscoll, C	MN	673
Oto	Duckert, L	WA	683
Oto	Feghali, J	NY	658
Oto	Jenkins, H	CO	679
Oto	Kveton, J	CT	656
Oto	Lambert, P	SC	667
Oto	Linstrom, C	NY	662
Oto	Miyamoto, R	IN	675
Oto	Roland, J	NY	663
Oto	Rubinstein, J	WA	685
Oto	Shelton, C	UT	679
Oto	Telian, S	MI	677
Oto	Wackym, P	OR	686
Oto	Wazen, J	FL	671
Oto	Wiet, R	IL	677
RadRO	Loeffler, J	MA	945

Acromegaly

Spec	Name	St	Pg
EDM	Biller, B	MA	204
EDM	Katznelson, L	CA	221
EDM	Klibanski, A	MA	205
EDM	Melmed, S	CA	221
Onc	Chang, S	CA	383

Acupuncture

Spec	Name	St	Pg
PM	Ngeow, J	NY	696
PMR	Borg-Stein, J	MA	832
PMR	Dillard, J	NY	833

Acute Coronary Syndromes

Spec	Name	St	Pg
Cv	Brindis, R	CA	114

Spec	Name	St	Pg
Cv	Eagle, K	MI	105
IC	Bach, R	MO	128
IC	Gibson, C	MA	123
IC	Henry, T	MN	128
IC	Holmes, D	MN	129

ADD/ADHD

Spec	Name	St	Pg
ChAP	Abright, A	NY	904
ChAP	Alessi, N	MI	907
ChAP	Biederman, J	MA	903
ChAP	Bird, H	NY	904
ChAP	Bogrov, M	MD	904
ChAP	Boxer, G	MO	907
ChAP	Coffey, B	NY	905
ChAP	Dulcan, M	IL	907
ChAP	Hertzig, M	NY	905
ChAP	Heston, J	TN	906
ChAP	Hirsch, G	NY	905
ChAP	Hudziak, J	VT	903
ChAP	Koplewicz, H	NY	905
ChAP	Kwon, H	WA	909
ChAP	Leventhal, B	NY	905
ChAP	Martini, D	UT	908
ChAP	Rostain, A	PA	906
ChAP	Russell, A	CA	909
ChAP	Slomowitz, M	IL	907
ChAP	Spencer, T	MA	904
ChAP	Turecki, S	NY	906
ChAP	Wilens, T	MA	904
ChiN	Nass, R	NY	146
N	Finkel, M	FL	519
Ped	Burgess, D	NJ	726
Ped	Hershorin, E	FL	727
Ped	Jacob, M	IL	728
Ped	Roizen, N	OH	728
Psyc	Hoffman, D	CO	895
Psyc	Keepers, G	OR	897

ADD/PTSD

Spec	Name	St	Pg
Psyc	Manevitz, A	NY	889

Addiction Psychiatry

Spec	Name	St	Pg
AdP	Anton, R	SC	901
AdP	Ciraulo, D	MA	900
AdP	Frances, R	NY	901
AdP	Galanter, M	NY	901
AdP	Greenfield, S	MA	900
AdP	Howell, E	UT	902
AdP	Kampman, K	PA	901
AdP	Kleber, H	NY	901
AdP	Kosten, T	TX	902
AdP	Nitenson, N	MA	900

Specialty & Special Expertise Index

Specialty & Special Expertise Index

Spec	Name	St	Pg
A&I	Wong, J	MA	84
A&I	Wood, J	MO	88

Allergy up to age 50

Spec	Name	St	Pg
PA&I	Bock, S	CO	732

Alopecia Areata

Spec	Name	St	Pg
D	Duvic, M	TX	197

Alzheimer's Disease

Spec	Name	St	Pg
Ger	Carr, D	MO	265
Ger	Gorbien, M	IL	265
Ger	Liem, P	AR	266
Ger	Morley, J	MO	265
Ger	Sachs, G	IN	265
GerPsy	Borson, S	WA	912
GerPsy	Burke, W	NE	911
GerPsy	Grossberg, G	MO	911
GerPsy	Kennedy, G	NY	910
GerPsy	Lyketsos, C	MD	910
GerPsy	Reisberg, B	NY	910
GerPsy	Rosen, J	PA	910
GerPsy	Rovner, B	PA	910
GerPsy	Small, G	CA	912
GerPsy	Streim, J	PA	910
GerPsy	Tune, L	GA	911
N	Ahern, G	AZ	530
N	Chui, H	CA	534
N	Cummings, J	NV	534
N	DeKosky, S	VA	518
N	Doody, R	TX	531
N	Farlow, M	IN	524
N	Feinberg, T	NY	509
N	Filley, C	CO	529
N	Gilman, S	MI	524
N	Henderson, V	CA	535
N	Longo, F	CA	536
N	Mesulam, M	IL	526
N	Miller, A	NY	513
N	Morris, J	MO	526
N	Petersen, R	MN	527
N	Relkin, N	NY	514
N	Sadowsky, C	FL	521
N	Zimmerman, E	NY	517
NS	Rezai, A	OH	485
Psyc	Arnold, S	PA	886
Psyc	Raskind, M	WA	898
Psyc	Weiner, M	TX	896

Amblyopia

Spec	Name	St	Pg
Oph	Gallin, P	NY	572
Oph	Miller, J	AZ	595
Oph	Tychsen, L	MO	592
Oph	Weiss, A	WA	601

Amblyopia & Vision Development

Spec	Name	St	Pg
Oph	Burke, M	OH	586

Amniocentesis

Spec	Name	St	Pg
MF	Grunebaum, A	NY	429
MF	McLaren, R	VA	431
MF	Nies, B	VA	431
MF	Philipson, E	OH	433
MF	Robinson, J	MA	427
MF	Strassner, H	IL	433

Amniotic Membrane Transplant

Spec	Name	St	Pg
Oph	John, T	IL	588

Amputation Surgery

Spec	Name	St	Pg
OrS	Pinzur, M	IL	635
OrS	Smith, D	WA	643

Amputee Rehabilitation

Spec	Name	St	Pg
PMR	Dillingham, T	WI	838
PMR	Esquenazi, A	PA	833
PMR	Gittler, M	IL	838
PMR	Kuiken, T	IL	839
PMR	Leonard, J	MI	839
PMR	Munin, M	PA	835
PMR	Richter, E	CT	832
PMR	Volshteyn, O	MO	840
PMR	Wilson, A	TX	842

Amyloid Heart Disease

Spec	Name	St	Pg
Cv	Young, J	OH	110

Amyloidosis

Spec	Name	St	Pg
Hem	Gertz, M	MN	318
Nep	Dember, L	MA	452
Onc	Davis, M	OH	365
Onc	Vescio, R	CA	391
Pul	Berk, J	MA	920

Amyloidosis/Joint Disease

Spec	Name	St	Pg
Rhu	Gorevic, P	NY	1024

Amyotrophic Lateral Sclerosis (ALS)

Spec	Name	St	Pg
N	Armon, C	MA	504
N	Barohn, R	KS	529
N	Engel, W	CA	534
N	Feldman, E	MI	524
N	Glass, J	GA	519
N	Graves, M	CA	535
N	Harati, Y	TX	531
N	Jones, H	MA	505
N	Lacomis, D	PA	512
N	McCluskey, L	PA	513
N	Mitsumoto, H	NY	513
N	Newman, D	MI	526
N	Pascuzzi, R	IN	526
N	Roos, R	IL	528
N	Shefner, J	NY	515

Spec	Name	St	Pg
N	Siddique, T	IL	528
N	Weiner, L	CA	537
N	Windebank, A	MN	529
PMR	Bach, J	NJ	833

Amyotrophic Lateral Sclerosis(ALS)

Spec	Name	St	Pg
N	Cudkowicz, M	MA	505
N	Rutkove, S	MA	506

Anal Cancer

Spec	Name	St	Pg
CRS	Dietz, D	OH	172
CRS	Fry, R	PA	168
CRS	Geisler, D	PA	168
CRS	Gorfine, S	NY	168
CRS	Nagle, D	MA	166
CRS	Welton, M	CA	177
DR	Coakley, F	CA	982
Onc	Berry, J	CA	383

Anal Disorders & Reconstruction

Spec	Name	St	Pg
CRS	Blatchford, G	NE	174
CRS	Gorfine, S	NY	168
CRS	Marcet, J	FL	170
CRS	Rafferty, J	OH	173

Anal Sphincter Repair

Spec	Name	St	Pg
CRS	Coutsoftides, T	CA	176
CRS	Lowry, A	MN	172

Anaphylaxis

Spec	Name	St	Pg
A&I	Castells, M	MA	84
A&I	Greenberger, P	IL	88
A&I	Korenblat, P	MO	88
A&I	Lieberman, P	TN	86
A&I	Metcalfe, D	MD	85
A&I	Sullivan, T	GA	87
PA&I	Burks, A	NC	730
PA&I	Ownby, D	GA	731

Anemia

Spec	Name	St	Pg
Hem	Blinder, M	MO	317
Hem	Isola, L	NY	311
Hem	Spivak, J	MD	313
Hem	Zuckerman, K	FL	316
PHO	Beyer, E	IL	768
PHO	Salvi, S	IL	772
PNep	Ault, B	TN	785

Anemia-Aplastic

Spec	Name	St	Pg
Hem	Dang, C	MD	310
Hem	Maciejewski, J	OH	319
Hem	Mangan, K	PA	311
Onc	Claxton, D	PA	335
PHO	Boxer, L	MI	768
PHO	Camitta, B	WI	768
PHO	Wang, W	TN	768

Specialty & Special Expertise Index

Specialty & Special Expertise Index

Spec	Name	St	Pg
IC	Diver, D	CT	123
IC	Feldman, T	IL	128
IC	Kleiman, N	TX	129
IC	Knopf, W	GA	127
IC	Laham, R	MA	123
IC	Matar, F	FL	127
IC	Morris, D	GA	128

Angioplasty & Restenosis

IC	Holmes, D	MN	129

Angioplasty & Stent Placement

IC	Chang, G	PA	124
IC	Dieter, R	IL	128
IC	Douglas, J	GA	127
IC	Ellis, S	OH	128
IC	Herrmann, H	PA	124
IC	Kandzari, D	GA	127
IC	Losordo, D	IL	129
IC	Margolis, J	FL	127
IC	Moses, J	NY	125
IC	Pichard, A	DC	125
IC	Reddy, B	GA	128
IC	Reiner, J	DC	125
IC	Rosenfield, K	MA	124
IC	Shani, J	NY	126
IC	Stone, G	NY	126
IC	Zelman, R	MA	124
VascS	Brewster, D	MA	1178
VascS	Kazmers, A	MI	1185
VIR	Kaufman, J	OR	997
VIR	McLean, G	PA	992

Angioplasty-Peripheral

VIR	Smith, S	IL	995

Angioplasty-Pulmonary Artery

PCd	Lock, J	MA	733

Ankle Reconstruction

OrS	Levine, D	NY	619

Ankle Replacement & Revision

OrS	DeOrio, J	NC	626
OrS	Greisberg, J	NY	616
OrS	Nunley, J	NC	627
OrS	Sangeorzan, B	WA	643

Ankle Surgery

SM	Paletta, G	MO	1039
SM	Scheller, A	MA	1036

Ankylosing Spondylitis

Rhu	Bobrove, A	CA	1031
Rhu	Chang, R	IL	1028
Rhu	Hugenberg, S	IN	1029

Spec	Name	St	Pg
Rhu	Kay, J	MA	1022
Rhu	Luthra, H	MN	1029

Anophthalmia

Oph	Bernardino, C	CA	596
Oph	Tse, D	FL	584

Anorectal Disorders

CRS	Abcarian, H	IL	171
CRS	Church, J	OH	171
CRS	Dietz, D	OH	172
CRS	Efron, J	MD	167
CRS	Eisenstat, T	NJ	167
CRS	Heppell, J	AZ	175
CRS	Lederman, E	MO	172
CRS	Procaccino, J	NY	169
CRS	Schoetz, D	MA	167
CRS	Senagore, A	CA	176
CRS	Shah, N	RI	167
CRS	Shellito, P	MA	167
CRS	Stein, D	PA	169
CRS	Trudel, J	MN	174

Anorectal Malformations

PS	Pena, A	OH	807
PS	Velcek, F	NY	804

Anorexia Nervosa-Severe

IM	Mehler, P	CO	420

Anterior Segment Surgery

Oph	Caprioli, J	CA	597
Oph	Dhaliwal, D	PA	571
Oph	Gaasterland, D	MD	572
Oph	Parrish, R	FL	583
Oph	Samuelson, T	MN	591
Oph	Shamie, N	CA	601

Anterior Segment Trauma/Reconstruction

Oph	Florakis, G	NY	572

Antibiotic Resistance

Inf	Edmond, M	VA	408
Inf	Patterson, J	TX	412
Inf	Scheld, W	VA	409
PInf	Alexander, K	IL	781
PInf	Long, S	PA	779
PInf	McCracken, G	TX	783

Antiphospholipid Syndrome (APS)

N	Hess, D	GA	519
Rhu	Belmont, H	NY	1023
Rhu	Lockshin, M	NY	1024

Spec	Name	St	Pg
Rhu	Petri, M	MD	1025

Anxiety & Depression

AdP	Ciraulo, D	MA	900
AM	Singh, N	MN	81
ChAP	Bird, H	NY	904
ChAP	Slomowitz, M	IL	907
GerPsy	Stein, E	CA	912
Psyc	Bronheim, H	NY	887
Psyc	Sadock, V	NY	890

Anxiety & Mood Disorders

AdP	Frances, R	NY	901
ChAP	Biederman, J	MA	903
ChAP	Hirsch, G	NY	905
ChAP	Koplewicz, H	NY	905
ChAP	Kwon, H	WA	909
Psyc	Appelbaum, P	NY	886
Psyc	Friedman, M	VT	884
Psyc	Levy, S	GA	892
Psyc	Locala, J	OH	894
Psyc	Price, L	RI	885
Psyc	Rosenthal, R	NY	890
Psyc	Roy-Byrne, P	WA	899
Psyc	Schatzberg, A	CA	899
Psyc	Scott, C	PA	891
Psyc	Sussman, N	NY	891
Psyc	Thase, M	PA	891
Psyc	Wait, S	MD	891

Anxiety Disorders

AM	Kaplan, D	CO	81
ChAP	Abright, A	NY	904
ChAP	Birmaher, B	PA	904
ChAP	Hagman, J	CO	908
ChAP	Riddle, M	MD	906
ChAP	Walkup, J	NY	906
Psyc	Bystritsky, A	CA	897
Psyc	Cohen, M	PA	887
Psyc	Eaton, W	DC	888
Psyc	Fyer, A	NY	888
Psyc	Hollander, E	NY	888
Psyc	McIntosh, J	UT	895
Psyc	Pi, E	CA	898
Psyc	Stein, M	CA	899

Aortic & Visceral Artery Surgery

VascS	Berguer, R	MI	1185
VascS	Hansen, K	NC	1184

Aortic Diseases & Dissection

Cv	Braverman, A	MO	104
Cv	Eagle, K	MI	105
Cv	O'Gara, P	MA	93
IC	Lasala, J	MO	129
IC	Schreiber, T	MI	129

Specialty & Special Expertise Index

Spec	Name	St	Pg
HS	Light, T	IL	300
HS	Melone, C	NY	297
HS	Putnam, M	MN	301
HS	Raskin, K	NY	297
HS	Rayan, G	OK	302
OrS	Bronson, M	NY	613
OrS	Buly, R	NY	613
OrS	Deland, J	NY	614
OrS	Gladstone, J	NY	615
OrS	Goodman, S	CA	641
OrS	Gorab, R	CA	641
OrS	Jiranek, W	VA	626
OrS	Kraay, M	OH	633
OrS	Nunley, J	NC	627
OrS	Stuchin, S	NY	624
OrS	Thornhill, T	MA	611
OrS	Vail, T	CA	644
OrS	Wapner, K	PA	624
PRhu	Goldsmith, D	PA	798
PRhu	Lehman, T	NY	799
PRhu	Wilking, A	TX	800
Rhu	Chang, R	IL	1028
Rhu	Fife, R	IN	1029
Rhu	Lipstate, J	LA	1031
Rhu	Mease, P	WA	1032
Rhu	Schubert, R	DC	1026
Rhu	Sessoms, S	TX	1031
Rhu	Solitar, B	NY	1026
Rhu	Starz, T	PA	1026

Arthritis-Hip & Knee

Spec	Name	St	Pg
OrS	Grelsamer, R	NY	616

Arthritis-Knee

Spec	Name	St	Pg
OrS	Leadbetter, W	MD	619

Arthritis-Septic

Spec	Name	St	Pg
Inf	Bayer, A	CA	413

Arthroplasty Imaging

Spec	Name	St	Pg
DR	Potter, H	NY	977

Arthroscopic Surgery

Spec	Name	St	Pg
HS	Atkinson, R	HI	303
HS	Beredjiklian, P	PA	295
HS	Greene, T	FL	298
HS	Slutsky, D	CA	303
OrS	Bauman, P	NY	612
OrS	Bigliani, L	NY	612
OrS	Cooper, D	TX	638
OrS	Glashow, J	NY	615
OrS	Green, A	RI	609
OrS	Hausman, M	NY	616
OrS	Johnson, D	KY	627
OrS	Kocher, M	MA	610
OrS	Lock, T	MI	633
OrS	Millett, P	CO	637
OrS	Minas, T	MA	610
OrS	Nicholas, S	NY	620

Spec	Name	St	Pg
OrS	Poehling, G	NC	628
OrS	Richmond, J	MA	611
OrS	Seltzer, D	AZ	639
OrS	Shelbourne, K	IN	635
OrS	Spindler, K	TN	629
OrS	Thomas, B	CA	644
SM	Altchek, D	NY	1036
SM	Byrd, J	TN	1038
SM	Ciccotti, M	PA	1037
SM	Fronek, J	CA	1040
SM	Gill, T	MA	1036
SM	Hershman, E	NY	1037
SM	Ho, S	IL	1039
SM	Jones, D	LA	1040
SM	Levine, W	NY	1037
SM	Ma, C	CA	1040
SM	Mirzayan, R	CA	1040
SM	Nisonson, B	NY	1037
SM	Sennett, B	PA	1038
SM	Speer, K	NC	1038
SM	Steiner, M	MA	1036
SM	Xerogeanes, J	GA	1038

Arthroscopic Surgery-Hip

Spec	Name	St	Pg
OrS	Kocher, M	MA	610
OrS	Mabrey, J	TX	639
OrS	McCarthy, J	OH	633
OrS	Padgett, D	NY	621
OrS	Westrich, G	NY	624
SM	Asnis, P	MA	1036

Arthroscopic Surgery-Knee

Spec	Name	St	Pg
OrS	Bartolozzi, A	PA	612
OrS	Fulkerson, J	CT	609
OrS	Nuber, G	IL	634
OrS	Padgett, D	NY	621
OrS	Westrich, G	NY	624

Arthroscopic Surgery-Wrist

Spec	Name	St	Pg
OrS	Goldner, R	NC	626

Artificial Heart Devices

Spec	Name	St	Pg
TS	Frazier, O	TX	1132
TS	Jeevanandam, V	IL	1127
TS	Kormos, R	PA	1114
TS	Samuels, L	PA	1116
TS	Tedder, M	TN	1124

Arts in the Healing Process

Spec	Name	St	Pg
Psyc	Avery, E	TX	895

Asbestos-related Lung Disease

Spec	Name	St	Pg
OM	Harber, P	CA	880
Pul	Rose, C	CO	935
TS	Krellenstein, D	NY	1114

Asherman's Syndrome

Spec	Name	St	Pg
RE	Odem, R	MO	1014
RE	Walmer, D	NC	1012

Asperger's Syndrome

Spec	Name	St	Pg
ChAP	Heston, J	TN	906
ChAP	Rostain, A	PA	906
ChAP	Volkmar, F	CT	904
Psyc	Brodkin, E	PA	887

Asthma

Spec	Name	St	Pg
A&I	Altman, L	WA	89
A&I	Benenati, S	FL	86
A&I	Bernstein, D	OH	87
A&I	Bernstein, J	OH	87
A&I	Bonner, J	AL	86
A&I	Busse, W	WI	87
A&I	Chandler, M	NY	84
A&I	Freeman, T	TX	88
A&I	Friedman, S	FL	86
A&I	Grammer, L	IL	88
A&I	Greenberger, P	IL	88
A&I	Henderson, W	WA	89
A&I	Korenblat, P	MO	88
A&I	Ledford, D	FL	86
A&I	Lewis, J	AZ	89
A&I	Lieberman, P	TN	86
A&I	MacLean, J	MA	84
A&I	Mazza, D	NY	85
A&I	Montanaro, A	OR	89
A&I	Pacin, M	FL	87
A&I	Routes, J	WI	88
A&I	Sanders, G	MI	88
A&I	Slankard, M	NY	85
A&I	Sullivan, T	GA	87
A&I	Sundy, J	NC	87
A&I	Tamaroff, M	CA	90
A&I	Umetsu, D	MA	84
A&I	Wasserman, S	CA	90
A&I	Wong, J	MA	84
A&I	Wood, J	MO	88
PA&I	Bahna, S	LA	732
PA&I	Burks, A	NC	730
PA&I	Ehrlich, P	NY	729
PA&I	Gelfand, E	CO	732
PA&I	Kelly, C	VA	731
PA&I	Klein, J	RI	729
PA&I	Lemanske, R	WI	731
PA&I	Leung, D	CO	732
PA&I	Ownby, D	GA	731
PA&I	Pongracic, J	IL	731
PA&I	Schuberth, K	MD	730
PA&I	Sly, R	DC	730
PA&I	Spergel, J	PA	730
PA&I	Strunk, R	MO	731
PA&I	Wolf, R	IL	731
PA&I	Wood, R	MD	730
Ped	Jacob, M	IL	728
PPul	Dozor, A	NY	793
PPul	Givan, D	IN	795
PPul	Kattan, M	NY	793

Specialty & Special Expertise Index

Spec	Name	St	Pg
Autoimmune Liver Disease			
Ge	Raiford, D	TN	241
Ge	Vierling, J	TX	252
Autoimmune Lung Disease			
Pul	Brown, K	CO	934
Autonomic Disorders			
Cv	Grubb, B	OH	106

B

Spec	Name	St	Pg
Baha Implant			
Oto	Young, N	IL	678
Balance Disorders			
ChiN	Eviatar, L	NY	146
Ger	Studenski, S	PA	263
N	Hain, T	IL	524
Oto	Gianoli, G	LA	681
Oto	Hammerschlag, P	NY	659
Oto	Hoffman, R	NY	659
Oto	Kartush, J	MI	675
Barrett's Esophagus			
Ge	Chang, K	CA	252
Ge	Cohen, J	NY	231
Ge	Eisen, G	OR	253
Ge	Estores, D	FL	240
Ge	Falk, G	PA	232
Ge	Fang, J	UT	249
Ge	Fleischer, D	AZ	251
Ge	Gerdes, H	NY	232
Ge	Gerson, L	CA	253
Ge	Ginsberg, G	PA	232
Ge	Greenwald, B	MD	233
Ge	Haber, G	NY	233
Ge	Infantolino, A	PA	233
Ge	Katz, P	PA	234
Ge	Lightdale, C	NY	235
Ge	Meiselman, M	IL	246
Ge	Ravich, W	MD	237
Ge	Reynolds, J	PA	237
Ge	Rothstein, R	NH	229
Ge	Savides, T	CA	255
Ge	Vargo, J	OH	248
Path	Montgomery, E	MD	710
S	Chand, B	OH	1071
S	Nava-Villarreal, H	NY	1056
S	Pellegrini, C	WA	1093
TS	Battafarano, R	MD	1109
TS	Ferguson, M	IL	1126

Spec	Name	St	Pg
Bartter's Syndrome			
Nep	Ellison, D	OR	461
Beckwith-Wiedemann Syndrome			
PlS	Napoli, J	DE	855
Behavioral Disorders			
AM	Ginsburg, K	PA	80
ChAP	Boxer, G	MO	907
ChAP	King, B	WA	908
ChAP	Ponton, L	CA	909
Psyc	Reus, V	CA	899
Behavioral Neurology			
N	Ahern, G	AZ	530
N	DeKosky, S	VA	518
N	Devinsky, O	NY	509
N	Heilman, K	FL	519
N	Kirshner, H	TN	520
Psyc	Neppe, V	WA	898
Behavioral Problems & Dementia			
GerPsy	Grossberg, G	MO	911
GerPsy	Rovner, B	PA	910
Behcet's Syndrome			
D	Fivenson, D	MI	193
Rhu	Spiera, H	NY	1026
Berger's Disease (IgA Nephropathy)			
PNep	Wyatt, R	TN	785
Beryllium-induced Lung Disease			
OM	Harber, P	CA	880
Pul	Balmes, J	CA	936
Pul	Rossman, M	PA	925
Biliary Cancer			
Onc	O'Reilly, E	NY	345
Onc	Patt, Y	NM	380
Onc	Posey, J	AL	359
Onc	Yen, Y	CA	391
S	Bouvet, M	CA	1088
S	Cameron, J	MD	1050
S	Chari, R	TN	1062
S	Drebin, J	PA	1052
S	Ellison, E	OH	1072
S	Heslin, M	AL	1064
S	Schulick, R	MD	1059
S	Yeo, C	PA	1061

Spec	Name	St	Pg
Biliary Disease			
Ge	Barnes, D	OH	243
Ge	Cunningham, J	AZ	250
Ge	Edmundowicz, S	MO	244
Ge	Elta, G	MI	245
Ge	Freiman, H	NY	232
Ge	Kowalski, T	PA	235
Ge	Lind, C	TN	241
Ge	Lindor, K	MN	246
Ge	Miskovitz, P	NY	236
Biliary Surgery			
PS	Meyers, R	UT	808
PS	Notrica, D	AZ	809
S	Ellison, E	OH	1072
S	Gower, R	AK	1091
S	Hebert, J	VT	1045
S	Levi, J	FL	1065
S	McAneny, D	MA	1046
S	Postier, R	OK	1086
S	Soper, N	IL	1078
Biochemical Genetics			
CG	Charrow, J	IL	158
CG	Craigen, W	TX	160
CG	Jonas, A	CA	161
CG	Northrup, H	TX	160
Bioterrorism Preparedness			
Path	Walker, D	TX	719
Bipolar/Mood Disorders			
ChAP	Birmaher, B	PA	904
ChAP	Hirsch, G	NY	905
ChAP	Slomowitz, M	IL	907
ChAP	Wilens, T	MA	904
Psyc	Benes, F	MA	884
Psyc	Black, D	IA	893
Psyc	Bowden, C	TX	895
Psyc	Calabrese, J	OH	893
Psyc	Davidson, J	TX	896
Psyc	DePaulo, J	MD	887
Psyc	Hirschfeld, R	TX	896
Psyc	Kupfer, D	PA	889
Psyc	Lawson, W	DC	889
Psyc	Levy, S	GA	892
Psyc	McIntosh, J	UT	895
Psyc	Nurnberger, J	IN	894
Psyc	Price, L	RI	885
Psyc	Reus, V	CA	899
Psyc	Roy-Byrne, P	WA	899
Psyc	Salloum, I	FL	892
Psyc	Strakowski, S	OH	894
Psyc	Sussman, N	NY	891
Psyc	Weiner, R	NC	892
Psyc	Weisler, R	NC	893

Specialty & Special Expertise Index

Specialty & Special Expertise Index

Spec	Name	St	Pg
RadRO	Ennis, R	NY	947
RadRO	Gejerman, G	NJ	948
RadRO	Grado, G	AZ	962
RadRO	Harrison, L	NY	948
RadRO	Henderson, R	FL	952
RadRO	Horwitz, E	PA	948
RadRO	Jhingran, A	TX	962
RadRO	Kaplan, I	MA	944
RadRO	Koh, W	WA	964
RadRO	Kudrimoti, M	KY	953
RadRO	Lee, W	NC	953
RadRO	Malcolm, A	TN	953
RadRO	Medbery, C	OK	963
RadRO	Nori, D	NY	949
RadRO	Toonkel, L	FL	956
RadRO	Vicini, F	MI	960
RadRO	Vijayakumar, S	MS	956
RadRO	Zelefsky, M	NY	951
U	Terris, M	GA	1158

Brain & Spinal Cord Tumors

NS	Bederson, J	NY	468
NS	Berger, M	CA	491
NS	Brem, H	MD	468
NS	Carson, B	MD	468
NS	Harsh, G	CA	493
NS	Jallo, G	MD	471
NS	Kaufman, B	WI	484
NS	Kobrine, A	DC	471
NS	Laske, D	PA	472
NS	Malik, G	MI	484
NS	Naff, N	MD	473
NS	Olivi, A	MD	473
NS	Piepmeier, J	CT	467
NS	Reid, W	TN	479
NS	Robertson, J	TN	480
NS	Thompson, R	TN	481
Onc	Friedman, H	NC	354
PHO	Dunkel, I	NY	758
PHO	Lange, B	PA	760
RadRO	Kleinberg, L	MD	949
RadRO	Lewin, A	FL	953
RadRO	Marcus, R	FL	954

Brain & Spinal Malformations

NS	Frim, D	IL	484

Brain & Spinal Tumors

N	Newton, H	OH	526
NRad	Tenner, M	NY	986
NS	Bilsky, M	NY	468
NS	Caputy, A	DC	468
NS	Chen, C	NY	468
NS	Chen, T	CA	492
NS	Frim, D	IL	484
NS	Lang, F	TX	489
NS	Penar, P	VT	467
NS	Sills, A	TN	480
NS	Swearingen, B	MA	467
RadRO	Flickinger, J	PA	947

Spec	Name	St	Pg
RadRO	Hartford, A	NH	944
RadRO	Regine, W	MD	950
RadRO	Wara, W	CA	966

Brain & Spinal Tumors-Pediatric

NS	Cohen, A	OH	483

Brain Cancer

RadRO	Cmelak, A	TN	952

Brain Development Abnormalities

NRad	Barkovich, A	CA	990
NRad	Barnes, P	CA	990

Brain Imaging

NRad	Osborn, A	UT	989
NuM	Mountz, J	PA	545

Brain Imaging-Pediatric

NRad	Provenzale, J	NC	987

Brain Infections

NuM	Alavi, A	PA	544
Path	Bollen, A	CA	719
PInf	Bradley, J	CA	783

Brain Injury

ChAP	Martini, D	UT	908
ChiN	Griesemer, D	MA	144
ChiN	Ichord, R	PA	146
ChiN	Noetzel, M	MO	149
N	Fellus, J	NJ	509
N	Jordan, B	NY	511
N	Kelly, J	CO	530
NP	Davis, J	MA	442
NP	Delivoria-Papadopoulos, M	PA	443
NRad	Burdette, J	NC	986
NS	Adelson, P	AZ	488
NS	Carson, B	MD	468
NS	Wilberger, J	PA	476
PS	Nance, M	PA	803

Brain Injury Rehabilitation

PMR	Bloch, R	MA	832
PMR	Flanagan, S	NY	834
PMR	Francisco, G	TX	841
PMR	Fried, G	PA	834
PMR	Glenn, M	MA	832
PMR	Ivanhoe, C	TX	841
PMR	Matthews, D	CO	840
PMR	Mayer, N	PA	835
PMR	Mysiw, W	OH	839
PMR	Ragnarsson, K	NY	835
PMR	Zafonte, R	MA	832

Brain Injury Rehabilitation-Pediatric

PMR	Massagli, T	WA	842

Brain Injury-Pediatric

NRad	Barnes, P	CA	990
NRad	Hunter, J	TX	989
NS	Ragheb, J	FL	479

Brain Injury-Traumatic

N	Diaz-Arrastia, R	TX	530
N	Filley, C	CO	529
N	Kelly, J	CO	530
NS	Luerssen, T	TX	490
NS	Maroon, J	PA	472

Brain Mapping

NRad	Faro, S	PA	985
NS	Silbergeld, D	WA	495

Brain Radiation Toxicity

N	Rogers, L	OH	527

Brain Tumor Imaging

NRad	Hesselink, J	CA	990
NRad	Koeller, K	MN	988
NRad	Loevner, L	PA	985
NRad	Murtagh, F	FL	987
NRad	Provenzale, J	NC	987

Brain Tumors

ChiN	Allen, J	NY	145
ChiN	Cohen, B	OH	148
ChiN	Duffner, P	NY	145
ChiN	Fisher, P	CA	151
ChiN	Keating, G	MN	149
ChiN	Packer, R	DC	147
ChiN	Phillips, P	PA	147
ChiN	Pomeroy, S	MA	144
DR	Elster, A	NC	979
N	Barger, G	MI	523
N	Batchelor, T	MA	504
N	Chamberlain, M	WA	534
N	Cloughesy, T	CA	534
N	Dalmau, J	PA	508
N	Gilbert, M	TX	531
N	Glass, J	PA	510
N	Kunschner, L	PA	511
N	Laterra, J	MD	512
N	Mikkelsen, T	MI	526
N	Moots, P	TN	520
N	Nabors, L	AL	520
N	Patchell, R	AZ	532
N	Posner, J	NY	514
N	Rogers, L	OH	527
N	Rosenfeld, M	PA	515
N	Rosenfeld, S	OH	528

Brain Tumors & Hemifacial Spasms

Specialty & Special Expertise Index

Spec	Name	St	Pg
Brain Tumors-Adult & Pediatric			
NS	Kondziolka, D	PA	472
NS	Mapstone, T	OK	490
RadRO	Shrieve, D	UT	961
RadRO	Suh, J	OH	960
RadRO	Woo, S	KY	956
Brain Tumors-Benign			
NS	Wilberger, J	PA	476
RadRO	Loeffler, J	MA	945
Brain Tumors-Complex			
NS	Lang, F	TX	489
Brain Tumors-Metastatic			
N	Phuphanich, S	CA	536
NS	Chen, T	CA	492
NS	Kondziolka, D	PA	472
NS	Laske, D	PA	472
NS	Olivi, A	MD	473
NS	Silbergeld, D	WA	495
Onc	Vredenburgh, J	NC	362
RadRO	Kleinberg, L	MD	949
Brain Tumors-Pediatric			
N	Janss, A	GA	520
NS	Edwards, M	CA	492
NS	Feldstein, N	NY	469
NS	Sandberg, D	FL	480
NS	Sanford, R	TN	480
NS	Selden, N	OR	495
NS	Souweidane, M	NY	475
NS	Sutton, L	PA	475
NS	Tomita, T	IL	486
NS	Wisoff, J	NY	476
RadRO	Merchant, T	TN	954
RadRO	Tarbell, N	MA	945
Brain Tumors-Recurrent			
PHO	Kuttesch, J	PA	760
Brain/Spinal Cord Injury			
PMR	Leslie, D	GA	837
Breast Augmentation			
PlS	Barone, C	TX	867
PlS	Meltzer, T	AZ	868
PlS	Stadelmann, W	NH	849
PlS	Young, V	MO	866
Breast Cancer			
CG	Rubinstein, W	IL	158
CG	Weitzel, J	CA	162
DR	Abbitt, P	FL	978
DR	Brem, R	DC	974
DR	Conant, E	PA	974

Spec	Name	St	Pg
DR	Dershaw, D	NY	975
DR	Edelstein, B	NY	975
DR	Evers, K	PA	975
DR	Feig, S	CA	983
DR	Freimanis, R	NC	979
DR	Helvie, M	MI	980
DR	Hricak, H	NY	975
DR	Huynh, P	TX	982
DR	Kopans, D	MA	973
DR	Lehman, C	WA	983
DR	Mitnick, J	NY	976
DR	Monsees, B	MO	980
DR	Otto, P	TX	982
DR	Parikh, J	WA	983
DR	Roth, S	PA	977
DR	Stough, R	OK	982
DR	Ulissey, M	TX	982
DR	Weinreb, J	CT	973
GO	Braly, P	LA	287
GO	Chambers, S	AZ	287
GO	Fiorica, J	FL	281
GO	Kelley, J	PA	278
GO	Runowicz, C	FL	283
Hem	Flynn, P	MN	318
Hem	Mears, J	NY	312
Hem	Schwartzberg, L	TN	316
Hem	Wisch, N	NY	314
IM	Rivlin, R	NY	419
NuM	Podoloff, D	TX	547
ObG	Goldman, M	CA	559
Onc	Abraham, J	WV	332
Onc	Albain, K	IL	363
Onc	Anderson, J	MI	363
Onc	Arteaga, C	TN	351
Onc	Arun, B	TX	376
Onc	Astrow, A	NY	333
Onc	Attas, L	NJ	333
Onc	Balducci, L	FL	351
Onc	Biggs, D	DE	334
Onc	Bitran, J	IL	363
Onc	Blackwell, K	NC	352
Onc	Brenin, C	VA	352
Onc	Brufsky, A	PA	334
Onc	Budd, G	OH	364
Onc	Burris, H	TN	352
Onc	Burstein, H	MA	326
Onc	Butler, W	SC	352
Onc	Buys, S	UT	373
Onc	Buzdar, A	TX	376
Onc	Camoriano, J	AZ	376
Onc	Carey, L	NC	353
Onc	Carlson, R	CA	383
Onc	Carpenter, J	AL	353
Onc	Celano, P	MD	335
Onc	Chabner, B	MA	327
Onc	Chang, J	TX	377
Onc	Chap, L	CA	383
Onc	Chew, H	CA	383
Onc	Chitambar, C	WI	364
Onc	Chlebowski, R	CA	383
Onc	Cobleigh, M	IL	365
Onc	Cohen, P	DC	335
Onc	Cohen, S	NY	336

Spec	Name	St	Pg
Onc	Colon-Otero, G	FL	353
Onc	Come, S	MA	327
Onc	Cowan, K	NE	373
Onc	Cristofanilli, M	PA	336
Onc	Daly, M	PA	336
Onc	Davidson, N	PA	336
Onc	Dickler, M	NY	337
Onc	Disis, M	WA	384
Onc	Dizon, D	RI	327
Onc	Doroshow, J	MD	337
Onc	Dutcher, J	NY	337
Onc	Elias, A	CO	374
Onc	Ellis, G	WA	384
Onc	Ellis, M	MO	365
Onc	Emens, L	MD	338
Onc	Erban, J	MA	327
Onc	Fabian, C	KS	374
Onc	Fitch, T	AZ	377
Onc	Fox, K	PA	339
Onc	Fracasso, P	VA	354
Onc	Ganz, P	CA	385
Onc	Garber, J	MA	328
Onc	Gaynor, E	IL	366
Onc	Geyer, C	PA	339
Onc	Glaspy, J	CA	385
Onc	Glick, J	PA	339
Onc	Goldstein, L	PA	339
Onc	Gradishar, W	IL	366
Onc	Graham, M	NC	355
Onc	Gralow, J	WA	385
Onc	Grana, G	NJ	340
Onc	Grossbard, M	NY	340
Onc	Haley, B	TX	377
Onc	Hammond, D	NH	328
Onc	Hayes, D	MI	367
Onc	Herbst, R	CT	329
Onc	Hoffman, P	IL	367
Onc	Holland, J	NY	341
Onc	Hollister, D	CT	329
Onc	Hudis, C	NY	341
Onc	Hutchins, L	AR	378
Onc	Ingle, J	MN	367
Onc	Isaacs, C	DC	341
Onc	Jahanzeb, M	FL	356
Onc	Kaufman, P	NH	329
Onc	Legare, R	RI	330
Onc	Limentani, S	NC	357
Onc	Lippman, M	FL	357
Onc	Livingston, R	AZ	379
Onc	Loprinzi, C	MN	368
Onc	Lyman, G	NC	357
Onc	Makhoul, I	AR	379
Onc	Marcom, P	NC	358
Onc	Matulonis, U	MA	330
Onc	McGuire, W	MD	343
Onc	Mintzer, D	PA	344
Onc	Moore, A	NY	344
Onc	Mortimer, J	CA	343
Onc	Muss, H	NC	358
Onc	Nabell, L	AL	358
Onc	Nissenblatt, M	NJ	344
Onc	Northfelt, D	AZ	379
Onc	Norton, L	NY	344

Specialty & Special Expertise Index

Specialty & Special Expertise Index

Specialty & Special Expertise Index

Specialty & Special Expertise Index

Specialty & Special Expertise Index

Spec	Name	St	Pg
Cardiac Surgery-Adult			
TS	Conte, J	MD	1110
TS	Diehl, J	PA	1110
TS	Joyce, L	MN	1127
TS	Krieger, K	NY	1114
TS	Merrick, S	CA	1136
TS	Panos, A	FL	1122
TS	Rastegar, H	MA	1107
Cardiac Surgery-Adult & Pediatric			
TS	Calhoon, J	TX	1131
TS	Christian, K	TN	1119
TS	Drinkwater, D	TN	1120
TS	Gundry, S	CA	1135
TS	Kirklin, J	AL	1121
TS	Mullett, T	KY	1121
TS	Spray, T	PA	1117
TS	Warner, K	MA	1108
Cardiac Surgery-Geriatric			
TS	Edwards, N	NY	1111
Cardiac Surgery-High Risk			
TS	Furukawa, S	PA	1111
TS	Gundry, S	CA	1135
Cardiac Surgery-Neonatal			
TS	Bichell, D	TN	1118
TS	Rosenkranz, E	FL	1123
TS	Walters, H	MI	1129
Cardiac Surgery-Neonatal & Pediatric			
TS	Brown, J	IN	1125
Cardiac Surgery-Pediatric			
TS	Bailey, L	CA	1134
TS	Bichell, D	TN	1118
TS	Fontana, G	CA	1135
TS	Harrell, J	TX	1132
TS	Turrentine, M	IN	1129
Cardiac Tumors, Myxomas			
TS	Grossi, E	NY	1112
Cardiac Tumors/Cancer			
TS	Reardon, M	TX	1133
Cardiomyopathy			
Cv	Elkayam, U	CA	114
Cv	Fonarow, G	CA	114
PCd	Driscoll, D	MN	738

Spec	Name	St	Pg
Cardiomyopathy-Hypertrophic			
IC	Bach, R	MO	128
IC	Heldman, A	FL	127
Cardiothoracic Surgery			
TS	Bains, M	NY	1109
TS	Bull, D	UT	1130
TS	Byrne, J	TN	1119
TS	Durham, S	MI	1125
TS	Galantowicz, M	OH	1126
TS	Girardi, L	NY	1112
TS	Glassford, D	TN	1120
TS	Lang, S	NY	1114
TS	Martin, T	FL	1121
TS	Moon, M	MO	1128
TS	Robbins, R	CA	1136
TS	Salerno, T	FL	1123
TS	Stuart, R	MO	1129
TS	Thistlethwaite, P	CA	1137
TS	Toyoda, Y	PA	1117
TS	Weiman, D	TN	1124
Cardiovascular Disease			
Cv	Abi-samra, F	LA	111
Cv	Andersen, H	NY	94
Cv	Anderson, J	UT	111
Cv	Armstrong, W	MI	104
Cv	Bairey, C	CA	113
Cv	Balady, G	MA	92
Cv	Ballantyne, C	TX	111
Cv	Bashore, T	NC	100
Cv	Bass, T	FL	100
Cv	Benjamin, I	UT	111
Cv	Blanchard, D	CA	113
Cv	Blumenthal, D	NY	94
Cv	Blumenthal, R	MD	95
Cv	Bonow, R	IL	104
Cv	Borer, J	NY	95
Cv	Borzak, S	FL	101
Cv	Bourge, R	AL	101
Cv	Bove, A	PA	95
Cv	Braverman, A	MO	104
Cv	Brindis, R	CA	114
Cv	Brozena, S	PA	95
Cv	Budoff, M	CA	114
Cv	Burket, M	OH	105
Cv	Byrd, B	TN	101
Cv	Cabin, H	CT	92
Cv	Califf, R	NC	101
Cv	Carabello, B	TX	111
Cv	Catherwood, E	NH	92
Cv	Cerqueira, M	OH	105
Cv	Chaitman, B	MO	105
Cv	Chizner, M	FL	101
Cv	Clements, S	GA	101
Cv	Cohen, H	NY	95
Cv	Connolly, H	MN	105
Cv	Cooper, C	OH	105
Cv	Coppola, J	NY	95
Cv	Corrigan, V	GA	101
Cv	Davidson, M	IL	105

Spec	Name	St	Pg
Cv	DeNofrio, D	MA	92
Cv	Devereux, R	NY	95
Cv	Dichek, D	WA	114
Cv	Eagle, K	MI	105
Cv	Edmundowicz, D	PA	95
Cv	Eisen, H	PA	96
Cv	Elkayam, U	CA	114
Cv	Fishbein, D	WA	114
Cv	Follansbee, W	PA	96
Cv	Fonarow, G	CA	114
Cv	Freeman, G	TX	111
Cv	French, W	CA	114
Cv	Friedman, S	NY	96
Cv	Fuster, V	NY	96
Cv	Gandy, W	GA	102
Cv	Gardin, J	NJ	96
Cv	Geltman, E	MO	106
Cv	Gibbons, R	MN	106
Cv	Gliklich, J	NY	96
Cv	Goldberg, N	NY	96
Cv	Gottdiener, J	MD	96
Cv	Gottlieb, S	MD	97
Cv	Gould, K	TX	112
Cv	Greenberg, M	NY	97
Cv	Grubb, B	OH	106
Cv	Halperin, J	NY	97
Cv	Hare, J	FL	102
Cv	Harrison, J	NC	102
Cv	Hauptman, P	MO	106
Cv	Hayes, S	MN	106
Cv	Herling, I	PA	97
Cv	Heroux, A	IL	106
Cv	Horn, E	NY	97
Cv	Hunt, S	CA	115
Cv	Hutter, A	MA	92
Cv	Inra, L	NY	97
Cv	Iskandrian, A	AL	102
Cv	Jaffe, A	MN	106
Cv	Jessup, M	PA	97
Cv	Johnson, A	CA	115
Cv	Johnson, M	WI	107
Cv	Johnson, P	MA	92
Cv	Judelson, D	CA	115
Cv	Katz, S	NY	98
Cv	Kaul, S	OR	115
Cv	Kereiakes, D	OH	107
Cv	Kirshenbaum, J	MA	92
Cv	Klein, L	IL	107
Cv	Kobashigawa, J	CA	115
Cv	Konstam, M	MA	93
Cv	Kostis, J	NJ	98
Cv	Krajcer, Z	TX	112
Cv	Kuvin, J	MA	93
Cv	Labovitz, A	MO	107
Cv	Landzberg, J	NJ	98
Cv	Lewis, S	OR	115
Cv	Liang, B	CT	93
Cv	Liebson, P	IL	107
Cv	Lindenfeld, J	CO	111
Cv	Linton, M	TN	102
Cv	Loscalzo, J	MA	93
Cv	Manning, W	MA	93
Cv	Massin, E	TX	112

Specialty & Special Expertise Index

Specialty & Special Expertise Index

Spec	Name	St	Pg
VascS	Kent, K	WI	1186
VascS	Kougias, P	TX	1187
VascS	Mackey, W	MA	1179
VascS	Marin, M	NY	1182
VascS	Mitchell, M	MS	1184
VascS	Perler, B	MD	1182
VascS	Ricotta, J	DC	1182
VascS	Riles, T	NY	1182
VascS	Todd, G	NY	1183
VascS	White, R	CA	1188
VascS	Zarins, C	CA	1188

Carotid Body Tumors

Spec	Name	St	Pg
VascS	LaMuraglia, G	MA	1179

Carpal Tunnel Syndrome

Spec	Name	St	Pg
HS	Abrams, R	CA	302
HS	Akelman, E	RI	294
HS	Carneiro, R	FL	298
HS	Carroll, C	IL	299
HS	Derman, G	IL	299
HS	Imbriglia, J	PA	296
HS	Kulick, R	NY	296
HS	Lane, L	NY	296
HS	Nagle, D	IL	301
HS	Raskin, K	NY	297
HS	Rosenwasser, M	NY	297
HS	Weiss, A	RI	294
NS	Taylon, C	NE	488
NS	Zager, E	PA	476

Cartilage Damage

Spec	Name	St	Pg
DR	Potter, H	NY	977
HS	Lee, W	MD	296
OrS	Anderson, L	CA	639
OrS	Chu, C	PA	613
OrS	Gladstone, J	NY	615
OrS	Hungerford, M	MD	618
OrS	Karas, S	GA	627
OrS	Mandelbaum, B	CA	642
OrS	Nuber, G	IL	634
OrS	O'Driscoll, S	MN	634
OrS	Zarins, B	MA	611
SM	Bush-Joseph, C	IL	1039
SM	Gambardella, R	CA	1040
SM	Ho, S	IL	1039
SM	Miniaci, A	OH	1039
SM	Rodeo, S	NY	1037
SM	Sennett, B	PA	1038

Cartilage Damage & Transplant

Spec	Name	St	Pg
OrS	Minas, T	MA	610
OrS	Plancher, K	NY	621
OrS	Williams, R	NY	625
SM	Jones, D	LA	1040

Castleman's Disease

Spec	Name	St	Pg
Onc	Camoriano, J	AZ	376
Onc	Sweetenham, J	OH	371

Cataract Surgery

Spec	Name	St	Pg
Oph	Afshari, N	NC	579
Oph	Boxer Wachler, B	CA	596
Oph	Caprioli, J	CA	597
Oph	Crandall, A	UT	593
Oph	Culbertson, W	FL	580
Oph	Feder, R	IL	587
Oph	Forster, R	FL	581
Oph	Foster, C	MA	568
Oph	Gibralter, R	NY	572
Oph	Goldberg, D	NJ	572
Oph	Gorovoy, M	FL	581
Oph	Holland, E	OH	588
Oph	John, T	IL	588
Oph	Koch, D	TX	594
Oph	Kornmehl, E	MA	568
Oph	Lane, S	MN	589
Oph	Lichter, P	MI	589
Oph	Liebmann, J	NY	574
Oph	Lindstrom, R	MN	589
Oph	Mackool, R	NY	575
Oph	Magramm, I	NY	575
Oph	Maloney, R	CA	599
Oph	Masket, S	CA	599
Oph	McCulley, J	TX	594
Oph	Orlin, S	PA	576
Oph	Parrish, R	FL	583
Oph	Pepose, J	MO	590
Oph	Pflugfelder, S	TX	595
Oph	Rosenberg, M	IL	591
Oph	Salz, J	CA	600
Oph	Samuelson, T	MN	591
Oph	Schein, O	MD	577
Oph	Schuman, J	PA	577
Oph	Seibel, B	CA	601
Oph	Serafano, D	CA	601
Oph	Shamie, N	CA	601
Oph	Shingleton, B	MA	569
Oph	Stark, W	MD	578
Oph	Steinert, R	CA	601
Oph	Stulting, R	GA	584
Oph	Wallace, R	LA	595
Oph	Wang, M	TN	584
Oph	Waring, G	GA	584
Oph	Zaidman, G	NY	579

Cataract Surgery Revision

Spec	Name	St	Pg
Oph	Masket, S	CA	599

Cataract Surgery-Lens Implant

Spec	Name	St	Pg
Oph	Cionni, R	UT	593
Oph	Dodick, J	NY	571
Oph	Greenfield, D	FL	581
Oph	Lass, J	OH	589
Oph	Miller, K	CA	599
Oph	O'Brien, T	FL	583
Oph	Osher, R	OH	590
Oph	Perez, V	FL	583
Oph	Wright, K	CA	602

Cataract-Pediatric

Spec	Name	St	Pg
Oph	Buckley, E	NC	580
Oph	Del Monte, M	MI	587
Oph	Hall, L	NY	573
Oph	Kerr, N	TN	582
Oph	Lambert, S	GA	582
Oph	Medow, N	NY	575
Oph	Plager, D	IN	590
Oph	Walton, D	MA	569
Oph	Wilson, M	SC	585

Catheter Ablation

Spec	Name	St	Pg
CE	Berger, R	MD	117
CE	Donahue, J	OH	120
CE	Epstein, A	PA	118
CE	Halperin, H	MD	118
CE	Lerman, B	NY	118
CE	Miller, J	IN	121
CE	Onufer, J	VA	120
CE	Prystowsky, E	IN	121
CE	Wilber, D	IL	122

Celiac Disease

Spec	Name	St	Pg
Ge	Di Marino, A	PA	231
Ge	Elliott, D	IA	244
Ge	Forsmark, C	FL	240
Ge	Green, P	NY	233
Ge	Kastenberg, D	PA	234
Ge	Murray, J	MN	246
Ge	Semrad, C	IL	247
PGe	Baldridge, A	NJ	749
PGe	Benkov, K	NY	749
PGe	Cohen, M	OH	751
PGe	Fasano, A	MD	749
PGe	Guandalini, S	IL	752
PGe	Hill, I	NC	751
PGe	Hoffenberg, E	CO	753
PGe	Leichtner, A	MA	748
PGe	Levy, J	NY	749
PGe	Newman, L	NY	749
PGe	Snyder, J	DC	750

Central Nervous System Cancer

Spec	Name	St	Pg
RadRO	Buatti, J	IA	957
RadRO	Markoe, A	FL	954
RadRO	Porrazzo, M	DC	949

Cerebral Palsy

Spec	Name	St	Pg
ChiN	Brunstrom, J	MO	148
ChiN	Darras, B	MA	144
ChiN	Edgar, T	WI	149
ChiN	Eviatar, L	NY	146
ChiN	Goldstein, E	GA	147
ChiN	Noetzel, M	MO	149
ChiN	Volpe, J	MA	145
HS	Carlson, M	NY	295
OrS	Sponseller, P	MD	623
OrS	Strongwater, A	NJ	623
Ped	Walker, W	WA	729

Specialty & Special Expertise Index

Specialty & Special Expertise Index

Spec	Name	St	Pg
CG	Pergament, E	IL	158
CG	Plon, S	TX	160
CG	Pyeritz, R	PA	156
CG	Randolph, L	CA	162
CG	Rimoin, D	CA	162
CG	Rosenbaum, K	DC	156
CG	Rubinstein, W	IL	158
CG	Saal, H	OH	158
CG	Saul, R	SC	157
CG	Seashore, M	CT	154
CG	Seaver, L	HI	162
CG	Shapiro, L	NY	156
CG	Shulman, L	IL	159
CG	Stevenson, R	SC	157
CG	Sutphen, R	FL	157
CG	Ward, J	TN	157
CG	Weaver, D	IN	159
CG	Weitzel, J	CA	162
CG	Whelan, A	MO	159
CG	Wilcox, W	CA	162
CG	Zackai, E	PA	156
MF	Watson, W	MN	433

Clinical Neurophysiology

N	Bertorini, T	TN	518

Clinical Trials

Spec	Name	St	Pg
AdP	Anton, R	SC	901
ChiN	Santos, C	DC	147
D	Bowen, G	UT	196
D	Gottlieb, A	MA	183
EDM	Riddle, M	OR	221
Ge	Araya, V	PA	230
Ge	Gish, R	CA	253
Ge	Greenwald, B	MD	233
Ge	Hanauer, S	IL	245
Ge	Okolo, P	MD	236
GO	Chan, J	CA	289
GO	Cornelison, T	MD	277
GO	Coukos, G	PA	277
GO	De Geest, K	IA	284
GO	Edwards, R	PA	277
GO	Follen, M	PA	278
GO	Ghamande, S	GA	281
GO	Odunsi, A	NY	279
GO	Stehman, F	IN	286
GO	Teng, N	CA	291
Hem	Djulbegovic, B	FL	315
Hem	Flynn, P	MN	318
Hem	Greer, J	TN	315
Hem	Grever, M	OH	318
Hem	Komrokji, R	FL	315
Hem	Kraut, E	OH	319
Hem	Maddox, A	AR	323
Hem	Maslak, P	NY	311
Hem	Nademanee, A	CA	325
Hem	O'Donnell, M	CA	325
Hem	Slease, R	DE	313
Hem	Streiff, M	MD	314
IC	Gibson, C	MA	123
IC	Kandzari, D	GA	127

Spec	Name	St	Pg
IM	Fischl, M	FL	419
Inf	Mildvan, D	NY	406
Inf	Saag, M	AL	409
N	Albers, G	CA	533
N	Chamberlain, M	WA	534
N	Janss, A	GA	520
N	Lipton, R	NY	513
N	Mitsumoto, H	NY	513
N	Newton, H	OH	526
N	Pennell, P	MA	506
N	Wolinsky, J	TX	532
NS	Brem, S	FL	477
NS	Markert, J	AL	478
NS	Sampson, J	NC	480
NS	Shaffrey, M	VA	480
NS	Yu, J	CA	496
Onc	Abbruzzese, J	TX	375
Onc	Advani, R	CA	382
Onc	Akerley, W	UT	373
Onc	Arun, B	TX	376
Onc	Berlin, J	TN	351
Onc	Bernard, S	NC	352
Onc	Birrer, M	MA	326
Onc	Blackwell, K	NC	352
Onc	Blobe, G	NC	352
Onc	Bunn, P	CO	373
Onc	Butler, W	SC	352
Onc	Carducci, M	MD	334
Onc	Chang, J	TX	377
Onc	Chapman, P	NY	335
Onc	Chu, E	PA	335
Onc	Cohen, R	PA	336
Onc	Disis, M	WA	384
Onc	Ellis, G	WA	384
Onc	Ensminger, W	MI	366
Onc	Estey, E	WA	384
Onc	Ettinger, D	MD	338
Onc	Fine, R	NY	338
Onc	Flaherty, K	MA	327
Onc	Friedberg, J	NY	339
Onc	Haas, N	PA	340
Onc	Hauke, R	NE	374
Onc	Hortobagyi, G	TX	377
Onc	Hwu, P	TX	378
Onc	Jurcic, J	NY	342
Onc	Kaminski, M	MI	367
Onc	Karp, J	MD	342
Onc	Kaufman, P	NH	329
Onc	Kraft, A	SC	356
Onc	Limentani, S	NC	357
Onc	Marcom, P	NC	358
Onc	Mortimer, J	CA	387
Onc	O'Connor, O	NY	345
Onc	O'Regan, R	GA	358
Onc	Orlowski, R	TX	379
Onc	Perez, E	FL	359
Onc	Perry, D	DC	346
Onc	Pinto, H	CA	388
Onc	Ready, N	NC	359
Onc	Remick, S	WV	346
Onc	Robert-Vizcarrondo, F	AL	360
Onc	Schilder, R	PA	347
Onc	Schuchter, L	PA	347

Spec	Name	St	Pg
Onc	Serody, J	NC	360
Onc	Shibata, S	CA	389
Onc	Sikic, B	CA	389
Onc	Sotomayor, E	FL	361
Onc	Triozzi, P	OH	371
Onc	Tripathy, D	CA	390
Onc	Wolchok, J	NY	350
Onc	Wolff, R	TX	381
Onc	Worden, F	MI	372
Oto	Weisman, R	CA	686
Path	Wilczynski, S	CA	722
PGe	Dubinsky, M	CA	754
PHO	Adamson, P	PA	756
PHO	Blaney, S	TX	774
PHO	Bruggers, C	UT	773
PHO	Croop, J	IN	769
PHO	Cunningham, J	IL	769
PHO	Goldman, S	IL	770
PHO	Halligan, G	PA	759
PHO	Jakacki, R	PA	760
PHO	Kreissman, S	NC	765
PHO	Maris, J	PA	761
PHO	Neuberg, R	SC	766
PHO	Razzouk, B	IN	772
PHO	Rheingold, S	PA	762
PHO	Rosenthal, J	CA	778
PHO	van Hoff, J	NH	756
PInf	Bryson, Y	CA	783
PInf	Edwards, K	TN	780
PInf	Flynn, P	TN	780
PPul	Borowitz, D	NY	793
Psyc	Mann, J	NY	890
Psyc	Weisler, R	NC	893
Pul	Brown, K	CO	934
RadRO	Blackstock, A	NC	951
RadRO	Bogart, J	NY	946
RadRO	Bradley, J	MO	957
RadRO	Koh, W	WA	964
RadRO	Kupelian, P	CA	964
RadRO	Le, Q	CA	965
RadRO	McGarry, R	KY	954
RadRO	Schild, S	AZ	963
RadRO	Senzer, N	TX	963
RadRO	Willett, C	NC	956
Rhu	Wofsy, D	CA	1032
S	Averbook, B	OH	1070
S	Julian, T	PA	1054
S	Leeming, R	OH	1074
S	Lowy, A	CA	1092
S	Meric-Bernstam, F	TX	1086
S	Olson, J	NC	1066
S	Pockaj, B	AZ	1086
S	Ramanathan, R	PA	1057
S	Sauter, E	ND	1081
S	Willey, S	DC	1061
S	Yang, J	MD	1061
TS	Pass, H	NY	1116
TS	Philpott, J	VA	1122
U	Keane, T	SC	1155
U	Moul, J	NC	1156
U	Shabsigh, R	NY	1151

Specialty & Special Expertise Index

Specialty & Special Expertise Index

D

Specialty & Special Expertise Index

E

Specialty & Special Expertise Index

Specialty & Special Expertise Index

Spec	Name	St	Pg
S	Farley, D	MN	1072
S	Gawande, A	MA	1045
S	Hanks, J	VA	1064
S	Howe, J	IA	1074
S	Kim, L	AR	1085
S	Livingston, E	TX	1086
S	McIntyre, R	CO	1080
S	Moore, F	MA	1047
S	Norton, J	CA	1092
S	Schlinkert, R	AZ	1087
S	Traynor, M	ND	1081
S	Weber, C	GA	1069
S	Weigel, R	IA	1079

Endocrine Tumors

Spec	Name	St	Pg
S	Carty, S	PA	1050
S	Fraker, D	PA	1053
S	Jackson, G	TX	1084
S	Lee, J	TX	1085
S	McAneny, D	MA	1046
S	Siperstein, A	OH	1078

Endocrinology

Spec	Name	St	Pg
EDM	Recker, R	NE	218
Ger	Gambert, S	MD	263
Ger	Morley, J	MO	265

Endocrinology & Joint Disorders

Spec	Name	St	Pg
Rhu	Lahita, R	NJ	1024

Endocrinology, Diabetes & Metabolism

Spec	Name	St	Pg
EDM	Abrahamson, M	MA	204
EDM	Ahmann, A	OR	219
EDM	Ain, K	KY	211
EDM	Axelrod, L	MA	204
EDM	Bahn, R	MN	214
EDM	Ball, D	MD	206
EDM	Barrett, E	VA	211
EDM	Beaser, R	MA	204
EDM	Bell, D	AL	212
EDM	Bergman, D	NY	207
EDM	Berkson, R	CA	220
EDM	Bhasin, S	MA	204
EDM	Bilezikian, J	NY	207
EDM	Biller, B	MA	204
EDM	Blum, C	NY	207
EDM	Bockman, R	NY	207
EDM	Braunstein, G	CA	220
EDM	Braverman, L	MA	204
EDM	Brennan, M	MN	214
EDM	Brillon, D	NY	207
EDM	Broadstone, V	IN	214
EDM	Burman, K	DC	207
EDM	Burmeister, L	MN	214
EDM	Buse, J	NC	212
EDM	Calvi, L	NY	207
EDM	Clore, J	VA	212
EDM	Clutter, W	MO	214

Spec	Name	St	Pg
EDM	Cohen, R	OH	214
EDM	Comi, R	NH	204
EDM	Cooper, D	MD	208
EDM	Cryer, P	MO	215
EDM	Cunningham, G	TX	218
EDM	Cushing, G	MA	205
EDM	D'Alessio, D	OH	215
EDM	Dalkin, A	VA	212
EDM	Daniels, G	MA	205
EDM	Davies, T	NY	208
EDM	Dobs, A	MD	208
EDM	Donner, T	MD	208
EDM	Earp, H	NC	212
EDM	Eckel, R	CO	218
EDM	Econs, M	IN	215
EDM	Edelman, S	CA	220
EDM	Ehrmann, D	IL	215
EDM	Emanuele, M	IL	215
EDM	Emanuele, N	IL	215
EDM	Feinglos, M	NC	212
EDM	Felig, P	NY	208
EDM	Fitzgerald, P	CA	220
EDM	Garibaldi, L	PA	208
EDM	Goodman, N	FL	212
EDM	Greene, L	NY	208
EDM	Greenspan, S	PA	208
EDM	Hammer, G	MI	215
EDM	Heber, D	CA	220
EDM	Herman, W	MI	215
EDM	Hirsch, I	WA	220
EDM	Hoffman, A	CA	220
EDM	Holick, M	MA	205
EDM	Hsueh, W	TX	218
EDM	Inzucchi, S	CT	205
EDM	Ipp, E	CA	220
EDM	Jacobs, T	NY	209
EDM	Jensen, M	MN	216
EDM	Kahn, B	MA	205
EDM	Kamdar, V	CA	221
EDM	Kandeel, F	CA	221
EDM	Katznelson, L	CA	221
EDM	Kennedy, L	OH	216
EDM	Khosla, S	MN	216
EDM	Kleinberg, D	NY	209
EDM	Klibanski, A	MA	205
EDM	Klonoff, D	CA	221
EDM	Kloos, R	OH	216
EDM	Koch, C	MS	212
EDM	Kopp, P	IL	216
EDM	Korytkowski, M	PA	209
EDM	Kronenberg, H	MA	205
EDM	Ladenson, P	MD	209
EDM	Larsen, P	MA	205
EDM	Lash, R	MI	216
EDM	Lavis, V	TX	219
EDM	LeBoff, M	MA	206
EDM	Lechan, R	MA	206
EDM	Levine, R	NH	206
EDM	Licata, A	OH	216
EDM	Lipson, A	DC	209
EDM	Mandel, S	PA	209
EDM	Marshall, J	VA	213
EDM	Mazzone, T	IL	217

Spec	Name	St	Pg
EDM	McConnell, R	NY	209
EDM	McGill, J	MO	217
EDM	McMahon, M	MN	217
EDM	Melmed, S	CA	221
EDM	Nathan, D	MA	206
EDM	Nestler, J	VA	213
EDM	Ober, K	NC	213
EDM	Orwoll, E	OR	221
EDM	Osei, K	OH	217
EDM	Ovalle, F	AL	213
EDM	Pearce, E	MA	206
EDM	Powers, A	TN	213
EDM	Quinn, S	FL	213
EDM	Reasner, C	TX	219
EDM	Recker, R	NE	218
EDM	Riddle, M	OR	221
EDM	Ridgway, E	CO	218
EDM	Robbins, R	TX	219
EDM	Roberts, M	PA	209
EDM	Rodbard, H	MD	210
EDM	Ross, D	MA	206
EDM	Rubenfeld, S	TX	219
EDM	Rushakoff, R	CA	221
EDM	Schutta, M	PA	210
EDM	Schwartz, S	PA	210
EDM	Seely, E	MA	206
EDM	Semenkovich, C	MO	217
EDM	Seplowitz, A	NY	210
EDM	Sherman, S	TX	219
EDM	Shuldiner, A	MD	210
EDM	Singer, P	CA	222
EDM	Siris, E	NY	210
EDM	Skyler, J	FL	213
EDM	Snyder, P	PA	210
EDM	Sowers, J	MO	217
EDM	Surks, M	NY	211
EDM	Swerdloff, R	CA	222
EDM	Tuttle, R	NY	211
EDM	Vance, M	VA	213
EDM	Waguespack, S	TX	219
EDM	Wartofsky, L	DC	211
EDM	Watts, N	OH	217
EDM	Weiss, R	IL	218
EDM	Weissman, P	FL	214
EDM	Werner, P	IL	218
EDM	Woeber, K	CA	222
EDM	Xing, M	MD	211
EDM	Young, I	NY	211

Endometriosis

Spec	Name	St	Pg
GO	Fiorica, J	FL	281
GO	Magrina, J	AZ	288
ObG	Einarsson, J	MA	552
ObG	Filip, S	NC	553
ObG	Goldstein, M	NY	553
ObG	Jenkins, T	AL	555
ObG	Merritt, D	MO	558
ObG	Pfeifer, S	PA	554
ObG	Steege, J	NC	556
RE	Adamson, G	CA	1016
RE	Agarwal, S	CA	1017
RE	Carson, S	RI	1006

Specialty & Special Expertise Index

Specialty & Special Expertise Index

Specialty & Special Expertise Index

Spec	Name	St	Pg	Spec	Name	St	Pg	Spec	Name	St	Pg
Ge	Gish, R	CA	253	Ge	Miskovitz, P	NY	236	Ge	Weinberg, D	PA	238
Ge	Glombicki, A	TX	251	Ge	Mittal, R	CA	254	Ge	Weinstock, J	MA	230
Ge	Goggins, M	MD	232	Ge	Munoz, S	PA	236	Ge	Wiesner, R	MN	248
Ge	Goldberg, M	IL	245	Ge	Murray, J	MN	246	Ge	Wilcox, C	AL	243
Ge	Gordon, S	NH	229	Ge	Navarro, V	PA	236	Ge	Wolfe, M	OH	249
Ge	Gostout, C	MN	245	Ge	Nunes, D	MA	229	Ge	Yanda, R	GA	243
Ge	Green, P	NY	233	Ge	Okolo, P	MD	236	Ge	Young, R	NE	249
Ge	Greenwald, B	MD	233	Ge	Ostroff, J	CA	254	Ge	Younossi, Z	VA	243
Ge	Haber, G	NY	233	Ge	Owyang, C	MI	247	Ge	Zaman, A	OR	255
Ge	Haluszka, O	PA	233	Ge	Pasricha, P	CA	254				
Ge	Han, S	CA	253	Ge	Peikin, S	NJ	236	**Gastroesophageal Reflux**			
Ge	Hanauer, S	IL	245	Ge	Pezzone, M	PA	237	**Disease (GERD)**			
Ge	Hawes, R	SC	240	Ge	Plevy, S	NC	241				
Ge	Herrine, S	PA	233	Ge	Pochapin, M	NY	237	Ge	Brazer, S	NC	239
Ge	Hillebrand, D	CA	254	Ge	Poordad, F	CA	254	Ge	Castell, D	SC	239
Ge	Hoffman, B	SC	240	Ge	Porayko, M	TN	241	Ge	Chey, W	MI	244
Ge	Hoops, T	PA	233	Ge	Proctor, D	CT	229	Ge	Cohen, L	NY	231
Ge	Hunter, E	ID	249	Ge	Raiford, D	TN	241	Ge	DeVault, K	FL	239
Ge	Infantolino, A	PA	233	Ge	Raju, G	TX	252	Ge	Di Marino, A	PA	231
Ge	Isaacs, K	NC	240	Ge	Ravich, W	MD	237	Ge	Feldman, E	CA	253
Ge	Itzkowitz, S	NY	233	Ge	Reddy, K	PA	237	Ge	Fennerty, M	OR	253
Ge	Jacobson, I	NY	234	Ge	Reichelderfer, M	WI	247	Ge	Freiman, H	NY	232
Ge	Jensen, D	IL	245	Ge	Reuben, A	SC	242	Ge	Gerson, L	CA	253
Ge	Kahrilas, P	IL	245	Ge	Rex, D	IN	247	Ge	Katz, P	PA	234
Ge	Kalloo, A	MD	234	Ge	Reynolds, J	PA	237	Ge	Levine, J	CT	229
Ge	Kantsevoy, S	MD	234	Ge	Roth, B	CA	255	Ge	Lind, C	TN	241
Ge	Kaplan, L	MA	229	Ge	Rothstein, R	NH	229	Ge	Lipshutz, W	PA	235
Ge	Kastenberg, D	PA	234	Ge	Sachar, D	NY	237	Ge	Markowitz, D	NY	236
Ge	Katz, P	PA	234	Ge	Sandborn, W	CA	255	Ge	Metz, D	PA	236
Ge	Kimmey, M	WA	254	Ge	Sartor, R	NC	242	Ge	Ravich, W	MD	237
Ge	Koch, K	NC	240	Ge	Savides, T	CA	255	Ge	Reynolds, J	PA	237
Ge	Kochman, M	PA	234	Ge	Schiano, T	NY	237	Ge	Roth, B	CA	255
Ge	Konicek, F	IL	245	Ge	Schiff, E	FL	242	Ge	Rothstein, R	NH	229
Ge	Korsten, M	NY	234	Ge	Schiller, L	TX	252	Ge	Schulze, K	IA	247
Ge	Kotler, D	NY	234	Ge	Schulze, K	IA	247	Ge	Shaker, R	WI	247
Ge	Kowalski, T	PA	235	Ge	Scudera, P	VA	242	Ge	Vaezi, M	TN	242
Ge	Kozarek, R	WA	254	Ge	Seidner, D	TN	242	NP	Gewolb, I	MI	446
Ge	Kurtz, R	NY	235	Ge	Semrad, C	IL	247	PGe	Baker, R	NY	749
Ge	Kwo, P	IN	246	Ge	Shaker, R	WI	247	PGe	Baker, R	NY	749
Ge	La Russo, N	MN	246	Ge	Sherman, S	IN	247	PGe	Gunasekaran, T	IL	752
Ge	Lambiase, L	TN	240	Ge	Shiffman, M	VA	242	PGe	Gupta, S	IN	752
Ge	Lashner, B	OH	246	Ge	Shike, M	NY	238	PGe	Heyman, M	CA	754
Ge	Lebwohl, O	NY	235	Ge	Siegel, C	NH	230	PGe	Levy, J	NY	749
Ge	Leighton, J	AZ	251	Ge	Silverman, W	IA	247	PGe	Mousa, H	OH	752
Ge	Lenz, H	CA	254	Ge	Slivka, A	PA	238	PGe	Schwarz, S	NY	750
Ge	Levine, J	CT	229	Ge	Smoot, D	DC	238	PGe	Snyder, J	DC	750
Ge	Lewis, B	NY	235	Ge	Sorrell, M	NE	249	PGe	Spivak, W	NY	750
Ge	Lichtenstein, G	PA	235	Ge	Speeg, K	TX	252	PS	Foglia, R	TX	809
Ge	Liddle, R	NC	241	Ge	Stump, D	TX	252	S	Ballantyne, G	CT	1044
Ge	Lightdale, C	NY	235	Ge	Surawicz, C	WA	255	S	Brunicardi, F	TX	1082
Ge	Lind, C	TN	241	Ge	Targan, S	CA	255	S	Chand, B	OH	1071
Ge	Lindor, K	MN	246	Ge	Te, H	IL	248	S	Crookes, P	CA	1089
Ge	Lipshutz, W	PA	235	Ge	Tobias, H	NY	238	S	Dempsey, D	PA	1052
Ge	Loftus, E	MN	246	Ge	Toskes, P	FL	242	S	Hunter, J	OR	1091
Ge	Lucey, M	WI	246	Ge	Tremaine, W	MN	248	S	Peters, J	NY	1057
Ge	Magun, A	NY	235	Ge	Vaezi, M	TN	242	S	Rattner, D	MA	1047
Ge	Markowitz, D	NY	236	Ge	Van Thiel, D	IL	248	S	Salky, B	NY	1058
Ge	Martin, P	FL	241	Ge	Vargo, J	OH	248	S	Soper, N	IL	1078
Ge	Mason, J	MA	229	Ge	Vege, S	MN	248	S	Sweeney, J	GA	1068
Ge	Mayer, L	NY	236	Ge	Vierling, J	TX	252	TS	Deschamps, C	MN	1125
Ge	Meiselman, M	IL	245	Ge	Wald, A	WI	248	TS	Landreneau, R	PA	1114
Ge	Mertz, H	TN	241	Ge	Waxman, I	IL	248	TS	Watson, T	NY	1118
Ge	Metz, D	PA	236	Ge	Waye, J	NY	238				

Specialty & Special Expertise Index

Specialty & Special Expertise Index

Spec	Name	St	Pg
Ger	Carr, D	MO	265
Ger	Ciocon, J	FL	264
Ger	Cooney, L	CT	262
Ger	Dale, L	MN	265
Ger	Duthie, E	WI	265
Ger	Dyer, C	TX	266
Ger	Finucane, T	MD	263
Ger	Flaherty, J	MO	265
Ger	Gambert, S	MD	263
Ger	Gorbien, M	IL	265
Ger	Greganti, M	NC	264
Ger	Hanson, L	NC	264
Ger	Kutner, J	CO	266
Ger	Lachs, M	NY	263
Ger	Landefeld, C	CA	267
Ger	Liem, P	AR	266
Ger	Lipschitz, D	AR	266
Ger	Lipsitz, L	MA	262
Ger	Lyles, K	NC	264
Ger	McCormick, W	WA	267
Ger	Meier, D	NY	263
Ger	Minaker, K	MA	262
Ger	Morley, J	MO	265
Ger	Oates, D	MA	262
Ger	Olson, J	IL	265
Ger	Palmer, R	VA	264
Ger	Resnick, N	PA	263
Ger	Reuben, D	CA	267
Ger	Ritchie, C	AL	264
Ger	Sachs, G	IN	265
Ger	Schwartz, R	CO	266
Ger	Studenski, S	PA	263
Ger	Supiano, M	UT	266
Ger	Tenover, J	CA	267
Ger	Thomas, D	MO	266
Ger	Tinetti, M	CT	262
Ger	Wei, J	AR	267

Geriatric Neurology

N	DeKosky, S	VA	518
N	Ferrendelli, J	TX	531

Geriatric Ophthalmology

Oph	Sterns, G	NY	578

Geriatric Psychiatry

GerPsy	Borson, S	WA	912
GerPsy	Burke, W	NE	911
GerPsy	Greenwald, B	NY	910
GerPsy	Grossberg, G	MO	911
GerPsy	Holroyd, S	VA	911
GerPsy	Kennedy, G	NY	910
GerPsy	Kramer, B	CA	912
GerPsy	Lyketsos, C	MD	910
GerPsy	Manepalli, J	MO	911
GerPsy	Mellow, A	MI	911
GerPsy	Reisberg, B	NY	910
GerPsy	Rosen, J	PA	910
GerPsy	Rovner, B	PA	910
GerPsy	Small, G	CA	912

Spec	Name	St	Pg
GerPsy	Stein, E	CA	912
GerPsy	Streim, J	PA	910
GerPsy	Tune, L	GA	911
GerPsy	Veith, R	WA	912
Psyc	Blazer, D	NC	891
Psyc	Ellison, J	MA	884
Psyc	Jenike, M	MA	885
Psyc	Marin, D	NY	890
Psyc	Nelson, J	CA	898
Psyc	Raskind, M	WA	898
Psyc	Salzman, C	MA	886
Psyc	Weiner, M	TX	896

Geriatric Rehabilitation

Ger	Allman, R	AL	264
PMR	Bloch, R	MA	832
PMR	Diamond, P	VA	836
PMR	Frost, F	OH	838
PMR	Lipkin, D	FL	837
PMR	Roth, E	IL	840

Germ Cell Tumors

Onc	Margolin, K	WA	387
PHO	Marina, N	CA	777
PHO	Olson, T	GA	766
PS	Morgan, W	TN	805

Gestational Trophoblastic Disease

GO	Burger, R	PA	276
GO	Curtin, J	NY	277
GO	Fromm, G	TX	287
GO	Giuntoli, R	MD	278
GO	Lurain, J	IL	284
GO	Muntz, H	WA	290
GO	Plaxe, S	CA	290
GO	Soper, J	NC	283

Gitelman's Syndrome

Nep	Ellison, D	OR	461

Glanzmann's Thrombasthenia

Hem	Coller, B	NY	310

Glaucoma

Oph	Alward, W	IA	585
Oph	Baerveldt, G	CA	596
Oph	Budenz, D	FL	580
Oph	Caprioli, J	CA	597
Oph	Crandall, A	UT	593
Oph	Gaasterland, D	MD	572
Oph	Gorovoy, M	FL	581
Oph	Greenfield, D	FL	581
Oph	Heuer, D	WI	588
Oph	Iwach, A	CA	598
Oph	Kaufman, P	WI	588
Oph	Kwon, Y	IA	588

Spec	Name	St	Pg
Oph	Lee, P	NC	582
Oph	Lichter, P	MI	589
Oph	Liebmann, J	NY	574
Oph	Myers, R	PA	576
Oph	Parrish, R	FL	583
Oph	Quigley, H	MD	576
Oph	Ritch, R	NY	577
Oph	Samuelson, T	MN	591
Oph	Schuman, J	PA	577
Oph	Sergott, R	PA	577
Oph	Sherwood, M	FL	584
Oph	Shingleton, B	MA	569
Oph	Smith, S	NY	578
Oph	Tsai, J	CT	569
Oph	Vajaranant, T	IL	592
Oph	Wallace, R	LA	595

Glaucoma-Pediatric

Oph	Del Monte, M	MI	587
Oph	Freedman, S	NC	581
Oph	Jaafar, M	DC	574
Oph	Medow, N	NY	575
Oph	Plager, D	IN	590
Oph	Traboulsi, E	OH	592
Oph	Walton, D	MA	569

Gliomas

N	Batchelor, T	MA	504
N	Mikkelsen, T	MI	526
N	Rosenfeld, S	OH	528
N	Taylor, L	WA	537
NS	Chen, T	CA	492
NS	Friedman, A	NC	477
NS	Lang, F	TX	489
NS	Weingart, J	MD	475
Onc	Friedman, H	NC	354
Onc	Vredenburgh, J	NC	362

Glomerulonephritis

Nep	Appel, G	NY	453
Nep	Berns, J	PA	453
Nep	Bolton, W	VA	455
Nep	Cho, K	CA	461
Nep	Cohen, D	NY	454
Nep	Falk, R	NC	456
Nep	Holzman, L	PA	454
Nep	Kasinath, B	TX	460
Nep	Rodby, R	IL	458
Nep	Winston, J	NY	455
PNep	Andreoli, S	IN	786
PNep	Benfield, M	AL	785
PNep	Eddy, A	WA	787
PNep	Fouser, L	WA	787
PNep	Mendley, S	MD	784

Gout

A&I	Sundy, J	NC	87
Rhu	Davis, W	LA	1030
Rhu	Fields, T	NY	1024
Rhu	Massarotti, E	MA	1022

Specialty & Special Expertise Index

Specialty & Special Expertise Index

Specialty & Special Expertise Index

Spec	Name	St	Pg	Spec	Name	St	Pg	Spec	Name	St	Pg
Onc	Algazy, K	PA	333	Hem	Gertz, M	MN	318	Hem	Rodgers, G	UT	321
Onc	Bashevkin, M	NY	334	Hem	Godwin, J	IL	318	Hem	Roodman, G	PA	313
Onc	Beatty, P	MT	373	Hem	Goldberg, J	PA	311	Hem	Rosenblatt, J	FL	315
Onc	Bergsagel, P	AZ	376	Hem	Gordon, L	IL	318	Hem	Rowley, S	NJ	313
Onc	Bolwell, B	OH	363	Hem	Greer, J	TN	315	Hem	Savage, D	NY	313
Onc	Claxton, D	PA	335	Hem	Gregory, S	IL	318	Hem	Saven, A	CA	325
Onc	Cohen, G	MD	335	Hem	Greipp, P	MN	318	Hem	Schiffman, F	RI	309
Onc	Colon-Otero, G	FL	353	Hem	Grever, M	OH	318	Hem	Schiller, G	CA	325
Onc	Deeg, H	WA	384	Hem	Habermann, T	MN	318	Hem	Schuster, M	NY	313
Onc	Druker, B	OR	384	Hem	Heinrich, M	OR	324	Hem	Schuster, S	PA	313
Onc	Erban, J	MA	327	Hem	Isola, L	NY	311	Hem	Schwartzberg, L	TN	316
Onc	Gabrilove, J	NY	339	Hem	Juckett, M	WI	319	Hem	Silverstein, R	WI	320
Onc	Mitsuyasu, R	CA	387	Hem	Kantarjian, H	TX	322	Hem	Singhal, S	IL	320
Onc	Rosen, S	IL	370	Hem	Keating, M	TX	322	Hem	Slease, R	DE	313
Onc	Rosove, M	CA	388	Hem	Kempin, S	NY	311	Hem	Snyder, D	CA	325
Onc	Schilder, R	PA	347	Hem	Kessler, C	DC	311	Hem	Sokol, L	FL	316
Onc	Shields, P	DC	347	Hem	Kipps, T	CA	324	Hem	Solberg, L	FL	316
Onc	Silver, S	MI	371	Hem	Klingemann, H	MA	308	Hem	Spitzer, T	MA	309
Onc	Strenger, R	RI	331	Hem	Komrokji, R	FL	315	Hem	Spivak, J	MD	313
PHO	Hord, J	OH	770	Hem	Kraut, E	OH	319	Hem	Stiff, P	IL	320
PHO	Ritchey, A	PA	762	Hem	Kuriakose, P	MI	319	Hem	Stone, R	MA	309
				Hem	Larson, R	IL	319	Hem	Strair, R	NJ	314
				Hem	Laughlin, M	VA	315	Hem	Strauss, J	TX	323
Hematology				Hem	Lazarus, H	OH	319	Hem	Streiff, M	MD	314
				Hem	Leung, L	CA	324	Hem	Tallman, M	NY	314
Hem	Abrams, C	PA	309	Hem	Levine, A	CA	324	Hem	Telen, M	NC	316
Hem	Adams-Graves, P	TN	314	Hem	Lill, M	CA	324	Hem	Uberti, J	MI	321
Hem	Allen, S	NY	309	Hem	Lin, W	TX	323	Hem	Van Besien, K	IL	321
Hem	Anderson, K	MA	308	Hem	Linenberger, M	WA	324	Hem	Vose, J	NE	321
Hem	Baer, M	MD	310	Hem	Litzow, M	MN	319	Hem	Williams, M	VA	316
Hem	Ballen, K	MA	308	Hem	Lyons, R	TX	323	Hem	Winter, J	IL	321
Hem	Barlogie, B	AR	321	Hem	Maciejewski, J	OH	319	Hem	Wisch, N	NY	314
Hem	Baron, J	IL	316	Hem	Maddox, A	AR	323	Hem	Yanovich, S	MD	314
Hem	Bigelow, C	MS	314	Hem	Mangan, K	PA	311	Hem	Yeager, A	AZ	323
Hem	Blinder, M	MO	317	Hem	Marks, P	CT	308	Hem	Zuckerman, K	FL	316
Hem	Bockenstedt, P	MI	317	Hem	Marks, S	PA	311				
Hem	Brenner, M	TX	321	Hem	Maslak, P	NY	311	**Hematopathology**			
Hem	Bricker, L	MI	317	Hem	Maziarz, R	OR	325				
Hem	Brodsky, R	MD	310	Hem	McGlave, P	MN	319	Hem	Rodgers, G	UT	321
Hem	Byrd, J	OH	317	Hem	Mears, J	NY	312	Path	Bagg, A	PA	707
Hem	Champlin, R	TX	322	Hem	Meehan, K	NH	308	Path	Banks, P	NC	712
Hem	Cheson, B	DC	310	Hem	Milhem, M	IA	320	Path	Behm, F	IL	714
Hem	Cobos, E	TX	322	Hem	Millenson, M	PA	312	Path	Chesney, C	TN	713
Hem	Coller, B	NY	310	Hem	Miller, M	MA	309	Path	Harris, N	MA	706
Hem	Comenzo, R	MA	308	Hem	Mitchell, B	CA	325	Path	Kinney, M	TX	718
Hem	Cooper, B	TX	322	Hem	Mosher, D	WI	320	Path	McCurley, T	TN	713
Hem	Copelan, E	OH	317	Hem	Munker, R	LA	323	Path	Morrow, J	CT	707
Hem	Cortes, J	TX	322	Hem	Nademanee, A	CA	325	Path	Nathwani, B	CA	721
Hem	Damon, L	CA	323	Hem	Nand, S	IL	320	Path	Orazi, A	NY	710
Hem	Dang, C	MD	310	Hem	Negrin, R	CA	325	Path	Swerdlow, S	PA	711
Hem	DeLoughery, T	OR	324	Hem	Nimer, S	NY	312	Path	Warnke, R	CA	722
Hem	Di Persio, J	MO	317	Hem	O'Donnell, M	CA	325	Path	Weisenburger, D	NE	717
Hem	Diuguid, D	NY	310	Hem	Ortel, T	NC	315	Path	Weiss, L	CA	722
Hem	Djulbegovic, B	FL	315	Hem	Palascak, J	OH	320				
Hem	Duffy, T	CT	308	Hem	Philipp, C	NJ	312	**Hemifacial Spasm**			
Hem	Emanuel, P	AR	322	Hem	Porcu, P	OH	320				
Hem	Erba, H	MI	317	Hem	Porter, D	PA	312	NS	Sen, C	NY	474
Hem	Farag, S	IN	317	Hem	Powell, B	NC	315				
Hem	Files, J	MS	315	Hem	Rai, K	NY	312	**Hemochromatosis**			
Hem	Filicko-OHara, J	PA	310	Hem	Rao, A	PA	312				
Hem	Flynn, P	MN	318	Hem	Raphael, B	NY	312	PHO	Wolfe, L	NY	763
Hem	Fonseca, R	AZ	322	Hem	Rapoport, A	MD	313				
Hem	Forman, S	CA	324	Hem	Richardson, P	MA	309				
Hem	Fruchtman, S	NY	310								

Specialty & Special Expertise Index

Specialty & Special Expertise Index

Specialty & Special Expertise Index

Spec	Name	St	Pg

Incontinence-Male & Female

| U | Nitti, V | NY | 1150 |
| U | Webster, G | NC | 1159 |

Incontinence/Pelvic Floor Disorders

CRS	Madoff, R	MN	173
CRS	Mutch, M	MO	173
CRS	Ramamoorthy, S	CA	176

Infant-Toddler Psychiatry

| ChAP | Zeanah, C | LA | 908 |

Infection Control

| Inf | Wallach, F | NY | 407 |

Infections in Cancer Patients

Inf	Freifeld, A	NE	412
Inf	Polsky, B	NY	407
Inf	Segal, B	NY	407
Inf	Sepkowitz, K	NY	407
Inf	Siegel, M	WA	414
PHO	Siegel, S	CA	778

Infections in Immunocompromised Patients

Inf	Cohen, M	NC	408
Inf	Cunha, B	NY	405
Inf	Edwards, J	CA	413
PInf	Alexander, K	IL	781
PInf	Emmanuel, P	FL	780
PInf	Flynn, P	TN	780
PInf	McKinney, R	NC	781
PInf	Michaels, M	PA	780

Infections in Int'l Adopted Children

| PInf | Krilov, L | NY | 779 |

Infections in Pregnancy

MF	Duff, W	FL	430
MF	Ismail, M	IL	432
ObG	Sweet, R	CA	560

Infections in Prosthetic Devices

| Inf | Brause, B | NY | 405 |
| Inf | Slama, T | IN | 411 |

Infections-CNS

| N | Simpson, D | NY | 515 |

Infections-Congenital

| ChiN | Bale, J | UT | 150 |

Infections-Emerging

| Path | Walker, D | TX | 719 |

Infections-Neonatal

| MF | Ismail, M | IL | 432 |
| NP | Davis, J | MA | 442 |

Infections-Neurologic

ChiN	Bale, J	UT	150
N	Coyle, P	NY	508
N	Roos, K	IN	527
NS	Rosenblum, M	MI	486

Infections-Respiratory

PInf	Krilov, L	NY	779
PInf	Wald, E	WI	782
Pul	Jacoby, D	OR	938
Pul	Niederman, M	NY	924

Infections-Surgical

Inf	Gumprecht, J	NY	405
Inf	Hammer, G	NY	405
Inf	Hartman, B	NY	406
Inf	O'Keefe, J	IL	411

Infections-Transplant

Inf	Alvarez-Elcoro, S	FL	408
Inf	Gorensek, M	FL	409
PInf	Green, M	PA	779

Infectious & Demyelinating Diseases

| N | Berger, J | KY | 518 |
| N | Cook, S | NJ | 508 |

Infectious Diarrhea

| Ge | Surawicz, C | WA | 255 |

Infectious Disease

A&I	Bonner, J	AL	86
D	Friedlander, S	CA	198
IM	Fischl, M	FL	419
Inf	Alvarez-Elcoro, S	FL	408
Inf	Auwaerter, P	MD	404
Inf	Bakken, J	MN	410
Inf	Ballon-Landa, G	CA	413
Inf	Bartlett, J	MD	404
Inf	Bayer, A	CA	413
Inf	Berkowitz, L	NY	404
Inf	Blumberg, H	GA	408
Inf	Brause, B	NY	405
Inf	Campbell, J	MO	410
Inf	Cancio, M	FL	408
Inf	Chaisson, R	MD	405
Inf	Cohen, M	NC	408

Inf	Cohn, S	IL	410
Inf	Corey, G	NC	408
Inf	Craven, D	MA	404
Inf	Cunha, B	NY	405
Inf	Daar, E	CA	413
Inf	DuPont, H	TX	412
Inf	Edmond, M	VA	408
Inf	Edwards, J	CA	413
Inf	Fauci, A	MD	405
Inf	Fichtenbaum, C	OH	410
Inf	Flaherty, J	IL	410
Inf	Flanigan, T	RI	404
Inf	Frank, I	PA	405
Inf	Freifeld, A	NE	412
Inf	Gorensek, M	FL	409
Inf	Gumprecht, J	NY	405
Inf	Hammer, G	NY	405
Inf	Hammer, S	NY	405
Inf	Hartman, B	NY	406
Inf	High, K	NC	409
Inf	Huitt, G	CO	412
Inf	Katner, H	GA	409
Inf	Keiser, P	TX	412
Inf	Longworth, D	OH	410
Inf	Lorber, B	PA	406
Inf	Louie, E	NY	406
Inf	Luby, J	TX	412
Inf	Maki, D	WI	410
Inf	Masur, H	MD	406
Inf	McGowan, J	NY	406
Inf	Mildvan, D	NY	406
Inf	Mildvan, D	NY	406
Inf	Nahass, R	NJ	406
Inf	O'Keefe, J	IL	411
Inf	Palefsky, J	CA	413
Inf	Patterson, J	TX	412
Inf	Patterson, T	TX	413
Inf	Pearson, R	VA	409
Inf	Pearson, R	VA	409
Inf	Perlman, D	NY	406
Inf	Perlman, D	NY	406
Inf	Polsky, B	NY	407
Inf	Quagliarello, V	CT	404
Inf	Rao, N	PA	407
Inf	Ratzan, K	FL	409
Inf	Richman, D	CA	413
Inf	Romagnoli, M	NY	407
Inf	Saag, M	AL	409
Inf	Salata, R	OH	411
Inf	Sax, P	MA	404
Inf	Scheld, W	VA	409
Inf	Schmitt, S	OH	411
Inf	Schooley, R	CA	414
Inf	Schooley, R	CA	414
Inf	Segal, B	NY	407
Inf	Sepkowitz, K	NY	407
Inf	Sha, B	IL	411
Inf	Siegel, M	WA	414
Inf	Slama, T	IN	411
Inf	Sobel, J	MI	411
Inf	Tomford, J	OH	411
Inf	Trenholme, G	IL	411
Inf	Van Der Horst, C	NC	409

Specialty & Special Expertise Index

Specialty & Special Expertise Index

Specialty & Special Expertise Index

Spec	Name	St	Pg
PCd	Ackerman, M	MN	737

Low Vision

Spec	Name	St	Pg
Oph	Sterns, G	NY	578

Lower Limb Arterial Disease

Spec	Name	St	Pg
VascS	Bandyk, D	FL	1183
VascS	Gloviczki, P	MN	1185
VascS	Howard, T	NE	1187
VascS	Kent, K	WI	1186
VascS	Mackey, W	MA	1179

Lower Limb Reconstruction

Spec	Name	St	Pg
PlS	Attinger, C	DC	850
PlS	Wilkins, E	MI	866

Lower Limb Surgery in Children

Spec	Name	St	Pg
OrS	McCarthy, J	OH	633

Lung Cancer

Spec	Name	St	Pg
DR	Austin, J	NY	974
DR	Black, W	NH	973
DR	Chiles, C	NC	978
DR	Erasmus, J	TX	982
DR	Henschke, C	NY	975
DR	Patz, E	NC	979
DR	Sagel, S	MO	980
DR	Swensen, S	MN	981
DR	Yankelevitz, D	NY	977
Hem	Maddox, A	AR	323
Hem	Schwartzberg, L	TN	316
Onc	Adelstein, D	OH	363
Onc	Aisner, J	NJ	332
Onc	Akerley, W	UT	373
Onc	Albain, K	IL	363
Onc	Algazy, K	PA	333
Onc	Antonia, S	FL	351
Onc	Argiris, A	PA	333
Onc	Axelrod, R	PA	333
Onc	Azzoli, C	NY	333
Onc	Belani, C	PA	334
Onc	Bitran, J	IL	363
Onc	Bonomi, P	IL	363
Onc	Bunn, P	CO	373
Onc	Butler, W	SC	352
Onc	Carbone, D	TN	353
Onc	Chachoua, A	NY	335
Onc	Chapman, R	MI	364
Onc	Clamon, G	IA	364
Onc	Cohen, R	PA	336
Onc	Cohen, S	NY	336
Onc	Conry, R	AL	353
Onc	Crawford, J	NC	353
Onc	Dowlati, A	OH	365
Onc	Dunphy, F	NC	354
Onc	Edelman, M	MD	337
Onc	Einhorn, L	IN	365
Onc	Ettinger, D	MD	338
Onc	Fossella, F	TX	377

Spec	Name	St	Pg
Onc	Gandara, D	CA	385
Onc	Garst, J	NC	354
Onc	Glisson, B	TX	377
Onc	Golomb, H	IL	366
Onc	Greco, F	TN	355
Onc	Grunberg, S	VT	328
Onc	Hageboutros, A	NJ	340
Onc	Herbst, R	CT	329
Onc	Hoffman, P	IL	367
Onc	Holland, J	NY	341
Onc	Hollister, D	CT	329
Onc	Hong, W	TX	377
Onc	Jahanzeb, M	FL	356
Onc	Johnson, B	MA	329
Onc	Johnson, D	TX	378
Onc	Kalemkerian, G	MI	367
Onc	Karp, D	TX	378
Onc	Kelly, K	CA	386
Onc	Khuri, F	GA	356
Onc	Kies, M	TX	378
Onc	Koczywas, M	CA	386
Onc	Kressel, B	DC	342
Onc	Kris, M	NY	342
Onc	Langer, C	PA	343
Onc	Lilenbaum, R	FL	357
Onc	Lippman, S	TX	378
Onc	Livingston, R	AZ	379
Onc	Lynch, J	FL	357
Onc	Lynch, T	CT	330
Onc	Martins, R	WA	387
Onc	Masters, G	DE	343
Onc	Miller, A	NC	358
Onc	Miller, D	KY	358
Onc	Miller, V	NY	344
Onc	Natale, R	CA	387
Onc	Northfelt, D	AZ	379
Onc	O'Brien, T	OH	368
Onc	Pao, W	TN	359
Onc	Pasmantier, M	NY	345
Onc	Perry, D	DC	346
Onc	Perry, M	MO	369
Onc	Pisters, K	TX	380
Onc	Ready, N	NC	359
Onc	Robert-Vizcarrondo, F	AL	360
Onc	Ross, H	AZ	380
Onc	Salgia, R	IL	370
Onc	Sandler, A	OR	389
Onc	Schiller, J	TX	380
Onc	Sherman, C	SC	360
Onc	Shin, D	GA	360
Onc	Simon, G	SC	360
Onc	Socinski, M	NC	361
Onc	Steen, P	ND	375
Onc	Stone, J	FL	361
Onc	Stoopler, M	NY	348
Onc	Strauss, G	MA	331
Onc	Tester, W	PA	349
Onc	Thigpen, J	MS	361
Onc	Vance, R	MS	362
Onc	Vinciguerra, V	NY	350
Onc	Vokes, E	IL	372
Onc	Wierman, A	NV	391
Path	Cagle, P	TX	717

Spec	Name	St	Pg
Path	Hammar, S	WA	720
Path	Katzenstein, A	NY	709
Path	Koss, M	CA	721
Path	Leslie, K	AZ	718
Path	Moran, C	TX	718
Path	Myers, J	MI	716
Path	Suster, S	WI	716
Path	Travis, W	NY	712
Path	Yousem, S	PA	712
Pul	Alberts, W	FL	927
Pul	Cooper, W	VA	928
Pul	Ernst, A	MA	920
Pul	Garver, R	AL	928
Pul	Goldman, A	FL	928
Pul	Guidry, G	LA	935
Pul	Kern, J	CO	934
Pul	King, E	PA	924
Pul	Libby, D	NY	924
Pul	Maxfield, R	NY	924
Pul	Silver, M	IL	933
Pul	Steinberg, H	NY	926
Pul	Sterman, D	PA	926
Pul	Teirstein, A	NY	926
Pul	Unger, M	PA	927
RadRO	Beitler, J	GA	951
RadRO	Blackstock, A	NC	951
RadRO	Bogart, J	NY	946
RadRO	Bonner, J	AL	952
RadRO	Bradley, J	MO	957
RadRO	Choi, N	MA	944
RadRO	Choy, H	TX	962
RadRO	Cox, J	TX	962
RadRO	Emami, B	IL	957
RadRO	Greenberger, J	PA	948
RadRO	Haffty, B	NJ	948
RadRO	Hahn, S	PA	948
RadRO	Halle, J	NC	952
RadRO	Haraf, D	IL	958
RadRO	Hayman, J	MI	958
RadRO	Heimann, R	VT	944
RadRO	Jose, B	KY	953
RadRO	Komaki, R	TX	963
RadRO	Kudrimoti, M	KY	953
RadRO	Le, Q	CA	965
RadRO	Lewin, A	FL	953
RadRO	Marks, L	NC	954
RadRO	McGarry, R	KY	954
RadRO	Morris, M	VA	954
RadRO	Movsas, B	MI	960
RadRO	Nori, D	NY	949
RadRO	Randolph-Jackson, P	DC	950
RadRO	Roach, M	CA	965
RadRO	Rosenman, J	NC	955
RadRO	Schild, S	AZ	963
RadRO	Seung, S	OR	966
RadRO	Streeter, O	DC	950
RadRO	Suntharalingam, M	MD	950
RadRO	Videtic, G	OH	961
RadRO	Werner-Wasik, M	PA	951
RadRO	Wilson, L	CT	946
TS	Altorki, N	NY	1109
TS	Bains, M	NY	1109
TS	Battafarano, R	MD	1109

America's Top Doctors® 11th Edition

Specialty & Special Expertise Index

Spec	Name	St	Pg	Spec	Name	St	Pg	Spec	Name	St	Pg
Onc	Fine, H	MD	338	Onc	Henry, D	PA	340	Onc	Levy, M	PA	343
Onc	Fine, R	NY	338	Onc	Herbst, R	CT	329	Onc	Lilenbaum, R	FL	357
Onc	Fisher, G	CA	385	Onc	Higano, C	WA	386	Onc	Lim, D	CA	386
Onc	Fisher, R	NY	338	Onc	Himelstein, A	DE	341	Onc	Limentani, S	NC	357
Onc	Fitch, T	AZ	377	Onc	Hochberg, E	MA	329	Onc	Lippman, M	FL	357
Onc	Flaherty, K	MA	327	Onc	Hochster, H	CT	329	Onc	Lippman, S	TX	378
Onc	Fleming, G	IL	366	Onc	Hoffman, P	IL	367	Onc	List, A	FL	357
Onc	Flinn, I	TN	354	Onc	Hogan, T	WV	341	Onc	Livingston, R	AZ	379
Onc	Flomenberg, N	PA	338	Onc	Holland, J	NY	341	Onc	Loehrer, P	IN	368
Onc	Forastiere, A	MD	339	Onc	Hollister, D	CT	329	Onc	Logothetis, C	TX	379
Onc	Ford, J	CA	385	Onc	Hong, W	TX	377	Onc	Loprinzi, C	MN	368
Onc	Forero, A	AL	354	Onc	Hortobagyi, G	TX	377	Onc	Lossos, I	FL	357
Onc	Forscher, C	CA	385	Onc	Horwitz, S	NY	341	Onc	Lyckholm, L	VA	357
Onc	Foss, F	CT	328	Onc	Hudes, G	PA	341	Onc	Lyman, G	NC	357
Onc	Fossella, F	TX	377	Onc	Hudis, C	NY	341	Onc	Lynch, J	FL	357
Onc	Fox, K	PA	339	Onc	Hurd, D	NC	355	Onc	Lynch, T	CT	330
Onc	Fracasso, P	VA	354	Onc	Hussain, M	MI	367	Onc	Makhoul, I	AR	379
Onc	Freedman, A	MA	328	Onc	Hutchins, L	AR	378	Onc	Maki, R	NY	343
Onc	Friedberg, J	NY	339	Onc	Hwu, P	TX	378	Onc	Maloney, D	WA	386
Onc	Friedman, H	NC	354	Onc	Ilson, D	NY	341	Onc	Marcom, P	NC	358
Onc	Fuchs, C	MA	328	Onc	Ingle, J	MN	367	Onc	Margolin, K	WA	387
Onc	Gabrilove, J	NY	339	Onc	Isaacs, C	DC	341	Onc	Markowitz, S	OH	368
Onc	Gandara, D	CA	385	Onc	Jacobs, C	CA	386	Onc	Marshall, J	DC	343
Onc	Ganz, P	CA	385	Onc	Jahanzeb, M	FL	356	Onc	Martins, R	WA	387
Onc	Garber, J	MA	328	Onc	Jillella, A	GA	356	Onc	Masters, G	DE	343
Onc	Garnick, M	MA	328	Onc	Johnson, B	MA	329	Onc	Mathew, P	MA	330
Onc	Garst, J	NC	354	Onc	Johnson, D	TX	378	Onc	Matulonis, U	MA	330
Onc	Gaynor, E	IL	366	Onc	Jonasch, E	TX	378	Onc	McGuire, W	MD	343
Onc	Gelmann, E	NY	339	Onc	Jurcic, J	NY	342	Onc	Meropol, N	OH	368
Onc	George, D	NC	354	Onc	Kalaycio, M	OH	367	Onc	Messersmith, W	CO	375
Onc	Gerson, S	OH	366	Onc	Kalemkerian, G	MI	367	Onc	Meyskens, F	CA	387
Onc	Geyer, C	PA	339	Onc	Kaminski, M	MI	367	Onc	Miller, A	NC	358
Onc	Glaspy, J	CA	385	Onc	Kane, M	CO	374	Onc	Miller, D	KY	358
Onc	Glick, J	PA	339	Onc	Kantoff, P	MA	329	Onc	Miller, T	AZ	379
Onc	Glisson, B	TX	377	Onc	Kaplan, L	CA	386	Onc	Miller, V	NY	344
Onc	Glode, L	CO	374	Onc	Karp, D	TX	378	Onc	Mintzer, D	PA	344
Onc	Gockerman, J	NC	355	Onc	Karp, J	MD	342	Onc	Mitsuyasu, R	CA	387
Onc	Godley, P	NC	355	Onc	Kaufman, P	NH	329	Onc	Moore, A	NY	344
Onc	Gold, P	WA	385	Onc	Kelly, K	CA	386	Onc	Moore, J	NC	358
Onc	Goldberg, R	NC	355	Onc	Kelly, W	PA	342	Onc	Morgan, D	TN	358
Onc	Goldstein, L	PA	339	Onc	Kelsen, D	NY	342	Onc	Mortimer, J	CA	387
Onc	Golomb, H	IL	366	Onc	Kemeny, N	NY	342	Onc	Motzer, R	NY	344
Onc	Goy, A	NJ	340	Onc	Kesari, S	CA	386	Onc	Muggia, F	NY	344
Onc	Gradishar, W	IL	366	Onc	Khuri, F	GA	356	Onc	Muss, H	NC	358
Onc	Graham, M	NC	355	Onc	Kies, M	TX	378	Onc	Nabell, L	AL	358
Onc	Gralow, J	WA	385	Onc	Kindler, H	IL	367	Onc	Nadler, L	MA	330
Onc	Grana, G	NJ	340	Onc	Kirkwood, J	PA	342	Onc	Nanus, D	NY	344
Onc	Greco, F	TN	355	Onc	Koczywas, M	CA	386	Onc	Natale, R	CA	387
Onc	Grem, J	NE	374	Onc	Kraft, A	SC	356	Onc	Nissenblatt, M	NJ	344
Onc	Grosh, W	VA	355	Onc	Kressel, B	DC	342	Onc	Northfelt, D	AZ	379
Onc	Grossbard, M	NY	340	Onc	Kris, M	NY	342	Onc	Norton, L	NY	344
Onc	Grossman, S	MD	340	Onc	Krishnamurthi, S	OH	368	Onc	O'Brien, S	TX	379
Onc	Gruber, S	MI	366	Onc	Kucuk, O	GA	356	Onc	O'Brien, T	OH	368
Onc	Grunberg, S	VT	328	Onc	Kuzel, T	IL	368	Onc	O'Connor, O	NY	345
Onc	Gulley, J	MD	340	Onc	Kvols, L	FL	356	Onc	O'Day, S	CA	387
Onc	Haas, N	PA	340	Onc	Kwak, L	TX	378	Onc	O'Regan, R	GA	358
Onc	Hageboutros, A	NJ	340	Onc	Lacy, J	CT	329	Onc	O'Reilly, E	NY	345
Onc	Haley, B	TX	377	Onc	Laheru, D	MD	343	Onc	O'Shaughnessy, J	TX	379
Onc	Hammond, D	NH	328	Onc	Langer, C	PA	343	Onc	Offit, K	NY	345
Onc	Hande, K	TN	355	Onc	Lawson, D	GA	356	Onc	Oh, W	NY	345
Onc	Hartmann, L	MN	366	Onc	Legare, R	RI	330	Onc	Olopade, O	IL	368
Onc	Hauke, R	NE	374	Onc	Lesser, G	NC	356	Onc	Oratz, R	NY	345
Onc	Hayes, D	MI	367	Onc	Levine, E	NY	343	Onc	Orlowski, R	TX	379

Specialty & Special Expertise Index

Spec	Name	St	Pg
D	Grichnik, J	FL	191
D	Halpern, A	NY	187
D	Johnson, T	MI	194
D	Johr, R	FL	191
D	Krunic, A	IL	194
D	Kupper, T	MA	183
D	Leffell, D	CT	183
D	Lowitt, M	MD	187
D	McDonald, C	RI	184
D	Mihm, M	MA	184
D	Miller, S	MD	187
D	Orengo, I	TX	197
D	Prioleau, P	NY	188
D	Rhodes, A	IL	195
D	Rigel, D	NY	188
D	Russell, M	VA	192
D	Shea, C	IL	195
D	Sober, A	MA	184
D	Swetter, S	CA	200
D	Taylor, R	TX	198
D	Tsao, H	MA	184
D	Wood, G	WI	196
D	Zitelli, J	PA	189
Hem	Milhem, M	IA	320
Onc	Albertini, M	WI	363
Onc	Atkins, M	MA	326
Onc	Biggs, D	DE	334
Onc	Borden, E	OH	364
Onc	Brockstein, B	IL	364
Onc	Chapman, P	NY	335
Onc	Chow, W	CA	383
Onc	Clark, J	IL	364
Onc	Cohen, G	MD	335
Onc	Cohen, S	NY	336
Onc	Conry, R	AL	353
Onc	Daud, A	CA	384
Onc	Dutcher, J	NY	337
Onc	Ernstoff, M	NH	327
Onc	Fay, J	TX	377
Onc	Glaspy, J	CA	385
Onc	Grosh, W	VA	355
Onc	Gruber, S	MI	366
Onc	Hutchins, L	AR	378
Onc	Hwu, P	TX	378
Onc	Kirkwood, J	PA	342
Onc	Kuzel, T	IL	368
Onc	Lawson, D	GA	356
Onc	Margolin, K	WA	387
Onc	Meyskens, F	CA	387
Onc	Miller, D	KY	358
Onc	O'Day, S	CA	387
Onc	Papadopoulos, N	TX	380
Onc	Pavlick, A	NY	345
Onc	Pecora, A	NJ	346
Onc	Richards, J	IL	370
Onc	Samlowski, W	NV	389
Onc	Schuchter, L	PA	347
Onc	Sosman, J	TN	361
Onc	Strauss, G	MA	331
Onc	Thompson, J	WA	390
Onc	Triozzi, P	OH	371
Onc	von Mehren, M	PA	350
Onc	Weber, J	FL	362

Spec	Name	St	Pg
Onc	Weiss, G	VA	362
Onc	Wolchok, J	NY	350
Oto	Califano, J	MD	657
Oto	Singer, M	CA	686
Path	Bastian, B	NY	708
Path	Cochran, A	CA	720
Path	Gottlieb, G	NY	709
Path	Prieto, V	TX	718
PlS	Chang, B	PA	851
PlS	Rees, R	MI	865
PlS	Yetman, R	OH	866
PlS	Zide, B	NY	858
RadRO	Wazer, D	RI	946
RadRO	Werner-Wasik, M	PA	951
S	Averbook, B	OH	1070
S	Bear, H	VA	1061
S	Brown, C	IL	1070
S	Byrd, D	WA	1089
S	Chang, A	MI	1071
S	Coit, D	NY	1051
S	Cusack, J	MA	1044
S	Daneker, G	GA	1063
S	Dooley, W	OK	1083
S	Eberlein, T	MO	1072
S	Edington, H	PA	1052
S	Edney, J	NE	1080
S	Edwards, M	OH	1072
S	Eisenberg, B	NH	1045
S	Essner, R	CA	1090
S	Fraker, D	PA	1053
S	Goodnight, J	CA	1090
S	Gray, R	AZ	1084
S	Johnson Miller, D	IN	1074
S	Kaufman, H	IL	1074
S	Kavanah, M	MA	1046
S	Kelley, M	TN	1064
S	Kim, J	OH	1074
S	Krag, D	VT	1046
S	Kuhn, J	TX	1085
S	Lee, J	TX	1085
S	Leitch, A	TX	1085
S	Lind, D	GA	1065
S	Loggie, B	NE	1080
S	Mansfield, P	TX	1086
S	McMasters, K	KY	1066
S	Moley, J	MO	1075
S	Nathanson, S	MI	1076
S	Neifeld, J	VA	1066
S	Olson, J	NC	1066
S	Pockaj, B	AZ	1086
S	Rosenberg, S	MD	1058
S	Roses, D	NY	1058
S	Ross, M	TX	1087
S	Schwartzentruber, D	IN	1077
S	Sener, S	CA	1094
S	Shapiro, R	NY	1059
S	Shen, P	NC	1067
S	Shenk, R	OH	1078
S	Sigurdson, E	PA	1059
S	Slingluff, C	VA	1068
S	Sondak, V	FL	1068
S	Talamonti, M	IL	1078
S	Tanabe, K	MA	1048

Spec	Name	St	Pg
S	Tyler, D	NC	1068
S	Urist, M	AL	1069
S	Wallace, A	CA	1095
S	White, R	NC	1069
S	Yeung, R	WA	1095

Melanoma Early Detection/Prevention

Spec	Name	St	Pg
D	Halpern, A	NY	187
D	Rhodes, A	IL	195
D	Schultz, N	NY	188
D	Swetter, S	CA	200

Melanoma Genetics

Spec	Name	St	Pg
D	Tsao, H	MA	184

Melanoma Risk Assessment

Spec	Name	St	Pg
D	Lessin, S	PA	187
D	Rhodes, A	IL	195

Melanoma-Advanced

Spec	Name	St	Pg
Onc	Albertini, M	WI	363
Onc	Flaherty, K	MA	327
Onc	O'Day, S	CA	387

Melanoma-Choroidal (eye)

Spec	Name	St	Pg
Oph	Abramson, D	NY	569
Oph	Augsburger, J	OH	586
Oph	Dutton, J	NC	580
Oph	Finger, P	NY	571
Oph	Grossniklaus, H	GA	581
Oph	Handa, J	MD	573
Oph	Harbour, J	MO	587
Oph	Schachat, A	OH	591
Oph	Shields, C	PA	578
Oph	Shields, J	PA	578
Oph	Wilson, M	TN	585
RadRO	Crocker, I	GA	952

Melanoma-Head & Neck

Spec	Name	St	Pg
D	Fewkes, J	MA	183
Oto	Bradford, C	MI	672
Oto	Myers, J	TX	682
PlS	Stadelmann, W	NH	849

Memory Disorders

Spec	Name	St	Pg
Ger	Ciocon, J	FL	264
Ger	Sachs, G	IN	265
GerPsy	Borson, S	WA	912
GerPsy	Small, G	CA	912
GerPsy	Stein, E	CA	912
N	Doody, R	TX	531
N	Heilman, K	FL	519
N	Henderson, V	CA	535
N	Jordan, B	NY	511
N	Kelly, J	CO	530
N	Relkin, N	NY	514

Specialty & Special Expertise Index

Specialty & Special Expertise Index

Spec	Name	St	Pg
OrS	Wang, J	CA	644
OrS	Wetzel, F	PA	624
Oto	Akervall, J	MI	671
Oto	Kennedy, D	PA	660
Oto	Orloff, L	CA	685
Oto	Rosenthal, E	AL	669
PS	Barksdale, E	OH	806
PS	Bensard, D	CO	808
PS	Black, C	TX	809
PS	Doody, D	MA	801
PS	Ford, H	CA	810
PS	Gaines, B	PA	802
PS	Holterman, M	IL	807
PS	Kane, T	DC	803
PS	Krummel, T	CA	810
PS	Liu, D	IL	807
PS	Lobe, T	CA	810
PS	Moss, R	OH	807
PS	Nakayama, D	GA	805
PS	Rodgers, B	VA	805
PS	Spigland, N	NY	803
PS	Voigt, R	MD	804
PS	Waldhausen, J	WA	811
RE	Falcone, T	OH	1013
RE	Isaacson, K	MA	1006
RE	Miller, C	IL	1014
RE	Petrozza, J	MA	1007
RE	Putman, J	TX	1016
RE	Sanfilippo, J	PA	1009
S	Bellows, C	LA	1082
S	Brunt, L	MO	1070
S	Cherqui, D	NY	1051
S	Courcoulas, A	PA	1051
S	Curcillo, P	PA	1051
S	Duh, Q	CA	1089
S	Duncan, M	MD	1052
S	Fahey, T	NY	1053
S	Fitzgibbons, R	NE	1080
S	Frantzides, C	IL	1072
S	Franz, M	MI	1072
S	Horvath, K	WA	1091
S	Ikramuddin, S	MN	1074
S	Koruda, M	NC	1064
S	Morton, J	CA	1092
S	Nissen, N	CA	1092
S	Ponsky, J	OH	1076
S	Ramanathan, R	PA	1057
S	Rattner, D	MA	1047
S	Rogers, S	CA	1094
S	Rosemurgy, A	FL	1067
S	Rosen, M	OH	1077
S	Schauer, P	OH	1077
S	Shibata, D	FL	1067
S	Simmons, R	NY	1059
S	Solorzano, C	TN	1068
S	Swanstrom, L	OR	1094
S	Sweeney, J	GA	1068
S	Tuttle, T	MN	1079
TS	Cohen, N	MD	1110
TS	Cohen, R	CA	1134
TS	Del-Nido, P	MA	1106
TS	Ferguson, M	IL	1126
TS	Fontana, G	CA	1135

Spec	Name	St	Pg
TS	Lazzaro, R	NY	1115
TS	Liao, K	MN	1127
TS	Mack, M	TX	1132
TS	Rice, D	TX	1133
TS	Rosengart, T	NY	1116
TS	Swistel, D	NY	1117
U	Balaji, K	NC	1153
U	Docimo, S	PA	1146
U	Irby, P	NC	1155
U	Kibel, A	MO	1162
U	McVary, K	IL	1163
U	Merguerian, P	NH	1143
VascS	Flanigan, D	CA	1188
VascS	Lumsden, A	TX	1187

Minimally Invasive Surgery-Pediatric

Spec	Name	St	Pg
U	Poppas, D	NY	1150

Minimally Invasive Thoracic Surgery

Spec	Name	St	Pg
TS	Brinckerhoff, L	MA	1106
TS	Bueno, R	MA	1106
TS	Demmy, T	NY	1110
TS	Fernando, H	MA	1106
TS	Howington, J	IL	1126
TS	Jones, D	VA	1120
TS	Krellenstein, D	NY	1114
TS	Maddaus, M	MN	1127
TS	Mason, D	OH	1127
TS	Nesbitt, J	TN	1122
TS	Rice, T	OH	1128
TS	Sonett, J	NY	1117
TS	Weksler, B	PA	1118

Minimally Invasive Urologic Surgery

Spec	Name	St	Pg
U	Andrews, P	AZ	1166
U	Assimos, D	NC	1153
U	Gill, I	CA	1170
U	Gluckman, G	IL	1161
U	Gomella, L	PA	1146
U	Hall, S	NY	1147
U	Kaouk, J	OH	1161
U	Kawachi, M	CA	1171
U	Lanteri, V	NJ	1148
U	Miller, S	GA	1156
U	Moul, J	NC	1156
U	Strup, S	KY	1158
U	Trabulsi, E	PA	1152
U	Uzzo, R	PA	1152
U	Wilson, T	CA	1173

Minimally Invasive Vascular Surgery

Spec	Name	St	Pg
VascS	Ahn, S	CA	1188
VascS	Benvenisty, A	NY	1180
VascS	Brener, B	NJ	1180

Spec	Name	St	Pg
VascS	Iafrati, M	MA	1178
VascS	McLafferty, R	IL	1186
VascS	Schneider, D	NY	1182
VascS	Todd, G	NY	1183

Miscarriage-Recurrent

Spec	Name	St	Pg
MF	Druzin, M	CA	436
MF	Landy, H	DC	429
MF	Lockwood, C	CT	427
MF	Paidas, M	CT	427
ObG	Ordorica, S	NY	554
ObG	Scher, J	NY	554
ObG	Young, B	NY	555
RE	Barnes, R	IL	1012
RE	DeVane, G	FL	1011
RE	Hill, J	NH	1006
RE	Kutteh, W	TN	1011
RE	Odem, R	MO	1014
RE	Ratts, V	MO	1014
RE	Stangel, J	NY	1010
RE	Walmer, D	NC	1012

Mitochondrial Disorders

Spec	Name	St	Pg
CG	Boles, R	CA	160
CG	Craigen, W	TX	160
ChiN	Cohen, B	OH	148
ChiN	Haas, R	CA	151
ChiN	Legido, A	PA	146

Mitral Valve Disease

Spec	Name	St	Pg
IC	Yeung, A	CA	130

Mitral Valve Prolapse

Spec	Name	St	Pg
Cv	Andersen, H	NY	94

Mitral Valve Robotic Surgery

Spec	Name	St	Pg
TS	Hargrove, W	PA	1112
TS	Murphy, D	GA	1122
TS	Smith, J	OH	1129
TS	Woo, Y	PA	1118

Mitral Valve Surgery

Spec	Name	St	Pg
TS	Adams, D	NY	1109
TS	Aklog, L	AZ	1131
TS	Alexander, J	IL	1124
TS	Bakhos, M	IL	1125
TS	Bolman, R	MA	1106
TS	Chitwood, W	NC	1119
TS	DeFilippi, V	CA	1135
TS	DeRose, J	NY	1110
TS	Filsoufi, F	NY	1111
TS	Fontana, G	CA	1135
TS	Fullerton, D	CO	1130
TS	Galloway, A	NY	1111
TS	Grossi, E	NY	1112
TS	Hashim, S	CT	1107
TS	Moon, M	MO	1128
TS	Naka, Y	NY	1115

Specialty & Special Expertise Index

Specialty & Special Expertise Index

Specialty & Special Expertise Index

Specialty & Special Expertise Index

Spec	Name	St	Pg	Spec	Name	St	Pg	Spec	Name	St	Pg
NS	Feldstein, N	NY	469	NS	Linskey, M	CA	493	NS	Sekhar, L	WA	495
NS	Fenstermaker, R	NY	469	NS	Liu, C	CA	494	NS	Sekhon, L	NV	495
NS	Fessler, R	IL	483	NS	Loftus, C	PA	472	NS	Selden, N	OR	495
NS	Foley, K	TN	477	NS	Luerssen, T	TX	490	NS	Selman, W	OH	486
NS	Frazee, J	CA	492	NS	Luken, M	IL	484	NS	Sen, C	NY	474
NS	Freeman, T	FL	477	NS	Lunsford, L	PA	472	NS	Shaffrey, C	VA	480
NS	Friedman, A	NC	477	NS	Madsen, J	MA	466	NS	Shaffrey, M	VA	480
NS	Frim, D	IL	484	NS	Malik, G	MI	484	NS	Shapiro, S	IN	486
NS	Giannotta, S	CA	493	NS	Mamelak, A	CA	494	NS	Shuer, L	CA	495
NS	Gokaslan, Z	MD	469	NS	Mapstone, T	OK	490	NS	Silbergeld, D	WA	495
NS	Golfinos, J	NY	469	NS	Markert, J	AL	478	NS	Sills, A	TN	480
NS	Goodman, R	NY	470	NS	Maroon, J	PA	472	NS	Sisti, M	NY	474
NS	Goumnerova, L	MA	466	NS	Martin, N	CA	494	NS	Sklar, F	TX	490
NS	Grady, M	PA	470	NS	Martuza, R	MA	467	NS	Solomon, R	NY	474
NS	Green, B	FL	477	NS	Mayberg, M	WA	494	NS	Souweidane, M	NY	475
NS	Greene, C	LA	489	NS	McCormick, P	NY	473	NS	Spencer, D	CT	467
NS	Grubb, R	MO	484	NS	McDermott, M	CA	494	NS	Spetzler, R	AZ	490
NS	Gupta, N	CA	493	NS	Menezes, A	IA	485	NS	Spinner, R	MN	486
NS	Guthikonda, M	MI	484	NS	Meyer, F	MN	485	NS	Steinberg, G	CA	495
NS	Guthrie, B	AL	478	NS	Mickey, B	TX	490	NS	Stieg, P	NY	475
NS	Gutin, P	NY	470	NS	Moore, F	NY	473	NS	Sun, P	CA	495
NS	Hadley, M	AL	478	NS	Morcos, J	FL	479	NS	Sundaresan, N	NY	475
NS	Haid, R	GA	478	NS	Murali, R	NY	473	NS	Sutton, L	PA	475
NS	Hankinson, H	NM	489	NS	Myseros, J	VA	479	NS	Swaid, S	AL	481
NS	Harbaugh, R	PA	470	NS	Naff, N	MD	473	NS	Swearingen, B	MA	467
NS	Harper, R	TX	489	NS	Nagib, M	MN	485	NS	Tamargo, R	MD	475
NS	Harrop, J	PA	470	NS	Nazzaro, J	KS	487	NS	Tatter, S	NC	481
NS	Harsh, G	CA	493	NS	Neuwelt, E	OR	494	NS	Taylon, C	NE	488
NS	Hartl, R	NY	470	NS	O'Rourke, D	PA	473	NS	Thompson, B	MI	486
NS	Heilman, C	MA	466	NS	Oakes, W	AL	479	NS	Thompson, R	TN	481
NS	Heros, R	FL	478	NS	Ojemann, J	WA	494	NS	Tomita, T	IL	486
NS	Hodes, J	KY	478	NS	Olivi, A	MD	473	NS	Traynelis, V	IL	487
NS	Hopkins, L	NY	470	NS	Olson, J	GA	479	NS	Turtz, A	NJ	475
NS	Huang, J	MD	470	NS	Origitano, T	MT	488	NS	Van Loveren, H	FL	481
NS	Jallo, G	MD	471	NS	Ott, K	CA	494	NS	Walker, M	UT	488
NS	Jho, H	PA	471	NS	Parent, A	MS	479	NS	Walsh, J	LA	491
NS	Jimenez, D	TX	489	NS	Park, T	MO	485	NS	Warnick, R	OH	487
NS	Johnson, S	CO	487	NS	Patel, S	SC	479	NS	Weiner, H	NY	475
NS	Judy, K	PA	471	NS	Penar, P	VT	467	NS	Weingart, J	MD	475
NS	Kaiser, M	NY	471	NS	Piatt, J	DE	473	NS	Welch, W	PA	476
NS	Kaplitt, M	NY	471	NS	Piepmeier, J	CT	467	NS	Wharen, R	FL	481
NS	Kassam, A	CA	493	NS	Pollack, I	PA	473	NS	Whiting, D	PA	476
NS	Kaufman, B	WI	484	NS	Quigley, M	PA	474	NS	Wilberger, J	PA	476
NS	Kestle, J	UT	487	NS	Raffel, C	OH	485	NS	Wilson, J	NC	481
NS	Khan, A	MD	471	NS	Ragheb, J	FL	479	NS	Wisoff, J	NY	476
NS	Kim, D	TX	489	NS	Reid, W	TN	479	NS	Yonas, H	NM	491
NS	Kim, D	TX	489	NS	Rezai, A	OH	485	NS	Yu, J	CA	496
NS	Kobrine, A	DC	471	NS	Rich, K	MO	485	NS	Zager, E	PA	476
NS	Kondziolka, D	PA	472	NS	Rigamonti, D	MD	474	NS	Zimmerman, C	ID	488
NS	Kotapka, M	PA	472	NS	Riina, H	NY	474				
NS	Krisht, A	AR	489	NS	Robertson, J	TN	480				
NS	Kuntz, C	OH	484	NS	Rock, J	MI	485		**Neurology**		
NS	Landy, H	FL	478	NS	Rodts, G	GA	480	N	Abou-Khalil, B	TN	517
NS	Lang, F	TX	489	NS	Rosenblum, M	MI	486	N	Adams, D	FL	517
NS	Laske, D	PA	472	NS	Rosenwasser, R	PA	474	N	Adams, H	IA	522
NS	Lavyne, M	NY	472	NS	Ruge, J	IL	486	N	Adams, R	SC	517
NS	Lemole, G	AZ	490	NS	Ryken, T	IA	486	N	Adornato, B	CA	533
NS	Levi, A	FL	478	NS	Sampson, J	NC	480	N	Ahern, G	AZ	530
NS	Levy, M	CA	493	NS	Samson, D	TX	490	N	Ahlskog, J	MN	522
NS	Liau, L	CA	493	NS	Sandberg, D	FL	480	N	Albers, G	CA	533
NS	Liker, M	CA	493	NS	Sanford, R	TN	480	N	Alberts, M	IL	522
NS	Lillehei, K	CO	487	NS	Sawaya, R	TX	490	N	Alexandrov, A	AL	517
NS	Link, M	MN	484	NS	Schwartz, T	NY	474	N	Amato, A	MA	504

Specialty & Special Expertise Index

Spec	Name	St	Pg	Spec	Name	St	Pg	Spec	Name	St	Pg
N	Aminoff, M	CA	533	N	Diaz-Arrastia, R	TX	530	N	Jordan, B	NY	511
N	Apatoff, B	NY	507	N	Dichter, M	PA	509	N	Josephson, D	IN	525
N	Armon, C	MA	504	N	Dodick, D	AZ	531	N	Kase, C	MA	506
N	Arnason, B	IL	522	N	Doody, R	TX	531	N	Kasner, S	PA	511
N	Ashizawa, T	FL	517	N	Elias, S	MI	524	N	Katirji, B	OH	525
N	Aurora, S	WA	533	N	Engel, W	CA	534	N	Kelly, J	CO	530
N	Azizi, S	PA	507	N	Engstrom, J	CA	534	N	Kent, T	TX	532
N	Balcer, L	PA	507	N	Fahn, S	NY	509	N	Kincaid, J	IN	525
N	Barger, G	MI	523	N	Farlow, M	IN	524	N	Kirshner, H	TN	520
N	Barkley, G	MI	523	N	Feinberg, T	NY	509	N	Klein, P	NJ	511
N	Barohn, R	KS	529	N	Feldman, E	MI	524	N	Kolodny, E	NY	511
N	Baser, S	PA	507	N	Feldmann, E	MA	505	N	Krauss, G	MD	511
N	Batchelor, T	MA	504	N	Fellus, J	NJ	509	N	Krumholz, A	MD	511
N	Bebin, E	AL	518	N	Ferrendelli, J	TX	531	N	Kula, R	NY	511
N	Becker, K	WA	533	N	Filley, C	CO	529	N	Kunschner, L	PA	511
N	Bell, R	PA	507	N	Fink, M	NY	509	N	Kurtzke, R	VA	520
N	Berger, J	KY	518	N	Finkel, A	NC	518	N	Kuzniecky, R	NY	512
N	Bergey, G	MD	507	N	Finkel, M	FL	519	N	Labar, D	NY	512
N	Bernstein, R	IL	523	N	Fisher, M	CA	535	N	Labiner, D	AZ	532
N	Bertorini, T	TN	518	N	Fisher, R	CA	535	N	Lacomis, D	PA	512
N	Blum, A	RI	504	N	Flaherty, A	MA	505	N	Langston, J	CA	535
N	Blumenfeld, H	CT	504	N	Foo, S	NY	509	N	Laterra, J	MD	512
N	Bourdette, D	OR	533	N	French, J	NY	510	N	Latov, N	NY	512
N	Bressman, S	NY	507	N	Frohman, E	TX	531	N	Lavin, P	TN	520
N	Brick, J	WV	508	N	Furie, K	MA	505	N	Levine, D	NY	512
N	Broderick, J	OH	523	N	Furlan, A	OH	524	N	Levine, S	NY	512
N	Bromberg, M	UT	529	N	Galetta, S	PA	510	N	Lew, M	CA	536
N	Brooks, B	NC	518	N	Gendelman, S	NY	510	N	Lewis, R	MI	525
N	Brown, R	MN	523	N	Gilbert, M	TX	531	N	Liporace, J	PA	512
N	Bruno, M	HI	533	N	Gilman, S	MI	524	N	Lipton, R	NY	513
N	Buchholz, D	MD	508	N	Gizzi, M	NJ	510	N	Lisak, R	MI	525
N	Burke, A	IL	523	N	Glass, J	PA	510	N	Liu, G	PA	513
N	Burns, R	AZ	530	N	Glass, J	GA	519	N	Logan, W	MO	525
N	Busis, N	PA	508	N	Goetz, C	IL	524	N	Logigian, E	NY	513
N	Calabresi, P	MD	508	N	Golbe, L	NJ	510	N	Longo, F	CA	536
N	Caplan, L	MA	504	N	Goldstein, L	NC	519	N	Lublin, F	NY	513
N	Cascino, T	MN	523	N	Goodgold, A	NY	510	N	Luders, H	OH	525
N	Chamberlain, M	WA	534	N	Goodin, D	CA	535	N	Lutsep, H	OR	536
N	Charles, A	CA	534	N	Goodwin, J	IL	524	N	Mahowald, M	MN	526
N	Charney, J	NY	508	N	Graves, M	CA	535	N	Maraganore, D	IL	526
N	Chelimsky, T	OH	523	N	Greer, D	CT	505	N	McArthur, J	MD	513
N	Chui, H	CA	534	N	Gress, D	VA	519	N	McCluskey, L	PA	513
N	Cloughesy, T	CA	534	N	Gross, P	MA	505	N	Mesulam, M	IL	526
N	Cohen, J	OH	523	N	Grotta, J	TX	531	N	Mikkelsen, T	MI	526
N	Cohen, J	NH	504	N	Guilleminault, C	CA	535	N	Miller, A	NY	513
N	Cole, A	MA	505	N	Hain, T	IL	524	N	Mitsumoto, H	NY	513
N	Cook, S	NJ	508	N	Haley, E	VA	519	N	Mohammad, Y	IL	526
N	Corbett, J	MS	518	N	Harati, Y	TX	531	N	Mohr, J	NY	514
N	Corey-Bloom, J	CA	534	N	Hauser, R	FL	519	N	Montgomery, E	AL	520
N	Cornblath, D	MD	508	N	Hauser, S	CA	535	N	Moots, P	TN	520
N	Couch, J	OK	530	N	Heck, C	CA	535	N	Morgenlander, J	NC	520
N	Coull, B	AZ	530	N	Hecox, K	WI	525	N	Morrell, M	CA	536
N	Coyle, P	NY	508	N	Heilman, K	FL	519	N	Morris, J	MO	526
N	Cudkowicz, M	MA	505	N	Henderson, V	CA	535	N	Nabors, L	AL	520
N	Cummings, J	NV	534	N	Hess, D	GA	519	N	Newman, D	MI	526
N	Cutrer, F	MN	524	N	Hiesiger, E	NY	510	N	Newman, L	NY	514
N	Dalmau, J	PA	508	N	Homer, D	IL	525	N	Newman, N	GA	521
N	De Angelis, L	NY	509	N	Hurtig, H	PA	510	N	Newton, H	OH	526
N	DeGiorgio, C	CA	534	N	Infante, E	TX	531	N	Nicholl, J	LA	532
N	DeKosky, S	VA	518	N	Jankovic, J	TX	532	N	Nolan, B	FL	521
N	DeLong, M	GA	518	N	Janss, A	GA	520	N	Nutt, J	OR	536
N	Devinsky, O	NY	509	N	Jobst, B	NH	505	N	Oaklander, A	MA	506
N	Dewberry, R	MD	509	N	Jones, H	MA	505	N	Oh, S	AL	521

Neurometabolic Disorders

Neuromuscular Disorder & Vision Problems

Neuromuscular Disorders

Neuropathology

Neurophysiology

Neurophysiology-Aging

Neurophysiology-Dementia

Neuroradiology

Specialty & Special Expertise Index

Occult Spinal Dysraphism (OSD)

Occupational Asthma

Occupational Lung Disease

Occupational Medicine

Occupational Musculoskeletal Disorders

Occupational Skin Diseases

Oculoplastic & Orbital Surgery

Oculoplastic Surgery

Ophthalmic Genetics

Ophthalmic Pathology

Ophthalmic Plastic Surgery

Ophthalmology

Specialty & Special Expertise Index

Specialty & Special Expertise Index

Specialty & Special Expertise Index

Specialty & Special Expertise Index

Specialty & Special Expertise Index

Spec	Name	St	Pg	Spec	Name	St	Pg	Spec	Name	St	Pg
Oto	Close, L	NY	658	Oto	Jacobs, J	NY	660	Oto	Pensak, M	OH	676
Oto	Corey, J	IL	673	Oto	Jenkins, H	CO	679	Oto	Persky, M	NY	662
Oto	Costantino, P	NY	658	Oto	Johnson, C	LA	681	Oto	Peters, G	AL	669
Oto	Couch, M	VT	655	Oto	Johnson, J	PA	660	Oto	Petruzzelli, G	IL	676
Oto	Courey, M	CA	683	Oto	Jones, P	IL	675	Oto	Piccirillo, J	MO	676
Oto	Davidson, B	DC	658	Oto	Josephson, J	NY	660	Oto	Picken, C	DC	662
Oto	Day, T	SC	666	Oto	Kang, D	OH	675	Oto	Pillsbury, H	NC	669
Oto	Denenberg, S	NE	679	Oto	Kaplan, M	CA	684	Oto	Pitman, K	MS	669
Oto	Deschler, D	MA	655	Oto	Kartush, J	MI	675	Oto	Poole, M	GA	669
Oto	Diaz, E	TX	680	Oto	Keane, W	PA	660	Oto	Postma, G	GA	669
Oto	DiNardo, L	VA	666	Oto	Keller, G	CA	684	Oto	Powell, N	CA	685
Oto	Donald, P	CA	683	Oto	Kennedy, D	PA	660	Oto	Pribitkin, E	PA	663
Oto	Donovan, D	TX	681	Oto	Kern, R	IL	675	Oto	Quatela, V	NY	663
Oto	Dornhoffer, J	AR	681	Oto	Kesser, B	VA	667	Oto	Randolph, G	MA	656
Oto	Driscoll, C	MN	673	Oto	Kingdom, T	CO	679	Oto	Rassekh, C	PA	663
Oto	Duckert, L	WA	683	Oto	Koch, W	MD	661	Oto	Rauch, S	MA	656
Oto	Edelstein, D	NY	658	Oto	Koufman, J	NY	661	Oto	Rebeiz, E	MA	656
Oto	Eisele, D	CA	684	Oto	Kraus, D	NY	661	Oto	Rice, D	CA	685
Oto	Epstein, J	FL	667	Oto	Krespi, Y	NY	661	Oto	Ries, W	TN	669
Oto	Farrior, E	FL	667	Oto	Kuhel, W	NY	661	Oto	Roland, J	NY	663
Oto	Farrior, J	FL	667	Oto	Kuhn, F	GA	667	Oto	Rosen, C	PA	663
Oto	Fee, W	CA	684	Oto	Kveton, J	CT	656	Oto	Rosenthal, E	AL	669
Oto	Feghali, J	NY	658	Oto	Lalwani, A	NY	661	Oto	Rubinstein, J	WA	685
Oto	Ferris, R	PA	658	Oto	Lambert, P	SC	667	Oto	Samant, S	TN	669
Oto	Flint, P	OR	684	Oto	Lanza, D	FL	668	Oto	Sasaki, C	CT	656
Oto	Ford, C	WI	673	Oto	Larrabee, W	WA	685	Oto	Sataloff, R	PA	663
Oto	Fried, M	NY	658	Oto	Lavertu, P	OH	675	Oto	Schaefer, S	NY	663
Oto	Friedman, M	IL	673	Oto	Lawson, W	NY	661	Oto	Schaitkin, B	PA	663
Oto	Funk, G	IA	673	Oto	Lebovics, R	NY	661	Oto	Schantz, S	NY	664
Oto	Futran, N	WA	684	Oto	Leonetti, J	IL	675	Oto	Schley, W	NY	664
Oto	Gantz, B	IA	674	Oto	Levine, P	VA	668	Oto	Senders, C	CA	686
Oto	Genden, E	NY	658	Oto	Linstrom, C	NY	662	Oto	Senior, B	NC	670
Oto	Gianoli, G	LA	681	Oto	Lustig, L	CA	685	Oto	Setzen, M	NY	664
Oto	Gliklich, R	MA	655	Oto	Lydiatt, D	NE	679	Oto	Shapshay, S	NY	664
Oto	Goebel, J	MO	674	Oto	Lydiatt, W	NE	679	Oto	Shelton, C	UT	679
Oto	Gold, S	NY	659	Oto	Macias, J	AZ	682	Oto	Shindo, M	OR	686
Oto	Goldenberg, D	PA	659	Oto	Mangat, D	KY	668	Oto	Shockley, W	NC	670
Oto	Goodwin, W	FL	667	Oto	Marentette, L	MI	675	Oto	Siegel, G	IL	677
Oto	Gosselin, B	NH	655	Oto	Mattox, D	GA	668	Oto	Sillers, M	AL	670
Oto	Graham, H	LA	681	Oto	McCaffrey, T	FL	668	Oto	Silverman, D	VT	657
Oto	Grandis, J	PA	659	Oto	McKenna, M	MA	656	Oto	Silverstein, H	FL	670
Oto	Grillone, G	MA	655	Oto	McMenomey, S	OR	685	Oto	Singer, M	CA	686
Oto	Grundfast, K	MA	656	Oto	Medina, J	OK	682	Oto	Sinha, U	CA	686
Oto	Hadlock, T	MA	656	Oto	Metson, R	MA	656	Oto	Smith, R	NE	680
Oto	Hammerschlag, P	NY	659	Oto	Miyamoto, R	IN	675	Oto	Snyderman, C	PA	664
Oto	Hanna, E	TX	681	Oto	Myers, J	TX	682	Oto	Song, J	CO	680
Oto	Har-El, G	NY	659	Oto	Naclerio, R	IL	676	Oto	Stankiewicz, J	IL	677
Oto	Harris, J	CA	684	Oto	Netterville, J	TN	668	Oto	Stasney, C	TX	682
Oto	Hartig, G	WI	674	Oto	Newkirk, K	DC	662	Oto	Stenson, K	IL	677
Oto	Haughey, B	MO	674	Oto	Niparko, J	MD	662	Oto	Stewart, M	NY	664
Oto	Hayden, R	AZ	681	Oto	Nuss, D	LA	682	Oto	Stringer, S	MS	670
Oto	Haynes, D	TN	667	Oto	O'Malley, B	PA	662	Oto	Strome, M	NY	664
Oto	Hicks, W	NY	659	Oto	Oghalai, J	CA	685	Oto	Strome, S	MD	664
Oto	Hilger, P	MN	674	Oto	Olsen, K	MN	676	Oto	Suen, J	AR	682
Oto	Hirsch, B	PA	659	Oto	Orloff, L	CA	685	Oto	Sulica, R	NY	665
Oto	Hoffman, H	IA	674	Oto	Osguthorpe, J	SC	668	Oto	Szachowicz, E	MN	677
Oto	Hoffman, R	NY	659	Oto	Ossoff, R	TN	668	Oto	Teknos, T	OH	677
Oto	Hogikyan, N	MI	674	Oto	Otto, R	TX	682	Oto	Telian, S	MI	677
Oto	Holliday, M	MD	660	Oto	Ozer, E	OH	676	Oto	Telischi, F	FL	670
Oto	Hopping, S	DC	660	Oto	Paparella, M	MN	676	Oto	Terris, D	GA	670
Oto	Hotaling, A	IL	674	Oto	Papel, I	MD	662	Oto	Toriumi, D	IL	677
Oto	Hurst, M	WV	660	Oto	Parisier, S	NY	662	Oto	Tucci, D	NC	670
Oto	Jackler, R	CA	684	Oto	Pelzer, H	IL	676	Oto	Tufano, R	MD	665

Specialty & Special Expertise Index

Specialty & Special Expertise Index

Specialty & Special Expertise Index

Specialty & Special Expertise Index

Pediatric & Adolescent Gynecology

Pediatric & Adolescent Sports Medicine

Pediatric & Adult Plastic Surgery

Pediatric Allergy & Immunology

Pediatric Cancers

Pediatric Cardiac Surgery

Specialty & Special Expertise Index

Spec	Name	St	Pg
PGe	Gunasekaran, T	IL	752
PGe	Gupta, S	IN	752
PGe	Heyman, M	CA	754
PGe	Hill, I	NC	751
PGe	Hoffenberg, E	CO	753
PGe	Jonas, M	MA	748
PGe	Kirschner, B	IL	752
PGe	Kleinman, R	MA	748
PGe	Krebs, N	CO	753
PGe	Leichtner, A	MA	748
PGe	Levy, J	NY	749
PGe	McDiarmid, S	CA	755
PGe	Molleston, J	IN	752
PGe	Mousa, H	OH	752
PGe	Murray, K	WA	755
PGe	Narkewicz, M	CO	753
PGe	Newman, L	NY	749
PGe	Novak, D	FL	751
PGe	Oliva-Hemker, M	MD	750
PGe	Piccoli, D	PA	750
PGe	Rhoads, J	TX	754
PGe	Rothbaum, R	MO	753
PGe	Rudolph, C	WI	753
PGe	Schwarz, K	MD	750
PGe	Schwarz, S	NY	750
PGe	Snyder, J	DC	750
PGe	Sokol, R	CO	754
PGe	Spivak, W	NY	750
PGe	Squires, R	PA	750
PGe	Suchy, F	CO	754
PGe	Ulshen, M	NC	751
PGe	Vanderhoof, J	NE	754
PGe	Whitington, P	IL	753
PGe	Wyllie, R	OH	753

Pediatric Gastrointestinal Surgery

CRS	Lavery, I	OH	172

Pediatric Glaucoma

Oph	Hodapp, E	FL	582

Pediatric Gynecology

AM	Emans, S	MA	80
ObG	Laufer, M	MA	552
ObG	Merritt, D	MO	558
PS	Velcek, F	NY	804
RE	Sanfilippo, J	PA	1009

Pediatric Hand Surgery

HS	Hentz, V	CA	303
HS	Koman, L	NC	299
HS	Lee, W	MD	296
HS	Mih, A	IN	301
PlS	Bentz, M	WI	862
PlS	Chang, J	CA	871
PlS	Sood, R	IN	866

Pediatric Hand/Arm Surgery

Spec	Name	St	Pg
HS	Carlson, M	NY	295

Pediatric Hematology-Oncology

PHO	Abromowitch, M	NE	773
PHO	Adamson, P	PA	756
PHO	Albritton, K	TX	774
PHO	Aledo, A	NY	756
PHO	Altman, A	CT	755
PHO	Andrews, R	WA	775
PHO	Angiolillo, A	DC	757
PHO	Arceci, R	MD	757
PHO	Arndt, C	MN	768
PHO	Banerjee, A	CA	775
PHO	Barredo, J	FL	763
PHO	Berg, S	TX	774
PHO	Bertolone, S	KY	763
PHO	Beyer, E	IL	768
PHO	Billett, A	MA	755
PHO	Blaney, S	TX	774
PHO	Blatt, J	NC	764
PHO	Blum, K	OH	768
PHO	Boxer, L	MI	768
PHO	Brecher, M	NY	757
PHO	Bruggers, C	UT	773
PHO	Buchanan, G	TX	774
PHO	Bussel, J	NY	757
PHO	Cairo, M	NY	757
PHO	Camitta, B	WI	768
PHO	Carroll, W	NY	757
PHO	Castellino, S	NC	764
PHO	Castle, V	MI	769
PHO	Chen, A	MD	757
PHO	Cheung, N	NY	757
PHO	Civin, C	MD	758
PHO	Coccia, P	NE	773
PHO	Cohen, K	MD	758
PHO	Cohn, S	IL	769
PHO	Corey, S	IL	769
PHO	Croop, J	IN	769
PHO	Cunningham, J	IL	769
PHO	Davies, S	OH	769
PHO	Diller, L	MA	755
PHO	Drachtman, R	NJ	758
PHO	Dreyer, Z	TX	774
PHO	Ducore, J	CA	776
PHO	Dunkel, I	NY	758
PHO	Fallon, R	IN	769
PHO	Felix, C	PA	758
PHO	Ferrara, J	MI	769
PHO	Finklestein, J	CA	776
PHO	Finlay, J	CA	776
PHO	Frangoul, H	TN	764
PHO	Frantz, C	DE	758
PHO	Friebert, S	OH	770
PHO	Friedman, A	MD	758
PHO	Friedman, D	TN	764
PHO	Furman, W	TN	764
PHO	Gajjar, A	TN	764
PHO	Garvin, J	NY	758
PHO	Geyer, R	WA	776
PHO	Giardina, P	NY	759

Spec	Name	St	Pg
PHO	Glader, B	CA	776
PHO	Godder, K	VA	764
PHO	Gold, S	NC	764
PHO	Goldman, S	TX	774
PHO	Goldman, S	IL	770
PHO	Graham, M	AZ	775
PHO	Green, D	TN	765
PHO	Greenberg, J	DC	759
PHO	Grupp, S	PA	759
PHO	Guarini, L	NY	759
PHO	Guinan, E	MA	755
PHO	Gururangan, S	NC	765
PHO	Halligan, G	PA	759
PHO	Halpern, S	NJ	759
PHO	Harris, M	NJ	759
PHO	Haut, P	IN	770
PHO	Hawkins, D	WA	776
PHO	Hayani, A	IL	770
PHO	Hayashi, R	MO	770
PHO	Helman, L	MD	759
PHO	Hetherington, M	MO	770
PHO	Hilden, J	CO	773
PHO	Homans, A	VT	755
PHO	Hoots, W	MD	760
PHO	Hord, J	OH	770
PHO	Horn, B	CA	776
PHO	Hudson, M	TN	765
PHO	Hutchinson, R	MI	770
PHO	Jakacki, R	PA	760
PHO	Johnston, J	GA	765
PHO	Kamen, B	NJ	760
PHO	Kane, J	TN	765
PHO	Kapoor, N	CA	776
PHO	Keller, F	GA	765
PHO	Kieran, M	MA	756
PHO	Kobrinsky, N	ND	773
PHO	Korones, D	NY	760
PHO	Kreissman, S	NC	765
PHO	Kung, F	CA	777
PHO	Kurtzberg, J	NC	765
PHO	Kushner, B	NY	760
PHO	Kuttesch, J	PA	760
PHO	Lange, B	PA	760
PHO	Laver, J	TN	766
PHO	Leung, W	TN	766
PHO	Link, M	CA	777
PHO	Lipton, J	NY	761
PHO	Loeb, D	MD	761
PHO	Luchtman-Jones, L	DC	759
PHO	Lusher, J	MI	771
PHO	Manco-Johnson, M	CO	774
PHO	Manera, R	IL	771
PHO	Marcus, J	NY	761
PHO	Marina, N	CA	777
PHO	Maris, J	PA	761
PHO	Matthay, K	CA	777
PHO	McLean, T	NC	766
PHO	Meyer, W	OK	775
PHO	Meyers, P	NY	761
PHO	Morgan, E	IL	771
PHO	Moscow, J	KY	766
PHO	Neglia, J	MN	771
PHO	Neuberg, R	SC	766

Specialty & Special Expertise Index

Spec	Name	St	Pg
NS	Nagib, M	MN	485
NS	Oakes, W	AL	479
NS	Ojemann, J	WA	494
NS	Parent, A	MS	479
NS	Park, T	MO	485
NS	Pollack, I	PA	473
NS	Raffel, C	OH	485
NS	Ragheb, J	FL	479
NS	Ruge, J	IL	486
NS	Sandberg, D	FL	480
NS	Sanford, R	TN	480
NS	Selden, N	OR	495
NS	Shuer, L	CA	495
NS	Sklar, F	TX	490
NS	Souweidane, M	NY	475
NS	Sun, P	CA	495
NS	Tomita, T	IL	486
NS	Walker, M	UT	488
NS	Walsh, J	LA	491
NS	Weiner, H	NY	475
NS	Wisoff, J	NY	476
NS	Zager, E	PA	476

Pediatric Nuclear Medicine

NuM	Dae, M	CA	547
NuM	Majd, M	DC	545

Pediatric Ophthalmology

Oph	Archer, S	MI	586
Oph	Azar, N	IL	586
Oph	Baker, J	MI	586
Oph	Borchert, M	CA	596
Oph	Buckley, E	NC	580
Oph	Burke, M	OH	586
Oph	Capo, H	FL	580
Oph	Caputo, A	NJ	570
Oph	Day, S	CA	597
Oph	Del Monte, M	MI	587
Oph	Demer, J	CA	598
Oph	Drack, A	IA	587
Oph	Eggers, H	NY	571
Oph	Ellis, G	LA	593
Oph	Eustis, H	LA	594
Oph	Freedman, S	NC	581
Oph	Gallin, P	NY	572
Oph	Granet, D	CA	598
Oph	Greenwald, M	IL	587
Oph	Guyton, D	MD	573
Oph	Hall, L	NY	573
Oph	Hess, J	FL	581
Oph	Hunter, D	MA	568
Oph	Isenberg, S	CA	598
Oph	Jaafar, M	DC	574
Oph	Katowitz, J	PA	574
Oph	Kerr, N	TN	582
Oph	Koller, H	PA	574
Oph	Kushner, B	WI	588
Oph	Lambert, S	GA	582
Oph	Lueder, G	MO	589
Oph	Magramm, I	NY	575
Oph	Mazow, M	TX	594

Spec	Name	St	Pg
Oph	McKeown, C	FL	582
Oph	Mets, M	IL	589
Oph	Miller, J	AZ	595
Oph	Mills, M	PA	575
Oph	Mims, J	TX	595
Oph	Mitchell, P	CT	569
Oph	Murphree, A	CA	600
Oph	Nelson, L	PA	576
Oph	Olitsky, S	MO	590
Oph	Paul, T	CA	600
Oph	Plager, D	IN	590
Oph	Pollard, Z	GA	583
Oph	Quinn, G	PA	576
Oph	Reynolds, J	NY	577
Oph	Richard, J	OK	595
Oph	Shields, C	PA	578
Oph	Shields, J	PA	578
Oph	Siatkowski, R	OK	595
Oph	Simon, J	NY	578
Oph	Traboulsi, E	OH	592
Oph	Tychsen, L	MO	592
Oph	Wang, F	NY	579
Oph	Weiss, A	WA	601
Oph	Wilson, M	SC	585
Oph	Wright, K	CA	602

Pediatric Orthopaedic Cancers

OrS	Lee, F	NY	619
OrS	O'Donnell, R	CA	642
OrS	Peabody, T	IL	635
OrS	Wurtz, L	IN	636

Pediatric Orthopaedic Surgery

OrS	Beaty, J	TN	625
OrS	Conrad, E	WA	640
OrS	Delahay, J	DC	614
OrS	Dormans, J	PA	614
OrS	Feldman, D	NY	615
OrS	Hensinger, R	MI	632
OrS	Herman, M	PA	617
OrS	Herzenberg, J	MD	617
OrS	Hyman, J	NY	618
OrS	Kasser, J	MA	610
OrS	Kocher, M	MA	610
OrS	Lee, F	NY	619
OrS	Malawer, M	MD	619
OrS	Marsh, J	CT	610
OrS	McCarthy, J	OH	633
OrS	Morcuende, J	IA	634
OrS	Oppenheim, W	CA	643
OrS	Paley, D	FL	627
OrS	Pizzutillo, P	PA	621
OrS	Rajacich, N	WA	643
OrS	Randall, R	UT	637
OrS	Roye, D	NY	622
OrS	Sponseller, P	MD	623
OrS	Strongwater, A	NJ	623
OrS	Tolo, V	CA	644

Pediatric Otolaryngology

Oto	Clark, K	OK	680
Oto	Grundfast, K	MA	656
Oto	Hotaling, A	IL	674
Oto	Jones, P	IL	675
Oto	Lalwani, A	NY	661
Oto	Naclerio, R	IL	676
Oto	Poole, M	GA	669
Oto	Senders, C	CA	686
PO	April, M	NY	788
PO	Arjmand, E	OH	790
PO	Arnold, J	OH	790
PO	Belenky, W	MI	790
PO	Bower, C	AR	791
PO	Casselbrant, M	PA	788
PO	Chan, K	CO	791
PO	Cotton, R	OH	790
PO	Crockett, D	CA	792
PO	Cunningham, M	MA	788
PO	Darrow, D	VA	790
PO	Dolitsky, J	NY	788
PO	Drake, A	NC	790
PO	Duncan, N	TX	792
PO	Eavey, R	TN	790
PO	Friedman, E	TX	792
PO	Geller, K	CA	792
PO	Goldsmith, A	NY	789
PO	Haddad, J	NY	789
PO	Harley, E	DC	789
PO	Holinger, L	IL	791
PO	Inglis, A	WA	792
PO	Jones, J	NY	789
PO	Katz, R	OH	791
PO	Kazahaya, K	PA	789
PO	Lusk, R	NE	791
PO	McGill, T	MA	788
PO	Miller, R	IL	791
PO	Myer, C	OH	791
PO	Parikh, S	WA	792
PO	Poe, D	MA	788
PO	Richardson, M	OR	792
PO	Rosbe, K	CA	793
PO	Rosenfeld, R	NY	789
PO	Tunkel, D	MD	789
PO	Ward, R	NY	789

Pediatric Pathology

Path	Faye-Petersen, O	AL	713
Path	Heller, D	NJ	709
Path	Triche, T	CA	722

Pediatric Plastic Surgery

PlS	Argenta, L	NC	858
PlS	Bartlett, S	PA	850
PlS	Beals, S	AZ	867
PlS	Bentz, M	WI	862
PlS	Boyajian, M	DC	850
PlS	Buchman, S	MI	863
PlS	Coleman, J	IN	863
PlS	Deleyiannis, F	CO	867
PlS	Gruss, J	WA	872

Specialty & Special Expertise Index

Specialty & Special Expertise Index

Specialty & Special Expertise Index

Spec	Name	St	Pg
PIS	Markowitz, B	CA	873
PIS	Marsh, J	MO	864
PIS	Marten, T	CA	873
PIS	Mast, B	FL	860
PIS	Matarasso, A	NY	854
PIS	Matthews, D	NC	860
PIS	Maxwell, G	TN	860
PIS	McCarthy, J	NY	854
PIS	McCraw, J	MS	860
PIS	Meara, J	MA	848
PIS	Medalie, D	OH	864
PIS	Mehrara, B	NY	854
PIS	Meltzer, T	AZ	868
PIS	Menick, F	AZ	869
PIS	Metzinger, S	LA	869
PIS	Miller, M	OH	864
PIS	Miller, T	CA	873
PIS	Molnar, J	NC	861
PIS	Morgan, R	VA	861
PIS	Moses, M	LA	869
PIS	Mulliken, J	MA	848
PIS	Mustoe, T	IL	864
PIS	Nahabedian, M	DC	854
PIS	Napoli, J	DE	855
PIS	Ness, J	MN	864
PIS	Neumeister, M	IL	865
PIS	Nichter, L	CA	873
PIS	Noone, R	PA	855
PIS	Olding, M	DC	855
PIS	Orgill, D	MA	849
PIS	Ousterhout, D	CA	874
PIS	Papay, F	OH	865
PIS	Patel, P	IL	865
PIS	Paul, M	CA	874
PIS	Persing, J	CT	849
PIS	Pitman, G	NY	855
PIS	Polley, J	IL	865
PIS	Posnick, J	MD	855
PIS	Price, G	MD	855
PIS	Puckett, C	MO	865
PIS	Rand, R	WA	874
PIS	Rappaport, N	TX	869
PIS	Rees, R	MI	865
PIS	Reinisch, J	CA	874
PIS	Ristow, B	CA	874
PIS	Robb, G	TX	869
PIS	Rockwell, W	UT	867
PIS	Rohrich, R	TX	869
PIS	Romano, J	CA	874
PIS	Rosenberg, H	CA	874
PIS	Sanger, J	WI	865
PIS	Schusterman, M	TX	869
PIS	Serletti, J	PA	855
PIS	Seyfer, A	MD	855
PIS	Sherman, R	CA	874
PIS	Siebert, J	WI	866
PIS	Siemionow, M	OH	866
PIS	Silver, L	NY	856
PIS	Singer, R	CA	875
PIS	Singh, N	MD	856
PIS	Slavin, S	MA	849
PIS	Slezak, S	MD	856
PIS	Smith, D	FL	861

Spec	Name	St	Pg
PIS	Smith, P	FL	861
PIS	Sood, R	IN	866
PIS	Spence, R	MD	856
PIS	Spinelli, H	NY	856
PIS	Stadelmann, W	NH	849
PIS	Staffenberg, D	NY	856
PIS	Stahl, R	CT	849
PIS	Stal, S	TX	870
PIS	Stevens, W	CA	875
PIS	Stotland, M	NH	849
PIS	Stuzin, J	FL	861
PIS	Sullivan, P	RI	849
PIS	Sultan, M	NY	856
PIS	Tabbal, N	NY	856
PIS	Taub, P	NY	857
PIS	Tebbetts, J	TX	870
PIS	Thaller, S	FL	861
PIS	Thorne, C	NY	857
PIS	Ting, J	NY	857
PIS	Tobin, G	KY	861
PIS	Topham, N	PA	857
PIS	Tufaro, A	MD	857
PIS	Urata, M	CA	875
PIS	Vander Kolk, C	MD	857
PIS	Vasconez, H	KY	861
PIS	Vogt, P	MN	866
PIS	Walton, R	IL	866
PIS	Wells, J	CA	875
PIS	Whitaker, L	PA	857
PIS	Wilcox, R	TX	870
PIS	Wilhelmi, B	KY	862
PIS	Wilkins, E	MI	866
PIS	Wolfe, S	FL	862
PIS	Yetman, R	OH	866
PIS	Young, V	MO	866
PIS	Yu, J	GA	862
PIS	Yuen, J	AR	870
PIS	Zide, B	NY	858
PIS	Zins, J	OH	867

Platelet Disorders

Hem	DeLoughery, T	OR	324
Hem	Lyons, R	TX	323
Hem	Marks, P	CT	308
PHO	Bussel, J	NY	757
PHO	Olson, T	GA	766
PHO	Parker, R	NY	761

Pleural Disease

Pul	Light, R	TN	929
Pul	Sahn, S	SC	929
TS	Friedberg, J	PA	1111

Pneumococcal Infections

PInf	Kaplan, S	TX	782

Pneumoconiosis

Pul	Rose, C	CO	935

Pneumocystis Carinii Pneumonia (PCP)

Pul	Huang, L	CA	937

Pneumonia

Inf	Craven, D	MA	404
Inf	Cunha, B	NY	405
Inf	Quagliarello, V	CT	404
Inf	Yu, V	PA	408
PPul	Wall, M	OR	798
Pul	Guidry, G	LA	935
Pul	Nash, T	NY	924
Pul	Niederman, M	NY	924

Pneumonia-Recurrent

PPul	Murphy, T	NC	795

Poison Control

PrM	Hoffman, R	NY	881

Polycystic Kidney Disease

Nep	Blumenfeld, J	NY	453
Nep	Perrone, R	MA	452
Nep	Rakowski, T	VA	456
Nep	Torres, V	MN	459
PNep	Brophy, P	IA	786
PNep	Kaplan, B	PA	784

Polycystic Ovarian Syndrome

EDM	Ehrmann, D	IL	215
EDM	Goodman, N	FL	212
EDM	Korytkowski, M	PA	209
EDM	Marshall, J	VA	213
EDM	Nestler, J	VA	213
RE	Azziz, R	GA	1011
RE	Barnes, R	IL	1012
RE	Cedars, M	CA	1017
RE	Chang, R	CA	1017
RE	Coutifaris, C	PA	1008
RE	Diamond, M	MI	1013
RE	Dumesic, D	CA	1017
RE	Friedman, C	OH	1013
RE	Jacobs, L	IL	1013
RE	Kazer, R	IL	1013
RE	Legro, R	PA	1008
RE	Ratts, V	MO	1014
RE	Richardson, M	KS	1015
RE	Session, D	GA	1012
RE	Smith, Y	MI	1014
RE	Soules, M	WA	1018
RE	Walmer, D	NC	1012
RE	Wilson, E	TX	1016

Polycythemia Rubra Vera

Hem	Fruchtman, S	NY	310
Hem	Spivak, J	MD	313
Hem	Streiff, M	MD	314

Specialty & Special Expertise Index

Specialty & Special Expertise Index

Specialty & Special Expertise Index

Spec	Name	St	Pg
Pul	Nardell, E	MA	921
Pul	Nash, T	NY	924
Pul	Nelson, J	NY	924
Pul	Niederman, M	NY	924
Pul	Pack, A	PA	924
Pul	Padilla, M	NY	925
Pul	Palevsky, H	PA	925
Pul	Parsons, P	VT	921
Pul	Patterson, J	OR	938
Pul	Perret, P	LA	936
Pul	Popovich, J	MI	932
Pul	Prakash, U	MN	932
Pul	Raghu, G	WA	938
Pul	Redlich, C	CT	921
Pul	Reilly, J	PA	925
Pul	Rennard, S	NE	935
Pul	Rizk, N	CA	938
Pul	Rochester, C	CT	922
Pul	Rose, C	CO	935
Pul	Rosenbluth, D	MO	933
Pul	Rossman, M	PA	925
Pul	Rubin, L	CA	938
Pul	Sahn, S	SC	929
Pul	Schluger, N	NY	925
Pul	Schwab, R	PA	925
Pul	Schwartz, D	CO	935
Pul	Schwarz, M	CO	935
Pul	Sharma, O	CA	939
Pul	Shellito, J	LA	936
Pul	Shore, B	MO	933
Pul	Silver, M	IL	933
Pul	Simon, R	MI	933
Pul	Staton, G	GA	929
Pul	Steiger, D	NY	925
Pul	Steinberg, H	NY	926
Pul	Sterman, D	PA	926
Pul	Stoller, J	OH	933
Pul	Stover-Pepe, D	NY	926
Pul	Strollo, P	PA	926
Pul	Sutherland, E	CO	935
Pul	Tapson, V	NC	930
Pul	Teirstein, A	NY	926
Pul	Tharratt, R	CA	939
Pul	Thomashow, B	NY	926
Pul	Tino, G	PA	926
Pul	Tobin, M	IL	933
Pul	Trulock, E	MO	933
Pul	Unger, M	PA	927
Pul	Vaughey, E	VA	930
Pul	Villanueva, A	MA	922
Pul	Voelkel, N	VA	930
Pul	Wallace, J	CA	939
Pul	Wanner, A	FL	930
Pul	Weissler, J	TX	930
Pul	Wenzel, S	PA	927
Pul	Wheeler, A	TN	930
Pul	White, D	MA	922
Pul	Wiedemann, H	OH	934
Pul	Young, K	PA	927

Pulmonary

Disease/Immunocompromised

Pul	Stover-Pepe, D	NY	926

Pulmonary Embolism

DR	Goodman, L	WI	980
DR	Sagel, S	MO	980
Pul	Arcasoy, S	NY	922
Pul	Palevsky, H	PA	925
Pul	Popovich, J	MI	932
S	Wakefield, T	MI	1079
TS	Jamieson, S	CA	1136

Pulmonary Fibrosis

Pul	Bascom, R	PA	922
Pul	Berk, J	MA	920
Pul	Brown, K	CO	934
Pul	Criner, G	PA	923
Pul	King, T	CA	938
Pul	Loyd, J	TN	929
Pul	Lynch, J	CA	938
Pul	Padilla, M	NY	925
Pul	Raghu, G	WA	938
Pul	Sahn, S	SC	929
Pul	Schwartz, D	CO	935
Pul	Schwarz, M	CO	935
Pul	Staton, G	GA	929

Pulmonary Hypertension

Cv	Bashore, T	NC	100
Cv	Bourge, R	AL	101
Cv	Horn, E	NY	97
Cv	Poon, M	NY	99
Cv	Rich, S	IL	108
Cv	Smart, F	LA	113
Cv	von der Lohe, E	IN	110
Cv	Wagoner, L	OH	110
NP	Steinhorn, R	IL	447
Pul	Arroliga, A	TX	935
Pul	Auger, W	CA	936
Pul	Criner, G	PA	923
Pul	Elliott, C	UT	934
Pul	Hertz, M	MN	931
Pul	Hill, N	MA	921
Pul	Krowka, M	MN	932
Pul	Loyd, J	TN	929
Pul	Mosenifar, Z	CA	938
Pul	Padilla, M	NY	925
Pul	Palevsky, H	PA	925
Pul	Rubin, L	CA	938
Pul	Steiger, D	NY	925
Pul	Tapson, V	NC	930
Pul	Trulock, E	MO	933
Pul	Voelkel, N	VA	930

Pulmonary Hypertension of Newborn (PPHN)

NP	Donn, S	MI	446
NP	Frantz, I	MA	442
NP	Seidner, S	TX	448

Spec	Name	St	Pg
NP	Van Marter, L	MA	442

Pulmonary Infections

Pul	Gibson, R	WA	937
Pul	Ingbar, D	MN	931
Pul	Metersky, M	CT	921
Pul	Rizk, N	CA	938
Pul	Shellito, J	LA	936
Pul	Stover-Pepe, D	NY	926
Pul	Wallace, J	CA	939

Pulmonary Pathology

Path	Cagle, P	TX	717
Path	Fishbein, M	CA	720
Path	Hammar, S	WA	720
Path	Katzenstein, A	NY	709
Path	Koss, M	CA	721
Path	Leslie, K	AZ	718
Path	Mark, E	MA	706
Path	Patchefsky, A	PA	710
Path	Travis, W	NY	712
Path	Yousem, S	PA	712

Pulmonary Rehabilitation

PPul	Warren, R	AR	797

Pulmonary Vascular Disease

Pul	Garrity, E	IL	931
Pul	Palevsky, H	PA	925
Pul	Rubin, L	CA	938
Pul	Schwarz, M	CO	935

R

Radiation Oncology

DR	Charboneau, J	MN	979
RadRO	Abrams, R	IL	956
RadRO	Ang, K	TX	961
RadRO	Anscher, M	VA	951
RadRO	Awan, A	IL	956
RadRO	Beitler, J	GA	951
RadRO	Ben-Josef, E	MI	957
RadRO	Berg, C	MD	946
RadRO	Blackstock, A	NC	951
RadRO	Bogart, J	NY	946
RadRO	Bonner, J	AL	952
RadRO	Bradley, J	MO	957
RadRO	Brizel, D	NC	952
RadRO	Buatti, J	IA	957
RadRO	Buchholz, T	TX	962
RadRO	Chakravarthy, A	TN	952
RadRO	Chao, K	NY	946
RadRO	Choi, N	MA	944
RadRO	Choy, H	TX	962
RadRO	Ciezki, J	OH	957

Specialty & Special Expertise Index

Spec	Name	St	Pg
RadRO	Cmelak, A	TN	952
RadRO	Constine, L	NY	946
RadRO	Cooper, J	NY	947
RadRO	Cox, J	TX	962
RadRO	Crocker, I	GA	952
RadRO	D'Amico, A	MA	944
RadRO	DeLaney, T	MA	944
RadRO	DeWeese, T	MD	947
RadRO	Dicker, A	PA	947
RadRO	Donahue, B	NY	947
RadRO	Donaldson, S	CA	964
RadRO	Dritschilo, A	DC	947
RadRO	Eifel, P	TX	962
RadRO	Eisbruch, A	MI	957
RadRO	Emami, B	IL	957
RadRO	Ennis, R	NY	947
RadRO	Fiveash, J	AL	952
RadRO	Flickinger, J	PA	947
RadRO	Forman, J	MI	957
RadRO	Formenti, S	NY	947
RadRO	Fowble, B	CA	964
RadRO	Freedman, G	PA	948
RadRO	Fuss, M	OR	964
RadRO	Gaffney, D	UT	961
RadRO	Gejerman, G	NJ	948
RadRO	Goodman, R	NJ	948
RadRO	Grado, G	AZ	962
RadRO	Greenberger, J	PA	948
RadRO	Grigsby, P	MO	957
RadRO	Haffty, B	NJ	948
RadRO	Hahn, S	PA	948
RadRO	Halberg, F	CA	964
RadRO	Halle, R	NC	952
RadRO	Halpern, H	IL	958
RadRO	Halyard, M	AZ	962
RadRO	Hancock, S	CA	964
RadRO	Haraf, D	IL	958
RadRO	Harari, P	WI	958
RadRO	Harris, J	MA	944
RadRO	Harrison, L	NY	948
RadRO	Hartford, A	NH	944
RadRO	Hayman, J	MI	958
RadRO	Heimann, R	VT	944
RadRO	Henderson, R	FL	952
RadRO	Herman, T	OK	962
RadRO	Hoppe, R	CA	964
RadRO	Horwitz, E	PA	948
RadRO	Isaacson, S	NY	949
RadRO	Jhingran, A	TX	962
RadRO	Johnstone, P	IN	958
RadRO	Jose, B	KY	953
RadRO	Kachnic, L	MA	944
RadRO	Kaplan, I	MA	944
RadRO	Kim, J	MI	958
RadRO	Kleinberg, L	MD	949
RadRO	Koh, W	WA	964
RadRO	Komaki, R	TX	963
RadRO	Konski, A	MI	958
RadRO	Kudrimoti, M	KY	953
RadRO	Kuettel, M	NY	949
RadRO	Kun, L	TN	953
RadRO	Kupelian, P	CA	964
RadRO	Kuske, R	AZ	963

Spec	Name	St	Pg
RadRO	Landry, J	GA	953
RadRO	Laramore, G	WA	965
RadRO	Larner, J	VA	953
RadRO	Larson, D	CA	965
RadRO	Lawrence, T	MI	958
RadRO	Le, Q	CA	965
RadRO	Lee, A	TX	963
RadRO	Lee, C	MN	959
RadRO	Lee, W	NC	953
RadRO	Lepanto, P	WV	949
RadRO	Lewin, A	FL	953
RadRO	Loeffler, J	MA	945
RadRO	Machtay, M	OH	959
RadRO	Macklis, R	OH	959
RadRO	Malcolm, A	TN	953
RadRO	Mansur, D	MO	959
RadRO	Marcus, R	FL	954
RadRO	Markoe, A	FL	954
RadRO	Marks, L	NC	954
RadRO	Martenson, J	MN	959
RadRO	Mauch, P	MA	945
RadRO	McCormick, B	NY	949
RadRO	McGarry, R	KY	954
RadRO	Medbery, C	OK	963
RadRO	Mendenhall, N	FL	954
RadRO	Mendenhall, W	FL	954
RadRO	Merchant, T	TN	954
RadRO	Meredith, R	AL	954
RadRO	Michalski, J	MO	959
RadRO	Minsky, B	IL	959
RadRO	Mittal, B	IL	959
RadRO	Morris, M	VA	954
RadRO	Morrison, W	TX	963
RadRO	Movsas, B	MI	960
RadRO	Mundt, A	CA	965
RadRO	Myerson, R	MO	960
RadRO	Nicolaou, N	PA	949
RadRO	Nori, D	NY	949
RadRO	Park, C	CA	965
RadRO	Peschel, R	CT	945
RadRO	Pezner, R	CA	965
RadRO	Pierce, L	MI	960
RadRO	Pollack, A	FL	955
RadRO	Porrazzo, M	DC	949
RadRO	Prosnitz, L	NC	955
RadRO	Quivey, J	CA	965
RadRO	Rabinovitch, R	CO	961
RadRO	Randall, M	KY	955
RadRO	Randolph-Jackson, P	DC	950
RadRO	Recht, A	MA	945
RadRO	Regine, W	MD	950
RadRO	Rich, T	VA	955
RadRO	Roach, M	CA	965
RadRO	Roberts, K	CT	945
RadRO	Rose, C	CA	966
RadRO	Rosenman, J	NC	955
RadRO	Rossi, C	CA	966
RadRO	Rotman, M	NY	950
RadRO	Russell, A	MA	945
RadRO	Russell, K	WA	966
RadRO	Sailer, S	NC	955
RadRO	Sandler, H	CA	966
RadRO	Schiff, P	NY	950

Spec	Name	St	Pg
RadRO	Schild, S	AZ	963
RadRO	Schomberg, P	MN	960
RadRO	Senzer, N	TX	963
RadRO	Seung, S	OR	966
RadRO	Shaw, E	NC	955
RadRO	Shina, D	NM	963
RadRO	Shrieve, D	UT	961
RadRO	Small, W	IL	960
RadRO	Smalley, S	KS	961
RadRO	Solin, L	PA	950
RadRO	Song, S	VA	955
RadRO	St Clair, W	KY	955
RadRO	Stea, B	AZ	963
RadRO	Stock, R	NY	950
RadRO	Streeter, O	DC	950
RadRO	Suh, J	OH	960
RadRO	Suntharalingam, M	MD	950
RadRO	Taghian, A	MA	945
RadRO	Tarbell, N	MA	945
RadRO	Taylor, M	MO	960
RadRO	Tepper, J	NC	956
RadRO	Thomas, C	OR	966
RadRO	Toonkel, L	FL	956
RadRO	Tripuraneni, P	CA	966
RadRO	Vicini, F	MI	960
RadRO	Videtic, G	OH	961
RadRO	Vijayakumar, S	MS	956
RadRO	Wara, W	CA	966
RadRO	Wazer, D	RI	946
RadRO	Weichselbaum, R	IL	961
RadRO	Weiss, M	PA	951
RadRO	Werner-Wasik, M	PA	951
RadRO	Wharam, M	MD	951
RadRO	Willett, C	NC	956
RadRO	Wilson, J	WI	961
RadRO	Wilson, L	CT	946
RadRO	Wolfson, A	FL	956
RadRO	Wong, J	CA	967
RadRO	Woo, S	KY	956
RadRO	Yahalom, J	NY	951
RadRO	Zelefsky, M	NY	951
RadRO	Zietman, A	MA	946

Radiation Therapy-Intraoperative

Spec	Name	St	Pg
RadRO	Harrison, L	NY	948

Radiofrequency Tumor Ablation

Spec	Name	St	Pg
DR	Charboneau, J	MN	979
S	Klimberg, V	AR	1085
TS	Cohen, N	MD	1110
VIR	Brown, K	NY	992
VIR	Kay, D	LA	996
VIR	McGahan, J	CA	997
VIR	Nemcek, A	IL	995
VIR	Soulen, M	PA	993
VIR	Wood, B	MD	993

Radioimmunotherapy of Cancer

Spec	Name	St	Pg
NuM	Carrasquillo, J	NY	544

Specialty & Special Expertise Index

Spec	Name	St	Pg
NuM	Wahl, R	MD	545
NuM	Wiseman, G	MN	546
RadRO	Macklis, R	OH	959
RadRO	Wong, J	CA	967

Radionuclide Therapy
RadRO	Meredith, R	AL	954

Rare Disorders
Ped	Morton, D	PA	727

Rare Genetic Disorders
CG	Wilcox, W	CA	162

Rare Lung Disease-Pediatric
PPul	Kim, Y	IN	796

Rare Skin Disorders
D	Shupack, J	NY	189

Rasmussen's Syndrome
N	Cole, A	MA	505
NS	Carson, B	MD	468
Ped	Vining, E	MD	727

Raynaud's Disease
D	Franks, A	NY	186
Rhu	Clements, P	CA	1031
Rhu	Medsger, T	PA	1025
Rhu	Wigley, F	MD	1027

Reconstructive Microvascular Surgery
HS	Hanel, D	WA	303
HS	Harris, G	IL	300
HS	Steinmann, S	MN	301
OrS	Hausman, M	NY	616
Oto	Burkey, B	OH	673
Oto	Day, T	SC	666
Oto	Teknos, T	OH	677
Oto	Valentino, J	KY	671
PlS	Levin, L	PA	853
PlS	Molnar, J	NC	861

Reconstructive Plastic Surgery
Oph	Lucarelli, M	WI	589
Oto	Toriumi, D	IL	677
PlS	Billmire, D	OH	862
PlS	Cutting, C	NY	851
PlS	Dagum, A	NY	851
PlS	Gottlieb, L	IL	863
PlS	Hultman, C	NC	860
PlS	Siemionow, M	OH	866
PlS	Thaller, S	FL	861
PlS	Tobin, G	KY	861

Spec	Name	St	Pg
PlS	Wilhelmi, B	KY	862
PlS	Zide, B	NY	858

Reconstructive Surgery
GO	Lele, S	NY	279
HS	Chung, K	MI	299
HS	Lee, W	MD	296
ObG	Hale, D	IN	557
Oph	Mawn, L	TN	582
Oph	Ng, J	OR	600
OrS	Bos, G	WA	639
OrS	Burke, D	MA	608
OrS	Cheng, E	MN	631
OrS	Cooper, D	TX	638
OrS	Ebraheim, N	OH	631
OrS	Goodman, S	CA	641
OrS	Greisberg, J	NY	616
OrS	Kraay, M	OH	633
OrS	Macaulay, W	NY	619
OrS	Manoli, A	MI	633
OrS	O'Keefe, R	NY	620
OrS	Parsons, T	MI	634
OrS	Thordarson, D	CA	644
OrS	Ward, W	NC	629
Oto	Baker, S	MI	672
Oto	Chalian, A	PA	657
Oto	Hicks, W	NY	659
Oto	Quatela, V	NY	663
Oto	Rosenthal, E	AL	669
PlS	Bentz, M	WI	862
PlS	Chang, J	CA	871
PlS	Cordeiro, P	NY	851
PlS	Ducic, I	DC	852
PlS	Dufresne, C	MD	852
PlS	Feldman, J	MA	848
PlS	Hagan, K	TN	859
PlS	Hardesty, R	CA	872
PlS	Hidalgo, D	NY	852
PlS	Hoffman, W	CA	872
PlS	Lee, R	IL	864
PlS	Lesavoy, M	CA	873
PlS	Loree, T	NY	853
PlS	MacKinnon, S	MO	864
PlS	Manson, P	MD	854
PlS	Sanger, J	WI	865
PlS	Serletti, J	PA	855
PlS	Seyfer, A	MD	855
PlS	Silver, L	NY	856
PlS	Smith, D	FL	861
PlS	Topham, N	PA	857
PS	Tuggle, D	OK	809
S	Edington, H	PA	1052
SM	Bradley, J	PA	1036
U	Atala, A	NC	1153
U	Brock, J	TN	1154
U	Davis, B	KS	1166
U	Foster, R	IN	1161
U	Griebling, T	KS	1166
U	Kaefer, M	IN	1161
U	Miller, S	GA	1156
U	Strand, W	TX	1168

Spec	Name	St	Pg

Reconstructive Surgery-Complex
OrS	Copp, S	CA	640
PlS	Brandt, K	MO	862
PlS	Patel, P	IL	865

Reconstructive Surgery-Face
Oto	Haughey, B	MO	674
Oto	Papel, I	MD	662
PlS	Baker, D	NY	850
PlS	Bartlett, S	PA	850
PlS	McCarthy, J	NY	854
PlS	Mehrara, B	NY	854
PlS	Menick, F	AZ	869
PlS	Smith, P	FL	861

Reconstructive Surgery-Skin
D	Brodland, D	PA	185
D	Cook, J	NC	190
D	Swanson, N	OR	200

Reconstructive Urologic Surgery
U	Assimos, D	NC	1153
U	Greenfield, S	NY	1147
U	Hemal, A	NC	1155
U	Koch, M	IN	1162
U	Rink, R	IN	1164
U	Thrasher, J	KS	1166
U	Webster, G	NC	1159

Rectal Cancer
CRS	Gorfine, S	NY	168
Ge	Aslanian, H	CT	228
Onc	Kemeny, N	NY	342
RadRO	Konski, A	MI	958
RadRO	Tepper, J	NC	956
RadRO	Weichselbaum, R	IL	961

Rectal Cancer/Sphincter Preservation
CRS	Abcarian, H	IL	171
CRS	Bailey, H	TX	175
CRS	Beart, R	CA	175
CRS	Delaney, C	OH	171
CRS	Geisler, D	PA	168
CRS	Guillem, J	NY	168
CRS	Ludwig, K	WI	172
CRS	Mantyh, C	NC	170
CRS	Rombeau, J	PA	169
CRS	Saclarides, T	IL	173
CRS	Stamos, M	CA	176
CRS	Thorson, A	NE	174
S	Skibber, J	TX	1087
S	Tyler, D	NC	1068

Rectovaginal Fistula
CRS	Birnbaum, E	MO	171
CRS	Hartmann, R	FL	170

Specialty & Special Expertise Index

Spec	Name	St	Pg
CRS	Lowry, A	MN	172
CRS	Mutch, M	MO	173

Reflex Sympathetic Dystrophy

Spec	Name	St	Pg
PM	Jain, S	NY	695

Reflex Sympathetic Dystrophy (RSD)

Spec	Name	St	Pg
N	Reder, A	IL	527
N	Schwartzman, R	PA	515
PM	Audell, L	CA	700
PM	Berde, C	MA	694
PM	Christo, P	MD	694
PM	Ferrante, F	CA	700
PM	Harden, R	IL	698
PM	Ngeow, J	NY	696
PM	Racz, G	TX	700
PM	Raja, S	MD	696
PM	Rosner, H	CA	701
PRhu	Sherry, D	PA	799

Refractive Surgery

Spec	Name	St	Pg
Oph	Cionni, R	UT	593
Oph	Dhaliwal, D	PA	571
Oph	Holland, E	OH	588
Oph	John, T	IL	588
Oph	Koch, D	TX	594
Oph	Krueger, R	OH	588
Oph	Lindstrom, R	MN	589
Oph	Maguire, L	MN	589
Oph	Maloney, R	CA	599
Oph	Mathers, W	OR	599
Oph	McDonnell, P	MD	575
Oph	Miller, K	CA	599
Oph	Orlin, S	PA	576
Oph	Pflugfelder, S	TX	595
Oph	Rosenberg, M	IL	591
Oph	Samuelson, T	MN	591
Oph	Stark, W	MD	578
Oph	Steinert, R	CA	601
Oph	Updegraff, S	FL	584
Oph	Wallace, R	LA	595

Rehabilitation for Rheumatic Diseases

Spec	Name	St	Pg
Rhu	Ehresmann, G	CA	1031

Reiter's Syndrome

Spec	Name	St	Pg
Rhu	Arnett, F	TX	1030
Rhu	Solitar, B	NY	1026

Relapsing Polychondritis

Spec	Name	St	Pg
Oto	Lebovics, R	NY	661
Rhu	Luthra, H	MN	1029

Relationship Problems

Spec	Name	St	Pg
Psyc	Bronheim, H	NY	887
Psyc	Levine, S	OH	893

Renal Artery Stenosis

Spec	Name	St	Pg
IC	Dieter, R	IL	128
Nep	Textor, S	MN	459
Nep	Townsend, R	PA	455
VascS	Calligaro, K	PA	1180
VascS	Mitchell, M	MS	1184

Renal Replacement Therapy

Spec	Name	St	Pg
PNep	Chandar, J	FL	785

Renovascular Disease

Spec	Name	St	Pg
Cv	Ramee, S	LA	112
IC	Petrossian, G	NY	125
IM	Weder, A	MI	420
VascS	Benvenisty, A	NY	1180
VascS	Cambria, R	MA	1178
VascS	Faries, P	NY	1181
VascS	Gewertz, B	CA	1188
VascS	Gusberg, R	CT	1178
VascS	Hansen, K	NC	1184
VascS	Stanley, J	MI	1186

Repetitive Motion Injuries

Spec	Name	St	Pg
HS	Derman, G	IL	299

Reproductive Endocrinology

Spec	Name	St	Pg
EDM	Bhasin, S	MA	204
EDM	Braunstein, G	CA	220
ObG	Berga, S	GA	555
ObG	De Cherney, A	MD	553
RE	Adamson, G	CA	1016
RE	Agarwal, S	CA	1017
RE	Azziz, R	GA	1011
RE	Barnes, R	IL	1012
RE	Bateman, B	VA	1011
RE	Blackwell, R	AL	1011
RE	Buster, J	MA	1006
RE	Carr, B	TX	1015
RE	Carson, S	RI	1006
RE	Cedars, M	CA	1017
RE	Chang, R	CA	1017
RE	Christman, G	MI	1012
RE	Clisham, P	LA	1015
RE	Coddington, C	MN	1012
RE	Copperman, A	NY	1008
RE	Coutifaris, C	PA	1008
RE	Crowley, W	MA	1006
RE	DeVane, G	FL	1011
RE	Diamond, M	MI	1013
RE	Dickey, R	LA	1016
RE	Dodds, W	MI	1013
RE	Dumesic, D	CA	1017
RE	Durso, N	VA	1011
RE	Falcone, T	OH	1013

Spec	Name	St	Pg
RE	Friedman, C	OH	1013
RE	Fritz, M	NC	1011
RE	Ginsburg, E	MA	1006
RE	Giudice, L	CA	1017
RE	Goldberg, J	OH	1013
RE	Gracia, C	PA	1008
RE	Grazi, R	NY	1008
RE	Grifo, J	NY	1008
RE	Grunfeld, L	NY	1008
RE	Haney, A	IL	1013
RE	Hill, J	NH	1006
RE	Hornstein, M	MA	1006
RE	Houmard, B	WA	1017
RE	Huang, J	TX	1016
RE	Isaacson, K	MA	1006
RE	Jacobs, L	IL	1013
RE	Johnson, J	MA	1007
RE	Kazer, R	IL	1013
RE	Kutteh, W	TN	1011
RE	Legro, R	PA	1008
RE	Licciardi, F	NY	1009
RE	Luciano, A	CT	1007
RE	Manganiello, P	NH	1007
RE	Marrs, R	CA	1017
RE	McClamrock, H	MD	1009
RE	McGovern, P	NJ	1009
RE	Milad, M	IL	1014
RE	Miller, C	IL	1014
RE	Moffitt, D	AZ	1016
RE	Molo, M	IL	1014
RE	Mukherjee, T	NY	1009
RE	Murphy, A	GA	1011
RE	Nagel, T	MN	1014
RE	Noyes, N	NY	1009
RE	Odem, R	MO	1014
RE	Ory, S	FL	1012
RE	Oskowitz, S	MA	1007
RE	Patrizio, P	CT	1007
RE	Paulson, R	CA	1017
RE	Petrozza, J	MA	1007
RE	Putman, J	TX	1016
RE	Ratts, V	MO	1014
RE	Richardson, M	KS	1015
RE	Rosenwaks, Z	NY	1009
RE	Sanfilippo, J	PA	1009
RE	Sauer, M	NY	1009
RE	Schenken, R	TX	1016
RE	Schlaff, W	CO	1015
RE	Seifer, D	NY	1010
RE	Session, D	GA	1012
RE	Smikle, C	CA	1018
RE	Smith, Y	MI	1014
RE	Sondheimer, S	PA	1010
RE	Soules, M	WA	1018
RE	Stangel, J	NY	1010
RE	Steinkampf, M	AL	1012
RE	Stewart, E	MN	1015
RE	Surrey, E	CO	1015
RE	Toth, T	MA	1007
RE	Van Voorhis, B	IA	1015
RE	Wallach, E	MD	1010
RE	Walmer, D	NC	1012
RE	Weiss, G	NJ	1010

Specialty & Special Expertise Index

Specialty & Special Expertise Index

Spec	Name	St	Pg

Running Injuries

SM	Metzl, J	NY	1037

S

Salivary Gland Tumors

Onc	Martins, R	WA	387
Oto	Blair, E	IL	672
Oto	Urken, M	NY	665
Oto	Weissler, M	NC	671
RadRO	Laramore, G	WA	965

Salivary Gland Tumors & Surgery

Oto	Clayman, G	TX	680
Oto	Deschler, D	MA	655
Oto	Eisele, D	CA	684
Oto	Goldenberg, D	PA	659
Oto	Hoffman, H	IA	674
Oto	Lydiatt, W	NE	679
Oto	Olsen, K	MN	676
Oto	Osguthorpe, J	SC	668
Oto	Rassekh, C	PA	663
Oto	Shockley, W	NC	670
Oto	Weber, R	TX	682
S	Shah, J	NY	1059

Sarcoidosis

Pul	Donohue, J	NC	928
Pul	King, T	CA	938
Pul	Padilla, M	NY	925
Pul	Raghu, G	WA	938
Pul	Rose, C	CO	935
Pul	Rossman, M	PA	925
Pul	Sharma, O	CA	939
Pul	Staton, G	GA	929
Pul	Teirstein, A	NY	926

Sarcoma

Hem	Heinrich, M	OR	324
Hem	Milhem, M	IA	320
Onc	Benjamin, R	TX	376
Onc	Borden, E	OH	364
Onc	Brockstein, B	IL	364
Onc	Chow, W	CA	383
Onc	Conry, R	AL	353
Onc	Demetri, G	MA	327
Onc	Ettinger, D	MD	338
Onc	Fitch, T	AZ	377
Onc	Grosh, W	VA	355
Onc	Hande, K	TN	355
Onc	Jacobs, C	CA	386
Onc	Kraft, A	SC	356
Onc	Maki, R	NY	343
Onc	Meyskens, F	CA	387

Onc	Patel, S	TX	380
Onc	Samuels, B	ID	375
Onc	Sandler, A	OR	389
Onc	Stewart, F	WA	390
Onc	Von Burton, G	LA	381
Onc	von Mehren, M	PA	350
OrS	Berrey, B	FL	625
OrS	Biermann, J	MI	630
OrS	Bos, G	WA	639
OrS	Conrad, E	WA	640
OrS	Healey, J	NY	616
OrS	Hornicek, F	MA	609
OrS	Lackman, R	PA	618
OrS	Malawer, M	MD	619
OrS	McDonald, D	MO	634
OrS	Scarborough, M	FL	628
OrS	Sim, F	MN	635
OrS	Ward, W	NC	629
OrS	Wurtz, L	IN	636
Path	Brooks, J	PA	708
Path	Fletcher, C	MA	706
Path	Goldblum, J	OH	715
Path	Patchefsky, A	PA	710
Path	Rubin, B	OH	716
Path	Triche, T	CA	722
Path	Weiss, S	GA	714
PHO	Albritton, K	TX	774
PHO	Arndt, C	MN	768
PHO	Marina, N	CA	777
PHO	Meyer, W	OK	775
PHO	Meyers, P	NY	761
PHO	Olson, T	GA	766
PHO	Williams, J	AZ	775
PlS	Rockwell, W	UT	867
RadRO	Brizel, D	NC	952
RadRO	Constine, L	NY	946
RadRO	DeLaney, T	MA	944
RadRO	Donaldson, S	CA	964
RadRO	Hahn, S	PA	948
RadRO	Herman, T	OK	962
RadRO	Michalski, J	MO	959
RadRO	Pollack, A	FL	955
RadRO	Prosnitz, L	NC	955
RadRO	Tepper, J	NC	956
RadRO	Wara, W	CA	966
RadRO	Wolfson, A	FL	956
S	Brennan, M	NY	1050
S	Brown, C	IL	1070
S	Dooley, W	OK	1083
S	Eilber, F	CA	1090
S	Eisenberg, B	NH	1045
S	Feig, B	TX	1083
S	Fraker, D	PA	1053
S	Leitch, A	TX	1085
S	Levine, E	NC	1065
S	Li, B	LA	1085
S	Lind, D	GA	1065
S	Nakakura, E	CA	1092
S	Nathanson, S	MI	1076
S	Pollock, R	TX	1086
S	Sondak, V	FL	1068
S	Weber, S	WI	1079
S	White, R	NC	1069

Sarcoma-Soft Tissue

Onc	Chow, W	CA	383
Onc	Forscher, C	CA	385
Onc	Maki, R	NY	343
Onc	Stockdale, F	CA	390
OrS	Benevenia, J	NJ	612
OrS	Healey, J	NY	616
OrS	Irwin, R	MI	632
OrS	Mayerson, J	OH	633
OrS	O'Donnell, R	CA	642
OrS	Randall, R	UT	637
OrS	Ready, J	MA	610
OrS	Schmidt, R	PA	623
OrS	Wittig, J	NY	625
PHO	Wexler, L	NY	763
RadRO	Landry, J	GA	953
RadRO	Pezner, R	CA	965
RadRO	Wharam, M	MD	951
S	August, D	NJ	1049
S	Hanna, N	MD	1053
S	Heslin, M	AL	1064
S	Hunt, K	TX	1084
S	Pisters, P	TX	1086
S	Singer, S	NY	1059
TS	Putnam, J	TN	1122

Scalp Disorders

D	Cotsarelis, G	PA	186

Scar Revision

D	Alster, T	DC	184
D	Lask, G	CA	199

Schizophrenia

ChAP	Rapoport, J	DC	906
ChAP	Russell, A	CA	909
Psyc	Adler, D	MA	884
Psyc	Benes, F	MA	884
Psyc	Boronow, J	MD	886
Psyc	Davidson, J	TX	896
Psyc	Freedman, R	CO	894
Psyc	Goff, D	MA	884
Psyc	Hirschfeld, R	TX	896
Psyc	Liberman, R	CA	898
Psyc	Marder, S	CA	898
Psyc	McIntosh, J	UT	895
Psyc	Weiner, R	NC	892

Schizophrenia-Clinical Trials

Psyc	McGlashan, T	CT	885

Schizophrenia-Early Detection/Treatment

Psyc	McGlashan, T	CT	885

Scleroderma

D	Falanga, V	RI	182

Specialty & Special Expertise Index

Specialty & Special Expertise Index

Specialty & Special Expertise Index

Specialty & Special Expertise Index

Spec	Name	St	Pg
OrS	Miller, M	VA	627
OrS	Millett, P	CO	637
OrS	Nicholas, S	NY	620
OrS	O'Driscoll, S	MN	634
OrS	Pettrone, F	VA	628
OrS	Pizzutillo, P	PA	621
OrS	Poehling, G	NC	628
OrS	Ramsey, M	PA	621
OrS	Rodosky, M	PA	622
OrS	Romeo, A	IL	635
OrS	Rosenberg, T	UT	637
OrS	Schafer, M	IL	635
OrS	Scott, W	NY	623
OrS	Seltzer, D	AZ	639
OrS	Souryal, T	TX	639
OrS	Spindler, K	TN	629
OrS	Steadman, J	CO	638
OrS	Taft, T	NC	629
OrS	Wickiewicz, T	NY	624
PMR	Borg-Stein, J	MA	832
PMR	Feinberg, J	NY	834
PMR	Herring, S	WA	842
PMR	Lutz, G	NY	834
PMR	Press, J	IL	840
PMR	Saal, J	CA	842
SM	Altchek, D	NY	1036
SM	Andrews, J	FL	1038
SM	Arendt, E	MN	1039
SM	Arendt, E	MN	1039
SM	Asnis, P	MA	1036
SM	Bradley, J	PA	1036
SM	Burke, C	PA	1037
SM	Bush-Joseph, C	IL	1039
SM	Bush-Joseph, C	IL	1039
SM	Byrd, J	TN	1038
SM	Ciccotti, M	PA	1037
SM	Estwanik, J	NC	1038
SM	Fronek, J	CA	1040
SM	Gambardella, R	CA	1040
SM	Garth, W	AL	1038
SM	Gill, T	MA	1036
SM	Harner, C	PA	1037
SM	Hershman, E	NY	1037
SM	Ho, S	IL	1039
SM	Jones, D	LA	1040
SM	Levine, W	NY	1037
SM	Ma, C	CA	1040
SM	Metzl, J	NY	1037
SM	Micheli, L	MA	1036
SM	Miniaci, A	OH	1039
SM	Mirzayan, R	CA	1040
SM	Nisonson, B	NY	1037
SM	Paletta, G	MO	1039
SM	Rodeo, S	NY	1037
SM	Saint-Phard, D	CO	1039
SM	Schechter, D	CA	1040
SM	Scheller, A	MA	1036
SM	Sennett, B	PA	1038
SM	Speer, K	NC	1038
SM	Steiner, M	MA	1036
SM	Teitz, C	WA	1040
SM	Xerogeanes, J	GA	1038

Sports Medicine Back Injuries

Spec	Name	St	Pg
OrS	Schuler, T	VA	628
OrS	Spivak, J	NY	623

Sports Medicine Radiology

Spec	Name	St	Pg
DR	Palmer, W	MA	973
DR	Pavlov, H	NY	977

Sports Medicine-Women

Spec	Name	St	Pg
OrS	Hannafin, J	NY	616
SM	Saint-Phard, D	CO	1039

Sports Neurology

Spec	Name	St	Pg
N	Jordan, B	NY	511

Staphylococcal Infections

Spec	Name	St	Pg
Inf	Corey, G	NC	408
Inf	Yu, V	PA	408

Steatohepatitis

Spec	Name	St	Pg
Ge	Raiford, D	TN	241

Stem Cell Therapy

Spec	Name	St	Pg
N	Phuphanich, S	CA	536
Onc	Kesari, S	CA	386

Stem Cell Therapy & Biosurgery

Spec	Name	St	Pg
TS	Boyd, W	CA	1134

Stem Cell Therapy in Heart Failure

Spec	Name	St	Pg
Cv	Hare, J	FL	102
IC	Heldman, A	FL	127
IC	Losordo, D	IL	129
IC	Mahmud, E	CA	130
IC	Perin, E	TX	130

Stem Cell Transplant

Spec	Name	St	Pg
Hem	Champlin, R	TX	322
Hem	Comenzo, R	MA	308
Hem	Damon, L	CA	323
Hem	Farag, S	IN	317
Hem	Files, J	MS	315
Hem	Greer, J	TN	315
Hem	Isola, L	NY	311
Hem	Klingemann, H	MA	308
Hem	Lazarus, H	OH	319
Hem	Lill, M	CA	324
Hem	Maciejewski, J	OH	319
Hem	Maslak, P	NY	311
Hem	Nimer, S	NY	312
Hem	Rowley, S	NJ	313
Hem	Savage, D	NY	313
Hem	Schwartzberg, L	TN	316

Spec	Name	St	Pg
Hem	Slease, R	DE	313
Hem	Uberti, J	MI	321
Hem	Van Besien, K	IL	321
Onc	Antin, J	MA	326
Onc	Bensinger, W	WA	383
Onc	Carabasi, M	PA	334
Onc	Cohen, G	MD	335
Onc	Erban, J	MA	327
Onc	Flomenberg, N	PA	338
Onc	Foss, F	CT	328
Onc	Freedman, A	MA	328
Onc	Gerson, S	OH	366
Onc	Pecora, A	NJ	346
Onc	Soiffer, R	MA	331
Onc	Sweetenham, J	OH	371
Onc	Wicha, M	MI	372
PA&I	Kamani, N	DC	729
PHO	Arndt, C	MN	768
PHO	Barredo, J	FL	763
PHO	Cairo, M	NY	757
PHO	Cunningham, J	IL	769
PHO	Davies, S	OH	769
PHO	Fallon, R	IN	769
PHO	Frangoul, H	TN	764
PHO	Godder, K	VA	764
PHO	Goldman, S	TX	774
PHO	Graham, M	AZ	775
PHO	Grupp, S	PA	759
PHO	Haut, P	IN	770
PHO	Horn, B	CA	776
PHO	Kurtzberg, J	NC	765
PHO	Laver, J	TN	766
PHO	Link, M	CA	777
PHO	Lipton, J	NY	761
PHO	Sondel, P	WI	772

Stem Cell Transplant in Lupus/Crohn's

Spec	Name	St	Pg
IM	Burt, R	IL	420

Stem Cell Transplant in MS

Spec	Name	St	Pg
IM	Burt, R	IL	420

Stem Cell Transplant-Fetal

Spec	Name	St	Pg
PA&I	Cowan, M	CA	733
PS	Flake, A	PA	802

Stem Cell Transplantation

Spec	Name	St	Pg
NS	Selden, N	OR	495

Stem Cells in Orthopedics

Spec	Name	St	Pg
OrS	Anderson, L	CA	639

Stereotactic Body Radiation Therapy

Spec	Name	St	Pg
RadRO	Fuss, M	OR	964
RadRO	Kupelian, P	CA	964

Specialty & Special Expertise Index

Specialty & Special Expertise Index

Specialty & Special Expertise Index

Specialty & Special Expertise Index

Specialty & Special Expertise Index

Specialty & Special Expertise Index

Specialty & Special Expertise Index

Urology

Specialty & Special Expertise Index

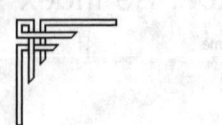

The Best in American Medicine
www.CastleConnolly.com

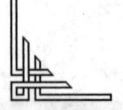
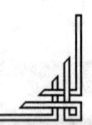

Alphabetical Listing of Doctors

Name	Specialty	Pg	Name	Specialty	Pg
A			Adams, Harold (IA)	N	522
			Adams, James (TX)	NP	447
Abaza, Mona (CO)	Oto	678	Adams, Reid (VA)	S	1061
Abbas, Fouad (MD)	GO	275	Adams, Robert (SC)	N	517
Abbitt, Patricia (FL)	DR	978	Adams-Graves, Patricia (TN)	Hem	314
Abbott, Richard (CA)	Oph	596	Adamson, G David (CA)	RE	1016
Abbruzzese, James (TX)	Onc	375	Adamson, Peter (PA)	PHO	756
Abcarian, Herand (IL)	CRS	171	Adashek, Joseph (NV)	MF	435
Abdu, William (NH)	OrS	608	Adelman, Mark (NY)	VascS	1179
Abecassis, Michael (IL)	S	1069	Adelson, P David (AZ)	NS	488
Abi-samra, Freddy (LA)	Cv	111	Adelstein, David (OH)	Onc	363
Abou-Khalil, Bassel (TN)	N	517	Adkins, Terrance (AZ)	CRS	174
Aboulafia, Albert (MD)	OrS	611	Adler, David (MA)	Psyc	884
Aboulafia, David (WA)	Onc	382	Adler, John (CA)	NS	491
Abouljoud, Marwan (MI)	S	1069	Adler, Ronald (NY)	DR	974
Abraham, Jame (WV)	Onc	332	Adornato, Bruce (CA)	N	533
Abrahamson, Martin (MA)	EDM	204	Advani, Ranjana (CA)	Onc	382
Abrahm, Janet (MA)	PM	694	Adzick, N Scott (PA)	PS	801
Abram, Stephen (WI)	PM	697	Afshari, Natalie (NC)	Oph	579
Abrams, Charles (PA)	Hem	309	Agarwal, Animesh (TX)	OrS	638
Abrams, Donald (CA)	Onc	382	Agarwal, Sanjay (CA)	RE	1017
Abrams, Gary (MI)	Oph	585	Agarwala, Brojendra (IL)	PCd	737
Abrams, Reid (CA)	HS	302	Aghajanian, Carol (NY)	Onc	332
Abrams, Ross (IL)	RadRO	956	Agress, Harry (NJ)	NuM	544
Abramson, David (NY)	Oph	569	Ahern, Geoffrey (AZ)	N	530
Abrass, Itamar (WA)	Ger	267	Ahlering, Thomas (CA)	U	1169
Abreu, Maria (FL)	Ge	238	Ahlgren, James (DC)	Onc	332
Abright, A Reese (NY)	ChAP	904	Ahlskog, J Eric (MN)	N	522
Abromowitch, Minnie (NE)	PHO	773	Ahmad, Amjad (IL)	Oph	585
Abu-Rustum, Nadeem (NY)	GO	276	Ahmad, Suhail (WA)	Nep	461
Abuhamad, Alfred (VA)	MF	430	Ahmann, Andrew (OR)	EDM	219
Accurso, Frank (CO)	PPul	796	Ahmann, Frederick (AZ)	Onc	375
Acker, David (MA)	MF	426	Ahn, Jung (NY)	PMR	833
Acker, Michael (PA)	TS	1109	Ahn, Sam (CA)	VascS	1188
Ackerman, Michael (MN)	PCd	737	Ahya, Vivek (PA)	Pul	922
Adam, Karolina (TX)	MF	434	Aiken, John (WI)	PS	806
Adams, David (FL)	N	517	Ain, Kenneth (KY)	EDM	211
Adams, David (NY)	TS	1109	Aisner, Joseph (NJ)	Onc	332
Adams, Elaine (IL)	Rhu	1028	Ajani, Jaffer (TX)	Onc	375

Alphabetical Listing of Doctors

Name	Specialty	Pg	Name	Specialty	Pg
Akelman, Edward (RI)	HS	294	Algazy, Kenneth (PA)	Onc	333
Akerley, Wallace (UT)	Onc	373	Allen, David (WI)	PEn	746
Akervall, Jan (MI)	Oto	671	Allen, Jeffrey (NY)	ChiN	145
Akhtar, Salman (PA)	Psyc	886	Allen, Nancy (NC)	Rhu	1027
Akins, Cary (MA)	TS	1106	Allen, Robert (SC)	PlS	858
Aklog, Lishan (AZ)	TS	1131	Allen, Steven (NY)	Hem	309
Al-Mefty, Ossama (MA)	NS	466	Allman, Richard (AL)	Ger	264
Alam, Daniel (OH)	Oto	671	Allon, Michael (AL)	Nep	455
Alavi, Abass (PA)	NuM	544	Allred, D Craig (MO)	Path	714
Alazraki, Naomi (GA)	NuM	545	Alster, Tina (DC)	D	184
Albain, Kathy (IL)	Onc	363	Altchek, David (NY)	SM	1036
Albala, David (NY)	U	1144	Alter, Craig (PA)	PEn	743
Albanese, Craig (CA)	PS	810	Alter, Gary (CA)	PlS	870
Albers, Gregory (CA)	N	533	Altman, Arnold (CT)	PHO	755
Albert, Daniel (WI)	Oph	585	Altman, Leonard (WA)	A&I	89
Albert, Daniel (NH)	Rhu	1022	Altorki, Nasser (NY)	TS	1109
Albert, Michael (DC)	Ge	230	Alvarez, Ronald (AL)	GO	280
Albert, Todd (PA)	OrS	611	Alvarez-Elcoro, Salvador (FL)	Inf	408
Albertini, Mark (WI)	Onc	363	Alward, Wallace (IA)	Oph	585
Alberts, David (AZ)	Onc	376	Amar, Arun (CA)	NS	491
Alberts, Mark (IL)	N	522	Amato, Anthony (MA)	N	504
Alberts, W Michael (FL)	Pul	927	Ambinder, Richard (MD)	Onc	333
Albertsen, Peter (CT)	U	1142	Amedee, Ronald (LA)	Oto	680
Albertson, Timothy (CA)	Pul	936	Ames, Christopher (CA)	NS	491
Albright, A Leland (WI)	NS	481	Ames, Frederick (TX)	S	1082
Albright, John (IA)	OrS	629	Amin, Mahul (CA)	Path	719
Albritton, Karen (TX)	PHO	774	Amin, Sandeep (IL)	PM	697
Aldea, Gabriel (WA)	TS	1134	Aminoff, Michael (CA)	N	533
Aledo, Alexander (NY)	PHO	756	Amling, Christopher (OR)	U	1169
Alessi, Norman (MI)	ChAP	907	Amonette, Rex (TN)	D	189
Alexander, Frederick (NJ)	PS	802	An, Howard (IL)	OrS	629
Alexander, H Richard (MD)	S	1048	Anand, Kanwaljeet (TN)	PCCM	741
Alexander, J Jeffrey (OH)	VascS	1184	Andersen, Glenna (VA)	ObG	555
Alexander, John (IL)	TS	1124	Andersen, Holly (NY)	Cv	94
Alexander, Joshua (NC)	PMR	836	Andersen, James (CA)	PlS	870
Alexander, Kenneth (IL)	PInf	781	Andersen, Peter (OR)	Oto	683
Alexander, Richard (MD)	U	1144	Anderson, Benjamin (WA)	S	1088
Alexander, Steven (CA)	PNep	787	Anderson, Jeffrey (UT)	Cv	111
Alexandrov, Andrei (AL)	N	517	Anderson, Joseph (MI)	Onc	363
Alfonso, Antonio (NY)	S	1049	Anderson, Karl (TX)	Ge	250
Alfonso, Eduardo (FL)	Oph	579	Anderson, Kenneth (MA)	Hem	308

Alphabetical Listing of Doctors

Name	Specialty	Pg	Name	Specialty	Pg
Aslanian, Harry (CT)	Ge	228	Babiera, Gildy (TX)	S	1082
Asnis, Peter (MA)	SM	1036	Bach, Bernard (IL)	OrS	630
Assimos, Dean (NC)	U	1153	Bach, John (NJ)	PMR	833
Aston, Sherrell (NY)	PlS	850	Bach, Richard (MO)	IC	128
Astrow, Alan (NY)	Onc	333	Back, Anthony (WA)	Onc	382
Atala, Anthony (NC)	U	1153	Backer, Carl (IL)	TS	1124
Athanasian, Edward (NY)	HS	294	Bacon, Bruce (MO)	Ge	243
Atkins, Michael (MA)	Onc	326	Bader, Thomas (PA)	ObG	552
Atkinson, John (MN)	NS	482	Badie, Behnam (CA)	NS	491
Atkinson, Robert (HI)	HS	303	Baer, Maria (MD)	Hem	310
Atlas, Scott (CA)	NRad	990	Baerveldt, George (CA)	Oph	596
Atnip, Robert (PA)	VascS	1180	Bagg, Adam (PA)	Path	707
Attas, Lewis (NJ)	Onc	333	Bagley, Demetrius (PA)	U	1144
Attinger, Christopher (DC)	PlS	850	Bahado-Singh, Ray (MI)	MF	431
Audell, Laura (CA)	PM	700	Bahn, Duke (CA)	DR	982
Auger, William (CA)	Pul	936	Bahn, Rebecca (MN)	EDM	214
Augsburger, James (OH)	Oph	586	Bahna, Sami (LA)	PA&I	732
August, David (NJ)	S	1049	Bahnson, Robert (OH)	U	1159
August, Phyllis (NY)	Nep	453	Baile, Walter (TX)	Psyc	895
Ault, Bettina (TN)	PNep	785	Bailes, Julian E (WV)	NS	467
Aurora, Sheena (WA)	N	533	Bailey, H Randolph (TX)	CRS	175
Austin, John (NY)	DR	974	Bailey, Leonard (CA)	TS	1134
Auwaerter, Paul (MD)	Inf	404	Bailey, Steven (TX)	IC	129
Averbook, Bruce (OH)	S	1070	Bailin, Philip (OH)	D	192
Avery, Eric (TX)	Psyc	895	Baim, Howard (IL)	Oto	671
Aviv, Jonathan (NY)	Oto	657	Bains, Manjit (NY)	TS	1109
Avram, Marc (NY)	D	185	Bairey, Cathleen Noel (CA)	Cv	113
Awan, Azhar (IL)	RadRO	956	Bajorin, Dean (NY)	Onc	334
Axelrod, Deborah (NY)	S	1049	Bakay, Roy (IL)	NS	482
Axelrod, Lloyd (MA)	EDM	204	Baker, Carol (TX)	PInf	782
Axelrod, Rita (PA)	Onc	333	Baker, Christopher (VA)	S	1061
Azar, Dimitri (IL)	Oph	586	Baker, Daniel (NY)	PlS	850
Azar, Nathalie (IL)	Oph	586	Baker, Emily (NH)	MF	426
Azizi, Sayed Ausim (PA)	N	507	Baker, James (MI)	A&I	87
Azodi, Masoud (CT)	GO	274	Baker, John (MI)	Oph	586
Azziz, Ricardo (GA)	RE	1011	Baker, Robert (NY)	PGe	749
Azzoli, Christopher (NY)	Onc	333	Baker, Shan (MI)	Oto	672
			Baker, Stephen (DC)	PlS	850
			Baker, Susan (NY)	PGe	749
			Bakhos, Mamdouh (IL)	TS	1125
			Bakken, Johan (MN)	Inf	410

B

Name	Specialty	Pg	Name	Specialty	Pg
Balady, Gary (MA)	Cv	92	Barksdale, Edward (OH)	PS	806
Balaji, K (NC)	U	1153	Barley, Christopher (NY)	IM	418
Balart, Luis (LA)	Ge	250	Barlogie, Bart (AR)	Hem	321
Balcer, Laura (PA)	N	507	Barnes, David (OH)	Ge	243
Baldassano, Robert (PA)	PGe	749	Barnes, Patrick (CA)	NRad	990
Balderston, Richard (PA)	OrS	612	Barnes, Randall (IL)	RE	1012
Baldridge, Alan (NJ)	PGe	749	Barnes, Willard (DC)	GO	276
Balducci, Lodovico (FL)	Onc	351	Barnett, Gene (OH)	NS	482
Bale, Allen (CT)	CG	154	Barohn, Richard (KS)	N	529
Bale, James (UT)	ChiN	150	Baron, Joseph (IL)	Hem	316
Balk, Robert (IL)	Pul	930	Baron, Todd (MN)	Ge	243
Balkany, Thomas (FL)	Oto	666	Barone, Constance (TX)	PlS	867
Ball, Douglas (MD)	EDM	206	Barredo, Julio (FL)	PHO	763
Ball, Edward (CA)	Onc	382	Barrett, Eugene (VA)	EDM	211
Ball, William (OH)	NRad	988	Barrow, Daniel (GA)	NS	476
Balla, Andre (IL)	Path	714	Bartelsmeyer, James (MO)	MF	431
Ballantyne, Christie (TX)	Cv	111	Barter, James (MD)	GO	276
Ballantyne, Garth (CT)	S	1044	Bartholomew, Deborah (OH)	ObG	556
Ballantyne, Jane (WA)	PM	700	Bartholomew, Dennis (OH)	CG	158
Ballard, Pamela (DC)	PMR	833	Bartlett, David (PA)	S	1049
Ballas, Zuhair (IA)	A&I	87	Bartlett, John (MD)	Inf	404
Ballen, Karen (MA)	Hem	308	Bartlett, Scott (PA)	PlS	850
Ballon-Landa, Gonzalo (CA)	Inf	413	Bartlett, Stephen (MD)	S	1049
Balmes, John (CA)	Pul	936	Bartolozzi, Arthur (PA)	OrS	612
Baltimore, Robert (CT)	PInf	778	Barton, Fritz (TX)	PlS	867
Baltuch, Gordon (PA)	NS	467	Basch, Samuel (NY)	Psyc	886
Bancalari, Eduardo (FL)	NP	444	Bascom, Rebecca (PA)	Pul	922
Bandyk, Dennis (FL)	VascS	1183	Baser, Susan (PA)	N	507
Banerjee, Anuradha (CA)	PHO	775	Bashevkin, Michael (NY)	Onc	334
Banks, Peter (NC)	Path	712	Bashore, Thomas (NC)	Cv	100
Bans, Larry (AZ)	U	1166	Baskin, Laurence (CA)	U	1169
Bar-Chama, Natan (NY)	U	1145	Basler, Joseph (TX)	U	1166
Barakat, Richard (NY)	GO	276	Bass, Theodore (FL)	Cv	100
Baratz, Mark (PA)	HS	295	Bassett, Lawrence (CA)	DR	982
Barbosa, Victoria (IL)	D	193	Bastian, Boris (NY)	Path	708
Bardot, Stephen (LA)	U	1166	Bastian, Robert (IL)	Oto	672
Barger, Geoffrey (MI)	N	523	Batchelor, Tracy (MA)	N	504
Barie, Philip (NY)	S	1049	Bateman, Bruce (VA)	RE	1011
Barkin, Jamie (FL)	Ge	239	Batjer, Hunt (IL)	NS	482
Barkley, Gregory (MI)	N	523	Batsford, William (CT)	CE	116
Barkovich, A James (CA)	NRad	990	Battafarano, Richard (MD)	TS	1109

Alphabetical Listing of Doctors

Name	Specialty	Pg	Name	Specialty	Pg
Bauer, Bruce (IL)	PlS	862	Belkin, Michael (MA)	VascS	1178
Bauer, Jerry (IL)	NS	482	Bell, David (AL)	EDM	212
Bauer, Stuart (MA)	U	1142	Bell, Debra (MN)	Path	715
Bauman, Phillip (NY)	OrS	612	Bell, Edward (IA)	NP	445
Baumann, Patricia (GA)	PM	696	Bell, Rodney (PA)	N	507
Bavaria, Joseph (PA)	TS	1109	Bellamy, Paul (CA)	Pul	937
Bayer, Arnold (CA)	Inf	413	Belldegrun, Arie (CA)	U	1169
Bayless, Theodore (MD)	Ge	230	Bellows, Charles (LA)	S	1082
Baylis, Henry (CA)	Oph	596	Belmont, H Michael (NY)	Rhu	1023
Bayliss, Susan (MO)	D	193	Belsito, Donald (NY)	D	185
Bazari, Hasan (MA)	Nep	452	Belsky, Mark (MA)	HS	294
Beall, Michael (VA)	U	1154	Belzberg, Allan (MD)	NS	468
Beals, Stephen (AZ)	PlS	867	Ben-Josef, Edgar (MI)	RadRO	957
Bear, Harry (VA)	S	1061	Benckart, Daniel (PA)	VascS	1180
Beart, Robert (CA)	CRS	175	Benedetti, Costantino (OH)	PM	697
Beaser, Richard (MA)	EDM	204	Benedetti, Enrico (IL)	S	1070
Beasley, Michael (NC)	PlS	858	Benedetti, Thomas (WA)	MF	435
Beatty, Charles (MN)	Oto	672	Benedetto, Pasquale (FL)	Onc	351
Beatty, Patrick (MT)	Onc	373	Benenati, James (FL)	VIR	993
Beaty, James (TN)	OrS	625	Benenati, Susan (FL)	A&I	86
Beauchamp, Robert (TN)	S	1062	Benes, Francine (MA)	Psyc	884
Beaudet, Arthur (TX)	CG	159	Benevenia, Joseph (NJ)	OrS	612
Bebin, E Martina (AL)	N	518	Benfield, Mark (AL)	PNep	785
Beck, David (LA)	CRS	175	Benjamin, Ivor (UT)	Cv	111
Beck, Sandra (KY)	CRS	170	Benjamin, Robert (TX)	Onc	376
Becker, Dorothy (PA)	PEn	743	Benkov, Keith (NY)	PGe	749
Becker, Ferdinand (FL)	Oto	666	Bennett, Richard (CA)	D	198
Becker, James (MA)	S	1044	Bennett, William (OR)	Nep	461
Becker, Kyra (WA)	N	533	Benninger, Michael (OH)	Oto	672
Becker, Yolanda (IL)	S	1070	Bensard, Denis (CO)	PS	808
Bederson, Joshua (NY)	NS	468	Bensinger, William (WA)	Onc	383
Beekman, Robert (OH)	PCd	737	Benson, Al (IL)	Onc	363
Beer, Tomasz (OR)	Onc	382	Benson, Carol (MA)	DR	973
Beerman, Lee (PA)	PCd	734	Benson, Mitchell (NY)	U	1145
Behm, Frederick (IL)	Path	714	Bentley, Frederick (AR)	S	1082
Behrens, Myles (NY)	Oph	569	Bentz, Michael (WI)	PlS	862
Behrns, Kevin (FL)	S	1062	Benvenisty, Alan (NY)	VascS	1180
Beitler, Jonathan (GA)	RadRO	951	Benzel, Edward (OH)	NS	482
Beitsch, Peter (TX)	S	1082	Benzon, Honorio (IL)	PM	697
Belani, Chandra (PA)	Onc	334	Berchuck, Andrew (NC)	GO	280
Belenky, Walter (MI)	PO	790	Berde, Charles (MA)	PM	694

Name	Specialty	Pg	Name	Specialty	Pg
Beredjiklian, Pedro (PA)	HS	295	Berrey, B Hudson (FL)	OrS	625
Berek, Jonathan (CA)	GO	289	Berry, Daniel (MN)	OrS	630
Berens, Pamela (TX)	ObG	559	Berry, J Michael (CA)	Onc	383
Berenstein, Alejandro (NY)	NRad	985	Bertolone, Salvatore (KY)	PHO	763
Berg, Christine (MD)	RadRO	946	Bertorini, Tulio (TN)	N	518
Berg, Daniel (WA)	D	198	Besinger, Richard (IL)	MF	432
Berg, Stacey (TX)	PHO	774	Bessey, Palmer (NY)	S	1049
Berga, Sarah (GA)	ObG	555	Bessler, Marc (NY)	S	1049
Berger, Joseph (KY)	N	518	Bettmann, Michael (NC)	VIR	994
Berger, Mitchel (CA)	NS	491	Betz, Randal (PA)	OrS	612
Berger, Ronald (MD)	CE	117	Beyer, Eric (IL)	PHO	768
Bergey, Gregory (MD)	N	507	Bhan, Atul (MA)	Path	706
Bergman, Donald (NY)	EDM	207	Bhasin, Shalender (MA)	EDM	204
Bergman, Ira (PA)	ChiN	145	Bhattacharyya, Neil (MA)	Oto	655
Bergsagel, Peter Leif (AZ)	Onc	376	Bialer, Martin (NY)	CG	155
Berguer, Ramon (MI)	VascS	1185	Biancaniello, Thomas (NY)	PCd	734
Berk, John (MA)	Pul	920	Bianchi, Diana (MA)	CG	154
Berke, Gerald (CA)	Oto	683	Bichell, David (TN)	TS	1118
Berkowitz, Carol (CA)	Ped	728	Bicher, Annette (VA)	GO	280
Berkowitz, Leonard (NY)	Inf	404	Bickers, David (NY)	D	185
Berkowitz, Richard (NY)	MF	428	Biederman, Joseph (MA)	ChAP	903
Berkowitz, Ross (MA)	GO	274	Bierbrauer, Karin (OH)	NS	482
Berkson, Richard (CA)	EDM	220	Bierman, Fredrick (NY)	PCd	734
Berl, Tomas (CO)	Nep	460	Bierman, Philip (NE)	Onc	373
Berland, Lincoln (AL)	DR	978	Biermann, J Sybil (MI)	OrS	630
Berlin, Cheston (PA)	Ped	726	Bigelow, Carolyn (MS)	Hem	314
Berlin, Jordan (TN)	Onc	351	Biggs, David (DE)	Onc	334
Berman, Brian (OH)	Ped	727	Bigliani, Louis (NY)	OrS	612
Berman, James (IL)	PGe	751	Bijwadia, Jagdeep (MN)	Pul	930
Berman, Michael (CA)	GO	289	Bilchik, Anton (CA)	S	1088
Bermudez, Ovidio (CO)	AM	81	Bilezikian, John (NY)	EDM	207
Bernard, Stephen (NC)	Onc	352	Biller, Beverly (MA)	EDM	204
Bernardino, Carlo (CA)	Oph	596	Billett, Amy (MA)	PHO	755
Bernardo, Jose (PA)	Nep	453	Billingsley, Kevin (OR)	S	1088
Berns, Jeffrey (PA)	Nep	453	Billmire, David (OH)	PlS	862
Bernstein, Daniel (CA)	PCd	740	Bilsky, Mark (NY)	NS	468
Bernstein, David (OH)	PInf	781	Biousse, Valerie (GA)	Oph	579
Bernstein, David (OH)	A&I	87	Bird, Hector (NY)	ChAP	904
Bernstein, Jonathan (OH)	A&I	87	Birmaher, Boris (PA)	ChAP	904
Bernstein, Richard (IL)	N	523	Birnbaum, Elisa (MO)	CRS	171
Bernstein, Robert (NY)	D	185	Birrer, Michael (MA)	Onc	326

Alphabetical Listing of Doctors

Name	Specialty	Pg	Name	Specialty	Pg
Bishop, Allen (MN)	HS	299	Blumberg, Henry (GA)	Inf	408
Bishop, Warren (IA)	PGe	751	Blume, Ralph (NY)	Rhu	1023
Bissell, Dwight (CA)	IM	421	Blumenfeld, Hal (CT)	N	504
Bitan, Fabien (NY)	OrS	612	Blumenfeld, Jon (NY)	Nep	453
Bitran, Jacob (IL)	Onc	363	Blumenfield, Michael (CA)	Psyc	896
Bittl, John (FL)	IC	126	Blumenkranz, Mark (CA)	Oph	596
Bjorkman, David (UT)	Ge	249	Blumenthal, David (NY)	Cv	94
Black, C Thomas (TX)	PS	809	Blumenthal, Roger (MD)	Cv	95
Black, Dennis (TN)	PGe	751	Boachie-Adjei, Oheneba (NY)	OrS	612
Black, Donald (IA)	Psyc	893	Bobrove, Arthur (CA)	Rhu	1031
Black, Keith (CA)	NS	492	Bock, Samuel (CO)	PA&I	732
Black, Kevin (MO)	Psyc	893	Bockenstedt, Paula (MI)	Hem	317
Black, William (NH)	DR	973	Bockman, Richard (NY)	EDM	207
Blackstock, A William (NC)	RadRO	951	Boden, Scott (GA)	OrS	626
Blackwell, Keith (CA)	Oto	683	Bodner, Donald (OH)	U	1159
Blackwell, Kimberly (NC)	Onc	352	Bodurka, Diane (TX)	GO	286
Blackwell, Richard (AL)	RE	1011	Bogart, Jeffrey (NY)	RadRO	946
Blaha, John (MI)	OrS	630	Boggan, James (CA)	NS	492
Blair, Elizabeth (IL)	Oto	672	Bogrov, Michael (MD)	ChAP	904
Blaivas, Jerry (NY)	U	1145	Boice, Charles (MD)	GO	276
Blakemore, Karin (MD)	MF	428	Bojrab, Dennis (MI)	Oto	672
Blanchard, Daniel (CA)	Cv	113	Boland, C Richard (TX)	Ge	250
Bland, Kirby (AL)	S	1062	Boles, Richard (CA)	CG	160
Blaney, Susan (TX)	PHO	774	Bolger, Graeme (AL)	Onc	352
Blatchford, Garnet (NE)	CRS	174	Bolger, William (FL)	Oto	666
Blatt, Julie (NC)	PHO	764	Boling, Peter (VA)	Ger	264
Blazer, Dan (NC)	Psyc	891	Bollen, Andrew (CA)	Path	719
Bleday, Ronald (MA)	CRS	166	Bolman, Ralph Morton (MA)	TS	1106
Bleiberg, Efrain (TX)	ChAP	908	Bologina, Jean (CT)	D	182
Blinder, Morey (MO)	Hem	317	Bolton, John (LA)	S	1082
Blitzer, Andrew (NY)	Oto	657	Bolton, W Kline (VA)	Nep	455
Blobe, Gerard (NC)	Onc	352	Bolwell, Brian (OH)	Onc	363
Bloch, Rina (MA)	PMR	832	Bond, Sheldon (KY)	PS	804
Block, Susan (MA)	Psyc	884	Bonner, James (AL)	A&I	86
Bloom, David (MI)	U	1159	Bonner, James (AL)	RadRO	952
Bloom, Patricia (NY)	Ger	262	Bono, James (MA)	OrS	608
Bloomer, Joseph (AL)	Ge	239	Bonomi, Philip (IL)	Onc	363
Bluemke, David (MD)	DR	974	Bonow, Robert (IL)	Cv	104
Blum, Andrew (RI)	N	504	Boone, Timothy (TX)	U	1166
Blum, Conrad (NY)	EDM	207	Boop, Frederick (TN)	NS	477
Blum, Kristie (OH)	PHO	768	Booth, Robert (PA)	OrS	613

Name	Specialty	Pg	Name	Specialty	Pg
Boraas, Marcia (PA)	S	1049	Bradley, James (PA)	SM	1036
Borchert, Mark (CA)	Oph	596	Bradley, Jeffrey (MO)	RadRO	957
Borden, Ernest (OH)	Onc	364	Bradley, John (CA)	PInf	783
Borer, Jeffrey (NY)	Cv	95	Bradley, Linda (OH)	ObG	556
Borg-Stein, Joanne (MA)	PMR	832	Bradshaw, Karen (TX)	ObG	559
Borgen, Patrick (NY)	S	1050	Braly, Patricia (LA)	GO	287
Borges, Lawrence (MA)	NS	466	Branch, Charles (NC)	NS	477
Borkowsky, William (NY)	PInf	779	Brandt, Fredric (NY)	D	185
Boronow, John (MD)	Psyc	886	Brandt, Harry (MD)	Psyc	887
Borowitz, Drucy (NY)	PPul	793	Brandt, Keith (MO)	PlS	862
Borson, Soo (WA)	GerPsy	912	Brandt, Lawrence (NY)	Ge	231
Borst, Matthew (AZ)	GO	287	Branham, Gregory (MO)	Oto	672
Borum, Marie (DC)	Ge	230	Brasington, Richard (MO)	Rhu	1028
Borzak, Steven (FL)	Cv	101	Braun, Martin (DC)	D	185
Bos, Gary (WA)	OrS	639	Braunstein, Glenn (CA)	EDM	220
Bosl, George (NY)	Onc	334	Braunstein, Seth (PA)	IM	418
Boston, Barry (TN)	Onc	352	Brause, Barry (NY)	Inf	405
Bostwick, David (VA)	Path	712	Bravender, Terrill (OH)	AM	80
Bourdette, Dennis (OR)	N	533	Braverman, Alan (MO)	Cv	104
Bourge, Robert (AL)	Cv	101	Braverman, Lewis (MA)	EDM	204
Bourgeois, Blaise (MA)	ChiN	144	Bray, Robert (CA)	NS	492
Boushey, Homer (CA)	Pul	937	Brazer, Scott (NC)	Ge	239
Bouvet, Michael (CA)	S	1088	Brecher, Martin (NY)	PHO	757
Bove, Alfred (PA)	Cv	95	Breidenbach, Warren (AZ)	HS	302
Bove, Edward (MI)	PS	806	Breitbart, William (NY)	Psyc	887
Bowden, Charles (TX)	Psyc	895	Brem, Henry (MD)	NS	468
Bowen, Glen (UT)	D	196	Brem, Rachel (DC)	DR	974
Bower, Charles (AR)	PO	791	Brem, Steven (FL)	NS	477
Boxer, Gary (MO)	ChAP	907	Brems, John (IL)	S	1070
Boxer, Laurence (MI)	PHO	768	Brendler, Charles (IL)	U	1159
Boxer Wachler, Brian (CA)	Oph	596	Brener, Bruce (NJ)	VascS	1180
Boxrud, Cynthia (CA)	Oph	597	Brenin, Christiana M (VA)	Onc	352
Boyajian, Michael (DC)	PlS	850	Brennan, Daniel (MO)	Nep	457
Boyd, Stuart (CA)	U	1169	Brennan, Michael (MN)	EDM	214
Boyd, Walter (CA)	TS	1134	Brennan, Murray (NY)	S	1050
Boyer, Thomas (AZ)	Ge	250	Brennan, Stephen (TX)	Nep	460
Boyle, Robert (VA)	NP	445	Brenner, Barry (MA)	Nep	452
Bozentka, David (PA)	HS	295	Brenner, Joel (MD)	PCd	734
Brackmann, Derald (CA)	Oto	683	Brenner, Malcolm (TX)	Hem	321
Braddom, Randall (NJ)	PMR	833	Brent, Burton (CA)	PlS	870
Bradford, Carol (MI)	Oto	672	Brent, David (PA)	ChAP	904

Name	Specialty	Pg	Name	Specialty	Pg
Bresalier, Robert (TX)	Ge	250	Brophy, Patrick (IA)	PNep	786
Bressler, Neil (MD)	Oph	570	Brown, Charles (IL)	S	1070
Bressler, Susan (MD)	Oph	570	Brown, Daniel (PA)	VIR	992
Bressman, Susan (NY)	N	507	Brown, Frederick (IL)	NS	482
Brewer, Molly (CT)	GO	274	Brown, Gary (PA)	Oph	570
Brewster, David (MA)	VascS	1178	Brown, John (IN)	TS	1125
Brick, Gregory (MA)	OrS	608	Brown, Karen (NY)	VIR	992
Brick, John (WV)	N	508	Brown, Kevin (CO)	Pul	934
Bricker, John (TX)	PCd	739	Brown, Kimberly (MI)	Ge	243
Bricker, Leslie (MI)	Hem	317	Brown, Robert (MN)	N	523
Bridges, Charles (NC)	TS	1119	Brown, Robert (NY)	Ge	231
Bridwell, Keith (MO)	OrS	630	Browne, J Dale (NC)	Oto	666
Brien, Earl (CA)	OrS	640	Browner, Bruce (CT)	OrS	608
Brillon, David (NY)	EDM	207	Brozena, Susan (PA)	Cv	95
Brinckerhoff, Laurence (MA)	TS	1106	Bruce, Jeffrey (NY)	NS	468
Brindis, Ralph (CA)	Cv	114	Brucker, Alexander (PA)	Oph	570
Bristow, Robert (CA)	GO	289	Bruera, Eduardo (TX)	Onc	376
Britt, L D (VA)	S	1062	Brufsky, Adam (PA)	Onc	334
Brizel, David (NC)	RadRO	952	Bruggers, Carol (UT)	PHO	773
Broadstone, Vasti Lima (IN)	EDM	214	Bruner, Janet (TX)	Path	717
Brock, John (TN)	U	1154	Brunicardi, F Charles (TX)	S	1082
Brockstein, Bruce (IL)	Onc	364	Bruno, Michiko (HI)	N	533
Broderick, Gregory (FL)	U	1154	Brunsting, Louis (OH)	TS	1125
Broderick, Joseph (OH)	N	523	Brunstrom, Janice (MO)	ChiN	148
Brodkin, Edward (PA)	Psyc	887	Brunt, L Michael (MO)	S	1070
Brodland, David (PA)	D	185	Brushart, Thomas (MD)	HS	295
Brodman, Michael (NY)	ObG	553	Bryson, Yvonne (CA)	PInf	783
Brodsky, James (TX)	OrS	638	Buatti, John (IA)	RadRO	957
Brodsky, Robert (MD)	Hem	310	Bubley, Glenn (MA)	Onc	326
Brody, Fred (DC)	S	1050	Bucciarelli, Richard (FL)	NP	445
Brody, Harold (GA)	D	189	Buch, Jeffrey (TX)	U	1167
Bromberg, Jonathan (MD)	S	1050	Buchanan, George (TX)	PHO	774
Bromberg, Mark (UT)	N	529	Buchbinder, Ellen (NY)	A&I	84
Bronheim, Harold (NY)	Psyc	887	Buchholz, David (MD)	N	508
Bronson, Michael (NY)	OrS	613	Buchholz, Thomas (TX)	RadRO	962
Brooks, Ari (PA)	S	1050	Buchman, Steven (MI)	PlS	863
Brooks, Benjamin (NC)	N	518	Buchman, Timothy (GA)	S	1062
Brooks, David (MA)	S	1044	Bucholz, Richard (MO)	NS	482
Brooks, John (PA)	Path	708	Bucholz, Robert (TX)	OrS	638
Brooks, Stuart (FL)	Pul	927	Buckley, Edward (NC)	Oph	580
Brophy, Colleen (TN)	VascS	1183	Buckner, Jan (MN)	Onc	364

Name	Specialty	Pg	Name	Specialty	Pg
Buckwalter, Joseph (IA)	OrS	630	Burt, Richard (IL)	IM	420
Bucky, Louis (PA)	PlS	851	Burt, Vivien (CA)	Psyc	897
Budd, George (OH)	Onc	364	Burton, Allen (TX)	PM	699
Budenz, Donald (FL)	Oph	580	Burton, Barbara (IL)	CG	158
Budoff, Matthew (CA)	Cv	114	Burton, Claude (NC)	D	190
Bueno, Raphael (MA)	TS	1106	Burton, John (MD)	Ger	262
Bulat, Robert (LA)	Ge	250	Busby, J Erik (AL)	U	1154
Bull, David (UT)	TS	1130	Buse, John (NC)	EDM	212
Bull, Marilyn (IN)	Ped	727	Bush-Joseph, Charles (IL)	SM	1039
Buly, Robert (NY)	OrS	613	Bushman, Wade (WI)	U	1160
Bumpous, Jeffrey (KY)	Oto	666	Busis, Neil (PA)	N	508
Bunn, Paul (CO)	Onc	373	Busse, William (WI)	A&I	87
Bunning, Robert (DC)	Rhu	1023	Bussel, James (NY)	PHO	757
Burchiel, Kim (OR)	NS	492	Buster, John (MA)	RE	1006
Burdette, Jonathan (NC)	NRad	986	Busuttil, Ronald (CA)	S	1088
Burger, Peter (MD)	Path	708	Butler, Charles (TX)	PlS	868
Burger, Robert (PA)	GO	276	Butler, David (TX)	D	196
Burgess, David (NJ)	Ped	726	Butler, John (CA)	S	1089
Burke, Allan (IL)	N	523	Butler, William (SC)	Onc	352
Burke, Charles (PA)	SM	1037	Butterly, David W (NC)	Nep	455
Burke, Dennis (MA)	OrS	608	Butterly, Lynn (NH)	Ge	228
Burke, Miles (OH)	Oph	586	Buxton, Alfred (MA)	CE	116
Burke, Peter (MA)	S	1044	Buyon, Jill (NY)	Rhu	1023
Burke, Redmond (FL)	TS	1119	Buys, Saundra (UT)	Onc	373
Burke, Thomas (TX)	GO	287	Buysse, Daniel (PA)	Psyc	887
Burke, William (NE)	GerPsy	911	Buzdar, Aman (TX)	Onc	376
Burket, Mark (OH)	Cv	105	Byrd, Benjamin (TN)	Cv	101
Burkey, Brian (OH)	Oto	673	Byrd, David (WA)	S	1089
Burks, A Wesley (NC)	PA&I	730	Byrd, H Stephenson (TX)	PlS	868
Burman, Kenneth (DC)	EDM	207	Byrd, J.W. (TN)	SM	1038
Burmeister, Lynn (MN)	EDM	214	Byrd, John (OH)	Hem	317
Burnett, Alexander (AR)	GO	287	Byrne, Janice (UT)	ObG	558
Burnett, Arthur (MD)	U	1145	Byrne, John G (TN)	TS	1119
Burns, A Jay (TX)	PlS	868	Bystritsky, Alexander (CA)	Psyc	897
Burns, James (MA)	Oto	655			
Burns, Richard (AZ)	N	530			
Burris, Howard (TN)	Onc	352	**C**		
Burschtin, Omar (NY)	Pul	922			
Burstein, Fernando (GA)	PlS	858	Cabin, Henry (CT)	Cv	92
Burstein, Harold (MA)	Onc	326	Cagle, Philip (TX)	Path	717
Burt, Randall (UT)	Ge	249	Cahill, John (NY)	PrM	880

Alphabetical Listing of Doctors

Name	Specialty	Pg	Name	Specialty	Pg
Cahill, Kenneth V (OH)	Oph	586	Cannistra, Stephen (MA)	Onc	326
Cahill, Kevin (NY)	PrM	881	Cannom, David (CA)	CE	122
Caillouette, James (CA)	OrS	640	Canterbury, Randolph (VA)	Psyc	892
Cain, Joanna (RI)	GO	274	Canto, Marcia (MD)	Ge	231
Cain, Mark (IN)	U	1160	Caplan, Louis (MA)	N	504
Cairns, Bruce (NC)	S	1062	Capo, Hilda (FL)	Oph	580
Cairo, Mitchell (NY)	PHO	757	Cappuccino, Andrew (NY)	OrS	613
Calabrese, Joseph (OH)	Psyc	893	Caprioli, Joseph (CA)	Oph	597
Calabresi, Peter (MD)	N	508	Caputo, Anthony (NJ)	Oph	570
Caldamone, Anthony (RI)	U	1142	Caputo, Thomas (NY)	GO	276
Caldarelli, David (IL)	Oto	673	Caputy, Anthony (DC)	NS	468
Caldwell, Randall (IN)	PCd	738	Carabasi, Matthew (PA)	Onc	334
Calhoon, John (TX)	TS	1131	Carabello, Blase (TX)	Cv	111
Califano, Joseph (MD)	Oto	657	Carbone, David (TN)	Onc	353
Califf, Robert (NC)	Cv	101	Cardenas, Diana (FL)	PMR	836
Callaghan, John (IA)	OrS	631	Cardenosa, Gilda (VA)	DR	978
Callahan, Eileen (NY)	Ger	263	Carducci, Michael (MD)	Onc	334
Callans, David (PA)	CE	117	Carey, John (MD)	Oto	657
Callen, Jeffrey (KY)	D	190	Carey, John C (UT)	CG	159
Callery, Mark (MA)	S	1044	Carey, Lisa (NC)	Onc	353
Calligaro, Keith (PA)	VascS	1180	Caritis, Steve (PA)	MF	428
Calvi, Laura (NY)	EDM	207	Carlson, Alan (NC)	Oph	580
Calvo, Benjamin (NC)	S	1062	Carlson, John (NJ)	GO	276
Cambria, Richard (MA)	VascS	1178	Carlson, Michelle (NY)	HS	295
Cameron, John (MD)	S	1050	Carlson, Robert (CA)	Onc	383
Cameron, Robert (CA)	TS	1134	Carneiro, Ronaldo (FL)	HS	298
Camisa, Charles (FL)	D	190	Carney, John (AR)	D	196
Camitta, Bruce (WI)	PHO	768	Carney, Michael (HI)	GO	289
Cammisa, Frank (NY)	OrS	613	Carpenter, Jeffrey (NJ)	VascS	1180
Camoriano, John (AZ)	Onc	376	Carpenter, John (AL)	Onc	353
Campbell, Bruce (WI)	Oto	673	Carr, Bruce (TX)	RE	1015
Campbell, David (CO)	TS	1130	Carr, David (MO)	Ger	265
Campbell, G Douglas (MS)	Pul	927	Carr, Stephen (RI)	MF	426
Campbell, J William (MO)	Inf	410	Carr-Locke, David (NY)	Ge	231
Campbell, Steven (OH)	U	1160	Carragee, Eugene (CA)	OrS	640
Campo, John (OH)	ChAP	907	Carrasquillo, Jorge (NY)	NuM	544
Campochiaro, Peter (MD)	Oph	570	Carraway, James (VA)	PlS	858
Cance, William (NY)	S	1050	Carroll, Charles (IL)	HS	299
Cancio, Margarita (FL)	Inf	408	Carroll, Peter (CA)	U	1169
Canellos, George (MA)	Onc	326	Carroll, William (NY)	PHO	757
Canning, Douglas (PA)	U	1145	Carson, Benjamin (MD)	NS	468

Name	Specialty	Pg	Name	Specialty	Pg
Carson, Culley (NC)	U	1154	Chamberlain, Marc (WA)	N	534
Carson, Donald (PA)	ObG	553	Chambers, Richard (CA)	OrS	640
Carson, Sandra (RI)	RE	1006	Chambers, Setsuko (AZ)	GO	287
Carter, H Ballentine (MD)	U	1145	Champlin, Richard (TX)	Hem	322
Carter, Keith (IA)	Oph	586	Chan, John (CA)	GO	289
Cartwright, Patrick (UT)	U	1165	Chan, Kenny (CO)	PO	791
Carty, Sally (PA)	S	1050	Chanan-Khan, Asher (NY)	Onc	335
Cascino, Terrence (MN)	N	523	Chancellor, Michael (MI)	U	1160
Casella, Samuel (NH)	PEn	742	Chand, Bipan (OH)	S	1071
Casselbrant, Margaretha (PA)	PO	788	Chandar, Jayanthi (FL)	PNep	785
Cassidy, Charles (MA)	OrS	608	Chandler, James (IL)	NS	483
Cassidy, Suzanne (CA)	CG	160	Chandler, Michael (NY)	A&I	84
Castell, Donald (SC)	Ge	239	Chandler, William (MI)	NS	483
Castellino, Sharon (NC)	PHO	764	Chandrasoma, Parakrama (CA)	Path	720
Castells, Maria (MA)	A&I	84	Chang, Alfred (MI)	S	1071
Caster, Andrew (CA)	Oph	597	Chang, Benjamin (PA)	PlS	851
Castle, Valerie (MI)	PHO	769	Chang, Gene (PA)	IC	124
Catalona, William (IL)	U	1160	Chang, Helena (CA)	S	1089
Catanzaro, Antonino (CA)	Pul	937	Chang, James (CA)	PlS	871
Cather, Jennifer (TX)	D	196	Chang, Jenny (TX)	Onc	377
Catherwood, Edward (NH)	Cv	92	Chang, Karen (CA)	Path	720
Caughey, Aaron (OR)	MF	436	Chang, Kenneth (CA)	Ge	252
Cedars, Marcelle (CA)	RE	1017	Chang, R Jeffrey (CA)	RE	1017
Cederbaum, Stephen (CA)	CG	161	Chang, Rowland (IL)	Rhu	1028
Cederna, Paul (MI)	PlS	863	Chang, Sam (TN)	U	1154
Celano, Paul (MD)	Onc	335	Chang, Stanley (NY)	Oph	570
Celli, Bartolome (MA)	Pul	920	Chang, Susan (CA)	Onc	383
Cello, John (CA)	Ge	252	Chang-Miller, April (AZ)	Rhu	1030
Cendales, Linda (GA)	HS	298	Chao, KS Clifford (NY)	RadRO	946
Cerfolio, Robert (AL)	TS	1119	Chao, Nelson (NC)	Onc	353
Cerqueira, Manuel (OH)	Cv	105	Chap, Linnea (CA)	Onc	383
Cetta, Frank (MN)	PCd	738	Chapman, Jens (WA)	OrS	640
Cha, Soonmee (CA)	NRad	990	Chapman, Paul (NY)	Onc	335
Chabner, Bruce (MA)	Onc	327	Chapman, Robert (MI)	Onc	364
Chabot, John (NY)	S	1050	Chapman, William (MO)	S	1071
Chachoua, Abraham (NY)	Onc	335	Char, Devron (CA)	Oph	597
Chaikof, Elliot (MA)	VascS	1178	Charboneau, J William (MN)	DR	979
Chaisson, Richard (MD)	Inf	405	Chari, Ravi (TN)	S	1062
Chaitman, Bernard (MO)	Cv	105	Chari, Suresh (MN)	Ge	243
Chakravarthy, Anuradha (TN)	RadRO	952	Charles, Andrew (CA)	N	534
Chalian, Ara (PA)	Oto	657	Charney, Jonathan (NY)	N	508

Alphabetical Listing of Doctors

Name	Specialty	Pg	Name	Specialty	Pg
Charrow, Joel (IL)	CG	158	Choy, Hak (TX)	RadRO	962
Chatham, W (AL)	Rhu	1027	Christenson, John (IN)	PInf	781
Cheatham, John (OH)	PCd	738	Christian, Karla (TN)	TS	1119
Chelimsky, Thomas (OH)	N	523	Christiani, David (MA)	Pul	920
Chen, Allen (MD)	PHO	757	Christie, Dennis (WA)	PGe	754
Chen, Chun (NY)	NS	468	Christie, Jason (PA)	Pul	923
Chen, David (PA)	U	1145	Christman, Brian (TN)	Pul	927
Chen, David (IL)	PMR	837	Christman, Gregory (MI)	RE	1012
Chen, Jonathan (NY)	TS	1110	Christo, Paul (MD)	PM	694
Chen, Mike (AL)	PS	804	Chu, Constance (PA)	OrS	613
Chen, Thomas (CA)	NS	492	Chu, Edward (PA)	Onc	335
Cheng, Edith (WA)	MF	436	Chui, Helena (CA)	N	534
Cheng, Edward (MN)	OrS	631	Chun, Jin (NY)	PlS	851
Cherny, W Bruce (ID)	NS	487	Chung, Daniel (MA)	Ge	228
Cherqui, Daniel (NY)	S	1051	Chung, Kevin (MI)	HS	299
Cherry, Kenneth (VA)	VascS	1183	Chung, Ki Young (SC)	Onc	353
Chesney, Carolyn (TN)	Path	713	Chung, Raymond (MA)	Ge	228
Cheson, Bruce (DC)	Hem	310	Church, James (OH)	CRS	171
Cheung, Nai-Kong V (NY)	PHO	757	Church, Joseph (CA)	PA&I	732
Cheville, Andrea (MN)	PMR	837	Chwals, Walter (MA)	PS	800
Chew, Helen (CA)	Onc	383	Ciancio, Gaetano (FL)	U	1154
Chey, William (MI)	Ge	244	Ciccotti, Michael (PA)	SM	1037
Childs, Stacy (CO)	U	1165	Ciezki, Jay (OH)	RadRO	957
Chiles, Caroline (NC)	DR	978	Ciocon, Jerry (FL)	Ger	264
Chinitz, Larry (NY)	CE	117	Cioffi, William (RI)	S	1044
Chiocca, E Antonio (OH)	NS	483	Cionni, Robert (UT)	Oph	593
Chitambar, Christopher (WI)	Onc	364	Ciraulo, Domenic (MA)	AdP	900
Chitwood, W Randolph (NC)	TS	1119	Cirigliano, Michael (PA)	IM	418
Chiu, David (NY)	PlS	851	Civantos, Francisco (FL)	Oto	666
Chiu, Yanek (CA)	CRS	176	Civin, Curt (MD)	PHO	758
Chizner, Michael (FL)	Cv	101	Clair, Daniel (OH)	VascS	1185
Chlebowski, Rowan (CA)	Onc	383	Clairmont, Albert (OH)	PMR	838
Chmait, Ramen (CA)	MF	436	Clamon, Gerald (IA)	Onc	364
Cho, Kathleen (MI)	Path	715	Clark, Joseph (IL)	Onc	364
Cho, Kerry (CA)	Nep	461	Clark, Keith (OK)	Oto	680
Cho, Kyung (MI)	VIR	994	Clark, Orlo (CA)	S	1089
Choi, Noah (MA)	RadRO	944	Clarke-Pearson, Daniel (NC)	GO	280
Choti, Michael (MD)	S	1051	Claxton, David (PA)	Onc	335
Chow, Warren (CA)	Onc	383	Clayman, Gary (TX)	Oto	680
Chowdhury, Khalid (CO)	Oto	679	Clayman, Ralph (CA)	U	1169
Choy, Andrew (CA)	Oph	597	Cleary, James (WI)	Onc	365

Name	Specialty	Pg	Name	Specialty	Pg
Clements, Philip (CA)	Rhu	1031	Cohen, Jonathan (NY)	Ge	231
Clements, Stephen (GA)	Cv	101	Cohen, Kenneth (MD)	PHO	758
Cliby, William (MN)	GO	283	Cohen, Lawrence (NY)	Ge	231
Clinton, Steven (OH)	Onc	365	Cohen, Mark (IL)	HS	299
Clisham, P Ronald (LA)	RE	1015	Cohen, Martin (NY)	CE	118
Cloherty, John (MA)	NP	442	Cohen, Michael (IA)	Path	715
Clohisy, Denis (MN)	OrS	631	Cohen, Mitchell (OH)	PGe	751
Cloninger, C Robert (MO)	Psyc	893	Cohen, Mitchell (PA)	Psyc	887
Clore, John (VA)	EDM	212	Cohen, Murray (PA)	S	1051
Close, Lanny (NY)	Oto	658	Cohen, Myron (NC)	Inf	408
Cloughesy, Timothy (CA)	N	534	Cohen, Neri (MD)	TS	1110
Clutter, William (MO)	EDM	214	Cohen, Philip (DC)	Onc	335
Cmelak, Anthony (TN)	RadRO	952	Cohen, Robbin (CA)	TS	1134
Coakley, Fergus (CA)	DR	982	Cohen, Robert (OH)	EDM	214
Cobleigh, Melody (IL)	Onc	365	Cohen, Roger (PA)	Onc	336
Coblyn, Jonathan (MA)	Rhu	1022	Cohen, Seymour (NY)	Onc	336
Cobos, Everardo (TX)	Hem	322	Cohen, Steven (CA)	PlS	871
Coccia, Peter (NE)	PHO	773	Cohn, Richard (IL)	PNep	786
Cochran, Alistair (CA)	Path	720	Cohn, Susan (IL)	PHO	769
Cockerell, Clay (TX)	D	197	Cohn, Susan (IL)	Inf	410
Cockerham, Kimberly (CA)	Oph	597	Coit, Daniel (NY)	S	1051
Coddington, Charles (MN)	RE	1012	Colachis, Samuel (OH)	PMR	838
Coe, Fredric (IL)	Nep	457	Colberg, John (CT)	U	1142
Coffey, Barbara (NY)	ChAP	905	Cole, Andrew (MA)	N	505
Coffman, Thomas (NC)	Nep	455	Cole, David (SC)	S	1063
Coggins, Cecil (MA)	Nep	452	Cole, Francis (MO)	NP	446
Cohen, Alan (OH)	NS	483	Coleman, Beverly (PA)	DR	974
Cohen, Arnold (PA)	MF	428	Coleman, John (IN)	PlS	863
Cohen, Bernard (FL)	D	190	Coleman, Morton (NY)	Onc	336
Cohen, Bernard (MD)	D	186	Coleman, R Edward (NC)	NuM	546
Cohen, Bruce (OH)	ChiN	148	Coller, Barry (NY)	Hem	310
Cohen, Burton (NY)	DR	974	Collins, Dale (NH)	PlS	848
Cohen, David (NY)	Nep	454	Collins, Evan (TX)	HS	302
Cohen, Gary (PA)	VIR	992	Colombani, Paul (MD)	PS	802
Cohen, Gary (MD)	Onc	335	Colon-Otero, Gerardo (FL)	Onc	353
Cohen, Gordon (WA)	TS	1134	Colquhoun, Steven (CA)	S	1089
Cohen, Harris (TN)	DR	978	Colvin, Edward (AL)	PCd	736
Cohen, Howard (NY)	Cv	95	Come, Steven (MA)	Onc	327
Cohen, Jeffrey (PA)	U	1145	Comenzo, Raymond (MA)	Hem	308
Cohen, Jeffrey (NH)	N	504	Comerota, Anthony (OH)	VascS	1185
Cohen, Jeffrey (OH)	N	523	Comi, Anne (MD)	ChiN	145

Alphabetical Listing of Doctors

D

Alphabetical Listing of Doctors

Name	Specialty	Pg	Name	Specialty	Pg
Dalmau, Josep (PA)	N	508	Day, Arthur (TX)	NS	488
Dalsing, Michael (IN)	VascS	1185	Day, Susan (CA)	Oph	597
Daly, Mary (PA)	Onc	336	Day, Terrence (SC)	Oto	666
Damiano, Ralph (MO)	TS	1125	Dayton, Merril (NY)	S	1051
Damon, Lloyd (CA)	Hem	323	De Angelis, Lisa (NY)	N	509
Dana, Reza (MA)	Oph	568	De Cherney, Alan (MD)	ObG	553
Daneker, George (GA)	S	1063	De Geest, Koen (IA)	GO	284
Daneshmand, Siamak (CA)	U	1170	De Juan, Eugene (CA)	Oph	597
Dang, Chi (MD)	Hem	310	De Lancey, John (MI)	ObG	557
Dang, Michael (HI)	TS	1134	De Las Morenas, Antonio (MA)	Path	706
Daniel, Rollin (CA)	PlS	871	De Lateur, Barbara (MD)	PMR	833
Danielpour, Moise (CA)	NS	492	De Lia, Julian (WI)	ObG	557
Daniels, Gilbert (MA)	EDM	205	De Luca, Francesco (PA)	PEn	744
Danoff, Dudley (CA)	U	1170	De Masters, Bette (CO)	Path	717
Darcy, Michael (MO)	VIR	994	De Meester, Tom (CA)	TS	1134
Darling, R Clement (NY)	VascS	1181	De Monte, Franco (TX)	NS	488
Darras, Basil (MA)	ChiN	144	De Simone, Philip (KY)	Onc	354
Darrow, David (VA)	PO	790	De Vivo, Darryl (NY)	ChiN	145
Das, Ananya (AZ)	Ge	250	Dea, Stanley (CA)	Ge	253
Dattilo, Jeffery (TN)	VascS	1183	Dean, Jonathan (UT)	PCCM	741
Daud, Adil (CA)	Onc	384	Deas, Deborah (SC)	ChAP	906
David, Carlos (MA)	NS	466	DeCamp, Malcolm (IL)	TS	1125
Davidoff, Andrew (TN)	PS	805	Decker, Gustav (AZ)	Ge	251
Davidson, Bruce (DC)	Oto	658	DeCross, Arthur (NY)	Ge	231
Davidson, Dennis (NY)	NP	442	Deeg, H Joachim (WA)	Onc	384
Davidson, Joyce (TX)	Psyc	896	DeFilippi, Vincent (CA)	TS	1135
Davidson, Michael (IL)	Cv	105	DeGiorgio, Christopher (CA)	N	534
Davidson, Nancy (PA)	Onc	336	Deitch, Edwin (NJ)	S	1052
Davidson, Richard (PA)	OrS	614	Deitz, Joel (PA)	Pul	923
Davidson, Susan (CO)	GO	286	DeKernion, Jean (CA)	U	1170
Davies, Stella (OH)	PHO	769	DeKosky, Steven (VA)	N	518
Davies, Terry (NY)	EDM	208	Del Giudice, Stephen (NH)	D	182
Davis, Bradley (KS)	U	1166	Del Monte, Monte (MI)	Oph	587
Davis, Gary (TX)	Ge	251	Del Priore, Giuseppe (IN)	GO	284
Davis, Glenn (NC)	PlS	859	Del Priore, Lucian (NY)	Oph	571
Davis, Janet (FL)	Oph	580	Del-Nido, Pedro (MA)	TS	1106
Davis, Jessica (NY)	CG	155	Delahay, John (DC)	OrS	614
Davis, Jonathan (MA)	NP	442	Delamarter, Rick (CA)	OrS	640
Davis, Mellar (OH)	Onc	365	Deland, Jonathan (NY)	OrS	614
Davis, William (LA)	Rhu	1030	Delaney, Conor (OH)	CRS	171
Dawson, Nancy (DC)	Onc	337	Delaney, Thomas (MA)	RadRO	944

Name	Specialty	Pg	Name	Specialty	Pg
DeLellis, Ronald (RI)	Path	706	Devinsky, Orrin (NY)	N	509
DeLeo, Vincent (NY)	D	186	DeVita, Vincent (CT)	Onc	327
DeLeon, Oscar (NY)	PM	695	Dewberry, Robert (MD)	N	509
Deleyiannis, Frederic (CO)	PlS	867	DeWeese, Theodore (MD)	RadRO	947
Delius, Ralph (MI)	TS	1125	Deziel, Daniel (IL)	S	1071
Delivoria-Papadopoulos, Maria (PA)		NP	Dhaliwal, Deepinder (PA)	Oph	571
443			Dhanireddy, Ramasubbareddy (TN)	NP	445
Della Rocca, Robert (NY)	Oph	571	Di Bisceglie, Adrian (MO)	Ge	244
Delmez, James (MO)	Nep	457	Di Giacinto, George (NY)	NS	469
DeLong, Mahlon (GA)	N	518	Di Lorenzo, Carlo (OH)	PGe	752
DeLoughery, Thomas (OR)	Hem	324	Di Marino, Anthony (PA)	Ge	231
DeLurgio, David (GA)	CE	119	Di Persio, John (MO)	Hem	317
Demarest, Gerald (NM)	S	1083	Di Saia, Philip (CA)	GO	289
DeMars, Leslie (NH)	GO	274	Diamond, Frank (FL)	PEn	745
Dember, Laura (MA)	Nep	452	Diamond, Michael (MI)	RE	1013
Demer, Joseph (CA)	Oph	598	Diamond, Paul (VA)	PMR	836
Demetri, George (MA)	Onc	327	Dias, Mark (PA)	NS	469
Demetris, Anthony (PA)	Path	708	Diaz, Angela (NY)	AM	80
Demmy, Todd (NY)	TS	1110	Diaz, Eduardo (TX)	Oto	680
Dempsey, Daniel (PA)	S	1052	Diaz, Fernando (MI)	NS	483
Dempsey, Robert (WI)	NS	483	Diaz-Arrastia, Ramon (TX)	N	530
Denenberg, Steven (NE)	Oto	679	Dichek, David (WA)	Cv	114
Dennery, Phyllis (PA)	NP	443	Dichter, Marc (PA)	N	509
Denny, Donald (NJ)	VIR	992	Dick, Gregory (MD)	PlS	852
DeNofrio, David (MA)	Cv	92	Dick, Macdonald (MI)	PCd	738
DeOrio, James (NC)	OrS	626	Dicker, Adam (PA)	RadRO	947
DePaulo, J Raymond (MD)	Psyc	887	Dickey, Richard (LA)	RE	1016
DePompolo, Robert (MN)	PMR	838	Dickler, Maura (NY)	Onc	337
DePriest, Paul (KY)	GO	280	Diduch, David (VA)	OrS	626
Derman, Gordon (IL)	HS	299	Diehl, James (PA)	TS	1110
DeRose, Joseph (NY)	TS	1110	Dienstag, Jules (MA)	Ge	228
Dershaw, D David (NY)	DR	975	Dieter, Robert (IL)	IC	128
Deschamps, Claude (MN)	TS	1125	Dieterich, Douglas (NY)	Ge	232
Deschler, Daniel (MA)	Oto	655	Diethrich, Edward (AZ)	TS	1131
DeShazo, Richard (MS)	A&I	86	Dietz, David (OH)	CRS	172
DeSilva, Stephen (MI)	HS	299	DiGiovanni, Christopher (RI)	OrS	608
Desnick, Robert (NY)	CG	155	Dillard, James (NY)	PMR	833
Desposito, Franklin (NJ)	CG	155	Dillehay, Gary (IL)	NuM	546
DeVane, Gary (FL)	RE	1011	Diller, Lisa (MA)	PHO	755
DeVault, Kenneth (FL)	Ge	239	Dillingham, Michael (CA)	OrS	641
Devereux, Richard (NY)	Cv	95	Dillingham, Timothy (WI)	PMR	838

Alphabetical Listing of Doctors

Name	Specialty	Pg	Name	Specialty	Pg
Dillon, Patrick (MO)	PS	807	Doody, Rachelle (TX)	N	531
Dillon, William (CA)	NRad	990	Dooley, Sharon (IL)	MF	432
DiMarco, John (VA)	CE	119	Dooley, William (OK)	S	1083
DiNardo, Laurence (VA)	Oto	666	Dorkin, Henry (MA)	PPul	793
Dines, David (NY)	OrS	614	Dormans, John (PA)	OrS	614
Dion, Jacques (GA)	NRad	986	Dornhoffer, John (AR)	Oto	681
DiPaola, Robert (NJ)	Onc	337	Doroshow, James (MD)	Onc	337
Disa, Joseph (NY)	PlS	852	Dorr, Lawrence (CA)	OrS	641
Disis, Mary (WA)	Onc	384	Dottino, Peter (NY)	GO	277
Diuguid, David (NY)	Hem	310	Doubilet, Peter (MA)	DR	973
Diver, Daniel (CT)	IC	123	Dougherty, Matthew (PA)	VascS	1181
Diwan, Sudhir (NY)	PM	695	Douglas, John (GA)	IC	127
Dixon, Sherwood (NV)	S	1089	Dover, Jeffrey (MA)	D	182
Dizon, Don (RI)	Onc	327	Dovey, Mark (PA)	PPul	793
Djulbegovic, Benjamin (FL)	Hem	315	Dowlati, Afshin (OH)	Onc	365
Dobs, Adrian (MD)	EDM	208	Downey, Robert (NY)	TS	1110
Docimo, Steven (PA)	U	1146	Dozor, Allen (NY)	PPul	793
Dodd, Gerald (CO)	DR	981	Drachtman, Richard (NJ)	PHO	758
Dodds, William (MI)	RE	1013	Drack, Arlene (IA)	Oph	587
Dodick, David (AZ)	N	531	Drake, Amelia (NC)	PO	790
Dodick, Jack (NY)	Oph	571	Drayer, Burton (NY)	NRad	985
Doghramji, Karl (PA)	Psyc	887	Drebin, Jeffrey (PA)	S	1052
Doherty, Dennis (KY)	Pul	928	Dreicer, Robert (OH)	Onc	365
Doherty, Gerard (MI)	S	1071	Dreyer, William (TX)	PCd	739
Dolgin, Stephen (NY)	PS	802	Dreyer, ZoAnn (TX)	PHO	774
Dolitsky, Jay (NY)	PO	788	Drinkwater, Davis (TN)	TS	1120
Domchek, Susan (PA)	Onc	337	Driscoll, Colin (MN)	Oto	673
Donahoe, Michael (PA)	Pul	923	Driscoll, Daniel (FL)	CG	157
Donahue, Bernadine (NY)	RadRO	947	Driscoll, David (MN)	PCd	738
Donahue, J Kevin (OH)	CE	120	Driscoll, Deborah (PA)	CG	155
Donald, Paul (CA)	Oto	683	Dritschilo, Anatoly (DC)	RadRO	947
Donaldson, Sarah (CA)	RadRO	964	Driver, Larry (TX)	PM	699
Donaldson, William (PA)	OrS	614	Droller, Michael (NY)	U	1146
Donehower, Ross (MD)	Onc	337	Drossman, Douglas (NC)	Ge	239
Donn, Steven (MI)	NP	446	Druker, Brian (OR)	Onc	384
Donner, Thomas (MD)	EDM	208	Druzin, Maurice (CA)	MF	436
Donohue, James (NC)	Pul	928	Dubeau, Louis (CA)	Path	720
Donohue, John (MN)	S	1071	Dubinsky, Marla (CA)	PGe	754
Donovan, Donald (TX)	Oto	681	Dubois, Michel (NY)	PM	695
Donovan, James (OH)	U	1160	Ducic, Ivica (DC)	PlS	852
Doody, Daniel (MA)	PS	801	Duckert, Larry (WA)	Oto	683

Name	Specialty	Pg	Name	Specialty	Pg
Ducore, Jonathan (CA)	PHO	776	Eason, James (TN)	S	1063
Duff, William (FL)	MF	430	Easter, David (CA)	S	1090
Duffner, Patricia (NY)	ChiN	145	Eaton, James (DC)	Psyc	888
Duffy, Thomas (CT)	Hem	308	Eavey, Roland (TN)	PO	790
Dufresne, Craig (MD)	PlS	852	Eberlein, Timothy (MO)	S	1072
Dufresne, Raymond (RI)	D	182	Ebraheim, Nabil (OH)	OrS	631
Dugoff, Lorraine (CO)	MF	434	Echeverri, Luis (TX)	TS	1131
Duh, Quan-Yang (CA)	S	1089	Eckardt, Jeffrey (CA)	OrS	641
Duhaime, Ann (MA)	NS	466	Eckel, Robert (CO)	EDM	218
Duker, Jay (MA)	Oph	568	Eckhardt, S (CO)	Onc	374
Dulcan, Mina (IL)	ChAP	907	Eckhoff, Devin (AL)	S	1063
Dulchavsky, Scott (MI)	S	1072	Eckler, Kristen (MA)	ObG	552
Dumesic, Daniel (CA)	RE	1017	Econs, Michael (IN)	EDM	215
Dumitru, Daniel (TX)	PMR	841	Eddleman, Keith (NY)	MF	428
Duncan, Mark D (MD)	S	1052	Eddy, Allison (WA)	PNep	787
Duncan, Newton (TX)	PO	792	Edelman, Martin (MD)	Onc	337
Dunkel, Ira (NY)	PHO	758	Edelman, Robert (IL)	DR	980
Dunphy, Frank (NC)	Onc	354	Edelman, Steven (CA)	EDM	220
Dunton, Charles (PA)	GO	277	Edelson, Richard (CT)	D	182
DuPont, Herbert (TX)	Inf	412	Edelstein, Barbara (NY)	DR	975
Durbin, William (MA)	PInf	779	Edelstein, David (NY)	Oto	658
Dure, Leon (AL)	ChiN	147	Edgar, Terence (WI)	ChiN	149
Durham, Janette (CO)	VIR	995	Edge, Stephen (NY)	S	1052
Durham, Samuel (MI)	TS	1125	Edington, Howard (PA)	S	1052
Durrie, Daniel (KS)	Oph	593	Edmond, Michael (VA)	Inf	408
Durso, Nancy (VA)	RE	1011	Edmundowicz, Daniel (PA)	Cv	95
Duska, Linda (VA)	GO	281	Edmundowicz, Steven (MO)	Ge	244
Dutcher, Janice (NY)	Onc	337	Edney, James (NE)	S	1080
Duthie, Edmund (WI)	Ger	265	Edwards, John (CA)	Inf	413
Dutton, Jonathan (NC)	Oph	580	Edwards, Kathryn (TN)	PInf	780
Duvic, Madeleine (TX)	D	197	Edwards, Michael (OH)	S	1072
Dyer, Carmel (TX)	Ger	266	Edwards, Michael (CA)	NS	492
Dzubow, Leonard (PA)	D	186	Edwards, Michael (NV)	PlS	871
			Edwards, Niloo (NY)	TS	1111
			Edwards, Paul (MI)	Oph	587
			Edwards, Robert (PA)	GO	277

E

Name	Specialty	Pg	Name	Specialty	Pg
			Edye, Michael (NY)	S	1052
Eagle, Kim (MI)	Cv	105	Efron, Jonathan (MD)	CRS	167
Eagle, Ralph (PA)	Oph	571	Eggers, Howard (NY)	Oph	571
Early, Dayna (MO)	Ge	244	Egleseder, W Andrew (MD)	HS	295
Earp, H Shelton (NC)	EDM	212	Ehrenkranz, Richard (CT)	NP	442

Alphabetical Listing of Doctors

Name	Specialty	Pg	Name	Specialty	Pg
Ehresmann, Glenn (CA)	Rhu	1031	Ellis, David (TX)	U	1167
Ehrlich, Paul (NY)	PA&I	729	Ellis, Demetrius (PA)	PNep	784
Ehrlich, Peter (MI)	PS	807	Ellis, George (LA)	Oph	593
Ehrmann, David (IL)	EDM	215	Ellis, Georgiana (WA)	Onc	384
Ehya, Hormoz (PA)	Path	708	Ellis, Jonathan (CA)	Ge	253
Eichelberger, Martin (DC)	PS	802	Ellis, Lee (TX)	S	1083
Eichenfield, Lawrence (CA)	D	198	Ellis, Matthew (MO)	Onc	365
Eichler, Craig (FL)	D	190	Ellis, Stephen (OH)	IC	128
Eidt, John (AR)	VascS	1187	Ellis, William (WA)	U	1170
Eifel, Patricia (TX)	RadRO	962	Ellison, David (OR)	Nep	461
Eilber, Frederick (CA)	S	1090	Ellison, E Christopher (OH)	S	1072
Ein, Daniel (DC)	A&I	85	Ellison, James (MA)	Psyc	884
Einarsson, Jon (MA)	ObG	552	Elmets, Craig (AL)	D	190
Einhorn, Lawrence (IN)	Onc	365	Elner, Victor (MI)	Oph	587
Einhorn, Thomas (MA)	OrS	609	Elster, Allen (NC)	DR	979
Eisbruch, Avraham (MI)	RadRO	957	Elta, Grace (MI)	Ge	245
Eisele, David (CA)	Oto	684	Emami, Bahman (IL)	RadRO	957
Eisen, Glenn (OR)	Ge	253	Emans, Sarah (MA)	AM	80
Eisen, Howard (PA)	Cv	96	Emanuel, Peter (AR)	Hem	322
Eisenberg, Burton (NH)	S	1045	Emanuele, Mary Ann (IL)	EDM	215
Eisenberg, Howard (MD)	NS	469	Emanuele, Nicholas (IL)	EDM	215
Eisenberger, Mario (MD)	Onc	338	Emens, Leisha (MD)	Onc	338
Eisendrath, Stuart (CA)	Psyc	897	Emerson, S Cameron (LA)	ObG	559
Eisenstat, Theodore (NJ)	CRS	167	Emery, Helen (WA)	PRhu	800
Eismont, Frank (FL)	OrS	626	Emmanuel, Patricia (FL)	PInf	780
El-Galley, Rizk (AL)	U	1154	Emond, Jean (NY)	S	1052
El-Youssef, Mounif (MN)	PGe	752	Emre, Sukru (CT)	S	1045
Elattrache, Neal (CA)	OrS	641	Emslie, Graham (TX)	ChAP	908
Elder, Jack (MI)	U	1160	Endrizzi, Donald (ME)	OrS	609
Elefteriades, John (CT)	TS	1106	Enelow, Richard (NH)	Pul	920
Elias, Anthony (CO)	Onc	374	Engel, William King (CA)	N	534
Elias, Sherman (IL)	CG	158	Engstrom, John (CA)	N	534
Elias, Stanton (MI)	N	524	Engstrom, Paul (PA)	Onc	338
Elkayam, Uri (CA)	Cv	114	Ennis, Ronald (NY)	RadRO	947
Ellenbogen, Kenneth (VA)	CE	119	Ensminger, William (MI)	Onc	366
Ellenbogen, Richard (WA)	NS	492	Epstein, Andrew (PA)	CE	118
Ellenhorn, Joshua (CA)	S	1090	Epstein, Jeffrey (FL)	Oto	667
Elliott, C Gregory (UT)	Pul	934	Epstein, Jonathan (MD)	Path	708
Elliott, David (IA)	Ge	244	Epstein, Leon (IL)	ChiN	149
Elliott, John (CA)	MF	436	Epstein, Michael (FL)	PCd	736
Elliott, Norman (GA)	Ge	239	Epstein, Stuart (CA)	PA&I	733

Alphabetical Listing of Doctors

Name	Specialty	Pg	Name	Specialty	Pg
Erasmus, Jeremy (TX)	DR	982	Fabian, Carol (KS)	Onc	374
Erba, Harry (MI)	Hem	317	Faddis, Mitchell (MO)	CE	120
Erban, John (MA)	Onc	327	Fadem, Stephen (TX)	Nep	460
Erdmann, Detlev (NC)	PlS	859	Fahey, Patrick (IL)	Pul	930
Eriksson, Elof (MA)	PlS	848	Fahey, Thomas (NY)	S	1053
Ernst, Armin (MA)	Pul	920	Fahn, Stanley (NY)	N	509
Ernstoff, Marc (NH)	Onc	327	Faigel, Douglas (AZ)	Ge	251
Errico, Thomas (NY)	OrS	615	Failla, Joseph (MI)	HS	299
Eschenbach, David (WA)	ObG	559	Fairman, Ronald (PA)	VascS	1181
Escobedo, Marilyn (OK)	NP	447	Falanga, Vincent (RI)	D	182
Esmaeli-Azad, Bita (TX)	Oph	594	Falco, Frank (DE)	PM	695
Esquenazi, Alberto (PA)	PMR	833	Falcone, Tommaso (OH)	RE	1013
Esquivel, Carlos (CA)	S	1090	Falk, Gary (PA)	Ge	232
Esserman, Laura (CA)	S	1090	Falk, Rena (CA)	CG	161
Essner, Richard (CA)	S	1090	Falk, Ronald (NC)	Nep	456
Estabrook, Alison (NY)	S	1053	Fallat, Mary (KY)	PS	805
Estes, N.A. Mark (MA)	CE	116	Fallon, Brian (NY)	Psyc	888
Estey, Elihu (WA)	Onc	384	Fallon, Michael (TX)	Ge	251
Estores, David (FL)	Ge	240	Fallon, Robert (IN)	PHO	769
Estwanik, Joseph (NC)	SM	1038	Famuyide, Abimbola (MN)	ObG	557
Eth, Spencer (FL)	Psyc	892	Fan, Leland (CO)	PPul	797
Ettenger, Robert (CA)	PNep	787	Fang, John (UT)	Ge	249
Ettinger, David (MD)	Onc	338	Fann, Jesse (WA)	Psyc	897
Eugster, Erica (IN)	PEn	746	Fanous, Yvonne (CA)	PA&I	733
Euhus, David (TX)	S	1083	Fanta, Christopher (MA)	Pul	920
Eustis, H Sprague (LA)	Oph	594	Fantini, Gary (NY)	VascS	1181
Evans, Douglas (WI)	S	1072	Farag, Sherif (IN)	Hem	317
Evans, Gregory (CA)	PlS	871	Farah, Tony (PA)	IC	124
Evans, James (PA)	NS	469	Farber, Martin (NY)	Rhu	1024
Evans, Mark (NY)	ObG	553	Faries, Peter (NY)	VascS	1181
Evans, Sarah (DC)	PMR	834	Farley, David (MN)	S	1072
Evers, Kathryn (PA)	DR	975	Farlow, Martin (IN)	N	524
Everson, Gregory (CO)	Ge	249	Farmer, Diana (CA)	PS	810
Eviatar, Lydia (NY)	ChiN	146	Faro, Scott (PA)	NRad	985
Ewalt, David (TX)	U	1167	Faro, Sebastian (TX)	ObG	559
Ewend, Matthew (NC)	NS	477	Farrar, William (OH)	S	1072
Ezaki, Marybeth (TX)	HS	302	Farraye, Francis (MA)	Ge	228
			Farrior, Edward (FL)	Oto	667
			Farrior, Joseph (FL)	Oto	667
			Fasano, Alessio (MD)	PGe	749
			Fauci, Anthony (MD)	Inf	405

F

Alphabetical Listing of Doctors

Name	Specialty	Pg	Name	Specialty	Pg
Fay, Joseph (TX)	Onc	377	Ferris, Robert (PA)	Oto	658
Faye-Petersen, Ona (AL)	Path	713	Fessler, Richard (IL)	NS	483
Feder, Robert (IL)	Oph	587	Fewkes, Jessica (MA)	D	183
Federle, Michael (CA)	DR	983	Fichtenbaum, Carl (OH)	Inf	410
Fee, Willard (CA)	Oto	684	Fidler, Jeff (MN)	DR	980
Feghali, Joseph (NY)	Oto	658	Fields, Abbie (DC)	GO	277
Feig, Barry (TX)	S	1083	Fields, Theodore (NY)	Rhu	1024
Feig, Stephen (CA)	DR	983	Fife, Rose (IN)	Rhu	1029
Feinberg, Joseph (NY)	PMR	834	Figlin, Robert (CA)	Onc	384
Feinberg, Todd (NY)	N	509	Files, Joe (MS)	Hem	315
Feinglos, Mark (NC)	EDM	212	Filicko-OHara, Joanne (PA)	Hem	310
Feins, Richard (NC)	TS	1120	Filip, Stanley (NC)	ObG	555
Feld, Gregory (CA)	CE	122	Filley, Christopher (CO)	N	529
Feldman, David (NY)	OrS	615	Filly, Roy (CA)	DR	983
Feldman, Edward (CA)	Ge	253	Filsoufi, Farzan (NY)	TS	1111
Feldman, Eva (MI)	N	524	Finan, Michael (AL)	GO	281
Feldman, Joel (MA)	PlS	848	Fine, Howard (MD)	Onc	338
Feldman, Joseph (IL)	PMR	838	Fine, Perry (UT)	PM	699
Feldman, Kenneth (WA)	Ped	728	Fine, Robert (TX)	IM	421
Feldman, Ted (IL)	IC	128	Fine, Robert (NY)	Onc	338
Feldmann, Edward (MA)	N	505	Finerman, Gerald (CA)	OrS	641
Feldon, Steven (NY)	Oph	571	Finger, Paul (NY)	Oph	571
Feldstein, Neil (NY)	NS	469	Fink, Matthew (NY)	N	509
Feliciano, David (GA)	S	1063	Finkel, Alan (NC)	N	518
Felig, Philip (NY)	EDM	208	Finkel, Michael (FL)	N	519
Felix, Carolyn (PA)	PHO	758	Finkel, Richard (PA)	ChiN	146
Fellus, Jonathan (NJ)	N	509	Finkel, Terri (PA)	PRhu	798
Feltes, Timothy (OH)	PCd	738	Finklestein, Jerry (CA)	PHO	776
Fennerty, M Brian (OR)	Ge	253	Finlay, Jonathan (CA)	PHO	776
Fenske, Neil (FL)	D	190	Finlayson, Christina (CO)	S	1080
Fenstermaker, Robert (NY)	NS	469	Finucane, Thomas (MD)	Ger	263
Ferguson, James (VA)	MF	430	Fiorica, James (FL)	GO	281
Ferguson, Mark (IL)	TS	1126	Firlit, Casimir (MO)	U	1161
Fernando, Hiran (MA)	TS	1106	First, Michael (NY)	Psyc	888
Fernhoff, Paul (GA)	CG	157	Fisch, Harry (NY)	U	1146
Ferrante, F Michael (CA)	PM	700	Fischbein, Lewis (MO)	IM	420
Ferrara, James (MI)	PHO	769	Fischer, Thomas (IN)	HS	300
Ferrell, Linda (CA)	Path	720	Fischl, Margaret (FL)	IM	419
Ferrendelli, James (TX)	N	531	Fish, Frank (TN)	PCd	736
Ferriero, Donna (CA)	ChiN	151	Fishbein, Daniel (WA)	Cv	114
Ferris, Frank (CA)	IM	421	Fishbein, Michael (CA)	Path	720

Name	Specialty	Pg	Name	Specialty	Pg
Fisher, Garth (CA)	PlS	871	Flickinger, John (PA)	RadRO	947
Fisher, George (CA)	Onc	385	Flinn, Ian (TN)	Onc	354
Fisher, Jonathan (CA)	S	1090	Flint, Paul (OR)	Oto	684
Fisher, Mark (CA)	N	535	Flomenberg, Neal (PA)	Onc	338
Fisher, Paul (CA)	ChiN	151	Florakis, George (NY)	Oph	572
Fisher, Richard (NY)	Onc	338	Flores, Raja (NY)	TS	1111
Fisher, Robert (PA)	Ge	232	Flowers, Franklin (FL)	D	190
Fisher, Robert (CA)	N	535	Flynn, Harry (FL)	Oph	580
Fisher, Rosemarie (CT)	Ge	228	Flynn, Joseph (WA)	PNep	787
Fisher, William (TX)	S	1083	Flynn, Michael (KY)	S	1063
Fishman, David (NY)	GO	278	Flynn, Patricia (TN)	PInf	780
Fishman, Elliot (MD)	DR	975	Flynn, Patrick (MN)	Hem	318
Fishman, Gerald (IL)	Oph	587	Flynn, Timothy (FL)	VascS	1183
Fishman, Henry (DC)	A&I	85	Fodor, Peter (CA)	PlS	871
Fishman, Scott (CA)	PM	700	Foglia, Robert (TX)	PS	809
Fitch, Tom (AZ)	Onc	377	Fogt, Franz (PA)	Path	708
Fitzgerald, Paul (CA)	EDM	220	Foley, Carmel (NY)	ChAP	905
Fitzgibbon, Dermot (WA)	PM	701	Foley, Eugene (WI)	CRS	172
Fitzgibbons, Robert (NE)	S	1080	Foley, Kevin (TN)	NS	477
Fitzpatrick, Richard (CA)	D	198	Follansbee, William (PA)	Cv	96
Fiveash, John (AL)	RadRO	952	Follen, Michele (PA)	GO	278
Fivenson, David (MI)	D	193	Fonarow, Gregg (CA)	Cv	114
Fivush, Barbara (MD)	PNep	784	Fong, Yuman (NY)	S	1053
Fix, R Jobe (AL)	PlS	859	Fonseca, Rafael (AZ)	Hem	322
Flaherty, Alice (MA)	N	505	Fontana, Gregory (CA)	TS	1135
Flaherty, John (IL)	Inf	410	Foo, Sun-Hoo (NY)	N	509
Flaherty, Joseph (MO)	Ger	265	Forastiere, Arlene (MD)	Onc	339
Flaherty, Keith (MA)	Onc	327	Forbess, Joseph (TX)	TS	1131
Flake, Alan (PA)	PS	802	Ford, Charles (WI)	Oto	673
Flamm, Scott (OH)	DR	980	Ford, Henri (CA)	PS	810
Flanagan, Steven (NY)	PMR	834	Ford, James (CA)	Onc	385
Flanders, Adam (PA)	NRad	985	Forero, Andres (AL)	Onc	354
Flanigan, D Preston (CA)	VascS	1188	Forman, Jeffrey (MI)	RadRO	957
Flanigan, Robert (IL)	U	1161	Forman, Stephen (CA)	Hem	324
Flanigan, Timothy (RI)	Inf	404	Formenti, Silvia (NY)	RadRO	947
Flatow, Evan (NY)	OrS	615	Fornari, Victor (NY)	ChAP	905
Fleischer, David (AZ)	Ge	251	Forscher, Charles (CA)	Onc	385
Fleming, Gini (IL)	Onc	366	Forsmark, Christopher (FL)	Ge	240
Fleshman, James (MO)	CRS	172	Forster, Richard (FL)	Oph	581
Fletcher, Christopher (MA)	Path	706	Fosko, Scott (MO)	D	193
Fletcher, Eugene (IN)	Pul	931	Foss, Francine (CT)	Onc	328

Alphabetical Listing of Doctors

Name	Specialty	Pg	Name	Specialty	Pg
Fossella, Frank (TX)	Onc	377	Freeman, Theodore (TX)	A&I	88
Fost, Norman (WI)	Ped	728	Freeman, Thomas (FL)	NS	477
Foster, C Stephen (MA)	Oph	568	Freemark, Michael (NC)	PEn	745
Foster, Carol (UT)	PEn	747	Freifeld, Alison (NE)	Inf	412
Foster, Harris (CT)	U	1142	Freiman, Hal (NY)	Ge	232
Foster, Richard (IN)	U	1161	Freimanis, Rita (NC)	DR	979
Foucar, M Kathryn (NM)	Path	718	Freischlag, Julie (MD)	VascS	1181
Fouser, Laurie (WA)	PNep	787	Freitag, Frederick (TX)	PM	699
Fowble, Barbara (CA)	RadRO	964	French, Jacqueline (NY)	N	510
Fowl, Richard (AZ)	VascS	1187	French, William (CA)	Cv	114
Fowler, Jeffrey (OH)	GO	284	Friberg, Thomas (PA)	Oph	572
Fowler, Wesley (NC)	GO	281	Fricker, Frederick (FL)	PCd	736
Fox, Harold (MD)	MF	428	Friebert, Sarah (OH)	PHO	770
Fox, James (PA)	PlS	852	Fried, Guy (PA)	PMR	834
Fox, Kevin (PA)	Onc	339	Fried, Marvin (NY)	Oto	658
Fracasso, Paula (VA)	Onc	354	Fried, Michael (NC)	Ge	240
Fraker, Douglas (PA)	S	1053	Friedberg, Jonathan (NY)	Onc	339
Frances, Richard (NY)	AdP	901	Friedberg, Joseph (PA)	TS	1111
Francis, Kathleen (NJ)	PMR	834	Frieden, Ilona (CA)	D	198
Francisco, Gerard (TX)	PMR	841	Friedlaender, Gary (CT)	OrS	609
Frangoul, Haydar (TN)	PHO	764	Friedlander, Sheila (CA)	D	198
Frank, Ian (PA)	Inf	405	Friedman, Aaron (MN)	PNep	786
Franklin, Morris (TX)	S	1083	Friedman, Alan (MD)	PHO	758
Franks, Andrew (NY)	D	186	Friedman, Allan (NC)	NS	477
Frantz, Christopher (DE)	PHO	758	Friedman, Barry (CA)	Psyc	897
Frantz, Ivan (MA)	NP	442	Friedman, Chad (OH)	RE	1013
Frantzides, Constantine (IL)	S	1072	Friedman, David (FL)	HS	298
Franz, Michael (MI)	S	1072	Friedman, Debra (TN)	PHO	764
Fraser, Charles (TX)	TS	1132	Friedman, Ellen (TX)	PO	792
Fraser, Lionel (MS)	U	1155	Friedman, Henry (NC)	Onc	354
Frassica, Frank (MD)	OrS	615	Friedman, Lawrence (MA)	Ge	229
Frazee, John (CA)	NS	492	Friedman, Lloyd (CT)	Pul	920
Frazier, O Howard (TX)	TS	1132	Friedman, Matthew (VT)	Psyc	884
Frazier, Thomas (PA)	S	1053	Friedman, Michael (IL)	Oto	673
Freedman, Arnold (MA)	Onc	328	Friedman, Nancy (NC)	PEn	745
Freedman, Barry (NC)	Nep	456	Friedman, Sanford (NY)	Cv	96
Freedman, Gary (PA)	RadRO	948	Friedman, Stuart (FL)	A&I	86
Freedman, Robert (CO)	Psyc	894	Friese, Randall (AZ)	S	1083
Freedman, Sharon (NC)	Oph	581	Frim, David (IL)	NS	484
Freeman, Gregory (TX)	Cv	111	Fritz, Marc (NC)	RE	1011
Freeman, Leonard (NY)	NuM	544	Frohman, Elliot (TX)	N	531

Alphabetical Listing of Doctors

Name	Specialty	Pg	Name	Specialty	Pg
Gebhardt, Mark (MA)	OrS	609	Gibbs, John (NY)	S	1053
Geffner, Mitchell (CA)	PEn	747	Gibbs, Ronald (CO)	MF	434
Gefter, Warren (PA)	DR	975	Gibralter, Richard (NY)	Oph	572
Geisler, Daniel (PA)	CRS	168	Gibson, C Michael (MA)	IC	123
Gejerman, Glen (NJ)	RadRO	948	Gibson, Ronald (WA)	Pul	937
Gelb, Bruce (NY)	PCd	734	Gigantelli, James (NE)	Oph	593
Gelberman, Richard (MO)	HS	300	Gilbert, Fred (NY)	CG	155
Gelfand, Erwin (CO)	PA&I	732	Gilbert, Mark (TX)	N	531
Geller, David (PA)	S	1053	Gilchrest, Barbara (MA)	D	183
Geller, Kenneth (CA)	PO	792	Gill, Harcharan (CA)	U	1170
Gellis, Stephen (MA)	D	183	Gill, Inderbir (CA)	U	1170
Gelmann, Edward (NY)	Onc	339	Gill, Thomas (MA)	SM	1036
Geltman, Edward (MO)	Cv	106	Gillette, Paul (TX)	PCd	739
Gendelman, Seymour (NY)	N	510	Gillman, Matthew (MA)	IM	418
Genden, Eric (NY)	Oto	658	Gilman, Sid (MI)	N	524
Gentile, Ronald (NY)	Oph	572	Gilsanz, Vicente (CA)	DR	983
George, Daniel (NC)	Onc	354	Ginsberg, David (CA)	U	1170
Georgiade, Gregory (NC)	PlS	859	Ginsberg, Gregory (PA)	Ge	232
Gerboth, Gregory (AK)	Pul	937	Ginsburg, Elizabeth (MA)	RE	1006
Gerdes, Hans (NY)	Ge	232	Ginsburg, Howard (NY)	PS	802
Geronemus, Roy (NY)	D	186	Ginsburg, Kenneth (PA)	AM	80
Gershenson, David (TX)	GO	287	Ginsburg, Mark (NY)	TS	1112
Gershwin, Merrill (CA)	Rhu	1032	Girardi, Leonard (NY)	TS	1112
Gerson, Lauren (CA)	Ge	253	Gish, Robert (CA)	Ge	253
Gerson, Stanton (OH)	Onc	366	Gitelis, Steven (IL)	OrS	631
Gertz, Morie (MN)	Hem	318	Gitelman, Stephen (CA)	PEn	748
Geschwind, Jean-Francois (MD)	VIR	992	Gitlin, Michael (CA)	Psyc	897
Gewertz, Bruce (CA)	VascS	1188	Gittes, George (PA)	PS	802
Gewitz, Michael (NY)	PCd	735	Gittler, Michelle (IL)	PMR	838
Gewolb, Ira (MI)	NP	446	Giudice, Linda (CA)	RE	1017
Geyer, Charles (PA)	Onc	339	Giuliano, Armando (CA)	S	1090
Geyer, J Russell (WA)	PHO	776	Giuntoli, Robert (MD)	GO	278
Ghamande, Sharad (GA)	GO	281	Giustra, Lawrence (GA)	Psyc	892
Gharagozloo, Farid (DC)	TS	1111	Givan, Deborah (IN)	PPul	795
Gharibo, Christopher (NY)	PM	695	Givner, Laurence (NC)	PInf	781
Gholam, Pierre (OH)	Ge	245	Gizzi, Martin (NJ)	N	510
Giannotta, Steven (CA)	NS	493	Glader, Bertil (CA)	PHO	776
Gianoli, Gerard (LA)	Oto	681	Gladstone, James (NY)	OrS	615
Giardiello, Francis (MD)	Ge	232	Glashow, Jonathan (NY)	OrS	615
Giardina, Patricia (NY)	PHO	759	Glaspy, John (CA)	Onc	385
Gibbons, Raymond (MN)	Cv	106	Glass, Jon (PA)	N	510

Alphabetical Listing of Doctors

Name	Specialty	Pg	Name	Specialty	Pg
Goodson, William (CA)	S	1091	Grammer, Leslie (IL)	A&I	88
Goodwin, James (IL)	N	524	Grana, Generosa (NJ)	Onc	340
Goodwin, Scott (CA)	VIR	996	Granai, Cornelius (RI)	GO	274
Goodwin, W Jarrard (FL)	Oto	667	Grandis, Arnold (NC)	MF	430
Gorab, Robert (CA)	OrS	641	Grandis, Jennifer (PA)	Oto	659
Gorbien, Martin (IL)	Ger	265	Granet, David (CA)	Oph	598
Gordon, Catherine (MA)	PEn	743	Grannis, Frederic (CA)	TS	1135
Gordon, Leo (IL)	Hem	318	Grant, Clive S (MN)	S	1073
Gordon, Marsha (NY)	D	186	Grant, Michael (TX)	S	1083
Gordon, Stuart (NH)	Ge	229	Grant, Richard (OH)	OrS	632
Gorensek, Margaret (FL)	Inf	409	Grasso, Michael (NY)	U	1146
Gorevic, Peter (NY)	Rhu	1024	Graver, L Michael (NY)	TS	1112
Gorfine, Stephen (NY)	CRS	168	Graves, Michael (CA)	N	535
Gorin, Michael (CA)	Oph	598	Gravett, Michael (WA)	MF	436
Gorovoy, Mark (FL)	Oph	581	Gray, Richard (AZ)	S	1084
Gospe, Sidney M (WA)	ChiN	151	Gray, William (NY)	IC	124
Gosselin, Benoit (NH)	Oto	655	Grazi, Richard (NY)	RE	1008
Gostout, Christopher (MN)	Ge	245	Greco, F Anthony (TN)	Onc	355
Gottdiener, John (MD)	Cv	96	Greden, John (MI)	Psyc	893
Gottlieb, Alice (MA)	D	183	Green, Andrew (RI)	OrS	609
Gottlieb, Geoffrey (NY)	Path	709	Green, Barth (FL)	NS	477
Gottlieb, Lawrence (IL)	PlS	863	Green, Carmen (MI)	PM	698
Gottlieb, Stephen (MD)	Cv	97	Green, Daniel (TN)	PHO	765
Gould, K Lance (TX)	Cv	112	Green, Howard (FL)	D	191
Goulet, Robert (IN)	S	1073	Green, Michael (PA)	PInf	779
Goumnerova, Liliana (MA)	NS	466	Green, Peter (NY)	Ge	233
Gourley, Mark (MD)	Rhu	1024	Green, Richard (NY)	VascS	1181
Govindarajan, Sugantha (CA)	Path	720	Green, Thomas (IL)	PPul	796
Gower, Roland (AK)	S	1091	Greenberg, Benjamin (RI)	Psyc	884
Goy, Andre (NJ)	Onc	340	Greenberg, Donna (MA)	Psyc	884
Gracia, Clarisa (PA)	RE	1008	Greenberg, Harly (NY)	Pul	923
Gradishar, William (IL)	Onc	366	Greenberg, Jay (DC)	PHO	759
Grado, Gordon (AZ)	RadRO	962	Greenberg, Mark (NY)	Cv	97
Grady, M Sean (PA)	NS	470	Greenberg, Richard (PA)	U	1147
Graf, Ben (WI)	OrS	631	Greenberg, William (MA)	Psyc	885
Graham, H Devon (LA)	Oto	681	Greenberger, Joel (PA)	RadRO	948
Graham, John (CA)	CG	161	Greenberger, Paul (IL)	A&I	88
Graham, Mark (NC)	Onc	355	Greene, Clarence (LA)	NS	489
Graham, Michael (AZ)	PHO	775	Greene, Frederick (NC)	S	1064
Graham, Thomas (OH)	HS	300	Greene, Graham (FL)	U	1155
Gralow, Julie (WA)	Onc	385	Greene, Loren Wissner (NY)	EDM	208

Name	Specialty	Pg	Name	Specialty	Pg
Greene, Michael (MA)	MF	426	Grogan, Thomas (AZ)	Path	718
Greene, Thomas (FL)	HS	298	Grosh, William (VA)	Onc	355
Greenfield, David (FL)	Oph	581	Gross, Ian (CT)	NP	442
Greenfield, Marjorie (OH)	ObG	557	Gross, Paul (MA)	N	505
Greenfield, Saul (NY)	U	1147	Gross, Susan (NY)	CG	156
Greenfield, Shelly (MA)	AdP	900	Grossbard, Michael (NY)	Onc	340
Greenhalgh, David (CA)	S	1091	Grossberg, George (MO)	GerPsy	911
Greenson, Joel (MI)	Path	715	Grossi, Eugene (NY)	TS	1112
Greenspan, Susan (PA)	EDM	208	Grossman, H Barton (TX)	U	1167
Greenwald, Blaine (NY)	GerPsy	910	Grossman, John (CO)	PlS	867
Greenwald, Bruce (MD)	Ge	233	Grossman, John (FL)	HS	298
Greenwald, Mark (IL)	Oph	587	Grossman, Melanie (NY)	D	186
Greenway, Hubert (CA)	D	199	Grossman, Stuart (MD)	Onc	340
Greenwood, Robert (NC)	ChiN	148	Grossniklaus, Hans (GA)	Oph	581
Greer, Benjamin (WA)	GO	290	Grotta, James (TX)	N	531
Greer, David (CT)	N	505	Grotting, James (AL)	PlS	859
Greer, John (TN)	Hem	315	Grubb, Blair (OH)	Cv	106
Greganti, Mac (NC)	Ger	264	Grubb, Robert (MO)	NS	484
Gregory, Richard (FL)	PlS	859	Gruber, Scott (MI)	S	1073
Gregory, Stephanie (IL)	Hem	318	Gruber, Stephen (MI)	Onc	366
Greiner, Carl (NE)	Psyc	894	Gruchalla, Rebecca (TX)	A&I	89
Greipp, Philip (MN)	Hem	318	Grum, Cyril (MI)	Pul	931
Greisberg, Justin (NY)	OrS	616	Grunberg, Steven (VT)	Onc	328
Greisler, Howard (IL)	VascS	1185	Grundfast, Kenneth (MA)	Oto	656
Grelsamer, Ronald (NY)	OrS	616	Grunebaum, Amos (NY)	MF	429
Grem, Jean (NE)	Onc	374	Grunfeld, Lawrence (NY)	RE	1008
Gress, Daryl (VA)	N	519	Grupp, Stephan (PA)	PHO	759
Grever, Michael (OH)	Hem	318	Gruss, Joseph (WA)	PlS	872
Gribetz, Michael (NY)	U	1147	Guandalini, Stefano (IL)	PGe	752
Grichnik, James (FL)	D	191	Guarda, Angela (MD)	Psyc	888
Griebling, Tomas (KS)	U	1166	Guarini, Ludovico (NY)	PHO	759
Griepp, Randall (NY)	TS	1112	Gugenheim, Joseph (TX)	OrS	638
Griesemer, David (MA)	ChiN	144	Guidry, George (LA)	Pul	935
Griffith, Bartley (MD)	TS	1112	Guillem, Jose (NY)	CRS	168
Grifo, James (NY)	RE	1008	Guilleminault, Christian (CA)	N	535
Grigsby, Perry (MO)	RadRO	957	Guinan, Eva (MA)	PHO	755
Grillone, Gregory (MA)	Oto	655	Gujral, Saroj (MN)	U	1161
Grimes, Pearl (CA)	D	199	Gulley, James (MD)	Onc	340
Griswold, John (TX)	S	1084	Gullquist, Scott (VA)	PCd	737
Grobelny, Thomas (IL)	NRad	988	Gumprecht, Jeffrey (NY)	Inf	405
Grody, Wayne (CA)	CG	161	Gunasekaran, T S (IL)	PGe	752

Alphabetical Listing of Doctors

Name	Specialty	Pg	Name	Specialty	Pg
Gunderson, John (MA)	Psyc	885	Hain, Timothy (IL)	N	524
Gundry, Steven (CA)	TS	1135	Haines, Kathleen (NJ)	PRhu	798
Gunter, Jack (TX)	PlS	868	Hakaim, Albert (FL)	VascS	1183
Gupta, Nalin (CA)	NS	493	Halberg, Francine (CA)	RadRO	964
Gupta, Prabodh (PA)	Path	709	Hale, Douglass (IN)	ObG	557
Gupta, Rajan (NH)	S	1045	Haley, Barbara (TX)	Onc	377
Gupta, Sandeep (IN)	PGe	752	Haley, Elliott (VA)	N	519
Gururangan, Sridharan (NC)	PHO	765	Halff, Glenn (TX)	S	1084
Gusberg, Richard (CT)	VascS	1178	Hall, Jesse (IL)	Pul	931
Gutai, James (MI)	PEn	746	Hall, Lisabeth (NY)	Oph	573
Guthikonda, Murali (MI)	NS	484	Hall, Simon (NY)	U	1147
Guthrie, Barton (AL)	NS	478	Halle, Jan (NC)	RadRO	952
Gutin, Philip (NY)	NS	470	Haller, Julia (PA)	Oph	573
Guy, John (FL)	Oph	581	Hallett, John (SC)	VascS	1184
Guyton, David (MD)	Oph	573	Halligan, Gregory (PA)	PHO	759
Guyton, Robert (GA)	TS	1120	Hallisey, Michael (CT)	VIR	991
			Halmi, Katherine (NY)	Psyc	888
			Halperin, Henry (MD)	CE	118
			Halperin, Jonathan (NY)	Cv	97
			Halperin, Allan (NY)	D	187

H

Name	Specialty	Pg	Name	Specialty	Pg
Haas, Eric (TX)	CRS	175	Halpern, Howard (IL)	RadRO	958
Haas, Naomi (PA)	Onc	340	Halpern, Steven (NJ)	PHO	759
Haas, Richard (CA)	ChiN	151	Haluszka, Oleh (PA)	Ge	233
Haas, Steven (NY)	OrS	616	Halyard, Michele (AZ)	RadRO	962
Haber, Gregory (NY)	Ge	233	Hamilton, Stanley (TX)	Path	718
Habermann, Thomas (MN)	Hem	318	Hammar, Samuel (WA)	Path	720
Hackford, Alan (MA)	CRS	166	Hammer, Gary (MI)	EDM	215
Hackney, David (MA)	NRad	984	Hammer, Glenn (NY)	Inf	405
Haddad, Joseph (NY)	PO	789	Hammer, Scott (NY)	Inf	405
Hadler, Nortin (NC)	Rhu	1027	Hammerschlag, Paul (NY)	Oto	659
Hadley, Mark (AL)	NS	478	Hammill, Stephen (MN)	CE	120
Hadlock, Theresa (MA)	Oto	656	Hammond, Denis (NH)	Onc	328
Haffty, Bruce (NJ)	RadRO	948	Hammond, Dennis (MI)	PlS	863
Hagan, Kevin (TN)	PlS	859	Hamra, Sameer (TX)	PlS	868
Hageboutros, Alexandre (NJ)	Onc	340	Hamvas, Aaron (MO)	NP	446
Hager, W David (KY)	ObG	555	Han, Steven-Huy (CA)	Ge	253
Hagman, Jennifer (CO)	ChAP	908	Hanauer, Stephen (IL)	Ge	245
Hahn, Stephen (PA)	RadRO	948	Hancock, Steven (CA)	RadRO	964
Haid, Regis (GA)	NS	478	Handa, James (MD)	Oph	573
Haig, Andrew (MI)	PMR	838	Hande, Kenneth (TN)	Onc	355
Haik, Barrett (TN)	Oph	581	Handy, John (OR)	TS	1135

Name	Specialty	Pg	Name	Specialty	Pg
Hanel, Douglas (WA)	HS	303	Harris, David (TX)	PMR	841
Haney, Arthur (IL)	RE	1013	Harris, Gerald (IL)	HS	300
Hanifin, Jon (OR)	D	199	Harris, Jay (MA)	RadRO	944
Hanke, C William (IN)	D	193	Harris, Jeffrey (CA)	Oto	684
Hankins, Gary (TX)	MF	434	Harris, Michael (NJ)	PHO	759
Hankinson, Hal (NM)	NS	489	Harris, Nancy (MA)	Path	706
Hanks, John (VA)	S	1064	Harrison, J Kevin (NC)	Cv	102
Hanley, Frank (CA)	TS	1135	Harrison, Louis (NY)	RadRO	948
Hanna, Ehab (TX)	Oto	681	Harrop, James (PA)	NS	470
Hanna, Nader (MD)	S	1053	Harsh, Griffith (CA)	NS	493
Hannafin, Jo (NY)	OrS	616	Hartford, Alan (NH)	RadRO	944
Hansen, Juliana (OR)	PlS	872	Hartig, Gregory (WI)	Oto	674
Hansen, Kimberley (NC)	VascS	1184	Hartl, Roger (NY)	NS	470
Hansen, Nora (IL)	S	1073	Hartman, Barry (NY)	Inf	406
Hansen, Ronald (AZ)	D	197	Hartmann, Lynn (MN)	Onc	366
Hansen-Flaschen, John (PA)	Pul	923	Hartmann, Rene (FL)	CRS	170
Hanson, Laura (NC)	Ger	264	Hashim, Sabet (CT)	TS	1107
Hanssen, Arlen (MN)	OrS	632	Haskal, Ziv (MD)	VIR	992
Haque, Waheedul (TX)	Psyc	896	Hastings, Hill (IN)	HS	300
Har-El, Gady (NY)	Oto	659	Hatch, Kenneth (AZ)	GO	287
Haraf, Daniel (IL)	RadRO	958	Haughey, Bruce (MO)	Oto	674
Harari, Paul (WI)	RadRO	958	Haughton, Victor (WI)	NRad	988
Harati, Yadollah (TX)	N	531	Hauke, Ralph (NE)	Onc	374
Harbaugh, Robert (PA)	NS	470	Hauptman, Paul (MO)	Cv	106
Harber, Philip (CA)	OM	880	Hauser, Robert (FL)	N	519
Harbour, J William (MO)	Oph	587	Hauser, Stephen (CA)	N	535
Harden, R Norman (IL)	PM	698	Hausman, Michael (NY)	OrS	616
Hardesty, Robert (CA)	PlS	872	Haut, Paul (IN)	PHO	770
Hardin, Joel (IL)	PCd	738	Havrilesky, Laura (NC)	GO	281
Hare, Joshua (FL)	Cv	102	Hawes, Robert (SC)	Ge	240
Hargrove, W Clark (PA)	TS	1112	Hawkins, Douglas (WA)	PHO	776
Harken, Alden (CA)	TS	1135	Hayani, Ammar (IL)	PHO	770
Harley, Earl (DC)	PO	789	Hayashi, Robert (MO)	PHO	770
Harman, Eloise (FL)	Pul	928	Hayden, Richard (AZ)	Oto	681
Harmon, William (MA)	PNep	783	Hayes, Daniel (MI)	Onc	367
Harner, Christopher (PA)	SM	1037	Hayes, David (MN)	CE	121
Harnsberger, Jeffrey (NH)	CRS	166	Hayes, Sharonne (MN)	Cv	106
Harper, Richard (TX)	NS	489	Hayman, James (MI)	RadRO	958
Harpole, David (NC)	TS	1120	Haynes, David (TN)	Oto	667
Harrell, James (TX)	TS	1132	Haynes, Johnson (AL)	Pul	929
Harrington, Elizabeth (NY)	VascS	1182	Healey, John (NY)	OrS	616

Alphabetical Listing of Doctors

Name	Specialty	Pg	Name	Specialty	Pg
Healey, Patrick (WA)	PS	810	Hergenroeder, Albert (TX)	AM	81
Heber, David (CA)	EDM	220	Hering, Bernhard (MN)	S	1073
Hebert, James (VT)	S	1045	Herling, Irving (PA)	Cv	97
Hecht, Andrew (NY)	OrS	616	Herman, Martin (PA)	OrS	617
Heck, Christianne (CA)	N	535	Herman, Terence (OK)	RadRO	962
Heckenlively, John (MI)	Oph	588	Herman, William (MI)	EDM	215
Hecox, Kurt (WI)	N	525	Heros, Roberto (FL)	NS	478
Hedges, Thomas (MA)	Oph	568	Heroux, Alain (IL)	Cv	106
Heffner, John (OR)	Pul	937	Herr, Harry (NY)	U	1147
Heffner, Linda (MA)	MF	426	Herrine, Steven (PA)	Ge	233
Heiden, Eric (UT)	OrS	637	Herring, Stanley (WA)	PMR	842
Heilman, Carl (MA)	NS	466	Herrmann, Howard (PA)	IC	124
Heilman, Kenneth (FL)	N	519	Herrmann, Virginia (SC)	S	1064
Heimann, Ruth (VT)	RadRO	944	Hersh, Peter (NJ)	Oph	573
Heinrich, Michael (OR)	Hem	324	Hershey, Andrew (OH)	ChiN	149
Heitmiller, Richard (MD)	TS	1112	Hershman, Elliott (NY)	SM	1037
Helderman, J Harold (TN)	Nep	456	Hershorin, Eugene (FL)	Ped	727
Heldman, Alan (FL)	IC	127	Hertz, Marshall (MN)	Pul	931
Helfet, David (NY)	OrS	617	Hertzig, Margaret (NY)	ChAP	905
Hellenbrand, William (CT)	PCd	733	Herzenberg, John (MD)	OrS	617
Heller, Debra (NJ)	Path	709	Herzog, David (MA)	ChAP	903
Hellstrom, Wayne (LA)	U	1167	Herzog, Thomas (NY)	GO	278
Helman, Lee (MD)	PHO	759	Heslin, Martin (AL)	S	1064
Helvie, Mark (MI)	DR	980	Hess, David (GA)	N	519
Hemal, Ashok (NC)	U	1155	Hess, J Bruce (FL)	Oph	581
Hemming, Alan (CA)	S	1091	Hesselink, John (CA)	NRad	990
Henderson, Randal (FL)	RadRO	952	Hester, T Roderick (GA)	PlS	859
Henderson, Victor (CA)	N	535	Heston, Jerry (TN)	ChAP	906
Henderson, William (WA)	A&I	89	Hetherington, Maxine (MO)	PHO	770
Hendricks-Munoz, Karen (NY)	NP	443	Heuer, Dale (WI)	Oph	588
Heney, Niall (MA)	U	1142	Heyl, Peter (GA)	MF	430
Henke, David (NC)	Pul	929	Heyman, Melvin (CA)	PGe	754
Henry, David (PA)	Onc	340	Hibbard, Judith (IL)	MF	432
Henry, Timothy (MN)	IC	128	Hicks, Terry (LA)	CRS	175
Henschke, Claudia (NY)	DR	975	Hicks, Wesley (NY)	Oto	659
Henshaw, Robert (DC)	OrS	617	Hidalgo, David (NY)	PlS	852
Hensinger, Robert (MI)	OrS	632	Hiesiger, Emile (NY)	N	510
Hensle, Terry (NJ)	U	1147	Higano, Celestia (WA)	Onc	386
Hentz, Vincent (CA)	HS	303	Higashida, Randall (CA)	NRad	990
Heppell, Jacques (AZ)	CRS	175	Higgins, Steven (CA)	CE	123
Herbst, Roy (CT)	Onc	329	High, Kevin (NC)	Inf	409

Name	Specialty	Pg	Name	Specialty	Pg
Hijazi, Ziyad (IL)	PCd	738	Hofkosh, Dena (PA)	Ped	727
Hilden, Joanne (CO)	PHO	773	Hogan, Thomas (WV)	Onc	341
Hilfiker, Mary (CA)	PS	810	Hogikyan, Norman (MI)	Oto	674
Hilger, Peter (MN)	Oto	674	Holcomb, John (TX)	S	1084
Hilibrand, Alan (PA)	OrS	617	Holden, Stuart (CA)	U	1171
Hill, Ivor (NC)	PGe	751	Holick, Michael (MA)	EDM	205
Hill, Joseph (NH)	RE	1006	Holinger, Lauren (IL)	PO	791
Hill, Nicholas (MA)	Pul	921	Holland, Edward (OH)	Oph	588
Hillebrand, Donald (CA)	Ge	254	Holland, James (NY)	Onc	341
Himelstein, Andrew (DE)	Onc	341	Hollander, Eric (NY)	Psyc	888
Hinkle, Andrea (NY)	PCCM	741	Holliday, Michael (MD)	Oto	660
Hinshaw, Daniel (MI)	S	1073	Holliday, Roy (NY)	DR	975
Hiotis, Spiros (NY)	S	1054	Hollier, Larry (LA)	VascS	1187
Hirsch, Barry (PA)	Oto	659	Hollingsworth, Alan (OK)	S	1084
Hirsch, Glenn (NY)	ChAP	905	Hollister, Dickerman (CT)	Onc	329
Hirsch, Irl (WA)	EDM	220	Holmes, David (MN)	IC	129
Hirsch, Joshua (MA)	NRad	984	Holmes, Gregory (NH)	ChiN	144
Hirschfeld, Robert (TX)	Psyc	896	Holmes, Lewis (MA)	CG	154
Ho, Allen (PA)	Oph	573	Holroyd, Suzanne (VA)	GerPsy	911
Ho, Sherwin (IL)	SM	1039	Holterman, Mark (IL)	PS	807
Hochberg, Ephraim (MA)	Onc	329	Holtzman, Ronald (NC)	NP	445
Hochberg, Marc (MD)	Rhu	1024	Holzman, Ian (NY)	NP	443
Hochschuler, Stephen (TX)	OrS	639	Holzman, Lawrence (PA)	Nep	454
Hochster, Howard (CT)	Onc	329	Homans, Alan (VT)	PHO	755
Hockstein, Steven (NY)	ObG	553	Homer, Daniel (IL)	N	525
Hoda, Syed (NY)	Path	709	Hong, Waun (TX)	Onc	377
Hodapp, Elizabeth (FL)	Oph	582	Hoops, Timothy (PA)	Ge	233
Hodes, Jonathan (KY)	NS	478	Hoots, William (MD)	PHO	760
Hodgson, Kim (IL)	VascS	1185	Hopewell, Philip (CA)	Pul	937
Hodin, Richard (MA)	S	1045	Hopkins, L Nelson (NY)	NS	470
Hoffenberg, Edward (CO)	PGe	753	Hoppe, Richard (CA)	RadRO	964
Hoffman, Andrew (CA)	EDM	220	Hopping, Steven (DC)	Oto	660
Hoffman, Brenda (SC)	Ge	240	Hord, Jeffrey (OH)	PHO	770
Hoffman, Daniel (CO)	Psyc	895	Horn, Biljana (CA)	PHO	776
Hoffman, Henry (IA)	Oto	674	Horn, Evelyn (NY)	Cv	97
Hoffman, John (PA)	S	1054	Hornicek, Francis (MA)	OrS	609
Hoffman, Lloyd (NY)	PlS	852	Hornstein, Mark (MA)	RE	1006
Hoffman, Philip (IL)	Onc	367	Horowitz, Ira (GA)	GO	281
Hoffman, Robert (NY)	PrM	881	Horowitz, Jed (CA)	PlS	872
Hoffman, Ronald (NY)	Oto	659	Horsager, Robyn (TX)	MF	435
Hoffman, William (CA)	PlS	872	Hortobagyi, Gabriel (TX)	Onc	377

Alphabetical Listing of Doctors

I

J

Alphabetical Listing of Doctors

Name	Specialty	Pg	Name	Specialty	Pg
Jensen, Donald (IL)	Ge	245	Jonas, Adam (CA)	CG	161
Jensen, Mary (VA)	NRad	987	Jonas, Maureen (MA)	PGe	748
Jensen, Michael (MN)	EDM	216	Jonas, Richard (DC)	TS	1113
Jessen, Michael (TX)	TS	1132	Jonasch, Eric (TX)	Onc	378
Jessup, Mariell (PA)	Cv	97	Jones, David (VA)	TS	1120
Jewell, Mark (OR)	PlS	872	Jones, Deryk (LA)	SM	1040
Jhingran, Anuja (TX)	RadRO	962	Jones, H Royden (MA)	N	505
Jho, Hae-Dong (PA)	NS	471	Jones, J (OH)	U	1161
Jillella, Anand (GA)	Onc	356	Jones, Jacqueline (NY)	PO	789
Jimenez, David (TX)	NS	489	Jones, Kenneth (CA)	Ped	729
Jimerson, David (MA)	Psyc	885	Jones, Marilyn (CA)	CG	161
Jiranek, William (VA)	OrS	626	Jones, Neil (CA)	PlS	872
Jobst, Barbara (NH)	N	505	Jones, Paul (IL)	Oto	675
Johanson, Norman (PA)	OrS	618	Jones, Robert (DC)	Path	709
John, Thomas (IL)	Oph	588	Jordan, Barry (NY)	N	511
Johnson, Allen (CA)	Cv	115	Jordan, Stanley (CA)	PNep	787
Johnson, Annette (NC)	NRad	987	Jorizzo, Joseph (NC)	D	191
Johnson, Bruce (MA)	Onc	329	Jose, Baby (KY)	RadRO	953
Johnson, Bruce (VA)	Pul	929	Joseph, David (AL)	U	1155
Johnson, Calvin (LA)	Oto	681	Joseph, Gregory (NC)	NRad	987
Johnson, Carl (MD)	OrS	618	Josephs, Shelby (MD)	PA&I	729
Johnson, Darren (KY)	OrS	627	Josephson, David (IN)	N	525
Johnson, David (TX)	Onc	378	Josephson, Jordan (NY)	Oto	660
Johnson, Eric (CA)	OrS	642	Josephson, Mark (MA)	CE	117
Johnson, Jonas (PA)	Oto	660	Josephson, Michelle (IL)	Nep	458
Johnson, Julia (MA)	RE	1007	Joyce, Lyle (MN)	TS	1127
Johnson, Maryl (WI)	Cv	107	Joyce, Michael (OH)	OrS	632
Johnson, Matthew (IN)	VIR	994	Juckett, Mark (WI)	Hem	319
Johnson, Paula (MA)	Cv	92	Judelson, Debra (CA)	Cv	115
Johnson, Ronald (PA)	S	1054	Judy, Kevin (PA)	NS	471
Johnson, Scott (TX)	TS	1132	Julian, Thomas (PA)	S	1054
Johnson, Stephen (CO)	NS	487	Jupiter, Jesse (MA)	OrS	610
Johnson, Timothy (MI)	MF	432	Jurcic, Joseph (NY)	Onc	342
Johnson, Timothy (MI)	D	194			
Johnson Miller, Denise (IN)	S	1074			
Johnston, Carolyn (MI)	GO	284	**K**		
Johnston, J Martin (GA)	PHO	765			
Johnston, James (PA)	Nep	454	Kachnic, Lisa (MA)	RadRO	944
Johnstone, Peter (IN)	RadRO	958	Kadmon, Dov (TX)	U	1167
Johr, Robert (FL)	D	191	Kaeding, Christopher (OH)	OrS	632
Jokl, Peter (CT)	OrS	609	Kaefer, Martin (IN)	U	1161

Name	Specialty	Pg	Name	Specialty	Pg
Kagan, Richard (OH)	S	1074	Kaplan, Michael (CA)	Oto	684
Kahn, Barbara (MA)	EDM	205	Kaplan, Sheldon (TX)	PInf	782
Kahn, Leonard (NY)	Path	709	Kaplan, Steven (NY)	U	1148
Kahrilas, Peter (IL)	Ge	245	Kaplitt, Michael (NY)	NS	471
Kaiser, Larry (PA)	TS	1113	Kapoor, Neena (CA)	PHO	776
Kaiser, Michael (NY)	NS	471	Kappy, Michael (CO)	PEn	747
Kalaycio, Matt (OH)	Onc	367	Kapur, Sandip (NY)	S	1054
Kalb, Robert (NY)	D	187	Karas, Spero (GA)	OrS	627
Kalemkerian, Gregory (MI)	Onc	367	Karasu, T Byram (NY)	Psyc	888
Kaliner, Michael (MD)	A&I	85	Karlan, Beth (CA)	GO	290
Kallmes, David (MN)	NRad	988	Karlan, Scott (CA)	S	1091
Kalloo, Anthony (MD)	Ge	234	Karp, Daniel (TX)	Onc	378
Kamani, Naynesh (DC)	PA&I	729	Karp, Judith (MD)	Onc	342
Kamdar, Vikram (CA)	EDM	221	Karpeh, Martin (NY)	S	1054
Kamelhar, David (NY)	Pul	923	Karram, Mickey (OH)	ObG	557
Kamen, Barton (NJ)	PHO	760	Karrer, Frederick (CO)	PS	808
Kaminski, Mark (MI)	Onc	367	Kartush, Jack (MI)	Oto	675
Kampman, Kyle (PA)	AdP	901	Karwande, Shreekanth (UT)	TS	1130
Kanal, Emanuel (PA)	DR	976	Kase, Carlos (MA)	N	506
Kanda, Louis (DC)	TS	1113	Kashtan, Clifford (MN)	PNep	786
Kandeel, Fouad (CA)	EDM	221	Kasinath, Balakuntalam S (TX)	Nep	460
Kandzari, David (GA)	IC	127	Kasiske, Bertram (MN)	Nep	458
Kane, Alex (TX)	PlS	868	Kasner, Scott (PA)	N	511
Kane, Javier (TN)	PHO	765	Kass, Evan (MI)	U	1161
Kane, Kay (MA)	D	183	Kassam, Amin (CA)	NS	493
Kane, Madeleine (CO)	Onc	374	Kasser, James (MA)	OrS	610
Kane, Timothy (DC)	PS	803	Kastenberg, David (PA)	Ge	234
Kanel, Gary (CA)	Path	720	Katirji, Bashar (OH)	N	525
Kang, Dong-Kyoo (OH)	Oto	675	Katner, Harold (GA)	Inf	409
Kantarjian, Hagop (TX)	Hem	322	Kato, Tomoaki (NY)	S	1054
Kanter, Kirk (GA)	TS	1120	Katowitz, James (PA)	Oph	574
Kantoff, Philip (MA)	Onc	329	Kattan, Meyer (NY)	PPul	793
Kantsevoy, Sergey (MD)	Ge	234	Kattwinkel, John (VA)	NP	445
Kaouk, Jihad (OH)	U	1161	Katz, Aaron (NY)	U	1148
Kaplan, Bernard (PA)	PNep	784	Katz, Nevin (MD)	TS	1113
Kaplan, David (CO)	AM	81	Katz, Philip (PA)	Ge	234
Kaplan, Frederick (PA)	OrS	618	Katz, Robert (OH)	PO	791
Kaplan, Irving (MA)	RadRO	944	Katz, Robert (IL)	Rhu	1029
Kaplan, James (KS)	Pul	934	Katz, Stuart (NY)	Cv	98
Kaplan, Lawrence (CA)	Onc	386	Katzen, Barry (FL)	VIR	994
Kaplan, Lee (MA)	Ge	229	Katzenstein, Anna-Luise (NY)	Path	709

Alphabetical Listing of Doctors

Name	Specialty	Pg	Name	Specialty	Pg
Katznelson, Laurence (CA)	EDM	221	Kelly, Karen (CA)	Onc	386
Kaufman, Bruce (WI)	NS	484	Kelly, Kevin (TN)	PlS	860
Kaufman, Cary (WA)	S	1091	Kelly, Thomas (CA)	MF	436
Kaufman, Howard (IL)	S	1074	Kelly, William (PA)	Onc	342
Kaufman, John (OR)	VIR	997	Kelsen, David (NY)	Onc	342
Kaufman, Paul (WI)	Oph	588	Kemeny, Nancy (NY)	Onc	342
Kaufman, Peter (NH)	Onc	329	Kemp, James (MO)	PPul	796
Kaufman, Richard (MA)	Path	706	Kempin, Sanford (NY)	Hem	311
Kaul, Sanjiv (OR)	Cv	115	Kenan, Samuel (NY)	OrS	618
Kavanah, Maureen (MA)	S	1046	Kendrick, Michael (MN)	S	1074
Kavey, Neil (NY)	Psyc	889	Kenkel, Jeffrey (TX)	PlS	868
Kavoussi, Louis (NY)	U	1148	Kennedy, David (PA)	Oto	660
Kawachi, Mark (CA)	U	1171	Kennedy, Gary (NY)	GerPsy	910
Kawamoto, Henry (CA)	PlS	873	Kennedy, Laurence (OH)	EDM	216
Kay, Dennis (LA)	VIR	996	Kennelly, Michael (NC)	U	1155
Kay, G Neal (AL)	CE	120	Kent, Kenneth (WI)	VascS	1186
Kay, Jonathan (MA)	Rhu	1022	Kent, Thomas (TX)	N	532
Kaye, Mitchell (MN)	Pul	931	Kenter, Keith (OH)	OrS	633
Kaysen, George (CA)	Nep	461	Kereiakes, Dean (OH)	Cv	107
Kazahaya, Ken (PA)	PO	789	Kern, Jeffrey (CO)	Pul	934
Kazer, Ralph (IL)	RE	1013	Kern, Robert (IL)	Oto	675
Kazmers, Andris (MI)	VascS	1185	Kernstine, Kemp (TX)	TS	1132
Keane, Thomas (SC)	U	1155	Kerr, Natalie (TN)	Oph	582
Keane, William (PA)	Oto	660	Kerrihard, Thomas (CA)	Psyc	897
Keating, Gesina (MN)	ChiN	149	Kesari, Santosh (CA)	Onc	386
Keating, Michael (TX)	Hem	322	Kesser, Bradley (VA)	Oto	667
Keen, Mary (IL)	PMR	839	Kessler, Craig (DC)	Hem	311
Keenan, Robert (PA)	TS	1113	Kestle, John RW (UT)	NS	487
Keens, Thomas (CA)	PPul	797	Ketcham, Douglas (MN)	VIR	995
Keepers, George (OR)	Psyc	897	Kevorkian, Charles (TX)	PMR	841
Keiser, Philip (TX)	Inf	412	Kezar, Laura (AL)	PMR	837
Kelepouris, Ellie (PA)	Nep	454	Khan, Agha (MD)	NS	471
Keller, Frank (GA)	PHO	765	Khandji, Alexander (NY)	NRad	985
Keller, Frederick (OR)	VIR	997	Khawaja, Shazib (GA)	IC	127
Keller, Gregory (CA)	Oto	684	Khosla, Sundeep (MN)	EDM	216
Keller, Steven (NY)	TS	1113	Khuri, Fadlo (GA)	Onc	356
Kelley, Joseph (PA)	GO	278	Kibel, Adam (MO)	U	1162
Kelley, Mark (TN)	S	1064	Kidwell, Earl (DC)	Oph	574
Kelly, Cynthia (CO)	OrS	637	Kieran, Mark (MA)	PHO	756
Kelly, Cynthia (VA)	PA&I	731	Kiernan, Paul (VA)	TS	1121
Kelly, James (CO)	N	530	Kies, Merrill (TX)	Onc	378

Alphabetical Listing of Doctors

Name	Specialty	Pg	Name	Specialty	Pg
Kiev, Jonathan (MD)	TS	1114	Klaas, Virginia (WA)	NuM	547
Kilmer, Suzanne (CA)	D	199	Klagsbrun, Samuel (NY)	Psyc	889
Kim, Choll (CA)	OrS	642	Klapheke, Martin (FL)	Psyc	892
Kim, Daniel (TX)	NS	489	Kleber, Herbert (NY)	AdP	901
Kim, Dong (TX)	NS	489	Kleiman, Martin (IN)	PInf	782
Kim, Edward (TN)	U	1155	Kleiman, Neal (TX)	IC	129
Kim, Jae Ho (MI)	RadRO	958	Klein, Andrew (CA)	S	1092
Kim, Jonathan (CA)	Oph	598	Klein, Eric (OH)	U	1162
Kim, Julian (OH)	S	1074	Klein, Lloyd (IL)	Cv	107
Kim, Lawrence (AR)	S	1085	Klein, Patricia (NJ)	N	511
Kim, Youn-Hee (CA)	D	199	Klein, Robert (RI)	PA&I	729
Kim, Young-Jee (IN)	PPul	796	Klein-Gitelman, Marisa (IL)	PRhu	800
Kimberly, Robert (AL)	Rhu	1027	Kleinberg, David (NY)	EDM	209
Kimmey, Michael (WA)	Ge	254	Kleinberg, Lawrence (MD)	RadRO	949
Kincaid, John (IN)	N	525	Kleinerman, Eugenie (TX)	Ped	728
Kindler, Hedy (IL)	Onc	367	Kleinman, Ronald (MA)	PGe	748
King, Aileen (ID)	ObG	558	Kleinman, William (IN)	HS	300
King, Andrew (CA)	Nep	462	Klibanski, Anne (MA)	EDM	205
King, Bryan (WA)	ChAP	908	Kliger, Alan (CT)	Nep	452
King, Earl (PA)	Pul	924	Klimberg, Vicki (AR)	S	1085
King, John (TX)	PMR	841	Kline, Mark (TX)	PInf	783
King, Richard (GA)	PMR	837	Kline, Richard (LA)	GO	288
King, Robert (CT)	ChAP	903	Klingemann, Hans-Georg (MA)	Hem	308
King, Stephanie (PA)	GO	278	Klingensmith, Georgeanna (CO)	PEn	747
King, Talmadge (CA)	Pul	938	Klonoff, David (CA)	EDM	221
Kingdom, Todd (CO)	Oto	679	Kloos, Richard (OH)	EDM	216
Kinkhabwala, Milan (NY)	S	1055	Klutke, Carl (MO)	U	1162
Kinney, Marsha (TX)	Path	718	Knechtle, Stuart (GA)	S	1064
Kipen, Howard (NJ)	OM	880	Kneisl, Jeffrey (NC)	OrS	627
Kipps, Thomas (CA)	Hem	324	Knopf, William (GA)	IC	127
Kirgan, Daniel (NV)	S	1091	Knudson, Mary (CA)	S	1092
Kirklin, James (AL)	TS	1121	Kobashigawa, Jon (CA)	Cv	115
Kirkwood, John (PA)	Onc	342	Kobrin, Sidney (PA)	Nep	454
Kirschenbaum, Alexander (NY)	U	1148	Kobrine, Arthur (DC)	NS	471
Kirschner, Barbara (IL)	PGe	752	Kobrinsky, Nathan (ND)	PHO	773
Kirschner, Kristi (IL)	PMR	839	Koch, Christian (MS)	EDM	212
Kirschner, Richard (OH)	PlS	863	Koch, Douglas (TX)	Oph	594
Kirshblum, Steven (NJ)	PMR	834	Koch, Kenneth (NC)	Ge	240
Kirshenbaum, James (MA)	Cv	92	Koch, Michael (IN)	U	1162
Kirshner, Howard (TN)	N	520	Koch, Wayne (MD)	Oto	661
Kirsner, Robert (FL)	D	191	Kocher, Mininder (MA)	OrS	610

Alphabetical Listing of Doctors

Name	Specialty	Pg	Name	Specialty	Pg
Kochman, Michael (PA)	Ge	234	Kotloff, Karen (MD)	PInf	779
Koczywas, Marianna (CA)	Onc	386	Kotloff, Robert (PA)	Pul	924
Kodner, Ira (MO)	CRS	172	Koufman, Jamie (NY)	Oto	661
Koeller, Kelly (MN)	NRad	988	Kougias, Panagiotis (TX)	VascS	1187
Koff, Stephen (OH)	U	1162	Koulos, John (NY)	GO	278
Koh, Jeffrey (OR)	PM	701	Kovitz, Kevin (IL)	Pul	932
Koh, Wui-Jin (WA)	RadRO	964	Kovnar, Edward (WI)	ChiN	149
Kohler, Matthew (SC)	GO	281	Kowalski, Thomas (PA)	Ge	235
Kokotailo, Patricia (WI)	AM	80	Kozarek, Richard (WA)	Ge	254
Koller, Harold (PA)	Oph	574	Kozin, Scott (PA)	HS	296
Kolodny, Edwin (NY)	N	511	Kozlowski, James (IL)	U	1162
Komaki, Ritsuko (TX)	RadRO	963	Kraay, Matthew (OH)	OrS	633
Koman, L Andrew (NC)	HS	299	Krackow, Kenneth (NY)	OrS	618
Komrokji, Rami (FL)	Hem	315	Kraft, Andrew (SC)	Onc	356
Kondziolka, Douglas (PA)	NS	472	Kraft, George (WA)	PMR	842
Konicek, Frank (IL)	Ge	245	Krag, David (VT)	S	1046
Konski, Andre (MI)	RadRO	958	Krajcer, Zvonimir (TX)	Cv	112
Konstam, Marvin (MA)	Cv	93	Kramer, Barry (CA)	GerPsy	912
Konstan, Michael (OH)	PPul	796	Krasna, Mark (MD)	TS	1114
Koo, John (CA)	D	199	Kraus, Dennis (NY)	Oto	661
Koos, Brian (CA)	MF	437	Kraus, Michael (IN)	Nep	458
Kopans, Daniel (MA)	DR	973	Krauss, Gregory (MD)	N	511
Kopf, Gary (CT)	TS	1107	Kraut, Eric (OH)	Hem	319
Koplewicz, Harold (NY)	ChAP	905	Krebs, Nancy (CO)	PGe	753
Koplin, Lawrence (CA)	PlS	873	Kreissman, Susan (NC)	PHO	765
Kopp, Peter (IL)	EDM	216	Kreitzer, Joel (NY)	PM	695
Korenblat, Phillip (MO)	A&I	88	Krellenstein, Daniel (NY)	TS	1114
Korf, Bruce (AL)	CG	157	Krespi, Yosef (NY)	Oto	661
Kormos, Robert (PA)	TS	1114	Kress, Douglas (PA)	D	187
Kornmehl, Ernest (MA)	Oph	568	Kress, Kenneth (GA)	OrS	627
Korones, David (NY)	PHO	760	Kressel, Bruce (DC)	Onc	342
Korsten, Mark (NY)	Ge	234	Kriegel, David (NY)	D	187
Koruda, Mark (NC)	S	1064	Krieger, Karl (NY)	TS	1114
Korytkowski, Mary (PA)	EDM	209	Krilov, Leonard (NY)	PInf	779
Kosofsky, Barry (NY)	ChiN	146	Kris, Mark (NY)	Onc	342
Koss, Michael (CA)	Path	721	Krishnamurthi, Smitha (OH)	Onc	368
Kosten, Thomas (TX)	AdP	902	Krisht, Ali (AR)	NS	489
Kostis, John (NJ)	Cv	98	Kron, Irving (VA)	TS	1121
Kotagal, Suresh (MN)	ChiN	149	Kronenberg, Henry (MA)	EDM	205
Kotapka, Mark (PA)	NS	472	Kronn, David (NY)	CG	156
Kotler, Donald (NY)	Ge	234	Krontiras, Helen (AL)	S	1064

Alphabetical Listing of Doctors

Name	Specialty	Pg
Krouse, Robert (AZ)	S	1085
Krowka, Michael (MN)	Pul	932
Krueger, Gerald (UT)	D	196
Krueger, Richard (NY)	Psyc	889
Krueger, Ronald (OH)	Oph	588
Krumholz, Allan (MD)	N	511
Krummel, Thomas (CA)	PS	810
Krunic, Aleksandar (IL)	D	194
Kucharczuk, John (PA)	TS	1114
Kucuk, Omer (GA)	Onc	356
Kudrimoti, Mahesh (KY)	RadRO	953
Kuettel, Michael (NY)	RadRO	949
Kuhel, William (NY)	Oto	661
Kuhn, Frederick (GA)	Oto	667
Kuhn, Joseph (TX)	S	1085
Kuiken, Todd (IL)	PMR	839
Kula, Roger (NY)	N	511
Kulick, Roy (NY)	HS	296
Kuller, Jeffrey (NC)	MF	431
Kumpe, David (CO)	VIR	996
Kun, Larry (TN)	RadRO	953
Kung, Faith (CA)	PHO	777
Kunkel, Elisabeth (PA)	Psyc	889
Kunschner, Lara (PA)	N	511
Kuntz, Charles (OH)	NS	484
Kupelian, Patrick (CA)	RadRO	964
Kupersmith, Mark (NY)	Oph	574
Kupfer, David (PA)	Psyc	889
Kupper, Thomas (MA)	D	183
Kurachek, Stephen (MN)	PPul	796
Kuriakose, Philip (MI)	Hem	319
Kurland, Geoffrey (PA)	PPul	794
Kurman, Robert (MD)	Path	710
Kurtin, Paul (MN)	Path	715
Kurtz, Alfred (PA)	DR	976
Kurtz, Robert (NY)	Ge	235
Kurtzberg, Joanne (NC)	PHO	765
Kurtzke, Robert (VA)	N	520
Kushner, Brian (NY)	PHO	760
Kushner, Burton (WI)	Oph	588
Kuske, Robert (AZ)	RadRO	963
Kutner, Jean (CO)	Ger	266
Kutteh, William (TN)	RE	1011
Kuttesch, John (PA)	PHO	760
Kuvin, Jeffrey (MA)	Cv	93
Kuzel, Timothy (IL)	Onc	368
Kuzniecky, Ruben (NY)	N	512
Kuzon, William (MI)	PlS	863
Kveton, John (CT)	Oto	656
Kvols, Larry (FL)	Onc	356
Kwak, Larry (TX)	Onc	378
Kwo, Paul (IN)	Ge	246
Kwolek, Christopher (MA)	VascS	1179
Kwon, Hower (WA)	ChAP	909
Kwon, Young (IA)	Oph	588

L

Name	Specialty	Pg
La Ban, Myron (MI)	PMR	839
La Gamma, Edmund (NY)	NP	443
La Quaglia, Michael (NY)	PS	803
La Russo, Nicholas (MN)	Ge	246
Labar, Douglas (NY)	N	512
Labiner, David (AZ)	N	532
Labovitz, Arthur (MO)	Cv	107
Lachs, Mark (NY)	Ger	263
Lackman, Richard (PA)	OrS	618
Lacomis, David (PA)	N	512
Lacy, Jill (CT)	Onc	329
Ladenson, Paul (MD)	EDM	209
Lage, Janice (SC)	Path	713
Laham, Roger (MA)	IC	123
Laheru, Daniel (MD)	Onc	343
Lahita, Robert (NJ)	Rhu	1024
Laks, Hillel (CA)	TS	1136
Lalwani, Anil (NY)	Oto	661
Lambert, H Michael (TX)	Oph	594
Lambert, Paul (SC)	Oto	667
Lambert, Scott (GA)	Oph	582
Lamberti, John (CA)	TS	1136
Lambiase, Louis (TN)	Ge	240

Alphabetical Listing of Doctors

Name	Specialty	Pg	Name	Specialty	Pg
Lamonica, Dominick (NY)	NuM	544	Lash, Robert (MI)	EDM	216
LaMuraglia, Glenn M (MA)	VascS	1179	Lashner, Bret (OH)	Ge	246
Lancaster, Johnathan (FL)	GO	282	Lask, Gary (CA)	D	199
Landefeld, Charles (CA)	Ger	267	Laske, Douglas (PA)	NS	472
Landers, Daniel (MN)	MF	432	Lass, Jonathan (OH)	Oph	589
Landon, Mark (OH)	MF	432	Latchaw, Laurie (NH)	PS	801
Landreneau, Rodney (PA)	TS	1114	Laterra, John (MD)	N	512
Landrigan, Philip (NY)	OM	880	Latov, Norman (NY)	N	512
Landry, Jerome (GA)	RadRO	953	Latson, Larry (FL)	PCd	737
Landy, Helain (DC)	MF	429	Lau, Christine (VA)	TS	1121
Landy, Howard (FL)	NS	478	Lauerman, William (DC)	OrS	619
Landzberg, Joel (NJ)	Cv	98	Laufer, Marc (MA)	ObG	552
Lane, Joseph (NY)	OrS	619	Laughlin, Mary (VA)	Hem	315
Lane, Lewis (NY)	HS	296	Laurencin, Cato (CT)	OrS	610
Lane, Stephen (MN)	Oph	589	Lavenstein, Bennett (VA)	ChiN	148
Lang, Frederick (TX)	NS	489	Laver, Joseph (TN)	PHO	766
Lang, Peter (MA)	PCd	733	Lavertu, Pierre (OH)	Oto	675
Lang, Samuel (NY)	TS	1114	Lavery, Ian (OH)	CRS	172
Lange, Beverly (PA)	PHO	760	Lavin, Patrick (TN)	N	520
Lange, Paul (WA)	U	1171	Lavis, Victor (TX)	EDM	219
Langer, Corey (PA)	Onc	343	Lavyne, Michael (NY)	NS	472
Langford, Carol (OH)	Rhu	1029	Lawrence, Theodore (MI)	RadRO	958
Langman, Craig (IL)	PNep	786	Lawry, George (CA)	Rhu	1032
Langston, J William (CA)	N	535	Lawson, David (GA)	Onc	356
Lannin, Donald (CT)	S	1046	Lawson, Edward (MD)	NP	443
Lansman, Steven (NY)	TS	1115	Lawson, William (NY)	Oto	661
Lanteri, Vincent (NJ)	U	1148	Lawson, William (DC)	Psyc	889
Lantos, John (MO)	Ped	728	Lazar, Harold (MA)	TS	1107
Lanza, Donald (FL)	Oto	668	Lazarus, Hillard (OH)	Hem	319
Lanza, Louis (AZ)	TS	1132	Lazzaro, Richard (NY)	TS	1115
Lapey, Allen (MA)	PPul	793	Le, Quynh-Thu Xuan (CA)	RadRO	965
Laramore, George (WA)	RadRO	965	Le Boit, Philip (CA)	Path	721
Larner, James (VA)	RadRO	953	Lea, Janice (GA)	Nep	456
Larrabee, Wayne (WA)	Oto	685	Leach, Steven (MD)	S	1055
Larsen, Christian (GA)	S	1065	Leadbetter, Wayne (MD)	OrS	619
Larsen, Donald (CA)	NRad	991	Leaf, Norman (CA)	PlS	873
Larsen, Philip Reed (MA)	EDM	205	LeBoff, Meryl (MA)	EDM	206
Larson, David (CA)	RadRO	965	Lebovics, Robert (NY)	Oto	661
Larson, Richard (IL)	Hem	319	Lebwohl, Mark (NY)	D	187
Larson, Steven (NY)	NuM	544	Lebwohl, Nathan (FL)	OrS	627
Lasala, John (MO)	IC	129	Lebwohl, Oscar (NY)	Ge	235

Name	Specialty	Pg	Name	Specialty	Pg
Lechan, Ronald (MA)	EDM	206	Leonetti, John (IL)	Oto	675
Leckman, James (CT)	ChAP	903	Lepanto, Philip (WV)	RadRO	949
Lederman, Eric (MO)	CRS	172	Lepor, Herbert (NY)	U	1148
Ledford, Dennis (FL)	A&I	86	Lerman, Bruce (NY)	CE	118
Lee, Andrew (TX)	RadRO	963	Lerner, Seth (TX)	U	1167
Lee, Andrew (TX)	Oph	594	Les, Kimberly (MI)	OrS	633
Lee, Cheryl (MI)	U	1162	Lesavoy, Malcolm (CA)	PlS	873
Lee, Chung (MN)	RadRO	959	Leshin, Barry (NC)	D	191
Lee, Francis (NY)	OrS	619	Leslie, Donald (GA)	PMR	837
Lee, Jeffrey (TX)	S	1085	Leslie, Kevin (AZ)	Path	718
Lee, Joon (PA)	IC	125	Leslie, Kimberly (IA)	MF	433
Lee, Kenneth (PA)	S	1055	Lesser, Glenn (NC)	Onc	356
Lee, Patrick (OR)	CRS	176	Lessin, Stuart (PA)	D	187
Lee, Paul (NC)	Oph	582	Leuchter, Andrew (CA)	Psyc	897
Lee, Raphael (IL)	PlS	864	Leung, Donald (CO)	PA&I	732
Lee, W P Andrew (MD)	HS	296	Leung, Lawrence (CA)	Hem	324
Lee, W Robert (NC)	RadRO	953	Leung, Wing (TN)	PHO	766
Leeming, Rosemary (OH)	S	1074	Levenback, Charles (TX)	GO	288
Leffell, David (CT)	D	183	Leventhal, Bennett (NY)	ChAP	905
Legare, Robert (RI)	Onc	330	Levi, Allan (FL)	NS	478
Legido, Agustin (PA)	ChiN	146	Levi, Joe (FL)	S	1065
Legro, Richard (PA)	RE	1008	Levin, David (OK)	Pul	936
Lehman, Constance (WA)	DR	983	Levin, Lawrence Scott (PA)	PlS	853
Lehman, Thomas (NY)	PRhu	799	Levine, Alexandra (CA)	Hem	324
Leichtner, Alan (MA)	PGe	748	Levine, David (NY)	N	512
Leighton, Jonathan (AZ)	Ge	251	Levine, David (NY)	OrS	619
Leipziger, Lyle (NY)	PlS	853	Levine, Edward (NC)	S	1065
Leitch, A Marilyn (TX)	S	1085	Levine, Elliot (IL)	ObG	558
Lele, Shashikant (NY)	GO	279	Levine, Ellis (NY)	Onc	343
Lem, Vincent (MO)	Pul	932	Levine, Joel (CT)	Ge	229
Lemanske, Robert (WI)	PA&I	731	Levine, Joseph (NY)	CE	118
Lemole, G Michael (AZ)	NS	490	Levine, Joshua (NY)	PlS	853
Lemons, James (IN)	NP	446	Levine, Laurence (IL)	U	1162
Lengyel, Ernst (IL)	ObG	558	Levine, Michael (PA)	PEn	744
Lenke, Lawrence (MO)	OrS	633	Levine, Paul (VA)	Oto	668
Lentz, Christopher (NM)	S	1085	Levine, Robert (NH)	EDM	206
Lentz, Samuel (NC)	GO	282	Levine, Stephen (OH)	Psyc	893
Lenz, Heinz (CA)	Ge	254	Levine, Steven (NY)	N	512
Leon, Martin (NY)	IC	125	Levine, William (NY)	SM	1037
Leonard, Ethan (OH)	PInf	782	Levitsky, Lynne (MA)	PEn	743
Leonard, James (MI)	PMR	839	Levy, Angela (DC)	DR	976

Alphabetical Listing of Doctors

Name	Specialty	Pg	Name	Specialty	Pg
Levy, Joseph (NY)	PGe	749	Lilenbaum, Rogerio (FL)	Onc	357
Levy, Michael (PA)	Onc	343	Lill, Michael (CA)	Hem	324
Levy, Michael (CA)	NS	493	Lillehei, Craig (MA)	PS	801
Levy, Moise (TX)	D	197	Lillehei, Kevin (CO)	NS	487
Levy, Richard (IL)	PEn	746	Lillemoe, Keith (MA)	S	1046
Levy, Steven (GA)	Psyc	892	Lim, Dean Wee (CA)	Onc	386
Lew, Mark (CA)	N	536	Lim, Henry (MI)	D	194
Lewin, Alan (FL)	RadRO	953	Lim Quan, Katherine (AZ)	D	197
Lewin, Mark (WA)	PCd	740	Limentani, Steven (NC)	Onc	357
Lewin, Neal (NY)	IM	419	Lin, Daniel (WA)	U	1171
Lewis, Blair (NY)	Ge	235	Lin, Jeffrey (DC)	GO	279
Lewis, Curtis (GA)	VIR	994	Lin, Weei-Chin (TX)	Hem	323
Lewis, John (AZ)	A&I	89	Lind, Christopher (TN)	Ge	241
Lewis, Richard (TX)	Oph	594	Lind, David (GA)	S	1065
Lewis, Richard (MI)	N	525	Lindenfeld, JoAnn (CO)	Cv	111
Lewis, Sandra (OR)	Cv	115	Lindor, Keith (MN)	Ge	246
Lewkowiez, Laurent (CO)	CE	122	Lindsay, Bruce (OH)	CE	121
Li, Benjamin (LA)	S	1085	Lindsey, Stephen (LA)	Rhu	1031
Li Volsi, Virginia (PA)	Path	710	Lindstrom, Richard (MN)	Oph	589
Liang, Bruce (CT)	Cv	93	Linenberger, Michael (WA)	Hem	324
Liao, Kenneth (MN)	TS	1127	Link, Mark (MA)	CE	117
Liau, Linda (CA)	NS	493	Link, Michael (CA)	PHO	777
Libby, Daniel (NY)	Pul	924	Link, Michael (MN)	NS	484
Liberman, Robert (CA)	Psyc	898	Linsenmeyer, Todd (NJ)	U	1148
Libertino, John (MA)	U	1143	Linskey, Mark (CA)	NS	493
Libutti, Steven (NY)	S	1055	Linstrom, Christopher (NY)	Oto	662
Licata, Angelo (OH)	EDM	216	Linton, MacRae (TN)	Cv	102
Licciardi, Frederick (NY)	RE	1009	Lipkin, David (FL)	PMR	837
Lichtenstein, Gary (PA)	Ge	235	Lipkowitz, George (MA)	S	1046
Lichter, Paul (MI)	Oph	589	Liporace, Joyce (PA)	N	512
Liddle, Rodger (NC)	Ge	241	Lippman, Marc (FL)	Onc	357
Lieberman, Michael (NY)	S	1055	Lippman, Scott (TX)	Onc	378
Lieberman, Phillip (TN)	A&I	86	Lipschitz, David (AR)	Ger	266
Liebmann, Jeffrey (NY)	Oph	574	Lipshultz, Larry (TX)	U	1168
Liebson, Philip (IL)	Cv	107	Lipshutz, William (PA)	Ge	235
Liem, Pham (AR)	Ger	266	Lipsitz, Lewis (MA)	Ger	262
Lieskovsky, Gary (CA)	U	1171	Lipson, Ace (DC)	EDM	209
Light, Richard (TN)	Pul	929	Lipstate, James (LA)	Rhu	1031
Light, Terry (IL)	HS	300	Lipton, Jeffrey (NY)	PHO	761
Lightdale, Charles (NY)	Ge	235	Lipton, Richard (NY)	N	513
Liker, Mark (CA)	NS	493	Lisak, Robert (MI)	N	525

Name	Specialty	Pg	Name	Specialty	Pg
Lisman, Richard (NY)	Oph	574	LoRusso, Thomas (VA)	Pul	929
List, Alan (FL)	Onc	357	Loscalzo, Joseph (MA)	Cv	93
Little, John (DC)	PlS	853	Losee, Joseph (PA)	PlS	853
Litzow, Mark (MN)	Hem	319	Losordo, Douglas (IL)	IC	129
Liu, Charles (CA)	NS	494	Lossos, Izidore (FL)	Onc	357
Liu, Donald (IL)	PS	807	Lott, Ira (CA)	ChiN	151
Liu, Grant (PA)	N	513	Loughlin, Gerald (NY)	PPul	794
Liu, Vincent (IA)	D	194	Loughlin, Kevin (MA)	U	1143
Livingston, Edward (TX)	S	1086	Louie, Eddie (NY)	Inf	406
Livingston, Robert (AZ)	Onc	379	Loulmet, Didier (NY)	TS	1115
Livingstone, Alan (FL)	S	1065	Love, Charles (OH)	CE	121
Ljung, Britt-Marie (CA)	Path	721	Love, Robert (IL)	TS	1127
Lloyd, L Keith (AL)	U	1155	Low, David (PA)	PlS	854
Lobe, Thom (CA)	PS	810	Lowe, Franklin (NY)	U	1149
Locala, Joseph (OH)	Psyc	894	Lowe, Lori (MI)	D	194
Lock, James (MA)	PCd	733	Lowenberg, David (CA)	OrS	642
Lock, Terrence (MI)	OrS	633	Lowitt, Mark (MD)	D	187
Lockey, Richard (FL)	A&I	86	Lowry, Ann (MN)	CRS	172
Lockhart, Jorge (FL)	U	1156	Lowy, Andrew (CA)	S	1092
Lockshin, Michael (NY)	Rhu	1024	Loyd, James (TN)	Pul	929
Lockwood, Charles (CT)	MF	427	Lu, Karen (TX)	GO	288
Loder, Elizabeth (MA)	PM	694	Lubahn, John (PA)	HS	296
Loeb, David (MD)	PHO	761	Lublin, Fred (NY)	N	513
Loeffler, Jay (MA)	RadRO	945	Luby, James (TX)	Inf	412
Loehrer, Patrick (IN)	Onc	368	Luby, Joan (MO)	ChAP	907
Loevner, Laurie (PA)	NRad	985	Lucarelli, Mark (WI)	Oph	589
Loewenstein, Richard (MD)	Psyc	889	Lucas, David (MI)	Path	716
Loftus, Christopher (PA)	NS	472	Lucci, Joseph (FL)	GO	282
Loftus, Edward (MN)	Ge	246	Lucente, Vincent (PA)	ObG	553
Logan, William (MO)	N	525	Lucey, Michael (WI)	Ge	246
Loggie, Brian (NE)	S	1080	Luchtman-Jones, Lori (DC)	PHO	761
Logigian, Eric (NY)	N	513	Luciano, Anthony (CT)	RE	1007
Logothetis, Christopher (TX)	Onc	379	Luck, James (CA)	OrS	642
Long, Sarah (PA)	PInf	779	Lucky, Anne (OH)	D	194
Longo, Frank (CA)	N	536	Luders, Hans (OH)	N	525
Longo, Walter (CT)	CRS	166	Ludwig, David (MA)	PEn	743
Longworth, David (OH)	Inf	410	Ludwig, Kirk (WI)	CRS	172
Loo, Marcus (NY)	U	1148	Lueder, Gregg (MO)	Oph	589
Loprinzi, Charles (MN)	Onc	368	Luerssen, Thomas (TX)	NS	490
Lorber, Bennett (PA)	Inf	406	Lugg, James (WY)	U	1166
Loree, Thom (NY)	PlS	853	Luggen, Michael (OH)	Rhu	1029

Alphabetical Listing of Doctors

Name	Specialty	Pg	Name	Specialty	Pg
Luken, Martin (IL)	NS	484	Mackey, William (MA)	VascS	1179
Lumsden, Alan (TX)	VascS	1187	MacKinnon, Susan (MO)	PlS	864
Lunsford, L Dade (PA)	NS	472	Macklis, Roger (OH)	RadRO	959
Lurain, John (IL)	GO	284	Mackool, Richard (NY)	Oph	575
Lusher, Jeanne (MI)	PHO	771	Maclaren, Noel (NY)	PEn	744
Lusk, Rodney (NE)	PO	791	MacLean, James (MA)	A&I	84
Lustig, Lawrence (CA)	Oto	685	Macones, George (MO)	MF	433
Lustig, Robert (CA)	PEn	748	Maddaus, Michael (MN)	TS	1127
Luterman, Arnold (AL)	S	1065	Maddox, Anne (AR)	Hem	323
Luthra, Harvinder (MN)	Rhu	1029	Madoff, Robert (MN)	CRS	173
Lutsep, Helmi (OR)	N	536	Madsen, Joseph (MA)	NS	466
Lutz, Gregory (NY)	PMR	834	Magid, Steven (NY)	Rhu	1025
Lyckholm, Laurel (VA)	Onc	357	Magovern, George (PA)	TS	1115
Lydiatt, Daniel (NE)	Oto	679	Magramm, Irene (NY)	Oph	575
Lydiatt, William (NE)	Oto	679	Magrina, Javier (AZ)	GO	288
Lyketsos, Constantine (MD)	GerPsy	910	Maguire, Joseph (PA)	Oph	575
Lyles, Kenneth (NC)	Ger	264	Maguire, Leo (MN)	Oph	589
Lyman, Gary (NC)	Onc	357	Magun, Arthur (NY)	Ge	235
Lynch, James (FL)	Onc	357	Mahler, Donald (NH)	Pul	921
Lynch, Joseph (CA)	Pul	938	Mahmud, Ehtisham (CA)	IC	130
Lynch, Thomas (CT)	Onc	330	Mahoney, Maurice (CT)	CG	154
Lynne, Charles (FL)	U	1156	Mahony, Lynn (TX)	PCd	740
Lyons, Roger (TX)	Hem	323	Mahowald, Mark (MN)	N	526
Lytle, Bruce (OH)	TS	1127	Mahvi, David (IL)	S	1075
			Majd, Massoud (DC)	NuM	545
			Makaroun, Michel (PA)	VascS	1182
M			Makhija, Sharmila (GA)	GO	282
			Makhoul, Issam (AR)	Onc	379
Ma, C (CA)	SM	1040	Maki, Dennis (WI)	Inf	410
Ma, Dong (NY)	PMR	835	Maki, Robert (NY)	Onc	343
Mabrey, Jay (TX)	OrS	639	Malawer, Martin (MD)	OrS	619
Macaulay, William (NY)	OrS	619	Malcolm, Arnold (TN)	RadRO	953
MacDonald, Kenneth (NC)	S	1065	Maldjian, Joseph (NC)	NRad	987
MacFadyen, Bruce (GA)	S	1065	Malik, Ghaus (MI)	NS	484
Machtay, Mitchell (OH)	RadRO	959	Malkowicz, S Bruce (PA)	U	1149
Macias, John (AZ)	Oto	682	Maloney, David G (WA)	Onc	386
Maciejewski, Jaroslaw (OH)	Hem	319	Maloney, Mary (MA)	D	183
Mack, Michael (TX)	TS	1132	Maloney, Robert (CA)	Oph	599
Mackay, Donald (PA)	PlS	854	Mamelak, Adam (CA)	NS	494
MacKenzie, Richard (CA)	AM	82	Mamounas, Eleftherios (OH)	S	1075
Mackey, Sean (CA)	PM	701	Manche, Edward (CA)	Oph	599

Name	Specialty	Pg	Name	Specialty	Pg
Manco-Johnson, Marilyn (CO)	PHO	774	Maris, John (PA)	PHO	761
Mancuso, Anthony (FL)	DR	979	Mark, Eugene (MA)	Path	706
Mandel, Eric (NY)	Oph	575	Markert, James (AL)	NS	478
Mandel, Susan (PA)	EDM	209	Markmann, James (MA)	S	1046
Mandelbaum, Bert (CA)	OrS	642	Markoe, Arnold (FL)	RadRO	954
Mandelbaum, David (RI)	ChiN	144	Markowitz, Bernard (CA)	PlS	873
Manders, Ernest (PA)	PlS	854	Markowitz, David (NY)	Ge	236
Manepalli, Jothika (MO)	GerPsy	911	Markowitz, Sanford (OH)	Onc	368
Manera, Ricarchito (IL)	PHO	771	Marks, Jeffrey (OH)	S	1075
Manevitz, Alan (NY)	Psyc	889	Marks, Lawrence (NC)	RadRO	954
Mangan, Kenneth (PA)	Hem	311	Marks, Peter (CT)	Hem	308
Manganiello, Paul (NH)	RE	1007	Marks, Stanley (PA)	Hem	311
Mangat, Devinder (KY)	Oto	668	Marmor, Michael (CA)	Oph	599
Mann, J John (NY)	Psyc	890	Maroon, Joseph (PA)	NS	472
Manning, Warren (MA)	Cv	93	Marrs, Richard (CA)	RE	1017
Mannis, Mark (CA)	Oph	599	Marsh, Christopher (CA)	U	1171
Manoli, Arthur (MI)	OrS	633	Marsh, James (PA)	S	1055
Mansfield, Paul (TX)	S	1086	Marsh, James (CT)	OrS	610
Manson, Paul (MD)	PlS	854	Marsh, Jeffrey (MO)	PlS	864
Mansur, David B (MO)	RadRO	959	Marshall, Fray (GA)	U	1156
Mantyh, Christopher (NC)	CRS	170	Marshall, John (VA)	EDM	213
Manzi, Susan (PA)	Rhu	1025	Marshall, John (DC)	Onc	343
Mapstone, Timothy (OK)	NS	490	Marshall, Margaret Blair (DC)	TS	1115
Maraganore, Demetrius (IL)	N	526	Marten, Timothy (CA)	PlS	873
Marcet, Jorge (FL)	CRS	170	Martenson, James (MN)	RadRO	959
Marchlinski, Francis (PA)	CE	119	Martin, Neil (CA)	NS	494
Marcom, Paul (NC)	Onc	358	Martin, Paul (FL)	Ge	241
Marcus, Carole (PA)	PPul	794	Martin, Richard (CO)	Pul	934
Marcus, Judith (NY)	PHO	761	Martin, Richard (OH)	NP	446
Marcus, Robert (FL)	RadRO	954	Martin, Tomas (FL)	TS	1121
Marder, Stephen (CA)	Psyc	898	Martinez, Fernando (MI)	Pul	932
Marentette, Lawrence (MI)	Oto	675	Martini, D Richard (UT)	ChAP	908
Margolin, Kim (WA)	Onc	387	Martins, Renato (WA)	Onc	387
Margolis, James (FL)	IC	127	Martuza, Robert (MA)	NS	467
Mari, Giancarlo (TN)	MF	431	Marx, Robert (NY)	OrS	619
Marin, Deborah (NY)	Psyc	890	Masaryk, Thomas (OH)	NRad	988
Marin, Michael (NY)	VascS	1182	Masket, Samuel (CA)	Oph	599
Marina, Neyssa (CA)	PHO	777	Maslak, Peter (NY)	Hem	311
Marini, John (MN)	Pul	932	Mason, David (OH)	TS	1127
Marino, Ralph (PA)	PMR	835	Mason, Joel (MA)	Ge	229
Marion, Robert (NY)	CG	156	Mason, Kristin (CO)	PMR	840

Alphabetical Listing of Doctors

Name	Specialty	Pg	Name	Specialty	Pg
Mason, Wilbert (CA)	PInf	783	Mazow, Malcolm (TX)	Oph	594
Masood, Shahla (FL)	Path	713	Mazza, David (NY)	A&I	85
Mass, Daniel (IL)	HS	301	Mazzone, Theodore (IL)	EDM	217
Massagli, Teresa (WA)	PMR	842	McAfee, Paul (MD)	OrS	620
Massarotti, Elena (MA)	Rhu	1022	McAneny, David (MA)	S	1046
Massin, Edward (TX)	Cv	112	McAninch, Jack (CA)	U	1171
Mast, Bruce (FL)	PlS	860	McArthur, Justin (MD)	N	513
Masters, Gregory (DE)	Onc	343	McCabe, Daniel (AZ)	S	1086
Mastrobattista, Joan (TX)	MF	435	McCaffrey, Thomas (FL)	Oto	668
Masur, Henry (MD)	Inf	406	McCall, William (NC)	Psyc	892
Matar, Fadi (FL)	IC	127	McCallum, Kimberli (MO)	Psyc	894
Matarasso, Alan (NY)	PlS	854	McCann, John (UT)	Oph	593
Matas, Arthur (MN)	S	1075	McCann, Merle (MD)	Psyc	890
Mather, Paul (PA)	Cv	98	McCann, Peter (NY)	OrS	620
Mathers, William (OR)	Oph	599	McCann, Richard (NC)	VascS	1184
Mathew, Paul (MA)	Onc	330	McCarthy, James (MN)	Nep	458
Mathisen, Douglas (MA)	TS	1107	McCarthy, James (OH)	OrS	633
Matsen, Frederick (WA)	OrS	642	McCarthy, Joseph (NY)	PlS	854
Matthay, Katherine (CA)	PHO	777	McCarthy, Patrick (IL)	TS	1128
Matthews, David (NC)	PlS	860	McCarthy, Paul (CT)	PRhu	798
Matthews, Dennis (CO)	PMR	840	McCarthy, Shirley (CT)	DR	973
Matthews, Jeffrey (IL)	S	1075	McClamrock, Howard (MD)	RE	1009
Mattox, Douglas (GA)	Oto	668	McClure, Robert (WA)	U	1171
Matulonis, Ursula (MA)	Onc	330	McCluskey, Leo (PA)	N	513
Matuschak, George (MO)	Pul	932	McComsey, Grace (OH)	PInf	782
Mauch, Peter (MA)	RadRO	945	McConnell, John (NC)	U	1156
Mauro, Matthew (NC)	VIR	994	McConnell, Robert (NY)	EDM	209
Mavroudis, Constantine (OH)	TS	1127	McCormick, Beryl (NY)	RadRO	949
Mawad, Michel (TX)	NRad	989	McCormick, Paul (NY)	NS	473
Mawn, Louise (TN)	Oph	582	McCormick, Wayne (WA)	Ger	267
Maxfield, Roger (NY)	Pul	924	McCoy, Karen (OH)	PPul	796
Maxwell, G Patrick (TN)	PlS	860	McCracken, George (TX)	PInf	783
Mayberg, Marc (WA)	NS	494	McCracken, James (CA)	ChAP	909
Mayer, John (MA)	TS	1107	McCraw, John (MS)	PlS	860
Mayer, Lloyd (NY)	Ge	236	McCulley, James (TX)	Oph	594
Mayer, Nathaniel (PA)	PMR	835	McCullough, Andrew (NY)	U	1149
Mayerson, Joel (OH)	OrS	633	McCune, W Joseph (MI)	Rhu	1029
Mayes, Maureen (TX)	Rhu	1031	McCurley, Thomas (TN)	Path	713
Maynard, Steven (DC)	ObG	554	McDermott, Michael (CA)	NS	494
Maytal, Joseph (NY)	ChiN	146	McDiarmid, Suzanne (CA)	PGe	755
Maziarz, Richard (OR)	Hem	325	McDonald, Charles (RI)	D	184

Name	Specialty	Pg	Name	Specialty	Pg
McDonald, Douglas (MO)	OrS	634	Meara, John (MA)	PlS	848
McDonald, Ruth (WA)	PNep	788	Mears, John Gregory (NY)	Hem	312
McDonnell, Peter (MD)	Oph	575	Mease, Philip (WA)	Rhu	1032
McDougal, W Scott (MA)	U	1143	Medalie, Daniel (OH)	PlS	864
McDougle, Christopher (MA)	ChAP	903	Medbery, Clinton (OK)	RadRO	963
McFadden, David (VT)	S	1047	Medich, David (PA)	CRS	168
McFarland, Edward (MD)	OrS	620	Medina, Jesus (OK)	Oto	682
McGahan, John (CA)	VIR	997	Medow, Norman (NY)	Oph	575
McGarry, Ronald (KY)	RadRO	954	Medsger, Thomas (PA)	Rhu	1025
McGill, Janet (MO)	EDM	217	Meehan, Kenneth (NH)	Hem	308
McGill, Trevor (MA)	PO	788	Megibow, Alec (NY)	DR	976
McGlashan, Thomas (CT)	Psyc	885	Mehler, Philip (CO)	IM	420
McGlave, Philip (MN)	Hem	319	Mehlman, David (IL)	Cv	107
McGovern, Francis (MA)	U	1143	Mehrara, Babak (NY)	PlS	854
McGovern, Peter (NJ)	RE	1009	Mehta, Davendra (NY)	CE	119
McGowan, Joseph (NY)	Inf	406	Meier, Diane (NY)	Ger	263
McGrath, Patrick (KY)	S	1066	Meiselman, Mick (IL)	Ge	246
Mcgrath-Morrow, Sharon (MD)	PPul	794	Mekhail, Nagy (OH)	PM	698
McGuire, Edward (MI)	U	1163	Melamed, Jonathan (NY)	Path	710
McGuire, William (MD)	Onc	343	Meller, Jose (NY)	Cv	98
McHenry, Christopher (OH)	S	1075	Mellow, Alan (MI)	GerPsy	911
McIntosh, J Michael (UT)	Psyc	895	Melmed, Shlomo (CA)	EDM	221
McIntyre, Robert (CO)	S	1080	Melone, Charles (NY)	HS	297
McKelvey, Robert (OR)	ChAP	909	Meltzer, Eli (CA)	A&I	89
McKenna, Michael (MA)	Oto	656	Meltzer, Toby (AZ)	PlS	868
McKeown, Craig (FL)	Oph	582	Melvin, W Scott (OH)	S	1075
McKinley, William (VA)	PMR	837	Mendenhall, Nancy (FL)	RadRO	954
McKinney, Ross (NC)	PInf	781	Mendenhall, William (FL)	RadRO	954
McLafferty, Robert (IL)	VascS	1186	Mendley, Susan (MD)	PNep	784
McLaren, Rodney (VA)	MF	431	Menezes, Arnold (IA)	NS	485
McLean, Gordon (PA)	VIR	992	Menick, Frederick (AZ)	PlS	869
McLean, Thomas (NC)	PHO	766	Menon, Mani (MI)	U	1163
McMahon, Marion (MN)	EDM	217	Menon, Ram (MI)	PEn	746
McMasters, Kelly (KY)	S	1066	Menter, M (TX)	D	197
McMenomey, Sean (OR)	Oto	685	Mentser, Mark (OH)	PNep	786
McMichael, Amy (NC)	D	191	Merchant, Thomas (TN)	RadRO	954
McPherson, David (TX)	Cv	112	Meredith, Ruby (AL)	RadRO	954
McVary, Kevin (IL)	U	1163	Meredith, Travis (NC)	Oph	582
Meacham, Lillian (GA)	PEn	745	Merguerian, Paul (NH)	U	1143
Meadow, William (IL)	NP	446	Meric-Bernstam, Funda (TX)	S	1086
Meals, Roy (CA)	HS	303	Meropol, Neal (OH)	Onc	368

Alphabetical Listing of Doctors

Name	Specialty	Pg	Name	Specialty	Pg
Merrick, Scot (CA)	TS	1136	Miller, Brent (MO)	Nep	458
Merritt, Diane (MO)	ObG	558	Miller, Charles (IL)	RE	1014
Mertz, Howard (TN)	Ge	241	Miller, D Craig (CA)	TS	1136
Mesrobian, Hrair-George (WI)	U	1163	Miller, D Douglas (GA)	Cv	102
Messersmith, Wells (CO)	Onc	375	Miller, Daniel (GA)	TS	1121
Mesulam, Marsel (IL)	N	526	Miller, David (TX)	GO	288
Metcalfe, Dean (MD)	A&I	85	Miller, Donald (KY)	Onc	358
Metersky, Mark (CT)	Pul	921	Miller, Joan (MA)	Oph	568
Mets, Marilyn (IL)	Oph	589	Miller, John (IN)	CE	121
Metson, Ralph (MA)	Oto	656	Miller, Joseph (AZ)	Oph	595
Metz, David (PA)	Ge	236	Miller, Karen (MA)	Ped	726
Metzinger, Stephen (LA)	PlS	869	Miller, Kenneth (MA)	Hem	309
Metzl, Jordan (NY)	SM	1037	Miller, Kevin (CA)	Oph	599
Meyer, Anthony (NC)	S	1066	Miller, Mark (VA)	OrS	627
Meyer, Fredric (MN)	NS	485	Miller, Michael (OH)	PlS	864
Meyer, William (OK)	PHO	775	Miller, Neil (MD)	Oph	575
Meyers, Bryan (MO)	TS	1128	Miller, Robert (IL)	PO	791
Meyers, Paul (NY)	PHO	761	Miller, Scott (GA)	U	1156
Meyers, Rebecka (UT)	PS	808	Miller, Stanley (MD)	D	187
Meyers, William (PA)	S	1055	Miller, Thomas (AZ)	Onc	379
Meyskens, Frank (CA)	Onc	387	Miller, Timothy (CA)	PlS	873
Michaels, Marian (PA)	PInf	780	Miller, Vincent (NY)	Onc	344
Michalski, Jeff (MO)	RadRO	959	Millett, Peter (CO)	OrS	637
Michelassi, Fabrizio (NY)	S	1055	Milley, J Ross (UT)	NP	447
Micheli, Lyle (MA)	SM	1036	Millis, J Michael (IL)	S	1075
Mickey, Bruce (TX)	NS	490	Millman, Richard (RI)	Pul	921
Mieler, William (IL)	Oph	590	Mills, Monte (PA)	Oph	575
Mies, Carolyn (PA)	Path	710	Mills, Stacey (VA)	Path	713
Mih, Alexander (IN)	HS	301	Milsom, Jeffrey (NY)	CRS	169
Mihm, Martin (MA)	D	184	Mims, James (TX)	Oph	595
Mikkelsen, Tommy (MI)	N	526	Minaker, Kenneth (MA)	Ger	262
Miknevich, Mary Ann (PA)	PMR	835	Minas, Tom (MA)	OrS	610
Milad, Magdy (IL)	RE	1014	Miniaci, Anthony (OH)	SM	1039
Milam, Douglas (TN)	U	1156	Minich, Lois (UT)	PCd	739
Mildvan, Donna (NY)	Inf	406	Mink, Jonathan (NY)	ChiN	146
Miles, Brian (TX)	U	1168	Minsky, Bruce (IL)	RadRO	959
Milhem, Mohammed (IA)	Hem	320	Mintzer, David (PA)	Onc	344
Mill, Michael (NC)	TS	1121	Mirmira, Raghu (IN)	PEn	746
Millenson, Michael (PA)	Hem	312	Mirvis, Stuart (MD)	DR	976
Miller, Aaron (NY)	N	513	Mirzayan, Raffy (CA)	SM	1040
Miller, Antonius (NC)	Onc	358	Mischel, Paul (CA)	Path	721

Alphabetical Listing of Doctors

Name	Specialty	Pg	Name	Specialty	Pg
Miskovitz, Paul (NY)	Ge	236	Montgomery, Erwin (AL)	N	520
Mistry, Bhargav (ND)	S	1081	Montgomery, Robert (MD)	S	1055
Mitch, William (TX)	Nep	460	Montie, James (MI)	U	1163
Mitchell, Beverly (CA)	Hem	325	Moodie, Douglas (TX)	PCd	740
Mitchell, Charles (FL)	PInf	781	Moon, Marc (MO)	TS	1128
Mitchell, James (ND)	Psyc	895	Moore, Anne (NY)	Onc	344
Mitchell, John (CO)	TS	1130	Moore, David (IN)	GO	284
Mitchell, Marc (MS)	VascS	1184	Moore, Ernest (CO)	S	1081
Mitchell, Max (CO)	TS	1131	Moore, Francis (MA)	S	1047
Mitchell, Michael (WI)	U	1163	Moore, Frank (NY)	NS	473
Mitchell, Paul (CT)	Oph	569	Moore, Joseph (NC)	Onc	358
Mitchell, Wendy (CA)	ChiN	152	Moore, Steven (IA)	Path	716
Mitnick, Hal (NY)	Rhu	1025	Moore, Thomas (CA)	MF	437
Mitnick, Julie (NY)	DR	976	Moore, Walter (GA)	Rhu	1028
Mitros, Frank (IA)	Path	716	Moossa, AR (CA)	S	1092
Mitsumoto, Hiroshi (NY)	N	513	Moots, Paul (TN)	N	520
Mitsuyasu, Ronald (CA)	Onc	387	Morady, Fred (MI)	CE	121
Mittal, Bharat (IL)	RadRO	959	Moran, Cesar (TX)	Path	718
Mittal, Ravinder (CA)	Ge	254	Moran, Christopher (MO)	NRad	989
Miyamoto, Richard (IN)	Oto	675	Moran, John (IL)	Cv	107
Mizen, Thomas (IL)	Oph	590	Morcos, Jacques (FL)	NS	479
Moder, Kevin (MN)	Rhu	1029	Morcuende, Jose (IA)	OrS	634
Modesitt, Susan (VA)	GO	282	Morgan, David (TN)	Onc	358
Modic, Michael (OH)	NRad	988	Morgan, Elaine (IL)	PHO	771
Moench, Louis (UT)	Psyc	895	Morgan, Linda (FL)	ObG	555
Moffitt, Drew (AZ)	RE	1016	Morgan, Mark (PA)	GO	279
Mohammad, Yousef (IL)	N	526	Morgan, Raymond (VA)	PlS	861
Mohl, Paul (TX)	Psyc	896	Morgan, Walter (TN)	PS	805
Mohler, James (NY)	U	1149	Morgan, Wayne (AZ)	PPul	797
Mohr, JP (NY)	N	514	Morgenlander, Joel (NC)	N	520
Moley, Jeffrey (MO)	S	1075	Morley, John (MO)	Ger	265
Molleston, Jean (IN)	PGe	752	Morrell, Martha (CA)	N	536
Molnar, Joseph (NC)	PlS	861	Morris, Colleen (NV)	CG	162
Molo, Mary (IL)	RE	1014	Morris, Douglas (GA)	IC	128
Mondino, Bartly (CA)	Oph	599	Morris, John (MO)	N	526
Moneim, Moheb (NM)	HS	302	Morris, Monica (VA)	RadRO	954
Money, Samuel (AZ)	VascS	1187	Morris, P Pearse (NC)	NRad	987
Monsees, Barbara (MO)	DR	980	Morris, Rohinton (PA)	TS	1115
Montague, Drogo (OH)	U	1163	Morrison, William (TX)	RadRO	963
Montanaro, Anthony (OR)	A&I	89	Morrow, Jon (CT)	Path	707
Montgomery, Elizabeth (MD)	Path	710	Morrow, Monica (NY)	S	1056

Alphabetical Listing of Doctors

Name	Specialty	Pg	Name	Specialty	Pg
Mortimer, Joanne (CA)	Onc	387	Murray, Joseph (MN)	Ge	246
Morton, D Holmes (PA)	Ped	727	Murray, Karen (WA)	PGe	755
Morton, John (CA)	S	1092	Murray, Pamela (WV)	AM	80
Moscow, Jeffrey (KY)	PHO	766	Murray, Timothy (FL)	Oph	582
Mosenifar, Zab (CA)	Pul	938	Murtagh, F Reed (FL)	NRad	987
Moses, Jeffrey (NY)	IC	125	Muschler, George (OH)	OrS	634
Moses, Michael (LA)	PlS	869	Muss, Hyman (NC)	Onc	358
Mosher, Deane (WI)	Hem	320	Mustoe, Thomas (IL)	PlS	864
Moskowitz, William (VA)	PCd	737	Mutasim, Diya (OH)	D	194
Moss, R Lawrence (OH)	PS	807	Mutch, David (MO)	GO	285
Mostwin, Jacek (MD)	U	1149	Mutch, Matthew (MO)	CRS	173
Mott, Michael (MI)	OrS	634	Muto, Michael (MA)	GO	275
Motzer, Robert (NY)	Onc	344	Myer, Charles (OH)	PO	791
Moul, Judd (NC)	U	1156	Myerburg, Robert (FL)	Cv	102
Mountz, James (PA)	NuM	545	Myers, Deborah (RI)	ObG	552
Mousa, Hayat (OH)	PGe	752	Myers, Jeffrey (TX)	Oto	682
Movsas, Benjamin (MI)	RadRO	960	Myers, Jeffrey (MI)	Path	716
Muggia, Franco (NY)	Onc	344	Myers, Jonathan (PA)	Oph	576
Mukherjee, Tanmoy (NY)	RE	1009	Myerson, Mark (MD)	OrS	620
Mukherji, Suresh (MI)	NRad	989	Myerson, Robert (MO)	RadRO	960
Muldoon, Thomas (NY)	Oph	576	Myones, Barry (TX)	PRhu	800
Mulhall, John (NY)	U	1149	Myseros, John (VA)	NS	479
Mullett, Timothy (KY)	TS	1121	Mysiw, W Jerry (OH)	PMR	839
Mulliken, John (MA)	PlS	848			
Mulvihill, John (OK)	CG	160			
Mulvihill, Sean (UT)	S	1081			
Mundt, Arno (CA)	RadRO	965	**N**		
Munin, Michael (PA)	PMR	835	Nabell, Lisle (AL)	Onc	358
Munker, Reinhold (LA)	Hem	323	Nabors, L Burt (AL)	N	520
Munoz, Jose (NY)	PInf	780	Naccarelli, Gerald (PA)	Cv	98
Munoz, Santiago (PA)	Ge	236	Naclerio, Robert (IL)	Oto	676
Muntz, Howard (WA)	GO	290	Nademanee, Auayporn (CA)	Hem	325
Murali, Raj (NY)	NS	473	Nadler, Lee (MA)	Onc	330
Muraskas, Jonathan (IL)	NP	446	Naff, Neal (MD)	NS	473
Murphree, A Linn (CA)	Oph	600	Nagel, Theodore (MN)	RE	1014
Murphy, Ana (GA)	RE	1011	Nagib, Mahmoud (MN)	NS	485
Murphy, Barbara (NY)	Nep	454	Nagle, Daniel (IL)	HS	301
Murphy, Douglas (GA)	TS	1122	Nagle, Deborah (MA)	CRS	166
Murphy, John (PA)	PCd	735	Nagler, Harris (NY)	U	1149
Murphy, Thomas (NC)	PPul	795	Nagorney, David (MN)	S	1076
Murphy, Timothy (RI)	VIR	991	Nagueh, Sherif (TX)	Cv	112

Name	Specialty	Pg	Name	Specialty	Pg
Nahabedian, Maurice (DC)	PlS	854	Ness, John (MN)	PlS	864
Nahass, Ronald (NJ)	Inf	406	Nestler, John (VA)	EDM	213
Naka, Yoshifumi (NY)	TS	1115	Netterville, James (TN)	Oto	668
Nakakura, Eric (CA)	S	1092	Neuberg, Ronnie (SC)	PHO	766
Nakayama, Don (GA)	PS	805	Neuburg, Marcelle (WI)	D	194
Nance, Michael (PA)	PS	803	Neumann, Donald (OH)	NuM	546
Nand, Sucha (IL)	Hem	320	Neumann, Ronald (MD)	NuM	545
Nanus, David (NY)	Onc	344	Neumeister, Michael (IL)	PlS	865
Napoli, Joseph (DE)	PlS	855	Neuwelt, Edward (OR)	NS	494
Nardell, Edward (MA)	Pul	921	Neuwirth, Michael (NY)	OrS	620
Narkewicz, Michael (CO)	PGe	753	Neville, Richard (DC)	VascS	1182
Nash, Thomas (NY)	Pul	924	Nevins, Thomas (MN)	PNep	786
Naslund, Michael (MD)	U	1149	New, Maria (NY)	PEn	744
Naslund, Thomas (TN)	VascS	1184	Newburger, Jane (MA)	PCd	733
Nass, Ruth (NY)	ChiN	146	Newell, Kenneth (GA)	S	1066
Natale, Ronald (CA)	Onc	387	Newkirk, Kenneth (DC)	Oto	662
Nathan, David (MA)	EDM	206	Newman, Daniel (MI)	N	526
Nathanson, S David (MI)	S	1076	Newman, Elliot (NY)	S	1056
Nathwani, Bharat (CA)	Path	721	Newman, Lawrence (NY)	N	514
Naunheim, Keith (MO)	TS	1128	Newman, Leonard (NY)	PGe	749
Nava-Villarreal, Hector (NY)	S	1056	Newman, Lisa (MI)	S	1076
Navarro, Victor (PA)	Ge	236	Newman, Nancy (GA)	N	521
Nazzaro, Jules (KS)	NS	487	Newton, Herbert (OH)	N	526
Neel, Victor (MA)	D	184	Ng, John (OR)	Oph	600
Neglia, Joseph (MN)	PHO	771	Ngeow, Jeffrey (NY)	PM	696
Negrin, Robert (CA)	Hem	325	Nghiem, Paul (WA)	D	199
Nehra, Ajay (MN)	U	1163	Nguyen, Dao (FL)	TS	1122
Neiberger, Richard (FL)	PNep	785	Nguyen, Ninh (CA)	S	1092
Neifeld, James (VA)	S	1066	Nicholas, Stephen (NY)	OrS	620
Nelson, Edward (UT)	S	1081	Nicholl, Jeffrey (LA)	N	532
Nelson, Heidi (MN)	CRS	173	Nicholson, H (OR)	PHO	777
Nelson, J Craig (CA)	Psyc	898	Nichter, Larry (CA)	PlS	873
Nelson, Joel (PA)	U	1149	Nicolaou, Nicos (PA)	RadRO	949
Nelson, Judith (NY)	Pul	924	Nicosia, Santo (FL)	Path	713
Nelson, Leonard (PA)	Oph	576	Niebyl, Jennifer (IA)	ObG	558
Nelson, Maureen (TX)	PMR	841	Nieder, Michael (FL)	PHO	766
Nemcek, Albert (IL)	VIR	995	Niederman, Michael (NY)	Pul	924
Nepola, James (IA)	OrS	634	Nielson, Dennis (CA)	PPul	797
Neppe, Vernon (WA)	Psyc	898	Nies, Barbara (VA)	MF	431
Nerad, Jeffrey (OH)	Oph	590	Nieshoff, Edward (MI)	PMR	839
Nesbitt, Jonathan (TN)	TS	1122	Nigra, Thomas (DC)	D	188

Alphabetical Listing of Doctors

Name	Specialty	Pg	Name	Specialty	Pg
Nimer, Stephen (NY)	Hem	312	Nurnberger, John (IN)	Psyc	894
Ninan, Mathew (TN)	TS	1122	Nuss, Daniel (LA)	Oto	682
Niparko, John (MD)	Oto	662	Nussbaum, Julian (GA)	Oph	583
Nishimura, Rick (MN)	Cv	107	Nussbaum, Robert (CA)	CG	162
Nisonson, Barton (NY)	SM	1037	Nutt, John (OR)	N	536
Nissen, Nicholas (CA)	S	1092			
Nissen, Steven (OH)	Cv	108			
Nissenblatt, Michael (NJ)	Onc	344			
Nitenson, Nancy (MA)	AdP	900			
Nitti, Victor (NY)	U	1150			
Nobunaga, Austin (OH)	PMR	839			
Nocero, Michael (FL)	Cv	102			
Noe, Carl (TX)	PM	699			
Noetzel, Michael (MO)	ChiN	149			

O

Name	Specialty	Pg	Name	Specialty	Pg
Nogee, Lawrence (MD)	NP	444	O'Brien, Joan (PA)	Oph	576
Nogueras, Juan (FL)	CRS	170	O'Brien, Susan (TX)	Onc	379
Nolan, Bruce (FL)	N	521	O'Brien, Terrence (FL)	Oph	583
Noone, R Barrett (PA)	PlS	855	O'Brien, Timothy (OH)	Onc	368
Norbash, Alexander (MA)	NRad	984	O'Connell, John (GA)	Cv	103
Norenberg, Michael (FL)	Path	714	O'Connor, Christopher (NC)	Cv	103
Nori, Dattatreyudu (NY)	RadRO	949	O'Connor, Owen (NY)	Onc	345
Norman, James (FL)	S	1066	O'Day, Steven (CA)	Onc	387
Norman, Kim (CA)	Psyc	898	O'Dell, James (NE)	Rhu	1030
Norris, Andrew (IA)	PEn	746	O'Donnell, Margaret (CA)	Hem	325
Northfelt, Donald (AZ)	Onc	379	O'Donnell, Michael (IA)	U	1164
Northrup, Hope (TX)	CG	160	O'Donnell, Richard (CA)	OrS	642
Norton, Jeffrey (CA)	S	1092	O'Dorisio, M Sue (IA)	PHO	771
Norton, Larry (NY)	Onc	344	O'Driscoll, Shawn (MN)	OrS	634
Norwitz, Errol (MA)	MF	427	O'Gara, Patrick (MA)	Cv	93
Notrica, David (AZ)	PS	809	O'Hea, Brian (NY)	S	1056
Nour, Nawal (MA)	ObG	552	O'Keefe, J Paul (IL)	Inf	411
Nouri, Keyvan (FL)	D	191	O'Keefe, Regis (NY)	OrS	620
Novak, Donald (FL)	PGe	751	O'Laughlin, Martin (KS)	PCd	739
Nowak, Eugene (NY)	S	1056	O'Leary, Michael (MA)	U	1143
Noyes, Nicole (NY)	RE	1009	O'Leary, Patrick (NY)	OrS	620
Nuber, Gordon (IL)	OrS	634	O'Malley, Bert (PA)	Oto	662
Nuchtern, Jed (TX)	PS	809	O'Neill, William (FL)	Cv	103
Nugent, William (NH)	TS	1107	O'Regan, Ruth (GA)	Onc	358
Nunery, William (KY)	Oph	583	O'Reilly, Eileen (NY)	Onc	345
Nunes, David (MA)	Ge	229	O'Reilly, Richard (NY)	PHO	761
Nunley, James (NC)	OrS	627	O'Rourke, Donald (PA)	NS	473
			O'Shaughnessy, Joyce (TX)	Onc	379
			Oakes, Daniel (CA)	OrS	642
			Oakes, W Jerry (AL)	NS	479
			Oaklander, Anne (MA)	N	506
			Oaks, Timothy (NC)	TS	1122

Alphabetical Listing of Doctors

Name	Specialty	Pg
Otto, Pamela (TX)	DR	982
Otto, Randal (TX)	Oto	682
Ousterhout, Douglas (CA)	PlS	874
Ovalle, Fernando (AL)	EDM	213
Ownby, Dennis (GA)	PA&I	731
Owyang, Chung (MI)	Ge	247
Oz, Mehmet (NY)	TS	1115
Ozer, Enver (OH)	Oto	676
Ozer, Howard (IL)	Onc	369

P

Name	Specialty	Pg
Pachter, H Leon (NY)	S	1056
Pacin, Michael (FL)	A&I	87
Pack, Allan (PA)	Pul	924
Packer, Roger (DC)	ChiN	147
Padgett, Douglas (NY)	OrS	621
Padilla, Maria (NY)	Pul	925
Pagani, Francis (MI)	TS	1128
Paget, Stephen (NY)	Rhu	1025
Pahl, Elfriede (IL)	PCd	739
Paidas, Charles (FL)	PS	805
Paidas, Michael (CT)	MF	427
Palacios, Igor (MA)	Cv	93
Palascak, Joseph (OH)	Hem	320
Palefsky, Joel (CA)	Inf	413
Paletta, George (MO)	SM	1039
Palevsky, Harold (PA)	Pul	925
Paley, Dror (FL)	OrS	627
Palfrey, Judith (MA)	Ped	726
Paller, Amy (IL)	D	195
Palmer, Jeffrey (MD)	PMR	835
Palmer, Robert (VA)	Ger	264
Palmer, William (MA)	DR	973
Panicek, David (NY)	DR	976
Panitch, Howard (PA)	PPul	794
Panos, Anthony (FL)	TS	1122
Pantilat, Steven (CA)	IM	421
Pao, William (TN)	Onc	359
Papadopoulos, Nicholas (TX)	Onc	380

Name	Specialty	Pg
Paparella, Michael (MN)	Oto	676
Papay, Francis (OH)	PlS	865
Papel, Ira (MD)	Oto	662
Pappas, Theodore (NC)	S	1066
Parent, Andrew (MS)	NS	479
Parikh, Jay (WA)	DR	983
Parikh, Manish (NY)	IC	125
Parikh, Sanjay (WA)	PO	792
Parisier, Simon (NY)	Oto	662
Park, Catherine (CA)	RadRO	965
Park, Julie (WA)	PHO	777
Park, Tae Sung (MO)	NS	485
Parker, Barbara (CA)	Onc	387
Parker, Robert (NY)	PHO	761
Parker, William (CA)	ObG	560
Parness, Ira (NY)	PCd	735
Parrillo, Joseph (NJ)	Cv	98
Parrish, Richard (FL)	Oph	583
Parry, Samuel (PA)	MF	429
Parsons, Polly (VT)	Pul	921
Parsons, Rosaleen (PA)	DR	976
Parsons, Theodore (MI)	OrS	634
Partain, Clarence (TN)	DR	979
Partin, Alan (MD)	U	1150
Parvizi, Javad (PA)	OrS	621
Pasche, Boris (AL)	Onc	359
Pascuzzi, Robert (IN)	N	526
Pasmantier, Mark (NY)	Onc	345
Pasricha, P Jay (CA)	Ge	254
Pass, Harvey (NY)	TS	1116
Passo, Murray (SC)	PRhu	799
Patchefsky, Arthur (PA)	Path	710
Patchell, Roy (AZ)	N	532
Patel, Pravin (IL)	PlS	865
Patel, Shreyaskumar (TX)	Onc	380
Patel, Sunil (SC)	NS	479
Patel, Vipul (FL)	U	1156
Pathria, Mini (CA)	DR	983
Patrinely, James (FL)	Oph	583
Patrizio, Pasquale (CT)	RE	1007
Patt, Yehuda (NM)	Onc	380

Name	Specialty	Pg	Name	Specialty	Pg
Patterson, Anthony (TN)	U	1156	Peng, Stanford (WA)	Rhu	1032
Patterson, G Alexander (MO)	TS	1128	Pennell, Page (MA)	N	506
Patterson, James (OR)	Pul	938	Pensak, Myles (OH)	Oto	676
Patterson, Jan E Evans (TX)	Inf	412	Penson, David (TN)	U	1157
Patterson, Marc (MN)	ChiN	149	Pepine, Carl (FL)	Cv	103
Patterson, Thomas (TX)	Inf	413	Pepose, Jay (MO)	Oph	590
Paty, Philip (NY)	S	1056	Perez, Edith (FL)	Onc	359
Patz, Edward (NC)	DR	979	Perez, Victor (FL)	Oph	583
Patzakis, Michael (CA)	OrS	643	Perez Fontan, J Julio (TX)	PCCM	742
Pauker, Susan (MA)	CG	154	Pergament, Eugene (IL)	CG	158
Paul, Malcolm (CA)	PlS	874	Perin, Emerson (TX)	IC	130
Paul, T Otis (CA)	Oph	600	Perkins, James (WA)	S	1093
Paulson, Richard (CA)	RE	1017	Perler, Bruce (MD)	VascS	1182
Pavlick, Anna (NY)	Onc	345	Perlman, David (NY)	Inf	406
Pavlov, Helene (NY)	DR	977	Perlman, Jeffrey (NY)	NP	444
Pawlik, Timothy (MD)	S	1057	Perlmutter, Joel (MO)	N	527
Payne, Christopher (CA)	U	1172	Perone, Jennifer (TX)	D	197
Paz, Isaac (CA)	S	1093	Perret, Philip (LA)	Pul	936
Peabody, Terrance (IL)	OrS	635	Perrone, Ronald (MA)	Nep	452
Peace, David (IL)	Onc	369	Perry, Arie (CA)	Path	721
Pearce, Elizabeth (MA)	EDM	206	Perry, David (DC)	Onc	346
Pearce, William (IL)	VascS	1186	Perry, Michael (MO)	Onc	369
Pearson, Richard (VA)	Inf	409	Perry, Stanton (CA)	PCd	740
Pearson, Thomas (NY)	PrM	881	Persing, John (CT)	PlS	849
Pecora, Andrew (NJ)	Onc	346	Persky, Mark (NY)	Oto	662
Pedley, Timothy (NY)	N	514	Peschel, Richard (CT)	RadRO	945
Peereboom, David (OH)	Onc	369	Pestronk, Alan (MO)	N	527
Peeters-Asdourian, Christine (MA)	PM	694	Petelin, Joseph (KS)	S	1081
Pegram, Mark (FL)	Onc	359	Peters, Glenn (AL)	Oto	669
Peikin, Steven (NJ)	Ge	236	Peters, Jeffrey (NY)	S	1057
Peitzman, Andrew (PA)	S	1057	Petersdorf, Stephen (WA)	Onc	388
Pejovic, Tanja (OR)	GO	290	Petersen, Michael (OH)	Oph	590
Pellegrini, Carlos (WA)	S	1093	Petersen, Ronald (MN)	N	527
Pellicci, Paul (NY)	OrS	621	Peterson, Bruce (MN)	Onc	369
Pello, Mark (NJ)	CRS	169	Peterson, Davis (AK)	OrS	643
Pelzer, Harold (IL)	Oto	676	Peterson, Laura (HI)	S	1093
Pemberton, John (MN)	CRS	173	Petito, Carol (FL)	Path	714
Pena, Alberto (OH)	PS	807	Petito, Frank (NY)	N	514
Penalver, Manuel (FL)	GO	282	Petras, Robert (OH)	Path	716
Penar, Paul (VT)	NS	467	Petri, Michelle (MD)	Rhu	1025
Pendergrass, Thomas (WA)	PHO	777	Petrossian, George (NY)	IC	125

Alphabetical Listing of Doctors

Name	Specialty	Pg	Name	Specialty	Pg
Petrozza, John (MA)	RE	1007	Pinzur, Michael (IL)	OrS	635
Petru, Ann (CA)	PInf	783	Piraino, Beth (PA)	Nep	454
Petruska, Paul (MO)	Onc	369	Pisters, Katherine (TX)	Onc	380
Petruzzelli, Guy (IL)	Oto	676	Pisters, Louis (TX)	U	1168
Petrylak, Daniel (NY)	Onc	346	Pisters, Peter (TX)	S	1086
Pettrone, Frank (VA)	OrS	628	Pitman, Gerald (NY)	PlS	855
Pevec, William (CA)	VascS	1188	Pitman, Karen (MS)	Oto	669
Pezner, Richard (CA)	RadRO	965	Pizzutillo, Peter (PA)	OrS	621
Pezzone, Michael (PA)	Ge	237	Plager, David (IN)	Oph	590
Pfeffer, Marc (MA)	Cv	93	Plancher, Kevin (NY)	OrS	621
Pfeifer, Samantha (PA)	ObG	554	Plante, Lauren (PA)	MF	429
Pfister, David (NY)	Onc	346	Platt, Lawrence (CA)	MF	437
Pflugfelder, Stephen (TX)	Oph	595	Platzker, Arnold (CA)	PPul	797
Philipp, Claire (NJ)	Hem	312	Plautz, Gregory (OH)	PHO	771
Philipson, Elliot (OH)	MF	433	Plaxe, Steven (CA)	GO	290
Phillips, Edward (CA)	S	1093	Plevy, Scott (NC)	Ge	241
Phillips, Harry (NC)	Cv	103	Plon, Sharon (TX)	CG	160
Phillips, Katharine (RI)	Psyc	885	Plotnick, Leslie (MD)	PEn	744
Phillips, Peter (PA)	ChiN	147	Plotz, Paul (MD)	Rhu	1025
Phillips, Robert (MA)	Cv	94	Pochapin, Mark (NY)	Ge	237
Phillips, S Michael (PA)	A&I	85	Pochettino, Alberto (PA)	TS	1116
Philosophe, Benjamin (MD)	S	1057	Pockaj, Barbara (AZ)	S	1086
Philpott, Jonathan (VA)	TS	1122	Podoloff, Donald (TX)	NuM	547
Phuphanich, Surasak (CA)	N	536	Poe, Dennis (MA)	PO	788
Pi, Edmond (CA)	Psyc	898	Poehling, Gary (NC)	OrS	628
Piatt, Joseph (DE)	NS	473	Pohl, Marc (OH)	Nep	458
Piccirillo, Jay (MO)	Oto	676	Pohlman, Brad (OH)	Onc	369
Piccoli, David (PA)	PGe	750	Poliakoff, Steven (FL)	GO	282
Pichard, Augusto (DC)	IC	125	Polin, Richard (NY)	NP	444
Picken, Catherine (DC)	Oto	662	Polisson, Richard (MA)	Rhu	1022
Picozzi, Vincent (WA)	Onc	388	Pollack, Alan (FL)	RadRO	955
Pienta, Kenneth (MI)	Onc	369	Pollack, Ian (PA)	NS	473
Piepmeier, Joseph (CT)	NS	467	Pollard, Zane (GA)	Oph	583
Pierce, Lori (MI)	RadRO	960	Polley, John (IL)	PlS	865
Pierson, Richard (MD)	TS	1116	Pollock, Raphael (TX)	S	1086
Pile-Spellman, John (NY)	NRad	986	Polly, David (MN)	OrS	635
Pillsbury, Harold (NC)	Oto	669	Polsky, Bruce (NY)	Inf	407
Pinckert, Thomas (MD)	MF	429	Pomeroy, John (NY)	ChAP	905
Pinson, C Wright (TN)	S	1066	Pomeroy, Scott (MA)	ChiN	144
Pinter, Joseph David (OR)	ChiN	152	Pomp, Alfons (NY)	S	1057
Pinto, Harlan (CA)	Onc	388	Pomposelli, Frank (MA)	VascS	1179

Name	Specialty	Pg
Pongracic, Jacqueline (IL)	PA&I	731
Ponn, Teresa (NH)	S	1047
Ponsky, Jeffrey (OH)	S	1076
Ponton, Lynn (CA)	ChAP	909
Poole, Michael (GA)	Oto	669
Poon, Michael (NY)	Cv	99
Poordad, Fred (CA)	Ge	254
Pope, John (TN)	U	1157
Pope, Richard (IL)	Rhu	1030
Popovich, John (MI)	Pul	932
Poppas, Dix (NY)	U	1150
Porayko, Michael (TN)	Ge	241
Porcu, Pierluigi (OH)	Hem	320
Porrazzo, Michael (DC)	RadRO	949
Portenoy, Russell (NY)	PM	696
Porter, Christopher (WA)	U	1172
Porter, David (PA)	Hem	312
Posey, James (AL)	Onc	359
Posner, Jerome (NY)	N	514
Posner, Marshall (NY)	Onc	346
Posner, Mitchell (IL)	S	1076
Posnick, Jeffrey (MD)	PlS	855
Posselt, Andrew (CA)	S	1093
Postier, Russell (OK)	S	1086
Postma, Gregory (GA)	Oto	669
Potenza, Bruce (CA)	S	1093
Potkul, Ronald (IL)	GO	285
Potter, Hollis (NY)	DR	977
Pow-Sang, Julio (FL)	U	1157
Powell, Bayard (NC)	Hem	315
Powell, Nelson (CA)	Oto	685
Powers, Alvin (TN)	EDM	213
Powers, Eric (SC)	Cv	103
Powers, Pauline (FL)	Psyc	892
Prados, Michael (CA)	Onc	388
Prager, Joshua (CA)	PM	701
Prakash, Udaya (MN)	Pul	932
Preminger, Glenn (NC)	U	1157
Press, Joel (IL)	PMR	840
Press, Oliver (WA)	Onc	388
Presti, Joseph (CA)	U	1172

Name	Specialty	Pg
Pribitkin, Edmund (PA)	Oto	663
Price, G Wesley (MD)	PlS	855
Price, Lawrence (RI)	Psyc	885
Pridjian, Gabriella (LA)	MF	435
Prieto, Victor (TX)	Path	718
Prinz, Richard (IL)	S	1076
Prioleau, Philip (NY)	D	188
Procaccino, John (NY)	CRS	169
Proctor, Deborah (CT)	Ge	229
Proctor, Monja (WA)	PS	810
Prosnitz, Leonard (NC)	RadRO	955
Provenzale, James (NC)	NRad	987
Pruthi, Raj (NC)	U	1157
Prystowsky, Eric (IN)	CE	121
Puccetti, Diane (WI)	PHO	771
Puckett, Charles (MO)	PlS	865
Pui, Ching-Hon (TN)	PHO	766
Pula, Thaddeus (MD)	N	514
Puliafito, Carmen (CA)	Oph	600
Pulido, Jose (MN)	Oph	591
Putman, John (TX)	RE	1016
Putnam, Joe (TN)	TS	1122
Putnam, Matthew (MN)	HS	301
Putterman, Allen (IL)	Oph	591
Putterman, Bart (TX)	ObG	559
Pyeritz, Reed (PA)	CG	156
Pynoos, Robert (CA)	Psyc	898

Q

Name	Specialty	Pg
Quaegebeur, Jan (NY)	PS	803
Quagliarello, Vincent (CT)	Inf	404
Quatela, Vito (NY)	Oto	663
Quencer, Robert (FL)	NRad	987
Quigley, Harry (MD)	Oph	576
Quigley, Matthew (PA)	NS	474
Quill, Timothy (NY)	IM	419
Quinn, David (CA)	Onc	388
Quinn, Graham (PA)	Oph	576
Quinn, Suzanne (FL)	EDM	213

Alphabetical Listing of Doctors

Name	Specialty	Pg
Quinones, Miguel (TX)	Cv	112
Quintessenza, James (FL)	TS	1123
Quittell, Lynne (NY)	PPul	794
Quivey, Jeanne (CA)	RadRO	965

R

Name	Specialty	Pg
Rabinovitch, Rachel (CO)	RadRO	961
Rabow, Michael (CA)	IM	421
Racz, Gabor (TX)	PM	700
Rader, Daniel (PA)	IM	419
Rader, Janet (WI)	GO	285
Radtke, Wolfgang (DE)	PCd	735
Raffel, Corey (OH)	NS	485
Rafferty, Janice (OH)	CRS	173
Ragheb, John (FL)	NS	479
Raghu, Ganesh (WA)	Pul	938
Ragnarsson, Kristjan (NY)	PMR	835
Rahko, Peter (WI)	Cv	108
Rai, Kanti (NY)	Hem	312
Raiford, David (TN)	Ge	241
Raja, Srinivasa (MD)	PM	696
Rajacich, Nicholas (WA)	OrS	643
Rajfer, Jacob (CA)	U	1172
Raju, Gottumukkala (TX)	Ge	252
Rakowski, Thomas (VA)	Nep	456
Ramamoorthy, Sonia (CA)	CRS	176
Ramamurthy, Somayaji (TX)	PM	700
Ramanathan, Ramesh (PA)	S	1057
Ramee, Stephen (LA)	Cv	112
Ramsay, David (NY)	D	188
Ramsey, Bonnie (WA)	PPul	798
Ramsey, Matthew (PA)	OrS	621
Ranawat, Chitranjan (NY)	OrS	621
Rand, Richard (WA)	PlS	874
Randall, Marcus (KY)	RadRO	955
Randall, R Lawrence (UT)	OrS	637
Randall, Thomas (PA)	GO	279
Randolph, Gregory (MA)	Oto	656
Randolph, Linda (CA)	CG	162

Name	Specialty	Pg
Randolph-Jackson, Pamela (DC)	RadRO	950
Rao, A Koneti (PA)	Hem	312
Rao, Nalini (PA)	Inf	407
Rao, Narsing (CA)	Oph	600
Rao, Vijay (PA)	DR	977
Raphael, Bruce (NY)	Hem	312
Rapoport, Aaron (MD)	Hem	313
Rapoport, Judith (DC)	ChAP	906
Rappaport, Leonard (MA)	Ped	726
Rappaport, Norman (TX)	PlS	869
Raptis, George (NY)	Onc	346
Rashid, Asif (TX)	Path	718
Raskin, Keith (NY)	HS	297
Raskin, Neil (CA)	N	536
Raskind, Murray (WA)	Psyc	898
Rasmussen, Steven (RI)	Psyc	885
Rassekh, Christopher (PA)	Oto	663
Rassman, William (CA)	S	1093
Rastegar, Hassan (MA)	TS	1107
Raszka, William (VT)	PInf	779
Ratain, Mark (IL)	Onc	370
Rattner, David (MA)	S	1047
Ratts, Valerie (MO)	RE	1014
Ratzan, Kenneth (FL)	Inf	409
Rauch, Paula (MA)	Psyc	885
Rauch, Steven (MA)	Oto	656
Rauck, Richard (NC)	PM	697
Rausen, Aaron (NY)	PHO	762
Ravich, William (MD)	Ge	237
Rayan, Ghazi (OK)	HS	302
Raz, Shlomo (CA)	U	1172
Razzouk, Bassem (IN)	PHO	772
Read, Thomas (MA)	CRS	167
Ready, John (MA)	OrS	610
Ready, Neal (NC)	Onc	359
Reaman, Gregory (DC)	PHO	762
Reardon, Michael (TX)	TS	1133
Reasner, Charles (TX)	EDM	219
Rebeiz, Elie (MA)	Oto	656
Reber, Howard (CA)	S	1093
Recht, Abram (MA)	RadRO	945

Name	Specialty	Pg	Name	Specialty	Pg
Recht, Michael (OR)	PHO	778	Rescorla, Frederick (IN)	PS	807
Rechtine, Glenn (NY)	OrS	622	Resnick, Neil (PA)	Ger	263
Recker, Robert (NE)	EDM	218	Resnik, Sorrel (FL)	D	192
Redberg, Rita (CA)	Cv	115	Reuben, Adrian (SC)	Ge	242
Redding, Gregory (WA)	PPul	798	Reuben, David (CA)	Ger	267
Reddy, Bhagat (GA)	IC	128	Reus, Victor (CA)	Psyc	899
Reddy, K Rajender (PA)	Ge	237	Reuter, Victor (NY)	Path	711
Reder, Anthony (IL)	N	527	Rex, Douglas (IN)	Ge	247
Redlich, Carrie (CT)	Pul	921	Reynolds, James (PA)	Ge	237
Reed, Carolyn (SC)	TS	1123	Reynolds, James (NY)	Oph	577
Reed, Eddie (AL)	Onc	359	Reynolds, Marleta (IL)	PS	808
Reed, Kathryn (AZ)	MF	435	Reynolds, R Kevin (MI)	GO	285
Reed, Robert (OH)	N	527	Rezai, Ali (OH)	NS	485
Rees, Riley (MI)	PlS	865	Rhee, Peter (AZ)	S	1087
Rege, Robert (TX)	S	1087	Rheingold, Susan (PA)	PHO	762
Regillo, Carl (PA)	Oph	577	Rhoads, J Marc (TX)	PGe	754
Regine, William (MD)	RadRO	950	Rhodes, Arthur (IL)	D	195
Reich, David (PA)	S	1057	Riba, Michelle (MI)	Psyc	894
Reich, Stephen (MD)	N	514	Ribeiro, Raul (TN)	PHO	767
Reichelderfer, Mark (WI)	Ge	247	Rice, Dale (CA)	Oto	685
Reid, Tony (CA)	Onc	388	Rice, David (TX)	TS	1133
Reid, William (TN)	NS	479	Rice, Henry (NC)	PS	805
Reilly, Donald (MA)	OrS	610	Rice, Laurel (WI)	GO	285
Reilly, John (PA)	Pul	925	Rice, Thomas (OH)	TS	1128
Reiner, Jonathan (DC)	IC	125	Rich, Keith (MO)	NS	485
Reiner, Mark (NY)	S	1057	Rich, Stuart (IL)	Cv	108
Reinisch, John (CA)	PlS	874	Rich, Tyvin (VA)	RadRO	955
Reinus, William (PA)	DR	977	Richard, James (OK)	Oph	595
Reis, Steven (PA)	Cv	99	Richards, Jon (IL)	Onc	370
Reisberg, Barry (NY)	GerPsy	910	Richards, William (AL)	S	1067
Reiss, Craig (MO)	Cv	108	Richardson, Marilyn (KS)	RE	1015
Reitz, Bruce (CA)	TS	1136	Richardson, Mark (OR)	PO	792
Relkin, Norman (NY)	N	514	Richardson, Paul (MA)	Hem	309
Remick, Scot (WV)	Onc	346	Richardson, William (NC)	OrS	628
Remmenga, Steven (NE)	GO	286	Richerson, George (IA)	N	527
Remzi, Feza (OH)	CRS	173	Richie, Jerome (MA)	U	1144
Rennard, Stephen (NE)	Pul	935	Richman, Douglas (CA)	Inf	413
Rennke, Helmut (MA)	Path	707	Richmond, John (MA)	OrS	611
Renz, John (IL)	S	1077	Richter, Edwin (CT)	PMR	832
Repke, John (PA)	MF	429	Ricketts, Richard (GA)	PS	805
Resar, Jon (MD)	IC	125	Ricotta, John (DC)	VascS	1182

Alphabetical Listing of Doctors

Name	Specialty	Pg	Name	Specialty	Pg
Riddle, Mark (MD)	ChAP	906	Robichaux, Alfred (LA)	MF	435
Riddle, Matthew (OR)	EDM	221	Robinson, Julian (MA)	MF	427
Ridge, John (PA)	S	1057	Robinson, Lary (FL)	TS	1123
Ridgway, E (CO)	EDM	218	Robinson, Lawrence (WA)	PMR	842
Ridker, Paul (MA)	Cv	94	Rocchini, Albert (MI)	PCd	739
Ries, W Russell (TN)	Oto	669	Rochester, Carolyn (CT)	Pul	922
Riew, K Daniel (MO)	OrS	635	Rock, Jack (MI)	NS	485
Rigamonti, Daniele (MD)	NS	474	Rockwell, William (UT)	PlS	867
Rigel, Darrell (NY)	D	188	Rodbard, Helena (MD)	EDM	210
Riina, Howard (NY)	NS	474	Rodby, Roger (IL)	Nep	458
Riles, Thomas (NY)	VascS	1182	Roddy, Sarah (CA)	ChiN	152
Riley, Laura (MA)	MF	427	Rodeo, Scott (NY)	SM	1037
Rilling, William (WI)	VIR	995	Rodgers, Bradley (VA)	PS	805
Rimoin, David (CA)	CG	162	Rodgers, George (UT)	Hem	321
Ringel, Steven (CO)	N	530	Rodosky, Mark (PA)	OrS	622
Rink, Richard (IN)	U	1164	Rodts, Gerald (GA)	NS	480
Riordan, John (CA)	Nep	462	Roehrborn, Claus (TX)	U	1168
Ristow, Brunno (CA)	PlS	874	Rogers, Douglas (OH)	PEn	747
Ritch, Robert (NY)	Oph	577	Rogers, Gary (OH)	Oph	591
Ritchey, A Kim (PA)	PHO	762	Rogers, James (TX)	PCd	740
Ritchie, Christine (AL)	Ger	264	Rogers, Joseph (NC)	Cv	103
Riviello, James (NY)	ChiN	147	Rogers, Lisa (OH)	N	527
Rivlin, Richard (NY)	IM	419	Rogers, Stanley (CA)	S	1094
Rizk, Norman (CA)	Pul	938	Roh, Mark (FL)	S	1067
Rizzo, Joseph (MA)	Oph	569	Rohrich, Rod (TX)	PlS	869
Roach, Mack (CA)	RadRO	965	Roizen, Nancy Jean (OH)	Ped	728
Robb, Geoffrey (TX)	PlS	869	Roland, J Thomas (NY)	Oto	663
Robbins, Larry (IL)	PM	698	Romagnoli, Mario (NY)	Inf	407
Robbins, Richard (TX)	EDM	219	Romaguera, Jorge (TX)	Onc	380
Robbins, Robert (CA)	TS	1136	Romano, James (CA)	PlS	874
Robert, Nicholas (VA)	Onc	359	Rombeau, John (PA)	CRS	169
Robert-Vizcarrondo, Francisco (AL)	Onc	360	Romeo, Anthony (IL)	OrS	635
Roberts, Barbara (RI)	Cv	94	Romond, Edward (KY)	Onc	360
Roberts, John (CA)	S	1094	Rood, Brian (DC)	PHO	762
Roberts, Kenneth (CT)	RadRO	945	Roodman, G David (PA)	Hem	313
Roberts, Michelle (PA)	EDM	209	Rook, Alain (PA)	D	188
Roberts, Patricia (MA)	CRS	167	Roos, Karen (IN)	N	527
Roberts, William (TX)	Path	719	Roos, Raymond (IL)	N	528
Robertson, Cary (NC)	U	1157	Roose, Steven (NY)	Psyc	890
Robertson, Jon (TN)	NS	480	Ropper, Allan (MA)	N	506
Robertson, Patricia (CA)	MF	437	Rosbe, Kristina (CA)	PO	793

Name	Specialty	Pg	Name	Specialty	Pg
Rose, Cecile (CO)	Pul	935	Roskes, Saul (MD)	PNep	784
Rose, Christopher (CA)	RadRO	966	Rosner, Howard (CA)	PM	701
Rose, Peter (OH)	GO	285	Rosoff, Philip (NC)	PHO	767
Rosemurgy, Alexander (FL)	S	1067	Rosove, Michael (CA)	Onc	388
Rosen, Charles (MN)	S	1077	Ross, Douglas (MA)	EDM	206
Rosen, Clark (PA)	Oto	663	Ross, Edgar (MA)	PM	694
Rosen, Jules (PA)	GerPsy	910	Ross, Helen (AZ)	Onc	380
Rosen, Michael (OH)	S	1077	Ross, Jeffrey (NY)	Path	711
Rosen, Steven (IL)	Onc	370	Ross, Lawrence (IL)	U	1164
Rosenbaum, Kenneth (DC)	CG	156	Ross, Merrick (TX)	S	1087
Rosenbaum, Richard (OR)	N	536	Rosse, Richard (DC)	Psyc	890
Rosenberg, Andrew (MA)	Path	707	Rosser, Tena (CA)	ChiN	152
Rosenberg, Howard (CA)	PlS	874	Rossi, Carl (CA)	RadRO	966
Rosenberg, Michael (IL)	Oph	591	Rossman, Milton (PA)	Pul	925
Rosenberg, Steven (MD)	S	1058	Rostain, Anthony (PA)	ChAP	906
Rosenberg, Thomas (UT)	OrS	637	Roth, Andrew (NY)	Psyc	890
Rosenblatt, Joseph (FL)	Hem	315	Roth, Bennett (CA)	Ge	255
Rosenblum, Marc (NY)	Path	711	Roth, Bruce (MO)	Onc	370
Rosenblum, Mark (MI)	NS	486	Roth, David (FL)	Nep	456
Rosenblum, Norman (PA)	GO	279	Roth, Elliot (IL)	PMR	840
Rosenbluth, Daniel (MO)	Pul	933	Roth, Jack (TX)	TS	1133
Rosenbush, Stuart (IL)	Cv	108	Roth, Susan (PA)	DR	977
Rosenfeld, Myrna (PA)	N	515	Rothbaum, Robert (MO)	PGe	753
Rosenfeld, Philip (FL)	Oph	584	Rothenberg, Russell (MD)	Rhu	1026
Rosenfeld, Richard (NY)	PO	789	Rothenberger, David (MN)	CRS	173
Rosenfeld, Steven (OH)	N	528	Rothman, Richard (PA)	OrS	622
Rosenfield, Kenneth (MA)	IC	124	Rothrock, John (AL)	N	521
Rosengart, Todd (NY)	TS	1116	Rothstein, Richard (NH)	Ge	229
Rosenkranz, Eliot (FL)	TS	1123	Rotman, Marvin (NY)	RadRO	950
Rosenman, Julian (NC)	RadRO	955	Rotmensch, Jacob (IL)	GO	285
Rosenquist, Richard (OH)	PM	698	Roubin, Gary (NY)	IC	126
Rosenthal, David (GA)	VascS	1184	Routes, John (WI)	A&I	88
Rosenthal, Eben (AL)	Oto	669	Rovner, Barry (PA)	GerPsy	910
Rosenthal, Joseph (CA)	PHO	778	Rowland, Randall (KY)	U	1157
Rosenthal, Norman (MD)	Psyc	890	Rowley, Howard (WI)	NRad	989
Rosenthal, Richard (NY)	Psyc	890	Rowley, Scott (NJ)	Hem	313
Rosenthal, Stephen (CA)	PEn	748	Roy-Byrne, Peter (WA)	Psyc	899
Rosenwaks, Zev (NY)	RE	1009	Roye, David (NY)	OrS	622
Rosenwasser, Melvin (NY)	HS	297	Rozbruch, S Robert (NY)	OrS	622
Rosenwasser, Robert (PA)	NS	474	Rubenfeld, Sheldon (TX)	EDM	219
Roses, Daniel (NY)	S	1058	Rubin, Brian (OH)	Path	716

Alphabetical Listing of Doctors

Name	Specialty	Pg	Name	Specialty	Pg
Rubin, Bruce (VA)	PPul	795	Sacco, Ralph (FL)	N	521
Rubin, Charles (IL)	PHO	772	Sachar, David (NY)	Ge	237
Rubin, Geoffrey (NC)	DR	979	Sachs, Greg (IN)	Ger	265
Rubin, Lewis (CA)	Pul	938	Saclarides, Theodore (IL)	CRS	173
Rubin, Mark (CA)	D	199	Sadda, SriniVas (CA)	Oph	600
Rubin, Peter (MA)	Oph	569	Sadeghi-Nejad, Hossein (NJ)	U	1150
Rubin, Stephen (PA)	GO	279	Sadock, Virginia (NY)	Psyc	890
Rubin, Susan (IL)	N	528	Sadowsky, Carl (FL)	N	521
Rubino, Francesco (NY)	S	1058	Saffle, Jeffrey (UT)	S	1081
Rubinstein, Jay (WA)	Oto	685	Safi, Hazim (TX)	TS	1133
Rubinstein, Wendy (IL)	CG	158	Safian, Robert (MI)	Cv	108
Rudnick, Michael (PA)	Nep	454	Sagalowsky, Arthur (TX)	U	1168
Rudolph, Colin (WI)	PGe	753	Sage, Jacob (NJ)	N	515
Ruge, John (IL)	NS	486	Sagel, Stuart (MO)	DR	980
Ruggiero, Joseph (NY)	Onc	346	Saha, Sukamal (MI)	S	1077
Rugo, Hope (CA)	Onc	389	Sahin, Aysegul (TX)	Path	719
Runowicz, Carolyn (FL)	GO	283	Sahin, Mustafa (MA)	ChiN	144
Rushakoff, Robert (CA)	EDM	221	Sahn, Steven (SC)	Pul	929
Rushton, H Gil (DC)	U	1150	Saif, M Wasif (NY)	Onc	347
Ruskin, Jeremy (MA)	CE	117	Saiki, John (NM)	Onc	380
Russell, Andrew (CA)	ChAP	909	Sailer, Scott (NC)	RadRO	955
Russell, Anthony (MA)	RadRO	945	Saiman, Lisa (NY)	PInf	780
Russell, Christy (CA)	Onc	389	Saint-Phard, Deborah (CO)	SM	1039
Russell, Kenneth (WA)	RadRO	966	Sakamoto, Kathleen (CA)	PHO	778
Russell, Mark (VA)	D	192	Salant, David (MA)	Nep	452
Russell, Stuart (MD)	Cv	99	Salata, Robert (OH)	Inf	411
Russo, Carolyn (AL)	PHO	767	Salem, Riad (IL)	VIR	995
Rutgers, Joanne (CA)	Path	721	Salem, Ronald (CT)	S	1047
Rutherford, Thomas (CT)	GO	275	Salerno, Tomas (FL)	TS	1123
Rutkove, Seward (MA)	N	506	Salgia, Ravi (IL)	Onc	370
Ryan, Colleen (MA)	S	1047	Salky, Barry (NY)	S	1058
Ryan, David (MA)	Onc	330	Sallan, Stephen (MA)	PHO	756
Ryken, Timothy (IA)	NS	486	Sallent, Jorge (FL)	PPul	795
			Salloum, Ihsan (FL)	Psyc	892
			Salo, Jonathan (NC)	S	1067
			Saltz, Leonard (NY)	Onc	347
S			Saltzman, Charles (UT)	OrS	637
Saag, Michael (AL)	Inf	409	Salvati, Eduardo (NY)	OrS	622
Saal, Howard (OH)	CG	158	Salvi, Sharad (IL)	PHO	772
Saal, Jeffrey (CA)	PMR	842	Salz, James (CA)	Oph	600
Sacchi, Terrence (NY)	IC	126	Salzman, Carl (MA)	Psyc	886

Name	Specialty	Pg	Name	Specialty	Pg
Samadi, David (NY)	U	1150	Saper, Joel (MI)	N	528
Samant, Sandeep (TN)	Oto	669	Sargent, Albert John (MA)	ChAP	903
Samberg, Eslee (NY)	Psyc	891	Sarnaik, Ashok (MI)	PCCM	741
Samii, Ali (WA)	N	537	Sarnoff, Deborah (NY)	D	188
Samlowski, Wolfram (NV)	Onc	389	Sarr, Michael (MN)	S	1077
Sampson, Christian (MA)	HS	294	Sartor, R Balfour (NC)	Ge	242
Sampson, John (NC)	NS	480	Sasaki, Clarence (CT)	Oto	656
Samson, Duke (TX)	NS	490	Sasson, Aaron (NE)	S	1081
Samuels, Brian (ID)	Onc	375	Sataloff, Dahlia (PA)	S	1058
Samuels, Louis (PA)	TS	1116	Sataloff, Robert (PA)	Oto	663
Samuels, Martin (MA)	N	506	Satava, Richard (WA)	S	1094
Samuels, Philip (OH)	MF	433	Sato, Thomas (WI)	PS	808
Samuelson, Thomas (MN)	Oph	591	Sauer, Mark (NY)	RE	1009
Sanborn, Timothy (IL)	Cv	108	Saul, Robert (SC)	CG	157
Sanchez, Luis (MO)	VascS	1186	Saunders, Elijah (MD)	Cv	99
Sanchez, Miguel (NJ)	Path	711	Saunders, John (MD)	S	1058
Sanda, Martin (MA)	U	1144	Sauter, Edward (ND)	S	1081
Sandberg, David (FL)	NS	480	Savage, David (NY)	Hem	313
Sandborn, William (CA)	Ge	255	Saven, Alan (CA)	Hem	325
Sanders, Georgiana (MI)	A&I	88	Saver, Jeffrey (CA)	N	537
Sanders, William (GA)	U	1157	Savides, Thomas (CA)	Ge	255
Sandhu, Harvinder (NY)	OrS	622	Savino, Peter (CA)	Oph	600
Sandler, Alan (OR)	Onc	389	Sawaya, Raymond (TX)	NS	490
Sandler, Eric (FL)	PHO	767	Sawczuk, Ihor (NJ)	U	1150
Sandler, Howard (CA)	RadRO	966	Sawin, Robert (WA)	PS	811
Sandler, Martin (TN)	NuM	546	Sax, Paul (MA)	Inf	404
Sandlow, Jay (WI)	U	1164	Saxena, Sanjaya (CA)	Psyc	899
Sandlund, John (TN)	PHO	767	Scandling, John (CA)	Nep	462
Sands, Jeff (GA)	Nep	457	Scantlebury, Velma (DE)	S	1058
Sanfilippo, Joseph (PA)	RE	1009	Scarborough, Mark (FL)	OrS	628
Sanford, Robert (TN)	NS	480	Scardino, Peter (NY)	U	1150
Sangeorzan, Bruce (WA)	OrS	643	Schachat, Andrew (OH)	Oph	591
Sanger, James (WI)	PlS	865	Schaefer, Steven (NY)	Oto	663
Sanger, Joseph (NY)	NuM	545	Schaeffer, Anthony (IL)	U	1164
Sankar, Raman (CA)	ChiN	152	Schafer, Michael (IL)	OrS	635
Santa-Emma, Philip (OH)	IM	420	Schaff, Hartzell (MN)	TS	1129
Santana, Victor (TN)	PHO	767	Schaffer, Randolph (CA)	S	1094
Santin, Alessandro (CT)	GO	275	Schaitkin, Barry (PA)	Oto	663
Santos, Cesar (DC)	ChiN	147	Schanberg, Laura (NC)	PRhu	799
Sanz, Luis (VA)	ObG	556	Schantz, Stimson (NY)	Oto	664
Saper, Clifford (MA)	N	506	Schatz, Lisa (CO)	CRS	174

Alphabetical Listing of Doctors

Name	Specialty	Pg	Name	Specialty	Pg
Schatz, Norman (FL)	N	521	Schmitt, Steven (OH)	Inf	411
Schatzberg, Alan (CA)	Psyc	899	Schnabel, Freya (NY)	S	1058
Schauer, Philip (OH)	S	1077	Schneider, Darren (NY)	VascS	1182
Schechter, David (CA)	SM	1040	Schnipper, Lowell (MA)	Onc	330
Scheff, Alice (CA)	NuM	547	Schnitt, Stuart (MA)	Path	707
Schein, Oliver (MD)	Oph	577	Schnittger, Ingela (CA)	Cv	116
Scheinberg, David (NY)	Onc	347	Schoen, Robert (CT)	Rhu	1022
Scheithauer, Bernd (MN)	Path	716	Schoenberg, Mark (MD)	U	1151
Schelbert, Heinrich (CA)	NuM	547	Schoetz, David (MA)	CRS	167
Scheld, W Michael (VA)	Inf	409	Schomberg, Paula (MN)	RadRO	960
Scheller, Arnold (MA)	SM	1036	Schooley, Robert (CA)	Inf	414
Schenken, Robert (TX)	RE	1016	Schorge, John (MA)	GO	275
Scher, Howard (NY)	Onc	347	Schottenfeld, Richard (CT)	AdP	900
Scher, Jonathan (NY)	ObG	554	Schraut, Wolfgang (PA)	S	1058
Scher, Mark (OH)	ChiN	150	Schreiber, Martin (OH)	Nep	458
Scherr, Douglas (NY)	U	1151	Schreiber, Theodore (MI)	IC	129
Schiano, Thomas (NY)	Ge	237	Schubert, Mark (AZ)	A&I	89
Schidlow, Daniel (PA)	PPul	794	Schubert, Richard (DC)	Rhu	1026
Schiff, David (VA)	N	521	Schuberth, Kenneth (MD)	PA&I	730
Schiff, Eugene (FL)	Ge	242	Schuchter, Lynn (PA)	Onc	347
Schiff, Peter (NY)	RadRO	950	Schuckit, Marc (CA)	AdP	902
Schiff, William (NY)	Oph	577	Schuger, Claudio (MI)	CE	121
Schiffer, Charles (MI)	Onc	370	Schulak, James (OH)	S	1077
Schiffman, Fred (RI)	Hem	309	Schuler, Thomas (VA)	OrS	628
Schiffman, Jade (TX)	Oph	595	Schulick, Richard (MD)	S	1059
Schild, Steven (AZ)	RadRO	963	Schulman, Steven (MD)	Cv	99
Schilder, Russell (PA)	Onc	347	Schultz, Neal (NY)	D	188
Schiller, Alan (NY)	Path	711	Schulze, Konrad (IA)	Ge	247
Schiller, Gary (CA)	Hem	325	Schuman, Joel (PA)	Oph	577
Schiller, Joan (TX)	Onc	380	Schuster, Michael (NY)	Hem	313
Schiller, Lawrence (TX)	Ge	252	Schuster, Stephen (PA)	Hem	313
Schilsky, Richard (IL)	Onc	370	Schusterman, Mark (TX)	PlS	869
Schink, Julian (IL)	GO	285	Schutta, Mark (PA)	EDM	210
Schirmer, Bruce (VA)	S	1067	Schwab, Frank (NY)	OrS	623
Schlaff, William (CO)	RE	1015	Schwab, Richard (PA)	Pul	925
Schlegel, Peter (NY)	U	1151	Schwartz, Allan (NY)	Cv	99
Schley, W Shain (NY)	Oto	664	Schwartz, Burton (MN)	Onc	370
Schlinkert, Richard (AZ)	S	1087	Schwartz, Cindy (RI)	PHO	756
Schluger, Neil (NY)	Pul	925	Schwartz, David (CO)	Pul	935
Schmalzried, Thomas (CA)	OrS	643	Schwartz, Gary (MN)	Nep	459
Schmidt, Richard (PA)	OrS	623	Schwartz, Herbert (TN)	OrS	628

Alphabetical Listing of Doctors

Name	Specialty	Pg	Name	Specialty	Pg
Schwartz, L Matthew (PA)	PMR	835	Sellke, Frank (RI)	TS	1108
Schwartz, Marshall (PA)	PS	803	Selman, Warren (OH)	NS	486
Schwartz, Michael (FL)	Onc	360	Seltzer, Dana (AZ)	OrS	639
Schwartz, Peter (CT)	GO	275	Selvaggi, Kathy (MA)	Onc	330
Schwartz, Robert (CO)	Ger	266	Selwyn, Peter (NY)	IM	419
Schwartz, Stanley (PA)	EDM	210	Semenkovich, Clay (MO)	EDM	217
Schwartz, Theodore (NY)	NS	474	Semrad, Carol (IL)	Ge	247
Schwartz, William (NY)	Cv	99	Sen, Chandranath (NY)	NS	474
Schwartzberg, Lee (TN)	Hem	316	Senagore, Anthony (CA)	CRS	176
Schwartzentruber, Douglas (IN)	S	1077	Sencer, Susan (MN)	PHO	772
Schwartzman, Robert (PA)	N	515	Senders, Craig (CA)	Oto	686
Schwarz, Adam (CA)	PCCM	742	Sener, Stephen (CA)	S	1094
Schwarz, Kathleen (MD)	PGe	750	Senior, Brent (NC)	Oto	670
Schwarz, Marvin (CO)	Pul	935	Sennett, Brian (PA)	SM	1038
Schwarz, Steven (NY)	PGe	750	Senzer, Neil (TX)	RadRO	963
Scott, C Paul (PA)	Psyc	891	Sepkowitz, Kent (NY)	Inf	407
Scott, Gwendolyn (FL)	PInf	781	Seplowitz, Alan (NY)	EDM	210
Scott, Richard (MA)	OrS	611	Serafano, Donald (CA)	Oph	601
Scott, W Norman (NY)	OrS	623	Sergent, John (TN)	Rhu	1028
Scott, Walter (PA)	TS	1116	Sergott, Robert (PA)	Oph	577
Scott-Conner, Carol (IA)	S	1078	Serletti, Joseph (PA)	PlS	855
Scudder, Sidney (CA)	Onc	389	Serody, Jonathan (NC)	Onc	360
Scudera, Peter (VA)	Ge	242	Serota, Ronald (PA)	AdP	901
Sculco, Thomas (NY)	OrS	623	Session, Donna (GA)	RE	1012
Seashore, Margretta (CT)	CG	154	Sessoms, Sandra (TX)	Rhu	1031
Seaver, Laurie (HI)	CG	162	Sethi, Kapil (GA)	N	522
See, William (WI)	U	1164	Seton, Margaret (MA)	Rhu	1022
Seely, Ellen (MA)	EDM	206	Setzen, Michael (NY)	Oto	664
Seftel, Allen (NJ)	U	1151	Seung, Steven (OR)	RadRO	966
Segal, Brahm (NY)	Inf	407	Sewell, C Whitaker (GA)	Path	714
Seibel, Barry (CA)	Oph	601	Sewell, Catherine (MD)	ObG	554
Seidner, Douglas (TN)	Ge	242	Sexson, Sandra (GA)	ChAP	907
Seidner, Steven (TX)	NP	448	Seyfer, Alan (MD)	PlS	855
Seifer, David (NY)	RE	1010	Sha, Beverly (IL)	Inf	411
Seiff, Stuart (CA)	Oph	601	Shaban, Stephen (NC)	U	1157
Seifter, Julian (MA)	Nep	453	Shabsigh, Ridwan (NY)	U	1151
Seitz, William (OH)	HS	301	Shabto, Uri (NY)	Oph	577
Sekhar, Laligam (WA)	NS	495	Shadick, Nancy (MA)	Rhu	1023
Sekhon, Lali (NV)	NS	495	Shaffrey, Christopher (VA)	NS	480
Selby, Robert (CA)	S	1094	Shaffrey, Mark (VA)	NS	480
Selden, Nathan (OR)	NS	495	Shah, Jatin (NY)	S	1059

Alphabetical Listing of Doctors

Name	Specialty	Pg	Name	Specialty	Pg
Shah, Nishit (RI)	CRS	167	Shenot, Patrick (PA)	U	1151
Shah, Prediman (CA)	Cv	116	Shepard, Alexander (MI)	VascS	1186
Shaked, Abraham (PA)	S	1059	Shepherd, Gillian (NY)	A&I	85
Shaker, Reza (WI)	Ge	247	Sherertz, Elizabeth (NC)	D	192
Shamberger, Robert (MA)	PS	801	Sherman, Carol (SC)	Onc	360
Shamie, Neda (CA)	Oph	601	Sherman, Frederick (PA)	PCd	735
Shani, Jacob (NY)	IC	126	Sherman, James (VA)	PPul	795
Shapiro, Amy (IN)	PHO	772	Sherman, Randolph (CA)	PlS	874
Shapiro, Charles (OH)	Onc	371	Sherman, Steven (TX)	EDM	219
Shapiro, Edward (MA)	Psyc	886	Sherman, Stuart (IN)	Ge	247
Shapiro, Eugene (CT)	PInf	779	Sherry, David (PA)	PRhu	799
Shapiro, Jerrold (IL)	Cv	109	Sherwood, Mark (FL)	Oph	584
Shapiro, Lawrence (NY)	CG	156	Shibata, David (FL)	S	1067
Shapiro, Richard (NY)	S	1059	Shibata, Stephen (CA)	Onc	389
Shapiro, Ron (PA)	S	1059	Shields, Carol (PA)	Oph	578
Shapiro, Scott (IN)	NS	486	Shields, Jerry (PA)	Oph	578
Shapiro, William (AZ)	N	532	Shields, Peter (DC)	Onc	347
Shapshay, Stanley (NY)	Oto	664	Shiffman, Mitchell (VA)	Ge	242
Sharkey, Peter (PA)	OrS	623	Shike, Moshe (NY)	Ge	238
Sharlip, Ira (CA)	U	1172	Shikora, Scott (MA)	S	1047
Sharma, Om Prakash (CA)	Pul	939	Shin, Dong Moon (GA)	Onc	360
Sharp, Gregory (AR)	ChiN	151	Shina, Donald (NM)	RadRO	963
Sharp, Kenneth (TN)	S	1067	Shindo, Maisie (OR)	Oto	686
Shaw, Dennis (WA)	DR	983	Shingleton, Bradford (MA)	Oph	569
Shaw, Edward (NC)	RadRO	955	Shinnar, Shlomo (NY)	ChiN	147
Shaywitz, Bennett (CT)	ChiN	145	Shlansky-Goldberg, Richard (PA)	VIR	993
Shaywitz, Sally (CT)	Ped	726	Shlofmitz, Richard (NY)	Cv	99
Shea, Christopher (IL)	D	195	Shochat, Stephen (TN)	PS	806
Shea, Richard (IN)	Cv	109	Shockley, William (NC)	Oto	670
Shea, Thomas (NC)	Onc	360	Shore, Bernard (MO)	Pul	933
Shearer, Patricia (FL)	PHO	767	Shorofsky, Stephen (MD)	IC	126
Shearer, William (TX)	PA&I	732	Short, Billie (DC)	NP	444
Shefner, Jeremy (NY)	N	515	Shortliffe, Linda (CA)	U	1172
Sheinfeld, Joel (NY)	U	1151	Shrager, Joseph (CA)	TS	1137
Shelbourne, K Donald (IN)	OrS	635	Shrieve, Dennis (UT)	RadRO	961
Shellito, Judd (LA)	Pul	936	Shuer, Lawrence (CA)	NS	495
Shellito, Paul (MA)	CRS	167	Shuldiner, Alan (MD)	EDM	210
Shelton, Clough (UT)	Oto	679	Shulman, Lawrence (MA)	Onc	331
Shemin, Richard (CA)	TS	1136	Shulman, Lee (IL)	CG	159
Shen, Perry (NC)	S	1067	Shulman, Lisa (MD)	N	515
Shenk, Robert (OH)	S	1078	Shulman, Stanford (IL)	PInf	782

Name	Specialty	Pg	Name	Specialty	Pg
Shupack, Jerome (NY)	D	189	Silverman, William (IA)	Ge	247
Siatkowski, R Michael (OK)	Oph	595	Silverstein, Herbert (FL)	Oto	670
Sibley, Richard (CA)	Path	721	Silverstein, Janet (FL)	PEn	745
Sicard, Gregorio (MO)	VascS	1186	Silverstein, Melvin (CA)	S	1094
Sicherer, Scott (NY)	PA&I	730	Silverstein, Roy (WI)	Hem	320
Sichting, Kay (IN)	PCCM	741	Silvestry, Frank (PA)	Cv	100
Siddique, Teepu (IL)	N	528	Sim, Franklin (MN)	OrS	635
Sidransky, David (MD)	Onc	347	Simeone, Diane (MI)	S	1078
Siebert, John (WI)	PlS	866	Simmons, Charles (CA)	NP	448
Siegel, Barry (MO)	NuM	546	Simmons, Rache (NY)	S	1059
Siegel, Corey (NH)	Ge	230	Simms, Robert (MA)	Rhu	1023
Siegel, Gordon (IL)	Oto	677	Simon, Daniel (OH)	Cv	109
Siegel, Herrick (AL)	OrS	628	Simon, George (SC)	Onc	360
Siegel, Martin (WA)	Inf	414	Simon, James (DC)	ObG	554
Siegel, Stuart (CA)	PHO	778	Simon, John (NY)	Oph	578
Siegelbaum, Marc (MD)	U	1151	Simon, Richard (MI)	Pul	933
Sielaff, Timothy (MN)	S	1078	Simpson, David (NY)	N	515
Siemionow, Maria (OH)	PlS	866	Simpson, Joe (FL)	ObG	556
Sigel, Eric (CO)	AM	81	Sinanan, Mika (WA)	S	1094
Sigman, Mark (RI)	U	1144	Singer, Carlos (FL)	N	522
Sigurdson, Elin (PA)	S	1059	Singer, Daniel (HI)	OrS	643
Sikic, Branimir (CA)	Onc	389	Singer, Mark (CA)	Oto	686
Sila, Cathy (OH)	N	528	Singer, Peter (CA)	EDM	222
Silber, Sherman (MO)	U	1164	Singer, Robert (CA)	PlS	875
Silbergeld, Daniel (WA)	NS	495	Singer, Samuel (NY)	S	1059
Silberstein, Stephen (PA)	N	515	Singh, Arun (RI)	TS	1108
Siller, Barry (TX)	GO	288	Singh, Dinesh (CT)	U	1144
Sillers, Michael (AL)	Oto	670	Singh, Nalini (DC)	PInf	780
Sills, Allen (TN)	NS	480	Singh, Navin (MD)	PlS	856
Sills, Edward (MD)	PRhu	799	Singh, Nimi (MN)	AM	81
Silva, Elvio (TX)	Path	719	Singhal, Seema (IL)	Hem	320
Silver, Julie (MA)	PMR	832	Sinha, Uttam (CA)	Oto	686
Silver, Lester (NY)	PlS	856	Siperstein, Allan (OH)	S	1078
Silver, Michael (IL)	Pul	933	Sirdofsky, Michael (DC)	N	515
Silver, Richard (SC)	Rhu	1028	Siris, Ethel (NY)	EDM	210
Silver, Samuel (MI)	Onc	371	Sisti, Michael (NY)	NS	474
Silverman, Damon (VT)	Oto	657	Sisung, Charles (IL)	PMR	840
Silverman, Gary (PA)	NP	444	Sivina, Manuel (FL)	VascS	1184
Silverman, Jan (PA)	Path	711	Sivit, Carlos (OH)	DR	981
Silverman, Lewis (NY)	Onc	348	Skibber, John (TX)	S	1087
Silverman, Paula (OH)	Onc	371	Skinner, Eila (CA)	U	1172

Alphabetical Listing of Doctors

Name	Specialty	Pg	Name	Specialty	Pg
Skinner, Kristin (NY)	S	1060	Smith, Lloyd (CA)	GO	290
Skinner, Michael (TX)	PS	809	Smith, Matthew (MA)	Onc	331
Sklar, Charles (NY)	PEn	744	Smith, Mitchell (PA)	Onc	348
Sklar, Frederick (TX)	NS	490	Smith, Paul (FL)	PlS	861
Skolnick, Alan (AK)	Cv	116	Smith, Peter (NC)	TS	1123
Skoner, David (PA)	PA&I	730	Smith, Ronald (CA)	Oph	601
Skyler, Jay (FL)	EDM	213	Smith, Russell (NE)	Oto	680
Slama, Thomas (IN)	Inf	411	Smith, Scott (NY)	Oph	578
Slankard, Marjorie (NY)	A&I	85	Smith, Sidney (NC)	Cv	104
Slap, Gail (PA)	AM	80	Smith, Steven (IL)	VIR	995
Slatkin, Neal (CA)	PM	701	Smith, Thomas (VA)	Onc	361
Slaughter, Mark (KY)	TS	1123	Smith, Thomas (MA)	Path	707
Slavin, Sumner (MA)	PlS	849	Smith, Wade (CA)	N	537
Slawin, Kevin (TX)	U	1168	Smith, Yolanda (MI)	RE	1014
Slease, Robert (DE)	Hem	313	Smoot, Duane (DC)	Ge	238
Sleasman, John (FL)	PA&I	731	Smythe, W Roy (TX)	TS	1133
Sledge, George (IN)	Onc	371	Snyder, David (LA)	CE	122
Slezak, Sheri (MD)	PlS	856	Snyder, David (CA)	Hem	325
Slingluff, Craig (VA)	S	1068	Snyder, Howard (PA)	U	1152
Slivka, Adam (PA)	Ge	238	Snyder, John (DC)	PGe	750
Sliwa, James (IL)	PMR	840	Snyder, Peter (PA)	EDM	210
Slomowitz, Marcia (IL)	ChAP	907	Snyderman, Carl (PA)	Oto	664
Slutsky, David (CA)	HS	303	Sobel, Jack (MI)	Inf	411
Sly, R Michael (DC)	PA&I	730	Sobel, Michael (WA)	VascS	1188
Small, Donald (MD)	PHO	762	Sobel, Stuart (FL)	D	192
Small, Eric (CA)	Onc	389	Sober, Arthur (MA)	D	184
Small, Gary (CA)	GerPsy	912	Soberman, Mark (DC)	TS	1116
Small, William (IL)	RadRO	960	Socinski, Mark (NC)	Onc	361
Smalley, Stephen (KS)	RadRO	961	Socol, Michael (IL)	MF	433
Smalling, Richard (TX)	IC	130	Soiffer, Robert (MA)	Onc	331
Smart, Frank (LA)	Cv	113	Soisson, Andrew (UT)	GO	286
Smedira, Nicholas (OH)	TS	1129	Sokol, Lubomir (FL)	Hem	316
Smikle, Collin (CA)	RE	1018	Sokol, Ronald (CO)	PGe	754
Smith, Barbara (MA)	S	1047	Sokol, Thomas (CA)	CRS	176
Smith, Craig (NY)	TS	1116	Sokoloff, Daniel (FL)	D	192
Smith, David (FL)	PlS	861	Solberg, Lawrence (FL)	Hem	316
Smith, Donna (IL)	GO	286	Solin, Lawrence (PA)	RadRO	950
Smith, Douglas (WA)	OrS	643	Solitar, Bruce (NY)	Rhu	1026
Smith, Joanne (IL)	PMR	840	Solomon, Gary (NY)	Rhu	1026
Smith, John (OH)	TS	1129	Solomon, Robert (NY)	NS	474
Smith, Joseph (TN)	U	1158	Solorzano, Carmen (TN)	S	1068

Name	Specialty	Pg	Name	Specialty	Pg
Soloway, Mark (FL)	U	1158	Sperling, Michael (PA)	N	516
Somerville, James (MN)	Nep	459	Spetzler, Robert (AZ)	NS	490
Sommer, Robert (NY)	PCd	735	Speyer, James (NY)	Onc	348
Sondak, Vernon (FL)	S	1068	Spiegel, David (CA)	Psyc	899
Sondel, Paul (WI)	PHO	772	Spiera, Harry (NY)	Rhu	1026
Sondheimer, Steven (PA)	RE	1010	Spigland, Nitsana (NY)	PS	803
Sonett, Joshua (NY)	TS	1117	Spindler, Kurt (TN)	OrS	629
Song, John (CO)	Oto	680	Spinelli, Henry (NY)	PlS	856
Song, Kit (WA)	OrS	644	Spinner, Robert (MN)	NS	486
Song, Shiyu (VA)	RadRO	955	Spitzer, Thomas (MA)	Hem	309
Sontheimer, Richard (UT)	D	196	Spivak, Jeffrey (NY)	OrS	623
Sood, Anil (TX)	GO	288	Spivak, Jerry (MD)	Hem	313
Sood, Rajiv (IN)	PlS	866	Spivak, William (NY)	PGe	750
Soparkar, Charles (TX)	Oph	595	Sponseller, Paul (MD)	OrS	623
Soper, John (NC)	GO	283	Spray, Thomas (PA)	TS	1117
Soper, Nathaniel (IL)	S	1078	Spriggs, David (NY)	Onc	348
Sorrell, Michael (NE)	Ge	249	Squires, Robert (PA)	PGe	750
Sorrentino, Matthew (IL)	Cv	109	St Clair, William (KY)	RadRO	955
Sorrentino, Robert (GA)	CE	120	Staats, Peter (NJ)	PM	696
Sosa, Julie (CT)	S	1047	Stadelmann, Wayne (NH)	PlS	849
Sosa, R Ernest (NY)	U	1152	Stadler, Walter (IL)	Onc	371
Soslow, Robert (NY)	Path	711	Stadtmauer, Edward (PA)	Onc	348
Sosman, Jeffrey (TN)	Onc	361	Staffenberg, David (NY)	PlS	856
Soter, Nicholas (NY)	D	189	Staggers, Barbara (CA)	AM	82
Sotereanos, Dean (PA)	HS	297	Stahl, Donna (OH)	S	1078
Sotomayor, Eduardo (FL)	Onc	361	Stahl, Richard (CT)	PlS	849
Soulen, Michael (PA)	VIR	993	Stainback, Raymond (TX)	Cv	113
Soules, Michael (WA)	RE	1018	Stal, Samuel (TX)	PlS	870
Souryal, Tarek (TX)	OrS	639	Staley, Charles (GA)	S	1068
Souweidane, Mark (NY)	NS	475	Stamos, Michael (CA)	CRS	176
Sowers, James (MO)	EDM	217	Stangel, John (NY)	RE	1010
Spack, Norman (MA)	PEn	743	Stankiewicz, James (IL)	Oto	677
Spann, Cyril (GA)	GO	283	Stanley, Charles (PA)	PEn	745
Speeg, Kermit (TX)	Ge	252	Stanley, James (MI)	VascS	1186
Speer, Kevin (NC)	SM	1038	Stanley, John (PA)	D	189
Spence, Robert (MD)	PlS	856	Staples, Edward (FL)	TS	1123
Spencer, Dennis (CT)	NS	467	Staren, Edgar (IL)	S	1078
Spencer, Thomas (MA)	ChAP	904	Stark, Walter (MD)	Oph	578
Spengler, Dan (TN)	OrS	628	Starnes, Vaughn (CA)	TS	1137
Spergel, Jonathan (PA)	PA&I	730	Starr, Arnold (CA)	N	537
Sperling, Mark (PA)	PEn	745	Starz, Terence (PA)	Rhu	1026

Alphabetical Listing of Doctors

Name	Specialty	Pg	Name	Specialty	Pg
Stasney, C Richard (TX)	Oto	682	Stevenson, Roger (SC)	CG	157
Staton, Gerald (GA)	Pul	929	Stevenson, William (MA)	CE	117
Stea, Baldassarre (AZ)	RadRO	963	Stewart, Allan (NY)	TS	1117
Steadman, J Richard (CO)	OrS	638	Stewart, Elizabeth (MN)	RE	1015
Steege, John (NC)	ObG	556	Stewart, Forrest (WA)	Onc	390
Steen, Preston (ND)	Onc	375	Stewart, Michael (NY)	Oto	664
Steen, Virginia (DC)	Rhu	1026	Stewart, Paula (AL)	PMR	837
Steers, William (VA)	U	1158	Stewart, Ronald (TX)	S	1087
Stefanyszyn, Mary (PA)	Oph	578	Stewart, William (OH)	Cv	109
Stehman, Frederick (IN)	GO	286	Stieg, Philip (NY)	NS	475
Steiger, David (NY)	Pul	925	Stiff, Patrick (IL)	Hem	320
Stein, David (PA)	CRS	169	Stiles, Alan (NC)	NP	445
Stein, Elliott (CA)	GerPsy	912	Stine, Susan (MI)	AdP	902
Stein, James (CA)	PS	811	Stock, Richard (NY)	RadRO	950
Stein, James (WI)	Cv	109	Stockdale, Frank (CA)	Onc	390
Stein, Murray (CA)	Psyc	899	Stolar, Charles (NY)	PS	804
Steinberg, Gary (CA)	NS	495	Stolier, Alan (LA)	S	1087
Steinberg, Gary (IL)	U	1165	Stoller, James (OH)	Pul	933
Steinberg, Harry (NY)	Pul	926	Stoller, Marshall (CA)	U	1173
Steiner, Hans (CA)	ChAP	909	Stone, Anthony (CA)	U	1173
Steiner, Mark (MA)	SM	1036	Stone, Edwin (IA)	Oph	591
Steinert, Roger (CA)	Oph	601	Stone, Gregg (NY)	IC	126
Steingart, Richard (NY)	Cv	100	Stone, Joel (FL)	Onc	361
Steinhagen, Randolph (NY)	CRS	169	Stone, Michael (NY)	Psyc	891
Steinherz, Laurel (NY)	PCd	735	Stone, Richard (MA)	Hem	309
Steinherz, Peter (NY)	PHO	762	Stoopler, Mark (NY)	Onc	348
Steinhorn, Robin (IL)	NP	447	Stopeck, Alison (AZ)	Onc	381
Steinkampf, Michael (AL)	RE	1012	Stotland, Mitchell (NH)	PlS	849
Steinmann, Scott (MN)	HS	301	Stough, Rebecca (OK)	DR	982
Stenson, Kerstin (IL)	Oto	677	Stout, J Timothy (OR)	Oph	601
Sterman, Daniel (PA)	Pul	926	Stover-Pepe, Diane (NY)	Pul	926
Stern, Jeffrey (CA)	GO	290	Stowe, Cary (FL)	TS	1124
Stern, Leonard (NY)	Nep	455	Strain, Eric (MD)	AdP	901
Stern, Matthew (PA)	N	516	Strair, Roger (NJ)	Hem	314
Stern, Peter (OH)	HS	301	Strakowski, Stephen (OH)	Psyc	894
Stern, Robert (MA)	D	184	Strand, William (TX)	U	1168
Sternberg, Paul (TN)	Oph	584	Strashun, Arnold (NY)	NuM	545
Sterns, Gwen (NY)	Oph	578	Strassner, Howard (IL)	MF	433
Stevens, W Grant (CA)	PlS	875	Stratta, Robert (NC)	S	1068
Stevenson, David (CA)	NP	448	Strauch, Eric (MD)	PS	804
Stevenson, Lynne (MA)	Cv	94	Strauch, Robert (NY)	HS	297

Name	Specialty	Pg	Name	Specialty	Pg
Straus, David (NY)	Onc	348	Summers, C Gail (MN)	Oph	591
Strauss, Gary (MA)	Onc	331	Sumpio, Bauer (CT)	VascS	1179
Strauss, H William (NY)	NuM	545	Sun, Peter (CA)	NS	495
Strauss, James (TX)	Hem	323	Sun, Weijing (PA)	Onc	349
Streeter, Oscar (DC)	RadRO	950	Sundaram, Chandru (IN)	U	1165
Streiff, Michael (MD)	Hem	314	Sundaram, Magesh (WV)	S	1060
Streim, Joel (PA)	GerPsy	910	Sundaresan, Narayan (NY)	NS	475
Strenger, Rochelle (RI)	Onc	331	Sundy, John (NC)	A&I	87
Stringer, Scott (MS)	Oto	670	Suntharalingam, Mohan (MD)	RadRO	950
Strollo, Patrick (PA)	Pul	926	Supiano, Mark (UT)	Ger	266
Strome, Marshall (NY)	Oto	664	Surawicz, Christina (WA)	Ge	255
Strome, Scott (MD)	Oto	664	Suresh, Santhanam (IL)	PM	698
Strong, Michael (PA)	TS	1117	Surks, Martin (NY)	EDM	211
Strongwater, Allan (NJ)	OrS	623	Surrey, Eric (CO)	RE	1015
Strouse, Thomas (CA)	Psyc	899	Sussman, Norman (NY)	Psyc	891
Strunk, Robert (MO)	PA&I	731	Suster, Saul (WI)	Path	716
Strup, Stephen (KY)	U	1158	Sutherland, Everett (CO)	Pul	935
Stryker, Steven (IL)	CRS	174	Sutherland, Richard (NC)	U	1158
Stuart, Richard (MO)	TS	1129	Sutphen, Rebecca (FL)	CG	157
Stubblefield, Michael (NY)	PMR	836	Sutton, John (NH)	S	1048
Stuchin, Steven (NY)	OrS	624	Sutton, Leslie (PA)	NS	475
Studenski, Stephanie (PA)	Ger	263	Sutton, Linda (NC)	Onc	361
Stulberg, S David (IL)	OrS	636	Svensson, Lars (OH)	TS	1129
Stulting, R Doyle (GA)	Oph	584	Swaid, Swaid (AL)	NS	481
Stump, David (TX)	Ge	252	Swain, Sandra (DC)	Onc	349
Stuzin, James (FL)	PlS	861	Swanson, David (TX)	U	1168
Stylianos, Steven (NY)	PS	804	Swanson, Jerry (MN)	N	528
Su, Li-Ming (FL)	U	1158	Swanson, Neil (OR)	D	200
Suarez, Jose (TX)	N	532	Swanson, Scott (MA)	TS	1108
Suchy, Frederick (CO)	PGe	754	Swanstrom, Lee (OR)	S	1094
Suen, James (AR)	Oto	682	Swarm, Robert (MO)	PM	698
Sugarbaker, David (MA)	TS	1108	Swartz, Richard (MI)	Nep	459
Sugarbaker, Paul (DC)	S	1060	Swearingen, Brooke (MA)	NS	467
Suh, John (OH)	RadRO	960	Sweeney, Christopher (MA)	Onc	331
Suki, Wadi (TX)	Nep	460	Sweeney, John (GA)	S	1068
Sulica, Radu Lucian (NY)	Oto	665	Sweet, Richard (CA)	ObG	560
Sullivan, Kathleen (PA)	PA&I	730	Sweetenham, John (OH)	Onc	371
Sullivan, Patrick (RI)	PlS	849	Swensen, Stephen (MN)	DR	981
Sullivan, Timothy (GA)	A&I	87	Swerdloff, Ronald (CA)	EDM	222
Sultan, Mark (NY)	PlS	856	Swerdlow, Charles (CA)	CE	123
Summergrad, Paul (MA)	Psyc	886	Swerdlow, Michael (NY)	N	516

Alphabetical Listing of Doctors

Name	Specialty	Pg
Swerdlow, Steven (PA)	Path	711
Swetter, Susan (CA)	D	200
Swiontkowski, Marc (MN)	OrS	636
Swisher, Stephen (TX)	TS	1133
Swistel, Alexander (NY)	S	1060
Swistel, Daniel (NY)	TS	1117
Szabo, Robert (CA)	HS	303
Szachowicz, Edward (MN)	Oto	677
Sze, Gordon (CT)	NRad	984

T

Name	Specialty	Pg
Tabbal, Nicolas (NY)	PlS	856
Tabsh, Khalil (CA)	MF	437
Taetle, Raymond (AZ)	Onc	381
Tafra, Lorraine (MD)	S	1060
Taft, Timothy (NC)	OrS	629
Tagawa, Scott (NY)	Onc	349
Taghian, Alphonse (MA)	RadRO	945
Takayama, Thomas (WA)	U	1173
Talamonti, Mark (IL)	S	1078
Tallman, Martin (NY)	Hem	314
Tamargo, Rafael (MD)	NS	475
Tamaroff, Marc (CA)	A&I	90
Tamborlane, William (CT)	PEn	743
Tanabe, Kenneth (MA)	S	1048
Taneja, Samir (NY)	U	1152
Tanner, Caroline (CA)	N	537
Tannous, Raymond (IA)	PHO	772
Taplin, Mary-Ellen (MA)	Onc	331
Tapson, Victor (NC)	Pul	930
Tarbell, Nancy (MA)	RadRO	945
Targan, Stephan (CA)	Ge	255
Tarraza, Hector (ME)	GO	275
Tartter, Paul (NY)	S	1060
Tatter, Stephen (NC)	NS	481
Taub, Peter (NY)	PlS	857
Tauber, Danna (PA)	PPul	795
Tayal, Ashis (PA)	N	516
Taylon, Charles (NE)	NS	488

Name	Specialty	Pg
Taylor, Frederick (MN)	N	528
Taylor, Lynne (WA)	N	537
Taylor, Marie (MO)	RadRO	960
Taylor, Peyton (VA)	GO	283
Taylor, R Stan (TX)	D	198
Taylor, Richard (TX)	PCCM	742
Tchou, Julia (PA)	S	1060
Tchou, Patrick (OH)	CE	121
Te, Helen (IL)	Ge	248
Teal, James (DC)	DR	977
Tebbetts, John (TX)	PlS	870
Tebbi, Cameron (FL)	PHO	767
Tedder, Mark (TN)	TS	1124
Teigland, Chris (NC)	U	1158
Teirstein, Alvin (NY)	Pul	926
Teirstein, Paul (CA)	IC	130
Teitel, David (CA)	PCd	740
Teitelbaum, George (CA)	NRad	991
Teitz, Carol (WA)	SM	1040
Teknos, Theodoros (OH)	Oto	677
Telen, Marilyn (NC)	Hem	316
Telian, Steven (MI)	Oto	677
Telischi, Fred (FL)	Oto	670
Tempero, Margaret (CA)	Onc	390
Tenenbaum, Joseph (NY)	Cv	100
Teng, Nelson (CA)	GO	291
Tenner, Michael (NY)	NRad	986
Tennison, Michael (NC)	ChiN	148
Tenover, Joyce (CA)	Ger	267
Teperman, Lewis (NY)	S	1060
Tepper, Joel (NC)	RadRO	956
Terr, Lenore (CA)	ChAP	909
Terris, David (GA)	Oto	670
Terris, Martha (GA)	U	1158
Tester, William (PA)	Onc	349
Tetrud, James (CA)	N	537
Tewari, Ashutosh (NY)	U	1152
Textor, Stephen (MN)	Nep	459
Thaller, Seth (FL)	PlS	861
Thames, Marc (AZ)	Cv	113
Tharratt, Robert (CA)	Pul	939

Name	Specialty	Pg	Name	Specialty	Pg
Thase, Michael (PA)	Psyc	891	Tomaselli, Gordon (MD)	CE	119
Thayer, Sarah (MA)	S	1048	Tomaszewski, John (PA)	Path	712
Thiers, Bruce (SC)	D	192	Tomford, J Walton (OH)	Inf	411
Thigpen, James (MS)	Onc	361	Tomich, Paul (NE)	MF	434
Thistlethwaite, J Richard (IL)	S	1079	Tomita, Tadanori (IL)	NS	486
Thistlethwaite, Patricia (CA)	TS	1137	Tomlinson, Gail (TX)	PHO	775
Thoder, Joseph (PA)	HS	297	Tonsgard, James (IL)	ChiN	150
Thomas, Bert (CA)	OrS	644	Toonkel, Leonard (FL)	RadRO	956
Thomas, Charles (OR)	RadRO	966	Topham, Neal (PA)	PlS	857
Thomas, Christie (IA)	Nep	459	Toppmeyer, Deborah (NJ)	Onc	349
Thomas, David (MO)	Ger	266	Toriumi, Dean (IL)	Oto	677
Thomas, Gregory (OR)	PHO	778	Tornetta, Paul (MA)	OrS	611
Thomas, Ronald (PA)	MF	429	Tornos, Carmen (NY)	Path	712
Thomashow, Byron (NY)	Pul	926	Torres, Vicente (MN)	Nep	459
Thompson, Ann Ellen (PA)	PCCM	741	Torti, Frank (NC)	Onc	361
Thompson, B Gregory (MI)	NS	486	Tortolani, Anthony (NY)	TS	1117
Thompson, Brad (IA)	DR	981	Toskes, Phillip (FL)	Ge	242
Thompson, George (OH)	OrS	636	Toth, Thomas (MA)	RE	1007
Thompson, Ian (TX)	U	1169	Toto, Robert (TX)	Nep	461
Thompson, John (WA)	Onc	390	Townsend, Raymond (PA)	Nep	455
Thompson, Reid (TN)	NS	481	Toyoda, Yoshiya (PA)	TS	1117
Thor, Ann (CO)	Path	717	Traboulsi, Elias (OH)	Oph	592
Thordarson, David (CA)	OrS	644	Trabulsi, Edouard (PA)	U	1152
Thorne, Charles (NY)	PlS	857	Tracy, Thomas (RI)	PS	801
Thornhill, Thomas (MA)	OrS	611	Tranbaugh, Robert (NY)	TS	1118
Thorp, John (NC)	MF	431	Trauner, Doris (CA)	ChiN	152
Thorson, Alan (NE)	CRS	174	Travis, William (NY)	Path	712
Thrasher, J Brantley (KS)	U	1166	Traynelis, Vincent (IL)	NS	487
Thulborn, Keith (IL)	NRad	989	Traynor, Michael (ND)	S	1081
Thurmond, Amy (OR)	DR	983	Treadwell, Marjorie (MI)	MF	433
Tinetti, Mary (CT)	Ger	262	Treadwell, Patricia (IN)	D	195
Ting, Jess (NY)	PlS	857	Tremaine, William (MN)	Ge	248
Tino, Gregory (PA)	Pul	926	Trenholme, Gordon (IL)	Inf	411
Tkaczuk, Katherine (MD)	Onc	349	Trento, Alfredo (CA)	TS	1137
Tobias, Hillel (NY)	Ge	238	Treon, Steven (MA)	Onc	331
Tobin, Gordon (KY)	PlS	861	Trerotola, Scott (PA)	VIR	993
Tobin, Martin (IL)	Pul	933	Trese, Michael (MI)	Oph	592
Tobis, Jonathan (CA)	Cv	116	Triche, Timothy (CA)	Path	722
Todd, George (NY)	VascS	1183	Triozzi, Pierre (OH)	Onc	371
Tolkoff-Rubin, Nina (MA)	Nep	453	Tripathy, Debasish (CA)	Onc	390
Tolo, Vernon (CA)	OrS	644	Tripuraneni, Prabhakar (CA)	RadRO	966

Alphabetical Listing of Doctors

Name	Specialty	Pg	Name	Specialty	Pg
Trisal, Vijay (CA)	S	1095	Ulissey, Michael (TX)	DR	982
Trobe, Jonathan (MI)	Oph	592	Ulshen, Martin (NC)	PGe	751
Troner, Michael (FL)	Onc	362	Umetsu, Dale (MA)	A&I	84
Trudel, Judith (MN)	CRS	174	Unger, Michael (PA)	Pul	927
True, Lawrence (WA)	Path	722	Ungerleider, Ross (NC)	TS	1124
Trulock, Elbert (MO)	Pul	933	Updegraff, Stephen (FL)	Oph	584
Trumble, Thomas (WA)	HS	303	Urata, Mark (CA)	PlS	875
Trump, Donald (NY)	Onc	349	Urba, Susan (MI)	Onc	371
Tsai, James (CT)	Oph	569	Urba, Walter (OR)	Onc	390
Tsangaris, Theodore (MD)	S	1060	Urist, Marshall (AL)	S	1069
Tsao, Hensin (MA)	D	184	Urken, Mark (NY)	Oto	665
Tse, David (FL)	Oph	584	Uzzo, Robert (PA)	U	1152
Tsokos, George (MA)	Rhu	1023			
Tucci, Debara (NC)	Oto	670			
Tucker, Rodney (AL)	IM	420	# V		
Tufano, Ralph (MD)	Oto	665			
Tufaro, Anthony (MD)	PlS	857	Vaccaro, Alexander (PA)	OrS	624
Tuggle, David (OK)	PS	809	Vaezi, Michael (TN)	Ge	242
Tulsky, James (NC)	IM	420	Vahdat, Linda (NY)	Onc	349
Tune, Larry (GA)	GerPsy	911	Vail, Thomas (CA)	OrS	644
Tunkel, David (MD)	PO	789	Vajaranant, Thasarat (IL)	Oph	592
Turecki, Stanley (NY)	ChAP	906	Valaitis, Sandra (IL)	ObG	558
Turek, Paul (CA)	U	1173	Valea, Fidel (NC)	GO	283
Turner, William (TX)	TS	1133	Valentine, Alan (TX)	Psyc	896
Turrentine, Mark (IN)	TS	1129	Valentino, Joseph (KY)	Oto	671
Turtz, Alan (NJ)	NS	475	Valentino, Leonard (IL)	PHO	772
Tuttle, R Michael (NY)	EDM	211	Valero, Vicente (TX)	Onc	381
Tuttle, Todd (MN)	S	1079	Valji, Karim (WA)	VIR	997
Tuxhorn, Ingrid (OH)	ChiN	150	Vallieres, Eric (WA)	TS	1137
Twardowski, Przemyslaw (CA)	Onc	390	Van Arsdalen, Keith (PA)	U	1152
Tychsen, Lawrence (MO)	Oph	592	Van Besien, Koen (IL)	Hem	321
Tyler, Douglas (NC)	S	1068	Van Der Horst, Charles (NC)	Inf	409
Tyson, Jon (TX)	NP	448	Van Dorsten, J Peter (SC)	MF	431
Tzakis, Andreas (FL)	S	1068	van Hoff, Jack (NH)	PHO	756
			Van Loveren, Harry (FL)	NS	481
			Van Marter, Linda (MA)	NP	442
# U			Van Nagell, John (KY)	GO	283
			Van Thiel, David (IL)	Ge	248
Uberti, Joseph (MI)	Hem	321	Van Voorhis, Bradley (IA)	RE	1015
Udelsman, Robert (CT)	S	1048	Van Zee, Kimberly (NY)	S	1061
Ulbright, Thomas (IN)	Path	717	Vance, Mary Lee (VA)	EDM	213

Name	Specialty	Pg
Vance, Ralph (MS)	Onc	362
Vander, James (PA)	Oph	578
Vander Kolk, Craig (MD)	PlS	857
Vander Salm, Thomas (MA)	TS	1108
Vanderhoof, Jon (NE)	PGe	754
Vapnek, Jonathan (NY)	U	1152
Varadhachary, Gauri (TX)	Onc	381
Vargo, John (OH)	Ge	248
Varma, Madhulika (CA)	CRS	176
Vas, George (NY)	N	516
Vasconez, Henry (KY)	PlS	861
Vaughan, William (AL)	Onc	362
Vaughey, Ellen (VA)	Pul	930
Vaughn, David (PA)	Onc	350
Vauthey, Jean (TX)	S	1087
Vege, Santhi (MN)	Ge	248
Veith, Richard (WA)	GerPsy	912
Velcek, Francisca (NY)	PS	804
Velvis, Harm (NY)	PCd	736
Venkat, K K (MI)	Nep	459
Venook, Alan (CA)	Onc	390
Verghese, Mohan (DC)	U	1153
Vernava, Anthony (FL)	CRS	171
Verrier, Edward (WA)	TS	1137
Verschraegen, Claire (VT)	Onc	332
Vescio, Robert (CA)	Onc	391
Vetrovec, George (VA)	Cv	104
Vetter, Thomas (AL)	PM	697
Vetto, John (OR)	S	1095
Vezina, L Gilbert (DC)	NRad	986
Vicini, Frank (MI)	RadRO	960
Vick, Nicholas (IL)	N	529
Vickers, Selwyn (MN)	S	1079
Videtic, Gregory (OH)	RadRO	961
Vierling, John (TX)	Ge	252
Vigneswaran, Wickii (IL)	TS	1129
Vignola, Paul (FL)	Cv	104
Vijayakumar, Srinivasan (MS)	RadRO	956
Vik, Terry (IN)	PHO	773
Villanueva, Andrew (MA)	Pul	922
Vinciguerra, Vincent (NY)	Onc	350

Name	Specialty	Pg
Vining, Eileen (MD)	Ped	727
Vining, Eugenia (CT)	Oto	657
Vinuela, Fernando (CA)	NRad	991
Visco, Anthony (NC)	ObG	556
Vitek, Jerrold (MN)	N	529
Vivino, Frederick (PA)	Rhu	1026
Vlahakes, Gus (MA)	TS	1108
Voelkel, Norbert (VA)	Pul	930
Vogelzang, Nicholas (NV)	Onc	391
Vogelzang, Robert (IL)	VIR	995
Vogt, Peter (MN)	PlS	866
Voigt, Roger (MD)	PS	804
Vokes, Everett (IL)	Onc	372
Volberding, Paul (CA)	Onc	391
Volgman, Annabelle (IL)	Cv	109
Volkmar, Fred (CT)	ChAP	904
Vollmer, Timothy (CO)	N	530
Volpe, Joseph (MA)	ChiN	145
Volpe, Nicholas (IL)	Oph	592
Volshteyn, Oksana (MO)	PMR	840
Von Burton, Gary (LA)	Onc	381
von der Lohe, Elisabeth (IN)	Cv	110
von Gunten, Charles (CA)	Onc	391
Von Hoff, Daniel (AZ)	Onc	381
von Mehren, Margaret (PA)	Onc	350
Von Roenn, Jamie (IL)	Onc	372
Voorhees, John (MI)	D	195
Vose, Julie (NE)	Hem	321
Vredenburgh, James (NC)	Onc	362

W

Name	Specialty	Pg
Wackym, P Ashley (OR)	Oto	686
Waggoner, Steven (OH)	GO	286
Wagman, Lawrence (CA)	S	1095
Wagner-Weiner, Linda (IL)	PRhu	800
Wagoner, Lynne (OH)	Cv	110
Waguespack, Steven (TX)	EDM	219
Wahl, Richard (MD)	NuM	545
Wain, John (MA)	TS	1108

Alphabetical Listing of Doctors

Name	Specialty	Pg	Name	Specialty	Pg
Waintraub, Stanley (NJ)	Onc	350	Walton, Robert (IL)	PlS	866
Wait, Susan (MD)	Psyc	891	Wamboldt, Marianne (CO)	ChAP	908
Wakefield, Thomas (MI)	S	1079	Waner, Milton (NY)	Oto	665
Wald, Arnold (WI)	Ge	248	Wang, Beverly (NY)	Path	712
Wald, Ellen (WI)	PInf	782	Wang, Frederick (NY)	Oph	579
Waldhausen, John HT (WA)	PS	811	Wang, Jeffrey (CA)	OrS	644
Waldo, Albert (OH)	CE	122	Wang, Ming (TN)	Oph	584
Walker, Alonzo (WI)	S	1079	Wang, Paul (CA)	CE	123
Walker, David (TX)	Path	719	Wang, Steven (CA)	Oto	686
Walker, Joan (OK)	GO	288	Wang, Winfred (TN)	PHO	768
Walker, Marion (UT)	NS	488	Wanner, Adam (FL)	Pul	930
Walker, R Dale (OR)	AdP	902	Wapner, Keith (PA)	OrS	624
Walker, William (WA)	Ped	729	Wapner, Ronald (NY)	MF	430
Walkup, John (NY)	ChAP	906	Wapnir, Irene (CA)	S	1095
Wall, Michael (OR)	PPul	798	Wara, William (CA)	RadRO	966
Wallace, Anne Marie (CA)	S	1095	Warady, Bradley (MO)	PNep	787
Wallace, Daniel (CA)	Rhu	1032	Ward, Barbara (CT)	S	1048
Wallace, Jeanne (CA)	Pul	939	Ward, Jewell (TN)	CG	157
Wallace, Mark (FL)	Inf	410	Ward, John (UT)	Onc	375
Wallace, Mark (CA)	PM	702	Ward, Robert (NY)	PO	789
Wallace, Richard (TX)	Inf	413	Ward, William (NC)	OrS	629
Wallace, Robert (LA)	Oph	595	Waring, George (GA)	Oph	584
Wallach, Edward (MD)	RE	1010	Warner, Ann (MO)	Rhu	1030
Wallach, Frances (NY)	Inf	407	Warner, Brad (MO)	PS	808
Wallen, Eric (NC)	U	1159	Warner, Kenneth (MA)	TS	1108
Waller, Edmund (GA)	Onc	362	Warnick, Ronald (OH)	NS	487
Walling, Arthur (FL)	OrS	629	Warnke, Roger (CA)	Path	722
Walmer, David (NC)	RE	1012	Warnock, David (AL)	Nep	457
Walsh, B Timothy (NY)	Psyc	891	Warren, Robert (SC)	PRhu	799
Walsh, Christine (NY)	PCd	736	Warren, Robert (AR)	PPul	797
Walsh, Edward (MA)	PCd	734	Warren, Robert (CA)	S	1095
Walsh, Garrett (TX)	TS	1133	Warren, Russell (NY)	OrS	624
Walsh, John (LA)	NS	491	Wartofsky, Leonard (DC)	EDM	211
Walsh, Joseph (NY)	Oph	579	Wasserman, Richard (TX)	PA&I	732
Walsh, Mary (IN)	Cv	110	Wasserman, Stephen (CA)	A&I	90
Walsh, Nicolas (TX)	PM	700	Watchko, Jon (PA)	NP	444
Walsh, Patrick (MD)	U	1153	Waters, Cheryl (NY)	N	516
Walsh, R Matthew (OH)	S	1079	Waters, Peter (MA)	HS	294
Walters, Henry (MI)	TS	1129	Watkins, Robert (CA)	OrS	644
Walters, Mark (OH)	ObG	558	Watson, Thomas (NY)	TS	1118
Walton, David (MA)	Oph	569	Watson, William (MN)	MF	433

Alphabetical Listing of Doctors

Name	Specialty	Pg	Name	Specialty	Pg
Watts, Nelson (OH)	EDM	217	Weiner, I David (FL)	Nep	457
Watts, Ray (AL)	N	522	Weiner, Kenneth (CO)	Psyc	895
Wax, Mark (OR)	Oto	686	Weiner, Leslie (CA)	N	537
Waxman, Alan (CA)	NuM	547	Weiner, Louis (DC)	Onc	350
Waxman, Harvey (PA)	Cv	100	Weiner, Michael (NY)	PHO	763
Waxman, Irving (IL)	Ge	248	Weiner, Myron (TX)	Psyc	896
Waye, Jerome (NY)	Ge	238	Weiner, Richard (NC)	Psyc	892
Wazen, Jack (FL)	Oto	671	Weiner, Richard (FL)	OrS	629
Wazer, David (RI)	RadRO	946	Weiner, William (MD)	N	517
Weaver, David (IN)	CG	159	Weinfeld, Steven (NY)	OrS	624
Weaver, W Douglas (MI)	Cv	110	Weingart, Jon (MD)	NS	475
Webb, Gary (OH)	Cv	110	Weinreb, Jeffrey (CT)	DR	973
Webb, Lawrence (GA)	OrS	629	Weinstein, Arthur (DC)	Rhu	1027
Weber, Collin (GA)	S	1069	Weinstein, Gregory (PA)	Oto	665
Weber, Jeffrey (FL)	Onc	362	Weinstein, Howard (MA)	PHO	756
Weber, Randal (TX)	Oto	682	Weinstein, James (NH)	OrS	611
Weber, Samuel (TX)	Oto	683	Weinstein, Sharon (UT)	PM	699
Weber, Sharon (WI)	S	1079	Weinstein, Stuart (IA)	OrS	636
Weber, Thomas (IL)	PS	808	Weinstock, Joel (MA)	Ge	230
Webster, George (NC)	U	1159	Weinstock, Robert (CA)	Psyc	899
Webster, Harry (MA)	PMR	832	Weintraub, Joshua (NY)	VIR	993
Wechsler, Daniel (NC)	PHO	768	Weisberg, Tracey (ME)	Onc	332
Wechsler, Lawrence (PA)	N	516	Weisenburger, Dennis (NE)	Path	717
Weder, Alan (MI)	IM	420	Weisler, Richard (NC)	Psyc	893
Wei, Jeanne (AR)	Ger	267	Weisman, Robert (CA)	Oto	686
Weichselbaum, Ralph (IL)	RadRO	961	Weisman, Steven (WI)	PM	699
Weig, Spencer (NC)	ChiN	148	Weiss, Arnold (RI)	HS	294
Weigel, Ronald (IA)	S	1079	Weiss, Avery (WA)	Oph	601
Weigel, Tracey (WI)	TS	1130	Weiss, Geoffrey (VA)	Onc	362
Weigelt, John (WI)	S	1080	Weiss, Gerson (NJ)	RE	1010
Weiland, Andrew (NY)	HS	297	Weiss, Lawrence (CA)	Path	722
Weiman, Darryl (TN)	TS	1124	Weiss, Marisa (PA)	RadRO	951
Wein, Alan (PA)	U	1153	Weiss, Robert (NJ)	U	1153
Weinberg, David (PA)	Ge	238	Weiss, Robert (CT)	U	1144
Weinberg, Harold (NY)	N	516	Weiss, Roger (MA)	AdP	900
Weinberg, Paul (PA)	PCd	736	Weiss, Roy (IL)	EDM	218
Weinberger, Michael (NY)	PM	696	Weiss, Sharon (GA)	Path	714
Weinblatt, Mark (NY)	PHO	762	Weissler, Jonathan (TX)	Pul	936
Weinblatt, Michael (MA)	Rhu	1023	Weissler, Mark (NC)	Oto	671
Weiner, George (IA)	Onc	372	Weissman, Peter (FL)	EDM	214
Weiner, Howard (NY)	NS	475	Weitz, Howard (PA)	Cv	100

Alphabetical Listing of Doctors

Name	Specialty	Pg	Name	Specialty	Pg
Weitzel, Jeffrey (CA)	CG	162	Whitlow, Patrick (OH)	IC	129
Weksler, Benny (PA)	TS	1118	Whitsett, Jeffrey (OH)	NP	447
Welch, William (PA)	NS	476	Whitworth, Pat (TN)	S	1069
Wells, Gretchen (NC)	Cv	104	Whyte, Richard (CA)	TS	1137
Wells, James (CA)	PlS	875	Wicha, Max (MI)	Onc	372
Wells, Robert (WI)	DR	981	Wickiewicz, Thomas (NY)	OrS	624
Wells, Winfield (CA)	TS	1137	Widra, Eric (DC)	RE	1010
Welton, Mark (CA)	CRS	177	Wiebke, Eric (IN)	S	1080
Wen, Patrick (MA)	N	506	Wiedemann, Herbert (OH)	Pul	934
Wener, Mark (WA)	Rhu	1032	Wierman, Ann (NV)	Onc	391
Wenstrom, Katharine (RI)	MF	427	Wiesel, Sam (DC)	OrS	625
Wenzel, Sally (PA)	Pul	927	Wiesenfeld, Harold (PA)	ObG	554
Werner, Phillip (IL)	EDM	218	Wiesner, Russell (MN)	Ge	248
Werner-Wasik, Maria (PA)	RadRO	951	Wiet, Richard (IL)	Oto	677
Werth, Victoria (PA)	D	189	Wigley, Frederick (MD)	Rhu	1027
West, Sterling (CO)	Rhu	1030	Wilansky, Susan (AZ)	Cv	113
Westrich, Geoffrey (NY)	OrS	624	Wilber, David (IL)	CE	122
Wetzel, F Todd (PA)	OrS	624	Wilberger, James (PA)	NS	476
Wetzler, Meir (NY)	Onc	350	Wilcox, C Mel (AL)	Ge	243
Wexler, Leonard (NY)	PHO	763	Wilcox, Christopher (DC)	Nep	455
Wexner, Steven (FL)	CRS	171	Wilcox, Robert (TX)	PlS	870
Weymuller, Ernest (WA)	Oto	687	Wilcox, William (CA)	CG	162
Wharam, Moody (MD)	RadRO	951	Wilczynski, Sharon (CA)	Path	722
Wharen, Robert (FL)	NS	481	Wilding, George (WI)	Onc	372
Wheeland, Ronald (MO)	D	195	Wilens, Timothy (MA)	ChAP	904
Wheeler, Arthur (TN)	Pul	930	Wiley, Joseph (MD)	PHO	763
Wheeler, Thomas (TX)	Path	719	Wilhelmi, Bradon (KY)	PlS	862
Whelan, Alison (MO)	CG	159	Wilking, Andrew (TX)	PRhu	800
Whelan, Richard (NY)	CRS	169	Wilkins, Edwin (MI)	PlS	866
Wheless, James (TN)	ChiN	148	Wilkins, Isabelle (IL)	MF	434
Whitaker, Linton (PA)	PlS	857	Wilkins, Ross (CO)	OrS	638
White, Charles (MD)	DR	977	Wilkins-Haug, Louise (MA)	MF	427
White, David (MA)	Pul	922	Wilkoff, Bruce (OH)	Cv	110
White, Jocelyn (OR)	IM	421	Willett, Christopher (NC)	RadRO	956
White, Neil (MO)	PEn	747	Willey, Shawna (DC)	S	1061
White, Richard (OH)	DR	981	Williams, David (MA)	IC	124
White, Richard (NC)	S	1069	Williams, George (MI)	Oph	592
White, Robert (CT)	VIR	991	Williams, Gerald (PA)	OrS	625
White, Rodney (CA)	VascS	1188	Williams, James (AZ)	PHO	775
Whiting, Donald (PA)	NS	476	Williams, Kim (MI)	Cv	110
Whitington, Peter (IL)	PGe	753	Williams, Mathew (NY)	TS	1118

Alphabetical Listing of Doctors

Name	Specialty	Pg	Name	Specialty	Pg
Williams, Michael (VA)	Hem	316	Wiviott, Lory (CA)	Inf	414
Williams, Riley (NY)	OrS	625	Wixson, Richard (IL)	OrS	636
Williams, Ronald (TX)	OrS	639	Wiznitzer, Max (OH)	ChiN	150
Williams, Shauna (ID)	CRS	174	Woeber, Kenneth (CA)	EDM	222
Willson, James (TX)	Onc	381	Wofsy, David (CA)	Rhu	1032
Wilson, Amy (TX)	PMR	842	Wolchok, Jedd (NY)	Onc	350
Wilson, Daniel (NE)	Psyc	895	Wolf, Gregory (MI)	Oto	678
Wilson, Darrell (CA)	PEn	748	Wolf, Raoul (IL)	PA&I	731
Wilson, David (OR)	Oph	602	Wolfe, Lawrence (NY)	PHO	763
Wilson, Ellen (TX)	RE	1016	Wolfe, M Michael (OH)	Ge	249
Wilson, J Frank (WI)	RadRO	961	Wolfe, S Anthony (FL)	PlS	862
Wilson, John (NC)	NS	481	Wolfe, Scott (NY)	HS	298
Wilson, Keith (OH)	Oto	678	Wolff, Antonio (MD)	Onc	351
Wilson, Lynn (CT)	RadRO	946	Wolff, Bruce (MN)	CRS	174
Wilson, Marion (SC)	Oph	585	Wolff, Robert (TX)	Onc	381
Wilson, Matthew (TN)	Oph	585	Wolfson, Aaron (FL)	RadRO	956
Wilson, Steven (OH)	Oph	592	Wolinsky, Jerry (TX)	N	532
Wilson, Timothy (CA)	U	1173	Wollmann, Robert (IL)	Path	717
Wilson, Walter (MN)	Inf	412	Woltering, Eugene (LA)	S	1087
Wilson, Wyndham (MD)	Onc	350	Wong, Brian (CA)	Oto	687
Winchell, Robert (ME)	S	1048	Wong, Carson (OH)	U	1165
Windebank, Anthony (MN)	N	529	Wong, Jeffrey (CA)	RadRO	967
Winer, Eric (MA)	Onc	332	Wong, Johnson (MA)	A&I	84
Winer, Sharon (CA)	RE	1018	Wong, Ronald (HI)	CRS	177
Winfield, Howard (AL)	U	1159	Woo, Howard (LA)	U	1169
Wingard, John (FL)	Onc	362	Woo, Peak (NY)	Oto	665
Winick, Naomi (TX)	PHO	775	Woo, Shiao (KY)	RadRO	956
Winn, Hung (MO)	MF	434	Woo, Y Joseph (PA)	TS	1118
Winston, Jonathan (NY)	Nep	455	Wood, Beverly (CA)	DR	984
Winter, Jane (IL)	Hem	321	Wood, Bradford (MD)	VIR	993
Wirth, Michael (TX)	OrS	639	Wood, David (MI)	U	1165
Wisch, Nathaniel (NY)	Hem	314	Wood, Douglas (WA)	TS	1138
Wise, Christopher (VA)	Rhu	1028	Wood, Gary (WI)	D	196
Wise, Paul (TN)	CRS	171	Wood, John (MO)	A&I	88
Wiseman, Gregory (MN)	NuM	546	Wood, R Patrick (TX)	S	1088
Wisoff, Jeffrey (NY)	NS	476	Wood, Robert (MD)	PA&I	730
Witman, Patricia (OH)	D	195	Wood, William (GA)	S	1069
Witt, Thomas (IL)	S	1080	Woodley, David (CA)	D	200
Witter, Frank (MD)	ObG	554	Woodson, B Tucker (WI)	Oto	678
Wittig, James (NY)	OrS	625	Woodson, Gayle (IL)	Oto	678
Wityk, Robert (MD)	N	517	Wooten, George (VA)	N	522

Alphabetical Listing of Doctors

Name	Specialty	Pg
Wooten, Virgil (OH)	Psyc	894
Worden, Francis (MI)	Onc	372
Wormser, Gary (NY)	Inf	407
Worsey, Michael (CA)	CRS	177
Wright, Cameron (MA)	TS	1109
Wright, Jackson (OH)	IM	420
Wright, Kenneth (CA)	Oph	602
Wright, Robert (IL)	N	529
Wurtz, L Daniel (IN)	OrS	636
Wyatt, Robert (TN)	PNep	785
Wyllie, Elaine (OH)	ChiN	150
Wyllie, Robert (OH)	PGe	753

X

Name	Specialty	Pg
Xerogeanes, John (GA)	SM	1038
Xing, Michael (MD)	EDM	211

Y

Name	Specialty	Pg
Yaddanapudi, Ravindranath (MI)	PHO	773
Yaffe, Bruce (NY)	IM	419
Yahalom, Joachim (NY)	RadRO	951
Yakes, Wayne (CO)	VIR	996
Yamada, Kelvin (MO)	ChiN	150
Yamaguchi, Ken (MO)	OrS	636
Yan, Albert (PA)	D	189
Yancovitz, Stanley (NY)	Inf	407
Yanda, Randy (GA)	Ge	243
Yang, James (MD)	S	1061
Yang, Stephen (MD)	TS	1118
Yankelevitz, David (NY)	DR	977
Yannuzzi, Lawrence (NY)	Oph	579
Yanovich, Saul (MD)	Hem	314
Yarbrough, Wendell (TN)	Oto	671
Yeager, Andrew (AZ)	Hem	323
Yeatman, Timothy (FL)	S	1069
Yeatts, R Patrick (NC)	Oph	585
Yee, Billy (CA)	RE	1018
Yee, Douglas (MN)	Onc	372
Yee, Jerry (MI)	Nep	459
Yen, Yun (CA)	Onc	391
Yeo, Charles (PA)	S	1061
Yetman, Randall (OH)	PlS	866
Yeung, Alan (CA)	IC	130
Yeung, Raymond (WA)	S	1095
Yonas, Howard (NM)	NS	491
Yoo, Jung (OR)	OrS	644
Yoon, Sydney (NY)	DR	978
York, Teresa (MD)	PHO	763
Young, Anne (MA)	N	507
Young, Bruce (NY)	ObG	555
Young, Iven (NY)	EDM	211
Young, James (OH)	Cv	110
Young, K Randall (PA)	Pul	927
Young, Ming-Lon (FL)	PCd	737
Young, Nancy (IL)	Oto	678
Young, Renee (NE)	Ge	249
Young, Robert (MA)	Path	707
Young, V Leroy (MO)	PlS	866
Younossi, Zobair (VA)	Ge	243
Yousem, David (MD)	NRad	986
Yousem, Samuel (PA)	Path	712
Yu, George (MD)	U	1153
Yu, Jack (GA)	PlS	862
Yu, John (CA)	NS	496
Yu, Victor (PA)	Inf	408
Yueh, Bevan (MN)	Oto	678
Yuen, James (AR)	PlS	870
Yung, WK Alfred (TX)	N	533
Yunus, Furhan (TN)	Onc	362
Yurt, Roger (NY)	S	1061

Z

Name	Specialty	Pg
Zach, Terence (NE)	NP	447
Zackai, Elaine (PA)	CG	156
Zacur, Howard (MD)	RE	1010
Zafonte, Ross (MA)	PMR	832

Name	Specialty	Pg	Name	Specialty	Pg
Zager, Eric (PA)	NS	476	Zubrow, Alan (PA)	NP	444
Zagoria, Ronald (NC)	DR	979	Zuckerman, Joseph (NY)	OrS	625
Zagzag, David (NY)	Path	712	Zuckerman, Kenneth (FL)	Hem	316
Zahn, Evan (FL)	PCd	737	Zusman, Randall (MA)	Cv	94
Zaidman, Gerald (NY)	Oph	579	Zwischenberger, Joseph (KY)	TS	1124
Zalud, Ivica (HI)	MF	437			
Zalzal, George (DC)	Oto	665			
Zaman, Atif (OR)	Ge	255			
Zannis, Victor (AZ)	S	1088			
Zarins, Bertram (MA)	OrS	611			
Zarins, Christopher (CA)	VascS	1188			
Zdeblick, Thomas (WI)	OrS	636			
Zeanah, Charles (LA)	ChAP	908			
Zeitels, Steven (MA)	Oto	657			
Zeitlin, Pamela (MD)	PPul	795			
Zelefsky, Michael (NY)	RadRO	951			
Zelenetz, Andrew (NY)	Onc	351			
Zelickson, Brian (MN)	D	196			
Zelman, Richard (MA)	IC	124			
Zeltzer, Lonnie (CA)	Ped	729			
Zeman, Robert (DC)	DR	978			
Zerbe, Kathryn (OR)	Psyc	900			
Zide, Barry (NY)	PlS	858			
Ziedonis, Douglas (MA)	AdP	900			
Ziemer, Gerhard (IL)	TS	1130			
Zietman, Anthony (MA)	RadRO	946			
Ziffer, Jack (FL)	NuM	546			
Zilleruelo, Gaston (FL)	PNep	785			
Zimmerman, Christian (ID)	NS	488			
Zimmerman, Donald (IL)	PEn	747			
Zimmerman, Earl (NY)	N	517			
Zimmerman, Jerry (WA)	PCCM	742			
Zimmerman, Robert (PA)	NRad	986			
Zinaman, Michael (MA)	RE	1007			
Zinner, Michael (MA)	S	1048			
Zinreich, S James (MD)	NRad	986			
Zins, James (OH)	PlS	867			
Zippe, Craig (OH)	U	1165			
Zitelli, Basil (PA)	Ped	727			
Zitelli, John (PA)	D	189			
Zoghbi, William (TX)	Cv	113			

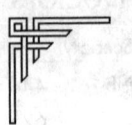

The Best in American Medicine
www.CastleConnolly.com

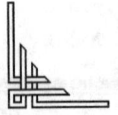
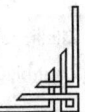

Acknowledgments

The publishers would like to thank the entire staff for their many hours and days of intense and precise work on this guide in order to further its goal of assisting consumers in making the best healthcare choices.

Castle Connolly Executive Management:

Chairman	John K. Castle
President & CEO	John J. Connolly, Ed.D.
Vice President, Chief Medical & Research Officer	Jean Morgan, M.D.
Vice President, Chief Strategy & Operations Officer	William Liss-Levinson, Ph.D.

Senior Research & Healthcare Associate — Maryann Hynd, RN

Senior Research Associate & Book Production Manager — Sara Sezer

Research Coordinators

Terysia Herbert
Jerville Weekes
Yuliya Nagdimova
Catherine Hoffman-Freiria

Book Layout, Database Management	Russell Hodgson
Office Manager	Marcie Samartino
Director of Client Relations	Jennifer Mojave
Corporate Services Manager	Alexander Salazar
Communications Manager	Nicki Hughes

We also would like to extend our gratitude to the American Board of Medical Specialties (ABMS) for allowing us to use excerpts, especially the descriptions of medical specialties and subspecialties, from the text of their publication "Which Medical Specialist for You?"

Other Publications from Castle Connolly Medical Ltd.:
America's Top Doctors® for Cancer; Top Doctors: New York Metro Area; Top Doctors: Chicago Metro Area; Cancer Made Easier: New York—Metro Area, Eldercare and others...

Order online at http://www.castleconnolly.com/books

The Best in American Medicine
www.CastleConnolly.com

Healthcare Solutions

Castle Connolly's Healthcare Solutions is designed to help your employees and their loved ones navigate through the healthcare system with less stress, faster service and better outcomes. It is a high touch service with a hands-on health advocate to serve as a guide and dedicated healthcare champion 24 hours a day, 7 days a week, 365 days a year. Why have your most valued employees, your most critical asset, spend their time -- and possibly company time –coping with difficult and complex medical issues they may know little about, when Castle Connolly's Healthcare Solutions professionals can resolve them quickly and expertly. With one phone call, your employees will gain priority access to a global network of best-in-class medical professionals, Castle Connolly Top Doctors™, and higher quality patient resources. Our professional staff coordinates the entire process to provide consistency and support during their time of need.

Services include, but are not limited to, the following:

» Identifying top physicians and hospitals (nationally)

» Identifying reputable non-physician providers, such as Dieticians, Physical and Occupational Therapists, etc.

» Facilitating second opinions

» Defining complex medical terminology and situations

» Providing a list of tailored questions to discuss with your medical team

» Conducting medical research on your health condition

» Navigating the healthcare system

» Assisting with medical record retrieval and/or arranging a medical record review

» Identifying and assisting with eldercare issues

» Coordinating a hospital transfer

» Arranging medical transport or evacuation for travelers

» Coordinating with the employers' other vendors for continuity of care

Corporate Products

Healthcare Solutions can be made available to your organization as a specific number of cases during the course of the year with the option to obtain more, or as a yearly retainer. Organizations may opt to make this service available for all of their employees, or to select groups such as high level executives or partners.

For further information on Healthcare Solutions, Corporate Membership, New Movers, and Doctor-Patient Advisor Program, please contact:

Alexander Salazar
Corporate Services Manager
212.367.8400, ext. 17
or
asalazar@castleconnolly.com

Services for Corporations & Organizations

This service enables an employer to assist employees in identifying Top Doctors to care for themselves and their families. It is a low-cost, non-intrusive service that will result in better care and, ultimately, lower healthcare costs. For as low as a few dollars per year, employees can have complete access to the Castle Connolly website and database of Top Doctors who were nominated by their peers and screened by the Castle Connolly physician-led research team.

Instead of simply choosing a doctor's name from the phone book or a plan directory, the employee can compare physician names to the Castle Connolly database of 30,000 plus Top Doctors and select from among the best doctors in the country. This will result in overall better care, lower costs and improved morale. Once an employee logs on to the Castle Connolly database, valuable background information is available on every Top Doctor such as: medical school, board certifications, fellowships, hospital affiliations, residencies and much more, to allow them to make the best informed decision they can make when selecting a doctor.

Top Doctors can have an enormous impact. For patients and their families, the value of receiving first-class medical care is great but unquantifiable – it is measured in quality and even length of life. Employers, however, can see the results in their bottom line. Faulty diagnoses and improper treatment take a toll in productivity and ripple out into higher workplace costs. No company should have to "make do" for weeks or months without a key employee or executive, when a Top Doctor may have solved the patient's problem quickly and efficiently. The effort to identify the best doctors from ordinary ones is justified by the money saved on incorrect treatments, unnecessary surgery and days lost from work.

The Corporate Membership is suited for employers of varying sizes and can also be of great value to professional, social, civic, fraternal and religious associations. Castle Connolly may also be able to adapt and tailor the presentation of the database to meet the specific corporate client's needs.

New Movers Program

The Castle Connolly New Movers Program is designed to alleviate that concern, or even fear, as well as the time-consuming struggle to identify the right – and best – doctors and hospitals in one's new community or region. The service can be provided on a family basis (those living in the household) or for a single client. The service includes identifying primary care physicians, including Pediatricians, OB/GYN's, Internists and Family Practitioners as well as other specialists that may be needed: for example, Ophthalmologists, Allergists, Endocrinologists, Surgeons or others as required.

Perhaps nothing is more challenging to a family that has relocated to a new community than finding appropriate healthcare resources, especially physicians. While they can turn to recommendations from new neighbors and friends, or select names from the phone book or a plan directory, that is hardly adequate, especially if there are special healthcare needs in the family.

A Castle Connolly Health Advisor will identify two or three recommendations for up to six different medical specialties. If, for some reason the client wishes to change doctors within two months, Castle Connolly will identify new physicians in the same specialty. After the selection process occurs, the Health Advisor will make an introductory phone call to the physician's office. This typically facilitates faster appointments.

Doctor-Patient Advisor Program for Corporations & Organizations

The Doctor-Patient Advisor is a focused, highly personalized advisory service providing one-on-one phone consultations to individuals who have serious or complex medical problems, or anyone who feels they need assistance in finding the right doctor. It is designed to assist people in identifying the best doctors to meet their complex medical needs. Patients or their family members can speak with a nurse practitioner regarding their condition. To assist in finding a doctor, Castle Connolly identifies two to three top specialists, based on the medical condition, patient needs and the patient's specific preferences regarding geographic location, hospital affiliation, gender, age and other considerations. Because Castle Connolly's corporate programs are not insurance, they are not covered by the Employee Retirement Income Security Act (ERISA) and may be offered to selected employee groups.

The program is not designed to answer general medical or health insurance questions. Because of the breadth and depth of our database - and the extensive healthcare experience of our staff – the identification of doctors can be limited to a given region or the search can focus on finding the very best anywhere in the nation. This high level service is available at a low cost of $3.00 per employee - per month. Each employee will need to go on to an indicated website and download their specific access code and use our toll-free number to call and consult with a Castle Connolly Health Advisor to ensure the process of finding a Top Doctor is efficient and effective. Our Health Advisors are available during regular business hours Monday through Friday 9:00am-5:00pm EST.

For further information on the following programs: Corporate Membership Program, New Movers Program and Doctor-Patient Advisor Program, contact:

Jennifer Mojave
Director of Client Relations
212.367.8400, ext. 35
or jmojave@castleconnolly.com

Strategic Partnerships

Castle Connolly Medical Ltd. has a number of strategic partnerships that may be of interest to consumers and physicians.

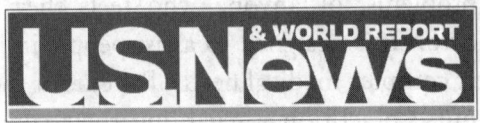

U.S. News & World Report and Castle Connolly created a strategic collaboration that will bring the Castle Connolly Top Doctors® database to online visitors to the U.S. News website. The online database went live on www.usnews.com in mid-July 2011 and will be linked with the U.S. News database of Best Hospitals. Consumers will be able to search the full database of Top Doctors across the nation, including all specialties and subspecialties. The detailed physician profiles, including designation of doctors affiliated with Castle Connolly's Partnership for Excellence hospital program, will be drawn from Castle Connolly's growing database of over 27,000 physicians currently accessible online at www.castleconnolly.com.

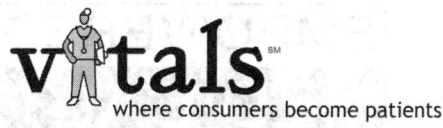

Vitals (www.vitals.com), an innovative online doctor review and comparison service from MDx Medical Inc., is the comprehensive source for vital information, peer evaluations and patient feedback on more than 700,000 doctors nationwide. Drawing upon prestigious information repositories, cutting-edge search and comparison technologies, and a robust patient feedback mechanism, Vitals has organized key information to help patients make an informed choice in their search for the right doctor. Castle Connolly and Vitals have a branding relationship in which those physicians who are Castle Connolly Top Doctors™ and appear on Vitals web sites have an icon indicating their status and recognition as a Castle Connolly Top Doctor.

In 2012, Castle Connolly will begin displaying insurance plans that are accepted by all physicians listed as Castle Connolly Top Doctors. An appointment scheduling feature will also appear on our site for those physicians who wish to participate in this feature. Additional information can be found at www.vitals.com.

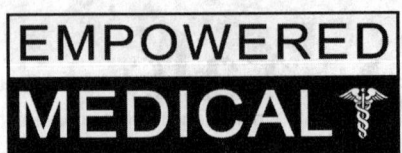

Empowered Doctor is a media, news and marketing service. Empowered Doctor produces syndicated consumer health reports. Its video and text news stories appear on major media websites, including CBS. Empowered Doctor also provides marketing services to hospitals, clinics and individual physicians by generating visibility in online search and social media. Empowered Doctor's clients benefit from the company's efficient methodologies for generating new patient referrals.

For more information call 888-333-1027 or visit www.empowereddoctor.com

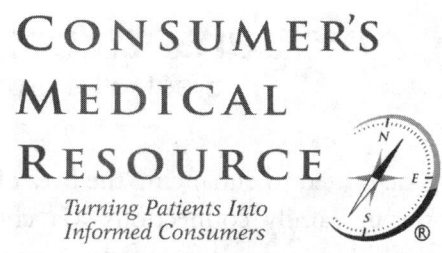

CONSUMER'S MEDICAL RESOURCE

Turning Patients Into Informed Consumers

Consumer's Medical Resource was started in 1996 to offer high-quality, high-impact employee benefit programs to help employees and their dependents, and has been a pioneer in Medical Decision Support® services. CMR addresses all medical conditions at any point within the continuum of care, by providing personalized, evidence-based medical research, information, access to genuine, in-person second opinions and support services to employees who face serious, complicated, and chronic illness, or would like to become well-informed healthcare consumers.

Leveraging a state-of-the-art integrated model of web, phone, and print-based services, CMR enables employees to fully understand and evaluate their options so they can make the most informed medical decisions possible with their doctors. The company is privately held and currently provides services to more than 600,000 Americans, achieving extremely high levels of user and customer satisfaction, improved clinical quality outcomes, and generated excellent ROI.

Castle Connolly and CMR are working together to provide Castle Connolly's various corporate services to CMR client companies and their employees.

For more information, please visit: http://www.consumersmedical.com.

grandparents.com®
it's great to be grand.

Grandparents.com is dedicated to enhancing the lives of America's 70 million grandparents by fostering family connections, via child- and grandparent-friendly activities, travel ideas, compelling lifestyle features, expert advice, gift ideas, recipes, and more. Visitors have access to a range of tools, including groups, discussions, a homepage blog, photo sharing, and a Facebook page and Twitter feeds. Through the Grandparents.com Benefits Club, catering to America's 120 million grandparents, Boomers and seniors, members benefit from discounts and incentives they can use every day, in categories like gifts, clothes, and vitamins, plus exclusive opportunities to save on hotels, cruises, auto rentals, theme park trips, theatrical productions, and insurance. Grandparents can share their membership benefits with four extended family and household members. In 2010, Grandparents.com was ranked as the No. 3 website for seniors, boomers, and grandparents, following the U.S. Government and AARP. Castle Connolly provides access to its Top Doctors' database, its Doctor-Patient Advisor and New Movers programs for Grandparents.com members.

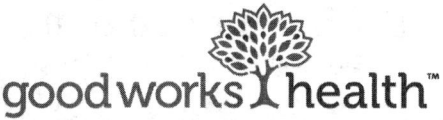

The Good Works Health government-approved platform - www.goodworkshealth.com - offers physicians the opportunity to direct donations, based on the fair market value of their time, to charities of their choice in exchange for participation in educational programs.

Participating physicians can choose from more than a million approved charities to designate as the recipients of these donations. Good Works Health's unique platform reaches a growing community of medical professionals in many specialties that are motivated by the opportunity to do good works. Castle Connolly actively works with Good Works Health to promote these opportunities to its Castle Connolly Top Doctors®

DrScore.com
PATIENTS SPEAK, DOCTORS LISTEN

Founded by Steven Feldman, M.D., DrScore.com is an interactive online survey site where patients can rate their physicians, as well as find a physician based on their service level preference.

The mission of DrScore.com is to improve medical care by giving patients a forum for rating their physician and by giving doctors an affordable, objective, non-intrusive means of documenting the quality of care that they provide. Visitors on Castle Connolly's website who are searching for "top doctors" have the option to also rate these and other physicians they have been to as patients, as well as to see if these physicians have been rated previously by other consumers on DrScore.com. Visitors to DrScore.com will be able to see if their doctors and/or other doctors are Castle Connolly "top doctors."

For more information, visit www.drscore.com.

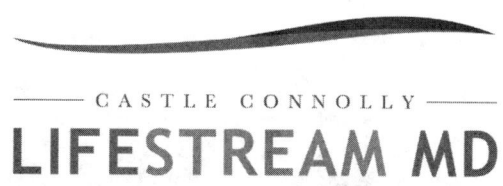

LIFESTREAM MD

Castle Connolly Medical Ltd. has a strategic relationship with Castle Connolly LifeStream MD to provide a unique health advisory service designed for families and executives, especially those who travel regularly or may have more than one residence.

Each client is assigned a Castle Connolly LifeStream MD physician who is available to them by phone 24/7/365. A client call from anywhere in the world is answered promptly and the client is connected with their Castle Connolly LifeStream MD physician advisor.

The Castle Connolly LifeStream MD physician acts as a health manager assisting in navigation of an increasingly complex health care environment. The Castle Connolly LifeStream MD physician does not replace the member's primary physician or specialists, but provides additional independent counsel and services that provide security to our members either at home or while traveling.

In the United States, the Castle Connolly LifeStream MD physician will use the Castle Connolly database of Top Doctors to assure that the client is cared for in the best medical facilities by the top doctors. Assistance in securing timely appointments with specialists and records transfers is facilitated as needed. Outside of the United States, Castle Connolly LifeStream MD has an affiliation with International SOS, the world's largest and leading provider of travel medical assistance to assure the LifeStream MD member is cared for by the best doctors and hospitals available in that region or, if necessary, is transported to a place where that care is available.

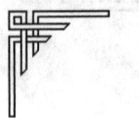

The Best in American Medicine
www.CastleConnolly.com

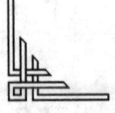

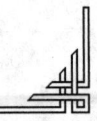

National Physician of the Year Awards

Castle Connolly Medical Ltd. proudly hosted its sixth annual *National Physician of the Year Awards* on March 28, 2011 at The Hudson Theatre New York City. It was a spectacular evening which allowed us to recognize both the outstanding honorees and the excellence of the many thousands of physicians throughout the nation.

The Genesis of the National Physician of the Year Award.

Each year we receive thousands of nominations from physicians and the medical leadership of major medical centers, specialty hospitals, teaching hospitals and regional and community medical centers across the United States as an integral part of our research, screening and selection process to identify *America's Top Doctors*®. The selected physicians, while spread across all fifty states and involved in more than 70 medical specialties and subspecialties, all share one distinguishing professional attribute: an unwavering dedication to their patients and to medicine as a whole. Each and every one of these outstanding medical professionals is a symbol of the clinical excellence that characterizes American medicine. In honor of these exemplary physicians, Castle Connolly Medical Ltd. has created the *National Physician of the Year Awards* to recognize the thousands of excellent, dedicated physicians across the United States. Our Medical Advisory Board selected the honorees from the hundreds nominated in a special nomination process conducted months before the event.

The honorees, Drs. Armando E. Giuliano, O. Wayne Isom, and David W. Kennedy are superb examples of excellence in clinical medical practice. In addition to these awards for Clinical Excellence, Castle Connolly Medical Ltd. honored Drs. George P. Canellos, and Matthew D. Davis for their lifetime achievement in medicine. Mrs. Evelyn H. Lauder is a tireless fundraiser for the Estee Lauder Companies' Breast Cancer Awareness Campaign and The Breast Cancer Research Foundation® organization and an exemplary recipient for the sixth National Health Leadership Award.

Each honoree received a beautiful and distinctive porcelain figurine created by the Boehm Porcelain Company exclusively for the National Physician of the Year Awards. The award features a golden caduceus, the symbol of the medical community, surrounded by a golden laurel wreath. Laurel wreaths were used by the ancients to crown and honor their leaders. The caduceus and laurel rest upon a column accented by the signature Castle Connolly logo. By combining the caduceus and the laurel wreaths, the award embodies the excellence in medical achievement that the National Physician of the Year Awards celebrates each year.

2011 National Physician of the Year Awards Honorees

"Doctors Make a Difference"

For Clinical Excellence

Armando E. Giuliano, M.D., FACS, FRCSED
Chief of Science and Medicine
John Wayne Cancer Institute at Saint John's Health Center,
Santa Monica, CA

O. Wayne Isom, M.D.
Chairman of the Dept. of Cardiothoracic Surgery
New York Presbyterian-Weill Cornell Medical College

David W. Kennedy, M.D.
Otorhinolaryngology Professor at the
University of Pennsylvania

For Lifetime Achievement

George P. Canellos, M.D.
Served as Founding Chief of Medical Oncology at
Dana-Farber Cancer Institute;

Matthew D. Davis, M.D.
University of Wisconsin Medical Center
Chair, UW Opthalmology

National Health Leadership

Evelyn H. Lauder
Chairman of The Breast Cancer Research Foundation®

Previous National Physician of the Year Award Honorees

2010

Clinical Excellence
John B. Buse, M.D., Ph.D.
Director of the Diabetes Care Center, Professor, Chief of the Division of
Endocrinology and Executive Associate Dean for Clinical Research,
University of North Carolina School of Medicine, Chapel Hill

Larry Norton, M.D.
Deputy Physician-in-Chief, Memorial Hospital, Memorial Sloan-Kettering
Cancer Center, for Breast Cancer Programs
Medical Director of the MSKCC's Breast and Imaging Center, Evelyn H.
Lauder Breast Center

Ching-Hon Pui, M.D.
Department Chair of Oncology, St. Jude Children's Research Hospital
Medical Director of the St. Jude International Outreach China Program,
holder of the Fahad Nassar Al-Rashid Chair of Leukemia Research

Lifetime Achievement
Basil I Hirschowitz, M.D.
Director, Gastroenterology Division, The University of Alabama
Receipient of the Kettering Medal from the General Motors Cancer
Foundation; Friedenwald Medal of the AGA; the Schindler Medal and the
Crystal Award for lifetime contributions to Endoscopy by the ASGE;
honorary doctorate of Gothenburg University; honorary fellow of the Royal
Society of Medicine

Leonard Apt, M.D.
Professor of Ophthalmology Emeritus; Director Emeritus and Founder of
the Division of Pediatric Opthalmology and Strabismus, and Co-Director of
UCLA's Center for Child Blindness

National Health Leadership
Alexandra Reeve Givens and Matthew Reeve
Trustees, The Christopher & Dana Reeve Foundation

2009

Clinical Excellence
Carol R. Bradford, M.D.,
Professor and Chair
Department of Otolaryngology
University of Michigan Medical System

Diane E. Meier, M.D.,
Director, Center to Advance Palliative Care
Mount Sinai School of Medicine

Judd W. Moul, M.D.,
Chief of Urology
Duke University Medical Center

Lifetime Achievement
Emil J. Freireich, M.D., D. Sc. (Hon.),
Ruth Harriet Ainsworth Chair, Distinguished Teaching Professor
Director, Special Medical Education Programs
Director, Adult Leukemia Research Program
The University of Texas M.D. Anderson Cancer Center

Thomas E. Starzl, M.D., Ph.D.
Professor of Surgery, Emeritus
Distinguished Service Professor
University of Pittsburgh Medical Center

National Health Leadership
Page Morton Black
Chairman of the Board, Parkinson's Disease Foundation

****

<u>2008</u>

Clinical Excellence
Robert W. Carlson, M.D.
Medical Oncology
Stanford University Medical Center

Stanley Chang, M.D.
Ophthalmology
New York-Presbyterian Hospital

L. Dade Lunsford, M.D.
Neurological Surgery
University of Pittsburgh Medical Center

Lifetime Achievement
Jacqueline A. Noonan, M.D.
Pediatric Cardiology
University of Kentucky Medical Center

Robert W. Schrier, M.D.
Nephrology
University of Colorado Health Sciences Center

National Health Leadership
Suzanne and Robert Wright
Vice-Chair of the Board, General Electric Company
Co-founders of Autism Speaks™

****

2007

Clinical Excellence
Delos M. Cosgrove, M.D.
Chairman, Board of Governors
CEO and President
The Cleveland Clinic

Joseph G. McCarthy, M.D.
Lawrence D. Bell Professor of Plastic Surgery
Director, The Institute of Reconstructive Plastic Surgery
NYU Medical Center

Patrick C. Walsh, M.D.
University Distinguished Service Professor and Director of Urology
The James Buchanan Brady Urological Institute
The Johns Hopkins Hospital

Lifetime Achievement
Maria Delivoria-Papadopoulos, M.D.
Director, The Neonatal Intensive Care Unit
St. Christopher's Hospital for Children;
Professor of Pediatrics, Physiology and Obstetrics/Gynecology
Drexel University College of Medicine

National Health Leadership
The Honorable Nancy G. Brinker
Founder of Susan G. Komen for the Cure
Former U.S. Ambassador to Hungary

****

<u>2006</u>

Clinical Excellence
Bart Barlogie, M.D., Ph.D.
Director, Myeloma Institute for Research Therapy
University of Arkansas for Medical Services

Marilyn J. Bull, M.D.
Morris Green Professor of Pediatrics
Riley Hospital for Children

Michael J. Zinner, M.D.
Moseley Professor of Surgery
Harvard Medical School
Surgeon-in-Chief, Brigham & Women's Hospital

Lifetime Achievement
Michael E. DeBakey, M.D.
Chancellor Emeritus, Baylor College of Medicine

National Health Leadership
Princess Yasmin Aga Khan
Honorary Vice Chair
Alzheimer's Association

Castle Connolly maintains Facebook, Twitter, LinkedIn and Sharecare accounts in an effort to keep consumers informed of the latest news not only regarding Castle Connolly Medical Ltd., its Top Doctors and Top Hospitals, but also reports on various health observances and events. A live Twitter feed can also be found on the homepage of www.castleconnolly.com.

Consumers who use our print guides, online database or refer to our regional magazine features can find up-to-date information about Castle Connolly, healthcare and medical news by logging onto these social networking sites:

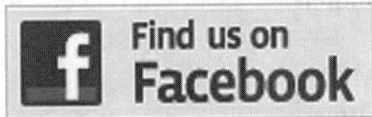

www.facebook.com/TopDoctors

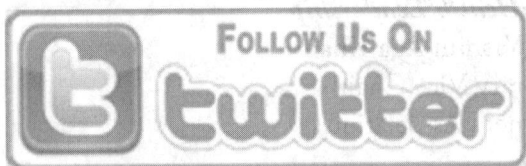

www.sharecare.com/group/castle-connolly-medical-ltd
or http://bit.ly/giuPHI (case sensitive)

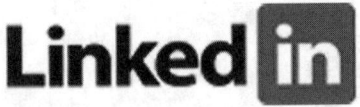

www.twitter.com/CastleConnolly

Linked in

http://linkd.in/mP4Lmb (case sensitive)

Do you have a story about a Castle Connolly Top Doctor or Top Hospital that you want to share? If so, please email a link to the article to:

Nicki Hughes
Communications Manager
nhughes@castleconnolly.com

Castle Connolly has developed a website and online database – www.AmericasTopCosmeticDoctors.com – to enable consumers to search and identify top cosmetic specialists who have been nominated by their peers through an extensive, annual survey process involving tens of thousands of American physicians. Nominated physicians' medical education, training, hospital appointments, disciplinary histories - and much more - are screened and reviewed by our physician-led research team. Those selected as top doctors may appear in a number of Castle Connolly guides/online databases, including www.AmericasTopCosmeticDoctors.com.

These doctors are specially trained in cosmetic procedures and spend the majority of their time in their medical practice doing cosmetic work. The Top Cosmetic Doctors whose profiles are included on this site are in one of only six medical specialties: Dermatology, Facial Plastic Surgery, Ophthalmology, Otolaryngology, Plastic Surgery or Surgery. The website also includes valuable information on how to select the right cosmetic doctor for you, as well as detailed information about some of the most common procedures.

For more information visit: www.AmericasTopCosmeticDoctors.com

Doctor-Patient Advisor for Individual Consumers

Doctor-Patient Advisor is a Castle Connolly Medical Ltd. service providing one-on-one consultations with a physician or nurse practitioner to individuals who have serious or complex medical problems or to anyone who feels he/she needs assistance finding the right physician for any purpose. Each client will receive personalized assistance in identifying the appropriate specialists for his/her condition, utilizing the Castle Connolly Medical Ltd. database of physicians and hospitals, as well as individual searches, to locate the best resources to meet the client's needs.

Fee: $375. For further information call (212) 367-8400 x 16.

Premium Membership at www.CastleConnolly.com

Reap the benefits of membership with Castle Connolly. Gain access to ALL online top doctor listings and get discounts on book purchases from our extensive catalog.

• Search among more than 28,000 Castle Connolly Top Doctor listings
• Search among select hospitals and centers of excellence
• Receive a 30% discount on all book purchases

Membership Levels:
• One year - $24.95
• Two years - $34.95

For more information visit: www.CastleConnolly.com/membership

Other Products From Castle Connolly

Castle Connolly Guides
Titles Include:
- *America's Top Doctors® for Cancer*
- *Top Doctors: New York Metro Area*

And Many More

To order other Castle Connolly guides at a 15% discount please visit
http://www.CastleConnolly.com/books
When ordering use discount code: **ATD11VAN**

Castle Connolly's Top Doctors Available Online
- Free Access to 20 -25% of Castle Connolly's Top Doctors
- Purchase Access to the entire database of more than 28,000 doctor profiles

http://www.castleconnolly.com/membership

Customer Feedback
We appreciate your comments regarding our guides. Please email us at
info@castleconnolly.com

The Best in American Medicine
www.CastleConnolly.com